A Call to Action

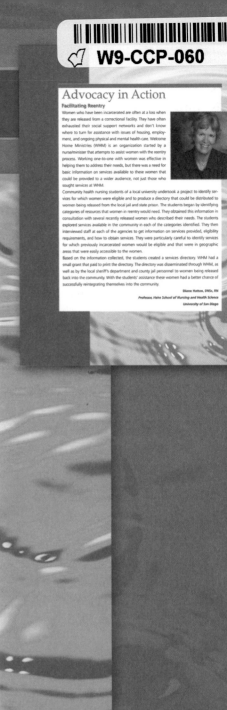

Advocacy in Action

Facilitating Reentry

Women who have been incarcerated are often at a loss when they are released from a correctional facility. They have often exhausted their social support networks and don't know where to turn for assistance with issues of housing, employment, and ongoing physical and mental health care. Welcome Home Ministries (WHM) is an organization started by a nurse/minister that attempts to assist women with the reentry process. Working one-to-one with women was effective in helping them to address their needs, but there was a need for basic information on services available to these women that could be provided to a wider audience, not just those who sought services at WHM.

Community health nursing students of a local university undertook a project to identify services for which women were eligible and to produce a directory that could be distributed to women being released from the local jail and state prison. The students began by identifying categories of resources that women in reentry would need. They obtained this information in consultation with several recently released women who described their needs. The students explored services available in the community in each of the categories identified. They then interviewed staff at each of the agencies to get information on services provided, eligibility requirements, and how to obtain services. They were particularly careful to identify services for which previously incarcerated women would be eligible and that were in geographic areas that were easily accessible to the women.

Based on the information collected, the students created a services directory. WHM had a small grant that paid to print the directory. The directory was disseminated through WHM, as well as by the local sheriff's department and county jail personnel to women being released back into the community. With the students' assistance these women had a better chance of successfully reintegrating themselves into the community.

Diane Hatton, DNSc, RN
Professor, Hahn School of Nursing and Health Science
University of San Diego

Dear Community Health Nurse Advocate,

This book is focused on the idea of nursing advocacy as a path to global health. It includes many true stories of community health nurses and their impact on their communities. The most important thing I hope you take away from reading this book is that we must all be advocates for the health of the population – locally, nationally, and globally. Whether or not you ever work in a community health setting, you need to keep your eyes on the big picture. You need to look beyond the care of individual clients to the needs of the populations from which those clients come. Not only do you need to be aware of that big picture, you need to be doing something about it!

Maybe your advocacy will take the form of political action at the local, state, or national level. Maybe it will mean working to support health promotion on campus or in your workplace or changing the conditions under which people live. Wherever you are, as an advocate for community health, you will be exhibiting nursing excellence. But you don't have to wait until you graduate to start working toward that goal. There are things you can do right now to improve the health of the population.

What are the needs of your community?

What are the big health issues?

What can you do about them?

Who can you link up with to deal with them?

Your textbook will help you answer these questions and start on the path to client advocacy. Reading assignments before class and applying what you've read through the activities on the Companion Website is the best way to get the most out of this book.

Each chapter is organized to help you understand the concepts and theories, with questions and exercises that will help you succeed in the classroom, in the clinical setting, and on course exams.

Prentice Hall and I value your opinions about this book. Please send feedback to us at nursing_excellence@prenhall.com.

I wish you success in your careers as nurses and as advocates. Together we can make a difference in our world!

Sincerely,

Mary Jo Clark, PhD, RN, PHN

Brief Contents

FIFTH EDITION

COMMUNITY HEALTH NURSING

Advocacy for Population Health

Mary Jo Clark

RN, MSN, PhD, PHN
Professor
Hahn School of Nursing and Health Science
University of San Diego
San Diego, California

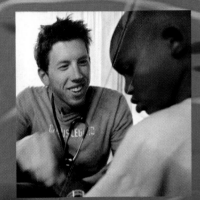

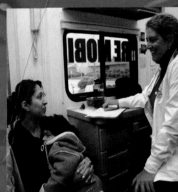

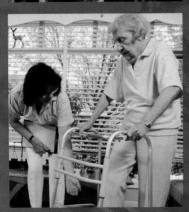

PEARSON

Prentice
Hall

Upper Saddle River, New Jersey 07458

Library of Congress Cataloging-in-Publication Data

Clark, Mary Jo Dummer.
  Community health nursing: advocacy for population health /
Mary Jo Clark.—5th ed.
    p. ; cm.
  Includes bibliographical references and index.
  ISBN 0-13-170982-8
  1. Community health nursing. I. Title.
  [DNLM: 1. Community Health Nursing. 2. Nursing Process.
WY 106 C594ca 2008]
  RT98.N88 2008
  610.73'43—dc22   2006023080

Publisher: Julie Levin Alexander
Assistant to Publisher: Regina Bruno
Editor-in-Chief: Maura Connor
Executive Acquisitions Editor: Pamela Lappies
Associate Editor: Michael Giacobbe
Development Editor: Elizabeth Tinsley
Managing Editor, Development: Marilyn Meserve
Editorial Art Manager: Patrick Watson
Media Product Manager: John J. Jordan
Director of Marketing: Karen Allman
Senior Marketing Manager: Francisco del Castillo
Marketing Coordinator: Michael Sirinides
Managing Editor, Production: Patrick Walsh
Production Editor: Trish Finley, GGS Book Services
Production Liaison: Anne Garcia
Media Project Manager: Stephen Hartner
Manufacturing Manager: Ilene Sanford
Manufacturing Buyer: Pat Brown
Senior Design Coordinator: Mary Siener
Printer/Binder: Courier Kendallville, Inc.
Composition: GGS Book Services
Interior Design: Janice Bielawa
Cover Design: Robert Aleman
Cover Illustration: Top, Corbis, Melanie Burford, *Dallas Morning News;*
Middle, George Dodson; Bottom, Photodisk; Background, Jupiter Images,
Biran Haglwara
Cover Printer: Phoenix Color

Pearson Education LTD.
Pearson Education Australia PTY, Limited
Pearson Education Singapore, Pte. Ltd
Pearson Education North Asia Ltd
Pearson Education Canada, Ltd.
Pearson Educación de Mexico, S.A. de C.V.
Pearson Education—Japan
Pearson Education Malaysia, Pte. Ltd
Pearson Education, Upper Saddle River, New Jersey

Notice: Care has been taken to confirm the accuracy of information presented in this book. The authors, editors, and the publisher, however, cannot accept any responsibility for errors or omissions or for consequences from application of the information in this book and make no warranty, express or implied, with respect to its contents.

The authors and publisher have exerted every effort to ensure that drug selections and dosages set forth in this text are in accord with current recommendations and practice at time of publication. However, in view of ongoing research, changes in government regulations, and the constant flow of information relating to drug therapy and reactions, the reader is urged to check the package inserts of all drugs for any change in indications or dosage and for added warning and precautions. This is particularly important when the recommended agent is a new and/or infrequently employed drug.

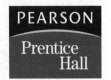

10 9 8 7 6 5 4 3 2

ISBN-13: 978-0-13-170982-9
ISBN: 0-13-170982-8

About the Author

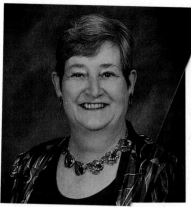

(Courtesy of Olan Mills)

Mary Jo Clark, PhD, RN, PHN, has been practicing and teaching community health nursing for 40 years. After completing her BSN degree at the University of San Francisco, she received her introduction to global community health nursing as a U.S. Peace Corps Volunteer in Vita, India, a rural town with a population of about 3,000. Returning to the United States, Dr. Clark employed her cross-cultural expertise as a Public Health Nurse in the Los Angeles County Department of Health Services. In 1973, she became a pediatric nurse practitioner, and later began teaching community health nursing at East Tennessee State University. She completed a master's degree in community health nursing at Texas Women's University and a PhD in nursing at the University of Texas at Austin. Moving with her Army nurse husband to Augusta, Georgia, she taught graduate and undergraduate community health at the Medical College of Georgia. For the past 20 years, Dr. Clark has taught at baccalaureate, master's, and doctoral levels at the University of San Diego, Hahn School of Nursing and Health Science. In addition to her full-time teaching and writing, Dr. Clark has maintained an active community health nursing practice. She is well known in the community health nursing field and has provided consultation and made presentations across the country and overseas. Her many and varied experiences in community health nursing in the United States and abroad form the core of the material presented in this book.

Dedication

This book is lovingly dedicated to Phil the elder, Phil the younger, and Heather, who are the wind beneath my wings, and to my fellow community health nursing faculty members: Connie Curran, Diane Hatton, and Linda Robinson, who embody the vision of advocacy that is the centerpiece of this book. We're making a difference, ladies.

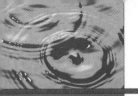

Thank You!

We would like to thank the hundreds of colleagues from schools and health facilities across the country who gave so generously of their time and attention. These individuals assisted in the development of this edition through one or more of the following activities—reviewed manuscript chapters, participated in focus groups, reviewed illustrations, and participated in surveys. This text has benefited immeasurably from your expertise.

Judith Alexander, University of South Carolina

Pam Ark, University of Central Florida

Tina Bayne, Washington State University

Sara Becker, South Dakota State University

Derryl Block, U Wisconsin Green Bay

Susan Boos, Fort Hays State University

Kathy Brewer-Smyth, University of Delaware

Cynthia Brown, College of St. Scholastica

Linda Bugle, Southeastern Missouri State University

Angeline Bushy, University of Central Florida

Beth Cameron, Wright State University, Miami Valley

Lucrinda Campbell, Houston Baptist University

Sharon Carlson, Otterbein College

Mary Carrico, West Kentucky Community and Technical College

Stephanie Chalupka, University of Massachusetts–Lowell

Rosemary Chaudry, Ohio State University

Deborah Chaulk, University of Massachusetts–Lowell

Melany Chrash, Waynesburg College

Barbara Courtney, East Carolina University

Gail Davidson, Cox College of Nursing

Liz Dietz, San Jose State University

Janice Edelstein, Marian College

Lori Edwards, Johns Hopkins University–School of Nursing

Karen Egenes, Loyola College

Bonnie Ewing, Adelphi University

Nancy Fahrenwald, South Dakota State University

Judy Frerick, Northern Kentucky University

Nancy S. Goldstein, The Johns Hopkins University School of Nursing

Vida Gorsegner, University of Missouri–Columbia

Ruth Grubesic, Texas Women's University–Houston

Connie Hall, Pennsylvania State University–Fayette

Sue Hayden, Troy University

Carole Heath, Sonoma State University

Carol Hoffman, University of Louisville

Brenda Hosley, Barea College

Katherine Howard, Raritan Bay Medical Center, Charles E Gregory School of Nursing

Esther Jacobs, Loyola College

Kathy Jenkins, Riverside School of Health Careers

Marie Louise Jorda, Florida International University

Irene Kalnins, St. Louis University

Janice Long, Kennesaw State University

Rita Lourie, Temple University

Carolyn Mason, Miami University of Ohio

Betty Mayer, University of Central Florida

Susan McMarlin, University of North Florida

Cynthia Mitchell, University of Missouri–St. Louis

Donna Mitchell, University of Rio Grande

Amy Moore, Texas Tech State University

Laurie Nagelsmith, Excelsior College

Virginia Nehring, Wright State University

Marianne Neighbors, University of Arkansas

Bridgit Pullis, Houston Baptist University

Becky Randall, South Dakota State University

Cindy Rieger, Oklahoma Baptist University

Sally Roach, University of Texas–Brownsville

Wanda Robinson, Oklahoma Baptist University

Connie Roush, University of North Florida

Jana Saunders, Texas Tech State University

Donna Shambley-Ebron, University of Cincinnati

Maria Smith, Georgia Southern University

Thomas Stenvig, South Dakota State University

Sheila Stroman, University of Central Arkansas

Donna Tilley, Texas Tech University Health Science Center–School of Nursing

Carol Torok, SUNY Institute of Technology

Kim White, Southern Illinois University–Edwardsville

Susan Williams, University of Alabama

Suzanne Yarborough, Excelsior College

Contributors

The Advocacy in Action vignettes that open each chapter, and are interspersed within some chapters, are stories of real advocacy by real nurses. Most were submitted by community health nursing students, faculty, and practicing nurses and highlight the real world of community health nursing and its emphasis on advocacy. Among them are the members of the executive board of the Association of Community Health Nursing Educators (ACHNE), for whose participation we are grateful: Derryl Block, University of Wisconsin, Green Bay; Susan Swider, Rush University; Joyce Krothe, Indiana University; Pamela A. Kulbok, University of Virginia; Julia Cowell, Rush University; Margaret Beaman, Indiana University. Wherever possible, we have included the names and pictures of the authors of contributed vignettes to give these often unsung heroes credit for their actions. We offer our appreciation to these contributors for their heartfelt expressions of nursing in the community and for their generosity in permitting us to tell their stories. The Advocacy in Action vignette that opens Chapter 3 describes the work of Susie Walking Bear Yellowtail, the first Native American registered nurse and an exemplary community health nurse advocate. The photograph that accompanies her story was graciously provided by Marina Weatherly, who has written a book about Ms. Yellowtail.

Many people were involved in the creation of the supplements that accompany and enhance this book. Denise Smart of Washington State University created the Instructor's Resource Manual material and the PowerPoint lecture slides. Pat Prechter and Teresa O'Neill, both of Our Lady of Holy Cross, wrote the review questions for the test bank. Four talented instructors wrote the content for the Companion Website. Katherine Magorian of Mount Marty College, Shelley Johnson of LaSalle University, and Claudia Stoffel of West Kentucky Community & Technical College wrote the questions, case studies, and exercises. Rita Lourie of Temple University recruited and managed the interviews with four women who have made a tremendous difference in ways that cannot yet be imagined for nurses and those they serve: Tine Hansen-Turton, Executive Director of the National Nursing Centers Consortium; Congresswoman Eddie Bernice Johnson, representing the 30th District of Texas; Vernice Ferguson, Senior Fellow Emeritus, University of Pennsylvania, and American Academy of Nursing "Living Legend"; and Sister Rosemary Donnelly, former executive vice president of Catholic University and former dean of the School of Nursing, and former president of Sigma Theta Tau International Honor Society. Our sincere thanks go out to them for their participation.

Historical photographs were provided courtesy of the Center for Nursing Historical Inquiry at the University of Virginia School of Nursing; the Center for the Study of the History of Nursing at the School of Nursing, University of Pennsylvania; the Louisiana Division of the New Orleans Public Library; and the National Library of Medicine. Other photographs were obtained from Image Works and Getty Images or are the work of the author.

Preface

This book represents the lessons learned and the progress made in more than 100 years of community health nursing in the United States. The year 1993 marked the 100th anniversary of the founding of the Henry Street Settlement, the acknowledged beginning of modern American community health nursing. Since then, the work of community health nurses and others has led to better health for individuals, families, and population groups. In this book, I have tried to distill the wisdom of early pioneers and present-day practitioners to guide and direct future generations toward nursing excellence.

Locally, nationally, and globally, society is in greater need of community health nursing services than at any time since our beginning. Although expected longevity has increased significantly in the last century, quality of life has not kept pace for a large portion of the world's population. Previously controlled communicable diseases are resurfacing, and new diseases are emerging to threaten the public's health. Malnutrition is a fact of life for many people. Chronic physical and emotional diseases are taking their toll on the lives of large numbers of people. Substance abuse and violence are rampant, and more and more frequently, environmental conditions do not support health. All of these are problems that community health nurses can and do help to solve.

Community health nurses must have the depth and breadth of knowledge that allows them to work independently and in conjunction with clients and others to improve the health of the world's populations. In part, this improvement occurs through care provided to individuals and families, but it must also occur on a larger scale through care provided to communities and population groups. *Community Health Nursing: Advocacy for Population Health* provides community health nurses with the knowledge needed to intervene at these levels. This knowledge is theoretically and scientifically sound, yet practical and applicable to society's changing demands.

NURSING EXCELLENCE THROUGH ADVOCACY

This edition focuses on the central facet of community health nursing—advocating for the health of the public. The theoretical concept of advocacy is introduced in Chapter 1 and is based on qualitative research by the author that examines the process of advocacy as it is performed by community health nurses. Practical application of the concept occurs in each of the subsequent chapters and is further emphasized in the two new features described on the following pages, "Advocacy in Action" and "Think Advocacy."

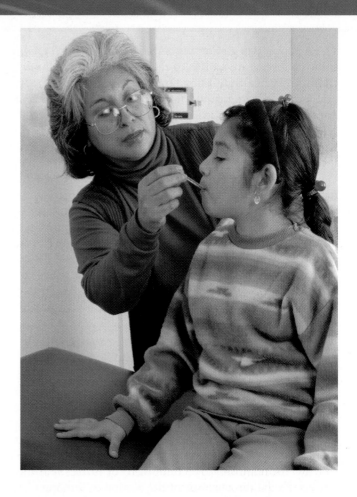

Community Health Nursing: Advocacy for Population Health, Fifth Edition, provides students with a strong, balanced foundation for community health nursing. The book is designed to help students first achieve excellence in the classroom through the many features and exercises that accompany the narrative. The additional tools and supplements will help students succeed at applying those concepts in clinical settings in the community, with the ultimate goal of preparing nurse generalists who will exhibit nursing excellence in any setting, providing care to individuals, families, communities, and population groups.

The underlying intent of this book is to convey to nursing students at the beginning of the 21st century the excitement and challenge of providing nursing care in the community. As we begin a new era of community health nursing, I believe that well-educated community health nurses can provide a focal point for resolution of the global health problems presented above. Early community health nurses changed the face of society; we can be a strong force in molding the society of the future by striving for nursing excellence through advocacy.

ORGANIZATION

This textbook is designed to present general principles of community health nursing and to assist students to apply those principles in practice. It is organized in five units. The first two units address general concepts of community health nursing practice, and the last three examine the application of those concepts to specific populations, settings, and community health problems.

UNIT I sets the stage for practice by describing community health nursing and the context in which it occurs. Readers are introduced to community health nursing as an area of specialized practice and to its emphasis on advocacy for the health of individuals, families, and population groups. The attributes and features that make community health nursing unique, standards for practice, and typical roles and functions of community health nurses are addressed. Then, the concept of populations as recipients of nursing care and the historical and theoretical underpinnings and development of community health nursing are presented.

A unique feature of this book is the consistent use of the Dimensions Model of Community Health Nursing to structure the discussion of principles of practice. The dimensions model is introduced in Chapter 4, which deals with several epidemiologic and community health nursing models, giving readers an overview of the theoretical foundations of community health nursing. Although the dimensions model is used as the basis for the rest of the book, readers also learn about other models that can be used to guide community health nursing practice. In Units II, III, IV, and V, elements of the dimensions model are used to examine the approaches used in community health nursing practice and the provision of care to selected populations, in particular settings, and with specific community health problems. The consistent use of the dimensions model permits students to readily identify commonalities and differences among processes, populations, settings, and health problems. Other chapters in this first unit explore the national and global health care, political, economic, cultural, and environmental contexts that influence the health of populations and the practice of community health nursing.

UNIT II examines approaches to community health nursing as a specialized area of practice. It highlights three specific approaches: health promotion and education, case management, and community empowerment. Aspects of other approaches to community health nursing (e.g., referral, social marketing, change processes, and leadership) are integrated into these and other chapters as appropriate.

UNIT III addresses community health care provided to special population groups. In each chapter, students are assisted to apply principles of care to individuals and families, as well as to these populations as aggregates. For example, Chapter 16 emphasizes community health nursing care for children and adolescents as population groups, as well as strategies for improving the health of individual children and adolescents. Similar approaches are taken to other population groups in the unit: families, communities, women, men, the elderly, and the poor and homeless.

UNIT IV presents community health nursing in specialized settings such as the home, school, work, correctional, and disaster settings. For example, Chapter 22 examines the role of the community health nurse in official and voluntary agencies as specialized settings. The local health department is used as an exemplar of official agencies, and parish or faith community nursing is the exemplar for community health nursing practice in a voluntary agency. In each chapter in the unit, students are guided in the use of the nursing process in the special practice setting. Consideration is given to factors influencing health in each of the six dimensions of health, and nursing interventions at the primary, secondary, and tertiary levels of prevention are discussed.

UNIT V focuses on community health nursing practice related to the control of common population health problems such as communicable diseases, chronic physical and mental health conditions, substance abuse, and societal violence. Again, students are assisted to apply the nursing process to identify factors contributing to problems in each of these areas and in designing nursing interventions at primary, secondary, and tertiary levels of prevention. Consideration is given to the care of individuals and families with these problems as well as to resolving common community health problems at the population level.

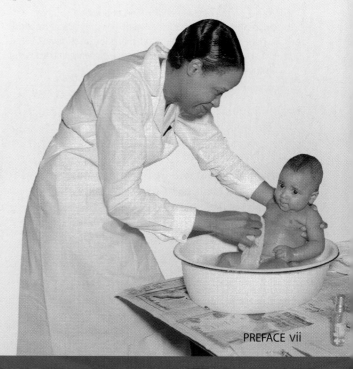

The boxes and charts in the fifth edition of *Community Health Nursing: Advocacy for Population Health* are tools to help you succeed in the classroom and in the community. They offer opportunities to consider specific aspects of providing nursing care in the community that you will encounter, offering you the chance to be better prepared to become an advocate.

Advocacy in Action

The vignettes at the beginning of every chapter and elsewhere in the text present real-life examples of advocacy by community health nurses. Contributed by students, faculty, and practicing community health nurses, these inspiring stories exemplify the advocacy role of the community health nurse to help you understand how you can work for change that will positively impact health.

Think Advocacy

These features help you to develop strategies for advocacy by thinking like community health nurses in practical, real-life situations. Following the scenario are questions that foster the use of critical thinking.

Think Advocacy

1. Talk with your classmates. What needs for advocacy with individual clients and families have arisen in your community health nursing clinical practice? Who were the participants in the advocacy situation? What actions were undertaken by the advocate? What were the consequences of those actions?
2. Based on the overall needs of the population you have witnessed in your community health nursing clinical rotation, where is advocacy needed at the population level? What risks might community health nurses experience in advocating in these areas?

Advocacy in Action

The Birth Certificate

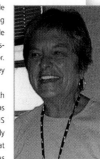

Navigating the U.S. social system can be a daunting task for people from other countries and cultures. A few years ago, a young Hmong woman found herself pregnant with her second child. She was able to obtain prenatal care and planned to call her husband for transportation to the hospital if he was at work when she went into labor. Most of their extended family had moved to North Carolina and they had few social supports remaining in the area.

Unfortunately, when she went into labor, she was home alone with her three-year-old daughter. The labor was rapid and the baby was born quite soon. The young woman knew to call 911 and EMS arrived to assist her shortly after the child was born. When the family went to obtain a birth certificate for the child, they were told that since it was a home birth, they needed proof that the baby was indeed theirs.

A local public health nurse was working with the family through a Parents as Teachers program to promote the development of preschool children in the community. The family took their problem to the nurse, who contacted the county vital statistics division and determined that a witness was needed to verify the birth to this mother. The only witness to the actual birth, however, was the three-year-old daughter, who was too young to provide verification. The nurse was told that if the EMS personnel, who arrived after the birth, had delivered the placenta and if they had documented that in the EMS record, the record would constitute verification. After more telephone calls, the community health nurse determined that the EMS personnel had indeed documented delivery of the placenta in the event record. She accompanied the parents to the EMS headquarters and assisted them in obtaining a copy of the record and then went with them to the vital statistics division to obtain the birth certificate. As a result of the nurse's advocacy and assistance, this family acquired its first U.S. citizen, a bright-eyed baby with a legal birth certificate.

Connie Curran, MSN, RN, PHN
Community Health Nurse
Bayside Community Center

Cultural Competence

In these boxes you will learn about cultural influences on health and illness and the effects of cultural beliefs and values on health care delivery. They encourage you to examine the effects of your own personal and professional cultural traditions, as well as those of clients, preparing you for clinical practice.

CULTURAL COMPETENCE

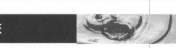

Some cultural groups traditionally think of people in the aggregate rather than as individuals. What cultural groups in your area have a community orientation? How might a community health nurse capitalize on this orientation? What aspects of traditional American culture make it more difficult to adopt aggregate thinking? What strategies by community health nurses might help people adopt a community orientation?

Healthy People 2010: Goals for Population Health

These boxes present relevant objectives from *Healthy People 2010* to familiarize you with these important government goals. You also learn about the current status of objectives here and on the Companion Website.

HEALTHY PEOPLE 2010
Goals For Population Health

OBJECTIVE	BASELINE	MOST RECENT DATA	TARGET
1-1. Increase the proportion of women with health insurance	84%	85%	100%
1-4c. Increase the proportion of women with an ongoing source of care	85%	86%	96%
2-9. Reduce the number of cases of osteoporosis	16%	NDA	8%
3-2. Reduce lung cancer deaths (per 100,000 women)	40.2	41.6	44.9*
3-3. Reduce breast cancer deaths (per 100,000 women)	26.6	25.6	22.3
3-4. Reduce cervical cancer deaths (per 100,000 women)	2.8	2.6	2.0
3-11a. Increase the proportion of women who have ever received a Pap test	92%	93%	97%
3-13. Increase the proportion of women aged 40 and over who have received a mammogram in the past 2 years	67%	70%	70%*
9-1. Increase the proportion of pregnancies that are intended	51%	NDA	70%
9-3. Increase contraceptive use among those who do not desire pregnancy	93%	NDA	100%
9-12. Reduce the proportion of married couples unable to conceive or maintain a pregnancy	13%	NDA	10%
9-13. Increase the proportion of health insurance policies that cover contraceptive services	NDA	NDA	NDA
15-34. Reduce the rate of physical assault by intimate partners (per 1,000 women)	4.4	2.6	3.3*
15-35. Reduce the rate of rape or attempted rape (per 1,000 women)	0.8	0.7	0.7*
16-4. Reduce maternal deaths (per 100,000 live births)	9.9	8.9	3.3
16-5. Reduce pregnancy complications (per 100 deliveries)	31.2	31.9	24#
16-6. Increase the proportion of pregnant women who receive early and adequate prenatal care	74%	75%	90%
16-17c. Increase abstinence from cigarette smoking by pregnant women	87%	89%	99%
19-2. Reduce the proportion of women who are obese	25%	33%	15%#
19-12c. Reduce iron deficiency anemia among females of childbearing age	11%	12%	7%#
22-1. Reduce the proportion of women with no leisure-time physical activity	43%	40%	20%
27-1. Reduce tobacco use by women	22%	20%	12%

NDA—No data available
* Objective has been met
# Objective moving away from target
Data from: Centers for Disease Control and Prevention. (2005). Healthy people data. Retrieved September 5, 2005, from http://wonder.cdc.gov/data2010

FOCUSED ASSESSMENT

Assessing the Policy Situation

Effective participation in policy formation requires the ability to assess the policy situation and determine factors that are operating in the situation. Here are some considerations that should guide policy assessment.

- What is the health problem or issue to be addressed? Why has the need for policy development or change arisen? What are the data related to the problem or issue?
- What is the appropriate policy arena? Where does jurisdiction lie?
- What is the goal or desired outcome of policy development?
- What are the potential alternative strategies for the problem? What are the advantages and disadvantages of each alternative? Which alternative(s) is most likely to achieve the goal or desired outcome?
- Are there strongly held values that will be supported or threatened by the proposed policy?
- Who will be affected by the policy? Who will support the policy? Who might oppose it? Why? What influence does the opposition wield? What is the power base of supporters of the proposed policy?
- Who should be involved in policy development? Implementation?
- Does the proposed policy adequately address the issue?
- Does the policy safeguard individual rights as much as possible?
- Are proposed implementation strategies fair and equitable?
- How easy or difficult will it be to implement the proposed policy?
- What will be the cost of policy implementation? What resources will be needed? How will these resources be obtained?

Focused Assessment

These boxes present a series of questions that assist you in conducting health assessments focused on a particular client, specific population groups, or particular aspects of care. They help you to tailor your nursing assessment to the specific needs of the client population, setting, or health problem addressed in the chapter.

Global Perspectives

This feature focuses on the relevance of global issues to local communities by presenting an international view of community health nursing practice. It helps you learn to look for links between events that may not be readily apparent.

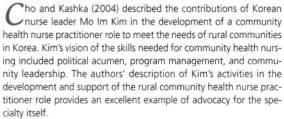

GLOBAL PERSPECTIVES

*C*ho and Kashka (2004) described the contributions of Korean nurse leader Mo Im Kim in the development of a community health nurse practitioner role to meet the needs of rural communities in Korea. Kim's vision of the skills needed for community health nursing included political acumen, program management, and community leadership. The authors' description of Kim's activities in the development and support of the rural community health nurse practitioner role provides an excellent example of advocacy for the specialty itself.

Explore how community health nursing practice has developed in another country. What events led to the development of the role? What factors have influenced how the community health nursing role is conceptualized in that country?

Evidence-Based Practice

These boxes present research findings related to chapter topics, helping you to examine the evidence base that underlies a specific aspect of community health nursing practice. They also pose questions that stimulate thinking about incorporating research into practice.

EVIDENCE-BASED PRACTICE

One of the criticisms of widespread use of complementary and alternative therapies is that many of them do not have a significant body of scientific evidence that supports their effectiveness. At the same time, there are conventional biomedical practices that are widely used without significant evidence for their efficacy (Park, 2002; Trachtenberg, 2002). Select one complementary or alternative health practice that interests you and examine the extent of the scientific basis for its practice. Then do the same for a relatively new conventional biomedical practice. How do the two practices compare with respect to the scientific evidence that supports them? In what areas is evidence lacking (e.g., overall effectiveness, effectiveness with specific population groups, etc.)? What additional evidence might be gleaned from research? How might you go about designing a study to develop that evidence?

Building Our Knowledge Base

These boxes encourage you to consider potential research questions related to chapter topics and to broaden your understanding of research principles and methods. It prods you to consider how you might be addressed by practicing community health nurses in preparation for your career.

BUILDING OUR KNOWLEDGE BASE

Design a study to determine what factors influence the participation of community members in community empowerment initiatives. What type of study would you conduct? What criteria would you use for selection of your subjects and how might you recruit people who meet those criteria to participate in your study? What data collection strategies would you use, and how would you analyze your data? What do you think your findings might indicate, and how could your findings be used to enhance community participation in empowerment activities?

Ethical Awareness

Presenting an ethical dilemma or issue related to the chapter, this box stimulates you to think about the course or courses of action you might take in a similar practice situation. You will be better prepared for clinical experiences that pose ethical dilemmas by considering possible courses of action to resolve the issues presented in these boxes.

ETHICAL AWARENESS

One of the major changes in the *Healthy People 2010* objectives is the shift from minimizing health disparities among various groups within the population to eliminating them altogether. What are the ethical implications of achieving this goal if it means reducing the level of service provided to groups with better health status in order to provide additional services to those with poorer health status? What models of ethical decision making would justify such an approach? What ethical arguments could be made against such reductions?

Special Considerations

Designed to promote critical thinking, these boxes highlight special information for you to contemplate.

SPECIAL CONSIDERATIONS	

PRINCIPLES OF PUBLIC HEALTH NURSING

Public health nursing is distinguished from other nursing specialties by its adherence to *all* of the following eight principles:

1. The client or "unit of care" is the population.
2. The primary obligation is to achieve the greatest good for the greatest number of people or the population as a whole.
3. The processes used by public health nurses include working with the client(s) as an equal partner.
4. Primary prevention is the priority in selecting appropriate activities.
5. The focus is selecting strategies that create healthy environmental, social, and economic conditions in which populations may thrive.
6. There is an obligation to actively identify and reach out to all who might benefit from a specific activity or service.
7. Optimal use of available resources to assure the best overall improvement in the health of the population is a key element of the practice.
8. Collaboration with a variety of other professions, populations, organizations, and other stakeholder groups is the most effective way to promote and protect the health of the people.

Reprinted with permission from the American Nurses Association. Public health nursing: Scope and standards of practice 2006. In press. Nursesbooks.org, Silver Spring, MD.

Client Education

These boxes identify important content for educating clients and the public regarding particular health issues and topics, equipping you for successful clinical encounters as you begin your career.

CLIENT EDUCATION	Use of Botanical Preparations

- Use of herbal remedies and dietary supplements should be reported to one's primary health care provider.
- "Natural" products do not have guaranteed safety or efficacy.
- Interactions of botanicals with prescription drugs may be dangerous.
- Lack of production standardization may result in differences in content and efficacy of products from batch to batch or from manufacturer to manufacturer.
- Lack of quality control in production may result in contamination, adulteration, or misidentification of botanical sources.
- Compounding errors may result in toxicity in custom-blended botanical preparations.
- Botanicals should not be used by pregnant or lactating women or those planning to become pregnant.
- Botanicals should not be taken in doses larger than those recommended.
- Some botanicals are known to have adverse effects.
- A small positive response to use of botanicals could be a result of a placebo effect.

Data from: American College of Obstetricians and Gynecologists. (2001). Use of botanicals for management of menopause symptoms. ACOG Practice Bulletin: Clinical Management Guidelines for Obstetrician-Gynecologists, 28, 1–15. Retrieved August 13, 2005, from http://www.acog.org/from_home/publications/misc/pb028.htm

HIGHLIGHTS	Attributes of Community Health Nursing
Population consciousness	Awareness of factors that impinge on the health of populations as well as that of individuals
Health orientation	Emphasis on health promotion and disease prevention rather than cure of illness
Autonomy	Greater control over health care decisions by both nurse and client than in other settings
Creativity	Use of innovative approaches to health promotion and resolution of health problems
Continuity	Provision of care on a continuing, comprehensive basis rather than a short-term, episodic basis
Collaboration	Interaction between nurse and client as equals; greater opportunity for collaboration with other segments of society
Intimacy	Greater awareness of the reality of client lives and situations than is true of other areas of nursing
Variability	Wide array of clients at different levels, from different ethnic backgrounds, and in different settings

Highlights

A feature intended to aid your review of content from the chapter, this bulleted summary of the main points or special focus appears periodically in the text.

Look for These Icons

The **MediaLink** logo appears in the margin next to related content on the Companion Website.

The *Healthy People 2010* icon appears in text after reference to *Healthy People 2010* objectives.

∞ The **cross-reference** icon appears in the text to refer you to other chapters.

The Community Assessment Reference Guide icon appears after references to assessment tools and inventories included in the *Community Assessment Reference Guide.*

Other Chapter Features to Help You Succeed

- **Chapter Objectives** at the beginning of each chapter summarize important points and help you identify key issues addressed in the chapter.

- **Key Terms** direct your attention to critical concepts included in a chapter by listing important vocabulary. At the point of definition within the chapter, each term is set in boldface type.

- **Case Studies** challenge you to apply the principles addressed in the chapter to realistic community health nursing practice situations. Each case study is followed by questions designed to promote critical thinking in nursing practice.

- **Test Your Understanding** assists you in evaluating your comprehension of concepts and principles presented in the chapter. These challenging review questions stimulate thought and discussion of important chapter concepts. Each question is followed by page references for a quick review of content addressed.

- **References** contained in each chapter present an up-to-date picture of principles and concepts related to the topic presented. References provide a balanced view of community health nursing, exploring a variety of issues from several perspectives, and provide a wide range of supplemental materials, including research reports, for the interested reader.

- **Appendices** A through D at the back of the book include four assessment tools to help you in clinicals. Those four appendices, along with six more, appear on the Companion Website that accompanies this book. These 10 tools and 18 more appear in the *Community Assessment Reference Guide*, a new book designed to accompany this text. It allows readers to photocopy immediately usable assessment tools and provides a greater number and selection of tools than was previously possible.

Resources for Students and Faculty

Companion Website

The Companion Website for the fifth edition of the textbook contains a variety of supplemental information and assessment tools that will be of immediate use to readers. The Web site includes the following features:

- **Case Studies:** Additional case studies are provided with thought-provoking questions that assist readers in applying content from the chapters. Case studies maintain a balance between application of practice concepts to individuals/families and population groups. Possible answers to case study questions are provided; however, readers may develop other, equally appropriate, responses.

- **Chapter Outlines:** Detailed chapter outlines assist readers to organize their learning of chapter content and to easily refer back to important portions of the chapter.

- **Advocacy Interviews:** Four video interviews with community health nurses and advocates who have made an impact on the health of the public tell their stories, showing how advocacy occurs in the lives of community health nurses and the populations they serve.

- **Chapter Objectives:** Chapter objectives assist readers in identifying key concepts contained in each chapter. They point out essential learning concepts, stimulate thought, and assist readers in reviewing chapter content.

- **Exam Review Questions:** Multiple-choice review questions are provided for each chapter to assist readers to evaluate their comprehension of chapter content.

- **Appendices:** Ten assessment tools aid students in evaluating individuals, families, and communities. Additional tools developed for use with specific populations or in particular settings are available in the *Community Assessment Reference Guide* designed to accompany this textbook.

- **Update *Healthy People 2010*:** This area of the Companion Website provides links to lead agencies where readers can obtain the latest figures on the status of selected *Healthy People 2010* national objectives.

Instructor Resource Manual

The Instructor Resource Manual is a wealth of helpful information for planning classroom activities. Included are learning objectives that provide instructors with student goals for each chapter. PowerPoint slides linked to chapter objectives can be used to structure class presentations. Suggested classroom and clinical activities promote student participation in learning and help bring community health nursing practice to life. A test bank with multiple-choice and alternate-format questions that test students' grasp of content is provided for each chapter.

Instructor Resource DVD-ROM

A test generator with electronic testbank is available on the Instructor Resource DVD-ROM, as well as PowerPoint lecture slides for each chapter and an Image Library with available images from the text.

Community Assessment Reference Guide

This collection of 38 assessment tools and inventories includes reproducible forms for providing nurse care for individuals, families, and population groups. A clinical tool kit, it offers you practical direction for the development of nursing diagnoses, planning, intervention, and evaluating the outcomes of care.

Guide to Special Features

Healthy People 2010

Special Considerations

Client Education

Highlights

Contents

The Context for Community Health Nursing

Advocacy in Action

Meeting Clients' Needs

Parkinson's disease is one of 45 incurable diseases for which the Japanese government covers medical expenses. Clients with Parkinson's disease in Nagaoka are followed by public health nurses through home visits and monthly meetings of a support group designed to provide socialization, problem-solving assistance, and emotional and spiritual support for clients and their families. The group is called "The Nettle Tree" and includes approximately 20 members. In the language of flowers, the blossom of the nettle tree means "cooperate and support."

In 2004, a major earthquake disrupted services and destroyed surrounding villages. Just after the temblor, the public health nurses worked hard to confirm the safety of their clients. Within two months, the support group was meeting again. The purpose of the first meeting was to allow members to "express their experiences as earthquake victims and to share their feelings with friends and acquaintances." They took time and talked to each other about their experiences. Many of them were still afraid of aftershocks, but they enjoyed the opportunity to talk about their experiences. They said "meeting the other members gave spiritual support," "I was anxious about other members' safety," "It was hard to control medication timing at the shelter because mealtimes were not regular," and "I had a terrible experience; I was buried under a chest and could not move."

Eleven subsequent meetings were held in 2005 as members of the community struggled to cope with the long-term effects of the earthquake. Members planned the theme of each meeting to address their needs. Some of the topics covered were "knowing the disease well" and "using public transportation even with a handicap." The ability to continue this service provided by public health nurses assisted the clients to cope with their disease even in the face of major social upheaval.

Yuko Uda (translated by Dr. Ariko Noji)
Public Health Nursing Supervisor, Nagaoka, Japan

Community Health Nursing as Advocacy

CHAPTER OBJECTIVES

After reading this chapter, you should be able to:

1. Define community health nursing.
2. Distinguish among community-based, community-focused, and community-driven nursing and describe their relationship to community health nursing.
3. Differentiate between district and program-focused community health nursing.
4. Describe the process of advocacy as enacted by community health nurses.
5. Identify at least five attributes of community health nursing.
6. Summarize the standards for community health nursing practice.
7. Identify the eight domains of competency for community health nursing.
8. Distinguish among client-oriented, delivery-oriented, and population-oriented community health nursing roles.
9. Describe at least five client-oriented roles performed by community health nurses.
10. Describe at least three delivery-oriented roles performed by community health nurses.
11. Describe at least four population-oriented roles performed by community health nurses.

KEY TERMS

 MediaLink
http//www.prenhall.com/clark

Additional interactive resources for this chapter can be found on the Companion Website. Click on Chapter 1 and "Begin" to select the activities for this chapter.

*I*n his 1916 address to Johns Hopkins Hospital Training School graduates, William H. Welch noted that America had "made at least two unique contributions to the cause of public health—the Panama Canal and the public health nurse" (Krampitz, 1987). According to figures collected by the Health Resources and Services Administration in 2000, public health nurses constituted 18% of the total nursing population in the United States, and the number of nurses employed in public health and community health settings increased 155% from 1980 to 2000 (Ray, 2003). Community health nurses constitute the largest single group of public health professionals in the United States (Sakamoto & Avila, 2004) and practice in state and local health departments, home health agencies, community health centers, and student and occupational health services as well as other settings. Who are they and what makes their practice unique? In this chapter we explore the features that set community health nursing apart from other nursing specialties and examine the roles and functions performed by community health nurses.

COMMUNITY HEALTH NURSING: WHAT'S IN A NAME?

Before we can explore this specialty area of nursing practice, we need to decide what to call it. There is considerable debate in this area. Some of the terms that have been used include *public health nursing, community health nursing, community-focused nursing, community-based nursing, community-driven nursing*, and *community-oriented health care* (Chen, Ervin, Kim, & Vonderheid, 1999; Nehls & Vandermause, 2004). This confusion regarding terminology characterizes the field in the United States as well as other parts of the world (Hamer, 2000; Murashima, Hatono, Whyte, & Asahara, 1999).

Both the terms *public health nursing* and *community health nursing* leave room for misinterpretation. Critics of the term *public health nursing* note that it implies the clientele of official public health agencies, who are often the underserved sick poor, as the primary recipients of care. In fact, the specialty addresses the needs of whole populations, including those who are well and affluent as well as those who are poor and sick. Although the Quad Council of Public Health Nursing Organizations (1999)—a coalition composed of the American Nurses Association (ANA) Council for Community, Primary, and Long-term Care Nursing Practice; the Public Health Nursing Section of the American Public Health Association; the Association of Community Health Nurse Educators (ACHNE); and the Association of State and Territorial Directors of Nursing—specified that although public health nursing can occur in either public or private agencies, the term *public health nurse* is often used for those nurses employed by official government health agencies such as state and local health departments. This is somewhat ironic since the term itself was coined by Lillian Wald, whose Henry Street Settlement, which gave birth to this nursing specialty in the United States, was certainly not an official government agency (Kuss, Proulx-Girouard, Lovitt, Katz, & Kennelly, 1997). Other authors distinguish between the two terms on the basis of focus. Public health nursing's perceived focus was one of environmental sanitation and control of communicable diseases, whereas community health nursing purportedly focused on health education and individual behavior change (Abrams, 2004).

Community health nursing, as a name for the specialty, also has the potential for inappropriate connotations. The term *community health nursing* was coined by the American Nurses Association as a general term for all nurses who worked outside of institutional settings such as hospitals (Kuss et al., 1997). Unless these nurses are engaged in population-focused nursing, however, they are not true community health nurses, but are nurses providing sick care in community settings. These nurses might be more appropriately described as engaged in "community-based" nursing (Nehls, Owen, Tipple, & Vandermause, 2001). "Community-focused" care is defined as the bringing of nursing knowledge and expertise to the community (Nehls & Vandermause, 2004), but such care may not have a population focus.

"Community-driven" care focuses on the needs of the community as a whole and emphasizes community participation in determining those needs (Nehls & Vandermause, 2004). This terminology, however, has the potential for limiting the focus of practice to those health needs identified by members of the community or population group. Although community involvement in the identification and resolution of health needs and issues is important, it is also true that part of community health nursing practice is raising community consciousness levels to the point where community members recognize the existence of health needs they may have previously ignored. Similarly, "community-oriented" care can be somewhat limiting, focusing program development on small aggregates while potentially ignoring health issues that affect larger population groups.

Despite the disagreement regarding labels, there is basic agreement that the defining characteristic of the specialty is population-focused nursing care directed toward the overall health of communities or population groups (Drevdahl, 2002; Grumbach, Miller, Mertz, & Finocchio, 2004). Some experts have suggested that the most appropriate title for the specialty is, indeed, "population-focused nursing." At this time, however, there appears to be considerable resistance within the specialty to such a major change in terminology. In the absence of a universally accepted term, we will use the term *community health nursing* throughout this book as most representative of the focus of the specialty.

DEFINING COMMUNITY HEALTH NURSING

In 1996, the Public Health Nursing Section of the American Public Health Association (APHA) defined public health nursing as "the practice of promoting and protecting the health of populations using knowledge from nursing, social, and public health sciences." The section further described public health nursing as a systematic process of assessing populations to identify groups in need of health promotion or at risk for disease, planning for community intervention, implementing the plan, evaluating outcomes, and using the resulting data to influence health care delivery.

The American Nurses Association (ANA) (1986) presented a similar definition, but used the term *community health nurse*, in the introduction to *Standards of Community Health Nursing Practice*. The 1999 definition by the Quad Council reinstated the term *public health nursing*, and the council currently defines the specialty as follows:

> Public health nursing is the practice of promoting and protecting the health of populations using knowledge from nursing, social, and public health sciences (American Public Health Association, Public Health Nursing Section, 1996). The practice is population-focused, with the goals of promoting health and preventing disease and disability for all people through the creation of conditions in which people can be healthy. (American Nurses Association, 2007)

A similar definition of community health nursing was provided by Nehls et al. (2001) as "a systematic process of delivering nursing care to improve the health of an entire community" (p. 305). For purposes of this book, **community health nursing** is a synthesis of nursing knowledge and practice and the science and practice of public health, implemented via systematic use of the nursing process and other processes to promote health and prevent illness in population groups.

THE MISSION OF COMMUNITY HEALTH NURSING

As we have seen, the defining characteristic of community health nursing is a focus on the health of population groups. The primary mission of community health nursing is improving the overall health of the population through health promotion, illness prevention, and protection of the public from a wide variety of biological, behavioral, social, and environmental threats (Berkowitz, 2002). In the words of one author, the purpose or mission of community health nursing is to "promote the good life" in all of its physical, social, psychological, cultural, and economic aspects (Uosukainen, 2001).

The focus of community health nursing care is the aggregate, a population with some common characteristics (e.g., pregnant adolescents, the elderly). The goal of care is the promotion of health and the prevention of illness and injury. Health promotion and illness prevention in the population may be achieved through interventions directed at the total population or at the individuals, families, and groups that constitute its members. Several authors have noted that community health nurses are most effective at the population level when they are grounded in knowledge of the needs of the individuals and families that comprise the populations with which they work (Smith & Bazini-Barakat, 2003; SmithBattle, Diekemper, & Leander, 2004b). The fact remains, though, that community health nurses provide care to individuals and families with an eye to how that care influences the health status of the population (Gebbie, 2002). Community health nursing practice is based on the expectation that improvement of population health will also benefit the individuals and families who constitute the population (Feenstra, 2000).

COMMUNITY HEALTH NURSING AND ADVOCACY

Achievement of the mission of community health nursing requires advocacy, usually at multiple levels. Advocacy in community health nursing involves striving for social justice, and one author likens advocacy efforts to the activities of a modern-day Robin Hood. Social justice requires "taking from the rich and giving to the poor [and] ambushing the public conscience and budget whenever possible" (Mullan, cited in Drevdahl, 2002, p. 162). This view of social justice highlights the fact that measures to achieve social justice are apt to be unpopular with the "rich" and will require concerted advocacy by community health nurses and others. The concept of social justice is based on the idea that social factors limit the distribution of goods and services throughout the population. Changing these social factors to promote more equitable distribution among members of society requires collective action (Drevdahl, 2002). Social justice, then, is defined as an equitable distribution of the burdens and benefits of society among its members (Drevdahl, Kneipp, Canales, & Dorcy, 2001). Health is one of the results of access to societal benefits, and it is incumbent on community health nurses to see that members of population groups have equitable access to all the societal benefits that promote health.

Defining Advocacy

Dictionary definitions of advocacy involve adoption of a cause or pleading in favor of a cause (Bassett, 2003). In nursing, advocacy was originally defined by the American Nurses Association in its 1976 *Code for Nurses with Interpretive Statements* as protecting clients from "incompetent, unethical, or illegal practice of any person" (p. 8). Over the years, the concept of advocacy by nurses has been expanded from protecting clients against harm to incorporate activities such as informing clients, protecting client rights, mediating between the client and members of the health care team, and supporting client autonomy (Chafey, Rhea, Shannon, & Spencer, 1998; Snowball, 1996). The *Guidelines for Professional Practice* in the United Kingdom suggest that nurse advocates should not act on personal assumptions of what is best for the client, but should inform the client and support his or her informed decisions. Similarly, the British *Guidelines for Mental Health and Learning Disabilities Nursing* defined advocacy as promoting self-determination and client empowerment (Wheeler, 2000). The revisions to *Public Health Nursing: Scope and Standards of Practice* (ANA, 2007) defined advocacy as "the act of pleading or arguing in favor of a cause, idea, or policy on someone else's behalf, with a focus on developing the community, system, individual, or family's capacity to plead their own cause or act on their own behalf."

Some authors have maintained that the essence of public health advocacy is "spreading the word," informing community members and decision makers regarding healthy behaviors (Avery & Bashir, 2003). This definition, however, puts the onus for health promotion on the individual, with community health nurses advocating for healthful behaviors and against unhealthful ones. Even when the focus is on developing policy related to healthful behavior (e.g., laws prohibiting smoking in public places), this limited definition of community health advocacy fails to address all of the other societal factors that may promote ill health, such as poverty, environmental hazards, and others. Other authors describe advocacy as developing "agency within groups and communities to co-create health through partnership, and intervening in the environment to support collective agency" (Kulbok, Gates, Vicenzi, & Schultz, cited in Westbrook & Schultz, 2000, p. 52). For community health nurses, then, **advocacy** can be defined as action taken on behalf of, or in concert with, individuals, families, or populations to create or support an environment that promotes health. Such actions may occur at the individual, family, community, or societal level and may include a variety of activities such as education for healthier behavior, promotion of access to health care services, or changes in societal conditions that endanger health.

Advocacy by Community Health Nurses

Drevdahl (2002) noted that advocacy has only recently become a focus of public health and that the mission of public health practice has shifted from an initial focus on epidemic control in the 1800s and early 1900s to one of disease prevention in the mid-1900s. Only recently has social justice become a major focus of the discipline. The current state of affairs for public health practitioners was described like this by one author: "Public health takes place in boardrooms, on street corners, in our homes, and in the legislature. So, too, does public health advocacy" (Bassett, 2003, p. 1204). Advocacy for healthful

living conditions for the general population has become a major public health focus in the United States as well as internationally.

Some authors trace the rise of a general nursing focus on advocacy to the beginning of the patient's rights movement of the 1970s (Foley, Minick, & Kee, 2002; Snowball, 1996). Advocacy in the acute care setting has been described as following one of four models: guardian of legal rights, preservation of patient values, champion of social justice and access to care, and client empowerment (Baldwin, 2003). Most of these models support the interests and welfare of individual clients. For community health nurses, on the other hand, advocacy for the health of populations, as well as individuals and families, has historically been a large part of their practice. As we will see in Chapter 3∞, community or public health nursing was synonymous with political activism and population advocacy for early nurse leaders such as Florence Nightingale, Clara Barton, Lillian Wald, Lavinia Dock, and Margaret Sanger (Drevdahl et al., 2001; Foley et al., 2002). Margaret Sanger, an early advocate of contraceptive rights for women, highlighted the need for continuing advocacy by community health nurses: "Though many disputed barricades have been leaped, you can never sit back smugly content, believing that victory is forever yours; there is always the threat of its being snatched from you" (Drevdahl et al., 2001, p. 28).

Advocacy for social justice is an essential aspect of the core mission of community health nursing, yet the last century has witnessed a decline in the social activist efforts of community health nurses. In part this decline has been attributed to a shift in control of community health nursing practice. In the early days of public health nursing, the practice of community health nurses was outside the control of the medical profession. After World War II, medicine began to dominate public health and community health nurses were less autonomous (Drevdahl et al., 2001). Another contributing factor, as we will see later, was the shift from a focus on health promotion and illness prevention to provision of direct care to individuals and families. Recently, however, community health nurses have begun to reclaim their population advocacy function, while still maintaining advocacy activities for individual clients and families.

The Advocacy Process

How does one engage in advocacy, particularly at the population level? There is a great deal in the literature about the need for advocacy and its importance as an element of nursing practice. There is very little discussion, however, of how advocacy occurs. Two qualitative research studies provide some information on the process involved in advocacy (Clark, 2001).

Advocacy arises out of a precipitating situation that results in vulnerability. Vulnerability may be experienced by clients at any level—individual, family, community, or population. Situations that may contribute to vulnerability may relate to health status (e.g., mentally retarded individuals or persons with HIV/AIDS), behavior (e.g., substance abuse), culture, social status (e.g., unemployment or poverty), environment, or other social factors that lessen people's abilities to promote and protect their health. Vulnerability is reflected in a loss of control over factors that impinge on health and that result in some kind of unmet need. Vulnerability prevents the person or group affected from acting on their own behalf and requires the efforts of an outside agent (the community health nurse) to act for or support action by the vulnerable person or group.

An advocacy situation involves three essential categories of participants: a recipient of the advocacy, an advocate, and an "adversary." The recipient of advocacy is the vulnerable individual, family, or population group who cannot act for themselves for a variety of reasons (e.g., fear, lack of knowledge, poverty). The advocate is the person or persons who act for or enable action by the recipient. The adversary may be a person, institution, or societal system that impedes action to address unmet needs. Individual clients may need advocacy with family members or health care professionals to meet their needs. For example, a community health nurse may have to intervene with overly protective parents who are not allowing a handicapped child to achieve his or her full potential. Similarly, advocacy may be needed with a physician who ignores a client's request for information about treatment options for breast cancer. A health department that charges fees for immunizations may be a health system adversary preventing access to preventive care for indigent segments of the population. Similarly, legislation prohibiting access to care for undocumented immigrants is a societal adversary impeding health promotion for this population.

One additional actor may also be present in an advocacy situation. This may be an "intermediary." Intermediaries may be of two types. Adversarial intermediaries interpret and support the adversary's position. For example, a nurse case manager may merely inform clients that their health insurance does not support a specific intervention rather than searching for a way to provide the desired intervention or discover an acceptable alternative. Unfortunately, adversarial intermediaries are often other nurses (Clark, 2001). Supportive intermediaries, on the other hand, support the efforts of the advocate to meet client needs. A legislator interested in changing eviction practices to protect vulnerable groups such as non-English-speaking residents would be an example of a supportive intermediary.

The research identified three major factors that influenced participants in an advocacy situation: knowledge, conviction, and emotion. Knowledge influenced all of the participants involved in a situation. For example, knowledge of current eviction regulations (or lack thereof) may lead unscrupulous landlords to evict tenants for complaints about unsafe housing conditions; conversely, lack of knowledge of appropriate channels for reporting housing violations may make tenants more vulnerable to coercion. Knowledge also influences the actions of the advocate when he or she knows what is allowable under the law.

Conviction was a factor that primarily influenced the advocates in the study situations. Advocates frequently voiced their conviction that their action was warranted. Often this conviction was upheld in the face of knowledge about possible consequences and even in the event of negative consequences for the advocate. Advocates repeatedly spoke of knowing they were doing "the right thing."

Emotion also plays a role in an advocacy situation. Emotions such as fear and anxiety may contribute to the vulnerability of the advocacy recipient. For example, fear of eviction may prevent tenants from filing complaints about unsafe housing conditions. The effect of both conviction and emotion can be seen in recent debates regarding gay marriage and granting spousal rights (e.g., to insurance coverage) to members of same-sex marriages.

In each advocacy situation, effective advocacy requires action on the part of the advocate. The type of action taken depends on the situation as well as on the personality of the advocate. Some actions are collaborative, with the advocate attempting to work cooperatively with the adversary to meet clients' needs. Other actions are more adversarial in nature. Types of actions that may be taken by advocates include adjusting (e.g., changing a therapeutic regimen or adjusting clinic hours to accommodate clients' schedules), connecting or "hooking up" clients with outside resources, supporting clients' decisions, helping (e.g., helping a sexually active adolescent to obtain contraceptives), and assuring (e.g., promoting access to care, assuring informed consent). Other approaches to advocacy include educating the advocacy recipient or adversary, confronting the adversary, requesting a change, showing (e.g., providing legislators with photographs of housing violations to promote effective legislation), explaining (e.g., explaining the effects of unprotected intercourse to sexually active adolescents), and enlisting the help of others (e.g., forming coalitions to promote legislation to enhance access to care for underserved segments of the population).

The last element of the advocacy process is its consequences. Advocacy has consequences for all of the participants in an advocacy situation. Generally the consequences are positive ones, but that is not always the case. Advocacy always carries an element of risk and may never be completely politically safe (Bassett, 2003; Mallik, 1998). In fact, some nursing literature actually cautions nurses against engaging in an advocacy role due to the lack of a clear definition of nursing advocacy and because of the potential for negative consequences. As stated by one author, "In many cases, they [nurses] would be well advised not to act as an advocate themselves. Rather they should attempt to empower the client to self-advocate" (Wheeler, 2000, p. 41). Although this may be sound advice in some areas of nursing practice, the extreme vulnerability of many underserved segments of the population make it less feasible for community health nurses. Frequently, community health nurses are the only persons knowledgeable about the needs of these groups. This firsthand knowledge of population needs makes it imperative for community health nurses to continue to engage in population advocacy. In fact, as some authors put it, "The future of PHN [public health nursing] depends on nursing's ability to recognize social, economic, and political aspects of the environment as they affect health and to intervene at the community level for structural change" (Drevdahl et al., 2001).

Community Health Nurse Functions in the Advocacy Role

As an advocate, the community health nurse engages in a number of activities or functions. These activities fit within a cycle of documentation, analysis, action, and documentation of effect (Bassett, 2003). The first nursing function is determining the need for advocacy and the factors that prevent clients from acting on their own behalf. Such factors can be quite varied. Some clients, for example, may not know how to go about making their needs known. Fear of reprisal might be another reason why clients do not speak for themselves. Other factors include apathy, feelings of hopelessness, and even language barriers.

A second function of the nurse as advocate is determining the point at which advocacy will be most effective. For example, should the nurse raise concerns of safety violations in rental housing with the landlord, with the housing authority, or with the media? Answers to such questions might be derived from knowledge of what has been tried previously and the effects of prior action. Related questions involve how the case should be presented. Should one, for example, ask for a meeting with interested parties, or stage a demonstration?

Collecting facts related to the problem is another advocacy-related function. An advocate is considerably less effective when he or she does not have all the facts about a situation. A community health nurse advocate should get a detailed chronological account of events related to the problem for which advocacy is needed. The nurse should also try to validate or verify the information obtained to support the claim that a problem exists and action is needed.

The fourth task in advocacy is presenting the client's case to the appropriate decision makers. This function requires tact and interpersonal skill. Threatening or confrontational behavior should be avoided whenever possible, as both can set up an adversarial relationship rather than a collaborative one, which may be detrimental to the client's cause. When other avenues fail, threats may have to be employed, but nurse and client must be committed to acting on them. For example, if the nurse threatens to report a landlord for safety code violations unless action is taken to remove hazards, he or she should actually be prepared to make the report.

The final function of the nurse as an advocate is to prepare clients to speak for themselves. The activities and functions of advocacy should not be carried out by the nurse alone, but should be a collaborative effort between nurse and client. In this way, clients learn how to develop and present a forceful argument for their own needs and may, in the future, be able to act without nursing intervention.

Advocacy necessitates involvement and commitment. The effective community health nurse cannot be content with the attitude "I'd like to help, but my hands are tied." Advocacy is not a popular concept. It frequently means frustration and argument. It is the antithesis of complacency and is essential to the practice of effective community health nursing. Community health nurses must speak for those who cannot speak for themselves and articulate their needs to those in power. Nurses must also assist members of the community to learn how to speak for themselves rather than remain dependent on the nurse. Advocacy is a twofold obligation to take the part of others and, in time, to prepare them to stand alone.

A final comment is necessary with respect to advocacy. Because advocacy promotes clients' right to self-determination, community health nurses must be prepared to support clients' decisions even when they run counter to health interests. For instance, the nurse may need to accept a community's decision not to act on an issue that the nurse believes to be important in favor of focusing on other issues of greater community concern.

TRENDS IN COMMUNITY HEALTH NURSING PRACTICE

Some trends in community health nursing are worth noting as a basis for describing the current practice of community health nurses. When community health nursing began with groups like the Henry Street Settlement in the United States, district nursing in England, and the Victorian Order of Nurses (VON) in Canada, community

Think Advocacy

1. Talk with your classmates. What needs for advocacy with individual clients and families have arisen in your community health nursing clinical practice? Who were the participants in the advocacy situation? What actions were undertaken by the advocate? What were the consequences of those actions?

2. Based on the overall needs of the population you have witnessed in your community health nursing clinical rotation, where is advocacy needed at the population level? What risks might community health nurses experience in advocating in these areas?

health nurses worked toward improvements in the health of the population both through services to individuals and families and through political activism at the aggregate level. This dual service level was most often accomplished through **district nursing**, a mode of service delivery in which each community health nurse was responsible for addressing all the health needs of a given population. Services included health promotion and education, and often illness care, for all the people residing in the nurse's "district" whatever their age, ethnicity, or economic level. Because of the broad spectrum of services provided across the age span, these nurses were required to engage in generalist practice and to have a broad knowledge base regarding a variety of community health problems, from prenatal diet to treatment for tuberculosis to substance abuse. A district nursing approach sometimes encouraged nurses to become focused on the needs of the specific individuals and families who made up their caseloads, losing sight of the bigger picture of health of the total population and the need for involvement in policy development as well as service delivery.

As funding sources for public health services became more categorical, community health nursing tended to adopt a program-focused approach and moved away from a population or systems focus (Kaiser, Barr, & Hays, 2003). **Program-focused nursing** is a service delivery system in which nurses focus their activities and efforts on specifically designated health problems or specific target populations. In program-focused nursing, community health nurses became specialists in a single program area—for example, tuberculosis screening and treatment or promotion of child development (May, Phillips, Ferketich, & Verran, 2003; Rafael, 1999a). Emphasis shifted from involvement with all segments of the population to specifically targeted high-risk groups (Chalmers, Bramadat, & Andrusyszyn, 1998).

Program-focused nursing also tended to place emphasis on group work, with fewer services to individuals and families, and was characterized by distance from clients. Community health nurses were no longer intimately involved in all health-related aspects of clients' lives but dealt only with their specialty areas (Rafael, 1999a).

In the wake of the Institute of Medicine report, *The Future of Public Health* (1988), which identified the core functions of public health, community health nursing groups have moved even more toward a focus on populations with less emphasis on direct care to individuals and families within those populations. Lack of emphasis on direct services, however, has resulted in the loss of connection with the community that was experienced by prior generations of community health nurses. This loss of connectedness, in turn, has made it more difficult for community health nurses to carry out the core functions. When community health nurses were intimately connected with community members, they were aware of the needs and problems faced by members of the population.

They also had access to data that allowed them to carry out their assurance function (one of the core public health functions, discussed in Chapter 5∞) and to evaluate the effectiveness of health care delivery systems (Rafael, 1999a; SmithBattle, Diekemper, & Leander, 2004b). Some research indicates that despite the resurgent emphasis on population health, most activities of public health nurses are related to the care of individuals and families. Similarly, nurse managers in these settings rated interventions directed at individuals and families as more important than activities directed to community and system levels (Grumbach et al., 2004). The authors also suggested that many public health nurses are poorly prepared for practice at the population level.

The point in discussing the dichotomous approaches to community health nursing exemplified by district nursing and program-focused nursing is to emphasize that community health nursing is not an either/or proposition. It is not a question of *either* providing direct services to individuals and families *or* engaging in population-focused activities, but a synthesis of the two. Services are provided to individuals and families as a means of improving the health of the overall population. The improvement of the health status of individuals and families is an admirable goal in itself, but appropriate to community health nursing only if it also leads to improved health of the total population. This perspective may lead to ethical dilemmas related to resource allocation when the good of the larger group is best served by denying certain services to individuals and families (Billings, 1998). Community health nursing in the future must address this dual mission of service to individuals and families and population health rather than dichotomize these two levels of service.

The community health nursing literature has often debated the related question of whether adequately prepared community health nurses should be generalists or specialists. It would seem that connectedness to communities requires visibility on the part of community health nurses that is served by multiple interactions with different types of clients with a wide array of health problems. These interactions would seem to necessitate a generalist background through which the community health nurse deals with multiple kinds of issues and problems (May et al., 2003). However, community health nursing also requires specialist preparation not possessed by nurses in other fields. This specialist preparation lies in the population skills required for population-focused practice. We will discuss some of these specialized skills needed by community health nurses later in this chapter.

PRINCIPLES OF COMMUNITY HEALTH NURSING

As noted earlier, the defining characteristic of community health nursing is its focus on the health of population groups. Community health nursing is also defined by its

GLOBAL PERSPECTIVES

*C*larke (2004) described public health nursing in Ireland, where nurses in the specialty must be qualified in three areas: general nursing, midwifery, and public health nursing. Public health nurses are attached to specific geographic areas or communities and engage in health promotion and illness prevention activities and care of the sick. The nurses interact with individual clients, families, and community groups. Recently, other general registered nurses without specific preparation in community health nursing have been introduced into the system to extend community access to community nursing services. There is some concern that the introduction of these nurses may lead to a weakening of the community health nursing role. How do these developments compare to recent changes in focus for community health nursing in the United States (e.g., a move away from individual/family-based care to population-focused care)?

adherence to eight principles of practice as delineated in the ANA *Public Health Nursing: Scope and Standards of Practice* (2007). Although other nursing specialties may incorporate one or more of these principles in their practice, public health nursing is distinguished from these other specialty areas by incorporation of all of them in practice. These defining principles are presented at right.

ATTRIBUTES OF COMMUNITY HEALTH NURSING

In addition to adherence to the principles discussed at right, community health nursing is characterized by a constellation of attributes that make it a unique field of nursing practice. These attributes include population consciousness, orientation to health, autonomy, creativity, continuity, collaboration, intimacy, and variability.

Population Consciousness

Community health nurses must have a consciousness beyond the needs of and services to individual clients and families. The nurse must develop an awareness of how information related to individual clients relates to the health status of the total population. Are this family's needs characteristic of the population, or unique to the family? Are the factors impinging on a particular client's health impinging on the health of the community at large?

Community health nurses must also have an awareness of what is taking place in the general population. What changes in the economic situation will affect the health of the population? What effect will closure of a major health care system have on community health? In short, community health nurses must see the big picture and be aware of the interactive nature of factors that influence health and well-being.

The centrality of this population focus was highlighted in two recent studies. In the first study, staff-level

public health nurses were asked to make recommendations for improving community health nursing practice. Their recommendations included increased system and organizational resources, improved visibility of public health, and enhanced collaboration as well as further education in concepts and skills needed for population-based practice (Zahner & Gredig, 2005b). The second study reflected improvements needed in community health nursing education from the perspective of nurses practicing in the specialty. Again, the nurses recommended a greater focus on population-based care and educational opportunities for clinical practice at this level (Zahner & Gredig, 2005a).

Orientation to Health

The 1988 Institute of Medicine report noted that the mission of public health is "fulfilling society's interest in assuring conditions in which people can be healthy." Promotion of health has also been a nursing function since the inception of district nursing with Florence Nightingale and was actively supported by Lillian Wald and the founders of the VON (Rafael, 1999b).

In other nursing specialties, health promotion is a facet of care, but one that is, of necessity, frequently given lower priority than health restoration needs. In community health nursing, on the other hand, the emphasis is on health promotion and maintenance rather than the cure of disease or disability. Although community health nurses frequently help clients resolve existing health problems, their major goal is to promote clients' highest level of physical, emotional,

SPECIAL CONSIDERATIONS

PRINCIPLES OF PUBLIC HEALTH NURSING
Public health nursing is distinguished from other nursing specialties by its adherence to *all* of the following eight principles:

1. The client or "unit of care" is the population.
2. The primary obligation is to achieve the greatest good for the greatest number of people or the population as a whole.
3. The processes used by public health nurses include working with the client(s) as an equal partner.
4. Primary prevention is the priority in selecting appropriate activities.
5. The focus is selecting strategies that create healthy environmental, social, and economic conditions in which populations may thrive.
6. There is an obligation to actively identify and reach out to all who might benefit from a specific activity or service.
7. Optimal use of available resources to assure the best overall improvement in the health of the population is a key element of the practice.
8. Collaboration with a variety of other professions, populations, organizations, and other stakeholder groups is the most effective way to promote and protect the health of the people.

Reprinted with permission from the American Nurses Association. *Public health nursing: Scope and standards of practice.* (2007). Silver Spring, MD: Nursesbooks.org.

and social well-being. Health promotion as practiced by community health nurses encompasses both promotion of self-care behaviors by clients and advocacy for social and environmental conditions that promote health (Uosukainen, 2001). For example, the health orientation of a community health nurse may lead to assistance with smoking cessation for individual clients as well as political activism to ban smoking in public places.

Autonomy

Autonomy, or self-direction, is a twofold attribute of community health nursing. Both the community health nurse and the client tend to be more self-directed than either might be in an institutional health care setting. Although all clients have the right and responsibility to make decisions about their health care, their autonomy in this regard tends to be eroded by the way health care and other social institutions operate. Because community health nursing care is typically provided in the client's home or neighborhood, the client is more likely to demand an active role in health care decision making, a situation the community health nurse should anticipate and foster. The same is true of community clients or population groups; community health nurses should actively involve these larger groups in the determination of health policy and planning for service delivery.

Community health nurses also exercise a considerable degree of professional autonomy. In some situations, community health nurses may be the only providers of health care available. They must then rely on their own judgment to choose an appropriate course of action, frequently without consultation with other providers (Rafael, 1999a). In this sense, the community health nurse is more autonomous in practice than is the institution-based nurse.

Creativity

Community health nurses deal with increasingly complex problems at both the individual/family and the population levels. Considerable creativity is required to develop solutions that fit within the constraints posed by client and community situations. Competition for resources by acute care delivery systems leaves little funding available for community health nursing activities, and that little funding must be used in ever more creative ways to achieve maximum benefit.

Continuity

Continuity of care is another hallmark of community health nursing. Whatever the setting in which community health nurses work, relationships between nurse and client tend to be of relatively long duration. Community health nurses often have the flexibility to work with most clients until both feel that services are no longer needed. Because of the extended nature of the relationship, community health nurses are able to evaluate long-term as well as short-term effects of nursing interventions. They are also able to provide care for a wider range of client needs than is usually possible in acute care nursing. Problems not addressed today can be dealt with in subsequent meetings, and changing circumstances can be evaluated over time. Continuity also occurs in community health nurses' interactions with communities and population groups. Involvement by the community health nurse in one initiative, for example, often leads to continuing involvement in efforts to address other community or population needs.

Collaboration

Because of the autonomy discussed earlier and the fact that interaction occurs in settings familiar to clients, nurse and client interact on a more equal footing than might otherwise be the case. This equality increases the potential for a truly collaborative relationship between nurse and client. Again, this collaborative essence of practice is reflected in the care of population groups as well as care of individuals and families. Community health nurses are often engaged in participatory action research in which members of the community or target population participate in the design and implementation of research identifying community needs and in the planning of services to meet those needs.

Community health nurses also have greater opportunity for interaction and collaboration with other providers of client services linked directly or indirectly to health. In the acute care setting, nurses frequently interact with other health and social services providers. Collaboration in community health nursing is described as both *intersectoral* and *multisectoral* (Kuss et al., 1997). It is intersectoral in that collaboration occurs with persons outside of the health care system. It is multisectoral in that community health nurses must usually collaborate with multiple other sectors of the population at the same time. For example, other sectors of society with which community health nurses might collaborate in addressing the problem of adolescent substance abuse might include police, school systems, and so on.

This multisectoral collaboration requires what have been referred to as *multilingual* and *multiperspectival* skills on the part of nurses (Diekemper, SmithBattle, & Drake, 1999a). Community health nurses must speak the languages not only of different ethnic groups, but also of other segments of society. They must be able to communicate in understandable terms with policy makers, funders, educators, and others with whom they collaborate. In addition, they must have an understanding of the multiple perspectives these groups bring to community health issues.

Intimacy

Another difference between community health nursing and other areas of nursing practice is the sphere of intimacy that typifies community health practice. Hospitals

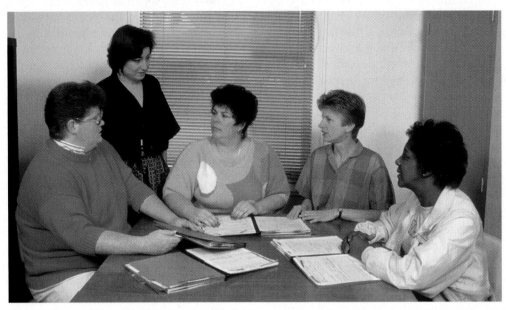

Community health nurses collaborate with people from widely varied segments of the population. (Cindy Charles/PhotoEdit Inc.)

and other institutional health care environments often modify a client's behavior, thus affecting the accuracy of the nurse's observations of clients, their families, and their problems. Practicing in the community setting, however, the nurse can get a more accurate picture of the factors that affect clients' health. The community health nurse may also become more intimately aware of everyday details of an individual client's normal life and environment. For example, the community health nurse might discover evidence of spouse abuse that might not be uncovered in other health care settings. Intrusion into the client's sphere of intimacy may provoke hostility, particularly in instances when care has not been sought but is mandated by circumstances (e.g., child abuse).

Effective community health nurses also become intimately involved with the community. More often than not, community health nursing is not circumscribed by specific working hours and community activities may impinge on other aspects of the nurse's life. For example, evenings may be devoted to meetings of community groups designed to address identified population health issues.

Variability

The last characteristic of community health nursing, one that is highly valued by practicing community health nurses, is variability. Community health nurses deal with diverse clients at different levels (individual, family, or population group) and ethnic backgrounds in a wide variety of settings. This variability necessitates a broad knowledge base and provides an exciting area of practice for those willing to accept the challenge.

All of these attributes are evidence of the unique status of community health nursing, which uses principles of both nursing and public health to prevent or alleviate health problems of groups of people as well as

individual members of society. Attributes characteristic of community health nursing are summarized on page 13.

STANDARDS FOR COMMUNITY HEALTH NURSING PRACTICE

One of the hallmarks of a profession is the establishment of standards of practice. Nursing, like other health-related professions, has set up standards for nursing practice and nursing service. The standards for nursing practice are further delineated in standards established for each of several specialty areas in nursing. Among these, and of particular interest to community health nurses, is the American Nurses Association's *Public Health Nursing: Scope and Standards of Practice* (2007).

The standards of care for community health nursing practice have been developed within the framework of the nursing process and the core functions of public health. They relate to the areas of assessment, diagnosis, outcomes identification, planning, implementation, and evaluation. Additional standards address expected levels of professional performance and deal with quality of practice, education, professional practice evaluation, collegiality, ethics, collaboration, research, resource utilization, leadership, and advocacy. Measurement criteria have been developed for each of the standards. The

CULTURAL COMPETENCE

*H*ow would you describe the culture of community health nursing? How does this culture differ from that of nurses in the acute care setting? What cultural features in both arenas might make communication difficult? How does the culture of community health nursing interface with that of client populations?

The public health nursing competencies incorporate expectations for care of individuals and families "within the context of population-focused practice" (p. 2), a unique feature compared to the COL competencies that deal only with population-focused practice. The

PUBLIC HEALTH NURSING: SCOPE AND STANDARDS OF PRACTICE

Standard 1. Assessment: The public health nurse collects comprehensive data pertinent to the health status of populations.

Standard 2. Population Diagnosis and Priorities: The public health nurse analyzes the assessment data to determine the population diagnoses and priorities.

Standard 3. Outcomes Identification: The public health nurse identifies expected outcomes for a plan that is based on population diagnoses or priorities.

Standard 4. Planning: The public health nurse develops a plan that reflects best practices by identifying strategies, action plans, and alternatives to attain expected outcomes.

Standard 5. Implementation: The public health nurse implements the identified plan by partnering with others.

Standard 5A. Coordination: The public health nurse coordinates programs, services, and other activities to implement the identified plan.

Standard 5B. Health Education and Health Promotion: The public health nurse employs multiple strategies to promote health, prevent disease, and ensure a safe environment for populations.

Standard 5C. Consultation: The public health nurse provides consultation to various community groups and officials to facilitate the implementation of programs and services.

Standard 5D. Regulatory Activities: The public health nurse identifies, interprets, and implements public health laws, regulations, and policies.

Standard 6. Evaluation: The public health nurse evaluates the health status of the population.

Standard 7. Quality of Practice: The public health nurse systematically enhances the quality and effectiveness of nursing practice.

Standard 8. Education: The public health nurse attains knowledge and competency that reflects current nursing and public health practice.

Standard 9. Professional Practice Evaluation: The public health nurse evaluates one's own nursing practice in relation to professional practice standards and guidelines, relevant statutes, rules, and regulations.

Standard 10. Collegiality and Professional Relationships: The public health nurse establishes collegial partnerships while interacting with representatives of the population, organizations, and health and human services professionals and contributes to the professional development of peers, students, colleagues, and others.

Standard 11. Collaboration: The public health nurse collaborates with representatives of the population, organizations, and health and human services professionals in providing for and promoting the health of the population.

Standard 12. Ethics: The public health nurse integrates ethical provisions in all areas of practice.

standards also serve as the basis for tools evaluating the quality of community health nursing care in the practice setting (Kaiser & Rudolph, 2003). The standards of practice for community health nursing are summarized at right.

COMMUNITY HEALTH NURSING COMPETENCIES

In 2003, the Quad Council developed a set of competencies for community health nursing at two levels of practice, the staff nurse/generalist and the manager/specialist/consultant. The competencies are intended to "facilitate education, orientation, training, and lifelong learning using an interdisciplinary model where appropriate" (p. 1). The competencies are based on those developed by the Council on Linkages between Academia and Public Health Practice (COL). The COL competencies incorporate the skills, knowledge, and attitudes required for effective public health practice in general. The Quad Council examined the applicability of the COL competencies specifically to community health nursing practice and developed performance expectations related to each competency for the two levels of practice. The generalist competencies are intended to reflect baccalaureate-level educational preparation, and the specialist competencies reflect master's-level preparation (Quad Council of Public Health Nursing Organizations, 2003).

(continued)

SPECIAL CONSIDERATIONS

Standard 13. Research: The public health nurse integrates research findings into practice.

Standard 14. Resource Utilization: The public health nurse considers factors related to safety, effectiveness, cost, and impact on practice and on the population in the planning and delivery of nursing and public health programs, policies, and services.

Standard 15. Leadership: The public health nurse provides leadership in nursing and public health.

Standard 16. Advocacy: The public health nurse advocates to protect the health, safety, and rights of the population.

Reprinted with permission from the American Nurses Association. Public health nursing: Scope and standards of practice. (2007). Silver Spring, MD: Nursesbooks.org.

competencies address eight domains of practice: (a) analytic assessment, (b) policy development and program planning, (c) communication, (d) cultural competence, (e) community dimensions of practice, (f) basic public health practice, (g) financial planning and measurement, and (h) leadership and systems thinking. The competencies are intended to reflect the practice of experienced community health nurses at both generalist and specialist levels, not novices, and expectations range from awareness through knowledge to proficiency on any given item. Any particular community health nursing position may incorporate components from some or all domains and from each level of practice. Appendix A∞ includes the competency domains and related skills as well as the expected level of performance for generalist and specialist community health nursing practice (Quad Council of Public Health Nursing Organizations, 2003).

ROLES AND FUNCTIONS OF COMMUNITY HEALTH NURSES

In their practice, community health nurses engage in a variety of roles and perform multiple functions. Although the emphasis on specific roles and functions varies from one practice setting to another, most community health nurses engage in some way in the roles described below. These roles are categorized on the basis of the primary focus of nursing care as client-oriented, delivery-oriented, or population-oriented roles.

ETHICAL AWARENESS

Your state is considering restricting the bulk of state health funding for health promotion and illness prevention services. This means that very little money would be available for assisting low-income clients with major health care expenditures (e.g., liver transplants). What would be your position on this issue? Why? To what extent is your position congruent with the standards for community health nursing practice?

Client-Oriented Roles

Client-oriented roles involve direct provision of services to individuals, families, and occasionally groups of people. As noted earlier, community health nursing does not entail exclusive provision of population-focused services, but instead uses services to individuals and families as one means of improving population health. Population-focused nursing is thus grounded in individual/ family-focused care (SmithBattle, Diekemper, & Leander, 2004b). Client-oriented community health nursing roles include those of caregiver, educator, counselor, referral resource, role model, primary care provider, and case manager.

Caregiver

The caregiver role involves applying the principles of epidemiology and the nursing process to the care of clients at any level—individual, family, group, or community. Some of the functions entailed in this role are assessing client needs, deriving nursing diagnoses, and planning appropriate nursing intervention. Implementing the plan of care may involve performing technical procedures or assuming one or more of the other client-oriented roles. Evaluating nursing care and its outcomes is another function performed in the caregiver role. This role is basic to all client encounters, and its functions are performed whether or not any of the other community health nursing roles are assumed.

In the care of individuals and families, the caregiver role may entail provision of delegated medical treatment as well as the provision of nursing care. In fact, in one study, 41% of California public health nurses reported that they engaged in delegated treatments to specific clients (Grumbach et al., 2004).

Community health nurses also engage in the caregiver role with populations as the recipients of care. Just as in the care of individuals and families, community health nurses assess the health status of the population, develop nursing diagnoses, and plan, implement, and evaluate care for the population. This usually entails the development of health care delivery programs to meet identified needs. The caregiver role with populations as clients is discussed in more detail in Chapters 13 and 15∞.

In some cases, the caregiver role may involve provision of primary care to individuals and families. **Primary care** is defined as essential health care services made universally accessible to all. It consists of initial care provided to clients at their point of entry into the health care system. The primary care function of most community health nurses involves health-promotive and illness-preventive interventions such as routine prenatal assessments, well-child care, and immunizations. Community health nurses also routinely deal with minor health problems such as constipation and diarrhea.

Other community health nurses, with advanced educational preparation, provide primary care as nurse practitioners. These nurses have assumed diagnostic and treatment services that were once the exclusive province of physicians. There has been some concern that the adoption of some aspects of medical practice by nurse practitioners might detract from the emphasis placed by community health nurses on health promotion and illness prevention. Although this is sometimes the case early in a nurse practitioner's career, most practitioners regain their nursing perspective fairly rapidly and provide both curative and health-promotive services.

Performance of the primary care role by community health nurses and other advanced practice nurses (APNs) enhances the accessibility and comprehensiveness of health care services available to the general public. APNs have been shown repeatedly to provide equal or better quality care than physicians in a cost-effective manner (Boyd, 2000).

Educator

Education is the process of facilitating learning that leads to positive health behavior. In the educator role, the community health nurse provides clients and others with information and insights that allow them to make informed decisions on health matters. The educator role may be performed at any client level. Community health nurses often provide educational services to individuals, families, and groups, and they are frequently involved in the development of population-based health education programs. Community health nurses, for example, educate individuals and their families about adequate nutrition. At the same time, they may educate the general public regarding the harmful effects, say, of a high-cholesterol, low-fiber diet. Similarly, community health nurses may educate legislators

and other policy makers regarding societal factors that impede population health.

Research with community health nurses has indicated that changes in the health care delivery system have made the role of educator of even greater importance. For example, in one study, nearly a third of California public health nurses engaged in community-level education, and nearly all provided health-related education to individuals and families (Grumbach et al., 2004). In the educator role, the nurse assesses the need for education and motivation for learning, develops and presents health-related information, and evaluates the effects of health education. We discuss these functions in greater detail in Chapter 11∞.

Although the educator role is primarily a client-oriented role, the community health nurse may also serve as an educator for his or her peers or other professionals, in keeping with the community health nursing performance standard for collegiality. The nurse may be involved, for example, in educating student nurses or students in other health-related disciplines. On occasion, the nurse may be called on to educate other health professionals as well. For example, in some jurisdictions community health nurses help educate private physicians regarding appropriate diagnostic, treatment, and reporting procedures for sexually transmitted diseases.

Counselor

Although many people do not distinguish between counseling and education, they *are* different. **Counseling** is the process of helping the client to choose viable solutions to health problems. In educating, one is presenting facts and developing attitudes and skills. In counseling,

Community health nurses provide health education to individuals, families, communities, and population groups. (Patrick J. Watson)

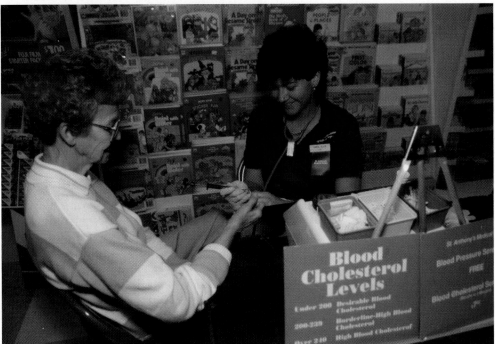

one is *not* telling people what to do but helping them to employ the problem-solving process and decide on the most appropriate course of action. In the role of counselor, community health nurses explain the problem-solving process and guide clients through each step. In this way, the nurse is not only helping the individual, family, or population to solve the immediate problem but also assisting in the development of problem-solving abilities. Community health nurses have indicated that they engage in the counseling role with individuals and families, communities, and at the systems level in the design of health care services (Grumbach et al., 2004).

Counseling involves several steps on the part of the community health nurse. The first step is to assist the client to identify and clarify the problem to be solved. The nurse and client together examine the factors that contribute to a problem and those that may enhance or impede problem resolution. At the second step of the counseling process, the community health nurse helps the client identify alternative solutions to the problem. If, for example, a large proportion of pregnant women in the population do not receive prenatal care, one could suggest an educational campaign, outreach efforts by lay health promoters, financial subsidies for care by available providers, or the use of nurse midwives.

Assisting the client to develop criteria for an acceptable solution to the problem is the third step in the counseling process. For example, an acceptable solution to the problem of poor nutrition among family members would need to fit the family's budget and might need to conform to cultural dietary preferences. A program to address nutritional needs at the population level would need to address the same constraints.

Next, the community health nurse would assist the client to evaluate each of the alternative solutions in terms of criteria established for an acceptable solution. The most appropriate alternative is one that best meets the acceptability criteria. This alternative is then implemented. Evaluation is the fifth step of the problem-solving process. If the alternative selected solves the problem, fine! If not, the process begins again. The problem-solving process is depicted in Figure 1-1.

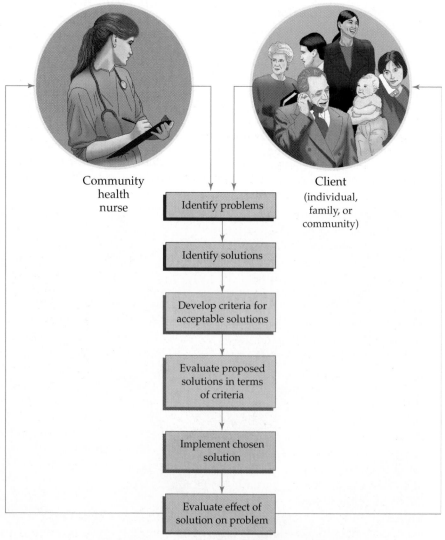

Community health nurse

Client (individual, family, or community)

Identify problems

Identify solutions

Develop criteria for acceptable solutions

Evaluate proposed solutions in terms of criteria

Implement chosen solution

Evaluate effect of solution on problem

FIGURE 1-1 Problem Solving in Community Health Nursing

Referral Resource

Referral is one of the key functions of community health nurses. **Referral** is the process of directing clients to resources required to meet their needs. These resources may be other agencies that can provide necessary services or sources of information, equipment, or supplies that the client needs and the community health nurse cannot supply.

A distinction must be made between the functions of referral and consultation. In a referral, the client is directed toward another source of services. In *consultation*, on the other hand, the nurse may seek assistance or information needed to help the client from another source, but the client does not receive services directly from the consultant. Community health nurses also provide consultation to other professionals and to policy-making bodies.

Referral is an important part of the role of the community health nurse in any practice setting. It is the nurse's responsibility to explore resources available to meet client needs and direct clients to them as appropriate. The degree of intervention required in a specific referral varies with the type of referral and the client situation. Sometimes it is sufficient to let a client know that a certain resource exists. On other occasions, the particular agency may require a written referral from the nurse or from a physician.

In some instances, the client may not be capable of following through on a referral. For example, the depressed client may not have the energy to phone for an appointment at the local mental health center, but may be able to keep an appointment made by the nurse. The nurse must determine in each situation the degree of dependence or independence needed by that client at that time, with the goal, of course, of gradually increasing the client's ability to function independently. Specific functions of the community health nurse in the referral role include determining the need for referral, identifying the appropriate referral resources, and making and following up on the referral. The referral process is discussed in more detail in Chapter 12∞.

Role Model

A **role model** is someone who consciously or unconsciously demonstrates behavior to others who will perform a similar role. Community health nurses serve as role models for a variety of people with whom they come in contact. Through their own behavior, nurses influence the behavior of others. For instance, the community health nurse's ability to deal with crisis without panic provides guidance for clients to do the same.

The community health nurse's role as a model is not confined solely to influencing the health-related behavior of clients. The nurse also serves as a role model for other health care professionals. One of the areas in which the role-modeling function is of primary importance is in the educational preparation of student nurses. The way the community health nurse treats

EVIDENCE-BASED PRACTICE

SmithBattle, L., Diekemper, M., & Leander, S. (2004a). Getting your feet wet: Becoming a public health nurse, Part 1. *Public Health Nursing, 21*, 3–11.

SmithBattle, L., Diekemper, M., & Leander, S. (2004b). Moving upstream: Becoming a public health nurse, Part 2. *Public Health Nursing, 21*, 95–102.

1. How well do the findings of the research study described in these two articles reflect your experience and that of your classmates in your community health nursing clinical rotations?
2. What interventions by your community health nursing faculty might make the transition to effective community health nursing practice easier for you?

clients, the type of activity in which the nurse engages, and the level of competence displayed may all influence students' attitudes and practice. This influence can be either positive or negative.

Case Manager

Although case management is a new concept for many nurses, it has long been an integral component of community health nursing. Indeed, the case manager role may be seen as a comprehensive role that encompasses many of the other client-oriented roles described here. A **case manager** is a health professional who coordinates and directs the selection and use of health care services to meet client needs, maximize resource utilization, and minimize the expense of care.

The Case Management Society of America (1995) defined case management as "a collaborative process which assesses, plans, implements, monitors, and evaluates options and services to meet an individual's health needs through communication and available resources to promote quality cost-effective outcomes." The aims of case management include identifying high-risk clients or those with the potential for high-cost service needs, making appropriate choices among available services and providers, controlling costs, and coordinating care to achieve optimal client outcomes.

Case management has been shown to be cost effective and to result in enhanced health outcomes in many settings (Bedell, Cohen, & Sullivan, 2000). Given this fact and community health nursing's long association with case management, it would seem appropriate to retain case management as an essential part of the community health nursing role. The process of case management will be addressed in more detail in Chapter 12∞.

Nursing functions in the case manager role and other client-oriented roles are summarized in Table 1-1♦.

Delivery-Oriented Roles

The **delivery-oriented roles** of community health nurses are those designed to enhance the operation of the health care delivery system, resulting in better care for

Role	Function
TABLE 1-1	**Client-Oriented Community Health Nursing Roles and Related Functions**
Caregiver	Assess client health status
	Derive nursing diagnoses
	Plan nursing intervention
	Implement the plan of care
	Perform delegated medical treatments or provide primary care as needed
	Introduce other supportive services as needed
	Teach and supervise others
	Teach clients self-care
	Coordinate health care services
	Serve as liaison between client and system
	Evaluate the outcome of nursing intervention and modify the plan of care as required
Educator	Assess client's need for education
	Develop health education plan
	Present health education
	Evaluate outcome of health education
Counselor	Identify and clarify problem to be solved
	Help client identify alternative solutions
	Assist client to develop criteria for solutions
	Assist client to evaluate alternative solutions
	Assist client to evaluate effects of solution
	Make client aware of problem-solving process
Referral resource	Obtain information on community resources
	Determine the need for and appropriateness of a referral
	Make the referral
	Follow up on the referral
Role model	Perform the behavior to be learned by clients or others
Case manager	Identify need for case management
	Assess and identify client health needs
	Design plan of care to meet needs
	Oversee implementation of care by others
	Evaluate outcome of care

clients. Roles in this category include coordinator or care manager, collaborator, and liaison.

Coordinator/Care Manager

Community health nurses frequently care for clients who are receiving services from a variety of sources. Because of their awareness of the needs of the client as a whole being, community health nurses are in an ideal position to serve as coordinators of care. **Coordination** is the process of organizing and integrating services to best meet client needs in the most efficient manner possible. Unlike the case manager, the coordinator does not plan the care to be carried out by other health care professionals, but organizes that care to meet clients' needs as effectively as possible. At the population level, coordination may be referred to as *care management,* or the grouping of people with similar needs in order to meet those needs more cost effectively (e.g., preschool children, persons with arthritis) (Michaels, 1997). This may involve the development of networks of providers and payers who combine efforts to provide services for specific population groups in a way that maximizes use of resources. Population care management provides a continuum of services to the designated population and facilitates information transfer between and among providers as well as easing client transfers between agencies (Williams, 2000). Community health nurses may be actively involved in initiating such systematic interorganizational coordination.

For individual clients, it is the community health nurse who most frequently enters the home or community and sees firsthand how the client is responding to a physical therapy program or how effective a roach-control program has been. She or he is also in the best position to transmit to other providers information regarding client needs, attitudes, and progress. The community health nurse is also best able to interpret to the client, in language he or she can understand, the purposes and procedures involved in programs instituted by other health care providers.

The community health nurse serving as a coordinator of client care performs a variety of functions. The first function involves determining who is providing care to the client, where services overlap, and where gaps in care may be occurring. The second function is to communicate with other providers regarding the particulars of the client situation and needs. Communication includes informing providers of other persons and agencies dealing with the client. Except in certain circumstances (e.g., child abuse or threat of harm to self or others), communication should be undertaken *only* with the consent of the client.

A simple example of coordinating services for an individual client might involve arranging for appointments in a prenatal clinic and a child health clinic on the same day, when both services are provided at the same location. Coordinating appointments in this way assists a pregnant woman with a 2-year-old and limited transportation to obtain needed health care for herself and her child without a second bus trip.

One additional function of the community health nurse in a coordinator role might be arranging a case conference to include nurse, client, and other providers of services. For example, the school nurse might arrange a meeting that would include not only the nurse but also the child, parents, teachers, and school psychologist to discuss the child's behavior problems in school.

At the population level, coordination might involve making a variety of agencies addressing similar health problems aware of what each is doing. Coordination at this level might also entail bringing similar agencies together to discuss service provision with the intent of eliminating gaps and overlaps in services.

Collaborator

Collaboration is "a dynamic, transforming process of creating a powersharing partnership" (Sullivan, 1998, p. 19), or, put more practically, a process of shared decision making by two or more people. As a collaborator, the community health nurse engages in joint decision making regarding action to be taken to resolve client health problems. Collaboration should always take place between nurse and client or a significant other. Collaborative efforts, however, may also include other providers.

Collaboration is frequently confused with the nurse's coordination role. Coordination is essentially a management function and involves making sure that efforts to provide services are consistent and occur without gaps or overlaps. Collaboration, on the other hand, entails joint decision making. Both collaboration and coordination, of course, necessitate working with clients and other professionals (and nonprofessionals) who contribute to the health care of clients. This contribution by others may be directly related to the client's (or population's) health status, as in the case of physicians, physical therapists, nutritionists, and other health care personnel. It may also be indirectly related, as are the services of police and firefighters, sanitation engineers, and city officials.

Collaboration is not a matter of each health care worker designing and providing a program in his or her area of expertise with a certain amount of coordination between efforts. Rather, it is a joint effort on the part of health care providers *and clients* to set mutual goals and to arrive at a mutually acceptable plan to achieve them. Collaboration is a relatively new function for most nurses and cannot take place without a mutual feeling of respect and collegiality among health team members.

The two primary functions of the community health nurse in a collaborative role are communication and joint decision making. In communicating, the nurse conveys to other team members his or her perceptions of client needs, factors influencing those needs, and ideas for problem resolution. In decision making, the community health nurse participates in joint problem-solving efforts, using the problem-solving process with the health care team to identify and evaluate alternative solutions to client problems and to select an appropriate alternative. Collaboration may also extend to joint activity to implement solutions selected and to evaluate the outcome.

Liaison

The liaison role of the community health nurse incorporates facets of the coordinator and referral resource roles and may even incorporate the advocacy role, depending on the client situation. A **liaison** provides a connection, relationship, or intercommunication. The community health nurse working with clients dealing with multiple health and social agencies may serve as that connection or liaison. In the referral resource role, the community health nurse may function as the initial point of contact between client and agency. The liaison role might involve continued communication between client and other providers via the nurse. Sometimes this communication includes the additional function of interpretation and reinforcement of provider recommendations to the client or advocacy for the client with the provider agency. At the population level, the community health nurse may serve as a liaison between community residents and policy makers. A summary of delivery-oriented roles and related functions is presented in Table 1-2◆.

Population-Oriented Roles

The client-oriented and delivery-oriented roles of community health nurses usually relate to the care of specific individuals or families. At times these roles may be extended to the care of communities or populations. As noted throughout this text, community health nurses are concerned primarily with the health of the population, and they perform a number of roles that are exclusively group oriented.

Population-oriented roles are those directed toward promoting, maintaining, and restoring the health of the population and include those of case finder, leader, and change agent. Additional population-oriented roles are policy developer, community organizer or mobilizer, coalition builder, social marketer, and researcher. Population-oriented roles are essential because the health of the population cannot be accomplished merely by changes in individual or family health status or behaviors, but also rests on changes in larger social and environmental factors that affect health (SmithBattle, Diekemper, & Drake, 1999).

Case Finder

Case finding has been described as basic to community health nursing. **Case finding** by the community health nurse involves identifying individual cases or occurrences of specific diseases or other health-related conditions requiring services. Why, then, is this considered a

TABLE 1-2	Delivery-Oriented Community Health Nursing Roles and Related Functions
Role	**Function**
Coordinator	Determine who is providing care to client
	Communicate with other providers regarding client situation and needs
	Arrange case conferences as needed
	Assist in development of care networks
Collaborator	Communicate with other health team members
	Participate in joint decision making
	Participate in joint action to resolve client problems
	Participate in joint activities to evaluate the outcome of care
Liaison	Serve as initial point of contact between client and agency
	Facilitate communication between client and agency personnel
	Interpret and reinforce provider recommendations
	Serve as client advocate as needed

population-oriented role? Despite the fact that case finding involves location of individual cases of a condition, the primary intent is the assessment and protection of the health of the general public. As we will see in Chapter 28∞, case finding is an important strategy in preventing the spread of communicable diseases in large population groups. Case finding is also a means of monitoring the health status of a group or community. For example, identifying more instances of child abuse may be an indication of a community health problem.

Case finding with respect to communicable disease also incorporates the community health nursing function of disease investigation. In this role, the community health nurse explores the factors contributing to the development of a communicable disease in a specific person. For example, investigation of cases of food poisoning may uncover unsanitary practices in a local restaurant or contamination of food supplies during processing, leading to modifications that will prevent illness in others.

Community health nurses have a relatively close and often prolonged association with clients and have the opportunity to detect changes in health status or early signs of health problems. During a visit to a hypertensive client, for example, the community health nurse may discover that the client's teenage daughter is pregnant and in need of prenatal care. Or the nurse may observe that members of a number of families who obtain water from a common source have had recent episodes of vomiting and diarrhea. If the nurse is dealing with clients as unified entities (whether individuals, families, or populations), he or she is in a position to detect potential or actual health problems early and intervene rapidly. The ability of community health nurses to conduct physical examinations has further enhanced their case-finding ability by giving them another avenue for detecting the presence of disease or disability.

Case-finding responsibilities include developing an index of suspicion, identifying instances of disease or other health-related conditions, and providing follow-up services. An **index of suspicion** is an estimation of the likelihood that a disease or problem may exist and is based on a broad foundation of knowledge of the signs and symptoms of a variety of health problems and their contributing factors. For example, to identify a potential outbreak of plague, the nurse must be familiar with the signs and symptoms of the disease and recognize these indicators of disease in the populations he or she serves.

The case-finder role necessitates use of the diagnostic reasoning process to identify potential cases of disease or instances of other health-related conditions (such as pregnancy or the need for immunizations) based on relevant cues. This diagnostic processing of relevant signs and symptoms into a probable diagnosis of the disease is the second function of the community health nurse as case finder.

The third community health nursing function related to case finding is the provision of follow-up care to the person or population with the identified condition. This usually entails referral of individual clients for further diagnostic services and for treatment if needed or initiation of population-based efforts to address the problem.

Leader

Leadership in the community health nursing context is a requisite skill for community health nurses. The leadership role may be enacted both with individual clients or families and with communities and populations; however, because this role demands knowledge of group dynamics as well as interpersonal skills, we deal with leadership as a population-oriented role.

Leadership is the ability to influence the behavior of others. Community health nurses may assume a leadership role with a variety of individuals, including clients, other health care professionals, members of other disciplines, public officials, and the general public. Because of the number of different types of followers that may be involved, the community health nurse as leader must be able to adapt a leadership style to fit the needs of the moment.

Community health nurse functions in the leadership role include identifying the need for action and leadership, assessing the leadership needs of followers, and selecting and executing a style of leadership appropriate to both the followers and the situation. The leadership function of the community health nurse is discussed in greater detail in Chapter 13∞.

Change Agent

Community health nurses also fill the role of change agent. A **change agent** is one who initiates and brings about change. Frequently, this role is performed in conjunction with the leadership role. Change is an unavoidable part of human existence, but when change is systematically planned, it can be controlled and used to enhance rather than undermine health. Specific functions of the community health nurse in the change agent role include recognizing the need for change, making others aware of the need for change, motivating others to change, and initiating and directing the desired change.

Community health nurses may serve as change agents working with individuals, families, groups, and communities or in health care delivery. For example, change may be required in the dietary patterns of individual clients or families. Or there may be a need to alter the way a community deals with the homeless or approaches sex education in its schools. Similar changes might be needed in the health care system. For example, services might need to be redesigned to meet the needs of ethnic minority groups moving into the area. Efforts to bring about changes in health care delivery to meet evolving societal needs have historically been an area of strength of community health nursing in the United States. If we are to continue to fulfill our role as community health nurses and achieve our purpose of improved health for all, we must renew our efforts as change agents at the population level. The change process and its implications for community health nursing are discussed in greater detail in Chapter 13∞.

Community Mobilizer

Community mobilization is defined as "a process by which community groups identify common goals and mobilize assets to implement strategies that address local concerns" (Berkowitz et al., 2001, p. 51). The key feature of community mobilization is participation by members of the community or population group in identifying population health needs and in developing, implementing, and evaluating strategies to meet those needs (Rattray, Brunner, & Freestone, 2002).

Community mobilization promotes the participation of members of population groups in the control of their own lives and gives them the power to enact changes in circumstances that affect their health. Functions of the community health nurse in the community mobilizer role include assisting communities to identify health issues of concern and to collect data related to the issue, mobilizing members to action, and assisting with coalition development within the community. Additional functions related to this role include helping community members to identify goals, assisting in the determination of plausible strategies to meet those goals, and participating in strategy implementation. Community mobilization will be discussed in more detail in Chapter 13∞.

Coalition Builder

As we will see in Chapter 7∞, coalition building is a strategy often used in political activism. **Coalition building** is the process of creating temporary or permanent alliances of individuals or groups to achieve a specific purpose. Coalitions have the advantage of fostering community-wide problem solving and collaborative policy and program development (Rattray et al., 2002). Functions of community health nurses as coalition builders include identifying potential coalition members, presenting the mutual benefit to be derived from alliance to potential coalition members, helping to delineate the goals of the coalition, assisting in the development of operating guidelines for the coalition, and participating in the selection and implementation of means to accomplish the goals of the alliance.

Policy Advocate

Policy development, as we will see in Chapter 2∞, is one of the core functions of public health practice, and community health nurses have a definite role in the execution of this function. A **policy advocate** is a person or group of people who work for and argue on behalf of policy formation or changes in policy that influence the health of population groups. Policy advocacy may occur at institutional, community, state, national, or international levels. Specific nursing functions involved in policy advocacy include determining the need for policy formation or change, developing policy goals, analyzing factors influencing the policy situation, identifying key decision makers involved in policy formation, assisting in the formulation of proposed policies, communicating the proposed policy to the general public and to policy makers, and monitoring the progress of policy formation (Center for Health Improvement, 2004). These functions will be discussed in more detail in Chapter 7∞.

Social Marketer

The most frequently quoted definition of **social marketing** in the literature is that provided by Andreasen (1995): "the application of commercial marketing technologies to the analysis, planning, execution, and evaluation of programs designed to influence the voluntary behavior of target audiences to improve their personal welfare or that of their society" (p. 7). Social marketing is consumer focused in that it responds to the needs, preferences, and lifestyle of the target population (Neiger, Thackeray, Barnes, & McKenzie, 2003) and is designed to address societal problems at the population level (Smith, 2000).

Behavior change, whether in terms of population health-related behaviors or policy formation by policy makers, is predicated on the basic marketing principle of beneficial exchanges in which all parties receive some desired benefit from the exchange (Maibach, 2003). For example, smokers may give up smoking in exchange for easier breathing. Similarly, politicians may support health-related legislation in return for anticipated voter allegiance at election time.

Social marketing is characterized by four interrelated concepts, often referred to as the four Ps: product, price, place, and promotion (Neiger et al., 2003). Community health nursing functions related to the social marketer role include identifying a needed change in societal behavior, analyzing behavioral motivations and perceived benefits and barriers to action, identifying particular target markets for interventions and determining the unique features of those markets, developing and testing strategies to promote the desired change, implementing those strategies, and evaluating their effectiveness. Concepts and principles of social marketing and related community health nursing functions are discussed in more detail in Chapter 11∞.

Researcher

A **researcher** explores phenomena observed in the world with the intent of understanding, explaining, and ultimately controlling them. The research role of the commu-

MediaLink Case Study: Empowerment Through Literacy

BUILDING OUR KNOWLEDGE BASE

1. What are some research questions you might ask about the practice of community health nurses in your local area?
2. How might you go about designing a study to answer one or more of those questions?

nity health nurse is sometimes seen as a relatively recent one; however, even at the beginnings of community health nursing in the United States, Lillian Wald and her contemporaries made use of carefully documented data to identify societal needs and fuel social reforms. The community health nurse's current research role may be carried out at several levels. Responsibilities of the community health nurse related to research include critically reviewing relevant research and its application to practice, identifying researchable problems, designing and conducting research studies, collecting data, and disseminating research findings. Functions related to the role of researcher and other population-oriented community health nursing roles are summarized in Table 1-3◆.

Community health nursing has as its primary goal the improvement of the health of the total population. This specialty area of nursing practice is characterized by attributes of population consciousness, orientation to health, autonomy, creativity, continuity, collaboration, intimacy, and variability. Community health nurses engage in client-oriented, delivery-oriented, and population-oriented roles. The degree of emphasis placed on the roles in each category, however, will vary from setting to setting.

TABLE 1-3	Population-Oriented Community Health Nursing Roles and Related Functions
Role	**Function**
Case finder	Develop knowledge of signs and symptoms of health-related conditions and contributing factors
	Use diagnostic reasoning process to identify potential cases of disease or other health-related conditions
	Carry out investigation of specific cases of disease as needed
	Provide follow-up care to identified cases
Leader	Identify the need for action
	Assess situation and followers to determine appropriate leadership style
	Motivate followers to take action
	Coordinate group member activities in planning and implementing action
	Assist followers to evaluate the effectiveness of action taken
Change agent	Recognize the need for change
	Alert others to the need for change
	Motivate others for change
	Initiate and direct change
Community mobilizer	Assist community members to identify health issues of concern
	Participate in data collection relevant to issues of concern
	Mobilize community members to take action
	Assist with coalition development to foster community action
	Assist community members to identify achievable goals
	Participate in the development of strategies to accomplish identified goals
	Participate in the implementation of community strategies to achieve goals
Coalition builder	Identify potential coalition members based on common interest, assets available, etc.
	Present potential coalition members with the benefits to be achieved through alliance
	Participate in the delineation of coalition goals
	Assist in the development of operating guidelines for the coalition
	Participate in the selection and implementation of strategies to accomplish coalition goals
Policy advocate	Determine the need for policy development
	Develop policy-related goals
	Analyze factors influencing the policy situation
	Identify key decision makers
	Assist in policy formulation
	Communicate the proposed policy
	Monitor the progress of policy development
Social marketer	Identify the need for societal behavior change
	Analyze motivation and perceived benefits and barriers to the desired change
	Identify target markets and their unique features
	Develop and test social marketing strategies appropriate to target markets
	Assist with implementation of strategies
	Evaluate the effectiveness of social marketing strategies in achieving the desired change
Researcher	Critically review research findings
	Apply research findings to practice as appropriate
	Identify researchable problems
	Design and conduct nursing research
	Collect and analyze data
	Disseminate research findings

Case Study

Transportation Services for Older Clients

Vista Hills is a small, low-income community within a major metropolitan area. In home visits to several older clients, the community health nurse assigned to the area discovers that they have not been able to keep medical appointments or get prescriptions filled due to lack of available transportation. There is a bus that traverses the area, but it only has stops on major thoroughfares, and most older community residents have difficulty walking from their homes to the bus stops. In the past, the community had access to a Dial-a-Ride service that provided door-to-door transportation for the elderly for 50 cents a ride (round trip). This service was discontinued several years ago because of escalating costs. Some residents use taxi services to meet their transportation needs, but find this very expensive given their limited incomes.

The city in which the community is located has some funds for transportation services for elderly clients, but the funds have not been allocated to this community because older residents comprise only 11% of the overall population.

1. What client-oriented, delivery-oriented, and population-oriented roles might the community health nurse perform in addressing this community health problem? Why are these roles appropriate to this situation?
2. Give examples of some specific activities the community health nurse might carry out in performing each role.

Test Your Understanding

1. What is community health nursing? How does it relate to community-based, community-focused, and community-driven nursing? (pp. 4–5)

2. How does district nursing differ from program-focused nursing? How do both relate to population-focused nursing? (pp. 8–9)

3. Describe an advocacy situation. Identify the principal actors in the situation. What actions may be needed to resolve the situation? (pp. 5–8)

4. Describe at least five attributes of community health nursing. Give an example of each attribute. (pp. 10–12)

5. Describe the standards of care for community health nursing practice. How do they differ from the standards of professional performance? (pp. 12–14)

6. What are the eight competency domains for community health nursing? Give an example of a community health nursing activity that might be involved in each domain. (pp. 13–14, Appendix A)

7. Distinguish among client-oriented, delivery-oriented, and population-oriented community health nursing roles. (pp. 14–22)

8. What are the client-oriented roles of community health nurses? Give an example of the performance of each role. (pp. 14–17)

9. Describe the three delivery-oriented roles performed by community health nurses. What functions are involved in each? How might you enact these roles with a population as client? (pp. 17–19)

10. What are the population-oriented roles of community health nurses? Give an example of the performance of each role. (pp. 19–22)

EXPLORE MediaLink

http://www.prenhall.com/clark
Resources for this chapter can be found on the Companion Website.

Audio Glossary
Appendix A: Quad Council PHN Competencies
Exam Review Questions

Case Study: Empowerment Through Literacy
MediaLink Applications: Lillian Wald, Nurse
  Advocate (Video)

Media Links
Challenge Your Knowledge
Advocacy Interviews

References

Abrams, S. E. (2004). From function to competency in public health nursing, 1931 to 2003. *Public Health Nursing, 21,* 507–510.

American Nurses Association. (1976). *Code for nurses with interpretive statements.* Kansas City, MO: Author.

American Nurses Association. (1986). *Standards of community health nursing practice.* Kansas City, MO: Author.

American Nurses Association. (2007). *Public health nursing: Scope and standards of practice.* Silver Spring, MD: Nursesbooks.org.

American Public Health Association, Public Health Nursing Section. (1996). The definition and role of public health nursing: A statement of the APHA Public Health Nursing Section. Washington, DC: Author.

Andreasen, A. R. (1995). *Marketing social change*. San Francisco: Jossey-Bass.

Avery, B., & Bashir, S. (2003). The road to advocacy—Searching for the rainbow. *American Journal of Public Health, 93*, 1207–1210.

Baldwin, M. (2003). Patient advocacy: A concept analysis. *Nursing Standard, 17*(21), 33–39.

Bassett, M. T. (2003). Public health advocacy. *American Journal of Public Health, 93*, 1204.

Bedell, J. R., Cohen, N. L., & Sullivan, A. (2000). Case management: The current best practices and the next generation of innovation. *Community Mental Health Journal, 36*, 179–194.

Berkowitz, B. (2002). Preserving our mission. *Public Health Nursing, 19*, 319–320.

Berkowitz, B., Dahl, J., Guirl, K., Kostelecky, B. J., McNeil, C., & Upenieks, V. (2001). *Public health nursing leadership: A guide to managing the core functions*. Washington, DC: American Nurses Association.

Billings, J. (1998). Public health: A long time coming. *Nursing Times, 94*(28), 30–31.

Boyd, L. (2000). Advanced practice nursing today. *RN, 63*(9), 57–62.

Case Management Society of America. (1995). *Standards of practice for case management*. Little Rock, AR: Author.

Center for Health Improvement. (2004). *Bringing policy change to your community*. Retrieved August 25, 2004, from http://www.healthpolicycoach.org/advocacy.asp?id=23

Chafey, K., Rhea, M., Shannon, A. M., & Spencer, S. (1998). Characterizations of advocacy by practicing nurses. *Journal of Professional Nursing, 14*(1), 43–52.

Chalmers, K. I., Bramadat, I. J., & Andrusyszyn, M. (1998). The changing environment of community health practice and education: Perceptions of staff nurses, administrators, and educators. *Journal of Nursing Education, 37*(3), 109–117.

Chen, S. C., Ervin, N. E., Kim, Y., & Vonderheid, S. C. (1999). Competency in community-oriented health care: Instrument development. *Evaluation & the Health Professions, 22*, 358–370.

Clark, M. J. (2001). Voicing their voice: The structure of advocacy. Unpublished raw data.

Clarke, J. (2004). Public health nursing in Ireland: A critical overview. *Public Health Nursing, 21*, 191–198.

Diekemper, M., SmithBattle, L., & Drake, M. A. (1999a). Bringing the population into focus: A natural development in community health nursing practice. Part I. *Public Health Nursing, 16*(1), 3–10.

Drevdahl, D. (2002). Social justice or market justice? The paradoxes of public health partnerships with managed care. *Public Health Nursing, 19*, 161–169.

Drevdahl, D., Kneipp, S. M., Canales, M. K., & Dorcy, K. S. (2001). Reinvesting in social justice: A capital idea for public health nursing? *Advances in Nursing Science, 24*(2), 19–31.

Feenstra, C. (2000). Community based and community focused: Nursing education in community health. *Public Health Nursing, 17*, 155–159.

Foley, B. J., Minick, M. P., & Kee, C. C. (2002). How nurses learn advocacy. *Journal of Nursing Scholarship, 32*, 181–186.

Gebbie, K. (2002). Applying your degree to public health practice: Academic nurse leader. In B. A. DeBuono & H. Tilson (Eds.), *Advancing healthy populations: The Pfizer guide to careers in public health* (pp. 178–184). New York: Pfizer Pharmaceutical Group.

Grumbach, K., Miller, J., Mertz, E., & Finocchio, L. (2004). How much public health is in public health nursing practice? *Public Health Nursing, 21*, 266–276.

Hamer, S. B. (2000). Public health nursing: Identifying priorities. *Nursing Standard, 14*(30), 31–32.

Institute of Medicine. (1988). *The future of public health*. Washington, DC: National Academy Press.

Kaiser, K. L., Barr, K. L., & Hays, B. J. (2003). Setting a new course for advanced practice community/public health nursing. *Journal of Professional Nursing, 19*, 189–196.

Kaiser, L., & Rudolph, E. J. (2003). Achieving clarity in evaluation of community/public health nurse generalist competencies through development of a clinical performance tool. *Public Health Nursing, 20*, 216–227.

Krampitz, S. D. (1987). The Yale experiment: Innovation in nursing education. In C. Maggs (Ed.), *Nursing history: The state of the art* (pp. 60–73). London: Croom Helm.

Kuss, T., Proulx-Girouard, L., Lovitt, S., Katz, C., & Kennelly, P. (1997). A public health nursing model. *Public Health Nursing, 14*, 81–91.

Maibach, E. W. (2003). Recreating communities to support active living: A new role for social marketing. *American Journal of Health Promotion, 18*(1), 114–119.

Mallik, M. (1998). Advocacy in nursing: Perceptions and attitudes of the nursing elite in the United Kingdom. *Journal of Advanced Nursing, 28*, 1001–1011.

May, K. M., Phillips, L. R., Ferketich, S. L., & Verran, J. (2003). Public health nursing: The generalist in a specialized environment. *Public Health Nursing, 20*, 252–259.

Michaels, C. (1997). Leading beyond traditional boundaries: A community nursing perspective. *Nursing Administration Quarterly, 22*(1), 30–37.

Murashima, S., Hatono, Y., Whyte, N., Asahara, K. (1999). Public health nursing in Japan: New opportunities for health promotion. *Public Health Nursing, 16*, 133–139.

Nehls, N., Owen, B., Tipple, S., Vandermause, R. (2001). Lessons learned from developing, implementing and evaluating a model of community-driven nursing. *Nursing & Health Care Perspectives, 22*, 304–307.

Nehls, N., & Vandermause, R. (2004). Community-driven nursing: Transforming nursing curricula and instruction. *Nursing Education Perspectives, 25*(2), 81–85.

Neiger, B. L., Thackeray, R., Barnes, M. D., & McKenzie, J. F. (2003). Positioning social marketing as a planning process for health education. *American Journal of Health Studies, 18*(2/3), 75–81.

Quad Council of Public Health Nursing Organizations. (1999). *Scope and standards of public health nursing practice*. Washington, DC: American Nurses Publishing.

Quad Council of Public Health Nursing Organizations. (2003). *Quad Council PHN Competencies*. Retrieved August 8, 2002, from http://www.uncc.edu/achne/quadcouncil/final_phn_competencies.doc

Rafael, A. R. F. (1999a). From rhetoric to reality: The changing face of public health nursing in Southern Ontario. *Public Health Nursing, 16*, 50–59.

Rafael, A. R. F. (1999b). The politics of health promotion: Influences on public health promoting nursing practice in Ontario, Canada from Nightingale to the nineties. *Advances in Nursing Science, 22*(1), 23–39.

Rattray, T., Brunner, W., & Freestone, J. (2002). *A new spectrum of prevention: A model for public health practice*. Martinez, CA: Contra Costa Health Services Public Health Division.

Ray, R. (2003). Everyday people. *NURSEweek, 16*(25), 13–15.

Sakamoto, S. D., & Avila, M. (2004). The public health nursing practice manual: A tool for public health nurses. *Public Health Nursing, 21*, 179–182.

Smith, K., & Bazini-Barakat, N. (2003). A public health nursing practice model: Melding public health principles with the nursing process. *Public Health Nursing, 21*, 42–48.

Smith, W. (2000). Social marketing: An evolving definition. *American Journal of Health Behavior, 24*, 11–17.

SmithBattle, L., Diekemper, M., & Drake, M. A. (1999). Articulating the culture and tradition of community health nursing. *Public Health Nursing, 165*, 215–222.

SmithBattle, L., Diekemper, M., & Leander, S. (2004a). Getting your feet wet: Becoming a public health nurse, Part 1. *Public Health Nursing, 21*, 3–11.

SmithBattle, L., Diekemper, M., & Leander, S. (2004b). Moving upstream: Becoming a public health nurse, Part 2. *Public Health Nursing, 21*, 95–102.

Snowball, J. (1996). Asking nurses about advocating for patients: "Reactive" and "proactive" accounts. *Journal of Advanced Nursing, 24*, 67–75.

Sullivan, T. J. (1998). Concept analysis of collaboration: Part I. In T. J. Sullivan (Ed.), *Collaboration: A health care imperative* (pp. 3–42). New York: McGraw-Hill.

Uosukainen, L. M. (2001). Promotion of the good life by public health nurses. *Public Health Nursing, 18*, 375–384.

Westbrook, L. O., & Schultz, P. (2000). From theory to practice: Community health nursing in a public health neighborhood team. *Advances in Nursing Science, 23*(2), 50–61.

Wheeler, P. (2000). Is advocacy at the heart of professional practice? *Nursing Standard, 14*(36), 39–41.

Williams, D. B. (2000). Population care management: What's in it for your organization? *Nursing Case Management, 5*, 1.

Zahner, S. J., & Gredig, Q.-N. B. (2005a). Improving public health nursing education: Recommendations of local public health nurses. *Public Health Nursing, 22*, 445–450.

Zahner, S. J., & Gredig, Q.-N. B. (2005b). Public health nursing: Practice change and recommendations for improvement. *Public Health Nursing, 22*, 422–428.

The Population Context

CHAPTER OBJECTIVES

After reading this chapter, you should be able to:

1. Distinguish among neighborhoods, communities, and aggregates as populations served by community health nurses.
2. Define population health.
3. Describe changes in approaches to population health.
4. Describe the three levels at which population health care occurs.
5. Describe trends in national health objectives for 1990, 2000, and 2010.

KEY TERMS

aggregates **27**
community **27**
communities of identity **27**
geopolitical community **27**
neighborhood **27**
population **27**
population-based practice **27**
population health **28**
primary prevention **30**
secondary prevention **30**
tertiary prevention **30**

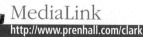

MediaLink
http://www.prenhall.com/clark

Additional interactive resources for this chapter can be found on the Companion Website. Click on Chapter 2 and "Begin" to select the activities for this chapter.

Advocacy in Action

Health Care in the County Jail

Jail and prison inmates are often overlooked as populations that need health care services. In part this may be because of their invisibility, yet this population often has far greater needs for health care than the general public. Jails and prisons are intended to be places of punishment for criminal behavior, and health care services are frequently secondary to the security and retribution aspects of incarceration. What the public and policy makers often do not recognize is that providing health care services in jails and prisons is cost-effective and benefits the entire community. Several years ago, a nursing faculty member whose husband was a deputy sheriff for the southern county in which she lived started providing volunteer

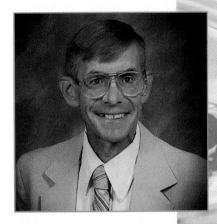

(Courtesy of Olan Mills)

health services in the county jail. She took several students with her on her forays into the jail and had an uphill battle convincing the county sheriff to permit them to have access to the inmates. Gradually, they were able to win the confidence of the sheriff and the jail personnel that they were not going to create a security risk and that they could assist personnel in dealing with problems for which the staff had no training or background.

After several months of volunteer work in the jail, the faculty member wrote a federal grant for a nursing clinic to be housed in the jail itself. Prior to that time, inmates with health needs that could not be addressed during the periodic visits by the volunteer faculty and students were sent to the local emergency department. The grant provided for one full-time nurse in the jail as well as for physician backup for health problems beyond the nurse's capabilities. One of the former student volunteers was hired as the nurse for the new clinic. The cost-effectiveness of the program was evaluated, and within six months of its initiation, the county's cost for health care services for inmates had decreased by 75%, primarily due to reduced emergency department visits and lost deputy time transporting inmates to the ED. With this information in hand, the sheriff was able to obtain county funding to continue the clinic after the grant period ended.

Philip Clark, RN, BSN

*T*he hallmark of community health nursing is that the primary client or recipient of care is a group of people, or population, rather than an individual or a particular family. Although nurses who engage in community health nursing practice may also provide services to individuals and families, they do so with the express purpose of improving the health of the overall population. As we saw in Chapter 1∞, the focus of their care is the population group, not the individuals and families who are its members. **Population-based practice** has been defined as practice that "focuses on entire populations, is grounded in community assessment, considers all health determinants, emphasizes prevention, and intervenes at multiple levels" (Keller, Strohschein, Lia-Hoagberg, & Schaffer, 2004).

DEFINING POPULATIONS AS A FOCUS FOR CARE

The population groups that form the focus for community health nursing can be many and varied. **Populations** are groups of people who may or may not interact with each other. Populations may refer to the residents of a specific geographic area, but can also include specific groups of people with some trait or attribute in common (e.g., a minority group, employees, the elderly) (Kindig & Stoddart, 2003). Three other commonly used, similar, but different terms for these smaller subgroups are *aggregate*, *neighborhood*, and *community*.

Aggregates are subpopulations within the larger population who possess some common characteristics, often related to high risk for specific health problems (Porche, 2004). School-aged children, persons with human immunodeficiency virus (HIV) infection, and the elderly are all examples of aggregates.

A **neighborhood** is a smaller, more homogeneous group than a community (Matteson, 2000) and involves an interface with others living nearby and a level of identification with those others. Neighborhoods are self-defined, and although they may be constrained by natural or man-made factors, they often do not have specifically demarcated boundaries. For example, a major highway may limit interactions between residents on either side, thus creating separate neighborhoods. Or a neighborhood may be defined by a common language or cultural heritage. Thus, non-Hispanic residents of a "Hispanic neighborhood" are not usually considered, nor do they consider themselves, part of the neighborhood.

A community may be composed of several neighborhoods (Matteson, 2000). Some authors define communities within geographic locations or settings (MacQueen et al., 2001), but the majority of writers have moved away from locale as a primary defining characteristic of communities. In addition to location, other potential defining aspects of communities include a social system or social institutions designed to carry out

specific functions; identity, commitment, or emotional connection; common norms and values; common history or interests; common symbols; social interaction; and intentional action to meet common needs. Although most of these characteristics are also true of neighborhoods, the critical distinction between neighborhoods and communities would appear to be a defined social structure containing institutions designed to accomplish designated community functions such as education, social support, and so on. For our purposes, then, a **community** is defined as a group of people who share common interests, who interact with each other, and who function collectively within a defined social structure to address common concerns. By this definition, geopolitical entities, such as the city of San Diego, a school of nursing, and a religious congregation can be considered communities. A **geopolitical community** is one characterized by geographic and jurisdictional boundaries, such as a city. All three communities (city, nursing program, and religious group), however, can be considered **communities of identity**—communities with a common identity and interests.

Community health nurses may work with any or all of these population groups—aggregates, neighborhoods, and communities—in their efforts to enhance the health status of the general public or overall population. Population health addresses the health needs of entire groups, and those health needs are affected by factors at individual, family, neighborhood, and societal levels (Northridge & Ellis, 2003).

DEFINING POPULATION HEALTH

Emphasis on the health of populations as a focus for care arose out of dissatisfaction with the limited effectiveness of individual-oriented care in improving the

MediaLink · Ruth Freeman Award

health of the general population (Szreter, 2003). The health of a population group goes beyond the health status of the individuals or groups who comprise it, but involves the collective health of the group (Frisch, George, Govoni, Jennings-Sanders, & McCahon, 2003). Several authors have noted the lack of a precise definition of population health (Friedman & Starfield, 2003; Kindig & Stoddart, 2003), but note that there are two basic approaches to defining population health: descriptive and analytic. Descriptive approaches focus on the health status of the population using a set of summary indicators of health (McDowell, Spasoff, & Kristjansson, 2004). In this approach, population health is viewed as the average level of health in the population and the distribution of health within the population (Friedman & Starfield, 2003). Analytic approaches define population health more broadly in terms of factors that influence health and are used to direct interventions to improving health status. Analytic approaches attempt to explain differences in the distribution of health (McDowell et al., 2004; Huttlinger, Schaller-Ayers, & Lawson, 2004).

Definitions of population health evolved from three conceptual models of health: a biomechanical model, a holistic model, and a dynamic model (McDowell et al., 2004). The biomechanical model focuses on health problems rather than on health per se and is present focused. From this perspective, a healthy population has low rates of illness and other health problems and has functioning systems equipped to deal with problems that arise. The holistic model incorporates the

concept of multiple factors influencing a positive state of health (as opposed to a negative state of absence of illness). In this view, a healthy population displays aggregated indicators of individual well-being. In the dynamic model, health is viewed as a process that improves the quality of life. This last perspective has been adopted by the World Health Organization in its 1984 conception of population health.

> To be healthy, in this conception, "an individual or group must be able to identify and to realize aspirations, to satisfy needs, and to change or cope with the environment. Health is, therefore, seen as a resource for everyday life, not the object of living. Health is a positive concept, emphasizing social and personal resources as well as physical capacities." (World Health Organization, as quoted in McDowell et al., 2004, pp. 390–391)

Population health can be defined as the attainment of the greatest possible biologic, psychological, and social well-being of the population as an entity and of its individual members. Health is derived from opportunities and choices provided to the public as well as the population's response to those choices (Wilcox & Knapp, 2000). Healthy populations provide their members with the knowledge and opportunities to make choices that improve health.

In large part, the health of a population is defined and determined by the perceptions, norms, and values of its members. Despite the resulting variability in definitions of health, there are certain characteristics that healthy populations have in common. In 1999, the

The primary focus of community health nursing is the health of total population groups. (David Grossman/The Image Works)

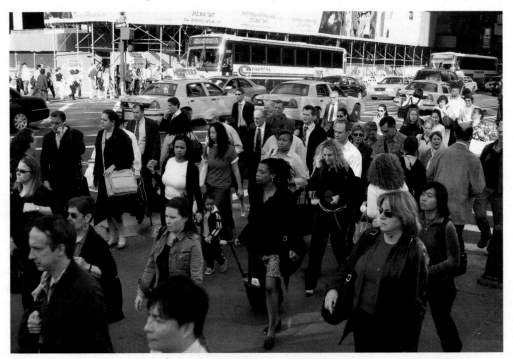

coalition for Healthier Cities and Communities, a national network of organizational partnerships dedicated to the improvement of population health, identified seven characteristics of healthy communities. Based on these characteristics, healthy communities:

- Foster dialogue among residents to develop a shared vision for the community
- Promote community leadership that fosters collaboration and partnerships
- Engage in action based on a shared vision of the community
- Embrace diversity among residents
- Assess both needs and assets
- Link residents to community resources, and
- Foster a sense of responsibility and cohesion among residents (Norris & Pittman, 2000).

Other characteristics of healthy communities include abilities to change and adapt to changing circumstances and manage conflict effectively (Duhl, 2000; Norris & Pitman, 2000).

Population health is fostered at the community level by the Healthy Cities and Healthy Communities programs. The Healthy Cities movement was initiated by the European region of the World Health Organization in 1984 (Awofeso, 2003) and was adapted as the Healthy Communities movement in the United States in the mid-1980s (Norris & Pittman, 2000). Both movements emphasize local involvement in creating conditions that support health through "a grassroots process, a way of addressing issues, making decisions, and setting policy involving the entire community" (Kesler, 2000, p. 238). They rest on the premise that healthy communities are the result of both personal choices regarding behavior and broad environmental conditions that affect health (e.g., housing, transportation, and education, as well as access to health services) (Norris & Pittman, 2000). Healthy Communities projects are based on the following eight basic principles:

- Health must be broadly defined to encompass quality-of-life issues (emotional, physical, and spiritual), not just the absence of disease.
- "Community" must also be broadly defined to encompass a variety of groups, not just populations defined by specific geographic boundaries.
- Action related to community health must arise from a shared vision derived from community values.

EVIDENCE-BASED PRACTICE

Clark et al. (2003) described a focus-group process used to incorporate the voices of underrepresented groups in a community assessment. Review the article and answer the following questions:

1. How does this study exemplify the principles of the Healthy Communities program?
2. If you were going to conduct a community assessment of your own community, what underrepresented groups would you want to include? Would a focus-group process, as described in the article, be culturally appropriate for these groups? Why or why not?

- Actions must address the quality of life for all residents, not just a select few.
- Widespread community ownership and diverse citizen participation are required for effective community action.
- The focus of action should be on systems change in the way decisions are made and community services are delivered.
- Community health rests on the development of local assets and resources to create an environment and infrastructure that support health.
- Effectiveness is measured on the basis of specific community indicators and outcomes and promotes accountability to community residents (Healthy Community Principles, 2000; Lee, 2000).

CHANGES IN APPROACHES TO POPULATION HEALTH

Over the years, a number of approaches have been taken within public health practice to promote population health. Changes in these approaches have coincided with shifts in the mission and focus of public health practice. In the 1800s and early 1900s, the focus was on control of epidemics. Starting in the mid-1900s, the focus of practice moved to disease prevention. At present, the emphasis in public health practice is one of social justice (Drevdahl, 2002). As we saw in Chapter 1∞, advocacy for social justice has always been a feature of community health nursing practice.

One author referred to these changes in the approaches to population health as the "three public health revolutions." The first revolution emphasized sanitation as a means of controlling communicable diseases. The second focused on personal behavior change to promote individual and population health. The third revolution emphasizes health as one dimension of quality of life, with a focus on "building healthy communities and healthy workplaces, strengthening the wide range of social networks for health, and increasing people's capabilities to lead healthy lives" (Kickbusch,

Children created a mural incorporating their views of the community. (Mary Jo Clark)

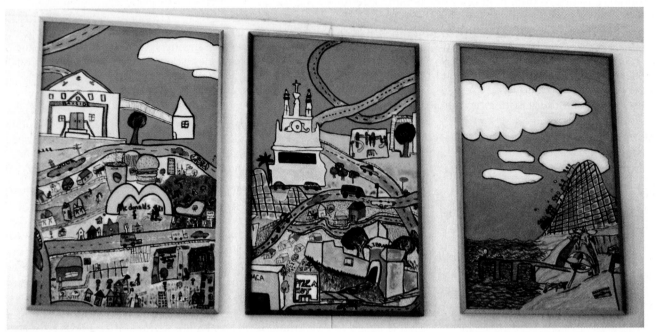

2003, p. 387). Public health practice will be discussed in more detail in Chapter 5∞.

LEVELS OF POPULATION HEALTH CARE

Health care for populations takes place at three levels, often referred to as the three levels of prevention. These three levels of care are primary prevention, secondary prevention, and tertiary prevention. **Primary prevention** was defined by the originators of the term as "measures designed to promote general optimum health or . . . the specific protection of man against disease agents" (Leavell & Clark, 1965, p. 20). Primary prevention is action taken prior to the occurrence of health problems and is directed toward avoiding their occurrence (Adams et al., 2001). Primary prevention may include increasing people's resistance to illness (as in the case of immunization), decreasing or eliminating the causes of health problems, or creating an environment conducive to health rather than health problems.

Secondary prevention is the early identification and treatment of existing health problems (Adams et al., 2001) and takes place after the health problem has occurred. Emphasis is on resolving health problems and preventing serious consequences. Secondary prevention activities include screening and early diagnosis, as well as treatment for existing health problems. Screening for hypertension is an example of secondary prevention. Secondary prevention would also include the actual diagnosis and treatment of a person with hypertension. Development of health care programs to diagnose and treat hypertension in the community would be an example of secondary prevention at the population level.

Tertiary prevention is activity aimed at returning the client to the highest level of function and preventing further deterioration in health (Adams et al., 2001). Tertiary prevention also focuses on preventing recurrences of the problem. Placing a client on a maintenance diet after the loss of a desired number of pounds constitutes tertiary prevention. Legislation to promote a living wage for all workers to prevent recurrent homelessness would be an example of tertiary prevention focused on populations rather than individuals.

OBJECTIVES FOR POPULATION HEALTH

The goals and desired outcomes for population health in the United States have been operationalized in several sets of national objectives. The first set of objectives was established in 1980 in the publication *Promoting Health/Preventing Disease: Objectives for the Nation* (U.S. Department of Health and Human Services, 1980) and targeted 15 priority intervention areas in three strategic action categories: preventive health, health protection, and health promotion. The primary goal of this initiative was to reduce mortality (Friedrich, 2000). Approximately one third of the 226 objectives were met by the target date of 1990 (National Center for Health Statistics, 1992).

A subsequent set of National Health Objectives, *Healthy People 2000: National Health Promotion and Disease Prevention Objectives*, was established for the year 2000 (U.S. Department of Health and Human Services, 1990). The broad goals for this second set of objectives were to (a) increase the span of healthy life (not just longevity), (b) reduce health disparities among subpopulations, and (c) achieve access to preventive health services for all (McAlearney, 2003). The year 2000 objectives differed

GLOBAL PERSPECTIVES

*T*he chapter describes the national health objectives for population health in the United States. What other countries have adopted a similar approach to population health? What other approaches to population health have been taken in the international community? For example, see Glouberman and Millar (2003) and Coburn, Denny, Mykhalovskiy, McDonough, Robertson, and Love (2003) for a discussion of the Canadian determinants-of-health approach to population health.

ETHICAL AWARENESS

*O*ne of the major changes in the *Healthy People 2010* objectives is the shift from minimizing health disparities among various groups within the population to eliminating them altogether. What are the ethical implications of achieving this goal if it means reducing the level of service provided to groups with better health status in order to provide additional services to those with poorer health status? What models of ethical decision making would justify such an approach? What ethical arguments could be made against such reductions?

from those for 1990 in several ways. First, priority intervention areas were increased from 15 to 22 to include cancer screening, HIV infection, and preventive services. Second, the focus of the objectives was moved beyond reduction of mortality to improving the quality of life. A third difference was the special attention given to the needs of high-risk populations such as the elderly and minority groups. Fourth, the year 2000 objectives reflected concern for access to basic health services for all. Finally, responsibility for overseeing and monitoring achievement in each priority area was delegated to a specific agency of the U.S. Public Health Service (U.S. Department of Health and Human Services, 1996). A report in June of 1999 indicated that 15% of the year 2000 objectives had been met and another 44% were moving toward the established targets. Unfortunately, another 18% of objectives were moving away from the targets, and others had not been assessed due to the lack of baseline and follow-up data (Friedrich, 2000).

The most recent set of objectives was published in January 2000 in *Healthy People 2010* (U.S. Department of Health and Human Services, 2000a)◆. This most recent set of national objectives was developed with input from the Healthy People Consortium, a coalition of more than 600 national and state health agencies, organizations, and experts (Davis, Okuboye, & Ferguson, 2000). The development of the objectives was based on a systematic approach consisting of four elements: goals, objectives, determinants of health, and health status (U.S. Department of Health and Human Services, 2000b). The goals provide direction for the development of more specific objectives. The two overarching goals are to increase quality and length of healthy life and to eliminate health disparities (Smith & Bazini-Barakat, 2003). The first goal continues the emphasis of *Healthy People 2000* on improved quality of life versus reduced mortality emphasized in the objectives for 1990. The second expands the year 2000 goal of reducing disparities to eliminating them altogether (McAlearney, 2003).

The objectives specify the amount of progress expected in improving the health status of the population in the next 10 years. The 2010 objectives have been expanded to cover 28 focus areas and 467 objectives. Some of the focus areas from the year 2000 objectives have been separated and others added. Table 2-1 ◆

provides a summary of focus areas included in the *Healthy People 2010* document with the agencies responsible for monitoring progress toward the objectives in each area. *Healthy People 2010* incorporates a common structure for each focus area that includes:

- Identification of the lead agency responsible for monitoring progress toward achievement of objectives.
- A concise goal statement for the focus area that delineates the overall purpose of the focus area.
- An overview of context and background for the objectives related to the focus area. This overview includes related issues, trends, disparities among population subgroups, and opportunities for prevention or intervention.
- Data on progress toward meeting related objectives for 2000.
- Objectives related to the focus area. These objectives are of two types: measurable outcome objectives and developmental objectives. Measurable objectives include baseline data, the target for 2010, and potential data sources for monitoring progress toward the target. Unlike the year 2000 objectives, which set separate targets for subpopulations, a single target is set for the entire population. The targets for each objective have been set at a level that is "better than the best," resulting in improved health status for all segments of the population (U.S. Department of Health and Human Services, 2000c). Developmental objectives relate to areas for which data systems do not exist and will direct the development of data systems related to emerging health issues.
- A standard data table, including a set of population variables by which progress will be monitored. The minimum set of variables includes race and ethnicity, gender, family income, and education level. Additional categories of variables will be incorporated where relevant and include geographic location, health insurance status, disability status, and other selected populations (e.g., school grade levels) (U.S. Department of Health and Human Services, 2000a).

The third element in the systematic approach to health improvement exemplified by the document is

MediaLink · Case Study: Seatbelt Safety

TABLE 2-1 Healthy People 2010: Focus Areas and Responsible Agencies

Focus Area	Responsible Agencies
Access to quality health services	Agency for Healthcare Research and Quality (AHRQ) (http://www.ahrq.gov) Health Resources and Services Administration (http://www.hrsa.gov)
Arthritis, osteoporosis, and chronic back pain	Centers for Disease Control and Prevention (http://www.cdc.gov) National Institutes of Health (http://www.nih.gov)
Cancer	Centers for Disease Control and Prevention (http://www.cdc.gov) National Institutes of Health (http://www.nih.gov)
Chronic kidney disease	National Institutes of Health (http://www.nih.gov)
Diabetes	Centers for Disease Control and Prevention (http://www.cdc.gov) National Institutes of Health (http://www.nih.gov)
Disability and secondary conditions	Centers for Disease Control and Prevention (http://www.cdc.gov) National Institute on Disability and Rehabilitation Research (http://www.ed.gov/about/offices/list/osers/nidr/index.html?src=mr) U.S. Department of Education (http://www.ed.gov)
Educational and community-based programs	Centers for Disease Control and Prevention (http://www.cdc.gov) Health Resources and Services Administration (http://www.hrsa.gov)
Environmental health	Agency for Toxic Substances and Disease Registry (http://www.atsdr.gov/atsdrhome.html) Centers for Disease Control and Prevention (http://www.cdc.gov) National Institutes of Health (http://www.nih.gov)
Family planning	Office of Population Affairs (http://opa.osophs.dhhs.gov)
Food safety	Food and Drug Administration (http://www.fda.gov) Food Safety and Inspection Service (http://fsis.usda.gov) U.S. Department of Agriculture (http://usda.gov)
Health communication	Office of Disease Prevention and Health Promotion (http://odphp.osophs.dhhs.gov)
Heart disease and stroke	Centers for Disease Control and Prevention (http://www.cdc.gov) National Institutes of Health (http://www.nih.gov)
HIV	Centers for Disease Control and Prevention (http://www.cdc.gov) Health Resources and Services Administration (http://www.hrsa.gov)
Immunization and infectious diseases	Centers for Disease Control and Prevention (http://www.cdc.gov)
Injury and violence prevention	Centers for Disease Control and Prevention (http://www.cdc.gov)
Maternal, infant, and child health	Centers for Disease Control and Prevention (http://www.cdc.gov) Health Resources and Services Administration (http://www.hrsa.gov)
Medical product safety	Food and Drug Administration (http://www.fda.gov)
Mental health and mental disorders	National Institutes of Health (http://www.nih.gov) Substance Abuse and Mental Health Services Administration (http://www.samhsa.gov)
Nutrition and overweight	Food and Drug Administration (http://www.fda.gov) National Institutes of Health (http://www.nih.gov)

Continued on next page

TABLE 2-1 Healthy People 2010: Focus Areas and Responsible Agencies *(continued)*

Focus Area	Responsible Agencies
Nutrition and overweight	Food and Drug Administration (http://www.fda.gov) National Institutes of Health (http://www.nih.gov)
Occupational safety and health	Centers for Disease Control and Prevention (http://www.cdc.gov)
Oral health	Centers for Disease Control and Prevention (http://www.cdc.gov) Health Resources and Services Administration (http://www.hrsa.gov) National Institutes of Health (http://www.nih.gov)
Physical fitness and activity	Centers for Disease Control and Prevention (http://www.cdc.gov) President's Council on Physical Fitness and Sports (http://www.fitness.gov)
Public health infrastructure	Centers for Disease Control and Prevention (http://www.cdc.gov) Health Resources and Services Administration (http://www.hrsa.gov)
Respiratory diseases	Centers for Disease Control and Prevention (http://www.cdc.gov) National Institutes of Health (http://www.nih.gov)
Sexually transmitted diseases	Centers for Disease Control and Prevention (http://www.cdc.gov)
Substance abuse	National Institutes of Health (http://www.nih.gov) Substance Abuse and Mental Health Services Administration (http://www.samhsa.gov)
Tobacco use	Centers for Disease Control and Prevention (http://www.cdc.gov)
Vision and hearing	National Institutes of Health (http://www.nih.gov)

Data from: U.S. Department of Health and Human Services. (2000). Healthy people 2010 (Conference edition, in two volumes). Washington, DC: Author. (Note: The Web address for Healthy People 2010 is http://www.health.gov/healthypeople.)

related to the determinants of health. These determinants are the "combined effects of individual and community physical and social environments and the policies and interventions used to promote health, prevent disease, and ensure access to quality health care" (U.S. Department of Health and Human Services, 2000b, p. 7).

Health status of the overall population, the fourth element of the approach, is the expected outcome and measure of success of the approach. Health status is reflected in the extent to which each of the 467 objectives is met, but is also reflected at a more general level in 10 leading health indicators (Sakamoto & Avila, 2004). These indicators are presented in Table 2-2◆ and are designed to reflect the major public health issues in the nation. A small set of two to three objectives is identified for each health indicator and will be used to track and report trends in the indicator. Information related to health indicators includes health impacts, trends, populations particularly affected, and related issues (U.S. Department of Health and Human Services, 2000a).

Figure 2-1 depicts the interrelationships among the four elements of the systematic approach taken to improving the health of the nation. Table 2-3◆ presents an overview of trends in the national objectives for

TABLE 2-2 Leading Health Indicators

Physical activity

Overweight and obesity

Tobacco use

Substance abuse

Responsible sexual behavior

Mental health

Injury and violence

Environmental quality

Immunization

Access to care

population health from 1990 to 2010. Information on the current status of specific *Healthy People* objectives is available from the *Healthy People* Web site at http://wonder.cdc.gov/data2010.

As we have seen in this chapter, the community or population group is the primary focus of care in community health nursing. Care is provided to individuals and families with an eye toward improving the health of the total population. National health objectives guide the provision of care and serve as a means of evaluating the effectiveness of population health care.

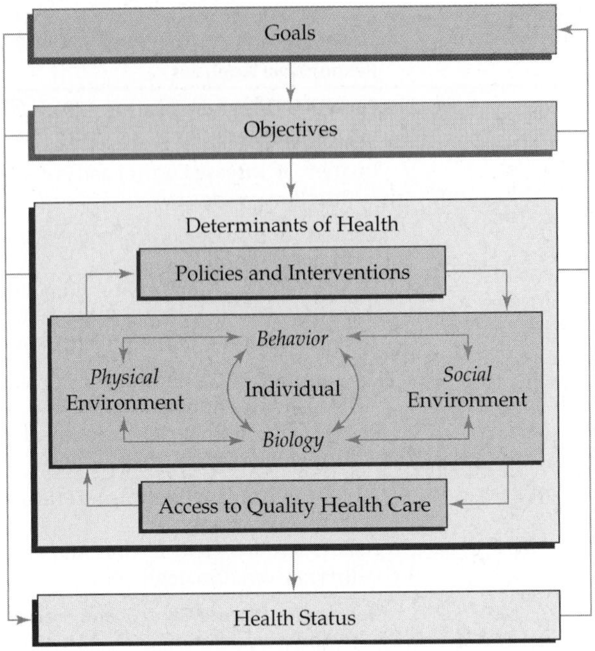

FIGURE 2-1 A Systematic Approach to Health Improvement
Data from: U.S. Department of Health and Human Services. (2000). *Healthy people 2010: Understanding and improving health* (2nd ed.). Washington, DC: Author.

TABLE 2-3 Trends in National Health Objectives: 1990, 2000, and 2010

Overall Goal

1990: Reduce mortality

2000: Increase the span of healthy life
       Reduce disparities in health status among
         subpopulations
       Achieve access to preventive health services for all

2010: Increase quality and years of healthy life
       Eliminate disparities in health status among
         subpopulations

Objective Categories

1990: Preventive health objectives
       Health protection objectives
       Health promotion objectives

2000: Health status objectives
       Risk reduction objectives
       Services and protection objectives

2010: Objectives promoting healthy behaviors
       Objectives promoting healthy and safe communities
       Objectives to improve systems for personal
         and public health
       Objectives to prevent and reduce diseases and
         disorders

Focus Areas

1990: 15 priority areas designated
2000: 22 priority areas designated
2010: 28 focus areas designated

Objectives

1990: 226 objectives identified
2000: 319 objectives identified
2010: 467 objectives identified

Progress Toward Achievement

1990: One third of objectives achieved by target date

2000: 15% of objectives achieved by target date
       44% making progress toward achievement
       18% moving away from the target
       23% untracked

2010: Not applicable

Other Changes

1990: Not applicable

2000: Lead agencies responsible for monitoring
         progress identified
       Emphasis placed on quality of life as well as longevity
       Special attention given to high-risk groups
       Emphasis given to access to health services
       Baseline data provided where available

2010: Widespread input into the development of
         the objectives
       Designation of leading health indicators
       Included a single target for each measurable
         objective, identified as "better than the best"
       Included developmental objectives
       Development of a common structure for each
         focus area
       Development of a standard data table for reporting
         progress toward achievement of objectives

Data from: U.S. Department of Health and Human Services. (2000). Healthy people 2010: Understanding and improving health *(2nd ed.). Washington, DC: Author.*

Case Study

Caring for Populations

1. Identify some of the neighborhoods in the area where your nursing program is located. What defines these neighborhoods—geographic boundaries, culture, or some other defining feature?
2. What kinds of neighborhoods make up the communities in the area? What similarities and differences are there among neighborhoods in a given community? What effects do differences among neighborhoods have on planning health

care services? Have these differences been taken into consideration in planning community health services?
3. What are some of the subpopulations or aggregates in your community? Select one of these aggregates and determine whether or not the health needs of that group are met within the community. If not, what health needs remain unmet? What could be done to meet the health needs of this aggregate?

Test Your Understanding

1. What is the difference between a neighborhood, a community, and an aggregate? (p. 27)

2. What is *population health*? What are some of the characteristics of healthy populations or healthy communities? (pp. 28–29)

3. What changes have occurred in approaches to population health over time? (pp. 29–30)

4. What are the three levels at which population health care occurs? Give an example of each in the care of an individual and the care of a population group. (p. 30)

5. Describe trends in national health objectives for 1990, 2000, and 2010. What are the overall goals of each document? What additional features have been added over time? (pp. 30–34)

EXPLORE MediaLink

http://www.prenhall.com/clark
Resources for this chapter can be found on the Companion Website.

Audio Glossary
Exam Review Questions
Case Study: Seatbelt Safety

MediaLink Applications: The Ruth Freeman
    Population Nursing Award
Media Links

Challenge Your Knowledge
Advocacy Interviews

References

Adams, M. H., Sherrod, R. A., Packa, D. R., Forte, L., Lammon, C. A. B., Stover, L., et al. (2001). Levels of prevention: Restructuring a curriculum to meet future health care needs. *Nurse Educator, 26*(1), 6–8.

Awofeso, N. (2003). The Healthy Cities approach—reflections on a framework for improving global health. *Bulletin of the World Health Organization, 81*, 222–223.

Clark, M. J., Cary, S., Diemert, G., Ceballos, R., Sifuentes, M., Atteberry, I., Vue, F., & Trieu, S. (2003). Involving communities in community assessment. *Public Health Nursing, 20*, 456–463.

Coburn, D., Denny, K., Mykhalovskiy, E., McDonough, P., Robertson, A., & Love, R. (2003). Population health in Canada. *American Journal of Public Health, 93*, 392–396.

Davis, L. J., Okuboye, S., & Ferguson, S. L. (2000). Healthy people 2010: Examining a

decade of maternal & infant health. *AWHONN Lifelines, 4*(3), 26–33.

Drevdahl, D. (2002). Social justice or market justice? The paradoxes of public health partnerships with managed care. *Public Health Nursing, 19*, 161–169.

Duhl, L. J. (2000). A short history and some acknowledgments. (Healthy communities.) *Public Health Reports, 115*, 116–117.

Friedman, D. J., & Starfield, B. (2003). Models of population health: Their value for US public health practice, policy, and research. *American Journal of Public Health, 93*, 366–369.

Friedrich, M. J. (2000). More healthy people in the 21st century? *JAMA, 283*, 37–38.

Frisch, N. C., George, V., Govoni, A. L., Jennings-Sanders, A., & McCahon, C. P. (2003). Teaching nurses to focus on the health needs of populations: A master's

degree program in population health nursing. *Nurse Educator, 28*, 212–216.

Glouberman, S., & Millar, J. (2003). Evolution of the determinants of health, health policy, and health information systems in Canada. *American Journal of Public Health, 93*, 388–392.

Healthy Community Principles. (2000). *Public Health Reports, 115*, 122.

Huttlinger, K., Schaller-Ayers, J., & Lawson, T. (2004). Health care in Appalachia: A population-based approach. *Public Health Nursing, 21*, 103–110.

Keller, L. O., Strohschein, S., Lia-Hoagberg, B., & Schaffer, M. A. (2004). Population-based public health interventions: Practice-based and evidence-supported. *Public Health Nursing, 21*, 453–468.

Kesler, J. T. (2000). Healthy communities and civil discourse: A leadership opportunity for public health professionals. *Public Health Reports, 115,* 238–242.

Kickbusch, I. (2003). The contribution of the World Health Organization to a new public health and health promotion. *American Journal of Public Health, 93,* 383–387.

Kindig, D., & Stoddart, G. (2003). What is population health? *American Journal of Public Health, 93,* 380–383.

Leavell, H. R., & Clark, E. G. (1965). *Preventive medicine for the doctor in his community: An epidemiologic approach* (3rd ed.). New York: McGraw-Hill.

Lee, P. (2000). Healthy Communities: A young movement that can revolutionize public health. *Public Health Reports, 115,* 114–115.

MacQueen, K. M., McLellan, E., Metzger, D. S., Kegeles, S., Strauss, R. P., Scotti, R., et al. (2001). What is community? An evidence-based definition for participatory public health. *American Journal of Public Health, 91,* 1929–1938.

Matteson, P. S. (2000). Preparing nurses for the future. In P. S. Matteson (Ed.), *Community-based nursing education* (pp. 1–7). New York: Springer.

McAlearney, A. S. (2003). *Population health management: Strategies to improve outcomes.* Chicago: Health Administration Press.

McDowell, I., Spasoff, R. A., & Kristjansson, B. (2004). On the classification of population health measures. *American Journal of Public Health, 94,* 388–393.

National Center for Health Statistics. (1992). *Health United States, 1991.* Washington, DC: Government Printing Office.

Norris, T., & Pittman, M. (2000). The healthy communities movement and the Coalition for Healthier Cities and Communities. *Public Health Reports, 115,* 118–124.

Northridge, M. E., & Ellis, J. A. (2003). Applying population health models. *American Journal of Public Health, 93,* 365.

Porche, D. J. (2004). *Public and community health nursing practice: A population-based approach.* Thousand Oaks, CA: Sage.

Sakamoto, S. D., & Avila, M. (2004). The public health nursing practice manual: A tool for public health nurses. *Public Health Nursing, 21,* 179–182.

Smith, K., & Bazini-Barakat, N. (2003). A public health nursing model: Melding public health principles with the nursing process. *Public Health Nursing, 20,* 42–48.

Szreter, S. (2003). The population health approach in historical perspective. *American Journal of Public Health, 93,* 421–431.

U.S. Department of Health and Human Services. (1980). *Promoting health/preventing disease: Objectives for the nation.* Washington, DC: Government Printing Office.

U.S. Department of Health and Human Services. (1990). *Healthy people 2000: National health promotion and disease prevention objectives.* Washington, DC: Government Printing Office.

U.S. Department of Health and Human Services. (1996). *Healthy people 2000: Fact sheet.* Washington, DC: Author.

U.S. Department of Health and Human Services. (2000a). *Healthy people 2010* (Conference edition, in two volumes). Washington, DC: Author.

U.S. Department of Health and Human Services. (2000b). *Healthy people 2010: Understanding and improving health* (2nd ed.). Washington, DC: Author.

U.S. Department of Health and Human Services. (2000c). Healthy people 2010: Understanding and improving health. *Prevention Report, 14*(4), 1–2, 4.

Wilcox, R., & Knapp, A. (2000). Building communities that create health. *Public Health Reports, 115,* 139–143.

The Historical Context

CHAPTER OBJECTIVES

After reading this chapter, you should be able to:

1. Describe the contributions of historical figures who influenced the development of community health nursing.
2. Discuss the contributions of community health nurses to social and health care reform.
3. List significant historical events in the development of community health nursing in the United States.
4. Describe evidence for a shift in public health policy toward a greater emphasis on health promotion.
5. Describe national and international events that are shaping current and future community health nursing practice.

KEY TERMS

diagnosis-related groups (DRGs) **54**
missionary nurses **45**
Nursing Interventions Classification (NIC) **55**
Nursing Outcomes Classification (NOC) **55**
variolation **44**
visiting nurse associations **45**

 MediaLink

http://www.prenhall.com/clark

Additional interactive resources for this chapter can be found on the Companion Website. Click on Chapter 3 and "Begin" to select the activities for this chapter.

Advocacy in Action

The Work of Susie Walking Bear Yellowtail

Born in 1903 on the Montana Crow Indian reservation, Susie Walking Bear Yellowtail was orphaned at the age of 12. In 1923, she became the first Native American registered nurse after graduating from the Boston City Hospital School of Nursing. Returning to the Montana Crow Agency, Ms. Yellowtail worked at the Bureau of Indian Affairs Hospital and later worked for the U.S. Public Health Service.

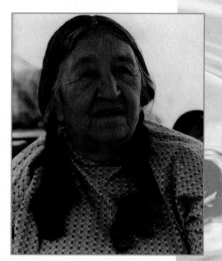

Experiences of Native American women sterilized without their consent and children dying on their mothers' backs while being carried 20 to 30 miles to a hospital led Ms. Yellowtail to a career of advocacy for Native American health care. Her advocacy activities encompassed 30 years of midwifery services in the Little Horn Valley and travel to many North American Indian reservations to evaluate health and health care. Through her membership on tribal councils and state health advisory boards, she became well known to health policy makers. She was appointed to the former U.S. Department of Health, Education, and Welfare's Council on Indian Health, the President's Special Council on Aging, and the President's Council on Indian Education and Nutrition, on which she served as an ambassador between her people and the federal government. She and her husband, Tom Yellowtail, also promoted understanding of American Indian culture in Europe and the Middle East as part of a U.S. cultural delegation in 1950. Throughout her life, she maintained her own cultural heritage, wearing Native American dress and engaging in the artistry of traditional Native American beadwork.

Ms. Yellowtail was also active in promoting the profession of nursing and was the founder of the Native American Nurses Association, which honored her as the "Grandmother of American Indian Nurses." Through her advocacy activities at tribal and federal levels, she was able to win funding for nursing education of Native American women.

In 1962 Ms. Yellowtail received the president's Award for Outstanding Nursing Health Care, and six years after her death her picture was included in the Outstanding Montanans Gallery at the Montana State Capitol. Ms. Yellowtail has been included among the 100 most influential Montanans of the 20th century and on July 1, 2002, became the first American Indian nurse admitted to the American Nurses Association Hall of Fame.

(*Sources:* http://www.ana.org/hof/yellowtail.htm;
http://www.minoritynurse.com/vitalsigns/jan03-4.html;
http://nsweb.nursingspectrum.com/NursesWeek/SusieWalkingBearYellowtail.htm;
http://www.nurses.info/personalities_susie_yellowtail.htm;
B. Cohen at http://missoulian.com/specials/100montanans/list/062.html;
S. Ridgeway at http://www.workingworld.com/magazine/viewarticle.asp?articleno=330&wn=1;
K. Rothwell at http://www.nursezone.com/Stories/SpotlightOnNurses.asp?articleID=6510)

*T*he history of public or community health nursing provides important insights into the events and factors that have shaped our practice. Knowledge of where we have been and how we got where we are gives us a sense of the present and future directions that community health nursing should take to achieve its goal—improved health for all people. Historical events that gave rise to a concern for the health of population groups influenced the development of both public health science and community health nursing. As noted by Rear Admiral Julia Plotnick (1994), former Chief Nurse of the U.S. Public Health Service:

> The profession of public health nursing was created in response to the social, political, and environmental forces that threatened the health of Americans a century ago. Previous generations of public health nurses saw the need for community-based programs that connected the work of health departments and the people at risk. They led many of the policy revolutions that helped bring family planning, workplace safety, and maternal child health services to people in need. (p. 1)

Her words are no less true today than they were a decade ago and set the stage for a discussion of our past in the context of our present and our future.

HISTORICAL ROOTS

The roots of modern public health and community health nursing practice go far back in history. For 5,000 years different cultural groups have developed a variety of approaches to dealing with common community health problems (Watts, 2003). Historical records provide evidence of concern for health and prevention of disease

Community health nurses visited clients in many different settings. (Photo courtesy of Center for Nursing Historical Inquiry, University of Virginia School of Nursing)

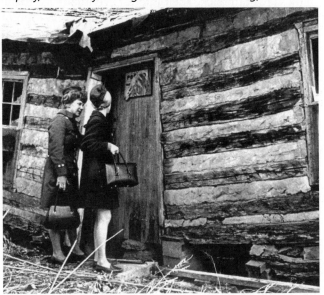

EVIDENCE-BASED PRACTICE

*C*onnolly (2004) presented a history of nursing historiography (the study of nursing history) and noted that research in nursing history, as in other fields of historical inquiry, has evolved in the last several decades. She pointed out that early nursing histories were "only weakly linked to the broader social, economic, and cultural contexts in which events unfolded" (p. 10) and tended to focus on the development of institutions in which nurses worked and the "great women" of nursing. These histories lauded nursing's accomplishments and recounted the profession's "purity, discipline, and faith [but] contained little about the less glorious aspects of the past" (p. 10).

Historians of this genre engaged in "political history," examining how public officials, legislation, and formal mechanisms of local, state, and federal government affected nursing. According to Connolly, history from this perspective assumed a coherence and unanimity in nursing that may not have truly existed. She maintained that early nursing political history, like much of history in general, was written from an elitist point of view and neglected the perspectives of other, less visible groups within and outside nursing.

During the 1960s and 1970s, historical research in general and nursing history in particular began to focus on those unheard voices, and a "social history" perspective was born. Connolly defined social history as "that which focuses on the experience, behavior, and agency of those at society's margins, rather than on its elite" (p. 5). Social historians examined nursing in the context of social factors influencing it (e.g., gender socialization, race relations, etc.).

Connolly recommended melding the two perspectives and examining political influences on nursing and nursing's influence on policy making in the context of social factors that influence both. For example, the Nurse Reinvestment Act could be examined in the light of the social factors that led to the shortage as well as the political history of legislative efforts to resolve past nursing shortages. Both perspectives can provide information that can direct policy development in ways that capitalize on past successes and avoid past mistakes.

How might you combine political and social history to examine some of the issues that affect community health nursing today? As an example, you might examine the nursing shortage in terms of the lack of ethnic diversity in the profession and how current legislation does or does not address this issue. What other issues can you think of that could be addressed from a combined political/social historical perspective?

in several ancient civilizations. Ancient Mesopotamia, the possible birthplace of humanity, and the Harappan civilization along the Indus River in what is now India employed sewage systems to prevent the spread of disease (Udwadia, 2000; Watts, 2003). Similarly, primitive tribes engaged in public health measures by not burying human wastes where they would contaminate water supplies (Association of State and Territorial Directors of Nursing, 2000). The Egyptians, Romans, and Aztecs were all known to emphasize the importance of clean water supplies. In fact, the Romans had water purification systems using settling basins and kept their drinking water separate from other water sources (Udwadia, 2000). The Romans also drained marshlands to minimize the spread of disease (Hancock, 2000).

The ancient Greeks spent a good deal of time theorizing about health and disease causation. Empedocles of Acragas, who lived from 493 to 433 CE, orginated the theory of imbalance among four "humors" as the cause of disease. These four humors (blood, bile, phlegm, and black bile) corresponded to the four elements believed to compose the world (fire, air, water, and earth) as well as to specific temperaments exhibited by individuals (sanguine, choleric, phlegmatic, or melancholic) (Kalisch & Kalisch, 2004).

Hippocrates, an eminent Greek physician, rejected the prior concept of disease as caused by supernatural intervention in favor of natural causation (Kalisch & Kalisch, 2004). He accepted the theory of the four humors, but believed they were influenced by environmental factors that shaped the physiologic response of people living in specific areas (Watts, 2003). There is some controversy regarding which of the writings on health and medicine ascribed to Hippocrates were actually composed by him. There is evidence, however, that he did write the famous treatise entitled *On Airs, Waters, and Places* as well as two books about epidemics in which he expounded on his theory of environmental contributions to disease (Udwadia, 2000).

The humoral theory, along with other selected elements of Hippocratic thinking, was adopted by the famous physician teacher, Galen. Galen's teachings were perpetuated in medical education until well into the Middle Ages, to the point that medical students would discard dissection evidence that did not support Galen's teachings as anatomic abnormalities. Despite his many other contributions, Galen has been credited by some authors with retarding the development of medical science for several hundred years through his erroneous concepts of causation (Watts, 2003).

Nursing of the sick at this period in history was primarily the function of the women of the family (Kalisch & Kalisch, 2004). In the case of large and wealthy households, the matron of the family cared for the health needs of both family members and servants or slaves. The care provided, however, was primarily palliative and was only slightly related to today's concept of nursing.

THE INFLUENCE OF CHRISTIANITY

Christianity, with its ethic of service to others, did a great deal to foster health care for particularly vulnerable populations such as lepers and the poor. Gradually that focus expanded to provision of care to other members of the population (e.g., in the many hospitals and other health-related institutions sponsored by Christian religious groups).

The Early Church

The advent of Christianity brought an emphasis on personal responsibility for the corporal and spiritual welfare of others. Care of the sick was seen as one means of fulfilling this responsibility, and early Christians employed their time and monetary wealth ministering to the sick. Such efforts were intended to provide comfort and material goods to the sick and suffering and bore little resemblance to modern nursing. Such services, although lacking an emphasis on prevention and health promotion or cure, did serve to bring about an awareness of illness within the population.

With the growth of Christianity and charitable giving by Christians, the wealth of the early Christian Church began to accumulate. A large portion of this wealth was used for organized care of the sick and needy through almshouses, asylums, and hospitals rather than through personal visitation to the sick. Hospitals or hospices of this time were not designed exclusively for care of the sick but ministered to all in need, including the sick, the poor, and travelers or pilgrims. The first hospital exclusively for the care of the sick was the Nosocomia, or "house for the sick," established by the Roman matron Fabia in the fourth century (Udwadia, 2000).

The Middle Ages

The mystical tradition of Christianity during the Middle Ages (500–1500 A.D.) led to a decline in population and personal health status. Castigation and neglect of the body to purify the soul resulted in a number of health problems. Many of the health-promotive activities of antiquity were abandoned in favor of fasting and the wearing of sackcloth and ashes.

The need for healthy warriors to fight in the Crusades sparked a slight renewal of interest in health. The Crusades also led to the development of the first hospitals, built in the Holy Land to care for Christian pilgrims and later for wounded Crusaders. The first of these was the Hospital of St. John in Jerusalem. Following the capture of Jerusalem in 1099 by the Christian forces, many Crusader knights were impressed with the care provided at the hospitals and sought to participate in the care of the sick. Their interest eventually led to the establishment of the Knights Hospitalers of St. John of Jerusalem, the first of the religious military orders that were to dominate the provision of nursing care for some time. The establishment of the Hospitalers was followed by the creation of the Knights Templar in 1118 and the Knights of the Teutonic Order in 1190. Interestingly, there were some women involved in the care of the sick under the auspices of female chapters of military orders, such as the Hospitaler Dames of the Order of St. John of Jerusalem (Kalisch & Kalisch, 2004).

Following the Crusades, other religious orders were formed to look after the sick. Groups of monks and nuns established hospitals to care for the ill. Initially, these hospitals provided care primarily for members of religious orders and their lay employees. For example, the Benedictine rule required each monastery to have a hospital for the care of ill brothers. Later, religious orders expanded the focus of their services to the sick poor. The Augustinian orders were particularly suited for nursing roles because their religious responsibilities were less burdensome than those of some other orders, leaving them more time to devote to the care of the sick (Kalisch & Kalisch, 2004).

In many instances, particular orders would focus on the care of specific groups or illnesses. For instance, the Antonites cared for persons with skin conditions, whereas Lazarites emphasized care of those with leprosy (Kalisch & Kalisch, 2004). Thus, the concept of specialization among health care providers is not as recent as one might believe.

Changes in social structure in the Middle Ages led to the development of cities, which increased the potential for the spread of disease. War and the attendant starvation and poor sanitation in cities have been described as the two most significant contributions to disease at this time. During the 14th century, recurring epidemics of plague killed nearly one fourth of the population of Europe. Periodic epidemics led to the establishment of some public health regulations, such as those related to burials and quarantine. Quarantine was first initiated in the city of Ragusa in 1347, then in Venice and Marseilles (Udwadia, 2000). It is interesting to note that the concept of quarantine was developed in Europe by town magistrates, not health care professionals. Similarly, an Egyptian Pasha instituted quarantine regulations in defiance of the recommendations of his French medical advisor (Watts, 2003).

OTHER RELIGIOUS INFLUENCES

Other religious groups contributed to the health of populations as well. In ancient times, the Jews developed a significant body of health regulations, incorporated into the Book of Leviticus (Association of State and Territorial Directors of Nursing, 2000). Similarly, Jewish physicians are credited with preserving scientific medicine through the Dark Ages by translating Greek and Arabic texts into Latin and promulgating Greco-Arabic medical knowledge in Europe. Similarly, Islamic medicine was a basis for the revival of the medical profession, embodied in the formation of the medical school at Salerno, Italy (Kalisch & Kalisch, 2004). Similarly, Ayurveda, based on traditional Indian philosophies, originated many of the alternative therapies gaining popularity today (Udwadia, 2000).

THE EUROPEAN RENAISSANCE

From 1500 to 1700, the European Renaissance gave rise to the beginnings of scientific thought. Also evident were the development of a social conscience and early recognition of social responsibility for the health and welfare of the population (Udwadia, 2000). England enacted the first Poor Law in 1601, making families financially responsible for the care of their aged and disabled members and creating publicly funded almshouses for those with no families. This development reflected the concept of "pauper stigma," under which the poor were believed to be responsible for their own condition due to lack of effort (Jonas, 2003). Another development in this period was the collection of vital statistics as a basis for public health policy decisions. Collection of vital statistics was pioneered by Johann Peter Sussmilch in the 1700s and systematized nationally in Sweden in 1748 and Britain in 1801 (Udwadia, 2000).

For most of the population, nursing was performed by family members. In 1610, however, Saint Francis DeSales and Madame de Chantal established a Parisian voluntary organization of well-to-do women to care for the sick in their homes. Care of the sick was institutionalized by some orders in the vows of consecration. For example, the Sisters of Charity, established in Paris in 1633 by Saint Vincent de Paul and Mademoiselle Louise Le Gras, and the Sisters of Bon Secours, established in 1822, took a fourth vow to care for the sick in addition to the traditional vows of poverty, chastity, and obedience (Kalisch & Kalisch, 2004).

A NEW WORLD

The discovery and colonization of the American continents led to different health issues and solutions to them. Communicable disease and poor health habits, for instance, traveled across the oceans in both directions. Native Americans were devastated by such diseases as measles and smallpox brought by European settlers (Graeme, 2002). Europeans, on the other hand, took tobacco back with them.

The Colonial Period

While new avenues of scientific thought were being opened in Europe, some of the ideas generated were being translated into a new way of life on a new continent. In the early colonial period in America, the health status of the colonists was good compared with that of their European counterparts, and longevity approached today's figures. The relative good health of the population was due primarily to low population density and, interestingly, poor transportation. Communities remained relatively isolated, and the spread of communicable diseases, the major health problem of the era, was curtailed by lack of movement between population groups (Fee, 2002).

Because doctors were few, health care was primarily a function of the family. Nursing care in the United States was provided by the women of the family, with assistance from neighbors where this was possible. The Sisters of Charity also provided services to the sick in the United States starting in 1809 under the direction of Mother Elizabeth Seton (Kalisch & Kalisch, 2004). In Canada, public health practice was carried out by Christian religious orders as early as the 17th century. One of the early Canadian public health activists was nurse

Jeanne Mance, who arrived in "New France" in 1659. Mance co-founded the Hôtel Dieu in Montreal and provided leadership for a variety of other community health efforts (Duncan, Leipart, & Mill, 1999).

Early Public Health Efforts

The growth of population centers led to concern for sanitation and vital statistics, the foci of early public health efforts in the colonies. In 1639, both Massachusetts and Plymouth colonies mandated the reporting of all births and deaths, instituting the official reporting of vital statistics in what would later become the United States. Environmental health and sanitation were also of concern in the early colonies. Concern for the spread of communicable diseases was manifested in the establishment of "pesthouses" for people with contagious conditions (Kalisch & Kalisch, 2004) as well as isolation and quarantine measures.

For the most part, health was seen as a personal responsibility with little governmental involvement. Temporary boards of health were established in response to specific health problems, usually epidemics of communicable disease, and were disbanded after the crisis had passed. Early public health efforts in Canada were also crisis oriented, and centralized action on public health issues was strongly resisted (Duncan et al., 1999).

Recognition of the need for a consistent and organized approach to health problems was growing, however, and in 1797, the state of Massachusetts granted local jurisdictions legal authority to establish health services and regulations. The following year, Congress passed the Act for Relief of Sick and Disabled Seamen to create hospitals for the care of members of the merchant marine. The group of hospitals created under this act was renamed the Marine Hospital Service in 1871 (Fee, 2002). Responsibility for quarantine was shifted to the Marine Hospital Service in 1878 as one of the first efforts to deal with health problems at a national, rather than state or local, level (Jonas, 2003).

Nursing during this period remained a function of the family. Although the care given was primarily palliative, the women of the house might also engage in some health-promotive practices, such as regular purging with castor oil. Treatment tended to consist of home remedies, and the literature of the era is replete with housewives' recipes for the treatment of a variety of ailments.

In 1813, the Ladies' Benevolent Society of Charleston, South Carolina, was established. This was the first organized approach to home nursing of the sick in the United States. This organization was initiated in response to a yellow fever epidemic and was completely nondenominational and nondiscriminatory in an era characterized by widespread racial discrimination. Care was provided to the sick in their homes by upper-class women. Because these women had no background in nursing, care focused on relieving suffering and providing material aid (Buhler-Wilkerson, 2001). With the

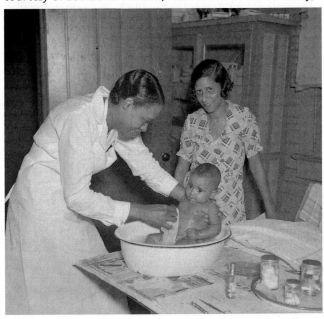

Community health nurses often demonstrated appropriate hygiene practices as well as teaching about them. (Photo courtesy of Louisiana Division, New Orleans Public Library)

exception of a 20-year period during and after the Civil War, the Ladies' Benevolent Society provided services until the 1950s.

A similar service was instituted in 1819 in Philadelphia's Jewish community by the Hebrew Female Benevolent Society of Philadelphia. This service was organized by Rebecca Gratz, a Jewish society woman believed to be the model for Sir Walter Scott's Rebecca (Benson, 1993).

Another early attempt at home care nursing also saw upper-class women visiting the homes of indigent women during childbirth. The Lying-in Charity for Attending Indigent Women in Their Homes was established in 1832 to assist poor women during and after delivery. Because of their lack of training, the services provided by these women emphasized social and emotional support for the woman in labor and assistance to her after delivery.

THE INDUSTRIAL REVOLUTION

The Industrial Revolution profoundly influenced health in both Europe and the United States. Movement on both continents from agricultural to industrial economies led to the development of large industrial centers and the need for a large workforce to labor under unhealthy conditions in mines, mills, and factories. By 1850, half of England's population lived in urban areas (Watts, 2003). The demand for manufactured goods and the necessity to get goods to market prompted advancements in transportation that increased mobility and the potential for spreading communicable diseases. In the United States, rural–urban migration and the presence of large contingents of poor immigrants led initially to the conversion of single-family dwellings in less affluent areas of town and then to the development of crowded tenement houses (Fee, Brown, Lazarus, & Theerman, 2002b). From 1820 to 1910, 30 million immigrants came to the United States, representing almost half of the populations of urban slums in major U.S. cities. By the mid-1890s, for example, two thirds of the population of New York City lived in 90,000 tenement houses (Kalisch & Kalisch, 2004). The plight of the immigrant population was compounded by the loss of traditional mechanisms of support from extended families and friends (Hamilton, 2001).

The poor were overworked and underpaid. Poor nutrition contributed to increased incidence of a variety of diseases, particularly tuberculosis. Recognition of tuberculosis as a growing problem among the poor led to the creation of the first tuberculosis hospital in England in 1840 (Zilm & Warbinek, 1995). The use of children in the workforce, coupled with low wages, inadequate food, and hazardous living and working conditions, led to many preventable illnesses and deaths among the children of the poor. In the 1870 census, more than 750,000 working children were recorded. This number does not include children of farm families who often worked alongside their parents. In 1930, the Fair Labor Standards Act abolished child labor (excluding farm labor) in the United States, but this practice remains rampant in other parts of the world (Helfand, Lazarus, & Theerman, 2001).

The 19th century saw a beginning recognition of the effects of these social and economic conditions on health, and the concept of social responsibility for public health began to take root. The growth of this concept was fostered by the publication in the mid-1800s of several landmark reports. The first of these publications was C. Turner Thackrah's treatise on occupational health, *The Effects of Arts, Trades, and Professions . . . on Health and Longevity.* In this document, Thackrah described the effects of working conditions on health.

In 1842, Edwin Chadwick's *Inquiry into the Sanitary Conditions of the Labouring Population of Great Britain* provided additional fuel for efforts to change the working and social conditions that contributed to disease. Chadwick's committee, however, drew the erroneous conclusion that disease caused poverty, not vice versa. Despite their mistaken notions of causality, Chadwick's report led to sanitary engineering solutions and annual local government spending for sanitary improvements that increased from £5 million in 1856–1871 to £30 million by 1910 (Watts, 2003). Chadwick's report heralded a shift in the view of public health from one of social reform to one of sanitary engineering (Berridge, 2000).

While Thackrah and Chadwick addressed the effects of working conditions on health and instigated reforms to prevent disease, Henry W. Rumsey focused on health promotion. Rumsey's *Essays on State Medicine* emphasized health promotion and illness prevention as social obligations of government. Some nations acted on this concept by establishing national health care systems. For example, Germany instituted a state-funded

Many families who received community health nursing services lived in a single room. (Photo courtesy of the Center for the Study of the History of Nursing, School of Nursing, University of Pennsylvania)

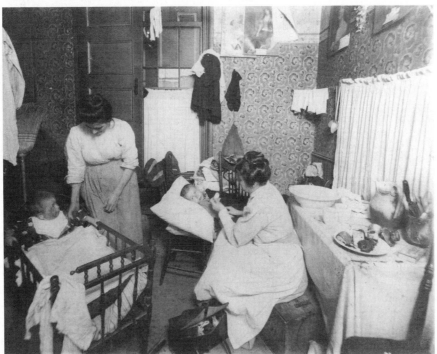

medical insurance program for working men and civil servants as early as 1869. Similar attempts were initiated in Britain in the 1860s, but the National Health Insurance Act was not passed until 1911 (Sigerist, 2003; Watts, 2003). In the United States, national health insurance was an element of Theodore Roosevelt's election platform in 1912 (Jonas, 2003).

Documents similar to those of Rumsey, Chadwick, and Thackrah were also published in the United States. The Massachusetts Sanitary Commission was established in response to concern over the effects of crowded living conditions, poverty, and poor sanitation on health. In 1850, Lemuel Shattuck drafted the commission's findings. The *Report of the Massachusetts Sanitary Commission* included recommendations for establishing state and local health departments, systematic collection of vital statistics, and sanitation inspections, and for instituting programs for school health and control of mental illness, alcohol abuse, and tuberculosis. Other recommendations included public education regarding sanitation, control of nuisances, periodic physical examinations, supervision of the health of immigrants, and construction of model tenements. In addition, the report recommended improved education for nurses and the inclusion of content on preventive medicine and sanitation in medical school curricula.

The publication of the *Report of the Massachusetts Sanitary Commission* marks the beginning of community health practice as we know it today (Epidemiology Program Office, 1999). Recommendations of the report form the basis for much of the present work of official state and local public health agencies. The eventual effect of the commission's report was the establishment of state boards of health. The first state board was established in Louisiana in 1855, but has been described as a "paper organization." In 1869, nearly 90 years after the advent of the first temporary boards of health and 19 years after the publication of Shattuck's report, Massachusetts established the first working board of health, followed by California in 1870 (Fee, 2002).

Collection of vital statistics at the national level was another activity undertaken in the latter half of the 19th century. The first national mortality statistics, for example, were published by the U.S. federal government in 1850 (Epidemiology Program Office, 1999).

During this period, great strides were made in the fledgling science of epidemiology. In 1854, without knowledge of the nature of the causative organism, John Snow determined the source of a London epidemic of cholera to be something in the water of the Broad Street pump (Centers for Disease Control and Prevention [CDC], 2004). Jacob Henle was the first to postulate microorganisms as a cause of disease rather than miasmas (harmful vapors) or humors (Udwadia, 2000). It was not, however, until 1876 that Louis Pasteur and Robert Koch, working independently, identified specific bacteria (Watts, 2003). These and other epidemiologic findings allowed more scientific measures to be applied to the control of communicable disease and contributed greatly to the armamentarium used by later community health nurses in preventing disease.

Another significant advance in public health practice was the development of vaccines for communicable diseases. As early as the 1700s India and the Ottoman Turks had developed a process of **variolation** in which material from smallpox lesions was inoculated into the skin, nose, or veins of a healthy person. In 1713, the Greek physician Timoni submitted a report on variolation to the Royal Society, but his conclusions were ignored until Lady Mary Montagu, wife of the British Ambassador to Turkey, wrote about her use of the practice for her children and recommended it to the British royal family. Variolation was practiced by some English physicians but was not widely accepted. Edward Jenner later used material from cowpox lesions to vaccinate people against smallpox, and this process was more widely adopted (Udwadia, 2000).

In 1890 the concept of immunization against diphtheria was tested in guinea pigs by Karl Fraenkel, and Emil Behring and Shibasaburo Kitasato used immune serum to provide protection against this disease. Tetanus antitoxin was introduced in 1915, and vaccines for other communicable diseases followed (Udwadia, 2000). Some of the significant events in the development of public health prior to the 20th century are summarized in Table 3-1◆.

Organized advocacy for the health of the population by public health professionals began in 1872 with the establishment of the American Public Health Association (APHA). APHA consists of members of more than 50 public health disciplines and is the oldest and largest association of public health professionals in the world (APHA, 2005a). Throughout its history, APHA has focused on the development of standards and policies

TABLE 3-1	Significant Public Health Events Prior to the 20th Century
Date	**Event**
1347	Quarantine first instituted in Ragusa, Italy.
1797	Jurisdiction to establish local boards of health first granted in Massachusetts.
1798	Marine Hospital Service, forerunner of the U.S. Public Health Service, created.
1854	Contaminated water demonstrated to be the cause of cholera by John Snow.
1869	State-funded medical insurance instituted for German workers. First modern state board of health established in Massachusetts.
1872	American Public Health Association established.
1876	Specific bacteria first isolated by Koch and Pasteur.
1890	Immune serum first used to prevent diphtheria.

that promote population health. APHA is organized in 24 discipline-based sections and seven special interest groups that cut across disciplines (APHA, 2005c). The APHA section of greatest interest to community health nurses is the Public Health Nursing Section, developed to provide leadership in community health nursing practice, policy development, and research (APHA, 2005b).

DISTRICT NURSING IN ENGLAND

The "three great revolutions" of the late 18th and early 19th centuries—the intellectual revolution, the French and American political revolutions, and the Industrial Revolution—set the stage for the development of community health nursing. In England, the same spirit that motivated industrial and prison reform led to concern for the health of large urban populations and the development of nursing practices to address these concerns.

In addition to being the acknowledged founder of modern hospital nursing, Florence Nightingale was instrumental in the development of community health or district nursing. Nightingale received her training in nursing at the school for deaconesses established by Theodor Fliedner. Fliedner's second wife, Caroline Bertheau, conceived the idea of extending the nursing services offered in the hospital to the sick in their homes. This concept influenced Nightingale, who endorsed the idea of health promotion as well as home care for illness (Falk Rafael, 1999).

In 1840, Elizabeth Frye, a Quaker woman, founded the Institute of Nursing in London. Members of the institute were called the Society of Protestant Sisters of Charity, but were later referred to as "nursing sisters" to avoid confusion with the prior Roman Catholic religious orders. These nursing sisters were laywomen who provided care to the sick poor in their homes and in prison (Udwadia, 2000). Frye was also actively involved in attempts by reformers to improve conditions in British prisons (Udwadia, 2000).

William Rathbone, another Quaker philanthropist, instituted professional home care for the sick poor in Liverpool in 1859 after seeing the effectiveness of a trained nurse in caring for his dying wife. Although the nurse hired for the experiment was often tempted to leave in its early days, the initiative was considered a success and spread to other cities in England (Kalisch & Kalisch, 2004). Unable to recruit sufficient trained nurses on his own, Rathbone turned to Florence Nightingale for assistance (Buhler-Wilkerson, 2001). Nightingale was instrumental in developing the concept of visiting nursing and viewed public health nursing as including specific nursing care for the sick poor as well as attention to environmental and sanitation issues (McDonald, 2000). The nursing services provided were organized in terms of local districts—hence the term *district nursing* (Buhler-Wilkerson, 2001).

The need to standardize community health nursing services was recognized early in the development of district nursing. A committee chaired by Rathbone undertook to conduct a study of district nursing services coordinated by Florence Lee, one of Nightingale's students. Lee's report, published in 1875, noted that many visiting nurses were not adequately trained, that their practice included responsibilities beyond hospital nursing, and that they required additional training. In addition, Lee recommended the employment of educated women for district nursing services. The report led to the formation in 1876 of the Metropolitan and National Nursing Association for Providing Trained Nurses for the Sick Poor (Buhler-Wilkerson, 2001). Prior to the employment of professional nurses to visit the sick poor, home visiting often provided the opportunity for proselytizing and attempts to convert the client to a specific religious persuasion or to redeem them from moral decrepitude.

VISITING NURSES IN AMERICA

In the United States, proselytizing was also part of the role of nurses who provided early home care to the sick poor; however, efforts had been made to incorporate the provision of nursing care in addition to proselytizing and providing for material needs. Wealthy women in several large cities hired trained nurses to visit the sick. For example, the Women's Branch of the New York City Mission first employed trained nurses to provide home visiting services in 1877 (Kalisch & Kalisch, 2004). The role of these and many other **missionary nurses** was to provide nursing care and religious instruction for the sick poor. Often, visiting of the sick was motivated by beliefs that poverty was a result of moral deficiency and that the poor needed exposure to the "elevating experience of their moral betters" (Buhler-Wilkerson, 2001, p. 18).

In 1878, the Ethical Culture Society of New York employed four nurses in dispensaries, inaugurating the ambulatory care role of the community health nurse. These nurses worked under the supervision of a physician and emphasized health teaching as well as illness care (Brainerd, 1985). In the next few years, **visiting nurse associations** were established in Buffalo (1885), and in Boston and Philadelphia (1886) (Center for the Study of the History of Nursing, n.d.). The Philadelphia agency was the first to institute a nurse's uniform, a fee for services, and a community nursing supervisor. The Boston Instructive District Nursing Association emphasized the community health nurse's educative function as well as her role in the care of the sick (Kalisch & Kalisch, 2004), signaling the beginning of the health promotion emphasis that now characterizes community health nursing. Similar events were taking place in Canada, with the establishment of the Victorian Order of Nurses (VON) in 1897 and the hiring of the first community health nurse in British Columbia in 1901 (Zilm &

Warbinek, 1995). This initiative was intended to provide midwifery services on the Northwest frontier, but medical opposition to nurse midwifery led to a shift in focus to home visiting services in urban areas (Richardson, 1998). By 1890, there were 21 visiting nursing organizations in the United States (Kalisch & Kalisch, 2004), and 22 years later, when the National Organization for Public Health Nursing (NOPHN) was founded, there were 3,000 visiting nurses in the United States (Winslow, 1993). Similarly, Alberta's District Nursing Service, founded in 1919 with three nurses, grew to encompass 13 nurses by 1935 and 35 by 1950 (Richardson, 1998).

NURSING AND THE SETTLEMENT HOUSES

The settlement movement was based on the belief espoused by Arnold Toynbee that educated persons could promote learning, morality, and civic responsibility in the poor by living among them and sharing certain aspects of their poverty. Groups of students from Oxford and Cambridge, acting on this belief, "settled" in homes in the London slums with the idea that their poor neighbors would learn through watching their behavior (Erickson, 1987).

In the United States, the settlement idea was adapted by nurses such as Lillian Wald, who believed that the most effective way to bring health care to the poor immigrant population was for nurses to live and work among them. Accordingly, Wald and her associate Mary Brewster established the forerunner of the Henry Street Settlement from their Jefferson Street tenement apartment in New York City in 1893 (Kalisch & Kalisch, 2004). The actual Henry Street establishment was purchased in 1895. The house on Henry Street differed from many other settlement houses of the era in its incorporation of visiting nurse services. In addition, visiting nurse services in the United States differed from those in England in their acceptance of the germ theory and its use as a foundation for many of their interventions. It has been noted by several authors that Florence Nightingale never did accept the germ theory and continued to hold to the theory of miasmas as the cause of disease (Udwadia, 2000; Watts, 2003).

The Henry Street Settlement is usually considered the first American community health agency because of its incorporation of modern concepts of community health nursing. At Henry Street, Wald redefined the basic principles of home care. She believed that access to the services of a nurse should be determined by the client and not based on a decision by a physician. In spite of the focus on health promotion at the Henry Street Settlement, Wald contended that the primary function of the visiting nurse was care of the sick in their homes, with health education as a secondary focus. She also felt that care of the poor should be equivalent to that available to the rich and that services provided should respect the client's individual dignity and independence (Buhler-Wilkerson, 2001). The latter principle led her to establish a 3-month probationary period for nurses employed at Henry Street to orient the nurses to the culture of the immigrant populations they served (Kalisch & Kalisch, 2004). Although the nurses were expected to view other cultures with tolerance, their activities were often based on myths and stereotypes that subsided as they were exposed to a variety of different cultures (Buhler-Wilkerson, 2001).

The nurses of the Henry Street Settlement did more than visit the sick in their homes. Lillian Wald coined the term *public health nurse* to reflect the focus on service to the whole community to improve both individual and societal conditions affecting health (Buhler-Wilkerson, n.d.). Health promotion and disease prevention were heavily emphasized, as was political activism. In Wald's words, "The call of the nurse is not only for bedside care of the sick, but to help in seeking out the deep-lying basic causes of illness and misery. That in the future, there may be less sickness to nurse and cure" (quoted in Buhler-Wilkerson, 2001, p. 98). Wald herself was a prime example of the political activist, supporting many changes in social conditions that would benefit the health of the public (National Association for Home Care, n.d.). In fact, the Henry Street Settlement served as the site for the opening reception of the 1909 National Negro Conference, one of the few places that would host an interracial gathering. This conference led to the establishment of the National Association for the Advancement of Colored People (NAACP) (Buhler-Wilkerson, 2001).

Other early community health nurses like Margaret Sanger, Clara Barton, and Dorothea Dix were also actively involved in promoting social change. Margaret Sanger's contributions to contraceptive services for women were touched on in Chapter 1∞ and are addressed in more detail in the *Think Advocacy* feature on page 47. Clara Barton and Dorothea Dix were both active in the provision of nursing care to both Federal and Confederate wounded in the American Civil War. Barton later served as the first woman to run a U.S. government office in her role locating missing Civil War soldiers with the Office of Correspondence with the Friends of the Missing Men of the United States Army (Behling, n.d.). Barton was also instrumental in the establishment of the American Red Cross in 1881 (Vinson, n.d.). Dix, in addition to her role in the Civil War, was actively involved in improving the plight of inmates in U.S. prisons (Kalisch & Kalsich, 2004).

The nurses of Henry Street, like other community health nursing pioneers, were able to accomplish more in the way of social activism than their hospital counterparts because their practice was essentially free of external control (Buhler-Wilkerson, n.d.). In fact, the Henry Street nurses have been described as "virtually independent practitioners in sick and preventive care,

Think Advocacy

Kalisch and Kalisch (2004) described the role of Margaret Sanger in promoting women's access to contraceptive services at the beginning of the 20th century. According to the authors, in 1912 Sanger cared for a 28-year-old mother of three who attempted a self-induced abortion of an unwanted pregnancy. The woman pleaded with Sanger to give her information to prevent subsequent pregnancies. Sanger, constrained by the 1873 Comstock Act, which classified contraceptive information as obscene, could not accede to her request and was later called by the woman's husband to attend her deathbed. This event was a catalyst for Sanger's activities to make contraceptive services available to women. She studied contraceptive technology in France and educated women by means of a journal she published entitled *The Woman Rebel*. In 1916, she opened a birth control clinic, which saw 150 women in its first day of operation. Arrested by an undercover policewoman posing as a client, Sanger was jailed. She publicly refused to abide by the law and was sentenced to 30 days in the workhouse. In spite of these sanctions, Sanger continued to promote access to contraceptive services for women and educate women in their use. She solicited the support of wealthy and influential women who were able to influence the policy makers of the day, and in 1921 instituted the American Birth Control League, the forerunner of the Planned Parenthood Federation.

- What community health issues in your community will require the level of commitment displayed by Margaret Sanger?
- How might you go about influencing those issues? What influential individuals and groups would you approach for support of your initiative?

CULTURAL COMPETENCE

Early community health nursing leaders were products of the culture and society of their times, yet many of them put aside cultural expectations of marriage and family to devote their energies to improving the health of the public. Explore the life and times of one of these leaders. What factors in her development led her to move outside of cultural prescriptions for women? In what ways did they continue to display their cultural heritage? Would these women face similar challenges today? Why or why not?

---

health, education, and school nursing" in an era when other nurses were experiencing medical domination (Roberts & Group, 1995, p. 82).

Other nursing settlement houses patterned on the Henry Street model were established. One particularly inspiring example was the Nurse's Settlement established in 1900 in Richmond, Virginia, by the graduating class of Old Dominion Hospital. These nurses had been exposed to the needs of Richmond's poor during student experiences with the Instructive Visiting Nurse Association of Richmond. The settlement they founded differed from the Henry Street Settlement in that it did not have any wealthy patrons to provide support and was initiated with the limited resources of the graduates themselves. Like Henry Street, the Richmond settlement focused on health promotion and education as well as care of the sick (Erickson, 1987).

EXPANDING THE FOCUS ON PREVENTION

The effectiveness of community health nurses in preventing sickness and death among the poor was recognized and became the basis for visiting nurse services offered by the Metropolitan Life Insurance Company.

This program was begun at the instigation of Lee Frankel and Lillian Wald. Wald convinced the Metropolitan board that providing nursing services to its policyholders would improve the public image of an industry tarnished by economic scandal. The compelling argument, though, was evidence that community health nursing reduced mortality and would limit the death benefits paid by the company. Services were begun on an experimental basis in 1909 with one of the Henry Street nurses (Buhler-Wilkerson, n.d.; 2001).

The 3-month experiment was such a success that the program was extended nationwide in 1911 (Buhler-Wilkerson, 2001) and continued to provide services until 1953. This association with the business world was an education for community health nurses, who had no conception of marketing or the economic bases for programs. The program was finally discontinued because of nursing's failure to grasp economic realities and the realization of diminishing returns by the insurance company.

The emphasis of community health nursing on health promotion began with health education in the home during visits to the poor in large cities. Gradually, however, the concepts of health promotion and illness prevention were expanded to other population groups to include services to mothers and young children, school-age youngsters, employees, and the rural population.

Concern for the health of mothers and children was growing, and the nurses of the Henry Street Settlement and other similar programs spent a large portion of their time in health promotion for this group of clients. Because they recognized that services to individual families would not overcome the effects of poverty, they worked actively to improve social conditions affecting health. Through the efforts of Lillian Wald and other social activists, the first White House Conference on Children was held in 1909. As a result of the conference, the U.S. Children's Bureau was established in 1912 to address the issue of child labor. Its efforts were later expanded to encompass a variety of initiatives related to child health (Helfand, Lazarus, & Theerman, 2000).

School nursing, another arena for health promotion, actually began in London in 1893 (Wolfe & Selekman, 2002) and was introduced in the United States by Lillian Wald in 1902. The initial impetus for school health

ETHICAL AWARENESS

*P*art of the impetus for the Children's Bureau was the use of child labor. This practice occurs today in underdeveloped countries and on U.S. farms. What are the ethical implications of child labor that allows families to meet basic survival needs? Are the implications similar or different for underdeveloped countries and U.S. farm families? Why or why not?

nursing was the high level of school absenteeism due to illness. In New York City in 1902, 15 to 20 children per school were being sent home daily. In response, Wald assigned Lina Struthers from the Henry Street Settlement to a pilot project in school nursing. Because of the overwhelming success of the project (a 90% decline in school exclusions in the first year), the New York Board of Health absorbed the program and hired additional nurses to continue the work (Kalisch & Kalisch, 2004).

The concept of school nursing spread to other parts of the country and to Canada. In 1904, Los Angeles became the first of many municipalities to employ nurses in schools (Gardner, 1952). In 1906, the Montreal Board of Health initiated medical inspections of schoolchildren, later appointing a VON nurse to a school nursing position. School nurses were also appointed in Hamilton in 1909 and Toronto in 1910 (Duncan et al., 1999).

Early school nursing focused on preventing the spread of communicable diseases and treating ailments related to compulsory school life. By the 1930s, however, the focus had shifted to preventive and promotive activities, including case finding, integrating health concepts into school curricula, and maintaining a healthful school environment (Igoe, 1980).

The first rural nursing service was established in 1896 in Westchester County, New York, by Ellen Morris Wood and was followed in 1906 by the initiation of a nursing service for both the poor and the well-to-do of Salisbury, Connecticut. Despite her usual sphere of activity in the city, Lillian Wald was also involved in the growth of rural community health nursing. She convinced the American Red Cross, founded in 1881, to direct its peacetime attention to expanding community health services in rural America. In 1912, the Red Cross established the Rural Nursing Service (later the Town and Country Nursing Service) to extend community health nursing services to rural areas (Kalisch & Kalisch, 2004). In Canada, rural nursing services were provided to large immigrant populations by such organizations as the Victorian Order of Nurses for Canada, the Canadian Red Cross Society, and the Women's Missionary Society (Bramadat & Saydak, 1993).

Another pioneer in the provision of health services in rural settings was Mary Breckenridge. In 1928, Breckenridge initiated the Frontier Nursing Service (FNS). The FNS provided midwifery services by nurses who traveled 700 square miles on horseback and served 1,000 families in a period of 5 years (Mary Breckenridge, n.d.). An assessment of its outcomes in the first 1,000 cases

In addition to school inspections, community health nurses made home visits to children excluded from school for communicable diseases. (Photo courtesy of the National Library of Medicine)

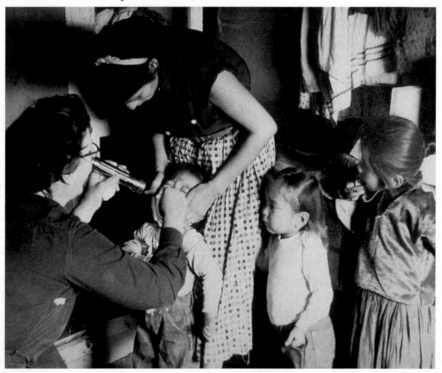

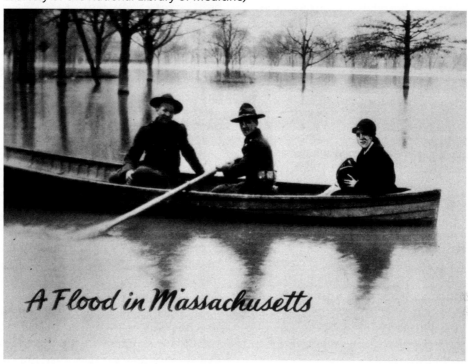

Community health nurses used varied means of transportation in their work. (Photo courtesy of the National Library of Medicine)

A Flood in Massachusetts

indicated no maternal mortality and fewer stillbirths and infant deaths than in the general population (Kalisch & Kalisch, 2004).

Other largely rural populations experiencing significant health problems were the Native American population on federal reservations and the African Americans in the South. Community health nursing services on the reservations arose out of a 1922 study of health conditions by the American Red Cross commissioned by the Bureau of Indian Affairs (Ruffing-Rahal, 1995). Nurses in this setting often found themselves breaking official rules in order to provide effectively for the needs of their clients (Abel, 1996). To meet the needs of black women in the South, some states co-opted local black midwives to work closely with public health nurses. As on the reservations, the rules imposed frequently violated accepted cultural health practices. For example, the nurses "forbade midwives to use any folk medicine or herbal remedies in their childbirth work" (Smith, 1994). In spite of the cultural insensitivity displayed, the partnership between public health nurses and midwives helped to create a modern public health system in the rural South.

Occupational health nursing provided another avenue for health promotion by community health nurses. This specialty area began in 1895 when Vermont's Governor Proctor employed nurses to see to the health needs of villages where employees of his Vermont Marble Company lived. These first employment-based services focused on care of the sick rather than prevention and care of occupation-related conditions (Kalisch & Kalisch, 2004). In 1897, the Employees' Benefit Association of John Wanamaker's department store in New York City hired nurses to visit employees' homes. These nurses soon expanded their role to include first aid and prevention of illness and injury in the work setting. The number of firms employing nurses increased rapidly from 66 in 1910 to 871 by 1919 (Brainerd, 1985).

STANDARDIZING PRACTICE

The need to standardize community nursing practice was recognized in both the United States and England. Early American attempts to standardize visiting nursing services included publications related to public health nursing and the development of a national logo by the Cleveland Visiting Nurse Association (VNA). This logo, or seal, was made available to any visiting nurse organization that met established standards. Both the Chicago (1906) and Cleveland (1909) VNAs published newsletters titled *Visiting Nurse Quarterly* to aid attempts to standardize care (Brainerd, 1985). Another attempt to standardize practice was the development of a list of standing orders for public health nurses by the Chicago Visiting Nurse Association in 1912 (Kalisch & Kalisch, 2004).

In 1911, a joint committee of the American Nurses Association (ANA) and the Society for Superintendents of Training Schools for Nurses met to consider the need for standardization. The result was a second meeting, held in 1912. Letters inviting representation were sent to 1,092 organizations employing visiting nurses at that time. These organizations included VNAs, city and state boards of health and education, private clubs and societies, tuberculosis leagues, hospitals and dispensaries, businesses, settlements and day nurseries, churches, and charitable organizations. A total of 69 agencies responded with their intent to send a representative to the meeting. The result of this second meeting was the formation of the National Organization for Public Health Nursing (NOPHN) (Brainerd, 1985). The objective of this organization was to provide for stimulation and standardization of public health nursing. This was the first professional body in the United States to include lay membership. Similar activity was undertaken in Canada, leading to the creation in 1920 of the public health section of the Canadian Association of Trained Nurses (Duncan et al., 1999).

The NOPHN was influential in maintaining public health nursing services at home during World War I and in the organization of the Division of Public Health Nursing within the U.S. Public Health Service in 1944. The NOPHN also provided advisory services regarding postgraduate education for public health nursing in colleges and universities. The NOPHN was incorporated into the National League for Nursing (NLN) in the restructuring of professional nursing organizations in the 1950s (Kalisch & Kalisch, 2004).

In 1986, the American Nurses Association developed the *Standards of Community Health Nursing Practice*. As we saw in Chapter 1 ∞, the standards are based on the use of the nursing process in community health nursing practice. In 1999, the standards were revised by the Quad Council of Public Health Nursing Organizations as the *Scope and Standards of Public Health Nursing Practice* and have recently undergone another revision (ANA, 2007).

Attempts were also made over the years to standardize the functions and competencies of community health nurses. These culminated in the Quad Council's 2003 adoption of the public health nursing competencies discussed in Chapter 1 ∞ (Quad Council, 2003, 2004), but began as early as 1931, when the Field Studies Committee of NOPHN developed functions and related objectives for generalized and specialized practice. These objectives were revised in 1936 and 1944 and again in 1949 in a document entitled *Public Health Nursing Responsibilities in a Community Health Program* (Abrams, 2004).

EDUCATING COMMUNITY HEALTH NURSES

As Steven Jonas (2003), noted public health author, has observed, whenever a new area of nursing practice is established, it is inevitably followed by the development of practice standards and related curricula. Public health nursing was no exception, and during the 1920s, nursing education was under study. The Goldmark Report, *Nursing and Nursing Education in the United States*, published in 1923, dealt with nursing education in general and pointed out the need for advanced

GLOBAL PERSPECTIVES

*C*ho and Kashka (2004) described the contributions of Korean nurse leader Mo Im Kim in the development of a community health nurse practitioner role to meet the needs of rural communities in Korea. Kim's vision of the skills needed for community health nursing included political acumen, program management, and community leadership. The authors' description of Kim's activities in the development and support of the rural community health nurse practitioner role provides an excellent example of advocacy for the specialty itself.

Explore how community health nursing practice has developed in another country. What events led to the development of the role? What factors have influenced how the community health nursing role is conceptualized in that country?

preparation for community health nursing. The report recommended that nursing education take place in institutions of higher learning (Kalisch & Kalisch, 2004). As a result, the Yale University School of Nursing and the Frances Payne Bolton School of Nursing at Western Reserve University opened in 1923. Canada's first baccalaureate program in nursing (also the first in the British Empire) was established in 1919 at the University of British Columbia (Duncan et al., 1999). The curricula of both U.S. and Canadian programs included community health nursing content.

Prior to the education of nurses in university settings, special postgraduate courses in public health nursing had been established by various agencies. The first of these in the United States was undertaken by the Instructive District Nursing Association of Boston in 1906 (Buhler-Wilkerson, 2001). In 1910, Teachers' College of Columbia University offered the first course in public health nursing in an institution of higher learning (Brainerd, 1985), and in 1927 the NLN curriculum document, *A Curriculum for Schools of Nursing*, emphasized the need for specific training for public health nursing (Kalisch & Kalisch, 2004). In Canada, the Canadian Red Cross Society instituted a 14-week certificate course for public health nurses in 1920 (Zilm & Warbinek, 1995). The first such course was offered by the University of Alberta in 1918 (Duncan et al., 1999).

In addition to witnessing the movement of community health nursing education to institutions of higher learning, the 1920s saw a shift in the employment of public health nurses. Before this time, most public health nursing services were provided by voluntary agencies such as the Red Cross and similar organizations. Although some local jurisdictions, such as Los Angeles, employed public health nurses in communicable disease control, no state recognized the role of this nursing specialty in an official health or education agency until 1907, when Alabama became the first state to approve public health nurse employment by government agencies. By 1924, a survey by NOPHN found that half of all nurses

Tuberculosis control has always been an important focus for community health nurses. (Photo courtesy of the National Library of Medicine)

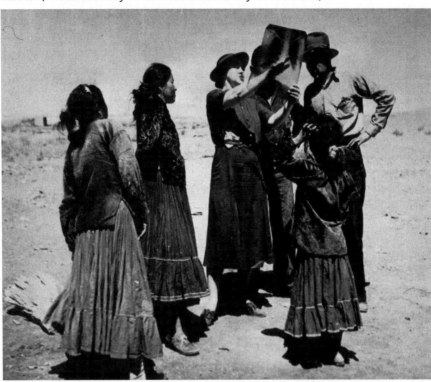

employed in public health nursing worked for official government agencies and approximately 41% of all U.S. counties had access to public health nursing services (Kalisch & Kalisch, 2004). By 1937, 67% of all community health nurses were employed by official public health agencies (Winslow, 1993). This same incorporation of public health nurses into governmental agencies began in Canada in the early 1900s (Matuk & Horsburgh, 1989).

The Brown Report of 1948, *Nursing for the Future*, reemphasized the need for nurses to be educated in institutions of higher learning to prepare them to meet community health needs (Kalisch & Kalisch, 2004). A similar, but earlier, report in Canada, *Survey of Nursing Education in Canada* (Weir, 1932), also known as the Weir Report, had recommended advanced educational preparation for community health nurses, particularly those practicing in rural areas. In 1964, the American Nurses Association (ANA) formally defined the public health nurse as a graduate of a baccalaureate program in nursing. In 1995, the Pew Health Professions Commission report, *Critical Challenges: Revitalizing the Health Professions*, reinforced baccalaureate education as the entry level for community-based practice. Today, in some states, such as California, only graduates from baccalaureate programs in nursing can be certified as public health nurses. Moreover, there are now master's and doctoral programs with a community health nursing focus. Table 3-2◆ presents a summary of significant events in the development of community health nursing practice.

FEDERAL INVOLVEMENT IN HEALTH CARE

For most of its history the federal government has left health matters to the states. It was not until 1879 that the United States established a National Board of Health in response to a yellow fever epidemic. This board continued to function until 1883, when it was dissolved. In 1912, the need for a permanent national agency responsible for the country's health was recognized, and the U.S. Public Health Service (USPHS) was created out of the reorganization of the Marine Hospital Service (Fee, 2002). In that same year, federal legislation created the office of the Surgeon General and mandated federal involvement in health promotion. It was not until 1953, however, that the need for advisement on health matters at the cabinet level was recognized with the creation of the Department of Health, Education, and Welfare. This department was reorganized in 1980 to create the present Department of Health and Human Services (DHHS).

Since the beginning of the 20th century, the federal government has become progressively more involved in health care delivery. Unfortunately, this involvement has been rather haphazard, dependent on the interests and concerns of different administrations. In the early years of the 20th century, the health needs of specific segments of the population began to be recognized, resulting in federal programs designed to enhance the health of mothers and children, the poor,

TABLE 3-2   Historical Events in the Development of Community Health Nursing

Date	Event
1813	Ladies' Benevolent Society of Charleston, South Carolina, organized as first home nursing service in the United States.
1819	Visiting nursing services organized through the Hebrew Female Benevolent Society of Philadelphia.
1832	Lying-in Charity for Attending Indigent Women in Their Homes established.
1840	Institute of Nursing in London founded by Elizabeth Frye to provide care in homes and prisons.
1859	District nursing initiated in Liverpool, England, by William Rathbone.
1876	Metropolitan and National Nursing Association for Providing Trained Nurses for the Sick Poor founded in England.
1877	Women's Branch of the New York City Mission is first to employ trained nurses for home visiting.
1880	Health promotion and education focus initiated by the Boston Instructive District Nursing Association.
1881	American Red Cross founded by Clara Barton.
1885–86	Visiting nurse associations established in Buffalo, Boston, and Philadelphia.
1893	First school nurse employed in London. Henry Street Settlement founded by Lillian Wald.
1896	First rural nursing service established (Westchester County, New York).
1897	Victorian Order of Nurses (VON) founded to pioneer community health nursing in Canada.
1899	International Council of Nurses established.
1900	Nurse's Settlement house founded in Richmond, Virginia.
1902	First school nursing program in the United States established by Henry Street Settlement.
1903	Henry Street Settlement school nursing program absorbed by New York City Department of Health.
1904	First school nurse is employed by a municipality (Los Angeles, California).
1906	The *Visiting Nurse Quarterly* first published (Chicago). First postgraduate course in public health nursing established by Instructive District Nursing Association of Boston.
1907	Public health nurse employment by government agencies first approved by Alabama.
1909	Metropolitan Life Insurance Company offers visiting nurse services to policyholders. Red Cross Nursing Service established.
1910	First postgraduate course in community health nursing in an institution of higher learning is established at Columbia University.
1911	Metropolitan Life Insurance visiting nurse services expanded nationwide.
1912	National Organization for Public Health Nursing (NOPHN) established. Red Cross Town and Country Nursing Service established. Standing orders for public health nursing activities adopted by Chicago Visiting Nurse Association.
1918	University of Alberta offered first Canadian course in public health nursing.
1919	Alberta District Nursing Service established to meet the needs of frontier families.
1920	Public health section of the Canadian National Association of Trained Nurses established.
1921	Maternity and Infancy (Sheppard–Towner) Act passed.
1923	Goldmark Report recommended education for nurses in institutions of higher learning and additional preparation for community health nursing.
1928	Frontier Nursing Service initiated by Mary Breckenridge.
1929	NOPHN established criteria and procedures for grading courses in public health nursing, initiating the accreditation process.
1931	Functions of public health nurses and related objectives first developed by the Field Studies Committee of NOPHN.
1932	Weir report on nursing education in Canada recognized need for advanced education for public health nurses and recommended an increase in the public health nurse workforce.
1933–1935	Nurses employed during the Depression in the Federal Emergency Relief Administration (FERA), Civil Works Administration (CWA), and Works Progress Administration (WPA).
1934	First public health nurse employed by USPHS.
1936	Public health nursing functions and objectives revised.
1944	Division of Public Health Nursing established in USPHS. Public health nursing functions and objectives revised.
1948	Brown Report reemphasized the need to educate nurses in institutions of higher learning and to include community health nursing content in curricula.

Continued on next page

TABLE 3-2	Historical Events in the Development of Community Health Nursing *(continued)*
Date	**Event**
1949	Public health nursing functions and objectives revised in *Public Health Nursing Responsibilities in a Community Health Program*.
1952	NOPHN absorbed into National League for Nursing (NLN).
1964	*Public health nurse* defined by American Nurses Association as a graduate of a baccalaureate program in nursing.
1973	Provision of home health services mandated for health maintenance organizations.
1986	*Standards of Community Health Nursing Practice* published by the American Nurses Association.
1988	Institute of Medicine report published, recommending restructuring of public health.
1993	National Center for Nursing Research established.
1995	Pew Health Professions Commission reinforced baccalaureate as entry level for community health nursing practice.
1999	Community health nursing standards revised by Quad Council of Public Health Nursing Organizations as *Scope and Standards of Public Health Nursing*.
2003	Public health nursing competencies established by the Quad Council of Public Health Nursing Organizations.
2007	*Public Health Nursing: Scope and Standards of Practice* revised.

those with sexually transmitted diseases, the mentally ill, and others. For example, in 1921, Congress passed the Sheppard–Towner Act to help state and local agencies meet the health needs of mothers and children. In addition to providing funds for maternity centers, prenatal care, and child health clinics, the legislation provided monies to enhance visiting nurse services (Kalisch & Kalisch, 2004). These funds allowed local agencies—for example, the San Diego County Health Department—to hire additional community health nurses, known as "Sheppard–Towner nurses" (Interview). In 1930, recognition of the need for federal support of health care research to address the health needs of mothers and children and other special groups led to the development of the National Institutes of Health.

As a result of the Great Depression of the 1930s, the federal government became even more active in health and social welfare programs. Jobs were created to employ thousands of the unemployed. Nurses were employed under Regulation 7 of the Federal Emergency Relief Act (1933), the Civil Works Administration (1933–34), and the Works Progress Administration (1935) to meet the health needs of the population (Kalisch & Kalisch, 2004). The first public health nurse was employed by the USPHS in 1934.

Recognition of the economic plight of the elderly led to passage of the Social Security Act in 1935, 60 years after the efforts of Lavinia Dock and others to provide health care to the elderly poor. This act established the Old-Age and Survivors Insurance (OASI, better known as Social Security) to improve the financial status of the elderly. Interestingly, the act also provided funds for the education of public health professionals, including public health nurses (Kalisch & Kalisch, 2004).

World War II also influenced health care delivery. Wage and price freezes and a dearth of skilled labor led industries to offer health insurance benefits in an attempt to compete for competent workers (McGuire &

Anderson, 1999). During the war, some 15 million U.S. service members were exposed to quality health care, some for the first time in their lives. Afterward, these veterans began to demand the same quality of care for themselves and their families in the civilian sector. This increased demand for care led to new arrangements for financing health care and the subsequent burgeoning of the health insurance industry. The growth in health insurance was further influenced by the 1954 inclusion of premiums as legitimate tax deductions. This development led to the use of insurance benefits as a tax-deductible substitute for higher wages in business and industry. Because such benefits were tax exempt for employees, they were readily accepted in lieu of salary increases by unions and other bargaining agents. Blue Cross hospitalization insurance was initiated at this time under the leadership of the American Hospital Association (Kalisch & Kalisch, 2004).

Increased demands for services also led to a lack of adequate facilities, especially in nonurban areas. In 1946, pressured by USPHS officials, Congress responded with passage of the Hill–Burton Act to finance hospital construction in underserved areas (Kalisch & Kalsich, 2004). Hospital construction and insurance coverage for care provided in the hospital further strengthened the national emphasis on curative rather than preventive care and widened the gap between bedside nursing and health promotion and prevention. In fact, a 1928 Bureau of Indian Affairs (BIA) circular directed BIA public health field nurses to promote the use of hospitals over home care (Abel, 1996). Hospitals became a major focus for health and illness care. Ironically, during this same period, the first hospital-based home care program was established at Montefiore Hospital in New York (Fondiller, n.d.), setting a precedent for the burgeoning home care industry of today. The present emphasis on cost containment has led to a shift away from institutional care and more home and community-based care.

This development has also resulted in a growing need for community health nurses to provide home health services.

THE LATTER HALF OF THE 20TH CENTURY

In 1966, the Social Security Act was amended to create the Medicare program to address the health care needs of older Americans. Medicaid, a program that funds health care for the indigent, was instituted in 1967. These two programs contributed to increased demands for health care services and resulted in rapid increases in the cost of health care. In 1965, when they were introduced as part of Lyndon Johnson's "Great Society" program, Medicare and Medicaid were seen by some as initial steps toward universal health care coverage in the United States, a vision that has yet to be fulfilled (Jonas, 2003).

Acknowledging the growing demand for health care and recognizing the differing abilities of certain areas of the country to meet those needs, the U.S. federal government responded with the Comprehensive Health Planning Act of 1966 and the National Health Planning and Resources Development Act of 1974. Both pieces of legislation were attempts to organize the planning of health care delivery to meet differing needs throughout the country (Jonas, 2003). Unfortunately, both efforts failed. One positive effect of the 1974 act was recognition of the contribution of nurse practitioners to the health status of the public, 9 years after the establishment of the first nurse practitioner program in 1965 (Jenkins & Sullivan-Marx, 1994).

The Child Health Act of 1967 and the Health Maintenance Organization Act of 1973 also recommended the use of nurses in extended roles. The 1971 publication of a report entitled *Extending the Scope of Nursing Practice* provided additional support for the use of nurses in expanded capacities (Kalisch & Kalisch, 2004). Subsequent legislation has led to the increased use of nurse practitioners in a variety of settings. Over the last few years, there has been increased use of community health nurses with advanced educational preparation as nurse practitioners providing primary care to selected populations.

While the United States was attempting to decentralize health care policy-making through health planning legislation, efforts were being made elsewhere to focus attention on risk factors for population health problems. The Lalonde Report, *New Perspectives for the Health of Canadians*, was published in Canada in 1974, identifying the importance of biological, environmental, and lifestyle risks as determinants of health and recommending greater attention to the elimination of risks in each of these areas. The Lalonde Report marked the initial shift away from a treatment paradigm to a health promotion focus at the national level in Canada (Scutch-

field & Last, 2003). As a result of the Lalonde report, the Health Promotion Directorate was formed in Canada in 1978 (Glouberman & Millar, 2003).

In 1978, at an international conference on primary health care, the Declaration of Alma Alta was developed, calling for access to primary health care for all. The resulting slogan for this campaign was "Health for all by the year 2000," a goal which has not yet been achieved (Watts, 2003). In 1984, the *Beyond Health Care* conference in Toronto established two key health promotion concepts: healthy public policy and healthy cities. These developments were followed by the adoption of health-for-all strategies in many nations, including the Canadian Epp report, *Achieving Health for All: A Framework for the Health of Canadians*, in 1986 (Glouberman & Millar, 2003).

The comparable movement in the United States is the focus on the achievement of the national health objectives discussed in Chapter 2∞. The need for systematic data collection relative to the achievement of the objectives was recognized in the introduction of the Behavioral Risk Factor Surveillance System (BRFSS). The system involves periodic surveys of the U.S. public to determine trends in specific health behaviors and health indicators (Mokdad, Stroup, & Giles, 2003).

The health-for-all concept was further developed in the World Health Organization's *Global Strategies for Health for All by the Year 2000*, published in 1981, and the *Ottawa Charter for Health Promotion*, developed at the First International Conference on Health Promotion in 1986. Both focused on social, economic, and political reform and empowerment as strategies for improving the health of the world's populations (Glouberman & Millar, 2003). The importance of health promotion at the global level was reinforced in the *Jakarta Declaration on Health Promotion into the 21st Century* (Fourth International Conference on Health Promotion, 1998).

Reform efforts in the United States in the late 20th century focused more on health care financing and the organization of services than on changes in social conditions affecting health. The Tax Equity and Fiscal Responsibility Act (TEFRA) of 1982 had a profound effect on health care and community health nursing. This act, passed in an effort to reduce Medicare expenditures, led to the development of **diagnosis-related groups (DRGs)** as a mechanism for prospective payment for services provided under Medicare (Kalisch & Kalisch, 2004). Basically, prospective payment means that health care institutions are paid a flat fee set in advance under Medicare. The fee is based on the client's diagnosis. The effect of this legislation has been earlier discharge of sicker clients and greater demand for home health and community health nursing services. Diagnosis-related groups and their effects have changed the role of community health nurses, who may need to return to the earlier role of care of the sick in their homes in addition to their roles in promoting health and preventing illness.

Public health practice, including community health nursing, is being restructured in light of the 1988 Institute of Medicine report, *The Future of Public Health*. This report identified the three core functions of public health as assessment, policy formation, and assurance (Scutchfield & Last, 2003). These functions will be discussed in more detail in Chapter 5∞. Similarly, the September 11, 2001, terrorist attacks on New York and the Pentagon and the development of new and reemerging communicable diseases, such as autoimmune deficiency syndrome (AIDS), later labeled acquired immunodeficiency syndrome, in 1981 and, more recently, severe acute respiratory syndrome (SARS), Ebola virus, and hantavirus, have highlighted inadequacies in the public health infrastructure here and internationally (CDC, 2002; Watts, 2003). These events are beginning to result in increased funding for public health efforts, including those related to terrorism.

Another event that could have a significant impact on community health nursing is the development of the **Nursing Interventions Classification (NIC)** system to categorize nursing services and facilitate their direct reimbursement (McCloskey & Bulechek, 2003). The NIC system should lend itself to direct reimbursement for nursing services under managed care, the new focus of the U.S. federal government. The **Nursing Outcomes Classification (NOC)** system is a parallel development that will allow nurses to document the effectiveness of intervention (Head et al., 2004).

At the close of the 20th century, a number of significant public health achievements had been accomplished. In the United States, the CDC identified the top 10 accomplishments of the century. These included routine immunization; improved motor vehicle safety; workplace safety; control of communicable diseases through sanitation, antibiotics, and surveillance measures; and decreased heart disease and stroke mortality. Additional accomplishments were safer and healthier foods and a decrease in the incidence of nutritional deficiency diseases, healthier mothers and babies, access to family planning services, fluoridation of drinking water, and recognition of tobacco as a health hazard (Schneider, 2000).

Another significant accomplishment was the international eradication of smallpox. The World Health Organization initiated its campaign to eradicate smallpox in 1966, and the last reported naturally occurring case in the world occurred in 1977. In 2002, the world marked the 25th anniversary of its freedom from this previously devastating disease (CDC, 2002). Significant events in American public health in the 20th century are presented in Table 3-3◆.

Table 3-4◆ summarizes recent international events related to global public health.

THE PRESENT AND BEYOND

The eradication of smallpox highlighted the effectiveness of international cooperation in health matters, which we will discuss in more detail in Chapter 6∞. Unfortunately, this accomplishment has had a negative consequence. The last case of smallpox in the United States occurred in 1949, prompting discontinuation of smallpox vaccination in 1971. This development has led to a generation of Americans who are vulnerable to the use of smallpox as a mechanism of bioterrorism and has prompted plans for preventive immunization of persons at greatest risk and mass immunization campaigns in the event of an attack.

Other advances of previous eras may also be undone in the current political climate. For example, in 2001, the U.S. Congress repealed the ergonomic standards put forth by the Occupational Safety and Health Administration under pressure from businesspeople who feared the cost of implementing measures to prevent repetitive motion injuries and other related conditions (Fee & Brown, 2001). Similarly, activities taken to prevent terrorist initiatives may undermine individual freedoms, and the focus on terrorism may serve to detract attention from other critical issues in public health, such as disparities in health status and societal conditions that affect the health of all. The current war also draws away resources that could be used to improve the overall health of the population. Community health nurses will need to reemerge as social activists to maintain a balance among these concerns that fosters the health of populations, both nationally and internationally.

Growing evidence indicates a shift to greater emphasis on health promotion and illness prevention in national and international health policy. The U.S. national health objectives, published first in 1980 and again in 1990 and 2000 and discussed in Chapter 2∞, are one sign of this shift. A second bit of evidence is the 1988 creation of the Center for Nursing Research (now the National Institute for Nursing Research) within the National Institutes of Health. One reason given in Senate testimony favoring the center was the health promotion and illness prevention focus in much of nursing research. Another somewhat encouraging sign is the passage of the Public Health Improvement Act of 2000, which provides funds for the development of public health activities at state and local levels (*The Nation's Health*, 2000).

In addition, one of the new focus areas for *Healthy People 2010* is the development of the public health infrastructure◆. The public health infrastructure includes the organizational structure of official government health agencies, the public health workforce, and the information systems employed in public health practice (U.S. Department of Health and Human Services, 2000).

MediaLink Case Study: Learning from the Past

TABLE 3-3	Significant 20th-Century Events in American Public Health
Date	**Event**
1906	Pure Food and Drug Act passed.
1912	Children's Bureau established to foster child health. Marine Hospital Service changed to U.S. Public Health Service.
1915	Tetanus antitoxin introduced.
1929	Blue Cross insurance instituted. Penicillin discovered by Alexander Fleming (discovery not acted on until World War II).
1930	National Institutes of Health established to conduct health-related research. Food and Drug Administration established. National Fair Labor Standards Act passed.
1935	Social Security Act established Old-Age and Survivors Insurance (OASI).
1938	Garfield/Kaiser Prepaid Group Practice established (forerunner of managed care).
1946	Hospital Survey and Construction (Hill–Burton) Act passed. Communicable Disease Center (CDC) established.
1953	U.S. Department of Health, Education, and Welfare (USDHEW) established.
1954	Health insurance premiums first allowed as tax deductions.
1955	Salk polio vaccine widely used.
1957	Nationalized Canadian health care system established.
1964	U.S. Surgeon General's report on smoking published.
1966	Comprehensive Health Planning and Public Health Services Act passed. Medicare program instituted to fund health care for the elderly.
1967	Medicaid program initiated to fund health care for the medically indigent.
1970	Occupational Safety and Health Administration established. Environmental Protection Agency established.
1974	National Health Planning and Resources Development Act passed. Lalone report, *New Perspectives for the Health of Canadians*, published.
1978	Canadian Health Promotion Directorate formed.
1979	*Healthy People: Surgeon General's Report on Health Promotion and Disease Prevention* published.
1980	USDHEW reorganized to form U.S. Department of Health and Human Services (USDHHS). *Promoting Health/Preventing Disease: Objectives for the Nation* published, creating the first set of national health objectives for the United States.
1981	Autoimmune deficiency syndrome (AIDS) identified (later labeled acquired immunodeficiency syndrome).
1982	Tax Equity and Fiscal Responsibility Act (TEFRA) passed.
1983	Prospective payment system based on diagnosis-related groups (DRGs) initiated.
1984	Behavioral Risk Factor Surveillance System (BRFSS) initiated.
1986	*Achieving Health for All: A Framework for the Health of Canadians* published.
1988	Institute of Medicine report, *The Future of Public Health*, published.
1989	*U.S. Public Health Services Task Force: Guide to Clinical Preventive Services* published, recommending standardized screening and prevention strategies for specific populations.
1990	*Healthy People 2000: National Objectives for Health Promotion and Illness Prevention* published.
1993	Health Plan Employer Data and Information Set (HEDIS) created.
1996	*Report on the Health of Canadians* identified environmental challenges to health.
2000	*Healthy People 2010* published. Public Health Improvement Act passed to assist state and local agencies in enhancing public health services.

In this chapter, we have seen how community health nursing grew to its present state. The future direction of community health nursing will be determined by the community health nurses of today and tomorrow. As noted by one historian of the Henry Street nurses, "We live in times not unlike those of the early Henry Street days. Our inner cities—cities within cities—are frightening, bleak places of despair. I am struck by the similarity of issues—poverty, sanitation, prostitution, pornography, . . . violence, drugs, communicable diseases, hopelessness" (Estabrooks, 1995). It may be time to return to the dual nature of the

TABLE 3-4	International Events Influencing Public Health
Date	**Event**
1902	Pan-American Health Organization (PAHO) founded.
1919	Health Organization of the League of Nations established.
1948	World Health Organization (WHO) established.
1977	Smallpox eradicated worldwide.
1979	Call for access to primary care for all established in Declaration of Alma Alta.
1981	Need for primary health care emphasized by World Health Organization report, *Global Strategies for Health for All by the Year 2000*.
1986	Prerequisites to and strategies for achieving health for all identified in *The Ottawa Charter for Health Promotion*.
1988	WHO goal for poliomyelitis eradication set.
1992	WHO goal for integration of hepatitis B vaccination into childhood immunization programs set.
1993	Global emergency declared by WHO in response to worldwide incidence of tuberculosis.
1994	Goal of measles elimination established by WHO Region of the Americas.
1998	Concepts of global health promotion reinforced in *Jakarta Declaration on Health Promotion into the 21st Century*.
2000	World Health Report 2000, *Health Systems: Improving Performance*, published.
2001	United Nations General Assembly Special Session on HIV/AIDS held.
2002	European Region of WHO declared polio-free. WHO goal of reducing worldwide measles mortality by 50% established.

BUILDING OUR KNOWLEDGE BASE

*I*t is important for community health nurses to understand the forces that shaped their practice in the past and continue to influence community health nursing today. Historical research can provide us with this understanding. Fee, Brown, Lazarus, and Theerman (2002a) described the career of Eugenia Broughton, an African American nurse who worked in South Carolina's Berkeley County Health Department, and the setting in which she worked. There may be similar information about public health nursing in your area that will help you understand the way the specialty is practiced today.

- When did community health nursing originate in your area? What was the impetus for its development? Who were the nurses who were influential in its development? How has local community health nursing changed with time? What factors prompted those changes?
- Where would you begin to look for answers to the questions posed above? What documents might provide information? Where might you find them?
- Are there people still living who might be able to shed light on those events? How would you go about finding them? What would you want to ask them? Why?

initial community health nursing role: personal care in conjunction with population-based health promotion and illness prevention. Perhaps then we can achieve the goal, set in 1923 but never accomplished, of one community health nurse to every 2,000 Americans (Winslow, 1993).

Advocacy in Action

The Shoestring Clinic

Upper East Tennessee is on the edge of the Appalachian region and shares a number of features of that region, including lack of access to health care for a significant portion of the population. Aware of this lack, community health nursing students and faculty created a weekly "clinic" to meet the health care needs of low-income residents of a federal housing project. The clinic was first held in a recreation room at the housing project, but this proved untenable as the landlord was not willing to permit regular use of the room. The clinic was moved to rooms provided by a nearby church, and members of the congregation became part of its clientele. Clinic services included health histories and physical examinations, blood pressure monitoring, health education, and referral for needed health care services.

During the academic year, the clinic was staffed one day a week by community health nursing faculty and students. Faculty members continued to staff the clinic during breaks and over the summer to assure continuity of services. Students were involved in planning the services and developing a record system, forms, and referral contacts in the larger community. In addition to the weekly clinic, students and faculty made home visits to clients needing additional follow-up. Local physicians were contacted to inform them of the availability of the clinic for low-income clients who needed monitoring or health education. Several physicians took advantage of the services to request follow-up for their clients regarding issues of medication compliance or health education.

Although the clinic was initiated long before the days of HIPPA, strict measures were taken to promote client confidentiality. Client records (and equipment) were not left at the clinic site, but were locked in the trunk of one faculty member's car and transported to the site each week. Over the course of several years, several hundred clients were seen and multiple referrals were initiated to obtain low-cost services for clients in need of them.

Case Study

Continuing the Focus on the Population's Health

Community health nursing in the United States arose in response to identified health needs among European immigrants. What recently arrived immigrant populations live in the area surrounding your nursing program? In what ways are these new immigrants similar to and different from those arriving in the United States at the end of the 19th century? How do their health needs compare to those encountered by the nurses on Henry Street?

Test Your Understanding

1. Who were some of the historical figures who influenced the development of community health nursing? What contributions did they make to its development? (pp. 45–51)

2. Describe some of the contributions made by early community health nurses to social and health care reform. (pp. 45–51)

3. List at least four major historical events that influenced the development of community health nursing in the United States. (pp. 45–57)

4. What evidence is there for a shift to greater emphasis on health promotion and illness prevention in the world? (p. 56)

5. What are some of the national and international events that are shaping current and future community health nursing practice? (pp. 55–57)

EXPLORE MediaLink

http://www.prenhall.com/clark
Resources for this chapter can be found on the Companion Website.

Audio Glossary
Exam Review Questions
Case Study: Applying Lessons Learned from the Past to the Present

MediaLink Applications: Public Health Nursing History (video)
Media Links

Challenge Your Knowledge
Advocacy Interviews

References

Abel, E. K. (1996). "We are left so much alone to work out our own problems": Nurses on American Indian reservations during the 1930s. *Nursing History Review, 4,* 43–64.

Abrams, S. E. (2004). From function to competency in public health nursing, 1931 to 2003. *Public Health Nursing, 21,* 507–510.

American Nurses Association. (2007). *Public Health Nursing: Scope and Standards of Practice.* Silver Spring. MD: Nursesbooks.org.

American Public Health Association. (2005a). *About APHA.* Retrieved December 14, 2005, from http://www.apha.org/about

American Public Health Association. (2005b). *APHA sections and special interest groups.* Retrieved December 14, 2005, from http://www.apha.org/sections/sectdesc.htm

American Public Health Association. (2005c). *Sections, SPIGs and caucuses.* Retrieved December 14, 2005, from http://www.apha.org/sections

Association of State and Territorial Directors of Nursing. (2000). *Public health nursing:*

A partner for healthy populations. Washington, DC: American Nurses Publishing.

Behling, S. (n.d.). Note on Clara Barton. Retrieved September 12, 2004, from http://www.rootsweb.com/~nwa/barton.html

Benson, E. R. (1993). Public health nursing and the Jewish contribution. *Public Health Nursing, 10*(1), 55–57.

Berridge, V. (2000). History in public health: Who needs it? *The Lancet, 356,* 1923–1925.

Brainerd, A. M. (1985). *The evolution of public health nursing.* New York: Garland. Reprinted from A. M. Brainerd (1922), *The evolution of public health nursing.* Philadelphia: Saunders.

Bramadat, I. J., & Saydak, M. I. (1993). Nursing on the Canadian Prairies, 1900–1930: Effects of Immigration. *Nursing History Review, 1,* 105–117.

Buhler-Wilkerson, K. (n.d.). *The call to the nurse: Our history from 1893 to 1943.* Retrieved September 12, 2004, from http://www.vnsny.org/mh_about_history_more.html

Buhler-Wilkerson, K. (2001). *No place like home: A history of nursing and home care in the United States.* Baltimore: Johns Hopkins University.

Center for the Study of the History of Nursing. (n.d.). Nursing in historic Philadelphia: A walk through time. Retrieved September 12, 2004, from http://www.upenn.edu/history/gallery.htm

Centers for Disease Control and Prevention. (2002). 25th anniversary of last case of naturally occurring smallpox. *Morbidity and Mortality Weekly Report, 51,* 952.

Centers for Disease Control and Prevention. (2004). 150th anniversary of John Snow and the Pump Handle. *Morbidity and Mortality Weekly Report, 53,* 783.

Cho, H. S. M., & Kashka, M. S. (2004). The evolution of the community health nurse practitioner in Korea. *Public Health Nursing, 21,* 287–294.

Connolly, C. A. (2004). Beyond social history: New approaches to understanding the state of and the state in nursing history. *Nursing History Review, 12,* 5–24.

Duncan, S. M., Leipart, B. D., & Mill, J. E. (1999). "Nurses as health evangelists"?: The evolution of public health nursing in Canada, 1918–1939. *Advances in Nursing Science, 22*(1), 40–51.

Epidemiology Program Office, Centers for Disease Control and Prevention. (1999). Changes in the public health system. *Morbidity and Mortality Weekly Report, 48,* 1141–1147.

Erickson, G. (1987). Southern initiative in public health nursing. *Journal of Nursing History, 3*(1), 17–29.

Estabrooks, C. A. (1995). Lavinia Lloyd Dock: The Henry Street years. *Nursing History Review, 3,* 143–172.

Falk Rafael, A. R. (1999). The politics of health promotion: Influences on public health promotion nursing practice in Ontario, Canada from Nightingale to the nineties. *Advances in Nursing Science, 22*(1), 23–39.

Fee, E. (2002). History and development of public health. In F. D. Scutchfield & C. W. Keck (Eds.), *Principles of public health practice* (pp. 11–30). Albany, NY: Delmar.

Fee, E., & Brown, T. (2001). Editor's note. *American Journal of Public Health, 91,* 1381.

Fee, E., Brown, T. M., Lazarus, J., & Theerman, P. (2002a). A dedicated public health nurse. *American Journal of Public Health, 92,* 565.

Fee, E., Brown, T. M., Lazarus, J., & Theerman, P. (2002b). Baxter Street then. *American Journal of Public Health, 92,* 753.

Fondiller, S. H. (n.d.). *The promise and the reality: Our history from 1944 to 1993.* Retrieved September 12, 2004, from http://www.vnsny.org/mh_about_history_more.html

Fourth International Conference on Health Promotion. (1998). The Jakarta Declaration on Health Promotion into the 21st Century. *Pan American Journal, 3*(1), 58–61.

Gardner, M. S. (1952). *Public health nursing* (3rd ed.). New York: Macmillan.

Glouberman, S., & Millar, J. (2003). Evolution of the determinants of health, health policy, and health information systems in Canada. *American Journal of Public Health, 93,* 388–392.

Graeme, K. (2002). *Smallpox's history in the world.* Retrieved July 25, 2006, from http://graemekennedy.name/science/2/immunoweb/bad/invaders/viruses/smallpox/history.html

Hamilton, A. (2001). The health of immigrants. *American Journal of Public Health, 91,* 1765–1767. (Reprinted from *Exploring the dangerous trades: The autobiography of Alice Hamilton, MD,* by A. Hamilton, 1943, Boston: Little, Brown)

Hancock, T. (2000). Healthy communities must also be sustainable communities. *Public Health Reports, 115,* 151–156.

Head, B. J., Aquilino, M. L., Johnson, M., Reed, D., Maas, M., & Moorhead, S. (2004). Content validity and nursing sensitivity of community-level outcomes from the Nursing Outcomes Classification (NOC). *Journal of Nursing Scholarship, 36,* 251–259.

Helfand, W. H., Lazarus, J., & Theerman, P. (2000). The Children's Bureau and public health at midcentury. *American Journal of Public Health, 90,* 1703.

Helfand, W. H., Lazarus, J., & Theerman, P. (2001). Night shift in a glass factory. *American Journal of Public Health, 91,* 1370.

Igoe, J. B. (1980). Changing patterns in school health and school health nursing. *Nursing Outlook, 28,* 486–492.

Interview with Harney M. Cordua, son of Dr. Olive Cordua, San Diego County Medical Officer. San Diego: San Diego Historical Society.

Jenkins, M. L., & Sullivan-Marx, E. M. (1994). Nurse practitioners and community health nurses: Clinical partnerships and future visions. *Nursing Clinics of North America, 29,* 459–470.

Jonas, S. (2003). *An introduction to the U.S. health care system* (5th ed.). New York, Springer.

Kalisch, P. A., & Kalisch, B. J. (2004). *American nursing: A history.* Philadelphia: Lippincott Williams & Wilkins.

Mary Breckenridge. (n.d.). Retrieved September 12, 2004, from http://www.angelfire.com/mo2/IllusionsPad.MBrekenridge.html

Matuk, L. Y., & Horsburgh, M. C. (1989). Rebuilding public health nursing: A Canadian perspective. *Public Health Nursing, 6,* 169–173.

McCloskey, J. C., & Bulechek, G. M. (Eds.). (2003). *Nursing interventions classification* (4th ed.). St. Louis: C. V. Mosby.

McDonald, L. (2000). Florence Nightingale and the foundations of public health care, as seen through her collected works. Retrieved July 18, 2002, from http://www.sociology.uoguelph.ca/fnightingale/online_papers/dalpaper.htm

McGuire, M. T., & Anderson, W. H. (1999). *The US healthcare dilemma: Mirrors and chains.* Westport, CT: Auburn House.

Mokdad, A. H., Stroup, D. F., & Giles, W. H. (2003). Public health surveillance for behavioral risk factors in a changing environment: Recommendations from the Behavioral Risk Factor Surveillance Team. *Morbidity and Mortality Weekly Report, 52*(RR-9), 1–11.

National Association for Home Care. (n.d.). Profiles in caring: Lillian Wald, 1867–1940. Retrieved September 12, 2004, from http://www.nahc.org/NAHC/Val/Volumns/SC10-4.html

The Nation's Health. (December 2000/January 2001). Legislation to benefit key public health issues. 1.

Pew Health Professions Commission. (1995). *Critical challenges: Revitalizing the health professions for the twenty-first century.* San Francisco, UCSF Center for the Health Professions.

Plotnick, J. (1994, March). *Public health components of the Health Security Act.* Paper presented at the meeting of the Public Health Nursing Division, San Diego County Department of Health Services, San Diego, CA.

Quad Council of Public Health Nursing Organizations. (1999). *Scope and standards of public health nursing practice.* Washington, DC: American Nurses Publishing.

Quad Council of Public Health Nursing Organizations. (2003). *Quad Council PHN competencies.* Retrieved August 8, 2002, from http://www.uncc.edu/achne/quadcouncil/final_phn_competencies.doc

Quad Council of Public Health Nursing Organizations. (2004). Public health nursing competencies. *Public Health Nursing, 21,* 443–452.

Richardson, S. (1998). Political women, professional nurses, and the creation of Alberta's District Nursing Service, 1919–1925. *Nursing History Review, 6,* 25–50.

Roberts, J. I., & Group, T. M. (1995). *Feminism and nursing: An historical perspective on power, status, and political activism in the nursing profession.* Westport, CT: Praeger.

Ruffing-Rahal, M. A. (1995). The Navajo experience of Elizabeth Foster, public health nurse. *Nursing History Review, 3,* 173–188.

Schneider, M.-J. (2000). *Introduction to public health.* Gaithersburg, MD: Aspen.

Scutchfield, F. D., & Last, J. M. (2003). Public health in North America. In R. Beaglehole (Ed.), *Global public health: A new era.* New York: Oxford University.

Sigerist, H. E. (2003). Medical care for all the people. *American Journal of Public Health, 93,* 57–59. (Reprinted from "Medical care for all people," by H. E. Sigerist, 1944, *Canadian Journal of Public Health, 35,* 253–267)

Smith, S. L. (1994). White nurses, black midwives, and public health in Mississippi, 1920–1950. *Nursing History Review, 2,* 29–49.

Udwadia, F. E. (2000). *Man and medicine: A history.* Oxford: Oxford University.

U.S. Department of Health and Human Services. (2000). *Healthy people 2010* (Conference edition, in two volumes). Washington, DC: Author.

Vinson, J. (n.d.). Clara Barton. Retrieved September 12, 2004, from http://www.rootsweb.com/~nwa/barton.html

Watts, S. (2003). *Disease and medicine in world history.* New York: Routledge.

Weir, G. M. (1932). *Survey of nursing education in Canada.* Toronto: University of Toronto Press.

Winslow, C. E. A. (1993). Nursing and the community. *Public Health Nursing, 10,* 58–63. (Reprinted from *The Public Health Nurse,* April 1938).

Wolfe, L. C., & Selekman, J. (2002). School nurses: What it was and what it is. *Pediatric Nursing, 28,* 403–407.

Zilm, G., & Warbinek, E. (1995). Early tuberculosis nursing in British Columbia. *Canadian Journal of Nursing Research, 27*(3), 65–81.

Advocacy in Action

The Birth Certificate

Navigating the U.S. social system can be a daunting task for people from other countries and cultures. A few years ago, a young Hmong woman found herself pregnant with her second child. She was able to obtain prenatal care and planned to call her husband for transportation to the hospital if he was at work when she went into labor. Most of their extended family had moved to North Carolina and they had few social supports remaining in the area.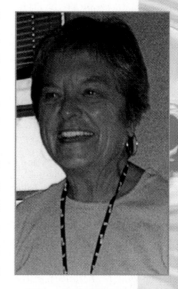

Unfortunately, when she went into labor, she was home alone with her three-year-old daughter. The labor was rapid and the baby was born quite soon. The young woman knew to call 911 and EMS arrived to assist her shortly after the child was born. When the family went to obtain a birth certificate for the child, they were told that since it was a home birth, they needed proof that the baby was indeed theirs.

A local public health nurse was working with the family through a Parents as Teachers program to promote the development of preschool children in the community. The family took their problem to the nurse, who contacted the county vital statistics division and determined that a witness was needed to verify the birth to this mother. The only witness to the actual birth, however, was the three-year-old daughter, who was too young to provide verification. The nurse was told that if the EMS personnel, who arrived after the birth, had delivered the placenta and if they had documented that in the EMS record, the record would constitute verification. After more telephone calls, the community health nurse determined that the EMS personnel had indeed documented delivery of the placenta in the event record. She accompanied the parents to the EMS headquarters and assisted them in obtaining a copy of the record and then went with them to the vital statistics division to obtain the birth certificate. As a result of the nurse's advocacy and assistance, this family acquired its first U.S. citizen, a bright-eyed baby with a legal birth certificate.

Connie Curran, MSN, RN, PHN
Community Health Nurse
Bayside Community Center

Theoretical Foundations for Community Health Nursing

CHAPTER OBJECTIVES

After reading this chapter, you should be able to:

1. Identify the need for a theoretical foundation for community health nursing.
2. Describe basic principles of epidemiology.
3. Apply selected epidemiologic and nursing models to community health nursing practice with individuals, families, and populations.

KEY TERMS

agent **64**
case fatality rate **63**
causality **62**
conceptual model **67**
determinants of health **66**
epidemiology **62**
host **64**
incidence **63**
metaparadigm **67**
morbidity **63**
mortality **63**
populations at risk **62**
prevalence **63**
risk **62**
social capital **71**
survival rate **63**
survival time **63**
target group **62**

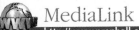

MediaLink
http://www.prenhall.com/clark

Additional interactive resources for this chapter can be found on the Companion Website. Click on Chapter 4 and "Begin" to select the activities for this chapter.

*E*ffective nursing practice is facilitated when nurses use a systematic approach to clients, their health status, and the nursing interventions needed to promote, maintain, or restore health. Conceptual or theoretical models provide such an approach. A conceptual model is defined as a "set of relatively abstract and general concepts that address the phenomena of central interest to a discipline, the nonrelational propositions that broadly define those concepts, and the relational propositions that state relatively abstract and general linkages between two or more concepts" (Fawcett & Gigliotti, 2001, p. 339). If used consistently, theoretical models assist community health nurses to evaluate health status and to plan, implement, and evaluate effective nursing care to improve health. The model used directs attention to relevant aspects of the client situation and to interventions that are apt to be most effective in that situation.

Generally two types of models are used by community health nurses, epidemiologic models and nursing models. Epidemiologic models provide a way of examining the factors that influence health and illness in the population, whereas nursing models go beyond this to suggest interventions that will protect, improve, or restore health.

EPIDEMIOLOGIC PERSPECTIVES

Epidemiology is the study of the distribution of health and illness within a population, factors that determine the population's health status, and use of the knowledge generated to control the development of health problems (Friis & Sellers, 2003). Epidemiologic perspectives on the factors that contribute to disease and illness have changed remarkably over time, and some authors describe four eras of epidemiologic thought. The first was the sanitary era, with interventions based on the ancient theory of miasmas discussed in Chapter 3∞. The second era was that of communicable diseases, in which interventions were based on the germ theory. Emphasis in the third or chronic disease era was on multiple layers of personal risk factors contributing to chronic diseases. The focus of the fourth era, at the beginning of the 21st century, remains to be seen, but the era may turn out to be what some have termed the "ecosocial" era (MacDonald, 2004), emphasizing the multiple interactions among biological, environmental, and social factors that lead to health or illness in population groups. An alternative direction for epidemiology in this fourth era might be molecular epidemiology, in which the contributions of genetics and DNA to disease "may become the germ theory of the new millennium" (MacDonald, 2004, p. 385).

Basic Concepts of Epidemiology

Before we examine epidemiologic models used by community health nurses in their practice, we should spend some time on the three basic concepts that underlie epidemiologic perspectives on health and illness: causality, risk, and rates of occurrence.

Causality

To control health problems, epidemiologists and community health nurses must have some idea of causality. The concept of **causality** is based on the idea that one event is the result of another event. Theories about the cause of disease have evolved over time. The main purpose of epidemiology is to identify causal links between contributing factors and resulting states of health and illness (Dicker, 2002). Over the years, concepts of causation have changed—from the earliest attempts to attribute health and illness to the will of the gods in early human history to belief in natural causes to identification of specific causes (e.g., a particular microorganism) that result in specific conditions. With the advent of single-cause/single-effect theories of disease causation, the scientific community began to look for specific causes for all health problems. Now, however, the concept of causality has become more complicated in view of the recognized interplay of a wide variety of factors in the development of both health and illness.

Risk

In addition to establishing the causes of health-related conditions, epidemiologists are interested in estimating the likelihood that a particular condition will occur. **Risk** is the probability that a given individual will develop a specific condition. One's risk of developing a particular condition is affected by a variety of physical, emotional, environmental, lifestyle, and other factors. When epidemiologists speak of **populations at risk**, they are referring to groups of people who have the greatest potential to develop a particular health problem because of the presence or absence of certain contributing factors. Some authors criticize the "risk factor epidemiology" characteristic of the chronic disease era of epidemiology, because they claim it ignores the role of social structure and social relationships in people's response to risk factors. Risk factor epidemiology also tends to assume that people are free to choose their responses, which may or may not be the case (Williams, 2003).

The population at risk becomes the target group for any intervention designed to prevent or control the problem in question. The **target group** includes those individuals who would benefit from an intervention program and at whom the program is aimed. The target group for an immunization campaign against pertussis, for example, would include unimmunized children under the age of 10 as well as college students whose immunity is waning.

Rates of Occurrence

The rate of occurrence of a health-related condition is also of concern to community health nurses. *Rates of occurrence* are statistical measures that indicate the extent of health problems in a group. Rates of occurrence allow comparisons between groups of different sizes with respect to the extent of a particular condition. For example, a community with a population of 1,000 may report 50 cases of syphilis this year, whereas another community of 100,000 persons may report 5,000 cases. On the surface, it would seem that the second community has a greater problem with syphilis than the first; however, both communities have experienced 50 cases per 1,000 population. In other words, both have a problem with syphilis of comparable magnitude.

Computing the statistical rates of interest in community health nursing involves dividing the *number of instances of an event* during a specified period by the *population at risk* for that event and *multiplying by 1,000* (or 100,000 if the numbers of the event are so small that the result of the calculation using a multiplier of 1,000 would be less than 1). The basic formula for calculating statistical rates of interest to community health nurses is presented below.

Both mortality and morbidity rates are of concern in community health nursing. **Mortality** is the ratio of the number of deaths in various categories to the number of people in a given population, whereas **morbidity** is the ratio of the number of cases of a disease or condition to the number of people in the population. Mortality rates describe deaths; morbidity rates describe cases of health conditions that may or may not result in death. For example, the number of people in a particular group who die as a result of cardiovascular disease is reflected in the mortality rate; however, the number of people experiencing cardiovascular disease is indicated by the morbidity rate.

Mortality and morbidity rates can be calculated for specific subsets of the population, for example, the rate of people who die in specific age groups or from specific diseases. Morbidity is further described in terms of the incidence and prevalence of a condition. **Incidence** reflects the number of *new* cases of a particular condition identified during a specified period of time. **Prevalence** is the *total number* of people affected by a particular condition at a specified point in time.

To illustrate the concepts of incidence and prevalence, consider a town with a population of 30,000 in which 15 new cases of hypertension were diagnosed in June. This is an indication of the incidence of hypertension. People who were diagnosed as hypertensive prior to June and who continue to live in the town still have hypertension. These additional cases of hypertension, however, are not reflected in the hypertension incidence rate for June, but are included in the prevalence, the total number of people in the community affected by hypertension.

Case fatality rates and survival rates are also of concern in community health. The **case fatality rate** for a particular condition reflects the percentage of persons with the condition who die as a result of it. For example, at present, most people with pancreatic cancer die because of the lack of an effective treatment. Relatively few people die of breast cancer, on the other hand, so breast cancer has a lower case fatality rate.

The converse of fatality is the **survival rate**, the proportion of people with a given condition remaining alive after a specific period (usually 5 years). For example, the 5-year survival rate for women with breast cancer is relatively high compared with the survival rate of those with pancreatic cancer. A related concept is **survival time**, or the average length of time from diagnosis to death. For example, given current medical technology, the survival time for children with Down syndrome is much longer today than at the beginning of the 20th century. Caution should be used in interpreting both survival rate and survival time information. Diagnostic technology has permitted earlier diagnosis of many conditions, increasing the time from diagnosis to death but not appreciably lengthening one's life (Gordis, 2004). Other rates that may be of interest to community health nurses include marriage and divorce rates, illegitimacy rates, employment rates, utilization rates for health care services and facilities, and rates for alcohol and drug use and abuse.

Community health nurses use morbidity and mortality data in assessing the health status of a population. Community morbidity and mortality rates that are generally high or higher than state or national rates usually indicate health problems that require intervention. For example, the nurse may note that local morbidity rates for childhood illnesses such as measles and rubella are twice those of the rest of the state. These differences indicate that a significant portion of the local child population is unimmunized. The nurse then uses these data to begin an investigation of the factors involved in the problem and to plan a solution. Is it a matter of inaccessibility of immunization services, lack of education on the need for immunization, or poor surveillance of immunization levels in the schools? The solution to the problem must be geared to the cause. Statistical data merely serve to indicate the presence of a problem; they do not delineate its specific nature.

Low morbidity and mortality rates do not indicate the absence of health problems in the community,

SPECIAL CONSIDERATIONS

BASIC FORMULA FOR CALCULATING STATISTICAL RATES

$$\text{Rate} = \frac{\text{Number of events over a period of time}}{\text{Population at risk at that time}} \times \begin{array}{l} 1{,}000 \text{ (or} \\ 100{,}000) \end{array}$$

as biostatistics are only one indicator of health status. Many health problems are not reported statistically, and their presence in the community is not reflected in morbidity and mortality rates. The nutritional status of the population is one area not addressed by biostatistics such as morbidity and mortality rates. Other indicators that the community health nurse employs in assessing a community's health status are discussed in Chapter 15∞.

Epidemiologic Models

Both nurses and epidemiologists use epidemiologic information to direct interventions to control health-related conditions. Determining appropriate control strategies often involves collecting large amounts of data about multiple factors that may be contributing to the condition. For this reason, it is helpful to have a model or framework to direct the collection and interpretation of these data. We explore three epidemiologic models here: the epidemiologic triad, the web of causation model, and determinants-of-health models.

The Epidemiologic Triad

Traditionally, epidemiologic investigation has been guided by the epidemiologic triad. In this model, data are collected with respect to a triad of elements: host,

agent, and environment (Dicker, 2002). The interrelationship of these elements results in a state of relative health or illness. The relationships among host, agent, and environment and specific considerations under each are depicted in Figure 4-1.

HOST The **host** is the client system affected by the particular condition under investigation. Community health nursing is concerned with the health of human beings, so, for our purposes, the host is a human being. A variety of factors can influence the host's exposure, susceptibility, and response to an agent. Host-related factors include intrinsic factors (e.g., age, race, and sex), physical and psychological factors, nutritional status, genetics, and the presence or absence of disease states or immunity, among others (Dicker, 2002). These and similar factors are addressed in more detail in the discussion of the dimensions model later in this chapter.

AGENT The **agent** is the primary cause of a health-related condition. The concept of agents of disease originated in the context of communicable diseases when specific microorganisms were found to cause specific diseases. Although the causes of some health problems may be so complex that no single agent can be identified, the concept of agent remains useful for exploring many health problems.

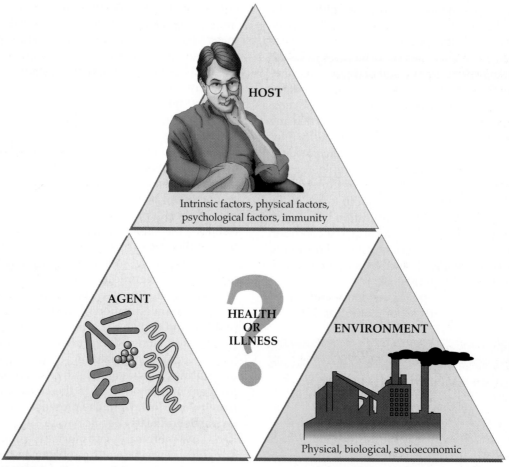

FIGURE 4-1 Elements of the Epidemiologic Triad Model

Agents can be classified into six types: physical agents, chemical agents, nutritive elements, infectious agents, genetic agents, and psychological agents. Physical agents include heat, trauma, and radiation. Chemical agents include various substances to which people may develop untoward reactions. Some plants such as poison ivy and ragweed can be considered chemical agents because they cause a chemical reaction resulting in an allergic response. An absence or an excess of a variety of nutritive elements is known to result in disease, as do the presence of and exposure to a number of infectious agents that cause communicable diseases. Genetic agents arise from genetic transmission from parent to child. Finally, psychological agents such as stress can produce a variety of stress-related conditions. The types of agents and examples of health conditions to which they contribute are listed in Table 4-1◆.

An agent's characteristics influence whether a given individual develops a particular health-related condition. These characteristics vary somewhat depending on the type of agent involved. Characteristics of infectious agents will be discussed in more detail in Chapter 28∞. Some noninfectious agents will be addressed in the context of the health problems to which they contribute (e.g., environmental contaminants in Chapter 10∞ and nutritional agents as they influence the health of children in Chapter 16∞ and older adults in Chapter 19∞).

TABLE 4-1	Agents and Selected Health Problems to Which They Contribute	
Type of Agent	**Example**	**Problems**
Physical	Heat	Burns, heat stroke
	Trauma	Fractures, concussion, sprains, contusions
	Radiation	Genetic changes
Chemical	Medications	Accidental poisoning, suicide
	Chlorine	Poisoning, asphyxiation (in gas form)
	Poison ivy	Rash and pruritus
Nutritive	Vitamin C	Scurvy (in absence of vitamin C)
	Iron	Anemia (in absence of iron)
	Vitamin A	Poisoning (in excess)
Infectious	Measles virus	Measles, measles encephalitis
	HIV	AIDS
	Varicella virus	Chickenpox
	Influenza virus	Influenza
Genetic	Genetic predisposition to disease	Sickle cell disease
	Genetic abnormality	Down syndrome, Turner's syndrome
Psychological	Stress	Ulcerative colitis, heart disease, suicide, asthma, alcoholism, drug abuse, violence

ENVIRONMENT The third element of the epidemiologic triad includes factors in the physical, biological, and socioeconomic environments that contribute to health-related conditions (Dicker, 2002). The physical environment consists of such factors as weather, terrain, and buildings. A variety of physical environment factors can influence health. For example, air pollution contributes to respiratory disease as well as other physiologic and psychological effects in human beings. Similarly, elements of community design such as walking trails have been shown to affect exercise behavior and health status (Richardson, 2004).

The biological environment, in the triad model, consists of all living organisms other than humans. Components of the biological environment include plants and animals as well as microorganisms, all of which can influence health.

The socioeconomic environment includes factors related to social interaction that may contribute to health or disease. For example, cultural factors, which are part of the social environment, can influence health behaviors. In a similar fashion, social norms may influence health and illness. For example, societal views of alcoholism and drug abuse as character weaknesses have hampered efforts to control these problems.

Factors in each of these three environments will be addressed in more detail in the discussion of the dimensions model later in this chapter. Because of its failure to address completely multiple causative factors, the triad model has not been as useful for chronic diseases or other health problems (e.g., societal violence) as it has for communicable diseases (Dicker, 2002).

The Web of Causation Model

The "web of causation" is a second model for exploring the influence of multiple factors on the development of a specific health condition. In this model, factors are explored in terms of their interplay, and both direct and indirect causes of the problem are identified (Friedman, 2003). The web of causation approach allows the epidemiologist to map the interrelationships among factors contributing to the development (or prevention) of a particular health condition. This approach also assists in determining areas where efforts at control will be most effective.

Some of the factors in a web of causation for the problem of adolescent tobacco use are depicted in Figure 4-2. It is obvious from the complexity of Figure 4-2 that multiple factors contribute to adolescent tobacco use. The interplay of these factors determines whether or not the problem occurs. The most direct causes are those linked directly to tobacco use—purchase of tobacco products and the decision to use them. Numerous other factors, however, contribute to the adolescent's decision to engage in the use of tobacco. These include perceptions of tobacco use as grown-up or "cool," peer pressure, and easy access to tobacco products. Perceptions of

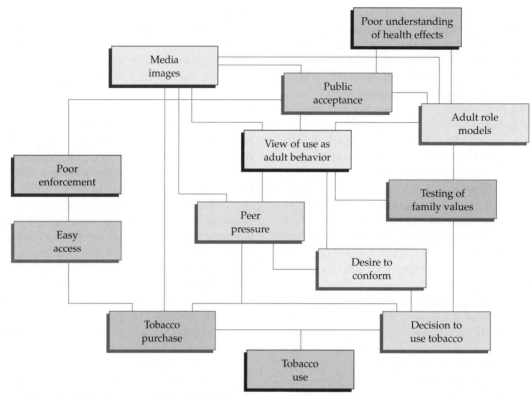

FIGURE 4-2 The Web of Causation for Adolescent Tobacco Use, Indicating the Interplay Between Multiple Direct and Indirect Causative Factors

tobacco use are influenced by media messages and adult role models as well as by peer perceptions. Easy access to tobacco products is influenced by poor enforcement of laws regarding the sale of tobacco products to minors, which is in turn influenced by public acceptance of tobacco use. Other contributing factors and their interrelationships are depicted in the figure. The web of causation has been criticized for its focus on factors exhibited by individuals rather than population patterns of contributing factors (MacDonald, 2004).

Determinants-of-Health Models

Because of the complexity of causal associations in many health problems, the triad and web of causation models have largely been replaced by models that focus on a variety of "determinants of health." **Determinants of health** are broad categories of factors that influence health and illness (Buijs & Olson, 2001). Emphasis on broad determinants of health and illness marks a change from individually focused explanations of disease to a focus on social and environmental contributions to health and illness. A focus on broad determinants of health acknowledges that individual behaviors are shaped by interaction with the environment (Merzel & Afflitti, 2003) and that contextual variables found in the environment probably interact in complex ways with individual variables to determine health and illness (Karpati, Galea, Awerbuch, & Levins, 2002).

The concept of determinants of health is not a new one, and was, in fact, the basis for the activities of mid-19th-century reformists (Williams, 2003). More recently, McKeown has been credited with coining the term *determinants of health*, which was incorporated into the Lalonde Report discussed in Chapter 3∞. The Lalonde Report incorporated the concept of four general determinants (human biology, health system, environment, and lifestyle) into the health field concept (Glouberman & Millar, 2003).

Over the years, the number and categories of determinants have varied among models. For example, Evans and Stoddart (2003) developed the Producing Health, Consuming Health Care (PHCHC) model in 1990, which included determinant categories such as social environment, physical environment, genetic endowment, individual biological and behavioral response, health and function, disease, health care, well-being, and prosperity. The Mandala model developed by Hancock and Perkins and embodied in the Ottawa Charter included only seven categories of determinants. The Population Health Promotion Model included nine categories (Evans & Stoddart, 2003) and other conceptualizations include as few as six categories (Dixon & Welch, 2000). Some of the models focus primarily on social determinants of health and illness, whereas others address biophysical, psychological, and environmental determinants as well (Marmot, 2000). More comprehensive models seek to "embrace population-level thinking without discarding biology or rejecting the notion of human agency, while at the same time rejecting the underlying assumptions of biomedical individualism"

(MacDonald, 2004, p. 387), namely that health and illness are the result of factors related to the individual alone and not to society as a whole. Figure 4-3 depicts a composite determinants-of-health model that reflects elements included in many of the models found in the literature.

GENERAL NURSING MODELS

One of the hallmarks of a scientific profession is the unique body of knowledge that it uses to direct professional practice. This body of knowledge is the result of systematic, scientific inquiry involving the formulation and testing of theory. As is the case with other scientific disciplines, professional nursing practice needs a sound theoretical foundation that describes the interrelationships among key concepts. These concepts form the metaparadigm for the discipline. A **metaparadigm** is a global overview or explanation of a discipline. The metaparadigm for nursing traditionally encompasses four related concepts of person, health, environment, and nursing (Parker, 2001).

Nurse theorists have developed unique perspectives on the relationships among the concepts of the nursing metaparadigm to create different conceptual models. A **conceptual model** is a schematic or verbal picture of the interrelationships that exist among concepts.

A number of conceptual models can be used in community health nursing. Five of these models will be discussed here.

Early conceptual models for nursing were developed to assist in the care of individual clients. Some of these models were adapted by community health nurses for use with families and communities or population groups. For example, previous community health nursing texts examined several of the traditional nursing conceptual models and demonstrated their application to community health nursing (Clark, 1984, 1992, 1996, 1999; Hanchett, 1988). Other authors have applied a single conceptual model in community health nursing practice (Melton, Secrest, Chien, & Andersen, 2001; Stepans & Knight, 2002; Wilson, 2000) or research (Bebe, 2003; Fawcett & Giangrande, 2001; Fawcett & Gigliotti, 2001). Of the general nursing models, the one most easily and often adapted for community health nursing is Betty Neuman's health systems model.

Neuman's health systems model involves a client system striving to prevent "penetration" or disruption of the system by a variety of stressors. Stressors are problems or conditions capable of causing instability in the system or "tension producing stimuli or forces occurring both with the internal and external environmental boundaries of the client system" (Neuman, 2002, p. 21). The client's state of health is

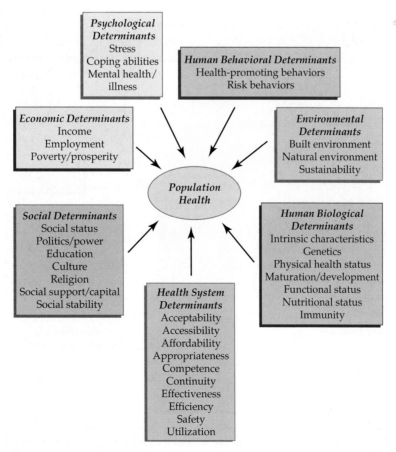

FIGURE 4-3 A Composite Determinants-of-Health Model

EVIDENCE-BASED PRACTICE

*E*xamine research studies related to community health nursing practice published in the last year. How many of them have had a specific theoretical or conceptual base? Which theoretical or conceptual frameworks were used as foundations for those studies that identified a theoretical base? Did the authors link the study findings back to the theoretical base to discuss whether or not the findings supported the relationships derived from the theory or model? Why is this important in community health nursing practice?

dependent on the degree of success achieved in preventing penetration of the client system by stressors or in effecting "reconstitution" of the system after penetration by stressors. Nursing intervention is indicated whenever the client is unable to prevent penetration or accomplish reconstitution without assistance (Aylward, 2001).

In Neuman's model, the client is viewed as a composite of a basic structure surrounded by three boundaries designed to protect the energy sources of the basic structure from environmental stressors (August-Brady, 2000). The core structure is an open system composed of five categories of variables: physiological, psychological, sociocultural, developmental, and spiritual (Gigliotti, 2003). The basic structure is an inner core that must be maintained to ensure survival. Penetration of the basic structure results in death. From Neuman's perspective, the client can be an individual, a family, a community, or a social issue (Fawcett & Gigliotti, 2001).

The protective boundaries are depicted as a series of layers around the core structure and include the lines of resistance and normal and flexible lines of defense (Stepans & Knight, 2002). These elements of the client are depicted in Figure 4-4. The *normal line of defense* is the client's usual state of wellness or the normal range of response to stressors. The *flexible line of defense* is a dynamic state of wellness that changes over time and is composed of factors that fluctuate (e.g., fatigue level). The flexible line of defense provides a protective cushion that prevents stressors from penetrating the normal line of defense (Fawcett & Gigliotti, 2001).

When the flexible line of defense is incapable of protecting the system, penetration of the normal line of defense occurs. Penetration by stressors leads to illness or other health problems when the energy required to stabilize the client system is beyond the system's capacity (Melton et al., 2001). The extent of penetration and the degree of reaction to penetration are influenced by physiological, psychological, sociocultural, developmental, and spiritual variables in the client situation. *Lines of resistance* are internal factors that act to return the client to a normal or improved state of health and

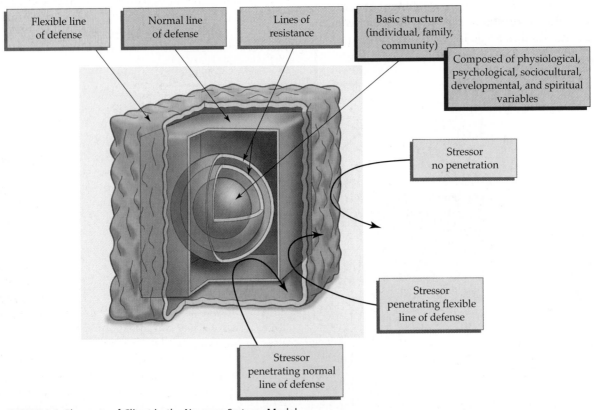

FIGURE 4-4 Elements of Client in the Neuman Systems Model

Adapted from Neuman, B. (2002). The Neuman systems model. In B. Neuman & J. Fawcett (Eds.), *The Neuman systems model* (4th ed.). Upper Saddle River, NJ: Prentice Hall.

protect against stressor penetration of the basic structure (Gigliotti, 2003).

Once stressor penetration of the client system occurs, the system engages in activities aimed at reconstitution. *Reconstitution* involves stabilization of the system and movement back toward the normal line of defense. The normal line of defense may be stabilized at a level either higher or lower than that prior to penetration (Fawcett & Gigliotti, 2001). For the client system to survive stressor penetration, reconstitution must take place before penetration of the basic structure can occur. Nursing intervention is indicated whenever a client system is unable to prevent penetration by a stressor or accomplish reconstitution on its own.

Intervention begins when a stressor is suspected or identified and may include primary, secondary, and/or tertiary prevention (August-Brady, 2000). Primary prevention occurs before stressor penetration and is designed to maintain wellness and prevent stressor penetration. Secondary prevention involves treatment of symptoms arising from penetration and includes interventions designed to strengthen the lines of resistance and regain system stability. Tertiary prevention is aimed at promoting reconstitution, supporting existing strengths, and conserving client energy (Fawcett & Gigliotti, 2001). Although Neuman's model has been widely used in community health nursing, it does not specifically identify the kinds of stressors that affect the health of individuals or population groups. Such identification aids in the development of primary prevention interventions to prevent stressor penetration at the population level. In addition, authors working with the model have identified a need to better delineate model concepts, including differentiating between the normal and flexible lines of defense (August-Brady, 2000).

COMMUNITY HEALTH NURSING MODELS

Although Neuman's health systems model has utility in community health nursing practice, models designed specifically for community health nursing practice may be more useful. Such models have been slow in coming, but there are now several models developed specifically for population-based practice in community health nursing. Four such models will be presented here: the dimensions model of community health nursing, the interventions wheel model, the Los Angeles County public health nursing practice model, and the community-as-partner model.

All four of these models have been designed to incorporate public health concepts into community health nursing practice models. Because the dimensions model of community health nursing provides the foundation for much of the rest of this book, it will be addressed in more detail than the other three models.

The Dimensions Model of Community Health Nursing

The dimensions model of community health nursing is a revision of the previously titled epidemiologic prevention process model (Clark, 1996). The dimensions model incorporates the nursing process and public health concept of levels of prevention. The model also, however, includes a determinants-of-health perspective on the factors that influence health and illness in populations and addresses relevant nursing activities within the dimensions of nursing that affect population health. The dimensions model consists of three elements: the dimensions of health, the dimensions of health care, and the dimensions of nursing practice. The dimensions of health guide the nurse's assessment of clients' health status, whether the client is an individual, a family, or a population. The dimensions of health care and the dimensions of nursing practice guide nursing interventions. Components of the dimensions model are depicted in Figure 4-5.

The Dimensions of Health

The dimensions of health are derived from the epidemiologic determinants-of-health perspective of public health, which acknowledges the interaction of multiple factors in population health and illness. The dimensions consist of six categories of factors that can be used to organize a community health assessment: the biophysical dimension, the psychological dimension, the physical environmental dimension, the sociocultural dimension, the behavioral dimension, and the health system dimension.

THE BIOPHYSICAL DIMENSION The biophysical dimension includes factors related to human biology that influence health. These factors may be related to age and developmental level, genetic inheritance, and physiologic function. Age can affect one's susceptibility to illness or the potential for exposure to other risk factors. Genetic inheritance encompasses gender and racial/ethnic characteristics as well as the specific gene pattern transferred by one's parents. Certain health problems (e.g., hemophilia and sickle cell disease) are more frequently associated with some gender or racial/ethnic groups than with others. The presence of

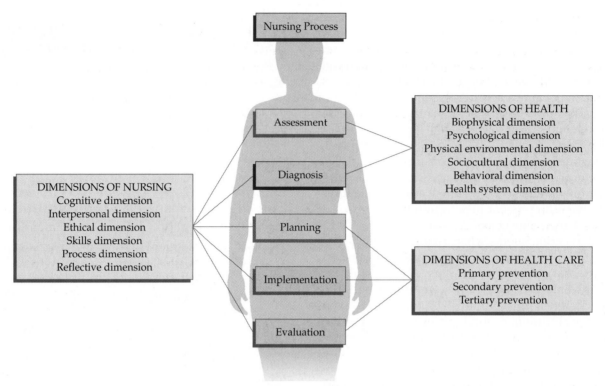

FIGURE 4-5 Elements of the Dimensions Model of Community Health Nursing

certain genetically transmitted traits also increases one's risk of developing some health problems, such as heart disease and some forms of cancer.

Factors related to physiologic function include one's basic state of health as it affects the probability of developing other health problems. Considerations in this area would include the presence or absence of other disease states. For example, obesity is a physiologic factor that contributes to a variety of health problems, including heart disease, diabetes, and stroke. Immunity is another aspect of physiologic function that affects susceptibility to disease. The concept of immunity is discussed in more detail in Chapter 28∞.

When assessing populations, rather than individuals, the age, gender, and racial/ethnic composition of the groups would be determined. Other information related to the components of the biophysical dimension include the prevalence of genetic traits for specific health conditions, the prevalence of specific physiologic conditions in the population (e.g., pregnancy, diabetes), and population levels of immunity.

THE PSYCHOLOGICAL DIMENSION The psychological dimension encompasses the health effects of both internal and external psychological environments. Depression and low self-esteem are two factors in one's internal psychological environment that contribute to a variety of health problems, including suicide, substance abuse, family violence, and obesity. External psychological factors can also influence the development of health problems. For example, a person who has a great deal of emotional support in a crisis is less likely to attempt

suicide than a person who faces a crisis without such support. Stress is another factor in the external psychological environment that is associated with a variety of health problems. The ability to cope with stress, on the other hand, is a factor in one's internal psychological environment. Coping styles also influence one's health status. For example, research has indicated that a distancing style of coping exhibited by some cultural groups is related to pre-term labor. For other women in the same study, the sheer number of life events with which they had to cope was a factor in early labor (Dole et al., 2004). In another study, the concept of *John Henryism*, or a "strong behavioral disposition to directly confront barriers to upward social mobility," was associated with better physical health in African American men (Bonham, Sellers, & Neighbors, 2004, p. 737).

Psychological dimension determinants at the population level would include the incidence and prevalence of psychiatric disorders, the amount of stress experienced by members of the population, and the extent of coping behaviors among individual members of the population. Another important factor to be assessed in the population is the capacity to deal with adverse events. For example, is the community able to cope with increased numbers of homeless individuals or with increasing unemployment?

THE PHYSICAL ENVIRONMENTAL DIMENSION While the psychological dimension addresses aspects of one's psychological environment, the physical environmental dimension encompasses the health effects of factors in the physical environment. The physical environment consists of weather, geographic locale, soil composition, terrain, temperature and humidity, and hazards posed by poor housing and unsafe working conditions. Additional elements of the physical environment that affect health include light and heat, exposure to pathogens and allergens, radiation, pollution, and noise. As an example of the effects of physical environmental factors, highway repair work has been associated with the potential for silicosis for workers and persons living along the highways in question (Valiante, Schill, Rosenman, & Socie, 2004). Similarly, elements of the built environment, such as areas to congregate or obtain exercise, have been shown to affect physical and psychological health in general (Leyden, 2003) and specific health conditions, such as obesity, in particular (Richardson, 2004).

The health effects of physical environmental factors will be addressed in greater detail in Chapter 10∞. Using the dimensions model, the community health nurse would assess the overall population, as well as individual clients, for the presence of environmental conditions detrimental to health. For example, poorly constructed highways may contribute to high rates of motor vehicle accidents for the population. At the individual level, poor lighting, stairs, and other hazards may increase the potential for falls in an elderly client.

THE SOCIOCULTURAL DIMENSION The sociocultural dimension consists of those factors within the social environment that influence health, either positively or negatively. Elements of the social structure such as employment, economics, politics, ethics, and legal influences all fall within this dimension of health. The sociocultural dimension also includes societal norms and culturally accepted modes of behavior. For example, meta-analyses of the effect of discrimination, a sociocultural factor, on health have indicated a relationship with generalized distress, depression, substance abuse, and psychosis, as well as diminished physical health and increased incidence of hypertension (Williams, Neighbors, & Jackson, 2003).

Another important factor in the sociocultural dimension is prevailing attitudes toward specific health problems. For example, the fear and stigma attached to HIV infection may seriously hamper efforts to control the spread of disease. Substance abuse, mental illness, family violence, and adolescent pregnancy are other examples of health problems in which social attitudes contribute to the problem or hinder the solution.

Societal action with respect to health behaviors also falls within this dimension. For example, legislation related to immunization in middle school children is credited with increasing vaccination rates for measles, mumps, and rubella vaccine and hepatitis B from 13% to 60% in one jurisdiction (Averhoff et al., 2004). Legislative action can also have negative effects on population health. For example, in Florida, repeal of a motorcycle helmet requirement for cyclists with at least $10,000 worth of health insurance led to a 48% increase in motorcycle fatalities the following year (Muller, 2004).

Social capital is an element of the sociocultural dimension of health that has been receiving increased attention in public health arenas. Social capital was first defined by Pierre Bourdieu, a French sociologist, as "the aggregate of the actual or potential resources which are linked to possession of a durable network of more or less institutionalized relationships of mutual acquaintance or recognition" (as quoted in Drevdahl, Kneipp, Canales, & Dorcy, 2001, p. 26). Put more simply, **social capital** is the extent of one's access to and participation in relationships that can provide one with the necessities for life. Social capital is comprised of two components: social relationships that permit claims to available resources and the actual resources received. Social capital, at the population level, is akin to the concept of social support networks available to individuals and families. As an example, the existence of and access to educational opportunities afforded a population group is one element of social capital that can affect health status in a number of ways.

The sociocultural dimension can also influence health in other ways. Congregating in large groups, particularly indoors during the winter, enhances the spread of certain diseases such as colds and influenza. Media portrayals of a variety of healthy and unhealthy behaviors are another way in which the sociocultural dimension influences health and illness. Occupation is another aspect of the sociocultural dimension that may influence health. Conversely, unemployment may have adverse effects on physical and emotional health (Artazcoz, Benach, Borrell, & Cortes, 2004). Many of the factors in the sociocultural dimension will be addressed further in the chapters related to economics, politics, and culture.

Community health nurses using the dimensions model with populations would assess the effects of sociocultural dimension factors on the health of the public. For example, the nurse might examine the unemployment rate in the population and the consequent effects on access to health care services.

THE BEHAVIORAL DIMENSION The behavioral dimension consists of personal behaviors that either promote or impair health. Behavioral factors are often those most amenable to change in efforts to prevent disease and promote health and, so, are of particular importance in community health nursing practice. Health-related behaviors include dietary patterns, recreation and exercise, substance use and abuse, sexual activity, and use of protective measures.

Dietary habits can either enhance or undermine health, and both leanness and obesity can predispose one to other health problems. Exercise patterns also influence health status, as do smoking, drinking, and drug use. For example, from 1995 to 1999 smoking was credited with 440,000 deaths and health-related costs of $157 billion for smokers themselves and $366 million for infants born to women who smoked during pregnancy (Office on Smoking and Health, 2002).

Recreational activities are another behavioral factor that may pose health risks, but may also improve both physical and emotional health. For example, boating and water skiing are recreational activities that promote exercise, but have also been shown to contribute to both fatal and nonfatal carbon monoxide poisoning for vacationers as well as employees at Arizona's Lake Havasu (Division of Surveillance, 2004). Sexual activity poses risks related to pregnancy and sexually transmitted diseases. Failure to use protective measures such as contraceptives or barrier devices during intercourse can also increase one's chances of health problems. Similarly, not wearing seat belts or motorcycle helmets increases the potential for serious injury.

THE HEALTH SYSTEM DIMENSION The final dimension of health to be considered is the health system dimension. The way in which health care services are organized and their availability, accessibility, affordability, appropriateness, adequacy, acceptability, and use influence the health of individual clients and population groups. Availability refers to the type and number of health services present in a community, and accessibility reflects the ability of clients to make use of those services. Affordability, the ability to pay for services, also influences health outcomes. Service appropriateness refers to a health care system's ability to provide those services needed and desired by its clientele. The adequacy of health services refers to the quality and amount of service provided relative to need, and acceptability reflects the level of congruence between services provided and the expectations, values, and beliefs of the target population. Finally, the extent to which members of the population actually make use of available health care services will influence health status.

Health system factors can influence health status either positively or negatively. For example, immunization services that are available and easily accessible to all community members promote control of communicable diseases such as measles, polio, and tetanus. Conversely, the failure of health professionals to take advantage of opportunities to immunize people contributes to increased incidence of these diseases. As another example, counseling by health care providers has been shown to increase rates of smoking cessation among clients, yet research indicates that many dentists do not incorporate routine smoking cessation education in their practice (Albert, Ward, Ahluwalia, & Sadowsky, 2002). Similar findings have been noted for members of other professional groups (National Center for Chronic Disease Prevention and Health Promotion, 2002).

As we will see in Chapter 5∞, some health care system contributions to health problems stem from the economics of health care delivery. The high cost of health services limits the ability of many individuals to take advantage of them. Continuity of care may also affect health outcomes for individuals and population groups. For example, persons with health insurance and a regular provider of care have been shown to be more likely to receive needed services than those without (DeVoe, Fryer, Phillips, & Green, 2003). Similarly, persons with diabetes who are able to receive care from a consistent site (not necessarily a particular provider), have been shown to have better control of their disease. Similar results have not been demonstrated for hypertension or lipid control, however (Mainous, Koopman, Gill, Baker, & Pearson, 2004).

In other instances, inappropriate actions on the part of health care providers may actually contribute to health problems. For example, inappropriate use of antibiotics has contributed to the development of antibiotic-resistant strains of gonorrhea and syphilis. Other health system activities may also contribute to disease. For example, rabies has been detected in recipients of organs from infected donors (Centers for Disease Control and Prevention [CDC], 2004), and transmission of the West Nile virus has been associated with blood transfusion (Division of Vector-borne Infectious Diseases, 2004).

Elements of the dimensions of health are summarized on page 73. The dimensions of health related to specific kinds of community health problems will also be discussed in the epidemiology sections of subsequent chapters of this book.

The community health nurse uses the dimensions of health to collect and organize data regarding client health status. Factors in each of the six dimensions may apply to clients at multiple levels, including individuals, families, groups, communities, and populations. From the data, the community health nurse derives community health diagnoses that guide the planning of nursing interventions. Table 4-2◆ summarizes the application of the dimensions of health to the problem of high incidence and prevalence of obesity in a university population.

The Dimensions of Health Care

Nursing interventions for identified health needs in the population are planned within the dimensions of health care. The dimensions of health care derive from the public health concept of levels of prevention and include primary prevention, secondary prevention, and tertiary prevention. Primary prevention was defined by the originators of the term as "measures designed to promote general optimum health or . . . the specific protection of man against disease agents" (Leavell & Clark, 1965, p. 20). Primary prevention involves action taken prior to the occurrence of health problems and encompasses

HIGHLIGHTS The Dimensions of Health

Biophysical Dimension

- Age and developmental level
- Genetics
- Physiologic function

Psychological Dimension

- Internal psychological environment
- External psychological environment

Physical Environmental Dimension

- Physical environment
- Environmental hazards

Sociocultural Dimension

- Social structure
- Societal norms
- Societal attitudes
- Social action

Behavioral Dimension

- Dietary practices
- Recreation and exercise
- Substance use and abuse
- Sexual activity
- Use of protective measures

Health System Dimension

- Availability
- Accessibility
- Affordability
- Appropriateness
- Adequacy
- Acceptability
- Use

screening and early diagnosis as well as treatment for existing health problems.

Tertiary prevention is activity aimed at returning the client (individual or population) to the highest level of function and preventing further deterioration in health. In community health nursing, tertiary prevention also focuses on preventing recurrences of the problem.

A particular nursing intervention may be viewed as a primary, secondary, or tertiary preventive measure depending on its relationship to the occurrence of a problem. If the intervention is designed to prevent the problem from occurring, it is primary prevention. For example, regular exercise can promote health. If the intent is to resolve an existing problem, the intervention involves secondary prevention. Exercise for the obese client as a way of losing weight would be secondary prevention. When the intervention is intended to prevent long-term consequences of an existing or former problem, it is tertiary prevention. For example, exercise after a broken leg is tertiary prevention designed to prevent muscle atrophy and contractures. The dimensions of health care are summarized on page 74.

The Dimensions of Nursing

The dimensions of nursing include the cognitive, interpersonal, ethical, skills, process, and reflective dimensions. The cognitive dimension of community health nursing practice encompasses the knowledge needed for the nurse to identify client health needs and to plan and implement care to meet those needs. This knowledge includes concepts drawn from multiple disciplines beyond nursing. The interpersonal dimension includes affective elements and interaction skills. Affective elements consist of the attitudes and values of the community health nurse that influence his or her ability to practice effectively with a variety of different people. Interaction skills and the abilities to collaborate and communicate effectively with others are additional elements of the interpersonal dimension.

aspects of health promotion and protection. In its health promotion aspect, primary prevention focuses on improving the overall health of individuals, families, and population groups. Health protection is aimed at preventing the occurrence of specific health problems. For example, immunization is a protective measure for certain communicable diseases. Health protection may also involve reducing or eliminating risk factors as a means of preventing disease.

Secondary prevention focuses on the early identification and treatment of existing health problems and occurs after the health problem has arisen. In community health practice at this stage, the major emphasis is on resolving health problems and preventing serious consequences. Secondary prevention activities include

TABLE 4-2 Application of the Dimensions of Health to the Problem of Obesity in a University Population	
Model Concept	**Application**
Biophysical dimension	Age composition of the population; prevalence of obesity in the population
Psychological dimension	Population attitudes to obesity; stress of college life; extent of use of food as stress reliever; extent of exposure to stressful circumstances; prevalence of eating disorders on campus
Physical environmental dimension	Weather conducive to outdoor exercise; facilities available for obese members of the population (e.g., size of classroom chairs)
Sociocultural dimension	Use of eating and drinking as social activities; extent of peer support for healthy lifestyles; availability of education for healthy lifestyles
Behavioral dimension	Dietary practices in campus population; availability of healthy foods in campus dining facilities; availability of recreational activities and equipment; extent of participation in physical activity among campus population; sedentary nature of university life
Health system dimension	Health center staff attention to weight problems among campus community members; availability of weight/diet counseling programs; availability of stress-reduction/counseling programs

In the ethical dimension, the community health nurse acts in accord with moral and ethical principles. Community health nurses must be able to make ethical decisions and be willing to act for the benefit of clients rather than for personal gain. Willingness to advocate for clients is another element of the ethical dimension, which we discussed in some detail in Chapter 1∞ and which forms a primary emphasis throughout the book. Aspects of the ethical dimension influence all of the other dimensions of nursing.

The skills dimension of community health nursing encompasses both manipulative and intellectual skills that are common to all areas of nursing practice. Manipulative skills include the ability to perform such activities as giving immunizations, providing tuberculin skin tests, and conducting hearing examinations and physical assessments. Intellectual skills include the capacity for critical thinking as well as the ability to examine data and draw inferences—in other words, diagnostic capabilities.

Community health nurses employ knowledge, attitudes, and skills in the application of several specific processes when providing care to individuals, families, and population groups. The most fundamental of these processes is, of course, the nursing process. Other processes used by community health nurses in their practice are the epidemiologic process, the health education process, the home visit process, and the case management process. Community health nurses also use change, leadership, group, and political processes in their care of clients. These processes and others compose the process dimension of community health nursing. Many of these processes are addressed in greater detail in later chapters of this book.

The reflective dimension is the final dimension of nursing in the model. In the reflective dimension, community health nurses reflect on their care through theory development, research, and evaluation. The creation of the dimensions model is itself an example of theory development in community health nursing. The importance of the other elements of the reflective dimension, research and evaluation of practice, is emphasized in each chapter of this book. The dimensions of nursing are summarized above right.

In the dimensions model, nursing actions occur in the context of the nursing process, as depicted in Figure 4-5. The dimensions of health, for example, are used to guide assessment of the client's health status and to derive nursing diagnoses. The dimensions of health care direct the planning, implementation, and evaluation of nursing interventions. For instance, the nurse may plan and implement a community immunization fair as a primary preventive measure and then evaluate the effects of the fair in terms of the resulting increase in community immunization levels and subsequent decrease in incidence rates for immunizable diseases.

The dimensions of nursing are employed in the context of the nursing process. For example, the nurse uses intellectual skills and cognitive knowledge of causative factors in health problems to assess health and derive nursing diagnoses. Similarly, the nurse might need to use interpersonal skills in collecting assessment data as well as in engaging members of the community in planning and implementing strategies to resolve identified health problems. Elements of the process dimension such as the health education process and the leadership process may also be required in implementing a plan of care. Finally, elements of the reflective dimension of nursing are used in the evaluation of nursing interventions and in the development of theory that provides the knowledge base for the cognitive dimension.

The dimensions model has the advantage over several of the other models discussed in this chapter in that it can be used to address more than health problems or conditions present in the population. For example, the model can be used to examine a proposed health policy or to study an ethical issue in community health nursing practice. As we will see in Chapter 9∞, the dimensions model is also useful in conducting a thorough cultural assessment. In addition, the model can be used to examine health and illness in specific settings and population groups.

The Interventions Wheel

The interventions wheel model, previously known as the Public Health Nursing Interventions model, was developed by the Minnesota Department of Health, Section of Public Health Nursing, and is based on input from expert community health nursing consultants and practicing public health nurses (Keller, Strohschein, Schaffer, & Lia-Hoagberg, 2004). The model, as depicted in Figure 4-6, consists of 17 identified community health nursing interventions that cross over three levels of population-based practice: individual-focused, community-focused, and systems-focused practice. Individual-level interventions are focused on change in individual health status, knowledge, or skills. Community-level interventions address changes in community norms, awareness, attitudes, and behaviors in an entire community or subgroups within a community. Systems-level interventions focus on changes in the organizations and health care delivery structures that serve individuals and communities (Naumanen-Tuomela, 2001). Interventions are defined as "actions public health nurses use to improve the health of populations" (Keller, Strohschein, Lia-Hoagberg, & Schaffer, 2004, p. 455). Many of the interventions included in the model were discussed in the context of the community health nursing roles presented in Chapter 1∞. Others are addressed in more detail in later chapters in this book. Table 4-3◆ applies the interventions to the three levels of community health nursing practice.

In the original model, the 17 interventions were displayed in alphabetical order. However, in a review of the interventions by community health nurses, it was determined that certain interventions were closely related, so they were grouped in terms of clusters or "wedges" of related functions. Also, during this exercise, community

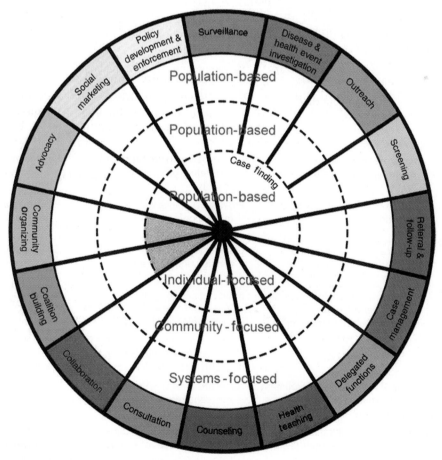

FIGURE 4-6 The Intervention Wheel

From Keller, L. O., Strohschein, S., Lia-Hoagberg, B., & Schaffer, M. A. (2004). Population-based public health interventions: Practice-based and evidence-supported. Part I. *Public Health Nursing, 21,* 453–468. Reprinted by permission of Blackwell Publishing, Inc.

health nursing experts determined that not all interventions were employed at all levels of practice. Specifically, case finding was found to occur only in relation to individual-focused practice, and so it is confined within the individual-focused ring in the figure. Similarly, community organizing and coalition building were found to occur only at community and systems levels and so are

"blacked out" in the individual-focused ring of the figure (Keller, Strohschein, Lia-Hoagberg, & Schaffer, 2004).

According to the originators of the model, the core functions of public health, assessment, policy development, and assurance are incorporated to some degree in each of the interventions at each level of practice. The model is also supposed to incorporate the concept of

TABLE 4-3 Examples of Nursing Interventions in Individual-, Community-, and System-Focused Practice

Interventions	Individual-focused	Community-focused	System-focused
Surveillance	Follow up on family members exposed to TB	Collect data on instances of family violence	Establish data systems that incorporate information on disease prevalence from private providers
Disease and health event investigation	Identify the source of infection in a child with TB	Advise nursing home coordinators on influenza prevention measures	Work with local health care providers to develop a computer-based communicable disease notification system
Outreach	Identify a pregnant family member on a home visit to a woman with hypertension	Arrange a referral system for school nurses who identify pregnant mothers of students	Develop a notification system for immunizations
Screening	Screen an adolescent for sexually transmitted disease	Arrange a community screening program for hypertension	Develop systems for screening, follow-up, and treatment for HIV infection
Referral and follow-up	Refer a family for financial help	Establish criteria for social service referrals	Develop a community referral network for prenatal care
Case management	Arrange home care for an elderly client	Develop a case management program for pregnant adolescents	Develop case management standards for local government agencies
Delegated functions	Provide directly observed therapy to a client with TB	Develop protocols for TB treatment services	Develop policies for TB treatment in local correctional facilities
Health teaching	Teach a mother about child development	Work with school and police officials to develop an antidrug education campaign in local schools	Develop a local health Web site to address health questions
Counseling	Assist a pregnant woman to explore prenatal care options	Help develop an eating-disorders counseling program in high schools	Engage in political activity to mandate insurance coverage for counseling services
Consultation	Assist a family in developing a nutritious diet	Provide assistance to local schools in developing school nutrition programs	Provide information to a state legislator on a health-related issue
Collaboration	Collaborate with a church to provide transportation for a client	Collaborate with local churches to provide homeless shelters	Collaborate in the development of a single application process for all forms of county assistance
Coalition building	Develop a family coalition to enact an intervention with a substance-abusing member	Build a coalition of police, school, and health personnel to prevent gang violence	Build a coalition to promote enforcement of local laws against tobacco sales to minors
Community organizing	Not relevant	Organize community members to request fee discounts from local health care providers	Develop a group to facilitate community organizing in several communities
Advocacy	Advocate for preschool enrollment for the child of a depressed mother	Advocate for recreation activities for teenagers	Advocate for services for substance-abusing adolescents
Social marketing	Distribute no-smoking buttons in local elementary school	Develop a teen theater campaign to address issues of conflict resolution	Write a grant to fund a media campaign to support smoke-free public spaces
Policy development and enforcement	Promote multilingual provider employment in area health	Participate in policy development in relation to dispensing	Engage in agency policy analysis and revision as needed

GLOBAL PERSPECTIVES

Shamsudin (2002) raised the issue of the applicability of theoretical models developed in the United States to the care of populations in other countries. She noted that because nursing is a social activity performed in the context of a particular social and cultural environment, conceptual models developed in one context might not be applicable in another. Other barriers to the adoption of U.S. models in other countries include the abstract language often used by nurse theorists and the educational level and facility with English of nurses in other countries. Of the theoretical models presented in this chapter, which ones do you think would be most applicable to other nations? Why?

determinants of health as all factors that influence health, not just clinical disease or health-related behaviors (Keller, Strohschein, Lia-Hoagberg, & Schaffer, 2004). However, it is not clear how determinants of health are to be incorporated into the context of the interventions contained in the wheel. Similarly, the authors indicate that the model emphasizes health promotion and illness prevention, yet a significant number of the interventions are directed primarily toward existing health problems (e.g., case finding, surveillance, disease and health event investigation, screening, delegated functions, and case management). Most of the other interventions, such as policy development and enforcement, advocacy, coalition building, community organizing, collaboration, counseling, and health education, might be directed toward health promotion and illness prevention, but could as easily be employed in addressing existing conditions. Although the model provides some guidance regarding the interventions that community health nurses employ in their practice, it does not assist in the identification of factors that are affecting the population's health and leading to the need to employ the interventions. Nor does the model really address the various levels of prevention at which community health nursing practice may occur.

The Los Angeles County Public Health Nursing Practice Model

The Los Angeles County Public Health Nursing (LAC PHN) practice model was developed by the Public Health Nursing division of the Los Angeles County Department of Health Services. The model is an attempt to link public health nursing with principles of public health practice (Sakamoto & Avila, 2004) with an overall goal of healthy people living in healthy communities. Like the dimensions model, the LAC PHN practice model incorporates public health concepts into the framework of the nursing process and is based on several underlying principles:

- Community or public health nursing is a multidisciplinary endeavor.
- Clients must be active participants in the endeavor.

- Community health nursing practice is population-based.
- Community health nursing practice is based on the core functions and essential services of public health.
- Community health nurses engage in the interventions described in the intervention wheel model (Smith & Bazini-Barakat, 2003).

The LAC PHN practice model, depicted in Figure 4-7, uses the concept of "health indicators" derived from the *Healthy People 2010* document rather than a more general array of health determinants to focus assessment of community health problems. The 10 health indicators are physical activity, overweight and obesity, tobacco use, substance abuse, responsible sexual behavior, mental health, injury and violence, environmental quality, immunization, and access to health care, as indicated in Chapter 2∞. Although the authors note that it is important to consider other indicators that may be of concern in a particular population, the model does not provide any guidance in what additional indicators should be assessed. The model also fails to provide direction in the assessment of factors that contribute to undesirable outcomes in leading indicators and other indicators of health. In particular, the model fails to acknowledge that health system factors may contribute to the existence of health problems.

The public health interventions derived from the interventions wheel model are incorporated into the planning and action components of the nursing process in the LAC PNH practice model. Like the interventions model, the LAC PHN practice model focuses on population-based practice that may focus at individual/family, community, and systems levels. The essential public health services are also incorporated within the elements of the nursing process in the model depicted in Figure 4-7. For example, the health monitoring function is incorporated into the assessment phase of the nursing process, whereas the diagnostic and investigative function is reflected in the diagnosis phase. These and other essential public health functions will be discussed in more detail in Chapter 5∞.

The Community-as-Partner Model

Anderson and McFarlane (2003) based their community-as-partner model (originally the community-as-client model) on Neuman's health systems model and the nursing process. In the community-as-partner model, the client for nursing care is the community or population group. The inner core consists of the people who make up the community along with their beliefs, values, and history. The core is surrounded by eight community subsystems that affect community members and are, in turn, affected by them. These subsystems include those related to the physical environment, education, safety and transportation, politics and government, health and social services, communication,

Public Health Nursing Practice Model*

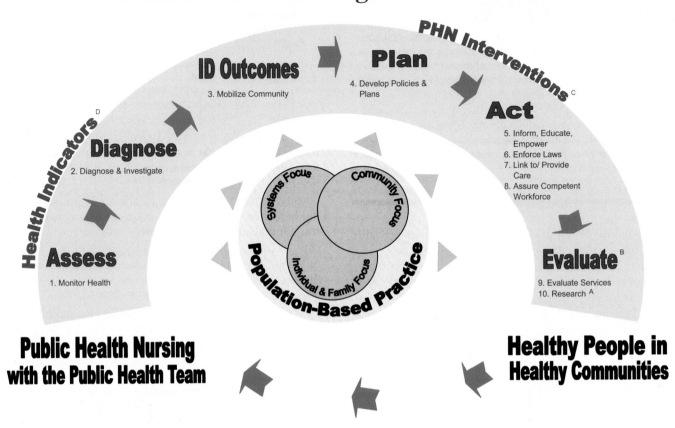

References:
(A) Public Health Functions Steering Committee. (1994, Fall). *Public Health in America.* Retrieved May 7, 2001, from the World Wide Web: http://health.gov/phfunctions/public.htm
(B) Quad Council of Public Health Nursing Organizations. (1999). *Scope and Standards of Public Health Nursing Practice.* Washington D.C.: American Nurses Association.
(C) Minnesota Department of Health, Public Health Nursing Section. (2000). P*ublic Health Nursing Practice for the 21st Century: National Satellite Learning Conference; Competency Development in Population-based Practice October 5, November 2, December 7, 2000.* St. Paul, MN: Minnesota Department of Health, Public Health Nursing Section. Retrieved May 7, 2001, from the World Wide Web: http://www.health.state.mn.us/divs/chs/phn/material.htm
(D) U.S. Department of Health and Human Services. (2000). *Healthy People 2010.* (Vol. 1). McLean, VA: International Medical Publishing, Inc.

*Created by Los Angeles County DHS, Public Health Nursing with input from CCLHDND-Southern Region. This model serves as the basis for the CCLHDND California PHN Practice Model (05-2002).
© 2002 Los Angeles County DHS Public Health Nursing

FIGURE 4-7 The Los Angeles County Public Health Nursing Practice Model

Reprinted by permission of Public Health Nursing, Los Angeles County Department of Health Services.

BUILDING OUR KNOWLEDGE BASE

Select a proposition suggested by one of the models discussed in the chapter. For example, you might select a proposition from the dimensions model that suggests that health system factors can actually contribute to health problems as well as resolve them or a proposition from Neuman's model that a particular element of the line of resistance, such as coping abilities, influences the effect of a stressor, like unemployment, on health.

- State the proposition that you have derived from the model.
- How might you go about testing the validity of your proposition?
- What variables would you measure? Where might you obtain your data, and how would you go about collecting it?
- What implications might the findings of your study have for community health nursing practice? Who should be apprised of the results of your study?

economics, and recreation. Factors in these subsystems may affect the flexible line of defense or the community's lines of resistance.

The normal line of defense in this model represents the community's usual level of wellness and its problem-solving or coping capacities. The flexible line of defense is a changing level of community health in response to stressors. As in the Neuman model, the client possesses lines of resistance or internal capacities to deal with stressor penetration.

The community health nurse using the community-as-partner model participates with members of the community to assess the health status of the community core and factors in the eight subsystems that affect health as well as the strength of the normal and flexible lines of defense and the lines of resistance. The nurse and community also assess for potential stressors

CULTURAL COMPETENCE

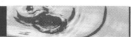

Which of the models described in this chapter could be applied to population groups with cultural heritages different from that of the mainstream American culture? Search the nursing literature to see if and how these models have been applied to different cultural groups. How successful was the application? Were there concepts from the models that needed to be adapted before they could be applied to the particular cultural group? How was the adaptation accomplished? How successful was the adaptation?

TABLE 4-4	Application of the Community-as-Partner Model to the Problem of Adolescent Tobacco Use
Model Concept	**Application**
Core	Adolescent population in the community; community attitudes toward tobacco use
Stressor	Increased tobacco use among adolescents
Normal line of defense	Community's usual response to tobacco use; prior history of ability to cope with similar problems
Flexible line of defense	Other factors impinging on the community's ability to deal with the problem (e.g., recent loss of local recreational resources for teens—recreational subsystem; current government instability due to recent political scandals—governmental subsystem)
Lines of resistance	Limited education on health effects of tobacco use—education subsystem; media images fostering tobacco use—communication subsystem; failure of police to enforce laws regarding tobacco sales to minors—safety subsystem
Primary prevention	Educational campaigns targeted to social perceptions of tobacco use aimed specifically at adolescents; enforcement of tobacco sales laws; initiation of adolescent social activities that preclude tobacco use (e.g., smoke-free rock concerts); removal of tobacco vending machines from public places
Secondary prevention	Identification and referral of adolescent tobacco users to smoking cessation programs

occurring from within or outside the community and the degree of community reaction when stressor penetration has occurred. Nurse and community together develop community health diagnoses and plan, implement, and evaluate interventions at the appropriate level of prevention (Anderson & McFarlane, 2003). Table 4-4◆ applies concepts of the community-as-partner model to the community health problem of increased tobacco use among adolescents.

In this chapter, we have explored several theoretical models that can be applied to community health nursing practice. Readers may choose to employ one of the models presented here or another model that is appropriate to community health nursing practice, or they may construct a personal model of practice. Whatever the option chosen, community health nursing is most effective when some kind of theoretical model is used as an organizing framework for care.

MediaLink Case Study: Theory Application

Case Study

Using Theory in Population-Focused Care

Sandville is a small community in Texas situated 5 miles from the U.S.–Mexico border. The primary industry in the area is cattle ranching. Most of the Anglo residents are descendants of the western cattle barons and make up about 40% of the town's population of 3,000. Another 25% of the population is composed of long-time Latino residents descended from wranglers who worked on the ranches in the past. Now many work in service occupations. Mexican immigrants who cross the border (legally or illegally) to obtain work make up about 10% of the population. Members of this group return frequently to Mexico, where extended family members continue to reside. The remainder of the town's population includes a group of newly arrived Asian engineers and their families who have come to staff the recently opened electronics plant and a small group of African Americans who have lived in the area since the end of the Civil War.

Most young people do not stay long in the area and those who do have few children, so the population (with the exception of the

Asian families) is aging. Cardiovascular disease and motor vehicle accidents on the two-lane highway passing through town create a booming business for the small local hospital. There are three primary care physicians in the community, one dentist, one pediatrician, and two family nurse practitioners. The county health department maintains a branch office in the town that is staffed by a public health nurse and a sanitation engineer 2 days a week.

Community health problems, in addition to cardiovascular disease and accidents, include arthritis and anemia. There is also a high rate of tuberculosis among the Mexican immigrants.

1. Select one of the models presented in the chapter and apply it to this case situation.
2. What elements of the model are exemplified by the information provided in the case study?
3. What problems might be present in the community other than those specified? What information in the case study led you to suspect the presence of these problems?
4. What nursing interventions would you employ as the community health nurse assigned to this community? Why?

Test Your Understanding

1. Why should community health nursing be based on a model or theory? (p. 62)

2. Examine the concept of causality as it affects a health problem with which you are familiar. What are the causative factors contributing to the problem? How are they interrelated? (p. 62)

3. What is meant by the term *risk*? How is the concept of risk used in community health nursing? (p. 62)

4. What is the difference between morbidity and mortality? (p. 63)

5. What are the major components of Neuman's health systems model? How might you apply this model to the care of a family? To a population group? (pp. 67–69)

6. What are the three elements of the dimensions model of community health nursing? What are the dimensions included in each element? Give an example related to the dimensions in each element that addresses the health of a population group? (pp. 69–74)

7. How do the nursing interventions presented in the interventions wheel model differ across levels of community health nursing practice? Give several examples of interventions at different levels. (pp. 75–77)

8. What are the elements of the LAC PHN practice model? Describe how the model might be used to direct community health nursing practice in your community. (pp. 77–78)

9. What are the elements of the community-as-partner model? Give an example that applies the model to a community health issue in your community. (pp. 77–79)

EXPLORE MediaLink

http://www.prenhall.com/clark
Resources for this chapter can be found on the Companion Website.

Audio Glossary
Exam Review Questions
Case Study: Theory Application

MediaLink Applications: The Population Focus
Media Links

Challenge Your Knowledge
Advocacy Interviews

References

Albert, D., Ward, A., Ahluwalia, K., & Sadowsky, D. (2002). Addressing tobacco in managed care: A survey of dentists' knowledge, attitudes, and behaviors. *American Journal of Public Health, 92,* 997–1001.

Anderson, E. T., & McFarlane, J. (2003). A model to guide practice. In E. T. Anderson and J. McFarlane (Eds.), *Community as partner: Theory and practice* (4th ed., pp. 165–176). Philadelphia: Lippincott.

Artazcoz, L., Benach, J., Borrell, C., & Cortes, I. (2004). Unemployment and mental health: Understanding the interactions among gender, family roles, and social class. *American Journal of Public Health, 94,* 82–88.

August-Brady, M. (2000). Prevention as intervention. *Journal of Advanced Nursing, 31,* 1304–1308.

Averhoff, F., Linton, L., Peddlecord, K. M., Edwards, C., Wang, W., & Fishbein, D. (2004). A middle school immunization law rapidly and substantially increases immunization coverage among adolescents. *American Journal of Public Health, 94,* 978–984.

Aylward, P. D. (2001). Betty Neuman: The Neuman systems model and global applications. In M. Parker (Ed.), *Nursing theories and nursing practice* (pp. 329–342). Philadelphia: Davis.

Bebe, L. H. (2003). Theory-based research in schizophrenia. *Perspectives in Psychiatric Care, 39*(2), 67–74.

Bonham, V. L., Sellers, S. L., & Neighbors, H. W. (2004). John Henryism and self-reported physical health among high socioeconomic status African American men. *American Journal of Public Health, 94,* 737–738.

Buijs, R., & Olson, J. (2001). Parish nurses influencing determinants of health. *Journal of Community Health Nursing, 18*(1), 13–23.

Centers for Disease Control and Prevention. (2004). Update: Investigation of rabies infections in organ donor and transplant recipients—Alabama, Arkansas, Oklahoma, and Texas, 2004. *Morbidity and Mortality Weekly Report, 53,* 615–616.

Clark, M. J. D. (1984). *Community nursing: Health care for today and tomorrow.* Reston, VA: Reston.

Clark, M. J. (1992). *Nursing in the community.* Norwalk, CT: Appleton & Lange.

Clark, M. J. (1996). *Nursing in the community* (2nd ed.). Stamford, CT: Appleton & Lange.

Clark, M. J. (1999). *Nursing in the community: Dimensions of community health nursing* (3rd ed.). Stamford, CT: Appleton & Lange.

DeVoe, J. E., Fryer, G. E., Phillips, R., & Green, L. (2003). Receipt of preventive care among adults: Insurance status and usual source of care. *American Journal of Public Health, 93,* 786–791.

Dicker, R. C. (2002). A brief review of the basic principles of epidemiology. In M. B. Gregg (Ed.), *Field epidemiology* (2nd ed., pp. 8–25). New York: Oxford University.

Division of Surveillance, Hazard Evaluations, and Field Studies, National Institute for Occupational Safety and Health. (2004). Carbon monoxide poisonings resulting from open air exposures to operating motorboats—Lake Havasu City, Arizona, 2003. *Morbidity and Mortality Weekly Report, 53,* 314–318.

Division of Vector-borne Infectious Diseases, National Center for Infectious Diseases. (2004). Transfusion-associated transmission of West Nile virus—Arizona, 2004. *Morbidity and Mortality Weekly Report, 53,* 842–844.

Dixon, J., & Welch, N. (2000). Researching the rural-metropolitan health differential using the "social determinants of health." *Australian Journal of Rural Health, 8,* 254–260.

Dole, N., Savitz, D. A., Siega-Riz, A. M., Hertz-Picciotto, I., McMahon, M. J., & Buekens, P. (2004). Psychosocial factors and preterm birth among African American and white women in central North Carolina. *American Journal of Public Health, 94,* 1358–1365.

Drevdahl, D., Kneipp, S., Canales, M., & Dorcy, K. S. (2001). Reinvesting in social justice: A capital idea for public health nursing? *Advances in Nursing Science, 24*(2), 19–31.

Evans, R. G., & Stoddart, G. L. (2003). Consuming research, producing policy? *American Journal of Public Health, 93,* 371–379.

Fawcett, J., & Giangrande, S. K. (2001). Neuman systems model-based research: An integrative review project. *Nursing Science Quarterly, 14,* 231–238.

Fawcett, J., & Gigliotti, E. (2001). Using conceptual models of nursing to guide nursing research: The case of the Neuman Systems Model. *Nursing Science Quarterly, 14,* 339–345.

Friedman, G. D. (2003). *Primer of epidemiology* (5th ed.). New York: McGraw-Hill.

Friis, R. H., & Sellers, T. A. (2003). *Epidemiology for public health practice* (3rd ed.). Sudbury, MA: Jones & Bartlett.

Gigliotti, E. (2003). The Neuman Systems Model Institute: Testing middle range theories. *Nursing Science Quarterly, 16,* 201–206.

Glouberman, S., & Millar, J. (2003). Evolution of the determinants of health, health policy, and health information systems in Canada. *American Journal of Public Health, 93,* 388–392.

Gordis, L. (2004). *Epidemiology* (3rd ed.). Philadelphia: Saunders.

Hanchett, E. S. (1988). *Nursing frameworks and community as client.* Norwalk, CT: Appleton & Lange.

Karpati, A., Galea, S. Awerbuch, T., & Levins, R. (2002). Variability and vulnerability at the ecological level: Implications for understanding the social determinants of health. *American Journal of Public Health, 92,* 1768–1772.

Keller, L. O., Strohschein, S., Lia-Hoagberg, B., & Schaffer, M. A. (2004). Population-based public health interventions: Practice-based and evidence-supported. Part I. *Public Health Nursing, 21,* 453–468.

Keller, L. O., Strohschein, S., Schaffer, M. A., & Lia-Hoagberg, B. (2004). Population-based public health interventions: Innovations in practice, teaching, and management. Part II. *Public Health Nursing, 21,* 469–487.

Leavell, H. R., & Clark, E. G. (1965). *Preventive medicine for the doctor in his community: An epidemiologic approach* (3rd ed.). New York: McGraw-Hill.

Leyden, K. M. (2003). Social capital and the built environment: The importance of walkable neighborhoods. *American Journal of Public Health, 93,* 1546–1551.

MacDonald, M. A. (2004). From miasma to fractals: The epidemiology revolution and public health nursing. *Public Health Nursing, 21,* 380–391.

Mainous, A. G. III, Koopman, R. J., Gill, J. M., Baker, R., & Pearson, W. S. (2004). Relationship between continuity of care and diabetes control: Evidence from the third National Health and Nutrition Examination Survey. *American Journal of Public Health, 94,* 66–70.

Marmot, M. (2000). Multilevel approaches to understanding social determinants. In L. F. Berkman & I. Kawachi (Eds.), *Social epidemiology.* London: Oxford University.

Melton, L., Secrest, J., Chien, J., & Andersen, B. (2001). A community needs assessment for a SANE program using Neuman's model. *Journal of the American Academy of Nurse Practitioners, 13,* 178–186.

Merzel, C., & Afflitti, J. (2003). Reconsidering community-based health promotion: Promise, performance, and potential. *American Journal of Public Health, 93,* 557–574.

Muller, A. (2004). Florida's motorcycle helmet repeal and fatality rates. *Journal of Public Health, 94,* 556–558.

National Center for Chronic Disease Prevention and Health Promotion. (2002). Prevalence of health-care providers asking older adults about their physical activity levels — United States, 1998. *Morbidity and Mortality Weekly Report, 51,* 412–414.

Naumanen-Tuomela, P. (2001). Finnish occupational health nurses' work and expertise: The client's perspective. *Journal of Advanced Nursing, 34,* 538–544.

Neuman, B. (2002). The Neuman systems model. In B. Neuman & J. Fawcett (Eds.), *The Neuman systems model* (4th ed., pp. 1–33). Upper Saddle River, NJ: Prentice Hall.

Office on Smoking and Health, National Center for Chronic Disease Prevention and Health Promotion. (2002). Annual smoking-attributable mortality, years of potential life lost, and economic costs—United States, 1995–1999. *Morbidity and Mortality Weekly Report, 51,* 300–303.

Parker, M. (2001). Introduction to nursing theory. In M. Parker (Ed.), *Nursing theories and nursing practice* (pp. 3–13). Philadelphia: Davis.

Richardson, K. (2004). Conference report: Highlights of obesity and the built environment: Improving public health through community design. *Medscape Diabetes & Endocrinology, 6*(2), 1–3. Retrieved August 31, 2004, from http://www/medscape.com/viewarticle/487906_print

Sakamoto, S. D., & Avila, M. (2004). The Public Health Nursing Practice Manual: A tool for public health nurses. *Public Health Nursing, 21,* 179–182.

Shamsudin, N. (2002). Can the Neuman Systems Model be adapted to the Malaysian nursing context? *International Journal of Nursing Practice, 8,* 99–105.

Smith, K., & Bazini-Barakat, N. (2003). A Public Health Nursing Practice Model: Melding public health principles with the nursing process. *Public Health Nursing, 20,* 42–48.

Stepans, M. B. F., & Knight, J. R. (2002). Application of Neuman's framework: Infant exposure to environmental tobacco smoke. *Nursing Science Quarterly, 15,* 327–334.

Valiante, D. J., Schill, D. P., Rosenman, K. D., & Socie, E. (2004). Highway repair: A new silicosis threat. *American Journal of Public Health, 94,* 876–880.

Williams, G. (2003). The determinants of health: Structure, context, and agency. *Sociology of Health & Illness, 25,* 131–154.

Williams, D. R., Neighbors, H. W., & Jackson, J. S. (2003). Racial-ethnic discrimination and health: Findings from community studies. *American Journal of Public Health, 93,* 200–208.

Wilson, L. (2000). Implementation and evaluation of church-based health fairs. *Journal of Community Health Nursing, 17*(1), 39–48.

Advocacy in Action

Getting an Appointment

A community health nursing student had been visiting with a woman who had had heart surgery 2 or 3 months prior to the start of the visits. While in the hospital for surgery, the woman had been diagnosed with diabetes. Although the doctors told her that she had diabetes, they did not fully explain to her what type she had nor how to manage it. Because of this her blood sugar was constantly above the normal range, and she experienced headaches daily.

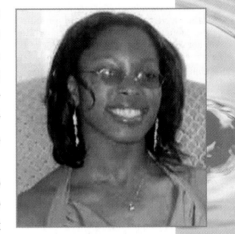

During the visits, the student established a couple of goals to achieve by the end of the visits. One of the goals was for the client to schedule a follow-up appointment since she had not had one since her surgery. The woman was having trouble contacting the clinic where she had been seen previously. Either the phone was busy or they would schedule her for an appointment that was months away.

At each visit, the student would ask if the client had been successful in contacting the clinic, but she could not get through to them. This situation went on for about 3 weeks. The 4th week, before visiting the woman, the student did some research, trying to find health care centers close to where the woman lived. The cost of the visit had to be affordable for the client—less than $40. During the next visit, the student suggested a health center that was a few blocks away and easily accessible by public transportation. The client seemed hesitant to call the center so the student initiated the call, explaining the woman's situation and emphasizing the need for an appointment in the near future. The center staff asked to speak to the client directly to get personal information and schedule a date and time that accommodated her busy schedule. The visit was scheduled for 2 to 3 weeks later. The client was put on a sliding fee scale, so the visit would cost less than $25. The client was very grateful but was nervous because she didn't like going to the doctor. The nursing student volunteered to go with her to the doctor's office to provide support and learn more about ways to meet her needs.

Kimesha Hammond

Nursing Student

5 CHAPTER

The U.S. Health System Context

CHAPTER OBJECTIVES

After reading this chapter, you should be able to:

1. Describe the popular health care subsystem.
2. Distinguish between the complementary and alternative subsystems of care.
3. Identify six fundamental obligations of official public health agencies.
4. Describe the organizational structure of the U.S. health care delivery system.
5. Compare and contrast official and voluntary health agencies.
6. Describe at least five functions performed by voluntary health agencies.
7. Identify ten essential public health services.
8. Discuss the involvement of local, state, and national governments in health care in the United States.
9. Identify outcomes of care at the primary, secondary, and tertiary levels of prevention.
10. Describe potential approaches to health system reform, including the possibility of a national health care system.

KEY TERMS

assessment **87**
assurance **88**
complementary/alternative
  health care subsystem **85**
core functions of public
  health **87**
health care system **85**
local public health system **91**
official health agencies **87**
passthrough funds **92**
personal health care
  sector **86**
policy development **88**
popular health care
  subsystem **85**

population health care
  sector (public health
  system) **86**
privatization **91**
public health
  practice **86**
scientific health care
  subsystem **86**
state public health
  system **93**
surveillance **88**
voluntary health
  agencies **89**

MediaLink
http://www.prenhall.com/clark

Additional interactive resources for this chapter can be found on the Companion Website. Click on Chapter 5 and "Begin" to select the activities for this chapter.

Community health nursing occurs in the context of a health care delivery system that creates constraints and provides opportunities for the practice of community health nursing. For example, lack of emphasis on health promotion in the health care delivery system increases the need for health promotion efforts by community health nurses but simultaneously limits funds available for health promotion activities.

Exploring the organization of health care delivery systems can help us to understand how these systems developed, how they work, and how and why they sometimes fail to work. Moreover, we can identify factors that positively or negatively influence community health nursing practice. Finally, we can identify areas where change is needed in the health care delivery system to best fulfill our goal as community health nurses, namely, the promotion of the public's health. The health care delivery system in the United States is a mixture of multiple sources of care at multiple levels that are affected by a variety of external forces.

FORCES INFLUENCING HEALTH CARE SYSTEMS

Health system observers have identified several forces that influence the organization and effectiveness of the U.S. health care system. Some of these factors include changing population demographics, growing numbers of uninsured residents, increasing demands for accountability, technological advances and innovation, professional labor issues, economic globalization, changes in delivery systems, and information management issues (Sultz & Young, 2004). The population in the United States, as in every other nation, is growing older, and older people tend to be the greatest users of health care services due to the prevalence of chronic disease in this population. In addition, the U.S. population is changing in terms of the ethnic groups represented, necessitating changes in health care delivery systems to accommodate clients from multiple cultures.

At the same time, there is a growing number of uninsured and underinsured individuals in the population,

particularly among members of ethnic and cultural minority groups. In Chapter 8∞ and Chapter 20∞ we will examine some of the factors leading to this growth, but the very existence of a large population of uninsured individuals results in unmet needs in the health care system as it currently exists. From 2003 to 2004, the number of uninsured people in the United States increased by nearly a million people (from 45 million to 45.8 million). In addition, the percentage of health insurance provided by employers decreased from 60.4% to 59.8%. For the most part, this loss was offset by increases in the number of people covered by government health insurance programs such as Medicaid and the State Children's Health Insurance Program (SCHIP), but proposed federal cuts in Medicaid funding will increase the number of uninsured persons even further (Families USA, 2004; 2005).

Lack of health insurance is equivalent to lack of access to health care services for many people. In addition to the loss of health of individuals, lack of access to care poses significant costs to society. These costs lie in the loss of productive citizens through early death and disability as well as higher health care costs due to increasingly serious diseases that could have been treated at lower cost early in their course. Overall these losses are estimated at $65 billion to $130 billion per year (Institute of Medicine [IOM], 2003a). Access to health care through affordable health insurance is perhaps the most important focus for advocacy to promote population health in the United States.

Another influence on health care systems is increasing public demand for accountability for both the quality of care provided and the use of resources to provide that care. Initiatives to assure standards of quality and limit the escalating costs of health care services have profoundly affected how health care is delivered. These and other economic influences on the health care system will be addressed in more detail in Chapter 8∞. Technological advances significantly influence the cost of health care and greatly affect health care delivery systems. Furthermore, the widespread availability of high-tech information sources, such as the Internet, allows the U.S. public to be better informed of technological advances in care and to increase their demands for costly, high-tech services.

The primary professional labor issue facing health care delivery systems is the shortage of health care personnel, particularly nurses. With many other occupational choices available to potential recruits, health care systems have had to make many changes to attract young people to health care occupations and to specific practice locales (e.g., rural or inner city areas). A second issue related to the professional workforce is the increasing need for advanced education for effective practice. The cost of educating providers and the need to provide the technology required to support the level of practice for which they are educated further increase the cost of

ETHICAL AWARENESS

Many people in the United States object to the use of tax dollars to fund care for people who have come into the country illegally. These objections have led to actions such as the passage of legislation in some states that prohibits the use of public funds to pay for health care for undocumented immigrants except in certain situations (e.g., life-threatening emergencies). Public health agencies and others receiving state funding have been directed to determine clients' citizenship or legal immigration status and to deny care to those who are not eligible. How would you respond to such a directive? Why?

health care services. In addition, health care systems are facing a need to change the ways they do business in order to attract providers (e.g., more flexible schedules, opportunities for job sharing, etc.).

Chapter 6∞ will address the effects of globalization on health and health care delivery. As we will see, these effects are both positive and negative. Changes in the organization of health care delivery systems also affect the operation and overall effectiveness of the U.S. health care system. For example, mergers of several institutions into large, for-profit organizations and competition among systems have a definite impact on health care delivery. Finally, changes in information management systems have led to changes in the completeness, accuracy, and transferability of information within and among health care organizations (Sultz & Young, 2004). For the most part this influence has been positive, leading to faster access to client care information, but it also raises issues of privacy and confidentiality.

All of these forces, as well as others that will be addressed elsewhere in this book (e.g., political activity and threats of terrorism), have contributed to the U.S. health care system as it presently exists and as it continues to evolve. Exploration of the health care system within the context of these forces can help us develop strategies to guide that evolution to greater effectiveness.

HEALTH CARE DELIVERY IN THE UNITED STATES

The World Health Organization (WHO) (2000) defined a **health care system** as "all the activities whose primary purpose is to promote, restore, or maintain health" (p. 5). No two health systems are alike, but many national health care systems share a number of commonalities. The major exception to this perception of commonality is the United States, which is the only developed nation in the world without a comprehensive approach to funding or providing health care services (Jonas, 2003). Health care delivery in the United States has been described as an "unsystematic system" (Budrys, 2001) because of its multicentric and uncoordinated nature. Despite the relative accuracy of this description, we can still examine U.S. health care delivery in terms of the structure depicted in Figure 5-1.

The organizational structure for health care delivery in the United States consists of three major elements or subsystems, depicted in Figure 5-1. These subsystems include the popular health care subsystem, the complementary or alternative health care subsystem, and the scientific health care subsystem.

The Popular Health Care Subsystem

Most health-related care is provided within the popular health care subsystem. The **popular health care subsystem** is the system in which care is provided by oneself, family members, or friends, in short by people who are

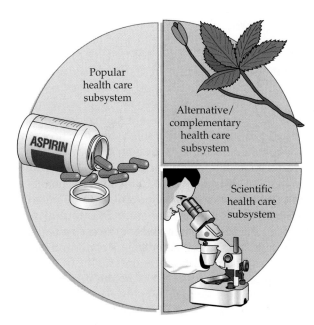

FIGURE 5-1 Organizational Structure of the U.S. Health Care Delivery System

not considered health care providers. It is estimated that 70% to 90% of illness care is provided within this system (WHO, 2000). The popular subsystem includes health care that each of us provides for ourselves and our families. When you have a headache, for example, you may take an over-the-counter analgesic. If you are constipated, you may either increase the bulk, fiber, and fluid in your diet or take a laxative. If your child has a mild fever, you might give him or her an antipyretic. All of these self-care or family care practices constitute popular subsystem health care.

Although health care in this subsystem is provided by oneself or by family members, community health nurses have an educational role in the popular subsystem. As we shall see in Chapter 11∞, one of the purposes of health education is to prepare clients to make informed self-care decisions. For example, a community health nurse might caution a client against overuse of laxatives and suggest dietary approaches to dealing with constipation, or the nurse may inform parents about the hazards of giving aspirin to children and recommend a nonaspirin substitute.

The Complementary/Alternative Health Care Subsystem

When self-care fails or seems inappropriate, people often turn to other sources of health care. Some of these sources might be folk health practitioners. The **complementary/ alternative health care subsystem** consists of providers and practices outside the scientific health care subsystem that are specifically focused on promotion of health and prevention of and care for illness. The terms *complementary* and *alternative* are often used interchangeably when discussing this subsystem, but actually differ in terms of their relationship to the scientific subsystem. Complementary health care practices are those that are used in conjunction with scientific care to *complement* and enhance its effects. Alternative practices, on the other hand, are used in place of, or as *alternatives* to, scientific interventions. Any given health practice may be considered complementary or alternative depending on its use in relation to scientific subsystem practices.

Practitioners in this subsystem are individuals who are believed to have special health-related knowledge or training above that provided to the average member of the society. Examples of alternative/complementary health care providers are the *curanderas* found among Latinos in the northeastern and southwestern regions of the United States and the herbalists found in these and other areas. The role of the community health nurse in the complementary/alternative health care subsystem is to assess the influence of this subsystem on health and to incorporate traditional health practices into the plan of care as appropriate. On occasion, the nurse may also need to caution clients against specific alternative practices that may be harmful to health (e.g., the use of traditional remedies that contain lead or other contaminants) or educate clients regarding the interactions between alternative and scientific therapies. We discuss the complementary/alternative health care subsystem in more detail in Chapter 9∞.

The Scientific Health Care Subsystem

The professional or **scientific health care subsystem** is the system of care based on scientific research-derived evidence. Health care provided in the scientific subsystem is based on knowledge derived from the biological, physical, and behavioral sciences and includes the services of nurses, physicians, pharmacists, social workers, and other health care professionals.

The scientific health care subsystem consists of two sectors that differ primarily in their focus of care. These sectors are the personal health care sector and the public, or population, health care sector.

The Personal Health Care Sector

The **personal health care sector** is the segment of the scientific health care subsystem that provides health-related services to individual clients. The primary emphasis in this sector is cure of disease and restoration of health, although individuals may also receive some health-promotive and illness-preventive services.

There are five major components to this sector of the health care system: health care institutions, personnel, health commodities firms, education/research institutions, and financing systems (Jonas, 2003). The institutional component consists of office settings, clinics, hospitals, nursing homes, and other places where care is dispensed to individual clients. The personnel component is composed of the professionals who provide services. Health commodities firms include indus-

tries that manufacture or supply the materials and equipment required to implement health care services. Some examples of commodities firms include pharmaceutical companies and manufacturers of durable medical equipment or health-related computer software.

Both educational and research institutions are components of the personal health sector in that they educate health professionals to provide individual client care services and conduct research related to therapeutic interventions and delivery systems. The final component of the sector is comprised of the systems that finance care, which include insurers, philanthropic institutions, and government agencies.

Any given element of the sector may embody several of these components. For example, a university hospital may provide services, educate providers, and conduct research. As we will see in Chapter 8∞, some health care organizations, such as managed care organizations (MCOs), also incorporate the financing element.

The personal health care sector may be further divided into for-profit and not-for-profit segments (Jonas, 2003). In the for-profit segment, health care services are provided with the intention of deriving monetary gain. Within this segment are the "proprietary" service providers, such as physicians and health care institutions designed to create revenue, and corporations that provide health care to employees (and occasionally their families) in order to limit the drain of health insurance costs on company revenue (Jonas, 2003).

The Population Health Care Sector

The **population health care sector** consists of both public and private organizations whose focus is the health of the total population. This sector is also referred to as the **public health system**, which has been defined as "all public, private, and voluntary entities that contribute to delivery of essential public health services within a state or local public health jurisdiction" (National Public Health Performance Standards Program [NPHPSP], n.d.a, p. i). Although this definition addresses only the state and local levels of health care, it can be extended to encompass the national public health system as well.

Public health practice is defined as "the art and science of preventing disease, promoting population health and extending life through organized local and global efforts" (McMichael & Beaglehole, 2003, p. 2). The Institute of Medicine (IOM) report on *The Future of*

GLOBAL PERSPECTIVES

*P*eople come to the United States from all over the world for many different purposes. Some intend only a short stay; others plan to relocate here permanently. What are some of the barriers within the U.S. health care system to obtaining care for those from other parts of the world? How might these barriers be eliminated or modified to improve their access to necessary care?

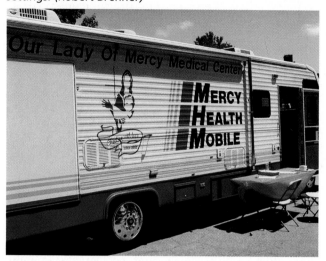

Community health services are provided in a variety of settings. (Robert Brenner)

Public Health defined the mission of public health practice as "fulfilling society's interest in assuring conditions in which people can be healthy" (quoted in Little Hoover Commission, 2003, p. 1). General goals for public health practice include improving population health, reducing health inequalities within the population, and developing environments that support health (McMichael & Beaglehole, 2003).

Several authors have noted that the U.S. health care system is poorly organized to achieve these goals (Studnicki et al., 2002). In part, this is due to the traditional U.S. cultural value of individualism. Other contributing factors include lack of funding for public health service (Patel & Rushefsky, 2002) and a focus by public health agencies on specific populations and conditions supported by categorical funding. The importance of public health is, however, highlighted by the assertion that the personal health care sector has little impact on population health. It has been said that even "lavish spending" in that sector will not result in substantial improvement in population health due to the influence of multiple factors that lie outside the province of personal health care services (Studnicki et al., 2002).

The Institute of Medicine (2003b) lists six areas of action and change that must be undertaken to assure effective population health in the United States:

- Adopting a population health approach that considers the multiple determinants of health;
- Strengthening the governmental and public health infrastructure, which forms the backbone of the public health system;
- Building a new generation of intersectoral partnerships that also draw on the perspectives and resources of diverse communities and actively engage them in health action;
- Developing systems of accountability to assure the quality and availability of public health services;
- Making evidence the foundation of decision making and the measure of success; and
- Enhancing and facilitating communication within the public health system (e.g., among all levels of the governmental public health infrastructure and between public health professionals and community members). (p. 4)

Care provided in the population health care sector has traditionally centered on promoting health and preventing disease, although some curative care does occur in this sector. Emphasis is on designing health care programs that meet the needs of population groups.

OFFICIAL PUBLIC HEALTH AGENCIES Official health agencies are agencies of local, state, and national governments that are responsible for the health of the people in their jurisdictions. Official agencies are supported by tax revenues and other public funding. They are accountable to the citizens of their jurisdiction, usually through an elected or appointed governing body. Many of the activities conducted by official agencies are mandated by law. For example, local health departments are required by state law to report cases of certain diseases. We will discuss specific functions of official agencies at local, state, and national levels in more detail later in this chapter. Generally speaking, however, official public health agencies are responsible for fulfilling six fundamental obligations to the public: preventing epidemics and the spread of disease, protecting the public from environmental hazards, preventing injury, promoting healthy behavior and good mental health, responding to disasters and assisting with recovery from their effects, and assuring the quality and accessibility of needed health care services (NPHPSP, n.d.b).

Core Public Health Functions These fundamental obligations are fulfilled in the context of three core public health functions identified by the IOM. The **core functions of public health** are its primary responsibilities and include assessment, policy development, and assurance (Mays, Halverson, Baker, Stevens, & Vann, 2004). These core functions form the foundation for public health practice and community health nursing activities (Keller, Strohschein, Lia-Hoagberg, & Schaffer, 2004; Missouri Department of Health, n.d.).

In their **assessment** function, public health agencies are expected to "regularly collect, assemble, analyze, and make available information on the health of the community, including statistics on health status, community health needs, and epidemiological and other studies of health problems" (IOM, quoted in Scutchfield & Last, 2003, pp. 107–108). Under this function public health agencies are responsible for assessing and monitoring the occurrence of health-related problems within the population, as well as identifying factors that contribute to, or prevent, those problems.

Some of the elements of the assessment function are performed in the context of **surveillance**, or the "ongoing (continuous or periodic) collection and analysis of population-based data to measure the magnitude of the problem (risk factors or disease) and trends over time" (Bonita, Winkelmann, Douglas, & de Courten, 2003, p. 11). Effective surveillance systems incorporate four essential elements. These include a theoretical base that posits causal connections and explanations for the development of health and illness and attention to time as a variable. Trends in problems and their associated risk factors must be developed over time rather than viewed at a particular point in time. Effective systems also use a systematic approach that provides "seamless interconnection" of data collection, analysis, interpretation, and data utilization activities (McQueen, 2003).

A variety of public health surveillance systems exist to monitor health problems and their causative factors in the United States. These include systems for collecting vital statistics such as births and deaths as well as risk factor surveillance systems such as the Behavioral Risk Factor Surveillance System (BRFSS) employed by all 50 states, the District of Columbia, and three U.S. territories. The BRFSS is used to track information on disease incidence and prevalence and the extent of health-related behaviors in the general population (Holtzman, 2003). A similar system, the Youth Risk Behavior Surveillance System (YRBSS), tracks health behaviors among high school students. Both systems are designed to address behaviors related to specific *Healthy People 2010* objectives (Brenner et al., 2004)◆.

When the BRFSS was initiated in 1984, the survey addressed six individual risk behaviors (cigarette smoking, alcohol use, physical inactivity, diet, hypertension, and safety belt use) (Mokdad, Stroup, & Giles, 2003). In its present form, the system includes a fixed core of nine factor categories related to incidence of chronic disease and health care access, as well as health-related behaviors. The system has also incorporated rotating core sections of three to six additional areas that are addressed in alternate years, emerging core sections to address new areas of concern, and 19 additional modules that can be included by specific jurisdictions to address health concerns particular to their areas (Holtzman, 2003).

The **policy development** function of public health involves advocacy and political action to develop local, state, and national policies conducive to population health. This may also include planning for health care delivery at the population level and assuring core funding for public health activities, as well as the use of scientific evidence as a basis for policy formation (Scutchfield & Last, 2003).

The third core function, **assurance**, reflects the responsibility of the public health sector to assure availability of and access to health care services essential to sustaining and improving the health of the population. This may involve the actual provision of services but

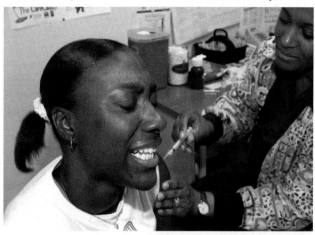

Assuring availability of health services is one of the core functions of public health. (Mario Villafuerte/Getty)

more often involves developing mechanisms whereby essential services are available within the community. For example, public health agencies may arrange for indigent members of the population to receive medical services from local providers rather than provide them directly. Assuring access means making sure not only that services are available to the population, but that they are provided at appropriate levels of care (Wimberley & Thai, 2002).

Performance of these functions requires the development of a public health infrastructure capable of supporting them. The public health infrastructure is defined as the "basic services or social capital of a country, or part of it, which makes economic and social activities possible" (Rutherford, as quoted in Powles & Comim, 2003, p. 160). Components of the public health infrastructure are similar to the components of the personal health care sector and include knowledge, the institutions and capacity required to respond to the public's health needs, and the resources required to produce health (e.g., personnel, commodities, and funding). The knowledge component of the infrastructure refers to both the professional knowledge possessed by health care providers and the knowledge and processes required for an informed populace. Requisite institutions include not only the agencies that monitor and

Think Advocacy

Your community includes a number of relatively large refugee populations from different war-torn areas of the world. Some members of these populations have been in the United States for 2 to 3 years and some have recently arrived. All of them have difficulty obtaining services to address health care needs they are currently experiencing. What might you do to address their lack of access to care? What other groups or agencies might you attempt to bring into a coalition to address the health needs of this population?

assure health services, but policy-making bodies (e.g., the legislature) and processes and health-related civic organizations. Similarly, required resources include not only health-related services but also systems to deal with sanitation, pollution, and other often invisible influences on the population's health (Powles & Comim, 2003).

Essential Public Health Services   The core public health functions have been operationalized in 10 essential public health services delineated by the Centers for Disease Control and Prevention in 1994 (NPHPSP, n.d.b). These services are:

- Monitoring health status to identify health problems
- Diagnosing and investigating health problems and hazards in the community
- Informing, educating, and empowering people regarding health issues
- Mobilizing community partnerships to identify and solve health problems
- Developing health policies and plans that support individual and community health efforts
- Enforcing laws and regulations that protect health and assure safety
- Linking people to needed personal health care services and assuring the provision of health care when otherwise unavailable
- Assuring a competent public health and personal health workforce
- Evaluating the effectiveness, accessibility, and quality of personal and population-based health services
- Conducting research to develop new insights and innovative solutions to health problems. (U.S. Department of Health and Human Services [USDHHS], 2000)

The statement of the essential functions of public health agencies led in 2001 to the development of core competencies for public health professionals performing these functions. These core competencies reflect eight domains of public health practice: analytic assessment skills, knowledge of basic public health sciences (e.g., epidemiology), cultural competence, communication skills, capacity for community-level practice, financial planning and management skills, leadership and systems thinking capabilities, and policy development and program planning skills (Council on Linkages Between Academia and Public Health Practice, 2001). As we saw in Chapter 1∞, the development of these general competencies led, in turn, to the development of the specific competencies for community health nursing practice presented in Appendix A∞.

Another development arising from identification of the essential functions of public health was the creation of three sets of performance standards to assess the effectiveness of state and local health agencies in carrying out the functions. The National Public Health Performance Standards were developed by a coalition of public and voluntary health agencies and designed to

EVIDENCE-BASED PRACTICE

May, Phillips, Ferketich, and Verran (2003) attempted to conduct a study of the effects of generalist community health nursing practice on improving population health. Interventions derived from a public health nursing model included those directed at personal prevention, organized indigenous caregiving, and community empowerment. The research team reported difficulties in implementing the program and in measuring its effectiveness due to conflicts between the research team and the local health care system in which the team attempted to implement the program. These conflicts centered around differences in philosophies of implementing care as they related to program financing, personnel, and organization and perceptions of the nature of nursing and the role of the public health nurse. With respect to implementing care, for example, the research team espoused a "one-stop shopping" approach, but found this difficult to actualize due to lack of administrative venues for obtaining sufficient supplies to support such needed services. The health department was also organized to support categorical services rather than "one-stop" services (e.g., immunizations on one day, family planning services on another). Similarly, employee productivity was defined administratively as product (e.g., number of clients seen) but by the research team as process (e.g., home visits or services, such as immunizations, provided outside of a categorically designated service such as an immunization clinic). Conflicts with respect to the nature of nursing and the role of public health nurses also reflected an emphasis on categorically funded programs and administrative demands for structured practice versus the more independent and autonomous practice demanded of the intervention program. The conclusion drawn by the authors was that "even in a progressive organization, organizational structures militated against the generalist role" and that "agency culture can constrain or enhance a professional role" (May et al., 2003, p. 257).

After reading the article, answer the following questions:

1. How might the difficulties encountered in implementing the planned nursing intervention have affected findings on its effectiveness?
2. What system changes would be required to successfully implement the planned intervention in order to evaluate its effectiveness?
3. Would implementing the planned intervention outside of an organized health care agency have contributed more to information on its effectiveness? Why or why not?

assess an optimal level of performance of state and local health agencies and capacities for public participation in public health governance as well as to promote quality improvement (NPHPSP, n.d.a).

VOLUNTARY HEALTH AGENCIES Voluntary health agencies are nonprofit organizations that provide adjuncts to services provided by government agencies. These may include institutional and personal services that address the needs of special groups, education for public health, or prevention, screening, health maintenance, rehabilitation, or terminal care services (Sultz & Young, 2004). They may focus on a specific disease entity, an organ system, or a population group. Voluntary agencies are funded primarily by donations. They are accountable to their supporters, and their activities are determined by supported interests rather than legal mandate. Their primary emphasis is on research, education, and policy development (primarily through legislative lobbying), although they may provide some direct health care services.

Voluntary agencies can be categorized on the basis of their source of funding. The first category consists of agencies supported by citizen contributions, such as the American Cancer Society. The first agency of this type in the United States was the Antituberculosis Society founded in Philadelphia in 1892. The focus of this type of agency frequently changes as health needs change. For example, the Antituberculosis Society is known today as the American Lung Association, indicating its broader focus on a variety of respiratory conditions. The second category consists of foundations established by private philanthropic contributions. An example of this type of voluntary organization would be the Kellogg Foundation, which provides funding for health care research. Today, more than 3,000 philanthropic foundations support health efforts. The third category of voluntary agency is funded by member dues. The American Public Health Association and the American Nurses Association are examples of this type of agency.

Integrating agencies, such as the United Way, coordinate the fund-raising activities of several voluntary agencies. A fifth type of voluntary agency includes religious organizations that derive their funds from contributions by members of a congregation. These groups often focus on local needs and are particularly effective because of their ability to draw on volunteers. The final category of voluntary health agency is the commercial organization that engages in health care activities. For example, the American Dairy Association provides literature and visual aids for nutrition education. Similarly, health insurance companies often put out literature on health promotion and illness prevention.

Voluntary agencies perform eight basic functions within the scientific health care subsystem. The first of these is *pioneering* activities. Voluntary agencies explore areas that are poorly addressed by the other components of the health care system. For example, research that culminated in the development of a vaccine for polio was the early focus of the March of Dimes. Now, polio immunization is largely a function of official agencies.

The second function of voluntary agencies is *demonstration* of pilot projects in health care delivery. For instance, the Planned Parenthood Association instituted clinics for contraceptive services long before most official health agencies became involved in this area of service. *Education* of the public and health professionals is the third function of voluntary agencies. For example, the American Cancer Society has spearheaded educational campaigns on the hazards of smoking. The fourth

function of voluntary agencies is *supplementation* of services provided by official health agencies. For instance, some voluntary agencies provide transportation to clinics, respite care, special equipment, and other ancillary services.

Fifth, voluntary agencies *advocate* for the public's health. For example, a voluntary agency may campaign against reduction of health care services due to budget cuts. The sixth function, promoting *legislation* related to health, is a closely related function. In one community, for example, a collaborative organization of residents and service providers was successful in promoting legislation to prevent tenants from being evicted without cause and to extend required eviction notice from 30 to 60 days.

The seventh function of voluntary agencies relates to health *planning and organization*. Voluntary agencies often assist official agencies in determining health care needs in the population and in planning programs to address those needs. The final function of voluntary agencies is *assisting official agencies* in developing well-balanced community health programs. For example, in 1915, when the San Diego Common Council passed an ordinance creating the position of Municipal Tuberculosis Visiting Nurse but could not afford to pay her salary, the State Tuberculosis Society agreed to fund the position for one year, allowing the city to hire its first community health nurse (Communication from the City Auditor, 1915). The functions of voluntary agencies are summarized below.

Relationships Between Personal and Population Health Sectors

The "appropriate" relationship between medicine and public health has been debated for more than a century (Brandt & Gardner, 2000). Although the Library of Medicine has defined public health as a "branch of medicine" (Little Hoover Commission, 2003), the two disciplines are quite distinct, but interrelated. Historically, public health has been identified with prevention

---

HIGHLIGHTS Functions of Voluntary Health Agencies

- Pioneering: exploring areas not addressed by other components of the health care system
- Demonstration: initiating and testing innovative strategies for health care delivery
- Education: educating both the public and health care professionals regarding health issues
- Supplementation: providing services that complement and strengthen those of official health agencies
- Advocacy: speaking for the public's benefit in the development of health policy
- Legislation: initiating and campaigning for health-related legislation
- Planning and organizing: assisting official health agencies in determining health care needs, priorities, policies, and programs
- Assisting official agencies: supporting the efforts of official health agencies in improving the health of the public

and health promotion, and medicine with the cure of existing health problems. This leads to a difference in thinking, with public health practice concerned with "upstream thinking" and prevention of adverse health events before they occur, and medicine involved in "downstream thinking" related to pathogenesis that already exists. As has already been stated, public health has a population focus, whereas medicine focuses on provision of care to individuals.

Other factors that separate the two disciplines include the rise of hospitals as the main venue for medical practice, whereas public health practice takes place outside of institutional settings, and the relative isolation of the educational preparation of each group from the other. As some authors noted, "population" as a concept for medicine is frequently perceived as "constructed by economic incentives, insurance plans, and carveouts" (Brandt & Gardner, 2000, p. 713) rather than as the totality of the populace, as perceived in public health. Generally speaking, the relationships between public health and medicine have been characterized by "critical differences in ideology, world view, politics, methods, and technologies—underlying questions about *where* and *how* to address problems associated with disease and its biological and social ramifications" (Brandt & Gardner, 2000, p. 713).

In the last several years, there has been significant crossover in the activities of agencies and organizations in the personal and public health care sectors. For example, public health care sector organizations have begun to provide more personal health care services to people with no other source of health care. In this respect, the public health care sector has provided a "safety net" for those who would otherwise not receive care.

Provision of personal health services is seen by many as undermining the fundamental responsibility of the public health sector (Drevdahl, 2002), and the burgeoning emphasis on a return to the core functions of public health has led many public health agencies to attempt to "privatize" personal health care services. **Privatization** is the movement of personal health care services from public health agencies to private organizations in the personal health care sector.

At the same time, many organizations in the personal health care sector are absorbing functions, such as immunization and treatment of sexually transmitted diseases, which have traditionally been the purview of public health agencies. Although there are calls for partnerships between managed care organizations and public health agencies to address population health problems, there are also concerns that such partnerships may result in an even greater shift to a "market perspective" by public health agencies in addressing primarily those health issues for which outside funding is available (Drevdahl, 2002). As we saw earlier, this type of categorical approach to public health needs is one of the elements of the public health system that has been criticized. It remains for the

BUILDING OUR KNOWLEDGE BASE

*L*iterature related to health economics and to medicine contains numerous articles comparing and contrasting various aspects of different health care delivery systems. As we have seen, there are research studies comparing relative costs, client satisfaction, and a variety of outcome measures. There are few, if any, studies, however, that examine the effects of health care delivery systems on nursing, yet nurses are the health professionals responsible for implementing a large segment of the care provided in any system.

- How would you design a study to examine the effects of different health care systems on nursing practice?
- What variables might you choose to examine? Why?
- Whom would you select as subjects for your study? Would you choose certain categories of nurses? Why or why not?
- What kind of data collection strategies would be most appropriate to the study variables you have identified? Are there tools already available that you might use?

ideal relationship between personal and population health care sectors to be determined and developed. Let us turn now, though, to a discussion of the levels at which health care services are provided.

Levels of Health Care Delivery in the United States

Health care delivery in the United States takes place on local, state, and national levels. Each level has certain responsibilities with respect to the health of the population. Both official and voluntary agencies exist at each level, but official agencies are the focus of this discussion. Public health agencies at each of the three levels—local, state, and national—perform the essential public health services, but the degree to which they are emphasized varies from level to level.

Although official health agencies at all three levels address public health needs, state governments hold primary responsibility for preserving and protecting the health of the public (Scutchfield & Last, 2003). This is because *police power*, or "power to provide for the health, safety, and welfare of the people" (Jonas, 2003, p. 115), is reserved to the states by the United States Constitution. In fact, any power not specifically delegated to the federal government by the Constitution remains within the purview of state governments. In the same way that the states, through the Constitution, have delegated certain responsibilities to the federal government, they may also delegate some health-related functions and responsibilities to agencies at the local level (Jonas, 2003).

The Local Level

A **local public health system** is defined as "all entities that contribute to the delivery of public health services within a community" (NPHPSP, n.d.a, p. i). The official agency at the local level is usually the *local health* *department.* Some local public health agencies are large health systems serving the populations of major jurisdictions such as New York City or Los Angeles County. Most, however, serve smaller populations that do not have the resources for performing all of the essential public health functions. The local health department's authority is derived, in part, from responsibilities delegated by the state. For example, the state delegates to the local level the responsibility for collecting statistics on births and deaths. Because this responsibility has been legally delegated, the local health department has the authority to ensure that a death certificate is filed for every death that occurs. The local agency also derives authority from local health ordinances. For instance, local government might pass an ordinance requiring all residential rental units to have functioning smoke detectors. Enforcement of this ordinance might then become the responsibility of the local health department.

Funding at the local level comes from both local taxes and state and federal subsidies. A portion of local public health agency funding comes from the state, including federal **passthrough funds**, money granted to the states by the federal government that is allocated to local government agencies. Other operating funds derive from local revenues, including local taxes. A small percentage of funding comes directly from federal monies (excluding Medicaid and Medicare funds). In recent years, local health departments have attempted to augment revenue sources by providing personal care services reimbursable under Medicare and Medicaid. Because many Medicare and Medicaid recipients are being enrolled in managed care organizations (MCOs) in the personal health care sector, these sources of revenue are being withdrawn from local health departments, in some cases jeopardizing their ability to subsidize services for other indigent populations (Drevdahl, 2002). Another small percentage of local health department funding is derived from client fees, private health insurance, regulatory fees, and so on.

Figure 5-2 depicts the typical organizational structure of a local health department. The staff and programs included will vary from place to place. In some areas, the district health officer might also fulfill the role of administrative officer. Small counties or districts may not be able to afford the full-time services of some types of personnel, and the services of nutritionists, social workers, dentists, and other personnel might be shared by several counties or provided at the state level. Nurses and clerical staff would be found in almost any health department. Other personnel who may be available include environmental specialists, physical therapists, psychologists, laboratory and X-ray technicians, and pharmacists.

Because delegation of specific responsibilities to local jurisdictions is the function of the state, the responsibilities assumed vary from state to state. Local responsibilities may also vary within regions of a particular state, depending on the local jurisdiction's capabilities and resources. Within the context of the core public health functions, local health agencies assess and monitor local health needs and resources, develop policies that foster local involvement in decision making and equitable allocation of resources, and assure availability of high-quality services to meet local health needs. The assurance function also includes educating the community on how to access available services (Scutchfield & Last, 2003). Typical responsibilities performed by local

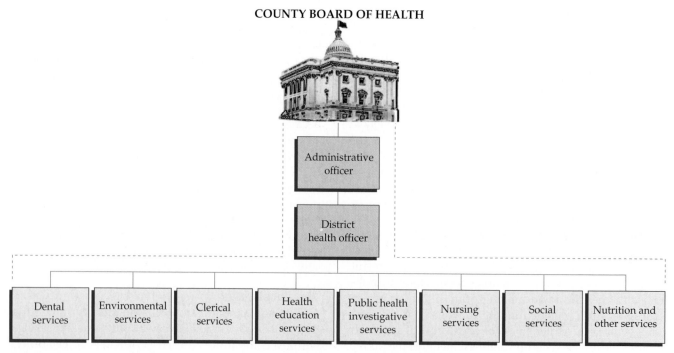

FIGURE 5-2 Typical Organizational Structure of a Local Health Department

health agencies include collection of vital statistics, communicable disease control, disease screening and surveillance, immunization, and health education. Other responsibilities include chronic disease control, sanitation, school health and maternal–child health programs, and public health nursing services. Local public health services may or may not include mental health services and primary care services for the indigent (Schneider, 2000). Specific services provided by local public health agencies will depend, in large part, on the needs of local populations.

The State Level

A **state public health system** is the "state public health agencies and other partners that contribute to public health services at the state level" (NPHPSP, n.d.a, p. i). The official agency at the state level has traditionally been a state department of health. As noted above, the state, not the federal government or the local jurisdiction, has primary authority in matters relating to health. The state retains the ultimate responsibility for the health of the public and possesses essential power to make laws and regulations regarding health. The responsibilities of the state with respect to health have been reinforced by what some have called the *new federalism*, a recent tendency by the federal government to return to the states responsibility for several formerly federally supported health and social services programs (Wimberley & Rubens, 2002).

The state health department derives funding from state tax revenues and may also receive monies from the federal government. A general organizational schema for a state department of health is depicted in Figure 5-3. The various divisions coordinate services at the state level and provide assistance to the local level.

Because of their primary responsibility for the health of the population, state public health agencies have more mandated functions related to health than the federal government (Sorenson, 2003). Based on the core public health functions, the Institute of Medicine has identified five key responsibilities of state health departments:

- Assessment of statewide health status and health care needs
- Development of statewide objectives related to health
- Assurance of adequate personnel and services to meet identified health care needs
- Guarantee of a minimum set of essential services to members of the population
- Assistance to local jurisdictions in health-related initiatives. (Scutchfield & Last, 2003)

Specific areas of responsibility, as defined by the Association of State and Territorial Health Officials, include personal health services, environmental health, health resources, laboratory services, support of local health departments beyond specific program areas, collection and analysis of health statistics, and licensing of health care providers and institutions (Jonas, 2003).

The National Level

Because the Constitution makes no reference to any responsibilities of the federal government regarding health, the federal government has no direct authority

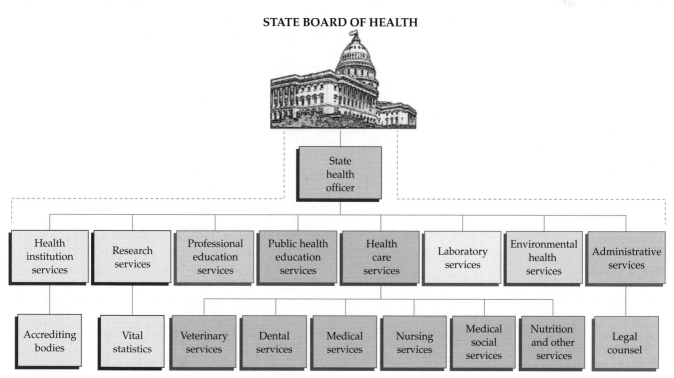

FIGURE 5-3 Typical Organizational Structure of a State Health Department

94   UNIT I / The Context for Community Health Nursing

to regulate health-related matters. The authority of the federal government with respect to health is derived indirectly from two other constitutional powers (Jonas, 2003). The first of these is the *power to regulate foreign and interstate commerce*. For example, because most cosmetics are transported across state lines, the federal Food and Drug Administration has the authority to establish standards of purity for the manufacture of cosmetics.

The second constitutional source of authority over health matters is the *power to levy taxes and spend to promote the general welfare*. For example, it can be argued that such programs as Medicaid and Medicare promote the general welfare and are therefore within the authority of the federal government.

The official health agency at the national level is the United States Department of Health and Human Services (USDHHS), created in 1980 with the division of the former Department of Health, Education, and Welfare into two separate departments. The head of the agency is the Secretary of Health and Human Services, who fills a Cabinet post and acts in an advisory capacity to the president in matters of health. The Office of the Secretary incorporates several offices. One of primary interest to community health nurses is the Office of Public Health and Science (OPHS), which was added to the division in 1996. The responsibilities of this agency include national public health needs assessment and leadership in population-based health care and preventive services. Agencies within OPHS are presented in Table 5-1◆. OPHS also oversees the provision

of services by the U.S. Public Health Services Commissioned Corps, an agency that provides health care personnel to meet the needs of specific underserved populations (Office of Public Health and Science, 2004).

Health-related agencies within the DHHS include the Administration on Aging, Administration for Children and Families, Agency for Healthcare Research and Quality, Agency for Toxic Substances and Disease Registry, Centers for Disease Control and Prevention, and the Centers for Medicare and Medicaid Services (formerly the Health Care Financing Administration) (USDHHS, 2004). Other health-related agencies in the department are the Food and Drug Administration, Health Resources and Services Administration, Indian Health Service, National Institutes of Health, Program Support Center, and the Substance Abuse and Mental Health Services Administration. These agencies, along with their primary functions and Internet addresses, are presented in Table 5-2◆.

Although the DHHS is the agency primarily responsible for national health, other agencies within the federal government are also involved in addressing health issues. For example, the Department of Defense provides health care for military personnel, dependents, and retirees, and the Department of the Interior addresses health concerns related to environmental pollution. Similarly, the Department of Labor is concerned with occupational health as well as other employment concerns, and the Treasury Department is actively involved in efforts to control drugs subject to abuse.

TABLE 5-1	Agencies within the Office of Public Health and Science
Agency	**Function**
National Vaccine Program Office (NVPO) http://www.hhs.gov/nvpo	Provide information on childhood, adolescent, and adult immunizations
Office of Disease Prevention and Health Promotion (ODPHP) http://odphp.osophs.dhhs.gov	Strengthen disease prevention and health promotion priorities of DHHS
Office of HIV/AIDS Policy (OHAP) http://www.osophs.dhhs.gov/aids/ohaphome.html	Advise HHS officials regarding HIV/AIDS policy, priorities, and program implementation
Office for Human Research Protections (OHRP) http://www.hhs.gov/ohrp	Provide leadership and oversight in the protection of human subjects in research
Office of Minority Health (OMH) http://www.cdc.gov/omh	Improve and protect the health of minority populations through development of policies and programs to eliminate disparities
Office of Population Affairs (OPA) http://opa.osophs.dhhs.gov	Advise HHS officials regarding reproductive and other population issues; oversee federal family planning and adolescent family life programs
Office of Research Integrity (ORI) http://ori.dhhs.gov	Promote integrity in federally funded biomedical and behavioral research
Office of the Surgeon General (OSG) http://www.surgeongeneral.gov	Oversee U.S. Public Health Service Commissioned Corps activities and provide support for other activities of the Surgeon General
Office on Women's Health (OWH) http://www.4woman.gov/owh	Redress inequities in research, health care services, and education for women
President's Council on Physical Fitness and Sports (PCPFS) http://www.fitness.gov	Promote population physical activity and sports participation
Regional Health Administrators (RHA) http://phs.os.dhhs.gov/ophs.rha.htm	Administer operations of 10 regional offices of the U.S. Public Health Services

TABLE 5-2 Agencies within the Department of Health and Human Services

Agency	Function
Administration for Children and Families (ACF) http://www.acf.hhs.gov	Promote the economic and social well-being of families, children, individuals, and communities
Administration on Aging (AoA) http://www.aoa.gov	Promote the dignity and health of older Americans and help society prepare for an aging population
Agency for Healthcare Research and Quality (AHRQ) http://www.ahrq.gov	Improve the quality, safety, efficiency, and effectiveness of health care for all Americans
Agency for Toxic Substances and Disease Registry (ATSDR) http://www.atsdr.cdc.gov	Prevent harmful exposures and disease related to toxic substances
Centers for Disease Control and Prevention (CDC) http://www.cdc.gov	Promote health and quality of life by preventing and controlling disease, injury, and disability
Centers for Medicare and Medicaid Services (CMS) (former Health Care Financing Administration—HCFA) http://www.cms.hhs.gov	Manage federal health care programs under Medicare and Medicaid
Food and Drug Administration (FDA) http://www.fda.gov	Protect the public health by assuring the safety, efficacy, and security of human and veterinary drugs, biological products, medical devices, national food supply, cosmetics, and products that emit radiation
Health Resources and Services Administration (HRSA) http://www.hrsa.gov	Improve and expand access to quality health care for all by eliminating barriers to care, eliminating health disparities, assuring quality of care, and improving public health and health care systems
Indian Health Service (IHS) http://www.ihs.gov	Raise the physical, mental, social, and spiritual health of American Indians and Alaska Natives to the highest level
National Institutes of Health (NIH) http://www.nih.gov	Acquire new knowledge to help prevent, detect, diagnose, and treat disease and disability
Program Support Center (PSC) http://www.psc.gov	Provide administrative support to operating divisions within DHHS to permit them to concentrate on their primary functions
Substance Abuse and Mental Health Services Administration (SAMHSA) http://www.samhsa.gov	Improve the lives of people with or at risk for mental and substance abuse disorders

Federal health-related agencies have a variety of responsibilities as outlined by the Institute of Medicine. These include supporting research and dissemination of health-related information, developing national objectives and priorities for health, and assurance related to actions and services in the interests of national public health. In addition, the federal government provides assistance to state agencies in the form of technical assistance and funding to support state health initiatives (Scutchfield & Last, 2003). One of the major ways in which the federal government enacts its knowledge development and dissemination function is through the activities of the National Institutes of Health (NIH). NIH consists of the Office of the Director, 19 research institutes, 7 centers, and the National Library of Medicine. The institutes and many of the centers fund and conduct research related to specific health problems, conditions, and susceptible populations. Figure 5-4 depicts the component parts of NIH.

OUTCOMES OF CARE

Outcomes achieved by health care delivery systems can be examined in terms of the level of care involved. In public health, practitioners use the concept of levels of prevention to examine levels of care and health care outcomes. The three levels of prevention are similar to those incorporated into the dimensions of health care within the dimensions model of community health nursing described in Chapter 4∞ and consist of primary, secondary, and tertiary prevention.

Access to health care, as an outcome of public health practice, is related to the core function of assurance as well as to all three levels of prevention. With respect to primary prevention, access involves the ability of the population to obtain goods and services necessary to promote health and prevent illness. For example, at this level access would include the availability of immunization services. Issues of access may also affect achievement of desired outcomes of secondary and tertiary prevention interventions. For example, if people in rural areas do not have access to prompt emergency services, a secondary prevention activity, the potential for surviving severe trauma or myocardial infarction declines. In addition to preventing these events from occurring, an effective health care system would limit the number of fatalities that accompany these events when they do occur. Similarly, lack of access to rehabilitative services at the tertiary level of prevention will lead to poor outcomes with respect to the prevalence of long-term consequences of trauma or the incidence of recurrent subsequent myocardial infarctions.

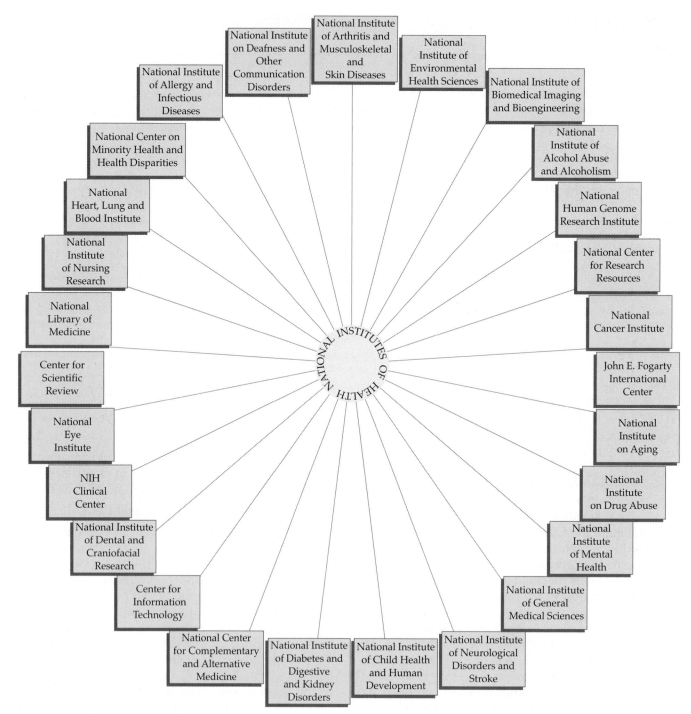

FIGURE 5-4 Major Components of the National Institutes of Health

Despite, or possibly because of, its complexity, the U.S. health care system does not achieve the level of favorable health outcomes at any of the three levels of prevention that one might expect given the proportion of the gross domestic product allocated to health care. For example, the World Bank has cited the United States as having the worst health outcomes relative to expenditures among developed nations (Studnicki et al., 2002). According to the World Health Organization, the United States ranks 20th in maternal mortality, with 20% of

pregnant women hospitalized for complications prior to delivery and 31% for complications sustained during labor and delivery (Snavely, 2004). Although some progress has been made in preventing illness and injury and in treating and preventing complications from existing health problems, much remains to be done at all levels of prevention. It is possible that accomplishing such progress will require significant changes in health care delivery in the United States, even to the point of moving toward establishing a national health care system.

MediaLink Case Study: Ideal Health Care System

A NATIONAL HEALTH CARE SYSTEM?

Given the failure of the current health care system to achieve desired outcomes at all three levels of prevention and its failure to provide care for significant segments of the population, there is a new call for health care reform. As one author noted, in comparison with other national health care systems that accomplish better outcomes with lower expenditures, "the US health care system is richly funded but designed so that it maximizes waste, inefficiency, and inequity" (Light, 2003, p. 25).

The Institute of Medicine (IOM) (2001) has suggested that a redesigned health care system in the United States should address six specific aims for improvement:

- Safety: avoiding injury resulting from the care provided
- Effectiveness: providing evidence-based services to those who can benefit from them and withholding services from those who are not likely to benefit
- Patient-centeredness: responding to individual preferences, values, and needs and ensuring that client values guide clinical decision making
- Timeliness: reducing waits and delays in services provided
- Efficiency: avoiding waste of resources
- Equity: providing care of the same quality to all people, regardless of gender, ethnicity, geographic location, or socioeconomic status. (p. 40)

Furthermore, the Institute's Committee on Quality of Health Care in America established a set of 10 rules that should guide redesign of health care processes. The first rule is that care should be based on continuous healing relationships in force 24 hours a day, 7 days a week, and provided in a variety of modalities, including the Internet and telephone, as well as in face-to-face interactions with providers. Second, care should be individualized based on client needs and values. Third, clients should control health care decisions that affect them. The fourth rule addresses the need for clients to have complete access to their own medical information and for clients and providers to communicate effectively and share information. Fifth, care should be based on "the best available scientific knowledge" and should not "vary illogically from clinician to clinician or from place to place." Sixth, as noted above, safety should be a consistent system property, with safeguards to prevent and mitigate errors. The seventh rule deals with the need for transparency and the availability of information that allows clients and families to make informed decisions in the selection of providers and health plans. Eighth, the health system should anticipate needs rather than react to their manifestation. The ninth rule reinforces the aim of efficiency noted above in that the system should not waste either resources or clients' valuable time. Finally, there should be effective communication and cooperation among providers and institutions to promote information exchange and coordination of care (IOM, 2001, pp. 8–9).

The present debate, as in the past, revolves around what direction health care reform should take to address the aims proposed by the IOM. Some nursing authors suggest that redesign could take one of two avenues, universal payment or universal care. Universal payment would make funds available for health services, assuming that services would then be available and would be used. Approaches to universal payment for health care might include a national tax similar to the current Social Security tax or a multiple-payer system with funding derived from a variety of sources including employer contributions, existing systems such as Medicare and Medicaid, and taxes and general revenues. The second avenue to universal coverage would be universal care, in which the actual provision of care would occur in a national health system or state-based systems (Gebbie, 2002).

Such proposals pose the main question: Should the United States move to a single-payer form of national health insurance, or engage in incremental reform? Many public health experts advocate a single-payer approach, which would mean radical change within the health care system. They describe key features of a single-payer (e.g., the federal government) system as:

- Universal and comprehensive coverage of the population
- No out-of-pocket costs for consumers
- Public administration at regional levels to minimize administrative duplication and waste and prevent two-class coverage between public and private insurance
- Global operating budgets for major health care institutions (e.g., hospitals, nursing homes, MCOs) with separate allocations for capital expenditures (e.g., building, major equipment purchases) to eliminate the cost and complexity of per-client billing procedures
- Free choice of providers and the ability to seek care from any licensed provider without penalty
- Public accountability and public involvement in policy development, but medical decisions reached between provider and client
- A ban on provision of health care on a for-profit basis
- Retraining and new positions for thousands of health care and insurance workers (e.g., insurance agents, billing clerks) who would be displaced by a single-payer plan. (Himmelstein & Woolhandler, 2003, p. 102)

Other authors advocate an incremental approach to health care reform that will "accommodate the realities of

CULTURAL COMPETENCE

What traditional features of the dominant American culture would make it difficult for much of the U.S. public to accept a single national health care system similar to that of some other nations? Might such a system be more easily accepted by members of ethnic minority groups residing in the United States than by the dominant population? Why or why not?

the American health care system and resist the temptation to propose radical restructuring" (Tooker, 2003, p. 106). They base their reasoning on what they label the seven "realities" of health care delivery in the United States. These realities include a perception that most Americans are satisfied with their current care and would be suspicious of major change and a recognition of partisan politics as impeding achievement of a single-payer program. These partisan political views derive from differences of opinion regarding the role that government should play in health affairs, with Democrats favoring a more active role than Republicans. A third reality is the geographic, ethnic, cultural, and medical diversity of the country and the perception that a single-payer plan could not address the resulting diversity of needs. Reluctance of the population to depend on large, government-run systems for vital services such as health is touted as a fourth reality. Fifth, consumers will expect to see a clear advantage for themselves in any change. Although a single-payer plan would address the needs of the nearly 46 million uninsured residents, it might not be viewed by the rest of the public as resulting in a personal improvement in care. A sixth reality is the necessity for any reform proposal to be clearly communicated to the public so that the overall effects can be anticipated. Finally, the author notes that strong leadership will be required for any level of reform in the health care system (Tooker, 2003). This author and others suggest a multifaceted approach to reform that "builds on the strengths of the current pluralistic system by combining the benefits of public health plans such as Medicaid and the State Children's Health Insurance Program (SCHIP) with a more competitive and affordable private insurance market" (Tooker, 2003, p. 107). They also suggest increasing insurance coverage by making it more affordable through expansion of public programs to selected groups and providing subsidies and tax credits for purchasing commercial insurance.

Whatever the approach taken to health care reform in the United States, it is clear that reform is needed. It is equally clear that reform should be based on specific principles and goals. The Rekindling Reform Steering Committee (2003), an affiliation of health policy makers from professional, governmental, and educational organizations, has developed a set of six principles and 24 goals to guide reform in establishing an equitable, humane, and cost-effective health care system. These principles and goals are summarized in Table 5-3◆.

TABLE 5-3 Principles and Goals of Health Care Reform

Principles of Health Care Reform

- Access to care should be provided to all without financial hardship.
- A full range of services needed to prevent illness and improve health should be available to all.
- Health care costs should be controlled and affordability assured through:
  - Distributing financial risk across the entire population
  - Reducing paperwork and administrative costs
  - Emphasizing prevention and community-based primary care
- Program administration should be simplified and sensibly organized.
- The system should be accountable and responsive to the health care needs of the public.
- The system should integrate a strong public health component that guarantees preventive and social services and creation of environments conducive to health.

Goals of Health Care Reform

- Guaranteed universal access to care
- Nondiscrimination based on race, gender, or sexual orientation
- Elimination of health disparities
- Provision of care to individuals and groups with special needs including underserved rural and urban populations
- Provision, in appropriate settings, of comprehensive benefits (medications, rehabilitation, dental and vision care, mental health services, occupational and long-term care, and complementary therapies) that preclude the need for supplemental insurance coverage
- Parity for mental health and other services

- Promotion of prevention and early intervention
- Continuity of coverage and continuity of care
- Consumer choice of providers
- Promotion of quality health care and achievement of better outcomes of care
- Elimination of duplication in coverage
- Affordability
- Progressive financing based on income
- Cost efficiency, with maximal expenditure on services and minimal expenditure on administrative costs
- Ease of use for both clients and providers
- Provision of an adequate health care workforce
- Structuring of the health care workforce to prevent fatigue and burnout
- Promotion of affirmative action in training and employing health care providers to address the needs of underserved populations
- Fair and equitable reimbursement for health care providers and other health workers
- Development of a strong network of nonprofit facilities, including safety net providers
- Effective consumer education regarding rights and responsibilities related to health
- Ongoing evaluation and planning to improve services, with input from clients, providers, and other stakeholders
- Public input and debate on policy development
- Publicly accountable mechanisms for organization and administration of services

Data from: Rekindling Reform Steering Committee. (2003). Rekindling reform: Principles and goals. American Journal of Public Health, 93, 115–117.

As we will see in Chapter 6∞, other nations have adopted approaches to health care delivery vastly different from that of the United States. Although the health care systems of these nations differ markedly from each other, they have in common universal coverage, reduced costs, and, in many instances, better outcomes than the U.S. system.

Case Study

The Ideal Health Care System

Design a health care delivery system that would meet the health needs of the American public. Diagram the organizational structure of the system, making sure that your system addresses the core functions of public health as well as the goals of medical care. Address the following questions:

1. What features (if any) would you incorporate from other national health care delivery systems (see Chapter 6∞) ?
2. How would you fund your system? How would health care providers be reimbursed? Why?
3. Would you offer comprehensive health care services? What would be included in the basic health services package? Would this basic coverage be available to all residents? Why or why not?
4. How would your system address the three levels of prevention? Would one level receive priority over the others? Why or why not?
5. What political, economic, and social changes would need to occur before your proposed system could be implemented in the United States?

Test Your Understanding

1. What is the popular health care subsystem? What is the role of the community health nurse with respect to this subsystem? (p. 85)

2. How do complementary and alternative subsystems of care differ? Give an example of each. (pp. 85–86)

3. What are the six fundamental obligations of official public health agencies? (p. 87)

4. Diagram the organizational structure of the U.S. health care delivery system. Describe the interactions between the component parts. (pp. 85–96)

5. Compare and contrast official and voluntary health agencies. What interactions occur between them? (pp. 87–90)

6. Describe five functions performed by voluntary health agencies. Give an example of each. (p. 90)

7. What are the 10 essential public health services? How might they be carried out differently by local, state, and national public health agencies? (p. 89)

8. How are local, state, and national governments involved in health care delivery? In what ways is this involvement similar? How does it differ between levels? (pp. 91–95)

9. Give at least one example of a primary, a secondary, and a tertiary prevention outcome of care. (pp. 95–96)

10. What are some of the approaches suggested for health system reform? What are the advantages and disadvantages of each approach? (pp. 97–98)

EXPLORE MediaLink

http://www.prenhall.com/clark
Resources for this chapter can be found on the Companion Website.

Audio Glossary	MediaLink Applications: Educating about	Challenge Your Knowledge
Exam Review Questions	Obesity (Video)	Advocacy Interviews
Case Study: Designing the Ideal Health	Media Links	
Care System		

References

Bonita, R., Winkelmann, R., Douglas, K. A., & de Courten, M. (2003). The WHO stepwise approach to surveillance (STEPS) of non-communicable disease risk factors. In D. V. McQueen & P. Puska (Eds.), *Global behavioral risk factor surveillance* (pp. 9–22). New York: Kluwer Academic/Plenum.

Brandt, A. M., & Gardner, M. (2000). Antagonism and accommodation: Interpreting the relationship between public health and medicine in the United States during the 20th century. *American Journal of Public Health, 90,* 707–715.

Brenner, N. D., Kann, L., Kinchen, S. A., Grunbaum, J. A., Whalen, L., Eaton, D., et al. (2004). Methodology of the Youth Risk Behavior Surveillance System. *Morbidity and Mortality Weekly Report, 53*(RR-12), 1–13.

Budrys, G. (2001). *Our unsystematic health system.* Lanham, MD: Rowman & Littlefield.

Communication from the City Auditor regarding tuberculosis nurse. (1915, August 20). San Diego, CA: City of San Diego Archives.

Council on Linkages Between Academia and Public Health Practice. (2001). *Core competencies for public health professionals.* Washington, DC: Public Health Foundation.

Drevdahl, D. (2002). Social justice or market justice? The paradoxes of public health partnerships with managed care. *Public Health Nursing, 19,* 161–169.

Families USA. (2004). *Census Bureau's uninsured number indicates third increase in a row.* Retrieved August 30, 2004, from http://familiesusa.org/site/PageServer?pagename=Media_Statement_Census2003

Families USA. (2005). *Census Bureau's uninsured number indicates fourth increase in a row.* Retrieved December 15, 2005, from http://familiesusa.org/site/resources/newsroom/statements/census-bureau-uninsured-number

Gebbie, K. M. (2002). Could a national health system work in the United States? In D. J. Mason, J. K. Leavitt, & M. W. Chaffee (Eds.), *Policy and politics in nursing and health care* (4th ed., pp. 214–217). St. Louis, MO: Saunders.

Himmelstein, D. U., & Woolhandler, S. (2003). National health insurance or incremental reform: Aim high or at our feet? *American Journal of Public Health, 93,* 102–105.

Holtzman, D. (2003). Analysis and interpretation of data from the U.S. Behavioral Risk Factor Surveillance System (BRFSS). In D. V. McQueen & P. Puska (Eds.), *Global behavioral risk factor surveillance* (pp. 35–46). New York: Kluwer Academic/Plenum.

Institute of Medicine, Committee on Quality of Health Care in America. (2001). *Cross the quality chasm: A new health system for the 21st century.* Washington, DC: National Academy Press.

Institute of Medicine. (2003a). *Hidden costs, value lost: Uninsurance in America.* Washington, DC: National Academies Press.

Institute of Medicine, Committee on Assuring the Health of the Public in the 21st Century. (2003b). *The future of the public's health in the 21st century.* Washington, DC: National Academies Press.

Jonas, S. (2003). *An introduction to the U.S. health care system* (5th ed.). New York: Springer.

Keller, L. O., Strohschein, S., Lia-Hoagberg, B., & Schaffer, M. A. (2004). Population-based public health interventions: Practice-based and evidence-supported. Part I. *Public Health Nursing, 21,* 453–468.

Light, D. W. (2003). Universal health care: Lessons from the British experience. *American Journal of Public Health, 93,* 25–30.

Little Hoover Commission, State of California. (2003). *To protect and prevent: Rebuilding California's public health system.* Sacramento, CA: Author.

May, K. M., Phillips, L. R., Ferketich, S. L., & Verran, J. (2003). Public health nursing: The generalist in a specialized environment. *Public Health Nursing, 20,* 252–259.

Mays, G. P., Halverson, P. K., Baker, E. L., Stevens, R., & Vann, J. J. (2004). Availability and perceived effectiveness of public health activities in the nation's most populous communities. *American Journal of Public Health, 94,* 1019–1026.

McMichael, T., & Beaglehole, R. (2003). The global context for public health. In R. Beaglehole (Ed.), *Global public health: A new era* (pp. 1-23). Oxford, UK: Oxford University.

McQueen, D. V. (2003). Perspectives on global risk factor surveillance: Lessons learned and challenges ahead. In D. V. McQueen & P. Puska (Eds.), *Global behavioral risk factor surveillance* (pp. 233–245). New York: Kluwer Academic/Plenum.

Missouri Department of Health. (n.d.). *Public health nurse's role in core functions.* Retrieved October 3, 2002, from http://www.state.mo.us/Publications/100-35.html

Mokdad, A. H., Stroup, D. F., & Giles, W. H. (2003). Public health surveillance for behavioral risk factors in a changing environment: Recommendations from the Behavioral Risk Factor Surveillance Team. *Morbidity and Mortality Weekly Report, 52*(RR-9), 1–11.

National Public Health Performance Standards Program. (n.d.a). *National Public Health Performance Standards.* Retrieved May 7, 2001, from http://www.phppo.cdc.gov/nphpsp

National Public Health Performance Standards Program. (n.d.b). *National Public Health Performance Standards Program home page.* Retrieved November 11, 2001, from http://www.phppo.cdc.gov/nphpsp/phdpp/10es.htm

Office of Public Health and Science. (2004). OPHS Offices. Retrieved October 7, 2004, from http://phs.os.dhhs.gov

Patel, K., & Rushefsky, M. E. (2002). The Canadian health care system. In K. V. Thai, E. T. Wimberley, & S. M. McManus (Eds.), *Handbook of international health care systems* (pp. 79–98). New York: Marcel Dekker.

Powles, J., & Comim, F. (2003). Public health infrastructure and knowledge. In R. D. Smith, R. Beaglehole, D. Woodward, & N. Drager (Eds.), *Global public goods for health: Health economic and public health perspectives* (pp. 159–173). Oxford, UK: Oxford University.

Rekindling Reform Steering Committee. (2003). Rekindling reform: Principles and goals. *American Journal of Public Health, 93,* 115–117.

Schneider, M. A. (2000). *Introduction to public health.* Gaithersburg, MD: Aspen.

Scutchfield, F. D., & Last, J. M. (2003). Public health in North America. In R. Beaglehole (Ed.), *Global public health: A new era.* New York: Oxford University.

Snavely, F. D. (2004, Spring). Maternal morbidity and mortality. *Prenatal Care Matters,* 1–2.

Sorenson, S. B. (2003). Funding public health: The public's willingness to pay for domestic violence prevention programming. *American Journal of Public Health, 93,* 1934–1938.

Studnicki, J., Murphy, F. V., Malvey, D., Costello, R. A., Luther, S. L., & Werner, D. C. (2002). Toward a population health delivery system: First steps in performance measurement. *Health Care Management Review, 27*(1), 76–95.

Sultz, H. A., & Young, K. M. (2004). *Health care USA: Understanding its organization and delivery* (4th ed.). Sudbury, MA: Jones and Bartlett.

Tooker, J. (2003). Affordable health insurance for all is possible by means of a pragmatic approach. *American Journal of Public Health, 93,* 106–109.

U.S. Department of Health and Human Services. (2000). *Healthy people 2010* (Conference edition, in two volumes). Washington, DC: Author.

U.S. Department of Health and Human Services. (2004). *About HHS.* Retrieved October 7, 2004, from http://dhhs.gov

Wimberley, E. T., & Rubens, A. J. (2002). Like plugging the holes in the colander: Health policy and provision in the United States circa the millennium. In K. V. Thai, E. T. Wimberley, & S. M. McManus (Eds.), *Handbook of international health care systems* (pp. 135–206). New York: Marcel Dekker.

Wimberley, E. T., & Thai, K. V. (2002). Introduction to international health systems: Themes and variations on themes. In K. V. Thai, E. T. Wimberley, & S. M. McManus (Eds.), *Handbook of international health care systems* (pp. 1–28). New York: Marcel Dekker.

World Health Organization. (2000). *The world health report 2000: Health systems: Improving performance.* Geneva, Switzerland: Author.

CHAPTER

The Global Context

CHAPTER OBJECTIVES

After reading this chapter, you should be able to:

1. Discuss the advantages of U.S. involvement in global health initiatives.
2. Identify at least five policy dilemmas faced by national health care systems.
3. Compare selected features of national health care systems.
4. Describe two types of international health agencies.
5. Distinguish between international and global health.
6. Discuss positive and negative health effects of globalization.
7. Identify elements of a global health policy agenda.
8. Describe community health nursing involvement with respect to international terrorism.

KEY TERMS

agroterrorism **129**
bilateral agencies **111**
Declaration of Alma Alta **119**
disability-adjusted life expectancy (DALE) **110**
disability-adjusted life years (DALYs) **125**
domestic terrorism **127**
elimination **120**
eradication **120**
global health **111**
global health policy **117**
globalization **103**
gross domestic product (GDP) **105**
"health for all by the year 2000" **119**
health-adjusted life expectancy (HALE) **109**
International Council of Nurses (ICN) **130**

international health **111**
international terrorism **128**
multilateral agencies **111**
non-governmental organizations (NGOs) **113**
Pan American Health Organization (PAHO) **112**
primary health care (PHC) **119**
sector-wide approaches (SWAPs) **114**
Sigma Theta Tau International **130**
terrorism **127**
World Health Organization (WHO) **111**

 MediaLink
http://www.prenhall.com/clark

Additional interactive resources for this chapter can be found on the Companion Website. Click on Chapter 6 and "Begin" to select the activities for this chapter.

Advocacy in Action

Cross-border Advocacy

A bilingual community health nurse received a referral to follow up on a 17-year-old immigrant who refused to go to a children's hospital to rule out a possible life-threatening disease. When the nurse visited, she discovered that the immigrant and her spouse had limited language and literacy skills as well as strong cultural and religious beliefs related to health and the use of herbal medicines and traditional healers. Both had little understanding of the disease and its treatment. They were experiencing economic difficulties and were living in an old trailer in the back of a house that lacked a bathroom or phone.

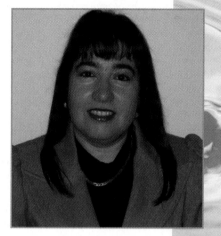

The couple were initially resistant to services. The nurse offered to help with the state Children's Services application, provided referrals for clothing, food, and a gift card, and scheduled an appointment with WIC. The following week the hospital wanted to schedule an appointment with a specialist. The PHN explained the need for medical care and the couple agreed to go. The hospital was contacted and arrangements were made, including transportation to the clinic. The PHN contacted Children's Services, and a community worker (CW) agreed to meet with the client at the clinic.

The next day the children's hospital was unable to contact the client concerning admission over the weekend, due to the client's lack of a telephone, and contacted the PHN for assistance. The nurse also called the client's consulate for help with required documents and transportation. Consulate staff agreed to follow up in the client's country for the necessary documentation and to locate the client's family in their remote village. Eventually the client was admitted to the children's hospital, and diagnosis and appropriate treatment were provided. Because of the client's precarious condition, the nurse continued to function as a liaison with all the agencies involved.

Claudia Pineda Benton, BSN, RN, BC

Public Health Nurse

We live in a small world that can be circumnavigated in a matter of hours, increasing the potential for the spread of disease, ideas, and technological advances. Today you are a nursing student in one country; 6 months or a year from now you may be working or vacationing in another. Or you may be caring for a client from a distant part of the world. Health problems cross national boundaries, and their solutions will need to cross boundaries as well. For all these reasons, community health nurses need to be well versed in the global context in which health problems arise and health care is delivered.

U.S. INVOLVEMENT IN GLOBAL HEALTH

Daily, the world is becoming more interconnected on many levels, and the rate of interconnection is increasing. This chapter addresses the global aspects of health, those that affect human beings across national boundaries and around the world. **Globalization** is defined as a "complex process of increasing economic, political, and social interdependence which takes place as capital, traded goods, persons, concepts, images, ideas, and values diffuse across states' boundaries" (Taylor, Bettcher, & Peck, 2003, p. 213). Globalization results in worldwide social interactions and is increasingly contributing to organizations and institutions that cross political boundaries. Increasing exchange related to economics, technology, and cultural attitudes, values, and practices has occurred as a result of the compression of time and space through technology

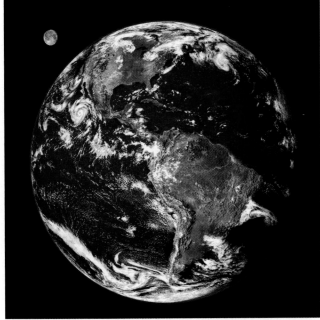

Many health concerns transcend national boundaries and require international cooperation. (© Photri/Topham/The Image Works)

(Doyal, 2004). More and more, global solutions must be sought to global problems of health and health care delivery.

The Centers for Disease Control and Prevention (CDC, 2003) has identified several reasons why the United States should be actively involved in global health initiatives. The first reason is to protect the U.S. public from the threat of communicable diseases, both at home and while traveling outside of the country. For example, in 2000 alone, 477 million people traveled into and out of the United States. At the same time, 127 million cars, 11.5 million trucks, and 5.8 million maritime containers entered the country, all of them posing the potential for the spread of a variety of communicable diseases (Fox & Kassalow, 2001). A second reason, and one that has motivated much of American involvement to date, is an interest in humanitarian efforts. Third, resolution of global health problems will lead to both economic and diplomatic benefits for the United States. Improved health will contribute to global prosperity through investment in the world's human capital and the ability of members of other nations to work more productively (Perkins, 2002b). This, in turn, will enhance the U.S. economy by opening markets for U.S.-produced goods. Similarly, U.S. participation in global health initiatives will improve international trust and reap diplomatic benefits. Finally, this increased trust and the defusing of hatreds among disadvantaged populations of the world is expected to enhance U.S. security, particularly in the face of growing threats of international terrorism (CDC, 2003). Threats to security may be conceptualized more broadly than threats of conflict or terrorist activity. As one author put it, "If one of the primary aims of the state is to protect the lives of its citizens, then risks to security can come in many forms other than those from conventional warfare" (Altman, 2003, p. 33). Such security risks include global health issues such as environmental degradation, refugee flows, and the spread of infectious diseases mentioned above, and there is a growing recognition of health issues as threats to national security broadly defined (Altman, 2003).

CDC's priorities for involvement in global health care initiatives include the following:

- Response to international disease outbreaks, with assistance in
  - Diagnostic capabilities
  - Epidemiologic analysis
  - Follow-up
- Global disease surveillance
- Research on global health problems
- Development and dissemination of new public health approaches
- Contributions to global disease control initiatives
- Training and capacity building for public health. (CDC, 2003)

ESSENTIAL PUBLIC HEALTH FUNCTIONS: AN INTERNATIONAL PERSPECTIVE

In Chapter 5∞, we examined the core functions and essential public health services developed for the U.S. health care system. Similar descriptions have been developed elsewhere in the world. For example, key areas of specialist public health practice in the United Kingdom have been identified as surveillance and assessment; health promotion and protection; quality and risk management assessment; collaboration; health program development, particularly to address health inequalities; and policy development. Additional key functions include community engagement, strategic leadership for health, research and development, and ethical management of oneself, personnel, and resources (Griffiths, 2003).

At a more international level, the Pan American Health Organization (PAHO, 2002) developed a list of essential functions based on the need for "collective intervention by the State and civil society to protect and improve the health of the people" (p. 3). Public health functions are defined by PAHO (2002) as "the set of functions that should be carried out specifically to achieve the central objective of public health: improving the health of populations" (p. 3). Public health functions can be *final*, those that contribute directly to the meeting of health goals, or *instrumental*, those that create the conditions that permit the achievement of health goals. The essential functions and related public health activities are presented in Table 6-1◆.

TABLE 6-1	Essential Public Health Functions of National Health Systems, Pan American Health Organization
Function	**Related Activities**
Monitoring, evaluation, and analysis of health status	▪ Identification of population health status and health needs and contributing factors ▪ Evaluation of health system performance ▪ Resource assessment ▪ Development of information technology
Surveillance, research, and control of risks and threats to public health	▪ Research and surveillance of disease patterns, outbreaks, and risk factors ▪ Development of infrastructure for population screening activities ▪ Provision of laboratory services ▪ Linking with international networks for rapid response
Health promotion	▪ Promotion of lifestyle changes and an environment conducive to a culture of health ▪ Education of the public for health ▪ Reorientation of the health system to a health promotion focus
Social participation in health	▪ Facilitation of community participation in policy formation
Development of policy and institutional capacity for planning and management in public health	▪ Definition of national and subnational health objectives ▪ Development, management, and assessment of health policy ▪ Capacity building for international cooperation for health
Strengthening of institutional capacity for regulation and enforcement in public health	▪ Development of regulatory and enforcement frameworks to protect the public's health ▪ Ensuring compliance with public health regulations
Evaluation and promotion of equitable access to necessary health services	▪ Promotion of equitable access to needed services ▪ Elimination or minimization of barriers to access ▪ Monitoring access to services
Human resources training and development in public health	▪ Development of the public health workforce profile needed to carry out essential functions ▪ Definition of licensure requirements ▪ Workforce education ▪ Assuring exposure to public health learning experiences ▪ Development of interdisciplinary and multicultural skills ▪ Provision of bioethics training
Quality assurance in personal and population-based health services	▪ Promotion of quality assessment systems ▪ Development of standards for quality assurance and improvement systems ▪ Development and assurance of user rights ▪ Development of satisfaction assessment systems
Research	▪ Development of knowledge to support policy-related decision making ▪ Development of innovative solutions to public health problems
Reduction of the impact of emergencies and disasters on health	▪ Policy development, planning, and implementation of activities to prevent, mitigate, respond to, and recover from disasters ▪ Development of integrated approaches to disaster management ▪ Increased participation and collaboration in disaster planning and response

Data from: Pan American Health Organization. (2002). Public health in the Americas: Conceptual renewal, performance assessment, and bases for action. Washington, DC: Author.

COMPARING NATIONAL HEALTH SYSTEMS

Nations throughout the world have developed unique organizational structures for delivering health care services to their peoples. Although no two health systems are alike, they tend to have certain commonalities. For example, all health systems are designed to address three major considerations: how services will be funded, how care will be organized and delivered, and how available resources will be channeled from payers to providers (Deber, 2003). In addition, national health systems have to address a number of policy dilemmas. These include balancing the need for regional or national coordination with the requirement to meet local health needs, distributing available resources equitably, providing necessary services without impeding the work of the voluntary health sector, balancing professional practice autonomy with accountability for population health outcomes, integrating primary care with hospital and specialty services, reconciling individual practice patterns with national standards and systems, and balancing individual client and population foci with limited resources (Light, 2003). Additional dilemmas faced by national health systems include assuring access to care in the face of cost constraints, balancing curative technology with allocations for prevention and promotion, maintaining a qualified health care workforce, ensuring community participation in policy making, and reaching hard-to-serve populations (Fried & Gaydos, 2002).

Unique features of selected health care systems in other countries indicate the many approaches that can be taken to address the considerations and dilemmas presented above. Features to be explored include the locus of decision making, expenditures, funding mechanisms, professional autonomy, coverage and access, health outcomes, and consumer satisfaction.

Locus of Decision Making

One area in which national health systems differ is the degree to which decision making is centralized or decentralized. In some countries (e.g., the United Kingdom, Japan), the health care system is highly centralized, with the majority of health care policy decisions made at the federal level (Gaydos & Fried, 2002). In Canada, on the other hand, the federal government sets general principles, which are then operationalized by each province as it sees fit (Deber, 2003; Patel & Rushefsky, 2002). Germany also has initiated a number of national principles that are implemented by the personal health care sector (Swami, 2002). In Australia, some components of the health system are administered by the central Commonwealth government, whereas others, such as hospitals, are operated by the states and territories (Davis & Lin, 2003). Japan, like the United Kingdom, has a highly centralized health care system, with the majority of policy

made at the national government level (Yajima & Takayanagi, 2002). The Russian Federation, which under communism had the epitome of a centralized system, has adopted a mandatory system of national health insurance. Although many institutions are still government owned and publicly financed, recent legislative changes permit regional decisions on resource allocation with central ministry approval (Bourhanskaia, Kubataev, & Paterson, 2002). In the United States, the foci for health care policy development are so many and varied that the health care system has been described as "hyperpluralist," with decisions made at local, state, and national government levels as well as at the level of the organization, provider, or client.

Recently, many European governments have looked to decentralize some portions of their health care systems, promoting decision making at regional or municipal levels. Decentralization has the advantage of tailoring health care delivery to meet the needs of differing populations. Centralization, on the other hand, can create impetus for more rational planning and cost control.

To a large extent, decisions about the centralization or decentralization of health care policy making are based on national attitudes and values. The hyperpluralism and lack of centralization of the U.S. health care system, for example, is largely a result of strongly held values of individualism and limited government involvement in everyday life. For this reason, any proposal for a centralized government-operated health care system is likely to encounter resistance from the U.S. population. Other nations place higher priority on communal obligations and solidarity. For example, cultural attitudes in many countries are characterized by a strong sense of mutual dependence and obligation between the sick and the well and across generations (Cruise, 2002; Rodwin, 2003). Health care systems, however they are designed, must support the values and beliefs of the populations served if they are to be effective in achieving established health goals.

Expenditures

Cost control has been a recent concern for health systems in all nations. Some countries, however, are more successful at controlling health care expenditures than others. For example, in 2002, Japan spent only 7.9% of its **gross domestic product (GDP)** (the total monetary value of all goods and services produced by a nation in a given period) on health care, whereas the United States expended 14.6% of its GDP, the highest percentage of any developed nation (World Health Organization [WHO], 2005c). To some extent, these higher expenditures are a result of greater incorporation of technology in health care practice, but also are due to limited control of health care costs. The economic aspects of the U.S. health care delivery system will be discussed in more detail in Chapter 8 ∞.

Most European countries and Canada lie between the United States and Japan in terms of their health care expenditures. Canada, for example, spent 9.6% of its GDP and France 9.7% on health care in 2002, whereas Germany spent 10.9%. The United Kingdom, on the other hand, spent even less than Japan, at 7.7% of the GDP in 1999. Figures for Australia and Russia are 9.5% and 6.2% of GDP, respectively (WHO, 2005c). Despite greater expenditures, health care outcomes are no better, and are sometimes worse, in the United States than elsewhere.

Another cost measure in which national health care systems differ is the percentage of health care expenditures paid out-of-pocket by consumers. Of the nations discussed here, the United Kingdom had the lowest out-of-pocket costs in 2002, at 9% of total health care expenditures, and Russia the highest at 28%. Out-of-pocket expenditures in Australia (20%) were somewhat higher than those in Japan and the United States (16% each) and Canada (15%), whereas those in France and Germany were somewhat lower (10% each) (WHO, 2005c).

Funding Mechanisms

Health care systems also vary widely in terms of the means by which services are funded and providers reimbursed. As we will see in Chapter 8∞, health care funding in the United States is derived from a number of sources, including out-of-pocket payment, private insurance, and federal and state tax dollars. Similarly, providers may be reimbursed on the basis of fee-for-service or flat rates per person or per service provided.

The majority of German health system funding is based on "sickness funds" provided by employers and employees. Statutory funds are of two types, primary funds and substitute funds. Primary funds cover two thirds of the population and include (a) craft funds that cover members of a particular trade or craft, (b) company funds that cover workers in a particular company, and (c) geographically based funds that cover employees of small companies, the unemployed, and those on welfare. Geographically based funds are derived from employers, employees, pension funds for retirees, and local government funds for the poor. Primary sickness funds are managed by employers or craft unions.

Substitute funds, on the other hand, are managed by the members themselves and are of two types. White-collar funds include clerical and professional occupations and managers, and blue-collar funds cover certain occupational categories and geographic regions. Funding for substitute funds is derived from equal contributions by employer and employee. Both primary and substitute funds contract with the regional Association of Sickness Fund Physicians for services based on an annual budget. The associations then reimburse providers based on a nationally determined fee schedule. The sickness funds also negotiate annual lump-sum budgets with local hospitals for operating costs, and capital costs are provided separately out of state budgets. Persons with annual incomes over a certain amount (about $25,000) can choose private insurance coverage, and many covered employees have supplemental private insurance plans. Ambulatory care physicians usually care for a panel of clients enrolled in specific sickness funds and are paid by their associations on a fee-for-service basis. Hospital physicians are salaried and cannot practice outside the hospital,

Many national health care systems incorporate advanced medical technology. (2005 AFP)

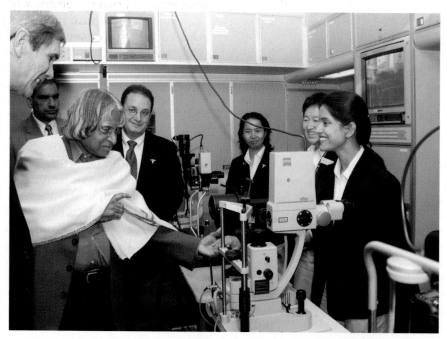

whereas primary care physicians cannot practice within them (Swami, 2002).

Like the U. S. Constitution, the Canadian Constitution assigned primary responsibility for the health of the population to the provinces rather than to the federal government (Deber, 2003). Initially, the Canadian national health care system "Medicare" was funded equally by federal and provincial revenues. Since 1977, however, the federal government has gradually reduced its contribution. For the most part, funds are derived from general tax revenues, although some provinces support the program by payroll taxes or insurance premiums. Hospitals are paid an annual lump sum by provincial governments, but physicians are reimbursed on a fee-for-service basis at rates negotiated between the provincial government and regional medical associations. There is a growing market for private insurance coverage and private for-profit hospitals, creating a "fast, deluxe service for those who pay" and a two-tiered delivery system (Patel & Rushefsky, 2002).

In the United Kingdom, health care system funding is largely derived from federal tax revenues (86%), and payroll taxes for employers and employees contribute another 12%; only 2% of funds are derived from user charges (Bloor & Maynard, 2002). System reforms in 1991 created General Practitioner (GP) fundholders (general practices with a certain number of clients) that were given a budget to provide services and/or contract for them with secondary providers. Changes also made hospitals independent trusts that contract with local health authorities and GP fundholders to provide hospital services. These changes, initiated to promote internal competition, have had somewhat limited success. More recent reforms increased the national health insurance tax to better fund services and organized GPs into geographically based primary care trusts that also provide community and public health services (Light, 2003).

One of the major criticisms of both the Canadian and British systems is the long wait for elective specialty care. However, private-sector care is available for those who can pay. Approximately 11.5% of the population has private health insurance. In 1999, only 7% of health care expenditures in the United Kingdom were spent on private care, whereas 86% of care was provided by the National Health Service. Physicians are primarily salaried, most on a capitated basis, with some fee-for-service payments and a basic practice allowance (Bloor & Maynard, 2002).

France's national health system was lauded by the World Health Organization as the most effective system in the world. It is part of a social security system that includes pensions, family allowances, and workplace accident coverage as well as health insurance. The system is administered by three main funds, one for salaried workers that covers 84% of the population, one for independent professionals, and one for farmers and other agricultural workers. Insurance plans differ somewhat for different occupation groups, but all conform to common national requirements. Actual care is provided through a mix of private and public institutions and providers. Approximately 90% of the population have supplementary insurance to cover other health services not provided under the national system (Rodwin, 2003), and 20% of hospital services are provided by for-profit institutions (Cruise, 2002).

Approximately half of the funds for the French national health system are derived from employer payroll taxes and another 35% from taxes on earnings. Special taxes (e.g., on liquor and tobacco), employee payroll taxes, and a general social contribution of 5.5% of all earnings provide additional funds. There is also a tax on the pharmaceutical industry (Rodwin, 2003). Ambulatory care services are paid for on a fee-for-service basis by clients, who are reimbursed by State Insurance Funds based on a nationally determined fee scale. Some physicians are permitted to bill clients for an additional sum (a practice called "balance billing"), as an incentive to participate in the system, but enrollment in this group has been discontinued due to increasing costs (Cruise, 2002). Proprietary hospitals are reimbursed on a negotiated per diem rate, but public and private nonprofit hospitals receive global budget allocations (Rodwin, 2003).

Funding for the Japanese health care system arises out of three compulsory social insurance plans, all of which provide the same benefits. The first type of plan is employment-based and covers approximately two thirds of the population. These plans consist of government-managed plans for employees of small companies, insurance societies for employees of large companies, a day laborers' insurance plan, Independent Seamans insurance, and a mutual aid insurance plan for government employees. Premiums in these plans are based on income and contributed by both employer and employee. The second type of plan is community health insurance and covers persons who are self-employed, unemployed, and farmers. These plans are administered by local governments with assistance from the federal government (Yajima & Takayanagi, 2002).

In 2000, Japan initiated the third type of plan, care insurance for the elderly and disabled to cover institutional or community-based care. Every person 40 years of age and older must contribute to this program. Half of program funding comes from general revenues (50% at the national level and 25% each from the prefecture and municipality) and half from premiums. Persons aged 40 to 64 years pay a supplement to their existing health insurance premium (about 0.9% of earnings). Those over 65 years of age have graduated premiums deducted from their public pensions based on income (Campbell & Ikegami, 2000).

Health care delivery in Japan takes place in a three-tiered system of physician-owned clinics, general hospitals in which physicians are salaried, and special function hospitals attached to universities or of large size. Independent physicians are reimbursed on a fee-for-service basis at fixed rates for specific services set at the national level. Japanese consumers pay relatively high out-of-pocket costs, with copayments (waived for the elderly) accounting for 12% of national health care expenditures (Yajima & Takayanagi, 2002).

The Australian "Medicare" system of universal health care insurance is a mix of public government-controlled financing and hospital services coupled with private professional practice and private for-profit and nonprofit hospitals. The public system is funded through general tax revenues and a specific income tax, but approximately 30% of the population has additional private insurance to pay the difference between the Medicare fee schedule and the costs of care. Private insurance also eliminates long waits for some services. Hospital care is provided in public hospitals, which may also care for privately insured clients. Physician services are reimbursed on a fee-for-service basis in the personal health care sector. Many providers bill the Medicare program directly. When providers do not engage in direct billing, clients may either pay the fee and be reimbursed for 85% by the system or take the bill for services to a Medicare office and have a check cut for 85% of the fee, which the client then sends to the provider along with the balance of the fee paid out-of-pocket. Providers who direct-bill the system must accept the Medicare reimbursement as payment in full and may not "balance bill" clients for the remainder of the fee (Lapsley, 2002).

Funding in the Russian health care system is provided by a 3.6% payroll deduction, which is administered by Territorial Insurance Funds that cover health services for the employed. Territorial government funds subsidize care for children, the elderly, and the unemployed. Reimbursement may take one of several avenues. Insurance companies that cover 30% of the population may serve as intermediaries between the funds and providers. In a second approach, providers are paid directly by the funds, or a combination of the two approaches may be used. Territories without established funds collect payroll taxes and providers are reimbursed by the prior regional health administrations (Bourhanskaia et al., 2002).

Consumer Choice and Professional Autonomy

National health systems also vary in terms of the degree of autonomy exercised by clients and providers within the system. In the U.S. system, the degree of autonomy of both clients and providers varies greatly depending on the source of health care funding, as we will see in Chapter 8∞. For example, clients enrolled in some managed care organizations may be constrained in their choice of provider or in their ability to seek the services of a specialist. Similarly, providers may be limited in their choice of treatment options, depending on the source of their funding. Some insurance plans, for instance, may cover certain procedures or medications and not others.

Expansion of consumer choice is one of the tenets of health care system reform in many European countries. In the Canadian, German, Japanese, Australian, and new Russian systems, clients have a choice in their primary providers. Choice of specialist care is constrained in Canada and the United Kingdom by limited availability and long waiting times in some areas (Light, 2003; Patel & Rushefsky, 2002). In other countries, such as Australia and managed care organizations in the United States, primary care physicians constitute "gatekeepers" who make decisions on when specialist care is warranted.

Providers may also be constrained in practice decisions either directly or by system factors. Providers in Japan and Germany are highly independent and there are few constraints on their practice. Health care professionals also have a high degree of autonomy in Canada and the United Kingdom, but are frequently constrained by the availability of special diagnostic or specialty care services. German providers are constrained by the amount of drugs that can be prescribed (Swami, 2002). Both French consumers and providers have a wide degree of choice and latitude. There are no gatekeepers to minimize access to specialty or hospital care (Rodwin, 2003), and consumers have wide choice in providers. Similarly, physicians are very autonomous in their practice. Both physician autonomy and free choice of provider are underlying principles of the French health care system (Cruise, 2002).

Finally, providers may be constrained in terms of their ability to access several revenue streams. In the United States, many providers are on the provider panels of several managed care organizations. As noted earlier, Japanese physicians who practice in clinic settings do not have hospital privileges and vice versa (Yajima & Takayanagi, 2002). Physicians in the United Kingdom have the ability to engage in private practice in addition to participation in the National Health System, and even public hospitals have a certain number of private-pay beds. Similarly, in the United Kingdom, Australia, and Germany, citizens have the option to purchase supplemental private insurance, yet German physicians are prohibited by law from advertising. In Canada, physicians can opt for private practice only if they choose not to participate in the national health care system, and private insurance companies are legally prohibited from offering coverage for any services covered under the national plan (Inglehart, 2000). In addition, Canada places some caps on physician income from the national health system (Patel & Rushefsky, 2002).

Access and Coverage

The United States is the only health care system in the developed world that does not provide universal access to health care for all citizens, and approximately 46 million people are uninsured (Families USA, 2005), compared to virtually none of the populations in other developed countries (Jonas, 2003). The other systems discussed here provide nearly, if not perfect, universal coverage. For example, in Russia, Germany, and Japan participation in the national program is compulsory (Bourhanskaia et al., 2002; Swami, 2002; Yajima & Takayanagi, 2002). Similarly, near-universal coverage in Canada and France follows citizens through relocation or periods of unemployment (Cruise, 2002; Patel & Rushefsky, 2002).

Although the bulk of the population is covered under all of the national health systems discussed, except that of the United States, that does not mean that all conceivable services are provided. For example, the Japanese system covers prescription drugs (Yoshikawa & Bhattacharya, 2002), as do many managed care plans in the United States. However, pharmaceuticals are covered only for the elderly in the Canadian system (Inglehart, 2000), although hospital and medical services are covered for all. The Australian system covers pharmaceuticals as well as medical and hospital care, but funding derives from different sources, with hospital funding from the states and territories and prescription drugs through the commonwealth government (Hall, 1999). In Japan, nursing care for the elderly is provided in the home or institutions, although few other national systems provide such coverage (Yoshikawa & Bhattacharya, 2002). Australia provides some government

subsidies for prescription drugs in outpatient settings, as well as hospitalization, general primary care, and most specialty care (Lapsley, 2002). The French and German systems provide the most comprehensive coverage. French participants are eligible for hospital and outpatient care, pharmaceuticals, nursing home care, cash benefits, and some dental and vision care. The French system is unique in that insurance coverage increases as individual costs rise, the reverse of most systems (Rodwin, 2003). The German national health system experiences frequent cost overruns due to the comprehensive package of services offered, including preventive, vision and dental, pharmaceutical, and outpatient and hospital services (Swami, 2002).

Health Outcomes

Another way of comparing national health care delivery systems is in terms of the outcomes achieved. One of the principal outcomes is that of life expectancy. Despite the level of health expenditures in the United States, life expectancy in 2003 lagged behind that in each of the other countries discussed here except the Russian Federation (WHO, 2005c).

Life expectancy, however, measures longevity as an outcome of health care, but does not measure the burden of disease and disability. A more reflective measure of health care outcomes is **health-adjusted life expectancy (HALE)**, or the number of years of healthy life that one can expect to attain. Again, the countries considered here vary considerably in terms of this outcome. According to 2002 estimates from WHO (2004b), Japan again ranked highest, with 75 years of expected disability-free life, followed by Australia (72.6), Canada and France (72.0), Germany (71.8), and the United Kingdom (70.6). The United States reported a healthy life expectancy of 69.3 years, and Russia achieved 68.4 years. Healthy life expectancy and longevity are compared for these nations in Table 6-2◆.

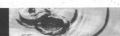

CULTURAL COMPETENCE

Fink (2002) described the efforts of some national health systems to incorporate traditional, complementary, and alternative therapies into the overall health system. Such efforts are motivated, in part, by the fact that significant portions of the world's population (including the U.S. population) use complementary and alternative therapies, often without acknowledging their use to scientific medical professionals. In fact, the worldwide market for traditional herbal remedies is estimated to reach $60 billion. In the United States, much use of traditional and complementary practices occurs in conjunction with the use of scientific medicine, although the two systems of care lack integration here and in most developed nations. In developing nations, on the other hand, the majority of people do not have access to scientific therapies, and traditional therapies are the only recourse available to them. In recognition of these factors, the World Health Organization developed a global strategy to promote safe and effective use of traditional therapies in the belief that lack of interaction between scientific and traditional systems is both dangerous and wasteful of opportunities to improve health. Traditional practitioners have the potential to reach people who might otherwise not be reached with health-related messages. Specific strategies that have been employed are the use of traditional birth attendants (TBAs) to promote maternal and child health and the incorporation of traditional healers to address psychological and palliative care for people with HIV/AIDS using a variety of traditional remedies. Drawbacks to such programs include the reluctance of many major donors to fund research on the effectiveness of traditional therapies and attitudes of superiority on the part of scientific providers. What kinds of interventions might be employed to change these perceptions and promote greater interaction between scientific and traditional health care systems in developed countries?

	Life Expectancy (years)*	Healthy Life Expectancy (years)#
TABLE 6-2 **International Comparisons of Life Expectancy, 2003, and Healthy Life Expectancy, 2002**		
Country		
Australia	81	72.6
Canada	80	72
France	80	72
Germany	79	71.8
Japan	82	75
Russia	65	58.4
United Kingdom	79	70.6
United States	77	69.3

*Data from: World Health Organization. (2005). The world health report, 2005: Make every mother and child count. Retrieved December 16, 2005, from http://www.who.int/whr/2005/annexes-en.pfd

#Data from: World Health Organization. (2004). The world health report 2004: Changing history. Geneva, Switzerland: Author.

TABLE 6-3 National Rankings for Health System Goal Attainment

Country	Overall Goal Attainment	DALE	Health Distribution	Fairness in Financial Distribution	Responsiveness
Australia	10	17	8	12	12
Canada	7	12	18	17	7
France	6	3	12	26	
Germany	14	22	20	6	5
Japan	1	1	3	8 (tied)	6
Russia	100	91	69	185	69
United Kingdom	9	14	2	8 (tied)	26
United States	15	24	32	54	1

Data from: World Health Organization. (2000). The world health report 2000: Health systems: Improving performance. Geneva, Switzerland: Author.

Goal attainment and overall system performance are other ways of assessing health system outcomes. WHO (2000) identified three goals of health care systems against which it has assessed the health care systems of its member nations. The first goal is the health of the population; the second is fairness of financial contribution to health. The third goal is responsiveness to people's expectations. With respect to overall goal attainment for the national health systems reviewed here, Japan was rated first of 191 member nations, followed by Canada, France, the United Kingdom, Australia, and Germany. The United States was rated 15th, and the Russian Federation 100th. Actual rankings for these countries are provided in Table 6-3◆.

The health goal is examined in terms of the overall level of health of the nation's population, as measured by years of **disability-adjusted life expectancy (DALE)** and the equity of distribution of health within the population. On this variable, France ranked 3rd among member nations with respect to DALE and 12th with respect to the distribution of health. Comparable rankings for the United States were 24th and 32nd (WHO, 2000). Rankings for the other comparison countries are included in Table 6-3◆.

On the variable of fairness of distribution of financial contributions to health, Germany was rated highest of the nations being compared here, at 6th among 191 nations, followed by the United Kingdom and Japan, Australia, Canada, and France. Only the Russian Federation, ranked 100th, fell below the ranking of the United States at 54th. Specific rankings for the seven comparison health care systems are provided in Table 6-3◆.

The United States ranked first in terms of the level of responsiveness of its health care system, with a rating of 8.10 of a possible 10 points. Responsiveness was measured by several variables related to respect for persons (dignity, autonomy, and confidentiality) and client orientation (prompt attention, quality of basic amenities, access to social support as part of care, and provider choice). Other nations' health care systems were rated less favorably, with Germany ranked 5th, Japan 6th, Canada tied for 7th position, Australia tied for 12th, the United Kingdom tied at 26th, and Russia tied at 69th

(WHO, 2000). National rankings on health system responsiveness are summarized in Table 6-3◆.

Overall health system performance was defined by WHO as the extent to which a system accomplished its goals compared to the most efficient system with the same level of resources. For this measure, top ratings were held by France, followed by Australia, Japan, the United Kingdom, Germany, Canada, the United States (at 37th), and Russia (WHO, 2000). System performance rankings are summarized in Table 6-4◆.

Child survival is another measure of the effectiveness of health care systems. According to 2003 WHO data (2005c), Malta and Iceland had infant mortality rates less than one per 1,000 live births, and Iceland and Singapore had the lowest mortality for children under 5 years of age (3 per 1,000). The worst infant mortality occurred in Burkina Faso, a poor West African nation, at 65 per 1,000 live births.

Health outcomes of national health systems do not seem to be linked to the extent of health care expenditures. As we saw earlier, the United States has the highest level of health expenditures in terms of percentage of GDP in the world but frequently poorer outcomes than other countries that spend less. Germany, for example, achieves longer overall life expectancy

TABLE 6-4 National Rankings for Overall and Health-related System Performance

Country	Overall System Performance	Health-related System Performance
Australia	9	15
Canada	30	35
France	1	4
Germany	25	41
Japan	10	9
Russia	130	127
United Kingdom	18	24
United States	37	72

Data from: World Health Organization. (2000). The world health report: Improving performance. Geneva, Switzerland: Author.

than the United States, but a shorter disability-adjusted life expectancy. Similarly, Germany exhibits lower cardiovascular disease mortality than the United States, but higher liver disease and cirrhosis death rates. In part, these differences are attributed to excessive alcohol consumption, particularly beer, in Germany (Swami, 2002). Health system outcomes for the United Kingdom are comparable to those of other countries spending far more on health services (Light, 2003). Similarly, health outcomes on some indicators are better in France than in the United States and many other countries (Rodwin, 2003).

Among the health systems discussed here, the Russian Federation achieves the worst health outcomes. For example, injury death rates in Russia are four times higher than in Western nations, in part due to alcohol use and lack of road and vehicle safety design factors present in the West. Russia also experiences high rates of cardiovascular disease mortality, particularly among young people with no history of heart disease. Russia also maintains extremely high lung cancer death rates and high rates of sexually transmitted disease incidence, primarily due to difficulties in obtaining barrier contraceptives. Since the breakup of the Soviet Union, com-

municable diseases have been on the rise, although there has been some success with vaccine-preventable diseases (McKee & Zatonski, 2003).

Consumer Satisfaction

Consumer satisfaction is another way in which health care systems can be compared. Satisfaction studies have been conducted for some of the national health care systems discussed here and not for others. Satisfaction ratings for several health care systems have declined in recent years, most noticeably Canada. For example, only 24% of Canadians rated their health care system as good or excellent in 1999 compared to 61% in 1991 (Inglehart, 2000). Australia also achieves high satisfaction ratings (Lapsley, 2002), as do Germany and France (Swami, 2002).

Table 6-5◆ summarizes information about the national health care systems discussed here related to locus of decision making, expenditures, funding mechanisms, autonomy, and coverage and access. As we have seen, national health care systems vary in a number of ways, and each system has both positive and negative features. No nation has yet developed a perfect health care delivery system. Community health nurses in all countries need to be actively involved in the development of systems that address the needs of the public.

INTERNATIONAL HEALTH VERSUS GLOBAL HEALTH

At this point, we need to make a distinction between international health activities and global health. **International health** involves health matters that affect two or more countries and is distinguished by the authority of the specific nation-states to address health issues that affect both (Lee, Fustukian, & Buse, 2002). **Global health**, on the other hand, involves multinational efforts to address health problems that cross national borders (Bunyanavich & Walkup, 2001); global health is also concerned with factors that affect the capacity of individual nation-states to deal with the determinants of health and illness (Lee et al., 2002). "International health becomes global health when the causes or consequences of a health issue circumvent, undermine, or are oblivious to the territorial boundaries of states and, thus, beyond the capacity of states to address effectively through state institutions alone" (Lee et al., 2002, p. 5).

Global/International Health Agencies

There are a variety of agencies that undertake global or international health efforts. These agencies can be loosely grouped as bilateral agencies, multilateral agencies, and non-governmental agencies. Bilateral and multilateral agencies tend to be associations of member nations represented by official government

GLOBAL PERSPECTIVES

*T*ollman and Pick (2002) described the failure of community-oriented primary care (COPC) strategies to achieve substantial improvements in health status in the population of South Africa. They note that although COPC lends itself to small-area needs assessments, the decentralized approach to health care adopted in South Africa has led to a lack of progress in translating national health policy into local and provincial practice. They identified a number of obstacles to doing so, including a lack of managerial capacity and limited community-based experience by local-level providers and administrators. Another barrier is excessive concern among staff for accountability to senior managers and an unwillingness to initiate independent activity related to local health concerns. In addition, health districts delineated in a decentralized structure do not fit well with local government boundaries, and there is confusion regarding the relative role of local and provincial governments with respect to specific aspects of care delivery. Local governments have also been focused on organizational structure and authority rather than health-related activity. The efforts of organizations such as the World Bank to promote primary care through public–private partnerships has led to disease-oriented programs with narrow foci that do not address broader social conditions that affect health. Another factor is the failure of providers (primarily nurses) to shift from an individual, curative-focused mode of practice to one of population health. One suggested remedy for this particular factor is the development of "midlevel workers" more qualified than community health workers to expand the services of nurse-based teams. Finally, an emerging market orientation focusing on cost-effectiveness and user fees impedes progress in achieving COPC goals.

What types of interventions might ameliorate the effects of these factors and enhance the effectiveness of COPC strategies in achieving improved health for South Africa's population?

TABLE 6-5   Comparison of Selected National Health System Features

Locus of Decision Making

Australia: Decentralized

Canada: Decentralized

France: Decentralized

Germany: Centralized

Japan: Highly centralized

Russian Federation: Decentralized

United Kingdom: Centralized, but becoming less so

United States: Hyperpluralistic

Expenditures[*]	Percent of GDP	Out-of-Pocket
Australia	9.5%	20%
Canada	9.6%	15%
France	9.7%	10%
Germany	10.9%	10%
Japan	7.9%	16%
Russian Federation	6.2%	28%
United Kingdom	7.7%	9%
United States	14.6%	14%

Funding Mechanisms

Australia: Tax revenues

Canada: Tax revenues (payroll tax in some provinces)

France: Payroll and income taxes

Germany: Payroll tax

Japan: Payroll tax, municipal revenues

Russian Federation: Payroll tax

United Kingdom: Tax revenues

United States: Variable

Provider Reimbursement

Australia: Fee-for-service

Canada: Fee-for-service

France: Fee-for-service, with about one third of providers able to "balance bill"

Germany: Fee-for-service

Japan: Fee-for-service

Russian Federation: Fee-for-service

United Kingdom: Fee-for-service, moving toward per-person flat fee

United States: Variable

Consumer Choice

Australia: Open choice of primary provider; gatekeeper for specialty services; can obtain supplemental private insurance if desired

Canada: Open choice of provider or specialist; supplemental insurance only for uncovered services

France: Open choice of provider

Germany: Open choice of provider and insurance company; private insurance available for higher-wage earners

Japan: Open choice of provider

Russian Federation: Open choice of provider and insurance company

United Kingdom: Open choice of primary provider within health authority

United States: Variable, often constrained in MCOs

Provider Autonomy

Australia: High

Canada: High in personal practice; specialty referrals often constrained by availability; MD cannot choose both private practice and participation in national program

France: High

Germany: High

Japan: High

Russian Federation: Unknown

United Kingdom: High in personal practice; specialty referrals often constrained by availability; MD able to engage in private practice as well

United States: Variable; often constrained in MCOs

Coverage

Australia: Universal

Canada: Universal; may have long waits for specialty or diagnostic services

France: Universal, but variability among insurance funds regarding specific services covered

Germany: Universal

Japan: Universal

Russian Federation: Universal, but resources not adequate to meet need

United Kingdom: Universal; may have long waits for specialty or elective services

United States: Approximately 46 million uninsured

[*]*2002 figures. Data from: World Health Organization. (2005). World health report 2005: Make every mother and child count. Retrieved December 16, 2005, from http://www.who.int/whr/2005/annexes-en.pdf*

health-related agencies. **Multilateral agencies** are those that involve several countries in joint activities related to health, whereas **bilateral agencies** usually involve only two countries in any single project.

Multilateral Agencies

The **World Health Organization (WHO)**, a specialized agency attached to the United Nations by formal agreement but not subordinate to the UN, is the primary agency dealing with global health issues. WHO was

established in 1948 to "direct and coordinate international health work by setting standards and guidelines and to provide technical assistance in cooperation with countries to strengthen national health programs" (Vonderheid & Al-Gasseer, 2002, p. 109). WHO is funded through subscription by member nations and focuses on health promotion and disease prevention, cure of illness, health systems and health resources development, and health-related international research (Thompson, 2002). The World Health Assembly is the governing body for WHO and sets global health policy (Vonderheid & Al-Gasseer, 2002).

The **Pan American Health Organization (PAHO)** is the multilateral agency that deals with health-related concerns in the Americas and provides an avenue for collective efforts to promote the health status of people in all nations in the Western Hemisphere. PAHO is the oldest of the global health organizations and celebrated its 100th anniversary in 2002. PAHO originated in 1902 as the International Sanitary Bureau. Its original focus was the development of uniform sanitary regulations and laws in North and South America. In 1958, the organization expanded its focus to address broader health issues and changed its name to the Pan American Health Organization (Fee & Brown, 2002).

One of PAHO's significant achievements is the development of the Regional Core Health Data Initiative with five components. These components include a basic indicators "brochure" that addresses information on 58 health indicators for 48 countries. The second component is a glossary of health indicators, and the third is a series of country health profiles that identify health-related strengths and weaknesses. The fourth component is a geographic information system, and the fifth is the list of essential public health functions discussed earlier. All of the components of the initiative provide direction for programs to enhance health status in member nations (Alleyne, 2002).

Other multilateral agencies include the health components of the North Atlantic Treaty Organization (NATO) and the Southeast Asia Treaty Organization (SEATO). The United Nations International Children's Emergency Fund (UNICEF) and the United Nations Educational, Scientific, and Cultural Organization (UNESCO) are two other agencies within the UN that provide assistance with matters of global health. The Food and Agricultural Organization (FAO) is a multilateral agency designed to enhance the world's food supply. Finally, the World Bank provides both funding and technical assistance in dealing with health problems around the world.

Bilateral Agencies

A number of bilateral organizations with health emphases exist throughout the world. Virtually all developed countries provide some form of health-related aid to underdeveloped countries, with the contribution of some countries far in excess of that provided by the United States. This section will focus on the bilateral organizations involving the United States. One of the federal agencies concerned with international health is the United States Agency for International Development (USAID), which administers all federally financed projects for foreign development, including those that are health related. This agency is housed in the U.S. State Department, and its twofold purpose is to promote U.S. foreign policy through expansion of democracy and free markets and to improve life in the developing world. To these ends, the agency supports economic growth, agriculture, and trade; global health; and democracy, conflict prevention, and humanitarian aid (USAID, 2005).

The Department of Health and Human Services includes the International Health Program Office within the CDC. This agency is concerned with cooperative projects for improving international health. The Fogarty International Center is housed in the NIH and focuses on international health. Other branches of the NIH (e.g., the Geographic Medicine Branch of the Institute of Allergy and Infectious Diseases) are involved in activities that are international in focus, as is the CDC. ACTION, the volunteer organization of the federal government, houses both the domestic assistance programs of VISTA (Volunteers in Service to America) and the international programs of the Peace Corps, many of which have a health focus. Federally chartered institutions such as the Institute of Medicine and the National Science Foundation are also concerned with problems of international health as well as with domestic problems.

Bilateral, or binational, initiatives are particularly needed along the U.S.–Mexican border. At present, there are 11.5 million people in 42 U.S. counties and 39 Mexican municipalities who live along the border, and this number is expected to double by 2020. A large majority (86%) of this population lives in "sister cities," cities that exist on both sides of the border. The North American Free Trade Agreement (NAFTA) has been perceived by some as a model for other areas of global endeavor in North America (Homedes & Ugalde, 2003).

There is a need for a variety of binational programs at the border. For example, populations on both sides of the U.S.–Mexican border are growing faster than other portions of either country, and health infrastructures are not keeping pace with this growth. Border areas experience a variety of health problems that do not respect national boundaries. For example, hepatitis A seropositivity is three times higher in border areas than in the rest of the United States and twice as high as in the rest of Mexico. Similarly, the incidence of salmonella infection is 26% higher in the border *colonias* than in the other parts of the United States and four times higher than in the rest of Mexico. Similar increases are also noted for shigella infection, and 9% of tuberculosis cases along the border are resistant to many antitubercular drugs. The spread of communicable disease is heightened by more than 1.1 million legal and untold illegal border crossings daily. There is also a need for binational efforts related to disaster preparedness and response, shared information systems, and referral systems to promote continuity of care, but collaboration is often difficult because of differences in the organization and financing of health care (Homedes & Ugalde, 2003).

Non-governmental Organizations

NGOs are the international or global counterparts of voluntary health agencies discussed in Chapter 5∞. **Non-governmental organizations (NGOs)** are agencies outside of the official government-sponsored agencies that work toward the public good. Examples of NGOs include religious groups, philanthropic foundations, corporations, and other organizations that engage in activities designed to address a variety of issues throughout the world, including health concerns. NGOs often have knowledge of local needs and can assist in the organization of grassroots activities that promote health initiatives (WHO, 2002). Recently NGOs have been assuming greater responsibility for dealing with global health issues, and private donors often prefer to work through NGOs rather than official government health agencies because they can sometimes move more rapidly to resolve problems without a lot of "red tape."

Exclusive use of NGOs to address health problems has a number of disadvantages, however. For example, NGOs tend to focus on specific initiatives rather than improvement of host-country health system infrastructure and capacity. There is also a growing number of NGOs operating in similar areas, which leads to a need for coordination of activities to prevent gaps and overlaps in functions and services. In addition, some NGOs may give little attention to local culture in attempts to create blanket solutions to global health issues. The major disadvantage of NGOs, however, is the potential loss of governmental ability or willingness to address health issues in the long term. Governments, whether state or national, are accountable to their citizens for the protection of health, and that responsibility cannot be relinquished to NGOs (Perkins, 2002a).

NGOs should align their priorities with national government priorities and design health-related activities in such a way that government will be able to sustain them without outside assistance. NGOs can use their influence to motivate government activity through grassroots organizations and are most effective when they are part of broad-based partnerships that include governments, academic and research institutions, private business, and civil society (WHO, 2002). NGOs can be involved in sector-wide approaches that provide a more lasting and effective solution to a variety of conditions that affect health.

Sector-wide approaches (SWAPs) are approaches to the resolution of health-related problems through attention to conditions in the broader social services sector that affect health. Components of this sector include health services and policies, water and sanitation, education, and social welfare services. As we saw in the discussion of determinants-of-health models in Chapter 4∞, a number of factors other than health services affect the health status of the population. Sector-wide approaches attempt to deal with those factors that

lie outside the purview of the health care delivery system. SWAPs are based on three premises:

- Development assistance is more effective when it is supported by government policies.
- Governments rarely change policies based on donor conditions.
- Donor-initiated projects may be poorly planned for local conditions, lie outside government priorities, and actually drain government capacity to deal with health issues.

The two aims of sector-wide approaches are (a) to interact with host-country governments, incorporating multiple sectors of government, to develop a nation's epidemiologic profile and understand priorities and (b) to promote donor assistance that allows the recipient government to build an effective health infrastructure that cuts across multiple sectors (Perkins, 2002a). Sector-wide approaches may also help to remedy situations in which considerable foreign assistance is provided to improve health in underdeveloped countries but does not achieve its full potential because of lack of capacity in some areas to engage in large-scale planning and management of broad social and health-related initiatives (Perkins, 2002c). There is a need to build on existing national strengths and to coordinate a broad spectrum of activities related to surveillance, health promotion, illness prevention, and treatment rather than the often fragmented approaches that exist currently. SWAPs may help to develop such coordinated initiatives since these activities require the efforts of social sectors other than the health care delivery system (Perkins, 2002d).

An example of a sector-wide approach might be efforts to provide access to safe, drinkable water in a developing nation. Assistance might be sought from an NGO to pay for building a water purification system, but local government initiatives will be required to support system maintenance. There may also be a need for cooperation from local agricultural business to prevent water contamination with agricultural runoff. At the same time, legislation might be needed that prohibits the dumping of human wastes within a prescribed distance of a water supply. For the safe water system to be developed and continue to function, activities will be required in several aspects of the health and social services sector. Focused assessment questions for examining the health system context in another country are provided on page 115.

GLOBALIZATION AND ITS EFFECTS ON HEALTH

Most of the literature on globalization tends to focus on economic interactions or cultural changes rather than health. One reason for this lack of attention is the fact that health care systems are traditionally focused

FOCUSED ASSESSMENT

Assessing a Health System Context

You are part of a group of health care professionals being sent to Botswana by an international NGO to provide assistance in developing a more effective health care system. The following are some of the questions you might use in an assessment to guide the group's efforts. The questions are based on the dimensions of health included in the dimensions model of community health nursing.

Biophysical Considerations

- What is the age and gender composition of the population of Botswana?
- What is the racial/ethnic composition of the population?
- Does the age, gender, and racial/ethnic composition vary in specific areas within the country?
- What physical health problems are prevalent in the population?
- What are the immunization levels within the population?

Psychological Considerations

- What stresses affect members of the population?
- How do members of the population typically cope with stress?
- What is the extent of mental illness within the population?

Physical Environmental Considerations

- What features of the natural environment affect the health of the population?
- What features of the built environment affect the health of the population?
- What effects do these environmental features have on health?

Sociocultural Considerations

- What is the economic level of the population? How equitably are economic resources distributed within the population?
- What are the typical occupations of members of the population? What potential health risks do these occupations pose?
- What is the level of employment/unemployment within the population? What is the average per capita income?
- What is the educational level of the population? Is there wide variation in educational level among subgroups in the population?

- What religious affiliations are represented in the population? What effect, if any, do these religious affiliations have on health?
- What ethnic cultural groups are represented in the population? What effects, if any, does cultural affiliation have on health?
- Are there areas of conflict between subgroups within the population? How are these conflicts manifested and what effects do they have on health?
- What is the level of social capital available to communities and individuals within the population? What are the sources of social capital?

Behavioral Considerations

- What is the typical dietary intake within the population? What are the health effects of the typical diet?
- What is the extent of food insecurity in the population? Who is affected by food insecurity?
- To what extent do members of the population use alcohol, tobacco, and other drugs?
- What types of physical and recreational activities do members of the population engage in?
- To what extent do members of the population engage in health promotion and illness prevention activities? What activities are performed?
- To what extent do members of the population engage in self-management of disease?

Health System Considerations

- How are health and health care services viewed in Botswana?
- What primary, secondary, and tertiary preventive health care services are available? How are they obtained? How are they funded?
- How equitable is access to health care services for various segments of the population?
- How are health care services organized? How effective are health care services in meeting the health needs of the population? How efficiently does the health care system utilize resources?
- What health care resources are available within the country (e.g., personnel, facilities, equipment)? What resources can be obtained from outside?
- What other resources are needed to effectively meet the health care needs of the population?

at national and subnational, rather than global, levels (Lee, 2003). Globalization was simply defined earlier in this chapter. Other definitions for globalization include:

[an] increasing interconnectedness of countries through cross-border flows of goods, services, money, people, information, and ideas; the increasing openness of countries to such flows; and the development of international rules and institutions dealing with cross-border flows. (McMichael & Beaglehole, 2003, p. 8)

the process of increasing economic, political, and social interdependence and global integration that takes place as capital, traded goods, persons, concepts, images, ideas, and values diffuse across state boundaries. (Hurrell & Woods, as quoted in Buse & Walt, 2002, p. 43)

These definitions approach globalization as a broad concept, but globalization is perceived somewhat differently by different groups. For example, economists view globalization as the development of a worldwide economy, whereas lawyers focus on the change in the legal status of nations and their citizens as more activities are constrained by international laws and attempts at global governance. Technologists, on the other hand, tend to see globalization as information exchange afforded by the Internet, and those interested in cultural studies view globalization as a movement to a more uniform global culture highly influenced by Western social mores (Lee, 2003).

The literature on globalization identifies four key processes that occur. The first of these is changes in the distribution of income (and poverty), with promotion of economic growth in many sectors accompanied by increasing inequalities within and between groups (e.g., among members of a particular ethnic minority group or between minority groups and members of the dominant society) (Doyal, 2004; Lee & Zwi, 2003). For example, the economic benefits of globalization are greater for wealthy nations than for poor nations, leading to growing economic disparities (Perkins, 2002b). Similar disparities may occur for people within countries experiencing economic growth, with the wealthy reaping greater benefits than other members of the population.

The second key process involves changes in production processes regarding when and how work is done and by whom. Again, the effects are mixed, with greater employment and initial entry into the labor market for some groups and loss of work for others. Changes in work processes may also lead to unhealthful working conditions in countries with limited occupational oversight. In addition, production changes have environmental effects that may be either positive or negative (e.g., environmental degradation or environmental improvements such as better water supplies) (Doyal, 2004).

Liberalization of trade is the third key process in globalization. Liberalization of trade is the effect of efforts by the World Trade Organization (WTO) and the North American Free Trade Agreement (NAFTA). Again, this process has both positive and negative effects. Positively, trade liberalization leads to greater financial prosperity and health in some areas. For example, dissemination of therapeutic technologies and vaccines can help to improve world health status. On the other hand, liberalization may lead to the global marketing and sale of products (e.g., tobacco) that are harmful to health. Liberalization of trade has also led to efforts promulgated by major producing nations, such as the United States, to protect intellectual property and patent rights. One example of this type of activity is the development of the World Trade Organization's Trade-related Intellectual Property (TRIPS) agreement. Such efforts have had the adverse effect of limiting access to antiretroviral drugs in poor countries with high rates of HIV infection (Gostin, 2003; Thomas, 2003). Some authors note that patents originated as rewards from the state to developers of innovative ideas and inventions precisely for the purpose of making the development available to the public. They argue that nations are obliged to place the welfare of their people over the rights of intellectual property holders (Heywood, 2004).

Another WTO initiative that has more positive health effects is the Agreement on the Application of Sanitary and Phytosanitary Measures to regulate animal and plant health and protect food safety (Koivusalo, 2003). The pervasive influence of economic initiatives on health status has led some authors to assert that the World Trade Organization and the World Bank have virtually replaced the World Health Organization as a health policy-making body (Poku & Whiteside, 2004). They also noted that economic globalization has resulted in a shift away from a global focus on social justice and equity to one emphasizing a market economy and efficiency.

The final process in globalization is the reshaping of nation-states. This is sometimes referred to as a "hollowing out" of nation-states, with a loss of influence in regulating activities. Hollowing may also occur when developing countries divert significant portions of their GDP to economic loan repayment, leading to reductions in health care expenditures (Doyal, 2004). Globalization results in an erosion of traditional boundaries that may lead to cross-border flows that strengthen state identity (e.g., international trade) or circumvent boundaries altogether (e.g., global warming, information technology) (Lee, 2003). Similarly, the leadership role of nation-states has been replaced, in some cases, by other actors such as NGOs and a proliferation of public–private partnerships (Poku & Whiteside, 2004).

In addition to key processes, there are three dimensions of globalization: spatial, temporal, and cognitive (Lee & Dodgson, 2003). The spatial dimension relates to one's experience and perception of physical space. Globalization contributes to perceptions of the world "as a single place" and results in changing territorial boundaries or the creation of cross-national organizations and entities. This dimension has a number of health effects, including the ease of spread of communicable diseases and changes in views of population health from national groups to subgroups that cut across national boundaries (e.g., women, minorities, adolescents, etc.). Changes in the spatial dimension have the positive effect of broader dissemination of health knowledge, but also reflect the expanding market for healthful and unhealthful products noted above (Lee, 2003). A related effect is the ease of illicit trade in harmful substances such as drugs and weapons (Taylor et al., 2003).

The temporal dimension of globalization reflects both a speeding up and a slowing down of time as we perceive it. Time is speeded up in terms of the accelerated pace with which events occur. People can circumnavigate the globe in a matter of hours and information can be transmitted instantaneously to multiple parts of

Think Advocacy

Many Mexican citizens are legally employed to work in the United States. They are sometimes employed in positions that provide health insurance benefits. Many of those who are eligible for health insurance prefer to obtain medical care from familiar providers in Mexico rather than from U.S. providers. Their insurance benefits, however, do not cover services provided in Mexico. What kind of advocacy would be required to encourage insurance companies to cover services on both sides of the border? What groups or coalitions might be able to engage in such advocacy? What might be the role of community health nurses in this kind of advocacy?

TABLE 6-6 Positive and Negative Effects of Globalization	
Positive Effects	**Negative Effects**
Promotion of economic growth	Increasing inequities between and within groups
Greater employment or entry into the workforce for some segments of the population	Job loss for some segments of the population
Positive environmental effects (e.g., safer water supplies)	Negative environmental effects (e.g., environmental degradation and increased resource consumption)
Greater financial prosperity and health for some	Creation of unhealthful working conditions
Rapid dissemination of health innovations and information	Marketing of unhealthful products (e.g., tobacco)
Development of global standards related to health (e.g., food safety standards)	Lack of access to available health innovations (e.g., antiretrovirals)
Changes in views of population health from a nation-specific perspective to a subgroup perspective across national boundaries	A shift away from the focus on social justice to an emphasis on market economies and efficiency
Positive effects of *geoculture* development (e.g., increasing autonomy for women)	Ease of spread of communicable diseases Ease of illicit trade in harmful substances Difficulty of keeping up with new developments and potential for information overload Increased time needed for decision making to incorporate input from diverse groups Negative effects of *geoculture* development (e.g., dissemination of poor health habits)

the world via the Internet (Lee & Dodgson, 2003). The health implications of this aspect of globalization include the rapid spread of disease, but also the equally rapid dissemination of surveillance and treatment information. Negative effects of this acceleration include the difficulty of keeping up with changes and the potential for information overload (Lee, 2003). On the positive side, the speed of Internet communication increases the potential for global cooperation to rapidly address emerging health crises (Taylor et al., 2003). Conversely, perceptions of time may slow. For example, because of the widespread nature of policy making involving diverse participants at a global level, decisions may require more time than in the past (Lee, 2003).

The cognitive dimension of globalization reflects changes in the creation and exchange of ideas, beliefs, values, and cultural practices that lead to changes in how we perceive ourselves and the world. Globalization also increases exponentially the number of groups that are attempting to influence those perceptions. Some authors refer to cultural changes that occur within this dimension as the development of a *geoculture* that may lead to changes in values, diet, and lifestyle practices that affect health (Lee, Fustukian, & Buse, 2002). The health implications of this dimension of globalization include greater sharing of health-related information, the potential for international adoption of health-related standards, and, as noted earlier, the dissemination of bad health habits (Lee, 2003). The transmission of ideas has the added effect of heightened consumer expectations (Wimberley & Thai, 2002) leading to increased production and consumption of goods and an increasing deficit of "environmental and ecological resources" and degradation of the natural environment as a global

"life-support system" (McMichael, Butler, & Ahern, 2003, p. 94). Positive and negative effects of globalization are summarized in Table 6-6◆.

GLOBALIZATION OF HEALTH CARE

Health is increasingly recognized as a global phenomenon that crosses national boundaries, in which events in one country affect the health status of people in other countries (Woodward & Smith, 2003). There has been little effort to date to globalize health initiatives, with the exception of some very focused projects (e.g., polio eradication). Globalization efforts have not yet promoted international, or even binational, policy cooperation in health activities similar to that being achieved in the economic arena (Homedes & Ugalde, 2003). There is a need for the development of health policies at the global level. Health policy is defined as "goals and means, environments and instruments, process and styles of decision making, implementation, and assessment" that affect health care delivery and health status (Leppo, as quoted in Lee et al., 2002, p. 10). **Global health policy** is "the ways in which globalization may be impacting on health policy and, alternatively, what health policies are needed to respond to the challenges raised by globalizing processes" (Lee et al., 2002, p. 10). Global health policy development implies *global governance*, which sees the world as a single place and involves movement toward "structures of international governance that manage a system of nation-states" or some form of "supraterritorial authority" (Lee & Dodgson, 2003, p. 138). One of the reasons that economic globalization has moved so much more rapidly than globalization in other sectors is the ability of the World Trade Organization to apply

BUILDING OUR KNOWLEDGE BASE

*B*use, Drager, Fustukian, and Lee (2002) described a research agenda for addressing the effects of globalization of health care initiatives. Areas included in the agenda are:

- Categorization of policy issues as either global or international
- Impact of globalization and global health policy on local populations
- Studies of transfer of responsibility between different policy-making levels
- New approaches to global health policy (understanding of cross-border health determinants and effects on health status)
- Study of effects of globalization in other sectors and influences on health
- Intersections of health policy making with other areas of policy
- Changes in global health governance, decision makers, best and bad practices

Select one of these areas and describe how you might design a related research study. What variables would you examine in your study? Where would your study take place? What is your rationale for the answers to these questions?

ETHICAL AWARENESS

*W*ikler and Cash (2003) identified the following ethical dilemmas in global public health:

1. Deciding whom to save
2. Balancing the health benefits with the risks of intervention strategies
3. Differences in priorities and values between providers and beneficiaries of interventions
4. Compromises with values such as privacy and self-determination
5. Concerns about lack of consensus on the "social contract" between researchers, subjects, sponsors, and society
6. Determining when to compromise ideals and standards to stay effective (e.g., when not to support particular ideologies)
7. Choices among serving the interests of the population, donors, sponsors, and selves

Select one of the national health systems described in this chapter and examine the literature to determine how well that system has addressed these dilemmas. Then compare your findings with how well they have been addressed in the U.S. health care system.

economic sanctions supported by global economic policies to nonconformist nations. At present, all global health initiatives are voluntary and there is no mechanism for sanctioning countries that fail to promote them, whereas WTO agreements are binding legal frameworks that affect world trade (Koivusalo, 2003).

Global Determinants of Health

Social determinants of health have become increasingly "supranational," often extending beyond the capacities of specific nations to address (Evans, 2004). A roundtable discussion among global health experts has identified a number of global health determinants. These determinants fell into the categories of psychosocial environment, socioeconomics, quality of and access to public health services, public policy, physical environment, behavior and lifestyle, preconception/in-utero influences, and biological factors (Perkins, 2002b). Psychosocial environmental factors included family, community, culture, and the effects of social exclusion. Socioeconomic factors included employment and education. Factors related to quality and access to services addressed services related to childcare, transportation, shopping, education, leisure, health care, and social services. Public policy factors related to the economy, welfare programs, crime, transportation, and health. Physical environmental factors included those related to air and water quality, housing, transportation, noise, and waste disposal. Behavioral and lifestyle determinants included diet, tobacco and alcohol use, exercise, and risk-taking behaviors. Maternal health and maternal nutrition were the two major preconception/in-utero factors that influence the health of infants and children. Finally, biological determinants included age, sex, and genetics. These cat-

egories of determinants are similar to those addressed in the determinants-of-health models and the dimensions model of community health nursing discussed in Chapter 4∞, but are clustered somewhat differently.

Challenges in the Globalization of Health

A number of challenges have been identified in the effort to develop global health policy and initiatives to address the multiple determinants of health presented above. One major challenge is dealing with vested interests such as tobacco companies and other industries that market products harmful to health (e.g., infant formulas to replace breastfeeding in developing countries) (Collin, 2003). Other challenges have been identified by different groups. In 2004, the *Journal of Nursing Scholarship* requested nursing input on the major challenges in improving the health of the world's population. Categories of challenges identified by the nursing membership included (a) improving societal conditions affecting health; (b) improving child and adolescent health; (c) improving family planning services; (d) reducing substance abuse incidence; (d) preventing the spread of communicable diseases; (e) managing physical and mental illness; (f) linking health systems and social processes, and (g) designing valid and economically feasible measures of health status (Hegvary, 2004). Specific foci needed to address each of these challenges are presented in Table 6-7◆.

The Gates Foundation and the National Institutes of Health have identified another similar set of challenges in global health, focused primarily on controlling communicable diseases. These challenges include improving childhood vaccines, creating new

TABLE 6-7 Nurse-identified Challenges in Improving Global Health and Associated Activity Foci

Challenge	Activity Foci
Improving social conditions affecting health	▪ Improving education levels for women ▪ Reducing poverty ▪ Interrupting cycles of violence ▪ Improving societal conditions that affect maternal mortality
Improving child and adolescent health	▪ Reducing infant and maternal mortality ▪ Reducing premature births ▪ Improving adolescent mental health ▪ Identifying and addressing childhood risks for adult health and illness
Improving family planning	▪ Assuring availability, accessibility, and affordability of family planning services
Reducing substance abuse	▪ Controlling access to drugs, alcohol, and tobacco ▪ Educating the public on the adverse effects of abused substances ▪ Curtailing marketing of harmful products
Preventing the spread of communicable diseases	▪ Promoting healthful physical environments ▪ Addressing global climate change as a factor in the development of communicable diseases ▪ Eliminating insect vectors ▪ Increasing immunization levels for vaccine-preventable diseases ▪ Promoting sanitation and personal hygiene
Managing physical and mental illness	▪ Reducing chronic disease incidence ▪ Engaging technology for health promotion ▪ Reducing the incidence of depression ▪ Improving pain management ▪ Reducing the incidence of pressure ulcers
Linking health systems and social processes	▪ Focusing on worldwide caring ▪ Redefining health as achieving maximum potential ▪ Incorporating indigenous health systems and practices ▪ Educating the public for health and health system participation ▪ Providing culturally sensitive, competent, and accountable health services ▪ Increasing access to care by decreasing barriers such as transportation, language, cultural differences, education, etc.
Designing valid and economically feasible methods of measuring health status	▪ Identifying desired health outcomes and targets ▪ Developing and testing valid and reliable health status indicators

vaccines (e.g., for HIV/AIDS), controlling insect vectors for disease, improving the treatment of communicable disease, curing latent and chronic infections, and measuring disability and health status accurately and economically (Hegvary, 2004).

Meeting these challenges requires development of a global health policy agenda. Components of one such agenda include aid to improve health and health infrastructures in all countries, aid in developing complementary health infrastructures at regional and global levels that address transborder determinants of health and foster global cooperation, and support for participation in health policy development by the disadvantaged. Additional elements of a desirable policy agenda include representation of health interests in other policy-making sectors (e.g., the economic sector) and use of communications technology to provide information needed for effective policy making (Buse, Drager, Fustukian, & Lee, 2002).

This policy agenda is reminiscent of the tenets of the "health for all by the year 2000" movement toward a global strategy of primary health care. Starting in 1977, the major emphasis in international health care has been the achievement of **"health for all by the year 2000,"** the outcome of the World Health Assembly of that year. The following year, the International Conference on Primary Health Care held in Alma Alta, in what was then the USSR, produced a report entitled *Primary Health Care*, otherwise known as the **Declaration of Alma Alta**. The central goal of the "health for all" movement was the provision of basic health care to all peoples of the world by the year 2000. Its three main objectives were promotion of healthy lifestyles, prevention of preventable conditions, and therapy for existing conditions. Although many nations have made progress in achieving these objectives, others have not, and considerable work remains to achieve the aims of the declaration.

Primary health care was the major strategy to be employed in achieving these objectives. **Primary health care (PHC)** is an approach to providing health care resources that focuses on provision of essential health care using socially acceptable and affordable methods and technology, accessibility, public participation in policy development, and intersectoral collaboration. The Declaration of Alma Alta proposed a set of core activities to be included in primary health care and tailored to the needs of a particular population. These activities included:

- Education to prevent and control major health problems in the area
- Promotion of nutrition and a safe and sufficient food supply
- Provision of safe water and basic sanitation
- Provision of maternal and child health care, including family planning services

- Immunization
- Prevention and control of endemic diseases
- Adequate treatment of common illnesses and injuries
- Provision of essential medications. (WHO, 2003b)

Unfortunately, in many areas the original PHC strategy has been subverted in *selective PHC*, targeted toward specific populations or conditions, rather than *comprehensive PHC*, which was designed to address a wide variety of determinants of health. Some authors have noted that this change in focus has been detrimental to a broader approach to global health and its social determinants (Sanders & Chopra, 2003).

Building Health Capacity

As we have noted several times throughout this chapter, many nations, particularly in the developing parts of the world, lack the capacity to engage in effective health care delivery. One of the particular challenges in addressing global health needs is to foster this capacity. In part this lack of capacity is due to economic factors. Some countries spend as little as $10 per person per year on health care services. In other developing countries, health resources are poorly distributed; as much as 60% of funds is used to care for the 10% of the population that lives in cities (WHO, 2002).

The World Health Organization has identified several strategies that will promote health care capacity in developing nations. The first strategy is debt relief. As noted earlier, many developing nations divert a significant portion of their income to repayment of economic debt. For example, some African nations spend as much as one third of their national budgets in debt repayment (WHO, 2002). For this reason, it has been recommended that financial assistance to these countries occur in the form of outright grants rather than loans that must be repaid (Perkins, 2002d). A second strategy involves coordination of aid to better match programs with needs, coupled with sector-wide approaches to problem resolution. Development of effective surveillance systems is another requirement for health care capacity. A fourth recommendation is the decentralization of services, with overall policy determination and monitoring by the central government. WHO also suggests intercountry initiatives when similar health problems are encountered and can be addressed by similar solutions. A further strategy for building health capacity is the creation of broad-based partnerships between government agencies, NGOs, academic and research institutions, the private sector, and civil society (groups of residents). Another recommendation is incorporation of NGOs and civil society as well as private practitioners in the development of health policy directions and their implementation. This will often require education of practitioners regarding public health practice and issues. Corporate involvement is another means of building capacity. Finally, listening to the poor and providing basic support services to empower them are necessary to develop a health structure in which people can eventually help themselves (WHO, 2002).

Global Health Issues and Initiatives

A number of problems have global effects for worldwide population health. Some of these problems include global environmental changes, communicable diseases, chronic disease and disability, tobacco consumption, and mental health problems. Other global health concerns include child health, women's health, war and civil unrest, and environmental issues. All of these problem areas lead to decreased life expectancy and an increased global burden of disease, and the severity of their effects differs between richer and poorer nations. For example, life expectancy differs 1.7-fold between women in developed nations (81.4 years) and men in sub-Saharan Africa (48.1 years). Average life expectancy at birth around the world is 65 years, but health-adjusted life expectancy (HALE), the length of time one can expect to live in good health, is only 56 years (Bonita & Mathers, 2003).

Causes of mortality also differ between developed and developing nations. HIV/AIDS, lower respiratory infections, perinatal conditions, diarrheal diseases, tuberculosis, malaria, and motor vehicle accidents are among the top 10 causes of death in developing countries, but not in developed countries. Conversely, cancers, self-inflicted injury, and diabetes are major causes of death in developed nations, but not in the developing world. Only ischemic heart disease, cerebrovascular disease, and chronic obstructive pulmonary disease (COPD) are common causes of death throughout the world (Bonita & Mathers, 2003).

Each of the categories of global health concerns contributing to worldwide morbidity and mortality listed above will be addressed briefly here, with the exception of global environmental changes, which will be discussed in Chapter 10∞.

Communicable Diseases

Considerable progress has been made with respect to control of some communicable diseases throughout the world. For example, global eradication of smallpox was certified in 1979 (UNICEF, 2002). Ironically, the last case of naturally occurring smallpox occurred in a smallpox vaccinator who received ineffective vaccine in Somalia in 1977 (Needham & Canning, 2003). **Eradication** is the reduction of the worldwide incidence of a disease to zero through specific efforts to control its spread. **Elimination** is the same phenomenon on a smaller scale; that is, the disease in question no longer occurs in one area of the world. Development of effective vaccines is not sufficient for successful disease eradication. There is also a need for systematic worldwide campaigns to deliver immunization services to susceptible individuals (Needham & Canning, 2003).

At present there are two perspectives regarding eradication efforts. From one perspective, eradication is an appropriate goal if it can be achieved. Feasibility is based on four primary premises:

- Eradication is biologically feasible (e.g., an effective vaccine or other strategy exists).
- Financial resources are sufficient to mount a worldwide campaign.
- Sufficient political will and commitment exist to implement the campaign.
- Social benefits go beyond the mere eradication of disease (e.g., improved economic productivity due to better health).

The second perspective is that eradication provides an avenue for later use of biologic agents as bioterrorist strategies and that global eradication campaigns divert resources away from other broader health and social problems (Needham & Canning, 2003). Recently, the United States has begun preparations for responding to the use of smallpox virus as a biological weapon to eliminate this potential threat (CDC, 2002a).

A study of the international poliomyelitis eradication campaign has indicated that the campaign resulted in a variety of positive effects other than near eradication of the disease. Among these are dissemination of vitamin A supplement, which has resulted in a 23% decrease in mortality of children 6 to 59 months of age; improved laboratory capacities; and better links between health workers and communities. Other program benefits include promotion of intersectoral collaboration, a new focus on delivery of services closer to communities, and a strengthening of local management capabilities and social mobilization efforts. The study also indicated that the program did not divert funds from other programs and, in fact, increased funding available for routine immunization.

Two slight disadvantages were also noted. The campaign did result in some slight disruption in other delivery services as personnel focused on poliomyelitis immunization activities and some missed opportunities to provide other immunizations. In addition, there was the possibility that the campaign resulted in expectations of house-to-house provision of other types of services. On balance, however, the effects of the campaign were exceptionally positive (Loevinsohn et al., 2002).

Diseases currently targeted for worldwide eradication include dracunculiasis (guinea worm disease), poliomyelitis, filariasis, mumps, rubella, and pork tapeworm. Several of these efforts will be discussed here. In 1986, the World Health Assembly adopted a resolution to eradicate dracunculiasis, a disease spread by ingestion of contaminated water that causes skin lesions on the lower extremities through which worms up to a meter long exit the host. These lesions often become secondarily infected, causing considerable disease burden. There is no cure for the disease, but it can be prevented by filtering drinking water or treating it with a larvicide

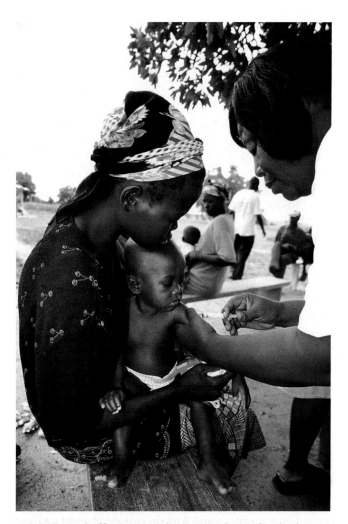

International efforts to eradicate measles and polio have been successful in some parts of the world. (© Sean Sprague/ The Image Works)

and encouraging infected persons to stay out of bodies of water when worms are emerging. At the time of the resolution, there were 3.5 million infected persons in 20 countries where the disease was endemic and 120 million people at risk for the disease. By 2002, only two major foci of disease remained (Sudan and Ghana), and by 2003, worldwide incidence had decreased by more than 99% (Division of Parasitic Diseases, 2002; 2004).

A similar initiative was undertaken in 1988 to eradicate poliomyelitis. The WHO strategy for polio eradication consisted of three aspects: (a) interruption of worldwide transmission of the disease, (b) global certification of eradication, and (c) preparation for the cessation of routine use of oral polio vaccine (Global Immunization Division, 2004a). From 1988 to 2001 the number of reported cases had decreased by 99%, from 350,000 to less than 1,000 cases per year. As of 2000, 82% of the world's children under 12 years of age had received three doses of oral polio vaccine (Division of Viral and Rickettsial Diseases, 2002). This figure had declined to 75% by 2002 due to the effects of war and civil conflict on efforts to reach unimmunized children in some areas and rumors of adverse vaccine effects (Division of Viral and Rickettsial Diseases, 2004b). By 2004, the number of countries with endemic polio had decreased from 125 to 6, with only 10 nonendemic countries reporting cases imported from other areas (Division of Viral and Rickettsial Diseases, 2004a). At present, three WHO regions have been declared polio-free—the Americas, Europe, and the Western Pacific—and interruption of transmission is thought to have been achieved in the African Region (Regional Office for Africa, 2003).

Reduction of measles mortality by 50% by 2005 is another global initiative related to communicable disease control. Measles is the leading cause of vaccine-preventable death in the world, resulting in 800,000 deaths each year (Division of Viral and Rickettsial Diseases, 2002). Mortality rates declined by 29% from 1999 to 2002 worldwide, but only by 19% in the Southeast Asia (SEA) region of WHO, where the number of cases of measles actually increased by 2.6% and immunization rates decreased by 5% compared to the prior 10 years (Department of Immunization and Vaccine Development, 2004). Southeast Asia accounts for 28% of global measles cases and 26% of deaths, and Africa accounts for 41% of cases and 58% of deaths (Global Immunization Division, 2003).

In 1994, the WHO Region of the Americas agreed on the goal of eliminating endemic measles by 2000, and the Pan American Health Organization set a goal of 95% vaccination coverage with two doses of measles vaccine among children in the Americas. By 2002, coverage had reached 92% of the child population (Global Immunization Division, 2004b; PAHO, 2003). Measles incidence decreased by 99% in the Americas from 1990 to 2001 due to high immunization rates. Communicable disease experts warn, however, that the potential for importation of new cases and possible epidemics remains high unless current immunization rates are maintained (Global Immunization Division, 2002).

Despite these impressive successes, communicable diseases remain a significant problem affecting global health status. For example, more than 600,000 deaths occur each year from hepatitis B infection, 93% of which are due to chronic infection, 21% to perinatally acquired disease, and 48% to infection acquired in early childhood. In 1992, WHO set a goal for the integration of hepatitis B vaccine into routine child immunization schedules by 1997. Unfortunately, by 2001, the initiative had only been implemented in 66% of member nations and only 31% of the world's children were effectively immunized (Division of Viral Hepatitis, 2003). Other diseases that contribute significantly to the global disease burden include HIV/AIDS, tuberculosis (TB), and malaria. These three diseases caused 5.7 million deaths worldwide in 2001 alone, and the World Health Organization's goal is to reduce mortality due to TB and malaria by 50% and HIV infection rates by 25% by 2012 (WHO, 2002).

In 2001, 36 million of the world's people were HIV-infected, 50% more than anticipated (WHO, 2002), and by the end of 2001 worldwide prevalence was expected to reach 40 million (Northridge, 2002). Of those infected, 14 million are women of childbearing age, and HIV/AIDS has led to 21 million deaths since the start of the epidemic and 4.3 million deaths among children. In addition, these deaths have created 13 million orphans. By 2020, it is anticipated that HIV/AIDS will have caused more deaths than any other disease epidemic in history (WHO, 2002). Worldwide, HIV/AIDS rose from the 28th to the 3rd leading cause of death between 1990 and 2000 and is the leading cause of disease burden in women (Bonita & Mathers, 2003).

Ninety-five percent of HIV infections occur in the developing world (WHO, 2002). The disease burden from HIV/AIDS is heaviest in sub-Saharan Africa. In 2000, for example, HIV/AIDS was responsible for 40% of deaths in adults 15 to 49 years of age, 20% of all adult deaths, and 25% of all deaths in South Africa. By 2010, the number of AIDS-related deaths is expected to be twice as high as all other causes of death combined. Since the start of the epidemic, 5 to 7 million deaths have occurred in South Africa alone. Based on seroprevalence figures among pregnant women, incidence rates for HIV infection in South Africa are also rising. In 1990, for example, less than 1% of pregnant South African women were HIV-infected. By 2000, that figure had risen to 25%. Similarly, infection rates in the general population had increased from 12.9% in 1998 to 19.9% in 2000 (Dorrington, Bourne, Bradshaw, Laubscher, & Timaeus, 2001).

In addition to the costs of suffering and death, the economic costs of HIV/AIDS are staggering. For example, infection resulted in an estimated 50% decline in sugar estate productivity from 1995 to 1997 in some sugar-producing nations due to lost productivity and overtime payments for employees filling in for those who were too ill to work. Similarly, maize production in Zimbabwe decreased 54% from 1992 to 1997 due to AIDS illness and death (WHO, 2002).

Experts have called for an integrated approach to dealing with the global problem of HIV/AIDS based

EVIDENCE-BASED PRACTICE

As noted in the chapter, Loevinsohn et al. (2002) reported a study of the overall effects of the poliomyelitis eradication campaign for the national health systems of participating countries. Examine the research literature to determine whether these findings hold true for other similar campaigns. If not, how do the findings regarding other campaigns differ from those related to the poliomyelitis campaign? What general conclusions might be drawn from the evaluation of these campaigns that might serve to help design effective eradication campaigns for other communicable diseases? Might these conclusions hold true for global campaigns to address health problems other than infectious diseases? Why or why not?

on five fundamental principles. These principles are as follows:

- Preventive activities are not sufficient to deal with the problem in countries with high prevalence of HIV infection.
- Treatment of infected persons preserves the human infrastructure of a country, improving economic productivity and prosperity.
- Treatment availability will increase screening and decrease silence about the disease.
- Treatment will reduce vertical (from mother to fetus) and horizontal (from person to person) transmission.
- Expanded HIV/AIDS treatment initiatives can help create infrastructures to support vaccine distribution and control of other communicable diseases. (Berkman, 2001)

Recent global efforts related to HIV/AIDS include the International AIDS Vaccine Initiative to promote the development and availability of a safe and accessible HIV vaccine. This effort has been under way since 1996 (WHO, 2002). Another global initiative related to HIV/ AIDS is a joint program sponsored by the Cooperative for Assistance and Relief Everywhere (CARE) and the U.S. Centers for Disease Control and Prevention. This project is intended to bring together scientific knowledge, surveillance capabilities, and years of experience in assisting people to help themselves to resolve many of the health and social problems affecting the world's poor. This interaction between a large federal agency and a global NGO has resulted in several lessons that might be applied in similar partnerships. These lessons include the following:

- Flexible funding is required for effective interagency cooperation.
- Continuing commitment from the top echelons of cooperating agencies is imperative.
- Dedication of an experienced staff to program activities is essential.
- Mechanisms are needed to pool and flexibly and quickly disburse project funds.
- Buy-in from host-country personnel is critical to the acceptance and success of new programs. (Bell & Stokes, 2001)

During the 20th century, the incidence of tuberculosis declined in most of the developed world. At the same time, it increased in the rest of the world to the point where the World Health Organization has declared an international emergency (WHO, 2005b). The global incidence of this disease is growing by 1.1% each year, and the number of cases is increasing by 2.4%. TB causes 2 million deaths per year and is the second leading cause of death in adults worldwide. Roughly one third of the world's population (2 billion people) is infected (CDC, 2002b), and approximately 8.8 million new cases of TB are diagnosed each year worldwide.

More than 99% of tuberculosis occurs in developing countries, and incidence has doubled or tripled in the last 10 years in some African countries. Not all TB occurs in poorer nations, however. In 2000, more than 100,000 cases occurred in Europe and North America as a result of international travel (WHO, 2002). Another significant portion of the tuberculosis in developed nations occurs in foreign-born individuals who migrate. For example, 58% of TB in Canada from 1990 to 1995 occurred among the foreign-born. It is estimated that only 14% of existing tubercular disease is detected by pre-emigration screening programs. TB imported from endemic countries is more often resistant to multiple drugs and more costly to treat (Cowie, Field, & Enarson, 2002).

Tuberculosis in general has high economic costs for the global community. For example, it is estimated that TB in a family breadwinner leads to a 20% to 30% drop in annual family income, and the worldwide economic costs are $12 billion (WHO, 2002). In 2000 a global initiative, the Global Alliance for TB Drug Development, was mounted to develop an affordable new drug for tuberculosis by 2010. Goals of the program include development of a drug that can be taken for a shorter period of time, that is more effective against multi-drug-resistant TB, and that prevents the development of latent tuberculosis into active disease (WHO, 2002). Treatment of tuberculosis is complicated by the growing incidence of HIV co-infection (WHO, 2004a), with approximately 10 million co-infected people throughout the world.

Anywhere from 300 to 500 million cases of malaria occur worldwide each year, and 1,200 cases occur in the United States. Forty-one percent of the world's population is exposed to malaria-bearing mosquitoes. Malaria results in 1 million deaths each year, 90% of which occur in sub-Saharan Africa. Despite higher standards of living and better medical care, the effects of malaria are felt in wealthy countries as well. Because of the limited incidence of malaria, residents in nonendemic areas such as the United States lack the protective immunity acquired from living in malaria-prone areas. In addition, providers are often unfamiliar with the diagnosis and treatment for the disease, leading to misdiagnosis or ineffective therapy (Barzolaski, 2004). Malaria was virtually eliminated in the United States in the 1950s, but is now reemerging as a condition of concern due to international travel, transport of mosquitoes via trade, and land use changes that have produced new mosquito breeding grounds (Needham & Canning, 2003).

Malaria interacts with malnutrition and common respiratory diseases to increase death rates, particularly among children. In 2000, for example, 906,000 children under 5 years of age died of malaria. Malaria also increases the risk of maternal and fetal deaths and low birth weight in infants. Elimination of malaria-causing mosquitoes or protection of the population from their bites is an effective preventive strategy for malaria, yet

MediaLink WHO and Malaria

less than 5% of those at risk for malaria sleep under insecticide-treated nets. Like HIV/AIDS and TB, malaria has economic effects. For example, over a 35-year period, malaria has been estimated to contribute to a 32% decrease in Africa's gross domestic product, for a loss of $100 billion per year. The cost of prevention would be far less. Insecticide-treated nets, for example, cost only $4 per net, with an additional cost of $1 a year for retreatment. Similarly, the cost of malarial treatment is approximately $2.50 per person ($1 per child), yet most of those infected throughout the world do not have access to effective drugs. The World Health Organization (2002) has estimated that targeted interventions addressing the problems of HIV/AIDS, tuberculosis, and malaria at a cost of $66 billion annually could save 8 million lives and generate revenues of $360 billion each year.

Much of the communicable disease burden in the world could be reduced by effective immunization programs. In fact, concentrated smallpox and poliomyelitis immunization campaigns are the basis for the successful control of these diseases. Despite the potential, however, approximately 37 million of the world's children remained unimmunized in 2000, and 11 million children die each year from vaccine-preventable diseases. For example, in spite of the elimination of neonatal tetanus in two thirds of countries, 200,000 infants and 30,000 mothers died of tetanus in 2000, and less than one third of women of childbearing age are immunized in some countries. Overall worldwide immunization rates approached 70% in the 1990s but varied widely from country to country, with a low of 18% coverage with diphtheria, tetanus, and pertussis (DTP) vaccine in war-torn Somalia compared with rates historically twice that. Immunization rates also differ significantly within countries. Children of wealthy residents of Niger are ten times more likely to be immunized than poor children and four times more likely to be immunized in Côte d'Ivoire, India, and Nigeria (UNICEF, 2002).

Discussion of one other recent communicable disease concern serves to highlight the health effects of globalization. Bovine spongiform encephalopathy (BSE) and its human variant, Creutzfeldt-Jakob disease (vCJD), are neurodegenerative diseases frequently causing death that are spread by infected animals and animal products. BSE and vCJD pose the dual threat of disease and jeopardization of food safety. There is an increasing concentration of world food production into megacorporations. For example, 10 major multinational corporations control most of the world's food industry, from agricultural production through processing and packaging to transport and sale. Widespread movement of contaminated animal products through these megacorporations increases the potential for the human spread of vCJD. Similarly, the addition of animal waste products such as bone and other animal parts to animal feed used around the world increases the potential for

infection of previously uninfected animals. Finally, global export of contaminated human blood and blood products for health-related uses may also spread the disease (Lee & Patel, 2003). The first two conditions are examples of possible effects of economic globalization on health, and the third is an example of a possible negative effect on globalization of health-related activities. Additional global effects of environmental modifications are discussed in Chapter 10∞.

Avian influenza (also called "bird flu") is another emerging communicable disease that is causing worldwide concern. Most avian influenza occurs, as the name suggests, in birds, but transmission to humans has occurred, primarily through contact with infected poultry but on rare occasions from person to person (CDC, 2006b). The primary area of concern is a highly pathogenic strain of avian influenza virus, H5N1, which has proved fatal in human beings (CDC, 2004b). Between January 2004 and April 2006, WHO documented human cases of H5N1 infection in nine countries (CDC, 2006a). At present there is no vaccine available for this condition; however, immunization with the annual influenza vaccine is recommended for health care providers likely to be exposed to prevent cross-strain interaction and development of a potential pandemic strain of the virus (CDC, 2004b). In the absence of an effective vaccine, global health measures are directed toward preventing the spread of disease through means such as isolation of persons with suspected disease and control of human exposure in work with poultry. H5N1 viral infection is resistant to treatment with the two most commonly used antiretroviral medications, amantadine and rimantadine, but other antiretroviral preparations (e.g., oseltamivir and zanamivir) should be effective in treating human infection (CDC, 2006a). Avian influenza is discussed in more detail in Chapter 28∞.

There is also increasing global concern for biological agents that might be used in bioterrorist attacks. Bioterrorism is discussed in more detail later in this chapter and in Chapter 27∞.

Chronic Disease and Disability

Although infectious diseases continue to be the primary health concern in several countries, many nations are experiencing a shift in health problems to encompass more chronic disease, injury, mental illness, nutritional problems, and environmentally caused disease. The rising incidence of chronic diseases in developing countries is a result of rising incomes, dietary changes, changes in exercise and substance use behaviors, and an aging population due to lower death rates and greater life expectancy. Chronic health problems already account for a significant portion of worldwide disease, and in 1999 noncommunicable diseases were responsible for 40% of world mortality and 43% of the global disease burden. By 2020, these figures are expected to increase to 73% and 60%, respectively.

These effects are expected to be experienced differentially by developed and developing nations. For example, in the next 30 years, the noncommunicable disease burden is expected to increase by 60% in developing and newly industrialized countries, compared to only a 10% increase in developed nations (Bonita, Winkelman, Douglas, & de Courten, 2003). In part, this is due to the fact that developed nations already experience a significant burden due to chronic diseases as a result of better control of communicable disease morbidity and mortality.

Chronic disease mortality is only one measure of its effects on health. Another measure of the international burden of chronic disease is **disability-adjusted life years (DALYs)**, or the number of years of disability-free healthy life lost due to disease. Causes of lost DALYs differ between developed and developing nations, as indicated in Table 6-8◆. In developed countries, unipolar depression causes the greatest loss of DALYs, followed by ischemic heart disease, alcohol-related disorders, cerebrovascular disease, Alzheimer's disease and other forms of dementia, motor vehicle accidents, lung cancer, osteoarthritis, COPD, and adult-onset hearing loss. In developing nations, the greatest number of DALYs are lost due to lower respiratory infections, perinatal conditions, HIV/AIDS, meningitis, and diarrheal diseases (Bonita & Mathers, 2003).

Economic growth brings about an increase in motor vehicle use and a concomitant increase in injury rates. The potential for injury from industrial accidents and toxic chemicals also increases with industrialization. Injury accounts for one in six years of life lived with disability worldwide and contributed to an estimated 5.1 million deaths in 1999. By far the greatest portion of these deaths (24%) were due to motor vehicle accidents, but 17% were self-inflicted, and 15% resulted from homicide, violence, and war (WHO, 2000).

TABLE 6-8	Percentage of DALYs Lost to Selected Conditions in Developed and Developing Nations
Developed Nations	**Developing Nations**
Unipolar depression 8.8%	Lower respiratory diseases 6.8%
Ischemic heart disease 6.7%	Perinatal conditions 6.7%
Alcohol-related diseases 5.4%	HIV/AIDS 6.6%
Cerebrovascular disease 4.9%	Meningitis 4.6%
Alzheimer's disease and other dementias 4.3%	Diarrheal diseases 4.6%
Motor vehicle accidents 3.1%	Unipolar depression 4%
Lung cancer 3%	Ischemic heart disease 3.5%
Osteoarthritis 2.7%	Malaria 3%
Chronic obstructive pulmonary disease 2.5%	Cerebrovascular disease 2.9%
Adult-onset hearing loss 2.5%	Motor vehicle accidents 2.8%

Data from: Bonita, R., & Mathers, C. D. (2003). Global health status at the beginning of the twenty-first century. In R. Beaglehole (Ed.), Global public health: A new era (pp. 24–53). Oxford, UK: Oxford University.

Tobacco Consumption

More than 4 million tobacco-related deaths occur worldwide each year, and this figure is expected to climb to 10 million by 2030 (Collin, 2003). In 1995, an estimated 29% of all people over 15 years of age (1.1 billion) smoked. Approximately 80% of these smokers live in low- and middle-income countries, and 80% are men, although the proportion of women smokers is increasing in many parts of the world (Jha, Ranson, Nguyen, & Yach, 2002).

Tobacco consumption is an area in which global health initiatives are critically important because of the transnational nature of the tobacco industry. Control of tobacco marketing and sales lies outside the jurisdiction of any single nation. New approaches to dealing with health issues such as tobacco and other drug use are required. Frequently, international efforts in this realm are patterned on agreements used for control of communicable diseases that have very different risk factors. In addition, these efforts, particularly those related to tobacco control, are often circumvented by vested economic interests (Collin, Lee, & Bissell, 2004). In May 2003, the World Health Assembly passed a resolution adopting the *WHO Framework Convention on Tobacco Control*, which called on member nations to undertake specific initiatives designed to promote national tobacco control strategies, reduce the demand for tobacco, protect populations from tobacco smoke, regulate the content of tobacco products, and educate the public on the hazards associated with tobacco use (World Health Organization, 2003c). After achieving the agreement of the required 40 WHO members, which did not include the United States, the convention went into effect in February 2005 (Late, 2005). In addition, several national initiatives related to tobacco control are serving as models for other countries in a *leapfrogging* process, in which a pilot project tested in one country is adopted elsewhere (Collin, 2003). For example, recent news highlighted a push to ban smoking in all public buildings in the United Kingdom, similar to the initial California legislation that eventually led to smoking bans in all places except residences.

Mental Health

A growing burden of mental illness is also being experienced worldwide. For example, major depression, schizophrenia, bipolar disorder, alcohol use disorders, and self-inflicted injury comprise five of the top ten leading causes of disability in the world. Mental health issues have been described as the "Cinderella" of global health concerns because of the higher visibility of other health-related issues such as HIV/AIDS and other communicable diseases (Patel & Thara, 2003, p. 2). As noted earlier, alcohol-related disorders, Alzheimer's disease, and depression are significant contributors to lost DALYs throughout the world.

Mental disorders creating global health concerns can be grouped into five major categories: severe disorders such as schizophrenia and bipolar affective disorder;

common disorders (e.g., depression, anxiety, and panic attacks); substance abuse disorders; mental disorders in the elderly (e.g., Alzheimer's disease and other forms of dementia); and mental disorders of childhood such as autism, attention deficit disorder, depression, and learning disability. In the 2001 WHO world health report, mental disorders accounted for 31% of all years lived with disability, and major depression alone accounted for 12% of lost years. In the age group of 15 to 44 years, mental disorders constituted four of the five leading causes of years lived with disability (major unipolar depression—16.4%, alcohol abuse—5.5%, schizophrenia—4.9%, and bipolar disorder—4.7%) (Patel & Thara, 2003).

Child Health

According to Needham and Canning (2003) in their book *Global Disease Eradication: The Race for the Last Child*, many of the efforts related to global health have been prompted by the plight of the world's children. In spite of millions of dollars of international assistance, however, children under 5 years of age in some parts of the world have a mortality rate of 91 per 1,000 live births compared to only 6 per 1,000 for developed nations. Even in developed countries, children living in poverty have worse outcomes than their wealthier counterparts. Causes of inequalities in child health include financial barriers to health care and other necessities and lack of access to quality care. Other contributing factors include low maternal education, lack of potable water and sanitation, and social determinants such as women's lack of access to resources and power and poor community resources (Wagstaff, Bustreo, Bryce, Cleason, & the WHO-World Bank Child Health and Poverty Working Group, 2004).

Some progress has been made in decreasing childhood mortality. For example, a Latin American or Caribbean child born in 1960 had 105 chances in 1,000 of dying before his or her first birthday. By 1990, this figure was down to 30 chances in 1,000 (Wagstaff et al., 2004). As noted earlier, considerable progress has been made in providing routine immunizations for the children of the world. However, 20% of 56 million deaths worldwide each year occur in children under 5 years of age, and 99% of these deaths occur in developing nations (Bonita & Mathers, 2003). More than half of child deaths are due to pneumonia, diarrheal diseases, malaria, measles, and HIV/AIDS. In addition, malnutrition is a contributing factor in 60% of these deaths (Wagstaff et al., 2004). Diarrheal disease is the leading cause of morbidity and mortality in children under 5 years of age, with an estimated 1.5 billion cases each year and 1.5 to 2.5 million deaths. Death rates have decreased somewhat due to the use of oral rehydration therapy, but this strategy has not been employed as widely as needed (King, Glass, Bresee, & Duggan, 2003). Diarrheal diseases are not likely to be well controlled, however, until improvements in water quality and sanitation are achieved worldwide. For example, 1.1 billion people in the world lack potable water and 2.4 billion lack adequate sanitation (CDC, 2002c).

Members of the WHO-World Bank Child Health and Poverty Working Group (Wagstaff et al., 2004) have suggested that a simple set of six preventive activities and two therapeutic activities could significantly decrease the extent of disease burden among children. Basic preventive activities include prenatal care, breastfeeding, birth spacing, hygiene, immunization, and insect control. Recommended therapeutic interventions include effective home management of illness and prompt medical attention when needed.

Women's Health

Women's health is another area of concern in global health care. Violation of women's rights and violence against women have been the subject of several recent international conferences. Violence is particularly apparent in refugee situations that occur with regularity in the modern world. Maternal mortality continues to be high in many parts of the world and now stands at 600,000

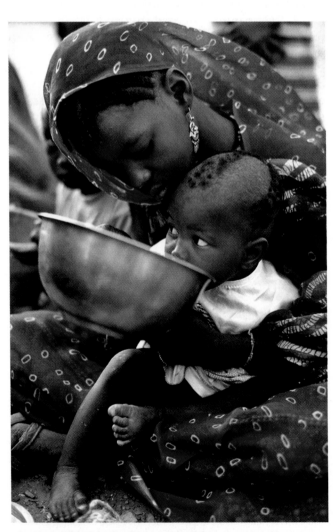

Malnutrition is a serious world health concern.
(© Lauren Goodsmith/The Image Works)

deaths per year. An additional 15 million women suffer complications of pregnancy and childbirth that lead to injury and disability (Doyal, 2004). Women also suffer high mortality rates from communicable diseases, with one third of deaths among women related to communicable disease (WHO, 2002).

Because of the biological effects of reproduction, women are more vulnerable to health problems (Doyal, 2004), but reproductive biology is only one of the reasons for poor health status among the women of the world. Gender inequities that contribute to discrimination and poverty are experienced by women throughout the world. For example, women constitute 70% of the world's population in extreme poverty (WHO, 2002), and more women than men in 12 of 15 developing countries and in 5 of 8 developed nations are in poverty. A variety of social conditions lead to differential health effects for men and women. Cultural norms regarding entitlement are less favorable for women than for men, and women are often employed in low-paying, high-risk jobs. In many countries, women retain responsibility for the care of homes and children while shouldering the additional burden of out-of-home labor. Increased participation in the labor force has the advantage of increased material and social support, but also leads to increased workload and greater potential for occupational exposures. Even women working in the home experience greater environmental risks due to increased use of carbon-based cooking fuels (Doyal, 2004).

Traditional gender roles may also place women at higher risk for HIV infection due to the inability to negotiate condom use or other elements of sexual activity. In 2000, for example, 1.3 million women died of AIDS-related conditions, and 16.4 million women were infected. In addition, women accounted for 47% of persons living with HIV infection (Doyal, 2004).

International trafficking in human beings, which affects primarily women and young girls and boys, is another area of growing international concern. An estimated 600,000 to 800,000 individuals are trafficked across international borders each year, and thousands more are enslaved in their own countries. More than 12 million people are believed to be enslaved in forced labor and sexual servitude throughout the world. Much of the human trafficking is for the purpose of sexual exploitation, but trafficking also involves involuntary servitude. Trafficking has been defined by the United Nations' *Protocol to Prevent, Suppress, and Punish Trafficking in Persons, especially Women and Children*, as

> the recruitment, transportation, transfer, harboring, or receipt of persons, by means of threat or use of force or other forms of coercion, of abduction, of fraud, or deception, or the abuse of power or of a position of vulnerability or the giving or receiving of payments or benefits to achieve the consent of the person having control over another person, for the purpose of exploitation. Exploitation shall include, at a minimum, the exploitation of the

prostitution of others or other forms of sexual exploitation, forced labor or services, slavery or practices similar to slavery, servitude or the removal of organs. (U.S. Department of State, 2005)

Trafficking in persons will be discussed in more detail in Chapter 32∞ .

Because of income differentials, new health-related products and effective treatments may not be available to women. Conversely, the use of medications of inferior quality, ones that cannot be sold in the countries where they are produced due to strict drug controls, may lead to ineffective treatment for HIV/AIDS and other conditions (Doyal, 2004). In addition, the high cost of HIV/AIDS drugs may contribute to inconsistent use and increased potential for development of drug resistance among both men and women worldwide. Women have also become a new global market for harmful products such as tobacco and products that undermine healthful behaviors, such as prepared formulas used in place of breastfeeding.

War and Civil Unrest

War and civil unrest are other global factors that have profound effects on health. For example, the conflict between Armenia and Azerbaijan in the early 1990s led to 600,000 internally displaced persons (those who have fled their homes but have not left the country) and 200,000 refugees. This displacement resulted in high rates of malnutrition and anemia, among other health problems. Similar effects have been noted in other war-torn areas (Division of Reproductive Health, 2004). War has myriad other health-related effects. An international physicians group, for example, projected possible health and environmental outcomes of war in Iraq. These included 268,000 to 480,000 deaths and economic costs related to the war and its aftermath of destabilization and reconstruction of $150 to $200 billion (Salvage, 2002).

War and civil unrest also increase the potential for terrorist activities. Terrorist activity creates intentional harm for individuals or for population groups. **Terrorism** is defined in the U.S. Code of Federal Regulations as "the unlawful use of force or violence against persons or property to intimidate or coerce a government, the civilian population, or any segment thereof, in furtherance of political or social objectives" (as quoted by the Federal Emergency Management Agency, [FEMA], 2004c, p. 1). Implied within this definition are four critical elements of terrorist activity. First, its purpose is to cause intimidation or engender fear. Second, terrorism involves the use of violence outside the ordinary. Third, terrorist violence is premeditated and carefully planned to achieve a purpose. That purpose or objective is the fourth element (Brauer, 2002). Terrorism is not random violence, but violence with a purpose.

Terrorist activity may be categorized as domestic or international, based on the origin of the person or group responsible. **Domestic terrorism** is perpetrated by individuals or groups within a given country without foreign direction or involvement. Domestic terrorism is directed against either the government or population segments of one's own country. White supremacist activities against African Americans, Jews, and other ethnic and religious groups are examples of domestic terrorism. **International terrorism**, on the other hand, is directed by foreign groups and may transcend national boundaries, affecting people in several countries or perpetrated by residents of one country against another (FEMA, 2004a).

Terrorists may have one of several motivations for their activities. These include religious, political, and ethnic/national motivations. The terrorist activities of Islamic groups such as al Qaeda and the Palestinian Islamic Jihad are examples of religiously motivated efforts. Reciprocal terrorist activities between ethnic Serbs and Albanians are primarily based on ethnic group conflicts. Single terrorists operating alone frequently also have a political motivation (Simon, 2002), as in the 2003 firebombing of sport utility vehicles in San Diego in protest of environmental degradation. Whatever their motivation, terrorists generally have several common goals. The first goal is to create fear in the populace, often to encourage the public to put pressure on officials to take actions desired by the terrorists. The second goal is to convey a sense of the powerlessness of government to deal with terrorist activities and protect the public, thereby undermining the credibility and authority of government bodies. Finally, terrorists wish to gain attention to their cause (FEMA, 2004a). Some authors suggest that terrorists may also have a fourth goal, to achieve some level of legitimacy with their own people, even among those who decry their methods (Nacos, 2002).

Although many of the effects of terrorism are similar to those experienced in war, they may be more far reaching and more devastating. The rules of war promulgated in the Geneva and Hague Conventions on Warfare in the late 19th and early to mid 20th centuries prohibited taking civilians hostage, maltreating prisoners of war, and engaging in reprisals against noncombatants and prisoners. Furthermore, the conventions recognized neutral territory and neutral parties. As is obvious from recent terrorist activities, these conventions are systematically violated by terrorists, which serves to enhance the fear their activities generate (Hoffman, 1998).

The terrorist attacks on the World Trade Center and the U.S. Pentagon on September 11, 2001, and the subsequent success in contaminating the U.S. mail suggest the increased sophistication of current world terrorist activities (Simon, 2002). The frequency of international terrorist activities has decreased somewhat since that time, with 41% fewer international terrorist attacks worldwide in 2003 than in 2001 (208 and 355 attacks, respectively). Terrorist attacks occur with differential frequency in various parts of the world. For example, from 1998 through 2003, 37% of all attacks occurred in Latin America, 25% in Asia, 12% in Western Europe, 11% in the Middle East,

and 9% in Africa, compared to less than 1% in North America. Likewise, attacks differ by type of target, with 63% of attacks targeting businesses and 23% targeting "other" facilities such as places of worship, transportation, and other places where people congregate. Only 2% and 4% of attacks targeted military installations and government facilities, respectively (U.S. Department of State, 2004). In part, the limited number of attacks against the latter two institutions derives from the enhanced security usually afforded them.

The devastation caused by terrorist attacks increases exponentially with the use of weapons of mass destruction (WMD). There are four categories of agents considered WMDs: nuclear, chemical, and biological weapons; and computers. Although the potential effects of nuclear, chemical, and biological weapons seem rather obvious, it may seem strange to think of computers as a possible weapon of mass destruction. Potential computer-mediated effects may range from the availability of information on the construction of homemade bombs (Simon, 2002) to dissemination of hate propaganda to the ability to shut down information systems vital to national defense or to health operations in times of emergency. Although most computer interference would not directly cause disease and death, it may hamper response to other crises that result in these effects.

Nuclear weapons, although potentially devastating in their effects, are unlikely to be used by terrorist groups because of the advanced technology needed and the high cost of materials. In the World Trade Center attacks, however, terrorists demonstrated that similar, if more localized, effects could be achieved with aviation fuel. Probably of greater concern, though, is the fact that both biological and chemical weapons are relatively inexpensive to develop and readily available to most terrorist groups. In addition, relatively small quantities of substances may cause considerable damage, and effects are often insidious and difficult to identify (Horton, 2003).

Biological weapons involve the use of microorganisms or their toxins to produce illness in people, animals, or plants (FEMA, 2004b). Human biological agents are considered weapons of mass destruction and are classified into three categories by the CDC (2004a). Category A diseases are those that can be easily disseminated, cause high mortality with significant public health impact, may lead to public panic and social disruption, and require special response preparation. These diseases include anthrax, botulism, plague, smallpox, tularemia, and viral hemorrhagic fever. Category B diseases include Q fever, brucellosis, glanders, ricin toxin, epsilon toxin, and *Staphylococcus B*, each of which can be transmitted with moderate ease, cause moderate morbidity and relatively low mortality, and require special diagnostic and surveillance capabilities. Category C diseases include emerging organisms that could be developed for mass dissemination and would have significant public health impact in terms of morbidity and mortality. Diseases in this category include Nipah virus, hantaviruses, tick-borne hemorrhagic fever and encephalitis viruses, yellow fever, and multi-drug-resistant tuberculosis. More information about several of these diseases is presented in Chapter 28∞ and in Appendix E on the Companion Website.

Agroterrorism is a subcategory of biological terrorism that is not considered use of a weapon of mass destruction because it does not directly affect people. **Agroterrorism** is "the deliberate introduction of a disease agent, either against livestock or into the food chain, for purposes of undermining stability and/or generating fear" (Cupp, Walker, & Hillison, 2004, p. 98). Bovine spongiform encephalitis, or BSE, discussed earlier, is a possible agroterrorist agent against animals; plant pathogens include wheat smut and a mildew that attacks corn crops. Like other bioterrorist agents, agroterrorist agents are classified based on their ability to disrupt food supplies and threaten food safety (Cupp et al., 2004).

Chemical warfare agents are highly toxic chemicals that can be disseminated as vapors, gases, liquids, or aerosols or adsorbed to dust particles (FEMA, 2004b). Chemical weapons are categorized by the major organ system affected. Categories include blister or vesicant agents, such as mustard, that affect the skin and lungs; chemicals that affect the blood such as arsine, hydrogen chloride, and hydrogen cyanide; and agents such as chlorine gas, nitrogen oxide, sulfur trioxide–chlorosulfonic acid, and zinc oxide that affect the respiratory system. Other categories of chemical agents include those that cause mental incapacitation, such as LSD and phenothiazines; those that affect the central and peripheral nervous systems, such as sarin and V-gas; those that are used for riot control, such as tear gas; and those that induce vomiting, such as adamsite and diphenylcyanoarsine (CDC, 2001).

Successful global efforts to deal with international terrorism must focus on five major objectives. The first objective is to limit death and suffering as a result of the terrorist activity. Special attention may need to be given to particularly vulnerable groups such as children, the elderly, and the physically compromised. A second objective is to preserve civil liberties by using the least restrictive strategies possible to curtail terrorist activities and the effects of those activities. Preservation of economic stability is a third objective, and prevention of scapegoating, hate crimes, and stigmatization of certain populations is the fourth. Finally, global strategies need to focus on enhancing the ability of individuals and groups to recover from terrorist attacks when necessary (Working Group on "Governance Dilemmas" in Bioterrorism Response, 2004).

Community health nurses may be involved in public health responses to terrorist attacks or in educating the public regarding preventive measures or actions to be taken in the case of exposure. In addition, community health nurses may be actively involved in prevent-

ing panic in the general public or in dealing with the psychological effects of a terrorist attack. In the case of biological attacks, community health nurses may be among the first to note symptoms of unusual illness in the population and should be familiar with the signs and symptoms of infection with the most likely biological agents (e.g., anthrax, smallpox, plague). Signs and symptoms of these diseases are included in Appendix E on the Companion Website. The effects of war and civil unrest as human-caused disasters will be addressed in more detail in Chapter 27∞.

NURSING AND GLOBAL HEALTH

Why should a nurse working in a particular country, such as the United States, be concerned about globalization and global health issues? The most obvious answer to this question, of course, is to be able to understand the effects of global health issues on the health status of the local population, but there are other reasons as well. Knowledge of effective elements of other national health care systems can assist nurses to advocate for appropriate health system reforms at home. Community health nurses can examine or conduct research on the effects of different national approaches to health care delivery that can be brought to the attention of health policy makers at state, national, and international levels.

In addition, nurses in most countries will encounter clients from a variety of other nations. These clients may need assistance in navigating the health system differences between their countries of origin and their current countries of residence. Knowledge of these other health systems will allow nurses to better educate clients with respect to similarities and differences between health systems and how to navigate the system in their country of residence. Similarly, knowledge of the health problems prevalent in their countries of origin can assist community health nurses in assessing the health status of individuals from other parts of the world.

At some point, community health nurses may work or travel in other countries, and knowledge of health systems and prevalent health problems can help them to better protect their own health or to better meet the health needs of their host countries. Finally, community health nurses may find themselves working with nurses from other countries, either at home or in international arenas, and knowledge of their health care systems will permit more effective collaboration in addressing the health care needs of all of the world's populations.

One of the primary global issues affecting nursing is the nursing workforce shortage. Although we in the United States have a relatively clear picture of the extent of the national nursing shortage, we often fail to realize that shortages in other nations may be even more acute. For example, although the United States has a nurse-to-population ratio of 97.2 nurses to every 10,000 people, 15 Latin American countries have fewer than 10 nurses per

10,000 people, and the regional average for Latin America is 30 nurses per 10,000 population. In addition, the nursing workforce is poorly distributed, with as many as 70% of nurses in some countries working exclusively in hospitals in large urban centers, leaving rural communities and public health centers with serious shortages (PAHO, 2005). WHO (2005a) has also noted the reluctance of health workers in many parts of the world, including nurses, to work in remote rural areas where needs may be far greater than in more popular urban centers. The U.S. health care system often exacerbates nursing shortages in other countries by recruiting foreign-educated nurses to the United States (PAHO, 2005). Community health nurses can actively advocate for education of nursing professionals in other countries and for restraints on foreign nurse recruitment in developed nations. They may also be involved in the development of training programs for community health nurses in global contexts.

Community health nurses are supported in their international activities by several agencies and organizations. WHO recognizes the importance of nursing (and midwifery) services to the accomplishment of global health objectives and so maintains a Nursing and Midwifery Services division to assist with nursing development throughout the world. The division has outlined five key areas for effort in its strategic directions document for 2002 to 2008: human resources planning to address the nursing shortage, personnel management, promotion of evidence-based practice, education for nursing practice, and stewardship of national health resources (WHO, 2003a). Information related to Nursing and Midwifery Services is available from the WHO Web site at http://www.who.int/health-services-delivery/nursing.

Another avenue for international involvement by community health nurses is the **International Council of Nurses (ICN)**. ICN is a federation of national nurses' associations, including the American Nurses Association, and represents nurses in more than 128 countries. The organization was established to address three primary goals:

- To promote worldwide nursing exchange
- To advance the nursing profession
- To influence global health policy

In its efforts to achieve these three goals, ICN works to standardize professional nursing practice worldwide and to improve the socioeconomic welfare of nurses (ICN, 2005a). ICN's mission is to lead the world to better health and to advocate for the health of populations (ICN, 1998). One of the major ways in which ICN works to achieve this mission is through the creation of nursing networks that serve as avenues for the exchange of nursing knowledge and expertise in specific areas. Some of the current networks supported by ICN focus on rural nursing, disaster preparedness and emergency care, leadership, and advanced nursing practice (ICN, 2005b).

Sigma Theta Tau International is another international nursing organization. Established in 1922 by six U.S. nursing students, Sigma Theta Tau's goal is to provide leadership and support scholarship related to nursing practice, education, and research. The organization was the first funder of nursing research in the United States and currently supports a variety of nursing education and research initiatives. In 1985, the organization was incorporated as Sigma Theta Tau International, Inc. to better connect the worldwide network of scholars who promote health worldwide (Sigma Theta Tau, 2005).

Community health nurses may also be actively involved in a wide variety of international nursing and multidisciplinary organizations that address special focus areas such as violence against women, menopause, child health, HIV/AIDS, family health, and so on.

As we have seen, a wide variety of health problems cross national boundaries, and global approaches must be taken to resolve them. As noted by one author, "Globalization could usher in a Golden Age of international cooperation—and with it, universal standards for work safety, improved infectious disease surveillance and control, more stringent environmental protection, greater equity in education, the freer exchange of expertise and the potential benefits of transnational food and drug regulation" (Hooey, 2001, p. 5). He continues, however, that this will require concerted cooperation on the part of the world's nation-states and questions whether such cooperation will occur. It remains to be seen whether such efforts can be undertaken and whether they will be successful.

Case Study

Cooperation for Polio Elimination

When I was a Peace Corps volunteer (PCV) in a small village in India, my site mate and I initiated a program for DTP and polio immunizations in the local primary health center and its five substations in outlying villages. We got funding for an initial supply of vaccines from the International Rotary Club. Vaccines were purchased in Bombay, a trip of 250 miles from the health center, and transported on ice to the village. This trip had to be made

every 6 weeks because of the limited shelf-life of the oral polio vaccine.

Since the health center possessed only two syringes, we acquired used disposable syringes and needles from Peace Corps headquarters in Bombay. This equipment was of the type that could be resterilized by boiling, and several hundred syringes were used each year to update immunizations for volunteers in the region. A very small fee was charged for each immunization. This revenue was used to pay for subsequent vaccine purchases, and the program was essentially self-funding.

We gave the immunizations ourselves, both in the health center itself and on specific immunization days in the subcenters, rather than involving our local nursing counterparts. Immunizations were also begun in the local school. Unfortunately, after the first dose of DTP in the school setting, many of the children developed mild inflammation and soreness at the injection sites. Their parents complained to the physician director of the health center, who put a stop to further immunization in the school setting. One member of the health center staff, whose daughter we had nursed through a life-threatening episode of typhoid, became a local proponent for immunization in the village. Many of her friends and family came to the health center requesting immunizations. Unfortunately,

she was of lower-class status and did not have influence with upper-class residents.

Just before we were scheduled to leave India, we took one of the host-country staff to Bombay and showed him where to purchase the vaccines. We left a supply of syringes and needles that could be used by the health center staff to continue the program. The program was sustained for a few years after we left, but then dwindled away. India remains one of the few countries in the world with endemic poliomyelitis.

1. What elements of a sector-wide approach did we incorporate in this project? What other elements might have improved the sustainability of the program?
2. How might we have benefited from knowledge of the lessons regarding NGO activities discussed in the chapter?

Test Your Understanding

1. What are three advantages to U.S. involvement in global health initiatives? (p. 103)

2. Identify at least five policy dilemmas faced by national health care systems. (p. 105)

3. Compare at least three different national health care systems on at least four criteria. In what ways are they similar? How do they differ? (pp. 105-111)

4. Differentiate between multilateral and bilateral international health agencies. Give examples of each and discuss when each might be most appropriate for solving a particular kind of health problem. (pp. 111–113)

5. What is the difference between international health and global health? (p. 111)

6. What are some of the positive and negative health effects of globalization? Give an example of each type of effect. (pp. 114–117)

7. What are the critical elements of a global health policy agenda? (pp. 118–119)

8. How can community health nurses be involved in the prevention of and response to international terrorism? (p. 129)

EXPLORE MediaLink

http://www.prenhall.com/clark
Resources for this chapter can be found on the Companion Website.

Audio Glossary
Exam Review Questions
Case Study: Bird Flu: A Global Health
   Issue

Appendix E: Information on Selected
   Communicable Diseases
MediaLink Applications: WHO Measures
   Against Malaria

Media Links
Challenge Your Knowledge
Advocacy Interviews

References

Alleyne, G. A. O. (2002). The Pan American Health Organization's first 100 years: Reflections of the Director. *American Journal of Public Health, 92,* 1890–1894.

Altman, D. (2003). Understanding HIV/AIDS as a global security issue. In K. Lee (Ed.), *Health impacts of globalization: Towards global governance* (pp. 33–46). New York: Palgrave Macmillan.

Barzolaski, B. (2004). The menace of malaria: Stay on your toes to keep malaria at arms length. *NURSEweek, 17*(17), 7–9.

Bell, P. D., & Stokes, C. C. (2001). Melding disparate cultures and capacities to create global health partnerships. *American Journal of Public Health, 91,* 1152–1154.

Berkman, A. (2001). Confronting global AIDS: Prevention and treatment. *American Journal of Public Health, 91,* 1348–1349.

Bloor, K., & Maynard, A. (2002). Universal coverage and cost control: The United Kingdom National Health Service. In K. V. Thai, E. T. Wimberley, & S. M. McManus (Eds.),

Handbook of international health care systems (pp. 261–286). New York: Marcel Dekker.

Bonita, R., & Mathers, C. D. (2003). Global health status at the beginning of the twenty-first century. In R. Beaglehole (Ed.), *Global public health: A new era* (pp. 24–53). Oxford, UK: Oxford University.

Bonita, R., Winkelmann, R., Douglas, K. A., & de Courten, M. (2003). The WHO stepwise approach to surveillance (STEPS) of noncommunicable disease risk factors. In D. V.

McQueen & P. Puska (Eds.), *Global behavioral risk factor surveillance* (pp. 9–22). New York: Kluwer Academic/Plenum.

Bourhanskaia, E. A., Kubataev, A., & Paterson, M. A. (2002). Russia's health care system: Caring in a turbulent environment. In K. V. Thai, E. T. Wimberley, & S. M. McManus (Eds.), *Handbook of international health care systems* (pp. 59–78). New York: Marcel Dekker.

Brauer, J. (2002). On the economics of terrorism. *Phi Kappa Phi Forum, 82*(2), 38–41.

Bunyanavich, S., & Walkup, R. B. (2001). US public health leaders shift toward a new paradigm of global health. *American Journal of Public Health, 91*, 1556–1558.

Buse, K., Drager, N., Fustukian, S., & Lee, K. (2002). Globalisation and health policy: Trends and opportunities. In K. Lee, K. Buse, & S. Fustukian (Eds.), *Health policy in a globalising world* (pp. 251–280). Cambridge, UK: Cambridge University.

Buse, K., & Walt, G. (2002). Globalisation and multilateral public-private health partnerships: Issues for health policy. In K. Lee, K. Buse, & S. Fustukian (Eds.), *Health policy in a globalising world* (pp. 41–62). Cambridge, UK: Cambridge University.

Campbell, J. C., & Ikegami, N. (2000). Long-term care insurance comes to Japan. *Health Affairs, 19*, 26–39.

Centers for Disease Control and Prevention. (2001). Agents/Diseases. Retrieved October 25, 2001, from http://www.bt.cdc.gov/agent/agentlist.asp

Centers for Disease Control and Prevention. (2002a). 25th anniversary of the last case of naturally acquired smallpox. *Morbidity and Mortality Weekly Report, 51*, 952.

Centers for Disease Control and Prevention. (2002b). World TB day, March 24, 2002. *Morbidity and Mortality Weekly Report, 51*, 229.

Centers for Disease Control and Prevention. (2002c). World water day, March 22, 2002. *Morbidity and Mortality Weekly Report, 51*, 237–238.

Centers for Disease Control and Prevention. (2003). Protecting the nation's health in an era of globalization: An introduction. *Phi Kappa Phi Forum, 83*(4), 38–41.

Centers for Disease Control and Prevention. (2004a). *Bioterrorism agents/diseases*. Retrieved April 25, 2006, from http://www.bt/cdc/gov/agent/agentlist-category.asp

Centers for Disease Control and Prevention. (2004b). *Interim recommendations for infection control in health-care facilities caring for patients with known or suspected avian influenza*. Retrieved May 9, 2006, from http://www.cdc.gov/flu/avian/infectcontrol.pdf

Centers for Disease Control and Prevention. (2006a). *Avian influenza: Current situation*. Retrieved May 9, 2006, from http://www.bt.cdc.gov/scripts/emailprint/print.asp

Centers for Disease Control and Prevention. (2006b). *Key facts about avian influenza (bird flu) and avian influenza A (H5N1) virus*. Retrieved May 9, 2006, from http://www.bt.cdc.gov/scripts/emailprint/print.asp

Collin, J. (2003). Think global, smoke local: Transnational tobacco companies and cognitive globalization. In K. Lee (Ed.), *Health impacts of globalization: Towards global governance* (pp. 61–85). New York: Palgrave Macmillan.

Collin, J., Lee, K., & Bissell, K. (2004). The framework convention on tobacco control: The politics of global health governance. In N. K. Poku & A. Whiteside (Eds.), *Global health and governance: HIV/AIDS* (pp. 75–92). New York: Palgrave Macmillan.

Cowie, R. L., Field, S. K., & Enarson, D. A. (2002). Tuberculosis in immigrants to Canada: A global problem which requires a global solution. *Canadian Journal of Public Health, 93*, 85–86.

Cruise, P. L. (2002). France's health care system. In K. V. Thai, E. T. Wimberley, & S. M. McManus (Eds.), *Handbook of international health care systems* (pp. 235–259). New York: Marcel Dekker.

Cupp, O. S., Walker, D. E. II, & Hillison, J. (2004). Agroterrorism in the US: Key security challenges for the 21st century. *Biosecurity & Bioterrorism, 2*(2), 97–105.

Davis, P., & Lin, V. (2003). Public health in Australia and New Zealand. In R. Beaglehole (Ed.), *Global public health: A new era* (pp. 190–208). Oxford, UK: Oxford University.

Deber, R. B. (2003). Health care reform: Lessons from Canada. *American Journal of Public Health, 93*, 20–24.

Department of Immunization and Vaccine Development, World Health Organization. (2004). Progress toward sustainable measles mortality reduction—South-East Asia Region, 1999–2002. *Morbidity and Mortality Weekly Report, 53*, 559–562.

Division of Parasitic Diseases. (2002). Progress toward global dracunculiasis eradication, June 2002. *Morbidity and Mortality Weekly Report, 51*, 810–811.

Division of Parasitic Diseases. (2004). Progress toward global eradication of dracunculiasis, 2002–2003. *Morbidity and Mortality Weekly Report, 53*, 871–872.

Division of Reproductive Health. (2004). Prevalence of anemia among displaced and nondisplaced mothers and children—Azerbaijan, 2001. *Morbidity and Mortality Weekly Report, 53*, 610–614.

Division of Viral and Rickettsial Diseases, National Center for Infectious Diseases. (2002). Measles—United States, 2000. *Morbidity and Mortality Weekly Report, 51*, 120–123.

Division of Viral and Rickettsial Diseases, National Center for Infectious Diseases. (2004a). Progress toward poliomyelitis eradication—Afghanistan and Pakistan, January, 2003–May, 2004. *Morbidity and Mortality Weekly Report, 53*, 634–637.

Division of Viral and Rickettsial Diseases, National Center for Infectious Diseases. (2004b). Progress toward global eradication of poliomyelitis—January 2003–April 2004. *Morbidity and Mortality Weekly Report, 53*, 532–535.

Division of Viral Hepatitis. (2003). Global progress toward universal childhood hepatitis B vaccination, 2003. *Morbidity and Mortality Weekly Report, 52*, 868–870.

Dorrington, R., Bourne, D., Bradshaw, D., Laubscher, R., & Timaeus, I. M. (2001). The impact of HIV/AIDS on adult mortality in South Africa. Retrieved December 20, 2001, from http://www.mrc.ac.za.bod

Doyal, L. (2004). Putting gender into health and globalization debates: New perspectives and old challenges. In N. K. Poku & A. Whiteside (Eds.), *Global health and governance: HIV/AIDS* (pp. 43–60). New York: Palgrave Macmillan.

Evans, T. (2004). A human right to health? In N. K. Poku & A. Whiteside (Eds.), *Global health and governance: HIV/AIDS* (pp. 7–25). New York: Palgrave Macmillan.

Families USA. (2005). *Census Bureau's uninsured number indicates fourth increase in a row*. Retrieved December 15, 2005, from http://familiesusa.org/siteresources/newsroom/statements/census-bureau-uninsured-number.

Federal Emergency Management Agency. (2004a). Backgrounder: Terrorism. Retrieved November 22, 2004, from http://www.fema/gov/hazards/terrorism/terror.shtm

Federal Emergency Management Agency. (2004b). Factsheet: Terrorism. Retrieved November 22, 2004, from http://www.fema/gov/hazards/terrorism/terrorf.shtm

Federal Emergency Management Agency. (2004c). Terrorism. Retrieved November 22, 2004, from http://www.fema/gov/hazards/terrorism

Fee, E., & Brown, T. (2002). 100 years of the Pan American Health Organization. *American Journal of Public Health, 92*, 1888–1889.

Fink, S. (2002). International efforts spotlight traditional, complementary, and alternative medicine. *American Journal of Public Health, 93*, 1734–1739.

Fox, D. M., & Kassalow, J. S. (2001). Making health a priority of US foreign policy. *American Journal of Public Health, 91*, 1554–1555.

Fried, B. J., & Gaydos, L. M. (2002). Preface. In B. J. Fried & L. M. Gaydos (Eds.), *World health systems: Challenges and perspectives* (pp. ix–xii). Chicago: Health Administration Press.

Gaydos, L. M. D., & Fried, B. J. (2002). The United Kingdom. In B. J. Fried & L. M. Gaydos (Eds.), *World health systems: Challenges and perspectives* (pp. 267–278). Chicago: Health Administration Press.

Global Immunization Division, National Immunization Program. (2002). Outbreak of measles, Venezuela and Colombia, 2001–2002. *Morbidity and Mortality Weekly Report, 51*, 757–760.

Global Immunization Division, National Immunization Program. (2003). Update: Global measles control and mortality reduction—Worldwide, 1991–2001. *Morbidity and Mortality Weekly Report, 52*, 471–474.

Global Immunization Division, National Immunization Program. (2004a). Global polio eradication initiative strategic plan, 2004. *Morbidity and Mortality Weekly Report, 53*, 107–108.

Global Immunization Division, National Immunization Program. (2004b). Progress toward measles elimination—Region of the Americas, 2002–2003. *Morbidity and Mortality Weekly Report, 53*, 304–306.

Gostin, L. O. (2003). Emerging issues in population health: National and global perspectives. *Journal of Law, Medicine, & Ethics, 31*, 476–481.

Griffiths, S. (2003). Public health in the United Kingdom. In R. Beaglehole (Ed.), *Global public health: A new era* (pp. 54–68). Oxford, UK: Oxford University.

Hall, J. (1999). Incremental changes in the Australian health care system. *Health Affairs, 18,* 95–110.

Hegvary, S. (2004). Working paper on grand challenges in improving global health. *Journal of Nursing Scholarship, 36,* 96–101.

Heywood, M. (2004). Drug access, patents and global health: "Chaffed and waxed sufficient." In N. K. Poku & A. Whiteside (Eds.), *Global health and governance: HIV/AIDS* (pp. 27–41). New York: Palgrave Macmillan.

Hoffman, B. (1998). *Inside terrorism.* New York: Columbia University Press.

Homedes, N., & Ugalde, A. (2003). Globalization and health at the United States-Mexico border. *American Journal of Public Health, 93,* 2016–2022.

Hooey, J. (2001). Global doubts. *Canadian Medical Association Journal, 165,* 5.

Horton, R. (2003). Bioterrorism: The extreme politics of public health. In R. Beaglehole (Ed.), *Global public health: A new era* (pp. 209–225). Oxford, UK: Oxford University.

Inglehart, J. K. (2000). Revisiting the Canadian health care system. *Health Policy Report, 342,* 2007–2012.

International Council of Nurses. (1998). *ICN's vision for the future of nursing.* Retrieved December 15, 2005, from http://www.icn.ch/visionstatement.htm

International Council of Nurses. (2005a). *About ICN.* Retrieved December 15, 2005, from http://www.icn.ch/abouticn.htm

International Council of Nurses. (2005b). *Nursing networks.* Retrieved December 15, 2005, from http://www.icn.ch/networks.htm

Jha, P., Ranson, K., Nguyen, S. N., & Yach, D. (2002). Estimate of global and regional smoking prevalence in 1995, by age and sex. *American Journal of Public Health, 92,* 1002–1006.

Jonas, S. (2003). *An introduction to the U.S. health care system* (5th ed.). New York: Springer.

King, C. K., Glass, R., Bresee, J. S., & Duggan, C. (2003). Managing acute gastroenteritis among children: Oral rehydration, maintenance, and nutritional therapy. *Morbidity and Mortality Weekly Report, 52,* (RR-16), 1–16.

Koivusalo, M. (2003). Assessing the health policy implications of WTO trade and investment agreements. In K. Lee (Ed.), *Health impacts of globalization: Towards global governance* (pp. 161–176). New York: Palgrave Macmillan.

Lapsley, H. M. (2002). The health care system in Australia. In K. V. Thai, E. T. Wimberley, & S. M. McManus (Eds.), *Handbook of international health care systems* (pp. 487–503). New York: Marcel Dekker.

Late, M. (2005, February). Historical international tobacco treaty to take effect this month. *The Nation's Health,* p. 1, 8.

Lee, K. (2003). Introduction. In K. Lee (Ed.), *Health impacts of globalization: Towards global governance* (pp. 1–10). New York: Palgrave Macmillan.

Lee, K., & Dodgson, R. (2003). Globalization and cholera: Implications for global governance. In K. Lee (Ed.), *Health impacts of globalization: Towards global governance* (pp. 123–143). New York: Palgrave Macmillan.

Lee, L., Fustukian, S., & Buse, K. (2002). An introduction to global health policy. In K. Lee, K. Buse, & S. Fustukian (Eds.), *Health policy in a globalising world* (pp. 3–17). Cambridge, UK: Cambridge University.

Lee, K. & Patel, P. (2003). Far from the maddening cows: The global dimensions of BSE and vCJD. In K. Lee (Ed.), *Health impacts of globalization: Towards global governance* (pp. 47–60). New York: Palgrave Macmillan.

Lee, K., & Zwi, A. (2003). A global political economy approach to AIDS; Ideology, interests, and implications. In K. Lee (Ed.), *Health impacts of globalization: Towards global governance* (pp. 13–32). New York: Palgrave Macmillan.

Light, D. W. (2003). Universal health care: Lessons from the British experience. *American Journal of Public Health, 93,* 25–30.

Loevinsohn, B., Aylward, B., Steinglass, R., Ogden, E., Goodman, T., Melgaard, B. (2002). Impact of targeted programs on health systems: A case study of the polio eradication initiative. *American Journal of Public Health, 92,* 19–23.

McKee, M., & Zatonski, W. (2003). Public health in eastern Europe and the former Soviet Union. In R. Beaglehole (Ed.), *Global public health: A new era* (pp. 87–104). Oxford, UK: Oxford University.

McMichael, T., & Beaglehole, R. (2003). The global context for public health. In R. Beaglehole (Ed.), *Global public health: A new era* (pp. 1–23). Oxford, UK: Oxford University.

McMichael, A. J., Butler, C. D., & Ahern, M. J. (2003). Global environment. In R. D. Smith, R. Beaglehole, D. Woodward, & N. Drager (Eds.), *Global public goods for health: Health economic and public health perspectives* (pp. 94–116). Oxford, UK: Oxford University.

Nacos, B. (2002). Terrorism, the mass media, and the events of 9–11. *Phi Kappa Phi Forum, 82*(2), 13–19.

Needham, C. A., & Canning, R. (2003). *Global disease eradication: The race for the last child.* Washington, DC: ASM Press.

Northridge, M. E. (2002). The global spread of HIV. *American Journal of Public Health, 92,* 335.

Pan American Health Organization. (2002). *Public health in the Americas: Conceptual renewal, performance assessment, and bases for action.* Washington, DC: Author.

Pan American Health Organization. (2003). Absence of transmission of the d9 measles virus—Region of the Americas, November, 2002–March, 2003. *Morbidity and Mortality Weekly Report, 52,* 228–229.

Pan American Health Organization. (2005). *Nursing shortage threatens health care.* Retrieved December 16, 2005, from http://www.paho.org/English/DD/PIN/ptoday18_sep05.htm

Patel, K., & Rushefsky, M. E. (2002). The Canadian health care system. In K. V. Thai, E. T. Wimberley, & S. M. McManus (Eds.), *Handbook of international health care systems* (pp. 79–98). New York: Marcel Dekker.

Patel, V., & Thara, R. (2003). *Meeting the mental health needs of developing countries: NGO innovations in India.* New Delhi: Sage.

Perkins, R. (2002a). Channeling aid. *The Pfizer Journal* (Global ed.), *III*(2), 19–27.

Perkins, R. (2002b). Global health and economic development. *The Pfizer Journal* (Global ed.), *III*(2), 4–9.

Perkins, R. (2002c). Health: A model for development. *The Pfizer Journal* (Global ed.), *III*(2), 10–14.

Perkins, R. (2002d). Targeting development assistance. *The Pfizer Journal* (Global ed.), *III*(2), 15–18.

Poku, N. K., & Whiteside, A. (2004). Global health and the politics of governance: An introduction. In N. K. Poku & A. Whiteside (Eds.), *Global health and governance: HIV/AIDS* (pp. 1–5). New York: Palgrave Macmillan.

Regional Office for Africa, World Health Organization. (2003). Progress toward poliomyelitis eradication—Southern Africa, 2001–March 2003. *Morbidity and Mortality Weekly Report, 52,* 521–524.

Rodwin, V. G. (2003). The health care system under French national health insurance: Lessons for health reform in the United States. *American Journal of Public Health, 93,* 31–37.

Salvage, J. (2002). *Collateral damage: The health and environmental costs of war on Iraq.* London: Medact.

Sanders, D., & Chopra, M. (2003). Globalization and the challenge of health for all: A view from sub-Saharan Africa. In K. Lee (Ed.), *Health impacts of globalization: Towards global governance* (pp. 105–119). New York: Palgrave Macmillan.

Sigma Theta Tau International Nursing Honor Society. (2005). *The society's vision and mission.* Retrieved December 15, 2005, from http://www.nursingsociety.org/about/overview.html

Simon, J. D. (2002). The global terrorist threat. *Phi Kappa Phi Forum, 82*(2), 10–12.

Swami, B. (2002). The German health care system. In K. V. Thai, E. T. Wimberley, & S. M. McManus (Eds.), *Handbook of international health care systems* (pp. 333–358). New York: Marcel Dekker.

Taylor, A. L., Bettcher, D. W., & Peck, R. (2003). International law and the international legislative process: the WHO framework convention on tobacco control. In R. D. Smith, R. Beaglehole, D. Woodward, & N. Drager (Eds.), *Global public goods for health: Health economic and public health perspectives* (pp. 212–229). Oxford, UK: Oxford University.

Thomas, C. (2003). Trade policy, the politics of access to drugs and global governance for health. In K. Lee (Ed.), *Health impacts of globalization: Towards global governance* (pp. 177–191). New York: Palgrave Macmillan.

Thompson, J. E. (2002). The WHO Advisory Group on Nursing and Midwifery. *Journal of Nursing Scholarship, 34,* 111–113.

Tollman, S. M., & Pick, W. M. (2002). Roots, shoots, but too little fruit: Assessing the contributions of COPC in South Africa. *American Journal of Public Health, 92,* 1725–1728.

Tooker, J. (2003). Affordable health insurance for all is possible by means of a pragmatic approach. *American Journal of Public Health, 93,* 106–109.

UNICEF. (2002). State of the world's vaccines and immunization. Retrieved February 3,

2003, from http://www.unicef.org/pubsgen/sowvi/sowvi-en02.pdf

U.S. Agency for International Development. (2005). *About USAID.* Retrieved December 16, 2005, from http://wwwusaid.gov/about_usaid

U.S. Department of State. (2004). *Patterns of global terrorism 2003.* Washington, DC: Author.

U.S. Department of State. (2005). *Trafficking in persons.* Retrieved December 16, 2005, from http://www.state.gov/documents/organization/47255.pdf

Vonderheid, S. C., & Al-Gasseer, N. (2002). World Health Organization and global health policy. *Journal of Nursing Scholarship, 34,* 109–110.

Wagstaff, A., Bustreo, F., Bryce, J., Cleason, M., & the WHO-World Bank Child Health and Poverty Working Group. (2004). Child health: Reaching the poor. *American Journal of Public Health, 94,* 726–736.

Wikler, D., & Cash, R. (2003). Ethical issues in global public health. In R. Beaglehole (Ed.), *Global public health: A new era* (pp. 226–252). Oxford, UK: Oxford University.

Wimberley, E. T., & Thai, K. V. (2002). Introduction to international health systems: Themes and variations on themes. In K. V. Thai, E. T. Wimberley, & S. M. McManus (Eds.), *Handbook of international health care systems* (pp. 1–28). New York: Marcel Dekker.

Woodward, D., & Smith, R. D. (2003). Global public goods and health: Concepts and issues. In R. D. Smith, R. Beaglehole, D. Woodward, & N. Drager (Eds.), *Global public goods for health: Health economic and public health perspectives* (pp. 1–23). Oxford, UK: Oxford University.

Working Group on "Governance Dilemmas" in Bioterrorism Response. (2004). Leading during bioattacks and epidemics with the public's trust and help. *Biosecurity & Bioterrorism, 2*(1), 25–40.

World Health Organization. (2000). *The world health report 2000: Health systems: Improving performance.* Geneva, Switzerland: Author.

World Health Organization. (2002). *Scaling up the response to infectious diseases.* Retrieved April 2, 2002, from http://www.who.int/infectious-disease-report/2002

World Health Organization. (2003a). *Nursing and midwifery services at the World Health Organization.* Retrieved December 15, 2005, from http://www.who.int/health-services-delivery/nursing

World Health Organization. (2003b). *Primary health care: A framework for future strategic directions.* Geneva, Switzerland: Author.

World Health Organization. (2003c). *World Health Assembly resolution 56.1.* Retrieved February 8, 2005, from http://tobacco/who.int

World Health Organization. (2004a). *Global tuberculosis control—Surveillance, planning, financing.* Retrieved April 28, 2004, from http://www.who.int/tb/publications/global_report/en

World Health Organization. (2004b). *The world health report 2004: Changing history.* Geneva, Switzerland: Author.

World Health Organization. (2005a). *Human resources for health.* Retrieved December 15, 2005, from http://www.wpro.who.int/sites/hrh/overview.htm

World Health Organization. (2005b). *TB emergency declaration issued by WHO Regional Office for Africa.* Retrieved December 16, 2005, from http://www.who.int/features_archive/tb_emergency_declaration/en

World Health Organization. (2005c). *World health report 2005: Make every mother and child count.* Retrieved December 16, 2005, from http://www.who.int/whr/2005/annexes-en.pdf

Yajima, R., & Takayanagi, K. (2002). The Japanese health care system: Citizen complaints and citizen possibilities. In K. V. Thai, E. T. Wimberley, & S. M. McManus (Eds.), *Handbook of international health care systems* (pp. 457–486). New York: Marcel Dekker.

Yoshikawa, A., & Bhattacharya, J. (2002). Japan. In B. J. Fried & L. M. Gaydos (Eds.), *World health systems: Challenges and perspectives* (pp. 249–266). Chicago: Health Administration Press.

CHAPTER 7

The Policy Context

CHAPTER OBJECTIVES

After reading this chapter, you should be able to:

1. Analyze potential community health nursing roles in policy development.
2. Discuss three avenues for public policy development.
3. Describe at least four aspects of the policy development process.
4. Apply criteria for health policy evaluation.

KEY TERMS

bill **143**
campaigning **151**
coalitions **148**
community organizing **150**
distributive policies **141**
electioneering **151**
executive orders **144**
governance **137**
judicial decisions **145**
laws **141**
legislative proposals **141**
lobbying **150**
networking **148**
pocket veto **144**
policy **137**
policy agenda **146**
political advocacy **150**
politics **137**
procedural policies **141**
public policy **137**
redistributive policies **141**
regulation **144**
regulatory policies **141**
substantive policies **141**

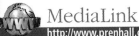
MediaLink

Additional interactive resources for this chapter can be found on the Companion Website. Click on Chapter 7 and "Begin" to select the activities for this chapter.

Advocacy in Action

National Advocacy for Local Problems

As part of a community health clinical, nursing students taught several health promotion classes to 6th graders at an urban middle school, focusing on healthy decision making. The 6th graders participated in lessons focused on goal setting, personal hygiene, female/male anatomy, pregnancy and fertilization, abstinence, sexually transmitted diseases, and finally contraception. An assessment of the community indicated that teenage pregnancy rates were high, much higher than the national average. The nursing students hypothesized that if a health promotion course such as the one they were teaching was to be successful, the curriculum needed to be comprehensive. However, the political climate in the country 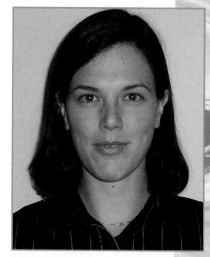 emphasized abstinence-only education, with little attention to healthy decision making or contraception. To bring attention to the need for and access to comprehensive health education, the nursing students went to Washington, DC.

The students spent several weeks preparing for their visit to Capitol Hill. They read about the debate between advocates of abstinence-only health education and advocates of comprehensive health education. They learned of an active bill in Congress to appropriate federal funds for states that promoted a comprehensive health education curriculum, and they located the committee responsible for the bill. Based on their geographical representation, the students decided on one particular senator on the committee who was a co-sponsor of the bill. Finally, they prepared talking points and a briefing packet for their meeting, including the pros and cons of comprehensive health education, national and state data on teenage pregnancy, and personal accounts of teaching health education in middle schools.

After the meeting, the students felt they had gained invaluable experience in the political process. They all agreed that as first-time advocates it was best to plan a visit with a member of Congress who was supportive of their cause and receptive to their ideas. One student stated, "Now I know it really is possible to call my representative and talk to him."

Amanda Slagle, MSN, MPH, RN

Clinical Instructor

Johns Hopkins University School of Nursing

*P*olicy decisions affect every aspect of our lives, including our access to health care and the way in which health care is provided. Policy arises from a demand for action, or inaction, in relation to a particular issue (Weissert & Weissert, 2002). Unfortunately, policy development often excludes those most knowledgeable about the area of concern (Partnership for the Public's Health, 2003). Community health nurses need an awareness of the political context in which their practice occurs and must possess the skills and abilities to influence health policy development to achieve their goal of improving the health of the public.

Policy is established by organizations and political units in both public and private sectors and reflects the values, beliefs, and attitudes of policy makers. Policy has been defined in several ways. Some of these definitions include:

- A "plan or course of action designed to define issues, influence decision-making, and promote broad community actions beyond those made by individuals" (Center for Health Improvement, 2004, p. 1).
- "A plan or course of action selected from alternatives and intended to influence or determine decisions, actions, and other matters" (Partnership for the Public's Health, 2003, p. 2).
- "The choices that a society, a segment of society, or organization makes regarding its goals and priorities and the ways it will allocate its resources to attain those goals" (Mason, Leavitt, & Chaffee, 2002, p. 8).

Although worded differently, these definitions have several common themes that can be incorporated into the following comprehensive definition. **Policy** is a set of principles determining the direction for action and allocation of resources to achieve an identified prioritized group or organizational goal.

As noted earlier, policy development takes place in both public and private sectors. **Public policy** is "policy made on behalf of the public, developed or initiated by government, and interpreted and implemented by public and private bodies" (Hanley, 2002, p. 55), whereas private policies are enacted to deal with problems in private-sector organizations. Public policies include laws or statutes, regulations, executive orders, and court rulings. Public policy is derived from **governance**, which is defined as "all the activities of government that affect society, such as the formulation of policies and regulations, the development of advice for citizens, and the passage of laws" (Keough, 2002, p. 105). Public policies arise from several interdependent sectors beyond that directly related to health, including housing, social security, education, and welfare services (Scott & West, 2001).

Public or private policy is created through the policy development process. Policy development was defined in Chapter 5∞ and has also been described as a "process by which society makes decisions, selects goals and the best means for reaching them, handles conflicting views about what should be done and allocates resources to address needs" (Center for Health Improvement, 2004, p. 1). **Politics**, on the other hand, is the mechanism by which policy development is influenced by those with a vested interest in its outcomes.

The extent to which the needs of the total population, or the group of people affected by a particular policy, are considered in policy development is reflected in the level of civil discourse that occurs in policy deliberation. Each of the five levels of discourse includes increasingly greater consideration of the needs of those affected. At the first level, policies are made by individuals, institutions, and interest groups, without much input from or consideration for the needs of those affected. In the second level of civil discourse, interested parties seek their own interests in the context of reciprocal endeavors. For example, nurses might agree to support a policy initiative of another group for an assurance of reciprocal support of nursing initiatives. At this level, people are focusing on their own rights with some consideration for the reciprocal rights of others. Level three involves the development of shared visions and consensus-oriented discourse. At level four, policy makers support principles of fairness and universal respect for others. Level five social discourse maintains this perspective on fairness and social justice but permits individuation to address the circumstances of each individual. At this level, policy making involves inclusive discourse among all involved in its development or affected by its outcomes (Kesler, 2000).

POLICY AND HEALTH

As noted above, policy in a variety of arenas can influence the health status of the population. Health policy, of course, has a direct impact on health in the population. The overall goal of health policy, as outlined by the World Health Organization (WHO), is to provide all people with opportunities to lead socially and economically productive lives (Kickbusch, 2003). In addition, several specific goals for health policy have been identified. The first of these goals is to prevent disease and injury and promote health; the second is to relieve pain and suffering. Caring for and curing illness and caring for those with incurable illness are additional health policy goals. Finally, health policy should attempt to avoid premature death or pursue a peaceful death when death is inevitable (Callahan, 2002). Development of health policy requires prioritization among these goals, resulting in promotion of some goals over others in any particular situation. Goal prioritization should be based on three policy directions: (a) goals that address the needs of underserved subpopulations, (b) goals that enhance population health in general, and (c) goals that promote equity in health care services (Callahan, 2002).

The effects of policies in many areas, including health, can be seen in the following examples. Welfare reform policies enacted as part of the Personal Responsibility and Work Opportunity Reconciliation Act of 1996 limited access to health care services for many welfare recipients by uncoupling Medicaid eligibility from welfare programs such as Temporary Assistance for Needy Families (TANF). The intent of the legislation was to reduce the numbers of people dependent on social welfare programs and promote employment opportunities. Although these intentions are laudable in themselves, they create other problems related to health and access to care for the families affected. Problems are also created for health care systems that carry a large burden of uncompensated care (Kullgren, 2003).

As another example, policy decisions on how seat belt legislation is enforced make a difference in seat belt use and, subsequently, in motor vehicle fatalities and serious injuries. Research has indicated that seat belt use is significantly higher in states that have primary seat belt legislation, which allows motorists to be stopped specifically for failure to use seat belts, than those with secondary legislation, in which citations can only be issued in the context of other traffic violations (Division of Unintentional Injury Prevention, 2004).

Similarly, a 1998 Master Settlement Agreement between the states and the tobacco industry led to an award of $200 billion over a period of 25 years. Although this money was intended to be used for tobacco education, many states have chosen to use the funds to meet other pressing needs, leaving less money available for anti-tobacco campaigns. This policy decision led, in turn, to a 23% increase in the number of adolescents who smoke (Office on Smoking and Health, 2004). Conversely, enactment of national legislation banning smoking in workplaces in Finland resulted in decreased exposure to environmental smoke for nonsmokers and decreased tobacco use and lower nicotine concentrations in smokers (Heloma, Jaakkola, Kahkonen, & Reijula, 2001).

A final example of the impact of policy development lies in the outcome of Oregon's attempt to ration health care funded with public monies. The intent of the Oregon legislation was to emphasize health promotion and illness prevention under the Medicaid program by prioritizing provision of funded services "according to their medical benefit and contribution to the population's overall health" in order to expand health care access to underserved populations (Oberlander, Jacobs, & Marmor, 2001, p. 209). The Oregon proposal created significant debate and resistance, particularly on the part of the U.S. Health Care Financing Administration (HCFA) (now the Centers for Medicare and Medicaid Services), which delayed granting of a waiver permitting the state to implement its rationing policy. In the meantime, however, state policy makers couched the issue in terms of the state's highly participative culture and achieved buy-in from broad segments of the population. What occurred in the end was not rationing as proposed but an unanticipated public willingness to approve higher taxes and other revenue sources to fund health care. Although the proposed rationing never took place, the state achieved its goal of expanded health care coverage for its population (Oberlander et al., 2001).

PROFESSIONAL ROLES IN POLICY DEVELOPMENT

Public health professionals, including community health nurses, perform a variety of roles in the development of health-related policy.

Public Health Professionals and Policy Development

Public health professionals should be involved in policy development at the population-based level. Such activity requires attention to four overarching ideals and five procedural principles for population-based care. The overarching ideals are improvement of the overall health of the population, reinvestment of cost savings in additional health services, trust that policy decisions are based on these two ideals, and self-determination and participation by members of the population in policy making. The overarching ideals provide the parameters within which policy development should occur, whereas the procedural principles address the way in which health care policies should be developed. The five procedural principles are fair consideration, openness, empowerment, appeal, and impartiality (Emanuel, 2002). These ideals and principles are summarized with relevant positive and negative examples in Table 7-1◆.

Community health nurses and other public health professionals should promote achievement of the overarching ideals and procedural principles. The Institute of Medicine has recommended that public health agencies and professionals engage in six specific roles in policy development that exemplify these ideals and principles (Partnership for the Public's Health, 2003). The first role is that of consciousness raising—making policy makers and the general public aware of issues and concerns that require policy development. For example, community health nurses might document housing code violations in local rental housing and disseminate findings to local residents and policy makers. The second role is that of initiating communication among policy makers and those affected by the issue. Continuing the previous example, community health nurses might help organize a town meeting between residents and policy makers to discuss code violations and what can be done about them. A third role involves promoting attention to long-range issues as well as current crises, and the fourth role emphasizes planning ahead for emerging issues as well as reacting to current ones. For

TABLE 7-1 Overarching Ideals and Procedural Principles for Population-Based Health Policy

Ideals

- Overall aim is improvement of the health of the population

  Example: Policies that support provision of health care to undocumented immigrants help protect the health of the general public.

- Cost savings derived should benefit the population by expanding the services offered or the number of persons served

  Negative example: Budget cuts to federal and state health care programs diminish access to needed health services.

- Trust that policy decisions are based on the two ideals above

  Negative example: A local mayor is found to promote housing policy decisions that benefit him as a landlord, to the detriment of his tenants.

- Self-determination and participation in policy making by members of the population

  Example: Public hearings are held regarding initiation of a local smoking ban in public places.

Procedural Principles

Principle	Description
Fair consideration	The needs of all individuals are given consideration. *Example: The rights of both affluent and poor neighborhoods are considered in decisions regarding the placement of "speed bumps" in residential neighborhoods.*
Openness	Decisions, and the rationale behind them, are made known to the public. *Example: Full city council meeting minutes are published and disseminated to community members.*
Empowerment	Members of the population have opportunities to participate in the policy-making process. *Example: Neighborhood Health Councils consistently identify health issues and bring them to the attention of policy makers for action.*
Appeal	Members of the population have opportunities to voice objections to decisions made. *Example: Community members organize a meeting with local transportation officials to protest changes in local bus routes.*
Impartiality	There should be no conflict of interest on the part of policy makers. *Negative example: Members of the local planning commission are the owners of a large percentage of local rental units and act against initiatives to construct new low-income housing.*

example, community health nurses might organize residents to address code violation issues, building an ongoing structure that will support similar action on future issues. The fifth role is one of advocacy, speaking for those who are not usually heard in policy deliberations,

and the final role is that of promoting fairness and balance in the design and implementation of health policy. For instance, community health nurses might present the housing issues of refugee tenants who are afraid of reprisals while also making sure that the viewpoints of landlords are represented in developing solutions.

The Nursing Profession and Policy Development

Florence Nightingale and other early community health nurses were adept at using the political process to promote the health of the population. We saw in Chapter 3 ∞ that Lillian Wald engaged in political activism to provide impetus for initiation of the Children's Bureau. She and other early nursing leaders were alert to the political culture of the times, using that knowledge to gain important changes in societal conditions. For example, Clara Barton and Florence Nightingale minimized their active support for women's suffrage issues in order to address what they considered more critical social issues. Others, such as Margaret Sanger and Lavinia Dock, were more confrontational in their political activism, but all achieved significant social changes. These early leaders in community health nursing realized that the political process was a means of achieving their goal of improved health for all and that, because of its focus on the health of population groups, community health nursing is, by definition, political in nature.

Stages of Nursing Involvement in Policy Development

Over the years, many nurses became uncomfortable with the idea of political involvement, with the possible exception of exercising the right to vote. Politics had an unfavorable aura that was seen as incompatible with nursing's altruistic philosophy. More recently, nurses have begun to realize the need to influence health care policy decisions.

Some nursing authors describe a series of stages in nursing involvement in political activity after the era of Lillian Wald and her cohorts. The initial stage was one of marginal participation in political activity, primarily in terms of voting. Later, nurses began to engage in collective policy development efforts to benefit the profession. A third stage was one of participation in coalitions to address societal health issues. Nursing, as a profession, is just beginning to enter a fourth stage, in which nurses provide leadership in mobilizing others to deal with health issues (Mason et al., 2002).

Spheres of Nursing Influence in Policy Development

Political writers in nursing have identified four spheres in which nurses influence policy development (Mason et al., 2002). The first sphere is in the workplace, where policies influence both health care delivery (e.g., policies related to fees for basic preventive services such as

EVIDENCE-BASED PRACTICE

Scott and West (2001) describe five reasons for nursing interest in the field of health policy:

- The need to examine the impact of health policy on people's lives
- The opportunity for nurses to be involved in setting research agendas and to conduct research related to health policy
- The close relationship between nursing policy and health policy
- Nursing's potential contribution to health policy formulation and implementation as the largest group of health care providers
- Lack of documentation of nurses' contribution to the policy process

How might these reasons provide impetus for nursing research on health policy formation and effects? What types of health policy research might derive from each?

immunizations) and health determinants (e.g., policies banning smoking in the workplace). The second sphere is the governmental policy arena, in which nurses advocate for public policies that support health. Note that public policies often "bleed" into the private sector. For example, the concept of diagnosis-related groups (DRGs) initiated for Medicare reimbursement has been adopted by some private-sector insurance carriers.

The third sphere of nursing influence in policy making is within professional organizations. Policy making in this sphere influences the regulation and education of the profession itself and provides impetus for public policy formation in the government sphere. The final sphere of influence is the community sphere, in which nurses influence the general public regarding health and health policy (Mason et al., 2002).

Community Health Nursing Roles in Policy Development

Community health nurses may engage in one or more of four roles in their efforts to influence policy development in areas that affect health. These roles include the roles of citizen, activist, politician, and researcher. In their role as citizens, nurses engage in traditional political activities such as staying informed; voting; speaking out on local issues; participating in public forums; becoming acquainted with local, state, and federal officials; and participating in politically active nursing organizations. In the activist role, nurses contact public officials, register others to vote, contribute to and work for political campaigns, and engage in other activities to educate and influence policy makers. In their role as politicians, some nurses become policy makers themselves through elected or appointed office (Chitty as cited in Leavitt, Chaffee, & Vance, 2002). In the researcher role, community health nurses involved in policy making carry out activities embodied in the Framework for Science and Technology Advice developed by the Canadian Council of Science and Technology. These activities include identifying policy

TABLE 7-2 Community Health Nursing Roles and Activities in Policy Development	
Role	**Related Nursing Activities**
Citizen	■ Voting ■ Staying informed ■ Speaking out on policy issues ■ Participating in public forums ■ Becoming acquainted with elected officials ■ Joining politically active professional nursing organizations
Activist	■ Contacting public officials ■ Registering members of the public to vote ■ Contributing to political campaigns ■ Working for political campaigns ■ Lobbying decision makers with relevant data ■ Forming or joining relevant coalitions ■ Writing letters to the editor ■ Inviting legislators to the workplace ■ Organizing media events to publicize issues ■ Providing testimony on health-related issues ■ Locating and soliciting grant funding
Politician	■ Running for public office ■ Seeking appointment to a regulatory body ■ Seeking appointment to a governing board of a public or private entity ■ Using nursing experience as a front-line policy maker
Researcher	■ Identifying health policy issues through research ■ Ensuring the inclusiveness of viewpoints in policy formation ■ Assuring the quality, integrity, and objectivity of data on which policy decisions are based ■ Recognizing and communicating uncertainty and risk (e.g., acknowledging when research evidence is equivocal) ■ Assuring transparency and openness regarding the bases for policy decisions ■ Reviewing policy decisions to assure that they reflect up-to-date knowledge

Data from: Keough, K. (2002). How science informs the decisions of government. Canadian Journal of Public Health, 93, 104–108; and Leavitt, J. K., Chaffee, M. W., & Vance, C. (2002). Learning the ropes of policy and politics. In D. J. Mason, J. K. Leavitt, & M. W. Chaffee (Eds.), Policy and politics in nursing and health care (4th ed., pp. 31–53). St. Louis, MO: Saunders.

issues; ensuring inclusiveness of viewpoints; assuring the quality, integrity, and objectivity of data and conclusions on which policies are based; recognizing and communicating uncertainty and risk; ensuring transparency and openness; and reviewing policy decisions to determine whether they are based on the most recent knowledge (Keough, 2002). Nursing activities in each of the four roles for policy involvement are summarized in Table 7-2◆. Actions related to the citizen, activist, and politician roles will be discussed in more detail in the section on strategies for implementing policy.

TYPES OF POLICIES

As noted earlier, health policies may be either public or private, depending on their source and focus. Policies may also be categorized as substantive or procedural

BUILDING OUR KNOWLEDGE BASE

*I*n the past, nurses as a professional group were less politically active than members of other groups. In today's society, political astuteness and involvement are critical to the development of health care delivery systems that support the primary goal of community health nursing: improved health for the public.

- What contribution might research make to understanding nursing's traditional lack of political involvement?
- What is the role of research in policy making?
- How would you go about determining what factors promote political activity by community health nurses?
- If you wanted to conduct a study of the extent of political activity among certain groups of students on your campus, what groups would you include? Why? How would you design your study?

(Weissert & Weissert, 2002). **Substantive policies** are those that dictate action to be taken. For example, a policy (in this case legislation) mandating helmet use by bicycle riders is a substantive policy, as is a policy funding health care services for the indigent. **Procedural policies** are those that determine how the action will occur. In the case of the helmet law, procedural policies would determine how the law would be implemented. In the health services funding policy, procedural policies would address who is eligible for services, how services are to be obtained, how providers will be reimbursed for services, and so on.

Policies can also be categorized as distributive, regulatory, or redistributive (Weissert & Weissert, 2002). **Distributive policies** allocate goods and services among members of the population. The Medicaid and Medicare programs are examples of distributive policies that determine who may receive care reimbursed by these funding sources. Similarly, Congressional funding decisions that promote specific research agendas over others (e.g., development of a vaccine for avian influenza) provide direction for allocation of federal research funds. **Regulatory policies** restrict or constrain behavior in some way. For example, nurse practice acts are regulatory policies that restrict the practice of nursing to people who meet identified criteria for licensure. Some policies are self-regulatory, as in the case of professional codes of ethics or standards for accreditation of schools of nursing. **Redistributive policies** take goods and services away from some members of the population and give them to others. For example, taxing the income of some citizens to fund services for others is a redistributive policy.

AVENUES FOR POLICY DEVELOPMENT

Health policy formation may take one of four major forms in the public sector: legislation and health programs created by legislation, rules and regulations for implementing legislation, administrative decisions, and judicial decisions (Hanley, 2002).

Legislation

Laws, or statutes, are public policy decisions generated by the legislative branch of government at the federal, state, or local level. Laws are created in a social system to express the collective values, interests, and beliefs of the society that generates them. As a society develops, so do its beliefs, values, and interests. Some laws enacted in earlier periods of a society's evolution eventually become obsolete. Sometimes laws are created or revised to address new problems that surface as society changes. Modifications or changes in laws are legislative attempts to correct discrepancies that may have arisen between past and current social practices. Although this description of the function of legislation is highly simplified, the point is that laws reflect societal needs and values and are subject to revision.

Policy formation via the legislative process is very similar at the federal and state levels. Figure 7-1 depicts the typical progress of a bill through the legislative process. The process is similar at federal and state levels, and the discussion here addresses both. The names of specific legislative bodies and committees will vary from one jurisdiction to another, however. A similar but more circumscribed process is used in the development of ordinances and policies by local government bodies (e.g., city council or county board of supervisors). Local communities may vary somewhat in the extent of and avenues for public input into policy decisions. The asterisks in Figure 7-1 indicate points in the state or federal process at which community health nurses might influence legislation.

Legislative proposals are statements of beliefs or interests that have been brought to the attention of a legislator. These interests may come to the legislator's attention through his or her constituents, personal experiences, or involvement on a legislative subcommittee dealing with specific issues. Community health nurses and nursing and other health-related organizations can

Federal legislation is only one way in which the political context influences health and health care services.
(© Andre Jenny/The Image Works)

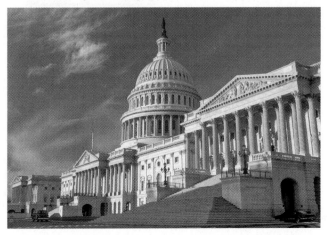

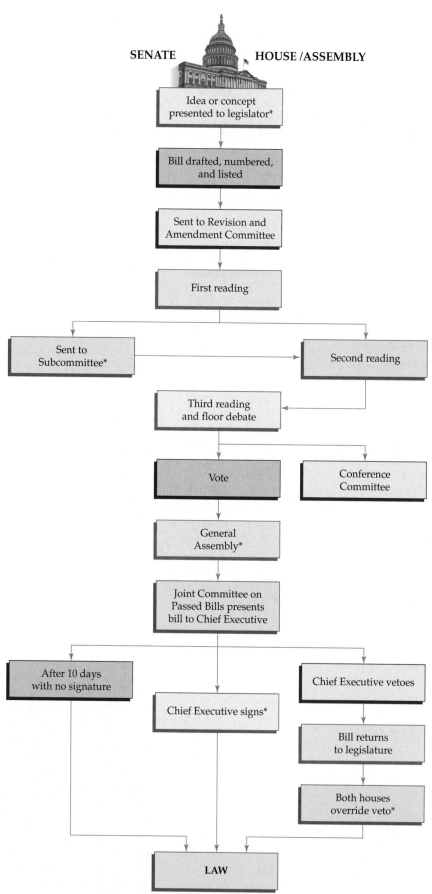

SENATE   HOUSE /ASSEMBLY

Idea or concept
presented to legislator*

Bill drafted, numbered,
and listed

Sent to Revision and
Amendment Committee

First reading

Sent to
Subcommittee*

Second reading

Third reading
and floor debate

Vote

Conference
Committee

General
Assembly*

Joint Committee on
Passed Bills presents
bill to Chief Executive

After 10 days
with no signature

Chief Executive vetoes

Chief Executive signs*

Bill returns
to legislature

Both houses
override veto*

LAW

* Points at which community health nurses can best influence the process

FIGURE 7-1 A Typical Legislative Process

influence the legislative process at this point by making lawmakers aware of the need to develop policy or to modify existing policies. After due consideration, constituents' beliefs or interests are drafted in a **bill**, which is a formally worded statement of the desired policy. Once a bill has been drafted, the sponsoring legislator submits it for identification, meaning that the bill will carry the legislator's name as sponsor. It is not unusual for a proposed bill to have multiple sponsors. Many state and national nursing and other health-related organizations (e.g., the American Nurses Association [ANA] or the American Public Health Association [APHA]) maintain a legislative focus that allows them to keep members informed of pending legislation with health implications. They also typically provide their members with information on how to access drafts of legislation for review and how to contact legislators and specific committees. Membership in such organizations is an important avenue for keeping up-to-date on legislative initiatives that may affect the health of the population.

The bill is assigned a number, listed by the clerk of the appropriate legislative body, and sent to a general committee for review. The committee may revise the language of the bill or amend it. In the normal course of events, the bill would then be sent on to the House or Senate floor for its "first reading." After its first reading, the bill might be referred to the appropriate committee for hearings. Some bills are sent to multiple committees. At the U.S. congressional level, there are six committees that deal with most health-related legislation: (a) the Senate Finance Committee, which establishes policy related to health programs supported by taxes and trusts, such as Medicare and Medicaid; (b) the House Ways and Means Committee, which oversees similar legislation for the House of Representatives; (c) the Senate Labor and Human Resources Committee; (d) the House Energy and Commerce Committee, both of which address matters related to programs administered by the Department of Health and Human Services; (e) the House Appropriations Committee; and (f) the Senate Appropriations Committee. The first four of these committees are legislative committees that deal with legislation establishing, modifying, or discontinuing health care programs. The House Appropriations and Senate Appropriations Committees are responsible for allocating the funds for the various federal programs. A third type of committee, budget committees, develop broad budgetary directions for the legislature (Center for Health Improvement, 2004). Similar committees exist at the state level.

Once bills are referred to a committee, it is not unusual for them to be sent to a subcommittee, which does the most thorough review of the proposed legislation. Functions of subcommittees include hearings, markup, and reporting. Subcommittees may hold public hearings on the issue addressed by the bill. "Markup" refers to modifications made in the proposal. Finally, the subcommittee makes a report regarding the intent of the bill, any amendments made in the committee, ramifications in terms of changes to current laws, the costs of implementation, and any dissenting views on the bill (Santa Anna, 2002). Community health nurses can influence the legislative process during subcommittee review by contacting lawmakers and making their views known on legislation pending before them. Such contacts may be made by individual nurses or by lobbyists employed by nursing and other health-related interest groups. Lobbying is discussed in more detail later in the chapter.

Committee members considering a particular piece of legislation can either review and modify a bill or decide not to report the bill out of committee, thus effectively killing it. Legislation can also bypass assignment to a standing committee and be assigned to a specially created ad hoc committee or advance directly to a second reading on the floor of the particular legislative chamber. The bill may then proceed to a third reading, be referred back to committee, or be sent to another committee for review and revision before advancing to the third and final reading. Following the third reading, the proposed legislation is placed on the calendar for floor debate and, finally, voted on. At this point in the legislative process, community health nurses can contact their own representatives and try to persuade them to support nursing's position on a particular bill.

If the legislation is passed in the chamber of Congress or the state legislature where it originated, it is sent to the other chamber for approval. In many cases, when a bill has advanced to this point, it is passed by the second chamber without further modification. The bill can, however, be sent to another committee for review and modification. Once a bill has passed the second chamber, it is returned to the house or chamber where it originated for final approval. At the state level, a bill must be signed by the leaders of both houses of the legislature as well as the secretary of state before it is forwarded for the governor's signature. After the bill is signed by the governor, it is renumbered according to the appropriate lawbook code number and filed with the secretary of state, and becomes law. A similar process occurs at the federal level after a bill is signed by the president.

In most states and in Congress, if the two chambers of the legislature cannot agree on a similar version of a given bill, a special committee composed of members of both chambers is formed. The purpose of this *joint conference committee* is to develop a compromise bill. It is highly unusual for a joint committee recommendation not to be passed. If, however, the committee cannot reach agreement, the bill dies. Once the compromise bill has passed both houses of the legislature, it is sent to the executive branch of the government (governor or president) for final approval.

The chief executive (governor or president) can either sign the bill or hamper its progress by not signing it or vetoing it. If the chief executive does not sign the bill, it automatically becomes law after 10 days, unless the legislative session ends in the interim. In that case, the bill dies. Holding a bill unsigned until the end of the session is called a **pocket veto**. Lobbying may also be used at this point to influence the chief executive's disposition of a particular bill. If the executive vetoes a bill, it is returned to the legislature. The legislature is then required to meet a constitutionally prescribed majority vote (usually a two-thirds majority) to override the veto and enact the bill into law. Any bill that does not complete the legislative process during the legislative session in which it is introduced is dead, and it must be reintroduced in a subsequent session if it is ever to become law.

Regulation

Policy decisions enacted as legislation are usually implemented by regulatory agencies charged with implementing specific types of legislation. For example, federal policies related to environmental issues are implemented by the Environmental Protection Agency (EPA); state health-related policies are usually implemented by a state board of health or a comparable agency.

These agencies develop regulations that determine how legislation will be implemented. A **regulation** is a rule or order having the force of law that deals with procedures to be followed in implementing a piece of legislation. Regulations are intended to promote individual accountability for actions and to protect the public health and welfare. Regulations specify how policies are realized in actual behavior.

Regulatory agencies exert a great deal of control over health-related activities by both professionals and the general public. State agencies such as boards of nursing, for example, regulate who may practice nursing and how nursing licensure is granted. These same agencies might also be responsible for determining which health care providers can write prescriptions for medication in those states where such practices are authorized for personnel other than physicians.

When a piece of legislation authorizing an activity such as prescription writing is passed, the legislature usually designates an existing agency or creates a new agency to implement the legislation. This agency develops the regulations that govern implementation of the law. In the case of prescription-writing privileges, the regulatory agency would determine who can write prescriptions and what additional qualifications might be required of those persons. For example, in California, nurses who are certified by the state as nurse practitioners may write prescriptions, but only if they have completed an approved course in pharmacology. Other regulations specify who is eligible for certification as a nurse practitioner in the state.

Another example of regulations that implement legislation is the procedures for handling hazardous substances in the workplace, which were developed by the Occupational Safety and Health Administration (OSHA). The enabling legislation mandated protection of employees from exposure to hazardous substances, but regulations developed by OSHA specify how certain substances should be handled. For example, certain types of ventilatory equipment are required in manufacturing processes using hazardous aerosols to minimize the risk of exposure to employees.

Regulations instituted by various agencies may dramatically influence the actual impact of a law. For example, when prescription writing by nurse practitioners was first instituted in Tennessee, one proposal was to restrict the privilege to nurse practitioners prepared at the master's level. As this requirement would have excluded many nurse practitioners in rural counties where physicians were scarce, it would have undermined the intent of the enabling legislation—to provide greater access to health care for underserved populations.

Community health nurses can have input into regulations that affect their professional practice as well as into the legislation that shapes public health policy. When a regulatory agency is in the process of formulating regulations, the public is informed that the process is being initiated. Generally, the agency formulates some preliminary regulations that are published for public review and comment. At the federal level, proposed regulations are published in the *Federal Register* as a *Notice of Proposed Rulemaking (NPRM)*; similar registers exist in each state. Interested parties are then allowed to comment on the proposed regulations and suggest changes.

When regulations deal with particularly sensitive areas, the regulatory body involved may hold public hearings to solicit input from interested parties. Community health nurses may either comment on proposed regulations in written communications to the regulatory agency or provide testimony at public hearings. Nursing input should be provided early in the development process. It should also be supported by data and identify how nursing's position on proposed regulations supports the intent of the legislation (Lorette & Jansto, 2002). The regulatory agency may use the input to refine the regulations, but is not required to do so. Regulations are published in the appropriate state or federal publication and promulgated among individuals affected by them. Once regulations are published and go into effect, they have the force of law.

Administrative and Judicial Decisions

Health policy development can also occur by means of administrative or judicial decisions. Administrative decisions are those made by an individual or agency that affect the implementation of health care policies or programs. For example, a state board of nursing or other similar agency would develop the processes by which one becomes licensed in that state. One specific type of administrative decision is an executive order. **Executive orders** are additions to legislation that an executive officer (president or governor) can make as long as they do not contravene the provisions of the legislation or contradict other existing laws. Former President Clinton, for example, used executive orders for achieving a number of health policy changes that were not originally included in legislation, such as instituting programs to promote Medicaid enrollment for eligible children. **Judicial decisions** are decisions within the court system regarding how laws are to be interpreted. As an example, the California courts ruled that the governor did not have the authority to delay implementation of legislation establishing nurse staffing ratios. Judicial decisions may also be referred to as *case law* or *common law* (Center for Health Improvement, 2004).

THE POLICY DEVELOPMENT PROCESS

Community health nurses can influence health-related policies at all levels. To do so, however, they must be conversant with the political process and its use. The ability of community health nurses to influence policy development is affected by their skill in assessing the policy situation, planning and implementing health care policy, and evaluating the effects of health policy development and the resulting health policies.

Models of Policy Development

A number of models have been developed to describe the policy-making process. Some of these models include the rational or rational-comprehensive model, the "garbage can" model, Kingdon's policy streams model, and the stage-sequential model. The rational model probably only describes policy formation in an ideal world that is

ETHICAL AWARENESS

*T*he resolution of ethical issues often requires political action. Conversely, policy development frequently has ethical ramifications or implications. Community health nurses engaged in policy development should analyze the ethical aspects of policy options. The Tavistock Group has suggested a framework of ethical principles in policy development. These principles include:

- Rights: All people have rights to health and to health care.
- Balance: There must be a balance between care of individual clients and care of populations.
- Comprehensiveness: Health policy should address health promotion, illness prevention, and mitigation of suffering and disability in addition to treatment of illness.
- Cooperation: Cooperation is needed between providers and clients, between providers, and between health and other sectors.
- Improvement: Improvement of health status should be an ongoing goal.
- Safety: Health care services and policies should not cause harm.
- Openness: Openness, honesty, and trustworthiness are required in health policy development. (Silva, 2002)

Select a health policy with which you are familiar and analyze the extent to which it conforms to these ethical principles. What might be done to address areas of nonconformity?

completely rational (Hanley, 2002). In this model the policy development process consists of defining a problem; identifying a goal for its resolution; determining and prioritizing the social values embedded in the goals; specifying criteria for problem resolution; examining alternative solutions in light of those criteria and selecting the alternative that best meets the identified goals; and implementing, monitoring, and evaluating the chosen alternative (Hanley, 2002; Weissert & Weissert, 2002).

As we can all readily attest, however, the world is not completely rational. The "garbage can" and stream models have been devised to explain policy making in a nonrational world. In the "garbage can" model, four independent streams flow into the "garbage can" and policies arise out of the mix of these streams as influenced by other situational variables (e.g., media coverage, etc.). The four streams identified are problems, solutions, participants, and opportunities for choice (Weissert & Weissert, 2002). Kingdon's model refined the "garbage can" model with three completely independent policy streams that interact to eventually create policy. The first is the problem stream, or the problems and issues to be addressed. The second is the policy stream, which consists of the goals and ideas of policy makers. The third stream is the political stream, or the conditions in the political environment that affect the policy agenda. Examples of conditions in this stream might be a change in administration or an event that heightens voters' concern regarding an issue. In this model, elements in each stream stir until linkages are made that result in policy. For example, a legislator may have a pet idea that suddenly seems appropriate to a specific problem (e.g., the idea of managed competition was linked to the problem of cost containment to create the concept of health maintenance organizations). When the political stream creates a window of opportunity in which the problem is of significance to a large segment of the population and to policy makers, the idea is advanced and becomes policy (Kingdon, 2002). Community health nurses can use the policy stream model to identify key opportunities to influence health policy development. To use this model, however, nurses need to stay attuned to what is happening in the policy arena. For example, community health nursing faculty supporting a proposed strengthening of smoking regulations on campus were able to point to pending city ordinances to prohibit smoking in all city parks and beaches. This was only possible because the faculty member was aware of what was being proposed at the City Council level.

The stage-sequential model is similar to the rational model, but incorporates elements of the streams models in its stages and goes beyond policy formulation to program implementation and evaluation. Stages of this model include agenda setting, formulation of goals and programs, program implementation, and evaluation (Hanley, 2002). Stages of the model, related activities, and outcomes are depicted in Table 7-3◆.

TABLE 7-3	Stages, Activities, and Outcomes of the Stage-Sequential Model of Policy Development	
Stage	**Related Activities**	**Outcome**
Agenda setting	▪ Problem perception ▪ Problem definition ▪ Mobilization of support	Government policy agenda
Formulation of goals and programs	▪ Data collection, analysis, and dissemination ▪ Alternative development ▪ Advocacy and coalition building ▪ Compromise, negotiation, and decision	Policy statement
Program implementation	▪ Resource acquisition ▪ Interpretation ▪ Planning ▪ Organizing ▪ Provision of benefits and services or coercion for required behavior	Program performance and impacts
Evaluation	▪ Evaluation of implementation ▪ Evaluation of performance ▪ Evaluation of impact	Direction for future policy decisions

Data from: Hanley, B. E. (2002). Policy development and analysis. In D. J. Mason, J. K. Leavitt, & M. W. Chaffee (Eds.), Policy and politics in nursing and health care (4th ed., pp. 55–69). St. Louis, MO: Saunders.

Agenda Setting

The first stage in policy development is setting the policy agenda. A **policy agenda** is the list of issues that become the focus for action by policy makers (Partnership for the Public's Health, 2003). For a particular issue to become a focus for action, policy makers often need to be made aware of the issue through issue analysis. Community health nurses may engage in issue analysis resulting in a formal policy issue paper. The elements of a policy analysis are included in Table 7-4◆. Tips for assessing a policy situation are presented on page 147.

Effective policy analysis requires collection, interpretation, and use of data, which may be of two types, primary data and secondary data. Primary data is information that the nurse him- or herself or affiliated groups collect. Secondary data is information from existing data sources. In an issue such as teenage pregnancy, adolescent pregnancy statistics collected by the local health department would be secondary data, whereas findings of a survey on why teens are sexually active collected by a teen pregnancy coalition would be primary data. Data have a variety of uses beyond validating a problem. For example, data can be used to convince others of the need for action, as a basis for developing policy goals and objectives, and to mark progress toward problem resolution (Center for Health Improvement, 2004).

Planning Health Care Policy

Planning health care policy involves a number of activities in which community health nurses can be involved. These activities include developing and evaluating

TABLE 7-4	Elements of an Issue Analysis
Element	**Explanation**
Problem identification	Description of the problem or issue, including information regarding causes and effects
Background	Description of factors affecting the problem; could be organized in terms of the dimensions of health; includes a description of past history of attempts at problem resolution
Political setting	Identification of the entities with jurisdiction over the problem
Issue statement	Statement of focus for policy development; usually couched in the form of a question on how the problem should be addressed
Stakeholders	Description of parties with an interest in the outcome of the issue (e.g., those affected by the problem, implementers of possible solutions, special interest groups, specific policy makers with an interest in the area)
Values assessment	Identification of underlying values shaping stakeholders' perspectives
Power analysis	Determination of power bases of stakeholders (both supporters and resisters of problem resolution)
Objectives	The desired outcome of the policy
Alternatives	Potential solutions to the problem
Evaluation criteria	Criteria for judging the appropriateness of alternative solutions in light of desired outcomes; typical criteria might include cost, equity, quality, feasibility, and resource needs
Alternative analysis and scoring	Analysis of the extent to which any given alternative meets established criteria for evaluation; may employ a scoring mechanism that ranks each alternative based on weighted criteria
Policy recommendation	Recommendation to select one or more alternatives based on the analysis

Data from: Hanley, B. E. (2002). Policy development and analysis. In D. J. Mason, J. K. Leavitt, & M. W. Chaffee (Eds.), Policy and politics in nursing and health care (4th ed., pp. 55–69). St. Louis, MO: Saunders; and Leavitt, J. K., Cohen, S. S., & Mason, D. J. (2002). Political analysis and strategies. In D. J. Mason, J. K. Leavitt, & M. W. Chaffee (Eds.), Policy and politics in nursing and health care (4th ed., pp. 71–91). St. Louis, MO: Saunders.

FOCUSED ASSESSMENT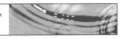

Assessing the Policy Situation

Effective participation in policy formation requires the ability to assess the policy situation and determine factors that are operating in the situation. Here are some considerations that should guide policy assessment.

- What is the health problem or issue to be addressed? Why has the need for policy development or change arisen? What are the data related to the problem or issue?
- What is the appropriate policy arena? Where does jurisdiction lie?
- What is the goal or desired outcome of policy development?
- What are the potential alternative strategies for the problem? What are the advantages and disadvantages of each alternative? Which alternative(s) is most likely to achieve the goal or desired outcome?
- Are there strongly held values that will be supported or threatened by the proposed policy?
- Who will be affected by the policy? Who will support the policy? Who might oppose it? Why? What influence does the opposition wield? What is the power base of supporters of the proposed policy?
- Who should be involved in policy development? Implementation?
- Does the proposed policy adequately address the issue?
- Does the policy safeguard individual rights as much as possible?
- Are proposed implementation strategies fair and equitable?
- How easy or difficult will it be to implement the proposed policy?
- What will be the cost of policy implementation? What resources will be needed? How will these resources be obtained?

---

alternative policy solutions for identified problems, delineating the policy, and planning strategies to garner support for the selected alternative.

Evaluating Policy Alternatives

There may be multiple policy alternatives to resolving a particular health problem, and policy makers must evaluate potential alternatives. The first step in evaluating alternatives is determining the criteria that will be used for evaluation. Some of the criteria that may be used include the relative cost of one alternative over another, the ease of implementing a particular alternative, the acceptability of the policy to those who will be affected, and so on. One particular area that should always be considered is the political feasibility of the policy alternative. Political feasibility reflects the anticipated ease or difficulty of getting the proposed policy accepted by policy makers. There are three sets of criteria regarding the political feasibility of a particular policy issue: issue-related factors, process factors, and institutional factors (Weissert & Weissert, 2002).

Issue-related factors include the comprehensiveness, complexity, and costliness of the proposed policy. Comprehensive policies that lead to massive change and those that are complex in their implementation are more difficult to achieve than those that result in modest or incremental change and are simple to implement.

Similarly, less costly alternatives usually receive greater support from policy makers than more costly ones. For example, moving to a national health system in the United States would be a sweeping change in the health care delivery system and would be extremely complex in its implementation. Incremental policies that cover smaller subpopulations (e.g., Medicare for the elderly) have historically been easier to enact.

Process factors relate to the situational context rather than the policy itself. Examples of process factors include the importance of the issue to the general public and to policy makers and the timing of the proposal in relation to other issues and factors, such as an election year or major focus on other events and issues (e.g., national security). Institutional factors reflect the political stream included in Kingdon's model and include such things as a landslide political victory or control of both houses of government by a single party.

Delineating the Policy

Once policy alternatives have been evaluated, an appropriate alternative or group of alternatives is selected and the policy itself is developed in detail. The program or plan should be made as clear and simple as possible. One of the reasons for the failure of the Health Security Act, proposed by former President Clinton, was its complexity and the inability of the general public, as well as legislators, to understand it (Mason et al., 2002). In addition, many details of the policy and its implementation, particularly with respect to program funding, had not been fully developed, leaving legislators with too many questions regarding the potential effectiveness of the program in addressing the need for health care reform.

An important consideration in outlining the details of the selected policy option is the identification of needed resources and their potential availability. What will be required to implement the planned policy? Is there a need for specially trained personnel? For equipment? Where will these resources be obtained, and how will they be financed? Where will funding for policy implementation be derived?

Strategies for Policy Adoption

When the proposed policy has been outlined, strategies are developed to promote its adoption by policy makers. In its *Health Policy Guide*, the Center for Health Improvement (2004) provides several overall suggestions for policy planning. These include developing a message, forming coalitions, mobilizing grassroots constituencies, and developing a specific action plan. The action plan should include long- and short-term goals, activity timeframes and areas of responsibility, strategies for developing community support, and identified target audiences and agents of change.

The message or issue should be framed in terms that are meaningful to stakeholders and target audiences (Leavitt, Cohen, & Mason, 2002). Different messages may be needed depending on the target. For example, messages designed for the general public might be different from those designed to enlist support from health professional organizations. Other specific strategies to promote adoption of a proposed policy by policy makers are discussed below.

STRATEGIES FOR CREATING SUPPORT Community health nurses alone cannot assure the development and implementation of effective health care policies. Although they may be actively involved in policy development, achieving policy approval and implementation usually requires broad-based support in many segments of society. Nurse policy makers can use a variety of strategies to create support for desired policy options. These include keeping informed of policy issues, communicating with policy makers, networking, coalition building, reciprocal action, creating media support, community organizing, lobbying, and providing testimony.

Staying Informed and Communicating with Policy Makers

Unlike the rest of the strategies for creating support for policy adoption, staying informed and communicating with policy makers are ongoing strategies that are not confined to a specific issue or policy. Community health nurses need to stay current on issues and problems related to health at local, state, national, and international levels. This can be accomplished through involvement in nursing and other health-related organizations and by keeping up with literature in public and professional domains (e.g., local news media and journal literature). For community health nurses, APHA is the single most effective advocacy group for public health policy in the United States and is also influential in international policy development. National and state nursing organizations (e.g., ANA and its state affiliates and nursing specialty organizations) also advocate for some health issues, but do not address population health issues with the breadth of APHA. As we saw in Chapter 6∞, the International Council of Nurses, composed of national nursing organizations, exerts a great deal of influence on international health policy, as do other international organizations.

To be seen as credible resources regarding specific issues, community health nurses need to become acquainted with policy makers at multiple levels. To do so, they should engage in regular contact with legislators and other policy makers, promote their visibility as issue experts, and provide clear, consistent messages. Community health nurses should develop strategies and tactics for becoming known to policy makers. *Strategies* are general approaches to be taken; *tactics* are the implementation details of strategy (Center for Health Improvement, 2004). Community health nurses may communicate with legislators through letters supporting a particular position or by presentation of data related to issues of interest to legislators or nurses. For example, a community health nurse may routinely send

new information regarding a particular topic to legislators who are supporting (or not supporting) a related piece of legislation. Similarly, nurses may make periodic visits to legislators who represent their state or district. On the local level, nurses may invite policy makers or members of their staffs to important community meetings or extend an invitation to participate in regular meetings of community-based organizations.

When communication relates to a particular issue, nurses or allied groups should create a clear public image and articulate key messages that are consistent and targeted to the intended audiences. Audiences may include the general public as well as legislators and other policy makers. Communication necessitates identifying the most appropriate means of reaching specific audiences. For example, members of an ethnic cultural group may be approached by means of ethnic radio and television stations or newspapers, whereas e-mail messages and telephone calls may be more appropriate for communicating with policy makers.

Networking, Coalition Building, and Reciprocal Action

Another group of related strategies for creating support for health policy initiatives includes networking, coalition building, and reciprocal action. **Networking** is a process of coming to know and becoming known to others with similar interests. Community health nurses can engage in networking by joining groups dedicated to addressing specific health-related issues or becoming involved in organizations that have a broader health focus. These groups or organizations may be local, regional, national, or international in their focus. At the local level, for example, a community health nurse might become a member of a community collaborative that addresses all kinds of community issues, including those that affect health. Or the nurse may become involved in the state nurses association or APHA. Nurses can also network by attending conferences related to specific areas of interest or by contacting authors who write about these areas.

Coalitions are alliances of individuals or groups who unite to address a common interest. Coalitions have several advantages in promoting adoption of a desired policy alternative. The first of these is the ability to pool resources and to achieve more extensive results than individuals or single agencies operating alone. Membership in coalitions may also lead to involvement in broader issues or similar issues at broader levels. Coalitions can make efficient use of resources and prevent duplication of effort. In addition, coalitions promote communication, cooperation, and idea generation and build a broader, more stable constituency than a single organization might have. Finally, all of these characteristics of coalitions build to a final advantage, greater political clout than independent action (Center for Health Improvement, 2004). It is critically important that coalitions include partnerships with groups of community residents as well as other groups and organizations working in the community.

In addition to their many advantages in supporting adoption of specific policy proposals, coalitions do have a few disadvantages. There is a need for staff time to carry out the work of the coalition that may draw staff of member agencies away from their usual responsibilities. There is also work needed to maintain the interactions of the coalition as well as to address the policy issue. For example, efforts must be undertaken to communicate among members. Another disadvantage is the increased time needed for group decisions and the potential for a weakened stance on an issue necessitated by the need to compromise to gain agreement among members. Finally, credit for the success of coalition endeavors must be shared among all members, which may make it more difficult for individual agencies to showcase their achievements to funders and other interested parties (Center for Health Improvement, 2004). Additional challenges posed by coalitions include getting the right participants, areas of distrust among members, and the need to protect one's own "turf" or agenda. One final difficulty is the potential for conflict among members posed by different perspectives on directions that should be taken to address policy issues or the strategies that should be employed to promote them (Rice, 2002).

Usually a few salient issues must be addressed for effective coalition formation. Three of these issues are coalition leadership, structure, and funding. Generally, two types of leadership are required for effective coalitions—motivational leadership and organizational leadership—and it is unusual for one person to embody both. The motivational leader has a bold vision and can motivate others to pursue that vision. The organizational leader deals with the day-to-day operation of the coalition. Issues related to coalition structure deal with governance and decision making. How should decisions be made, and by whom? Finally, there is the issue of funding. Some coalitions acquire operating funds from dues paid by members, but many have to seek outside funding through grants and other sources. The need to actively seek funds adds to the work of the coalition (Rice, 2002).

Coalition formation occurs in a series of steps, the first of which is determining whether or not a coalition is an appropriate approach to a given policy issue. If so, the next task is determining who should be invited to participate. Once participation has been solicited, the group must develop consensus on the goals to be achieved and the strategies used to achieve them. The coalition then engages in activities designed to achieve the designated goals and evaluates goal accomplishment. Throughout this process, the coalition must engage in activities that maintain its forward momentum (Center for Health Improvement, 2004).

Networking and coalition building may necessitate reciprocal action. This usually involves providing support for the issues and projects of interest to other members of the network or coalition in return for their support on issues of interest to nursing. For example, nurses may agree to support bond issues to expand police and fire services in return for the support of these groups in issues related to housing code violations.

Creating Media Support Much of the information regarding policy issues received by the general public is transmitted by the media. To create public support for a policy initiative, community health nurses must carefully select and orchestrate media coverage. Again, this was one of the flaws in the campaign to pass the Health Security Act. The news media focused more on the politics behind the legislation than on its content, diminishing the U.S. public's understanding of the proposed program and thereby diminishing their support. Another problem was the well-organized media campaign mounted by the opposition (Mason et al., 2002).

Nurses need to help assure that policy debate is framed in the interests of the public's health while accounting for contextual factors that influence the policy situation. For example, a policy should not be

Advocacy in Action

Sweet, Sweet Lead

Because of its location on the U.S.–Mexico border, many products are imported for sale in San Diego. Several brands of Mexican candy with high concentrations of lead were one import that was enjoying great popularity among children in the area.

The community health nurse for the local area, who was herself Hispanic, became aware of the dangers posed by these products. She brought her concerns to the Collaborative, an informal organization of local residents and health and social services personnel. Through the Collaborative and its alliances with other social activist groups, an initiative was undertaken to discourage the sale of these candies in several small local stores frequented by the Hispanic population. In addition, the danger posed by the candies was the focus of one of the health-related exhibits at the community's annual multicultural fair. The community health nurse and other concerned community residents helped to educate children and parents about the lead hazards posed by the candy. Eventually, because of the work of this nurse and others, Mexican candy manufacturers agreed to stop exporting the lead-laced candies to the San Diego area.

perceived to unduly advantage one segment of the population to the disadvantage of others. Policy makers should seek out media that are favorable to the particular issue, and media messages should be targeted to specific audiences to create support for a given policy initiative (Center for Health Improvement, 2004). Media messages should be designed not only to inform the public, but also to encourage them to mobilize to support the initiative. Public support is only effective when it is visible to policy makers through organized efforts such as contacting legislators, and so on.

Community Organizing Another way community health nurses create support for policy directions is community organizing. **Community organizing** is the process of mobilizing community resources in support of planned change within the community. It is a systematic process of assessment, analysis, and planning, conducted within the context of the political process. Steps in the community organization process include locality development, social planning, and social action. Locality development involves promoting the ability of community members to help themselves. Training community members for leadership roles and promoting their ability to interact with policy makers would be examples of locality development. Social planning involves the collection of data that later informs social action. Community health nurses can be actively involved and provide a leadership role in data collection activities. Social action includes specific activities by members of the community to address problems and create change (Christopher, Miller, Beck, & Toughill, 2002).

Lobbying and Advocacy Lobbying and advocacy are additional means for promoting adoption of a particular policy alternative. In the political context, these terms have different legal definitions. **Lobbying** refers to

"actions in support or opposition to legislation (and sometimes administrative action, such as the issuance of regulations) that are governed by one or more federal, state, or local laws" (Partnership for the Public's Health, 2003, p. 4). **Political advocacy** is defined as "all (unregulated) activities designed to influence public policy that do not fall under the lobbying definition" (p. 5). The critical difference between lobbying and political advocacy is that lobbying occurs as an attempt to influence policy makers to take a *particular action with respect to specific legislation*. Political advocacy, on the other hand, involves communicating with policy makers regarding an issue *without* requesting specific action (Partnership for the Public's Health, 2003).

Both lobbying and advocacy may occur directly or through grassroots efforts. Direct lobbying involves contacting legislators or other policy makers directly to discuss an issue. Lobbyists employed by nursing and other health-related interest groups (e.g., ANA, APHA) engage in direct lobbying. Grassroots lobbying is directed toward influencing public opinion with respect to an issue (Center for Health Improvement, 2004). Again, lobbying is involved when a specific course of action with respect to particular legislation is promoted. For example, a nursing organization may initiate efforts to educate the general public regarding the potential health effects of proposed state or federal budget cuts and promote a campaign of public letter writing. Advocacy, on the other hand, involves presenting information without suggesting a particular response by the audience.

Lobbying by nonprofit organizations is controlled by Internal Revenue Service regulations that limit the extent of lobbying permitted and require lobbying activities to be reported. Some state regulations have similar requirements for nonprofit organizations and may also require nonprofit groups to register as lobbyists. Government agencies may or may not be permitted to engage in lobbying activities, but lobbying may be restricted to specific individuals within the organization. The federal Hatch Act specifically prohibits government employees of agencies receiving federal monetary support from engaging in any partisan political activity (Partnership for the Public's Health, 2003). Political advocacy is much less restrictive and is usually a safer avenue for influencing policy makers for individual nurses and coalitions. Nurse lobbyists may meet directly with legislators or staff members to present nursing's perspective on an issue. They may also provide policy makers with position statements or fact sheets related to specific issues or arrange for policy makers to meet with nurses who have expertise in the area of interest.

Think Advocacy

Tsoukalas and Glantz (2003) described the efforts of health advocacy groups to promote clean air legislation in Duluth, Minnesota. After passage of an initial weak ordinance, the advocacy groups analyzed strategies used by the tobacco industry to oppose the ordinance. Strategies that led to initial tobacco industry success included framing the issue as one of individual rights, recruiting support from third-party groups such as the National Smokers Alliance and manufacturers of ventilation equipment, and promulgating claims of lost revenue among members of the Minnesota Licensed Beverage Association and the Duluth Hospitality Association. Knowledge of these tactics allowed the health advocacy coalition to mount a successful campaign for a stronger ordinance.

1. What principles of political activism described in the chapter did the tobacco industry successfully employ?
2. How might community health nurses have been involved in the health coalition's advocacy effort?

Presenting Testimony Policy makers sometimes hold public hearings or meetings to gather background information on an issue before attempting to draft legislative proposals or regulations. On occasion, such meetings are held by legislative subcommittees to explore the potential impact of a proposed piece of legislation. Writing and presenting testimony in a public hearing is another method community health nurses can use to influence policy makers.

Testimony presented by community health nurses should specifically address the issue in question and be brief, factual, and well documented. Legislative representatives are not usually health care providers, so testimony should avoid medical jargon and be clearly understandable. A copy of the testimony should be given to the legislative representatives and staff either immediately preceding or at the time of the hearing. Documentation of sources of data permits later verification by legislators or their staff members. Community health nurses should also be conversant with the format for hearings and the rules governing presentation of testimony. In addition, it is helpful to identify potential questions that might be asked by policy makers in order to be prepared to answer as fully as possible. On no account, however, should data be invented if the answer to a question is not known (Ray & Roberts, 2002).

TRADITIONAL POLITICAL STRATEGIES   Community health nurses can also influence policy development and implementation through more traditional political activities. These activities influence the selection of

GLOBAL PERSPECTIVES

Cho and Kashka (2004) described the political efforts of Mo Im Kim to establish a national community health nurse practitioner program in Korea. The intent of the program was to combine the skills of community health nurses with those of nurse practitioners to meet the health care needs of rural Koreans. Dr. Kim began by instituting a 6-month community health nurse practitioner program at Yon Sei University. The program addressed health policy formation, implementation and evaluation of community health programs, program management, and community development strategies as well as skills in physical assessment, prevention and detection of disease, and disease management. Dr. Kim and her associates made use of a number of political opportunities, including a government coup, to promote the concept of the CHNP to meet population health needs. Some of her strategies included capitalizing on the reform goals of the new regime, informing officials of the work of the CHNPs and inviting them to nursing seminars where firsthand stories of practice were shared, lobbying legislators and government officials, and publishing a collection of CHNP cases. Dr. Kim herself also held a congressional office. Dr. Kim used research data regarding the public popularity of the CHNP program to sway legislators and defuse resistance from vested interests such as physicians and obtained external assistance from the Asian Foundation and WHO. She also engaged in specific initiatives to educate government officials, such as arranging for the chair of the Congressional Health Policy Committee to visit the United States and observe community health nursing roles.

1. How might Dr. Kim's political strategies be adapted for use in another country or culture?
2. Would Dr. Kim's strategies be likely to be successful in the United States? Why or why not?

policy makers and issues to be addressed and include voting, campaigning, and holding office.

Voting   Voting is perhaps the easiest means of influencing health care policy formation at governmental levels. Nurses can themselves vote and motivate others to vote to support policy directions that enhance public health. One vote alone may not seem important, but it may be a key factor in determining the outcome on an important issue. Because lawmakers in the United States are elected, they are susceptible to the power their constituents hold through the ballot box. Thus, voting is a vital component of the political process in which all nurses can participate.

In addition to voting, nurses can educate others regarding the need to vote. Legislative networks among nurses are intended to keep members informed of health-related issues and the need for support or lack of support of certain policy directions. Nurses can also educate the general public on legislative issues that come up for public vote. Finally, nurses can participate in voter registration programs that motivate the general public to exercise their constitutional right to influence policy formation.

Campaigning   **Campaigning** is a process designed to influence the public to vote in a particular way on an issue or a candidate. An issue or candidate is presented in a favorable light with the intent of influencing voters. Campaigning can be implemented via media presentations, in group meetings or rallies, or in face-to-face contacts with the public.

Campaigning for an issue involves presenting information related to the issue that persuades people to support nursing's position. Campaigning for a specific candidate can help ensure the election of policy makers who support nursing's position on important issues. Campaigning is an opportunity for nurses to become personally known to a candidate and other campaign workers. It is also an opportunity to become known as a reliable source of information about health and health care issues. Campaigning for a candidate also creates a debt on the part of an elected official that may result in future support for a position promoted by community health nurses.

Much of the work of political action committees (PACs) is designed to support the candidacy of specific individuals. The American Nurses Association Political Action Committee (ANA-PAC) was created in response to nursing's perceived lack of influence in the formulation of health care policy. The purpose of ANA-PAC is to promote constructive national health care legislation through the political "electioneering" process. **Electioneering** is the active process of endorsing candidates and contributing time and money to their campaigns. ANA-PAC and similar political action committees supported by nurses seek to enhance the political influence of nurses by supporting the election of candidates who back the profession and its position on significant health-related issues.

There are some constraints on campaign involvement for certain groups of nurses. For example, nurses employed by government agencies (whether part-time or full-time, permanently or temporarily) are prohibited by the Hatch Act (also known as the Act to Prevent Pernicious Political Activities) from soliciting campaign contributions (even anonymously by telephone) or engaging in campaign activities while on duty, in uniform, or using an agency vehicle. They are also prohibited from running for office in a partisan election. The provisions of the Hatch Act cover all federal employees, employees of the District of Columbia, employees of state or local agencies funded by the federal government, and Commissioned Officers in the U.S. Public Health Service (Malone & Chaffee, 2002).

Holding Office A final means of creating support for policy directions promoted by community health nurses is to become a policy maker oneself. This may involve running for elective office or being appointed to a specific position. In either case, the community health nurse must first become politically active in some of the other ways described in this chapter to be sufficiently well known to be elected or appointed to a policy-making position (Dickson, Wyrsch, & Chaffee, 2002).

One may also work in the background in policy making by becoming a legislative staff person or a lobbyist for an organized group. Again, such positions require familiarity with the political process and well-developed interpersonal relationships with legislators and other policy makers. Strategies to influence policy development and implementation are summarized in Table 7-5◆.

Evaluating Policy Development

Community health nurses should be involved in evaluating the policy development process. In evaluating the process itself, the nurse would consider the extent to which all stakeholders, including those affected by a given policy, have been involved in policy development. In addition, the nurse would assess the adequacy of strategic management of the policy development process, gaining insights into what worked and what did not for application in future policy development efforts.

Community health nurses should also evaluate the adequacy of health policies developed. Criteria for evaluating health policies include their adequacy in meeting the health needs of the public, safeguards for the rights of individuals, equitable allocation of resources, their capacity for implementation, and the effects of the policy on the target population.

Health policies must be developed that effectively address the health needs of the affected population, and identification of needs must derive from population-based data. For example, a local government policy allowing homeless persons to sleep in city-owned buildings addresses only one small part of the plight of the homeless population. In this case, a more comprehensive policy that addresses both short-term and long-term solutions to the problems of homelessness is needed.

TABLE 7-5	Strategies for Promoting Policy Adoption
Strategy	**Description of Strategy**
Strategies for creating support	
Staying informed	Keeping current on health-related issues at local, state, national, and international levels
Communicating with policy makers	Becoming known to policy makers Establishing credibility as a source of information
Networking	Becoming aware of and known to groups and individuals with similar policy-related interests
Coalition building	Creating a temporary alliance among individuals or groups to work toward common goals
Reciprocal action	Supporting the policy efforts of others in return for support of issues of interest to nursing
Creating media support	Selecting appropriate media and designing targeted media messages for specific audiences
Community organizing	Mobilizing community resources in favor of planned change or a proposed policy
Lobbying	Engaging in personal communications with policy makers in an attempt to elicit a specific action with respect to a specific policy
Presenting testimony	Providing information on an issue to policy makers at a public hearing
Traditional political strategies	
Voting	Exercising one's personal right to vote Encouraging others to vote Participating in voter registration drives
Campaigning	Providing endorsements or monetary support for specific policy proposals or candidates with the intent of influencing voters' responses
Holding office	Assuming a position as a policy maker by virtue of election or appointment to a specific office

Safeguarding individual rights is another criterion for sound health care policy development. As an example, a policy that would require homeless individuals to surrender personal belongings to meet communal needs when admitted to a shelter would violate their property rights. There are circumstances, however, in which the good of society supersedes individual rights (Stallworth & Lennon, 2003). For example, homeless persons may be prohibited from smoking in a shelter to prevent exposing others to smoke or to prevent a fire. Whenever possible, though, health policies should be written so that they do not violate the rights of individuals affected by them.

Health care policies should also promote equitable distribution of health care resources. This means that policies should not discriminate against certain subgroups within the population. For example, open

CULTURAL COMPETENCE

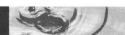

*T*he voices of many members of ethnic groups in the United States are not heard in the policy-making process. For example, members of many refugee groups are fearful of attracting notice to themselves by speaking out, based on their past experiences with repressive and authoritarian regimes. Similarly, many immigrants, even those admitted to the United States legally, are open to exploitation or do not receive services for which they are eligible because of fears of repercussions and possible deportation. What might community health nurses do to make sure these voices are heard? What culturally appropriate strategies might be used to promote political involvement among these groups?

housing policies in homeless shelters may inadvertently discriminate against women and children who may be subjected to force to make them give way to adult males who desire shelter. Sex-segregated shelters that ensure access for both males and females provide for a more equitable allocation of resources.

For a specific health policy to be effective in promoting health or preventing illness, it must be capable of being implemented or enforced. For example, a local government might adopt a policy encouraging houses of worship to provide overnight shelter for homeless individuals. But unless the houses of worship are willing to cooperate, the policy cannot be implemented.

Community health nurses planning to influence health care policy formation should assess proposed policies or modifications of existing policies in light of these five criteria. Policies that do not meet the criteria should be redesigned, if possible, before they are presented to policy makers. If a proposed policy continues not to meet one or more criteria, its supporters should be prepared to justify the need for the policy. For example, nurses should be prepared to convince policy makers that a smoking ban in shelters for the homeless is warranted despite the violation of the individual's personal freedom of choice.

Community health nurses may also be actively involved in assessing the effects of health care policies on meeting the needs of the particular target group. Community health nurses could assist in collecting data related to the outcomes of programs put into operation. For example, data might be gathered on the incidence of health problems among the homeless to evaluate the effects of policies designed to promote primary and secondary prevention activities in this population. In addition, information could be collected regarding the number of persons who continue to be homeless despite assistance from established programs.

Effective community health nurses use the political process to attain their primary objective, enhancing the health of the populations with which they work. Political activity by community health nurses may occur at the institutional or societal level and often involves efforts to influence legislation related to health issues.

MediaLink

Case Study: Political Action

Case Study

Case Study: Influencing Housing Policy

In focus groups conducted to determine local health needs, residents of a low-income, culturally diverse neighborhood repeatedly voiced concerns about intimidation of tenants by landlords. Because of housing shortages, many tenants were (justifiably) worried that reporting inadequacies to landlords would result in evictions. With limited low-income housing available, people were not willing to take the risk of making complaints about needed repairs or noisy neighbors.

Cultural differences, the tenants' lack of facility with English, and the fact that most owners of rental units were absentee landlords complicated the situation. More than half of the residents in the community were members of ethnic cultural groups, including many relatively recent refugees from Southeast Asia and the Middle East. Long-time area residents were primarily older persons on fixed incomes who also could not afford to antagonize landlords.

There was a fledgling landlord/tenant association in the neighborhood, but few of the absentee landlords were active participants. There was also a neighborhood collaborative that had successfully mounted some initiatives to improve conditions for residents, including decreasing drug dealing in selected areas of the neighborhood and putting up anti-tobacco billboards. The collaborative had developed relatively close relationships with

city council members and county supervisors in the wider community, although recently several political positions had been filled by new electees. One or two long-time residents were particularly influential with local politicians. The nearby university law school provided landlord/tenant mediation services to individuals in the community. Other agencies and associations active in the neighborhood included local schools, the community center, Boys and Girls Club, the community health center, the local health department office, the university school of nursing, a Lao-Hmong Association, the Vietnamese Federation, and several programs geared toward children and the elderly.

1. What steps might the local community health nurses take to address the problem of intimidation by landlords?
2. What community groups might be appropriate coalition partners in resolving this problem? Why?
3. What approaches might be taken in terms of policy development to deal with intimidation?
4. Are there particular government agencies that should become involved? If so, what are they and how would you promote their involvement?
5. How might local residents become actively involved in resolving the issue?
6. What cultural considerations have relevance for this situation and its resolution?

Test Your Understanding

1. What potential roles can community health nurses play in policy development? (pp. 139–140)

2. What are the main avenues for public policy formation? (pp. 141–145)

3. Outline the legislative and regulatory processes. Identify strategies by which community health nurses might influence these processes and points at which those strategies might be most effective. (pp. 141–144)

4. Describe the policy development process. How might community health nurses be involved in this process? (pp. 145–153)

5. Identify four criteria for evaluating health policy development. Give an example of the application of each criterion. (pp. 152–153)

EXPLORE MediaLink

http://www.prenhall.com/clark

Resources for this chapter can be found on the Companion Website.

Audio Glossary
Exam Review Questions
Case Study: Political Action: New State Bill to Increase RN-to-patient Ratios

MediaLink Applications: Preparing Effective Testimony
Media Links
Challenge Your Knowledge

Update *Healthy People 2010*
Advocacy Interviews

References

Callahan, D. (2002). Ends and means: The goals of health care. In M. Danis, C. Clancy, & L. R. Churchill (Eds.), *Ethical dimensions of health policy* (pp. 3–18). New York: Oxford University Press.

Center for Health Improvement. (2004). *Health policy guide*. Retrieved August 25, 2004, from http://www.healthpolicycoach.org/advocacy.asp?id=5207

Cho, H. S. M., & Kashka, M. S. (2004). The evolution of the community health nurse practitioner in Korea. *Public Health Nursing, 21*, 287–294.

Christopher, M. A., Miller, J. L., Beck, T. L., & Toughill, E. H. (2002). Working with the community for change. In D. J. Mason, J. K. Leavitt, & M. W. Chaffee (Eds.), *Policy and politics in nursing and health care* (4th ed., pp. 687–696). St. Louis, MO: Saunders.

Dickson, B. R., Wyrsch, S. J., & Chaffee, M. W. (2002). Political appointments. In D. J. Mason, J. K. Leavitt, & M. W. Chaffee (Eds.), *Policy and politics in nursing and health care* (4th ed., pp. 543–550). St. Louis, MO: Saunders.

Division of Unintentional Injury Prevention, National Center for Injury Prevention and Control. (2004). Impact of primary laws on adult use of safety belts—United States, 2002. *Morbidity and Mortality Weekly Report, 53*, 257–260.

Emanuel, E. J. (2002). Patient vs. population: Resolving the ethical dilemmas posed by treating patients as members of populations. In M. Danis, C. Clancy, & L. R. Churchill (Eds.), *Ethical dimensions of health policy* (pp. 227–245). New York: Oxford University Press.

Hanley, B. E. (2002). Policy development and analysis. In D. J. Mason, J. K. Leavitt, & M. W. Chaffee (Eds.), *Policy and politics in nursing and health care* (4th ed., pp. 55–69). St. Louis, MO: Saunders.

Heloma, A., Jaakkola, M. S., Kahkonen, E., & Reijula, K. (2001). The short-term impact of national smoke-free workplace legislation on passive smoking and tobacco use. *American Journal of Public Health, 91*, 1416–1418.

Keough, K. (2002). How science informs the decisions of government. *Canadian Journal of Public Health, 93*, 104–108.

Kesler, J. T. (2000). Healthy communities and civil discourse: A leadership opportunity for public health professionals. *Public Health Reports, 115*, 238–242.

Kickbusch, I. (2003). The contribution of the World Health Organization to a new public health and health promotion. *American Journal of Public Health, 93*, 383–387.

Kingdon, J. W. (2002). The reality of public policy making. In M. Danis, C. Clancy, & L. R. Churchill (Eds.), *Ethical dimensions of health policy* (pp. 97–116). New York: Oxford University Press.

Kullgren, J. T. (2003). Restrictions on undocumented immigrants' access to health services: The public health implications of welfare reform. *American Journal of Public Health, 93*, 1630–1633.

Leavitt, J. K., Chaffee, M. W., & Vance, C. (2002). Learning the ropes of policy and politics. In

D. J. Mason, J. K. Leavitt, & M. W. Chaffee (Eds.), *Policy and politics in nursing and health care* (4th ed., pp. 31–53). St. Louis, MO: Saunders.

Leavitt, J. K., Cohen, S. S., & Mason, D. J. (2002). Political analysis and strategies. In D. J. Mason, J. K. Leavitt, & M. W. Chaffee (Eds.), *Policy and politics in nursing and health care* (4th ed., pp. 71–91). St. Louis, MO: Saunders.

Lorette, J., & Jansto, C. L. (2002). How regulations are shaped: The rules of the game. In D. J. Mason, J. K. Leavitt, & M. W. Chaffee (Eds.), *Policy and politics in nursing and health care* (4th ed., pp. 467–470). St. Louis, MO: Saunders.

Malone, T. A., & Chaffee, M. W. (2002). Political activity of government-employed nurses. In D. J. Mason, J. K. Leavitt, & M. W. Chaffee (Eds.), *Policy and politics in nursing and health care* (4th ed., pp. 583–587). St. Louis, MO: Saunders.

Mason, D. J., Leavitt, J. K., & Chaffee, M. W. (2002). Policy and politics: A framework for action. In D. J. Mason, J. K. Leavitt, & M. W. Chaffee (Eds.), *Policy and politics in nursing and health care* (4th ed., pp. 1–18). St. Louis, MO: Saunders.

Oberlander, J., Jacobs, L. R., & Marmor, T. R. (2001). The politics of health care rationing: Lessons from Oregon. In R. B. Hackey & D. A. Rochefort (Eds.), *The new politics of state health policy* (pp. 207–226). Lawrence, KS: University Press of Kansas.

Office on Smoking and Health, National Center for Chronic Disease Prevention and

Health Promotion. (2004). Effect of ending an antitobacco youth campaign on adolescent susceptibility to cigarette smoking—Minnesota, 2002–2003. *Morbidity and Mortality Weekly Report, 53*, 302–304.

Partnership for the Public's Health. (2003, April). Improving public health through policy advocacy. *Community-based Public Health Policy & Practice, 8*, 1–8.

Ray, M. M., & Roberts, S. (2002). Lobbying policymakers: Individual and collective strategies. In D. J. Mason, J. K. Leavitt, & M. W. Chaffee (Eds.), *Policy and politics in nursing and health care* (4th ed., pp. 551–561). St. Louis, MO: Saunders.

Rice, R. (2002). Coalitions: A powerful political strategy. In D. J. Mason, J. K. Leavitt, & M. W. Chaffee (Eds.), *Policy and politics in nursing and health care* (4th ed., pp. 121–140). St. Louis, MO: Saunders.

Santa Anna, Y. (2002). Legislative and regulatory processes. In D. J. Mason, J. K. Leavitt, & M. W. Chaffee (Eds.), *Policy and politics in nursing and health care* (4th ed., pp. 451–462). St. Louis, MO: Saunders.

Scott, C., & West, E. (2001). Nursing in the public sphere: Health policy research in a changing world. *Journal of Advanced Nursing, 33*, 387–395.

Silva, M. C. (2002). Ethical issues in health care, public policy, and politics. In D. J. Mason, J. K. Leavitt, & M. W. Chaffee (Eds.), *Policy and politics in nursing and health care* (4th ed., pp. 177–184). St. Louis, MO: Saunders.

Stallworth, J., & Lennon, J. L. (2003). An interview with Dr. Lester Breslow. *American Journal of Public Health, 93*, 1803–1805.

Tsoukalas, T., & Glantz, S. A. (2003). The Duluth Clean Indoor Air ordinance: Problems and success in fighting the tobacco industry at the local level in the 21st century. *American Journal of Public Health, 93*, 1214–1221.

Weissert, C. S., & Weissert, W. G. (2002). *Governing health: The politics of health policy* (2nd ed.). Baltimore, MD: Johns Hopkins University.

Advocacy in Action

Affordable Medicine

St. Agnes Nurses Center is a free nurse-managed center in West Chester, Pennsylvania, that provides health care to uninsured and underinsured men, women, and children in the area on a part-time basis. Students from Villanova University go to St. Agnes as part of their Health Promotion clinical experience.

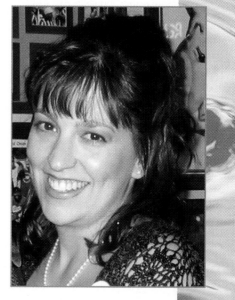

One of the clients at St. Agnes, Manny, was a 57-year-old gentleman from Puerto Rico with long-term cardiac problems related to diabetes. Manny required many medications to manage his health, medications he could not afford on his limited salary.

We referred Manny to a nearby clinic that offered more comprehensive care, but he would not go because he had developed trust in the nursing staff at St. Agnes. In order to assist Manny and other patients in similar circumstances with obtaining their much-needed medications, I explored pharmaceutical patient assistance programs and developed a system to make it easier for patients to take advantage of this service. With Manny's limited command of English and lack of telephone/Internet access, navigating the process on his own would have been very difficult and perhaps impossible.

Michelle Gallagher, BSN, RN

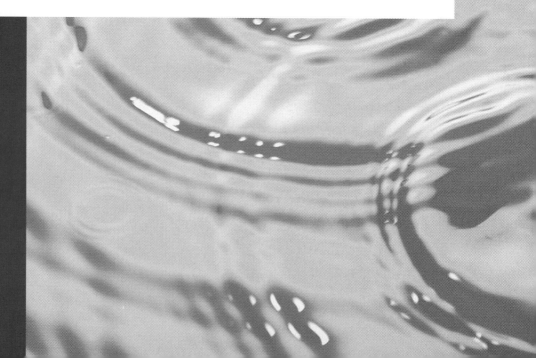

CHAPTER 8

The Economic Context

CHAPTER OBJECTIVES

After reading this chapter, you should be able to:

1. Analyze interrelationships among economic conditions, health care services, and health status.
2. Discuss factors contributing to escalating health care costs.
3. Discuss the effects of economic factors on the provision of public health services.
4. Distinguish among selected approaches to financing health care services.
5. Analyze the effects of selected health care reimbursement mechanisms.

KEY TERMS

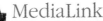
MediaLink
http://www.prenhall.com/clark

Additional interactive resources for this chapter can be found on the Companion Website. Click on Chapter 8 and "Begin" to select the activities for this chapter.

*E*conomics can be defined as the study of the ways in which societies make choices in how they address problems of scarcity (Pfoutz, Price, & Chang, 2002). Scarcity results when there are insufficient resources to satisfy the wants and desires of the population (Price, Pfoutz, & Chang, 2001). Currently, the federal government and the states are experiencing an economic crisis that affects the health of the population as well as the health care services that are provided. This crisis is the result of several factors, including recent tax cuts, poor economic performance, and increased expenditures in areas such as defense and national security. These factors are unlikely to change in the near future for a number of reasons. Congress is unlikely to reduce federal spending and likely to extend tax cuts under pressure from many constituencies. These factors will maintain expenditures while at the same time reducing revenues that could fund them. Although tax cuts and low interest rates will stimulate the economy in the short run, they are likely to cause a long-term imbalance, leading to increasing deficits, lower rates of national savings, higher interest rates, and a slowed economy as well as reductions in government-supported services (Bass, Irons, & Taylor, 2003). All of these factors will lead to a greater scarcity of health resources and more severe effects on the health of the population.

When we consider the economic context of health, we often think of the effects of poverty on health status or the increasing cost of health care. However, there are many different aspects to the economic context in which community health nursing takes place. The two major considerations in this area are the interrelationships between economics and health and the financing of health care services. Each of these aspects will be discussed here.

INTERRELATIONSHIPS AMONG ECONOMIC FACTORS AND HEALTH

Three fundamental economic principles must be considered in examining the effects of economic conditions on health and health care services. The first principle is that resources are always more limited than what is needed for desired levels of consumption. Second, resources have alternative uses. Third, different people will have differing ideas as to what those uses should be. Based on these principles, the basic question related to health care economics is how limited resources should be used. What types of health services should consume the resources available? Two related questions address the methods by which those services should be produced and how they should be distributed within the population (Price et al., 2001).

The interrelationships among economic factors and health status are many and varied. In this chapter,

we will discuss three specific relationships: (a) the relationship between health and societal productivity and stability, (b) health care spending and rising costs, and (c) the effects of socioeconomic factors on health status.

Societal Productivity and Stability

As we noted earlier, we often think of the effects of economic factors on health status. What we tend to forget, however, is that health also affects a nation's economic welfare. A healthy population is more productive than an unhealthy one and is better able to learn and to use education effectively to increase society's overall productivity. When people are unable to work due to health deficiencies, society loses their productive capability. In addition, the productive capacity of other family members may also be lost (Perkins, 2002). For example, diseases leading to disability result in lost productivity for those affected and for family members who must leave work to care for them. As we saw in Chapter 6∞, productivity in some industries declined by nearly half in some highly affected countries (World Health Organization [WHO], 2002). Even in countries with good control of disabilities caused by chronic illness, less than half of people with chronic diseases work until the usual retirement age (Huey, 2001).

Poverty and ill health lead to lower income and slowed economic growth as well as social instability and conflict. For example, approximately 70% of persons with large medical bills depleted their savings, two thirds borrowed money from friends or family, and one quarter took out loans or mortgaged their homes to pay them, weakening the overall economy as well as a given family's economic status (Alliance for Health Reform, 2003). Conversely, nations with strong economies are better able to afford health care and other determinants of health, and recently national expenditures for both education and health have been viewed as investments in human capital that will increase economic strength (Perkins, 2002).

Health care programs may also have a more direct effect on the economy than that seen in increased capacity for production. For example, a report by Families USA (Klein, Stoll, & Bruce, 2004) indicated that state Medicaid programs actually generate revenue for states far beyond the costs of the programs. This revenue comes from a number of sources, including federal block grants that would otherwise not come to the states, new business, and new jobs. A **block grant** is a lump sum made available to the states by the federal government to be used as each state sees fit within certain broadly defined parameters. Medicaid provides 43% of all federal funding to the states. Each state dollar spent by states will generate $1.92 to $6.22 in federal aid, depending on the funding formula, which varies from state to state. The more state dollars spent on Medicaid, the greater the federal financial contribution, which makes Medicaid revenues an important source of state funding. In addition, every $1 million spent by states on Medicaid services is estimated to generate $3.35 million in new business as that money circulates in the population. Finally, in 2005, Medicaid programs were expected to generate 3.3 million new jobs with salaries amounting to $133 billion. Overall, the anticipated $132 billion Medicaid expenditure by the states will generate more than $367 billion in revenues (Klein et al., 2004). Similarly, health care services in general generate revenues that support the overall economy.

Health Care Spending

The amount of money spent on health care services in the United States has been increasing at an alarming rate for the last several years. There are two theories of how general economic factors influence the economics of health care delivery: the demand-pull theory and the cost-push theory. According to the demand-pull theory, health care inflation or the increasing cost of health services is fueled by increased demand for services and a supply of services insufficient to meet the demand. In the cost-push theory, on the other hand, health care inflation is the result of higher costs in providing services due to provider wage increases, malpractice costs, increasingly expensive technology, and so on (Pfoutz

et al., 2002). In reality, as we will see, increasing health care costs are due to both types of factors.

Overall, health care spending has risen from 5.1% of the gross domestic product (GDP) in 1960 to 15.3% in 2003, and is expected to rise to 18.7% by 2014 (Centers for Medicare and Medicaid Services [CMS], 2005d). U.S. per capita expenditures for health care in 1960 were $143, but increased to $5,671 in 2003, the most recent year for which data are available (National Center for Health Statistics [NCHS], 2005). **Per capita expenditures** reflect the average amount spent on health care per person per year. Health care expenditures have increased consistently from one year to the next since 1960. From 1960 to 2003, personal health care expenditures increased by an average of 10% each year (NCHS, 2005).

Factors that have contributed to increasing health care spending include an aging population, greater use of technology, emphasis on costly specialty care, costs of care for the uninsured, and the labor-intensive nature of health care delivery (Sultz & Young, 2004). An aging population contributes to greater demand for and use of services, particularly as the prevalence of chronic diseases with high costs for disease management increases in older age groups. The size of the older population relative to other age groups in the United States has increased consistently over the last several decades. In 1950, for example, people over the age of 65 years comprised only 8.1% of the U.S. population; by 2030 the proportion of the population over 65 years of age is expected to increase to 21.8%, half of them over 75 years of age. By 2050, an estimated 25% of all those over 65 will be more than 85 years old. People over age 65 consume a large portion of the health care services provided each year. For example, they account for one third of all hospitalizations, the most costly form of health care, and half of all hospital days. People over 45 years of age also use more health services than those at younger ages (Sultz & Young, 2004).

Greater use of technology, particularly in response to fears of malpractice, and greater use of specialty care have also contributed to increased health care spending. Nearly two thirds of U.S. physicians are specialists, who tend to command higher reimbursement than generalists and employ more expensive technology. In addition, specialists have been associated with more inappropriate use of costly therapies. Greater use of technology also creates a demand for a better prepared health care

GLOBAL PERSPECTIVES

The Organization for Economic Cooperation and Development (OECD) is an organization composed of 30 member states. Since 1984, data have been collected from each of these nations regarding their health care spending. In 2000, U.S. per capita spending was more than twice the OECD median ($4,631 per person vs. $1,983). U.S. spending was 44% higher than that of the next highest country, which was Switzerland at $3,222. In most of the OECD countries, the majority of health care spending is financed by government expenditures, with a median of only 26% privately funded compared to 56% in the United States. U.S. privately funded per capita health care spending ($2,580) was five times the OECD median ($451). A significant portion of U.S. spending is for pharmaceuticals. Per capita spending on pharmaceuticals in the United States in 2000 was $556, more than twice the median OECD spending ($262). Despite the higher expenditures for care, Americans do not seem to receive more services than their counterparts in OECD countries. For example, Americans receive slightly fewer physician visits per capita than the OECD median, spend shorter-than-median stays in the hospital when hospitalized, and have fewer per capita days in the hospital. Americans are, however, exposed to more technology than people in OECD nations. For example, the United States has 72% more MRI units and 11% more CT scanners per 1 million population than the OECD median, performs 92% more coronary angioplasties per 100,000 population than the next most prolific country, and has more than twice as many individuals undergoing kidney dialysis as the OECD median (Anderson, Reinhardt, Hussey, & Petrosyan, 2003). One could conclude from these findings that the high cost of health care in the United States compared to other developed nations is due to high drug costs, expensive technology use, and duplication of services rather than greater provision of services.

ETHICAL AWARENESS

Some health care policy makers have proposed that government funding should be used to provide health promotion and illness and injury prevention services rather than to treat existing health problems. What are the ethical implications of such proposals? What approaches to ethical decision making would support such proposals? What approaches would argue against them?

workforce at all levels, thereby increasing the costs of its use (Sultz & Young, 2004).

Health care spending differs for different elements of the health care system. For example, in 2003, 31% of health care dollars was spent on hospital care, 23% on other services (e.g., dental and home health services), 22% on provider services (physicians and others), 7% on nursing home care, 11% on prescription drug costs, and 7% on program administration (CMS, 2005e). This breakdown of health care expenditures is depicted in Figure 8-1. Health care delivery is a labor-intensive segment of the economy, requiring 24-hour-a-day and 7-day-a-week coverage in some settings. By 2010, the health care workforce is expected to account for 13% of all wage and salary jobs (Sultz & Young, 2004) and will comprise a large portion of national health care costs in the future.

Costs of uncompensated care for the uninsured and increasing prescription drug prices are two other factors implicated in rising health care costs. **Uncompensated care** is that proportion of care for which the provider receives no reimbursement and includes both charity care and bad debt. A large segment of the population is uninsured or underinsured, resulting in large amounts of uncompensated care provided by health care institutions and providers. A study by the U.S. Government Accountability Office (GAO) (2005) found that the extent of uncompensated care ranged from 3.2% to 18% of all patient operating costs in hospitals in

five states. For-profit hospitals generally provided less uncompensated care than nonprofit hospitals, and nonfederal government hospitals in all five states provided the highest levels of uncompensated care. According to a study by Pricewaterhousecooper's Health Research Institute (2005), the extent of uncompensated care in the United States increased 20% from 1999 to 2003, to $24.9 billion. Bad debt was seen to increase from 7.6% to 9.9% of total net revenues in the same period. In addition, major for-profit hospital chains reported a 60% to 70% increase in the amount of charity care provided from 2002 to 2004. Uncompensated care leads to a phenomenon known as **cost shifting**, the passing on of the cost of uncompensated care to those who do pay for care, either those who pay out-of-pocket or those covered by health insurance. Cost shifting leads in turn to higher insurance premiums and higher overall costs for health care.

U.S. drug prices have risen considerably more than the consumer price index. The **consumer price index (CPI)** is the estimated cost of all goods and services purchased by a typical household (Chang, 2001b). In 2003, U.S. prescription drug costs amounted to $179.2 million (NCHS, 2005), and prescription drug spending increased 15.3% in 2002 alone, with one third of this increase due to higher drug prices (Mahan, 2004). The price of the 30 brand-name drugs most often prescribed for the elderly, who consume most prescription drugs, increased an average of 6.5% in 2003, 4.3 times the rate of inflation. Over a period of 3 years, prices on these drugs increased by 22% overall, but prices on some drugs (e.g., Combivent, used for asthma control) increased by as much as 56%. Some of these drugs increased in price several times in the 3-year period. For example, the price of Toprol XL, a beta-blocking agent, increased 7 times from 2001 to 2004 (Mahan, 2004).

Many Americans pay much of the cost of prescription medications out-of-pocket. From 1977 to 1996, for example, out-of-pocket drug spending increased by 150%, and out-of-pocket costs have continued to rise since then, reaching $103.4 billion in 2003 (CMS, 2005d). These increased costs force many people, particularly those in lower income groups, to spend higher and higher percentages of their income on health products. In 1996, for example, 43% of people in the lowest income quartile spent more than 10% of their income on prescription drugs and other health care products (American Association of Retired Persons [AARP], 2002). Increased drug costs are also one of the most consistent explanations given for increased insurance premiums (Bauman, 2002). Pharmaceutical companies cite the high costs of research and development (R&D) of new drugs as the primary cause of higher drug prices, yet the U.S. pharmaceutical industry puts only 12.5% of revenue into R&D, compared to the 20% spent by British companies. In addition, the pharmaceutical industry consistently achieves high returns on its investments,

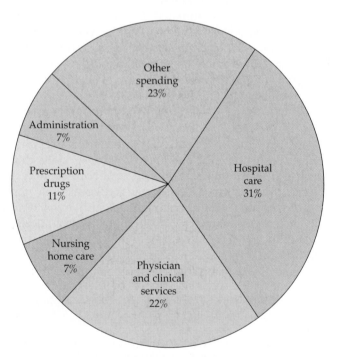

FIGURE 8-1 Distribution of National Health Care Expenditures, United States, 2003

Data from: Centers for Medicare and Medicaid Services. (2005). The nation's health dollar, Calendar year 2003, Where it came from, Where it went. *Retrieved December 23, 2005, from http://www.cms.gov/ nationalhealthexpenddata/downloads/piechartSourcesExpenditures2003.pdf*

anywhere from 3 to 8 times those of any other industrial sector in the United States (Barry, 2002).

Many authors have suggested allowing U.S. citizens to purchase less expensive prescription drugs from international markets or discounted drugs from U.S. manufacturers. The Veterans Administration (VA), for example, very successfully negotiates for drug discounts with U.S. pharmaceutical companies (Mahan, 2004). Certain providers, such as federally qualified health centers (FQHCs), migrant centers, and AIDS assistance programs, qualify for prescription drug discounts under section 340B of the United States Public Health Service Act (Mitchem, 2002).

Some state and local jurisdictions have begun to purchase prescription medications from outside the United States, even though the federal government prohibits such purchases. For example, Burlington, Vermont, saved $54,000 in one year because of its purchase contract with a Canadian pharmacy, and Montgomery, Alabama, counted $200,000 in savings in 2002, enough to waive copayments and deductibles on medications for its employees. The federal rationale for not permitting out-of-country purchases is a diminished quality of medications, but many of the drugs purchased were manufactured in the United States, and then sold abroad (Wiebe, 2004).

A large proportion of Americans are without any assistance in paying for prescription medications. With increasing costs, many employers are reducing or eliminating prescription coverage from health care plans or requiring higher copayments by beneficiaries. As a result, many people fail to take medications as directed due to the costs. For example, in one study, 18% of chronically ill adults cut back on medications and 14% used less medication than prescribed due to cost and lack of insurance coverage (Piette, Heisler, & Wagner, 2004).

Those most seriously affected by rising prescription drug costs have been the elderly who live on fixed incomes that do not rise with rising inflation rates. Some effort has been made to improve prescription drug access for Medicare beneficiaries through the Medicare Prescription Drug, Improvement, and Modernization Act of 2003. This legislation initiated Medicare Prescription Drug Coverage to assist older Americans with drug costs. This program was implemented in January 2006 (CMS, 2005a) and will be discussed in more detail in the section related to the Medicare program.

Socioeconomic Factors and Health Status

Socioeconomic status affects health directly, in terms of access to health care, as well as indirectly, through factors such as social and educational opportunities, knowledge of health promotion and prevention, and shaping health behaviors (Santelli, Lowry, Brener, & Robin, 2002). Despite the relatively high standard of living in the United States, the point has been made that "there are considerable pockets of the population for whom access to care and the effects on health status are much more similar to those of poorer and less successful Third World countries than they are to the rest of the industrial world" (Vladek, 2003, p. 16). This statement was supported by the findings of *Crossing the Quality Chasm*, an Institute of Medicine report published in 2001.

Socioeconomic factors have a variety of effects on the health status of the population. Two major factors that will be discussed here are welfare reform and diminishing access to health care. Questions for assessing the economic status of a population are provided in the focused assessment below.

Welfare Reform

Due to spiraling increases in public assistance programs, the U.S. Congress enacted the Personal Responsibility and Work Opportunity Reconciliation Act (PRWORA) of 1996, more commonly known as the welfare reform act. Welfare reform consisted of a number of provisions that reduced eligibility for public assistance, limited the time people could receive assistance, and divorced eligibility for Medicaid from assistance programs. The intent of the new program was to move people from the welfare rolls to become involved in gainful employment. PRWORA terminated the Aid to Families with Dependent Children (AFDC) program and replaced it with Temporary Assistance for Needy Families (TANF). This change has several ramifications for eligibility for health care assistance. Children in families receiving AFDC were automatically eligible for Medicaid, but the welfare reform provisions divorced welfare assistance from health care assistance (Waitzkin et al., 2002). PRWORA also imposed a 5-year maximum on receipt of cash assistance over one's lifetime (Hildebrandt, 2002). In addition, welfare reform prohibited access of immigrants (except those in refugee or asylum categories) to public

---

FOCUSED ASSESSMENT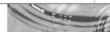

Assessing the Economic Status of a Population

- What is the average income of the group?
- What proportion of the group has incomes at or below poverty level?
- What subpopulations are included in the low-income group?
- What proportion of low-income families receives some form of public assistance? Are all those eligible for assistance receiving it? If not, why not?
- What is the level of unemployment in the population? For those who are employed, what are the typical salaries?
- What proportion of the population receives employment-based health insurance benefits? Why do others not receive benefits (e.g., part-time employment, cannot afford premiums, etc.)?
- How are most health care services for the population funded?
- What revenue sources fund public health services for the population? Are these revenues adequate to provide needed services?

assistance for the first 5 years of U.S. residence and gave states the option to consider a ban on assistance beyond the 5-year limit (Kullgren, 2003).

Although the health impact of welfare reform is not yet known, there are several indicators that it has had both positive and negative effects. On the positive side, one study of women in welfare-to-work programs reported an increased sense of self-esteem among the participants. At the same time, all of the women in the study voiced feelings of increased anxiety and depression and difficulty juggling work, family responsibilities, and health care activities (Hildebrandt, 2002). The findings of one study of Latina women in New York City, California, and Texas indicated that welfare reform had little effect on access to prenatal care or pregnancy outcomes (Joyce, Bauer, Minkoff, & Kaestner, 2001). Another study with similar populations, however, indicated that Latina women in California, even those who were not immigrants, were afraid to apply for Medicaid assistance during pregnancy even though their eligibility for care was not affected by PRWORA. No similar findings were noted in New York or Florida, and the authors attributed the differences to the immigrant-unfriendly political atmosphere generated in California by several pieces of legislation aimed at restricting the access of undocumented immigrants to public services (Bauer, Collins, Doyle, Fuld, & Fuentes-Afflick, 2002). These latter findings suggest an interaction between social environmental and economic factors in California that did not occur in the other states.

A longitudinal study of welfare recipients in Illinois affected by PRWORA indicated that some of the goals of the legislation were achieved, but not to the extent anticipated. For example, although the overall rate of employment increased from 46% to 49% in the first 2 years after implementation, only 18% of the sample was employed consistently through the 6 years of the study. Similarly, increased family income was achieved by 35% of the subjects, but 76% of them remained below the federal poverty level even with the increase. Finally, the number of families who fell behind on rent or were evicted increased by 13 percentage points (Glenn, 2002). Because welfare reform uncoupled Medicaid eligibility from public assistance programs, a significant number of children had discontinuous health insurance coverage. As we will see later in this chapter, breaks in the continuity of insurance coverage have negative implications for health status. TANF is not the only source of monetary and other assistance to poor people in the United States. Federal, state, and local jurisdictions provide other sources of assistance that are discussed in Chapter 20∞.

Access to Health Care and Health Disparities

The second major way in which economic factors affect health is through diminished access to health care. Access to health care is defined as "the timely use of needed, affordable, convenient, acceptable, and effective personal health care services" (Chang, 2001a, p. 336). Diminished access occurs as a result of the mixed effects of poverty and lack of health care insurance. Access to health care is such an important issue that it has been selected as one of the 10 leading health indicators of population health in the United States and is the focus of the first set of national health objectives included in *Healthy People 2010* (U.S. Department of Health and Human Services [USDHHS], 2000). Leading indicator objectives and other objectives relevant to health care access are presented below♦. Additional information about *Healthy People 2010* objectives is available at the *Healthy People 2010* data Web site at http://wonder.cdc.gov/data 2010.

POVERTY Poverty is measured in terms of one's income relative to the current federal or state income guidelines. The poverty level is defined in terms of both household income and size. In 2005, for example, the poverty level for a family of four was an annual income less than

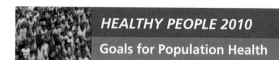

HEALTHY PEOPLE 2010
Goals for Population Health

Critical Indicator Objectives

1-1	Increase the proportion of persons with health insurance.
1-4a	Increase the proportion of persons who have a specific source of ongoing care.
1-16a	Increase the proportion of pregnant women who begin prenatal care in the first trimester of pregnancy.

Other Relevant Access to Health Care Objectives

1-2	Increase the proportion of insured persons with coverage for clinical preventive services.
1-3	Increase the proportion of persons appropriately counseled about health behaviors.
1-5	Increase the proportion of persons with a usual primary care provider.
1-6	Reduce the proportion of families that experience difficulties or delays in obtaining health care or do not receive needed care for one or more family members.
1-10	Reduce the proportion of persons who delay or have difficulty getting emergency medical care.
1-11	Increase the proportion of persons who have access to rapidly responding prehospital emergency medical services.
1-13	Increase the number of Tribes, States, and the District of Columbia with trauma care systems that maximize survival and functional outcomes of trauma patients and help prevent injuries from occurring.
1-15	Increase the proportion of persons with long-term care needs who have access to the continuum of long-term care services.

Data from: U.S. Department of Health and Human Services. (2000). Healthy People 2010 (Conference ed., Vol. 1). Washington, DC: Author.

$19,350 in all states except Alaska and Hawaii, which had slightly higher income levels defining poverty (Center for Medicaid and State Operations, 2005). According to the U.S. Census Bureau (2004), 12.5% of the U.S. population, or 35.9 million people, were living in poverty in 2003. This was an increase from 12.1% in 2002. The poverty rate in 2003 was nearly 10 percentage points below the peak rate in 1959, but is the result of increases over the previous 3 years. Increases were also noted in specific population groups. For example, the rate of children (those under 18 years of age) living in poverty increased from 16.7% in 2002 to 17.6% in 2003, to include 12.9 million children. Poverty rates in 2003 among people aged 18 to 64 years and over 65 years of age were 10.8% and 10.2%, respectively (U.S. Census Bureau, 2004).

Blacks and Hispanics are more likely to be poor or near poor in every age category than Whites or Asian/Pacific Islanders (National Center for Health Statistics, 2003). Overall, in 2003, 24.4% of African Americans and 22.5% of Hispanics were poor compared to only 11.8% of Asians and 8.2% of non-Hispanic Whites. When the near poor are considered, approximately half of all African Americans and Hispanics in the U.S. population are included (NCHS, 2005).

Poverty contributes to a variety of disparities related to health among segments of the population. **Health disparities** are differences in measures of health status or access to health services associated with gender, race, ethnicity, education, income, disability, place of residence (e.g., urban or rural), or sexual orientation (USDHHS, 2000). Disparities occur with respect to morbidity and mortality as well as access to preventive health services. For example, in 2003, only 76% of children aged 19 to 35 months with family incomes below poverty level were fully immunized with the routine series of immunizations, compared to 83% of children in families at or above poverty level. Similar disparities between poor and nonpoor children were noted across racial and ethnic groups, but poor African American and Hispanic children were somewhat less likely to receive the complete immunization series than poor White children. Poor children were also less likely to have any kind of health care visit (84.7%) than nonpoor children (92.3%), and poor children were more than three times as likely as nonpoor children to lack a regular source of health care, or "medical home." Due to the lack of a regular source of care, poor children were more likely to receive care in an emergency department (ED). Twenty-seven percent of poor children had at least one ED visit compared to only 18.3% of nonpoor children, and poor children were more than twice as likely as their nonpoor counterparts to have two or more ED visits in 2003 (NCHS, 2005).

Similar figures are noted for adults. For example, in 2002–2003, 22.7% of poor adults under 65 years of age had no regular source of health care, compared to only 14% of the nonpoor. As was the case with children, poor adults make greater use of ED services than nonpoor adults. In 2003, 22.6% of poor adults had at least one ED visit, compared to only 5.4% of nonpoor adults (NCHS, 2005).

Disparities are even greater for dental care. In 2003, less than half of all poor people over 2 years of age had a dental visit in the past year, compared to 73.4% of the nonpoor. At all ages, nearly one fourth to one third of the poor experienced untreated dental caries, compared to 11% to 16% of the nonpoor in various age groups (NCHS, 2005).

The poor are also less likely than the nonpoor to receive health promotion and screening services. For example, in 2003, only 55.4% of poor women over 40 years of age had had a mammogram in the preceding 2 years, compared to 74.3% of nonpoor women. Similarly, only 70.5% of poor women over 18 years of age had received a Papanicolaou smear in the previous 3 years, whereas 83% of nonpoor women had been screened (NCHS, 2005).

Poverty is also associated with poorer health status. Among people over age 50, for instance, half of those with chronic conditions have incomes below 200% of poverty level (AARP, 2002). Poverty leads to malnutrition, poor housing, lack of health care, and lack of adequate childcare, all of which have negative health implications. In addition, poverty is associated with low literacy levels, which limit earning power and access to health care (Darling, 2004).

Individual poverty is not the only economic factor that has health-related effects. Research has indicated that income inequity within the population has been linked to increased incidence and prevalence of acute and chronic diseases, poor social cohesion, and violence (Drevdahl, Kneipp, Canales, & Dorcy, 2001). Overall neighborhood socioeconomic status has also been linked to poorer health status independent of personal income. For example, living in a low-socioeconomic-status neighborhood

BUILDING OUR KNOWLEDGE BASE

There is considerable research that indicates that economic factors have a direct effect on access to and use of health care services. There is also some research, however, suggesting that even when economic factors are equalized, some subpopulations have lower utilization rates for health care services and poorer health status. This is particularly true of ethnic cultural groups.

- How would you design a study to separate economic from noneconomic factors influencing use of health care services?
- What subpopulations might you want to study? Why? How would you recruit members of that population for participation in your study?
- How might you go about gathering information from your study participants? What information would you want to gather? What data collection methods might you use?

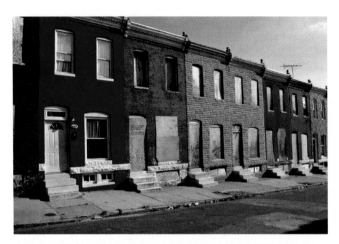

Research has shown that low-income neighborhoods affect the health of even those of moderate income who live in them. (© Rachel Epstein/The Image Works)

has been linked to a twofold risk of homicide victimization after adjusting for individual status (Cubbin, LeClere, & Smith, 2000). Similarly, living in a low-socioeconomic-status area has been associated with an increased risk of mortality from various causes (Winkleby & Cubbin, 2003).

LACK OF HEALTH INSURANCE Access to care is further impeded by lack of health care insurance. Lack of insurance coverage is so important that it has been identified as one of the national surveillance indicators for chronic disease risk (Centers for Disease Control and Prevention [CDC], 2004). The number of uninsured people in the United States increased from 41.2 million in 2001 to 45.8 million in 2004 (Families USA, 2005). When those who are uninsured for part of the year are considered, this figure rises even higher. For example, 82 million people were uninsured for at least 3 months in 2002. Of these, two thirds were uninsured for 6 months or more, and half for 9 months or longer (Stoll & Jones, 2004). Lack of health insurance is most common among younger adults; 23.5% of people aged 18 to 44 years were uninsured in 2003, compared to only 9.8% of children and 12.5% of those 45 to 64 years of age. Only 1.1% of U.S. elderly persons are not covered by some form of health insurance (NCHS, 2005).

There are a number of reasons for lack of health insurance in such a large portion of the population. Nearly two thirds of people under 65 years of age who have insurance receive it as an employment-based benefit. Those without insurance may be unemployed or work in jobs that do not provide insurance coverage. Others may lose coverage due to job loss; loss of eligibility for Medicaid or State Child Health Insurance Programs (SCHIP); or loss of coverage through a spouse due to death, separation, or divorce (Committee on Rapid Advance Demonstration Projects, 2003). Even those eligible for employment-based health insurance

may not be covered due to inability to pay the beneficiary portion of premiums or competing priorities for limited incomes (Diamant et al., 2004). In one report, for instance, 40% of uninsured persons reported that they would have to cut food, rent, and utilities in order to be able to afford health insurance (Stoll & Jones, 2004). In addition, people with chronic conditions who retire prior to age 65 may not be eligible for employer-provided retirement health benefits (AARP, 2002).

Lack of insurance disproportionately affects some segments of society. For example, even though steadily employed, minority group members are less likely to be employed in jobs that provide health insurance coverage. In 2003, approximately 35% of Native Americans and Hispanics were uninsured; 18% of African Americans and Asians lacked health insurance compared to only 12% of White Americans (NCHS, 2005).

Lack of health insurance is associated with a variety of health effects. For example, the uninsured are less likely than those with insurance to receive cancer screening and other preventive services, and they tend to receive less adequate care and have consistently worse outcomes for chronic diseases such as diabetes, cardiovascular disease, end-stage renal disease, HIV infection, and mental illness. They are also less likely to comply with medication regimens for hypertension and HIV due to costs, are at greater risk for hospital deaths, and display earlier cancer mortality due to late diagnosis (Institute of Medicine [IOM], 2002). These adverse health effects seem to be associated with both complete and intermittent lack of health insurance (Stoll & Jones, 2004; Sudano & Baker, 2003).

Having health insurance is associated with better health status, a regular source of care, and more appropriate use of health care services. In addition, people with insurance are more likely to receive health-promotive and illness-preventive services (IOM, 2002; Stoll & Jones, 2004). For example, in 2003, uninsured children were more than three times as likely as insured children not to have received at least one health visit during the past year, and uninsured children were nine times less likely to have a regular source of care. Insured children, particularly those with Medicaid coverage, were slightly more likely than uninsured children to have one or more ED visits. These figures suggest that even with government insurance, children may have difficulty obtaining the services of a regular health care provider, possibly due to the reluctance of some providers to accept Medicaid clients because of poor reimbursement rates. Uninsured adults were five times less likely than insured adults to have a regular source of care. With respect to preventive services, uninsured women were less likely than those with insurance to receive mammograms and Papanicolaou smears as well as other services (NCHS, 2005).

According to another Institute of Medicine report (IOM, 2003), lack of health insurance has implications

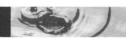

Members of ethnic cultural groups have been shown to have poorer health care outcomes than others in the U.S. population. In part, this is due to lack of access to care due to financial constraints. Even when members of these groups have health insurance, however, their health outcomes tend to be less favorable than among Caucasian members of the population with similar forms of health care coverage. What other factors might be contributing to these differential outcomes? Which of these factors arise out of ethnic cultures and which arise out of the dominant culture or the culture of the health care system?

for society as well as for the individuals involved. For example, lack of insurance leads to premature death and loss of social productivity. In addition, the uncompensated care related to high numbers of uninsured individuals in the population may lead to health system closure and loss of providers, resulting in decreased community health care capacity. Because health problems have been allowed to escalate due to the inability to afford care, the ultimate societal costs for treatment are much higher than they would be if treatment was initiated earlier. In fact, it is estimated that annual societal losses due to lack of insurance for the total U.S. population range from $55 billion to $130 billion and that the additional cost of insuring the entire population would be only $34 billion to $69 billion per year beyond the $99 billion already being spent (IOM, 2003).

FINANCING HEALTH CARE SERVICES

The second major way in which the economic context influences health care delivery is in the ways in which health care services are financed. In this section, we will look briefly at financing for public health services and then in more detail at payment for personal health care services in the United States.

Financing Public Health Services

Poor funding of public health services is another long-term trend that affects the health of the population. In 2003, for example, total health care expenditures in the United States amounted to more than $1.6 trillion, yet only $53.8 billion (3.2%) was spent for public health services (NCHS, 2004). This amount included personal health care services (e.g., well-child care and family planning services) provided by government health agencies as well as public health activities (NCHS, 2005).

Many public health agencies have relied on government funding sources for personal care services to subsidize other traditional health services as well as care for uninsured populations, with public health agencies serving as safety-net providers. As we will see later in this chapter, there is a growing emphasis on shifting

Medicaid and Medicare recipients into mainstream managed care organizations, which may significantly decrease the revenue on which many public agencies have come to depend. The loss of revenues as more Medicaid enrollees move to managed care plans may jeopardize the ability of public agencies to meet their public health obligations (Drevdahl, 2002). Curtailment of services by safety-net agencies will also result in the loss of services to clients who have no other source of health care and are not eligible for publicly funded insurance programs.

The public health infrastructure has received greater attention (and some funding) in response to the terrorist attacks of September 11, 2001. Concerns for potential bioterrorism have led to the creation of a Cabinet-level post related to Homeland Security with ties to many existing public health agencies. There has also been more attention to funding for bioterrorist response capabilities at the state and local levels (Sultz & Young, 2004). Some concerns have been expressed that the antiterrorism emphasis has decreased attention to and funding for routine public health endeavors.

In addition, public health funding has taken on something of the market approach displayed by the private economic sector, with services being tailored to funding availability rather than to the needs of the population. Conversely, private-sector managed care organizations (MCOs) have taken over many traditional public health functions, such as immunizations, child health, and Medicaid services. There are questions of the extent to which managed care is capable of addressing population-level needs, particularly in a for-profit setting (Drevdahl, 2002).

Financing Personal Health Services

In 2003, personal health care services accounted for $1.4 trillion in health expenditures in the United States, or nearly 86% of all health-related funding. Personal health services include hospitalization, professional services (physicians, dentists, and other health care providers), nursing home and home health care, and medical products, including prescription drugs (NCHS, 2005). The two major aspects of financing personal health services are financing approaches (general approaches to paying for health care services) and financing mechanisms (specific methods for reimbursing institutions and professionals that provide care). Figure 8-2 depicts the relative percentage of health care funding from different sources.

Approaches to Financing Health Care Services

Approaches to financing health care services are categorized based on the source of risk bearing for health care costs (Kongstvedt, 2002). The four approaches that we will review here are personal payment, government programs, commercial insurance, and self-funded insurance.

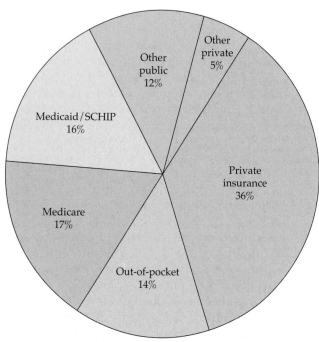

FIGURE 8-2 Sources of Health Care Funding, United States, 2003
Data from: Centers for Medicare and Medicaid Services. (2005).
The nation's heath dollar, Calendar year 2003, Where it came
from, Where it went. *Retrieved December 23, 2005, from*
http://www.cms.gov/nationalhealthexpenddata/downloads/
piechartSourcesExpenditures2003.pdf

PERSONAL PAYMENT Perhaps the easiest to understand
and least often used approach to financing health care is
personal payment. In a personal payment system, when
you see a provider for care, you pay him or her directly
out of your pocket. Personal payment tends to be used by
the very wealthy, by the uninsured (if they can afford any
payment at all), or for certain specific goods and services
that are not covered under an insurance plan. For example, if you do not have vision coverage in your health
insurance plan, you would personally pay for your eye
examination, new glasses, and so on. The entire risk for
the costs of health care rests on the recipient of care.

Personal payment for health care services and
products comprises part of the 14% of health care funds
derived from out-of-pocket funds depicted in Figure 8-2.
Insurance premiums, deductibles, and copayments are
the other components of out-of-pocket funding.
Premiums are the monthly amount paid by a recipient of
care for health insurance benefits. A **deductible** is the
amount of money that you must pay before the insurance plan begins to pay for any care. A **copayment** is a
fixed amount or percentage that the client pays for each
visit or service provided (Chang, Price, & Pfoutz, 2001).

Personal payment is also the funding approach used
in flat-rate medical clinics that are becoming more common in the United States. Flat-rate clinics charge clients a
fixed or flat rate for "emergent" care services for illness,
sometimes on an annual basis (e.g., $500 for all visits in a
year) or on a per-visit basis (e.g., a flat rate of $30 for each
visit). These clinics initially began as elite and expensive

sources of immediate care for the wealthy, charging as
much as $10,000 a year for personalized services with a
variety of "extras" (e.g., home prescription delivery). The
concept is being revamped, however, to provide more
accessible care to the general population. Many of the
recipients of care at flat-rate clinics have health insurance
coverage for hospitalization, but use the clinics to address
routine illness needs (Bluestein, 2005). In flat-rate clinics,
the risk for the cost of care is borne by the clinic.

GOVERNMENT PROGRAMS In government-funded health
programs, the risk for the costs of care is borne by the
government, and ultimately by taxpayers. In 2003, government funding sources contributed 43.8% of all personal health care expenditures in the United States. One
third of all personal health care was funded by the federal government and 10.5% by state governments
(NCHS, 2005). These funds primarily fall into the
Medicare and Medicaid/SCHIP sources of funding
depicted in Figure 8-2. The remainder of government
programs (e.g., Department of Veterans Affairs, state
and local public health spending, Department of
Defense, and so on) fall into the "other public" category
in the figure. In 2004, slightly more than 27% of the U.S.
population was covered by government health insurance programs (Families USA, 2005).

Federal, state, and local governments have a variety
of programs that finance health care. The two major federal government programs are Medicare and Medicaid.
Medicare is designed to provide care for the elderly and
certain individuals who are disabled. The Medicaid program is jointly financed by federal and state funds and
was developed to address the health care needs of the
poor. Other federal health care programs include the
Department of Veterans Affairs, military programs
including Department of Defense facilities and the
TRICARE program, the Federal Employee Health Benefits Program (FEHBP), the Indian Health Service, and the
National Health Service Corps (Pulcini, Neary, &
Mahoney, 2002). The Department of Veterans Affairs and
the Indian Health Service provide services for selected
population groups, military veterans and Native Americans, respectively. Both Department of Defense and TRI-
CARE programs provide services to active-duty members of the military, retirees, and their dependents.
Department of Defense facilities are managed and staffed
by the military. TRICARE, on the other hand, is a program by which members of the military, retirees, and
their dependents receive care in the civilian sector with
funding provided by the federal government. TRICARE
functions much like traditional commercial health insurance or managed care plans, both of which will be discussed later. A similar type of program, FEHBP, serves
employees of federal agencies outside of the military. In
this program, the federal government functions primarily
as an employer purchasing employment-based health
insurance for employees, just as in the private sector

(Kongstvedt, 2002). The National Health Service Corps is designed to provide health care services in underserved areas of the country. Like Medicaid, the State Child Health Insurance Program (SCHIP) is funded by the federal government but administered by the states. The SCHIP program was initiated to provide care for poor children who did not meet eligibility requirements for Medicaid. Medicare, Medicaid, and SCHIP are discussed in more detail below. Local jurisdictions, such as counties, often have programs that fund health services for indigent persons who are not eligible for Medicaid.

Medicare Medicare is part of the social insurance program arising from provisions of the Social Security Act. Under Medicare, people over 65 years of age who are eligible for Social Security benefits receive partial coverage of health services. Certain other individuals, such as the disabled, are eligible for Medicare coverage before age 65 (Jonas, 2003). In 2004, Medicare enrolled 4.7 million people. Federal expenditures for Medicare in 2004 amounted to $308.9 billion and are expected to more than double to $746.8 billion by 2014 (CMS, 2005d).

At its inception in 1965, Medicare was intended to protect the elderly against expensive hospitalizations. The optional Medicare Part B was added to cover physician expenses. Medicare Part C, or Medicare + Choice, was instituted in 1997 to provide beneficiaries with a choice of options among traditional fee-for-service practices and managed care plans (Sultz & Young, 2004). Medicare + Choice has since been replaced by the Medicare Advantage Plans and other Medicare Health Plans that provide a managed care option for Medicare enrollees. Medicare Part D, Medicare Prescription Drug Coverage, was initiated under the Medicare Prescription Drug, Improvement, and Modernization Act of 2003 and was fully implemented in 2006. In the interim, prescription drug coverage was provided under a temporary program that enabled Medicare beneficiaries to purchase drug discount cards at an average cost of $30 per month. These cards provided a 10% to 25% discount on specified brand-name drugs (Mahan, 2004). Each of the components of Medicare will be discussed briefly. Elements of each component are summarized in Table 8-1◆.

TABLE 8-1 Components of Medicare

Medicare Component	Services	Premiums (2006)	Deductible (2006)	Copayment
Part A	▪ Hospitalization ▪ Skilled nursing facility ▪ Home health ▪ Hospice ▪ Blood (given in an inpatient setting)	▪ None for 99% of Medicare beneficiaries ▪ $216/month for people with 30–39 quarters of covered employment ▪ $393/month for others	$952/benefit period	Hospitalization ▪ None for first 60 days ▪ $238/day for days 61–90 ▪ $476/day for days 91–150 ▪ All costs after 150 days SNF ▪ None for first 20 days ▪ $119/day for days 21–100 Blood ▪ Cost of replacing first 3 pints
Part B	▪ Physician services ▪ Outpatient services ▪ Some home health care ▪ Durable medical equipment ▪ Screening/preventive services	$88.50/month	$124/year	▪ 20% of cost for most approved services ▪ 50% of outpatient mental health services ▪ Cost of replacing first 3 pints of blood provided in outpatient setting, then 20% ▪ None for home health or clinical laboratory services
Medicare Advantage Plans	▪ Replaces Medicare A & B for enrollees ▪ May include additional services	Based on plan	Based on plan	Based on plan
Medicare Part D	Prescription drug services	Based on plan (expected average $32/month)	$250/year	▪ 25% of drug costs from $250 to $2,250 ▪ 100% of costs up to $5,100 ▪ 5% or a small copayment for the rest of the year

Data from: Centers for Medicare and Medicaid Services. (2005). Medicare & you, 2006. Retrieved December 21, 2005, from http://www.medicare.gov/publications/pubs/pdf/10050.pdf; Centers for Medicare and Medicaid Services. (2005). Medicare premiums and coinsurance rates for 2006. Retrieved December 21, 2005, from http://questions.medicare.gov/cgi-bin/medicare.cfg/php/enduser/std_alp.php?p_sid=vrTlxDXh; and Centers for Medicare and Medicaid Services. (2005). Medicare premiums and deductibles for 2006. Retrieved December 23, 2005, from http://new.cms.hhs.gov/apps/media/press/release.asp?Counter=1557

Medicare Part A covers medically necessary hospitalization, care in a skilled nursing facility (SNF), some home health care, hospice services, and blood administered in an inpatient setting. Part A coverage is available to all participants in the Social Security program and is provided without additional premiums to those who have 40 or more quarters of Medicare-covered employment or whose spouse meets this criterion (CMS, 2005b). Funding for Medicare Part A is derived from nonvoluntary Social Security payroll taxes on one's income with a matching payment from the employer. People who do not meet the employment criterion may enroll in Medicare Part A with payment of a monthly premium. The maximum premium for 2006 was $393 per month, but was somewhat less ($216 per month) for people with 30 to 39 quarters of covered employment (CMS, 2005b). Only 1% of U.S. elderly persons pay a premium for Part A coverage.

Part A benefits begin after the beneficiary has incurred otherwise covered expenses of $952 (the 2006 deductible amount). Benefits are paid within a *benefit period*. A benefit period begins with admission to a hospital or SNF and ends when no further hospital or SNF care has been received for 60 consecutive days. One may have several benefit periods within a given year and must pay the deductible for each benefit period. Within each benefit period, Medicare pays all covered costs for the first 60 days. For hospitalizations longer than 60 days, the beneficiary pays a copayment for each additional day ($238 a day for days 61 to 90 and $476 a day for days 91 to 150 for 2006). Medicare does not pay anything for additional days of hospitalization beyond 150 days. There is no copayment for the first 20 days of SNF care, but a copayment ($119 a day in 2006) is required for each day thereafter (CMS, 2005b). A copayment to replace the first three pints of blood administered in an inpatient setting is also required unless replacement blood is donated in the client's name (CMS, 2005a). Information on current Medicare premiums and copayments is available from the CMS Web site at http://www.cms.hhs.gov.

Medicare Part B covers medically necessary provider services, outpatient care, some home health care, and other services that are not covered under Part A (CMS, 2005a) (a full listing of services covered under Medicare Parts A and B is available on the CMS Web site). Part B also covers a variety of preventive services including colorectal, breast, cervical, and prostate cancer screening; osteoporosis screening; immunizations; and so on.

Part B coverage is optional and entails payment of an additional premium similar to that paid for private health insurance, but much less costly. By law, the Medicare Part B premium must be sufficient to cover 25% of the program's costs, so the premium increases each year as health care costs increase. For 2006, the monthly premium was $88.50 (CMS, 2005c). Part B

premiums may be slightly higher for Medicare beneficiaries who did not enroll in Part B when they first became eligible (10% per year not covered) (CMS, 2005a). Beneficiaries with incomes less than 135% of the federal poverty level may receive assistance with their Part B premiums, and about one fourth of Medicare enrollees receive some such assistance (CMS, 2005c). For some Medicare enrollees, the Medicaid program pays their Medicare Part B premiums.

Like Part A, there is a deductible amount that must be paid before Part B coverage begins ($124 in 2006), but unlike Part A, the Part B deductible is paid only once a year. In addition to the monthly premiums and annual deductible, beneficiaries pay a 20% copayment for Medicare-approved services or supplies. Higher copayments are required for some specific services such as outpatient mental health services (50%) or blood administered in an outpatient setting (cost of replacing the first three pints). No copayment is required for Medicare-approved home health or clinical laboratory services.

If health service providers accept Medicare assignment, beneficiaries do not have any additional costs for Medicare-approved services. **Assignment** is an agreement whereby the Medicare beneficiary agrees to allow the service provider to bill Medicare directly for services or goods (e.g., a walker or ventilator) provided. In return, the provider agrees to accept the Medicare reimbursement amount as full payment. If providers do not accept assignment, the most that the beneficiary can be charged for a Medicare-approved service or product is 15% above the Medicare-approved amount for that service or product. This is called the **limiting charge**.

As noted earlier, Medicare Part C, or Medicare + Choice, was intended to permit Medicare enrollees to exercise the same options with respect to their health care as others in the U.S. population. Specifically, the program allowed beneficiaries to apply their Medicare funding to enrollment in a Medicare-approved managed care plan. Medicare + Choice was replaced by the Medicare Advantage Plans that accomplish the same purpose. These plans again allow choices among health care plans and include Medicare health maintenance organizations (HMOs), Medicare preferred provider organizations (PPOs), Medicare special needs plans, and Medicare private fee-for-service plans. Medicare HMOs and PPOs are similar to those discussed in the section on employment-based group health plans. Medicare special needs plans provide coverage to select groups of people, such as nursing home residents, those who are eligible for both Medicare and Medicaid, and those with certain chronic or disabling conditions. Medicare private fee-for-service plans allow recipients to choose any provider that accepts the plan, and the plan determines what the recipients' share of the cost will be. Some Medicare Advantage Plans also include prescription drug coverage and services not included under the Original Medicare Plan (Parts A & B) (CMS, 2005a).

In 2006, the major provisions of the Medicare Prescription Drug, Improvement, and Modernization Act of 2003 were implemented as Medicare Part D, Medicare Prescription Drug Plans. This drug subsidization program requires beneficiaries to enroll in one of many Medicare Prescription Plans offered by private insurance companies. Although described as a "voluntary" plan, Medicare beneficiaries who chose not to enroll in a prescription plan will be required to pay increased premiums of 1% for every month that they delay coverage, if they decide to enroll at a later time. Plans vary in terms of costs, drugs covered, and pharmacies participating (CMS, 2005a). Premiums were expected to average $32 per month in 2006. Medicare beneficiaries with incomes below 135% of poverty level can get assistance with Part D premiums, and those between 135% and 150% of poverty level can receive partial assistance (CMS, 2005c).

Plan beneficiaries pay the first $250 of annual drug costs (the deductible amount). After the deductible is paid, the beneficiary pays a copayment (typically 25% of the cost) for each prescription for the next $2,000 in annual drug costs. Once total drug costs have reached $2,250, the beneficiary pays 100% of all drug costs until total drug expenditures for the year reach $5,100, at which point the beneficiary resumes paying a small copayment (about 5% of drug costs) (CMS, 2005a). Drug costs between $2,250 and $5,100 are referred to as the "doughnut hole," or gap in prescription drug care coverage, under Medicare. It is anticipated that deductibles, premiums, and the gap in coverage will increase, with a projected coverage gap of more than $5,000 in 2013 (from the initial gap of $2,850). Some experts predict that the program will not significantly alleviate seniors' difficulty in affording medications due to the yearly increase in drug costs and the increasing gap in coverage (Mahan, 2004).

Although the Medicare program has provided significant assistance to the elderly population with respect to hospitalization and, to a lesser extent, provider services, it does not provide adequate coverage in a number of areas. For example, mental health services are only partially covered, and long-term custodial health care is not addressed at all by the program; as we saw earlier, prescription drug coverage will be inadequate even with Medicare Part D (AARP, 2002).

Medicare has begun to provide for some preventive services such as influenza and pneumonia immunization and mammography, but these are generally considered insufficient to meet the health promotion needs of the elderly population (Pulcini, Neary, & Mahoney, 2002). For instance, Medicare covers only half of the preventive services recommended for the elderly, yet covers other services without scientific evidence for their value (Partnership for Prevention, 2003). Due to limited coverage for prescription medication and other services, many Medicare beneficiaries also carry supplemental insurance

policies to cover what Medicare does not (Kongstvedt, 2002). These supplemental policies are often referred to as *Medigap policies* because they cover gaps in services not provided under Medicare (CMS, 2005a). Although some research indicates that seniors with supplemental insurance achieve better health outcomes in some areas (Fang & Alderman, 2004), the cost of such "wraparound" policies is becoming prohibitive for many seniors who live on fixed incomes.

Medicaid   The Medicaid program was established in 1965 to provide health care services to a large segment of the population who could not otherwise afford care. Its original purpose was to integrate the indigent into mainstream health care services. In 2003, Medicaid covered services for approximately 30.9 million people, including low-income families, low-income seniors who need assistance with Part B Medicare premiums and prescription drug coverage, many nonelderly adults with disabilities, and low-income women who were pregnant. Medicaid expenditures in 2003 were $160.9 billion (NCHS, 2005). Despite the number of people enrolled, Medicaid only covers 40% of children in low-income families, 70% of poor children with disabilities, and 41% of the working-age poor with disabilities (Klein et al., 2004).

Medicaid is a means-tested program, which means that eligibility for services is based on one's income (Jonas, 2003). Under the program, the federal government provides block grants to the states that are combined with matching funds from the states. The Medicaid program is administered by the states, but state programs must provide a minimum set of federally defined benefits. Beyond that, states are free to determine the level of service provided as well as eligibility requirements for the program, and both benefits and requirements differ drastically from state to state. Due to rising costs in recent years, many states have engaged in cost-control mechanisms in their Medicaid programs, including reducing program eligibility, freezing or actually reducing provider reimbursements (which may lead providers to refuse to see Medicaid clients), reducing benefits, and increasing prescription drug copayments for beneficiaries (Kaiser Family Foundation, 2003).

The Medicaid program funds health care services for three categories of people: the categorically needy, the medically needy, and certain special groups such as low-income persons eligible for Medicare, working individuals with disabilities, women with breast cancer, and people with tuberculosis (TB). For the latter group, Medicaid pays only for TB treatment, not for other health-related services. In 2005, all but one state provided services for women with breast cancer, but only nine states, the District of Columbia, and Puerto Rico included people with TB.

The categorically needy are people who are considered needy because of their membership in certain

MediaLink   Case Study: Medicare Plan D

groups or categories. The categorically needy include the following:

- Pregnant women and children under 6 years of age with incomes at or below 133% of the federal poverty level
- Children 6 to 19 years of age with family incomes below poverty level and their caretakers
- Families who meet the prior eligibility requirements for AFDC
- Recipients of Supplemental Security Income (SSI), an income subsidization program for low-income Social Security recipients
- Individuals or couples living in medical institutions with incomes below 300% of the SSI income standard. (Center for Medicaid and State Operations, 2005)

The medically needy are people who do not fit in the categorically needy category but cannot afford health insurance coverage on their own. Not all states have medically needy programs as part of their Medicaid program, but those that do must cover low-income pregnant women and children, and certain blind persons. States may also choose to include other groups of people as medically needy. In 2005, 34 states and the District of Columbia had medically needy programs (Center for Medicaid and State Operations, 2005). Information on specific populations and services covered under Medicaid programs in individual states is available from the CMS Web site.

In the past, Medicaid covered most prescription drug costs for enrollees. Now prescription drug costs for "dual eligibles," persons eligible for both Medicare and Medicaid, will be covered under a Medicare Prescription Drug Plan (CMS, 2005a). Medicaid will cover the costs of Medicare Prescription Drug Plan premiums, but it is anticipated that the change will increase copayments for prescription drugs from those previously paid under the Medicaid program.

Because both Medicare and Medicaid are programs that arise out of federal legislation, they are often confusing. Table 8-2◆ provides characteristic features that may help differentiate the two programs.

State Children's Health Insurance Program
The State Children's Health Insurance Program (SCHIP) was authorized by Congress in 1997 to address the health insurance needs of low-income children who do not meet the income eligibility requirements for Medicaid (Center for Medicaid and State Operations, 2005). By 1999, all 50 states had received approval for their SCHIP programs (Ullman & Hill, 2001). The enacting legislation gave states the option of either expanding existing Medicaid programs or creating separate SCHIP programs to include the 10 million uninsured children who were eligible for Medicaid but unenrolled, or with family incomes too high for Medicaid eligibility but too low to afford commercial insurance coverage. Most SCHIP

TABLE 8-2	Differentiating Features of Medicare and Medicaid	
Feature	Medicare	Medicaid
Funding source	Social Security contributions	General tax revenues (federal and state)
Program administration	Federal	State
Beneficiaries	Elderly and disabled persons	Medically indigent
Benefits	Standardized for each component Hospitalization, primary care (under Part B only), prescription drugs, selected preventive services, no dental services	Vary from state to state Primary care, preventive services, prescription drug coverage, hospitalization, may include dental services

programs provide services to children in families with incomes at or below 200% of the federal poverty level (Center for Medicaid and State Operations, 2005). The SCHIP program gave the states extraordinary latitude in determining how to deal with the problem of uninsured children and is an example of a phenomenon called **devolution**, or the transfer of responsibility for an area from federal to state governments (Brandon, Chaudry, & Sardell, 2001).

In 1999, 2 million children were enrolled under a SCHIP. By 2002, this number had increased to 5.3 million (Sultz & Young, 2004). In addition to covering previously uninsured children, SCHIP appears to have been effective in reducing health care needs among children enrolled. For example, in its first year the Kansas CHIP decreased the unmet health needs of enrolled children from 51% to 16.5% and increased the number of children with a regular source of health care from 92% to 95.6% (Fox, Moore, Davis, & Heintzelman, 2003).

COMMERCIAL INSURANCE Commercial or private insurance provides coverage of the costs of health care by an insurance company based on payment of premiums designed to cover costs. This source of funding is represented by the private insurance segment of the pie chart in Figure 8-2. In this approach to health care financing, the risk of health care costs is borne by the insurance company. Commercial insurance companies are unregulated by the federal government except for regulations under the Health Insurance Portability and Accountability Act (HIPAA), which permits continuation of group health coverage on termination of employment and prohibits denial of insurance under certain conditions (Wimberley & Rubens, 2002). Commercial insurance is, however, regulated by complex state regulations, usually including laws that mandate certain types of coverage (Kongstvedt, 2002). In 2003, 68.9% of the American public was covered by some form of commercial health insurance (NCHS, 2005).

Commercial insurance is of three general types: individual health insurance, wraparound or supplemental plans, and group health plans. Wraparound plans were discussed in the context of Medicare supplementation, but may also be used to supplement coverage of other types of insurance. The wraparound policy covers services that are not covered under other forms of insurance (Kongstvedt, 2002).

Individual Insurance   Individual health insurance is purchased by an individual directly from an insurance company. It tends to be expensive because the individual does not have the bargaining power of a large entity such as a corporation that can guarantee the insurance company a number of subscribers. In fact, individual insurance may cost twice as much as employer-sponsored group plans (Bauman, 2002). Individual policies also tend to have limited coverage, again because of the expense. Some people may not be eligible for such policies because of existing health conditions that make them a poor economic risk for the insurance company. Under the Consolidated Omnibus Reconciliation Act (COBRA), individuals who have been insured under an employment-based group plan may continue individual coverage at the group premium rate for 18 months after termination of employment (Wimberley & Rubens, 2002). This legal provision is available whether or not there is a preexisting medical condition, but the individual is responsible for the entire cost of the premium, which makes it unaffordable for many people following a job loss (Kongstvedt, 2002).

Employment-Based Group Health Plans   By far the greatest number of people with commercial insurance obtain it by way of employment. Because of the number of people they insure, employers are able to obtain insurance for whole groups of employees at discounted rates not available to individual purchasers. Employment-based insurance is popular because it is purchased with pretax dollars. Employee health benefits are a pretax deduction for the employer and are not considered taxable income for employees (Bauman, 2002), although this may change with proposed changes in income tax regulations. In 2003,

Think Advocacy

National studies have found that immigrants, both legal and undocumented, have lower rates of insurance coverage than native-born Americans and that immigrants who are noncitizens are less likely to have health insurance than those who are citizens (Prentice, Pebley, & Sastry, 2005). Yet immigrants, particularly those who are refugees, may have significant health care needs that go unmet because of their lack of health insurance. What programs exist in your local area to address these needs? How adequate are these programs? How might community health nurses engage in initiatives to better address the health needs of these groups?

63.3% of the total U.S. population received employment-based insurance, down slightly from 65% the previous year (NCHS, 2005). By 2004, this figure had decreased to 59.8% (Families USA, 2005).

As we saw earlier, however, significant segments of the population are not eligible for employment-based health insurance. In 2003, only 19.9% of people with incomes below poverty level had employment-based health insurance (NCHS, 2005). That same year, only half of firms with fewer than 10 employees offered health insurance benefits (Alliance for Health Reform, 2003). In addition, the cost of group health plan premiums, while not as expensive as individual insurance coverage, has continued to escalate. In 2005, health insurance benefits constituted more than 10% of employees' total compensation, compared to slightly less than 7% in 1991 (NCHS, 2005).

Employers are faced with one of several unpalatable options due to rising premium costs: (a) pay the increased premiums, thereby reducing their profit margins, (b) reduce the level of benefits covered, (c) pass a larger share of health insurance costs on to employees (e.g., a greater percentage of premiums), or (d) discontinue coverage altogether (Nolin & Killackey, 2005). These decisions have led to a proliferation of types of employment-based coverage in an effort to reduce costs to employers.

There are several approaches to employment-based group health insurance: defined benefits plans, defined contribution plans, fixed contribution plans, and consumer-driven plans. In defined benefits plans, employers select a predetermined set of benefits that are covered by the plan. Differing sets of benefits may be available under different plans or from different companies. For example, benefits may or may not cover reproductive services such as contraception. Similarly, dental insurance plans may or may not cover any amount for orthodontics. Employees of large companies may have a choice among several different defined benefits plans. In a defined contribution plan, the employer provides a set amount of money to each employee, which the employee can use to purchase whatever type of insurance plan is desired. Defined contribution plans have more advantages for employers than employees. Employers' health insurance costs remain constant, but employees may find that the amount provided does not go far to cover the costs of a desirable health insurance plan. In a fixed contribution plan, the employer chooses a specific benefits package and provides a fixed amount toward the premiums for that package, with the expectation that the employee will pay the difference in the cost of the plan (Kongstvedt, 2002).

A fourth approach is a consumer-driven plan, in which the employer usually provides a defined catastrophic coverage for serious illness or injury as well as a flexible health care spending account. The employee can then use the amount in the health spending account to pay directly for any other health care expenses incurred. Health spending accounts are similar to the health savings accounts allowed by the Internal Revenue Service. A health savings account is money contributed by the employee through payroll deduction prior to taxes that is available for certain health care expenses not covered by insurance plans. The health spending account included in a consumer-driven health plan differs in that the contribution is made by the employer rather than the employee. In many such plans, monies left in a health spending account can be carried over in subsequent years; in others, whatever money is not spent in a given year is forfeited (Nolin & Killackey, 2005).

Consumer-driven plans have the advantage of covering catastrophic events, the most expensive area of health care, with flexibility for addressing other health care needs. They have the disadvantage of controlling only the small portion of health care expenditures outside of catastrophic coverage. In addition, there is concern that ill-informed consumers may make poor health choices that later lead to the need for more costly services. Attempts to prevent this from occurring include the incorporation of online access to health-related information and nurse counseling and coaching. There is also the possibility that if many people who receive employment-based health care coverage opt for consumer-driven plans, it will reduce the number of people with traditional commercial insurance, driving prices beyond the capacity of many to afford. In the words of one health economic observer, such a migration would "destroy the social contract on which health insurance depends: the willingness of those who do not need much health care to pay for those who do" (Taylor, cited in Nolin & Killackey, 2005, p. 252).

The options available to most employees whose employers provide health insurance benefits include some form of managed care plan. Managed care has no single definition but refers to a set of principles that govern provider/payer/recipient relationships (Sultz & Young, 2004). In managed care, the payer and provider functions of health care are combined in the same organization. This is in contrast to more traditional indemnity insurance, in which the insurance company pays for care but does not actually provide the care given. **Managed care organizations (MCOs)** are "delivery systems or health-care entities that are willing to be clinically and financially accountable for the health outcomes of a group of individuals for predetermined capitation payments" (Chang et al., 2001, p. 302). They are characterized by integration of funding and delivery systems and a comprehensive array of services. In 2003, 34% of the U.S. population under 65 years of age and 10% of the elderly population were enrolled in managed care plans (NCHS, 2005). For most of the elderly, MCO coverage was provided under one of the Medicare Advantage Plans.

Despite a wide and growing variety, managed care plans usually have two elements in common. First, they generally require some form of authorization for services, particularly specialty services, and second, they usually include some restriction on choice of providers (Kongstvedt, 2002). The types and forms of MCOs create a veritable alphabet soup and include open- and closed-panel health maintenance organizations (HMOs), preferred provider organizations (PPOs), point of service (POS) plans, and others. Managed care organizations are usually characterized by a specific enrolled population, a designated set of covered services (usually including a variety of health-promotive and illness-preventive services), and a fixed subscription or enrollment premium that covers all designated services. Table 8-3◆ summarizes key features of some of the more common forms of MCOs. Figure 8-3 depicts the general funding approach of employment-based health insurance with MCO enrollment.

SELF-FUNDED INSURANCE Some of the approaches used by employers to minimize the costs of commercial insurance benefits for employees and their families,

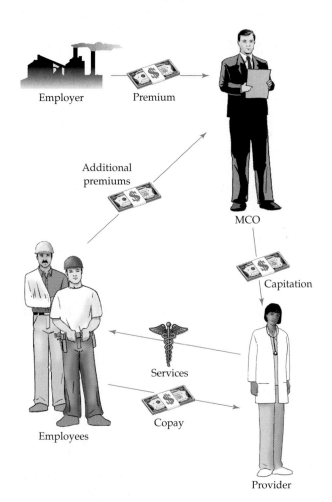

FIGURE 8-3 Health Care Funding Through Employment-Based Managed Care Plan Enrollment

TABLE 8-3 Key Features of Common Forms of Managed Care Organizations

Type of MCO	Key Features
All MCOs	Provide comprehensive health care to an enrolled group for a specified fee (premium). Emphasize health promotion and illness prevention as means of minimizing costs. Attempt to minimize costs by providing care in the least expensive environment with the least expensive provider.
Health maintenance organization (HMO)	Depends on subtype (see below). Members are generally restricted to services from providers within the plan. Services provided outside the plan are not covered and the member is liable for the full cost of outside services. Primary care providers (PCPs) function as "gatekeepers" preventing members from seeking specialty care without authorization.
Open-panel HMO	HMO contracts with groups of providers who may see clients from other MCOs as well as fee-for-service clients. ■ Direct contract — HMO contracts directly with independent physicians for service for its members ■ Individual Practice Association (IPA)— HMO contracts with groups of physicians
Closed-panel HMO	Providers see only members of the particular HMO, usually in facilities provided by the HMO. ■ Group model — HMO contracts with a group of providers and hospitals separately to provide services exclusively for HMO members (also known as an exclusive provider organization, EPO) ■ Staff model — HMO employs providers on a salaried basis
Network model HMO	HMO contracts with several large multispecialty groups of providers that operate independently of each other.
Mixed model HMO	Same HMO incorporates two or more of the above types of arrangements. So a given HMO might have separate closed-panel and open-panel segments that usually operate independently of each other.
Individual Practice Association (IPA)	Group of independent providers (usually physicians) forms an association to contract with managed care organizations to provide services to MCO enrollees.
Preferred provider organizations (PPOs)	MCO includes a group of independent "preferred providers" (hospitals, physicians, and other providers) that provide services at a discounted rate to MCO members. If members choose to obtain services outside the plan, they are covered at a reduced rate, and the member must pay the difference (usually 20% of costs).
Point of service (POS) plans	Plan members choose a participating PCP who serves as a gatekeeper for specialty care. Specialty care requires a referral, but the member may choose to see a specialist outside the plan and pay a higher deductible, copayment, or both. Differentials may be as high as 20% to 40% of the cost of services.
Integrated delivery systems (IDSs)	Coordinated network of health care organizations that provide a continuum of services to a defined population. Characterized by a defined population, a defined set of services, clinical and administrative integration of services and information systems, a capitated payment system, and pooled revenues from several sources. Emphasizes centralized planning and management and a shared mission and vision. Includes hospital beds and at least one long-term-care service. May include contracts with several HMOs for the provision of services.
Other weird arrangements (OWAs)	Because of the proliferation and combination of features of many different models of MCOs, there are other types of plans that defy description. These models are collectively referred to as OWAs.

Data from: Chang, C. F., Price, S. A., & Pfoutz, S. K. (2001). The impact of managed care. In C. F. Chang, S. A. Price, & S. K. Pfoutz (Eds.), Economics and nursing: Critical professional issues (pp. 297–334). Philadelphia: F. A. Davis; Jonas, S. (2003). An introduction to the U. S. health care system (5th ed.). New York: Springer; and Kongstvedt, P. R. (2002). Managed care: What it is and how it works. Gaithersburg, MD: Aspen.

such as increasing copayments and decreasing benefits, were discussed earlier. Self-funded insurance and self-insurance are more radical approaches taken by some large employers and unions. In a self-funded insurance plan, a large employer collects pooled premiums from its employees and pays for the costs of care provided to employees and their dependents. Self-insured programs are similar, but the employing organization hires a third party (often a commercial insurance company) to administer the program and process claims (Sultz & Young, 2004). Self-funded insurance is one component of the "other private" source of health care funding depicted in Figure 8-2.

Self-funded plans have a number of advantages for employers allowed under the Employee Retirement Income Security Act (ERISA). They avoid the third party that increases premium costs. In addition,

costs are based on the level of pooled risk of the company's employees, not all participants in an insurance program. The employer or union also collects interest on the pooled premiums until they are used to fund health care services. Self-funding avoids the premium tax collected by state governments as a percentage of commercial insurance premiums, and self-funded programs are exempt from state insurance regulations. Although they are regulated by the U.S. Department of Labor, they do not have to meet the minimum benefits requirements of commercial plans (Kongstvedt, 2002).

In self-funded plans, the risk for excessive health care costs is borne by the employer or union. However, these organizations often get around this disadvantage by purchasing corporate insurance protecting them against catastrophic losses (Kongstvedt, 2002).

CHARITY CARE The other component of the "other private" source of health care funding depicted in Figure 8-2 is charity care or philanthropy. **Charity care** is defined as care that is provided free of charge to individuals who meet established financial criteria and that was never expected to generate revenue. There is no reliable estimate of the amount of charity care provided in the United States, because the costs for charity care are accounted for in different ways in health care organizations' accounting systems. A 1995 survey of U.S. hospitals, however, indicated that approximately 5% of net operating income is expended in charity care (Pricewaterhousecooper's Health Research Institute, 2005).

Charity care may be provided by individual health care organizations or funded by a wide variety of voluntary organizations and philanthropic foundations, as we saw in Chapter 5∞. For example, the Gates Foundation has funded a massive international immunization campaign. Other organizations and foundations fund similar health care programs as well as providing services or funding services for individual needy clients and families. The National Center for Charitable Statistics (2005) included 30,009 tax-exempt public charities with a health focus in 2004. In addition, 102,881 private foundations, many of which have health-related interests, hold tax exemptions. According to the Center's 2005 statistics, health-related public charities received $703.6 billion in donations. The Center's National Taxonomy of Exempt Entities classification system includes 21 category codes for tax-exempt nonprofit organizations related to health care. These include hospitals, research institutes, community health systems, adult day care centers, and other health-related entities.

A number of organizations provide tips on selecting reputable charities to which one might wish to give donations. These include the Better Business Bureau (BBB) Wise Giving Alliance (2003) (http://www.give.org/tips/giving.asp), the Federal Trade Commission

(FTC) (2003) (http://www.ftc.bcp/conline/pubs/tmarkg/charity.htm), and the Metropolitan Life Insurance Company (2003-05) (http://www.metlife.com/Applications/Corporate/WPS/CDA/PageGenerator/0,,P1971~AP,00.html). In addition, the BBB Wise Giving Alliance has promulgated standards for charity accountability against which a potential donor can judge a charity's worthiness. The Alliance also publishes reports about major charity organizations that are available to the general public at the Web site listed above.

Reimbursement Mechanisms

In addition to the general approaches to financing health care services, there are several approaches to reimbursing providers for health care services provided to specific clients. The two general categories of financing or reimbursement mechanisms are out-of-pocket payments and third-party payments.

OUT-OF-POCKET PAYMENTS Out-of-pocket payments are the monies that health care recipients pay "out of their own pockets" for services received. Out-of-pocket payments occur in several forms. One form is the direct payment for services discussed earlier. When you purchase health care services that are not covered by your health insurance plan (e.g., vision care), you may write checks for the eye examination, prescription lenses, and so on. The portion of your health insurance premiums that you pay is another form of out-of-pocket payment. Premiums for wraparound insurance for Medicare beneficiaries are another example. As much as 26% of out-of-pocket spending by Medicare enrollees over age 65 goes for supplemental insurance (AARP, 2002).

Commercial insurance plans and some government plans frequently include other forms of out-of-pocket payments referred to as "cost sharing." Through these payments, you "share" the costs of the services with the insurer. There may be two kinds of cost sharing required—deductibles and copayments. The amount of the deductible may be several hundred dollars and must usually be paid each year before insurance benefits begin. Deductibles are a fixed amount for a given time period. Once they have been satisfied, no further deductible amount is due until the beginning of a new time period.

Copayments may be a fixed amount per service or a percentage of the cost of services (Chang et al., 2001). Until recently, copayments have been relatively small, at $5 to $10 per office visit or prescription. More recently, however, copayments have escalated in an effort by insurers to shift some of the rising cost of health care, particularly prescription drugs, to consumers. In 2003, out-of-pocket spending accounted for nearly 14% of all personal health care expenditures. During the previous year, out-of-pocket expenses accounted for nearly 28% of nursing home spending and nearly 30% of prescription drug costs.

EVIDENCE-BASED PRACTICE

The discussion in this chapter shows that economic forces, health care delivery, and health status are inextricably interwoven. Avenues for redesigning that relationship might include development of a national health insurance program similar to that in several other nations (e.g., Britain). Such redesign, however, should be based on scientific evidence. If you were going to look at the overall costs and benefits of such an initiative, what categories of costs would you examine? Try to think of all the potential costs that might be involved (e.g., loss of jobs in the health insurance industry). What categories of benefits might you address? Again, think broadly in terms of the benefits that might accrue from such a program. After you have listed all of the potential costs and benefits that might occur, look for studies in the literature that address them. What overall conclusions, if any, can you draw from this literature? What categories of factors remain unexplored? How might you study those factors?

(The latter figure is expected to decline to roughly 20% of prescription drug costs by 2014, primarily due to the implementation of Medicare Part D.) On average, overall out-of-pocket expenditures in 2003 were $778 per person in the United States. These per capita costs are expected to nearly double to $1,327 by 2014, and per capita drug costs are expected to increase by 176% in the same period in spite of the decreased percentage of out-of-pocket costs represented by prescription drugs (CMS, 2005d).

THIRD-PARTY REIMBURSEMENT Third-party payment mechanisms were designed to protect the average citizen from the financial devastation of serious illness and to supplement client payment. In a third-party reimbursement system, payment for health care services is made by someone or some agency other than the individual receiving service, usually some form of public or private insurance. Third-party reimbursement may be either retrospective or prospective. **Retrospective reimbursement** is payment for services rendered based on the cost of those services; cost is determined after the fact. Forms of retrospective reimbursement include fee-for-service payment, discounted fee-for-service payment, and per diem payments. In a fee-for-service system, providers are paid for each service rendered after that service has been provided (Chang et al., 2001). Fee-for-service payment is based on the unit of service as a single visit to a provider or a single procedure. Discounted fee-for-service mechanisms are used in PPOs and other similar forms of managed care as discussed earlier.

Per diem payment is a similar arrangement in which an inpatient facility is paid retrospectively, at a flat rate per day, for the number of days a client was hospitalized (Ling, 2000). Per diem reimbursement is usually used for institutional providers such as hospitals, skilled nursing facilities, and long-term-care facilities.

Retrospective reimbursement has the disadvantage of encouraging health care providers to give services that may not be necessary, merely because they are reimbursable. A provider who can be reimbursed for each office visit may be tempted to see a client three times when two visits would suffice. Or tests and treatments may be given that are not strictly necessary. For example, a surgeon might suggest a hysterectomy to a woman when other, less expensive measures would be equally effective.

In 1983, prompted by rising costs, the federal government instituted prospective reimbursement for services provided under Medicare. **Prospective reimbursement** is payment at a predetermined, fixed rate for a specific health care program or set of services (Chang et al., 2001). Forms of prospective payment include diagnosis-related groups (DRGs), the Resource-Based Relative Value Scale (RBRVS), and capitation. Both the DRG and RBRVS systems are based on payment for each episode of illness.

Prospective payment for services provided under the Medicare program is based on clients' diagnoses, with set fees for care of clients who fall into specific diagnosis-related groups. DRGs are categories of client diagnoses for which typical costs of care have been calculated, based on the cost of specific services required. In the DRG system, providers are paid a set fee based on clients' diagnoses and the typical costs of care for someone with that diagnosis.

A similar prospective payment system, the **Resource-Based Relative Value Scale (RBRVS),** was initiated in 1992 for physician services provided to Medicare clients. In this system, the typical costs of a given health service have been calculated based on the prevailing cost for that service in a particular locale. Physicians providing a given service are paid a flat fee based on the estimated cost of the service. Costs are categorized into more than 7,000 Current Procedural Terminology (CPT) codes that are used for Medicare billing purposes.

Capitation is "a prospective payment system that pays health plans or providers a fixed amount per enrollee per month to provide a defined set of health services based on enrollee needs" (Chang et al., 2001, p. 303). The net effect is a fixed budget for the program that must cover all services provided. Capitation is a prominent feature of many managed care plans.

Prospective reimbursement eliminates the incentive to overtreat clients. Because providers are paid at a fixed rate, extending the services provided to a client does not result in additional revenue. Indeed, continued service may be to the provider's disadvantage if the costs of service exceed the fixed rate paid for them. Providers, then, have an incentive to minimize the costs of care. Implementation of DRGs has led to shorter hospital stays and movement of many services to outpatient settings to cut costs (Abood, 2000).

Prospective payment systems also have disadvantages. Health care institutions may attempt to avoid caring for the very sick or provide inadequate care to minimize costs. For example, under the DRG system, a hospital would be paid the same rate for Medicare recipients hospitalized for diabetes whether their hospital stays were 3 days or 30 days. Those who are very ill and who require more than the average stay for their diagnostic group may be discharged from services before they are actually ready for discharge. In the long run, such practices may lead to subsequent readmissions and to increased health care costs.

FUTURE DIRECTIONS

Several conclusions can be drawn from our discussion thus far. First, health status and economics have a dynamic relationship in which each influences the other. Second, given the number of people in poverty and who are uninsured and the effects of poverty and lack of insurance on health and access to health care, the current mechanisms for financing health care delivery are inadequate to meet the needs of the U.S. population. Third, some sort of change is needed to address these problems for the future.

Several suggestions have been made for future directions in health care financing. These include tax credits for the purchase of private or group health insurance and similar credits to enable displaced workers to extend insurance coverage under COBRA. It is unlikely that either of these approaches will have much effect on the problem of the uninsured, since many of this group are not working, and those who are do not receive incomes high enough to afford health insurance coverage even with tax credits (Alliance for Health Reform, 2003).

Another approach would be to expand Medicaid and SCHIP to other vulnerable segments of the population. For example, coverage could be extended to parents of children enrolled in these programs. This approach might help and could be expected to extend coverage to about one third of uninsured adults with chronic conditions, those most in need of services (Tu & Reed, 2002).

Many authorities argue that the problems of health care costs and lack of access to care will not be resolved without some form of universal health care coverage

(Alliance for Health Reform, 2003; Vladek, 2003). Again, there are a number of approaches that could be taken to create a universal system in the United States. For example, Medicare could gradually be expanded to cover the entire population. Another option would be to require employers to provide insurance for all their employees or to require all persons to carry health insurance similar to the requirement for driver's licenses. Finally, a comprehensive system could be developed that would be government financed and managed and funded with tax revenues. This would necessitate development of a more simplified, fair, and efficient tax system than is currently in place (Bass et al., 2003), as well as considerable planning to develop a viable health care system.

Whatever approaches are taken to controlling the costs of health care and developing new payment mechanisms, community health nurses should be actively involved in relevant policy decisions. Community health nurses may also be involved in research to determine the outcomes and cost-effectiveness of various modes of health care delivery. Future financing mechanisms must support a balance between cost control and access to and quality of health care services, and community health nurses must help to assure that such a balance is maintained.

Case Study

Financing Care for the Underserved

You have been appointed to the mayor's task force on health care in the midsize community in which you work as a community health nurse. The assessment of community health and economic status conducted by the task force indicates that most of the population's health care needs are adequately met at all three levels of prevention. The exception to this, however, is the population of the migrant farm camp at the edge of town.

This group consists primarily of male Mexican workers who have entered the United States on legal work visas. Very few of the workers have brought their families with them. Most of this population receives no health care except for treatment in the emergency room of the community hospital. Usually, this care is provided for work-related injuries or serious illness. Members of this group receive no primary preventive care and do not seek care for minor illnesses because of their inability to pay.

Because most of these people are in the United States legally, they would be eligible for county medical assistance (CMA); however, very few have applied for this program because of language barriers, lack of transportation to the social services office, and inability to afford to take the time off work to submit an application. Even if they did receive assistance, they would be unlikely to find a regular health care provider who has a contract with the county to provide services under CMA reimbursement.

Only one community clinic and one independent nurse practitioner, in addition to the community hospital, have county contracts. Local physicians receive adequate income from private paying clients and those with private health insurance. Because of the extended time between provision of services and receipt of reimbursement, these physicians no longer accept county assistance clients.

The rest of the population is well off when compared with average state and national incomes. With the exception of the migrant workers, most residents are employed by three large industries and receive salaries that are quite adequate to meet the cost of living. Because of the industry present in the community, the local tax base is more than adequate. The community does not budget any public funds for health care as the majority of the population is adequately served by private providers. There is no local health department, but the county offers public health services in a town 50 miles away.

1. What factors are influencing the health status of the migrant group?
2. How would you finance health care for this population group?
3. Would fee-for-service care or managed care arrangements be more appropriate for providing care to the migrant population? Why?

Test Your Understanding

1. Describe the interrelationships among economics, health care services, and health status. (pp. 158-165)

2. What are some of the factors contributing to escalating health care costs? What effects do escalating costs have on access to care? What effects do they have on population health status? (pp. 159–161)

3. What effects have economic factors had on the provision of public health services? (p. 165)

4. What is the difference between prospective and retrospective reimbursement? What are the advantages and disadvantages of each? (p. 175)

5. What characteristics do managed care programs have in common? How do types of managed care plans differ? (pp. 172-173)

EXPLORE MediaLink

http://www.prenhall.com/clark

Resources for this chapter can be found on the Companion Website.

Audio Glossary
Exam Review Questions
Case Study: Helping Seniors
  with Medicare Plan D

MediaLink Applications: Universal Health
  Care in Massachusetts
Media Links
Challenge Your Knowledge

Update *Healthy People 2010*
Advocacy Interviews

References

Abood, S. (2000). Why care about Medicare reimbursement? *American Journal of Nursing, 100*(6), 70–72.

Alliance for Health Reform. (2003). *Cover the uninsured week: On-campus resource guide.* Washington, DC: Author.

American Association of Retired Persons. (2002). *Beyond 50.02: A report to the nation on trends in health security.* Washington, DC: Author.

Anderson, G. F., Reinhardt, U. E., Hussey, P. S., & Petrosyan, V. (2003). It's the prices, stupid: Why the United States is so different from other countries. *Health Affairs, 22*(3), 89–105.

Barry, P. (2002, June). Drug profit vs. research. *AARP Bulletin*, pp. 7–9.

Bass, G. D., Irons, J. S., & Taylor, E. (2003). Moving toward long-term action on tax and budget issues. Retrieved April 30, 2004, from http://www.ombwatch.org

Bauer, T., Collins, S., Doyle, J., Fuld, J., & Fuentes-Afflick, E. (2002). *Challenges associated with applying for health insurance among Latina mothers in California, Florida, and New York.* Retrieved February 3, 2003, from http://www.nyam.org/divisions/healthscience/childhealth/pdf/latinomedicaidpolicyreport.pdf

Bauman, N. L. (2002). *A gathering storm in California health care? Trends in managed care costs, accountability, and quality.* Retrieved February 3, 2003, from http://www.thelatinocoalition.com/issues/pdf/Californiahealthcarestudy.pdf

Better Business Bureau Wise Giving Alliance. (2003). *Investigate before you donate.* Retrieved December 28, 2005, from http://www.give.org

Bluestein, G. (2005). *Flat-fee medical clinics come to rural America.* Retrieved December 27, 2005, from http://www.msnbc.com/id/9354279

Brandon, W. P., Chaudry, R. V., & Sardell, A. (2001). Launching SCHIP: The states and children's health insurance. In R. B. Hackey & D. A. Rochefort (Eds.), *The new politics of state health policy* (pp. 142–185). Lawrence, KS: University Press of Kansas.

Center for Medicaid and State Operations. (2005). *Medicaid at a glance.* Retrieved December 21, 2005, from http://www.cms/hhs.gov/MedicaidEligibility/downloads/MedGlance05.pdf

Centers for Disease Control and Prevention. (2004). Indicators for chronic disease surveillance. *Morbidity and Mortality Weekly Report, 53*(RR-11), 1–114.

Centers for Medicare and Medicaid Services. (2005a). *Medicare & you, 2006.* Retrieved December 21, 2005, from http://www.medicare.gov/publications/pubs/pdf/10050.pdf

Centers for Medicare and Medicaid Services. (2005b). *Medicare premiums and coinsurance rates for 2006.* Retrieved December 21, 2005, from http://questions.medicare.gov/cgi-bin/medicare.cfg/php/enduser/std_alp.php?p_sid=vrTlxDXh

Centers for Medicare and Medicaid Services. (2005c). *Medicare premiums and deductibles for 2006.* Retrieved December 23, 2005, from http://new.cms.hhs.gov/apps/media/press/release.asp?Counter=1557

Centers for Medicare and Medicaid Services. (2005d). *National health care expenditures projections: 2004–2014.* Retrieved December 23, 2005, from http://www.cms.hhs.gov/NationalHealthExpendituresData/03_NationalHealthAccountsProjected.asp

Centers for Medicare and Medicaid Services. (2005e). *The nation's health dollar, Calendar year 2003, Where it came from, Where it went.* Retrieved December 23, 2005, from http://www.cms.gov/nationalhealthexpenddata/downloads/piechartSourcesExpenditures2003.pdf

Chang, C. F. (2001a). Access to health care. In C. F. Chang, S. A. Price, & S. K. Pfoutz (Eds.), *Economics and nursing: Critical professional issues* (pp. 335–363). Philadelphia: F. A. Davis.

Chang, C. F. (2001b). Why does health care cost so much? In C. F. Chang, S. A. Price, & S. K. Pfoutz (Eds.), *Economics and nursing: Critical professional issues* (pp. 68–96). Philadelphia: F. A. Davis.

Chang, C. F., Price, S. A., & Pfoutz, S. K. (2001). The impact of managed care. In C. F. Chang, S. A. Price, & S. K. Pfoutz (Eds.), *Economics and nursing: Critical professional issues* (pp. 297–334). Philadelphia: F. A. Davis.

Committee on Rapid Advance Demonstration Projects: Health Care Finance and Delivery

Systems. (2003). *Fostering rapid advances in health care: Learning from system demonstrations.* Washington, DC: National Academies Press.

Cubbin, C., LeClere, F. B., & Smith, G. S. (2000). Socioeconomic status and injury mortality: Individual and neighborhood determinants. *Journal of Epidemiology and Community Health, 54,* 517–524.

Darling, S. (2004). Family literacy: Meeting the needs of at-risk families. *Phi Kappa Phi Forum, 84*(2), 18–21.

Diamant, A. L., Hays, R. D., Morales, L. S., Ford, W., Calmes, E., Asch, S., et al. (2004). Delays and unmet need for health care among adult primary care patients in a restructured urban public health system. *American Journal of Public Health, 94,* 783–789.

Drevdahl, D. (2002). Social justice or market justice? The paradoxes of public health partnerships with managed care. *Public Health Nursing, 19,* 161–169.

Drevdahl, D., Kneipp, S. M., Canales, M. K., & Dorcy, K. S. (2001). Reinvesting in social justice: A capital idea for public health nursing? *Advances in Nursing Science, 24*(2), 19–31.

Families USA. (2005). *Census Bureau's uninsured number indicates fourth increase in a row.* Retrieved December 15, 2005, from http://www.familiesusa.org/resources/newsroom/statements/census-bureau-uninsured-number-indicates-fourth-increase-in-a-row.html

Fang, J., & Alderman, M. H. (2004). Does supplemental private insurance affect care of Medicare recipients hospitalized for myocardial infarction? *American Journal of Public Health, 94,* 778–782.

Federal Trade Commission. (2003). *Charitable donations: Give or take?* Retrieved December 28, 2005, from http://www.ftc.gov/bcp/conline/pubs/tmarkg/charity.htm

Fox, M. H., Moore, J., Davis, R., & Heintzelman, R. (2003). Changes in reported health status and unmet need for children enrolling in the Kansas Children's Health Insurance Program. *American Journal of Public Health, 93,* 579–582.

Glenn, D. (2002). What the data actually show about welfare reform. *Chronicle of Higher Education, XLVIII*(41), A14–A16.

Hildebrandt, E. (2002). The health effects of work-based welfare. *Journal of Nursing Scholarship, 34,* 363–368.

Huey, F. L. (2001). A global perspective on the human and economic burdens of chronic disease. *Pfizer Journal (Global ed.), 11*(2), 10–16.

Institute of Medicine. (2001). *Crossing the quality chasm.* Washington, DC: National Academies Press.

Institute of Medicine. (2002). *Care without coverage: Too little, too late.* Washington, DC: National Academies Press.

Institute of Medicine. (2003). *Hidden costs, value lost: Uninsurance in America.* Washington, DC: National Academies Press.

Jonas, S. (2003). *An introduction to the U. S. health care system* (5th ed.). New York: Springer.

Joyce, T., Bauer, T., Minkoff, H., & Kaestner, R. (2001). Welfare reform and the perinatal health and health care use of Latino women in California, New York City, and Texas. *American Journal of Public Health, 91,* 1857–1864.

Kaiser Family Foundation. (2003, September 23). *Kaiser daily health policy report.* Retrieved April 28, 2004, from http://www.kaisernetwork.org

Klein, R., Stoll, K., & Bruce, A. (2004). *Medicaid: Good medicine for state economies, 2004 update.* Retrieved August 30, 2004, from http://www.familiesusa.org

Kongstvedt, P. R. (2002). *Managed care: What it is and how it works.* Gaithersburg, MD: Aspen.

Kullgren, J. T. (2003). Restrictions on undocumented immigrants' access to health services: The public health implications of welfare reform. *American Journal of Public Health, 93,* 1630–1633.

Ling, C. (2000). Managed care: Its origins, today's picture—and what's ahead. *NurseWeek, 13*(14), 20–21.

Mahan, D. (2004). *Sticker shock: Rising prescription drug prices for seniors.* Retrieved August 30, 2004, from http://www.familiesusa.org

Metropolitan Life Insurance Company. (2003-05). *Making charitable contributions.* Retrieved December 28, 2005, from http://www.metlife.com/Applications/Corporate/WPS/CDA/PageGenerator/0,,-1971~AP,00.html

Mitchem, F. (2002). Providing pharmaceutical services in a tumultuous environment. *Community Health Forum, 3*(3), 7–11.

National Center for Charitable Statistics. (2005). *Nonprofit organizations.* Retrieved December 28, 2005, from http://nccsdataweb.urban.org

National Center for Health Statistics. (2003). *Health United States, 2003 with chartbook on trends in the health of Americans.* Washington, DC: Author.

National Center for Health Statistics. (2004). *Health United States, 2004 with chartbook on trends in the health of Americans.* Washington, DC: Author.

National Center for Health Statistics. (2005). *Health, United States, 2005 with chartbook on trends in the health of Americans.* Retrieved December 23, 2005, from http://www.cdc.gov/nchs/data/hus/hus05.pdf

Nolin, J., & Killackey, J. (2005). Redirecting health care spending: Consumer-directed health care. *Nursing Economics, 22,* 251–253.

Partnership for Prevention. (2003). *A better Medicare for healthier seniors: Recommendations to modernize Medicare's prevention policies.* Retrieved July 25, 2003, from http://www.prevent.org

Perkins, R. (2002). Global health and economic development. *The Pfizer Journal (Global ed.), III*(2), 4–9.

Pfoutz, S. K., Price, S. A., & Chang, C. F. (2002). Health economics. In D. J. Mason, J. K. Leavitt, & M. W. Chaffee (Eds.), *Policy and politics in nursing and health care* (4th ed., pp. 229–239). St. Louis, MO: Saunders.

Piette, J. D., Heisler, M., & Wagner, T. (2004). Cost-related medication underuse among chronically ill adults: The treatments people forgo, how often, and who is at risk. *American Journal of Public Health, 94,* 1782–1787.

Prentice, J. C., Pebley, A. R., & Sastry, N. (2005). Immigration status and health insurance coverage: Who gains? Who loses? *American Journal of Public Health, 95,* 109–116.

Price, S. A., Pfoutz, S. K., & Chang, C. F. (2001). The economics of nursing and health care. In C. F. Chang, S. A. Price, & S. K. Pfoutz (Eds.), *Economics and nursing: Critical professional issues* (pp. 3–36). Philadelphia: F. A. Davis.

Pricewaterhousecooper's Health Research Institute. (2005). *Acts of charity: Charity care strategies for hospitals in a changing landscape.* Retrieved December 27, 2005, from http://healthcare.pwc.com/cgi-local/hcregister.cgi?link=reg/charitycare.pdf&update=true

Pulcini, J. A., Neary, S. R., & Mahoney, D. F. (2002). Health care financing. In D. J. Mason, J. K. Leavitt, & M. W. Chaffee (Eds.), *Policy and politics in nursing and health care* (4th ed., pp. 241–265). St. Louis, MO: Saunders.

Santelli, J. S., Lowry, R., Brener, N. D., & Robin, L. (2002). The association of sexual behaviors with socioeconomic status, family structure, and race/ethnicity among US adolescents. *American Journal of Public Health, 90,* 1582–1588.

Stoll, K., & Jones, K. (2004). *One in three: Nonelderly Americans without health insurance, 2002–2003.* Retrieved August 30, 2004, from http://www.familiesusa.org

Sudano, J. J., & Baker, D. W. (2003). Intermittent lack of health insurance coverage and use of preventive services. *American Journal of Public Health, 93,* 130–137.

Sultz, H. A., & Young, K. M. (2004). *Health care USA: Understanding its organization and delivery* (4th ed.). Sudbury, MA: Jones and Bartlett.

Tu, H. T., & Reed, M. C. (2002). *Options for expanding health insurance coverage for people with chronic conditions.* Retrieved August 13, 2002, from http://www.hschange.org/CONTENT/414/?topic=topic06

Ullman, F., & Hill, I. (2001). Eligibility under State Children's Health Insurance Programs. *American Journal of Public Health, 91,* 1449–1451.

U.S. Census Bureau. (2004). *Poverty: 2003 highlight.* Retrieved September 30, 2004, from http://www.census.gov

U.S. Department of Health and Human Services. (2000). *Healthy people 2010* (Conference ed., Vol. I). Washington, DC: Author.

U.S. Government Accountability Office. (2005). *Nonprofit, for-profit, and government hospitals: Uncompensated care and other community benefits.* Retrieved December 23, 2005, from http://www.gao.gov/new.items/d05743t.pdf

Vladek, B. (2003). Universal health insurance in the United States: Reflections on the past, the present, and the future. *American Journal of Public Health, 93,* 16–19.

Waitzkin, H., Williams, R. L., Bock, J. A., McCloskey, J., Willging, C., & Wagner, W. (2002). Safety-net institutions buffer the impact of Medicaid managed care: A multimethods assessment in a rural state. *American Journal of Public Health, 92,* 598–610.

Wiebe, C. (2004). Drug import programs defy federal warnings, reap benefits. Retrieved October 13, 2004, from http://www.medscape.com/viewarticle/490299

Wimberley, E. T., & Rubens, A. J. (2002). Like plugging the holes in the colander: Health policy and provision in the United States circa the millennium. In K. V. Thai, E. T. Wimberley, & S. M. McManus (Eds.), *Handbook of international health care systems* (pp. 135–206). New York: Marcel Dekker.

Winkleby, M. A., & Cubbin, C. (2003). Influence of individual and neighborhood socioeconomic status on mortality among black, Mexican-American, and white women and men in the United States. *Journal of Epidemiology and Community Health, 57*, 444–452.

World Health Organization. (2002). *Scaling up the response to infectious diseases*. Retrieved April 2, 2002, from http://www.who.int/infectious-disease-report/2002

Advocacy in Action

No Cause for Referral

A registered nurse student enrolled in a community health nursing course was assigned to a Hispanic family who had a newborn infant with multiple congenital anomalies. The family had been referred to a number of services to deal with the infant's many needs. There was some question that the child was blind in addition to the other problems identified at birth, and the family had been referred for diagnostic services. The family was also referred to the public health nursing service of the county health department in which the student was obtaining her clinical experience.

Because the student was a native Spanish-speaker, she was able to communicate effectively with the family. When she went to visit them, she discovered that they had not followed up on the vision screening referral although they were keeping all of the child's other health-related appointments. When the student reported back to the public health nurse, who was also Hispanic, the nurse was quite adamant that the family be reported to Child Protective Services (CPS) for medical neglect. The student tried to explain that the family intended to comply with the referral, but did not yet have the money to do so. They were extremely proud and did not want to accept what they considered to be "charity" to pay for the needed services. They were paying for other services that were not covered by their insurance out-of-pocket. The public health nurse continued to insist that they were guilty of neglect.

Distressed by the nurse's failure to acknowledge the family's beliefs and values, the student brought the matter to the attention of her instructor. Together she and the instructor discussed the issue with the public health nursing supervisor, who upheld the student's point of view. The supervisor later met with the public health nurse to inform her that a CPS referral was not warranted in this case.

The student's advocacy for this family is perhaps even more remarkable in light of the fact that her own baby was born at the same time as this infant, also with congenital anomalies, and the two infants were in the neonatal intensive care unit at the same time. The student's baby died and this baby lived. When asked why she did not tell the instructor and request another assignment, the student said she at first thought she could deal with it. She later found that the assignment was a painful reminder of her own child's death, but by then she was committed to doing what she could to help this family. It was not until the end of the semester that she felt able to share this information with the instructor.

CHAPTER 9

The Cultural Context

CHAPTER OBJECTIVES

After reading this chapter, you should be able to:

1. Differentiate among culture, race, nationality, and ethnicity.
2. Discuss direct and indirect influences of culture on health and health care.
3. Describe cultural competence.
4. Identify barriers to cultural competence.
5. Conduct a cultural assessment of an individual, family, group, or health system.
6. Design, implement, and evaluate culturally competent care and health care delivery systems.

KEY TERMS

 MediaLink
http://www.prenhall.com/clark

Additional interactive resources for this chapter can be found on the Companion Website. Click on Chapter 9 and "Begin" to select the activities for this chapter.

Why study culture? The most obvious answer, of course, is to enable us to provide effective care for the increasingly diverse populations that we serve. There are, however, other reasons as well. Each of us is the product of a cultural background that influences, often unconsciously, our thoughts, beliefs, values, attitudes, and behaviors. When we are unaware of the influences of culture on our own behaviors, we are less able to recognize how our attitudes and behaviors influence others. The more we know about culture in general, and our own culture in particular, the better able we are to modify our interactions with others to provide effective care. In addition, as nurses, we are immersed in a biomedical culture, the influences of which are again often unrecognized. Awareness of the influences of biomedical culture on our practice can assist us to modify elements of that culture that impede effective health care. Finally, as nurses, we generally work with health care institutions and organizations that have their own distinct cultures. If we are to work effectively within these organizations, we must conform to the cultural expectations others have of us. Similarly, recognition of organizational culture and its influence on practice can help us modify health care systems to better meet the needs of clients from diverse cultural backgrounds.

The principles of cultural assessment and cultural competence can be applied in client care situations as well as professional interactions within nursing and between nursing and other disciplines. Throughout this chapter, we will examine cultural principles as they relate to traditional ethnic cultures, the dominant U.S. culture, biomedical culture, and organizational culture.

CULTURE, RACE, AND ETHNICITY

Culture is often equated with ethnicity, nationality, or race. As we saw above, however, groups other than ethnic minorities or national populations are influenced by culture. Similarly, culture may cut across racial or ethnic groups. For example, both White nurses and nurses of color are imbued with the culture of nursing, which cuts across racial boundaries. Similarly, Arab Muslims and African American Muslims subscribe to similar aspects of culture derived from their adherence to Islam, but display other cultural beliefs and behaviors unique to their ethnic heritage. As an example of the interaction of race and ethnicity, the population categories included in the most recent census subdivided racial categories of Black and White into subcategories of Black/Hispanic, Black/non-Hispanic, White/Hispanic, and White/non-Hispanic, combining features of race and ethnicity to create more informative categories.

Culture has been defined as "a shared system of meaning, the way that people experience, perceive, and interpret their world" (Becker, Gates, & Newsom, 2004,

p. 2066) or the "practices, beliefs, values, and norms which can be learned or shared, and which guide the actions and decisions of each person in the group" (Weibert, 2002, p. 1). In more practical terms, culture is the way in which a group of people makes sense of the world around them and that directs their interactions and behaviors within that world. For our purposes, **culture** is defined as the ways of thinking and acting developed by a group of people that permit them to interact effectively with their environment and to address concerns common to the human condition. A group's **worldview**, which shapes culture, is their way of looking at the universe and their relationship to that universe.

Ethnicity, on the other hand, is defined as "the aggregate of cultural practices, social influences, religious pursuits, and racial characteristics shaping the distinctive identity of a community" (Paisley et al., 2002, p. 138). An ethnic group usually has a relatively homogenous social culture (Gesler & Kearns, 2002). **Nationality** usually refers to one's country of birth, but may also refer to a country adopted for permanent residence. Again, nationality may cut across ethnic and racial designations. For example, citizens of the United States consider themselves Americans (nationality), but

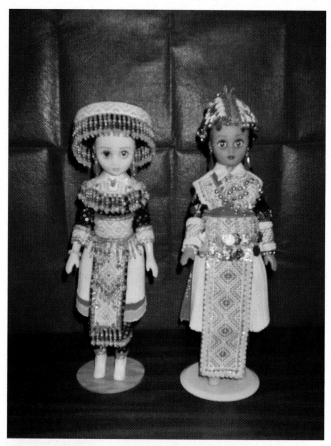

Hmong residents in the United States maintain their cultural heritage with traditional New Year's costumes and celebrations. (Mary Jo Clark)

include members of all three racial groups (White, Black, and Asian) as well as multiple ethnicities (e.g., German Americans, Irish Americans, African Americans).

Race is an artificial categorization of people based on genetic inheritance and physical characteristics such as skin color, blood type, hair color and texture, and eye color (Purnell & Paulanka, 2005). Much of the demographic and other information used for planning health care delivery services (e.g., census data, morbidity and mortality data) is categorized on the basis of race. Recently, however, many authors have indicated that racial categorization does not fully convey the differences among groups, particularly those related to disparities in health status (Kressin, Chang, Hendricks, & Kazis, 2003). In a 1999 report, the Institute of Medicine (IOM) noted that racial categorization no longer adequately addresses the diversity of the U.S. population and suggested the substitution of ethnicity for race as a means of categorizing health-related data. The IOM based this recommendation on their contention that ethnicity provides a greater "appreciation of the range of cultural and behavioral attitudes, beliefs, lifestyle patterns, diets, environmental living conditions, and other factors" than does the concept of race (IOM, cited in Oppenheimer, 2001, p. 1053).

Societal or ethnic culture is most often learned within the family, but is also transmitted in one's day-to-day interactions with other members of the group. Biomedical and professional cultures, on the other hand, are learned in the context of specific educational preparation and through interactions with others in professional practice. Similarly, the organizational culture of the workplace is transmitted through both formal and informal mechanisms in the workplace (e.g., through formal orientation programs and through everyday interactions with supervisors and coworkers).

Culture is characterized by universality, largely unconscious influence, uniqueness, stability as well as dynamism, and internal variability. Culture is a universal experience. All people engage in culturally prescribed behavior patterns, although these patterns vary from group to group. Even though culture affects virtually every aspect of life, its influence is largely unconscious. The influence of culture is rarely consciously noted, unless one purposefully undertakes a study of one's own culturally determined behavior. It is for this reason that nurses need to become aware of their own cultural beliefs, biases, and behaviors in order to understand their influence on interactions with clients and with members of other health care disciplines.

Moreover, the culture of any particular group is unique. Although several cultures may exhibit certain commonalities, no two cultures, like no two individuals, are exactly alike. The beliefs and behaviors that constitute a particular culture arise from the unique constraints faced by a given group of people in dealing with problems common to humanity. These unique situational constraints are the source of cultural variation among groups of people. For example, the arid nature of the southwestern United States has led to water conservation practices among residents of the region that would not be seen in other parts of the country. Similarly, although the cultures of nursing and medicine have some commonalities, they also have many distinct differences. Likewise the organizational culture of one health care institution may differ markedly from that of another institution even though both exist for the same basic purpose.

Another characteristic of culture is its stability. Cultural characteristics tend to endure across generations. Culture, however, is neither static nor immutably fixed; it is dynamic and subject to change. Culture is "continually being socially produced by people as they struggle to achieve power and meaning" in their lives (Gesler & Kearns, 2002, p. 13). Although the superficial aspects of culture can change relatively easily, basic cultural values and beliefs change slowly and may provide the basis for strong resistance to change. Changes within cultural groups may also lead to conflict, particularly intergenerational conflict.

Finally, the degree to which members of a cultural group adhere to cultural beliefs, values, and customs varies considerably. For example, you may not always believe or act in ways typical of nursing's culture. Similarly, not all members of an ethnic population exhibit the beliefs and behaviors typical of the group. Adherence to the values and behaviors of a particular culture is influenced by the extent of one's acculturation. **Acculturation** or cultural assimilation is the acquisition of at least some of the beliefs, values, and behaviors of another culture. Acculturation usually occurs because such adaptation is required for survival in a new environment. For members of ethnic groups, acculturation is usually considered in terms of their acquisition of beliefs, values, and behaviors typical of the dominant societal culture. Acculturation also takes place, however, in other venues. Your nursing education, for example, is designed to promote your

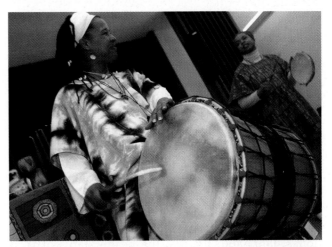

Traditional music enables some cultural groups to maintain their heritage. (© E.A. Kennedy III / The Image Works)

TABLE 9-1	Characteristics of Culture
Characteristic	**Description**
Universality	Culture is a pervasive phenomenon that influences all human interactions.
Unconscious influence	Expression of cultural meaning through beliefs, values, attitudes, and behaviors often occurs without conscious awareness.
Uniqueness	All cultures are different, and although similarities may exist among cultural groups, no two cultures are exactly alike.
Stability	Culture is lasting and endures through generations.
Dynamism	Culture changes over time. Superficial aspects of culture change more readily than deeply held beliefs and values.
Variability	The degree of adherence to cultural beliefs, values, and behaviors varies with individual members of the culture and depends on a variety of factors.

acculturation to the nursing profession and its unique culture. In the same way, you are becoming acculturated to the overall biomedical culture. You will also need to become acculturated to a certain extent to the health care institution or agency that employs you, if you are to be successful there. In all of these examples, acculturation may have both positive and negative effects. We will discuss some of these effects throughout the chapter. Characteristics of culture are summarized in Table 9-1◆.

CULTURE AND HEALTH

Culture, whether it is that of an ethnic group, the dominant society, a professional discipline, or health professionals as a group, has both positive and negative health consequences. For example, the dominant U.S. culture values cure of disease, often through the use of expensive technology. This cultural value results in extensive expenditures for expensive high-technology therapies and little attention to health promotion and illness prevention needs. At the same time, the dominant culture values an attractive physical appearance, which may lead people to engage in more exercise activities than they would if uninfluenced by this value.

Ethnic/Societal Culture and Health

Ethnic minority cultures and the dominant societal culture have both direct and indirect effects on health. Direct effects stem from specific culturally prescribed practices related to diet and food or to health and illness. For example, all cultures have prescribed practices intended to promote health and prevent illness or to restore health when illness occurs. Similarly, all cultures have particular dietary practices that influence nutritional status and, thereby, the health status of their members. For example, the typical diets of many ethnic minority groups are basically healthful, but some

dietary practices (e.g., the preponderance of fried food in the southern United States) have negative health effects. Similarly, the prevalence of fast food and "super sizing" in the dominant culture contributes to obesity and other adverse health effects.

Ethnic and societal cultures also affect health indirectly. Some of these indirect effects result from cultural definitions of health and illness, acceptability of health care programs and providers, and cultural influences on compliance with suggested health or illness regimens. Cultural definitions of health and illness determine what kinds of health problems are considered worthy of attention and what conditions are likely to be disregarded. If, for example, certain behaviors that are perceived as evidence of mental illness by health professionals are considered normal in the client's culture, then the client is unlikely to take any action to deal with those behaviors. Similarly, minor illnesses may be ignored if health is defined in terms of one's ability to work or to perform other social roles. In general, people are likely to disregard any type of condition that is not defined as illness in their own culture. This cultural propensity can lead to serious health consequences.

Cultural factors may also determine the acceptability of both health programs and health providers. For example, cultures that eschew scientific medicine in favor of healing based on faith in God may view immunization programs as inimical to their beliefs. In other cultures, health care providers may be considered lower-class persons not to be associated with, effectively preventing people from taking advantage of many health opportunities. For example, nursing has been considered a lower-class occupation in India, and nurses have had limited opportunity to influence the health of their clients for the better because of their low social status.

Cultural factors often determine whether clients will comply with recommendations when they do seek professional help. Culture gives rise to certain expectations regarding treatment. If health care providers' recommendations are too far removed from these expectations, the provider loses credibility, and the client is unlikely to comply with those recommendations (Flaskerud, 2000). For example, in the dominant U.S. culture, clients have come to expect health care providers to address most health problems with prescription medications. When no prescription is provided, even though the health problem doesn't really require medication, clients may be dissatisfied with care and fail to follow through on other more appropriate recommendations, such as dietary changes, weight loss, and so on.

Biomedical Culture and Health

Health culture has been defined as

> All the phenomena associated with the maintenance of well-being and problems of sickness with which people cope in traditional ways within their own social

networks. It is a general term that includes both the cognitive and social aspects of [health traditions]. The cognitive dimension involves values and beliefs, the blueprints for health action, and requires us to understand theories of health maintenance, disease etiology, prevention, diagnosis, treatment and cure. The social system dimension refers to the organization of health care or the health care delivery system. It requires understanding of the structure and functioning of any organized set of health-related social roles and behaviors. (Weidman, quoted in Gesler & Kearns, 2002, p. 30)

Although this definition was developed to address the health aspects of ethnic cultures, it applies no less to the culture of biomedicine and those of the health care professions.

Like ethnic and dominant societal cultures, the overall biomedical culture and the cultures of professional health disciplines and organizations may have both positive and negative influences on the health of population groups. The emphasis on the provider as an authority and the client as subordinate that pervades the biomedical culture may lead clients to forgo health care in an effort to control their own lives and health or to fail to accept responsibility for health actions on their own behalf. Unfortunately, health professionals often fail to recognize the influence of the biomedical culture and the dominant societal culture on their practice, and may see biomedicine as having been "purged" of cultural influences by its reliance on objective scientific evidence. As one author noted, "because medicine tends to be blind to the mythological, ritualized, and culturally embedded aspects of its philosophy and praxis, it generally denies the role these dynamics play in healing" (Wolpe, 2002, p. 168).

Authors in the health professions and other disciplines give a variety of examples of the cultural rituals and artifacts embedded in the biomedical culture. For example, the use of the hospital gown in biomedically oriented hospitals is a ritual that conveys the dependence of the client on the institution and their loss of autonomy with respect to even their own apparel (Hillier, 2003). Similar rituals include meals served at specific times whether clients are hungry or not and the need to schedule an appointment to receive services in most biomedical organizations. These cultural rituals within the biomedical and health professional community are primarily based on dominant cultural values of efficiency and time consciousness. Although generally harmless, except in the level of discomfort experienced by clients, some of these rituals may have negative health effects. For example, time consciousness, the resulting expectation that things will occur rapidly, and an unwillingness to let labor progress at its natural pace have been cited as contributing factors in the frequency of cesarean sections in the United States (Hillier, 2003).

The biomedical culture in the United States has also been characterized by vacillation between risk taking and risk avoidance. There is a tendency to want to try new things, such as experimental therapies, while at the same time trying to protect oneself from the possible consequences (e.g., through conservative practice to avoid malpractice claims) (Hillier, 2003). Negative health effects can result from either perspective. For example, clients may be pressured to agree to new treatments with undetermined efficacy or may be subjected to the discomfort and possible expense of diagnostic tests or therapeutic interventions that are not really warranted.

Culture may also have adverse effects on the health professions themselves. For example, some nurse authors have cited the lack of cultural sensitivity in the NCLEX-RN exam as a contributing factor in the dearth of nurses representative of ethnic minority groups and in the exacerbation of the nursing shortage. In addition, the cost of preparing for and taking the examination itself may disadvantage minority nurses. This may be particularly true for nurses prepared in other countries whose programs may not include some of the content tested on the examination. For example, psychiatric conditions may not be addressed in some curricula due to the cultural stigma attached to mental illness in some cultures. Even the format of the test may not be culturally appropriate to nurses whose education has not included multiple-choice testing formats (Wessling, 2003).

ETHNIC DIVERSITY IN THE UNITED STATES

As we noted earlier, one of the primary reasons for becoming knowledgeable about culture and its effects on health lies in the ethnic and cultural diversity of the clients that we serve. Beyond the period of early colonization of North America by settlers primarily from England, the United States has always been ethnically and culturally diverse. Even in the early colonial periods, there were cultural differences in the groups that settled here. For example, many of the first settlers were members of specific religious groups seeking religious freedom that brought their own cultures with them. Later immigrant groups came from other Western European countries, particularly Ireland and Germany, but from other parts of the world as well. Although possessed of their own distinct cultures, these groups had more in common than many later immigrant groups.

Today the United States is more ethnically and culturally diverse than ever before. For example, the Latino/Hispanic population, 35.3 million people in 2002 or 12.5% of the total U.S. population, is expected to comprise 25% of the population by 2050. African Americans constituted 12% of the population, and Asians comprised another 4% of the population. In addition, there were 561 recognized American Indian/Alaska Native tribes speaking 200 indigenous languages (U.S. Department of Health and Human Services [USDHS], 2002). By 2050, racial and ethnic minorities are expected to constitute 50% of the U.S. population (Centers for Disease Control and Prevention [CDC], 2004).

Even these figures do not give a full picture of the extent of diversity in the population because of the different ethnicities represented within each of these large groups. For example, an estimated 4 million Arabs live in the United States, with more than 80 different ethnicities represented in this group alone (Taylor, 2004). Similarly, the Asian population consists of Chinese, Japanese, Filipino, Korean, Pacific Islander, Southeast Asian (which is further subdivided), and persons from the Indian subcontinent (Gomez, Kelsey, Glaser, Lee, & Sidney, 2004). Vietnamese and Cambodians constitute 12% of the overall Asian population (Division of Adult and Community Health, 2004), and Koreans are the fifth largest Asian group in the United States (1.2 million persons in 2000) (Moskowitz, Kazinets, Tager, & Wong, 2004). The Hispanic population includes people from Spain, Mexico, Puerto Rico, and a variety of central and South American countries, each with its own unique culture and different health problems and service needs.

Even among the Anglo population of the United States, there are distinct cultural groups. For example, Southern Whites and Blacks often have more in common, particularly with respect to diet and other consumption patterns, than Southern Whites have with Caucasian groups in other areas of the country (e.g., midwestern German Americans or Italian Americans in the Northeast) (Sharpless, 2002). Gypsies, or the Roma, are another distinct cultural group found in the United States (Vivian & Dundes, 2004).

Diversity also exists within cultural groups, and people "may move between cultures while simultaneously inhabiting a relatively unique coculture (or subculture) with its own concepts, rules, and social organization" (Becker et al., 2004, p. 266). Members of a given cultural group may exhibit various levels of adherence to the beliefs, values, and behaviors of that group. Some people, for example, maintain a traditional cultural stance, adhering strongly to the culture of their family of origin. Others are bicultural, and are equally at home in traditional and dominant cultures. Still others are acculturated, having given up their original culture and subscribing almost completely to the new culture. Acculturation is not only seen in movement from ethnic cultural traditions to those of the dominant culture, but also reflected in the degree to which gay and lesbian individuals subscribe to the mores of those subcultural groups. Finally, some people may be marginal in their cultural affiliations, with little interaction with either a culture of origin or the dominant culture. Many homeless individuals may be considered culturally marginalized (McLaurin, 2002).

The United States is not the only country to experience cultural diversity, yet diversity may be even less well recognized in other nations than in the United States. For example, a group of Japanese nursing students visiting the United States to study social and health care cultures were amazed to note the cultural diversity present there. When they were asked about cultural diversity in their own country, they indicated that there was no diversity. They were unable to recognize the cultural diversity posed by the Ainu, the original population of Japan, and the large resident Korean population as well as the wide variety of foreign visitors to Japan.

ASSESSING CULTURAL INFLUENCES ON HEALTH AND HEALTH CARE

As noted earlier, community health nurses must incorporate cultural concepts into the care of individuals and their families as well as the development and implementation of health care programs for population groups. In addition, nurses must be able to function effectively within the biomedical, professional, and organizational cultures in which they work and to modify those cultures to improve population health care. To accomplish these tasks, nurses must have knowledge of the cultural groups with which they interact. Such knowledge is derived from a cultural assessment, including assessment of the group to determine typical beliefs, values, and behaviors and assessment of individual group members in terms of their adherence to those beliefs, values, and behaviors.

Principles of Cultural Assessment

Four basic principles should guide the study of a culture. First, view the culture in the context in which it developed. As noted earlier, cultural practices arise out of a need to meet common human problems in a particular human setting. That setting must be considered in exploring culture.

Second, examine the underlying premise of culturally determined behavior. What was the intended purpose for the behavior when it originated? Does the behavior still fulfill this purpose? When one knows the underlying reason for behaviors that seem strange, the behaviors may not seem quite so strange after all. Third, the nurse examines the meaning of behavior in the cultural context. The meaning of certain behaviors from the perspective of the nurse may be very different from the behavior's meaning to others. Using the previous example of the hospital gown, its original purposes were to minimize spread of microorganisms via clothing brought in from the outside, promote ease of access to clients for therapeutic procedures, and prevent ruin of clients' personal clothing by blood and other substances. With the advent of washing machines, however, the first and third purposes are really no longer relevant in many situations. In fact, given the rate of nosocomial infection in hospitals, wearing one's personal clothing might actually be safer than wearing a hospital gown.

Similarly, when faced with the potential meaning attached to the practice from a client perspective of dependence and loss of autonomy, is the advantage of the hospital gown to providers outweighed by its disadvantages in the provider–client relationship? Using another example, the dominant U.S. cultural values of independence and self-sufficiency make sense in the light of the historical development of the United States, but do they still serve their underlying purpose in the context of an increasingly interdependent global society?

Finally, there is the need to recognize intracultural variation. Not every member of any given cultural group displays all of the beliefs and behaviors typical of that culture. Subgroups within a cultural group may exhibit different behavior patterns. Or individuals may be more or less adherent to the beliefs, values, attitudes, and behaviors typically expected by members of the culture. Not all Mexican Americans, for example, will demonstrate a belief in the "evil eye." Similarly, not all perinatal providers believe that an enema is a necessary part of preparation for birth. Another term used to denote the degree of adherence or nonadherence to elements of a culture is *heritage consistency*, or "the degree to which one's lifestyle reflects his or her respective tribal culture" (Estes & Zitzow, quoted in Spector, 2004, p. 8). Although this concept was obviously developed in relation to ethnic cultural heritages, it is equally applicable to the "tribal culture" of nursing or biomedicine. Principles of cultural assessment are summarized below.

Obtaining Cultural Information

How does one become knowledgeable about a culture? Perhaps the best way to begin is to recognize the influences of culture on one's own life and behavior. Personal insights regarding culture will enable the nurse to recognize and accept cultural beliefs and behaviors that may differ from his or her own. Once familiar with his or her own cultural heritage, the nurse can begin to read literature related to other cultures of interest. In reading, the community health nurse should examine the qualifications of the authors writing. Was the book or article written by a member of the culture? Is it based on empirical data derived from research, on personal experience with a particular culture, or on stereotypes? Information about a culture from the perspective of nonmembers of the culture can also be instructive. For example, some of the sociological and social anthropological research on

professional cultures can assist us to see the elements of culture that are embedded in biomedicine or in nursing practice that we might not have identified viewing them from inside the culture.

A second means of acquainting oneself with a culture is to interview colleagues who are members of that culture. Explore with them their concepts of health and illness and attitudes and practices affecting health. Discover how these concepts may differ from those held by previous generations or other members of their family. Health care professionals, by virtue of their knowledge of health matters, are likely to have achieved a greater degree of acculturation and conformity with the dominant U.S. culture with respect to health practices than nonprofessionals from the same group. These individuals, however, remain a valid source of information regarding cultural health beliefs and practices. You can also employ this strategy when newly employed or considering employment in a particular health care organization. Talk to people who are already members of the organization about the organizational culture. How are clients viewed? How are employees viewed? How are employees expected to interact with each other? With clients? If the organizational culture seems to be too alien to your own personal culture, you may not want to work there. Clients' perspectives on biomedical culture can also be enlightening. How do they perceive some of the attitudes and behaviors typical of the culture? Do these perceptions enhance or impede effective health care delivery?

One of the best ways to become familiar with a particular culture is to spend time living within it. For example, prospective nurses may be encouraged to engage in volunteer work or to shadow practicing nurses to explore the culture of nursing as a career option. Similarly, one might spend time living within an ethnic cultural group. This approach, however, is not always feasible. Alternatives include home visits to families within the group to observe daily living in the cultural context and questioning clients and families regarding health-related beliefs and practices. Another possible approach is observing activities and interactions at health facilities and community or religious functions.

When assessing another culture directly, whether it is an ethnic cultural group or the organizational culture of a health care institution, the community health nurse should follow a few general guidelines. First, look and listen before asking questions or taking action. Observation aids in asking pertinent and timely questions and forestalls actions that may be inappropriate. Second, explore how the group feels about being studied. Explain that your reasons for studying the culture are practical and do not arise out of idle curiosity. Third, discover any special protocols. Should one speak to a local leader or agency supervisor before beginning to observe a group? Is there a council or leadership group

---

HIGHLIGHTS   **Principles of Cultural Assessment**

- View all cultures in the context in which they developed.
- Examine underlying premises for culturally determined beliefs and behaviors.
- Interpret the meaning and purpose of behavior in the context of the specific culture.
- Recognize the potential for intracultural variation.

who should grant permission for participation in group activities? Fourth, foster human relations, putting them before the need to obtain information. Information will not assist the nurse to provide care or function effectively in a work setting if he or she alienates members of the group. Social amenities are important in many cultures and should be attended to before the "business" of information gathering begins in earnest. In fact, information about social amenities is part of the data needed by the nurse.

Many people, in exploring another culture, look for differences from their own culture. The nurse, however, should also look for cultural similarities to use as a foundation in aiding clients to accept and use health care services. Cultural differences should be accepted as normal.

Locate group leaders and respected residents, those considered wise, "ordinary" group members, and clients who can converse knowledgeably about the culture. Critics of the traditional aspects of the culture may also be interviewed to provide a balanced picture.

Participate as well as observe. The nurse must assess each situation as it occurs to determine whether participation or observation is the more appropriate activity. Participation conveys an openness to cultural differences and a willingness to engage in culturally prescribed activities rather than ridicule them. Some activities, however, are closed to outsiders, and the community health nurse's participation would not be welcomed.

When exploring another culture, the nurse should also consider the feelings of group members about questions asked. The nurse should ascertain what types of questions are acceptable or offensive in a particular culture. For example, U.S. Peace Corps volunteers in India found it difficult to adjust to frequent questions about their salary or how much their clothes cost. Such questions were perfectly acceptable in Indian society, but considered impolite or "nosy" in the United States. Similarly, there may be certain questions that can safely be asked within the biomedical culture. For example, some physicians may respond readily to questions about a particular element of their practice or the plan of care for a client, whereas others would perceive questions as threatening to their authority. The same may be true in the employment setting, where certain questions are acceptable and others are not.

A little forethought as to the phrasing and timing of questions can prevent serious mistakes. Ask questions positively without implying value judgments. For example, "I notice you put garlic on a string around the baby's neck; can you tell me what it's used for?" is far more acceptable than "Why in the world do you hang garlic around the baby's neck?" Nurses might ask the same questions of themselves and gauge their own emotional reaction to the questions. A nurse can also try out questions on colleagues who are members of the culture being explored. Suggested modes of cultural exploration are summarized at right.

HIGHLIGHTS   Modes of Cultural Exploration

- Become conversant with your own culture and its influences on your life.
- Review the existing literature on beliefs, values, and behaviors of specific cultural groups.
- Interview colleagues who are members of the cultural group in question.
- Immerse yourself in the culture to be studied.
- Observe members of specific cultural groups.
- Interview members of cultural groups, particularly group leaders.
- Interview other persons who are conversant with the culture.

Considerations in Cultural Assessment

General areas to be considered in a cultural assessment based on the dimensions model of community health nursing include factors in the biophysical, psychological, physical environmental, sociocultural, behavioral, and health system dimensions.

Biophysical Considerations

Biophysical considerations in cultural assessment include those related to maturation and aging, genetics, and physiologic function. Each of these areas will be explored with respect to ethnic cultures and the dominant U.S. culture. Where appropriate, biomedical and professional cultures and organizational culture are also discussed.

MATURATION AND AGING Cultural groups may display different attitudes toward age. For example, the dominant U.S. culture is oriented toward youth, and youth is valued over age. A significant proportion of the gross domestic product is expended each year on trying to look, feel, and act young. In many traditional ethnic cultures, on the other hand, older persons tend to be highly respected and influential within the family and social group.

Biomedical and organizational cultures may also display differential attitudes toward age. For example, many health care providers are of the opinion that older clients are reaching the end of their lives and health promotion interventions are unwarranted because they will have little effect. Research, however, indicates that health promotion activities with the elderly can have profound, positive effects on health status and self-care capacity. As we will see in Chapter 19∞, ageism and stereotypes of the elderly significantly affect the type of health care services provided to older clients. Similarly, age may be viewed differently in different organizational cultures. How are older employees treated in the organization? Is their expertise valued, or are they expected to move aside in favor of younger employees?

In addition to the attitudes of the cultural group toward aging and people of different age groups, the community health nurse would want to consider the age composition of the cultural group because this information will help to identify potential age-related health concerns. For example, if a large percentage of the cultural group is young children, different types of services will be required. Similarly, if a large portion of the workforce in the organization is close to retirement age, consideration needs to be given to finding replacements. This is currently a problem for health care professions in general and nursing in particular.

GENETICS Considerations related to genetics would be more relevant in the assessment of ethnic cultural groups than for biomedical or organization cultures. Generally, ethnic groups differ with respect to several physical characteristics with genetic components: body build and structure, skin color, enzymatic variations, and susceptibility to disease (Spector, 2004).

Physical differences that derive from genetic inheritance in some ethnic groups have implications for nursing, and nurses need to be conversant with these physiologic variations. For example, WHO has created specific Asia-Pacific guidelines for overweight and obesity due to differences in body size and composition between Asians and Europeans (Division of Nutrition and Physical Activity, 2004). African American youth, on the other hand, tend to exceed standard Caucasian heights and weights at all ages except birth. Different ethnic groups also experience enzymatic variations such as the lactose intolerance of many Asian and Native American groups.

Genetic inheritance may also play a part in the types of health problems commonly seen in members of some ethnic groups. For example, Afghanis experience high rates of glucose-6-phosphate dehydrogenase (G-6-PD) deficiency, sickle cell disease, and thalassemia (Giger & Davidhizar, 2002). Knowledge of the prevalence of these diseases in certain population groups can promote accurate diagnosis and treatment. Similarly, heart disease, although prevalent throughout the world, may occur at younger ages in India than in other ethnic groups. Ethnic groups may also vary in their capacity to metabolize drugs, resulting in the need to adjust dosages to accommodate these differences (Purnell & Paulanka, 2005). There may also be differences among groups with respect to their susceptibility to adverse health effects of environmental hazards.

PHYSIOLOGIC FUNCTION Considerations related to physiologic function are the third component of the biophysical dimension of health addressed in a cultural assessment. Areas to be considered include health problems prevalent in a particular group (beyond those with a genetic component discussed above), attitudes to body parts and functions, perceptions of health and illness and disease causation, and culture-bound syndromes. Community health nurses should be familiar with the kinds of health problems experienced by a particular ethnic

cultural group. This permits the development of health delivery programs targeted to meeting specific needs in the population. At the same time, such knowledge may lead to stereotyping and inappropriate individual diagnosis and treatment within the biomedical culture. Uncertainty about a clinical diagnosis on the part of a professional provider may lead him or her to rely on probability to make a diagnosis. Knowing that a certain ethnic group has a high prevalence of a specific condition may lead to a diagnosis of that condition, when the symptoms are actually the result of some other disease (Escarce, 2005).

Attitudes toward Body Parts and Physiologic Functions

There may be considerable difference in the attitudes toward body parts and physiologic functions among ethnic cultural groups and between these groups and the dominant U.S. culture. For example, Muslims are extremely modest and may be reluctant to bare their bodies to health care providers, particularly a provider of the opposite gender (Yosef, 2004). In India, it is common for women to bare their midriff, but in village society in many parts of the country, baring the shoulders is considered indecent. Similarly, the head is considered sacred in many Asian cultures (Purnell & Paulanka, 2005), and touching the head of another may be considered threatening or insulting. The Roma consider the upper body to be more pure that the lower body and may take special precautions to prevent cross-contamination (e.g., using two separate bars of soap for bathing, covering the legs completely, and cleansing the body in the shower rather than a bath) (Vivian & Dundes, 2004).

Clothing and exposure of different body parts is an area of culture that may show drastic change. It was not so very long ago that women wore floor-length skirts, and to show even as much as an ankle was considered "fast" behavior in the dominant U.S. culture. Today, short skirts or shorts and bare legs and midriffs are common among youth in the United States and other parts of the world, but may be shocking to older people, even within the dominant culture. Among many Muslim groups, modest women are expected to be completely covered, including their hair and face.

Different ethnic cultural groups also have different attitudes toward specific physiologic functions. In many cultures, menstruating women are considered unclean and are expected to remove themselves from the flow of daily life. Among the Roma, for example, the clothing of menstruating women is washed separately from the clothing of other family members (Vivian & Dundes, 2004). In the previous century in the United States, menstruation was sometimes viewed as a time of weakness and vulnerability in the dominant culture, and women were expected to rest and not engage in strenuous activity during their menstrual periods. Today, most menstruating women continue their normal life activities. Breastfeeding, urination, defecation, and sexual activity are other bodily functions that are viewed differently by different cultural groups.

Many members of the dominant U.S. societal culture are embarrassed to see women breast-feeding in public, yet this is a commonly accepted practice in many ethnic cultural groups. Similarly, urinating, defecating, and spitting in public are practices that are generally frowned upon in "polite" U.S. society, but may be common, or even necessary, in places without private sanitation facilities. Groups may also differ with respect to the position assumed for defecation or cleansing themselves afterwards. For example, most American homes are equipped with sit-down flush toilets. Even in some areas in rural America that still use "outhouses," a seating area is provided. In other countries, such as Japan and India, even some modern toilets are designed for squatting rather than sitting. Similarly, most people in the United States would use toilet paper to cleanse themselves after urinating or defecating. This practice, however, is considered very unsanitary by those in other cultures (e.g., rural India) who wash themselves with water using the left hand. The left hand is then considered contaminated and is not used for clean activities such as eating.

Different groups also differ with respect to the types of touch that are permissible in public and who may touch whom. In the dominant U.S. culture, kissing and holding hands is permissible between men and women, but may be less so in certain settings and situations (e.g., in church). In other cultural groups, such intimate behaviors are not condoned between members of opposite genders, but may be acceptable between members of the same gender without connoting a same-sex sexual orientation.

In biomedical culture, providers usually think nothing of baring whatever body part needs to be examined or treated. Often there is scant concern for clients' modesty and the embarrassment that results. Although nurses are taught to respect clients' privacy and to protect their modesty during procedures, often the pace of the work setting leads nurses to forget these "amenities." Similarly, biomedical culture often undertakes invasive procedures (e.g., shaving the head for surgery) that may have very negative connotations in other cultures.

Perceptions of Health and Illness and Disease Causation

Cultural groups also differ in their perceptions of what constitutes health and illness and what causes disease. These perceptions derive from a group's need to devise health interventions that ensure the survival of the group (Holroyd, Twinn, & Shia, 2001). To protect or restore health, one must be able to identify health and illness and devise interventions that address their causes. Based on their perceptions of health and disease, cultural groups develop explanatory models that address causation, symptomatology, pathological processes, the course of the disease, and appropriate treatment (Gesler & Kearns, 2002). For many Asians and

some Latinos, health is a balance between the forces of yin and yang, and intervention is directed toward restoring that balance (Steefel, 2003). Many African Americans view individual health as closely linked to community and spiritual life (Becker et al., 2004). In one study, older African Americans viewed health as the ability to stay active and to participate in desired activities and functions (Walcott-McQuigg & Prohaska, 2001). Native Hawaiians may subscribe to *ola `pono*, a holistic explanatory model in which health is perceived as harmony in three domains—the physical world, social relationships, and spiritual life—and illness is the result of imbalance among them (Ka`opua, 2003). For the Roma, on the other hand, health is good luck and is manifested in increasing weight, and disease is due to impurities and filth (Vivian & Dundes, 2004).

For some groups, disease may have natural or supernatural causes (de Rios, 2002). For example, among the Navajo, dreams of the dead may be associated with illness or death due to a claim on the dreamer by a spirit (Napoli, 2002). Some gypsies, or Roma, believe that epilepsy is caused by the devil (Vivian & Dundes, 2004). Among some Japanese, disease may be perceived as punishment for one's own wrongdoing or that of one's ancestors (Avery & Bashir, 2003). Similar beliefs have been noted among other Asian groups (Wong-Kim, Sun, & DeMattos, 2003). A variety of beliefs about disease causation are seen in the dominant U.S. culture, where illness may be thought to occur as a result of exposure to cold, wrong living (e.g., drinking, sexual activity), pathogens, poor diet, and so on. In the past, in the biomedical culture, disease was perceived to have a discrete external causative agent (e.g., a microorganism, exposure to environmental carcinogens). More recently, greater attention is being given to mind–body interactions in psychoneuroimmunology and to concepts of multiple causation.

One forceful example of the variety of disease causation perceptions lies in a study of beliefs about cancer causation among different cultural groups. In this study, some Spanish-speaking and Chinese participants thought cancer was caused by eating high-temperature foods. Chinese participants also saw stress management and relaxation as having value in preventing cancer. Similarly, Russians perceived emotional control and positive thinking as protective against cancer. Somali and Spanish-speaking subjects viewed spirituality as a mediating factor in the development of cancer, and Somalis subscribed to praying for Allah's blessing as a form of cancer prevention (Paisley et al., 2002).

Cultural groups may also develop complex disease taxonomies such as the Kamba system of Kenya, which characterizes disease by causal systems, appropriate treatment system, disease characteristics, and characteristics of the victim of disease. The International Classification of Disease (ICD-9) is the biomedical culture's comparable classification system (Gesler &

Kearns, 2002). Cultural conceptions of disease causation and treatment will be discussed in more detail in the section on health care systems.

Culture-Bound Syndromes In addition to differences in definitions of health and disease, cultural groups may differ in the conditions that are recognized as illnesses by group members. Many ethnic cultural groups recognize recurrent patterns of behavior or symptoms that lie outside the biomedical system. These culturally recognized illnesses are called **culture-bound syndromes** or folk illnesses (Purnell & Paulanka, 2005). They are often unique to a given culture, although similar conditions may be seen in several cultural groups.

African Americans recognize a number of culture-bound mental illnesses, including *zar*, spirit possession characterized by shouting, weeping, laughing, singing, or hitting one's head against the wall; "falling out," a sudden collapse preceded by dizziness; or "rootwork," illness caused by a hex or sorcery (Spector, 2004). Among the Amish, folk illnesses include *abnemme*, or failure to thrive in a child, and *aagwaschse*, a condition of crying and abdominal discomfort caused by a rough buggy ride. Many Latino cultural groups recognize a variety of culture-bound illnesses such as *susto, empacho, caida de mollera*, and *mal de ojo* (evil eye) (Purnell & Paulanka, 2005). Belief in the evil eye as a cause of illness is fairly widespread and may be encountered among people of Italian, German, Greek, Iranian, Mexican, Polish, and Turkish origin and others (Hatfield, 2004; Purnell & Paulanka, 2005; Spector, 2004).

Culture-bound syndromes can be found among some Asian groups as well. *Hwa Byung, koro, Qi-gong psychotic reaction*, and *taijin kyofusho* are Asian culture-bound syndromes that result in psychiatric rather than physical symptoms (Spector, 2004). *Ch'eena* is a similar condition of sadness that may be experienced by Native Americans when they leave their homeland (Napoli, 2002), and *tosca* is a nervous disease recognized by the Roma (Vivian & Dundes, 2004). These and other culture-bound syndromes are described in Appendix B, Table B-1 ∞.

Culture-bound syndromes are not unique to ethnic cultural groups, but may also be seen in the dominant U.S. and biomedical cultures. For example, *anorexia nervosa* is a recognized illness in Western cultures, particularly in the United States, that is not seen in many other cultural groups (Flaskerud, 2000). Similarly, *herzinsuffizienz*, the most common cardiovascular diagnosis in Germany, is not recognized in many other Western cultures including France, England, and the United States (Wolpe, 2002). Herzinsuffizienz, which literally translated means "heart weakness," is a medical diagnosis that seems to incorporate a constellation of more widely recognized cardiac conditions and is related to several *International Classification of Disease (ICD)-10* codes (Herzinsuffizienz, n.d.).

Similarly, seasonal affective disorder, a form of depression recognized by the biomedical culture and believed to be caused by diminished light in winter, is not seen in some countries such as Norway that experience severe winters (Stuhlmiller, 1998). Tips for a focused assessment of biophysical factors in cultural assessment, including the type and prevalence of culture-bound syndromes, are included below.

Psychological Considerations

Areas to be considered in assessing the psychological dimension as it relates to health and culture include the importance of group versus individual goals, attitudes toward change, and attitudes toward mental health and mental illness. The importance of culture in relation to mental health is highlighted by findings that treatment programs specifically designed for certain ethnic groups have better outcomes than generalized mental health programs.

The extent of stress experienced by the cultural group also affects their health status. As we will see later, stressful interactions with the dominant culture in the form of prejudice and discrimination affect health both directly and indirectly. Members of ethnic cultural groups may also experience stress related to intergenerational

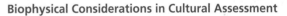

FOCUSED ASSESSMENT

Biophysical Considerations in Cultural Assessment

Maturation and Aging

- What is the age composition of the cultural group?
- What attitudes toward age and aging are prevalent in the culture? How do these attitudes affect health and health care?
- At what age are members of the culture considered adults?
- Are there cultural rituals associated with coming of age?

Genetics

- What is the gender composition of the cultural group? Are there differences in the cultural value given to one gender over the other?
- Does gender play a role in the acceptability of health care providers?
- Do members of the cultural group display genetically determined physical features or physiologic differences?
- Do group members display differences in normal physiologic values (e.g., hematocrit, height)?
- What genetically determined illnesses, if any, are prevalent in the cultural group?

Physiologic Function

- What physical health problems are common within the cultural group?
- What are the cultural attitudes to body parts and physiologic functions? How do these attitudes affect health and health care delivery?
- How do members of the cultural group define health and illness? What do they perceive as the cause(s) of disease?
- How does the cultural group classify disease?
- Does the group recognize any culture-bound syndromes? If so, what are they? What are their characteristic features?

conflict as some generations become more acculturated to the dominant culture while others attempt to retain traditional cultural orientations. Similarly, members of the gay, lesbian, bisexual, and transgender cultures may experience estrangement from family or at least diminished emotional support. Membership in the biomedical culture can itself be a source of stress given the life-and-death decisions that are sometimes required of members of this cultural group. Similarly, members of professional cultures may experience stress and frustration in situations in which they are unable to achieve desired outcomes for their clients. This stress may be exacerbated by the relative loss of control of one's own practice that has accompanied the move to managed systems of health care.

PRIMACY OF INDIVIDUAL VERSUS GROUP GOALS Cultural groups differ with respect to the priority given to individual goals versus those of the larger group, and may be characterized as either collectivist or individualist societies. Collectivist societies emphasize the good of the group, harmonious relationships, traditional values, and group loyalty. Individualist societies are characterized by the belief that people have "a right to think for themselves, to live their lives as they saw fit, and to express themselves on the basis of their own opinions" (Hillier, 2003, p. 75). Individualist societies emphasize individuality, confrontation, frankness, challenge of existing assumptions and knowledge, and personal responsibility for oneself and one's immediate family (Hillier, 2003).

The dominant U.S. culture is highly individualistic. Many traditional ethnic cultures, on the other hand, have a collectivist perspective. For example, in many Asian and Latino cultural groups, family goals take precedence over the personal goals of members. Many Native American tribal cultures are community oriented, and illness may be perceived as resulting from estrangement from the community. For these reasons, community members are important participants in many Native American healing practices.

Medicine as a culture has some elements of collectivism. For example, the previous taboo against advertising medical services and the reluctance to criticize the medical practice of others might be seen as attempts to protect the professional group. Certainly, much political activity undertaken by medical groups has collectivist underpinnings in promoting the welfare of the medical profession. Nursing, on the other hand, although also a collectivist culture, has worked more often for the benefit of the collective society than for the profession itself. A move away from individualism in medicine can also be seen in the dwindling number of independent practitioners and the expansion of group practice and managed care.

ATTITUDES TOWARD CHANGE Group attitudes toward change also influence the psychological environment and health care for members of cultural groups. The dominant U.S. culture is positively oriented toward change, which is frequently considered "progress." As we saw earlier, biomedical culture tends to vacillate between the desire for change and the tendency to stick to traditional forms of care. In the biomedical culture, change is often linked to technological advances, and more particularly, to public knowledge of and demand for care based on those advances. One of the interesting areas of change in biomedical culture that is occurring primarily in response to public demand is the incorporation of what were once considered traditional "folk" health practices, now termed complementary and alternative medicine (CAM). We will discuss CAM in more detail later in this chapter.

The culture of nursing is also characterized by a certain degree of ambiguity with respect to attitudes toward change. On the one hand, nursing is attempting to move toward evidence-based practice. On the other, many nurses are unwilling to give up practices that have no demonstrated therapeutic effectiveness or that are no longer practical in the current health care system because they learned to provide care that way. Nursing education has been criticized for its willingness to "jump on every bandwagon that comes by" but cannot agree on a single mechanism for entry into the profession. Changes in nursing education often lack a sound basis in student and societal needs and evidence of effectiveness of specific educational activities.

Ethnic cultural groups vary with respect to their eagerness to engage in change, but many tend to hold to traditional ways of doing things. Attitudes toward change also differ within cultural groups (and within professional groups, as well), based on the level of acculturation to the dominant culture.

Closely allied to group attitudes toward change are culturally based attitudes of resignation and acceptance. In many areas of the world, notably underdeveloped countries but also among the poor of the developed world, people have little access to the means to change the circumstances of their lives. Over many years or generations, people in such groups may become resigned to their condition. Widespread resignation within a cultural group can hinder health promotion and disease prevention initiatives, and may even affect willingness to seek care for existing health problems.

ATTITUDES TOWARD MENTAL HEALTH AND ILLNESS Cultural groups also differ in their definitions of what constitutes mental health and mental illness and their attitudes toward mental illness. For example, in some groups, symptoms that would be construed as mental illness in the biomedical culture are considered normal behavior or a fact of life. As we saw earlier, ethnic cultural groups may also recognize a variety of emotional conditions that are not documented in the *Diagnostic and Statistical Manual* (DSM-IV), which serves as the compendium of mental illness in the biomedical culture.

In many cultural groups, including segments of the dominant U.S. culture, mental illness carries an unpalatable stigma, leading members of the group to avoid seeking care. Mental illness may also be seen as a stigma for the family as well as for the individual involved. In one study of the mental health status of refugee women, for example, the women did not voice emotional distress except through concerns for their children, due to fears of stigma (Drennan & Joseph, 2005). Similarly, in the dominant U.S. culture, those with a history of mental illness or substance abuse may encounter difficulty with employment or election to public office, among other social effects. Among some Arabs, Vietnamese, and Haitians, mental illness may be perceived as possession by an evil spirit or failure to honor good spirits, warranting religious intervention rather than psychotherapy. Psychological distress may be concealed or expressed psychosomatically due to perceptions of stigma attached to mental illness. Other cultural groups are more tolerant of mental health problems. For example, among the Amish, children with mental health problems are expected to attend school and to receive assistance from other students and parents. Similarly, the Irish may care for mentally ill family members at home out of a sense of family solidarity, and home care may be preferred by Arab clients because hospitalization for mental illness is often considered abandonment by one's family. Stigma is not usually attached to mental illness in Italian culture, since it is believed to be caused by God. Similarly, mental impairment is readily accepted in Appalachian culture (Purnell & Paulanka, 2005).

In the dominant U.S. culture, and even in the biomedical and professional cultures, mental illness also continues to carry a stigma, although much progress has been made in this area. The degree of stigma varies with the type of condition and is less severe for problems like depression than for chronic mental health problems such as schizophrenia in which bizarre behavior may be displayed. As we have seen, factors in the psychological dimension of culture may have profound effects on the health of population groups. Tips for a focused assessment of psychological factors in cultural assessment are included at right.

Physical Environmental Considerations

Cultural groups differ in their perceptions of relationships between people and the environment. The dominant U.S. culture seeks mastery over the environment. Many traditional ethnic cultures, on the other hand, seek harmonious relationships with the external physical environment. For example, traditional African American cultural groups have often perceived a need for cooperation with a powerful natural environment in order to promote survival. Similarly, some cultural groups also view seasonal changes as directly affecting human health and behavior. Again, seasonal affective disorder is an example recognized in biomedical culture.

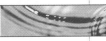

FOCUSED ASSESSMENT

Psychological Considerations in Cultural Assessment

- Does the culture have an individualist or collectivist perspective?
- How do members of the cultural group prioritize individual, family, and group welfare and goals?
- What is the extent of stress experienced by members of the cultural group? What are the usual sources of stress? How do group members typically cope with stress?
- Is there intergenerational conflict within the cultural group that contributes to stress?
- How do members of the cultural group perceive change? How do they adapt to change?
- Do members of the cultural group exhibit attitudes of resignation and fatalism? If so, what effect does this have on the use of health care services?
- What attitudes toward mental health and illness are held by members of the cultural group? Is there stigma attached to mental illness for the individual? For the family?

Other aspects of relationships to the external environment include perceptions of space and time. With respect to time, some cultural groups, such as the dominant culture in the United States and African American culture, are future oriented, whereas others are past or present oriented. Many Asian cultures, for example, attach great importance to the past and are considered past oriented. Native American and Latino groups, on the other hand, tend to be oriented to the present moment (Spector, 2004). Both past- and present-oriented cultural groups may have difficulty in long-range planning for future events.

Other perceptions related to time may also be of importance in planning nursing care for individual clients or for population groups. Care of a Muslim client, for example, may need to be planned to prevent interference with specified times for prayer (Taylor, 2004). At the group level, effective health programs targeted to Jewish clients or Seventh Day Adventists would not be scheduled on Saturday. Similarly, many cultural groups have fluid concepts of time that make appointment-based health care delivery, a biomedical cultural norm, less effective.

Cultural groups also have differing attitudes to space. Most community health nurses in the United States subscribe to European American notions of acceptable personal space in certain situations. Preferred distance between people in European American culture can be described as follows:

- Public distance: greater than 12 feet
- Social distance: 4 to 12 feet
- Personal distance: 1.5 to 4 feet
- Intimate distance: within 1.5 feet (Spector, 2004)

European Americans are frequently uncomfortable when their perceived personal space is invaded by another person. Among other cultural groups, however, there is considerable variation in what is perceived as one's personal space, leading to the potential for discomfort and conflict.

One final consideration with respect to the physical environment relates particularly to immigrant and refugee groups. The change in their physical environment may lead to a variety of health problems not encountered in their homelands. For example, the heavy traffic patterns in most U.S. cities have contributed to traffic fatalities in Hmong children whose parents are not accustomed to having to teach traffic safety. Similarly, exposure to a variety of household cleaning products common in U.S. households has led to a number of accidental poisonings among refugees. In addition, research has indicated that refugee children may experience elevated blood lead levels several months after coming to the United States due to the need to find housing in older run-down areas with a high degree of lead contamination (National Center for Environmental Health, 2005). Tips for assessing elements of the physical environmental dimension of culture as they affect health are presented below.

Sociocultural Considerations

Elements of the sociocultural dimension of health can have profound effects on health and health-related behaviors. Each cultural group has norms that govern the interaction of its members. Considerations to be addressed in assessment include relationships with the supernatural, interpersonal roles and relationships, relationships with health care providers and the larger society, socioeconomic status, and life experiences such as those related to sexuality and reproduction, coming of age, marriage, immigration, and death.

RELATIONSHIPS WITH THE SUPERNATURAL Human psychological health is often intertwined with spiritual health, particularly among many ethnic cultural groups. Even in the dominant societal culture, spiritual interventions, such as prayer, are commonly invoked in health promotion and restoration. Attitudes and behaviors with respect to the supernatural world are often exhibited in the form of religious affiliation and magical practices.

Spirituality and Religion Spirituality and religion may have profound consequences for health. Religion, or religiosity, has been defined as "organized worship involving services and structured activities" (Holt, Kyles, Wiehagen, & Casey, 2003, p. 38). Religion is a community-based activity in which the individual acts as a member of a group. Spirituality, on the other hand, is more of an individual perspective, and has been defined as a "search for meaning and purpose in life, involving a higher being, that may or may not involve religiosity" (Holt et al., 2003, p. 38).

The influences of religion and spiritual beliefs may be seen in three areas. First, specific religious beliefs or practices may influence health, either positively or negatively. Second, religious groups may be involved in the provision of health care. Finally, the type and quality of interactions between religious leaders and the health care system can profoundly influence the acceptability and use of health care services.

Both the dominant U.S. culture and many ethnic minority cultures see religion or spirituality as an important factor in health and illness. For many cultural groups, faith and prayer serve as sources of strength in

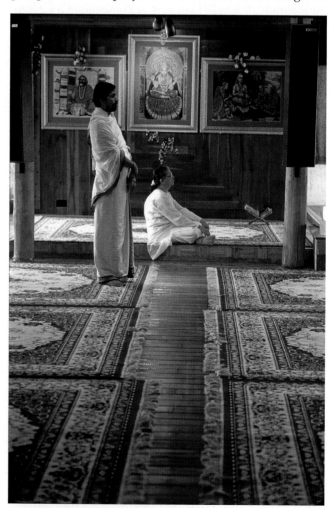

Religion is an important aspect of a group's culture.
(© David Wells / The Image Works)

FOCUSED ASSESSMENT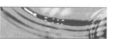

Physical Environmental Considerations in Cultural Assessment

- How do members of the cultural group perceive their relationship to the environment?
- How do members of the cultural group perceive personal space?
- What is the orientation of the cultural group to time?
- What changes in their physical environment have members of the cultural group experienced? What influence do these changes have on the health status of the group?

adversity, including ill health. In fact, in a 2004 survey, 45% of respondents reported using prayer for health reasons, and 10% had participated in prayer groups related to health (National Center for Complementary and Alternative Medicine [NCCAM], 2005a). Religion is an aspect of culture that influences health and health-related behavior and may have both positive and negative effects on health. For example, church attendance by African Americans provides avenues for social support, and prayer is seen as improving one's ability to cope with adversity (Holt et al., 2003). African American churches also function as informal service providers related to primary care, mental health, health promotion, and health policy formation, even though they often have few links to the formal health care system (Blank, Mahmood, Fox, & Guterbock, 2002). For Native Americans, health is intimately tied to interactions with the spirit world (Napoli, 2002), and Islam, the third largest religion in the United States (Esposito, 2003), provides guidance in the maintenance of health and prevention of illness. Handwashing, physical fitness, oral hygiene, moderation in diet, and prohibition of intoxicants are all health-related practices promoted by Islam (Yosef, 2004). As a practical example, the Islamic prayer ritual, practiced at daybreak, noon, midafternoon, sunset, and evening, combines elements of movement, recitation, meditation, and cleanliness (Esposito, 2003; Taylor, 2004). An example of negative health effects of religious practices lies in the use of mercury in some Afro-Caribbean religious rituals.

Religion may also deter healthful behaviors. Although *Islam* is literally interpreted as "surrender to the will of Allah, God" (Esposito, 2003), the concept of fatalism that may be engendered is actually a misinterpretation of faith teachings. Instead, Islam teaches that Allah has given people their bodies with the intent that they care for them and that part of that caring lies in promoting health (Yosef, 2004). Members of the Islamic faith are not alone in sometimes perceiving health promotion activities as violating the will of God. For example, many Latinos also see illness as ordained by God (Domian, 2001) and may not seek care for that reason. Similarly, members of the Netherlands Reformed Church and the Reformed Congregation of North American Dutch, among other religious groups, view immunization as challenging God's will and disease as the result of sinful behavior (Kulig et al., 2002).

In the dominant U.S. culture, religion and spirituality are perceived by many as influencing health. For example, many U.S. Roman Catholics engage in prayer to saints specifically associated with illness, pilgrimage to shrines within and outside the United States, and charismatic healing. Other faith groups also believe in principles of prayer, anointing of the sick, and faith healing. Religious approaches to healing in various faith traditions can be grouped into four categories: spiritual healing, inner healing, physical healing, and deliverance

or exorcism. Spiritual healing addresses illness of the spirit due to personal sin and involves repentance and forgiveness. Inner healing is used for emotional illness and seeks to heal one's memories. Physical healing is employed for physical disease or injury and usually involves prayer and laying-on of hands. Finally, exorcism is used when disease is perceived to be the result of possession by evil spirits (Spector, 2004).

Biomedical culture tends to separate health care and religion or spirituality as distinct and unrelated fields, despite evidence that religious practices may enhance well-being. For example, studies in the general U.S. population have indicated that religious attendance is associated with improvement of functional disability, an outcome that has been called "religious coping." Similarly, people with mobility limitations have been shown to engage in prayer as a form of intervention more often than those without limitations (Hendershot, 2003). Religious participation has also been linked to better overall health (Gesler & Kearns, 2002).

Magic   Religion and magic are closely intertwined in many cultures. Distinctions between the two are based on the agent of action. Religion is viewed as supplicative; the person typically conciliates personified supernatural powers, requesting specific action on their part. For example, a particular client may make an offering to gods or spirits or pray for a cure for his or her illness or relief from suffering. Magic, on the other hand, is considered manipulative. In using magic, an individual manipulates impersonal powers to achieve a desired result (Watson, 1998). Beliefs in magic as a means of causing or curing disease are common in many traditional ethnic cultures, including African American, Italian, Native American, and Latino groups (Spector, 2004).

ROLES AND RELATIONSHIPS   Culturally defined roles and relationships are learned first within the family, and may differ by family type, age, and gender. The predominant family form in U.S. societal culture remains the two-parent nuclear household, with loose relationships with kin in both parents' families of origin. As we will see in Chapter 14∞, however, this family form is being supplanted by a variety of other family forms, including single-parent families, nuclear dyads, extended families, and cohabiting couples. In many ethnic cultural groups, the extended family remains the predominant family type, but in many countries this is changing as younger family members move away from the family of origin in search of employment opportunities.

Roles within the family are frequently defined by age, gender, and family position. In the traditional U.S. culture of the past, men were considered the family providers and women were responsible for care of the home and family, except in families that were dependent on women's income to replace or supplement that of male family members. Gender role expectations in the dominant culture, however, have experienced a number of changes due to the number of women living alone and those who have never been married, more single-parent households, more out-of-wedlock births, and older age at marriage and childbearing (Hillier, 2003). In addition, with many women now in the workforce, by choice or out of necessity, family roles are less stringently delineated along the lines of gender.

In many traditional ethnic cultures, on the other hand, gender roles are more specifically defined. Men are often considered the head of the family and the primary decision maker on major family issues. For example, in traditional Afghan families, the father, oldest son, or an older uncle serves as the family spokesperson. Women have authority for decisions within the home (Giger & Davidhizar, 2002), but in some cultures these are also the province of male family members. In other ethnic cultural groups (e.g., some Native American tribes), women are the primary decision makers. Although Muslim women are expected to be subservient to men, men have a reciprocal responsibility to provide for all dependent females (even divorced wives). Muslim women who work outside the home retain their earnings as personal wealth, although many choose to spend this money on family needs (Taylor, 2004).

Asian Indian women's traditional role is defined in terms of childbearing. They are expected to give selflessly to their families and to put the needs of other family members before their own (Choudry et al., 2002). Similarly, in many Chinese families, the power of women lies in their ability to conceive and perpetuate the male line. They are expected to be obedient and unassuming and to follow the practice of *sam shung* (thrice obeying: father, husband, and son) (Holroyd et al., 2001). In traditional Latino families, parents are seen as the caretakers and educators of their children, and only other family members are acceptable substitutes as caretakers (Domian, 2001). Gender roles may also entail strict separation of men from women except within the immediate family, as occurs in many Muslim groups (Esposito, 2003).

Age may also play a role in family decision making. For example, in most cultural groups, including the dominant U.S. culture, parents often make decisions related to their children. In the dominant culture, however, adolescents are often given more decision latitude regarding their own behavior than their counterparts in other cultural groups. Among the Roma, medical decisions for a wife are often made by her husband's parents rather than by her husband or herself. The husband's mother also makes decisions regarding her son's children since children are considered to belong to the husband's family. For this reason, the consent of the grandmother, rather than the mother, may be critical to health promotion decisions such as those related to immunization (Vivian & Dundes, 2004).

Children in many ethnic cultural groups are expected to respect and obey their parents without question (Giger & Davidhizar, 2002). Children in the dominant U.S. culture, however, are generally given more latitude to question parents' decisions or the rationale for those decisions. As we saw earlier, the dominant culture is youth oriented, and the elderly are not as well respected as may be the case in many ethnic cultural groups.

Age and gender also influence roles within the biomedical and health professional cultures. Traditionally, as a largely female profession, nurses were expected to be subservient to physicians, and only recently have nurses begun to be respected as equally expert providers of care. An interesting twist to this hierarchy is seen in the military health care culture, where respect and authority are based on rank, not professional affiliation. The influence of age in the biomedical and professional cultures is less forthright. Older professionals have greater experience than their younger counterparts, but in many instances, this advantage is offset by better education among younger practitioners.

Appropriate Demeanor Roles and positions within a cultural group, as well as directives for general interpersonal behavior, lead to rules regarding appropriate and inappropriate demeanor within the group. Behaviors acceptable in one culture are not necessarily acceptable in another. For example, looking someone in the eye is considered forthright and honest in most segments of the dominant U.S. culture, but would be considered rude or threatening in other cultural groups. Community health nurses need to consider how their typical behaviors are perceived by clients as well as how clients' behavior should be interpreted. Community health nurses should be aware of and validate their interpretations of client behavior. They must also recognize that clients are using a similar process to assign meaning to the behavior of the nurse. Therefore, it is important to understand the usual meaning of a given behavior in the client's culture to avoid misunderstanding or giving offense. Appendix B, Table B-2∞ presents examples of acceptable and unacceptable behaviors for several ethnic cultural groups.

There are similar behavioral expectations in the biomedical and professional cultures. Some of these may make it difficult for clients from other cultural groups to interact effectively with health care professionals. For example, Western psychotherapy relies on clients gaining insight into their own behaviors. Many Asian clients, on the other hand, expect health care providers to be authoritative and direct them in what to do to resolve their health problems rather than guide them in introspection. Similarly, physicians may have expectations of nurses' demeanor in their interactions with them, and vice versa, that complicate interdisciplinary communication and interactions.

Communication Communication plays a significant role in one's interaction with other members of one's own culture and with those of other cultures. In assessing cultures, community health nurses attend to all types of communication, including oral and written communication, the language spoken, forms of nonverbal communication, speed of speech and intonation, slang, and culturally inappropriate words, phrases, and topics (Batts, 2002).

The language spoken by members of ethnic cultural groups and group members' facility with the language of the dominant culture will affect intercultural interactions, particularly as they influence health. Differences in dialects among cultural groups may also impede communication. In the United States, 46 million people do not speak English, and another 21 million do not speak it well. Non-English-speakers have been found to be less likely to have a regular source of health care or to get preventive care (Jacobs, Shepard, Suaya, & Stone, 2004). Ideally, health care providers should be able to speak a client's native tongue, but this is not always possible or practical. In such cases, interpreters or other linguistic services may be needed to assist with communication.

Linguistic services generally consist of four components: oral services, interpretation services, written services, and translation services (Batts, 2002). Interpretation services are used in the context of oral communication. Interpretation is not a word-for-word rendering of what is said, but involves conveying meaning-for-meaning. Translation, on the other hand, is the rendering of the written word in another language (Partnership for the Public's Health, n.d.). Interpretation services are not always available in many health care settings due to their cost (approximately $35 per visit), yet research has shown that clients who receive interpretation services made more visits to providers, received more preventive services, and were given more prescriptions than those who needed, but did not receive, interpretation services. It is hypothesized that ultimate health care costs may be decreased enough, due to prevention and earlier intervention, to warrant the added cost of interpretation services.

Approaches to interpretation in health care settings range from the ideal of bilingual and bicultural providers to using family members as interpreters. Unfortunately, the lack of qualified bicultural providers and the cultural diversity encountered in many health care settings often prohibits this solution to problems of interpretation. Even when providers speak the same language as the client, there may be difficulties related to dialect or socioeconomic status that make communication difficult. Health care agencies may also employ other bilingual staff who serve as interpreters. This approach is most effective, but also most costly, when staff are used exclusively for interpretation rather than being pulled away from other responsibilities to provide interpretation services. Another option is the use of outside interpreters or telephone interpretation. These approaches usually need to be arranged in advance and so are not particularly useful in emergency situations. In addition, these services tend to be expensive, and the interpreter may not be conversant with medical terminology. Telephone interpretation also has the disadvantage of the loss of communication through body language. Family members should be a last resort in meeting interpretation needs. Use of family members to interpret runs the risk of violating client confidentiality

Advocacy in Action

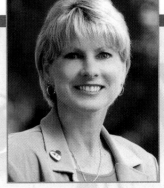

Learning English

Maria was a young Hispanic woman who came to the United States from Mexico. She had a 10-year-old son who was being raised by her mother back in Mexico and whom she had not seen in 5 years. Maria was working two jobs, earning minimum wage, in order to send money to her mother in Mexico, where she said the living conditions were very bad. Because she was undocumented, she had no health insurance. The area clinic that provides care to the working poor had reached its quota of Spanish-speaking patients. Maria came to the Nurses Center at St. Agnes because she was very tired and feeling sick. She was eventually diagnosed with severe renal disease.

A nurse practitioner at the center initiated a referral to an agency that cared primarily for Spanish-speaking individuals and provided the comprehensive care Maria needed. Maria did not have a car and did not speak English. One of the community health nurses at the center contacted the clinic, made Maria's appointment, facilitated the development of a payment plan for services, and drove her to her appointments. The nurse did not speak Spanish, so she began listening to tapes in order to teach herself. On their rides to the clinic over nearly a year, Maria and the nurse would teach each other their languages. Maria received the care that she needed, developed a beginning understanding of English, and began to network with other members of the Hispanic community.

Maryanne Lieb, RN, MSN
Director, Nurses Center at St. Agnes
Clinical Professor, Villanova University

and creates the potential for family conflict or other adverse effects (Batts, 2002). Tips for assessing the need for interpretation services with a particular client are provided below.

Interpretation and translation are usually considered in terms of communication between providers and members of ethnic cultural groups. It is wise to keep in mind, however, that both interpretation and translation may be required to render biomedical terminology intelligible to clients and other members of the lay public. U.S. statistics indicate that 20% of adults and 40% of those over age 65 years and members of ethnic minority groups read at or below a 5th grade level. In addition, the average reading level of all U.S. adults is at the 8th to 9th grade. Most health education materials, on the other hand, are written at a 10th grade level or higher (Doak & Doak, n.d.). There may also be difficulties in communication within the biomedical culture itself due to the different languages employed by many health care disciplines. For example, how well do members of other disciplines understand the language of nursing diagnosis?

In addition to the words used, paralanguage variations may be important in communication between cultures. *Paralanguage* includes the tone of voice, volume, and inflection typically used in verbal communication (Purnell & Paulanka, 2005). For example, many Afghanis tend to use a loud volume for urgent messages and repeat messages for emphasis (Giger & Davidhizar, 2002). Many African American clients may routinely use a louder voice and more rapid speech in ordinary conversation than some other cultural groups. In contrast, in the dominant U.S. culture, a loud voice may convey an emergency but may also be interpreted as anger. Inflections also signal meaning in conversation. For example, in English, a question is indicated with an upswing in tone at the end of the sentence. In other languages, such as Marathi, an Asian Indian language, questions may be indicated by appending a word to the end of the sentence or by means of an interrogative word at the beginning of the sentence (similar to English).

Nonverbal communication also varies among cultural groups. For example, hospitalized Filipino clients may expect nurses to evaluate their level of pain based on nonverbal cues such as grimacing and moaning. Failure to do so may be interpreted as a lack of concern for the client (Pasco, Morse, & Olson, 2004). Gestures are another element of nonverbal communication that may differ among cultural groups. For example, when you want someone to come closer to you in the dominant U.S. culture, you might crook your finger. In India, on the other hand, you would use a sweeping motion of the fingers toward you with the hand held prone. In yet other cultures (e.g., among some Vietnamese), beckoning in any form is considered rude.

Another aspect of communication to be considered in a cultural assessment is the level of prescribed reticence within the group—the extent to which people are expected or willing to share private information. In the dominant U.S. culture, it is not uncommon for people to tell much of their life story during a chance encounter in the grocery store. Yet there are certain things that one does not ask. For example, it would be considered rude to ask a chance acquaintance how much money they make or whether they are sexually active. Yet these kinds of questions are routinely asked by health care professionals and may insult even members of the dominant culture if the reason for them is not carefully explained. Among many other cultural groups, there may be even greater reluctance to provide personal or family information, particularly when it relates to emotions.

RELATIONSHIPS WITH HEALTH CARE PROVIDERS Another aspect of the sociocultural dimension as it affects health is expectations of interactions between clients and health care providers. In many ethnic cultural groups, as well as in the dominant U.S. and biomedical cultures, the provider is seen as dominant and the client as subordinate (Holroyd et al., 2001). In some respects, this expectation is changing as many members of the dominant U.S. culture gain knowledge of health-related matters from the Internet and are exposed to marketing initiatives by health-related vendors such as pharmaceutical companies.

Many Native Americans and members of other cultural groups expect providers to spend time in casual conversation or even to share meals before addressing intimate health issues. Providers working with Native Americans may need to be comfortable with self-disclosure and participation in tribal ceremonies in order to establish trusting relationships (Napoli, 2002). In the biomedical culture, however, the focus is on obtaining health-related information rather than on observing social amenities. Similarly, health care providers are taught to withhold personal information, which may make it difficult for clients from other cultural groups to develop a trusting relationship. Among

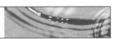

FOCUSED ASSESSMENT

Assessing Interpretation Needs

- What language does the client speak in the home?
- How long has the client been speaking the language of the dominant culture?
- What is the client's level of literacy in the language of origin? In the language of the dominant culture?
- What types of things does the client read in each language?
- When does the client prefer an interpreter?
- Can the client rephrase instructions to staff in the language of the dominant culture?

Data from: McLaurin, J. A. (2002). Assimilation, acculturation, and alternative medicines. MCN Streamline: The Migrant Health News Source, 8(6), 1–3.

Filipino clients, for example, there may be an expectation that relationships with health care providers move from the provider being considered *ibang tao* (not one of us) to *hindi ibang tao* (one of us), and that until such a trust relationship has been developed, clients may not directly communicate their needs to providers, but may prefer to have their needs communicated by family members (Pasco et al., 2004).

RELATIONSHIPS WITH THE LARGER SOCIETY The relationship between ethnic cultural groups and the dominant society may also have significant effects on health status. Many people in the dominant U.S. culture display **xenophobia**, an irrational fear of strangers (Spector, 2004), particularly those who are significantly different from oneself in appearance or behavior. When this fear centers on those of different sexual orientations, it is termed *homophobia*. Xenophobia, homophobia, and other negative reactions to persons of another cultural group may lead to racism, prejudice, and discrimination. **Racism** is the belief that people can be classified on the basis of biophysical traits into groups that differ in terms of mental, physical, and ethical capabilities, with some groups being intrinsically superior or inferior to other groups. **Prejudice** is the holding of negative attitudes or feelings toward members of another group. It is an internal perspective, and may or may not be acted upon. **Discrimination**, on the other hand, is a behavioral demonstration of racism or prejudice involving differential treatment of an individual or group based on unfavorable attitudes toward the group.

Discrimination has been shown to have negative effects on health through both direct and indirect mechanisms. Discrimination by health care providers leads to inappropriate and ineffective care. Discrimination may be seen in response to members of ethnic cultural groups, but also in response to other individuals as well. For example, gay, lesbian, bisexual, and transgender individuals report significant discrimination against them by members of the dominant U.S. society, as well as among health care providers. Discrimination may have indirect effects in terms of willingness to seek health care services or via the stress caused by exposure to culturally related discrimination or harassment. For example, lifetime experiences in five interpersonal domains (work, getting a job, school, health care, and service in a store or restaurant) has been associated with preterm labor and low-birth-weight infants among African American women, suggesting a cumulative effect of discriminatory experiences (Collins, David, Handler, Wall, & Andes, 2004; Mustillo et al., 2004).

Response to negative experiences with the larger society can also have adverse influences on health. For example, in one study, preschool children of parents who denied experiencing racism reported higher levels of problem behaviors. Conversely, the children of parents who took action through confrontation experienced

less anxiety and depression. Similarly, research has indicated an association between racial harassment and tobacco use among African American young adults, with those reporting harassment more than twice as likely as those who do not to engage in tobacco use (Bennet, Wolin, Robinson, Fowler, & Edwards, 2005). These findings were consistent with a larger body of research on the effects of discrimination on mental and physical health status among adults (Caughy, O'Campo, & Muntaner, 2004).

Members of the biomedical culture also experience different relationships with the larger societal culture. In most ethnic cultures and in the dominant U.S. culture, health care providers are held in high esteem by the society in which they function. In the dominant U.S. culture, this can be seen in the incomes of physicians and in the trust placed in nurses. Nursing has not always been as highly valued as a profession, however. In the early days of the history of modern nursing, for example, nursing was seen as an occupation of lower-class women that most families would not want to see their daughters enter. This was also true on the Indian subcontinent as little as 30 years ago and may still be true in some parts of the world. Even in cultures in which nursing is esteemed, the profession may not be valued as highly as medicine. Although the status of nursing is changing within the biomedical culture, nursing has not usually been as highly valued as medicine and some other health professional disciplines. In fact, nursing is still viewed in some settings and by some members of other professional disciplines as a handmaiden group.

SOCIOECONOMIC STATUS The socioeconomic status of a cultural group also influences its health status. Generally speaking, most members of the biomedical culture are of relatively high socioeconomic status. Even within this group, however, there is considerable variation, with physicians and dentists more often included in the upper to upper middle class and nursing and other health care disciplines considered to be middle- to lower-middle-class occupations. Members of many ethnic minority groups in the United States, on the other hand, tend to have relatively low socioeconomic status, but even that status varies among groups. For example, Cambodians and Vietnamese tend to have lower education and income levels than other Asian groups or the general U.S. population (Division of Adult and Community Health, 2004).

Income, education, and the resulting lower socioeconomic status are some of the major contributing factors in health disparities noted in the United States. For example, American Indian and Alaska Native populations have been found to have worse outcomes for all of the health behaviors measured in the Behavioral Risk Factor Surveillance System (BRFSS) (Denny, Holtzman, & Cobb, 2003). Similarly, late diagnosis of cancer occurs more frequently in minority populations than in the general U.S. population (Wong-Kim et al., 2003). Health disparities are particularly prevalent among immigrant and refugee populations, who tend to have lower education and economic levels than the general population (Kogut, 2004). Chapter 8∞ presented a general discussion of poverty and health insurance and their influence on health disparities. Specific health disparities and their underlying causes are discussed in relevant chapters throughout this book.

LIFE EXPERIENCES Cultural groups may differ significantly in the ways they address life experiences common to human existence. Although all cultural groups deal with these common life experiences, cultural beliefs and behaviors related to them can vary considerably. Life experiences that will be addressed here include experiences related to sexuality and reproduction, coming of age, marriage, death, and immigration.

Sexuality and Reproduction Different cultures have differing perspectives on and attitudes toward human sexuality and sexual activity. Some groups (e.g., fundamentalist Muslims and Christians) perceive sexual activity as inherently sinful and to be tolerated only within the bounds of marriage (Yosef, 2004). Other groups are more tolerant of sexual activity outside of marriage, but may differ in terms of their application of this norm to men and women. For example, among Latinos, extramarital sexual activity is accepted for men but not women. "Good" women are not sexually experienced or knowledgeable and may not be willing to discuss sexual issues with their partners for fear of being thought prostitutes. These cultural attitudes place Latinas at risk for sexually transmitted diseases and cervical cancer since sexual beliefs have been found to influence willingness to obtain Pap smears. Similarly, discussion of sexual matters is inappropriate in traditional Chinese culture, and women who express curiosity or knowledge of sexual matters may be considered *ahm suup*, a derogatory term meaning inappropriately sexual. Such attitudes may also lead Chinese women to forgo Pap smears because to request them would be seen as socially inappropriate (Holroyd et al., 2001).

Attitudes toward homosexuality are another area that should be explored by the community health nurse engaged in a cultural assessment of a group of people. Homosexuality may be defined and perceived differently in some cultures than in the dominant U.S. culture. For example, Cuban men may perceive same-sex encounters as evidence of virility, but a gay lifestyle is usually stigmatized. Muslims and traditional Christians and Jews generally consider homosexuality sinful. In some Asian cultures, homosexuality can be viewed as expressing disdain for societal norms that include expectations for marriage and children and brings shame to the family of the homosexual individual. China and Iran are particularly repressive of homosexual behavior, and such attitudes may accompany recent immigrants (Purnell & Paulanka, 2005).

Cultural groups also vary with respect to attitudes and behaviors related to contraception. In societies where childbearing is an expectation, contraception is not approved and abortion is not to be considered. Nonetheless, even in these cultures, there may be a variety of methods employed to induce abortion, some of which can be extremely dangerous. For example, poisoning with pennyroyal, a common abortifacient that is highly toxic, occurs periodically in the United States and Britain. Other common abortifacients include gin with juniper (known by the name *bastard killer* in Tudor England) and raspberry leaf tea (Hatfield, 2004).

Many ethnic cultural groups also engage in a variety of behaviors designed to prevent conception, some of which are based on traditional explanatory models for conception. For example, some African Americans believe that one is more apt to get pregnant if one has intercourse during menses and is "safe" at midcycle or that it is impossible to become pregnant until one has had a menstrual period following delivery of a baby. This latter belief may also be seen among some Italians (Purnell & Paulanka, 2005) and members of other cultural groups. Members of cultural groups may also engage in a variety of behaviors to promote conception. Selected cultural beliefs and behaviors related to menstruation, conception, and contraception are presented in Appendix B, Table B-3∞.

All cultural groups have prescribed and proscribed behaviors to be performed when pregnancy does occur, as well as during labor and delivery. Some authors have noted the relatively positive birth outcomes among immigrant women, particularly Latinas, compared to other low-income women, suggesting that healthful behaviors and social support arising out of cultural beliefs about pregnancy should be emulated by other groups. This advantage seems to be lost with increasing acculturation to the dominant U.S. culture (McGlade, Saha, & Dahlstrom, 2004).

Birth rituals, which occur in some form in all cultures, "convey symbolic messages that speak of a culture's most deeply held values and beliefs" (Hillier, 2003, p. 8). Birthing systems usually prescribe a specific locale for the birth event to take place, as well as specific practices to be employed. Generally speaking, the technocratic society of the United States and other developed nations advocates birth in a specialized locale, usually a delivery room within a hospital setting. Some authors have noted that this locale is designed to make the birth easy for the birth attendants rather than the mother and is intended to promote organizational efficiency (Hillier, 2003). The second locale specified for births is the woman's local sphere. In many ethnic cultural groups, this is the home. For others (e.g., the Roma), birth should take place outside of the home because it is an unclean event and would contaminate the home (Vivian & Dundes, 2004).

Cultural groups also forbid some practices during pregnancy and engage in a number of others to promote a positive pregnancy outcome. For example, Chinese women may perceive pregnancy as a hot condition and, thus, refuse prenatal vitamins, a hot medication. In Malaysia, one part of the role of the traditional midwife is to instruct the pregnant woman on the cultural taboos to be observed. In addition, the midwives supervise a variety of precautionary measures, "roast" the body to replenish the heat lost during delivery, and engage in postpartum massage (Hillier, 2003). Another example of an ethnic cultural birthing practice is the use of dates by women of Islamic heritage to strengthen uterine contractions during labor (Elgindy, 2005).

Biomedical culture is not exempt from birthing rituals, many of which have little scientific basis or evidence of effectiveness. For example, the practice of performing an episiotomy to keep the perineum from tearing has no scientific evidence of its efficacy and may be a function of the dominant U.S. cultural value for trying to speed up a natural process. Similarly, the routine practices of fetal monitoring and giving an enema prior to delivery have not demonstrated any difference in pregnancy outcomes (Hillier, 2003). Selected cultural beliefs and behaviors related to the perinatal period are presented in Appendix B, Table B-4∞.

Coming of Age   Some ethnic cultural groups have specific ceremonies that mark the movement of children into adulthood. For Jewish children, for example, the *bar mitzvah* for boys and the *bat mitzvah* for girls mark their entry into adult life. Similarly, in the southern United States, some groups still hold debutante parties as a rite of passage for young girls. Initiation of dating may be seen as a coming-of-age ritual in some segments of the dominant U.S. culture. In rural India, this change is typically signaled by a change in female clothing from a short dress or skirt and blouse to the traditional sari.

Female genital mutilation (FGM) is an extreme coming-of-age ritual for young girls in some cultural and religious groups in which portions of the female genitalia (clitoris and possibly the labia) are excised to promote chastity. Some authors suggest that immigrant women may be at greater risk for FGM in resettlement areas than in their country of origin due to attempts by the group to maintain their cultural identity. Although FGM is illegal in the United States and other countries, it does still occur. Community health nurses should be alert to the possible practice of FGM in client populations with whom they work because of the serious physical and psychological health effects, including infection and difficulties with fertility, pregnancy, and delivery.

Marriage   Typical age at marriage, who is considered an appropriate marriage partner, how marriages are contrived, and the roles and rights of the partners in marriage are some of the issues that may affect health. In cultural groups where marriage takes place soon after a woman's

You are a community health nurse working with clients in a predominantly Asian Indian community. In India, young children are frequently given the responsibility of watching even younger siblings while parents work, and it is not uncommon to find an 8-year-old girl supervising two or three younger children. In your community, both parents in most Indian families work in order to meet the high cost of living, and you have encountered a number of children under the age of 10 left home alone with younger siblings. Your nursing supervisor recently issued a directive indicating that such incidents are to be reported to the local Child Protective Services as child neglect and endangerment. What will you do about this situation?

first menstrual period, the potential for complications of pregnancy increase. Conversely, in the dominant U.S. society, marriage is occurring at later ages, and women may be nearing the end of their childbearing years when a first pregnancy occurs, which may also increase the risk of adverse maternal and infant outcomes.

Who is considered an appropriate spouse within the cultural group is also a consideration. In some societies, excessive consanguinity may result in a high prevalence of genetically determined diseases (Giger & Davidhizar, 2002). In others, marriage to an "outsider" is not considered acceptable and may cause significant stress for the couple and their children. Finally, the nurse should consider the attitude of the cultural groups to same-sex couples. In the dominant U.S. culture, for instance, this is a current issue that is being hotly debated, and cultural attitudes and family reactions to same-sex couples have been shown to create increased stress on the marriage and for the participants.

In the dominant U.S. culture, most marriages are "love matches," but in other parts of the world and in some ethnic groups within the United States, marriages may still be arranged by parents. Such marriages do not create negative health effects unless one party or the other resents being forced to marry, which may lead to individual as well as family stress. Pressure to marry may also occur in some groups when a girl becomes pregnant out-of-wedlock, although such pressure is less likely to occur today with the increasing number of single-parent families. Cultural attitudes toward divorce may also lead to stigma for couples who become divorced. Although this is not usually a problem in the dominant U.S. culture today, it may create family conflict in cultural groups that have a more traditional concept of the permanence of marriage.

Finally, one would assess the roles and responsibilities expected of marital partners within the cultural group. Is the wife expected to be subservient to her husband? Is she allowed to own property in her own right? What are either partner's rights in the event of abuse? Answers to all of these questions have implications for the physical and emotional health of the couple as well as other family members.

MediaLink   Appendix B: Cultural Influences on Health and Health-related Behaviors

Death All cultural groups have beliefs and practices related to death and dying that may vary considerably from those of other groups. Culture influences attitudes toward death and dying in a number of ways. One area of influence is the need for comfort experienced by the dying client. In those cultures in which death is seen as a normal part of life, there may be less need to comfort the dying and his or her family; conversely, in cultures in which death is feared, comfort may be needed and appreciated. Members of the biomedical culture, because of their focus on cure and promoting longevity, tend not to deal well with the concept of death and may need assistance in dealing with the death of a client or a loved one. They may also need to be encouraged to accede to clients' requests to die with dignity and without heroic lifesaving measures.

The community health nurse should assess whether those he or she is dealing with have a cultural belief in an afterlife. Some non-Western religions, including Hinduism, believe in reincarnation until the soul has achieved perfection and passes to Nirvana. Do religious beliefs regarding death and afterlife offer a source of comfort to clients and families, or do they engender fear and anxiety?

Culture also influences the selection and perception of health care providers when death is imminent. People from some cultures, including a growing body of mainstream Americans, believe that death should occur at home and are therefore unlikely to seek medical care for a dying client for fear that he or she will be removed from the home and placed in a hospital to die. For many people, going to the hospital means that death is inevitable. For example, Asian, Native American, African American, and Appalachian clients may equate hospitalization with imminent death.

Care of the body following death, and funeral and burial practices, are also influenced by culture, as are expectations regarding grief and mourning and practices to be observed during this period. Mourning is a cultural expression of grief following death, and mourning practices may vary from group to group.

Finally, culture influences communication regarding death, particularly with respect to children and their knowledge of and participation in the rites that accompany a death. For example, for African Americans on the Sea Islands, preparation for death involves holding a "prewake" for several months before an anticipated death, during which friends and family discuss the person's life and contributions to society (Blake, 1998). Appalachians are usually quite open in their communication about death, and Native American and Latino children may help with the care of the dying family member and participate in funeral and grieving practices. Despite this participation, members of many cultural groups may resist telling the client or others regarding imminent death (Purnell & Paulanka, 2005).

Similarly, some cultural groups may resist the discussion or use of advance directives for fear that such a discussion implies a belief that death is near and may cause the ill client to lose hope. For these groups, discussion of death is avoided. Use of advance directives may also be resisted in some cultures because of a perceived lack of need for them. For example, among African Americans, the family usually makes end-of-life decisions (Purnell & Paulanka, 2005).

Other questions relate to who should attend the dying client. The eldest son of a Chinese client is often expected to be present with his dying parent, whereas in some Native American tribes, the maternal aunt is the more important figure. Some members of other tribes believe that the spirit cannot leave the body until family members are present.

Nurses should be familiar with the death rites of specific cultural groups so they can assist the family through their time of grief. Should the nurse wash and prepare the body, or is a family member responsible for this? Should personal belongings be left with the body or given to the family? The nurse should learn the answers to such questions when working with clients from other cultures. Death rites and the presence of family members may violate institutional policies in some health care settings, and nurses may need to function as advocates for culturally competent care in these instances.

Members of many Native American tribes see the body as a "seed to be planted" and believe that the body must be disposed of in its entirety. Thus, family members may request amputated limbs to be kept until death and disposal of the body. They may also resist having an autopsy performed. Resistance to autopsy may also be noted among the Roma, who believe all body parts must be present for the soul to retrace its steps in the first year after death (Vivian & Dundes, 2004). Autopsy may also be resisted by members of some Orthodox Jewish and Christian groups. In a similar vein, some Native Americans may request the return of hair or nail clippings from hospitalized clients to prevent their use by witches. Disposal of the body can vary among tribes and may include burning, burial, or exposure to the elements.

Mourning can be very emotional in some cultural groups (Vivian & Dundes, 2004) and very subdued in others and may last for varying periods of time. For instance, following four days of mourning, the Cheyenne and Quechan cease grieving, as do members of some other tribes. In some tribes, the name of the deceased is never spoken again, and memory of the deceased is actively suppressed. Among Hmong clans, mourning may last until the following New Year celebration (which usually occurs in late December).

Clothing may assume special meanings in relationship to death. The clothing of a deceased Chinese person, for instance, is believed to contain evil spirits. Family members of hospitalized clients should be encouraged to take clothing home until the client is discharged. If the client should die, the family may be reluctant to accept the deceased's personal effects. Clothing is also used to symbolize mourning, and mourning garments are worn for varying lengths of time in different cultures. The color of mourning can also vary. For example, black is the color of mourning for many cultures, including the dominant U.S. culture, but among the Hmong and Vietnamese, white signifies mourning and black is worn for weddings and other celebrations.

Non-Anglo cultural groups often celebrate death in a way that is foreign to many members of the dominant U.S. culture. The dominant culture, and particularly biomedical culture, is more likely to try to defy death. In traditional African American culture, death is perceived as a passage from one realm of life to another. Funerals are generally occasions for celebration despite the grief of family members left behind. As is true in the larger society, funerals and wakes are seen as a psychosocial mechanism that facilitates grieving. Funerals for many Latinos are evidence of their deep religious belief in an afterlife. Among the Hmong, funerals are very elaborate functions that may last for several days. As we have seen, beliefs and behaviors regarding death and dying vary among different cultures. Appendix B, Table B-5∞ presents selected cultural behaviors related to death and dying.

Immigration Many members of ethnic minority groups have experienced immigration as a significant life event. Some authors distinguish among categories of immigrants as refugees, sojourners, and immigrants, who may be legal or undocumented. A **refugee** is "any person who is outside his or her country of nationality who is unable or unwilling to return to that country because of persecution or a well-founded fear of persecution" based on race, religion, or other social categorization (e.g., political affiliation) (Spector, 2004, p. 35). A **sojourner** is someone who is in a country other than the country of origin but who expects to remain there only a short time (Purnell & Paulanka, 2005). An **immigrant** is usually a permanent resident of the new host country (Spector, 2004).

In the 2000 U.S. census, there were more than 31 million immigrants in the United States. This is three times as many as resided there in 1970 and twice as many as were counted in the 1980 census. One in five children in the United States is a child of immigrant parents (Kogut, 2004). Nine percent of U.S. families with children are mixed-status families in which at least one member is a noncitizen, and 85% of immigrant families include children who are U.S. citizens. Approximately 85% of immigrants in the United States are there legally, so total numbers of immigrants may be slightly underestimated. Among undocumented immigrants, 28% enter the country legally but overstay their visa limits. Despite the national furor over the drain that immigrants, particularly undocumented immigrants, are perceived to put on social systems, a report by the National Research Council indicated that immigration generally benefits the overall U.S. economy and has little effect on job opportunities for citizens (Lillie-Blanton & Hudman, 2001).

The United States is not the only country to experience significant immigration, particularly of refugees. For example, in 2001, there were 70,000 refugees in the United Kingdom (Drennan & Joseph, 2005), and many other refugees can be found in Canada and other relatively stable countries as well as in many countries adjacent to refugees' countries of origin.

Immigrants, and particularly refugees, tend to exhibit poorer health status than the general population and are more likely to number among the working poor than the general population (Lillie-Blanton & Hudman, 2001). Many refugees arrive in the host country in relatively good health, but experience a decline in health status soon afterwards due to communicable diseases prevalent in their countries of origin, traumatic experiences that led to their status as refugees, and the experience of being a refugee itself. Refugees may be isolated from the mainstream society and have difficulty obtaining needed services due to the complexity of bureaucratic systems. In addition, they may have little trust of health care providers because of a general distrust of authorities and the misunderstandings that occur with a diversity of cultures and languages (Drennan & Joseph, 2005).

Immigrants may experience an increased risk of chronic diseases due to changes in their dietary patterns with acculturation to the host culture or the unavailability of many staple foods from their country of origin (Lockyear, 2004). When immigration is associated with trauma, pain, and suffering, there is also an increased prevalence of mental health problems. For example, an increase in the number of Chinese immigrants with depressive disorders who lacked social support was noted 10 to 12 months after arrival in the host country. Post-migration stress may be exacerbated by unemployment or underemployment and may result in depression, post-traumatic stress disorder (PTSD), alcohol abuse, and poor general health status (Fogel, 2004). Immigrants and refugees may experience varying degrees of hostility from members of the dominant culture that increase their stress. Hostility may be mutual, as exemplified in the riots among refugees in France in 2005, which were motivated by frustration with poor social and economic conditions.

In the biomedical and professional cultures, one could examine the extent of experience in working with immigrants and refugees and the comfort of members of these cultural groups in working with them. Members of these cultures may be descended from early (or more recent) immigrants to the United States, and may perceive the immigration experience through the lens of their parents or grandparents in a time when opportunities for immigrants were more obvious. They may also fail to recognize the extent of psychological trauma that may have been experienced by present-day immigrants and refugees compared to those of the past.

MediaLink · Appendix B: Cultural Influences on Health and Health-related Behaviors

Immigrant nurses and other health care providers also face challenges when they attempt to work in a foreign milieu. This occurs whether the nurse is a Peace Corps volunteer working overseas or a nurse emigrating from Canada or the Philippines to the United States. Some authors suggest that two of the most difficult issues for nurses emigrating to the United States are functioning in a litigious society and serving as a patient advocate when advocacy by nurses is not a part of their culture of origin. Many nurses from other cultural groups are not accustomed to having responsibility for identifying and correcting inappropriate or incorrect physician medication and other orders. These nurses may also have difficulty understanding the legal implications of their practice, which may be vastly different from those in their countries of origin (Priest, 2005). Similarly, the confrontational approach often required for client advocacy may be culturally foreign to nurses from other ethnic cultural groups. As we noted earlier, immigrant nurses and other health care providers may experience difficulties in becoming licensed in some highly biomedical cultures such as the United States. Tips for a focused assessment of sociocultural dimension factors in cultural assessment, including the effects of immigration, are provided below.

FOCUSED ASSESSMENT

Sociocultural Considerations in Cultural Assessment

Relationships with the Supernatural

- What are the perceptions of members of the cultural group with respect to supernatural forces?
- What roles, if any, do supernatural forces have in health and illness?
- What are the religious affiliations of members of the cultural group? What are the major tenets of the religion(s)?
- What influence does religious affiliation or spirituality have, if any, on health care beliefs and practices?
- Do religious leaders have a role with respect to health and illness within the cultural group? If so, what is that role?
- Do magical influences play a part in health and illness within the cultural group?

Roles and Relationships

- What are the gender roles expected within the cultural group?
- What roles are expected of family members in various positions (e.g., parent, child, elder)?
- What is the typical family structure within the cultural group? Has this structure changed with recent life events? If so, what are the health effects of change in family structure?
- Who is responsible for decisions within the family? Within the larger cultural group?
- What behaviors are expected in interactions with others within the cultural group? Outside the group?
- What is the primary language of the cultural group? What is the level of fluency with the language of the dominant culture among members of the group?
- What other forms of communication are employed by members of the cultural group?
- What is the level of prescribed reticence expected of members of the cultural group?

Relationships with Health Care Providers

- What do members of the cultural group expect in relationships with health care providers?
- What do providers expect in terms of relationships with clients?
- How congruent are provider and client expectations of their relationship?

Relationships with the Larger Society

- What is the quality of interaction between the larger society and members of the cultural group?

- What is the attitude of members of the dominant culture toward the cultural group? What is the attitude of members of the cultural group toward the dominant culture?
- To what extent are members of the cultural group subjected to or perceive prejudice, discrimination, hostility, or harassment?

Socioeconomic Status

- What is the attitude of members of the cultural group toward material wealth and possessions?
- What is the education level typical of members of the cultural group? What is the group's attitude toward education?
- What is the socioeconomic status typical of members of the cultural group? What effect does socioeconomic status have on health and access to health care services?

Life Experiences

- What attitudes and beliefs do members of the cultural group hold toward sexuality?
- What are the attitudes of group members toward differences in sexual orientation?
- What attitudes and practices related to conception and contraception are displayed by members of the cultural group?
- What are the attitudes, beliefs, and practices of the cultural group related to pregnancy, birth, and the postpartum period?
- Are there specific coming-of-age rituals within the cultural group? What are the health effects of these rituals and practices, if any?
- How is marriage perceived within the cultural group? At what age does marriage usually occur?
- Who is considered an appropriate spouse for a member of the cultural group? How are marriages contracted?
- What are the expected roles and responsibilities of couples? How are they expected to interact with other family members?
- What are the attitudes, beliefs, and practices of the group with respect to death?
- Is there a cultural belief in an afterlife? If so, what effect does this belief have on attitudes toward death and dying?
- What cultural practices are typical of the group in its care of dying members, mourning, and funeral rites?
- Have members of the cultural group experienced other significant life events, such as immigration? If so, was immigration voluntary or forced? What are the effects of the immigration experience on the health of group members?

Behavioral Considerations

Culturally determined lifestyle patterns and related behaviors may also influence the health status of members of a cultural group. Aspects of the behavioral dimension to be addressed in a cultural assessment include dietary practices, other consumption patterns, and other health-related behaviors.

DIETARY PRACTICES Apparel and dietary practices are some of the more obvious differences among ethnic cultural groups, with dietary practices having significant implications for health and illness. Some dietary practices have a religious basis. For example, for both Jews and Muslims, pork is eschewed on religious grounds, and both groups follow strict butchering practices. Other religiously motivated dietary practices among Muslims include not eating bloody meat and not drinking alcoholic beverages (Elgindy, 2005; Norman, 2002). Muslims also fast during the month of Ramadan, eating and drinking nothing between sunrise and sunset. Among Orthodox Jews who keep kosher, separate utensils are used for preparing meat and dairy products, and these foods are not eaten together. In addition, only mammals with cloven hooves and fish with fins and scales are eaten (Elgindy, 2005). Jains, a religious group found primarily on the Indian subcontinent, are strict vegetarians because of their beliefs in the sanctity of all life. For Jains and other cultural groups, including the dominant U.S. culture, food is a way of establishing community, particularly in a new place. Food may have religious connotations aside from specifically prescribed and proscribed foods. For instance, Southeast Asian Buddhists may make a practice of feeding monks to earn merit for themselves and their ancestors (Norman, 2002).

Among other ethnic cultural groups, food preferences and dietary practices are more a function of foods available than of religious beliefs and practices. For example, due to poverty and climate the three staple items of Southern Black diets were corn, pork, and syrup (Sharpless, 2002). As we saw earlier, immigration and acculturation to the dominant culture may have a negative effect on the healthier aspects of some traditional diets. For example, in one study, more highly acculturated Hispanic women ate more convenience foods, salty snacks, and fatty foods and fewer vegetables and fruits than their less acculturated counterparts. Similarly, several Asian groups increased consumption of dairy products, and more acculturated subjects ate more fats and sweets, bagels and pizza, and were more likely to drink soda than less acculturated women. They were also more likely to skip breakfast. Among South Korean immigrants, acculturation led to higher fat intake and consumption of more bread, cereal, spaghetti, pizza, green salads, sweets, and soda (Lockyear, 2004). In other studies, Somali, Chinese, and Spanish-speaking subjects perceived their traditional diets as compatible with scientific recommendations for fruit and vegetable consumption (Paisley et al., 2002), but Cambodians and Vietnamese were somewhat less likely to consume as many fruits and vegetables as they did in their countries of origin, perhaps because of the relatively high cost of produce in the United States (Division of Adult and Community Health, 2004).

Ethnic cultural groups are not the only ones to experience changes in dietary patterns. For example, the move from home-cooked meals to fast foods in the dominant U.S. and other cultures is widely recognized as a contributing factor in the increasing prevalence of obesity. Patterns of food consumption have also

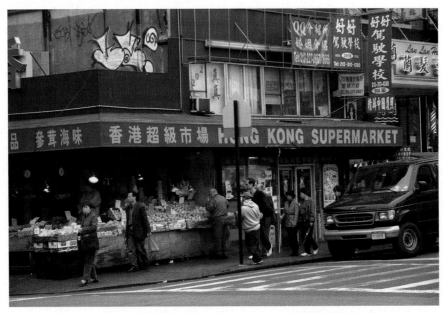

Ethnic markets support cultural food preferences. (Patrick J. Watson)

changed, with fewer meals eaten as a family group and more special family occasions celebrated with dinner in a restaurant than a celebratory home-cooked meal (Pillsbury, 2002). Generally speaking, the health impact of these and other similar changes in dietary patterns is a negative one.

In addition to considering the food preferences and meal patterns of a particular cultural group, the nurse may also want to assess the meaning of food (and specific food items) within the culture. Other considerations relate to what constitutes food for a cultural group (e.g., snails or hamburger, tomatoes or dandelion greens), who does the cooking and how, and the uses of food for specific health purposes. For example, corn is used for religious ceremonies in some Native American groups, and turkey is the traditional Thanksgiving meat in the dominant U.S. culture. With respect to cooking practices, some groups (e.g., some Asian cultures) use stir-fry methods that preserve vitamins; others (e.g., Southern U.S. Whites and Blacks) eat a lot of fried foods that increase fat intake. Still other groups may boil vegetables until vitamins are lost. Finally, some foods (for example, the classic chicken soup or Jell-O in the dominant U.S. culture), are used to promote or restore health.

OTHER CONSUMPTION PATTERNS AND HEALTH-RELATED BEHAVIORS Other consumption patterns within the cultural group are part of the behavioral dimension of a cultural assessment. Areas that the community health nurse might explore are the extent of tobacco use, alcohol consumption, attitudes toward and use of prescription and nonprescription medications, caffeine consumption, and so on. Additional considerations include use of safety precautions, leisure-time pursuits, and exercise.

As we saw in Chapter 6∞, U.S. tobacco companies have particularly targeted ethnic minority groups, immigrants, and residents of developing countries as new markets for their products. Many Asian men, for example, smoke, and Cambodian and Vietnamese men are more likely than those in other cultural groups to smoke (Division of Adult and Community Health, 2004). Cultural groups also vary with respect to physical activity. For instance, large segments of the dominant U.S. culture and many ethnic cultural groups do not engage in the recommended level of physical activity. Cultural fatalism may influence safety behaviors such as seat belt or helmet use.

Use of and attitudes toward alcohol are other areas in which cultural groups may vary. For example, French and Italian groups usually include wine with most meals, yet experience low prevalence of alcohol abuse. In other groups, however, where drinking alcohol is seen to be a sign of adulthood or manliness, alcohol abuse is more prevalent. Ease of access to controlled substances is an area of concern in the biomedical culture. Cultures also vary in their perceptions of alcohol and other substance abuse, with some cultures perceiving

it as a disease (biomedical culture) and others as a character weakness (e.g., some fundamentalist religious groups).

Another area for assessment with respect to behavioral factors influencing the health of cultural groups is the use of health-related and safety practices. Among many Hmong immigrants, for example, the use of child car seats is limited due to the number of children in the family and the cost of car seats. Members of the biomedical culture may also vary in the degree to which they engage in safety practices such as the use of gloves during routine procedures such as immunization.

Culturally determined behaviors and attitudes toward health-related behaviors can have a profound effect on a group's health status. Tips for a focused assessment of behavioral considerations in cultural assessment are included below.

Health System Considerations

Factors related to health systems also affect the health of population groups. In assessing cultural groups, one would address health system factors related to the design of health systems, health care providers, and health care practices.

HEALTH CARE SYSTEMS Considerations related to health care systems address the perceptions of members of the cultural group with respect to health care and the design and philosophical underpinnings of the

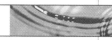

FOCUSED ASSESSMENT

Behavioral Considerations in Cultural Assessment

- What dietary practices are typical of members of the cultural group? What are the preferred foods? How are they typically prepared? Are any foods proscribed?
- Do certain foods or dietary practices (e.g., fasting) have religious significance for members of the cultural group?
- What is the effect of acculturation on dietary practices?
- What are the other consumption patterns of the cultural group (e.g., tobacco and alcohol use, caffeine consumption)?
- To what extent do members of the cultural group engage in health and safety behaviors?

health care system. Health systems may differ in their focus and their perspectives on individual responsibility for health and illness (Purnell & Paulanka, 2005). The biomedical culture and many health professional cultures focus heavily on curative practices. The dominant U.S. culture emphasizes restoration of health rather than health promotion and illness prevention, as seen in the level of funding provided for these various activities. As noted earlier, the health system in the biomedical culture is technocratic and focused on disease entities. Only recently has there been somewhat greater attention paid to health promotion and illness prevention in the biomedical culture. Health and illness tend to be seen as individual or family responsibilities, with less attention to societal factors influencing health. Illness is often seen as the result of personal behaviors over which the client has considerable control. As we saw in Chapter 4∞, it is only relatively recently that attention has been given to the effects of social determinants of health.

Many ethnic cultural health systems, on the other hand, place significant emphasis on health promotion and illness prevention. Health is viewed holistically, and in some cultural groups, health and illness may have significant implications for the group or community in terms of both cause and resolution. Naturopathy is a health system that places special emphasis on illness prevention, and therapeutic interventions in this system often focus on promoting healthy lifestyles and controlling risk factors for illness (Budrys, 2001).

Recent biomedical literature abounds with references to "alternative health systems." **Alternative health systems** are defined as health care systems that include theories, philosophies, and practices that differ from those of biomedicine or allopathic medicine

(Anumolo et al., 2004). Alternative health systems have also been referred to as *ethnomedicine* or *folk medicine* (Northridge, 2002). The Institute of Medicine (IOM) (2005) identified several alternative health systems, including:

- Ayurveda, a traditional system of the Indian subcontinent
- Homeopathy, a system based on the conception that "like cures like" and that employs small amounts of toxic substances to stimulate the body's own capacity for healing
- Mind–body medicine, which focuses on the interactions of mind and body
- Orthomolecular medicine, which employs large doses of vitamins and minerals in an effort to rebalance one's individual biochemistry
- Spiritual healing, which incorporates healing energy derived from spiritual sources
- Traditional Chinese (or Oriental) medicine (TCM), which is a complete system of diagnostic and therapeutic approaches
- Naturopathic medicine, a holistic system that supports the natural healing capacity of the person

Other alternative health care systems include Shamanism (de Rios, 2002), Christian Science, and chiropractic (Silenzio, 2002). *Ola `pono* is a traditional Hawaiian paradigm of health (Ka`opua, 2003). Each of these health care systems, including the biomedical or allopathic system, includes basic theoretical and philosophical concepts, perceptions of disease causation, and specific diagnostic and therapeutic practices. Table 9-2◆ describes salient features of some of these health care systems.

TABLE 9-2	Selected Health Care Systems
System	**Description**
Ayurveda	**Source:** India
	Basic Concepts:
	All matter is composed of five elements: ether, air, fire, water, and earth.
	Human beings are composed of body (*dhatus*—body tissues, *malas*—waste products, and *doshas*—physiologic elements) and soul (*atma*— soul or spirit, and *nana*, mood, cognition).
	Doshas are the embodiment of the five elements in the body:
	Vata dosha: composed of ether and air; controls functions of the central and sympathetic nervous systems; regulates feelings and emotions; prevalent after age 55 years
	Pitta dosha: composed of fire and water; controls heat production and metabolism, vision, skin texture; influences intellect and cheerfulness, anger, hate, and jealousy; prevalent from puberty to middle age
	Kapha dosha: composed of water and earth; influences strength, cell reproduction, memory, emotional bonding, greed, and envy; prevalent in childhood
	Individuals differ in the preponderance of each element in the body, giving rise to seven different "constitutions" that influence physical and behavioral aspects of the individual.
	Cause of Disease: Disease is caused by imbalance among elements of mind and body or ineffective functioning of one or more elements.
	Diagnosis: Diagnostic processes include observation, touch, questioning, assessment of pulses; examination of urine, stool, tongue, bodily sounds, eyes, skin, and total appearance; and assessment of digestive capacity, personal habits, and individual resilience.

Continued on next page

TABLE 9-2	Selected Health Care Systems *(continued)*	

System	Description
	Treatment: Treatment entails four types of therapies: *Shodan:* cleansing by means of five *panchakarma*: intestinal cleansing, cleansing of the stomach and duodenum, medicinal enemas, medicinal nasal oils, and, occasionally, bloodletting *Shaman:* palliation through burning toxic wastes, fasting, yoga, lying in the sun, breathing exercises, and meditation *Rasayan:* rejuvenation through herbal remedies and dietary supplements *Satwajaya:* stress reduction, mental nurturing, and spiritual healing
Biomedicine (allopathy)	**Source:** Cartesian worldview of mind–body separation
	Basic Concepts: The body functions mechanically, based on complex physical and chemical interactions and independent of the influence of the mind.
	Cause of Disease: Disease causation is perceived from a mechanistic perspective, that is, changes in structure or function of the human "machine" in response to specific factors (e.g., microorganisms, fat intake, genetics) result in disease.
	Diagnosis: Diagnosis tends to rely on symptom presentation, invasive tests, and technological processes.
	Treatment: Treatment focuses on repair or replacement of bodily processes by means of pharmaceutical, immunological, and surgical interventions.
Chinese Medicine	**Source:** Originated in China, but has spread throughout much of Asia
	Basic Concepts: The human body is composed of several vital substances: Qi (pronounced "chee") is the body's vital energy force, responsible for effective physiologic function. It forms the basis for the other bodily substances. Blood moistens and nourishes the body. Jing (essence) is a specific hereditary energy force contained in the kidney that determines constitution and regulates growth, development, and reproduction. Body fluids such as saliva, mucus, sweat, urine, and excretory fluids may be deficient or stagnant. Shen encompasses the mental, emotional, and spiritual aspects of the individual. Qi flows through a network of 12 principal meridians or channels within the body and can be adjusted through acupuncture. All life is composed of male and female aspects of yang and yin. Yin is related to the water element and has properties of moistness, coolness, and substance. Yang is related to fire and has properties of warmth, dryness, and lack of substance.
	Cause of Disease: Disease is caused by an imbalance between forces of yin and yang and among the five elements of wood, fire, earth, metal, and water. Yin/yang imbalance may be related to deficiency, stagnation, counterflow, or sinking Qi.
	Diagnosis: Diagnosis relies on two primary mechanisms: examination of the depth and quality of pulses in multiple locations, and examination of the color, shape, coating, and moistness of the tongue, which indicates the nature of imbalance between yin and yang.
	Treatment: Traditional treatments in Chinese medicine include: Acupuncture: insertion of slender needles at specific points on the meridians to influence the flow of Qi within the body Qigong: meditative movements and breathing exercises to improve the flow of Qi Herbal preparations
Chiropractic	**Source:** Roots in ancient Chinese and Greek writings; promoted in the United States with the establishment of a chiropractic professional organization by Daniel David Palmer in 1895 and the Palmer School of Chiropractic in 1897
	Basic Concepts: Natural and conservative methods are best used to promote and restore health. The human body has a vast capacity to heal itself. Adjustment and manipulation of musculoskeletal articulations, particularly in the area of the spine, and adjacent tissues can be used to treat functional disorders.
	Cause of Disease: Disease is caused by misalignment of body parts.
	Diagnosis: Based on perceptions of misalignment, may include specific measures of alignment through physical examination or X-ray.
	Treatment: Treatment focuses on manipulation of body parts.
Homeopathy	**Source:** Developed by a German allopathic physician, Samuel Hahnemann, who was disenchanted with 19th-century biomedicine
	Basic Concepts: One's vital force can promote self-healing. Stimulation of vital force promotes the body's healing response. Based on the law of similars—"like cures like"—and the law of infinitesimals—disease can be cured by use of very dilute doses of substances that are similar to the disease and would produce symptoms similar to those of the disease in a healthy person.

Continued on next page

TABLE 9-2	Selected Health Care Systems *(continued)*
System	**Description**
	Small doses of substances cure; larger doses damage the body's ability to heal itself. The smaller the dose, the more effective in healing. Hering's laws of cure: 　Healing occurs from head to foot. 　Healing occurs from internal to external. 　Healing progresses from more vital to less vital organs. 　Symptoms disappear in the reverse order of their appearance.
	Cause of Disease: Disease is caused by an imbalance or disruption in vital energy.
	Diagnosis: Diagnosis occurs by means of case taking or an interview to determine the client's problem and all symptoms experienced, and involves categorizations of the client's constitutional type.
	Treatment: Treatment is individualized and holistic, considering lifestyle as well as emotional state and other factors. Treatment involves prescription of remedies that are akin to the symptoms experienced, based on the *Materia Medica*, a compendium of remedies and their uses. Remedies may be derived from plant, mineral, or animal sources and are regulated by the FDA.
Ho`oponopono	**Source:** Hawaii
	Basic Concepts: 　*Ho`oponopono* is a traditional Hawaiian healing practice designed to restore balance in three domains: physical, social, and spiritual. 　It is used in combination with herbal treatments. 　Prayer is included at the beginning and end of the healing process and at times of particular challenge.
	Cause of Disease: Imbalance in the physical, social, or spiritual domains causes disease.
	Treatment: Treatment occurs in four stages: 　Foundation building: establishes processes for discussing sensitive topics, pools family's spiritual strengths, identifies issues of concern 　Understanding meaning: explores meaning of event to the individual and family and promotes shared feelings 　Resolution of concerns and acceptance of responsibility for one's part in them: seeking forgiveness, making amends, releasing negative emotions 　Closure: prayer and celebration of family unity in a meal (may include music)
Native American Healing	**Source:** North American tribes
	Basic Concepts: 　Health is a reflection of harmony between the individual and nature, supernatural beings, and other people. 　Body and spirit are one entity. 　Health and disease have both physical and spiritual aspects.
	Cause of Disease: Disease results from disharmony and may be caused by: 　internal factors, such as negative thinking or disturbance in life energy 　external factors, such as: 　　pathogenic forces (e.g., microorganisms, sorcery, or supernatural beings) 　　environmental poisons (e.g., pollution, alcohol abuse, poor diet) 　　traumatic physical, emotional, or spiritual events 　　breach of taboo and inharmonious relationships with nature, other people, or spiritual beings
	Diagnosis: Diagnostic approaches vary from group to group and may include hand trembling, crystal gazing, dream interpretation, divination, questioning, and observation.
	Treatment: Treatment also varies among groups, but may include prayer, music and chanting, purification rituals and ceremonies, herbs, massage, counseling, and fasting. Family and community are frequently intimately involved in healing practices.
Naturopathy	**Source:** Initiated in the United States by Benjamin Lust, a proponent of hydrotherapy
	Basic Concepts: 　The body has the ability to heal itself. 　Natural substances have healing properties. 　Treatment should encompass the whole person. 　Prevention and health promotion are important to health.
	Cause of Disease: Disease results from alterations in the mechanisms by which the body heals itself.
	Diagnosis: Diagnosis is made by history and physical examination.
	Treatment: Treatments include a variety of therapies such as nutrition, botanicals, fasting, heat, cold, exercise, counseling, and lifestyle modification.
Shamanism	**Source:** Siberia and Central and Southeast Asia. Possibly began as a religion in western China and Russia; variations also found in cultural groups in North and South America, Africa, the South Pacific, and Australia

Continued on next page

TABLE 9-2	Selected Health Care Systems *(continued)*
System	**Description**
	Basic Concepts: Shamanism distinguishes between disease and illness. Disease is a pathological state; illness is the personal experience of the victim. Health and illness result from the interventions of spirits or supernatural beings. **Cause of Disease:** Disease results from an imbalance between the individual and the spiritual world and may be due to loss of one or more of one's souls or the malignant intervention of evil spirits. **Diagnosis:** Diagnosis occurs by means of a trance during which the shaman's soul leaves the body and travels to the spirit world to seek information from the spirits responsible for the illness. **Treatment:** Treatment entails two major foci: returning power to the client (e.g., restoring a lost soul) removing harmful powers (e.g., removing the influence of evil spirits) Treatment entails intervention through trances, communication with spirit helpers to intercede on behalf of clients, and removal of "magical darts" or evil spirits (usually by sucking them out of the client's body).
Traditional African Healing	**Source:** African tribal, Native American, and White colonial practices **Basic Concepts:** Human beings are composed of body and spirit (which includes mind). The balance between hot and cold in the body is important for health. **Cause of Disease:** Disease may be caused by natural and supernatural causes or an imbalance between hot and cold. **Treatment:** Treatment varies with the identified cause of disease and may employ spiritual or magic practices, herbs and diet therapy, massage, and dermabrasive practices such as cupping, pinching, rubbing, and burning.

Data from: American Cancer Society, 2005; American Chiropractic Association, 2004a; 2004b; Anumolo, Miller, Popoola, Talley, Rushing, Huebscher, & Shuler, 2004; Budrys, 2001; de Rios, 2002; Fee, Brown, Lazarus, & Theerman, 2002; Horstman, 2005; Ka`opua, 2003; National Center for Complementary and Alternative Medicine, 2003; 2004b; 2005b; Schneirov & Geczik, 2003. (See References in this chapter for full citations.)

HEALTH CARE PROVIDERS Each of the health care systems described in Table 9-2◆ makes use of a cadre of providers who function in accord with the precepts of that system. There are also a few independent providers who do not subscribe to a particular system of care as the basis for their activities. Health care providers within cultural health systems vary with respect to how they enter their profession, the type of training they receive, their degree of specialization and focus of care, the health-promotive and curative practices they employ, and the way in which they are viewed by members of the culture.

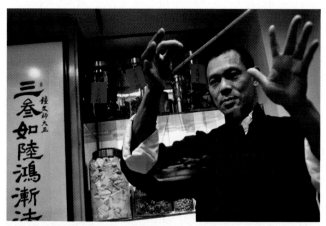

Members of many cultural groups seek the services of traditional practitioners. (© Justin Guariglia / The Image Works)

Health practitioners may come to their calling in several ways, including inheritance, family position, birth portents, revelation, apprenticeship, self-study, and formal education. Healing skills are sometimes believed to be passed down in families from generation to generation. Among the Hmong, for example, healers may inherit a *neng*, or healing spirit, from another clan member (Bankston, 1995). One's position within the family may also indicate special abilities, for instance, a seventh or ninth child or a child born after twins. In some ethnic cultures, the elderly are also considered to have special powers due to their closeness to death. Unusual occurrences during pregnancy or at birth, such as being born with a "caul," or amniotic membrane over the face, may also herald healing skills. Other practitioners may be called in a dream or vision or after recovering from a life-threatening illness themselves. Others show an aptitude for healing and may be apprenticed to an experienced healer (Snow, 1998). A few practitioners learn their calling on their own because of a personal interest. In the biomedical culture, professional health care providers receive specific training in their discipline, most often in a recognized institution for post-secondary education. Even within the biomedical culture, however, there are variations in educational preparation for practice in a specific discipline (e.g., diploma, associate degree, and bachelor's degree preparation for entry into the nursing profession versus post-baccalaureate education for physicians and dentists).

There is also wide variation in the types of people who provide health care in different cultural groups, from the family member or friend with expertise in dealing with illness to the specialist practitioner. Many people first seek advice on health from knowledgeable family members or friends before seeking more professional assistance. These family members and friends practice what may be called "domestic care" (Stowe, 2003). In less serious illnesses, for example, Hmong family members may act as "soul callers" to recall the wandering soul of the ill person. For more serious illness, however, the professional skills of a shaman are sought (Bankston, 1995). In the dominant U.S. culture, as well, people may rely on the wisdom and expertise of family members and friends for the care of minor illnesses or in making the decision to seek the assistance of a professional health care provider.

Professional assistance may be sought from a variety of different practitioners, depending on one's cultural background. There is also a growing tendency among the general public to seek health care from providers in non-biomedical health systems (IOM, 2005). Many clients with back pain or headache, for example, are seeking pain relief through acupuncture and the use of chiropractic services. In fact, some health insurance plans are even beginning to cover some more traditional alternative healing practices. In 1999, for example, two thirds of managed care organizations and insurance companies responding to a survey indicated that they covered the services of at least one alternative health care provider (IOM, 2005). There is also a growing body of scientific research attesting to the efficacy of many traditional forms of healing. For example, one study indicated a 73% decline in recurrent urinary tract infections among women experiencing acupuncture compared to 52% in the control group (Alraek, Soedal, Fagerheim, Digranes, & Baerheim, 2002).

Some cultural groups include a wide array of health providers, many of whom are highly specialized. Zuni healers, for example, are divided into several highly secret medicine societies, each of which specializes in the treatment of specific conditions. Specialization is also an emphasis in biomedicine, and there is a variety of specialty areas of practice in medicine and in nursing. Community health nursing is one area of specialization in nursing. Among the Navajo, healers may be divided into medicine men or women and diagnosticians. The function of the diagnostician is to determine the cause of illness through divination, whereas the medicine man or woman treats it (Spector, 2004). Singers are considered the most specialized practitioners among the Navajo and cure by means of specific songs and ceremonies (Purnell & Paulanka, 2005). Asian practitioners are often divided into the categories recognized in Chinese medicine, including acupuncturists and herbalists. Herbalists are also found among African American, Latino, and Appalachian cultural groups.

Religious healers, faith healers, or spiritualists are found among many cultural groups, including Asians, Latinos, African Americans, and Appalachians. Religion as a source of healing is common, and prayer and other religious rituals may accompany more scientific forms of healing for many. The charismatic healing tradition of the Roman Catholic Church is another example of the use of religious practices in healing. Other cultural groups embrace the practice of psychic healers thought to possess healing energy that can be transmitted to others, usually by some form of touch. Belief in this transfer of energy underlies the practice of therapeutic touch as a nursing intervention.

Practitioners of healing magic may also be found in a number of ethnic cultural groups. For example, *espiritistas* in the Latino alternative health tradition of spiritualism specialize in the treatment of illness caused by witchcraft (Purnell & Paulanka, 2005). Spiritual healers may also be seen among African American cultural groups, and the voodoo priest or priestess found among some African American groups is another example of magic used in healing (Spector, 2004).

Another group of health practitioners found in many cultures specializes in massage and is exemplified by the *sabador* in some Latino cultures. Massage and manipulation of body parts are also employed in chiropractic practice. Finally, many cultural groups include midwives as recognized health practitioners. In fact, midwifery as a specialized practice is a growing phenomenon in nursing that is gaining in popularity throughout the United States.

In assessing any cultural group, the nurse explores several areas related to health care providers. Among these are the types of practitioners recognized by the group, the health-related services provided, and the methods employed. Who and where are the practitioners? Is there a recognized hierarchy among practitioners? Who uses what type of provider, and what is the prevailing attitude of community members toward different types of providers? Finally, the nurse explores the expectations involved in the client–provider relationship discussed earlier in this chapter.

HEALTH CARE PRACTICES Individual members of ethnic and dominant U.S. cultures and practitioners of different health care systems employ a wide variety of practices to promote health, prevent illness, and restore health or cope with the consequences of ill health. Some practices are unique to the biomedical culture or to ethnic cultural groups, and some cut across several cultural groups. Health care practices that are not part of the array of interventions commonly employed in biomedical care may be referred to as *complementary or alternative medicine* (CAM) or therapies. Because not all of these therapies lie within the purview of the discipline of medicine, we will use the terminology *complementary or alternative therapies* (CAT) here.

The category of complementary and alternative therapies is generally defined by its exclusion as

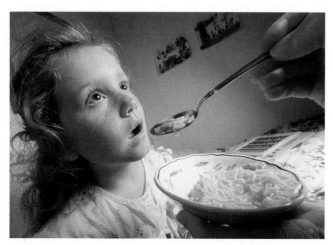

Chicken soup remains a common feature of illness care in mainstream U.S. culture. (Mark Richards)

biomedical therapy (Wolpe, 2002), but the definition of CAT is inconsistent and fluid, in part because of the number of these therapeutic approaches that are being incorporated into biomedicine. The National Center for Complementary and Alternative Medicine (2004a) defined CAM as a "group of diverse medical and health care systems, practices, and products that are not presently considered to be part of conventional medicine" (p. 1). Complementary and alternative therapies are often distinguished based on their relationship to biomedicine (Hess, 2002). Initially, the term *alternative therapies* was used to describe those with an origin outside the Western biomedical tradition. *Complementary,* on the other hand, was a term used in Britain for therapies that complemented the body's healing capabilities (Trachtenberg, 2002). Today, **complementary therapies** are those that are used in conjunction with biomedicine, whereas **alternative therapies** are substituted for or used in exclusion of biomedical therapies.

Approximately 80% of people in the world's poorest countries employ CAT as their only avenue of health care (Northridge, 2002). In one study in Turkey, almost half of elderly women (48%) reported using herbal remedies, particularly if they experienced some form of disability related to activities of daily living (Gozum & Unsal, 2004). The use of CAT is increasing in industrialized nations, and more biomedical providers are incorporating CAT into their routine practice. In the 2002 National Health Interview Survey (NHIS), for example, 36% of the U.S. adult population reported using CAT. Total annual visits to CAT providers in the United States exceed those made to primary providers in the biomedical system. Approximately half of the CAT users in the United States use these therapies as self-care, whereas the other half visit CAT providers. Overall use of CAT in the United States increased 25% from 1990 to 1997, but use of herbal preparations increased 380% and high-dose vitamin use increased by 130%. In some studies, CAT use is higher among members of ethnic minority

groups than among the dominant U.S. population. In others, CAT use is associated with female gender, higher education levels, hospitalization in the previous year, and smoking cessation (IOM, 2005). Scholars of health-related print media suggest that the use of CAT and other approaches to self-care is not a new phenomenon in the United States, and that the first settlers brought books of remedies with them when they emigrated to the New World (Rosenberg, 2003). Interest in self-care became even more prevalent after the American Civil War, with people seeking greater control over their own morbidity and mortality (Silver-Isenstadt, 2003).

In a 2001 survey of U.S. hospitals, 15% offered at least one CAT in response to consumer demand. Two thirds of U.S. managed care organizations surveyed in 1999 covered at least one form of CAT (usually chiropractic or acupuncture) through insurance riders for additional benefits (IOM, 2005). Similarly, 39% of Scottish primary care providers in one study reported using CAT and conventional biomedical therapies concurrently (Featherstone, Godden, Gault, Emslie, & Took-Zozaya, 2003), and in 1998, 2.2 million visits were made to practitioners of CAT in the United Kingdom (Richardson, 2004). Another indication of the growing interest in and use of CAT is the fact that in 2001, 47% of state boards of nursing permitted nurses to function as CAT providers, and an additional 13% were considering doing so. In another study, more than half of medical, nursing, and pharmacy students and faculty at a major medical school reported that they would provide CAT or refer clients to CAT providers (IOM, 2005).

Most expenditures for CAT are out-of-pocket expenses and included $21.2 billion dollars to CAT providers and an additional $8 billion for herbs and vitamins. Reasons given for use of CAT include failure of biomedical therapies, dissatisfaction with client–provider interactions and mistrust of the biomedical system,

GLOBAL PERSPECTIVES

Although traditional Chinese medicine is gaining greater acceptance and use in the United States, its use is declining in China. Some of the reasons for its decline are an increased emphasis on profit, decentralization, and movement to a fee-for-service and private insurance system for health care. In addition, there are a growing number of for-profit Western hospitals in China and greater emphasis on Western medicine in the education of younger providers. Another reason for the decline is the increasingly busy lifestyle of modern Chinese, who no longer have the time for frequent provider visits or preparation of herbal teas and other remedies. These pressures to move to a Westernized approach to health care are viewed by some as a threat to the cultural significance of traditional Chinese medicine, a reduction in the availability of low-cost services, and loss of a valuable source of care for major segments of the population (Burke, Wong, & Clayson, 2003). How might the principles of integrative health care discussed in this chapter help to prevent this loss?

advertising, interest in health promotion, and lack of access to biomedical care. Other reasons for CAT use are the opportunity to make a "lifestyle statement," congruence with personal values, recommendation from a biomedical provider, avoidance of aging, and failure to recognize that one is using CAT (Bodeker & Kronenberg, 2002; IOM, 2005; NCCAM, 2004a).

The Institute of Medicine (2005) has defined 127 modalities or systems of CAT, some of which (e.g., Kegel's exercises) have long been considered part of modern nursing practice. The National Institutes of Health has grouped CAT into the seven categories described in Table 9-3◆. Tataryn (2002), however, has noted that this categorization is based on similarities among therapies within each category and has suggested classifying CAT into four categories based on their underlying assumptions related to health and illness. The classification system is also capable of categorizing biomedical therapies. The categories thus produced are hierarchical, with each subsequent level incorporating the assumptions of previous levels. Complex therapies that contain the assumptions of two or more categories are placed in the higher-level category (Tataryn, 2002).

At the first level of the classification are therapies based on the body paradigm. The underlying assumption for this paradigm is that disease is primarily the result of changes in the biochemistry and structure of the body due to contact with disease-causing agents. Two basic types of interventions lie within this category: physical substances and physical manipulation. Physical substances (e.g., prescription medications, herbs) exist on a continuum of "naturalness" ranging from natural substances such as herbs at one end, through extracts and concentrates derived from natural substances, to synthetic substances at the other end. Physical manipulative therapies also occur on a continuum from natural to invasive and include interventions such as massage, surgery, chiropractic, and so on (Tataryn, 2002).

The second category is related to the mind–body paradigm, which assumes that the mind affects the body. The effects of the mind may be indirectly or directly causal. In the dualism assumption of this paradigm, mind and body are assumed to be separate entities and the mind affects the body by means of three mechanisms: (a) interpretation and the degree of attention paid to symptoms or other events, (b) emotional reaction to the meaning of illness, or (c) lifestyle and other behavioral choices that affect health. Under the unity assumption, mind and body are assumed to be intimately connected and mind exerts a direct causal effect in health and illness. Examples of therapies included in this category include counseling, dream interpretation, hypnosis, and art therapy.

The body–energy paradigm views health and illness as the result of the balance, flow, or interplay of energy. Interventions in this paradigm are aimed at regaining an energy balance so the body can heal itself and include therapies such as homeopathy, therapeutic touch, acupuncture, yoga, and magnetic therapy. Finally, the body–spirit paradigm "assumes the existence of nonlocal, nonphysical being or beings or states of consciousness, that is/are transcendental to but able to act on the material universe" (Tataryn, 2002, p. 886). Therapies focus on seeking intervention from one of two sources: outside supernatural agencies or a personal higher self that can enter into a healing state of consciousness. Examples of therapies in this paradigm include prayer, exorcism, laying-on of hands, and magical interventions. Table 9-4◆ provides a summary of these four paradigms, the underlying assumptions, and associated therapeutic practices.

A number of concerns have been raised regarding the increasing use of CAT in the United States, particularly herbal preparations. These concerns deal with

TABLE 9-3	National Institutes of Health Categories of Complementary and Alternative Therapies	
Category	**Description**
Mind–body medicine	Behavioral, psychosocial, social, and spiritual approaches to health care *Examples: mind–body systems, mind–body methods, religion, spiritualism*
Alternative medical systems	Systems of theory and practice developed outside of the Western biomedical tradition *Examples: see Table 9-2*
Lifestyle and disease prevention	Prevention of illness, risk factor modification, or support of healing and recovery *Examples: lifestyle therapies, health promotion strategies*
Biologically based therapies	Natural and biologically based practices, interventions, and products *Examples: phytotherapy or herbalism; diet therapies; orthomolecular medicine; pharmacologic, biological, and instrumental interventions*
Manipulative and body-based systems	Systems based on manipulation or body movement *Examples: chiropractic, massage and body work, unconventional physical therapies*
Biofield therapies	Use of energy fields for health-related purposes *Examples: healing/therapeutic touch*
Bioelectromagnetics	Unconventional use of electromagnetic fields

Data from: Parkman, C. A. (2002). CAM therapies and nursing competency. Journal for Nurses in Staff Development, 18(2), 61–67.

TABLE 9-4	Paradigmatic Classification of Therapeutic Interventions	
Paradigm	**Assumptions**	**Therapies Included**
Body paradigm	Disease results from contact with disease-causing agents that cause changes in body structure or biochemistry.	*Physical substances:* Herbs, extracts, synthetic substances (pharmaceuticals, chemotherapeutic agents, synthetic vitamins) *Physical manipulation:* Massage, surgery, colonic irrigation, chiropractic, radiotherapy, enema
Mind–body paradigm	The mind affects the body to produce health or illness. *Dualism assumption:* the mind only interprets what is going on in the body and is only an indirect cause of illness *Unity assumption:* the mind exerts a causative effect in health and illness (psychoneuroimmunology, or psychoneuroendocrinology)	Counseling, dream interpretation, art therapy, hypnosis, imagery, psychotherapy, support groups, stress reduction
Body–energy paradigm	Health and illness result from an imbalance in energy.	Homeopathy, therapeutic touch, acupressure, acupuncture, crystal therapy, magnetic therapy, *Qigong*, reflexology, Reiki, *T`ai chi*, yoga
Body–spirit paradigm	Internal or external spiritual forces cause health and illness.	Prayer, rituals, exorcism, faith healing, laying-on of hands, magic, psychic diagnosis and intervention, sacramental rites, Shamanic healing

Data from: Tataryn, D. J. (2002). Paradigms of health and disease: A framework for classifying and understanding complementary and alternative medicine. Journal of Alternative and Complementary Medicine, 8, 877–892.

issues of regulation, standardization, quality, safety, and efficacy (Boehringer, 2003). Because herbals are considered dietary supplements by the U.S. Food and Drug Administration (FDA), they must carry labels indicating that they are not intended for use to prevent or treat illness. Unfortunately, herbals are often used by the public for these purposes without FDA evaluation of their safety or efficacy. In addition, there is no standardization regarding the strength of active ingredients or their biological activity, which often vary from batch to batch due to differences in plants and growing conditions. Quality is an issue in that preparations do not always contain what they are supposed to, possibly due to incorrect plant identification, contamination and adulteration, inability to disintegrate completely in the body, or misleading product information. Safety is another area of concern. Herbals are considered "natural substances," so people may not be aware of potential side effects, allergic reactions, or adverse events. In addition, the safety of many herbals for children and pregnant women has not been determined. Finally, although many herbals are the basis for many pharmaceuticals, there is limited information about the efficacy of many other herbs.

One other area of concern is the potential for interaction with prescription medications and the fact that most clients who use CAT do not disclose that use to biomedical providers. It is estimated that 63% to 72% of CAT users do not inform their providers of their use. Reasons given for nondisclosure include failure of the provider to ask, lack of importance, lack of understanding by providers, and fear that providers would disapprove of or discourage CAT use (IOM, 2005).

Complementary and alternative therapies may be used for primary, secondary, and tertiary preventive purposes. Appendix B (Tables B-6 and B-7)∞ presents an array of cultural approaches to primary and secondary prevention. Many of the primary preventive strategies could also be used as tertiary prevention to prevent recurring health problems. Assessment of the use of cultural health care practices can be guided by the focused assessment questions provided on page 215.

INTERACTIONS AMONG HEALTH CARE SYSTEMS Another component of cultural assessment is the exploration of relationships and interactions between and among health care systems. Do members of an ethnic cultural group use the services of both biomedical and traditional health systems? If so, what is the effect of this dual

EVIDENCE-BASED PRACTICE

One of the criticisms of widespread use of complementary and alternative therapies is that many of them do not have a significant body of scientific evidence that supports their effectiveness. At the same time, there are conventional biomedical practices that are widely used without significant evidence for their efficacy (Park, 2002; Trachtenberg, 2002). Select one complementary or alternative health practice that interests you and examine the extent of the scientific basis for its practice. Then do the same for a relatively new conventional biomedical practice. How do the two practices compare with respect to the scientific evidence that supports them? In what areas is evidence lacking (e.g., overall effectiveness, effectiveness with specific population groups, etc.)? What additional evidence might be gleaned from research? How might you go about designing a study to develop that evidence?

FOCUSED ASSESSMENT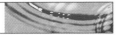

Assessing Health Care Practices

- What practices does the client/cultural group employ to promote health and prevent illness?
- What home remedies, if any, do clients/members of cultural groups employ to treat health problems? For what problems are they used? How are they used?
- What over-the-counter remedies are used by the client/cultural group? For what and how are they used?
- What provider-prescribed medications and treatments are used by the client/cultural group? By whom are they prescribed? If therapies are prescribed by multiple providers, are all providers aware of this?
- What are the client's/cultural group's preferences with respect to the type of treatment modalities prescribed (e.g., massage, medications in liquid or tablet form)?
- What measures are used by the client/cultural group to deal with the consequences of long-term health problems (e.g., pain relief, mobility limitation)?
- Are any of the health practices or therapies employed by the client/cultural group potentially harmful?

usage? Another area for consideration lies in the attitudes of providers in one system toward providers in other systems. To what extent do providers in different systems interact with each other? What is the character of that interaction? For example, is it collaborative or adversarial?

Providers in one system may fail to see the value of practices of another system. This attitude is not restricted to biomedical practitioners. In one study of immunization practices in Alberta, Canada, for example, some alternative providers supported the concept of immunization and referred their clients for immunization services. Others, however, did not perceive the children of their clients as at risk for immunizable diseases most often associated with residents of third-world countries. Many of these providers also believed that having the disease would provide life-long immunity superior to that conferred by immunization (Kulig et al., 2002). Similarly, biomedical providers may perceive spiritual or magico-religious health practices employed in some traditional health systems as evidence of superstition.

Varying degrees of interaction occur between and among health care systems. In this discussion, we will focus primarily on interactions between the biomedical system and other systems of health care. Some of the failure of interactions among systems is the result of repression of traditional systems of health care. For example, the Hawaiian system of *ho`oponopono* was forbidden by early colonial laws (Ka`opua, 2003). Similarly, the practice of lay midwives attending births was actively discouraged by the medical community in the United States, and many practiced their calling outside the law. On the other hand, interaction between systems may be

encouraged. For example, biomedical providers in the Peruvian social security system are permitted to refer clients to traditional providers for care, which is reimbursed by the system (Fink, 2002). Similarly, CAT has been integrated into the national health systems of China, North and South Korea, and Vietnam (Northridge, 2002). Referrals between health systems may be somewhat uneven, however, rather than equally reciprocal. For example, in the United States, 97% of chiropractors in one study would refer clients to biomedical physicians as needed, yet only 50% of biomedical physicians would make a referral to a chiropractor (Smith & Carber, 2002).

Lack of interaction between and among health care systems may lead to a variety of problems for their users. As we saw earlier, for example, failure to tell providers of one system that one is using the services of another may contribute to health problems such as drug–drug interactions. Many CAT users believe that biomedical physicians are prejudiced against herbals and other traditional practices or that they know little about them (Parkman, 2002). In some instances, reliance on traditional health care practices may lead to delay in seeking care and more severe illness when biomedical care is sought.

People in ethnic cultural groups may encounter a variety of barriers to obtaining care in the biomedical system, resulting in a preference for seeking care in traditional systems. Racial and cultural biases and inappropriate services, philosophical differences, language

BUILDING OUR KNOWLEDGE BASE

*T*he Institute of Medicine (2005) recommended that the National Institutes of Health (NIH) and other agencies and organizations fund research to examine:

- Outcomes and costs of combining CAM and conventional medical treatments
- Outcomes and costs of delivery systems that combine CAM and conventional medical treatments
- Outcomes (including reproducibility, safety, and cost-effectiveness) of models of care delivery involving solo CAM providers or solo conventional providers and integrated models that incorporate both CAM and conventional providers in the same system
- Factors that lead to decisions for CAM use
- Adherence to CAM instructions and guidelines among clients and providers
- Effects of CAM on wellness and disease prevention
- How the public obtains and evaluates information on CAM modalities
- Adverse events related to CAM use
- Interactions between CAM and conventional medicine

Discuss how you might design a study to address one of these recommendations. What forms of CAM could reasonably be studied in your local area? Are there health systems in the area that integrate both CAM and conventional medicine that can be studied? Is there already research going on in those systems to address the IOM recommendations? If so, how are nurses involved in these studies, if at all? If not, how might nurses become involved?

barriers, and a lack of knowledge of available biomedical services are some of the reasons given for not seeking care in the biomedical system. In addition, some members of ethnic cultural groups report their perceptions of "language discrimination," being treated unfairly because of their language or accent. In one study, for example, people reporting language discrimination were more than twice as likely to use informal services and to seek help from family and friends (Spencer & Chen, 2004). This is particularly true with respect to mental health services.

Some authors have noted that Eastern and Western systems of mental health care are "incommensurable," due to their different philosophical traditions and conceptualizations of mental illness. Differences in interpersonal boundaries and language issues also complicate the use of conventional mental health services by members of some cultural groups. In addition, nonlinear thinking patterns typical of some cultural groups may be interpreted by Western practitioners as confusion or resistance to treatment, and culturally unfamiliar behaviors may be viewed as pathological. Similarly, key concepts (e.g., death, rape, suicide) may have significantly different meanings in different cultural contexts, resulting in different emotional responses. All of these factors may lead to inappropriate diagnoses and treatment approaches in the Western mental health tradition (Kozuki & Kennedy, 2004). Tips for a focused assessment of the use of cultural and biomedical health care providers and systems are presented below.

FOCUSED ASSESSMENT

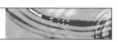

Assessing the Use of Health Care Providers and Systems

- From whom does the client/cultural group seek advice on health promotion and illness prevention?
- From whom does the client/cultural group first seek assistance with health care problems?
- For what types of health issues is assistance sought by the client/members of the cultural group?
- Do clients/members of the cultural group seek assistance from different types of providers for different problems? If so, whom do they seek for what kinds of problems? What is the rationale for the types of providers selected?
- Who are the recognized providers of health care within the cultural group? What types of care do they provide? What is the extent of their use by members of the group?
- Do members of the cultural group voice a preference for providers with certain characteristics (e.g., nurse practitioners over physicians, providers of a specific gender, herbalists over biomedical providers)? If so, on what beliefs and attitudes are these preferences based?
- Are there barriers to the use of specific types of health care providers? If so, what are they?
- If members of the cultural group use multiple providers, are the providers aware of this? If not, why?

As we have seen, cultural assessment includes exploration of factors in each of the six dimensions of health that influence health and health care practices. A comprehensive tool for cultural assessment based on the dimensions of health can be found in the *Community Assesssment Reference Guide* designed to accompany this book.

PLANNING CULTURALLY COMPETENT CARE AND DELIVERY SYSTEMS

Providers in all health systems should engage in culturally competent care. Doing so requires that providers be culturally competent in their care of individual clients and that care delivery systems also be culturally competent. The need for culturally competent care and care systems lies in the increasing diversity of populations throughout the world, the increasing provision of care in the home setting where cultural factors are more influential, and the increasing disparities in health status among many ethnic cultural minorities (Johnson, 2005). Benefits of culturally competent care include promoting more appropriate and accurate diagnoses of health problems and compliance with treatment recommendations, reducing delays in care seeking and use of services, enhancing client/provider communication, and enhancing the compatibility of biomedical and traditional health care systems (Health Resources and Services Administration [HRSA], 2001).

Cultural Competence

Cultural competence has been defined as "a dynamic fluid, continuous process whereby an individual, system, or health care agency finds meaningful and useful care delivery strategies based on knowledge of the cultural heritage, beliefs, attitudes, and behaviors of those to whom they render care" (Giger & Davidhizar, 2002, p. 81). Another widely accepted definition is that put forth by the U.S. Health Resources and Services Administration: "Cultural and linguistic competence is a set of congruent behaviors, attitudes, and policies that come together in a system, agency, or among professionals that enables work in cross-cultural situations" (HRSA, 2001, p. 1). Several models of cultural competence have been developed that delineate the critical elements of the concept. Elements of three of those models, the ASKED, BE SAFE, and Culturally Competent Community Care models, are presented in Table 9-5◆. As noted in the table, cultural competence goes beyond cultural sensitivity and awareness to develop a plan or system of care that "incorporates the client's values, beliefs, lifeways, and practices into mutually acceptable care" and is "built on experiential knowledge gained in encounters with clients that recognizes intraethnic variation within cultural groups" (Cioffi, 2004, p. 437).

TABLE 9-5 Elements of Selected Models of Cultural Competence

ASKED Model	BE SAFE Model	Culturally Competent Community Care Model
Model Elements	**Model Elements**	**Model Elements**
A: Cultural awareness based on examination of one's own prejudices and biases, leading to cultural humility	B: Barriers to use of biomedical care such as prejudice, socioeconomic status, ethnicity, stigma, mistrust, geography, and so on	Interpersonal caring: Attitudes, judgments, and actions in support of another culture
S: Cultural skill in collecting relevant cultural data and conducting a culturally based examination	E: Ethics: consideration of differences in ethical conceptualizations in the culture (e.g., third-party notification, confidentiality, truth telling, death, professionalism)	Cultural sensitivity: Respectful attitudes toward other cultures based on awareness of one's own culture
K: Cultural knowledge of differences and similarities among cultural groups	S: Sensitivity: lack of provider bias, stigma, cultural imposition	Cultural knowledge: Cognitive understanding of elements of another culture
E: Cultural encounters in face-to-face cross-cultural interactions	A: Assessment of physical, emotional, spiritual, social, mental, and occupational factors affecting health	Cultural skill: Roles and functions required for cultural competence, including abilities to conduct cultural assessments, determine health needs within a cultural context, and serve as an advocate
D: Cultural desire and personal motivation to practice in a culturally competent manner	F: Facts about the cultural beliefs, values, practices, worldview, and so on	
	E: Encounters: Knowledge of behavioral dos and don'ts, communication	

Data from: ASKED Model: Campinha-Bacote, 2002; BE SAFE Model: McNeil, 2002; Culturally Competent Community Care Model: Kim-Godwin, Clarke, & Barton, 2001. (See References in this chapter for full citations.)

Characteristics of Cultural Competence

Individual cultural competence reflects several inherent characteristics. First among these is an awareness of one's own culturally determined perspectives without letting them influence one's interactions with others. Cultural competence is also characterized by knowledge and understanding of another culture and by acceptance of and respect for other cultures. The culturally competent health care provider does not assume that other cultures are similar to his or her own and is nonjudgmental in examining the beliefs, values, attitudes, and practices of other cultural groups. In addition, the competent provider displays an openness to and comfort with encounters with persons from other cultural heritages. Finally, cultural competence is characterized by a conscious process of adaptation of care to the cultural context (Purnell & Paulanka, 2005).

At the health system level, culturally competent health care programs also display certain characteristic traits. These include a broad definition of culture beyond considerations of race, language, and ethnicity, and recognition of value in clients' cultural heritage. Culturally competent systems are also characterized by a recognition of the complexities involved in language interpretation and an awareness of the need to consider linguistic variation within cultural groups (including professional cultures), cultural variation within language groups (e.g., among the multiple cultural groups that speak Spanish), and variation in literacy levels among members of a particular cultural group. Culturally competent systems of care facilitate learning between providers and communities and involve communities in defining and addressing their health care needs. They also foster interagency collaboration and take steps to institutionalize cultural competency

within the system (HRSA, 2001). Characteristics of cultural competence at the individual provider and health system level are summarized in Table 9-6◆.

Challenges in Developing Cultural Competence

A number of challenges have been identified that may impede the development of cultural competence in individual providers or in health care systems. The first challenge is the recognition of clinical differences among cultural groups. Providers may be "culturally blind" and fail to recognize the differences among cultures (including biomedical culture) and the influence of culture on health and health care. Communication among cultural groups may also be a challenge in developing cultural competence, even among those that share a common language, because of the differences in the

TABLE 9-6 Individual and System-Level Characteristics of Cultural Competence

Individual Characteristics	System Characteristics
■ Awareness of personal perspectives	■ Broad definition of culture
■ Knowledge and understanding of other cultures	■ Value attributed to cultural beliefs
■ Not assuming similarity to one's own culture	■ Recognition of complexity in language interpretation
■ Nonjudgmental view of other cultures	■ Facilitation of learning between providers and cultural communities
■ Openness to and comfort with cultural encounters	■ Involvement of cultural communities in defining and addressing health needs
■ Conscious adaptation of care to the cultural context	■ Interagency collaboration
	■ Institutionalization of cultural competence

way that words are used, their particular meanings, and the interpretation of paralanguage and nonverbal aspects of communication. A third challenge is developing a sense of ethics and recognizing when it is appropriate to incorporate elements of culture in the plan of care and when those elements of culture may be harmful and should be eliminated or modified. Developing trust between members of a cultural group and those of the biomedical culture may be another challenge in developing cultural competence (Johnson, 2005). As we will see in Chapters 17 and 18∞, many members of the gay, lesbian, bisexual, and transgender cultures have reason to distrust health care providers. Distrust of biomedical providers is also a relatively common occurrence among members of African American and Roma cultures (Vivian & Dundes, 2004).

Cultural competence may also be impeded by stereotypes held by providers. Development of culture-specific knowledge has both benefits and disadvantages. On the plus side, knowledge of other cultures leads to recognition of cultural differences, opens the mind to alternative viewpoints, and serves as a starting point for cultural assessment of individual clients or subgroups within the population. However, such knowledge may give providers a false sense of security in working with members of other cultures and may lead to stereotyping (HRSA, 2002). **Stereotyping** involves "processes by which people use social categories (e.g., race or gender), in acquiring, processing, and recalling information about others" (Escarce, 2005, p. 2). Stereotyping is a useful cognitive strategy for organizing information about the complex world in which we live, and is not necessarily associated with negative attitudes toward members of other cultural groups. It is when providers fail to assess individuals or segments of a population group to see how closely they conform to beliefs and behaviors typical of the cultural group that stereotyping interferes with culturally competent care.

Other barriers to the provision of culturally competent care include viewing cultures as "them," not "me," without recognizing the influence of culture on one's own life; confusing race, culture, and ethnicity; and misdiagnosing ethnic-specific medical concerns due to lack of knowledge or communication difficulties (HRSA, 2002). Cultural mismatches may also impede culturally competent care. Ideally, both an ethnic match and a language match exist between provider and client (Fogel, 2004). An ethnic match occurs when both client and provider have the same ethnic identity. Given the dearth of biomedical providers from many ethnic cultural minority groups, ethnic matches are often difficult to obtain. In a language match, the client's native language is one of the five languages best spoken by the provider. Ethnic and language match seem to be particularly important in the area of mental health. For example, both ethnic and language match have been associated with longer retention in mental health treatment

and better treatment outcomes for some ethnic cultural groups (Fogel, 2004).

Modes of Culturally Competent Care

Three modes of providing culturally competent care were identified by Leininger in her theory of transcultural nursing (Cioffi, 2004). These include preservation, accommodation, and repatterning. Each of these modes is briefly discussed below.

Preservation

Preservation involves attempts to maintain cultural resources that may promote health or assist in recovery of health when illness occurs. Preservation may occur when community health nurses support and encourage traditional health care practices. Encouraging retention of healthier ethnic diets rather than acculturation to fast foods is an example of preservation. Preservation activities require an assessment of the value of traditional cultural practices to the client and development of a plan of care that incorporates those values and associated practices (McLaurin, 2002). For example, clients may be encouraged to participate in traditional healing rituals if this is their desire. Or the nurse may modify a therapeutic diet to include cultural food preferences. As another example, the nurse may assist a client to see how exercise might be increased without interfering with a busy work schedule in the dominant U.S. culture.

Accommodation

In the accommodation mode, emphasis is placed on adjusting or adapting the actions of either client or provider to facilitate interaction designed to positively influence health. Many routine practices in the biomedical culture can be modified to accommodate the cultural beliefs and practices of other cultural groups. For example, midwives serving Chinese clients accommodated their belief that delivery causes a loss of heat by providing warm drinks and using a handheld shower for episiotomy care. They also encouraged breast-feeding for twenty minutes, followed by bottle feeding to accommodate the cultural belief that colostrum does not provide sufficient nutrition for newborn infants. They also accommodated Islamic needs for modesty by limiting the exposure of women in labor to male attendants and wrapped newborns warmly to give to their fathers immediately after delivery to whisper a traditional prayer in the infant's ear (Cioffi, 2004). Similarly, group therapy for Native American women with diabetes, arthritis, or alcohol problems employed culturally appropriate practices such as storytelling, yoga, retreats, and time in a sweat lodge, as well as health education to address their health problems (Napoli, 2002). In another example, a program for cancer education for African American women incorporated spiritually based educational materials, capitalizing on the strong spirituality of most African American culture (Holt et al., 2003).

The incorporation of CAT into biomedical practice through "integrative medicine" is another means of accommodation. Integrative medicine "describes a clinical philosophy in which the most appropriate CAM, conventional medical treatments, or both are employed to address patients and their diseases from the most holistic, mind-body-spirit perspective possible" (Scherwitz et al., 2003, p. 549). The intent of integrative medicine is to deal with symptoms of illness as well as causes, whether those causes are mental, physical, or spiritual or a combination of these.

The World Health Organization's *Traditional Medicines Strategy 2002–2005* identified four areas for action to promote the integration of CAT into biomedicine. These included strategies to address needs related to policy; safety, efficacy, and quality; access; and rational use (Bodeker & Kronenberg, 2002). Table 9-7◆ highlights each strategy and the related actions needed for effective integration of CAT into biomedical practice.

Integration of CAT into biomedical practice has been found to be highly effective in many areas. For example, in one survey of the use of alternative therapies with the seriously mentally ill, 86% of participants reported the use of these therapies as beneficial (Russinova, Wewiorski, & Cash, 2002). In another study, acupressure at the Sanyinjiao point (above the ankle), initially by trained providers and then by clients, significantly reduced pain, but not anxiety, associated with dysmenorrhea (Chen & Chen, 2004). Similarly, massage therapy has been found to reduce the frequency and duration (but not intensity) of chronic tension headaches (Quinn, Chandler, & Moraska, 2002).

The combination of CAT and biomedical therapy has also been found to be helpful in dealing with some conditions. For example, Chinese herbal medicine used in combination with interferon alpha was found to be more effective than either therapy alone in dealing with chronic hepatitis B (McCulloch, Broffman, Gao, & Colford, 2002). Similarly, auricular acupuncture and education together were more effective in promoting smoking cessation than either therapy in isolation (Bier, Wilson, Studt, & Shakleton, 2002).

Some authors have called for caution in the integration of CAT in biomedical practice from the perspective of both types of practitioners. For example, some have noted that "American medicine has a history of delegitimizing lay healers and then assimilating their knowledge" (Wolpe, 2002, p. 169), and that the incorporation of CAT into biomedicine is typical of a long history of co-opting other practices in order to control them. There is also a fear that incorporation of CAT and its "scientization" will cause a loss of features of CAT that made it attractive to clients to begin with (e.g., the close provider–client relationship inherent in most CAT) (Wolpe, 2002). At the same time, there is concern that biomedical providers are being asked to step outside their areas of expertise to evaluate the appropriateness of CAT for their clients or even to provide CAT themselves (Tataryn, 2002).

The Institute of Medicine (2005) has suggested a systematic process for evaluating the appropriateness of incorporating CAT into biomedical health systems. The process should begin with a determination of the persons responsible for gathering information about various forms of CAT and for making incorporation decisions. Both the informal and formal mandates affecting the system should be examined, as should the system's mission and values and their congruence with various forms of CAT. In addition, an assessment of the internal and external environments as they affect incorporation of CAT in the institution should also be conducted. For example, are qualified practitioners of desired CAT available to the system? What forms of CAT are covered by insurance plans among the system's clientele? All of this information can lead to an informed decision on whether or not to incorporate CAT in the setting.

Repatterning

Repatterning involves changing the attitudes and behaviors of providers or members of a specific cultural group. A significant amount of repatterning has already

TABLE 9-7	WHO-defined Areas for Action in Integrating CAT in Biomedical Practice
Area for Action	**Specific Needs**
Policy	▪ Official recognition of CAT providers and practices ▪ Regulatory mechanisms for CAT ▪ Integration of CAT in national health systems ▪ Equitable distribution of CAT benefits ▪ Resources for CAT development and capacity building
Safety, efficacy, quality	▪ Evidence base regarding efficacy ▪ International standards for safety, efficacy, and quality ▪ Regulation of herbal preparations ▪ Registration of CAT providers ▪ Support for research on CAT safety, efficacy, and quality ▪ Development of appropriate research methodologies
Access	▪ Data on levels of access to and affordability of CAT ▪ Official recognition of CAT providers ▪ Identification of safe and effective practices ▪ Increased cooperation between CAT and biomedical providers ▪ Consideration of sustainability of plant resources
Rational use	▪ Training for CAT providers ▪ Training in CAT for biomedical providers ▪ Communication between CAT and biomedical providers ▪ Public education on the rational use of CAT

Data from: Bodeker, G., & Kronenberg, F. (2002). A public health agenda for traditional, complementary, and alternative medicine. American Journal of Public Health, 92, 1582–1591.

occurred among many biomedical providers, resulting in a willingness to employ CAT in their practices. Similarly, repatterning has taken place in the insurance world, leading to coverage for some complementary and alternative therapies. As more such therapies are integrated into the biomedical system, it is anticipated that the system itself may be repatterned in ways that will change the overall delivery of care to a more humanistic, less mechanistic perspective.

Repatterning may also be warranted for members of ethnic cultural groups to be able to function effectively within the dominant culture. For example, there may be a need to explain host country laws regarding childcare and neglect to immigrants whose cultural practice is to have older siblings care for younger children. Similarly, refugee women exposed to rape and trauma may need assistance in adjusting to the need for invasive screening techniques such as Pap smears (Drennan & Joseph, 2005).

The presence of lead and other toxic substances in some traditional remedies is another area in which repatterning may be required. For instance, 4% of adults with elevated blood lead levels in 27 states could trace their ingestion of lead to contaminated foods or remedies. Similarly, in 2002–2003, twelve cases of lead poisoning reported to the Centers for Disease Control and Prevention were attributed to Ayurvedic medicines such as *guglu* tablets, *sundari kapp* pills or liquid, *jambrulin*, and other pills, powders, and tablets (Hazard Evaluations and Field Studies, 2004a; 2004b).

Clients from ethnic cultural groups, particularly immigrants, may need nursing assistance dealing with intergenerational conflicts arising from different levels of acculturation among family members. For example, traditional foodways may create difficulty, conflict, and guilt for younger women who do not have time to prepare traditional cultural dishes due to changes in their roles (e.g., work outside the home) (Norman, 2002). Similarly, Asian Indian women immigrants to Canada in one study found it difficult to bridge the intergenerational culture gap between their children and their parents. Difficulties were compounded when elders or the mothers did not speak English. The change to more nuclear family patterns following immigration also meant fewer social supports and less assistance with tasks available to these women, increasing their personal stress. Conversely, the expectation that children would be well educated and highly successful in their new environment placed stress on the children that often led to negative consequences (Choudry et al., 2002). Culturally competent community health nurses could engage in interventions that could assist families experiencing these and other stresses of relocation.

Education regarding appropriate and inappropriate use of CAT is another way in which community health nurses may assist with repatterning for members of ethnic cultural groups as well as members of the dominant culture. The World Health Organization (2004) has identified several considerations in educating the public regarding safe and effective use of CAT. Categories of education needed include general considerations, such as the need to be informed consumers and for both CAT and biomedical providers to be conversant with CAT; knowledge of how to find reliable information; information about specific therapies; information regarding providers; and information about the costs of and insurance coverage for CAT. Specific areas of public education related to CAT are delineated in the client education box below.

Designing Culturally Competent Delivery Systems

In addition to providing culturally competent care for individual clients, families, and population groups, community health nurses can contribute to the development of culturally competent health care delivery systems. Some authors have identified a continuum of cultural competence in organizations that ranges from

---

CLIENT EDUCATION   Safe Use of Complementary and Alternative Therapies

General Considerations
- Use of CAT by informed consumers, knowledgeable about appropriate uses and safety considerations
- Extent of provider knowledge regarding CAT including knowledge of CAT use by particular clients

Finding and Identifying Reliable Information Regarding CAT
- Credibility and objectivity of information sources
- Purpose of the information source (e.g., if product sales are the primary purpose, information may be slanted)
- Relevance and accuracy of information presented
- Frequency with which information is updated

Information Regarding Specific Therapies
- Claims and evidence supporting them
- Product quality information regarding active ingredients, recognition of quality standards, storage information, expiration date, quality control of raw materials
- Precautions for use
- Adverse events/potential toxicity
- Interactions and contraindications
- Information regarding dose, time, frequency, duration, method of administration, preparation instructions
- Safety for use with children, pregnant women, the elderly

Information Regarding CAT Practitioners
- Qualifications for practice, education and experience related to the therapy
- Certification, if relevant
- Surveillance and monitoring

Cost/Insurance Coverage
- Typical costs of CAT
- What forms of CAT are covered under insurance

Data from: World Health Organization. (2004). Guidelines on developing consumer information on proper use of traditional, complementary and alternative medicine. *Geneva, Switzerland: Author.*

TABLE 9-8	Levels of Cultural Competence in Organizations
Level of Competence	**Description**
Cultural destructiveness	Members of the organization believe in the inferiority of other cultures and the reservation of rights and privileges to members of the dominant culture. No attempt is made to promote cultural diversity in the workforce, and members of the organization lack cultural knowledge.
Cultural incapacity	The organization employs a token minority staff and engages in discrimination and paternalization. There is no attempt to engage in cross-cultural training.
Cultural blindness	The organization attempts to be "color blind" and ignore cultural differences, claiming to "treat everyone alike."
Cultural pre-competence	The organization makes plans to become culturally competent, but may display complacence based on minimal effort toward that goal.
Cultural competence	The organization displays acceptance and respect for other cultures. Its mission and policies support services for diverse populations, and adherence to the mission and policies is monitored.
Cultural proficiency	The organization is proactive with respect to diversity and engages in research on ways to effectively incorporate culture into the delivery of care.

Data from: Johnson, L. D. (2005, Winter). The role of cultural competency in eliminating health disparities. Minority Nurse, pp. 52–55.

cultural destructiveness through cultural competence to cultural proficiency (Cross, Bazron, Dennis, & Isaacs, cited in Johnson, 2005). The levels of cultural competence across the continuum are described in Table 9-8◆.

Movement toward the cultural proficiency end of the continuum requires that a health system provide care with an understanding of and respect for culture and its influences on health and that the care provided incorporates community participation in its planning and delivery. In addition, it requires staff who respect the cultures of others and who reflect and respond to the values and demographics of the community served. Finally, movement toward cultural proficiency requires policies that assure a consistent response to cultural differences in the population served (HRSA, 2001).

In 1997, the U.S. Office of Minority Health developed the *National Standards for Culturally and Linguistically Appropriate Services in Health Care*, which can be used to guide the development of culturally competent health care systems (Spector, 2004). These standards, sometimes referred to as CLAS standards, include the following:

- Provision of effective, understandable, and respectful care consistent with cultural beliefs, practices, and preferred language by all staff
- Recruitment, retention, and promotion of a diverse staff representative of the population served
- Ongoing training of staff in culturally and linguistically appropriate care
- Provision of language assistance at no cost to clients at all points of contact at all hours
- Assurance of the competence of language assistance
- Provision of easily understood client education materials and signs
- Development of clear goals, policies, plans, and mechanisms of accountability for culturally competent and linguistically appropriate care
- Periodic assessment of system cultural competence and incorporation into quality improvement systems

- Collection and updating of client data on race, ethnicity, and spoken and written language
- Maintenance of an up-to-date demographic, cultural, and epidemiologic profile of the community served
- Development of organization/community partnerships for the design and implementation of culturally relevant services
- Development of culturally and linguistically sensitive grievance processes capable of identifying, preventing, and resolving cross-cultural conflicts
- Notification of the public regarding the progress made in implementing these standards

The creation of culturally competent delivery systems that adhere to these standards requires a comprehensive and systematic strategy. Some of the considerations in such a strategy include the recognition of the difficulty and incremental nature of such changes in systems and of the need to learn from both successes and failures. Conversion to a culturally competent system begins with an assessment of the status quo to determine the context and environment for change, the resources for and obstacles to change, and readiness for change. The actual change requires creation of an infrastructure

CULTURAL COMPETENCE

Many large health care organizations employ a culturally diverse staff and serve several different cultural population groups. In some organizations, staff whose first language is other than English are prohibited from speaking to each other in their native language in front of clients.

- In what ways does this prohibition demonstrate or not demonstrate culturally competent organizations?
- What interventions might these organizations employ to demonstrate respect and acceptance of the cultural values and behaviors of both clients and staff?

that supports cultural competence, from buy-in by decision makers to the support of staff to the identification of external supporters. Key elements in the infrastructure include cultural knowledge, a planning group and point person, data, and resources. Once the infrastructure for a culturally competent system has been built, the organization can move forward to identify objectives, goals, actions, timelines, and current and future resource needs and their availability (Freeman, 2002).

Community health nurses can be involved in the development of culturally and linguistically appropriate health care services in a number of ways. If they are employed in the particular organization that needs to adopt more culturally and linguistically appropriate approaches to health care, they can assess current practices and the barriers to CLAS that they represent. They can also be involved in the development of policies and procedures that promote CLAS in the organization. In addition, community health nurses can help the agency to conduct an assessment of the cultural groups served by the agency and assist in the development of agency–community partnerships to better meet the needs of community members. If the nurse is not an employee of an agency that needs to improve the cultural

HEALTHY PEOPLE 2010
Goals for Population Health

Physical Activity

Objective 22-2. Increase the percentage of adults with daily moderate physical activity for 30 minutes to 50%. (2002 data)

	BASELINE	MOST RECENT DATA	TARGET
Native American	27%	25%	50%#
Asian/Pacific Islander	27%	N/A	50%
African American	24%	25%	50%
Latino	23%	23%	50%
White	33%	33%	50%

Tobacco Use

Objective 27-1a. Reduce adult cigarette smoking to 12%. (2002 data)

Native American	35%	34%	12%
Asian	13%	13%	12%
African American	25%	22%	12%
Latino	19%	16%	12%
White	25%	23%	12%

Injury and Violence

Objective 15-15. Reduce deaths due to motor vehicle accidents to 9.2 per 100,000 population. (2002 data)

Native American	26.9	28.1	9.2#
Asian/Pacific Islander	8.1	8.2	9.2#
African American	15.6	14.8	9.2
Latino	13.9	14.9	9.2#
White	14.8	15.5	9.2#

Objective 15-32. Reduce homicides to 3 per 100,000 population. (2002 data)

Native American	9.1	8.4	3
Asian/Pacific Islander	3.0	2.9	3
African American	20.1	21.0	3#
Latino	7.6	7.3	3
White	3.8	3.7	3

Immunization

Objective 14-24. Increase the proportion of children with complete immunizations to 80%. (2002 data)

Native American	65%	62%	80%#
Asian/Pacific Islander	73%	77%	80%
African American	66%	69%	80%
Latino	69%	73%	80%
White	74%	77%	80%

Access to Health Care

Objective 1-1. Increase the proportion of persons with health insurance to 100%. (2002 data)

Native American	62%	61%	100%#
Asian	81%	83%	100%
African American	80%	81%	100%
Latino	66%	66%	100%
White	84%	85%	100%

Objective 1-4a. Increase the proportion of persons with a regular source of health care to 96%. (2002 data)

Native American	82%	87%	96%
Asian	84%	82%	96%#
African American	86%	87%	96%
Latino	79%	77%	96%#
White	88%	89%	96%

Objective 16-6a. Increase the proportion of pregnant women who receive prenatal care in the first trimester to 90%. (2002 data)

Native American	69%	70%	90%
Asian/Pacific Islander	83%	85%	90%
African American	73%	75%	90%
Latino	74%	77%	90%
White	85%	85%	90%

Objective moving away from target

Data from: U.S. Department of Health and Human Services. (2004). DATA2010: The Healthy People 2010 Base. Retrieved February 21, 2005, from http://wonder.cdc.gov/scripts/broker.exe

and linguistic appropriateness of its services, he or she can bring to the attention of agency administrators the concerns of members of local cultural groups regarding the services provided. Community assessment and policy development may also be areas of involvement for nonemployee community health nurses. The process used in the development of culturally competent health care systems is essentially the same process used to develop any kind of health care program, and is discussed in greater detail in Chapter 15∞.

EVALUATING CULTURAL COMPETENCE

Evaluation of care provided to clients from another cultural group should focus on both the outcomes of care and the delivery processes employed. In terms of outcomes, nurses should examine indicators of health status for individual clients and for subcultural groups. For example, has the nurse been able to improve the client's nutritional status without changing his or her cultural dietary pattern? Has the frequency of successful pregnancy outcomes been increased for members of a given cultural group? Have inappropriate biomedical practices been modified to promote better care?

Health care delivery systems should also be examined in terms of their cultural competence. Congruence with the standards for CLAS is one way to assess the cultural competence of health care systems. At the population level, the extent to which disparities in health among ethnic minority populations have been decreased is another way of evaluating the cultural competence of the national health care system. Some of the *Healthy People 2010*◆ objectives that might be examined and data on their current national status are presented on page 222. As indicated, none of the objectives has been met for any of the minority (or majority) populations, and, for some groups, movement has actually been away from 2010 targets. A particular health system could look at the extent of disparities among its clientele as one measure of its cultural competence.

Case Study

Culture and Care

Apple Valley is a rural agricultural community approximately 100 miles from the U.S.–Mexico border. Because of the mild climate, there are crops to be tended and harvested much of the year, and many Latino migrant workers are involved in this work. Although there is work for a significant portion of the year, many of the laborers have extended families still in Mexico. They frequently work for several months, then return to Mexico to share their earnings and visit with family members. When they return to the United States, they often come as nuclear family groups, and both parents work in the fields. Children may or may not attend school while in Apple Valley.

There are high infant and maternal mortality rates among this group as the women do not usually receive care during their pregnancies. In part this is because of the high cost of care, but it also results from lack of facility with English and inability to take time from work to receive care. Although most of the workers are legal immigrants, they are not eligible for financial assistance or care at the local health department prenatal clinic. Complicated deliveries often take place in the local hospital, however, and contribute to the burden of "uncompensated care" since the migrant families are usually unable to pay the hospital bills. According to some of the workers, there is a Latino woman living year-round in Apple Valley who serves as a midwife for some of the women.

1. What cultural factors are operating in this situation? What other circumstances, not necessarily cultural in origin, complicate the situation?
2. What interventions by the community health nurse could help to reduce the infant and maternal mortality rates?
3. Who else should be involved in efforts to resolve the problem? Why?
4. How could the community health nurse motivate involvement by other segments of the population?

Test Your Understanding

1. How does culture differ from race, nationality, and ethnicity? (pp. 182–183)

2. How does culture influence health? Give some examples of dominant, ethnic, and biomedical cultural influences on the health of individuals or populations. (pp. 184–185)

3. Define cultural competence. What are some barriers to cultural competence? How can these barriers be overcome? (pp. 216–223)

4. Describe some of the considerations in a cultural assessment. Describe how you might go about obtaining cultural assessment data. (pp. 186–216)

5. What are some of the characteristics of culturally competent health care systems? What strategies can be used to develop culturally competent systems? (pp. 220–223)

EXPLORE MediaLink

http://www.prenhall.com/clark
Resources for this chapter can be found on the Companion Website.

Audio Glossary
Appendix B: Cultural Influences on Health
and Health-related Behaviors
Exam Review Questions
Case Study: Care of the African American
Muslim Patient

MediaLink Application: Racism and
Powerlessness (video)
Media Links
Challenge Your Knowledge

Update *Healthy People 2010*
Advocacy Interviews

References

Acevedo-Garcia, D., Barbeau, E., Bishop, J. A., Pan, J., & Emmons, K. M. (2004). Undoing the epidemiological paradox: The tobacco industry's targeting of U.S. immigrants. *American Journal of Public Health, 94,* 2188–2193.

Alraek, R., Soedal, L. I., Fagerheim, S. U., Digranes, A., & Baerheim, A. (2002). Acupuncture treatment in the prevention of uncomplicated recurrent lower urinary tract infections in adult women. *American Journal of Public Health, 92,* 1609–1611.

American Cancer Society. (2005). *Shamanism.* Retrieved December 29, 2005, from http://cancer.org/docroot/ETO/contnet/ETO_5_3X_Shamanism.asp?sitearea=ETO

American Chiropractic Association. (2004a). *History of chiropractic care.* Retrieved December 29, 2005, from http://www.acatoday.com/media/whatis/history_chiro.shtml

American Chiropractic Association. (2004b). *What is chiropractic?* Retrieved December 29, 2005, from http://www.acatoday.com/media/whatis

Anumolo, A. K., Miller, H., Popoola, M. M., Talley, B., Rushing, A., Huebscher, R., et al. (2004). Alternative health care systems. In R. Huebscher & R. A. Shuler (Eds.), *Natural and complementary health care practices* (pp. 715–761). St. Louis: Mosby.

Avery, B., & Bashir, S. (2003). The road to advocacy — Searching for the rainbow. *American Journal of Public Health, 93,* 1207–1210.

Bankston, C. L. III. (1995). Hmong Americans. In J. Galens, A. Sheets, & R. V. Young (Eds.), *Gale encyclopedia of multicultural America* (pp. 670–681). Detroit, MI: Gale Research.

Batts, F. (2002). Cultural competence and linguistically appropriate services in the clinical setting. In *Bridging Cultures & Enhancing Care: Approaches to Cultural and Linguistic Competency in Managed Care* (pp. 12–18). Washington, DC: Health Resources and Services Administration.

Becker, G., Gates, R. J., & Newsom, E. (2004). Self-care among chronically ill African Americans: Culture, health disparities, and health insurance status. *American Journal of Public Health, 94,* 2066–2073.

Bennett, G. G., Wolin, K. Y., Robinson, E. L., Fowler, S., & Edwards, C. L. (2005). Perceived racial/ethnic harassment and tobacco

use among African American young adults. *American Journal of Public Health, 95,* 238–240.

Bier, I. D., Wilson, J., Studt, P., & Shakleton, M. (2002). Auricular acupuncture, education, and smoking cessation: A randomized, sham-controlled trial. *American Journal of Public Health, 92,* 1642–1647.

Blake, J. H. (1998). "Doctor can't do me no good": Social concomitants of health care attitudes among elderly blacks in isolated rural populations. In W. H. Watson (Ed.), *Black folk medicine: The therapeutic significance of faith and trust* (pp. 33–40). New Brunswick, NJ: Transaction.

Blank, M., Mahmood, M., Fox, J. C., & Guterbock, T. (2002). Alternative mental health services: The role of the Black church in the South. *American Journal of Public Health, 92,* 1668–1672.

Bodeker, G., & Kronenberg, F. (2002). A public health agenda for traditional, complementary, and alternative medicine. *American Journal of Public Health, 92,* 1582–1591.

Boehringer, S. K. (2003). Herbal medicines: Nurses must help public evaluate pros and cons. *NurseWeek, 16*(8), 15–16.

Budrys, G. (2001). *Our unsystematic health care system.* Lanham, MD: Rowman & Littlefield.

Burke, A., Wong, Y., & Clayson, Z. (2003). Traditional medicine in China today: Implications for indigenous health systems in a modern world. *American Journal of Public Health, 93,* 1082–1083.

Campinha-Bacote, J. (2002). A culturally conscious approach to the delivery of healthcare services. In *Bridging Cultures & Enhancing Care: Approaches to Cultural and Linguistic Competency in Managed Care* (pp. 24–26). Washington, DC: Health Resources and Services Administration.

Caughy, M. O., O'Campo, P. J., & Muntaner, C. (2004). Experiences of racism among African American parents and the mental health of their pre-school age children. *American Journal of Public Health, 94,* 2118–2124.

Centers for Disease Control and Prevention. (2004). Health disparities experienced by racial/ethnic minority populations. *Morbidity and Mortality Weekly Report, 53,* 755.

Chen, H., & Chen, C. (2004). Effects of acupressure at the Sanyinjiao point on primary dysmenorrhea. *Journal of Advanced Nursing, 48,* 380–387.

Choudry, U. K., Jandu, S., Mahal, J., Singh, R., Sohi-Pabla, H., & Mutta, B. (2002). Health promotion and participatory action research with South Asian women. *Journal of Nursing Scholarship, 34,* 75–81.

Cioffi, J. (2004). Caring for women with culturally diverse backgrounds: Midwives experiences. *Journal of Midwifery and Women's Health, 49,* 437–442.

Collins, J. W., David, R. J., Handler, A., Wall, S., & Andes, S. (2004). Very low birthweight in African American infants: The role of maternal exposure to interpersonal racial discrimination. *American Journal of Public Health, 94,* 2132–2138.

Denny, C. H., Holtzman, D., & Cobb, N. (2003). Surveillance for health behaviors of American Indians and Alaska Natives: Findings from the Behavioral Risk Factor Surveillance System, 1997–2002. *Morbidity and Mortality Weekly Report, 52*(SS-7), 1–13.

de Rios, M. D. (2002). What we can learn from Shamanic healing: Brief psychotherapy with Latino immigrant clients. *American Journal of Public Health, 92,* 1576–1578.

Division of Adult and Community Health, National Center for Chronic Disease Prevention and Health Promotion. (2004). Health status of Cambodians and Vietnamese—Selected communities, United States, 2001–2002. *Morbidity and Mortality Weekly Report, 53,* 760–765.

Division of Nutrition and Physical Activity, National Center for Chronic Disease Prevention and Health Promotion. (2004). Physical activity among Asians and Native Hawaiian or other Pacific Islanders — 50 states and the District of Columbia, 2001–2003. *Morbidity and Mortality Weekly Report, 53,* 756–760.

Doak, L. G., & Doak, C. C. (Eds.). (n.d.). *Pfizer health literacy principles: A handbook for creating patient education materials that enhance understanding, promote health outcomes.* Retrieved December 1, 2003, from http://www.pfizerhealthliteracy.com/4548_Health_literacy_all.pdf

Domian, E. W. (2001). Cultural practices and social support of pregnant women in a northern New Mexico community. *Journal of Nursing Scholarship, 33,* 331–336.

Drennan, V. M., & Joseph, J. (2005). Health visiting and refugee families: Issues in professional practice. *Journal of Advanced Nursing, 49*, 155–163.

Elgindy, G. (2005, Winter). Meeting Jewish and Muslim patient's dietary needs. *Minority Nurse*, pp. 56–58.

Escarce, J. J. (2005). How does race matter, anyway? *Health Services Research, 40*(1), 1–7.

Esposito, J. L. (2003). Islam: FAQs. *Saudi Aramco World, 54*(5), 12–18.

Featherstone, C., Godden, D., Gault., C., Emslie, M., & Took-Zozaya, M. (2003). Prevalence study of concurrent use of complementary and alternative medicine in patients attending primary care services in Scotland. *American Journal of Public Health, 93*, 1080–1083.

Fee, E., Brown, T. M., Lazarus, J., & Theerman, P. (2002). Exploring acupuncture: Ancient ideas, modern techniques. *American Journal of Public Health, 92*, 1592.

Fink, S. (2002). International efforts spotlight traditional, complementary, and alternative medicine. *American Journal of Public Health, 92*, 1734–1739.

Flaskerud, J. H. (2000). Ethnicity, culture, and neuropsychiatry. *Issues in Mental Health Nursing, 21*, 5–29.

Fogel, J. (2004). *Conference report: Culture and mental health: Highlights of the 54th meeting of the Canadian Psychiatric Association.* Retrieved December 8, 2004, from http://www.medscape.com/viewarticle/493073

Freeman, C. (2002). Building cultural competence in organizations: Focus on promoting and sustaining change. In *Bridging Cultures & Enhancing Care: Approaches to Cultural and Linguistic Competency in Managed Care* (pp. 10–12). Washington, DC: Health Resources and Services Administration.

Gesler, W. M., & Kearns, R. A. (2002). *Culture/place/health.* London: Routledge.

Giger, J. N., & Davidhizar, R. (2002). Culturally competent care: Emphasis on understanding the people of Afghanistan, Afghanistan Americans, and Islamic culture and religion. *International Nursing Review, 49*, 79–86.

Gomez, S. L., Kelsey, J. L., Glaser, S. L., Lee, M. M., & Sidney, S. (2004). Immigration and acculturation in relation to health and health-related risk factors among specific Asian subgroups in a health maintenance organization. *American Journal of Public Health, 94*, 1977–1984.

Gozum, S., & Unsal, A. (2004). Use of herbal therapies by older, community-dwelling women. *Journal of Advanced Nursing, 46*, 171–178.

Hatfield, G. (2004). *Encyclopedia of folk medicine.* Santa Barbara, CA: ABC-CLIO.

Hazard Evaluations and Field Studies, National Institute for Occupational Safety and Health. (2004a). Adult blood lead epidemiology and surveillance—United States, 2002. *Morbidity and Mortality Weekly Report, 53*, 578–582.

Hazard Evaluations and Field Studies, National Institute for Occupational Safety and Health. (2004b). Lead poisoning associated with Ayurvedic medications—Five states, 2002–2003. *Morbidity and Mortality Weekly Report, 53*, 582–584.

Health Resources and Services Administration. (2001). *Cultural competence works.* Merrifield, VA: Author.

Health Resources and Services Administration. (2002). *Bridging cultures and enhancing care: Approaches to cultural and linguistic competency in managed care.* Retrieved May 9, 2003, from http://www.hrsa.gov/financeMC

Hendershot, G. (2003). Mobility limitations and complementary and alternative medicine: Are people with disabilities more likely to pray? *American Journal of Public Health, 93*, 1079–1080.

Herzinsuffizienz. (n.d.). (translation from German). Retrieved May 10, 2006, from http://de.wikipedia.org/wiki/herzinsuffizienz

Hess, D. J. (2002). Complementary or alternative? Stronger vs weaker integration policies. *American Journal of Public Health, 92*, 1579–1581.

Hillier, D. (2003). *Childbirth in the global village: Implications for midwifery education and practice.* London: Routledge.

Holroyd, E., Twinn, S. F., & Shia, A. T. Y. (2001). Chinese women's experiences and images of the Pap smear examination. *Cancer Nursing, 24*(1), 68–75.

Holt, C. L., Kyles, A., Wiehagen, T., & Casey, C. (2003). Development of a spiritually based breast cancer education booklet for African American Women. *Cancer Control, 10*(5), 37–44.

Horstman, J. (2005). *Homeopathy.* Retrieved December 29, 2005, from http://www.arthritis.org/resources/arthritistoday/2000_archives/2000_03_04_homeopathy

Institute of Medicine. (2005). *Complementary and alternative medicine in the United States.* Washington, DC: Author.

Jacobs, E. A., Shepard, D. S., Suaya, J. A., & Stone, E. (2004). Overcoming language barriers in health care: Costs and benefits of interpreter services. *American Journal of Public Health, 94*, 866–869.

Johnson, L. D. (2005, Winter). The role of cultural competency in eliminating health disparities. *Minority Nurse*, pp. 52–55.

Ka`opua, L.S.I. (2003). Training community practitioners in a research intervention: Practice examples at the intersection of cancer, western science and native Hawaiian healing. *Cancer Control, 10*(5), 5–12.

Kim-Godwin, Y. S., Clarke, P. N., & Barton, L. (2001). A model for the delivery of culturally competent community care. *Journal of Advanced Nursing, 35*, 918–925.

Kogut, B. H. (2004). Why adult literacy matters. *Phi Kappa Phi Forum, 84*(2), 26–28.

Kozuki, Y., & Kennedy, M. G. (2004). Cultural incommensurability in psychodynamic psychotherapy in Western and Japanese traditions. *Journal of Nursing Scholarship, 36*, 30–38.

Kressin, N. R., Chang, B., Hendricks, A., & Kazis, L. E. (2003). Agreement between administrative data and patients' self-reports of race/ethnicity. *American Journal of Public Health, 93*, 1734–1739.

Kulig, J. C., Meyer, C. J., Hill, S. A., Handley, C. E., Lichtenberger, S. M., & Myck, S. J. (2002). Refusals and delay of immunization within Southwestern Alberta: Understanding alternative beliefs and religious perspectives. *Canadian Journal of Public Health, 93*, 109–112.

Lillie-Blanton, M., & Hudman, J. (2001). Untangling the web: Race/ethnicity, immigration, and the nation's health. *American Journal of Public Health, 91*, 1736–1738.

Lockyear, P. L. B. (2004). Cultural differences in diet and heart health among women. *Medscape Ob/Gyn & Women's Health, 9*(2). Retrieved October 13, 2004, from http://www.medscape.com/viewarticle/490343

McCulloch, M., Broffman, M., Gao, J., & Colford, J. M. (2002). Chinese herbal medicine and interferon in the treatment of chronic hepatitis B: A meta-analysis of randomized, controlled trials. *American Journal of Public Health, 92*, 1619–1627.

McGlade, M. S., Saha, S., & Dahlstrom, M. E. (2004). The Latina paradox: An opportunity for restructuring prenatal care delivery. *American Journal of Public Health, 94*, 2062–2065.

McLaurin, J. A. (2002). Assimilation, acculturation, and alternative medicines. *MCN Streamline: The Migrant Health News Source, 8*(6), 1–3.

McNeil, J. (2002). Model of cultural competency for working with African American patients infected with HIV. In *Bridging Cultures & Enhancing Care: Approaches to Cultural and Linguistic Competency in Managed Care* (pp. 26–28). Washington, DC: Health Resources and Services Administration.

Moskowitz, J. M., Kazinets, G., Tager, I. B., & Wong, J. (2004). Breast- and cervical-cancer screening among Korean women—Santa Clara County, California, 1994 and 2002. *Morbidity and Mortality Weekly Report, 53*, 765–767.

Mustillo, S., Krieger, N., Gunderson, E. P., Sidney, S., McCreath, H., & Kiefe, C. I. (2004). Self-reported experiences of racial discrimination and black-white differences in preterm and low-birthweight deliveries: The CARDIA study. *American Journal of Public Health, 94*, 2125–2131.

Napoli, M. (2002). Holistic health care for native women: An integrated model. *American Journal of Public Health, 92*, 1573–1575.

National Center for Complementary and Alternative Medicine. (2003). *Questions and answers about homeopathy.* Retrieved December 29, 2005, from http://www.nccam.nih.gov/health/homeopathy/index.htm

National Center for Complementary and Alternative Medicine. (2004a). *The use of complementary and alternative medicine in the United States.* Retrieved August 30, 2004, from http://www.nccam.nih.gov/news/camsurvey.pdf

National Center for Complementary and Alternative Medicine. (2004b). *Whole medical systems: An overview.* Retrieved December 29, 2005, from http://www.nccam.nih.gov/health/backgrounds/wholemed.htm

National Center for Complementary and Alternative Medicine. (2005a). *Prayer and spirituality in health: Ancient practices, modern science.* Retrieved December 29, 2005, from http://www.nccam.nih.gov/news/newsletter/2005_winter/prayer.htm

National Center for Complementary and Alternative Medicine. (2005b). *What is Ayurvedic medicine?* Retrieved December 29, 2005, from http://www.nccam.nih.gov/health/ayurveda

National Center for Environmental Health. (2005). Elevated blood lead levels in refugee children—New Hampshire, 2003–2004. *Morbidity and Mortality Weekly Report, 54,* 42–45.

Norman, C. E. (2002). Savoring the sacred: Understanding religion through food. *Phi Kappa Phi Forum, 82*(3), 19–23.

Northridge, M. (2002). Integrating ethnomedicine into public health. *American Journal of Public Health, 92,* 1561.

Oppenheimer, G. M. (2001). Paradigm lost: Race, ethnicity, and the search for a new population taxonomy. *American Journal of Public Health, 91,* 1049–1055.

Paisley, J. A., Haines, J., Greenberg, M., Makarchuk, M., Vogelzang, S., & Lewicki, K. (2002). An examination of cancer risk beliefs among adults from Toronto's Somali, Chinese, Russian, and Spanish-speaking communities. *Canadian Journal of Public Health, 93,* 138–141.

Park, C. M. (2002). Diversity, the individual, and proof of efficacy: Complementary and alternative medicine in medical education. *American Journal of Public Health, 92,* 1568–1571.

Parkman, C. A. (2002). CAM therapies and nursing competency. *Journal for Nurses in Staff Development, 18*(2), 61–67.

Partnership for the Public's Health. (n.d.). *Tips and tools: Working effectively across languages.* Oakland, CA: Author. (also available from http://www.partnershipph.org).

Pasco, A. C., Morse, J. M., & Olson, J. K. (2004). Cross-cultural relationships between nurses and Filipino Canadian patients. *Journal of Nursing Scholarship, 36,* 239–246.

Pillsbury, R. (2002). Thoroughly modern dining: A look at America's changing celebration dinner. *Phi Kappa Phi Forum, 82*(3), 24–27.

Priest, C. (2005). Held liable. *Reflections on Nursing Leadership, 31*(1), 20–22.

Purnell, L. D., & Paulanka, B. J. (2005). *Guide to culturally competent health care.* Philadelphia: F. A. Davis.

Quinn, C., Chandler, C., & Moraska, A. (2002). Massage therapy and frequency of chronic tension headaches. *American Journal of Public Health, 92,* 1657–1661.

Richardson, J. (2004). What patients expect from complementary therapy: A qualitative study. *American Journal of Public Health, 94,* 1049–1053.

Rosenberg, C. E. (2003). Health in the home: A tradition of print and practice. In C. E. Rosenberg (Ed.), *Right living: An Anglo-American tradition of self-help medicine and*

hygiene (pp. 1–20). Baltimore, MD: Johns Hopkins University.

Russinova, Z., Wewiorski, N. J., & Cash, D. (2002). Use of alternative health care practices by persons with serious mental illness: Perceived benefits. *American Journal of Public Health, 92,* 1600–1603.

Scherwitz, L., Stewart, W., McHenry, P., Wood, C., Robertson, L., & Cantwell, M. (2003). An integrative medicine clinic in a community hospital. *American Journal of Public Health, 93,* 549–552.

Schneirov, M., & Geczik, J. D. (2003). *A diagnosis for our times.* Albany, NY: State University of New York.

Sharpless, R. (2002). Traditional Southern cooking—Not gone with the wind. *Phi Kappa Phi Forum, 82*(3), 10–14.

Silenzio, V. M. B. (2002). What is the role of complementary and alternative medicine in public health? *American Journal of Public Health, 92,* 1562–1564.

Silver-Isenstadt, J. (2003). Passions and perversions: The radical ambition of Dr. Thomas Low Nichols. In C. E. Rosenberg (Ed.), *Right living: An Anglo-American tradition of self-help medicine and hygiene* (pp. 186–205). Baltimore, MD: Johns Hopkins University.

Smith, M., & Carber, L. (2002). Chiropractic health care in health professional shortage area in the United States. *American Journal of Public Health, 92,* 2001–2009.

Snow, L. F. (1998). *Walkin' over medicine.* Detroit: Wayne State University Press.

Spector, R. E. (2004). *Cultural diversity in health and illness* (6th ed.). Upper Saddle River, NJ: Prentice Hall.

Spencer, M. S., & Chen, J. (2004). Effect of discrimination on mental health service utilization among Chinese Americans. *American Journal of Public Health, 94,* 809–814.

Steefel, L. (2003). No cookie cutter approach to postpartum culture care. *Nursing Spectrum* (Western ed.), 4(6), 8–9.

Stowe, S. (2003). Conflict and self-sufficiency: Domestic medicine in the American South. In C. E. Rosenberg (Ed.), *Right living: An Anglo-American tradition of self-help medicine and hygiene* (pp. 147–169). Baltimore, MD: Johns Hopkins University.

Stuhlmiller, C. M. (1998). Understanding seasonal affective disorder and experiences in northern Norway. *Image: Journal of Nursing Scholarship, 30,* 151–156.

Tataryn, D. J. (2002). Paradigms of health and disease: A framework for classifying and understanding complementary and alternative medicine. *Journal of Alternative and Complementary Medicine, 8,* 877–892.

Taylor, T. (2004). Promises and possibilities: Images of Islam in America. *Saudi Aramco World, 55*(5), 16–31.

Trachtenberg, D. (2002). Alternative therapies and public health: Crisis or opportunity? *American Journal of Public Health, 92,* 1566–1567.

U.S. Department of Health and Human Services. (2002). Culture counts in mental health services and research. *Prevention Report, 16*(2), 1–3. Retrieved March 5, 2002, from http://odphp.osophs.dhhs.gov/pubs/prevrpt/02spring/pr.htm

U.S. Department of Health and Human Services. (2004). *DATA2010: The Healthy People 2010 Base.* Retrieved February 21, 2005, from http://wonder.cdc.gov/scripts/broker.exe

Vivian, C., & Dundes, L. (2004). The crossroads of culture and health among the Roma (gypsies). *Journal of Nursing Scholarship, 36,* 86–91.

Walcott-McQuigg, J. A., & Prohaska, T. R. (2001). Factors influencing participation of African American elders in exercise behavior. *Public Health Nursing, 18,* 194–203.

Watson, W. H. (Ed.). (1998). *Black folk medicine: The therapeutic significance of faith and trust.* New Brunswick, NJ: Transaction.

Weibert, S. (2002). Cultural diversity and breastfeeding. San Diego County Breastfeeding Coalition. *Breastfeeding Update, 2*(3), 1,3.

Wessling, S. (2003, Winter). Does the NCLEX-RN® pass the test for cultural sensitivity? *Minority Nurse,* pp. 46–50.

Wolpe, P. R. (2002). Medical culture and CAM culture: Science and ritual in the academic medical center. In D. Callahan (Ed.), *The role of complementary and alternative medicine: Accommodating pluralism* (pp. 163–171). Washington, DC: Georgetown University.

Wong-Kim, E., Sun, A., & DeMattos, M. C. (2003). Assessing cancer beliefs in a Chinese immigrant community. *Cancer Control, 10*(5), 22–28.

World Health Organization. (2004). *Guidelines on developing consumer information on proper use of traditional, complementary and alternative medicine.* Geneva, Switzerland: Author.

Yosef, A-R.. (2004). Male Arab-Muslim's health and health promotion perceptions and practices. (Unpublished manuscript.)

The Environmental Context

CHAPTER OBJECTIVES

After reading this chapter, you should be able to:

1. Analyze the interrelationships among environmental factors and human health.
2. Discuss elements of the natural, built, and social environments that affect population health.
3. Analyze the role of the community health nurse with respect to environmental health issues at the individual/family and population levels.
4. Identify factors in the natural, built, and social environments that influence the health of an individual/family or a selected population group.
5. Analyze the role of community health nurses in primary prevention measures for environmental issues that affect population health.
6. Identify secondary and tertiary prevention measures for individuals or populations affected by environmental health problems and the role of the community health nurse in their implementation.

KEY TERMS

built environment **234**
ecological footprint **235**
environmental health **229**
land use mix **235**
natural environment **229**
social disorganization **238**
sustainable development **229**
urban sprawl **235**

MediaLink
http://www.prenhall.com/clark

Additional interactive resources for this chapter can be found on the Companion Website. Click on Chapter 10 and "Begin" to select the activities for this chapter.

Advocacy in Action

An Environment for Health

A group of undergraduate community health nursing students developed strong advocacy skills in their work with seniors living in a subsidized housing complex in an impoverished part of the city. An assessment of the population revealed five problems: inadequate disease self-management, lack of transportation, minimal health promotion, poor lighting near the building, and high risk for lead exposure in the older building. All interventions required advocacy skills, but clearly the transportation and high-risk environment would be the greatest challenges. The nursing students developed partnerships with 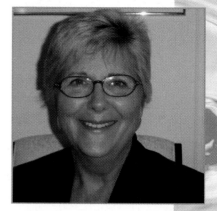 the residents, presented their assessment findings, and led a discussion regarding potential solutions at a regular monthly resident meeting. To address the transportation problem, the clinical instructor, two student representatives, and two resident managers met with the transportation authority to present the assessment data regarding transportation. The group recommended relocation of the bus stop near the entrance to the housing complex. Students assisted residents with petitions and presentations at the TA office. Within 6 months the bus stop was built and appointment-keeping behavior increased 25%.

To promote a healthier lifestyle, the clinical instructor encouraged the health education department to develop a clinical rotation at the high-rise. Interdisciplinary student teams developed regular exercise and nutrition classes for the residents.

Requests to the housing authority (HA) regarding inadequate exterior lighting and high lead content throughout the building were ignored for several months. A lead poisoning program provided by the public health nursing students escalated the residents' frustration with potential lead exposure for their grandchildren. The lighting problem could wait. The students assisted the resident managers with a request that the local health department conduct environmental lead testing. The HA was surprised by the results and lead abatement began within 6 weeks.

These clinical experiences enhanced both the advocacy skills of the public health nursing students and the self-advocacy skills of the residents.

Margaret L. Beaman, PhD, RN-BC

Professor Emeritus, IUE School of Nursing

Concerns for environmental effects on human health were documented nearly 2,500 years ago when Hippocrates wrote his famous treatise, *On Airs, Waters, and Places* (Hancock, 2000). Although Hippocrates and his contemporaries mistakenly believed illness resulted from *miasmas,* or unhealthy vapors, in specific locales, their conception of environmental effects on health was correct in the light of modern scientific information. Nursing, as a profession, has also had an abiding concern for the effects of environment on health. Florence Nightingale's campaign for cleanliness in the surroundings of wounded British soldiers in the Crimean War is a legendary example of this concern. What is less well known is her support for reforestation (McDonald, 2000) and a paper she presented in 1887 to the International Congress of Hygiene and Demography castigating the British government for the unsanitary conditions found in India. This last activity is particularly interesting since Miss Nightingale did not believe that diseases such as cholera, often seen in India, were contagious and perceived quarantine measures as "evil" (Watts, 2003).

Other early community health nurses were equally concerned about the contribution of the environment to human disease. Lillian Wald and her compatriots were concerned about both physical and social environmental effects on health, and much of their work was directed to changing social conditions that contributed to disease and illness. Community health nurses remain concerned with the effects of environmental factors on health and regularly engage in interventions related to environmental concerns that affect individuals, families, and population groups. To engage in effective action at all levels, community health nurses must have an understanding of environmental influences on health.

ENVIRONMENT AND HEALTH

The World Health Organization (WHO) has defined **environmental health** as

> those aspects of human health and disease that are determined by factors in the environment. It includes both the direct pathological effect of chemicals, radiation, and some biological agents, and the effects on health and well-being of the broad physical, psychological, social, and aesthetic environment, which includes housing, urban development, land use, and transportation. (WHO, quoted in Uosukainen, 2001, p. 378)

According to WHO data, approximately 25% to 33% of the global burden of disease is due to environmental exposures (Butterfield, 2002), and environmental conditions are responsible for roughly one fourth of the preventable illnesses in the world (U.S. Department of Health and Human Services [USDHHS], 2002). In recent years, greater attention has been given to the health risks posed by environmental conditions. This attention

is evident in the number of national health objectives that focus on environmental health issues. Sixteen objectives related to environmental health were included in the objectives for the year 2000 (U.S. Department of Health and Human Services, 1991), and an additional 14 objectives were added to the 2010 objectives (U.S. Department of Health and Human Services, 2000). These objectives can be found at the Healthy People◆ Web site, http://www.healthypeople.gov.

Many environmental forces influence human health. Microorganisms such as bacteria, viruses, and fungi cause communicable diseases, and animals contribute to the spread of these diseases. Plants may contribute to accidental poisoning or to allergic reactions. Industry, vehicles, and buildings add to air and water pollution and excess noise. Climate and terrain contribute to natural disasters, which are discussed in Chapter 27∞. In addition, climate and terrain may promote air and water pollution, which have long-term effects on health. Community design and the incorporation of walking and biking areas influence opportunities for healthy physical activity, and the quality of interpersonal interactions within the population influence people's willingness to take advantage of these opportunities. All of these facets of the environment give rise to environmental hazards that affect human health. Some of the environmental components that produce health hazards are presented in Figure 10-1.

The environment has been described as a "global life-support system" (McMichael, Butler, & Ahern, 2003). Human health requires a viable environment that incorporates the local ecosystem, including the air, water, and soil, and the availability of safe and adequate food. In addition, a viable environment requires **sustainable development**, which has been defined as "development that meets the needs of the present without compromising the ability of future generations to meet their own need" (*The Brundtland Report*, quoted in Uosukainen, 2001, p. 377).

COMPONENTS OF THE HUMAN ENVIRONMENT

The environmental context that influences human health incorporates a number of components. These include the natural and constructed, or built, environments, as well as the social and psychological environments. In this chapter we will deal with aspects of the natural, built, and social environments. Other elements of the social environment and the psychological environment are addressed in other chapters throughout this book.

The Natural Environment

The **natural environment** consists of those features of the environment that exist in a natural state, unmodified in any significant way by human beings. Elements

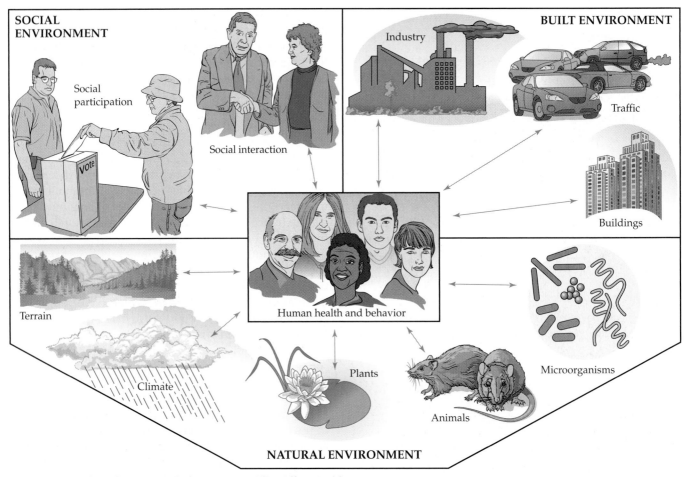

FIGURE 10-1 Selected Environmental Components That Affect Health

of the natural environment include weather and climate, terrain (e.g., mountains, rivers, oceans), natural flora and fauna (plants and animals), biological agents, and natural resources (air, wood, water, fuel). As we will see in Chapter 27∞, the natural environment contributes to a variety of human health hazards in the form of disasters related to high winds, precipitation, earthquakes, and so on. Weather and climate also have positive effects on human health. For example, a moderate level of precipitation (both rain and snow) is required for crop growth and adequate water supplies for human consumption. Some of the concerns related to the natural environment include air and water pollution, global climate change and its consequences, radiation and temperature extremes, biological hazards, and the depletion of natural resources. As we will see, many of these concerns are interrelated and are connected to features of the social and built environments.

Climate has multiple effects on human health. For example, from 1979 to 1999, more than 8,000 deaths occurred in the United States as a result of exposure to heat, nearly half due to the weather (Division of Environmental Hazards and Health Effects, 2003). Conversely, from 1979 to 2002, hypothermia, primarily due to cold weather, accounted for an average

of 689 deaths per year, mostly among elderly persons (Division of Environmental Hazards and Health Effects, 2005). In addition, poor weather conditions contribute to 28% of motor vehicle accidents in the United States each year, at a cost of 7,000 deaths, 800,000 injuries, and $42 billion (Eisenberg & Warner, 2005). Although there have always been deaths due to hypo- and hyperthermia and motor vehicle accidents caused by weather conditions, the potential for illness and injury due to temperature extremes and adverse weather conditions has increased recently as a result of global climate changes. Community health nurses can educate individuals, families, and communities to prevent weather-related mortality. For example,

CULTURAL COMPETENCE

*T*he World Health Organization (2003) provides several examples of the abrogation of the water rights of indigenous peoples. These include elimination of fishing lifestyles and alteration of traditional cultural gathering places by dam construction and elimination of ground water in wells and springs due to coal extraction in Native American territories. What might community health nurses do to prevent this type of exploitation? What strategies might be used? What alliances might need to be created?

education tips for preventing heat-related deaths are provided at right.

Global climate changes result from several inter-related mechanisms. These include ocean oscillations, greenhouse gases, and stratospheric ozone depletion that result in global warming, polar meltdown, rising sea levels, and increased tectonic and volcanic activities (Diaz, 2004). Ocean oscillations refer to periodic changes in five major ocean currents (e.g., El Niño, La Niña) that affect weather and storm patterns and cause increased or decreased precipitation and the resulting flooding, droughts, and prolonged wildfire seasons (Diaz, 2004). El Niño is a disruption of the tropical Pacific ocean-atmosphere system that results in warmer water temperatures than usual. La Niña, on the other hand, results in cooler water temperatures (National Oceanic and Atmospheric Administration [NOAA], n.d.a; n.d.b). These oscillations are also responsible for changes in weather, plankton growth, and reproduction of microorganisms. For example, the El Niño/Southern Oscillation (ENSO) has been associated with increased incidence of cholera due to warmer sea temperatures (Aron & Glass, 2001), and warmer oceans are expected to contribute to other pathogenic growth and increased prevalence of infectious diseases (Knowlton, 2004).

Greenhouse gases are a collection of gases released naturally and as a by-product of human industrial processes that accumulate in the troposphere (the portion of the earth's atmosphere that reaches from the earth's surface to the tropopause, where the stratosphere begins). Greenhouse gases absorb infrared radiation from the earth and trap solar heat, leading to increased tropospheric temperatures. Carbon dioxide (CO_2) is the primary greenhouse gas contributing to this phenomenon, and atmospheric CO_2 levels are expected to have increased by 66% between 1850 and 2050.

CLIENT EDUCATION	Preventing Heat-related Deaths

During heat waves:

- Check on elderly, disabled, or homebound persons frequently.
- Never leave children alone in cars and ensure that they cannot lock themselves in an enclosed space.
- Evaluate persons at risk for heat-related death frequently for heat-related hazards and illnesses, and take appropriate preventive action.
- Seek air-conditioned environments.

If exposure to heat cannot be avoided:

- Reduce, eliminate, or reschedule strenuous activities.
- Drink water or nonalcoholic fluids frequently.
- Take showers regularly.
- Wear lightweight and light-colored clothing.
- Avoid direct sunlight.

Data from: Division of Environmental Hazards and Health Effects, National Center for Environmental Health. (2003). Heat-related deaths—Chicago, Illinois, 1996–2001, and United States, 1979–1999. Morbidity and Mortality Weekly Report, 52, 610–612.

Approximately three fourths of the CO_2 buildup results from the burning of fossil fuels (Diaz, 2004).

The loss of the ozone layer in the stratosphere also contributes to global warming. Stratospheric ozone forms a protective layer around the earth's atmosphere that prevents a significant portion of ultraviolet light from reaching the earth's surface. Although the production of chlorofluorocarbons (CFCs) responsible for the depletion of the ozone layer has been halted by international agreement, it is anticipated that it will take approximately 50 years for any noticeable benefit to occur. In the

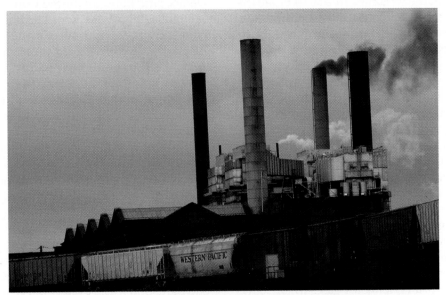

Uncontrolled industrial processes may contribute to a variety of environmental health concerns. (Patrick J. Watson)

meantime, global temperatures continue to rise and exposure to increasing levels of ultraviolet radiation result in increased prevalence of skin cancers, particularly malignant melanomas, and cataracts (Diaz, 2004).

The rise in global temperatures resulting from these environmental changes will have multiple effects, such as increased precipitation, melting of polar ice caps, and rising sea levels. Increased precipitation is likely to occur during both summer and winter, primarily in the form of ice and rain rather than snow. This will result in faster runoff and less water reserve for use during hot seasons. Polar meltdown will cause higher sea levels and a greater potential for flooding, erosion, avalanches, and rockslides. Since more than 70% of the world's population lives within 100 miles of a coastal area, higher sea levels could put a significant number of people at risk for flooding in these areas. Changing weather patterns will also contribute to drought in other areas and lead to crop failure and increasing world hunger (Diaz, 2004).

Polar meltdown and rising sea levels will have other consequences as well. For example, decreased cooling and reduced pressure by heavy ice masses in the polar areas are expected to result in the uncapping of many currently dormant volcanoes. Eruptions will endanger populations in local areas where they occur, but smoke and fumes will have more far-reaching consequences through air pollution carried on thermal currents throughout major parts of the world. At the same time, increased pressure from growing water bodies will causes changes in the tectonic plates that cover the earth, resulting in more frequent and more intense earthquakes (Diaz, 2004).

Many of these effects are already being noted throughout the world. For example, the average surface temperature of the earth has increased by 1° since 1950, and the level of the earth's seas has risen 4 to 8 inches in the last century. The estimated increase of 5.5° F in global temperature and 18 inches in sea level anticipated by 2100 will cause repeated floods and droughts. In addition, rising CO_2 levels will cause changes in growing seasons, leading to increased pollen production and possibly higher allergenic content in plants that will in turn result in greater prevalence and severity of asthma and other allergic responses (Patz et al., 2004). Warmer temperatures will also lead to increases in insect populations (McMichael, 2001).

Global efforts have been initiated to address the reduction in CO_2 emissions within the context of the Kyoto Protocol, which went into effect in February 2005. The Kyoto Protocol amends the United Nations Framework Convention on Climate Change to control emissions of CO_2 and five other greenhouse gases. Unfortunately, the protocol remains unsupported by the United States, which contributes a significant proportion of the world's CO_2 emissions (Leaders prepare for Kyoto Protocol to take effect, 2005), and 25% of all greenhouse gases (Diaz, 2004).

The safety and adequacy of the world's water supply is another concern related to the natural environment. According to the World Health Organization (2003), 1.1 billion people throughout the world do not have access to safe drinking water supplies, and 2.4 billion have inadequate sanitation facilities (Mintz, Bartram, Lochery, & Wegelin, 2001). These conditions are worst for Afghanis, among whom only 19% of urban and 11% of rural residents have access to improved water sources (sources not taken directly from a stream or other natural body of water). In addition, less than 10% of the rural populations of Afghanistan, the Democratic Republic of the Congo, Eritrea, Ethiopia, Mongolia, Niger, the Republic of Korea, and Rwanda have access to improved sanitation (WHO, 2004). Approximately one third of urban water systems in Africa and Latin America and half of those in Asia operate only intermittently, and two thirds of urban sewage generated worldwide is dumped untreated into lakes, rivers, and coastal waters (Population Information Program, 2002).

Water quality is also impaired in industrialized countries. For example, a study of water samples in major U.S. cities found frequent contamination with a variety of pollutants including lead and other heavy metals, pathogens, chlorination by-products, medications, and other carcinogens and toxins. Water is contaminated by sewage, storm water, or snowmelt in urban and suburban areas; agricultural runoff, including pesticides, fertilizers, and animal wastes; mining and industrial wastes; hazardous wastes; petroleum and chemical leaks; and natural contaminants, such as radiation (Natural Resources Defense Council, 2003).

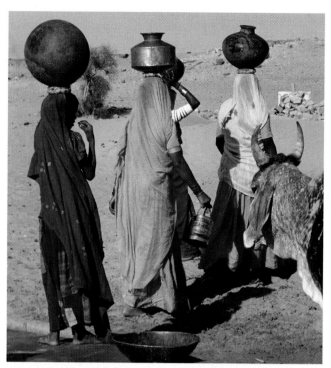

Much of the world's population does not have access to potable water sources. (© Alison Wright/The Image Works)

SPECIAL CONSIDERATIONS

WATER ACCESS AND HEALTH IMPLICATIONS

Access Level	Distance/Time	Health Implications
None	More than 1 kilometer or more than 30 minutes round trip	Inadequate water for consumption and effective hygiene
Basic	Within 1 kilometer or 30 minutes round trip	Adequate water for consumption, not for effective hygiene
Intermediate	Water provided on-plot by at least one tap	Probably adequate for consumption and hygiene
Optimal	Multiple taps within house	Adequate for consumption and hygiene

Data from: World Health Organization. (2003). Right to water. Geneva, Switzerland: Author.

Internationally, adverse health effects related to poor water quality include water-transmitted pathogens, water-washed diseases due to poor personal hygiene, water-based diseases due to parasites in the water, and water-related diseases due to insect vectors that breed in water. In addition, collecting and carrying water often accounts for significant time and effort, particularly for the poor of the world. Water is often costly, as well, consuming as much as 20% of the income of poor families in developing countries (Mintz et al., 2001).

In the United States, 61 disease outbreaks occurred as a result of recreational water contamination from 2001 to 2002 (Yoder et al., 2004), and 31 outbreaks were related to contaminated drinking water during that same period. Of the drinking water outbreaks, pathogenic organisms caused 80%, and 20% were related to chemical contamination (Blackburn et al., 2004). In 2003, pathogenic microorganisms contaminated more than 5,500 bodies of water in the United States (Gaffield, Goo, Richards, & Jackson, 2003). Looking back to our discussion on the effects of global warming, extremely heavy precipitation due to climate changes has been linked with waterborne disease outbreaks. Surface water sources are contaminated within a month of heavy rains, and area groundwater sources within 2 months (Curriero, Patz, Rose, & Lele, 2001).

Lead and other heavy metals also contaminate water supplies. As we will see later, lead contamination is often related to features of the built environment, such as older lead pipes and newer brass fittings, as are some other types of metal poisoning. Several metals (e.g., arsenic and mercury) are naturally occurring contaminants as well as hazards contributed by the built environment (Zierold, Knobeloch, & Anderson, 2004). Frequent fish consumption, for example, has been found to be related to higher mercury levels in hair samples due to contamination of the food chain (McDowell et al., 2004). Urban runoff, in particular, contaminates not only water supplies but also shellfish

GLOBAL PERSPECTIVES

According to the World Health Organization (2003), 1.1 billion of the world's 6 billion people are without adequate water, and one child dies every 15 minutes from diarrheal diseases caused by poor water supplies and lack of sanitation. WHO has taken the stance that access to safe and sufficient water supplies should be considered a basic human right. This right would include access to the following:

■ Sufficient water to prevent dehydration, for cooking, for adequate hygiene, for agricultural use to grow needed food, for cultural uses, for securing livelihoods, and for adequate housing
■ Water that is safe and acceptable and does not carry the risk of water-related disease
■ Water that is accessible (preferably available at housing sites)
■ Water that is affordable to the world's populations (WHO, 2003)

Cultural uses of water entail protection of traditional water sources, such as sacred springs and other bodies of water that have cultural or religious significance. In addition, traditional water-related occupations should be protected (e.g., not destroying fishing as a traditional occupation by building dams).

beds, causing infectious diseases such as hepatitis A and Norwalk virus (Gaffield et al., 2003).

Hazardous air quality is also an issue of concern at both national and global levels. For example, in 1998 alone, 1.2 billion pounds of neurotoxic chemicals were discharged into the air and water in the United States, and 1.4 million urban dwellers worldwide are exposed to poor air quality (Butterfield, 2002). In 2000, an extended heat wave killed 15,000 people in France and 2,000 in England and Wales. Approximately one fourth of these deaths were attributed to ambient air levels of ozone and particulate pollution exacerbated by the heat (Patz et al., 2004). We will consider the problem of air pollution in greater depth in the context of the built environment.

CLIENT EDUCATION   Air Quality and Health Implications

Code	Air Quality	Health Implications
Green	Good	Continue routine activity
Yellow	Moderate	Limited outdoor exertion for highly sensitive people
Orange (advisory)	Unhealthy for sensitive groups	Limited outdoor exertion for active children, adults, and people with respiratory conditions
Red (alert)	Unhealthy	Avoid outdoor exertion by active children, adults, and people with respiratory conditions; limited outdoor exertion by all others
Purple (health alert)	Very unhealthy	Avoid outdoor exertion by active children, adults, and people with respiratory conditions; limited outdoor exertion by all others

AIRNow. (2006). Air Quality Guide for Ozone. Retrieved May 23, 2006, from <http://www.airnow.gov/index.cfm?action=static.consumer>http://www.airnow.gov/index.cfm?action=static.consumer

The Built Environment

The **built environment** includes "all buildings, spaces, and products that are created or modified by people" (*Health Canada*, quoted in Srinivasan, O'Fallon, & Dearry, 2003, p. 1446). Elements of the built environment include homes, schools, workplaces, roads, and features such as urban sprawl and air pollution. Public health experts have broadened the concept of the built environment to incorporate public policy, political action, and the commercial and sociocultural environments (Richardson, 2004), but we will address those factors under the social environment, separate from the built environment.

The built environment has both direct and indirect effects on health. Direct effects derive from exposure to hazardous conditions arising from the built environment (Hancock, 2000). Indirect effects are the result of the effects of the built environment on the natural environment (e.g., contamination of air and water) or on human health-related behaviors (Wang et al., 2004). Examples of direct health effects include lead poisoning arising from ingestion or inhalation of lead from older structures painted with lead-based paints or respiratory disease due to air pollution. In the United States, approximately 42 million dwellings and 52% of all residential units pose the risk of exposure to lead. In addition, 1.8 million children, those likely to suffer the most serious effects of lead exposure, live in homes with deteriorating lead paint or lead water pipes (Potula, Hegarty-Steck, & Hu, 2001). From 1999 to 2002, for example, 2.2% of U.S. children 1 to 5 years of age included in the National Health and Nutrition Examination Surveys (NHANES) (434,000 children) had blood lead levels greater than 10 μg/dL. Although the number of cases of lead poisoning declined by 43% from 1997 to 2001, the national objective of zero cases has not been achieved (Meyer et al., 2003). Similarly, in 2001, the mean state prevalence of blood lead levels above 25 μg/dL among working adults was 12.5 per 100,000 population (Roscoe et al., 2003). Tips for assessing the potential for lead exposure are presented below.

Air pollution, urban sprawl, and resource use are some of the other concerns related to the built environment. A significant portion of air pollutants arise from industrial sources, in particular coal-fired power plants. For example, it is estimated that fine particle emissions from power plants contribute to 24,000 deaths per year (2,800 due to lung cancer), more than 38,000 nonfatal heart attacks, and 554,000 asthma attacks. Approximately 90% of deaths due to particulate matter could be avoided with reductions in sulfur dioxide (SO_2) and nitrous oxide (NO) emissions from power plants. Power plants also contribute to ambient air levels of mercury, CO_2, and ozone. Unfortunately, older power plants, those that are most likely to contribute to these emissions, are exempted from compliance with environmental regulations that apply to newer plants (Schneider, 2004). These effects are likely to be compounded by an anticipated 42% increase in electricity generation by 2020, increasing CO_2 emissions by 800 million tons, mercury emissions by 4 tons, and NO and SO_2 emissions by 100,000 and 2 million tons, respectively (U.S. General Accounting Office [GAO], 2002).

Similarly, many plywood manufacturers and users of industrial and commercial boilers are exempted from new Environmental Protection Agency (EPA) regulations because of the undue financial burden of compliance on the industries. These exemptions were allowed in spite of government estimates that the boiler exemption will increase hazardous air pollutants by 13,300 tons, fine particle emissions by 24,000 tons, volatile organic compounds (which cause smog) by 13,000 tons, and SO_2 by 60,000 tons and will cost $1.7 billion a year in health-related expenditures. In addition, these exemptions will result in an estimated 230 avoidable deaths, 720 hospitalizations, and 18,000 asthma attacks, while saving the boiler industry $170 million (8% of the costs to the public's health). Similarly, the plywood manufacturer exemptions will cost an estimated $300

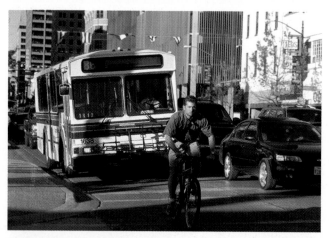

Both natural and built environments affect human health. (© Bob Daemmrich/The Image Works)

FOCUSED ASSESSMENT

Assessing Lead Exposure Risk

- Do you live in an area where 25% or more of the houses were built before 1950?
- Do you live in or regularly visit a house built before 1950?
- Is anyone you know (family member, neighbor's child, child's playmate) being treated for lead poisoning?
- Do any jobs or hobbies of family members involve exposure to lead?
- Do you live near an active lead smelter or battery recycling plant?

Data from: California Department of Health Services. (1998). Interim childhood lead poisoning targeted screening guidelines. Sacramento, CA: Author.

MediaLink · Lead Poisoning Prevention Video

EVIDENCE-BASED PRACTICE

*E*xamine the literature on "green buildings." What health effects, if any, have been demonstrated for this type of architectural design? What are the implications for future building design, if any?

million a year to save the industry $66 million (Environmental Integrity Project, 2004).

Urban sprawl is another feature of the built environment that has drawn considerable attention in recent years. **Urban sprawl** has been defined as "low density development that outpaces population growth" (Schmidt, 2004, p. A620) and is characterized by low population density (fewer than 3,500 people per square mile, the point beyond which nonautomobile travel usually begins) (Lopez, 2004), loss of open spaces, automobile dependence due to low connectivity between destinations, air and water pollution, and limited opportunities to walk or bicycle to work or school. Other characteristic features of urban sprawl include poor land use mix, limited activity centers and downtown areas, "leap-frogging" development, and employment dispersion (Frumkin, 2003; Lopez, 2004; Schmidt, 2004).

Land use mix is "the degree to which the environment has a mix of commercial, residential, and other noncommercial uses" (Richardson, 2004, p. 3). Poor land use mix has a long historical tradition in the United States, dating from 1785 federal legislation mandating a rectangular grid pattern for public lands in the West (including towns and cities) and segregated land use for residential and commercial purposes. Although such regulations led to improved traffic flow, they limited opportunities for social interaction and increased the reliance on vehicles for transportation (Semenza, 2003). Leap-frogging development is the practice of developing distant parcels of land while skipping over those closer to developed areas (Lopez, 2004).

All of the characteristic features of urban sprawl lead to increased resource use. The extent of resource use is conceptualized in terms of humanity's **ecological footprint,** which has been defined as "the area of biologically productive space required per person in order to maintain the current lifestyle" (Hancock, 2000, p. 152). An ecological footprint is usually measured in hectares per person (one hectare is 10,000 square meters or 2.47 acres). Worldwide, the current ecological footprint is 2.3 hectares per capita, but there are only 1.7 hectares per person available, suggesting that we are outpacing our resources by more than 35%. The ecological footprint of industrialized nations is even greater, at 10.3 hectares per person in the United States, 7.7 in Canada, and 5.9 in Sweden (Hancock, 2000). Earlier in this chapter, we referred to the need for sustainable development. In this context, a sustainable or ecological community is one that "does not erode the natural capital (air, water, land, renewable and nonrenewable resources) of the earth, and whose structure and function result in a harmonious relationship with the local, regional, and global ecosystems" (Hancock, 2000, p. 152)—in other words, communities with acceptable ecological footprints.

Urban sprawl not only wastes available land and converts valuable agricultural land to other uses, it increases energy use and contributes to pollution. Globally, transportation uses 60% of the world's oil production, and urban sprawl contributes to greater vehicle use. This rate of use is expected to climb to 73% between 1990 and 2030 (Hancock, 2000). Increased vehicle use also contributes to a variety of health effects. In addition to air pollution, each hour spent in a car has been found to result in a 6% increase in the risk of obesity due to lack of physical activity. Similarly, each kilometer walked results in a 4.8% decrease in one's risk (Frank, cited in Richardson, 2004). In part, the greater risk of illness may also be attributable to traffic stress in areas relying on automobile travel (Gee & Takeuchi, 2004).

Conditions in the built environment affect health behaviors, an indirect effect. For example, building renovation and the installation of materials with potential

Advocacy in Action

Not in Our Backyard!

Nurses are often so involved in the care of individual clients and their families or in addressing issues related to their access to care that they may be unaware of the relevance of environmental issues that affect health. That was not the case for one RN student returning to school for her baccalaureate and master's degrees.

The student worked as a staff nurse in a small local hospital situated near a vacant piece of property. Through the local news media, the student became aware of a proposal to locate a solid waste management operation next to the hospital. Concerned about the possible effects of such a facility on the health of already ill patients, the student mobilized hospital staff, administration, and community residents to protest the location of the facility so close to the hospital. As a result of their activities, the waste management facility was built elsewhere. Because of her involvement in initiating the protest campaign, the student received an award for civic activism from the local government.

BUILDING OUR KNOWLEDGE BASE

*F*rumkin (2003) described four aspects of the built environment that should be studied:

- The effects of human contact with nature (both positive and negative)
- The effects of buildings on human health (the effects of designs to improve indoor air quality, conserve energy, conserve environmental resources, promote physical activity, and make use of natural lighting)
- The effects of public places as venues for social interaction and physical activity, traffic control, and the use and effects of open spaces
- The effects of urban form (e.g., urban sprawl, declining center city areas)

Select one of these areas of study and describe how you might design a study to explore that aspect of the built environment.

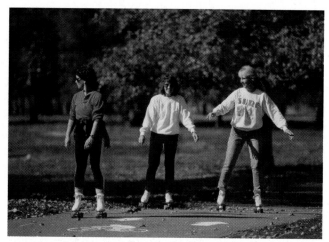

Aspects of the built environment strongly influence health-related behaviors such as exercise. (Patrick J. Watson)

chemical emissions have been linked to increased frequency of asthma attacks (Jaakkola, Parise, Kislitsin, Lebedeva, & Spengler, 2004). On the other hand, the built environment may enhance health. Well-designed communities that encourage physical activity, for instance, promote health. In a U.S. national survey in 1999, only 19% of children reported walking to school and 6% rode their bicycles. Barriers to walking or biking were reported as long distances, traffic, bad weather, crime danger, and school policies against such modes of transportation. Children without reported barriers were six times more likely to walk or ride a bike to school than those with barriers (Division of Unintentional Injury Prevention, 2002). Activity levels within communities are also associated with other features of the built environment such as adequate lighting and available recreation areas (Addy et al., 2004). In addition, features such as "traffic calming" physical structures (e.g., speed bumps) that self-enforce traffic regulations have been associated with reductions in the frequency of traffic accidents and injuries to children in neighborhoods in which they are installed (Tester, Rutherford, Wald, & Rutherford, 2004).

The Social Environment

Throughout this book, we discuss the effects of several elements of the social environment on the health of populations. For example, Chapter 8∞ addressed the economic aspect of the social environment, and Chapter 9∞ dealt with the cultural aspects. In this chapter, we will focus on two additional aspects of the social environment as they affect health: social capital and neighborhood quality.

A basic definition of social capital was presented in Chapter 4∞. Social capital has also been defined as "resources, which vary in terms of both quantity and quality, embedded in social networks that help individuals achieve goals that would otherwise be less attainable" (Reisig, Holtfreter, & Morash, 2002, p. 169). The World Bank conceptualized social capital as "the norms and networks that enable collective action" (quoted in Henderson & Whiteford, 2003, p. 505). Social capital is derived from relationships that make resources available to members of a group and depends on the overall level of resources available to the group (Reisig et al., 2002).

There is considerable confusion in the literature regarding whether social capital is considered a feature of individuals and their families or of the larger social group (Carlson & Chamberlain, 2003). At the community level, social capital is conceptualized as "the network of associations, activities, or relations that bind people together as a community via certain norms and psychological capacities, notably trust, which are essential for civil society and productive of future collective action or goods" (Farr, 2004, p. 9). Social capital incorporates three elements: form, norms, and resources (Monkman, Ronald, & Theramene, 2005).

Form reflects the nature and structure of social ties, their breadth, depth, and any gaps in those relationships. Relationships among group members may be strong or weak, based on the degree of intimacy in the relationship, and may also be horizontal or vertical. Horizontal relationships occur among social equals, whereas vertical relationships link people to others who are differentially situated (Monkman et al., 2005). The former are sometimes called bonding relationships, and the latter bridging relationships (Altschuler, Somkin, & Adler, 2004). In a community, horizontal relationships lead to the development of trust and mutual assistance. Vertical relationships permit group action to influence or tap into resources outside the group itself (Wallerstein, 2002).

Norms include attitudes of trust and expectations of reciprocal assistance. Generalized norms of reciprocity result in information sharing, favor trading, participation in voluntary groups, cooperation, and provision or acceptance of assistance. Reciprocity norms also eliminate the need to negotiate and balance social exchanges (Arnold, 2003), and save time and effort on transaction costs because relationships do not require formal contracts or monitoring for repayment (Streeten, 2002).

Resources, in the context of social capital, include those available to individual members of the group as well as to the group as a whole. Because of the relationships among group members, resources available to one member become available to others. The extent of social capital in a community or population group depends on the resources available to the group as well as the relationships that permit access to those resources.

A qualitative study identified the following features of social capital: movement toward common goals by individuals as well as formal institutions, multidimensional relationships that foster trust, awareness of and action related to the needs of others, advocacy, and awareness of the bigger social picture (Looman, 2004). Communities with high levels of social capital have also been characterized by collective efficacy, a sense of community, neighborhood cohesion, and community competence (Henderson & Whiteford, 2003).

The level of social capital within a population has been linked to both positive and negative effects. Positive health influences may derive from a number of hypothesized relationships between social capital and health. For example, available social capital may promote a sense of mastery and reduced stress, greater ability to influence outside resources, and openness and tolerance among group members (Looman, 2004). Whatever the causative factors in the relationship, lower levels of social capital have been linked to increased mortality (even after controlling for the effects of poverty) (Carlson & Chamberlain, 2003), less effective reentry into society for former female inmates (Reisig et al., 2002), and higher rates of sexually transmitted diseases. In one study, social capital levels predicted 10 of 14 behavioral variables among adolescents, including sexual activity, early sexual debut, and number of sex partners (Lower degrees of "social capital" predict higher rates of STDs, 2002). High social capital, on the other hand, has been linked to economic growth, increased participation in community decisions, improved government performance, and decreased crime (Brody & Lovrich, 2002; Scott, 2002). Social capital, in the form of a sense of belonging, has been associated with better physical and mental health among older women as well as with increased physical activity levels, decreased stress, and better social support (Young, Russell, & Powers, 2004). Social capital expressed as participation in social and civic organizations and reciprocity among neighbors has been linked to decreased risk of hunger among families after adjustment for socioeconomic status (Martin, Rogers, Cook, & Joseph, 2004).

Some authors, however, note the potential for disadvantages to social capital. These disadvantages lie in the group norms and in the relationship of the group to the outside world. Group norms can, in some instances, promote "antisocial capital"—that is, social capital put to inappropriate uses. Examples given include social norms and behaviors related to drug rings, nepotism, cronyism, and crime. The purpose of some social groups, such as the Ku Klux Klan, is to suppress other groups. In such instances, social capital may lead to social isolation for some members of the group as strong subsegments of the population direct group activity (Streeten, 2002). Expectations of conformity to social norms in communities with high levels of social capital may lead to group opposition to conventional norms in the case of criminal activity (Reisig et al., 2002) or to exclusion, and even scapegoating, of nonconformists (Brody & Lovrich, 2002). In one study, for example, increased social capital was linked to a decrease in constitutional protections for those who violated group norms (Brody & Lovrich, 2002). As these authors noted, "We must not overlook the sad fact that communities of exclusion and homogeneity are much easier to build than are inclusive, accepting, forgiving, and socially heterogeneous communities" (p. 128).

Another area for consideration is the differential effects of social capital on some subgroups within the population. For example, young people in the community may not have access to some elements of community social capital because of hostility on the part of some adults and perceptions of their rights to the use of communal spaces and resources (Morrow, 2000). As another example, homeless individuals are denied access to community social capital when they are prohibited from using public facilities such as parks.

With respect to interactions with the larger society, some authors have warned that an emphasis on building social capital within groups and communities may be used as an excuse not to redistribute economic resources to address structural inequalities in access to resources. A focus on building social capital may also result in "blaming the community" due to perceptions that if the community "could get its act together, they could solve their own problems" (Muntaner, Lynch, & Smith, 2000; Wallerstein, 2002).

The other aspect of the social environment to be considered here is that of neighborhood quality. A neighborhood effect is an independent causal effect on a health or social outcome. Neighborhood effects may be of two types: contextual and integral. Contextual effects arise from the relationships attendant on social capital or its absence. Integral effects arise from features of the built environment such as toxic dumps, parks, and so on (Oakes, 2004).

Neighborhood quality is related to social capital as well as to the built environment, but encompasses other features of the community as well. Neighborhood quality includes such characteristics as socioeconomic status (SES) apart from that of individual community members, deterioration, social organization or disorganization, safety, and noise (Lee & Cubbin, 2002). **Social disorganization** is a community's "inability to realize the common values of its residents and to maintain social control" (Jozefowicz-Simbeni & Allen-Meares, 2002, p. 127). Social disorganization within a community is often related to population mobility, unemployment, rental housing, large numbers of female-headed households, and high rates of divorce (Lee & Cubbin, 2002).

Neighborhood quality has been found to be related to a number of health effects. For example, in one study, low neighborhood SES and social disorganization were found to be linked to poor dietary habits, but not to physical activity or youth smoking (Lee & Cubbin, 2002). In another study in England, women living in wards characterized by high deprivation scores had a 27% higher risk of coronary heart disease than women in areas with deprivation scores below the median (Lawlor, Smith, Patel, & Ebrahim, 2005). Similarly, children from low-SES neighborhoods have been found to be exposed to more noise, crowding, and environmental toxins than those in more affluent neighborhoods, regardless of their own family incomes (Evans & Marcynyszyn, 2004).

Aspects of neighborhood quality such as cohesion, community problems (e.g., trash, gangs, and drinking), and safety have been linked to several child mental health outcomes, including conduct disorder, hyperactivity, and emotional distress, as well as physical outcomes such as injuries (Curtis, Dooley, & Phipps, 2004). Parental perceptions of neighborhood quality have also been associated with childhood asthma (Wind, Van Sickle, & Wright, 2004). In addition, neighborhood problems such as traffic, noise, crime, trash, poor lighting, and limited access to public transportation have been linked to increased loss of functional ability in the elderly. For example, reported functional loss among elderly residents was 50% higher in neighborhoods with one identified problem and 2.5 times higher in neighborhoods with two or more problems. Neighborhood characteristics have also been associated with social isolation, hearing loss, depression, and cognitive impairment among the elderly (Balfour & Kaplan, 2002). Caution should be used, however, in interpreting the causal nature of such associations, due to the difficulties in sorting out the effects of neighborhood variables from other variables affecting health and illness (Oakes, 2004).

INTERACTIONS AMONG ENVIRONMENTAL COMPONENTS

Although we have discussed the natural, built, and social environments as if their effects on health are independent of one another, they are actually intimately related. For example, industrial and human wastes deposited into the ocean from the built environment have polluted waters and altered the marine food chain.

Overfishing of coastal waters has, in turn, led to an increasing dependence on farmed fish, which have been shown to have significantly higher levels of contaminants than wild fish, thereby increasing the potential for human health effects (Knowlton, 2004). Similarly, ozone levels that contribute to air pollution peak during traffic rush hours (part of the built environment) and with increasing temperatures during the day (the natural environment) (Patz et al., 2004). Surprisingly, ozone levels are worse in less densely populated areas due to increased vehicle use as a result of urban sprawl. For example, high-population-density areas have been found to have ozone levels averaging 51 ppb less than low-density areas (Schmidt, 2004).

Elements of the natural environment also interact with human development, human behavioral factors, and elements of the social environment to contribute to health problems. For instance, the effects of severe heat waves are associated with increased age, decreased SES, poor housing quality, and lack of air conditioning, as well as with the use of alcohol and some medications (Center for Climatic Research, 2004). Another example of the interactions between built and natural environments lies in the aging water systems in most U.S. cities. Most water systems in the United States are, on average, 100 years old. Aging pipes and equipment are not adequate to handle the contaminant loads contributed by other elements of the built environment, leading to breakdowns and contamination of natural water supplies (Natural Resources Defense Council, 2003).

Elements of the built environment designed to enhance food production also affect the natural environment. Much agriculture in the United States has become highly industrialized. For example, most food animals are now raised in concentrated feeding operations (CFOs) that result in more animals housed in less space and the production of manure wastes far above that needed to meet the nutritional needs of traditional croplands. In addition, CFOs require far more feed than can be supplied in-house, contributing to extensive transportation of feed with the attendant use of oil resources and toxic emissions. CFOs also use significant amounts of antibiotics in animal feed to offset the potential for communicable disease in animals in crowded conditions. This leads to increased antibiotic contamination of water sources and growing resistance to antibiotics among human pathogens. Finally, the confined nature of CFOs contributes to air pollution, particularly for employees in these indoor operations (Osterberg & Wallinga, 2004). Lack of adequate sanitation, another element of the built environment, also leads to outbreaks of infectious diseases due to foods contaminated in the growing and packing process. This is particularly true of Mexican produce imported to the United States, especially such commodities as onions and strawberries that have complex surfaces to which viral and fecal particles adhere (Epidemiology Program Office, 2003).

Think Advocacy

If access to water is a basic human right, how should community health nurses deal with the practice of cutting off access to water sources when clients are not able to pay their water bills or purchase bottled water for family members who are immunocompromised?

We noted before the effects of the built environment on human health-related behaviors such as walking. Community design also affects the natural environment. Urban development, for example, increases the amount of impervious surfaces that do not absorb rain water, leading to greater storm water volume and runoff, which have the potential to contaminate water sources (Gaffield et al., 2003). The built environment also affects levels of social capital through its effects on opportunities for people to congregate and interact with each other (Cohen et al., 2003). Research has demonstrated that communities with walkable, mixed-use neighborhoods exhibit higher levels of social capital than automobile-dependent ones (Leyden, 2003).

In addition to diminishing social capital, urban sprawl disturbs the natural environment. For instance, in one study in New York, 75% of plant and animal species affected by urban sprawl were in decline. The remaining 25% tended to be pests and weeds rather than more desirable flora and fauna. Whitefooted mice that transmit Lyme disease and West Nile virus, for example, thrive in the context of urban sprawl (Schmidt, 2004).

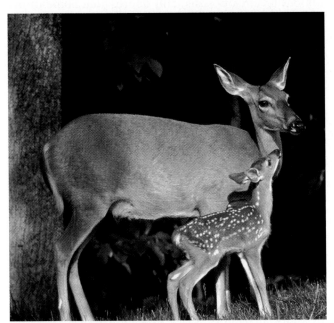

Increased interaction between wild animals and human beings increases the potential for transmission of zoonoses such as Rocky Mountain spotted fever. (© Tom Brakefield/The Image Works)

On occasion, human illness may have effects on the environment. We saw in Chapter 6∞ how high rates of HIV infection and AIDS can affect a country's economic productivity, but illness may have other effects, sometimes even beneficial ones. For example, seasonal hay fever was responsible for the growth in tourism among sufferers who frequented low-pollen areas such as the White Mountains of New Hampshire. This growth was also related to the social environmental element of social capital, since it was only the wealthier classes who were able to travel to escape hay fever season (Mitman, 2003). Socioeconomic status also influences who will be affected by toxic exposures from such activities as ski boating (Division of Environmental Hazards and Health Effects, 2002).

Social environmental changes such as the move to smaller, nuclear families requires more housing, uses more natural resources, and creates a larger ecological footprint (Population Information Program, 2002). These effects, as well as those of global climate change in the natural environment, are anticipated to result in major social upheavals such as water wars and environmental refugees, drought, and malnutrition (Diaz, 2004).

COMMUNITY HEALTH NURSING AND ENVIRONMENTAL HEALTH

Because of their consistent presence in the community, community health nurses are some of those most likely to become aware of environmental health problems, yet they are often unprepared to recognize and deal with them. Protection of the environment is one of the essential functions of public health, and the participation of community health nurses in this function is critical. Community health nursing activity related to environmental health issues occurs at both the level of the individual/family client and the population.

Standards and competencies for occupational and environmental health nursing practice have been developed and are discussed in Chapter 24∞. In addition, a number of national initiatives support the role of nursing with respect to environmental health issues. The first of these initiatives was an offshoot of the Agency for Toxic Substances and Disease Registry (ATSDR). ATSDR, part of the Superfund legislation passed in 1980, was created to prevent or minimize public exposure to hazardous substances. In 1994, ATSDR established the Environmental Health Nursing Initiative to promote research, collaboration, and educational opportunities related to environmental health (Larsson & Butterfield, 2002). The ATSDR initiative was designed to promote a more active role for the nursing profession in addressing environmental health with a goal of making environmental health "an integral component of nursing practice, education, and research" (ATSDR, n.d., p. 1). To that end, the initiative has developed a series of education resources and training programs and roundtable discussions around nursing involvement in environmental health.

In 1995, the Institute of Medicine report, *Nursing, Health and the Environment* (Pope, Snyder, & Mood, 1995), promulgated four general competencies for nursing with respect to environmental health. The first of these competencies addressed knowledge related to mechanisms for environmental exposure, prevention and control strategies, and the need for evidence-based approaches to dealing with environmental issues. The second competency dealt with the ability to take an environment exposure history and make appropriate referrals for health care services as well as informing the public regarding environmental hazards. The third competency underscored the need for advocacy to support environmental justice in resolving environmental health problems, and the fourth reflected knowledge and use of legislative and regulatory processes to address environmental conditions that jeopardize health.

Concurrent with these two initiatives, the National Institute of Nursing Research (NINR) undertook a third initiative to emphasize nursing's role in environmental health research. Foci for this endeavor included reducing environmental hazards for vulnerable populations, targeting specific settings for environmental research (e.g., the workplace), and identifying infrastructure needs to support environmental health research by nurses (Larsson & Butterfield, 2002).

Community health nurses can make use of the dimensions model of community health nursing to address environmental health problems. Use of the model focuses on assessment, intervention planning, and evaluation of environmental interventions.

Assessing Environmental Health in Populations

The first step in ameliorating environmental health problems is an assessment of the factors contributing to them and their effects on human health. In addition to identifying environmental factors in the community that may affect health, community health nurses assess the population for factors that may increase the risk or severity of the health effects of environmental conditions. The age composition of the population is one such factor. For example, children's higher metabolic rate increases the rate of absorption of toxins, and very young children are closer to the floor, where air pollutants, in particular, accumulate. In addition, the rapid rate of growth and cell differentiation in children fosters genetic alteration and carcinogenesis. Older adults, because of changes in their cardiovascular, renal, pulmonary, and immune systems, are less able to detoxify environmental toxins and, consequently, have a higher risk of adverse health effects.

Existing genetic and physiologic conditions may also increase the potential for health effects of environmental factors. For example, levels of environmental toxins that might not harm an adult may be harmful to the fetus in a pregnant woman. A higher prevalence of chronic respiratory conditions, such as asthma, increases the adverse health effects of plant pollens and air pollution.

Community health nurses also assess individual clients and population groups for evidence of environmentally caused disease. Air pollution, for example, affects the respiratory system primarily, but may also produce cardiovascular, central nervous system, or hematopoietic effects. Air pollution also irritates the eyes and mucous membranes of the respiratory system. Water pollution can affect the gastrointestinal system, skin, liver, and reproductive, hematopoietic, lymphatic, cardiovascular, and genitourinary systems. Pesticides can adversely affect the central nervous system and produce kidney damage, a variety of cancers, and chromosomal changes. Radiation can cause skin cancer, visual impairment, cataracts, and genetic mutations, as well as lung and other cancers. Lead poisoning damages the central nervous system as well as the gastrointestinal system and can impair growth and development. Other metals and hazardous chemicals may cause cancers or central nervous system, gastrointestinal, and metabolic damage. High levels of noise not only compromise human hearing, but can contribute to gastrointestinal, dermatologic, central nervous system, cardiovascular, and psychological problems. Finally, built environments that hinder physical activity contribute to obesity, osteoporosis, and depression. Some of the effects of these environmental hazards are presented in Figure 10-2.

Occupational settings give rise to multiple opportunities for exposure to environmental hazards, and community health nurses should assess the potential for exposure to hazardous environmental conditions created by local occupations and industries. Other social factors, such as socioeconomic status, may influence exposure to environmental hazards. For example, children in families with lower income levels and living in housing of lower economic value are at higher risk for lead poisoning (Kim, Staley, Curtis, & Buchanan, 2002).

Policies related to environmental hazards are another area for consideration. A significant proportion of environmental policy at the national level arises from and is implemented by the United States Environmental Protection Agency (EPA). The EPA was established in 1970, and its focus is the protection of human health and the environment. Some of the functions of the EPA are developing and enforcing environmental regulations, supporting state environmental programs and environmental education, conducting environmental research, and promoting environmental partnerships and

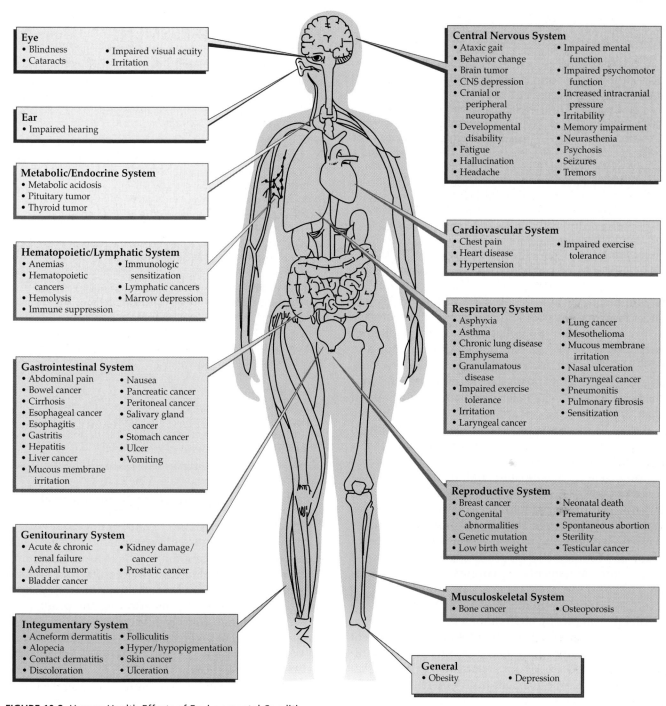

Eye
- Blindness
- Cataracts
- Impaired visual acuity
- Irritation

Ear
- Impaired hearing

Metabolic/Endocrine System
- Metabolic acidosis
- Pituitary tumor
- Thyroid tumor

Hematopoietic/Lymphatic System
- Anemias
- Hematopoietic cancers
- Hemolysis
- Immune suppression
- Immunologic sensitization
- Lymphatic cancers
- Marrow depression

Gastrointestinal System
- Abdominal pain
- Bowel cancer
- Cirrhosis
- Esophageal cancer
- Esophagitis
- Gastritis
- Hepatitis
- Liver cancer
- Mucous membrane irritation
- Nausea
- Pancreatic cancer
- Peritoneal cancer
- Salivary gland cancer
- Stomach cancer
- Ulcer
- Vomiting

Genitourinary System
- Acute & chronic renal failure
- Adrenal tumor
- Bladder cancer
- Kidney damage/ cancer
- Prostatic cancer

Integumentary System
- Acneform dermatitis
- Alopecia
- Contact dermatitis
- Discoloration
- Folliculitis
- Hyper/hypopigmentation
- Skin cancer
- Ulceration

Central Nervous System
- Ataxic gait
- Behavior change
- Brain tumor
- CNS depression
- Cranial or peripheral neuropathy
- Developmental disability
- Fatigue
- Hallucination
- Headache
- Impaired mental function
- Impaired psychomotor function
- Increased intracranial pressure
- Irritability
- Memory impairment
- Neurasthenia
- Psychosis
- Seizures
- Tremors

Cardiovascular System
- Chest pain
- Heart disease
- Hypertension
- Impaired exercise tolerance

Respiratory System
- Asphyxia
- Asthma
- Chronic lung disease
- Emphysema
- Granulamatous disease
- Impaired exercise tolerance
- Irritation
- Laryngeal cancer
- Lung cancer
- Mesothelioma
- Mucous membrane irritation
- Nasal ulceration
- Pharyngeal cancer
- Pneumonitis
- Pulmonary fibrosis
- Sensitization

Reproductive System
- Breast cancer
- Congenital abnormalities
- Genetic mutation
- Low birth weight
- Neonatal death
- Prematurity
- Spontaneous abortion
- Sterility
- Testicular cancer

Musculoskeletal System
- Bone cancer
- Osteoporosis

General
- Obesity
- Depression

FIGURE 10-2 Human Health Effects of Environmental Conditions

programs (U.S. Environmental Protection Agency, n.d.). As we saw earlier, the activities of the EPA are sometimes hampered by concessions given to major businesses and industry.

Similar agencies exist at the state level, and community health nurses should become familiar with state and local agencies and their functions. For example, the California Environmental Protection Agency (Cal/EPA) includes departments and boards that address environmental concerns related to toxic substances, waste management, air and water quality,

pesticide regulation, and environmental health hazard assessment (Cal/EPA, 2003).

Certain personal behaviors prevalent in the population may interact with elements of the physical environment to cause or exacerbate health problems. Smoking, for example, increases lead absorption levels for both smokers and their children. Similarly, reliance on biomass fuels for cooking and heating creates indoor air pollution, which contributes to 600,000 deaths per year (Population Information Program, 2002). Recreational activities are also affected by

ETHICAL AWARENESS

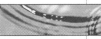

*I*n a review of the ethical and scientific aspects of studies submitted to the Environmental Protection Agency to support pesticide reregistration, Lockwood (2004) noted that several had violated acceptable guidelines for informed consent, failed to manage financial conflicts of interest, and provided distorted results. He also noted that while all of the studies reviewed were approved by human subjects committees, the committees were part of the research organizations paid by the study sponsors, creating a potential conflict of interest. He maintains that the current level of knowledge on the health effects of pesticide exposure should result in a moratorium on human testing of pesticides and that EPA decisions on reregistration of pesticide products should be based on other forms of evidence (e.g., epidemiologic studies of the effects of naturally occurring pesticide exposures).

FOCUSED ASSESSMENT

Assessing Environmental Influences on Population Health

- What natural, built, and social environmental conditions have the potential to influence the health of the population? How do these conditions affect health? What is the extent of their influence on health at the present time?
- What segments of the population are most likely to be adversely affected by environmental conditions? Why?
- What factors contribute to the presence and influence of environmental conditions within the population?
- To what extent do environmental conditions arise from or are influenced by individual behavior (e.g., smoking, use of aerosols and cleaners)?
- What are the attitudes of members of the population to environmental health issues? What priority is given to resolution of environmental health issues?
- What barriers exist to improving environmental conditions?
- What is the potential for eliminating hazardous environmental conditions? What is the potential for limiting human exposure if hazardous environmental conditions cannot be eliminated?
- What actions will be required to address environmental health concerns within the population?
- Does the health care system contribute to environmental health hazards? If so, how?
- Is the health care system adequate to address environmentally caused disease in the population?
- Are health care providers prepared to recognize and treat environmentally caused diseases in individual clients?

environmental factors. For example, after-school sports and after-work physical activity at times of peak ozone levels increase the potential for respiratory health effects (Patz et al., 2004). Similarly, swimming and other water-related recreational activities increase the potential for exposure to microorganisms and chemical agents when water is contaminated (Gaffield et al., 2003).

Finally, health system factors may contribute to or exacerbate environmental health problems. For example, despite federal and state mandates to screen children for lead exposure and inclusion of lead screening in covered Medicaid services, less than 20% of California children have been tested (Ross, Walker, & Wiles, 2000). Health care providers have little knowledge of the manifestations or treatment of many environmentally caused diseases. Tips to assist you in your assessment of environmental health issues are presented at right.

Some environmental assessment data can be obtained primarily by observation in the home or community. For example, elements of the built environment such as traffic safety hazards or recreational opportunities are easily observed. Data related to environmental health effects may be available from local health departments or environmental protection agencies or from state agencies. Information on human behaviors that contribute to environmental health problems (e.g., smoking) is best obtained by asking family members or in community surveys. Information on environmental policy can be obtained from local government, environmental protection agencies, and local businesses and industries. Other elements of environmental assessment are addressed in relevant chapters in this book (e.g., community assessment in Chapter 15∞ and school and occupational settings in Chapters 23 and 24∞, respectively, as well as in assessment tools included in the *Community Assessment Reference Guide* 🗒 designed to accompany this text.

Planning to Improve Environmental Health

Community health nurses assess for environmental hazards present in the community, the factors contributing to them, and the health effects that result. They then use this information to plan interventions to address environmental health problems affecting the population. These interventions can occur at the primary, secondary, or tertiary level of prevention.

Primary Prevention

Primary prevention directed toward the natural environment focuses on the protection and preservation of natural resources. For example, energy conservation and development of new energy resources and industrial processes can minimize emission of greenhouse gases and reduce the effects of global warming. Countries with large coastal areas should take precautions in anticipation of coastal flooding and engage in better surveillance of global weather and geologic activity as well as measures for arthropod and rodent vector control related to global warming (Diaz, 2004). Community health nurses can advocate energy conservation and other forms of environmental conservation as well as educate the public in conservation measures. For example, nurses can initiate recycling campaigns within the community or in health care facilities. They can also educate the public regarding vector control measures that do not jeopardize human health (e.g., care in use of rodenticides or pesticides).

Primary prevention within the built environment would include the development of well-designed communities that minimize urban sprawl, limit resource use, promote mixed land use and the development of social capital, and foster healthy behaviors such as walking and bicycling. Principles of smart growth that would contribute to healthier community design are summarized below. In addition, the contributions of the built environment to degradation of the natural environment could be minimized by investing in more effective water systems that make use of newer technological approaches that are more effective and more environmentally friendly. For example, use of ozone or ultraviolet light to purify water eliminates more hazardous elements without creating potentially harmful chlorination by-products. Use of granulated activated carbon would further reduce the amount of disinfection by-products in water. Finally, upgrading systems to incorporate membrane filtration treatment would eliminate virtually all contaminants (Natural Resources Defense Council, 2003). Community health nurses can advocate for water treatment systems that do not damage the natural environment and yet provide safe water for human consumption. They can also educate clients on inexpensive water treatment measures when more technologically advanced systems are not available (e.g., in underdeveloped countries or on a camping trip).

Developing countries that will not be able to initiate water treatment systems in the near future can encourage point-of-use water treatment systems that incorporate use of dilute solutions of sodium hypochlorite (laundry bleach), solar disinfection by means of ultraviolet light projected through clear plastic bottles or bags, and safe water storage in narrow-mouth containers that require pouring or the use of a spigot to prevent recontamination of the water by dipping. Use of such systems will require access to the needed supplies and public motivation to offset the added costs in terms of time and money (Mintz et al., 2001).

HIGHLIGHTS   Principles of Smart Growth

- Mixed land use
- Compact building design
- A range of housing options and opportunities
- Walkable neighborhoods
- Attractive communities that engender a sense of place
- Preservation of open space and critical environmental features
- Available transportation choices
- Predictable, fair, and cost-effective development decisions
- Community collaboration in development decisions

Data from: Schmidt, C. W. (2004): Sprawl: The new manifest destiny? Environmental Health Perspectives, 112, A620–A627. Retrieved August 26, 2004, from http://www.medscape.com/viewarticle/487573

Public education and social support will be required for all of these initiatives, and many of them will require political advocacy as well (USDHHS, 2002). For example, there is a need for additional lead poisoning prevention legislation, funding for programs, and public education to foster identification of risk groups and intervention to reduce exposure risks (Meyer et al., 2003). Similarly, developers and community development agencies will need to be convinced of the need for smart growth and for provision of affordable mass transit located near schools, homes, and workplaces in those communities already affected by urban sprawl (Schmidt, 2004). Community health nurses can be actively involved in all of these activities. For example, they may organize local residents to work with developers to plan mixed-use communities and community designs that promote fitness and exercise. Other examples of primary prevention activities by community health nurses directed at promoting environmental health for individuals/families and for populations are presented in Table 10-1◆.

Secondary Prevention

Secondary prevention with individuals and their families would be geared to identifying and resolving existing health problems caused by environmental conditions. For example, community health nurses might be involved in screening for elevated lead levels or for hearing loss. They might also make referrals for testing of water supplies for clients who are concerned about potential contamination. When possible environmentally caused health conditions are identified, community health nurses might make referrals for medical diagnosis and treatment as needed. They might also make referrals for assistance with eliminating environmental hazards. For example, the nurse might be aware of lead-based paint in dwellings in some parts of town. He or she can screen young children in the area for elevated blood lead levels (BLLs) and make referrals for treatment for children with positive test results. The nurse might also make a referral for assistance in removing lead-based paint from the homes of affected children. Finally, the nurse might monitor children's responses to therapy and the potential for continued exposure to lead.

At the population level, community health nurses might promote targeted screening programs to identify the prevalence of risk factors in the community. For example, although the 2010 objective sets a goal of radon testing in 20% of all U.S. homes (USDHHS, 2000), initial testing can be targeted to homes in areas that have high natural radon levels. Community health nurses can encourage policy makers to adopt targeted screening practices for appropriate populations in the community.

Political activity by community health nurses might also be needed to influence health policy makers

MediaLink   Case Study: Advocacy in Environmental Health

TABLE 10-1   Primary Preventive Measures for Selected Environmental Hazards for Individuals, Families, and Populations

Environmental Hazard	Individual/Family	Population
Radiation	Refer for assistance with testing and sealing a home against radon leaks.	Educate the public on the hazards of radon exposure and preventive measures. Encourage targeted screening of homes for high radon levels.
	Encourage spending most of one's time in higher levels of the home.	Engage in political activity to promote building standards that safeguard occupants in areas with high levels of natural radiation.
	Discourage overuse of diagnostic x-rays.	Educate public about the hazards of overuse of diagnostic x-rays.
	Encourage adequate cleaning of door seals on microwave ovens and maintenance of safe distance while microwave is in operation.	Engage in political activity to promote and enforce safety standards for nuclear reactors.
	Discourage sunbathing. Encourage use of sunscreen and protective clothing when outdoors.	Educate the public about the hazards of exposure to ultraviolet radiation.
	Discourage smoking in home, refer for smoking cessation assistance.	Promote availability of smoking cessation services.
Lead and heavy metals	Encourage families to remove lead-based paint from older homes.	Encourage communities to remove lead-based paint from older homes.
	Encourage covering surfaces on which paint is peeling.	
	Encourage families to wash small children's hands as well as toys to remove lead-contaminated dust.	Promote legislation to reduce air pollution and acid rain to prevent pollution of water with heavy metals.
	Encourage close supervision of small children. Encourage calcium intake to limit lead absorption.	Encourage policy makers to set and enforce standards for solid waste sites to prevent metal contamination in waters.
	Encourage families to use cold water to drink and cook with and to allow the tap to run for a few minutes.	
Noise	Encourage families to limit noise in the home. Encourage use of ear protection in high-noise areas.	Promote noise abatement ordinances.
Infectious agents	Promote routine immunization for all ages.	Educate the public on the need for immunizations. Encourage policy makers to provide low-cost immunization services.
	Encourage good hygiene. Encourage washing fruits and vegetables before eating.	Encourage enforcement of regulations for food processing and food handlers.
	Encourage adequate refrigeration of food. Encourage susceptible individuals to boil water for cooking and drinking in areas with unsafe water.	Promote adequate sanitation, waste disposal, and water treatment.
Insects and animals	Encourage immunization of family pets.	Encourage development and enforcement of immunization and leash laws.
	Refer for assistance in eliminating insects, rats, and other pests from the home.	Promote ordinances controlling insect breeding areas.
	Encourage use of insect repellent and protective clothing when outdoors.	
Plants	Eliminate poisonous houseplants. Eliminate poisonous plants from the yard. Eliminate other hazardous plants (e.g., poison ivy, plant allergens) from home environment. Encourage close supervision of small children.	Eliminate poisonous plants from recreation areas.
Poisons	Educate families on proper use and storage of household chemicals and medications. Encourage close supervision of children.	Educate public on hazards of household chemicals and medications.
	Encourage proper disposal of hazardous wastes.	Promote legislation to limit use of hazardous chemicals in home and industry. Promote hazardous waste disposal services.
Air pollution	Encourage limiting physical activity on days with high air-pollutant levels.	Promote legislation to prevent air pollution.
	Encourage carpooling.	Promote incentives for carpooling.
	Discourage use of space heaters in poorly ventilated areas.	Promote legislation to develop safety standards for home heating devices.

Continued on next page

TABLE 10-1	Primary Preventive Measures for Selected Environmental Hazards for Individuals, Families, and Populations *(continued)*	
Environmental Hazard	**Individual/Family**	**Population**
	Encourage frequent cleaning of heater and air-conditioning filters.	Promote building standards that ensure adequate ventilation.
	Encourage opening doors and windows to permit air exchange.	
	Encourage replacing asbestos insulation as needed.	Promote replacement of hazard-producing industrial processes.
	Encourage installation of CO monitors in home.	
	Educate for use of household products with adequate ventilation.	
Water pollution	Encourage use of bottled water by high-risk persons in areas with heavily polluted water.	Promote legislation to prevent water pollution.
	Encourage use of fewer polluting products.	Promote replacement of hazard-producing industrial processes.
	Educate about water purification techniques as needed.	Promote filtration of water sources for newer pathogens, etc.
Energy conservation	Educate regarding interventions to conserve electricity, water, etc.	Advocate for policies that conserve resources, promote smart growth, and limit urban sprawl.
	Promote recycling.	

to provide adequate access to diagnostic and treatment facilities for people with health problems caused by environmental conditions. Or a nurse might campaign for stricter standards for pollutant emissions in air and water. Table 10-2◆ provides additional examples of secondary prevention measures that might be taken to improve environmental health in families and population groups.

TABLE 10-2	Secondary Preventive Measures for Selected Environmental Hazards for Individuals, Families, and Populations	
Environmental Hazard	**Individual/Family**	**Population**
Radiation	Look for signs of health problems that may be caused by radiation among clients and members of their families.	Monitor incidence of health problems caused by radiation.
	Refer for diagnosis and treatment as needed.	Promote accessibility of diagnostic and treatment facilities.
	Monitor effectiveness of treatment.	Monitor longevity to determine effects of treatment in groups of people.
Lead and heavy metals	Screen for elevated blood levels of heavy metals in persons at risk.	Promote accessibility of screening services.
		Promote compliance with Medicaid lead screening guidelines.
		Promote adequate reimbursement for lead screening services.
	Observe for signs of heavy metal poisoning.	Monitor incidence of heavy metal poisoning.
	Refer for diagnosis and treatment as needed.	Promote accessibility of diagnostic and treatment facilities.
	Monitor effects of treatment.	Monitor prevalence of complications due to heavy metal poisoning.
Noise	Screen for hearing loss in persons at risk.	Promote accessibility of screening services.
	Refer for diagnosis and treatment as needed.	Promote accessibility of diagnostic and treatment services.
	Monitor effects of treatment.	
Infectious agents	Screen for selected communicable diseases in high-risk persons.	Promote accessibility of screening services.
	Observe for signs of communicable diseases.	Monitor incidence of communicable diseases.
Insects and animals	Educate families about first aid for insect and animal bites.	Promote accessible treatment facilities for animal bites.
	Observe for signs and symptoms of diseases caused by insects or animals.	Monitor the incidence of diseases caused by insects or animals.
	Refer for medical assistance as needed.	Promote accessibility of diagnostic and treatment services for diseases caused by insect and animal bites.

Continued on next page

TABLE 10-2 Secondary Preventive Measures for Selected Environmental Hazards for Individuals, Families, and Populations *(continued)*

Environmental Hazard	Individual/Family	Population
Plants	Inform families of poison control center activities. Refer families for poison control center services as needed. Refer for treatment of allergies and other conditions caused by plants.	Educate the public about poison control activities. Promote community support of poison control centers.
Poisons	Educate families about first aid for poisoning. Observe for signs and symptoms of poisoning. Refer families for poison control services as needed.	Educate the public about first aid for poisoning. Monitor the incidence of accidental poisoning. Promote access to poison control center services.
Air pollution	Observe for signs and symptoms of diseases caused by air pollution. Refer for diagnosis and treatment as needed.	Promote legislation to reduce pollutant emissions. Promote access to diagnostic and treatment services.
Water pollution	Observe for signs and symptoms of water-related diseases. Refer for diagnosis and treatment of water-related diseases.	Promote legislation to control water pollution. Promote availability of diagnostic and treatment services for water-related diseases.

Tertiary Prevention

Community health nurses may need to work with individuals or families to prevent recurrence or complications of environmentally caused health problems. For example, a community health nurse might assist a family to find housing where exposure to lead is not a problem. Or the nurse might provide parents with referrals for assistance in coping with the mental effects of longstanding lead poisoning in their children. Another tertiary preventive measure might involve suggestions for decreasing noise levels in the home to prevent further impairment of hearing.

Tertiary prevention might also be needed to deal with environmental problems at the aggregate or group level. An example might be political activity to mandate standards that prevent the recurrence of a leak at a nuclear power plant or to pass a bond issue to renovate a water treatment plant and prevent recontamination of drinking water with sewage. Advocacy for funds to remove lead hazards from older homes or legislation mandating lead removal in rental units are other possible community health nursing interventions.

Table 10-3◆ presents several tertiary prevention interventions related to environmental health in the care of individuals/families and populations.

Evaluating Environmental Health Measures

Community health nurses are also involved in evaluating the effectiveness of environmental control measures. Evaluation would focus on the effectiveness of primary, secondary, and tertiary preventive measures related to individuals, families, and population groups. For example, the nurse might monitor blood lead levels of children in housing with lead-based paint to determine whether primary preventive measures have prevented initial elevation. For those children who already

have elevated blood lead levels, evaluation would focus on the effects of chelating agents in reducing blood levels and the prevention of symptoms of lead poisoning. Evaluation of tertiary measures would be aimed at the effectiveness of abatement procedures in preventing blood lead levels from rising again after treatment. Similar approaches to evaluation of primary, secondary, and tertiary preventive interventions could be used for each of the environmental health problems addressed in this chapter. Evaluation at the aggregate level would focus on the extent to which national objectives for environmental health have been achieved. The status of selected national health objectives related to the environmental health of the U.S. population is summarized on page 247.

TABLE 10-3 Tertiary Preventive Measures for Selected Environmental Health Hazards for Individuals, Families, and Populations

Individual/Family	Population
Monitor for long-term effects of environmentally caused illnesses.	Monitor effects of environmental changes on incidence of environmentally caused disease.
Promote adjustment to the long-term effects of environmentally caused illness.	Promote availability of services for members of the population affected by environmentally caused illness.
Refer families to personal or environmental health services for dealing with consequences of adverse environmental conditions.	
Promote changes in environmental conditions to prevent recurrence of environmentally caused disease.	Promote environmental policies to prevent recurrence of environmental health problems.

HEALTHY PEOPLE 2010

Goals for Population Health

OBJECTIVE	BASELINE	MOST RECENT DATA	TARGET
8-1. Reduce the proportion of people exposed to harmful air pollutants			
Ozone	43%	41%	0%
Particulate matter	12%	11%	0%
Carbon monoxide	20%	13%	0%
Nitrogen dioxide	5%	0%	0%*
Sulfur dioxide	2%	1%	0%
Lead	<1%	0%	0%*
8-5. Increase the proportion of people receiving safe drinking water from community water systems	85%	DNA	95%
8-6. Reduce waterborne disease outbreaks	6	DNA	2
8-7. Reduce daily per capita water withdrawals	101 gal	DNA	90.9 gal
8-11. Eliminate elevated BLLs in children	4.4%	2.2%	0%
8-13. Reduce pesticide exposures resulting in visits to health care facilities (per 1,000 pop)	21.156	DNA	13.5
8-15. Increase recycling of municipal solid waste	27%	DNA	38%
8-18. Increase the proportion of homes tested for radon	17%	DNA	20%
8-22. Increase the proportion of pre-1950s homes tested for lead-based paint	16%	DNA	50%
8-23. Reduce the proportion of substandard homes	6.2%	DNA	3%
8-29. Reduce the global burden of disease deaths due to poor water quality, sanitation, and personal/domestic hygiene	2.6 mil	DNA	2.1 mil

DNA = Data not available

*Objective has been met

Data from: Centers for Disease Control and Prevention. (2005). Healthy people data. Retrieved September 6, 2005, from http://wonder.cdc.gov/data2010

Case Study

Environmental Advocate

Janice Wu, a community health nurse, is visiting a new client in a nursing home in an inner-city area in Los Angeles. As she enters the nursing home, she notices that several of the residents are doing calisthenics in the yard. Some of the residents are sitting on the sidelines and appear quite short of breath. When Janice checks to make sure they are all right, they tell her that they usually have a hard time breathing when they exercise on smoggy days like today. The residents say that they usually try to continue their exercises because it is one of the few activities that gets them out of the building. They also enjoy the social aspects of the exercise sessions. Many of them state that they have always been active and want to maintain their strength and mobility as long as possible. They express fears of being bedridden and unable to care for themselves.

After Janice is sure that all of the residents will be all right, she goes on to see her client. When she enters the building, she notices that it is quite hot inside, even though all the windows and doors are open. Although it is only 10 A.M., it promises to be one of L.A.'s scorching summer days. After seeing her client, Janice talks to the director about the heat in the building. The director tells her that the building is always hot and that the air conditioning has never worked properly. The last time the service people came to fix the air-conditioning unit, they said it could not be repaired and would have to be replaced. The nursing home is run by a large national corporation, and the director says she has been told they will have to wait until the next budget year (October) before money will be available for a new air conditioner. Fortunately, the heating system is separate, so there will be heat when the colder weather starts. The director says that staff members have been particularly careful about maintaining hydration in the residents during the hot weather, but many of the residents seem fatigued and listless with the heat.

1. What hazards are present in the natural, built, and social environments in this situation? What health effects, if any, are these hazards causing?

2. What level(s) of prevention is (are) warranted in this situation? What might Janice do to intervene?

Test Your Understanding

1. What are some ways that environmental factors affect human health? Give examples of this relationship. (pp. 229, 240–241)

2. Discuss elements of the natural, built, and social environments that affect population health. Identify factors in each of these three components of the environment that are influencing the health of an individual, family, or population with which you are familiar. (pp. 229–239)

3. Analyze the role of the community health nurse with respect to environmental health issues at the individual/family and population levels. (pp. 239–246)

4. Identify primary prevention measures for environmental issues that affect population health. Give examples of related community health nursing interventions. (pp. 242–243)

5. Identify secondary and tertiary prevention measures for individuals or populations affected by environmental health problems and describe possible community health nursing interventions related to each. (pp. 243–246)

EXPLORE MediaLink

http://www.prenhall.com/clark
Resources for this chapter can be found on the Companion Website.

Audio Glossary
Exam Review Questions
Case Study: Advocacy in Environmental
  Health

MediaLink Application: Lead Poisoning
  Prevention (video)
Media Links
Challenge Your Knowledge

Update *Healthy People 2010*
Advocacy Interviews

References

Addy, C. L., Wilson, D. K., Kirtland, K. A., Ainsworth, B. E., Sharpe, P., & Kimsey, D. (2004). Associations of perceived social and physical environmental supports with physical activity and walking. *American Journal of Public Health, 94*, 440–443.

Agency for Toxic Substances and Diseases Registry. (n.d.). *The ATSDR environmental health nursing initiative.* Retrieved May 10, 2006, from http://www.atsdr.cdc.gov/EHN

AIRNow. (2006). *Air Quality Guide for Ozone.* Retrieved May 23, 2006, from http://www.airnow.gov/index.cfm?action=static.consumer

Altschuler, A., Somkin, C. P., & Adler, N. E. (2004). Local services and amenities, neighborhood social capital, and health. *Social Science & Medicine, 59*, 1219–1229.

Arnold, M. (2003). Intranets, community, and social capital: The case of Williams Bay. *Bulletin of Science, Technology, and Society, 23*(2), 78–87.

Aron, J. L., & Glass, G. E. (2001). Geographic information systems. In J. L. Aron & J. A. Patz (Eds.), *Ecosystem change and public health: A global perspective* (pp. 60–99). Baltimore, MD: Johns Hopkins University Press.

Balfour, J., & Kaplan, G. A. (2002). Neighborhood environment and loss of physical function in older adults: Evidence from the Alameda County study. *American Journal of Epidemiology, 155*, 507–515.

Blackburn, B. G., Craun, G. E., Yoder, J. S., Hill, V., Calderon, R. L., Chen, N., et al. (2004). Surveillance for waterborne-disease outbreaks associated with drinking water—United States, 2001–2002. *Morbidity and Mortality Weekly Report, 53*(SS-8), 23–45.

Brody, D. C., & Lovrich, N. P. (2002). Social capital and protecting the rights of the accused in the American states. *Journal of Contemporary Criminal Justice, 18*, 115–131.

Butterfield, P. G. (2002). Upstream reflections on environmental health: An abbreviated history and framework for action. *Advances in Nursing Science, 25*(1), 32–49.

California Department of Health Services. (1998). *Interim childhood lead poisoning targeted screening guidelines.* Sacramento, CA: Author.

California Environmental Protection Agency. (2003). *The history of the California Environmental Protection Agency.* Retrieved December 31, 2005, from http://www.calepa.ca.gov/about/History01

Carlson, E. D., & Chamberlain, R. M. (2003). Social capital, health, and health disparities. *Journal of Nursing Scholarship, 35*, 325–331.

Center for Climatic Research, University of Delaware. (2004). Impact of heat waves on mortality—Rome, Italy, June–August, 2003. *Morbidity and Mortality Weekly Report, 53*, 369–371.

Centers for Disease Control and Prevention. (2005). *Healthy people data.* Retrieved September 6, 2005, from http://wonder.cdc.gov/data2010

Cohen, D. A., Mason, K., Bedimo, A., Scribner, R., Basolo, V., & Farley, T. A. (2003). Neighborhood physical conditions and health. *American Journal of Public Health, 93*, 467–471.

Curriero, F. C., Patz, J. A., Rose, J. B., & Lele, S. (2001). The association between extreme precipitation and waterborne disease outbreaks in the United States, 1948–1994. *American Journal of Public Health, 51*, 1194–1199.

Curtis, L. J., Dooley, M. D., & Phipps, S. A. (2004). Child well-being and neighborhood quality: evidence from the Canadian National Longitudinal Survey of Children and Youth. *Social Science & Medicine, 58*, 1917–1927.

Diaz, J. H. (2004). The public health impact of global climate change. *Family and Community Health, 27*, 218–229.

Division of Environmental Hazards and Health Effects, National Center for Environmental Health. (2002). Carbon-monoxide poisoning resulting from exposure to ski-boat exhaust—Georgia, June 2002. *Morbidity and Mortality Weekly Report, 51*, 829–830.

Division of Environmental Hazards and Health Effects, National Center for Environmental Health. (2003). Heat-related deaths—Chicago, Illinois, 1996–2001, and United States, 1979–1999. *Morbidity and Mortality Weekly Report, 52*, 610–612.

Division of Environmental Hazards and Health Effects, National Center for Environmental Health. (2005). Hypothermia-related deaths—United States, 2003–2004. *Morbidity and Mortality Weekly Report, 54*, 173–175.

Division of Unintentional Injury Prevention. (2002). Barriers to children walking and biking to school—United States, 1999. *Morbidity and Mortality Weekly Report, 51*, 701–704.

Eisenberg, D., & Warner, K. E. (2005). Effects of snowfalls on motor vehicle collisions, injuries, and fatalities. *American Journal of Public Health, 95*, 120–124.

Environmental Integrity Project. (2004). Stacking the deck: How EPA's new air toxics rules gamble with the public's health to benefit industry. Retrieved August 30, 2004, from http://www.environmentalintegrity.org

Epidemiology Program Office. (2003). Hepatitis A outbreak associated with green onions at a restaurant—Monaca, Pennsylvania, 2003. *Morbidity and Mortality Weekly Report, 52*, 1155–1157.

Evans, G. W., & Marcynyszyn, L. A. (2004). Environmental justice, cumulative environmental risk, and health among low- and middle-income children in upstate New York. *American Journal of Public Health, 94*, 1942–1944.

Farr, L. (2004). Social capital: A conceptual history. *Political Theory, 32*(1), 6–33.

Frumkin, H. (2003). Healthy places: Exploring the evidence. *American Journal of Public Health, 93*, 1451–1456.

Gaffield, S. J., Goo, R. L., Richards, L. A., & Jackson, R. J. (2003). Public health effects of inadequately managed stormwater runoff. *American Journal of Public Health, 93*, 1527–1533.

Gee, G. C., & Takeuchi, D. T. (2004). Traffic stress, vehicular burden and well-being: A multilevel analysis. *Social Science & Medicine, 59*, 405–414.

Hancock, T. (2000). Healthy communities must also be sustainable communities. *Public Health Reports, 115*, 151–156.

Henderson, S., & Whiteford, H. (2003). Social capital and mental health. *The Lancet, 362*, 505–506.

Jaakkola, J. J. K., Parise, H., Kislitsin, V., Lebedeva, N. I., & Spengler, J. D. (2004). Asthma, wheezing, and allergies in Russian schoolchildren in relation to new surface materials in the home. *American Journal of Public Health, 94*, 560–562.

Jozefowicz-Simbeni, D. M. H., & Allen-Meares, P. (2002). Poverty and schools: Intervention and resource building through school-linked services. *Children & Schools, 24*, 123–136.

Kim, D. Y., Staley, F., Curtis, G., & Buchanan, S. (2002). Relation between housing age, housing value, and childhood lead levels in children in Jefferson County, Ky. *American Journal of Public Health, 92*, 769–772.

Knowlton, N. (2004). Ocean health and human health. *Environmental Health Perspectives, 112*.

Retrieved April 28, 2004, from http://www.medscape/viewarticle/473216

Larsson, L. S., & Butterfield, P. (2002). Mapping the future of environmental health and nursing: Strategies for integrating national competencies into nursing practice. *Public Health Nursing, 19*, 301–308.

Lawlor, D. A., Smith, F. D., Patel, R., & Ebrahim, S. (2005). Life-course socioeconomic position, area deprivation, and coronary heart disease: Findings from the British women's heart and health study. *American Journal of Public Health, 95*, 91–97.

Leaders prepare for Kyoto Protocol to take effect. (2005, February). *The Nation's Health*, p. 11.

Lee, R. E., & Cubbin, C. (2002). Neighborhood context and youth cardiovascular health behaviors. *American Journal of Public Health, 92*, 428–436.

Leyden, K. M. (2003). Social capital and the built environment: The importance of walkable neighborhoods. *American Journal of Public Health, 93*, 1546–1551.

Lockwood, A. H. (2004). Human testing of pesticides: Ethical and scientific considerations. *American Journal of Public Health, 94*, 1908–1915.

Looman, W. S. (2004). Defining social capital for nursing: Experiences of family caregivers of children with chronic conditions. *Journal of Family Nursing, 10*, 412–428.

Lopez, R., (2004). Urban sprawl and risk for being overweight or obese. *American Journal of Public Health, 94*, 1574–1579.

Lower degrees of "social capital" predict higher rates of STDs. (2002, August 6). *TB & Outbreaks Week*, p. 6.

Martin, K. S., Rogers, B. L., Cook, J. T., & Joseph, H. M. (2004). Social capital is associated with decreased risk of hunger. *Social Science & Medicine, 59*, 2645–2654.

McDonald, L. (2000). Florence Nightingale and the foundations of public health care, as seen through her collected works. Retrieved July 18, 2002, from http://www.sociology.uoguelph.ca/fnightingale/online_papers/dalpaper.htm

McDowell, M. A., Dillon, C. F., Osterloh, J., Bolger, M., Pellizzari, E., Fernando, R., et al. (2004). Hair mercury levels in U.S. children and women of childbearing age: Data from NHANES 1999–2000. *Environmental Health Perspectives, 112*, 1165–1171.

McMichael, A. J. (2001). Global environmental change as "risk factor": Can epidemiology cope? *American Journal of Public Health, 91*, 1172–1174.

McMichael, A. J., Butler, C. D., & Ahern, M. J. (2003). Global environment. In R. D. Smith, R. Beaglehole, D. Woodward, & N. Drager (Eds.), *Global public goods for health: Health economic and public health perspectives* (pp. 94–116). Oxford, UK: Oxford University.

Meyer, P. A., Pivetz, T., Dignam, T. A., Homa, D. M., Schoonover, J., & Brody, D. (2003). Surveillance for elevated blood lead levels among children—United States, 1997–2001. *Morbidity and Mortality Weekly Report, 52* (SS-10), 1–21.

Mintz, R., Bartram, J., Lochery, P., & Wegelin, M. (2001). Not just a drop in the bucket: Expanding access to point-of-use water treatment

systems. *American Journal of Public Health, 91*, 1565–1570.

Mitman, G. (2003). Hay fever holiday: Health, leisure, and place in gilded-age America. *Bulletin of the History of Medicine, 77*, 600–635.

Monkman, K., Ronald, M., & Theramene, F. D. (2005). Social and cultural capital in an urban Latino school community. *Urban Education, 40*(1), 4–33.

Morrow, V. M. (2000). 'Dirty looks' and 'trampy places' in young people's accounts of community and neighbourhood: Implications for health inequalities. *Critical Public Health, 10*, 141–152.

Muntaner, C., Lynch, J., & Smith, G. D. (2000). Social capital and the third way in public health. *Critical Public Health, 10*, 107–124.

National Oceanic and Atmospheric Administration. (n.d.a). *What is El Niño?* Retrieved May 10, 2006, from http://www.pmel.noaa.gov/tao/elnino/el-nino-story.html

National Oceanic and Atmospheric Administration. (n.d.b). *What is La Niña?* Retrieved May 10, 2006, from http://www.pmel.noaa.gov/tao/elnino/la-nina-story.html

Natural Resources Defense Council. (2003). *What's on tap?: Grading drinking water in U.S. cities.* Retrieved September 25, 2003, from http://www2.nrdc.org

Oakes, J. M. (2004). The (mis)estimation of neighborhood effects: Causal inference for a practicable social epidemiology. *Social Science & Medicine, 58*, 1929–1952.

Osterberg, D., & Wallinga, D. (2004). Addressing externalities from swine production to reduce public health and environmental impacts. *American Journal of Public Health, 94*, 1703–1708.

Patz, J. A., Kinney, P. L., Bell, M. L., Ellis, H., Goldberg, R., Hogrefe, C., et al. (2004). *Heat advisory: How global warming causes more bad air days.* Natural Resources Defense Council. Retrieved September 30, 2004, from http://www.nrdc.org/globalwarming/heatadvisory/heatadvisory.pdf

Pope, A. M., Snyder, M. A., & Mood, L. H. (Eds.). (1995). *Nursing, health, and environment: Strengthening the relationship to improve the public's health.* Washington, DC: National Academy Press.

Population Information Program, Center for Communication Programs. (2002). Meeting the urban challenge. *Population Reports.* Retrieved July 25, 2003, from http://www.jhucpp.org

Potula, V., Hegarty-Steck, M., & Hu, H. (2001). Blood lead levels in relation to paint and dust lead levels: The lead-safe Cambridge program. *American Journal of Public Health, 12*, 1973–1974.

Reisig, M. D., Holtfreter, K., & Morash, M. (2002). Social capital among women offenders: Examining the distribution of social networks and resources. *Journal of Contemporary Criminal Justice, 18*, 167–187.

Richardson, K. (2004). Highlights of obesity and the built environment: Improving public health through community design. *Medscape Diabetes and Endocrinology, 6*(2). Retrieved August 31, 2004, from http://www.medscape.com/viewarticle/487906

Roscoe, R. J., Ball, W., Curran, J. J., DeLaurier, C., Falken, M. C., Fitchett, R., et al. (2003). Adult blood lead epidemiology and surveillance, United States, 1998–2001. *Morbidity and Mortality Weekly Report, 52* (SS-11), 1–10.

Ross, Z., Walker, B., & Wiles, R. (2000). *Lead astray: California's broken promise to protect children from lead poisoning.* Environmental Working Group. Retrieved January 9, 2002, from http://www.ewg.org/reports/leadastray

Schmidt, C. W. (2004). Sprawl: The new manifest destiny? *Environmental Health Perspectives, 112,* A620–A627. Retrieved August 26, 2004, from http://www.medscape.com/viewarticle/487573

Schneider, C. G. (2004). *Dirty air, dirty power: Mortality and health damage due to air pollution from power plants.* Boston, MA: Clean the Air. Retrieved August 30, 2004, from http://cta.policy.net

Scott, J. D. (2002). Assessing the relationship between police-community coproduction and neighborhood-level social capital. *Journal of Contemporary Criminal Justice, 18,* 147–166.

Semenza, J. C. (2003). The intersection of urban planning, art, and public health: The Sunnyside piazza. *American Journal of Public Health, 93,* 1439–1441.

Srinivasan, S., O'Fallon, L. R., & Dearry, A. (2003). Creating healthy communities, healthy homes, healthy people: Initiating a research agenda on the built environment and public health. *American Journal of Public Health, 93,* 1446–1450.

Streeten, P. (2002). Reflections on social and antisocial capital. *Journal of Human Development, 3*(1), 7–22.

Tester, J. M., Rutherford, G. W., Wald, Z., & Rutherford, M. W. (2004). A matched case-control study evaluating the effectiveness of speed bumps in reducing child pedestrian injuries. *American Journal of Public Health, 94,* 646–650.

Uosukainen, L. M. (2001). Promotion of the good life by public health nurses. *Public Health Nursing, 18,* 375–384.

U.S. Department of Health and Human Services. (1991). *Healthy people 2000: National health promotion and illness prevention objectives.* Washington, DC: Author.

U.S. Department of Health and Human Services. (2000). *Healthy people 2010* (Conference edition, in two volumes). Washington, DC: Author.

U.S. Department of Health and Human Services. (2002). Environmental health: Promoting health for all through a healthy environment. *Prevention Report, 16*(3), 1–11. Retrieved May 30, 2002, from http://odphp.osophs.dhhs.gov/pubs/prevrpt/02volume16/issue3pr.htm

U.S. Environmental Protection Agency. (n.d.). *About EPA.* Retrieved December 31, 2005, from http://www.epa.gov/cgi-bin/epaprintonly.cgi

U.S. General Accounting Office. (2002). Air pollution: Meeting future electricity demand will increase emissions of some harmful substances. Retrieved January 30, 2003, from http://www.gao.gov

Wallerstein, N. (2002). Empowerment to reduce health disparities. *Scandinavian Journal of Public Health, 30,* 72–77.

Wang, G., Macera, C. A., Scudder-Socie, B., Schmid, T., Pratt, M., Buchner, D., & Health, G. (2004). Cost analysis of the built environment: The case of bike and pedestrian trails in Lincoln, Neb. *American Journal of Public Health, 94,* 549–553.

Watts, S. (2003). *Disease and medicine in world history.* New York: Routledge.

Wind, S., Van Sickle, D., & Wright, A. L. (2004). Health, place, and childhood asthma in southwest Alaska. *Social Science & Medicine, 58,* 75–88.

World Health Organization. (2003). *Right to water.* Geneva, Switzerland: Author.

World Health Organization. (2004). *World Health Report 2004.* Geneva, Switzerland: Author.

Yoder, J. S., Blackburn, B. G., Craun, G. E., Hill, V., Levy, D. A., Chen, N., et al. (2004). Surveillance for waterborne-disease outbreaks associated with recreational water—United States, 2001–2002. *Morbidity and Mortality Weekly Report, 53*(SS-8), 1–21.

Young, A. F., Russell, A., & Powers, J. R. (2004). The sense of belonging to a neighborhood: Can it be measured and is it related to health and well being in older women? *Social Science & Medicine, 59,* 2627–2637.

Zierold, K. M., Knobeloch, L., & Anderson, H. (2004). Prevalence of chronic diseases in adults exposed to arsenic-contaminated drinking water. *American Journal of Public Health, 94,* 1936–1937.

Approaches to Community Health Nursing

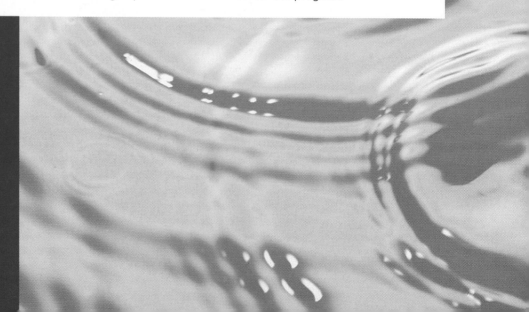

Advocacy in Action

Fit and Healthy

Obesity is a serious concern in community health. Healthy food and exercise habits begin in childhood and need to be fostered throughout life. A collaborative organization of local residents and health and social services providers had written a grant to provide a health and fitness program for school-aged children to prevent obesity and promote health. Unfortunately, the grant was not funded. One of the criticisms was that the grant writers had not identified a specific curriculum to be used in the program. Over the next two years, several groups of community health nursing students undertook to write a nutrition and fitness curriculum for third-, fourth-, and fifth-grade students. Each student subgroup addressed either nutrition or exercise and fitness for a specific grade level.

The curricula developed were age appropriate for the particular grade level and were designed to be taught by people without a health background. In order to make the curriculum more acceptable for incorporation into the regular school routine, the nursing students developed content and learning activities that would meet state-mandated curricular standards. For example, in the lesson on body mass index, schoolchildren used math skills to calculate their own BMI based on their height and weight. Other lessons on cultural foods and their nutrients supported achievement of social studies objectives. Each lesson included an overview of the content for the teacher, preparatory setup and materials needed, and activities to get the children actively involved in their learning. The curricula also included approaches to measuring effectiveness that addressed both knowledge and health-related behaviors and indicators.

Copies of the curricula have been shared with a committee of public health officials and school district officials working on the problem of obesity in the community. In addition, the curricula are being implemented by a nursing faculty member as part of a research study, and portions of the curricula are being implemented in an after-school program.

Health Promotion

CHAPTER OBJECTIVES

After reading this chapter, you should be able to:

1. Define health promotion.
2. Distinguish health promotion from health education.
3. Apply selected models for health promotion practice.
4. Identify three strategies for health promotion.
5. Describe the four Ps of social marketing.
6. Analyze the significance of empowerment for health promotion.
7. Describe the health education process.
8. Design and implement a health education program for a selected population.
9. Analyze the implications of language and health literacy for health promotion.
10. Identify criteria for evaluating health information on the Internet.
11. Discuss criteria for evaluating health promotion programs.

KEY TERMS

empowerment **259**
health education **263**
health literacy **269**
health promotion **255**
learning domain **264**

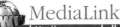

MediaLink
http://www.prenhall.com/clark

Additional interactive resources for this chapter can be found on the Companion Website. Click on Chapter 11 and "Begin" to select the activities for this chapter.

Six distinct approaches have been taken to public health over time (Awofeso, 2004). The first approach involved health protection by means of social structures and lasted from ancient times until the 1830s. These social structures included rules of behavior, usually enforced by means of religious, political, or cultural sanctions. "Miasma control" was the second approach to fostering the health of the public. Miasmas were harmful mists or vapors in the air. This era of public health, from the 1840s through the 1870s, was exemplified by the sanitary movement and gained impetus from Chadwick's 1842 *Inquiry into the Sanitary Conditions of the Labouring Population of Great Britain*. From approximately 1880 to 1940, public health practice focused on contagion control based on the germ theory. During the 1940s to 1960s, emphasis was placed on preventive medicine, which expanded the germ theory to consider other disease vectors and nutritive factors in illness. Public health activity in this era was focused on populations at high risk for specific conditions. The 1970s and 1980s saw the rise of the primary health care movement, based on the Declaration of Alma Alta, and recognized the effects of social factors on health. Finally, from 1990 to the present, the focus has been on the "new public health," which emphasizes health promotion based on the ability of members of the population to make informed health decisions. This new focus retains many of the features of prior eras, including regulation of some aspects of health via legislation, sanitation, immunization, a focus on risk modification, and recognition of the effects of social conditions on health. The eras and foci of public health practice over time are summarized in Table 11-1◆. The emphasis on health promotion in the new public health focus highlights the importance of this role for community health nurses.

TABLE 11-1	Eras of Public Health Practice and Related Foci	
Era	Time Period	Focus
Health protection	Ancient times–1830s	Regulation of behavior enforced by religious, political, or cultural sanctions
Miasma control	1840s–1870s	Sanitation
Contagion control	1880s–1930s	Immunization, disinfection
Preventive medicine	1940s–1960s	Risk factor modification
Primary health care	1970s–1980s	Modification of social and other factors that influence health
Health promotion	1990s–present	Development of capacity for informed health decisions

HEALTH PROMOTION AND POPULATION HEALTH

Each year chronic diseases cause 1.7 million deaths in the United States, and two thirds of all deaths are due to five conditions: heart disease, cancer, stroke, chronic obstructive pulmonary diseases, and diabetes. Chronic conditions result in major activity limitations for 30 million Americans. In addition, chronic conditions and their risk factors result in a significant economic burden for society. For example, cardiovascular disease and stroke cost an estimated $351.8 billion in 2003 in direct (medical care) and indirect (lost productivity) costs. Similarly, the 2002 cost of cancer in the United States was $171.6 billion, and diabetes had total estimated costs of $132 billion. In addition to the costs of care from health providers, medications, and necessary supplies and equipment (the direct costs), these conditions lead to lost productivity for those affected, for family members, and for employers. For example, the client may need to take time from work for follow-up visits with health care providers, or a family member may need to quit work to care for a client who is disabled by his or her condition. Similarly, work productivity may be lost due to diminished attentiveness at work when one is worried about one's own health or that of a family member or one's condition poses physical limitations that impair one's ability to work effectively. The aggregate costs of medical care also result in higher insurance premiums for employers and those covered. These costs and others make for a considerable financial burden on the individuals affected, their families, and society at large.

Risk factors for these and other chronic diseases also have serious economic costs. For example, direct and indirect costs related to smoking amount to $155 billion per year, and the annual costs of poor nutrition in the United States are estimated at $42 billion. In 2002 alone, health care costs attributable to physical inactivity amounted to $76 billion. It is clear from these figures that the United States can no longer support the personal and financial costs of chronic diseases, which account for 75% of all health care expenditures (U.S. Department of Health and Human Services [USDHHS], 2003b). Nor can we afford the burden of communicable disease or other health problems such as substance abuse, societal violence, and mental illness. The obvious answer to these problems is health promotion and disease prevention. In spite of the common sense of this response, however, only 5% of the $1.4 trillion spent on health in the United States is spent for health promotion and illness prevention (USDHHS, 2003a). In the United Kingdom, only 1% of the National Health Service budget is spent for health promotion (Whitehead, 2003).

Like public health practice, health promotion practice has undergone changes in its approach over time. Health promotion began with a medical approach focusing on immunization and screening for existing diseases, then shifted to a focus on changing individual risk behaviors. An educational approach, often taken in health promotion, assumed that knowledge of healthy behavior would lead to behavior change in the public. Unfortunately, research has shown repeatedly that this is not the case. More recently, health promotion approaches have focused on empowerment, through the growth of individuals or groups, and on change in the social and environmental conditions that impede healthy behavior (Uys, Majumdar, & Gwele, 2004). This latter change has been described as a shift from behavioral models of health promotion to social-ecological models that are "based on the premise that an individual's behavior is shaped by a dynamic interaction with the social environment, which includes influences at the interpersonal, organizational, community, and policy levels" (Merzel & D'Afflitti, 2003, p. 557).

As defined by the World Health Organization, health promotion is a "process of enabling people to increase control over, and to improve, their health" (quoted in Laverack, 2004, p. 9), a much more general approach than risk behavior modification. As noted by one author, health promotion "should be linked to a reformation of the social structures, conditions, and policies that contribute to illness and disease in communities" (Whitehead, 2003, p. 670). Again, according to WHO, health promotion is more than changing behaviors, but involves public policy formation, development of environments that support health, and promotion of community action to create conditions conducive to good health (Buijis & Olson, 2001). As defined from this sociopolitical perspective, **health promotion** is

> The process by which the ecologically driven sociopolitical-economic determinants of health are addressed as they impact on individuals and the communities within which they interact. This serves to counter social inaction and social division/inequality. It is an inherent political process that draws on health policy as a basis for social action that leads to community coalitions through shared radical consciousness. Health promotion seeks to radically transform and empower communities through involving them in activities that influence their public health—particularly via agenda setting, political lobbying and advocacy, critical consciousness-raising and social education programmes . . . Health promotion looks to develop and reform social structures through developing participation between representative stakeholders in different sectors and agencies. (Whitehead, 2004, p. 314)

Health promotion has been a WHO emphasis since the 1996 Ottawa Charter contributed to a new conceptualization of health promotion based on the WHO philosophy of "Health for All." The Ottawa Charter emphasized health as a "resource for living" rather than an end in itself and marked an international shift from disease prevention to capacity building, improving the capability of nations and communities to provide environments that support health and healthy behaviors (Kickbusch, 2003). The Charter identified three strategies to promote global health: advocacy for conditions favorable to health, development of environments that support health as well as personal information and skills to make health decisions, and mediation between groups (Tones & Green, 2004). In addition, five action areas were identified: development of healthy public policy, creation of supportive environments, facilitation of community action, development of personal skills, and reorientation of health services to a health promotion focus (Evans & Stoddart, 2003).

The foci of the Ottawa Charter were further expanded in 1997 in the *Jakarta Declaration on Leading Health Promotion into the 21st Century*. The Jakarta Declaration viewed health promotion as increasing health expectancy by means of increasing health gains throughout populations, reducing inequities, promoting human rights, and enhancing social capital. The Declaration also established four priorities for health promotion in the 21st century: promoting social and individual responsibility for health, increasing investment in health development, increasing partnerships for health, and developing a global infrastructure for health promotion (Tones & Green, 2004). In Sweden, the National Committee for Public Health operationalized these priorities in six strategic areas that provide the focus for health promotion in that nation. The strategic areas addressed improved social capital, child development in satisfactory environments, better workplace conditions, improved physical environments, motivation for health-promoting behaviors, and development of the health promotion infrastructure (Kickbusch, 2003).

In the United States, health promotion efforts tend to continue to be focused on behavior modification and prevention of specific health conditions (termed *vertical health promotion*), rather than on changing broader factors that influence health (*horizontal health promotion*) (Tones & Green, 2004). In 2003, however, the United States Department of Health and Human Services (USDHHS, 2003b) launched the *Steps to a Healthier US* initiative, which focuses on promoting behavior change and improving policy and environmental conditions that support healthy behavior and illness prevention. The *Steps* initiatives focus on reducing the burden of five specific conditions—asthma, cancer, diabetes, heart disease and stroke, and obesity—and employ both vertical and horizontal health promotion strategies. The vertical strategies focus on behavior modification and prevention of the five conditions. The horizontal strategies address the policies and environmental conditions that influence health, such as insurance coverage for smoking cessation and incentives for schools to include physical activity in the curriculum. The *Steps* programs will be discussed in more detail in Chapter 29∞.

MODELS FOR HEALTH PROMOTION

A number of models have been developed to guide health promotion practice. These include the Precaution Adoption Process model (Weinstein & Sandman, 2002), the Information-Motivation-Behavioral Skills (IMB) Model (Fisher & Fisher, 2002), the Theory of Reasoned Action and the related Theory of Planned Behavior (Butler, 2001), and the Health Belief Model (Tones & Green, 2004). Additional models include the Representational Approach (Donovan & Ward, 2001), Pender's Health Promotion Model (Pender, Murdaugh, & Parsons, 2001), and the PRECEDE-PROCEED model (Erkel, 2002). Each of these models is an attempt to explain why people do or do not engage in health-promoting activity. These explanations assist community health nurses to understand the motivations and factors involved in such decisions and help them to select appropriate strategies for promoting health in the population. Although it is not possible to discuss all of these models here, the reader is referred to the literature cited for a description of the models. In this chapter, we will briefly explore the Precaution Adoption Process model, the Theory of Reasoned Action, the Health Belief Model, Pender's Health Promotion Model, and the PRECEDE-PROCEED model. In addition, the Representational Approach is described below.

The Precaution Adoption Process Model

The Precaution Adoption Process model is a stage model that describes the stages that occur in decisions to adopt or not adopt a health-related behavior (whether or not to take a specific precautionary action) (Weinstein & Sandman, 2002). In stage 1, the person is unaware of the health-related issue and the need to adopt any particular health-related behavior. In the second stage, one is aware of the issue but is unengaged by it and is not considering any action. In stage 3, the person is deciding whether or not to act. He or she has considered the possibility of action but has not yet made a decision whether or not to adopt the behavior. Stage 3 may be followed by either stage 4 or stage 5. In stage 4, the person has decided not to act. Conversely, in stage 5, the person has decided to act but has not yet taken action. The process may stop at stage 4 for those who decide not to adopt the behavior in question. People in stages 4 and 5 are more resistant to persuasion than those in stage 3 who have not yet made a decision. Given human tenacity, it is more difficult to influence someone to change his or her mind than it is to persuade someone who has not yet made a decision to do so. Persons in stage 5 who have decided to adopt the behavior proceed to stage 6, in which they act to engage in the behavior, and hopefully to stage 7, in which the behavior becomes a routine part of their lifestyle. This process explaining the adoption or nonadoption of the health-related behavior of exercise is depicted in Figure 11-1.

We can apply this model using a community-based example of installing speed bumps in residential areas. The decision to employ speed bumps to slow traffic must be adopted by the City Council. In the first stage of the decision adoption process, the Council is unaware of the extent of and potential for injury and death due to drivers exceeding the speed limit in residential areas. In stage 2, Council members may have become aware of the high frequency of pedestrian injuries in these areas, but is not considering taking any action to remedy the situation. At stage 3, the Council may be presented with a petition from local residents for the installation of speed bumps, but has not decided whether or not to authorize their installation. If the City Council proceeds to stage 4, they will decide not to install speed bumps based on the cost of installation, which they believe would outweigh the benefits to be gained in terms of injuries and deaths prevented. If, on the other hand, they vote to install the speed bumps, but have not yet authorized the City Accounting Office to put out bids for their installation, they are in stage 5 of the adoption process. At stage 6, all

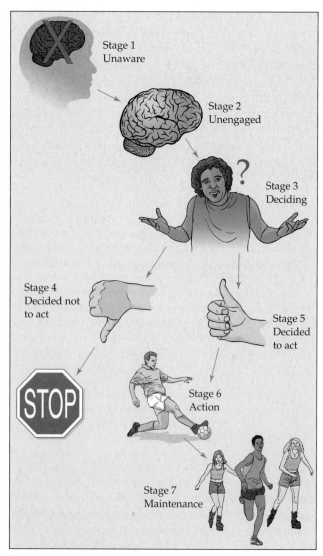

FIGURE 11-1 Stages of Adoption of Exercise Behavior

processes are in place, and speed bumps are being installed in identified residential areas. The City Council may then proceed to stage 7, in which construction of all new residential developments within the city limits must include speed bumps.

The Theory of Reasoned Action

The Theory of Reasoned Action, developed by Ajzen and Fishbein, is based on two premises. First, attitudes toward a health-related behavior reflect a person's attitudes toward the expected consequences of the behavior. For example, if you expect that exercise will result in a more desirable figure, and if you value that more desirable shape, you are likely to value, and engage in, exercise. The second premise is that attitudes are the product of subjective norms influenced by others. In the theory, the intention to act is based on one's own attitude toward the behavior, one's perceptions of the attitudes of others (subjective norms), and the value placed on others' judgments (Butler, 2001). Action is also influenced by perceptions of one's ability to control behavior. For example, if you want to quit smoking and perceive that significant others in your life want you to quit, but you think stopping smoking will be too difficult, you will probably not attempt to quit even though your attitudes and those of people who matter to you support quitting.

Using the previous population-level example of the speed bumps, if City Council members expect the installation of the barriers to reduce speeds on residential streets and subsequently reduce the frequency of pedestrian injuries and deaths, they may approve their installation. Action to install the speed bumps is even more likely if City Council members believe that failure to take action will anger voters to the point they will not be reelected. Both the perceived consequences of installing speed bumps and perceptions of voters' attitudes will influence their decision to take a health-promoting action on the part of the city.

The Health Belief Model

The Health Belief Model was developed by Becker, Rosenstock, and their colleagues several years ago and has been widely used in research and program development related to health-promoting behaviors. Elements of the model include individual perceptions of susceptibility and seriousness, modifying factors (demographic, sociopsychologic, and structural variables), perceptions of benefits and barriers to action, and cues to action. In the model, health-promotive action is based on four basic premises or beliefs. First, one believes that one is susceptible to, or at risk for, a particular health problem. Second, one believes that the health problem can have serious consequences. Third, one believes that the problem can be prevented, and fourth, that the benefits of action outweigh the costs or barriers (Butler, 2001; Tones & Green, 2004). For example, you may believe that, never

having had chickenpox as a child, you are susceptible to chickenpox (perceived susceptibility). You also believe that chickenpox may cause serious consequences (perceived severity). This perception is confirmed when one of your classmates is hospitalized with complications of chickenpox (cue to action). In addition, you know that varicella immunization will virtually eliminate your risk of developing chickenpox (perceived benefit to action). Even though you know the possibility of an adverse reaction to the vaccine exists and you have to skip lunch to visit the student health center (perceived costs), you decide the benefits outweigh the barriers, and you get immunized.

Examining our community-level example of installing speed bumps in the light of this model, perceptions of susceptibility would relate to City Council members' perceptions of the potential for injuries on residential streets. The perceived severity of the problem would reflect their knowledge of the number of deaths and serious injuries that have occurred. Perceived benefits might include reduced frequency of pedestrian injuries and satisfied voters. The cost of installing the speed bumps and, possibly, the loss of revenue from speeding tickets, might constitute perceived barriers to the project. Finally, the fact that the mayor's son was nearly hit by a speeding car in front of his house may serve as a cue to action that motivates Council members to authorize the installation of speed bumps.

Pender's Health Promotion Model

Nola Pender has developed a nursing model that directs nursing intervention for health promotion. In the Health Promotion Model, behavior is influenced by individual characteristics and behavior-specific cognitions and affect (emotion) that result in a commitment to action. Commitment to action results in actual behavior but may be modified by competing demands and preferences (Pender et al., 2001). Individual characteristics include personal biological, psychological, and sociocultural factors that are relevant to the behavior involved. Prior behavior in this area is another individual characteristic that influences health-promoting behavior. For example, a client who was physically active prior to pregnancy will be more likely to engage in exercise after delivery than one who was not.

Behavior-specific cognitions and attitudes include the perceived benefits of and barriers to health-promoting activity as well as one's perceived self-efficacy. For example, the community that does not perceive itself as able to cope with the problem of inadequate housing will probably not take any action to resolve the problem. Activity-related affect or feeling states related to the behavior, to oneself, or to the situation are also important in motivating health-promoting behavior. Interpersonal and situational influences are additional factors related to cognition and affect that influence behavior. For example, if family members support weight loss, a client is more likely to stick to a diet. Conversely, low income, a situational influence, might adversely affect the client's weight loss options.

Individual characteristics and behavior-specific cognitions and affect may lead to a commitment to health-promoting activity. Commitment includes both the intention to act and a specific plan of action. Commitment to action should lead to performance of the actual health-promoting behavior unless there is interference from competing demands and preferences. For example, the client's intention to diet may be subverted by a family member's serious illness and the need to eat in fast food restaurants near the hospital.

Although Pender's model was developed to be used to enhance health-promoting behavior with individual clients, it can also be applied to population groups. Using the speed bump example, individual characteristics might relate to members of the City Council or of the community. For example, if members of the City Council have young children or live on busy residential streets, they may be more inclined to take action than if they do not. Conversely, if the area of the city requesting speed bumps is composed largely of immigrants who rarely vote in local elections, they may be less likely to respond. Prior action may also have a bearing on the Council's decision. For example, if they have taken other "traffic calming" actions (approaches to traffic control that are self-enforcing) such as installing cameras on traffic lights at busy intersections, they may be inclined to install speed bumps as well. If, however, the City Council perceives itself to have little control over traffic violations, their perceived lack of self-efficacy may lead them to decide that speed bumps will have little impact.

Emotional reactions to the problem may have an influence on the Council's decision as well. If, for example, the most recent death of a child led to rioting or demonstrations outside City Hall, or if one of the Council members has had a child injured by a speeding driver, action may be forthcoming. Again, the City Council would weigh the perceived benefits of installing speed bumps (voter satisfaction and fewer injuries) against the perceived costs (financial costs of installing the speed bumps, need to delay construction of a city park, etc.) to decide whether or not to commit to installing the speed bumps. Even if the Council votes to install the bumps, installation may be sidetracked by a subsequent financial crisis or by torrential rains that delay construction, both of which would reflect situational constraints that impede action to implement the Council's decision.

The PRECEDE-PROCEED Model

The PRECEDE-PROCEED model has been widely used in health education practice and consists of two components. The PRECEDE component reflects diagnostic activities that take place prior to planning health promotion activities. Diagnostic elements include **P**redisposing, **R**einforcing, and **E**nabling constructs (C) in the educational (E) diagnosis (D) and evaluation (E) that occur as a precursor to health promotion interventions (Erkel, 2002). Predisposing factors are personal factors that motivate one to change behavior (Tones & Green, 2004) and include knowledge, attitudes, and perceptions related to the behavior. Using our previous example, predisposing factors might include the willingness of the City Council to act on citizen complaints or the fact that a speeding driver has hit one of their own children. Reinforcing factors are the positive and negative consequences of the behavior that promote or hinder its performance (e.g., voter approval and cost to the city). Enabling factors are the skills and resources needed to engage in the behavior or barriers that impede the behavior. In our speed bump example, perhaps the city has previous experience with installing speed bumps or city engineers are aware of a new process that slows deterioration of speed bumps after installation, making periodic replacement less necessary.

At the level of individual health promotion, perhaps you know that exercise is good for you and you would like to fit more exercise into your daily routine (predisposing factors). When you did exercise regularly, you felt better, were better able to concentrate on your studies, and were better able to prevent excess weight gain (reinforcing factors). Unfortunately, it is winter and too cold to exercise outdoors, the university gym closes before you get home from your clinical assignments, and you cannot afford to belong to a private exercise club. In this instance, you lack the enabling factors that would encourage you to get more exercise. The PRECEDE component of the model determines the factors or environmental conditions that would need to be changed for you to engage in this health-related behavior.

The PROCEED component of the model focuses on the development of health promotion interventions that will enhance the potential for healthy behavior. The **P** in this component of the model stands for policy, the **R** for regulatory, and the **O** for organizational constructs (C) in educational (E) and environmental (E) development (D), or the areas in which intervention might be undertaken to promote adoption of the desired behavior (Erkel, 2002). Returning to the example of your exercise behaviors, the university could require all students to take a one-unit physical education course each semester. This is a regulatory intervention that would require you to have some physical activity. On the other hand, a policy intervention changing the hours that the gym is open could achieve the same effect. Finally, organizationally, the School of Nursing could reschedule clinical experiences for other days and times to permit you to use the gym during its current hours of operation.

In our population-based speed bump example, the City Council could adopt a policy of using traffic calming strategies, including speed bumps, rather than hiring

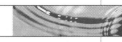

additional police officers for traffic control in residential areas. They might also pass a city ordinance that mandates speed bumps on every residential street with a population density of more than 20 school-aged children. Organizational constructs would relate to the process implemented to obtain bids for speed bump construction, deciding where to install them first, and so on.

STRATEGIES FOR HEALTH PROMOTION

Use of a health promotion model permits the community health nurse to identify factors involved in the health promotion situation and to design health promotion programs that address these factors. Use of a model also focuses attention on all of the factors that influence health promotion, not just personal behaviors, and leads to a more horizontal approach to health promotion. Whatever the model used to direct health promotion activities, accomplishment of health promotion goals rests on one of three views of responsibility (Tones & Green, 2004). In the first view, people themselves determine whether or not the goals are met, through their behavioral choices. In the second view, the environment constrains people's abilities to meet health promotion goals. In the third view, goal accomplishment is a function of the interaction between environmental conditions and individual abilities and motivation. This latter view is the most effective in facilitating horizontal health promotion efforts that encompass all of the factors in the health promotion situation.

Different strategies for health promotion affect goal accomplishment in different ways. Three particular

FOCUSED ASSESSMENT

Assessing the Health Promotion Situation

- What are the expectations of the population with respect to health and health promotion? What is the attitude of health care providers to health promotion activities? What is the level of motivation for health promotion among various segments of the population?
- What factors in the population affect the ability of its members to promote their health? To what extent are these factors related to personal behavior or attributes (e.g., education level, SES)? To environmental factors?
- What facilitates health promotion in the population? What barriers to health-promoting activities exist?
- What health-promoting behaviors do members of the population currently use? What additional health promotion activities are needed?
- What resources are available within the health system to support health promotion?
- Who determines health promotion policies and priorities?
- What societal changes are needed to create an environment conducive to health and health promotion? What barriers exist to these changes?

strategies will be discussed here: empowerment, social marketing, and health education. Empowerment focuses on the environmental conditions that affect people's abilities to act in ways that promote health. Giving residents a voice in designing communities that promote physical activity is an example of empowerment. Social marketing, on the other hand, emphasizes enhancing people's motivation to act and reflects the view of personal agency. Motivating people to actually take advantage of opportunities for physical activity present in the community exemplifies social marketing. Health education provides the information and skills that underlie the other two strategies. For example, empowerment requires knowledge of political process and advocacy skills that can be provided through health education endeavors. Similarly, social marketing to change people's attitudes to health-related behaviors is of little use unless they have information on which to base new attitudes. Specific skills derived from health education are also required to carry out health behaviors even in the context of positive attitudes. For example, you may believe that condom use is an effective and desirable means of preventing sexually transmitted diseases, but unless you know how to correctly put on a condom, your positive attitude and behavioral intention are of little value. The assessment tips provided above may guide selection of a specific health promotion strategy in a particular situation.

Empowerment

As we noted earlier, the primary focus of health promotion should be on empowering people and improving their capacity to make informed, healthy decisions. **Empowerment** involves "enabling communities to

GLOBAL PERSPECTIVES

*A*ccording to the World Health Organization (WHO, 2002), 10 risk factors contribute to most of the global burden of disease: underweight; unsafe sex; high blood pressure; tobacco use; alcohol use; unsafe water, sanitation, and hygiene; iron deficiency; indoor smoke from use of solid fuels; high cholesterol; and obesity. The prevalence of these risk factors, however, varies between developed and developing countries, as depicted below.

Developing Nations	Developed Nations
Underweight	Obesity
Unsafe sex	Tobacco use
Unsafe water, sanitation, and hygiene	Alcohol use
Iron deficiency	High blood pressure
Indoor air pollution	High cholesterol

These risk factor differences necessitate risk analysis, defined as "a systematic approach to estimating the burden of disease and injury due to different risks" (WHO, 2002, p. 8), to determine the appropriate foci for health promotion and illness prevention programs in different parts of the world. In global health promotion, as in many other areas, one size does **NOT** fit all.

acquire the knowledge and skills to make informed decisions and allowing communities to make those decisions" (MacDonald, 2002, p. 99). The first half of this definition reflects the previous emphasis on providing information, but the key feature of empowerment is allowing individuals and groups to act, for better or worse, on that information and creating the physical, socioeconomic, and cultural conditions in which they are able to do so (Tones & Green, 2004). Empowerment requires emancipatory approaches to health promotion that focus on "increasing one's capacity to act rather than be acted upon" (Vanderplaat, 2002, p. 89). Emancipatory approaches to health promotion are characterized by

- Rejection of the "individual deficit" concept embedded in traditional social programs. People are not deficient; their environments are.
- Rejection of attempts to manipulate behavior change through transfer of knowledge and skills and recognition that structural, as well as behavioral, change is required to promote health and well-being.
- Recognition of people's capacity to create knowledge and solutions from their own experience rather than from "expert knowledge" (Vanderplaat, 2002).

Community empowerment (also viewed as community participation, community competence, community capacity, or community development) addresses "new forms of social organization and collective action to redress inequalities of the distribution of power (decision-making authority) and resources" (Laverack, 2004, p. 13). Community empowerment has been described as occurring along a five-point continuum that addresses

- Empowering individuals for personal action
- Empowering individuals to form small mutual assistance groups
- Empowering groups to create community organizations
- Empowering community organizations to form partnerships
- Empowering communities to take social and political action to improve environmental conditions that affect health (Laverack, 2004)

As the last point on the continuum, health promotion as empowerment is an essentially political activity that affects communities, not just individuals (Whitehead, 2004).

If we use smoking cessation as an example, a community health nurse might refer an individual client to a smoking cessation program or suggest other strategies that will help him or her stop smoking. At the second point on the continuum, a community health nurse in an occupational setting might suggest to employees who want to stop smoking that they form a smoking cessation support group. At the third point, the same occupational health nurse might assist the smoking cessation support groups and other nonsmokers to band together to request a ban on smoking in the organization. Businesses and industries with smoking bans might form partnerships to advocate with health insurers for lower insurance rates at the fourth point on the continuum. Finally, at the fifth point, the community health nurse might assist several partnerships and other interested parties to lobby for statewide legislation prohibiting smoking in all public places.

For health promotion practice to empower communities, several key requisites must be met. First, practitioners must possess analytic and communication skills needed to motivate community participation. Second, peer and organizational norms must support empowering health promotion practice. Third, managers of community agencies must be empowerment-oriented, and, finally, agencies that wish to promote health must have internal policies that permit and encourage empowerment of community members (Laverack, 2004). The critical nature of these requisites is reflected in the experience of a graduate student working with a health agency to conduct a community health needs assessment. The assessment was framed in the context of the Dimensions Model of Community Health Nursing described in Chapter 4∞. The student conducted a series of focus groups with community residents to identify their perceptions of community needs and indicated to participants that the data generated would be used to improve health-related conditions in the community. Unfortunately, the community agency with which the student was working was not prepared for the breadth of community concerns generated and the fact that those concerns lay outside of the agency's usual parameters (dealing with physical health conditions). Because the organizational norms and policies and management orientation within the agency did not support empowering health promotion practice, nothing was done with the results of the assessment, leaving both the student and the community members frustrated by the lack of action.

Community empowerment can be integrated into traditional health promotion programs with the intent of producing a general outcome of increased community control over factors that influence their health. Specific outcomes will be unique to the community or group empowered and the purpose of the health promotion initiative (Laverack, 2004). Community empowerment will be addressed in more detail in Chapter 13∞.

Social Marketing

According to the Institute of Medicine, decisions regarding health-related behaviors occur within a social and cultural context. Changes in health behavior require an understanding of the influences exerted by that context (Kreuter et al., 2003). These social influences on behavior tend to exist in a hierarchy; one is influenced in turn by one's peer group, one's nuclear and extended family, community norms, and national norms promulgated via mass media (Tones & Green, 2004). Multiple factors arising from these contextual levels have been found to influence health-related behaviors. For example, in one meta-analysis of 37 studies, factors such as loneliness, social support, perceived health status, self-efficacy, future time perspective, self-esteem, hope, and depression were predictive of health-promoting behaviors in the populations studied (Yarcheski, Mahon, Yarcheski, & Cannella, 2004). Other authors have found religion, religiosity, church attendance, and spirituality to be strongly related to health-related behaviors in some populations (Holt, Kyles, Wiehagen, & Casey, 2003). Social marketing, as a health promotion strategy, uses information about the factors that influence behavior in specific population groups to promote adoption of health-related behaviors or elimination of unhealthy behaviors.

Social marketing involves "the application of commercial marketing technologies to the analysis, planning, execution, and evaluation of programs designed to influence the voluntary behavior of target audiences in order to improve their personal welfare or that of their society" (Andreasen, quoted in Neiger, Thackeray, Barnes, & McKenzie, 2003, p. 75). The aim of social marketing is to use commercial marketing principles to address social problems rather than generate profit (Smith, 2000). In essence, social marketing, as it relates to health promotion, involves conveying a health-related message in a way that is relevant and of interest to a particular target audience. For example, successful anti-smoking campaigns for young people have been based on social marketing principles. Teenagers value being part of the group and being attractive to others. Social marketing campaigns were directed toward making nonsmoking the social norm by emphasizing the unattractive aspects of smoking.

Social marketing is characterized by the concept of exchange, the use of research to direct action, and the development of a "marketing mix" and a positioning strategy (Smith, 2000). Each of these characteristics will be addressed briefly using the example of smoking among adolescents. In social marketing, adolescents are being asked to exchange something, in this case smoking, for a more healthful behavior, not smoking. The central issue is to determine what exchange will satisfy the target audience. For adolescents, being accepted by

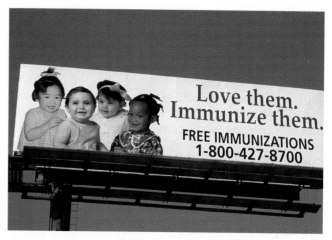

Health promotion campaigns may make use of media advertising. (Michael Newman)

the group or being more attractive to others might be benefits for which they would exchange smoking.

Social marketing is based on research that occurs in three phases (Black & Blue, 2001). The first stage is the preproduction or prepromotion stage of a health promotion initiative. In this stage, research focuses on describing the target population, their attributes, interests, and concerns. Using our adolescent smoking example, researchers at this stage would be interested in exploring what motivates behavior in teenagers and, particularly, why they decide whether or not to use various forms of tobacco. The second stage involves research to develop and test marketing messages and strategies with the target population. In this stage, the planning group would design and test the effectiveness of specific anti-smoking messages with adolescents. The design of these messages might make use of another marketing research strategy, focus groups of adolescents to develop and/or react to anti-smoking messages. In the final stage, research methods are used to study the application and effectiveness of the marketing interventions. At this point, anti-smoking messages would be widely disseminated and their effectiveness in deterring adolescent smoking studied.

A marketing mix is established through research strategies in the prepromotion phase and is based on the four Ps of social marketing: product, price, place, and promotion (Neiger et al., 2003). Some authors add a fifth P for policy (Turning Point, n.d.). The product is the need, service, or desired behavior that the target audience is being asked to adopt (e.g., not smoking). Price reflects the cost of or barriers to adopting the desired behavior or giving up an unhealthy behavior (e.g., possible weight gain, irritability, or being thought "uncool"). The place element of social marketing is the location where the product or service can be obtained (e.g., where smoking cessation programs or nicotine patches are available) as well as the places where members of the target group can be reached. In our adolescent smoking example, this might

CULTURAL COMPETENCE

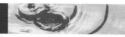

*I*n many Asian cultural groups, it is considered polite to give the person to whom you are speaking the answer they wish to hear, whether or not this answer reflects your true beliefs or feelings. Similarly, a student who does not learn reflects poorly on the teacher and causes him or her to "lose face." How might these cultural values and expectations affect a health education situation? How might you overcome any adverse influences on the effectiveness of health education?

include junior and senior high schools, sporting events, or rock concerts. Promotion refers to the communication strategies and messages used to motivate members of the target audience to act. This might include posters or radio or television messages that present the less attractive aspects of smoking (e.g., smoker's breath, discolored hands and teeth). Policy refers to laws and regulations that influence the behavior at issue (Turning Point, n.d.). For example, enforcement of laws prohibiting tobacco sales to minors would make smoking more difficult. Prosecuting the parents of minors who smoke might be even more effective, but would most likely give rise to questions of fairness.

A positioning strategy addresses the price or costs of the behavior vis-à-vis the competing behavior. Developing a positioning strategy involves identifying the benefits of the desired behavior and its costs and comparing them to the benefits and costs of the competing behavior (Smith, 2000). For example, smoking and non-smoking are competing behaviors. The primary cost of smoking, of course, is death. However, if the target audience is youth for whom death is a distant event, focusing on this cost will not prove very effective. Focusing on the unattractive aspects of smoking highlights elements of the price of smoking that are apt to get the attention of young people, who are very conscious of personal appearance and attractiveness to others.

Critical elements of social marketing include understanding the competition, understanding the target market (through prepromotion research), creation of a mutually beneficial exchange, and segmenting the market and targeting interventions to the specific interests of particular market segments. Segmentation is the "process of using consumer research to identify groups of people (i.e., target markets stratified by age, income, geography, etc.) who share certain relevant attributes such that they are likely to respond to a given offer in a similar manner" (Maibach, 2003, p. 116). Using the smoking example, targeting specific health promotion messages to youth reflects audience segmentation. Other strategies would be used for other segments of the population, such as adult Asian men who smoke. Segmentation leads to decisions about the most effective use of resources and promotion strategies for a particular segment of a target population.

The Turning Point Social Marketing National Excellence Collaborative, one of five national collaboratives working to strengthen public health in the United States, has described six phases in the social marketing process (Turning Point, n.d.). The first phase is describing the problem to be resolved. The second phase involves conducting market research to determine the characteristics of the target audience. The third phase involves creating a marketing strategy or plan of action for the social marketing program. In this phase, the health promotion practitioner identifies the target audience to be reached and influenced by the intervention.

More than one target audience may be identified based on market segmentation. Behavioral goals and strategies to achieve them are developed for each target market. For example, the goal of an anti-tobacco campaign for adults might be smoking cessation by current smokers. This goal might be expanded in a campaign for youth to include cessation by current smokers and noninitiation of smoking by nonsmokers. Similarly, different promotion strategies would be devised for each group based on group characteristics and circumstances that influence smoking behaviors. The last element in creating the marketing strategy is identifying and allocating resources.

In the fourth phase of the social marketing process, the actual intervention is planned. For example, billboards might be designed to convey the message and located where they will be seen by specific targeted audiences. Graphic flyers and posters might be placed in school settings, and so on. The fifth phase involves planning strategies for monitoring and evaluating the intervention, and the sixth phase involves actually implementing the interventions and evaluating their effects. This last phase may also include revising the campaign based on consumer feedback (Kennedy & Crosby, 2002). The phases of social marketing are summarized in Table 11-2◆. The focused assessment below can help to guide development of a social marketing plan.

Health Education

The third health promotion strategy to be addressed is health education. Health education is a participatory learning process that enables people to make informed decisions about health. In the past, health education was seen primarily as provision of information based on the assumption that merely having the information would motivate people to act on it. Health education was also based on an "authority model," in which the health care professional was seen as the authority. In more recent

---

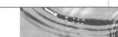

FOCUSED ASSESSMENT

Strategic Questions for Social Marketing Design

- What is the problem to be addressed?
- What actions will address the problem?
- Who must take the action to resolve the problem?
- What does the audience want in exchange for adopting the desired behavior?
- What is the competition for the desired behavior?
- What is the best time and place to reach the target audience?
- How often and from whom should the intervention be received to be effective?
- How can we integrate a series of interventions to act, over time, in an integrated fashion, to influence the behavior?
- Do we have the resources needed for the interventions?

Data from: Turning Point Social Marketing National Excellence Collaborative. (n.d.). The basics of social marketing. Retrieved September 28, 2004, from http://www.turningpointprogram.org

TABLE 11-2	Phases of the Social Marketing Process
Phase	**Description**
1. Problem description	▪ Identification of the health problem or issue to be resolved, including contributing factors and the target audience for intervention
2. Market research	▪ Determination of characteristics of the target audience
3. Strategy development	▪ Creation of a tailored marketing strategy or plan of action for each segment of the target audience ▪ Identification and allocation of resources
4. Intervention design	▪ Development of actual marketing messages
5. Monitoring plan	▪ Development of strategies for monitoring intervention effectiveness
6. Implementation	▪ Dissemination of marketing messages ▪ Evaluation of the effectiveness of marketing messages

Data from: Turning Point Social Marketing National Excellence Collaborative. (n.d.). The basics of social marketing. Retrieved September 28, 2004, from http://www.turningpointprogram.org

conceptualizations, health education is perceived as an approach to changing the environment to one conducive to healthy behavior (Whitehead, 2001). Formally defined from this newer perspective, **health education** is

> an activity that seeks to inform the individual on the nature and causes of health/illness and that individual's personal level of risk associated with their lifestyle-related behavior. Health education seeks to motivate the individual to accept a process of behavioral change through directly influencing their value, belief, and attitude systems, where it is deemed that the individual is particularly at risk or has already been affected by illness/disease or disability. (Whitehead, 2004, p. 313)

Purposes and Goals of Health Education

The primary purpose of health education is to assist clients in making health-related decisions. Health education may equip clients to make any of three types of health-related decisions: decisions about self-care, decisions about the use of health resources, and decisions about societal health issues. The Joint Commission on Accreditation of Healthcare Organizations (JCAHO) has identified six goals of health education in the acute care setting. These goals can also be applied to health education of individuals and groups in community settings. The goals are:

- Client participation in health decision making
- Increased potential to comply with health recommendations
- Development of self-care skills
- Improved client and family coping
- Increased participation in continuing care for specific conditions
- Adoption of healthier lifestyles (Habel, 2002)

Think Advocacy

The Healthy People Curriculum Task Force has recommended incorporation of a common curriculum framework related to health promotion and illness prevention in clinical practice for the education of all health professionals (Allan et al., 2004). Suggested curricular elements include the following:

- Evidence base of practice
  Epidemiology and biostatistics
  Evaluation of health-related literature
  Outcome measurement
  Health surveillance measures
  Determinants of health
- Clinical preventive and health promotion services
  Screening
  Counseling
  Immunization
  Chemoprevention
- Health systems and health policy
  Health system organization
  Health services financing
  Health workforce
  Health policy formation
- Community aspects of practice
  Communicating with the public
  Environmental health
  Occupational health
  Global health issues
  Cultural dimensions of practice
  Community services

To what extent are these areas reflected in your nursing curriculum? What might you do to advocate adoption of this common curriculum framework in your nursing program?

With the exception of the fifth goal, participation in continuing care, which reflects secondary and tertiary prevention for existing health problems, all of these goals can also be related to health promotion.

Domains of Health Learning

As we saw earlier, health education may be required for empowerment or social marketing strategies to be effective. Different types of learning may be required to support each of these strategies or in specific health promotion situations. Types of health learning have been classified into four learning domains: the cognitive,

ETHICAL AWARENESS

Children are sometimes punished by their parents for behaviors enacted "when they know better." Some people have suggested similar sanctions for people who "know better" but continue to engage in unhealthful behaviors. For example, it has been suggested that smokers should be ineligible for public assistance for health problems related to smoking or that motorcycle riders who fail to wear helmets should bear responsibility for the consequences of their actions. Are such attitudes justified? Why or why not?

affective, psychomotor, and social interaction skills domains (Tones & Green, 2004). A **learning domain** is a category or type of learning desired as a result of the health education encounter. The classic taxonomy of learning domains included the cognitive, affective, psychomotor, and perceptual domains (Bloom, Englehart, Furst, Hill, & Krathwohl, 1956). The cognitive domain encompasses intellectual skills related to factual information and its application. In the affective domain, the focus of learning is on attitudes and values. Emphasis in the psychomotor domain is on the learning of physical manipulative skills (Bastable, 2003). Finally, in the perceptual domain, emphasis is on learning to perceive and extract information from stimuli. More recent authors have added the social interaction skills domain to address learning that is required for communication, persuasion, and influencing others (including policy makers) (Butler, 2001; Tones & Green, 2004).

Taxonomies of learning tasks classify tasks within each of the established domains in a hierarchical fashion. In the cognitive and psychomotor domains, learning tasks are arranged in order of increasing complexity of intellectual or physical skill involved. For example, it requires greater intellectual skill to apply a fact to a particular decision-making situation than simply to recall the fact. Similarly, less skill is required to follow printed knitting instructions than to create one's own pattern. Hierarchies of learning tasks in the cognitive and psychomotor domains are presented in Table 11-3◆.

Tasks in the affective domain are organized in terms of the degree to which an attitude or value has been internalized by the learner (Krathwohl, Bloom, & Masia, 1964). For example, the student who consistently displays empathy for clients is operating at a higher level of internalization than one who merely discusses the importance of empathy in nursing. The taxonomy of the affective domain is also presented in Table 11-3◆.

Finally, learning tasks in the perceptual domain are arranged in terms of the extent to which the learner is able to extract information from a situation by way of perceptual skills. For example, a nursing student might notice a few salient characteristics of a family during a first home visit (e.g., cleanliness of the home, character of mother–child interactions), whereas an experienced community health nurse would derive much more information from the same encounter. The levels of a proposed taxonomy for the perceptual domain are listed in Table 11-3◆.

Principles of Learning

A number of principles of learning have been identified that apply to health education as well as to other forms of learning encounters. These principles can be grouped as general principles of learning and principles related to the health education message and its delivery. The first, and possibly most important, general principle is that effective learning takes place in a "shame-free"

environment (Public Health Group, 2002). Second, time, resources, and creativity are required to develop health education presentations that are appropriate to the target audience. When that audience is a culturally diverse group, the health education program should be developed by a culturally diverse team, and the curriculum written as a team effort. Similarly, when the audience involves members of previously disenfranchised communities, time will be required to create trust and rapport between the target audience and the health educators. Including community members in planning health education programs will enhance the development of trust and rapport as well as make the program more culturally appropriate. In addition, there is a need to recognize the culturally specific history of the group and how it influences health behaviors and readiness for health education (Burhansstipanov et al., 2003). These general principles as well as self-explanatory principles related to the health education message and its delivery are summarized in Table 11-4◆.

Assessing Health Education Needs

The health education process begins with an assessment of the audience, their health education needs, and the learning environment. A needs assessment is a "planned process that identifies the reported needs of an individual or group" (Butler, 2001, p. 259). When the client is a group or a community, the first task in assessment is to identify the target audience. Selection of the target audience may be based on level of need, resources available, or probability of success. Assessment then proceeds to identifying characteristics of the audience that influence the learning situation. The assessment can be conducted in terms of the dimensions model of community health nursing, addressing biophysical, psychological, physical environmental, sociocultural, behavioral, and health system factors that influence the health education situation. When members of the target audience participate in conducting the assessment, the accuracy of the assessment and its relevance to their needs are enhanced.

Biophysical considerations influence both the learning needs and the learning capabilities of individual clients or populations. To learn effectively, clients may need to have reached a certain level of physical or psychological maturation. For example, small children who have not yet developed abilities for abstract thought will need concrete examples of concepts to be learned. Similarly, a child who still has poorly developed eye–hand coordination will have difficulty learning insulin injection techniques, so teaching will most likely involve parents as well. At the other end of the age spectrum, changes associated with aging may lead to sensory impairment that influences health education with older populations. Age or maturation level also affects the client's need for education. For instance, preschool children do not need information about menstruation, but preadolescent girls do. In addition, clients'

TABLE 11-3 Taxonomy of Learning Tasks in the Cognitive, Psychomotor, Affective, and Perceptual Domains

Domain	Learning Tasks and Description
Cognitive	▪ Knowledge: Recall of facts, methods, or processes *Sample learning objective*: Learners will be able to list elements of the food pyramid. ▪ Comprehension: Basic understanding of the meaning of facts *Sample learning objective*: Learners will be able to describe elements of the food pyramid in terms of recommended servings. ▪ Application: Use of abstractions in concrete situations *Sample learning objective*: Learners will be able to evaluate their diet in light of the servings recommended for elements of the food pyramid. ▪ Analysis: Ability to break concepts down into component parts *Sample learning objective*: Learners will be able to identify the nutrients provided by selected elements of the food pyramid. ▪ Synthesis: Ability to combine parts into a new pattern or whole *Sample learning objective*: Learners will be able to incorporate food preferences of a specific ethnic group into a food pyramid tailored to that group. ▪ Evaluation: Judgment about the value of information and processes for specific purposes *Sample learning objective*: Learners will be able to describe the relative importance of incorporating elements of the food pyramid in diets designed for primary or secondary prevention of obesity.
Affective	▪ Receiving: Sensitization to the existence of a phenomenon *Sample learning objective*: Learners will describe protections for the civil rights of gay and lesbian members of the community. ▪ Responding: Low level of commitment to behaviors embodying a value, performance of the behavior because of outside constraint *Sample learning objective*: Learners will adhere to legally mandated protections afforded to gay and lesbian members of the community. ▪ Valuing: Ascribing worth to a thing, behavior, or value accompanied by fairly consistent performance of related behaviors *Sample learning objective*: Learners will usually refrain from actions discriminating against gay and lesbian members of the community. ▪ Organization: Organization of values in hierarchical relationships *Sample learning objective*: Learners will be able to apply the value of nondiscrimination to other segments of the population. ▪ Characterization: Person can be characterized by consistent behavior in keeping with a specific set of values *Sample learning objective*: Learners will consistently refrain from discriminatory actions against "undesirable" segments of the population.
Psychomotor	▪ Perception: Awareness of objects and the relationships among them *Sample learning objective*: Learners will be able to discuss items needed for insulin injection. ▪ Set: Physical, mental, and emotional readiness to act *Sample learning objective*: Learners will express willingness to learn insulin injection technique. ▪ Guided response: Performance of an action with instructor input and guidance *Sample learning objective*: Learners will demonstrate correct insulin injection technique with instructor coaching. ▪ Mechanism: Performance of task as a habit *Sample learning objective*: Learners consistently demonstrate correct insulin injection technique. ▪ Complex overt response: Performance of task with a high degree of skill *Sample learning objective*: Learners demonstrate correct insulin injection technique smoothly and rapidly. ▪ Adaptation: Ability to adjust the skill to meet the needs of new situations *Sample learning objective*: Learners are able to adjust insulin dosage to accommodate increased exercise. ▪ Origination: Ability to create new acts or ways of manipulating materials *Sample learning objective*: Learners are able to switch to use of an insulin pump with little difficulty.
Perceptual	▪ Sensation: Awareness of differences, or change, in stimuli *Sample learning objective*: Nursing students can distinguish an abnormal tympanic membrane from a normal one. ▪ Figure perception: Awareness of an object or phenomenon as a distinct entity *Sample learning objective*: Nursing students can identify the light reflex on a tympanic membrane. ▪ Symbol perception: Identification of pattern or form, ability to name or classify an object or phenomenon *Sample learning objective*: Nursing students can distinguish a bulging tympanic membrane from a retracted one. ▪ Perception of meaning: Awareness of significance of symbols, ability to interrelate symbols *Sample learning objective*: Nursing students can recognize a bulging tympanic membrane as evidence of possible middle ear infection. ▪ Perceptive performance: Complex decisions with multiple factors, ability to change behavior based on its effectiveness *Sample learning objective*: Nursing students can combine evidence of a bulging tympanic membrane, loss of typical tympanic membrane landmarks, fever, and ear pain to derive a diagnosis of probable middle ear infection.

TABLE 11-4 General, Message-related, and Delivery-related Principles of Learning

General Principles of Learning

- Effective learning requires a shame-free environment.

- Time, resources, and creativity are required to develop health education programs appropriately targeted to specific audiences.

- Time will be required to develop trust with disenfranchised communities before effective health education can occur.

- Culturally diverse teams should participate in the development of health education programs for culturally diverse audiences.

- Curricula for health education programs should be developed as a team effort.

- Curriculum development should acknowledge and incorporate the distinct culturally specific history of the target audience.

- Curriculum development should capitalize on lessons learned from similar projects.

Message-related Principles of Learning

- Messages personalized to the audience will be more effective than global or generalized messages suitable for mass dissemination.

- Health education messages should include content most relevant to the target audience, rather than trying to cover all of the related information.

- The message should highlight important concepts.

- Messages should give high priority to client action and motivation.

Delivery-related Principles of Learning

- Information should be linked to existing knowledge.

- Information should be presented in fun and interactive ways to promote integration of concepts.

- Modes of presentation should allow sufficient time for group members to assimilate and interact with it.

- Messages should be presented in clear, simple language, and should avoid professional jargon.

- Materials should generally be developed at grade levels one to two grades below the highest grade completed in school and should employ short sentences and simple, one- and two-syllable words.

- Information should be reinforced and repeated as needed, using illustrations as appropriate.

- Written materials should use large type fonts and a mix of upper- and lower-case letters and should employ ample white space to prevent readers from being overwhelmed by content.

- Information in written materials should be bulleted when possible.

- Written materials should be reinforced verbally.

- Multiple approaches should be used to assess understanding of content (e.g., questioning, demonstration, etc.).

maturational levels may influence existing knowledge of a particular subject. For example, a group of third graders will probably have a broader knowledge of nutrition concepts than preschoolers.

Assessing aspects of physiologic function in the population may reveal special needs for health education or impediments to learning. For example, a high prevalence of diabetes in the population suggests a need for diabetes self-care education, whereas high incidence rates for sexually transmitted diseases among adolescents indicate other needs for prevention education. Inadequate physiologic function can also give rise to impediments to learning. For example, the presence of physical disabilities may require specialized approaches to health education. Pain, another biophysical factor, may also impede learning.

Elements of the psychological dimension can profoundly influence willingness and ability to learn. Attitudes toward health and health behaviors can either enhance or detract from the motivation to learn. Among clients attending a series of parenting classes, for example, those parents who attend only because of a court mandate related to child abuse usually benefit less than those who attend because they perceive a need for help.

Psychological factors such as stress and anxiety can also impede learning, even for those who are motivated to learn. Nurses can limit the negative effects of the psychological dimension by actions designed to decrease stress and anxiety. For example, the nurse can create a climate in which clients do not feel threatened and in which the nurse educator is seen as a source of support rather than a

threat. The nurse who has children and who teaches parenting classes for abusive parents might create such a climate by beginning the first session with a description of the frustration the nurse sometimes feels as a parent.

The physical environment should also be considered in terms of its effects on learning. Is there adequate lighting for the tasks to be accomplished? Is there too much noise? Will clients be distracted by other activities occurring in the learning environment? During a home visit, for example, the nurse might ask that the television be turned off before attempting to educate a hypertensive client about his or her medication.

Physical environmental factors may also give rise to the need for health education. For example, population groups affected by natural disasters may need education on how to purify their drinking water to prevent communicable diseases. Similarly, health education efforts might be targeted to persons with chronic respiratory conditions in areas with significant air pollution.

The sociocultural dimension is particularly influential in shaping attitudes about health and health-related behaviors. Examples and attitudes of those around us influence our willingness to engage in self-care behaviors in addition to affecting our attitudes to health issues at the societal level.

Elements of the sociocultural dimension also influence one's exposure to health-related information. People with lower education levels are less likely than those with more formal education to have been exposed to prior health education. The education level of the population and of specific target audiences necessarily influences the nurse's choice of teaching strategies and content to be presented.

Cultural influences on health education with population groups include typical communication styles, concepts of time and personal space, values, and perceptions of environmental control. Client life roles and role expectations, which are culturally defined, are other factors that may affect interest in health education and motivation to learn. When content is perceived to be relevant to the roles one is expected to fulfill, one's motivation to learn is likely to be high. Roles may also influence one's ability to attend to health messages. For example, if members of the audience are responsible for the care of children, they are unlikely to be able to attend educational presentations unless childcare is arranged.

Culture may also influence the effectiveness of health education in terms of the trust placed in health professionals. Many culturally diverse audiences may distrust health professionals as a result of past experiences or cultural misunderstandings. Language is another sociocultural factor that might hamper learning abilities unless the nurse allows for language differences in planning health education. The implications of language will be addressed in more detail in the discussion of planning for health education programs.

Occupation is another social dimension factor that can give rise to health education needs. Trash collectors, for example, might require education related to body mechanics and techniques for lifting heavy objects, whereas nurses require information about how to handle contaminated needles and other equipment.

Behavioral factors influence needs for health education. For example, the extent of obesity in the United States suggests the need for intensive dietary education. Similarly, smokers may need help with smoking cessation and education on alternative ways to meet needs satisfied by smoking. As another example, sexually active clients may need education regarding contraceptives and safe sexual practices.

In the health system dimension, preventive and therapeutic recommendations may precipitate a need for health education. For example, clients may need to be educated on the correct use of medications or how to keep a sprained ankle immobilized to promote healing. Elements of the health care regimen may also influence clients' abilities to learn. For example, pain medication may make a client drowsy and inhibit the ability to learn material presented. The degree of emphasis placed on health education by health care providers and providers' expertise in using the health education process are other health care system factors that influence clients' health-related knowledge and attitudes. Tips for assessing a health education situation are presented on page 268. In addition, an assessment tool is provided in the *Community Assessment Reference Guide* designed to accompany this book.

Planning and Implementing Health Education Programs

In the context of health education, planning involves a "process of making decisions as to what topic to address, what problems to attack and/or where to direct time and resources" (Butler, 2001, p. 259). Elements of the planning process include prioritizing learning needs, developing goals and objectives, and selecting content and teaching/learning strategies. Other considerations in planning and implementing health education programs include language and health literacy and the use of the Internet as a teaching medium.

PRIORITIZING LEARNING NEEDS Planning health education programs begins with prioritizing learning needs. Generally speaking, a health education needs assessment will indicate several areas of need, not all of which can be addressed in a single health education program. Prioritization involves determining the relative effects of behaviors and risk factors present in the population and the benefits to be achieved by changing them. Another consideration in prioritizing health education needs is the ease with which contributing factors can be changed. For example, members of the population may not use seat belts, get too little exercise, and fail to obtain periodic mammograms. A change to using seat belts would result in the most immediate and dramatic benefit to the community and be the easiest of the three behaviors to change. For these reasons, the community health nurse might first begin with health education efforts in this area. Members of the community can also help determine priorities, ensuring that topics of greatest interest and relevance to the target audience are addressed.

DEVELOPING GOALS AND OBJECTIVES Goal identification involves specifying the broad purpose of the health education encounter. Some authors distinguish between

BUILDING OUR KNOWLEDGE BASE

*D*onovan and Ward (2001) noted that two decades of research have indicated five consistent themes in illness representations: identity, cause, timeline, consequences, and cure or control. Identity refers to the labels that one associates with the symptoms of a health problem. Cause reflects one's perceptions of the source of the problem or its origins. The timeline component of a disease representation refers to conceptualizations of a problem as acute, chronic, or cyclic in nature. Consequences reflect beliefs about the short- and long-term outcomes of the problem; and, finally, the theme of cure or control addresses one's perceptions of the extent to which the problem is amenable to cure or to control.

These themes are found consistently in representations of illness. How would you conduct a study to determine if these same themes would be found in representations of states of health? Might the themes uncovered vary among cultural and ethnic groups? How would you discover whether the themes vary?

FOCUSED ASSESSMENT

Assessing the Health Education Situation

Biophysical Considerations

- What is the age composition of the target audience? What learning needs arise from the age and developmental level of the audience? Will the developmental level of the audience affect the ability to learn or the teaching strategies used?
- Do physical health problems in the population give rise to the need for health education or pose any impediments to learning?

Psychological Considerations

- Is the target population aware of the need for health education? What is the level of motivation to learn? Will population attitudes toward health and health behaviors enhance or detract from learning ability?
- Does the target audience exhibit levels of stress or anxiety that will interfere with learning?

Physical Environmental Considerations

- Are there conditions in the physical environment that give rise to a need for health education? What effects, if any, will the physical environment have on learning?

Sociocultural Considerations

- What effects will the learners' peers have on motivation to learn?
- What is the current education level of the learners? What prior exposure to health information has the population received?

- What is the primary language spoken by members of the target audience?
- Are there cultural beliefs and practices that are likely to influence learning?
- Do the occupations of group members give rise to a need for health education?
- Are there other facets of the social situation (e.g., SES, time for or transportation to educational opportunities) that may influence health education? What effect do these facets have on the health education situation?

Behavioral Considerations

- Do health behaviors prevalent in the population give rise to the need for health education?

Health System Considerations

- Do local health care providers emphasize health education? Do members of the population have access to health care services where they might receive health education?
- Does the population have a need for education regarding the use of health care services?
- Do health care recommendations give rise to a need for health education? Are there elements of the health care regimen that may influence learning abilities (e.g., medications)?
- Will attitudes toward health care services and providers influence the ability to learn?

---

program goals—the intended purpose of the overall health education program—and educational goals—the learning outcome expected for the audience. For example, the program goal for a nutrition program might be to prevent obesity in school-age children. The educational goal, on the other hand, might be for parents to become knowledgeable regarding appropriate nutrition for their children.

Objectives describe specific outcomes to be achieved as a result of the health education program. Using the prior example, an objective related to the program goal might be that the community incidence (number of new cases) of childhood obesity will decline by 50% within 2 years. An educational objective might be that parents are able to correctly describe the number of servings of each element of the food pyramid required by an elementary school student.

Objectives should be stated in measurable terms that allow one to evaluate whether the expected results have been achieved. Evaluability of outcomes also requires that they be specific. For example, an outcome objective such as "reduce adolescent tobacco use" is somewhat vague. If one adolescent smoker stops smoking, have we met our objective? Similarly, an objective to "stop adolescent tobacco use" is not particularly realistic. No matter what interventions are employed, it is unlikely that we will ever prevent all adolescents from using tobacco. A more realistic, and more measurable, objective for tobacco education might be to "reduce the prevalence of tobacco use among high school seniors by 50% within

1 year." As stated, the objective provides a target measure for accomplishment (a 50% decline in the number of seniors who use tobacco) as well as a time frame for expected accomplishment (1 year from program initiation).

SELECTING CONTENT AND TEACHING STRATEGIES The content selected for inclusion in a health education program will depend on its relevance to the target population. Audiences are more likely to attend to information that they perceive as highly relevant to their own situations (Kreuter et al., 2003). One must be selective in planning the content because no audience needs or wishes to learn everything about a particular topic that the health educator may know. Going back to the general principles discussed earlier, an effective educator chooses the content that is most relevant to the target audience.

Selection of teaching strategies will depend on a number of factors, including characteristics of the audience, the content and objectives to be achieved, program budget, time available, cultural appropriateness, and the environment for health education (Gilbert & Sawyer, 2000). In educating individual clients, health education messages may make use of tailored or "customized communication in which specific messages are provided to specific individuals, based on unique characteristics of each person as gathered through a personal assessment" (Kreuter et al., 2003, p. 70). This process is akin to the social marketing approach described earlier for use with population groups.

In some studies, tailored messages have been found to be more effective than generalized messages in motivating behavior change. In other studies, the effects of tailored messages have been mediated by cultural characteristics. For example, in one study, religiosity and racial pride affected the degree of attention given to tailored health education messages among African American women (Kreuter et al., 2003).

Recently, a number of authors have suggested using highly graphic messages in health education initiatives to motivate healthful behaviors. For example, in one study, use of graphic package labeling on cigarettes led to decreased tobacco use among 20% of the population exposed. Negative emotions generated by graphic package labeling, such as fear and disgust, were associated with stopping smoking, attempts to stop smoking, and reduced smoking (Hammond, Fong, McDonald, Brown, & Cameron, 2004). Similarly, truth advertising—focusing on making adolescents aware of the tobacco industry's special efforts to target them for smoking initiation—has been associated with an increase in antitobacco attitudes and beliefs (Farrelly et al., 2002). Another study by the same authors indicated that "truth" campaigns also accounted for approximately 22% of the decline in smoking prevalence among youth (Farrelly, Davis, Haviland, Messeri, & Healton, 2005).

LANGUAGE AND LITERACY IN HEALTH EDUCATION

Language is a particularly important consideration in health education initiatives in the United States, where approximately 46 million people do not speak English and another 21 million do not speak it well. Research has indicated that non-English-speakers are less likely than their English-speaking counterparts to have a regular source of health care and to receive preventive care and may be at higher risk for medical error. Similarly, studies show that, although relatively few people have access to interpretation services, those who do, receive more preventive services, more prescriptions, and more office visits. These effects may actually lower the overall cost of services due to earlier receipt of care and greater emphasis on health promotion and prevention (Jacobs, Shepard, Suaya, & Stone, 2004). The use of interpreter services was discussed in more detail in Chapter 9∞.

Health literacy is closely related to language in its effects on health education initiatives. **Health literacy** is defined as "the ability of individuals to obtain, interpret, and understand basic health information and services *and* to use such information and services in ways that enhance health" (Public Health Group, 2002, p. 3). Health illiteracy, according to the American Medical Association, is an inability to read, comprehend, or act on medical instructions. Approximately 48% of the U.S. population that speaks English as their native language does not have adequate health literacy skills. Ninety million U.S. adults have difficulty understanding health information, and 40 to 44 million of them are functionally illiterate (Darling, 2004), meaning that they read below a fifth-grade level. Another 50 million people are marginally literate (Public Health Group, 2002). Overall, one in five U.S. adults "lacks sufficient literacy skills to meet daily needs in their families, their workplaces, and their communities" (Kogut, 2004, p. 26)

Health illiteracy affects some groups more than others. For example, approximately one third of Medicare recipients are unable to understand basic health-related materials, which may explain why about 30% of hospitalizations among the elderly are due to

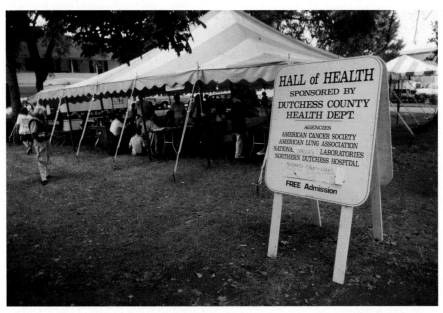

Community fairs provide excellent opportunities for health education activities by community health nurses. (Patrick J. Watson)

medication errors. Close to 40% of all people in the United States with chronic conditions are functionally illiterate, which impairs their ability to engage in effective self-care. Persons with low literacy have been shown to be less likely to receive preventive care, more likely to be hospitalized, and more likely to have poor health outcomes than those with adequate literacy skills (Public Health Group, 2002). Lack of health literacy has also been linked to poor health knowledge, particularly related to cancer, low cancer screening rates, late diagnosis, and poor self-reported health status (Bennet, Kripalani, Weiss, & Coyne, 2003).

Five basic principles address health literacy considerations in health education. These principles are as follows:

- The content of health-related materials should be based on written objectives for the health education encounter.
- Reader involvement with the materials is critical.
- Materials should be easy to read and understand.
- Health-related materials should *look* easy to read.
- Visual features of health-related materials should clarify content and motivate reader action. (DeBuono, 2002)

These principles and related tasks in the development of materials for low-literacy populations are presented in Table 11-5◆. Including members of the target population in the development of health education materials

helps to ensure that materials are culturally and linguistically appropriate to the audience.

THE INTERNET IN HEALTH EDUCATION The Internet is often used by individual clients, the general public, and health care providers as a source of health-related information (Fogel, 2003). Using the Internet as a medium for health education has both advantages and disadvantages. Two general problems that may be encountered are inaccurate information and biased information (Kiley, 2003). To address these problems, the National Center for Complementary and Alternative Medicine has developed a set of criteria for evaluating health-related Web sites that has been suggested for international use by the World Health Organization (WHO, 2004). Evaluative elements include the reputability of the owner of the site, sources of financial support for the site, the purpose of the site, the sources of information provided, evidence provided to support the information given, the existence of an editorial group that oversees selection of content, and the currency of information provided. Additional criteria include the selection of links to other sites, whether the site collects personal data from users or requires subscription, and the ability to contact the owner of the site. Other authors suggest additional criteria for evaluating Internet information, including the point of view or political stance of the site owner/organization, the relationship of the author of selected information to the owner of the site, acknowledgment of controversial issues, and information regarding the regularity with which information on the site is updated (Kirk, cited in Gilbert & Sawyer, 2000).

Visitors to a particular Internet site can also look for the display of approval logos on the Web site's home page. Three organizations currently evaluate health-related Web sites, and their logos indicate their credibility. The organizations are:

- Health on the Net (http://www.hon/ch/HONcode): Logo indicates that the site abides by an 8-point code of honesty for medical Web sites.
- American Accreditation Healthcare Commission (URAC) (http://urac.org/websiteaccreditation/portal/Business/Index.asp): Approved sites meet a set of 50 quality standards.
- MedCIRCLE (http://www.medcircle.info): Provides standard information regarding medical Web sites (e.g., owner, sponsoring organization, etc.)

In addition, Internet users can visit one of several sites that monitor health-related quackery on the Internet. These sites include:

- Quackwatch (http://quackwatch.com)
- National Council Against Health Fraud (http://www.ncahf.org)
- Health Care Reality Check (http://www.hcrc.org)
- American Council on Science and Health (http://www.acsh.org) (Kiley, 2003)

TABLE 11-5	Health Literacy Principles and Related Tasks
Principle	**Related Tasks**
Base content on written objectives	▪ Explain the purpose and benefits of content from the reader's perspective. ▪ Use objectives to limit content to essential material. ▪ Outline the sequence of topics. ▪ Emphasize desired outcome behaviors.
Involve the reader	▪ Create interaction between the reader and the content. ▪ Provide examples relevant to the reader. ▪ Make materials age, gender, and culture appropriate.
Make content easy to read	▪ Assess the education level of the audience and adjust the reading level accordingly. ▪ Use a conversational style to present information. ▪ Break up complex topics into more simple components.
Make content *look* easy to read	▪ Use plenty of white space. ▪ Cue the reader to important concepts. ▪ Use sharp contrast colors and large type fonts.
Use visuals that clarify and motivate	▪ Use realistic visuals without distracting details. ▪ Use active captions for material. ▪ Explain how to use concepts covered and give examples.

Data from: DeBuono, B. A. (2002). *Pfizer Health Literacy Initiative. New York:* Pfizer Graphic.

EVALUATING HEALTH PROMOTION PROGRAMS

Like all community health nursing activities, the effectiveness of health promotion initiatives should be evaluated. Several authors have noted the difficulty involved in such an evaluation, primarily because it is difficult to determine when an event does not occur if it would have occurred without the intervention. Another area of difficulty lies in the fact that the unit of analysis in community-based health promotion evaluation should be the community, but resource constraints in both programs and program evaluations rarely allow participation by an entire community. Therefore one has the problem of identifying who in the community was exposed to the program and who was not. In addition, the quasi-experimental nature of most program evaluations leads to selection effects among participants, with those most interested in a program and possibly more highly motivated regarding the particular topic, involved. Similarly, evaluation measures may focus on complete avoidance of a negative behavior (or always engaging in a positive one) and, thus, may miss small gains (e.g., reduction in the number of cigarettes smoked versus stopping smoking altogether) (Merzel & D'Afflitti, 2003; Twinn, 2001).

In spite of these difficulties, however, health promotion programs can and should be evaluated. This evaluation may occur at different levels. For example, diagnostic evaluation assesses the accuracy of the needs assessment on which the health promotion program was based. Formative evaluation, also called process evaluation, examines the way in which the program was carried out. Finally, summative evaluation may focus on program outcome, impact, or both (Butler, 2001; MacDonald, 2002).

EVIDENCE-BASED PRACTICE

Some authors have noted that evaluating the effects of population-based health promotion programs is difficult because the programs are not evenly applied to all members of the population. In programs designed for individuals, on the other hand, one can compare persons who were exposed to the health promotion intervention to a matched group of people who were not. Population-based programs are usually targeted to large segments of the population, and any given individual may or may not have been exposed to the program.

- How might you design a study to evaluate the effects of a population-based media campaign to prevent family violence that would address this type of difficulty?
- What outcome measures would you use?
- Who would your study population include? How would you recruit them?
- What kind of data would you collect? How and when might you collect it?

Health promotion programs may also be evaluated in terms of the extent to which they achieve criteria of empowerment, participation, holism, intersectoral collaboration, equity, use of multiple strategies, and sustainability (Tones & Green, 2004). First and foremost, programs should be empowering, allowing beneficiaries to assume control of the program. They should also foster participation of the target population at all stages of development, implementation, and evaluation. Third, they should be holistic, with a focus on multiple aspects of health. They should also involve participation and collaboration by multiple community sectors to achieve desired ends and should be guided by concerns for equity and social justice. Effective health promotion programs also employ a variety of approaches to achieving change. Finally, the results of effective health promotion programs are sustainable, with changes that can be maintained beyond the initial period of funding.

A number of the *Healthy People 2010* ◆ objectives reflect health promotion efforts, and the relevant targets can be used to evaluate the effectiveness of specific health promotion initiatives. Many of the objectives related to all 10 of the leading health indicators emphasize health promotion. For example, objectives related to injury and violence prevention include reductions in pedestrian deaths on public roads, an objective in keeping with our speed bump example earlier in the chapter, as well as increased use of seat belts. Similarly, objectives related to nutrition and overweight include increasing the percentage of people who eat sufficient fruits and vegetables and decreasing fat intake, both of which reflect health promotion. Specific objectives and the degree of progress toward their accomplishment are included in relevant chapters throughout this book. The complete set of objectives and data on accomplishment may be obtained from the *Healthy People* data Web site at http://wonder.cdc.gov/data2010.

Community health nurses are actively involved in health promotion and health education efforts with individuals, families, and population groups. Table 11-6◆ describes the elements of a health education program and considerations related to assessing the health education situation, planning the program, and evaluating its effectiveness. In the table, the assessment of factors influencing the health education situation is framed in the context of the dimensions of health. The program described is an actual population-based health education initiative undertaken by community health nursing students in a culturally diverse community.

As we have seen, health promotion is more than promoting behavior change among individuals or population groups. It also involves activity to change the social, political, economic, and/or physical environment in ways that are conducive to health. Achieving changes at these levels requires advocacy and empowerment as well as information giving and motivation.

TABLE 11-6 Elements of a Community Health Education Program for Disaster Preparedness

Element	Considerations
Assessment	**Biophysical factors** ▪ Many elderly and families with young children live in the community. ▪ There are several disabled community members. **Psychological factors** ▪ There is apathy regarding family disaster preparedness among community residents. ▪ Residents do not believe disasters are likely to affect them. **Physical environmental factors** ▪ The community sits on a major geologic fault. ▪ The community is surrounded by dry canyons with potential for wildfires. ▪ The community is in a coastal area that could be subjected to tsunamis. ▪ Many residences are old and might be heavily damaged in an earthquake. ▪ Most of the residences are older homes and rental units. Few of them are equipped with smoke alarms. **Sociocultural factors** ▪ The community includes several large groups of Hispanic immigrants and Asian refugees as well as small groups of African Americans, Sudanese and Somali refugees, and older white residents. ▪ Many residents do not speak English. Major languages spoken are English, Spanish, Vietnamese, and Hmong. ▪ Community income levels are low and many community residents have less than a high school education. ▪ Most families in the community have little knowledge of disaster preparedness. ▪ Several homeless individuals live in makeshift shelters in the canyons. ▪ Fire department services are central to the community and respond rapidly to emergency calls. **Behavioral factors** ▪ Homeless persons living in the canyons often cook over open fires, posing a wildfire hazard. ▪ Many people in the community smoke, increasing the potential for house fires. ▪ Many of the Hmong population cook over open braziers in their homes, increasing the potential for house fires. ▪ Few families in the community have gathered supplies in the event of potential disasters. **Health system factors** ▪ Health care providers in the community do not routinely educate clients regarding disaster preparedness. ▪ The local health department has concentrated on community response to possible bioterrorist attacks and has not actively promoted preparation for other types of disasters.
Purpose/goal	To increase disaster preparedness among families in the community
Levels of prevention	*Primary prevention*: Prevent disasters from occurring *Secondary prevention*: Preparation for and effective response to a disaster
Objectives	**Affective domain** ▪ Community residents will demonstrate an understanding of the need for smoke detectors in homes. ▪ Community residents will demonstrate an understanding of the need for disaster preparedness. **Cognitive domain** ▪ Community residents will be able to identify critical supplies needed for disaster preparedness. ▪ Community residents will demonstrate appropriate responses to specific emergencies.
Content	▪ Content was chosen to address the two types of disasters most likely to occur in the community: fire and earthquake. ▪ Information about preventing fires, responding to fires and earthquakes, and needed disaster supplies was gathered from a variety of sources (e.g., local fire officials, the Internet, Red Cross, and county health department disaster divisions). ▪ Content was reviewed to pick out the five or six most salient pieces of information.
Teaching strategies/materials	▪ The project was planned to be implemented as an exhibit at the multicultural fair held annually in the community. This fair attracts approximately 10,000 people each year, most of whom are community residents. ▪ Because of the fair venue, messages were developed for the limited time people were likely to spend at the booth. ▪ According to community informants, many of the Hmong population were not literate, even in Hmong (which did not have a written form until recently), so information brochures were developed in English, Spanish, and Vietnamese, and pictorial messages were used for the Hmong population. ▪ Pictures and samples of necessary disaster supplies were exhibited. ▪ Fire prevention and response coloring books were obtained from the local fire department and crayons were purchased and wrapped in sets of three to give out with the coloring books. ▪ Posters indicating needed disaster supplies and information families should have were created and hung in the booth. Key information was transferred to refrigerator magnets that were handed out to participants. ▪ Donations were solicited for raffle prizes related to disaster prevention and preparedness (e.g., smoke alarms, flashlights) and raffles were held throughout the day to attract fair participants to the booth.

Continued on next page

Element	Considerations

TABLE 11-6 Elements of a Community Health Education Program for Disaster Preparedness *(continued)*

Element	Considerations
Evaluation	■ Visitors to the booth were asked to select pictures from a collection of items that they would include in disaster preparedness supplies and attach them to a felt board. This was a highly popular activity and although it was designed primarily for children, many adults participated as well. Most participants were able to select correct items. ■ Visitors were also asked what they would do in the event of an earthquake (get outside or under a sturdy doorway or table) or a fire (e.g., stop, drop, and roll) and how to prevent fires. Most participants answered correctly. ■ Ideally, a community survey would be conducted after the fair to determine how many community residents actually collected disaster preparedness supplies or installed smoke detectors, but this was not possible in the time frame available for the project.

Case Study

Promoting Population Health

New state legislation has mandated that the majority of funds allocated for public health efforts be devoted to health promotion activities rather than to care of clients with existing health problems. Some of the major health problems encountered in the state at this time include heart disease, family violence, and social isolation among the elderly.

1. Which of these issues would be most amenable to health promotion efforts? Why?

2. Choose one of the three problems and design a set of interventions to address it. How might you employ empowerment strategies to address the problem selected?

3. Discuss the four Ps of social marketing related to the problem selected. How might you segment your target audience?

4. What role would health education play in addressing the problem selected?

Test Your Understanding

1. How would you define health promotion? (p. 255)

2. How does health promotion differ from health education? (p. 255)

3. Compare and contrast two of the models for health promotion discussed in the chapter. (pp. 256–259)

4. What are three possible strategies that may be used to promote health? Which of these strategies are primarily focused on individuals and which on population groups? (pp. 259–263)

5. What are the four Ps of social marketing? Give an example of each. (pp. 261–262)

6. What is the significance of empowerment for health promotion? (pp. 259–260)

7. What are the elements of the health education process? How would a community health nurse go about designing a population-based health education program? (pp. 262–271)

8. What are the implications of language and health literacy for health education and health promotion? (pp. 269–270)

9. What are some of the criteria for evaluating health information available on the Internet? Give examples of Web sites that meet the criteria and those that do not. (p. 270)

10. What are some of the difficulties of evaluating health promotion programs? Give an example of each difficulty. (p. 271)

11. What are some criteria for evaluating health promotion programs? Give examples of programs that do and do not meet the criteria. (p. 271)

EXPLORE MediaLink

http:/www.prenhall.com/clark
Resources for this chapter can be found on the Companion Website.

Audio Glossary	MediaLink Application: Celebrity Health	Update *Healthy People 2010*
Exam Review Questions	Promotion (video)	Advocacy Interviews
Case Study: Health Promotion through	Media Links	
Education	Challenge Your Knowledge	

References

Allan, J., Barwick, T. A., Cashman, S., Cawley, J. F., Day, C., Douglass, C. W., et al. (2004). Clinical prevention and population health: Curriculum framework for health professions. *American Journal of Preventive Medicine, 27*, 471–476.

Awofeso, N. (2004). What's new about the new public health? *American Journal of Public Health, 94*, 705–709.

Bastable, S. B. (2003). *Nurse as educator: Principles of teaching and learning for nursing practice* (2nd ed.). Sudbury, MA: Jones and Bartlett.

Bennet, I. M., Kripalani, S., Weiss, B. D., & Coyne, C. A. (2003). Combining cancer control information with adult literacy information: Opportunities to reach adults with limited literacy skills. *Cancer Control, 10*(5), 81.

Black, D. R., & Blue, C. L. (2001). Using social marketing to develop and test tailored health messages. *American Journal of Health Behavior, 25*, 260–271.

Bloom, B. S., Englehart, M. D., Furst, E. J., Hill, W. F., & Krathwohl, D. R. (1956). *Taxonomy of educational objectives: The classification of educational goals: Handbook 1: The cognitive domain.* New York: David McKay.

Buijis, R., & Olson, J. (2001). Parish nurses influencing determinants of health. *Journal of Community Health Nursing, 18*(1), 13–23.

Burhansstipanov, L., Krebs, L. U., Bradley, A., Gamito, E., Osborn, K., Dignan, M. B., et al. (2003). Lessons learned while developing "Clinical Trials Education for Native Americans" curriculum. *Cancer Control, 10*(5), 29–36.

Butler, J. T. (2001). *Principles of health education and health promotion* (3rd ed.). Stamford, CT: Wadsworth.

Darling, S. (2004). Family literacy: Meeting the needs of at-risk families. *Phi Kappa Phi Forum, 84*(2), 18–21.

DeBuono, B. A. (2002). *Pfizer health literacy initiative, 2002.* New York: Pfizer Graphic.

Donovan, H. S., & Ward, S. (2001). A representational approach to patient education. *Journal of Nursing Scholarship, 33*, 211–216.

Erkel, E. (2002). Principles of planning effective community programs. In C. C. Clark (Ed.), *Health promotion in communities: Holistic and wellness approaches* (pp. 47–68). New York: Springer.

Evans, R. G., & Stoddart, G. L. (2003). Consuming research, producing policy? *American Journal of Public Health, 93*, 371–379.

Farrelly, M. C., Davis, K. C., Haviland, M. L., Messeri, P., & Healton, C. G. (2005). Evidence of a dose-response relationship between "truth" antismoking ads and youth smoking prevalence. *American Journal of Public Health, 95*, 425–431.

Farrelly, M. C., Healton, C. G., Davis, K. C., Messeri, P., Hersey, J. C., & Haviland, M. L. (2002). Getting to the truth: Evaluating national tobacco countermarketing campaigns. *American Journal of Public Health, 92*, 901–907.

Fisher, J. D., & Fisher, W. A. (2002). The information-motivation-behavioral skills model. In R. J. DiClemente, R. A. Crosby, & M. C. Kegler (Eds.), *Emerging theories in health promotion practice and research: Strategies for improving public health* (pp. 40–70). San Francisco: Jossey-Bass.

Fogel, J. (2003). Internet use for cancer information among racial/ethnic populations and low literacy groups. *Cancer Control, 10*(5), 45–51.

Gilbert, G. G., & Sawyer, R. G. (2000). *Health education: Creating strategies for school and community health* (2nd ed.). Boston: Jones and Bartlett.

Habel, M. (2002). Patient education: Helping patients, families take charge of their health. *NurseWeek, 15*(1), 21–22.

Hammond, D., Fong, G. T., McDonald, P. W., Brown, K. S., & Cameron, R. (2004). Graphic Canadian cigarette warning labels and adverse outcomes: Evidence from Canadian smokers. *American Journal of Public Health, 94*, 1442–1445.

Holt, C. L., Kyles, A., Wiehagen, T., & Casey, C. (2003). Development of a spiritually based breast cancer education booklet for African American Women. *Cancer Control, 10*(5), 37–44.

Jacobs, E. A., Shepard, D. S., Suaya, J. A., & Stone, E. (2004). Overcoming language barriers in health care: Costs and benefits of interpreter services. *American Journal of Public Health, 94*, 866–869.

Kennedy, M. G., & Crosby, R. A. (2002). Prevention marketing: An emerging integrated framework. In R. J. DiClemente, R. A. Crosby, & M. C. Kegler (Eds.), *Emerging theories in health promotion practice and research: Strategies for improving public health* (pp. 255–284). San Francisco: Jossey-Bass.

Kickbusch, I. (2003). The contribution of the World Health Organization to a new public health and health promotion. *American Journal of Public Health, 93*, 383–387.

Kiley, R. (2003). *Medical information on the Internet: A guide for health professionals* (3rd ed.). Edinburgh: Churchill Livingstone.

Kogut, B. H. (2004). Why adult literacy matters. *Phi Kappa Phi Forum, 84*(2), 26–28.

Krathwohl, D. R., Bloom, B. S., & Masia, B. B. (1964). *Taxonomy of educational objectives: The classification of educational goals: Handbook 1: The affective domain.* New York: David McKay.

Kreuter, M. W., Steger-May, K., Bobra, S., Booker, A., Holt, C. L., Lukwago, S. N., et al. (2003). Sociocultural characteristics and responses to cancer education materials among African American women. *Cancer Control, 10*(5), 69–80.

Laverack, G. (2004). *Health promotion practice: Power and empowerment.* Thousand Oaks, CA: Sage.

MacDonald, S. (2002). Evaluating community health programs. In C. C. Clark (Ed.), *Health promotion in communities: Holistic and wellness approaches* (pp. 96–110). New York: Springer.

Maibach, E. W. (2003). Recreating communities to support active learning: A new role for social marketing. *American Journal of Health Promotion, 18*(1), 114–119.

Merzel, C., & D'Afflitti, J. (2003). Reconsidering community-based health promotion: Promise, performance, and potential. *American Journal of Public Health, 93*, 557–574.

Neiger, B. L., Thackeray, R., Barnes, M. D., & McKenzie, J. F. (2003). Positioning social marketing as a planning process for health education. *American Journal of Health Studies, 18*(2/3), 75–81.

Pender, N. J., Murdaugh, C. L., & Parsons, M. A. (2001). *Health promotion in nursing practice* (4th ed.). Upper Saddle River, NJ: Prentice Hall.

Smith, W. A. (2000). Social marketing: An evolving definition. *American Journal of Health Behavior, 24*(1), 11–17.

Tones, K., & Green, J. (2004). *Health promotion: Planning and strategies.* Thousand Oaks, CA: Sage.

Turning Point Social Marketing National Excellence Collaborative. (n.d.). *The basics of social marketing.* Retrieved September 28, 2004, from http://www.turningpointprogram.org

Twinn, S. (2001). The evaluation of the effectiveness of health education interventions in clinical practice: A continuing methodological challenge. *Journal of Advanced Nursing, 34*, 230–237.

U.S. Department of Health and Human Services. (2003a). Focus: Now is the Time for Prevention. *Prevention Report, 17*(4). Retrieved September 15, 2003, from http://odphp.osophs.dhhs.gov/pubs/prevrpt

U.S. Department of Health and Human Services. (2003b). *The power of prevention.* Retrieved July 25, 2003, from http://www.healthierus.gov/steps

Uys, L. R., Majumdar, B., & Gwele, N. (2004). The Kwazulu-Natal health promotion model. *Journal of Nursing Scholarship, 36*, 192–196.

Vanderplaat, M. (2002). Emancipatory politics and health promotion practice: The health professional as social activist. In L. E. Young & V. E. Hayes (Eds.), *Transforming health promotion practice: Concepts, issues, and applications* (pp. 87–98). Philadelphia: F. A. Davis.

Weinstein, N. D., & Sandman, P. M. (2002). The precaution adoption process model and its application. In R. J. DiClemente, R. A. Crosby, & M. C. Kegler (Eds.), *Emerging theories in health promotion practice and research: Strategies for improving public health* (pp. 16–39). San Francisco: Jossey-Bass.

Whitehead, D. (2001). Health education, behavioral change and social psychology: Nursing's contribution to health promotion? *Journal of Advanced Nursing, 34*, 822–832.

Whitehead, D. (2003). Incorporating socio-political health promotion activities in clinical practice. *Journal of Clinical Nursing, 12*, 668–677.

Whitehead, D. (2004). Health promotion and health education: Advancing the concepts. *Journal of Advanced Nursing, 47*, 311–320.

World Health Organization. (2002). *The world health report 2002: Reducing risks, promoting healthy life.* Retrieved January 30, 2003, from http://www.int/whr/2002/en

World Health Organization. (2004). *Guidelines on developing consumer information on proper use of traditional, complementary and alternative medicine.* Geneva, Switzerland: Author.

Yarcheski, A., Mahon, N. E., Yarcheski, T. J., & Cannella, B. L. (2004). A meta-analysis of predictors of positive health practices. *Journal of Nursing Scholarship, 36*, 102–108.

Case Management

CHAPTER OBJECTIVES

After reading this chapter, you should be able to:

1. Identify client-centered and system-centered goals of case management.
2. Discuss standards and principles of case management practice.
3. Analyze legal and ethical issues related to case management.
4. Identify criteria for selecting clients in need of case management.
5. Assess the need for case management and factors influencing the case management situation.
6. Discuss aspects of developing a case management plan.
7. Identify advantages and disadvantages of clinical pathways.
8. Describe at least three considerations in delegation.
9. Describe the benchmarking process and its use in case management.

KEY TERMS

abandonment **282**
benchmarking **292**
case management **278**
clinical pathway **283**
delegation **288**
discharge planning **286**
disease management **285**
negligence **282**
negligent referral **283**
population case management **277**
resource file **290**
utilization review **293**
variances **283**

MediaLink
http://www.prenhall.com/clark

Additional interactive resources for this chapter can be found on the Companion Website. Click on Chapter 12 and "Begin" to select the activities for this chapter.

Advocacy in Action

Promoting a Peaceful Death

As an Air Force nurse and case manager at Eglin AFB in Florida, I was blessed to have an opportunity to serve an 87-year-old retired lieutenant colonel, a former Air Force pilot. The client's history of progressive idiopathic neuropathy had left him wheelchair bound, unable to speak or swallow, and with no bowel or bladder control. He required total care from his elderly wife. The patient's family described this once-robust pilot as being trapped in his deteriorating body, even though his mind remained sharp. He was unable to effectively communicate his needs or desires to his family, and the situation was frustrating for all involved.

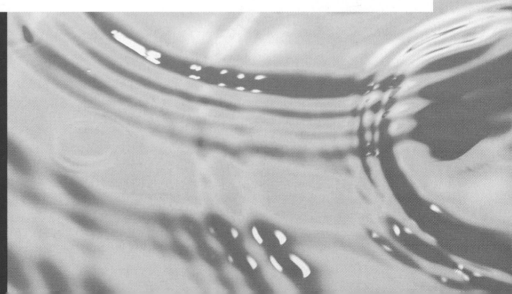

After visiting him in his home, I facilitated referrals to hospice, occupational therapy, and speech therapy. In an amazingly short time, the client improved dramatically, and the anxiety level among the family members dropped almost overnight. He was able to communicate his love to his wife and children before he died. His wife called me 20 minutes after he died peacefully at home. I went immediately to his home and was embraced by the family. In the days that followed, I made arrangements with mortuary and casualty affairs. In addition, I ensured that the client received full military honors. I presided as the officer in charge of the honor guard, where I presented the American flag to the client's wife on behalf of a grateful nation.

My purpose in sharing this story is not to talk about me but to spotlight the importance of community health nurses. To be honest, I had been skeptical of the value of community health until I began practicing it. Now I'm a strong advocate and wish to spread the word wherever I go.

Don L. Smith, Capt., USAF, NC

*C*ase management has been a focus of care since the 1860s (Reel, Morgan-Judge, Peros, & Abraham, 2002) and was first practiced in the settlement houses discussed in Chapter 3∞. When community health nursing was initiated at the Henry Street Settlement in 1893, case management became an integral part of the services provided. This focus on case management was continued in the home visiting services provided by the Metropolitan Life Insurance Company, begun in 1911 with the aim of minimizing payment of death benefits and of providing service to the enrolled community. Case management was primarily used to eliminate "useless cases" for which participating Visiting Nurse Associations were not reimbursed. These early efforts at case management, as we know it today, focused on:

- Proper case selection, including exclusion of chronic disease. Services primarily addressed acute illness and pregnancy. Pregnancy services were later reduced with the introduction of Sheppard-Towner legislation supporting maternal child services.
- Discharge when services were no longer needed.
- Early referral to limit the number of visits and duration of care (Buhler-Wilkerson, 2001).

Until recently, case management continued to be practiced more informally as coordination of care provided to clients of community health nurses and a few other health care providers. Now, case management is perceived as a formal discipline with principles that cut across multiple settings (Cudney, 2002).

The case management process is employed at two levels, that of the individual or family and that of population groups. The latter is sometimes referred to as *population care management* or *population management* (Schroeder, Trehearne, & Ward, 2000; Williams, 2000). Individual or family case management is a one-to-one endeavor in which the case manager develops a relationship with a particular client and his or her family (Lantz, Keeton, Romano, & DeGroff, 2004). **Population case management** is the development of systems of care, across multiple agencies, for specific groups of people with similar needs (Williams, 2000). Population case management may address episodes of illness or cut across the wellness/illness continuum (Schroeder et al., 2000). Epidemiologic findings can be used by community health nurses and others to provide a foundation for the development of systems of care that meet the health needs of a given population. For example, knowing that a large percentage of clients with uncontrolled hypertension live in certain areas of a community can help target case management services directed toward hypertension control in those areas.

Case management may focus on individual clients or population groups; however, one study indicated that individually focused case management was the most

frequently reported activity, with 91% of California public health nurses reporting that they engaged frequently or extensively in case management at this level (Grumbach, Miller, Mertz, & Finocchio, 2004). Case management activities may be performed by community health nurses as employees of the agency providing services to the client, as self-employed case managers, or as employees of case management services. In the latter two instances, case management activity is referred to as "external case management" (Cesta & Tahan, 2003).

DEFINING CASE MANAGEMENT

The case management literature includes a number of definitions for the concept. The most frequently encountered definition is that developed by the Case Management Society of America (n.d.), "a collaborative process of assessment, planning, facilitation and advocacy for options and services to meet an individual's health needs through communication and available resources to promote quality cost-effective outcomes" (p. 1). Other sources define case management as

- "a process that aims to coordinate the provision of client support systems and services. Whenever possible, the process involves the client, their carer(s) and family in decisions that affect their care. Case management will often involve the development of a plan that sets out goals to be achieved and the role of service providers, the client, their carer(s) and family in achieving these goals" (Commonwealth of Australia, 2000, p. 1).
- "a collaborative process [that] directs, links, and coordinates with clients, family, healthcare professionals, service providers, and others to assess, plan, implement, advocate, coordinate, educate, monitor, and evaluate options and delivery of community health services and community resource [sic]" (Capital Health Region of British Columbia, quoted in Gallagher, Alcock, Diem, Angus, & Medves, 2002, p. 86).
- "an entity (usually a person) that coordinates, integrates, and allocates care within limited resources" (Rapp & Goscha, 2004, p. 320).
- "a process where a single person takes responsibility for maintaining a long-term supportive relationship with a patient, regardless of where the patient is and

MediaLink Penalizing Obesity and Smoking (video)

regardless of the number of agencies involved. Its function is to assist patients to identify, secure and sustain the range of internal and external resources they need to live as independently [sic] a life as possible in the community" (Wilson, quoted in Askey, 2004, p. 12).

Many of these definitions address individual-focused case management, whereas community health nurses are often involved in population-focused case management activities. For that reason, the definition of **case management** selected for use in this text is "a patient care delivery system that focuses on meeting outcomes within identified timeframes using appropriate resources" (Cesta & Tahan, 2003, p. 413). This definition addresses the key features of case management, achievement of designated outcomes within a specific time period with the most cost-effective use of available resources.

CASE MANAGEMENT MODELS

Case management programs may be based on a variety of different models. For example, case management models have been characterized as full-service models, broker models, and hybrid models (Bedell, Cohen, & Sullivan, 2000). Full-service models provide most of the services needed by a given client within the organization. Full-service models may also be called clinical models because of the actual provision of some care by the case manager (Askey, 2004). Broker models, on the other hand, provide very few direct client services, referring clients to other agencies for care. Hybrid models provide some direct services, but refer clients for others. Research with psychiatric clients has indicated that full-service models demonstrated consistent positive effects on treatment compliance, hospital readmissions, cost of care, symptom management, and client satisfaction, but had little effect on client quality of life and functional level and actually increased the use of community-based services. Patient outcomes were consistently better in full-service models than in broker models. Hybrid models that more closely resembled full-service models were more effective than those that incorporated more elements of broker models (Bedell et al., 2000).

Case management services may also be episode-based or longitudinal. Episode-based programs provide care for individuals and their families across an episode of illness, usually a hospitalization. Longitudinal programs provide care across a continuum of health or developmental needs (Reel et al., 2002). Case management for clients with chronic conditions, such as diabetes, tends to be longitudinal in nature, whereas case management for a pregnant woman would usually be confined to the episode of pregnancy.

Case management models can also be characterized as minimal, coordination, or comprehensive mod-

els. In the minimal model, the case manager focuses on outreach, assessment, planning, and referral. In a coordination model, the case manager provides these services in addition to personal advocacy, direct care, and reassessment. In a comprehensive model, which is similar to a full-service model as described above, the case manager adds additional services such as advocacy for resource development, crisis intervention, and public education (Lantz et al., 2004). These last services tend to occur at the population level. For example, a community health nurse might organize community members to advocate for recreational facilities to meet the needs of members of the population with physical disabilities.

Another way to categorize case management models is as generalist or specialist models. In generalist models, a single case manager works to meet the needs of the client. For example, community health nursing practice with individuals and families is an example of a generalist model in which the community health nurse coordinates multiple services for the client. In specialist or team models, the client interacts with a multidisciplinary team (Lantz et al., 2004). As an example, team model case management for a population of clients with HIV/AIDS might include nutritionists or dieticians, social workers, psychologists, and members of the clergy, as well as nurses and physicians. Finally, case management models may be categorized based on the setting for practice. Hospital-based models address case management needs during hospitalization and shortly after discharge. Community-based models focus on care after hospital discharge. Combination hospital- and community-based models are again longitudinal in nature in that they provide a continuum of care across settings (Stanton, Walizer, Graham, & Keppel, 2000).

When case management systems are designed, developers are faced with the question of what type of model to adopt. The focused assessment questions presented below indicate some of the considerations in this decision.

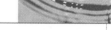

FOCUSED ASSESSMENT

Considerations in Developing a Case Management System

- Who will function as the case manager?
- What role functions will the case manager perform?
- What effects will the case management program have on other departments in the system?
- Is there a need for a specific case management department within the system?
- Will a case management system result in the potential for eliminating other roles in the system?
- Who will supervise the case manager?

Data from: Cesta, T. G. (2002). The politics of case management. In D. J. Mason, J. K. Leavitt, & M. W. Chaffee (Eds.), Policy and politics in nursing and health care (4th ed., pp. 319–324). St. Louis, MO: Saunders.

GOALS OF CASE MANAGEMENT

Case management programs are generally designed to accomplish two types of goals: client-centered goals and system-centered goals (Gallagher et al., 2002). Client-centered goals include promoting optimal health and independence and client satisfaction with care. Additional client-centered goals are enhanced quality of life, prevention of deterioration in health status, decreased need for acute care services, empowerment and advocacy, and promotion of optimal health through resource acquisition (Cesta & Tahan, 2003; Fraser & Strang, 2004; Schifalacqua & O'Hearn, 2004). For the client, case management ensures effective coordination of care and helps to reduce the confusion and complexity of the health care system. The case manager can assist the client to obtain needed services in the most acceptable and affordable settings. Case management, if effectively performed, should also result in improved client health outcomes in most instances. Effective case management also results in attention to all of the client's health needs to minimize the development of other health problems. In addition, case management provides clients with continuity of care and a regular and consistent source of assistance with health needs (Blaha, Robinson, Pugh, Bryan, & Havens, 2000).

At the health system level, case management also emphasizes service delivery in the least expensive setting possible, thereby limiting the overall costs of health care. System-centered goals focus on equitable resource allocation, decreased utilization, and cost containment while maintaining service quality (Cesta & Tahan, 2003). Additional system-centered goals include decreased fragmentation of care and cost-efficiency with the best possible care provided in the most efficient manner (Fraser & Strang, 2004; Schifalacqua & O'Hearn, 2004).

Effective case management minimizes hospitalization for needs that can be dealt with in community practice settings. For those clients who do need hospitalization, case management may shorten the length of stay and prevent subsequent readmissions by adequately addressing continuing health care needs after discharge. The cost of health care is also minimized when case management eliminates duplication of services. Population case management arrangements among several agencies provide a consistent flow of clients and limit overlapping services. In addition, the transfer of clients, ease of access to services, and communication between providers are also facilitated by population case management arrangements. When payers are included in the design of population case management systems, paperwork and waits for authorization for services are also reduced (Williams, 2000). Table 12-1◆ summarizes the client-centered and system-centered goals and benefits of case management.

FUNCTIONS OF CASE MANAGERS

The role functions of case managers vary to a certain extent, based on the case management model employed; however, there are some generalizations that can be made regarding the roles played and skills required by case managers across systems. Typical functions of case managers and examples of related activities for both individual- and population-level case management are summarized in Table 12-2◆. Skills required by case managers include the ability to judge clients' needs in the context of available resources, advocacy skills, and skills in collaboration, assessment, planning, delegation, referral, and negotiation. Case managers also need the ability to predict outcomes based on client condition and interventions employed and skills related to cost

TABLE 12-1 Client-centered and System-centered Goals and Benefits of Case Management	
Client-centered Goals/Benefits	**System-centered Goals/Benefits**
▪ Access to quality sources of needed care over a continuum of services	▪ Cost containment and cost-efficiency
▪ Access to acceptable and affordable health care services	▪ Minimization of hospitalization and rehospitalization
▪ Continuity of care and consistent source of assistance	▪ Reduced duplication and fragmentation of services
▪ Better coordination of care	▪ Elimination of inappropriate care and decreased service utilization
▪ Assistance in negotiating a complex health care system	▪ Effective resource allocation
▪ Attention to multiple health needs	▪ Earlier discharge
▪ Attainment of positive health outcomes	▪ Better communication among agencies and providers
▪ Ability to function independently	▪ Integrated service delivery and ease of transfer among agencies
▪ Prevention of deterioration	▪ Increased access to services
▪ Reduced risk and need for acute care services	▪ Decreased paperwork
▪ Adjustment of client and family to illness states	▪ Reduced time for authorization of services
▪ Improved quality of life	▪ Increased client satisfaction
▪ Increased satisfaction with care	▪ Increased professional satisfaction
▪ Empowerment	▪ Financial viability

TABLE 12-2	Case Manager Role Functions
Role Function	**Description**
Clinical expert	Is knowledgeable regarding clinical conditions and best, evidence-based practice *Individual example:* Recognizes effect of increased exercise in diabetic client's increasing frequency of episodes of hypoglycemia *Population example:* Is knowledgeable regarding the psychological implications of asthma in a school-age population
Consultant	Provides assistance to clients and other health care professionals regarding client needs and available services *Individual example:* Assists mother of a child with asthma to identify environmental triggers in the home *Population example:* Provides consultation to a school district in the development of a case management system for children with asthma
Coordinator of care	Arranges seamless care across systems and agencies to meet client needs; makes referrals to needed services; serves as liaison to community agencies *Individual example:* Arranges for transfer of client records from primary care provider and hospital to home health agency *Population example:* Helps to negotiate provision of counseling services by the County Mental Health Agency for clients with HIV/AIDS receiving care at a local hospice
Manager of care	Controls use of resources and activities of care team members to assure quality outcomes *Individual example:* Suggests home health aide services rather than nursing home placement for an older client recovering from a broken arm *Population example:* Helps develop an assessment protocol to be used by all team members in providing services to children with asthma
Educator	Educates clients, families, health care providers, and the public regarding health issues and interventions *Individual example:* Educates parents of a child with asthma on reducing environmental triggers *Population example:* Educates teachers and school administrators on behavior modification strategies for children with ADHD
Negotiator/broker	Negotiates appropriate care to meet client needs in the most cost-effective settings *Individual example:* Negotiates an extension of home care services for a woman who is not yet able to function independently *Population example:* Negotiates with a local high school student association for assistance with household tasks for low-income elderly in the community
Advocate	Serves as liaison between client and health care system and advocates for services to meet client needs *Individual example:* Advocates for delayed discharge of a homeless client with no place to go *Population example:* Advocates for development of case management services for pregnant teenagers
Outcome and quality manager	Monitors and evaluates client care outcomes and quality of care provided *Individual example:* Asks clients referred for prenatal services about their experiences of care *Population example:* Collects data on the number of pregnant clients who obtain prenatal care in the first trimester
Researcher	Engages in research related to interventions and outcomes, as well as the case management role *Population example:* Conducts research on the effects of a specific clinical pathway in terms of expected health-related outcomes
Risk manager	Minimizes financial risk to the organization by identifying and dealing with threats to client or staff safety in the care situation *Individual example:* Arranges for a lift in the home of an obese client to prevent injury to family and staff caretakers *Population example:* Promotes changes in medication documentation to prevent duplication of doses
Change agent	Promotes change in client behaviors and/or health care delivery systems *Individual example:* Refers a client who smokes for smoking cessation services *Population example:* Promotes changes in staff scheduling to provide 24-hour emergency response capabilities
Holistic care provider	Provides care to address the client's needs holistically rather than in a fragmented way *Individual example:* Identifies needs related to all dimensions of health and incorporates interventions addressing all needs in the case management plan *Population example:* Considers all of the factors influencing the client population in the design of case management systems
Counselor	Addresses the emotional and spiritual needs of clients and their families *Individual example:* Assists a client's caretaker to deal with the emotional burden of care; refers for counseling as needed *Population example:* Arranges for provision of counseling as part of case management services for clients with HIV/AIDS
Utilization manager	Reviews services to determine medical necessity, appropriateness of setting, and quality of care *Individual example:* Reviews a client's functional status to determine the need for continued physical therapy *Population example:* Collects data to determine the need for continued home schooling for pregnant adolescents

Continued on next page

TABLE 12-2   Case Manager Role Functions *(continued)*

Role Function	Description
Transition/discharge planner	Assists with smooth transition between elements of the health care system *Individual example:* Develops a discharge plan for an elderly woman leaving the hospital after repair of a hip fracture *Population example:* Develops procedures and processes for transferring clients from acute to home care services
Ethicist	Brings ethical dilemmas to the attention of the health care team and facilitates their resolution *Individual example:* Brings to the attention of the care team the competing needs of an older woman and her daughter caretaker *Population example:* Disseminates information to policy makers on the probable adverse effects of discontinuing local health department well-child services

Data from: Cesta, T. G., & Tahan, H. A. (2003). The case manager's survival guide: Winning strategies for clinical practice (2nd ed.). St. Louis: Mosby.

analysis and the collection and evaluation of outcome data (Fraser & Strang, 2004).

STANDARDS AND PRINCIPLES OF CASE MANAGEMENT PRACTICE

In 1995, the Case Management Society of America (CMSA, 1995) developed standards for case management practice in U.S. health care systems. Those standards were updated in 2002 (CMSA, 2002). The standards of practice are similar to those for community health nursing presented in Chapter 1∞. They include standards related to identifying and assessing cases, identifying problems, planning, monitoring implementation of the case management plan, evaluating the effects of intervention, and modifying the plan to achieve appropriate, cost-effective outcomes.

In addition, research on case management programs with mentally ill individuals has identified a set of principles that contribute to effective case management (Rapp & Goscha, 2004; Simpson, Miller, & Bowers, 2003). Most of these principles are also relevant to case management with clients in other health care settings and with a variety of health problems. General principles of effective case management are as follows:

- People do not need to be "case managed"; the services and resources they receive are the object of case management.
- Assertive outreach to identify clients in need of case management fosters program effectiveness.
- Whenever possible, case managers should provide services themselves rather than refer clients to other sources. The therapeutic relationship between case manager and client has been shown to be key to the success of case management.
- Natural community resources (e.g., employers, schools, community health agencies) are the primary partners for effective case management.
- Most effective case management activity occurs in the community rather than in institutional settings.
- Both individual (generalist) and team (specialist) models of case management are effective, and each has advantages and disadvantages. A team approach

provides support and backup, as well as additional expertise, for the primary case manager, but is more time consuming and labor intensive than individual case management models.

- Case managers should have primary responsibility for services provided to clients.
- Case managers can be paraprofessionals, but require expert professional supervision.
- Caseload size should be small to allow frequent contact with clients.
- Case management services should be time-unlimited, if possible.
- Case management should provide clients with access to assistance 24 hours a day, 7 days a week, to deal with emergency situations.
- Case managers should foster choice and self-determination among clients and families.
- Members of the case management team should receive training and supervision as needed.
- Case management services should address a variety of client needs, including social needs and support for daily living.
- Case managers should work with families and caregivers as well as the client.
- Case managers should remain informed regarding available community services and resources.
- Case management plans should be flexible enough to address changing client needs and circumstances.

ETHICAL AND LEGAL ISSUES IN CASE MANAGEMENT

A study of case managers identified several categories of ethical concerns related to their practice. These included equity-related concerns; beneficence-related concerns; non-maleficence-related concerns; concerns related to autonomy, consent, and living at risk; and other concerns. Equity-related concerns involved the fair allocation of resources based on elements such as age, gender, socioeconomic status, and so on. Beneficence is the ethical principle of doing good for another. Beneficence-related concerns included issues related to providing care over an appropriate time frame. For example, case managers found themselves rationing care to allow them to provide services over a longer period of time, based on anticipated client needs. Non-maleficence is the converse ethical principle of doing no harm. Concerns related to non-maleficence centered around the need to provide clients with choices and the need to prevent harm to clients or to others providing care to clients. Concerns related to autonomy, consent, and living at risk dealt with clients' rights to engage in risk-related behaviors if they chose to do so and the right to refuse services. Other concerns in these areas focused on needing to violate system rules to meet clients' needs, balancing client autonomy with the case manager's responsibility to protect them from harm, and providing services appropriate to client needs given resource constraints (Gallagher et al., 2002).

Although many of the legal and ethical issues in case management are common to other aspects of community health nursing, some warrant special attention. These issues include confidentiality, denial of services, breach of contract, negligence, failure to follow clinical pathways or, conversely, failure to individualize care, and reportable events. The issue of confidentiality has two aspects in case management. The first is the need for client permission to make contacts and arrangements for services on the client's behalf. The case management plan should be presented to and agreed upon by the client before any further action is taken. The second aspect of confidentiality relates to unauthorized disclosure of information about the client (Powell, 2000). To avoid a breach of confidentiality in this area, the community health nurse case manager should inform clients of the need to share information with others and obtain client authorization before doing so.

Denial of services includes failure to authorize services due to lack of justification of medical necessity or appropriateness of services (Cesta & Tahan, 2003). Wrongful denial of services involves decisions not to provide care that are arbitrary and are not based on medical information related to need. Community health nurses often find themselves in the position of advocating for clients who have been denied services. For example, a school nurse may need to convince school officials of the need for a learning disability assessment for a student who is performing poorly in school. At the population level, the same school nurse may advocate for changes in referral procedures that make disability assessment more accessible to all children in need. In the latter instance, the school nurse is engaging in population case management, whereas advocacy for a specific child would be part of individual case management.

Abandonment occurs when the case manager terminates services to a client with continuing needs without notifying the client or arranging for services from another provider. Although community health nurse case managers may encounter situations in which services need to be terminated (e.g., in the face of client failure to comply with the treatment plan), the nurse should make every effort to avoid abandonment. It may be helpful to develop a contract with clients indicating both case manager and client responsibilities with respect to the case management plan. In addition, the case manager should carefully document both positive and negative aspects of the client's response to case management services and continued efforts to enlist client cooperation. Although *abandonment* is a term that has legal implications in the care of individual clients, the concept of abandonment may also apply to population groups. For example, community health nurses may need to assist communities to find ways to meet the needs of low-income families for childcare when after-school program budgets are cut.

Breach of contract occurs when a managed care organization drops a client from the plan without adequate justification or when the system fails to pay for care that should be covered by a plan. Breach of contract, in the legal sense, applies to care of individual clients, although communities might be said to breach an unwritten contract with citizens when they discontinue needed service programs.

Several types of negligence also pose legal and ethical issues in case management. **Negligence** is the failure to act in a situation as a reasonably prudent nurse would if faced with the same situation. Wrongful denial of services could be considered a form of negligence on the part of the system (Williams, 2000). Other types of negligence include negligent actions on the part of the case manager or other providers and negligent referrals. Four conditions must exist for negligence to occur (Case, 2004). First, there must be a duty to provide care based on accepted standards. Second, there must be a breach of duty in which the case manager or other provider does not provide the care or does not provide care in keeping with the standards. Third, an injury must result from the breach of duty, and, finally, the injury must result in some form of quantifiable damage to the client (Aiken & Aucoin, 2003). Failure of a local health department to provide effective communicable disease control programs could be considered an example of negligence at the population level.

ETHICAL AWARENESS

Clients may reach the limits of their health insurance coverage for certain types of services before their health needs have been fully met. When this occurs, health care providers may terminate services if the client does not have another means of paying for them. Obviously this is not in the client's best interests. Continuing to provide uncompensated services, however, may lead to failure of the health organization, jeopardizing care to many other clients. What ethical arguments can be brought to bear for either action (continuing services without payment or discontinuing services)? What might the role of the nurse case manager be in such an ethical dilemma?

Although designed to promote standardization of patient care and limit legal liability, legal issues can arise from the use of or failure to use clinical pathways. A **clinical pathway** is "a tool for achieving coordinated care and desired health outcomes within an anticipated time frame, by using the appropriate resources available. A clinical pathway is a blueprint that guides the clinician in the provision of care" (Commonwealth of Australia, 2005, p. 2). Clinical pathways are frequently used as standards against which actions may be judged in a malpractice or negligence suit. Failure to adhere to a clinical pathway can be considered negligence if the clinical pathway is appropriate to the client situation. Conversely, case managers and other care providers may be found negligent for failing to take the individual client situation into account and deviating from the clinical pathway as needed. Deviations from the typical path are called **variances** (Cesta & Tahan, 2003). Legal challenges can be avoided with careful documentation of implementation of the clinical pathway and client variance that warrants deviation from the path. Periodic update of clinical pathways based on new best-practices information can also forestall legal action. Clinical pathways are discussed in more detail later in this chapter.

Nurse case managers may also be held legally liable for negligent referrals. A **negligent referral** may be (a) a referral that results in harm or injury to the client because the case manager has not adequately assessed the competency of the provider, or (b) a failure to make a referral when one is warranted (Williams, 2000). Case managers can prevent negligent referrals by investigating the providers or agencies to which they refer clients in terms of licensure and relevant accreditation, client outcomes data, billing practices, insurance coverage, and malpractice information. A second tactic to prevent negligent referrals is to provide the client with several provider options rather than making a single referral. Finally, the case manager should follow up on the outcomes of referrals made.

The last legal issue to be addressed here is reportable events. Like all nurses, nurse case managers have a legal mandate to report the occurrence, or even the suspicion, of certain kinds of events. These include child and elder abuse and, in some jurisdictions, intimate partner violence. Other reportable events include violent injuries, specific communicable diseases, and coroners' cases. Nurse case managers should be aware of what events (particularly what communicable diseases) are considered reportable in their area and should also let clients know of the need to report such events when they occur.

DESIGNING CASE MANAGEMENT SYSTEMS

Development of a case management system involves case finding (identifying clients or populations in need of case management or disease management), determining the level of risk in the target population, and designing case management services to address the identified level of risk (Hillegass, Smith, & Phillips, 2002). Case finding may occur through one of three mechanisms: provider referral, population-based screening, or screening during health events. For example, if health care providers are referring a number of clients with diabetes for case management services, a focused diabetes case management system may be needed for this population. Similarly, if population-based diabetes screening or screening in the context of events like community health fairs indicates a high prevalence of undiagnosed diabetes, population-based diabetes case management services may be needed.

Screening, in this context, should be distinguished from assessment. Screening involves risk identification. Assessment, on the other hand, involves identification of the need for case management services among those revealed by screening tests to be at high risk for health problems (Hillegass et al., 2002).

Case-finding activities result in the identification of the target population for the case management system. The second task in developing case management systems is determining the level of risk present in the population. The level of risk for specific health problems determines the focus of the case management program. In populations with low levels of risk, case management activities are directed toward prevention and education and occur primarily at the group level. When populations exhibit a moderate level of risk, case management may be added to the prevention, education, and group interventions. Case management will be needed for those persons at risk who exhibit comorbidity (the presence of other disease processes), limitations in two or more activities of daily living, or indications of cognitive impairment. Populations at high risk require more intensive case management activities that may involve chronic care activities and risk management or specialty care management for specific populations (e.g., the elderly at risk for abuse) (Hillegass et al., 2002).

Once the target population and level of risk have been identified, goals and outcome indicators for the case management program need to be established and

---

EVIDENCE-BASED PRACTICE

A number of health agencies, organizations, and institutions have developed clinical pathways for specific populations and conditions. An Internet search for "clinical pathways" will provide access to a wide variety of clinical pathways. Select one condition of interest and examine the clinical pathways related to that condition for similarities and differences. Examine the extent to which various pathways are supported by credible research findings. Based on the evidence available, can you create a composite pathway that incorporates the best supported interventions included in the pathways reviewed?

Think Advocacy

There is a high rate of adolescent pregnancy in your community. The large majority of pregnant teenagers choose to keep their babies. Most of them end up dropping out of school, and approximately half become pregnant again within a year. You think case management services might help improve outcomes for these girls and their children, but no such services are available in the community. How would you go about initiating such services? What community partners should be involved in advocating for and developing case management services for pregnant adolescents? How would you get these community partners involved?

key stakeholders identified. Key stakeholders are those who would have an interest in the outcomes of the program and might include recipients of care and their families, health care providers, third-party payers, regulatory agencies, and others. Then core interventions can be developed based on the goals to be accomplished and the outcomes to be achieved. These interventions are then implemented and their effects monitored and evaluated (Lamb, Shelton, & Zazworsky, 2003). As an example, a group of community health nurses may notice that they are receiving large numbers of requests for home visits to clients with HIV/AIDS. Assessment of this population may indicate several common unmet needs. These needs may include financial assistance with the cost of medications, management of fatigue and opportunistic diseases, and care for psychosocial effects of HIV/AIDS, such as isolation and depression. The nurses might initiate community-wide efforts to develop a case management system to address the needs of this population. Steps involved in actually planning such a system are similar to those involved in planning any health program and are discussed in detail in Chapter 15∞.

THE CASE MANAGEMENT PROCESS

The process of case management involves case selection, assessment, plan development and implementation, and evaluation. Each of these components of the process will be addressed briefly.

Case Selection

Not all clients encountered by community health nurses will need case management services, so the nurse must identify those clients who do need services and can benefit most from them (Cesta & Tahan, 2003). Case selection may involve identifying certain population groups for whom case management systems should be developed (population case management) and identifying individual clients and families in need of case management services. Both population groups and individual clients can be identified on the basis of several indicators. Indicators for population groups that need case

management services include those with high-cost diagnoses, high-volume resource utilization, and poor coordination of services (Schifalacqua & O'Hearn, 2004). Clients with HIV/AIDS, diabetes, cancer, and asthma are all examples of populations with high-cost diagnoses. These diseases also result in high-volume resource use that may warrant development of case management services. Case management services might also be developed for pregnant women or children with asthma for whom services are often poorly coordinated and for whom case management has been shown to have significant positive effects.

Individual client indicators of the need for case management can be categorized as personal indicators, health-related indicators, and social indicators. Personal indicators may include diminished functional status, a history of substance abuse or mental illness, poor cognitive abilities, prior noncompliance with treatment plans, age over 65 years, experience of a major life change or significant change in self-image, potential for severe emotional response to illness, or unrealistic expectations of potential outcomes of care. Health-related factors include the presence of specific medical conditions or diagnoses (e.g., Alzheimer's disease, AIDS, eating disorders, severe burns, trauma), multiple diagnoses, history of prolonged recovery or increased potential for complications, recent or frequent hospital readmissions or emergency department use, intentional or unintentional drug overdose, and involvement of multiple health care providers, agencies, or funding sources. Social indicators are living alone or with a person who is disabled, being uninsured, evidence of family violence, homelessness or an unhealthy home environment, lack of support systems or financial resources, single parenthood, or living in an area where services are lacking. The presence of one or more of these indicators does not necessarily mean that the client is in need of case management services, but it should alert the community health nurse to that possibility. The nurse would then further explore the client situation to determine an actual need for services.

Assessing the Case Management Situation

To develop an effective case management plan for an individual client or a case management system for a specific population group, the community health nurse

BUILDING OUR KNOWLEDGE BASE

Select a client group you have encountered in your community health clinical experience that might benefit from case management (e.g., adolescent mothers, clients with hypertension). How would you design a case management system to meet the needs of this client group? How would you evaluate the effectiveness of case management in meeting their needs?

case manager must assess the client's (or group's) health status and identify factors in the situation that affect health and are likely to affect the case management plan and achievement of planned health outcomes. Assessment should also validate the need for case management and may be organized in terms of the dimensions of health. For example, biophysical considerations such as age and physiological health status or functional ability may indicate problems that need to be addressed by the case manager or constraints that will affect interventions selected. Arthritic deformities may complicate the ability of a diabetic client to draw up and give an insulin injection, so the case management plan will need to account for these limitations. At the population level, extensive cardiovascular comorbidity in the population with diabetes will necessitate the development of a case management system that addresses problems related to both diseases.

Similarly, mental health status, coping abilities, and anxiety are psychological dimension factors that may affect case management needs and activities with individual clients. In terms of population case management, a high incidence of suicide among disabled residents would be an indication of the need for case management programs. Physical environmental considerations that may influence the case management situation include clients' living conditions or neighborhood social capital, as well as the influences of environmental pollution. For example, population case management for persons with asthma would need to address control of environmental triggers, possibly even at the level of advocating legislation for better control of air pollutants, as well as education for individuals on reducing triggers in the home or work setting.

Sociocultural factors will also influence the types and extent of services to be included in the case management plan. Some factors to consider are the client's education level, support systems, economic status, occupation, transportation, and cultural beliefs and behaviors. Changes in social roles should also be considered in assessing the case management situation. Unemployment and financial status are examples of two sociocultural factors that might influence population case management for persons with HIV/AIDS. Behavioral considerations such as substance abuse, lack of physical activity, or poor diet may also give rise to the need for case management or influence development of the case management plan. Using the HIV/AIDS example, population case management systems might be developed differently for men who have sex with men (MSM) than for heterosexual women.

Considerations related to the health care system include assessment of the types of health care services that the client is likely to need. The nurse case manager assesses the availability of those services in the client's community as well as influences related to the type and level of insurance coverage the client has. Client

attitudes toward health services and health care providers are another important element of this dimension affecting case management. At the population level, the nurse case manager might assess the cluster of services available to meet the needs of specific populations (e.g., those with HIV/AIDS). The nurse could also explore existing interactions between service organizations and the need and desire for closer coordination of services. A tool for assessing case management situations from the perspective of the dimensions of health can be found in the *Community Assessment Reference Guide* designed to accompany this text.

Developing the Case Management Plan

A case management plan is "a timeline of patient care activities and expected outcomes of care that address the plan of care of each discipline involved in the care of a particular patient" or population group (Cesta & Tahan, 2003, p. 413). Effective case management plans are interdisciplinary, outcomes-based, clinically specific (addressing a particular clinical issue rather than a diagnosis), and flexible, and include avenues for provider documentation of their implementation (Cesta & Tahan, 2003).

Activity may focus on case management or disease management. In case management, the case manager addresses all of the client's identified needs, or as many of them as can be addressed given the resources available. **Disease management**, on the other hand, is "the process of intensively managing a particular disease across different care settings and levels of care using a population-based complex and sophisticated program that places a heavy emphasis on health risk identification, prevention, and maintenance" (Cesta & Tahan, 2003, p. 414). Assisting a client with diabetes to control his or her disease is an example of disease management. Assisting the same client to meet a wide variety of health and social needs is case management. A similar distinction can be made at the population case management level. For example, services to a diabetic population that focus on control of their disease involve disease management. Services to the same population that address a wider array of needs, not just those related to diabetes control, exemplify case management.

Case management plans are often based on clinical pathways (also called critical pathways or multidisciplinary action plans, or MAPs) (Cesta & Tahan, 2003). As noted earlier, clinical pathways are multidisciplinary plans that incorporate best practices for use with specific groups of clients with specific health problems. Essential components of clinical pathways include a timeline, categories of care activities or interventions to be employed, identification of intermediate and long-term outcomes, and a variance record (St. Vincent's Hospital Sydney, n.d.). The variance record documents deviations from the interventions and outcomes delineated in the clinical

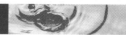
pathway and may be either positive or negative (Commonwealth of Australia, 2005).

In using a clinical pathway, the case manager conducts a generic assessment of the client and then selects the appropriate pathway(s) based on the assessment. A particular pathway may include one or more specific assessment tools to be used. Implementation of the pathway involves identifying appropriate outcome measures, performing a path-specific assessment, identifying individual needs that may necessitate modifications in the pathway, developing a plan of care with the client and other providers, and determining the reassessment data required and how it will be collected. Use of pathways also requires documentation, which usually consists of recording the assessment, the treatment plan, and variances from the pathway. The pathway is then adjusted based on analysis of variances (Commonwealth of Australia, 2005).

Clinical pathways may also be used in designing population case management systems. For example, a clinical pathway for care of populations with HIV/AIDS may be modified for use with a population comprised mainly of MSM. Clinical pathways can be used for health promotion as well as for disease management. Table 12-3◆ presents goals and activities that might be included in a clinical pathway for pregnant women. The pathway is intended for use by community health nurses working in an agency that provides pregnancy-monitoring services in the home but does not provide on-site prenatal care. Ideally, care activities would take place in each trimester of the pregnancy and the postpartum period, as indicated. When prenatal care is initiated late in the pregnancy, however, the timeline for accomplishing care activities is compressed. When no prenatal care is received and a referral is made after delivery, only the postpartum section of the pathway and selected elements from previous sections would be implemented. Use of the clinical pathway would usually include completion of assessment forms and a written treatment plan that includes goals and activities similar to those included in Table 12-3◆ as well as projected and actual dates of goal achievement. In addition, use of many clinical pathways entails completion of a discharge plan if additional services are needed. For example, a discharge plan for a pregnant woman might include periodic home visits to address child health issues, success with contraceptive methods

selected, and continued guidance with parenting skills, if needed.

Discharge planning is a special application of the case management process and involves identifying follow-up needs and arranging for care after discharge from a hospital or other institutional setting (Sultz & Young, 2004). Discharge planning has been described as laying the foundation for case management and is intended to ease the transition from one level of care to another (Hubber & McClelland, 2003). Indicators of the need for discharge planning are similar to those for case management in general, but studies suggest that, at least for older clients, functional dependence is the best predictor of readmission and a significant indicator of the need for discharge planning.

The Nursing Interventions Classification (NIC) schema (McCloskey & Bulechek, 2000) identifies 17 separate activities involved in discharge planning:

- Assisting in preparation for discharge
- Collaborating in planning for continuity of care
- Coordinating health provider activities to promote timely discharge
- Assessing client and caregiver knowledge regarding care after discharge
- Identifying teaching needs
- Monitoring readiness for discharge
- Communicating discharge plans
- Documenting the plan
- Developing a post-discharge follow-up plan
- Assisting in the development of a supportive environment for implementing aftercare
- Developing a plan congruent with the client's health care, social, and financial needs
- Arranging for post-discharge evaluation
- Encouraging self-care
- Arranging the discharge process
- Arranging caregiver support if needed
- Discussing financial resources for health care after discharge
- Coordinating appropriate referrals

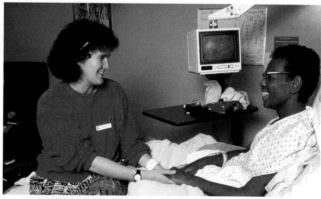

Case management often begins with discharge planning for hospitalized clients. (Cindy Charles/PhotoEdit)

TABLE 12-3   Clinical Pathway Goals and Activities: Pregnancy

Goal	Activity
First trimester	
▪ Pregnancy is confirmed (within 1 week)	▪ Refer for pregnancy test
▪ Client situation/health status is assessed (within 1 week)	▪ Assess client situation/health status by ▪ Obtaining past pregnancy history ▪ Obtaining personal and family medical history ▪ Obtaining social history ▪ Obtaining prepregnancy and baseline weight ▪ Obtaining baseline blood pressure ▪ Assessing fetal heart tones and fetal movement when pregnancy is far enough advanced ▪ Assessing for edema ▪ Checking hematocrit ▪ Assessing for normal discomforts of pregnancy
▪ High-risk pregnancy is identified (within 1 week)	▪ Analyze assessment data for evidence of high-risk pregnancy
▪ Prenatal care is obtained (within 1 month)	▪ Refer for ▪ Routine or high-risk prenatal care ▪ Medicaid or other form of assistance as needed
▪ Client is knowledgeable regarding pregnancy (within 2 months)	▪ Educate client regarding ▪ Interventions for normal discomforts of pregnancy ▪ Signs of complications of pregnancy and what to do ▪ Continuing sexual activity
▪ Existing health problems are controlled (throughout)	▪ Monitor status of existing health problems (e.g., glucose monitoring for diabetes, medication use) ▪ Refer for medical care as needed
Second trimester	
▪ Pregnancy complications are prevented or detected as early as possible	▪ Assess (at each visit) ▪ Fundal height ▪ Blood pressure ▪ Fetal heart tones and fetal movement ▪ Edema ▪ Proteinuria
▪ Existing health problems remain controlled	▪ Monitor status of existing health problems (e.g., glucose monitoring for diabetes, medication use) ▪ Refer for medical care as needed
▪ Client is knowledgeable regarding pregnancy	▪ Educate client regarding ▪ Braxton-Hicks contractions ▪ Fetal development ▪ Progression of pregnancy ▪ Sexual activity
Third trimester	
▪ Pregnancy complications are prevented or detected as early as possible	▪ Continued assessment as in second trimester
▪ Existing health problems remain controlled	▪ Monitor status of existing health problems (e.g., glucose monitoring for diabetes, medication use) ▪ Refer for medical care as needed
▪ Client is prepared for birth of child	▪ Assess preparations made for new baby ▪ Assist with preparations as needed (e.g., baby supplies, sleeping arrangements, childcare for other children, etc.) ▪ Discuss possible effects of new baby on family members (e.g., sibling rivalry, relationship with father)
▪ Client is knowledgeable regarding labor and delivery	▪ Educate client (or refer for childbirth classes) regarding ▪ Signs of labor ▪ Progression of labor
▪ Client is knowledgeable regarding childcare	▪ Assess level of childcare knowledge and educate as needed or refer for childcare classes
▪ Client is knowledgeable regarding contraceptive options	▪ Educate client regarding contraceptive options and their availability, as needed
Postpartum period	
▪ Normal involution occurs	▪ Assess ▪ Fundal height ▪ Amount, color, and character of lochia ▪ Blood pressure ▪ Refer for any abnormal findings

Continued on next page

TABLE 12-3	Clinical Pathway Goals and Activities: Pregnancy *(continued)*
Goal	**Activity**
▪ Episiotomy, if any, heals without infection	▪ Check episiotomy ▪ Educate client regarding episiotomy care
▪ Client receives postpartum examination	▪ Refer for postpartum examination
▪ Client obtains contraceptive services, if desired	▪ Refer for contraceptive services, if needed
▪ Client returns to prepregnancy weight	▪ Educate regarding diet and exercise
▪ Newborn's umbilical cord is healing	▪ Assess umbilical cord ▪ Educate mother regarding cord care ▪ Refer for any abnormal findings
▪ Newborn is developing normally and gaining weight	▪ Assess height and weight ▪ Conduct physical examination ▪ Conduct developmental assessment
▪ Mother is successfully breast- or bottle-feeding infant	▪ Assess feeding practices ▪ Assess breasts ▪ Discuss maternal and infant diet

▪ Mother is coping effectively with motherhood	▪ Assess
	  ▪ Maternal–infant bond
	  ▪ Postpartum depression
	  ▪ Coping
	▪ Promote coping skills as needed

▪ Infant receives primary immunizations	▪ Educate mother and refer for immunization services
▪ Infant is in a safe environment	▪ Assess infant's environment ▪ Provide safety education ▪ Refer for infant car seat, if needed
▪ Family is adjusting to presence of infant	▪ Assess adjustment ▪ Educate family members regarding infant needs ▪ Refer family members for counseling, if needed

Implementing the Case Management Plan

Implementation of the case management plan involves communicating the plan, delegating, initiating referrals, and monitoring plan implementation. Each of these aspects of implementing the plan will be discussed briefly.

Communicating the Plan

Clients and their significant others should be involved in the development of the case management plan. Once the plan is in place, they will need to be informed of arrangements made for care and expectations of them in following through on the management plan. For example, clients may need to call to make a specific appointment with a provider even though care has been arranged by the case manager. Clients will also need to know about any payments required and the names of contact persons in agencies to which they have been referred. Additional information to be conveyed to clients relates to the expected duration and outcome of services.

The case manager also needs to communicate the case management plan to the providers who will be giving the necessary care. Client needs and expectations of the provider should be addressed as well as any previous plans and their effects, expectations for continued care, and any other information relevant to the client's situation. The case manager should be careful to obtain the consent of the client before providing such information.

Finally, the payer should be informed of and approve the management plan. The nurse case manager should confirm and document that referral agencies and payers have received the information sent. He or she should also confirm that clients and family members understand the information provided.

Delegation

Delegation has been defined by the National Council of State Boards of Nursing as "transferring to a competent individual the authority to perform selected tasks in a selected situation" (quoted in Case, 2004, p. 17). Several considerations guide the nurse case manager in making delegation decisions. The first consideration is the stability of the client. Care of unstable clients should not be delegated to unlicensed assistive personnel, but should be retained by the case manager or other qualified provider. A second consideration is the competence of the person to whom the task is being delegated. Competence is closely linked to the scope of responsibility of the delegatee, as well as the frequency with which the person performs the delegated task. Potential for harm to the client is another consideration in delegation. Tasks that pose significant potential for harm should not be delegated unless the case manager can be assured that delegation will not result in harm to the client.

Other considerations in delegation include the level of decision making and problem solving required. In making delegation decisions, the nurse case manager should differentiate between hands-on tasks and those involving use of the nursing process. Tasks requiring high levels of decision making should not be delegated to unlicensed personnel or family members who are unprepared for making such decisions. The ability of the client for self-care is another consideration, as is the predictability of the outcome of the task. Interventions with unpredictable outcomes should be performed by the nurse case manager or other qualified personnel rather than ancillary personnel or family members (Case, 2004).

In addition to determining whether delegation is appropriate in a given situation and deciding to whom a task should be delegated, the case manager also needs to supervise delegated tasks. The community health nurse case manager should provide clear instructions to the delegatee and provide oversight for task performance and client outcomes (Case, 2004). Although tasks are delegated, the case manager retains responsibility for their performance and outcomes. Criteria for determining effective delegation include the five "rights" in the box below.

Initiating Referrals

The case manager may not be able to provide all of the services needed by a client or a group of clients. In this case, the case manager makes referrals to other sources of service to meet client needs. Referral involves directing a client to another source of information or assistance. It differs from delegation in that the nurse case manager relinquishes responsibility for the implementation of the portions of the plan of care for which the client is referred, although he or she retains overall responsibility for the quality of care provided. Referrals to a variety of health care and related services may be part of case management for an individual client and his or her family. Similarly, case management systems for groups of clients may make use of an identified set of agencies to address most needs of the population group. Four basic considerations enter into the decision to refer clients to particular providers, agencies, or services: the acceptability of the referral, eligibility for services, constraints operating in the situation, and community resources available.

ACCEPTABILITY The first consideration in making a referral is the acceptability of the referral to the client. Some clients may be unwilling to obtain help if they perceive it

as "charity." In other cases, clients may have philosophies different from those of the referral resource. For example, a Southern Baptist client may be reluctant to accept assistance from an agency supported by the Roman Catholic Church. Barriers to acceptability of a specific referral may include fear of a strange agency or provider, prior negative experiences, lack of faith in the referral resource, failure to acknowledge a problem requiring referral, and concerns about costs. Finally, reaching out for assistance may be counter to the client's culture or frame of reference, or following up on a referral may be preempted by client concerns with higher priorities.

ELIGIBILITY The second consideration in referral is the client's eligibility for the service provided. There are many determinants of eligibility for service. Sometimes eligibility is based on financial need, and clients may need to provide evidence of income and expenditures. In other instances, eligibility might be based on residence within a particular jurisdiction or membership in a particular group. For example, nonresidents are not usually eligible for state-supported medical assistance, or a particular agency may provide services only to members of a specific religious or ethnic group. Eligibility can also be based on age. As an example, senior citizens' groups usually do not provide services for anyone under the age of 55. Finally, eligibility is sometimes based on the existence of a particular condition. For instance, certain shelter services might be available only to abused women rather than to homeless people in general.

SITUATIONAL CONSTRAINTS The presence of situational constraints, or factors in the client's situation that would prevent him or her from following through on a referral, is a third consideration. For example, does the client have transportation available to go to the appropriate place of care? If clients do not speak English, will they be able to find an interpreter to help them, or are interpretation services provided by the agency? The nurse making the referral should assess any situational constraints present and then take action to eliminate or minimize the effects of those constraints. The nurse case manager may also need to coordinate funding benefits among multiple agencies to prevent barriers to timely access to care.

RESOURCE AVAILABILITY Information related to each of the three previous referral considerations will be readily available if the nurse has thoroughly assessed each of the dimensions of health prior to developing the case management plan. Resource availability information, on the other hand, will be obtained through assessment of the community. The community health nurse case manager needs to be familiar with health care and other support services available in the community. Information on community resources can be obtained in a number of ways. Two major sources of information are the local health department and the yellow pages. Other

SPECIAL CONSIDERATIONS

THE FIVE "RIGHTS" OF DELEGATION
- Right task
- Right circumstances
- Right person
- Right communication
- Right supervision

Data from: Case, N. (2004). Delegation skills: Critical thinking strategies you can apply to the challenges of delegating. Advance for Nurses, 1(4), 17–22.

resources are neighborhood information and referral centers, local government offices and chambers of commerce, and police and fire departments. The local library is also a source of information and may even have a directory of local resources.

It is not sufficient for the community health nurse to merely be aware of the existence of community resources. The nurse must know where these resources are located and understand the requirements for referral to each resource. The nurse should systematically collect information on the types of services a referral resource provides, criteria for eligibility for services, and whether any fee is involved. Information to be sought also includes indicators of the quality of services provided and the credentials and competencies of providers. The community health nurse case manager may want to establish a **resource file** or database to systematically organize and store information on area resources. Figure 12-1 depicts a sample resource file entry. The resource file can be organized by category of services. A particular agency with more than one type of service could be entered in several different categories, or a cross-reference system could be used. The resource described in Figure 12-1 deals with transportation.

Information about the resource's funding source can be useful in tracking service availability. For example, if tax revenues have declined in the area, the community health nurse case manager may want to contact agencies funded by public money to determine whether services have been cut prior to making a specific referral. Also, it may be important to some clients to know that the services they receive from an agency are provided by tax dollars rather than "charity."

Of course, the resource file entry includes the referral resource's full name, address, and telephone number. The business hours notation may refer to when the agency is open or times when a particular service is offered. For example, the entry might read "Family planning: Monday, 9:00 A.M.–noon, Prenatal: Tuesday, 1:00–4:00 P.M."

It is helpful to have the name of a contact person in the agency as well. Referrals are facilitated when agency personnel are familiar with the person making the referral. Unfortunately, situations do occur in which some agency employees are more inclined to accommodate professional colleagues than clients. When the case manager refers a client to an agency and gives that individual the name of a contact person who knows the nurse, the client who mentions that he or she was referred by the

Resource category: _Transportation_	Funding source: _Voluntary_
Agency name: _St. Martha's Catholic Church_	
Address: _3710 Montebank Rd, Otenada, Mississippi_	
Phone number: _817-3421_	Business hours: _Mon-Fri 8-4_
Contact person: _Mrs. Jefferson_	Title: _receptionist / secretary_
Source of referral: _self or other_	
Eligibility: _anyone without transportation - need not be members of church_	
Fee: _none_	
Services: _Provides transportation to church services as well as other services such as Dr.'s office, grocery shopping, etc. on periodic basis_	
Access: _call to arrange transportation_	
Other comments: _1) Do not provide transportation on long-term basis, i.e., to work or school_	
2) depends upon availability of volunteer drivers	
3) drivers trained to assist disabled riders	

FIGURE 12-1 Sample Resource File Entry

nurse may get a more prompt response than the client who does not have a specific person to contact. Having a specific contact person within the agency may also facilitate requests for services when the request is made by the nurse case manager rather than the client.

"Source of referral" in Figure 12-1 refers to the preferred originator of the referral. Some agencies accept referrals only from specific persons, usually physicians. If a professional referral is required, the nurse should specifically inquire about the acceptability of referrals from nurse practitioners, if they are available in the area. In the example in Figure 12-1, no specific referral source is required. Clients may request services on their own or be referred by anyone else.

As noted previously, information related to the eligibility of clients for services is very important. To make appropriate referrals, the nurse must know who is eligible for a particular service and who is not. This helps to minimize client frustration in being referred for services for which they do not qualify. The importance of a notation regarding fees is obvious. Clients need to know beforehand if they will be charged for services provided by the referral resource. The nurse should also be familiar with the types of insurance coverage accepted by the resource. For example, does the agency accept clients covered by Medicaid but not TriCare? An additional notation might indicate whether the agency can help clients with financial arrangements for out-of-pocket expenses. The nurse should also know whether payment is expected at the time of services or if the client will receive a bill later.

Notation should also be made regarding the types of services provided by the resource. The entry regarding access refers to the means by which the client gains entry to the system. In the example in Figure 12-1, the client needs to call ahead to arrange transportation. Additional information under this entry would indicate any supporting documentation the client must provide to be eligible for services. Should he or she bring health insurance papers, or just the policy number? Will the client need proof of residence, monthly expenditures, or medical expenses?

Finally, the nurse should obtain and store information regarding the competency of providers to whom referrals are made. Information about the credentials of providers, prior client complaints, malpractice actions, and so on can be recorded in the comments section as indicated in the third comment in Figure 12-1.

The type of information included in the sample resource file entry allows the community health nurse case manager to make appropriate referrals that do not waste clients' time and energy. It also allows the nurse to prepare clients for what they will encounter in following through on a referral. The file should be updated on a regular basis and as circumstances in various agencies change. Having a specific contact person in each agency may help to ensure that the nurse is notified of program changes. Experiences and reactions of clients following the use of a particular resource can also be used to update resource information and to evaluate the quality of service provided. A copy of the resource file entry form is included in the *Community Assessment Reference Guide* designed to accompany this text.

Monitoring Plan Implementation

Monitoring is another important aspect of implementing the case management plan. Once the plan is developed, the community health nurse case manager does not simply let the plan proceed to unfold on its own or close the case to case management services. Rather, the nurse case manager monitors the implementation of the plan and progress toward achievement of identified goals. Specific areas to be addressed at this stage include monitoring changes in the client's medical status (either positive or negative), social circumstances, and the quality of care provided; observing for changes in functional ability or mobility; and identifying evolving education needs. In addition, the nurse will assess the effectiveness of pain management if relevant and monitor changes in client or family satisfaction with services and their outcomes (Powell, 2000).

Evaluating the Process and Outcomes of Case Management

Evaluation is an integral component of the case management process. The community health nurse case manager focuses on three areas in evaluating case management: client outcomes, quality of care, and system outcomes.

Evaluating Client Outcomes

Some authors note that client-related outcomes may be of three types: non-health-related outcomes, health-related outcomes, and variances (Cesta & Tahan, 2003). Client satisfaction would be a non-health-related outcome. Health-related outcomes would include avoidance of adverse effects. For example, the case management plan may include influenza immunization for an adolescent with asthma. The teen's continued freedom from influenza infection would indicate success in this element of the plan. Similarly, education of a client with diabetes for self-care may be planned as a means of avoiding common complications of diabetes.

A second type of health-related outcome might be improved physiological status, such as improved blood pressure control in a hypertensive client. Improvement in signs and symptoms of chronic conditions is another category of client outcome used to evaluate the effectiveness of case management services. For example, better pain control for clients with arthritis would be an indicator of a positive health-related outcome. Finally, improved functional status and quality of life are other categories of client-related outcomes that can be used to evaluate the effectiveness of case management. As an example, a client with chronic obstructive pulmonary disease (COPD) may be able to return to some of his or her former activities as a result of care provided through case management.

Case management services have been found to be effective in achieving client health-related outcomes in a number of situations. For example, community health nurse case management has been found to be of help in promoting social adjustment and improving mood for mood-disordered single parents. Case management in this program also resulted in cost savings due to clients' lower use of social assistance services (Markle-Reid, Browne, Roberts, Gafni, & Byrne, 2002). Similarly, case management resulted in shorter length of stay, lower critical care utilization, lower mortality, lower costs, and fewer readmissions for clients experiencing coronary artery bypass (Cudney, 2002). On the other hand, case management did not affect hospital readmission rates for clients with a history of self-harm (Clarke et al., 2002). Prevention case management, however, did result in changes in attitudes toward condom use and avoidance of injection drug use and intentions to practice safer sexual practices among incarcerated women (Bauserman et al., 2003). Case management has also been found to result in positive client outcomes with high-risk elderly clients (Newcomer, Maravilla, & Graves, 2004), HIV-infected clients (Gasiorowicz et al., 2005; Massachusetts Department of Public Health, 2004), and children with asthma (Taras, Wright, Brennan, Campana, & Lofgren, 2004).

Health-related outcomes can also be evaluated at the case management system level. Using our pregnancy clinical pathway as an example, we can evaluate both interim and ultimate outcomes. The proportion of women who obtain prenatal care in the first trimester is one example of an interim health-related outcome, as is the percentage of women who develop anemia or toxemia during pregnancy. Ultimate health-related outcomes for this clinical pathway would include the rate of pregnancy-related maternal complications or the number of healthy babies born.

As noted earlier, a variance is a deviation from the plan or from expected outcomes. Variance analysis is the analysis of trends in variance data that can be used to evaluate case management outcomes for individual clients and population groups (Commonwealth of Australia, 2005). Variance may be either positive, with greater than anticipated outcomes, or negative, with deviations from the plan or poorer outcomes. For example, one expected outcome of a population case management program for people with diabetes might be a 25% decrease in hospitalizations. A 50% decrease would be a positive variance. A negative variance would be a modest 10% decline in hospitalization rates or no change at all. Similarly, the program might be intended to provide annual dilated eye examinations to 75% of those with

diabetes, one of the *Healthy People 2010*◆ objectives. Annual eye examinations in 90% of the population would be an example of a positive variance, and achievement of the objective for only 60% of those with diabetes would be a negative variance.

Variance may result from several different types of factors: client/family factors, clinical factors, system factors, and community factors (Commonwealth of Australia, 2000). The most common client/family factor is failure to comply with the management plan, but clients may also be more advanced than the clinical pathway suggests, leading to positive variances in outcomes or to a lack of need for specific services. Clinical factors include adverse events (e.g., development of medication side effects necessitating a change in regimen) or an exacerbation of the client's condition. Typical system factors include lack of needed equipment, failure to perform planned interventions, or delay in referral for needed services. Finally, community factors may reflect the unavailability of relevant practitioners or services, funding cutbacks, and so on.

Evaluating the Quality of Services

As noted earlier, the case manager is responsible for monitoring and evaluating the quality of services provided in implementing the case management plan. To obtain evaluative data in this area, the nurse might periodically visit providers to observe and discuss the quality of care given. For example, the nurse might ask an oncologist about the breadth of options usually presented to women with breast cancer. An oncologist who presents only one option to clients may not be the most appropriate referral for the case manager to make. The community health nurse case manager might also contact clients or family members to obtain their perceptions of the quality of services provided. The nurse should be particularly alert to situations in which clients discontinue services from one or more providers before goals are achieved. Exploration of the client's reasons for discontinuing services may indicate poor quality of care.

Quality of care should also be assessed in population case management. Evaluating the quality of care may involve the use of benchmarks. **Benchmarking** is a process of comparing processes and outcomes among competing organizations to identify performance levels that a particular agency wants to exceed (Cesta & Tahan, 2003). Clinical benchmarking reflects not only the best outcome actually achieved for a given group of clients or diagnosis, but should be based on the evidence of the best possible outcome (Ellis, 2000). Steps in the benchmarking process are presented on page 293.

Evaluation of quality of care may also make use of one or more sets of national quality indicators. Such indicators include the Health Plan Employer Data and Information Set (HEDIS), developed by the National Committee for Quality Assurance, and the Outcome-based

SPECIAL CONSIDERATIONS

STEPS IN THE BENCHMARKING PROCESS

- Identify the area of practice involved (e.g., control of blood pressure in hypertensive clients).
- Identify a patient-focused outcome (e.g., blood pressures consistently lower than 140/90).
- Identify factors and processes that affect the outcome (e.g., medication compliance).
- Identify benchmarks for the best practice for each factor (e.g., medication education provided on the initial visit and reinforced at each visit thereafter).
- Construct a scoring continuum for practice (e.g., medication education consistently provided on first visit, education delayed to subsequent visits, no education provided).
- Score current practice with comments on why scores were assigned (e.g., medication education delayed beyond first visit in 60% of cases).
- Compare results with the identified best practice.
- Share the results with others involved (e.g., physicians, nurse clinicians, etc.).
- Develop a plan of action for improving practice (e.g., identify and modify factors preventing medication education on initial visits).

Data from: Ellis, J. (2000). Sharing the evidence: Clinical practice benchmarking to improve continuously the quality of care. Journal of Advanced Nursing, 32(1), 215–225.

Quality Indicators (OBQI) for home health agencies, based on the federal government's Outcome and Assessment Information Set (OASIS). Quality indicators have also been developed by the American Accreditation Healthcare Commission (formerly the Utilization Review Accreditation Commission [URAC]) (Cesta & Tahan, 2003).

Evaluating System Outcomes

System outcomes reflect the effects of case management on the health care system. Elements that might be evaluated in this area include staff satisfaction, length of stay (or frequency and duration of care), costs of care, and the adequacy of interdepartmental or interdisciplinary communication (Cesta & Tahan, 2003). Other system outcome variables that might be examined include the number of days that clients did not meet established outcome criteria, reimbursement denial amounts or rates, readmissions, emergency department visits, and costs per case for case management versus cost savings resulting from case management services (Cudney, 2002).

Evaluating system outcomes may also entail utilization review. **Utilization review** is a process of monitoring the necessity of care and the resources used and may involve preadmission review, concurrent review,

retrospective review, or telephonics (Powell, 2000). In a preadmission review, the nurse case manager determines the appropriateness of the requested services before they are given. Areas for consideration include the need for the service and the appropriateness of the setting and level of services proposed. For example, the case manager may determine that a requested nursing home admission is not appropriate because the client can be effectively cared for at home for far less cost. Concurrent review takes place while services are being provided to determine client progress toward goals and the need to continue services. Telephonics is a form of concurrent review in which the information needed to determine the appropriateness of service continuation is obtained by telephone. In retrospective review, the case manager determines the need for and appropriateness of services after they have been provided with the intent of approving or denying reimbursement for those services. Utilization review is generally performed by case managers who have an identified role in reimbursement decisions and may or may not be required of community health nurse case managers.

Other approaches to evaluating system outcomes for case management systems include quality outcomes measurement and the development and testing of a program theory or logic model. Quality outcomes measurement involves the identification of measures of quality in system performance and collection of data related to those measures. An example of a quality indicator might be reduction in pain levels in home care clients within a specified number of hours after intervention. Measurement of the indicator would require a follow-up contact with the client within that time frame to determine whether the pain has been controlled at an acceptable level. At the system level, the percentage of clients whose pain is effectively controlled would be the quality indicator. Benchmarking, as discussed earlier, may be used to establish measures for quality indicators.

In the use of a program theory, the community health nurse would develop a pictorial model of interventions included in the case management plan or system and the expected results of those interventions. Evaluation would then include collection of data to determine the extent to which the interventions actually resulted in the expected outcomes. Program theories are discussed in more detail in Chapter 15∞.

Case management has been shown to be an effective nursing intervention used since the beginning of community health nursing practice. Community health nurses can improve their practice with more systematic use of the case management process with individuals as well as population groups.

Case Study

Population Case Management in Action

As a community health nurse working in an elementary school in a small town, you notice a significant increase in both school absences related to asthma and children who are coming to your office with difficulty breathing during the school day. Although each child's situation is unique, they seem to share a number of common characteristics. Most of them are from low-income families in which both parents work. They all live in the neighborhood surrounding the school. There is considerable construction occurring in the neighborhood that keeps everything coated with dust. The school yard is a home for pollen-producing weeds. The school is old and previous water leaks have led to widespread mold and mildew in some of the classrooms and in the heating vents.

Most of the children are using albuterol inhalers when they have difficulty breathing, but few of them are using nasal steroids on a regular basis or using their albuterol prior to activities in the school yard. Many of the children tell you that their doctors have prescribed nasal steroids, but their families cannot afford to have the prescriptions filled. In talking with some of the primary care providers in the community, you find that they are frustrated with their inability to control asthma in many of the children and that their practices are inundated with children with mild to severe attacks.

1. Does this situation warrant development of a case management system? Why or why not?
2. What are the children's health needs in this situation? How do biophysical, psychological, physical environmental, sociocultural, behavioral, and health system factors influence those needs?
3. What desired outcomes would you establish for a case management system? Do these outcomes reflect primary, secondary, or tertiary prevention?
4. How would you involve members of the community in developing the case management plan? Who should be involved?
5. What referrals would be appropriate for many of the children? What is the expected outcome of these referrals? How would you go about making the referrals?
6. How would you evaluate the case management system for this population? Be specific about the evaluative criteria you would use and how you would obtain the information to evaluate care.

Test Your Understanding

1. Identify at least three client-centered and three system-centered goals of case management. How might these goals conflict? (p. 279)

2. Give examples of the use of at least three of the general principles of case management. (p. 281)

3. Describe the four elements that must be present for negligence to occur. Give an example of each. (p. 282)

4. What are some of the criteria used to determine the need for population case management systems? How do they differ from indicators of the need for case management for individual clients or families? (p. 284)

5. What types of considerations should be included in assessing a case management situation? Give examples of how factors in each area could affect the case management situation. (pp. 284–285)

6. What are the major aspects of developing the case management plan? Give an example of each. (pp. 285–286)

7. What three areas should be considered in implementing the case management plan? (pp. 288–291)

8. What are three areas to be considered in evaluating case management? (pp. 291–293)

EXPLORE MediaLink

http://www.prenhall.com/clark
Resources for this chapter can be found on the Companion Website.

Audio Glossary
Exam Review Questions
Case Study: Health Promotion through
  Case Management

MediaLink Application: Penalizing Obesity
  and Smoking (video)
Media Links
Challenge Your Knowledge

Advocacy Interviews

References

Aiken, T. D., & Aucoin, J. W. (2003). Legal issues in case management. In T. G. Cesta & H.A. Tahan, *The case manager's survival guide: Winning strategies for clinical practice* (2nd ed., pp. 304–52). St. Louis: Mosby.

Askey, R. (2004). Case management: A critical review. *Mental Health Practice, 7*(8), 12–16.

Bauserman, R. L., Richardson, D., Ward, M., Shea, M., Bowlin, C., Tomoyasu, N., et al. (2003). HIV prevention with jail and prison inmates: Maryland's prevention case management program. *AIDS Education and Prevention, 15,* 465–480.

Bedell, J. R., Cohen, N., & Sullivan, A. (2000). Case management: The current best practices and the next generation of innovation. *Community Mental Health Journal, 36,* 179–194.

Blaha, C., Robinson, J. M., Pugh, L. C., Bryan, Y., & Havens, D. S. (2000). Longitudinal nursing case management for elderly heart failure patients: Notes from the field. *Nursing Case Management, 5,* 32–36.

Buhler-Wilkerson, K. (2001). *No place like home: A history of nursing and home care in the United States.* Baltimore: Johns Hopkins University.

Case, N. (2004). Delegation skills: Critical thinking strategies you can apply to the challenges of delegating. *Advance for Nurses, 1*(4), 17–22.

Case Management Society of America. (n.d.). *Definition of case management.* Retrieved April 5, 2005, from http://www.cmsa.org/About-UsDefinition.aspx

Case Management Society of America. (1995). *Standards of practice for case management.* Little Rock, AR: Author.

Case Management Society of America. (2002). *Standards of practice for case management* (rev.). Little Rock, AR: Author.

Cesta, T. G. (2002). The politics of case management. In D. J. Mason, J. K. Leavitt, & M. W. Chaffee (Eds.), *Policy and politics in nursing and health care* (4th ed., pp. 319–324). St. Louis, MO: Saunders.

Cesta, T. G., & Tahan, H. A. (2003). *The case manager's survival guide: Winning strategies for clinical practice* (2nd ed.). St. Louis: Mosby.

Clarke, T., Baker, P., Watts, C. J., Williams, K., Feldman, R. A., & Sherr, L. (2002). Self-harm in adults: A randomized controlled trial of nurse-led case management versus routine care only. *Journal of Mental Health, 11,* 167–176.

Commonwealth of Australia, Department of Veteran's Affairs. (2005). *Introduction to the revised clinical pathway documentation suite.* Retrieved January 3, 2006, from http://www.dva.gov.au/health/provider/community_nursing/pathways/word_docs/clinical_pathway_introduction.doc

Commonwealth of Australia, Department of Veteran's Affairs. (2000). *Clinical pathways manual.* Retrieved April 10, 2005, from http://www.dva.gov.au/health/provider/community_nursing/pathways/prelims.pdf

Cudney, A. E. (2002). Case management: A serious solution for serious issues. *Journal of Healthcare Management, 47,* 149–152.

Ellis, J. (2000). Sharing the evidence: Clinical practice benchmarking to improve continuously the quality of care. *Journal of Advanced Nursing, 32*(1), 215–225.

Fraser, K. D., & Strang, V. (2004). Decision-making and nurse case management: A philosophical perspective. *Advances in Nursing Science, 27*(4), 32–43.

Gallagher, E., Alcock, D., Diem, E., Angus, D., & Medves, J. (2002). Ethical dilemmas in home care case management. *Journal of Healthcare Management, 42,* 85–97.

Gasiorowicz, M., Llanas, M. R., DiFranceisco, W., Benotsch, E. G., Brondino, M. J., Catz, S. L., et al. (2005). Reductions in transmission risk behaviors in HIV-positive clients receiving prevention case management services: Findings from a community demonstration project. *AIDS Education and Prevention, 17*(Suppl. A), 40–52.

Grumbach, K., Miller, J., Mertz, E., & Finocchio, L. (2004). How much public health is in public health nursing practice? *Public Health Nursing, 21,* 266–276.

Hillegass, B. E., Smith, D. M., & Phillips, S. L. (2002). Changing managed care to care management: Innovations in nursing practice. *Nursing Administration Quarterly, 26*(5), 33–46.

Hubber, D. L., & McClelland, E. (2003). Patient preferences and discharge planning transitions. *Journal of Professional Nursing, 19,* 204–210.

Lamb, G., Shelton, P. S., & Zazworsky, D. (2003). Disease management. In T. G. Cesta & H. A. Tahan, *The case manager's survival guide: Winning strategies for clinical practice* (2nd ed., pp. 134–152). St. Louis: Mosby.

Lantz, P. M., Keeton, K., Romano, L., & DeGroff, A. (2004). Case management in public health screening programs: The experience of the National Breast and Cervical Cancer Early Detection Program. *Journal of Public Health Management Practice, 10,* 545–555.

Markle-Reid, M., Browne, G., Roberts, J., Gafni, A., & Byrne, C. (2002). The 2-year costs and effects of a public health nurse case management intervention on mood-disordered single parents on social assistance. *Journal of Evaluation in Clinical Practice, 8*(1), 45–59.

Massachusetts Department of Public Health. (2004). Voluntary HIV testing as part of routine medical care—Massachusetts, 2002. *Morbidity and Mortality Weekly Report, 53,* 523–526.

McCloskey, J. C., & Bulechek, G. M. (2000). *Nursing interventions classification* (3rd ed.). St. Louis: Mosby.

Newcomer, R., Maravilla, V., & Graves, M. T. (2004). Outcomes of preventive case management among high-risk elderly in three medical groups. *Evaluation & the Health Professions, 27,* 323–348.

Powell, S. K. (2000). *Case management: A practical guide to success in managed care* (2nd ed.). Philadelphia: Lippincott.

Rapp, C. A., & Goscha, R. J. (2004). The principles of effective case management of mental health services. *Psychiatric Rehabilitation Journal, 27,* 319–333.

Reel, S. J., Morgan-Judge, T., Peros, D. S., & Abraham, I. L. (2002). School-based rural case management: A model to prevent and reduce risk. *Journal of the American Academy of Nurse Practitioners, 14,* 291–296.

St. Vincent's Hospital Sydney. (n.d.). *What are clinical pathways?* Retrieved April 4, 2005, from http://wwwsvh.stvincents.com.au/qi/Clin_Pathways/cp_what.htm

Schifalacqua, M. M., & O'Hearn, P. (2004). How to make a difference in the health care of a population—One person at a time. *Nursing Administration Quarterly, 28*(1), 29–35.

Schroeder, C. A., Trehearne, B., & Ward, D. (2000). Expanded role of nursing in ambulatory managed care, Part II: Impact on outcomes of costs, quality, provider, and patient satisfaction. *Nursing Economics, 18,* 71–78.

Simpson, A., Miller, C., & Bowers, L. (2003). Case management models and the care programme approach: How to make the CPA effective and credible. *Journal of Psychiatric and Mental Health Nursing, 10,* 472–483.

Stanton, M. P., Walizer, E. M., Graham, J. I., & Keppel, L. (2000). Case management: A case study. *Nursing Case Management, 5,* 37–45.

Sultz, H. A., & Young, K. M. (2004). *Health care USA: Understanding its organization and delivery* (4th ed.). Sudbury, MA: Jones and Bartlett.

Taras, H., Wright, S., Brennan, J., Campana, J., & Lofgren, R. (2004). Impact of school nurse case management on students with asthma. *Journal of School Health, 74,* 213–219.

Williams, D. B. (2000). Population care management: What's in it for your organization? *Nursing Case Management, 5,* 1.

Advocacy in Action

Asian Women's Co-op

A nurse educator working in Southeast Asia spent a year with her clinical nursing students conducting a community survey of the surrounding villages in Ward 13. After completing an assessment and analysis, she concluded that an intervention was necessary to combat the excessive amount of drinking by the village men in this particular community. Her goal was to establish a program similar to Alcoholics Anonymous (AA) that would help the men become sober and therefore more productive members of society. She met with the ward officer and his colleagues to discuss her idea. They all agreed that the men drank excessively but did not agree that these men 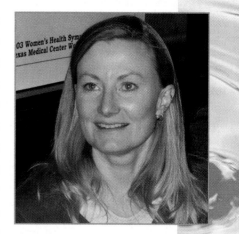 would be interested in an AA-type program. They felt the time and money might be better spent working with the women in this community.

A meeting was scheduled with several women who were leaders in the community and women interested in discussing an intervention plan. During this meeting, the women were very excited to find someone who was concerned with their needs and had access to the resources they needed. They wanted to learn skills for knitting and sewing to make articles of clothing to sell to tourists. This activity would provide them with their own income and their families with food and other essentials not affordable to them with the money provided by their husbands. They wanted to be self-sufficient and provide a better life for their children.

The nurse educator, community women, and ward officer submitted a proposal to a non-governmental organization for funding. The proposal was approved and funded, and the women were given sewing and knitting equipment and supplies. The ward office provided access to a meeting room for the women, and trainers were provided through a local handicraft business. During the training, the women expressed interest in learning about proper nutrition for their children. They also wanted to learn to read and write. Resources were found to provide these services, and the women met in weekly training sessions. Upon successful completion of the training, each woman received a certificate of completion. Thirty women in the district completed the first training in 1994.

Since 1994, the women have continued to learn to sew and knit. They have bought three more sewing machines to supplement the original three from the grant. They have rented their own space in the town to conduct the training, and now training is provided twice daily, 6 days a week. A little bit of money and a lot of motivation changed the lives of many people; these women only needed someone to believe they could fulfill their goals and provide them with the resources to do so. As of 2001, they have been self-sustaining in their women's skills training center.

Ruth Grubesic

Assistant Professor, Director International Nursing Affairs

Texas Woman's University

Community Empowerment

CHAPTER OBJECTIVES

After reading this chapter, you should be able to:

1. Discuss the relationship of community empowerment to other similar concepts.
2. Identify levels of community empowerment.
3. Apply selected models for community empowerment.
4. Describe the process of community empowerment.
5. Apply criteria to evaluate community empowerment.
6. Analyze the role of community health nurses in community empowerment.

KEY TERMS

MediaLink
http://www.prenhall.com/clark

Additional interactive resources for this chapter can be found on the Companion Website. Click on Chapter 13 and "Begin" to select the activities for this chapter.

Throughout this book, we emphasize the advocacy role of the community health nurse. Community health nurses act on behalf of individuals, families, and population groups that, for whatever reason, cannot act for themselves. The ultimate outcome of advocacy by community health nurses, however, is the ability of the client to act independently. Community empowerment, as discussed in this chapter, endeavors to accomplish that outcome, to enable communities to identify community health problems and take steps to resolve them independently of or in concert with health care professionals and others. Just as successful nursing education programs prepare graduates to function effectively on their own in the practice milieu, so too does effective community health nursing, as community empowerment, prepare communities to deal with their own health problems and issues.

Although some authors trace the beginnings of community organization and empowerment to the settlement house activities of the late 1800s (Minkler & Wallerstein, 2005), the nurses of the Henry Street Settlement did not engage in community organization or empowerment activities as we know them today. Those nurses certainly functioned as advocates for the health and social welfare needs of the immigrant populations they served, but they did not work to enable those populations to act on their own behalf. On the contrary, they tried to work within the existing power structure to benefit these populations, rather than attempting to redistribute power in their favor. Today's social change professionals, also called "conscious contrarians" (Minkler, 2005) or "civic revolutionaries" (Henton, Melville, & Walesh, 2004), are characterized by a worldview of people and society that rejects the dominant distribution of social power and chooses community organization or empowerment to foster a redistribution of power (Minkler, 2005).

EMPOWERMENT AND RELATED CONCEPTS

Community empowerment, the topic of this chapter, is closely related to a number of similar concepts. Empowerment is defined as "an enabling process through which individuals or communities take control over their lives and their environment" (Minkler & Wallerstein, 2005, p. 26) or as "the development of understanding and influence over personal, social, economic, and political forces impacting life situations" (Schultz, Israel, Zimmerman, & Checkoway as quoted in Ogilvie, Allen, Laryea, & Opare, 2003, p. 114). Similarly, the World Health Organization (WHO) has defined empowerment as "a social action process by which individuals, communities, and organizations gain mastery over their lives in the context of changing

ETHICAL AWARENESS

Minkler and Pies (2005) described a number of ethical issues and practical dilemmas involved in community organizing or empowerment. Some of these issues include conflicting loyalties, funding sources, promoting real participation by community members, cross-cultural issues, the unanticipated consequences of organizing, and questions of the common good.

- Conflicting loyalties may arise when promoting community empowerment is in conflict with the best interests of the health professional's employing agency. For example, in one community, residents wanted to create another source of health care services. Some of the people assisting with community development were employed by a local health care agency that might lose part of its clientele if new services were initiated.
- Available funding sources may mean that community efforts cannot be directed to areas of real interest to the community, but to those that have potential for funding. For example, in one community, the most pressing issues were those affecting senior citizens, but the initiatives for which grant funding was available addressed the needs of children and youth.
- Community participation is often difficult to elicit, particularly in low-income communities where people may work several jobs to make ends meet, leaving them little time to engage in community development initiatives. The health professional is then faced with the necessity to proceed with identified initiatives with less actual community resident participation than desired.
- Multiple cultural orientations within the community and between community members and health professionals provide the potential for cultural misunderstandings and perceptions of racism. Many ethnic groups are not vocal in community organizing processes, and health professionals need to be cognizant of the need to elicit and incorporate their perspectives as well as those of more vocal groups.
- Community organizing efforts may occasionally lead to unanticipated negative consequences. For example, recent news coverage of the campaign to immunize against polio, initiated 50 years ago, had the unintended effect of stigmatizing persons with polio as disabled and focusing negative attention on their disabilities.
- Finally, the "common good" may be defined differently by different segments of the community. For example, local government may see upscale housing as a means of increasing tax revenue to support public services, yet affordable housing may be a greater need for the majority of residents. The question then becomes one of who defines what the common good entails.

How might these ethical considerations influence community organizing activities in your area? What strategies might help address them?

their social and political environment to improve equity and quality of life" (as quoted in Wallerstein, 2002, p. 73). **Community empowerment** is the process of "enhancing capacity of communities to control their own lives, effect change, mobilize and use resources, and obtain services to address health problems and collectively counter health risk behaviors and conditions that produce and support them" (May, Phillips, Ferketich, & Verran, 2003, p. 254).

Community empowerment arises from activities related to community development, community organizing, community mobilization, and community building. Empowerment, in turn, leads to increased community capacity and competence. The relationships among these concepts are depicted in Figure 13-1. **Community development** is often the term used to refer to the rejuvenation of communities through housing and business development (Rubin, 2000). Community development may also be conceived more generally as promoting group action and providing a voice in decision making for disadvantaged groups within the population (Billings, 2000). This perspective on community development is more akin to the concept of community empowerment as discussed in this chapter than to the more traditional view of community development as economic development.

The concept of community organization was presented in Chapter 7∞ and reflects a process "by which community groups are helped to identify common problems or goals, mobilize resources, and develop and implement strategies for reaching the goals they have collectively set" (Minkler & Wallerstein, 2005, p. 26). Community mobilization, a similar term, was defined as a community health nursing role in Chapter 1∞, and involves "working with individuals and groups to provide population-based community driven assessments, interventions, and evaluations" (Westbrook, as quoted in Westbrook & Schultz, 2000, p. 53). Both of these processes tend to be more problem-specific than community empowerment, which is designed to develop overall community abilities to deal with a variety of problems. Community building is another similar, but more general, process that leads to community empowerment. **Community building** is defined as "continuous, self-renewing efforts by residents and professionals to engage in collective action, aimed at problem solving and enrichment, that creates new or strengthened social networks, new capacities for group action and support, and new standards and expectations for the life of the community" (Blackwell & Colmenar, 2005, p. 436). Community building efforts frequently lead to increases in community social capital as described in Chapter 10∞. Another related term is *capacity building*, which may occur at three levels. The first level of capacity building is that of developing the capabilities of the health infrastructure to deliver needed health care services. The second level is the capacity to maintain and sustain programs when initial funding (usually external funding) is withdrawn. The third level is that of community abilities to address a variety of health-related issues (Labonte & Laverack, 2001).

Community empowerment results in increased community competence and capacity, as depicted in Figure 13-1. **Community competence** is defined as "the ability of the community to engage in effective problem solving" (Anderson, Guthrie, & Schirle, 2002, p. 43).

Community capacity is the "abilities, behaviors, relationships, and values that enable individuals, groups, and organizations at any level of society to carry out tasks or functions and to achieve their development objectives over time" (Morgan, as quoted in Ogilvie et al., 2003, p. 113). The community empowerment literature identifies several domains of community capacity. These include:

- An articulated and shared value system
- Active participation by community residents
- Assumption of leadership roles by community members
- Empowering organizational structures and rich social support networks that provide structures and mechanisms for community dialogue
- Ability to achieve consensus on goals and actions to reach them
- A variety of skills, knowledge, and resources
- The ability to critically reflect on community circumstances and to identify factors underlying community problems
- A sense of community cohesion, commitment, and trust
- The ability to mobilize resources to address community problems
- An understanding of community history and its influence on community action or inaction
- Access to power
- Links to others as resources outside the community
- Equitable relationships both within and outside the community
- Community control over decisions and programs
- The ability to engage in strategic planning for future development (Eng & Parker, 2002; Norton, McLeroy, Burdine, Felix, & Dorsey, 2002; Tones & Green, 2004; Wallerstein, 2002)

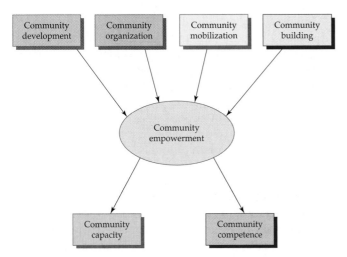

FIGURE 13-1 The Relationship of Community Empowerment to Other Similar Concepts

MediaLink Grassroots Organizing Video

LEVELS OF EMPOWERMENT

Empowerment may occur at a variety of levels. Two of the possible levels are those of the individual community member and of the community at large. Individual empowerment focuses on improving individual skills and self-esteem as a precursor to taking control of one's own life. Community empowerment focuses on increased civic participation and preparation for collective action to address common concerns or achieve common goals (Anderson et al., 2002). Individual empowerment is a process of increasing one's power to take action to improve one's own life (Askey, 2004). Individual empowerment may address one or more of three areas of personal development: (a) intrapersonal components, such as perceived control and self-efficacy; (b) interactional components related to transactions between people and with the environment; and (c) behavioral components related to the development of specific actions and skills (Ogilvie et al., 2003).

Community health nurses may be involved in both individual and community empowerment. For example, a nurse may assist an abused woman to obtain job training and to request a restraining order against her abuser, empowering her to leave the abusive situation. At the community level, a community health nurse might assist residents of a low-income neighborhood to collect information on gang-related criminal activity and present a petition to the City Council requesting a greater police presence in the neighborhood.

Community empowerment may also occur at horizontal and vertical levels (Wallerstein, 2002). Horizontal empowerment is internal to the community and is reflected in the community's ability to solve problems by mobilizing its own resources. This level is related to what is termed "locality development" or the empowerment of local communities to make change (Drevdahl, 2002). For example, a community health nurse might help neighborhood residents to form a neighborhood watch group to help control gang activity. Vertical empowerment involves efforts to change power structures outside the community and to leverage outside power and resources to address community concerns and may involve organizing marginalized groups to make demands on the larger society. Vertical empowerment is reflected in the previous example of petitioning the City Council for better police coverage. Finally, community empowerment may be conceived as occurring along a continuum from personal empowerment to the development of small mutual support groups, to the development of community organizations, to the creation of coalitions and linking with outside resources to address community concerns (Laverack, 2004; Uys, Majumdar, & Gwele, 2004). At the level of personal empowerment, a community health nurse might help a homeless man with a substance abuse problem find work and enroll in a recovery program. At the next level, the nurse might assist a group of homeless individuals to form a support group that permits them to share knowledge of resources. Helping to create an organization composed of homeless individuals and families and members of the social services community to address the health care needs of the homeless population would be an example of the third level of empowerment. Finally, at the fourth level, the community health nurse might assist the community organization to link with legal advocates and others to promote legislation to protect the civil rights of homeless individuals.

MODELS FOR COMMUNITY EMPOWERMENT

The dominant framework for community organizing or empowerment work is Rothman's work in the 1970s addressing three levels of practice: locality development, social planning, and social action. Locality development involves development of a sense of community and a group identity. Social planning focuses on the resolution of specific problems identified in the community, and social action is geared toward increasing the problem-solving ability of the community in general. Most models on which community empowerment activities are based involve a combination of these levels (Minkler & Wallerstein, 2005). Some of the models to be discussed here include the Community Action Model (Lavery et al., 2005), the Nursing Model of Community Organization for Change (Anderson et al., 2002), the Community Organization Model (Tones & Green, 2004), and the Planned Approach to Community Health (PATCH) model (Butler, 2001). Elements of each of these models are compared in Table 13-1◆. As can be seen in Table 13-1◆, each of the models incorporates components similar to those of the nursing process, usually addressing some sort of community assessment, diagnosis, or analysis; goal development; selection and implementation of appropriate intervention strategies; and evaluation of the outcomes achieved. The table also includes examples of ways in which community health nurses could be involved in community empowerment in the context of each model.

TABLE 13-1 Elements of Selected Community Empowerment Models and Examples of Community Health Nursing (CHN) Involvement

Community Action Model	Nursing Model of Community Organization for Change	Community Organization Model	PATCH Model
Step 1 • Train a few essential community members • Identify the issue • Choose a meaningful focus for the issue *CHN involvement: Help identify community members for training; assist community members to collect assessment data, identify relevant issues, prioritize issues, and select one for action.* **Step 2** • Conduct community diagnosis of root causes of the issue • Assess the extent of the effect on the community *CHN involvement: Assist community members to develop data categories and collection methods regarding factors contributing to the issue and the effect of the issue on the community.* **Step 3** • Analyze diagnostic results *CHN involvement: Assist community members to analyze data and identify key contributing factors as a target for action.* **Step 4** • Select, plan, and implement actions to address the issue • Identify desired outcomes to be achieved *CHN involvement: Assist community members to identify and evaluate possible alternative approaches to issue resolution and*	**Assessment/reassessment** • Identify felt needs, assets from community perspective and with community involvement *CHN involvement: Assist community members to design and conduct community needs/asset assessment.* **Planning/design** • Establish goals to be achieved • Design interventions to achieve them *CHN involvement: Assist community members to determine desired outcome of action, to identify and evaluate possible alternative approaches to action, and to develop specific strategies for the alternative selected.* **Implementation** • Implement the actions designed to achieve the identified goals *CHN involvement: Educate community members, as needed, on how to implement selected actions; assist community members to develop mechanisms to monitor implementation and progress toward goal achievement.* **Evaluation/dissemination** • Identify successful and unsuccessful elements • Disseminate information to community to promote decision making	**Community analysis** • Define community • Develop a community profile • Assess community capacity • Assess barriers to action • Assess readiness for change *CHN involvement: Assist community members to design and conduct community needs/asset assessment.* **Design initiation** • Develop an organizational structure • Develop a core planning group and identify a coordinator • Recruit members • Define goals • Clarify roles and responsibilities • Provide training and get recognition *CHN involvement: Help identify potential planning group members; educate planning group members in group process and guide progression in the steps of group development; assist community members to develop and disseminate information messages related to planning.* **Implementation** • Develop interventions • Develop timeline • Generate broad community participation • Plan media coverage • Obtain financial and other support • Develop evaluation plans *CHN involvement: Assist community members to determine desired outcome of action, to identify and evaluate possible alternative approaches to action, and to develop specific strategies for the alternative(s) selected and timelines for their implementation; help to identify additional community members who can be asked to participate; link community members to media contacts and assist them in the development of media messages.*	**Mobilize the community** *CHN involvement: Help to identify appropriate community members as participants.* **Collect and organize data related to the issue** *CHN involvement: Assist community members to design and conduct community needs/asset assessment.* **Choose health priorities** *CHN involvement: Assist community members to prioritize issues and select one for action.* **Develop a comprehensive intervention plan with multisectoral collaboration** *CHN involvement: Assist community members to determine desired outcome of action, to identify and evaluate possible alternative approaches to action, and to develop specific strategies for the alternative selected.* **Evaluate the effectiveness of interventions** *CHN involvement: Assist community members in the development of criteria to measure success and data collection methods and in analyzing evaluative data in light of desired outcomes.*

Continued on next page

TABLE 13-1 Elements of Selected Community Empowerment Models and Examples of Community Health Nursing (CHN) Involvement *(continued)*

Community Action Model	Nursing Model of Community Organization for Change	Community Organization Model	PATCH Model
to identify the desired outcome of action. **Step 5** • Enforce or maintain the action or activity *CHN involvement: Assist community members to develop mechanisms to monitor ongoing activity and results (e.g., changes in the issue or its effects on the community); link community members to agencies or organizations that will enforce action (e.g., housing authority or City Planning Commission).*	*CHN involvement: Assist community members in developing criteria to measure success and data collection methods, in analyzing evaluative data in light of desired outcomes, in selecting mechanisms for disseminating information, and in writing messages for dissemination.*	**Maintenance/consolidation** • Sustain activities as part of community structure • Retain staff and volunteers • Recruit additional participants • Acknowledge contributions *CHN involvement: Assist community members to recognize successful endeavors and progress toward achieving outcomes; assist with writing grant proposals to sustain community activities; help to identify and recruit additional participants; assist community members to plan events to recognize contributions made.* **Dissemination/reassessment** • Update community analysis • Assess effectiveness of interventions • Summarize and disseminate findings *CHN involvement: Assist community members to develop criteria to measure success, to select data collection methods, to analyze evaluative data in light of desired outcomes, to develop strategies to disseminate evaluation findings and to determine directions for future action based on findings.*	

One additional type of model that may be employed is the natural helper model. This model differs from those presented in Table 13-1◆ in that it is not a process model but focuses on the use of natural helpers within the community to promote community empowerment. *Natural helpers* are "particular individuals to whom others naturally turn for advice, emotional support, and tangible aid" (Eng & Parker, 2002, p. 126). Several types of informal helpers may exist in a community. Among these are family, friends, and neighbors, natural helpers, role-related helpers, people with similar problems, and volunteers. The role of friends, family, and neighbors as informal helpers is well understood, and the category of natural helpers has been defined above. Role-related helpers are people who, because of their role in the community, can provide help in certain circumstances. For example, educated shopkeepers could assist clients to make healthy food choices or could be sources of information and referral in other health-related areas. People who have similar kinds of problems can form self-help and support groups and share group resources, knowledge, and skills. Volunteers are people who are willing to provide their time and energy to specific initiatives or program efforts. Natural helpers are not the same as community health workers (CHWs), who are members of a community with some training hired by community agencies to work directly with their fellow residents. We will discuss the use of community members as health workers later in this chapter.

ORGANIZING FOR COMMUNITY EMPOWERMENT

As we can see, based on the models included in Table 13-1◆, the process of community empowerment is very similar to the nursing process. In this chapter, we will address some of the aspects of that process, focusing on assessment, planning, strategies for implementation, and evaluation.

Assessing Communities

Community organizing and empowerment initiatives may take one of two approaches or a combination of both. The first, and more traditional, approach is to focus on community needs and needs-oriented solutions. The second approach is capacity-focused and involves developing individual and group capacities or assets as the first step in community rejuvenation (McKnight & Kretzmann, 2005). A combined approach examines both community needs and community assets.

Community assessment, in the context of community empowerment, has two general purposes. The first is to provide information for change—facts about the current situation, contributing factors, and assets that may be brought to bear to facilitate change. The second purpose is to provide information for empowerment.

As the old adage states, "knowledge is power," and communities need knowledge in order to assess the situation and take action (Hancock & Minkler, 2005). The same elements of community assessment data can contribute to the achievement of both purposes. Community assessment may also result in several other indirect effects for community empowerment, including the creation of social cohesion among community members, encouragement of self-help within the community, persuasion for change, and identification and development of local leadership. Additional effects of community assessment may include development of civic consciousness and a sense of responsibility for community welfare, identification of professional and technical support for local initiatives, better coordination of existing services to meet local needs, and training in democratic processes, leading to decentralization of some government functions (Clinard, cited in Kennedy & Crosby, 2002).

The actual assessment of the community can be framed in terms of the dimensions of health from the dimensions model, examining factors in each of the six dimensions that reflect community assets or that contribute to community needs. The specifics of such an assessment are addressed in detail in Chapter 15∞. Some of the areas that might be examined in a community empowerment assessment are quality-of-life indicators, "provocative indicators," community processes and their effects on health, and formal and informal leadership within the community. Provocative indicators are those for which there may not be valid and reliable data, but that make people think and take notice of an issue (Hancock & Minkler, 2005). In one community assessment, for example, community members repeatedly expressed perceptions of poor care provided by a local community clinic. Although these perceptions were not accurate, they forced clinic administrators to examine how their services were perceived in the community and to make changes in service delivery to improve their image among community members.

In the context of community empowerment, asset data from the community assessment can be organized in terms of three levels of "building blocks" that contribute to community regeneration. At the first level are the primary building blocks, those that are under the direct control of the community. Primary building blocks include the talents of individual community members, personal income, local businesses (including in-home businesses), and community associations and organizations and their capacities. These may include business, religious, cultural, citizens', communications, and other organizations and associations within the community (McKnight & Kretzmann, 2005).

Secondary building blocks are located within the community but controlled by outsiders. These may include private and nonprofit organizations (e.g., a private university or hospital, banks), public institutions and services (e.g., the local health department), and the physical resources of the community (e.g., vacant land). The third level of building blocks includes potential building blocks located outside the community and controlled by outsiders. Examples of potential building blocks are welfare funding, capital improvement funds, and public information (McKnight & Kretzmann, 2005).

Community health nurses can help members of the community to conduct an assessment as a first step in community empowerment. For example, the nurse can assist community members to identify relevant categories and sources of data needed and to develop effective data collection strategies. In addition, the nurse can help community members analyze assessment data and identify factors that impede and facilitate community empowerment. Clark et al. (2003) provided an example of a community health nurse facilitating resident involvement in a community assessment. In this process, the community health nurse assisted community members to conduct focus groups among multiple segments of the community to identify community needs and assets. The findings of the assessment were shared with the wider community and became the impetus for a variety of community-initiated efforts to improve living conditions in the community.

Planning Considerations

Capacity-oriented community empowerment planning is characterized by three elements. First, it incorporates as many internal community resources as possible. Second, it is based on the results of a community capacity inventory or assessment of community assets. Finally, community building strategies will build on community assets (McKnight & Kretzmann, 2005).

Community empowerment planning also poses several challenges to the social change professional or community health nurse. These challenges include:

- Reconciling individual and community needs by creating common purposes, values, and complementary roles.
- Reconciling trust and accountability. Community members must trust each other and outside assistance, yet demand that persons responsible for action on behalf of the community are accountable for their actions.
- Reconciling economic and social goals by creating a cycle of renewal in which strengthening local business and economic interests also strengthens the social fabric of the community and vice versa.
- Reconciling people and place by recognizing and addressing diversity among community members whose needs may not all be the same despite their residence in the same community.
- Reconciling change and continuity by moving from expectations of stability to acceptance of change as a *given*. There is a need to recognize and accept that

turnover will occur among participants in community organizing activities and to work to maintain stability of function in spite of turnover.

- Reconciling idealism and practicality by supporting the core values of the community in the context of the constraints imposed by the reality of the situation. Community members need to continually strive toward the ideal, but be willing to accept incremental changes in achieving it (Henton et al., 2004).

Specific elements in the process of planning for community empowerment are similar to those in planning any community initiative or program and are addressed in more detail in Chapter 15∞. Here we will focus on three aspects of planning that are particularly relevant for empowerment planning: issue selection, team building, and coalition development.

Issue Selection

Issue selection is a critical element in planning for community empowerment. **Issue selection** involves "identifying winnable and specific targets of change that unify and build community strength" (Minkler & Wallerstein, 2005, p. 35). Issues in community empowerment are selected not only on the basis of community needs but also for their value in fostering community leadership development (Staples, 2005). Potential criteria for issue selection are reflected in the focused assessment questions below.

There are four basic considerations in developing the initial outline of an issue (Staples, 2005). The first of these is constituency. Who are the constituents or parties

---

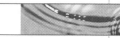

FOCUSED ASSESSMENT

Selecting an Issue for Community Empowerment

- Is the issue simply and easily explained by community members?
- Will the issue unite community members and involve them in problem resolution?
- Does the issue provide greater visibility and credibility for the community or for the organizing group within the community?
- Is the issue consistent with the long-range goals of the community or organization?
- Does the issue have potential for promoting growth of the group?
- Will the issue provide educational or training experiences for community leaders?
- How will the issue affect community or organizational resources?
- Does the issue have potential for creating new community allies? New enemies?
- Does the issue focus on direct action?
- Will the issue result in victory?

Data from: Minkler, M., & Wallerstein, N. (2005). Improving health through community organization and community building. In M. Minkler (Ed.), Community organizing and community building for health (2nd ed., pp.26–50). New Brunswick, NJ: Rutgers University Press; Staples, L. (2005). Selecting and cutting the issue. In M. Minkler (Ed.), Community organizing and community building for health (2nd ed., pp. 173–192). New Brunswick, NJ: Rutgers University Press.

interested in the issue? What is the source of their interest? The second consideration is the goals of constituents with respect to the issue. What do constituents hope to accomplish in addressing the issue? Potential targets for action are the third consideration in framing an issue. Who will decide the issue? Who can influence those who will decide the issue? The final consideration addresses the question of how leverage can be gained with respect to the issue and suggests direction for the empowerment effort. For example, is legislation the best approach to resolving the issue, or are there other avenues for addressing the issue that would be more effective than legislation? Continuing with the example from Clark et al. (2003), the community health nurse reported the assessment findings to members of the community at large at a community forum. Housing was one issue that cut across all of the focus groups participating in the assessment. The constituency for this issue included most of the members of the community. Potential targets for action, in this case City Council members, members of the County Board of Supervisors, and representatives of the housing authority, were also invited to the community forum. As a result of the forum, a community group was formed, with the support of public officials, to address local housing issues in several ways, including passage of city ordinances that protected tenants from intimidation and exploitation by landlords.

Team Building

Community empowerment is a group effort that requires activity by a team of committed individuals. Team members must not only be committed to the effort but must also have the ability to work effectively as a team. Two aspects of team building involve motivating community participation and actual development of the group.

MOTIVATING COMMUNITY PARTICIPATION Community empowerment, of necessity, requires participation by community members in all facets of issue identification and action to resolve identified issues. Authors have identified eight levels of community participation. The first two levels, manipulation and therapy, actually reflect nonparticipation, in which clients and communities are passive targets of interventions without having input into decisions regarding those interventions. The next three levels reflect token participation: informing the community regarding potential actions or interventions, consulting with members of the community in designing actions, and placating community members by listening to their input but not necessarily incorporating it into decisions. The three last levels of participation are considered true participation and reflect reallocation of power to community members. The first of these is partnership, in which community members and decision makers have joint authority for decisions and action. The second is delegated power, in which the

decision-making authority has delegated power for certain decisions to community members. At the highest level, citizen power, community members have control over the issue and all decisions or intervention programs related to it (Arnstein, cited in Broadnax, 2000). A similar continuum of participation has been identified for consumer involvement in health care delivery from information giving to true empowerment (McKenna & Keeney, 2004).

From an empowerment perspective, the last level of community participation is the most desirable, and movement toward this level should be an ultimate goal of empowerment activity. Participation by community members even at lower levels, however, may be difficult to achieve for a number of reasons (Merzel & D'Afflitti, 2003). Community members may have other competing concerns or uses for their time. For example, one community empowerment initiative centered on the development of community health councils, grassroots groups charged with identifying community health concerns and bringing them to the community collaborative for collective action. In this impoverished community, however, almost all of the adults were working, many at

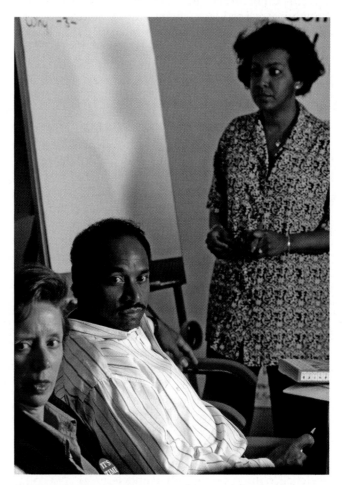

Community empowerment requires participation by diverse segments of the community. (Mark Richards/ PhotoEdit)

BUILDING OUR KNOWLEDGE BASE

*D*esign a study to determine what factors influence the participation of community members in community empowerment initiatives. What type of study would you conduct? What criteria would you use for selection of your subjects and how might you recruit people who meet those criteria to participate in your study? What data collection strategies would you use, and how would you analyze your data? What do you think your findings might indicate, and how could your findings be used to enhance community participation in empowerment activities?

multiple jobs, and had little time to spare for work in the health councils.

Community members may also have different priorities from those of community organizers or health care professionals. If the community empowerment initiative, however, is based on a sound assessment of community needs and assets, social change professionals will be able to identify community priorities and incorporate them into issue selection as discussed earlier.

Another deterrent to community participation may be perceived lack of community control of decisions and resources. This rather fatalistic attitude may be a cultural factor or the result of past experience trying to influence factors affecting community health status. Community members may also have experiences of exploitation by outsiders, which may limit their enthusiasm for community participation activities (Markens, Fox, Taub, & Gilbert, 2002). Use of asset assessment data may help to convince community members of their ability to make changes through participation. Successful resolution of community issues, based on the criteria for issue selection addressed above, will also help to reduce this barrier to participation in subsequent community initiatives. Fears of exploitation will only be resolved by the development of trust and seeing that activities do indeed benefit, rather than exploit, the community.

The volunteer nature of community participation is another factor to be considered. People may agree to participate in initiatives related to specific personal interests but not be interested in continuing to participate in other initiatives. This is why it is particularly important to address the challenge of stability versus change in community empowerment activities. Participants are likely to change over time, and that change must be accommodated without losing the momentum of community empowerment activities.

Finally, widespread participation may be hampered by the lack of sufficient time to engage multiple stakeholders with competing priorities. As noted earlier, one of the challenges in community empowerment is to create shared purposes and values and develop complementary, rather than competing, roles for participating segments of the community. However, this effort takes time that may

not be available in addressing time-sensitive issues. As we noted in Chapter 7∞, there may be a window of opportunity for addressing an issue that requires rapid movement and action within the available time frame.

Even when community members are willing and able to participate in community empowerment activities, they often lack the requisite skills and abilities to do so. There is frequently a need to engage in specific team-building activities to meld a cohesive community group prior to initiating any action. Effective teamwork requires a shared team culture, open communication, and mutual respect and value for the opinions and contributions of others. Development of such a milieu requires the nurturing of group process and the development of group dynamics outside the context of community action related to specific issues (Scholes & Vaughan, 2002). Returning to the housing example, the local neighborhood committee joined forces with a citywide organizing project to work on the issue of safe and affordable housing. At the same time, community residents were invited to participate in a course popularly called "Community Organizing 101," offered by the local university to develop community organizing and empowerment skills. Community health nurses participated as part of the multidisciplinary faculty for the course, assisting residents to identify and strategize to resolve other community health-related issues.

STAGES OF GROUP DEVELOPMENT Group development occurs in a series of stages: orientation, accommodation, negotiation, operation, and dissolution. These stages parallel the components of the nursing process, as indicated in Table 13-2◆. Specific tasks must be accomplished during each stage of group development for the group to function effectively.

Orientation The orientation stage of group development, sometimes referred to as the "forming stage" (Drinka & Clark, 2000), is when group members come to know each other and assess their ability to function as a group. Tasks of this stage include selection of group members, training them for group participation, and identification of group goals and purposes. Also during this stage, the group assesses community empowerment needs and community assets.

Development of group-related skills in the context of community empowerment includes cognitive and

CULTURAL COMPETENCE

*W*hat cultural groups are represented in your community? How might cultural factors affect their participation in community empowerment endeavors? How might you go about motivating the participation of culturally diverse segments of the community in community empowerment activities?

TABLE 13-2   Tasks of Group Development by Stage and Related Nursing Process Component

Nursing Process Component	Stage of Group Development	Group Development Tasks
Assessment and diagnosis	Orientation (forming)	1. Selection of group members 2. Training for group participation 3. Identification of goals and purposes
Planning	Accommodation (norming)	1. Establishment of modes of decision making 2. Development of mechanisms for conflict resolution 3. Development of communication network 4. Development of climate conducive to group collaboration
	Negotiation (norming)	1. Negotiation of member roles 2. Development of methods of task assignment
Implementation	Operation (performing)	1. Assignment of specific tasks to accomplish group goals 2. Performance of actions to accomplish goals
Evaluation	Dissolution (leaving)	1. Planning of evaluative mechanisms for outcomes of action taken 2. Assignment of member roles and tasks in evaluation 3. Data collection 4. Analysis of evaluative findings 5. Possible group dissolution

social interaction skills (Tones & Green, 2004). Cognitive skills required for community members to be empowered include literacy skills and decision-making and problem-solving skills, as well as knowledge of political processes. Requisite social interaction skills include life skills and assertiveness skills as well as skill in talking to policy makers and motivating others. Community health nurses who possess these skills can assist other group members in their development. In addition, community health nurses can educate group members regarding group processes and guide members through the stages of effective group development.

Accommodation   The accommodation (or "norming") stage of group development focuses on the development of group dynamics, the ways in which the group will carry out its group-related functions. This does not relate to activities the group will undertake to resolve any identified community issues, but to the ways in which the group itself will operate. Tasks in this stage include developing an atmosphere conducive to group collaboration and establishing modes of group decision making, conflict resolution, and communication.

Group action requires group decisions, and decisions must be made after careful consideration by group members. To facilitate decision making, group members should agree on the method by which decisions will be made. Because most people are not familiar with group processes or the deliberate need to select a decision-making strategy, the community health nurse may need to guide the group in this task.

Decisions can be made in one of six ways: by default, by the leader, by a subgroup, by majority vote, by consensus, or by unanimous consent. Decisions made by default result from a lack of response by the group. The second method of decision making, in which decisions are made by the leader, is appropriate when a decision cannot wait on the slow-moving democratic process (e.g., when there is an emergency). The group may decide to give the group leader authority to make independent decisions in certain circumstances, but should decide in advance what those circumstances will be. In an effective group, this is not the method used for making most of the group's decisions.

In the third approach to group decision making, group decisions are made by a subgroup. This might involve "railroading," in which the subgroup uses its power and influence to force a decision on other group members. Conversely, the larger group may purposefully delegate the making of certain decisions to a subgroup. Many nursing organizations, for example, delegate authority to an executive board for decisions regarding everyday operation and make only major decisions as a total group.

Majority vote by group members, the fourth method of decision making, is already familiar to us. The fifth method involves consensus or agreement by all group members despite any reservations that individual members might have. Finally, decisions may be made by unanimous consent, in which all group members agree without reservation. In both the consensus and unanimous consent methods, the group may take a relatively long time to reach a decision because of the need for all members to agree. For the purposes of community empowerment, majority vote, consensus, and unanimous consent are the most appropriate methods for group decision making.

Establishing modes of group conflict resolution is the second task in the accommodation stage of group development. Breakdowns in the decision-making process are one source of conflict within the group. Other potential sources of conflict are unclear expectations, poor communication, differing values or attitudes, and competition for scarce resources (Habel, 2000). Lack of clear jurisdiction among group members and conflicts of interest may also be sources of conflict within the group. Additional sources of conflict are interdependence when needs are not met and the existence of prior unresolved conflict between members or subgroups.

Conflict is a normal component of group effort and is to be expected. In fact, many group behavior theorists include a conflict or "storming" stage in describing the development of groups over time (Drinka & Clark, 2000). If the group has developed mechanisms for conflict resolution before conflicts arise, conflict can often be a positive rather than divisive experience for the group.

Recognition of conflict as a normal phenomenon is essential if the group is to plan ahead for conflict resolution. Again, many groups do not anticipate conflict, and when conflict occurs they are unprepared to deal with it. Strategies for resolving conflict constructively involve creating a climate conducive to discussion, identifying and eliminating sources of conflict, capitalizing on areas of agreement, and rationally considering alternative solutions to conflict. The community health nurse can explore these approaches to conflict resolution with members of the group and assist members to select the most appropriate approach.

Creating a climate in which disagreement is acceptable can minimize or resolve conflict. Conflict resolution requires that all parties be fully able to express their perspectives through open communication. Open communication cannot take place when there is pressure to conform and lack of acceptance of different opinions. Lack of communication hampers conflict resolution as well as contributing to conflict. As a group leader, the community health nurse may need to encourage group members to express thoughts and opinions that may not be congruent with those of other members. Through the use of interpersonal skills, the nurse can ensure that communications within the group are not accusatory, but deal with issues rather than personalities.

Recognizing the existence of conflict and identifying its sources and possible solutions are strategies for constructive use of conflict. A conflict that is ignored in the hope that it will resolve itself is likely to become worse. The community health nurse can encourage other group members to acknowledge that a conflict exists and help them explore the reasons for conflict. Again, the nurse should be alert to covert signs of conflict and bring them to the attention of the rest of the group. For example, a nurse working with a group trying to determine budget allocations among health care

programs within the county may notice that representatives of programs for the elderly are maintaining a stony silence during the discussion. The nurse may comment on the fact that they have not participated in the discussion and ask why. In the ensuing discussion, it may be learned that these group members feel that too much money is being allocated to maternal–child health programs and that the elderly are being shortchanged. Once this conflict has been exposed, the group can begin work to resolve it.

Another strategy for resolving conflict involves identifying small areas of trust and agreement between group members that can be expanded. For example, although two group members may disagree on the "appropriate" approach to a problem, they can capitalize on their shared concern for clients' welfare. Finally, rational consideration of alternative solutions to a particular conflict using the group's decision-making process and the problem-solving process can result in conflict becoming a valuable learning experience in group problem solving. The community health nurse can assist the group to explore a variety of alternative solutions to a conflict and to select an approach that is agreeable to all members.

Developing group communication strategies is another task in planning group operation. The importance of an effective communication network cannot be overemphasized. The group must develop a common language that facilitates communication, and members should refrain from using jargon familiar only to members of their own discipline. When it is necessary to use terminology unfamiliar to others, efforts should be made to translate it into the common language. The nurse in this situation can either play the part of the translator or ask other members for clarification. For example, some members of a group may use acronyms unfamiliar to others, such as CMS. The nurse should then explain to the group that this stands for the Centers for Medicare and Medicaid Services. If the nurse does not recognize the acronym, he or she would ask for an explanation of its meaning.

The group should also agree on the form that communication will take. For example, communications may be verbal, written, or a combination of both, depending on the situation. Perhaps the group will decide that communication with sponsoring institutions should take the form of formal written memoranda, whereas communications between group members should be more informal verbal messages.

Consideration should also be given to the fact that communication takes place outside of regular group sessions. The content of these informal encounters between group members should not undermine group function or provide a forum for airing grievances or denigrating other members. The community health nurse who encounters unproductive communication outside of group meetings can bring relevant issues to the attention of the entire group so open discussion can take place and conflict can be avoided or resolved.

Establishing a climate in which group members feel respected and in which differences are accepted contributes to an effective communication network. This means that all group members should be encouraged to participate and should receive positive reinforcement for their contribution whether or not others agree with it. In the beginning of the group's operation, the nurse group leader may need to ask reluctant group members for their ideas and opinions. As their participation is received positively, they will begin to volunteer remarks.

Negotiation Tasks of the negotiation stage of group development include role negotiation and methods of task assignment. Professional roles often overlap, and role negotiation is crucial to effective group function. In addition, social change professionals working in a community empowerment context need to be careful not to usurp roles that should be performed by community members. The goal of community organizing and empowerment is to develop leadership within the community, not to provide that leadership (Pilisuk, McAllister, Rothman, & Larin, 2005). When two or more group members possess similar skills, the group must decide who will be responsible for exercising those skills. These decisions may be made as a general rule of thumb, so that one member always has responsibility for certain activities, or may change with the needs of the situation.

One particular group role that must be negotiated is the role of leader. This position incorporates functions related to group administration, liaison with outside groups, teaching, and coordination of group effort. Additional team leadership roles may include providing information for group decision making, clarifying issues, refocusing the group's attention, and playing "devil's advocate" to promote exploration of alternative ideas. The leadership role may be assigned to one member, may shift with the situation, or may reside with the group as a whole. In the last instance, no one member acts as the leader, and leadership functions are performed by the group as a unit.

Operation and Dissolution The operation stage of group development is analogous to the implementation stage of the nursing process. It is during this stage that the group assigns and performs specific roles and tasks to achieve group-designated goals and objectives.

The dissolution stage of group development focuses on evaluation of the group's accomplishments and decisions regarding the continuation or dissolution of the group. Depending on the focus of group empowerment initiatives, the group may shift its focus to address other community issues after achieving its original purpose. Or it may dissolve to reform with other participants to address additional issues. Tasks of the dissolution stage of group development include

planning evaluative mechanisms related to both the process and outcomes of community empowerment, assignment of member roles in evaluation, data collection and analysis, and dissemination of findings. Evaluation of community empowerment activities will be discussed in more detail later in this chapter.

Coalition Development

The advantages and disadvantages of coalitions and the steps in their development were presented in Chapter 7∞. A coalition is "an organization of individuals representing diverse organizations, factions, or constituencies who agree to work together in order to achieve a common goal" (Wandersman, Goodman, & Butterfoss, 2005, p. 293). In the context of community empowerment, coalition development consists of four components: resource acquisition, development of a maintenance subsystem, production, and goal attainment (Prestby & Wandersman, as cited in Wandersman et al., 2005). Resource acquisition involves recruiting coalition members as well as acquiring external resources. The maintenance subsystem consists of the organizational control structure described in Chapter 7∞ and strategies to maintain member commitment and mobilize members' resources. The production component involves action strategies to facilitate community empowerment and maintenance of the coalition's internal structure (e.g., disseminating meeting minutes, promoting communication between members). The goal attainment component is relatively self-explanatory except that it also includes development of a "track record" of successes in community empowerment.

Because of their varied interests and interactions in the community, community health nurses can be particularly helpful in identifying potential coalition members and initiating contacts with potential members. For example, because of her role as a member of the advisory committee for a home health agency, the community health nurse may be acquainted with individuals and organizations that would be interested in collaborating on efforts to provide transportation services for disabled individuals.

Implementation Strategies

Implementation of community empowerment activities encompasses the basic principles of implementing any community program. These principles will be discussed in detail in Chapter 15∞. Here we will briefly address two possible strategies that may be used in implementation, media advocacy and the use of community workers.

Media Advocacy

According to the U.S. Department of Health and Human Service (USDHHS), **media advocacy** is defined as "strategic use of mass media to advance a social or public policy agenda" (Wallack, 2005, p. 423). Media advocacy was discussed in the context of public policy development in Chapter 7∞. It is appropriate to make a few more comments about media advocacy as it relates to community empowerment. Media advocacy fulfills the function of drawing attention to an issue and promoting its inclusion in a policy agenda. Attention may also be drawn to the power inequities among segments of society, setting the stage for empowerment initiatives.

A second function of media advocacy is to focus attention on factors contributing to issues of concern (Wallack, 2005). In the context of community empowerment, media coverage may also highlight causal factors in power inequities and suggest ways to empower communities. Finally, media advocacy may be used to advance a particular strategy as a solution to an identified problem. In the case of community empowerment, that might entail policy strategies that empower communities. For example, media coverage might highlight the lack of community involvement in community planning decisions and advocate appointment of community representatives as members of the local planning board as a strategy for addressing the problem. As another example, a community health nurse might help to organize a "tent city" media event with tents pitched in local parks to highlight the plight of low-income renters being displaced by high-income condominium conversions. Community health nurses can cultivate media contacts and identify areas of interest of specific media. Then when an issue requires media attention, the nurse can assist community residents to develop newsworthy perspectives to be shared with radio, television, or newspaper personnel.

Using Community Workers

The concept of community member participation in all facets of community empowerment, from assessment to evaluation, was presented earlier. Community

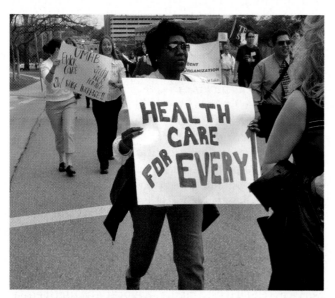

Protests or marches may be one way of raising consciousness regarding important health issues. (© Bob Daemmrich/The Image Works)

> ## Think Advocacy
> Gunther (2005) described 10 principles for effective advocacy campaigns. These principles are:
>
> - Communicate values underlying the advocacy initiative.
> - Frame discourse in an oppositional framework in which people can be *against* something.
> - Focus on winning over those who are undecided regarding an issue.
> - Project confidence and take the high moral ground to persuade the undecided.
> - Aggressively confront opposition. Identify them and attack their motives.
> - Convince target audiences that they, as individuals, can make a difference.
> - Minimize campaign costs by focusing on opinion leaders who will further disseminate your position to others.
> - Project responsible extremism, rather than reasonable moderation, to influence the media.
> - Don't stop with passage of the law or problem resolution; your position will most likely need to be reiterated and defended on an ongoing basis.
> - Strategic diversity in approaches is critical to successful advocacy, with multiple independent advocacy campaigns focused on the same issue (e.g., within different cultural or ethnic groups or other target audiences).
>
> Examine a community organization issue in your area. How might these principles of effective advocacy be implemented in the process?

participation in the implementation phase of empowerment activities may be particularly critical to their success. Many times this participation may involve using natural helpers, as described earlier in the chapter, or training and using community health workers (CHWs). As we saw earlier, community members often do not have the time to participate in community empowerment activities on a volunteer basis. However, when community members have paid employment as community workers, the dual goals of community empowerment and personal economic development can be achieved.

Community health workers are "carefully chosen community members who participate in training that enables them to promote health in their own communities" (Farquhar, Michael, & Wiggins, 2005, p. 597). Use of CHWs in community empowerment, as well as in health care delivery programs, necessitates training them as resources for peers, linking them to service providers and community leaders, and supporting them in actions to resolve community problems (Eng & Parker, 2002). Use of CHWs has been found to be effective in a variety of situations outside of community empowerment activities. For example, in one study, use of CHWs led to a reduction in asthma symptom days and urgent-care service use and improved quality-of-life scores for children with asthma (Krieger, Takaro,

Song, & Weaver, 2005). Similarly, CHWs have been found to be effective in both Latino and African American communities in promoting a variety of health-related initiatives (Farquhar et al., 2005).

Community health workers can serve a variety of functions in community empowerment. They can be instrumental in conducting assets and needs assessments, particularly in eliciting the perspectives of usually silent segments of a community (e.g., ethnic minority group members, immigrants, and refugees, as well as the elderly). They can also help identify other potential community leaders and recruit them to participate in community empowerment activities. Community health workers can help to educate community members and mobilize support for empowerment activities during the implementation stage of community empowerment initiatives. Finally, they can be actively involved in the design, implementation, and analysis of evaluative findings related to the effectiveness of community empowerment activities.

Evaluating Community Empowerment

Evaluation of community empowerment is another area that should involve community members as participants in all phases, from conceptualizing the evaluation, to data collection and analysis, to dissemination and use of evaluative findings. Community participation in evaluation helps to continue to build community competence while assessing the outcomes of prior activities. **Participatory evaluation** is defined as "a partnership approach to evaluation that engages those who have a stake in the project, program, or initiative in all aspects of evaluation design and implementation" (Coombe, 2005, pp. 368–369).

Participatory evaluation has several benefits. First, it tends to help overcome resistance to the evaluation among those whose activities are being evaluated. Second, participatory evaluation enhances the integration of both qualitative and quantitative evaluation methods because of the broader backgrounds, expertise, and interests of multiple participants. Participatory evaluation also promotes innovation in methods because community members often view evaluative questions or data collection from a different perspective than health care professionals or evaluation experts. In addition, participatory evaluation enhances the ability of the community to systematically collect and make sense of data. Finally, participatory evaluation links community members and evaluation professionals in partnerships that foster mutual learning (Coombe, 2005). Basic principles of participatory evaluation include the following:

- Community participation and ownership of the evaluation activity
- Collaboration among all stakeholders with commensurate responsibility for the evaluation
- Findings that promote change on multiple levels
- Transforming power relationships with community members in control of the evaluation (Cousins & Whitmore, as cited in Coombe, 2005)

Steps in participatory or empowering evaluation are similar to those in any evaluation process except that community participation is integral in each step. The basic steps are: (a) taking stock of community status, resources, capacities, challenges, and programs resulting from empowerment activities; (b) setting goals for the evaluation; (c) developing evaluation strategies; and (d) documenting the evaluation process and findings (Roe, Roe, Carpenter, & Sibley, 2005).

Given sufficient time and resources, both the process and the outcomes of empowerment should be evaluated. Evaluation can focus on the internal dynamics of the empowerment process, the abilities of community members to partner with others and bring in resources, and/or the direct or indirect health effects of empowerment (Minkler & Wallerstein, 2005). Since increased community capacity or competence is one of the anticipated outcomes of empowerment, one can examine several different levels of capacity indicators: population indicators, program-specific indicators, and community capacity indicators (Labonte & Laverack, 2001). Population indicators might be such things as access to health care services as a result of community empowerment efforts, or the election of one or more community members to decision-making bodies. Program-specific indicators will differ depending on the issues selected as vehicles for community empowerment. For example, if the issue selected relates to access to and use of immunization services, community immunization levels would be an appropriate program-related indicator. Community capacity indicators would be measures of the domains of community capacity discussed earlier in the chapter. For example, what is the extent of participation in community initiatives as a result of empowerment activities? Have community members stepped forward to assume leadership roles in community initiatives? How well are they performing in a leadership role? Are there organizational structures present in the community whereby community members can provide input into decisions that affect their community and their lives? To what extent are

---

EVIDENCE-BASED PRACTICE

*I*n the chapter, we noted two studies of the use of community health workers (CHWs) and their effectiveness in achieving community health-related goals (Farquhar et al., 2005; Krieger et al., 2005). Seek out additional literature related to the use of CHWs. Do the balance of studies indicate their effectiveness or their ineffectiveness? If the research literature supports the effectiveness of CHWs as described in the chapter, how might the CHW concept be incorporated into community health initiatives in your community?

community members able to mobilize internal and external resources to address areas of concern? These and other questions can be used to assess community progress in each of the domains of community capacity.

A final measure of the effectiveness of community empowerment efforts would be the extent to which community members are included in policy making. The ultimate goal of effective community organizing and empowerment should be the inclusion of community members in every aspect of policy making (Blackwell, Minkler, & Thompson, 2005).

COMMUNITY HEALTH NURSING AND COMMUNITY EMPOWERMENT

Community health nurses can be active proponents of and participants in community empowerment. Unfortunately, in the past, community health nurses and other health professionals have been guilty of imposing their values and perceptions of need on communities rather than empowering communities to act for their own benefit (Broadnax, 2000). In a British study of general practitioners (GPs), community health nurses, and the general public, 100% of GPs and members of the public and 97% of community health nurses agreed that work toward community empowerment was a critical role for community health nurses, but one for which they are largely unprepared. Study recommendations included the need for community health nurses to ask community members what they want with respect to their health. The authors also recommended work by community health nurses to increase public involvement in the planning and delivery of health services, involve consumers in community capacity building, and motivate policy makers to include community members as equal participants in decision making (McKenna & Keeney, 2004).

Health care professionals, including community health nurses, play an advisory and facilitative role in community empowerment. This role is temporary and catalytic (Anderson et al., 2002). As noted earlier, the purpose of community empowerment is to develop leadership within the community rather than to lead. The influence of community health nurses in community empowerment lies in enactment of three roles: discovery, decision, and drive (Henton et al., 2004). The discovery role involves making community members aware of the need for empowerment and building a compelling case for change in the status quo. Because of their visibility in and knowledge of the community, community health nurses are admirably situated to identify community problems and to promote community participation in their resolution. In the decision role, community health nurses assist community members to determine potential alternative strategies, to evaluate them, and to select the strategies most likely to contribute to achievement of community-identified goals. In the drive role, community health nurses assist in mobilizing the community for change.

Core functions of community empowerment practice for community health nurses include initiating dialogue, building community capacity, connecting community groups to larger organizations, promoting media advocacy, and promoting group cohesion (Pilisuk et al., 2005). Additional functions include consciousness raising, assistance in policy formation, and political advocacy. In essence, the community health nurse acts as "a motivational catalyst to initiate or precipitate a desire to bring about community-endorsed health reform" (Whitehead, 2003, p. 671). As we saw at the beginning of this chapter, effective community empowerment is the ultimate outcome of community health nursing advocacy.

Case Study

Indigent Health Care

You have been given a referral to visit Mrs. Esparza, who lost her baby after a premature delivery. The address you have been given is located in a poor neighborhood that houses a large number of migrant workers. When you arrive at the home, you discover that it is a two-bedroom apartment occupied by three couples and their five children. Both Mrs. Esparza and her husband are present when you arrive, and both are obviously grieving the loss of their third child. In talking with them, you discover that Mrs. Esparza did not receive any prenatal care and was admitted to the delivery unit of the local hospital after going to the emergency room when she experienced heavy contractions in the 29th week of her pregnancy. Mr. Esparza becomes angry when you ask about prenatal care, shouting that they tried to get an appointment at the health department's prenatal clinic but were

told there was a 2-month wait for new appointments. At that time Mrs. Esparza was in the 5th month of her pregnancy. In tears, he informs you that they did not have the money to see a private doctor. Even though most of the migrant workers are in the United States legally, they are not eligible for any financial assistance. Your state does not provide Medicaid pregnancy coverage for nonresident women. Mrs. Esparza reminds her husband that they are not alone in their suffering. When you inquire further into her comment, she tells you that seven other women in the apartment complex have lost babies at some point in their pregnancies in the last 2 years. You comfort the family as best you can, make arrangements for Mrs. Esparza to receive a postpartum examination at the health department, and refer the three families to the immunization clinic because all of the children in the home are behind on their immunizations. You explain that both postpartum services and immunizations are free to those who do not have money to pay for them, even for nonresidents.

When you return to the office, fellow community health nurses describe similar visits to families in the area. In checking county vital statistics, you note that the census track where the Esparzas live and two adjacent areas that house large migrant populations have a fetal death rate three times that of the rest of the county.

1. How would you begin to empower the migrant worker community to address the issue of lack of access to prenatal care?
2. What assets might you look for within the migrant community to address the issue?
3. What allies might you find in the nonmigrant community to assist you?
4. How can you motivate participation by community members in the initiative?

Test Your Understanding

1. What is the relationship of community empowerment to similar concepts such as community organization, community building, community competence, and community capacity? (pp. 298–299)

2. What are the levels at which community empowerment occurs? (p. 300)

3. What are the similarities and differences among the community empowerment models discussed in the chapter? Select one of the models discussed and describe how it might be used to foster community empowerment in your own community. (pp. 300–303)

4. What are the elements in the process of organizing for community empowerment? Give an example of each element as it might apply to your own community. (pp. 303–309)

5. What criteria might you use to evaluate the effectiveness of community empowerment in your community? (pp. 311–312)

6. What is the role of the community health nurse in community empowerment? (p. 312)

EXPLORE MediaLink

http://www.prenhall.com/clark
Resources for this chapter can be found on the Companion Website.

Audio Glossary
Exam Review Questions
Case Study: Planned Change

MediaLink Application: Grassroots
  Organizing (video)
Media Links

Challenge Your Knowledge
Advocacy Interviews

References

Anderson, D., Guthrie, T., & Schirle, R. (2002). A nursing model of community organization for change. *Public Health Nursing, 19,* 40–46.

Askey, R. (2004). Case management: A critical review. *Mental Health Practice, 7*(8), 12–16.

Billings, J. R. (2000). Community development: A critical review of approaches to evaluation. *Journal of Advanced Nursing, 31,* 472–480.

Blackwell, A. G., & Colmenar, R. A. (2005). Principles of community building. In M. Minkler (Ed.), *Community organizing and community building for health* (2nd ed., pp. 436–437). New Brunswick, NJ: Rutgers University Press.

Blackwell, A. G., Minkler, M., & Thompson, M. (2005). Using community organizing and community building to influence policy. In M. Minkler (Ed.), *Community organizing and community building for health* (2nd ed., pp. 405–418). New Brunswick, NJ: Rutgers University Press.

Broadnax, P. A. (2000). *Integrating a systems perspective into leadership development of senior nursing students in community-based health care environments.* Columbus, MS: Institute for Nursing Leadership.

Butler, J. T. (2001). *Principles of health education and health promotion* (3rd ed.). Stamford, CT: Wadsworth.

Clark, M. J., Cary, S., Diemert, G., Ceballos, R., Sifuentes, M., Atteberry, I., Vue, F., & Trieu, S. (2003). Involving communities in community assessment. *Public Health Nursing, 20,* 456–463.

Coombe, C. M. (2005). Participatory evaluation: Building community while assessing change. In M. Minkler (Ed.), *Community organizing and community building for health* (2nd ed., pp. 368–385). New Brunswick, NJ: Rutgers University Press.

Drevdahl, D. (2002). Social justice or market justice? The paradoxes of public health partnerships with managed care. *Public Health Nursing, 19,* 161–169.

Drinka, T. J. K., & Clark, P. G. (2000). *Health care teamwork: Interdisciplinary practice and teaching*. Westport, CT: Auburn House.

Eng, E., & Parker, E. (2002). Natural helper models to enhance a community's health and competence. In R. J. DiClemente, R. A. Crosby, & M. C. Kegler (Eds.), *Emerging theories in health promotion practice and research: Strategies for improving public health* (pp. 126–156). San Francisco: Jossey-Bass.

Farquhar, S. A., Michael, Y. L., & Wiggins, N. (2005). Building on leadership and social capital to create change in 2 urban communities. *American Journal of Public Health, 95*, 596–601.

Gunther, H. C. (2005). Ten principles of effective advocacy campaigns. In M. Minkler (Ed.), *Community organizing and community building for health* (2nd ed., pp. 462–463). New Brunswick, NJ: Rutgers University Press.

Habel, M. (2000). *Developing your leadership potential*. Sunnyvale, CA: NurseWeek.

Hancock, T., & Minkler, M. (2005). Community health assessment or healthy community assessment: Whose community? Whose health? Whose assessment? In M. Minkler (Ed.), *Community organizing and community building for health* (2nd ed., pp. 138–157). New Brunswick, NJ: Rutgers University Press.

Henton, G., Melville, J., & Walesh, K. (2004). *Civil revolutionaries: Igniting the passion for change in America's cities*. San Francisco, Jossey-Bass.

Kennedy, M. G., & Crosby, R. A. (2002). Prevention marketing: An emerging integrated framework. In R. J. DiClemente, R. A. Crosby, & M. C. Kegler (Eds.), *Emerging theories in health promotion practice and research: Strategies for improving public health* (pp. 255–284). San Francisco: Jossey-Bass.

Krieger, J. W., Takaro, T. K., Song, L., & Weaver, M. (2005). The Seattle-King County Healthy Homes Project: A randomized, controlled trial of a community health worker intervention to decrease exposure to indoor asthma triggers. *American Journal of Public Health, 95*, 652–659.

Labonte, R., & Laverack, G. (2001). Capacity building in health promotion, Part I: For whom? And for what purpose? *Critical Public Health, 2*, 111–127.

Laverack, G. (2004). *Health promotion practice: Power and empowerment*. Thousand Oaks, CA: Sage.

Lavery, S. H., Smith, M. L., Esparza, A. A., Hrushow, A., Moore, M., & Reed, D. F. (2005). The community action model: A community-driven model designed to address disparities in health. *American Journal of Public Health, 95*, 611–616.

Markens, S., Fox, S. A., Taub, B., & Gilbert, M. L. (2002). Role of black churches in health promotion programs: Lessons from the Los Angeles Mammography Promotion in Churches Program. *American Journal of Public Health, 92*, 805–810.

May, K. M., Phillips, L. R., Ferketich, S. L., & Verran, J. A. (2003). Public health nursing: The generalist in a specialized environment. *Public Health Nursing, 20*, 252–259.

McKenna, H., & Keeney, S. (2004). Community nursing: Health professional and public perceptions. *Journal of Advanced Nursing, 48*, 17–25.

McKnight, J. L., & Kretzmann, J. P. (2005). Mapping community capacity. In M. Minkler (Ed.), *Community organizing and community building for health* (2nd ed., pp. 158–172). New Brunswick, NJ: Rutgers University Press.

Merzel, C., & D'Afflitti, J. (2003). Reconsidering community-based health promotion: Promise, performance, and potential. *American Journal of Public Health, 93*, 557–574.

Minkler, M. (2005). Introduction to community organizing and community building. In M. Minkler (Ed.), *Community organizing and community building for health* (2nd ed., pp. 1–21). New Brunswick, NJ: Rutgers University Press.

Minkler, M., & Pies, C. (2005). Ethical issues and practical dilemmas. In M. Minkler (Ed.), *Community organizing and community building for health* (2nd ed., pp. 116–137). New Brunswick, NJ: Rutgers University Press.

Minkler, M., & Wallerstein, N. (2005). Improving health through community organization and community building. In M. Minkler (Ed.), *Community organizing and community building for health* (2nd ed., pp. 26–50). New Brunswick, NJ: Rutgers University Press.

Norton, B. L., McLeroy, K. R., Burdine, J. N., Felix, M. R. J., & Dorsey, A. M. (2002). Community capacity: Concept, theory, and methods. In R. J. DiClemente, R. A. Crosby, & M. C. Kegler (Eds.), *Emerging theories in health promotion practice and research: Strategies for improving public health* (pp. 194–227). San Francisco: Jossey-Bass.

Ogilvie, L., Allen, M., Laryea, J., & Opare, M. (2003). Building capacity through a collaborative international nursing project. *Journal of Nursing Scholarship, 35*, 113–118.

Pilisuk, M., McAllister, J., Rothman, J., & Larin, L. (2005). New contexts of organizing: Functions, challenges, and solutions. In M. Minkler (Ed.), *Community organizing and community building for health* (2nd ed., pp. 97–115). New Brunswick, NJ: Rutgers University Press.

Roe, K, M, Roe, K., Carpenter, C. G., & Sibley, C. B. (2005). Community building through empowering evaluation. In M. Minkler (Ed.), *Community organizing and community building for health* (2nd ed., pp. 386–404). New Brunswick, NJ: Rutgers University Press.

Rubin, H. J. (2000). *Renewing hope within neighborhoods of despair: The community-based development model*. Albany, NY: State University of New York Press.

Scholes, J., & Vaughan, B. (2002). Cross-boundary work: Implications for the multiprofessional team. *Journal of Clinical Nursing, 11*, 399–408.

Staples, L. (2005). Selecting and cutting the issue. In M. Minkler (Ed.), *Community organizing and community building for health* (2nd ed., pp. 173–192). New Brunswick, NJ: Rutgers University Press.

Tones, K., & Green, J. (2004). *Health promotion: Planning and strategies*. Thousand Oaks, CA: Sage.

Uys, L. R., Majumdar, B., & Gwele, N. (2004). The Kwazulu-Natal health promotion model. *Journal of Nursing Scholarship, 36*, 192–196.

Wallack, L. (2005). Media advocacy: A strategy for empowering people and communities. In M. Minkler (Ed.), *Community organizing and community building for health* (2nd ed., pp. 419–432). New Brunswick, NJ: Rutgers University Press.

Wallerstein, N. (2002). Empowerment to reduce health disparities. *Scandinavian Journal of Public Health, 30*, 72–77.

Wandersman, A., Goodman, R. M., & Butterfoss, F. D. (2005). Understanding coalitions and how they operate as organizations. In M. Minkler (Ed.), *Community organizing and community building for health* (2nd ed., pp. 292–313). New Brunswick, NJ: Rutgers University Press.

Westbrook, L. O., & Schultz, P. (2000). From theory to practice: Community health nursing in a public health neighborhood team. *Advances in Nursing Science, 23*(2), 50–61.

Whitehead, D. (2003). Incorporating sociopolitical health promotion activities in clinical practice. *Journal of Clinical Nursing, 12*, 668–677.

Unit III

Care of Special Populations

Advocacy in Action

Reconnecting Family

Steve had been estranged from his family for a long time for reasons that were unclear to us. When he came to the Nurses Center at St. Agnes for health care, we found him to be a very gracious, polite young man in his 30's. Steve presented complaining of hemoptysis, and soon after examining him we concluded that he needed extensive diagnostics and treatment. Steve did not realize that he had health insurance through Medicare, nor did he know how to access it. With the help of center staff, Steve was connected with a physician who accepted his insurance and welcomed Steve as a patient. Although we discontinued our treatment of Steve at that time, he periodically stopped in at the Nurses Center to

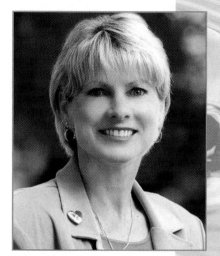

express his gratitude and give us updates on his condition. Steve was diagnosed with lung cancer, and although the prognosis was poor, he was accepting treatment. At the time, Steve was living in the homeless shelter system. One of the community health nurses facilitated contact with his uncle, who took Steve in and cared for him until he died a couple of months later. Over that period Steve became reacquainted with other family members. The staff at the Nurses Center never lost touch with Steve and sent him many get-well cards with their thoughts and good wishes. Steve died having been given the opportunity to reunite with his family.

After his death, a note with a check enclosed arrived at the Center from Steve's sisters. They thanked the nurses for caring for their brother and communicated how grateful Steve was for having come in contact with the Nurses Center. The check was a donation made in Steve's memory to help us continue to help individuals and families such as Steve's.

Maryanne Lieb, RN, MSN

Director, Nurses Center at St. Agnes

Clinical Professor, Villanova University

Care of Families

CHAPTER OBJECTIVES

After reading this chapter, you should be able to:

1. Describe at least five family types and their characteristic features.
2. Describe elements of at least one theoretical model applied to families.
3. Identify family assessment considerations in the biophysical, psychological, physical environmental, sociocultural, behavioral, and health system dimensions.
4. Differentiate between formal and informal family roles.
5. Differentiate between situational and maturational crises.
6. Discuss family-focused intervention at the primary, secondary, and tertiary levels of prevention.

KEY TERMS

binuclear family **319**
cohabiting family **320**
crisis **331**
dual-earner family **318**
ecomap **325**
extended family **318**
family **318**
family development **323**
family life cycle **323**
family resilience **330**
foster families **320**
gay or lesbian family **320**
genogram **325**
grandparent-headed family **320**
hardiness **330**
maturational crisis **332**
nuclear conjugal family **318**
nuclear dyads **318**
role conflict **333**
role overload **333**
roles **333**
single-parent family **319**
situational crisis **332**
stepfamily **319**

 MediaLink
http://www.prenhall.com/clark

Additional interactive resources for this chapter can be found on the Companion Website. Click on Chapter 14 and "Begin" to select the activities for this chapter.

The family is the oldest and most persistent of all social institutions, but it has changed radically in the last few decades in terms of its structure and role functions (Giorgianni, 2003). Family has been defined as "a group of two or more persons who are related by birth, marriage, or adoption" (Hofferth, 2003b, p. 71), but this definition does not encompass some of the nontraditional family forms. For our purposes, a **family** is a social system consisting of two or more people who define themselves as a family and who share bonds of emotional closeness (Friedman, Bowden, & Jones, 2003).

This broad definition of family suggests that the principles of community health nursing applied to family clients must be flexible enough to meet the needs of many different family forms.

TYPES OF FAMILIES

Families come in multiple sizes and configurations, each characterized by certain structural features and facing certain unique stresses. The role and structure of the family has evolved over time to meet the needs of the current environment (Giorgianni, 2003). Factors underlying these changes include delayed age at marriage, increasing cohabitation, increasing single parenthood, the movement of women into the workforce, and delayed and declining fertility and mortality, with fewer children born and more older persons living longer (Casper & Bianchi, 2002). Critical attributes of families include existence as a system or unit, a sense of commitment or attachment that results in obligation among members, and performance of basic caregiving functions of protection, nourishment, and socialization. Attributes previously considered integral to the concept of family, such as the presence of children and being related or living together, may or may not be found in today's varied family structures (Wright & Leahy, 2005). Among the family forms encountered by community health nurses in today's world are the traditional nuclear family, extended families, single-parent families, stepfamilies, cohabiting families, gay and lesbian families, grandparent-headed families, foster families, and fragmentary families. Each of these family types will be briefly discussed here.

Nuclear Conjugal Families

The **nuclear conjugal family**, or, more simply, the nuclear family, is composed of husband, wife, and children (Casper & Bianchi, 2002). Husband and wife are joined by marriage and their children are either biological offspring or adopted. The nuclear family is found in all ethnic and socioeconomic groups and is sanctioned by all religions. In the past, this type of family has been accepted as a social institution necessary to raise children properly. Today, the nuclear conjugal family is becoming less common in response to societal changes.

In 2003, for example, there were more than 75.5 million families in the United States. Only 34% of those households consisted of a married couple with children under 18 years of age. Slightly over 40% of U.S. families are **nuclear dyads**, married couples without children under 18 years of age living in the home (U.S. Census Bureau, 2005). Nuclear dyads may result from choice, infertility, or movement of grown children out of the household.

Nuclear families may also include adopted children. Children may be adopted because a couple is unable to have children of their own or in addition to the children born to the couple. In some cases, adopted children were part of the extended family of one partner or the other (e.g., children of a brother or sister who is deceased or unable to care for them). In other instances, the adopted children have no previous relationship to the adoptive family. Any addition of a new family member will require adaptation and changes in family relationships and roles. When children are adopted beyond infancy, however, there may be additional stresses faced as the child adapts to vastly changed circumstances and the family accommodates to a virtual stranger in their midst. Biracial adoptive families may face even more stresses if the culture in which the family exists attaches stigma to racial intermingling. These families may be in particular need of advocacy on the part of the community health nurse to help them deal with the effects of racial prejudice. For example, the community health nurse might link the family to other biracial families who can provide support.

Another variant of the nuclear family is the **dual-earner family**, which consists of two working parents with or without children. Dual-earner families may exist because of the need for increased income or as a result of women marrying later and developing a commitment to careers that continue after initiating a family (Casper & Bianchi, 2002). In 2000, for example, both parents worked in 64% of two-parent families with children (Fellmeth, 2003).

Extended Families

The **extended family** includes family members other than spouses and children, such as grandparents, aunts, uncles, and cousins. Extended families may also include stepkin in the case of stepfamilies (Wright & Leahy, 2005). Traditionally, extended families either shared household expenses and tasks or lived in close proximity and provided mutual support. Many extended families live in multigenerational households, but the extent of multigenerational living varies considerably by race and ethnicity. For example, during 1997 to 1999, the percentage of men in multigenerational households ranged from 12% among white men to 23% among black men, with Hispanic men in between at 21%. Among women, percentages of persons living in multigenerational households were 11.5%, 22%, and 21%, respectively (Casper & Bianchi, 2002).

Like the nuclear family, the extended family has been affected by societal change. In the past, members of extended families often lived in close proximity to the nuclear family. But owing to increased mobility and the enticement of better jobs in other areas, families are more likely to live away from their extended kin network. Thus, the extended family is now more likely to be a long-distance unit with whom the nuclear family corresponds and visits. This phenomenon has limited the social, economic, and emotional support formerly available to members of a nuclear family from older and more experienced relatives.

As time passes and circumstances change, the nuclear family may take extended family members into the home. This typically occurs as a consequence of the early marriage of children, where the newlyweds must live with parents or when adult children return home following a divorce, an economic setback, or some other life crisis. Some adult children remain in the home due to economic constraints and older age at marriage. New living arrangements to incorporate extended family members into the nuclear family can also occur when aging parents can no longer live alone. The parent of a grown child may present adjustment problems for the nuclear family that has been separated from the parent for some time.

Single-Parent Families

Single-parent families are among the most common family units encountered by community health nurses. A **single-parent family** consists of an adult woman or man and children. Single-parent families result from divorce, nonmarital pregnancies, the absence or death of a spouse, or adoption by a single person. In 2003, 28% of U.S. households with children under 18 years of age were single-parent households. Most of these households (81%) were headed by women, although the number of single-parent families headed by men is increasing each year and has more than tripled since 1980. The relative proportion of single-parent households varies among ethnic groups. In 2003, for example, 22% of White families in the United States were single-parent families, compared to 58% of African American families

and 30% of Hispanic families. Women as single parents outnumber men by at least four to one in each of the three groups (U.S. Census Bureau, 2005).

Single-parent families are characterized by increasing poverty and role changes, role overload, and role conflict for the single parent. Research has indicated that children in single-parent families are generally worse off than their counterparts in two-parent families, particularly with respect to behavior problems (Giorgianni, 2003). In 2003, 28% of female-headed and 13.5% of male-headed single-parent families had incomes below federal poverty levels (U.S. Census Bureau, 2004). Single mothers, in particular, often work for low wages and have difficulty working in full-time positions because of childcare demands (Ellwood & Jencks, 2004).

Single parenthood occurs in other nations as well. For example, the extent of single-mother households in Europe ranges from 21% in the United Kingdom to 5% in Spain and Italy. Several of these countries, unlike the United States, have systems designed to support these mothers and their families. In these countries, social transfer funding (welfare) often contributes a significant portion of the income of single-parent families (Rainwater & Smeeding, 2004). As we will see later in this chapter, welfare reform strategies have placed an even greater burden on these families in the United States.

Stepfamilies

Stepfamilies are increasingly evident in American society. A **stepfamily** is composed of two adults, at least one of whom has remarried following divorce or the death of a spouse and at least one of whom has children from a prior relationship. Stepfamilies can include children from either adult's previous marriage, as well as offspring from the new marriage. In 2001, nearly four of every 1,000 persons in the United States sought a divorce (U.S. Census Bureau, 2005), and approximately 75% of divorced persons remarry. It is estimated that 43% of marriages include at least one spouse who has been married before (Wright & Leahy, 2005).

The propensity for divorce and remarriage creates large numbers of new stepfamilies each year. Other terms used for stepfamilies include *blended, remarried,* or *reconstituted* families. The extended kin network of a stepfamily can include stepgrandparents, stepaunts, stepuncles, and stepcousins, as well as an ex-spouse who is the biological parent of some of the children but no longer a part of the household. The existence of stepfamilies may also contribute to the creation of a **binuclear family**, in which a child is a member of two nuclear households as a result of a joint-custody arrangement or visitation rights following the divorce of the child's parents.

Stepfamilies face a number of unique challenges related to limited family loyalty, complexity of family interactions, preexisting parent–child coalitions, differences in the balance of power, multiple parental figures

---

BUILDING OUR KNOWLEDGE BASE

A study of the effects of multigenerational families in Japan found that women living in multigenerational families had more caregiving concerns but fewer concerns about finances and future health status than women in nuclear families. Women in multigenerational families also drank less and were less likely to smoke, but were more sedentary than other women. For men, living in multigenerational families was associated with increased smoking (Takeda et al., 2003). How would you design a study to determine if multigenerational family living has similar effects in other cultural groups? What other outcome variables might you explore in your study? What contributions might your findings make to community health nursing practice with families?

for children, and ambiguous family boundaries (Wright & Leahey, 2005). Complex relationships with extended kin networks and former spouses and unrealistic expectations of family relationships may further complicate life for members of stepfamilies.

Cohabiting Families

A **cohabiting family** consists of a man and a woman living together without being married. Individuals who choose cohabitation range in age from teens to retired elderly persons. The reasons cited for preferring this arrangement include the desire for a "trial marriage," the increased safety of living with another, and financial necessity. Cohabitation is becoming more prevalent in the United States. During the mid-1990s, for example, 56% of first marriages were preceded by cohabitation. From 1978 to 1998, the number of women cohabiting at any given point in time tripled from 3% to 9%, and the number of cohabiting men more than doubled to 12% (Casper & Bianchi, 2002). In 2000, there were 5.4 million unmarried partner households in the United States (U.S. Census Bureau, 2005).

The extent of cohabitation is also increasing in most European countries. For example, in one multinational study, 45% of older women and 79% of younger women in France were involved in cohabitation arrangements. Many of these families include children. The percentage of cohabiting households with children under 15 years of age ranged from 1% in Greece to 62% in Britain (Kiernan, 2004). In the United States, 10% of all births occur to cohabiting couples, and an estimated 40% of U.S. children will live in a cohabiting family at some point in their lives (Giorgianni, 2003).

Like stepfamilies, cohabiting families are faced with multiple stressors. Cohabiting couples who marry, for example, have higher rates of divorce than other couples (Casper & Bianchi, 2002). Approximately one third of cohabiting couples in Europe separate within 5 years and about half become married. Both figures are slightly higher for U.S. couples who cohabit (Kiernan, 2004). Rates of child abuse and child fatality are also higher in cohabiting families than in other families (Giorgianni, 2003).

Gay and Lesbian Families

A **gay or lesbian family** is a form of cohabitation in which a couple of the same sex live together and share a sexual relationship. In the United States, in 2000, approximately 10% of unmarried-partner households included partners of the same sex. About half of these households were formed by gay partners and half by lesbian partners (U.S. Census Bureau, 2005). The gay or lesbian family might include children and might resemble the traditional nuclear family in terms of the mutual support and sexual and economic interdependence of the couple involved. In addition to the usual stresses of family life, gay and lesbian families experience the added stresses created by the lack of societal and legal sanction and the stigmatization that accompany known homosexuality. Issues related to same-sex orientations are discussed in more detail in Chapters 17 and 18∞.

Grandparent-headed Families

Approximately 70% of people over 50 years of age in the United States are grandparents (Casper & Bianchi, 2002). Although 19% of all U.S. family households include members 65 years of age or older (U.S. Census Bureau, 2005), many of these families are ones in which older family members have been absorbed into nuclear families as a result of economic or care needs. A **grandparent-headed family**, on the other hand, is one in which the older person or grandparent is the head of the household. Approximately 7% of all U.S. households are headed by grandparents. In some of these households, nuclear families or single-parent families have moved back into the households of their families of origin due to divorce or economic crises. In 1998, for example, 17% of unmarried mothers and their children lived with the mother's family of origin.

In a growing number of these families, however, grandparents are raising their grandchildren on their own. An estimated 2% of all children under age 18 are being raised by their grandparents (Casper & Bianchi, 2002). This amounts to 5.5 million children (Giorgianni, 2003). Contributing factors in the increase in grandparents with responsibility for raising grandchildren include drug abuse, child abuse, divorce, AIDS, and nonmarital births (Casper & Bianchi, 2002).

Both children and grandparents in this situation tend to have worse health outcomes than members of other families. Asthma, poor nutrition, poor sleep patterns, disability, hyperactivity, and weakened immune systems have been noted in families where grandparents are raising grandchildren. These families are also likely to be poorer than other families (Casper & Bianchi, 2002). Parenting by grandparents is also complicated by the potential for intrusion by the children's biological parents, raising the levels of stress encountered by all family members (Giorgianni, 2003).

Foster Families

Foster families consist of at least one adult and one or more foster children placed by the court system. Foster families may also include the adults' own biological or adopted children. Foster family composition may change frequently, and many foster children have experienced multiple foster home placements over time. The extent of foster care increased by 79% from 1982 to 1994 to include more than 468,000 children (dos Rets, Zito, Safer, & Soeken, 2001). Foster children constitute 1% to 3% of all children receiving Medicaid assistance, but account for 4% to 8% of overall Medicaid expenditures (Rosenbach, Lewis, & Quinn, 2003).

Studies indicate that foster children have a higher incidence of mental disorders (57%) than other children receiving public assistance (4%). Most common diagnoses include attention deficit hyperactivity disorder, depression, and developmental disorders, all of which contribute to stress within the foster family (dos Rets et al., 2001). The family types presented here are summarized in Table 14-1◆.

Fragmentary Households

The U.S. Census Bureau distinguishes between families and "households." A household consists of the people living within a single housing unit. Households may include more than one family group, but may also consist of single persons living alone or persons living with others who are not related to them in any way. Roommates, for example, would be considered a household, but not a family unit. These living arrangements may be referred to as *fragmentary households* (Casper & Bianchi, 2002). In 2003, approximately 13% of the U.S. population 15 years of age and older lived alone. More women than men live alone, particularly among the elderly. Among people 65 years of age or older, women are nearly three times more likely than men to live alone (U.S. Census Bureau, 2005). Living alone can contribute to social isolation and deteriorating health.

TABLE 14-1	Types of Families and Their Characteristic Features
Family Type	**Characteristic Features**
▪ Nuclear conjugal family	Mother and father who are married with one or more biological or adopted children
▪ Extended family	Kin network of the adult male and female of a nuclear family (e.g., grandparents, aunts, uncles, cousins)
▪ Single-parent family	One adult male or female with biological or adopted children
▪ Stepfamily	Reconstituted or blended family created by a marriage in which one or both spouses have children from a previous relationship(s) and possibly children of the new union
▪ Binuclear family	A child (or children) who is part of two nuclear households as a result of divorce and joint custody
▪ Cohabiting couple	A male and a female living together without marriage, with or without children
▪ Gay or lesbian family	A cohabiting couple of the same sex, with or without children
▪ Grandparent-headed family	One or both grandparents and one or more children in a household in which the grandparent is head of household; may also include children's biological parents and other family members
▪ Foster family	One or more adults and one or more court-designated foster children, with or without other biological or adopted children

THEORETICAL APPROACHES TO FAMILY NURSING

Many disciplines provide care and services to families and have developed theoretical models for dealing with families. Three types of social science models will be discussed here: systems models, developmental models, and structural–functional models. Other social science family models, such as transactional theory, stress theory, and family change theory, are useful in addressing selected family problems, but do not provide the broad scope of understanding required for community health nursing care of families.

Systems Approaches

Systems models conceive of families as open systems in which the whole of the system is more than the sum of its component parts or members, but also includes the interactions among them. The health of the family as a unit is influenced by interactions among members and between the family system and larger outside systems. The basic concepts of systems theory are derived from the work of biologist Ludwig von Bertalanffy and sociologist Talcott Parsons, working independently to describe biological and social systems, respectively (Friedman et al., 2003). Systems theory incorporates basic principles that can be applied to any kind of system, from an automobile engine, to the human body, to families, to organizations, to communities, and so on (von Bertalanffy, 1973). A *system* is defined as "a complex of elements in interaction" with each other in which the interaction is ordered rather than random (von Bertalanffy, 1981). The "elements" that make up a system are also known as *subsystems*. Systems are hierarchical in nature, with some systems in turn constituting subsystems within more complex systems. For example, the cardiovascular system is a subsystem in the human body, a system that is itself a subsystem in the totality of an individual, who is a subsystem in a family system, and so on. In a family, the subsystems are the family members.

Another concept of systems theory is the *suprasystem* or the context in which a given system functions. The next higher order system in the hierarchy is one aspect of the suprasystem for a lower-order system. For example, the family is part of the suprasystem of an individual system, and the community is a suprasystem element for the family system. The concept of hierarchical systems is depicted in Figure 14-1. The system of interest in any given situation is sometimes referred to as the *focal system* and other systems within the suprasystem as *interacting systems* (Friedman et al., 2003).

Any system is more than the sum of the parts or subsystems of which it is made and also incorporates reciprocal interactions among its parts. This systems principle means that whatever affects one portion of a system will affect other portions because of their interdependence. The interrelationships between subsystems within the system, between subsystems and the

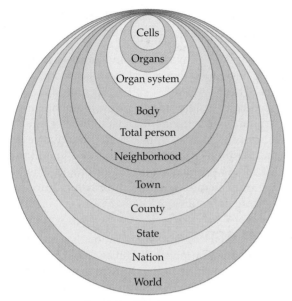

FIGURE 14-1 Hierarchical Systems

suprasystem, and between the suprasystem and the system as a whole are important determinants of health and are one of the major foci in using a systems approach to community health nursing.

All systems have *boundaries* that define what is part of the system and what is not. For example, a community may have geographic boundaries such as city limits; whereas a family's boundaries are often (but not always) determined by blood and legal ties. The permeability of the system boundary determines whether one is dealing with an open or closed system. An *open system* is one that exchanges matter, energy, or information with the environment; a closed system does not. All of the systems of interest to community health nurses (individuals, families, and population groups) are open systems.

All systems also have two mutual goals—the maintenance of a steady state and system growth—and engage in three categories of processes designed to accomplish these goals. The first category includes those processes needed to regulate exchanges with the environment. These processes are the input, throughput, and output processes. *Input* is the process whereby energy, matter, or information enter the system from outside the system's boundaries. *Throughput* is the process by which the material received into the system is transformed in some way, and *output* is what the system discharges back into the environment. In a family system, for example, input might be a report of a child's misbehavior in school. Throughput involves the processes by which the family acts on the report. The family might choose to ignore it, to criticize the child, or to explore and modify the child's reasons for misbehavior. Output would be the result of the processes used. If the family chooses to ignore the report, the behavior is likely to continue. If the family criticizes and punishes the child, the behavior may change, but the

child's self-esteem may be damaged. If, on the other hand, the family attempts to explore the child's behavior and modify it, the behavior is likely to change, but the child's self-esteem will be left intact.

The second category, processes involved in system operation, includes those processes designed to limit expenditures of system energy, provide for organization, and prevent overload. Using these processes, a system may refuse to accept input. For example, the family may choose to suspend nonessential family tasks while one member is hospitalized.

Internal processes, the third category of system processes, include subsystems change processes and adaptive processes. In subsystems change processes, a change in one subsystem results in changes in related subsystems. For example, when a new child is born into the family, relationships among family members must adapt to accommodate the new member. The teenage son or daughter, for instance, may need to assume more household responsibilities to free parents for care of the infant.

Adaptive processes, the second type of internal processes, involve the systems concepts of entropy, negentropy, and feedback. *Entropy* is a state of system disorganization resulting from the demands of continual readjustment of subsystem interrelations. A certain level of entropy is necessary for the system to continue to function and to avoid stasis or cessation of activity. However, as entropy rises above optimal levels, the system's ability to work toward its goals decreases proportionately. For example, the number of family members' outside activities may increase beyond the capacity of the designated chauffeur to accommodate, and adjustments will need to be made to ensure effective family function.

Negentropy relates to an increase in order and organization, which allows energy to be used to meet system goals. Negentropy is necessary for maintenance of the steady state, but the system must periodically move away from this steady state in order for growth to occur. If, for example, the family refuses to adjust family roles to adapt to the increasing independence of adolescent members, family function and individual development are impeded.

Feedback is the process whereby the system output returns as input. Negative feedback tends to minimize changes in the system and contributes to maintenance of the steady state. Negative feedback, in essence, plays down any discrepancies between the desired state of affairs and things as they are. Using the school misbehavior as an example, if the outcome of action is improved behavior, feedback from the school will not provoke further family action; this negative feedback indicates that the actual and desired behaviors are congruent. Awareness of discrepancies often results in system changes contributing to growth. In the example, positive feedback indicates that discrepancies remain between actual and desired states and would suggest that the child's behavior still does not meet expectations. In this case, the family system would probably take additional actions to improve the child's behavior.

Developmental Approaches

Developmental approaches to family nursing are based on the supposition that human beings and social units, such as families, develop in a logical fashion with predictable stages or milestones along the way. At each stage of development, the client is expected to accomplish specific tasks that provide a foundation for accomplishing the tasks of the next stage. Some authors distinguish between family development and family life cycle. In this context, **family development** is the unique path taken by any given family in its movement through the stages of growth. **Family life cycle**, on the other hand, is

the typical path expected of most families (Wright & Leahy, 2005).

According to family developmental theory, families, like individuals, pass through predictable developmental or family life stages first described by Duvall (Duvall & Miller, 1990). There are differing expectations in each stage of family development. As the expectations change, so do interactions among family members. The term used for these stage expectations is *family developmental tasks*. The developmental tasks of each stage necessitate certain changes within the family in the roles of its members in order for the family to fulfill its functions.

Duvall divided the family life cycle into the eight stages presented in Table 14-2◆. More recent family theorists such as Carter and McGoldrick (1999) have expanded the conceptualization of family stages, as

TABLE 14-2	Duvall's and Carter and McGoldrick's Stages of Family Development with Associated Developmental Tasks	
Duvall's Stages of Family Development	**Carter and McGoldrick's Stages of Family Development**
	Stage I: Single Young Adult Tasks: 1. Accept self-responsibility 2. Differentiate self from family of origin 3. Develop intimate peer relationships 4. Develop a career and financial independence
Stage I: Beginning Family Tasks: 1. Establish a mutually satisfying marriage 2. Develop new relationships with kin networks 3. Engage in family planning	**Stage II: New Couple** Tasks: 1. Achieve commitment to the new relationship 2. Form the marital relationship 3. Realign relationships with families and friends
Stage II: Early Childbearing Family Tasks: 1. Establish a stable family unit 2. Reconcile conflict in family and individual developmental tasks 3. Facilitate accomplishment of members' developmental tasks	**Stage III: Family with Young Children** Tasks: 1. Adjust the marriage to the presence of children 2. Distribute child-rearing, household, and financial tasks 3. Develop new relationships with family members (parenting and grandparenting)
Stage III: Family with Preschool Children Tasks: 1. Integrate second or third child 2. Socialize children to familial and societal expectations and roles 3. Begin separation from children	
Stage IV: Family with School-Age Children Tasks: 1. Separate from children to a greater degree 2. Foster education and socialization 3. Maintain the stability of the marriage	
Stage V: Family with Teenage Children Tasks: 1. Maintain the stability of the marriage 2. Develop new communication channels 3. Maintain family standards	**Stage IV: Family with Adolescents** Tasks: 1. Adapt to growing independence of adolescent family members 2. Adjust to increasing frailty of own parents 3. Change parent–child relationships 4. Address marital and career issues
Stage VI: Launching Center Family Tasks: 1. Promote independence of children 2. Integrate spouses of children into the family 3. Restore the marital relationship 4. Develop outside interests 5. Assist aging parents	**Stage V: Launching Children and Moving On** Tasks: 1. Accept multiple entries and exits from family structure 2. Renegotiate the marital dyad 3. Adapt relationships to accommodate in-laws and grandchildren 4. Deal with disability and death of one's own parents

Continued on next page

TABLE 14-2 Duvall's and Carter and McGoldrick's Stages of Family Development with Associated Developmental Tasks (continued)	
Duvall's Stages of Family Development	**Carter and McGoldrick's Stages of Family Development**
Stage VII: Family of Middle Years Tasks: 1. Cultivate leisure activities 2. Provide a healthful environment 3. Sustain satisfying relationships with own parents and children	**Stage VI: Family in Later Life** Tasks: 1. Accept the change in generational roles 2. Maintain function 3. Explore new roles 4. Assure support for middle and older generations 5. Deal with the death of others and one's own approaching death
Stage VIII: Family in Retirement and Old Age Tasks: 1. Maintain satisfying living arrangements 2. Adjust to decreased income 3. Adjust to loss of spouse, relatives, and friends	

Data from: Carter, B., & McGoldrick, M. (1999). Overview: The expanded family life cycle: Individual, family and social perspectives. In B. Carter & M. McGoldrick (Eds.), The expanded family life cycle: Individual, family and social perspectives (3rd ed., pp. 1–26). Boston: Allyn & Bacon; and Duvall, E., & Miller, B. (1990). Marriage and family development (6th ed.). New York: Harper College.

depicted in Table 14-2◆. In either model, each stage involves the accomplishment of specific tasks. At the same time that the family is engaged in accomplishing these tasks, family members are involved in accomplishing their own individual developmental tasks, which may parallel family tasks or conflict with them. The family must foster accomplishment of both family and individual tasks in order to function as an effective unit. Thus, there may be conflict or stress when the accomplishment of a family task is in direct opposition to task achievement by the individual. The family must develop healthy mechanisms for dealing with this type of conflict when it arises.

Families generally experience some stress as they pass from one stage to the next, since the transition usually involves one or more role changes. The family needs to negotiate these changes and respond by reevaluating roles and goals. For example, in Duvall's stage II, when the first child is born, the family enters a new stage that necessitates changes in the roles of both husband and wife and in their interactions with each other. The developmental tasks of each stage of family development are included in Table 14-2◆.

One of the criticisms of Duvall's developmental model is that it applies primarily to the traditional nuclear family. Carter and McGoldrick (1999) have identified developmental stages for divorced families and families resulting from remarriage. These stages are depicted in Table 14-3◆. In applying developmental models, the focus of care is on identifying the family stage of development, assessing the degree to which the family has achieved the developmental tasks of that and previous stages, and engaging in action to promote accomplishment of developmental tasks.

Structural–Functional Approaches

A structural–functional approach to family nursing is based on the principle that all families possess structure designed to allow them to perform specific functions. The health of the family is dependent on performance of these necessary functions.

The two basic concepts of a structural–functional approach are structure and function. *Structure* is the pattern of organization of the interdependent parts of a whole. Structural elements of a family include family members and family interaction patterns related to roles,

TABLE 14-3 Developmental Stages of Divorced and Remarried Families
Developmental Stages of Divorced Families
Stage I: Decision to Divorce Task: Accepting the failure of the marriage
Stage II: Planning System Breakup Tasks: 1. Addressing custody/property allocation issues 2. Dealing with extended family responses to the divorce
Stage III: Separation Task: Adjusting relationships among family members
Stage IV: Divorce Task: Overcoming hurt, anger, and other emotions precipitated by divorce
Stage V: Postdivorce Tasks: 1. Functioning as a single-parent household or maintaining a noncustodial parental role and meeting financial responsibilities for former spouse and children 2. Maintaining relationships with kin networks 3. Rebuilding social networks
Stages of Remarriage
Stage I: Entering a New Relationship Task: Making a commitment to the new relationship
Stage II: Conceptualizing and Planning the New System Tasks: 1. Developing new relationships 2. Realigning prior relationships
Stage III: Remarriage and Reconstruction Task: Accepting a new model of the family

Data from: Carter, B., & McGoldrick, M. (1999). Overview: The expanded family life cycle: Individual, family and social perspectives. In B. Carter & M. McGoldrick (Eds.), The expanded family life cycle: Individual, family and social perspectives (3rd ed., pp. 1–26). Boston: Allyn & Bacon.

values, communication patterns, and power structure (Friedman et al., 2003).

Family structure may be identified and assessed by means of genograms and ecomaps. A **genogram** is a diagram of a family tree incorporating information regarding family members and their relationships over at least three generations. Information that may be included in a genogram includes dates of birth, deaths, marriages, separations, and divorces; health status (including presence of acute and chronic illness); ethnicity; genetic inheritance; occupation or unemployment; retirement; and significant family problems such as trouble with the law, family violence, or incest. Creation of a genogram is an excellent method of family engagement when the community health nurse first encounters the family (Wright & Leahey, 2005). A sample genogram is included in Figure 14-2.

By convention, certain symbols have certain meanings in a genogram. For example, females are represented by circles and males by squares. Squares and circles marked with an "X" indicate deceased family members. A double circle or square indicates the *index person,* or identified client. The lines connecting persons in the diagram indicate the character of relationships between them. Broader lines indicate stronger relationships, broken lines reflect distant or tenuous ones, and cross-hatched lines indicate conflictual relationships (Wright & Leahey, 2005).

An **ecomap** is a visual representation of relationships both within and outside the family (Wright & Leahey, 2005). An ecomap can be used to depict the relationships of family members with each other and with outside forces such as health care providers, employers, and extended family members (Ray & Street, 2005). The segment of the genogram including the household of interest may be contained within the larger central circle of the ecomap. Outside forces are represented by smaller

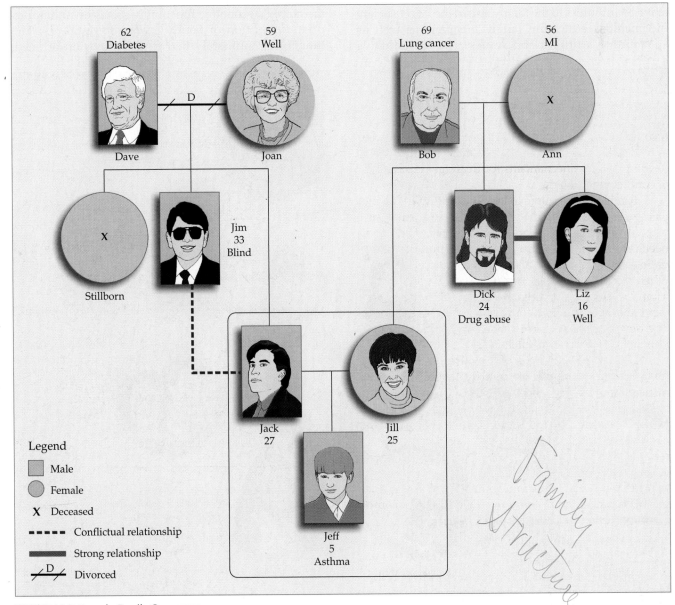

FIGURE 14-2 Sample Family Genogram

circles on the periphery. Again, relationships are represented by the types of lines connecting the circles in the diagram. Figure 14-3 presents a sample ecomap in which there are strong supportive relationships between the wife and the community health nurse and between the son and his teacher and conflictual relationships between the husband and his employer and between the family and the next-door neighbor. There is also a tenuous relationship with the extended family.

Structural elements affect families' abilities to perform functions that ensure continued survival and influence health. A *function* is one of a group of related actions that lead to accomplishment of specific goals, the goals of interest in family nursing being survival and health. Family functions fall into the five categories depicted in Table 14-4◆. The affective function of the family reflects its ability to meet the emotional and belonging needs of its members. The socialization function is designed to assist family members to become active contributors to the family and to the larger society and includes educating family members as well as transmitting attitudes and values. The reproductive

TABLE 14-4	Family Functions and Related Goals
Function	**Goals**
Affective	Meet the emotional needs of family members.
Socialization	Educate family members as contributing members of society.
	Instill family attitudes and values in members.
Reproductive	Ensure survival of family and society.
	Regulate sexual activity.
	Provide for sexual satisfaction.
Economic	Provide financial resources sufficient to meet family needs.
Provision of needs	Meet family members' needs for food, shelter, clothing, health care, etc.

function ensures continuity of the family and of society (Friedman et al., 2003). Another aspect of this function is control of sexual behavior and reproduction. The goal of the family's economic function is provision and appropriate allocation of family economic resources. This function is intimately tied to the provision of needs

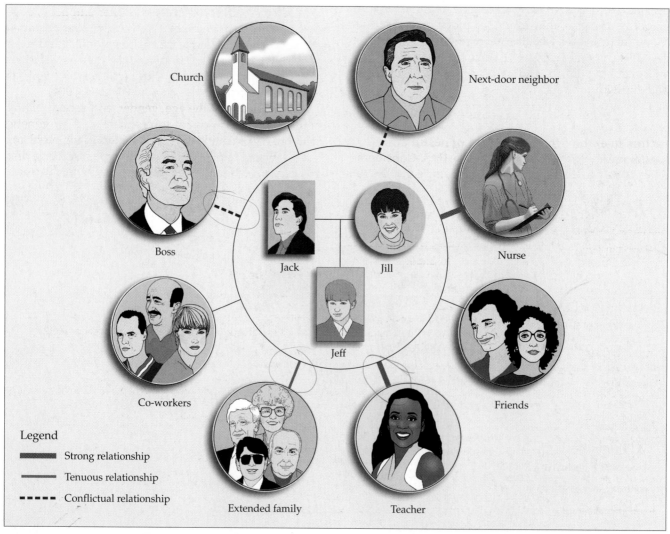

FIGURE 14-3 Sample Family Ecomap

function, which reflects the family's ability to meet members' needs for food, shelter, health care, and so on. The relationship of structural and functional elements in families is presented in Table 14-5◆.

Family structural elements may influence abilities to carry out required functions, thereby undermining family health. The community health nurse using a structural–functional approach to care first assesses how effectively the family performs expected functions and identifies any problems in functional areas. The nurse then identifies structural elements that are contributing to functional difficulties. Intervention using a structural–functional model is designed to improve functional performance. For example, ineffective communication patterns and fixed family roles are structural elements that may interfere with the family's ability to meet the affective needs of its members. In this case, nursing intervention would focus on improving family communication and redefining roles.

CARE OF FAMILIES

Community health nurses work with individual families and with families as an aggregate within the population. In doing so, they examine epidemiologic factors that influence family health status and use the nursing process to assess family health, diagnose needs for care, and plan, implement, and evaluate care for families at both individual and societal levels.

The Epidemiology of Family Health

Factors in each of the dimensions of health affect the health status and health needs of families. Considerations related to the biophysical, psychological, physical environmental, sociocultural, behavioral, and health system dimensions of family health will be briefly addressed here.

Biophysical Considerations

When the community health nurse first encounters a family, assessment begins with the gathering of data to identify the physical needs of family members. It is important to note that the physical status of each family member should be explored as a biophysical consideration in family assessment. The physical health status of each member affects how the family functions and how members relate to each other. As expressed by one author, "Illness is superimposed on each family member's often fragile balance between personal, mutual, financial, and social needs" (Giorgianni, 2003, p. 7). For example, if a child has a chronic disease, the entire family must make adjustments to accommodate the youngster's special needs. The parents have to adjust their schedules to care for the child and ensure that the child is seen by appropriate health care providers. Siblings may assume household chores or provide some measure of care for their ill brother or sister. Other family members can assist with care and offer emotional support for the parents and children. As another example, chronic back pain due to occupational injury has been shown to cause restructuring of family roles, relationships, and interpersonal interactions, as well as increased family stress (Strunnin & Boden, 2004).

Knowledge of the age, gender, and race of family members, as well as information related to genetic inheritance, can guide the nurse in identifying problems and planning family care. For example, knowing that there are several young children in the home, the nurse

TABLE 14-5	Interrelationships Among Functional and Structural Elements in Families
Functional Element	**Structural Elements**
Affective function	*Role:* Who provides support, reassurance, encouragement? *Values:* How, when, and where is affection displayed? *Communication:* How are affective messages conveyed? By whom? *Power:* Do affective bonds confer power? Diminish power?
Socialization function	*Role:* Who socializes children? *Values:* How, when, and where are children socialized? *Communication:* How are standards communicated? Are accepted standards and behavior congruent? *Power:* Is socialization one-way or two-way? Is power maintained or diminished by socialization?
Reproductive function	*Role:* Who engages in reproductive functions? With whom? *Values:* When, where, and how are reproductive functions carried out? *Communication:* How is information about sexuality conveyed? How are sexual desires conveyed? By whom? Does reproductive activity also convey affection? *Power:* Is manipulation of the reproductive function used to confer power?
Economic function	*Role:* Who earns? Who spends? *Values:* How, when, and where are expenditures made? For what? *Communication:* How are economic needs communicated? To whom? *Power:* Who makes economic decisions? How?
Provision of necessities function	*Role:* Who provides what? *Values:* What should be provided? When? Where? How? To whom? *Communication:* How are needs communicated? To whom? *Power:* Who makes decisions about allocation of resources? How?

may emphasize safety precautions when interacting with the family. An elderly family is more likely to have members with chronic, debilitating illnesses and may need closer scrutiny for evidence of these problems. The presence of older family members may contribute to *filial crises* in which they and their adult children are faced with acknowledging their mortality and accommodating role reversals. Multiple generations in the household may also result in the *sandwich generation* phenomenon in which younger adult members are caught between meeting the needs of their children and their aging parents (Casper & Bianchi, 2002). Or, a family's race may increase its members' risks for certain diseases such as sickle cell disease among African Americans and peoples of Eastern Mediterranean descent.

The developmental status of individual family members is also an important determinant of family health. For example, parents who have not accomplished developmental tasks of adolescence and young adulthood may have difficulty focusing on the needs of their children. Achievement of the developmental tasks of the family unit discussed earlier in this chapter will also affect family health status.

Psychological Considerations

Psychological considerations are a particularly important component of family health since "families set the foundation for self-worth, resilience, and the ability to form healthy and caring relationships" (Martin, as quoted in Giorgianni, 2003, p. 6). Areas for consideration include communication patterns, relationships and dynamics, coping and emotional strengths, child-rearing practices, family goals, the presence or absence of emotional problems, and the existence of family crises.

COMMUNICATION PATTERNS Communication patterns are an important indicator of functioning in the psychological dimension. Family communication occurs through two basic channels, a digital channel and an analog channel. The digital channel communicates verbal messages, and the analog channel addresses nonverbal communication and artistic expression (Wright & Leahey, 2005). An example of artistic expression as a means of communication might be a child's drawing of the family that incorporates perceptions of family problems. Both analog and digital communication should be considered in family assessment, as should the listening ability of family members. How do members communicate values and ideas? When one family member talks, do others listen? Do they show anger or boredom while listening?

Communication within dyadic relationships in the family is characterized by degrees of symmetry and complementarity. In a symmetrical relationship, the two parties communicate as equals. In a complementary relationship, they communicate as superior and inferior. Both types of relationships are appropriate in certain situations (Wright & Leahey, 2005). For example, one would expect communication in a parent–child dyad to be complementary when children are young, but to exhibit a greater degree of symmetry as children grow older.

The feeling tone expressed in communication is another indicator of the psychological environment. Family communications may contribute to interpersonal difficulties or facilitate cohesion and problem resolution. Sarcastic and resentful statements could block further communication between family members. For example, "When are you ever going to use your head?" does not facilitate communication. Other types of one-way communication include repeated complaints, manipulation through covert requests, insulting remarks, lack of validation, and inability to focus on one issue (Friedman et al., 2003).

Communication patterns can influence the effectiveness of parenting, particularly in the area of discipline. Praise enhances the development of self-worth in the child, whereas negative or condescending communications restrict the child's development. More about communications and child discipline can be found in Chapter 16∞.

The nurse should be aware of several dysfunctional communication patterns that may be employed within families. For instance, messages may be passed from one family member to another in a chainlike fashion that does not allow for reciprocal discussion, or communication may isolate a family member, as when the mother and children exclude the father from their discussions. Another problematic pattern is the wheel in which a central person directs what communication will be passed between family members. By way of comparison, a successful pattern of communication is the "switchboard" in which there is reciprocal communication among all family members. Figure 14-4 illustrates these patterns of communication.

A final consideration is the degree of communication between the family and the suprasystem. Is the family open to new ideas and opinions from people outside the family? Are outsiders invited to participate in family discussions or are they expected to "mind their own business"?

FAMILY RELATIONSHIPS AND FAMILY DYNAMICS Family relationships and family dynamics are other areas in the family's psychological environment that influence health. *Family relationships* are those bonds between family members that create identifiable patterns, such as subgroups and isolated members. Family relationships that are close, cohesive, and supportive of individual members contribute to individual health and to the health of the family as a whole. Excessively close relationships, however, may inhibit individual development and be detrimental to both individual and family health. Distant, nonsupportive, or conflictual relationships increase stress within families and contribute to poor physical and mental health in family members.

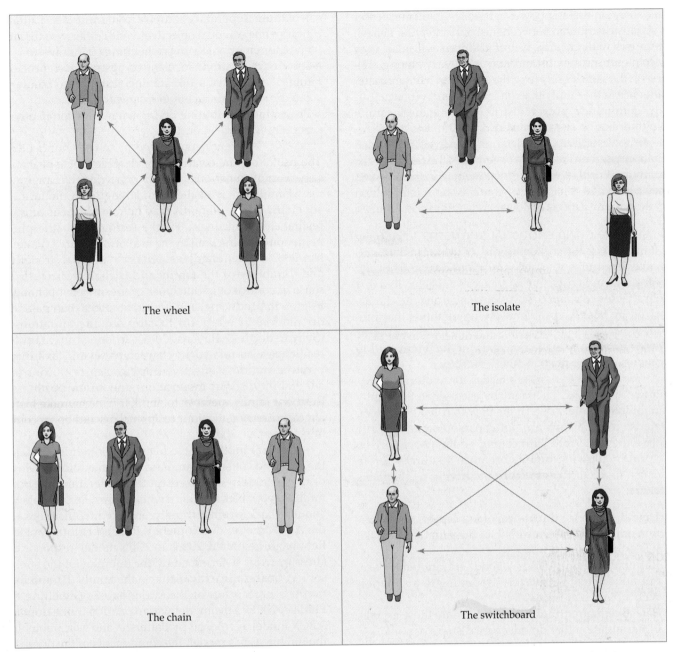

The wheel

The isolate

The chain

The switchboard

FIGURE 14-4 Family Communication Patterns

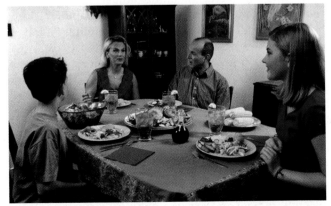

Meals can be a time of family sharing. (© Bob Daemmrich/ The Image Works)

Family dynamics describes the hierarchical patterns within the family. Power and leadership within the family are central elements of family dynamics. Power should be appropriately distributed within the family based on circumstances. For example, young children generally have little power and influence in families; but as children age, they should have increasing power and influence with respect to family decisions, particularly those that affect themselves. In some families, however, family life may revolve around the needs of one member, often to the detriment of the health of other family members. This may be particularly true in families with disabled members.

Power within families is often culturally determined. For example, in some cultural groups, adult men hold decision-making power in families. In others, power is equally distributed between husband and wife. The relative power and influence of children will also vary within cultural groups and may even vary among children in the same family (e.g., the eldest son having greater influence in the family than other children). When culturally determined power distribution enhances family health or has no specific impact on health, it is appropriate. If, however, culturally determined power distribution no longer serves the family or impedes the health of the family unit or that of individual members, intervention may be needed. Chapter 9∞ contains more information on the cultural aspects of power and authority in families.

FAMILY COPING AND EMOTIONAL STRENGTHS Identifying a family's coping strategies and defense mechanisms enables the nurse to assist families to deal realistically with stress and crisis. *Coping strategies* are behaviors that help a family to adapt to stress or change and are characterized by positive problem-solving methods that prevent or resolve crisis situations. Coping involves specific actions taken to manage demands on the family and to bring resources to bear on family problems.

Defense mechanisms are tactics for avoiding recognition of problems. They may be used when the family cannot immediately determine how to solve a problem. Defense mechanisms are not considered problematic unless they interfere with coping and may actually be helpful in allowing time to organize resources before facing a problem. Common family defense mechanisms include:

- **Denial:** ignoring threat-provoking aspects of a situation or changing the meaning of the situation to make it less threatening
- **Rationalization:** giving a "good" or rational excuse, but not the real reason for responding to a situation with a particular behavior
- **Selective inattention:** attending to only those aspects of the situation that do not cause distress or pain

ETHICAL AWARENESS

You are working with Mrs. Rhodes, who is pregnant with her third child. She has not yet told her husband that she is pregnant, because he beat her several times during each of her previous pregnancies. She is afraid that he will beat her again when he learns that she is pregnant. He doesn't believe that either of the other two children is his, even though Mrs. Rhodes says she has never been unfaithful to him. He tends to take his anger out on the older child, a 9-year-old boy, by yelling at him and telling him what a "piece of crap" he is. Mrs. Rhodes assures you that her husband has never physically abused either of the two children. Mrs. Rhodes tells you that she does not want to leave her husband because she still loves him and believes that he loves her. She does not want you to share the information she has given you with anyone, including the nurse midwife. What would you do in this situation?

- **Isolation:** separating emotion from content in a situation so one can deal objectively with otherwise threatening or emotionally overwhelming conditions
- **Intellectualization:** focusing on abstract, technical, or logical aspects of a threatening situation to insulate oneself from painful emotions generated
- **Projection:** attributing one's own motivation to other people

The use of coping strategies or defense mechanisms is seen most often when the family is faced with change.

Families may also exhibit strengths in the face of adversity. These strengths may be referred to as family resilience or hardiness. **Family resilience** is "the phenomenon of doing well in the face of adversity" (Patterson, 2002, p. 349). **Hardiness** refers to "internal strengths and durability of the family and is characterized by a sense of control over outcomes of life, a view of change as growth producing, and an active rather than passive orientation in adapting to stressful life situations" (Svavarsdottir & Rayens, 2005). In one study, family resilience was related to characteristics of flexibility, positive outlook, effective coping, sense of control, adaptability, social integration, and resourcefulness. Resilient families are also characterized by cohesion, effective communication, commitment, and connectedness (Lee et al., 2005).

Several models have been developed to explain the resilience of some families rather than others. Most of these models are based on the understanding that multiple variables influence whether families are able to "bounce back" from adversity, and are modifications of the ABCX model developed by Reuben Hill (Saloviita, Italinna, & Leinonen, 2003). In Hill's model, response to stressors (X) is determined by the interplay of the stressor (A), the resources available to the family (B), and the family's perception of the situation (C) (Zwelling & Phillips, 2001). This model was expanded in the double ABCX model developed by Patterson and McCubbin. In the double ABCX model, the components of the original model interact to create a response to a stressful situation. After the event, the family adjusts to the cumulative effect of multiple stressors (aA) by employing new and existing resources (bB) and by redefining their perception of the original stressful event (cC) (Han, 2003). The result is a level of post-crisis adaptation (or maladaptation) (xX) (Saloviita et al., 2003).

McCubbin and McCubbin (1993) later modified the model to indicate two stages of family response to stress, adjustment and adaptation. In the short-term adjustment stage, the family attempts to manage the stressor without major changes in family functional patterns. Adaptation is a long-term goal in which the family is able to cope with the stressor on an ongoing basis using both new and existing patterns of function. Family resources that facilitate adjustment and adaptation may be internal to the family (e.g., characteristics and capabilities of family members) or external (e.g., social support networks) (McCubbin, Thompson, & McCubbin, 2001). As an example, when a child is hospitalized with a new diagnosis of diabetes, the family must adjust to the hospitalization while still maintaining family function. Parents may alternate staying with the hospitalized child and caring for other children. Grandparents or friends may function as family resources, assisting in the maintenance of family function (e.g., picking other children up after school, providing meals). If the family perceives itself as able to cope with the hospitalization and later with the ongoing demands of the diagnosis, it will be more resilient than a family that perceives the difficulties of the situation as insurmountable.

When the child is discharged from the hospital, the family must adapt to the ongoing care demands posed by the diagnosis of diabetes. Again a resilient family with effective support systems and positive perceptions regarding the situation will adapt more readily than another family might. The extent of other stressors affecting the family, or stressor buildup, will also affect the family's resilience.

CHILD-REARING AND DISCIPLINE PRACTICES Another consideration in the psychological dimension of family health is the child-rearing and discipline practices employed to socialize children. Although such practices are usually derived from culture, a sociocultural factor, they are addressed as a psychological consideration because of their potential to cause psychological problems among family members or to strengthen a sense of right and wrong in each child.

Child-rearing attitudes and practices in the family often reflect cultural attitudes toward children and children's place in the world. Cultural mores also define prescribed behaviors of parents in socializing their children as well as behaviors expected of the child. Harsh and punitive interactions with children and severe disciplinary measures can undermine children's physical and psychological health. On the other hand, lax, permissive, or inconsistent parenting also causes problems for children in terms of confusion regarding appropriate behavior or later inability to control their own behavior to conform to societal dictates. Discipline should be fair and relevant and should be linked to explanations of what was done wrong and how the behavior can be corrected in the future. A more detailed discussion of discipline is included in Chapter 16∞.

FAMILY GOALS Family goals are a function of family values and reflect a family's cultural background. Family goals also vary with a family's developmental stage, economic status, and the physical health of family members. Problems arise when there is disagreement on family goals. For example, an immigrant family worked hard to send their son to college (a family goal). Before his sophomore year, the son refused to return to school,

preferring instead to work as a plumber's apprentice. The discrepancy between the son's personal goals and those of the family created a stressful situation for all family members.

Conflict may also occur between the goals of the family unit and societal goals and expectations. For example, a common societal goal is to provide children and young people with an education that will allow them to be more productive members of society. Family goals of economic security, however, may conflict with this societal goal when gainful employment by adolescent family members is given higher priority than educational attainment. Similarly, family goals of economic security conflict with societal goals of child safety when young children are left to supervise younger siblings while parents work.

PRESENCE OF MENTAL ILLNESS Another element of the psychological dimension of family health is the presence or absence of mental or emotional illness among family members. Such illnesses not only affect the health status of individual family members, but can profoundly influence the health of the family unit. For example, families with a schizophrenic member may not progress through the stages of family development as effectively as other families. In particular, they have been shown to have difficulties with the task of child separation from the family. In many families, schizophrenia has had the effect of "making parenthood permanent and lifelong parental support necessary" (Jungbauer, Stelling, Dietrich, & Angermeyer, 2004, p. 605). The presence of schizophrenia in these families has required parents to revise their expectations for their child and for their own lives.

As another example, postpartum depression in male spouses has been linked to maternal postpartum depression. In fact, men whose wives experience postpartum depression are approximately 25 times more likely to be depressed themselves than men whose wives are not depressed (Goodman, 2004). Consider the effect on the family of two spouses who are depressed and may be unable to carry out their normal spousal and parental roles.

FAMILY CRISIS Family exposure to stress may lead to the development of a crisis situation. A family can view any situation as a crisis. What is a crisis for one family may not be a crisis for another. Moreover, some families function and thrive on daily crises and would deteriorate if crisis situations were eliminated from their lives. Crisis assessment and intervention, then, must be based on the family's perception of a crisis event.

A **crisis** occurs when a family faces a problem that is seemingly unsolvable. None of their methods of problem solving work. The problem becomes psychologically overwhelming, and anxiety and tension increase until the family becomes disorganized and unable to cope (Friedman et al., 2003). A crisis state is unlikely to be sustained for more than 6 weeks because it is difficult to endure the high stress and tension associated with crisis without breakdown or change. The result of a crisis can be either resolution, resulting in a healthier, more positive state of being, or loss of well-being and a higher potential for recurrent crisis. Temporary relief can be gained from the use of defense mechanisms, environmental action, or both. Resolution and more permanent relief and growth require appropriate coping mechanisms. During periods of crisis, families are more susceptible to change and are usually more open to help when it is offered. This receptivity affords the nurse the opportunity to produce change with modest intervention.

Families experience two types of crises: maturational and situational. A **maturational crisis** is viewed as a "normal" transition point where old patterns of communication and old roles must be exchanged for new patterns and roles (Friedman et al., 2003). Every family experiences maturational crisis points, whether or not a crisis is actually experienced. Examples of transition periods when maturational crises may occur are adolescence, marriage, parenthood, and one's first job. Such periods in life are usually predictable, so families can be prepared to use coping mechanisms that assist them through each transition period.

All the transitional periods experienced by families have in common a change in roles or the addition of new roles, and crises occur when a family is unable or unwilling to accept new roles. There may be a history of poor role modeling from parents that leaves children unprepared for new roles and unable to leave home successfully. There may be family members who are unable or unwilling to view one member in a new role. For example, it is sometimes difficult for parents to acknowledge that their teenage children need to make decisions for themselves.

A **situational crisis** can occur when the family experiences an event that is sudden, unexpected, and unpredictable. Such events threaten biological, psychological, or social integrity and lead to disorganization, tension, and severe anxiety. Examples include illness, accidents, death, and natural disasters.

Some crises may arise that contain elements of both situational and maturational crisis events. For example, a young girl may be going through the maturational transition of adolescence and encounter the situational crisis of an unwanted pregnancy. The multiplicity of crisis events further impairs the family's ability to cope.

Why do some families go into crisis while others do not? Four categories of factors seem to play a part in determining whether or not a crisis will occur. These factors relate to (a) the stressor itself and the family's perceptions of the stressor, (b) other stressors impinging on the family, (c) family coping ability, and (d) the extent of family resources. Factors related to the stressor and

how it is perceived by the family include the extent of the impact of the stressor on the family and the severity of that impact, the duration of the stressor and whether its onset was sudden or gradual, and the degree of perceived control the family has over the stressor. A stressor that is perceived as manageable is less likely to cause a crisis situation than one that is seen as uncontrollable. The cause and predictability of the stressor may also influence the occurrence of crisis. Stressors with unknown causes or unpredictable effects create greater anxiety and greater potential for crisis.

The family's perception of the stressor may be distorted by previous experience with crises that were not growth producing. For example, there are crisis-prone families who have a chronic inability to perceive or solve existing problems. Their inability to cope with problems results in an exaggerated response to new changes, and crises occur for them that would be averted by other families.

The extent of other concurrent stressors affecting the family may also be a determining factor in the development of a crisis. Multiple stressors may have additive effects that precipitate crises. As noted earlier, maturational and situational crises may occur simultaneously, stretching family coping abilities beyond their limits. Existing family problems such as illness, unemployment, and marital strife may make a seemingly minor stressor a precipitating factor in a crisis. Situational demands created by the stressor may also increase the potential for crisis. Unfortunately, situational demands created by the health care system may enhance the potential for crisis. For example, the illness of a child is a stressor; if taking the child to the clinic necessitates losing work time and money, this creates an additional burden for the family.

The family's coping mechanisms represent internal family resources important to crisis resolution. Among these resources are cohesion or closeness among family members, open communication, use of humor, control of the meaning of the problem, and role flexibility. The family's ability to cope lessens the impact of any crisis event. It is important to assess what degree of success has been achieved using these mechanisms in the past and whether the family is aware of the mechanisms used.

Situational support arises from external resources such as the extended family, community agencies, churches, neighbors, and friends of the family. The degree of security felt by family members in relationships with these support systems may be sufficient to avert crises. A tool to assess family risk for experiencing a crisis is provided in the *Community Assessment Reference Guide* designed to accompany this text.

Physical Environmental Considerations

Physical environmental factors within and outside the home also affect the health of families. Within this setting, the family develops either functional or dysfunctional relationships. A chaotic, crowded, unsanitary, or unsafe home can contribute to physical and psychological health problems among family members. Considerations within the home include space available to family members, both for family interactions and for individual privacy. Another consideration is the presence of safety hazards in the home. What constitutes a safety hazard depends, in part, on the ages and health status of family members. For example, uncovered electrical outlets would be a safety hazard in homes with young children, and dangling cords and loose throw rugs would be safety hazards for both young children and elderly family members.

The family's external environment includes the neighborhood in which they live and the larger environment. Physical environmental characteristics at this level include the types of homes in the area, degree of industrialization, crime rate, and level of sanitation. Other important considerations include population density, common occupations of neighbors, availability of transportation, shopping facilities, health services, churches, schools, and recreational facilities. Each of these areas is assessed in relation to the specific needs of individual family members and of the family as a whole.

Sociocultural Considerations

The sociocultural dimension of family health shares some of the influences of the psychological environment. For instance, relationships outside the family are the basis for a portion of personality development. The leadership ability of individual family members is developed in school and in cultural, social, and political organizations where family members have the opportunity to interact with others and to contribute to community endeavors. Family discussions of social, cultural, and political issues help to develop social awareness as children grow and encourage the children to become involved in community, county, state, and national politics or social movements. Areas for consideration in the sociocultural dimension include family members' roles, culture and religion, social class and economic status, employment and occupational factors, and external resources. An additional special consideration for some families is their status as refugees.

FAMILY ROLES One of the most interesting aspects of the sociocultural dimension is role enactment within families. **Roles** are socially expected behavior patterns that are determined by a person's position or status within a family. Each person in a family occupies several roles by virtue of his or her position. For example, the adult woman in a family typically has the roles of wife, mother, cook, and confidante. Roles can take two forms: formal and informal. Formal roles are expected sets of behaviors associated with family positions such as husband, wife, mother, father, and child. Examples of formal roles are those of breadwinner, homemaker, house repairperson, chauffeur, child caretaker, financial manager, and cook. Informal roles are those expected behaviors not associated with a particular position.

Informal roles influence the psychological dimension within the family by determining whether, how, and by whom emotional needs are met.

Family roles may be complementary or conflictual in nature. **Role conflict** occurs when the demands of a single role are contradictory or when the demands attending several roles contradict or compete with each other. For example, a mother who works will experience role conflict when a business meeting she is expected to attend conflicts with her child's school play. Role conflict can also occur when one individual's definition of a role does not correspond with someone else's definition of the same role. For example, a husband may expect his wife to be responsible for all the cooking for the family, but the wife may work late and expect the husband to prepare an evening meal.

Role overload is another phenomenon that occurs in families when members assume multiple roles. **Role overload** occurs when an individual is confronted with too many role expectations at one time, even though these expectations do not contradict each other. For example, a mother with four children who returns to school and also has a part-time job may experience role overload in trying to meet the demands of housekeeping, cooking family meals, performing well on the job, and making straight As. Role overload may give rise to what has been called "spill-over stress," stress that accumulates and takes a toll on the person experiencing it and may then affect relationships with other family members. For example, a single parent experiencing role overload may begin to neglect an elderly parent who depends on his or her care.

Role overload is particularly apparent with respect to family caregiver roles and may result in diminished health for the person caring for ill or disabled family members. The estimated value of care provided by families to disabled and chronically ill family members and friends is $196 billion (Navaie-Waliser et al., 2002). In 2001, 20% of Americans reported that they or their spouses provided daily assistance to a disabled family member or friend (American Association of Retired Persons [AARP], 2002), and half of U.S. women will be asked to perform a caregiver role for a disabled family member at some time in their lives (Giorgianni, 2003). Caregiver effects are also noted in other countries. For example, Italian families caring for family members with Alzheimer's disease have reported changed relationships with the care recipient and other family members, changes in lifestyle, difficulty in providing care due to lack of knowledge, and concerns about the future (Vellone, Sansoni, & Cohen, 2002). In Japan, the effects of caregiving roles are highly gendered, with women providing most of the care for disabled family members. In fact, an estimated 85% of care to older family members is provided by women in spite of recent changes in social thinking on the role of women within the family (Takeda et al., 2003).

Advocacy in Action

There's a Father in the Delivery Room

Not too many years ago, it was unusual for fathers or other family members to be admitted to the delivery room when a woman was in labor. During this period, some hospitals were beginning to allow fathers to be present during delivery, but that was not the case at one major medical center hospital. At that time, women who were seen in prenatal clinics run by the County Department of Health Services delivered at the medical center. Public health nurses followed these clients during their pregnancies and made periodic home visits to monitor the pregnancy and provide prenatal education.

One family that was being followed by a public health nurse was very interested in having the father present in the delivery room, but this was contrary to hospital policy. At the request of the family, the public health nurse contacted the head of the labor and delivery unit at the hospital, and after much negotiation, the hospital agreed to allow the father to be present when his wife went into labor and delivered. They would only agree to this, however, if the father received instruction on how to gown, glove, and conduct himself in the delivery room. The public health nurse agreed to provide this instruction to both husband and wife, and they became the first couple to have the father present during a delivery at the hospital.

Potential effects of caregiving on caregivers include social isolation (Aldred, Gott, & Gariballa, 2005), depression (Flaskerud & Lee, 2001), increased susceptibility to illness, anxiety, interpersonal strain, and neglect of one's own health (Chang, Nitta, Carter, & Markham, 2004). The type of coping behavior exhibited by caregivers has also been linked to drinking behavior in dementia caregiving (Mjelde-Mossey, Barak, & Knight, 2004). Caregiving over a period of time has also been associated with poor mental health (McCann, Herbert, Bienias, Morris, & Evans, 2004).

The effects of caregiving may be different based on the overall level of function of the family. For example, caregivers for stroke survivors in lower functioning families were found to have poorer mental health than those in higher functioning families. Mental health effects were also affected by the degree of memory loss and behavior change exhibited by the care recipient (Clark et al., 2004). Similarly, studies of caregiving for persons with HIV/AIDS and age-related dementias have shown that the caregiver burden is greater when care recipients exhibit anger and depression or have poorer functional status (Flaskerud & Lee, 2001). Personality traits of caregivers may also affect the influence of caregiving on both caregivers and recipients. For instance, pessimistic caregivers have been found to experience greater depression and worse physical health than caregivers who were more optimistic (Lyons, Stewart, Archbold, Carter, & Perrin, 2004).

The greater the amount of time spent in caregiving activities, the greater the potential for caregiver stress and negative effects on family caregivers. For example, in one study women who provided more than 36 hours of care a week to a disabled spouse were six times more likely than noncaregivers to experience depression or anxiety. When care was provided to a disabled parent, women were twice as likely to report depression (Cannuscio et al., 2002). These adverse effects were seen whether or not the caregiver was employed or socially integrated or isolated (Cannuscio et al., 2004). Even when others in the family help with caretaking responsibilities, increased strain on the primary caregiver may occur due to different expectations regarding care recipients' levels of independence and needs (Usita, Hall, & Davis, 2004).

Flexibility of family roles and mutual respect for individuality are other aspects of the sociocultural dimension of family health. Family roles often change when a family member is absent, ill, or incapacitated and cannot fulfill his or her usual roles. It is important to

CULTURAL COMPETENCE

Asahara, Momose, Murashima, Okubo, and Magilvy (2001) described the effects of *sekentei*, a Japanese cultural consciousness of being observed by others with the expectation of conforming to cultural norms such as care of family members. Increased perceptions of *sekentei* were found to be related to increased caregiver burden, but not to decreased use of or willingness to use outside assistance. Are there parallel concepts in other cultural groups that might influence the effects of caregiving on family members? To what extent are members of the dominant U.S. culture expected to provide for the care of their parents? How do these expectations affect family caretaking and caretaker burden?

EVIDENCE-BASED PRACTICE

Several studies have shown that persons caring for family members with disabilities or chronic illness often experience caregiver burden with consequent physical and psychological health effects. Conduct a literature search for studies related to the positive and negative effects of family caregiving. Based on the literature, can you identify factors that would place family caregivers at particular risk for caregiver burden and its subsequent effects? How might knowledge of these risk factors enhance community health nursing interventions to prevent or minimize burden among family caretakers?

assess the ability of family members to take on these unfilled roles and make the necessary role adjustments. When the ill or absent member is ready to resume roles, a readjustment may again be necessary. For example, when Frank had his heart attack, Beth had to go to work and assume the breadwinner role. Now Frank is recovered and can return to work. Beth likes her job and does not want to quit. Assistance in adjusting to changes in roles can alleviate conflict and stress in this and similar situations.

Role adjustments may also be required as the family progresses through its various developmental stages. For example, the parental role should be enacted differently with an adolescent child than with a preschooler.

CULTURE AND RELIGION Family cultural information is essential to building relationships and designing family interventions that will not conflict with cultural values. Does the family engage in cultural practices related to health? If so, are these practices helpful or harmful? What cultural factors will affect attempts to resolve family health problems?

Cultural factors may support or impede a family's abilities to adapt to changing environmental circumstances and may influence the health of individual members. As we said earlier, cultural factors play a large part in determining family caregiver roles, how those roles are performed and by whom, and the effect of those roles on the health of caregivers.

One specific aspect of culture that may influence family health is that of religious affiliation or spirituality. The influence of religious beliefs and practices on the health of the family can be assessed by asking specific questions about the importance of religion in family interactions and decision making and the role of religion for the family as a whole. For example, strong religious beliefs may prohibit the use of contraceptives, or health teaching may need to be modified in keeping with the family's religious convictions. Or religious beliefs and practices may promote health. For example, the proscription of alcoholic beverages can have health-promotive effects for Muslim families (Yosef, 2004). Close affiliation with an organized church may also provide a source of emotional and/or material support for family members in time of need.

SOCIAL AND ECONOMIC STATUS The social class and economic status of a family can profoundly affect its health. Lack of financial resources can mean that the family does not have enough nutritious food, adequate shelter, or access to health care. Social class delineations involve groupings of people based on financial status, race, occupation, education, lifestyle, and language. In America, the lower social class consists of people with less money, less education, and less access to resources such as health care.

The family's social class is important to the extent that it affects lifestyle, interactions with the external environment, and the structural and functional characteristics of the family. Economic status is closely tied to social class and education level.

Homelessness among families is often the result of economic factors. For example, 28% of family homelessness is attributed to housing difficulties and 20% to economic hardship. From 1991 to 1997, there was a 12% increase in what is termed *worst-case housing*, in which families with incomes at half or less of the median income in the community are not receiving federal housing assistance. The extent of worst-case housing status increased even more in some subgroups within the population. For example, an increase of 29% was noted for families with children, 31% for African American families, and 74% for Hispanic families. In 2000, requests for shelter increased by 15% from the previous year, the largest increase noted to date. Among families, shelter requests increased by 17% (Sherman & Redlener, 2003).

The loss of Aid to Families with Dependent Children (AFDC), a result of welfare reform in the United States, has forced many poor mothers to work, reducing their ability to provide reciprocal assistance with childcare and other family supports previously available to them. Welfare reform occurred as a result of passage of the Personal Responsibility and Work Opportunity Reconciliation Act of 1996. The act limited the amount of time that families can receive welfare funding, implemented mandatory job training, and promoted movement from public assistance to employment (Casper & Bianchi, 2002).

Unfortunately, welfare reform may not have achieved its primary goal of allowing families to be self-sufficient. For example, although employment is high at exit from welfare, family income is often not improved due to employment in low-paying jobs. In addition, former welfare recipients now need to pay full amounts for housing, childcare, health care, and transportation,

GLOBAL PERSPECTIVES

Chiu, Shyu, and Liu (2001) conducted a study in Taipei, Taiwan, to determine the relative costs of care provided to severely impaired stroke survivors through hospital chronic care units, nursing home placement, home health services, and family care. They found that caring for clients in their homes was both more expensive and less effective in improving functional status than nursing home and chronic hospital care. Nursing home care was slightly less expensive than hospital care. In large part, these results were due to the cost of lost labor and income when family members cared for a stroke victim at home. For each family member involved in care, costs amounted to the equivalent of U.S. $1,244 per month. This figure did not take into account lost earnings if family members stopped work to care for the stroke survivor. In addition, family care has social and emotional, as well as financial, costs. Do you think a similar study conducted in the United States would result in similar findings? Why or why not?

further limiting the availability of usable income. An estimated third of former welfare recipients in states participating in one study returned to public assistance rolls within 2 years. In states where mothers of young children were required to work, mothers were 2.5 times more likely to return to welfare. For families that stayed off welfare, family income increased by only 30%. Half of these families were poor when they exited public assistance programs and 40% were still poor after 2 years (Hofferth, 2003a).

EMPLOYMENT OR OCCUPATIONAL FACTORS Job-related factors that influence family health may present in three forms. First, the job might produce stress for the adult that results in illness. Second, the adult might be exposed to hazards that he or she brings home to other family members. Third, job-related problems and time constraints might interfere with family commitments.

Occupational or workplace stress can lead to a number of stress-related illnesses. Safety hazards within the work setting may cause injury and disability to the family breadwinner(s). The financial burden and stress of an occupation-related illness have led to divorce and the dissolution of families, among other problems. Similarly, job-related stress may lead to reduced energy for effective parenting and for maintaining the marital bond, if one exists (Polatnick, 2000).

Sometimes hazardous substances to which a working parent is exposed not only threaten the parent, but may also inadvertently be brought home to other family members. For example, nurses and other health care workers need to be aware that some infectious diseases may be transmitted to young children via clothing and shoes. Working with lead or other hazardous substances may also result in exposure of family members through contaminated clothing and other articles worn on the job (National Institute for Occupational Health and Safety, 2001).

Job-related family problems also might arise if a family member's work commitment conflicts with family commitments. Out of financial necessity, more parents are working, and they are working more hours than in the past. In 2000, for example, 78.5% of all single female parents worked outside the home, and in 64% of married couple families, both parents worked. These figures give rise to extensive childcare needs for American families.

Approximately 62% of U.S. children under 6 years of age (13 million children) and 45% of those under 1 year of age are in some form of childcare arrangement. Among children under 5 years of age, 39% are cared for in someone's home and 26% in childcare facilities. Childcare costs are escalating sharply and can range from a low of $3,536 per year for a California school-age child cared for in a home setting to as much as $9,412 for an infant in a day care center. For a family with a median income, childcare costs for one infant and one preschool child may amount to 30% of the family's total income (Fellmeth, 2003).

Employment may have other indirect effects on family health status and effective family function. For example, in one survey of more than a thousand large employers, 95% offered family health insurance and 87% paid at least part of the premium for family coverage. Fourteen percent also provided health insurance coverage for cohabiting partners. Many low-wage or part-time jobs, however, do not provide this employment benefit. In the same survey, 80% of employers allowed time off for family needs, and 65% allowed flexible schedules. Another 49% allowed time off for care of sick children over and above paid employee sick time. Nearly one fourth of the employers surveyed offered educational workshops on family issues, and 23% provided elder care resources and referrals. Far fewer employers (12%) provided childcare or had childcare resources nearby (Giorgianni, 2003).

EXTERNAL RESOURCES As we saw in Chapter 10∞, both personal or family social capital and community social capital influence health and illness in the population. Individual family capital may include extended family members, churches, or other social organizations in which a family participates that can provide support in times of adversity. The form of that support may be emotional, material, or instrumental. For example, being able to discuss one's worries related to one or more children with friends or extended family members may provide a mother with emotional support. Suggestions from the community health nurse on how to handle a rebellious adolescent are an example of instrumental support, and obtaining a short-term loan from one's parents is an example of material support.

External family resources may also be derived from community social capital. This would include the availability of social services to families in need. For example, the availability of the Temporary Assistance to Needy Families (TANF) to some low-income families is one form of community social capital. Other examples include American Red Cross Disaster Relief Services for families affected by natural or human-precipitated disasters and crisis counseling centers for low-income families.

Think Advocacy

In conducting an assessment of families in your community, you find that there are a number of families with older members in which all other adult members are employed. Many of these older family members feel socially isolated because their children are not available to take them to participate in local activities designed for senior citizens. There is a local senior citizens center that has a variety of activities these individuals might enjoy, but there is no public transportation to allow them to reach the center. How might you begin to address this problem within the community?

REFUGEE STATUS One factor that profoundly affects the health and functional ability of many families is their status as refugees or immigrants. Immigration restrictions may result in lengthy separations for families that create *ambiguous losses.* Family members are not permanently lost, as they would be in death, but the uncertainty regarding the length of separation does not permit families to acknowledge and work through the loss. Coping strategies for family members may include *memory work* that idealizes the missing family members. When family members are reunited, idealization may make it difficult to reincorporate returned individuals who do not conform to one's memories of them. In addition, family roles will have been adapted to their absence and will need to be renegotiated with their return. Individual family members will have changed, and the recognition of those changes (e.g., aging, loss of roles) may affect self-image. In addition, most family members will need to address their emotional responses to the separation (e.g., guilt for leaving others behind, feelings of betrayal and abandonment). Finally, achievement of balance during separation may have necessitated the use of surrogates that may be questioned in family reunification (Rousseau, Rufagari, Bagilishya, & Measham, 2004). For example, an uncle or family friend may have served as a surrogate father in the father's absence, and the appropriateness of this surrogate may be questioned when the father is reunited with the family.

Behavioral Considerations

Health-related behavior is the fifth area for consideration in the epidemiology of family health. As noted by one author, "Families establish the patterns of preventive care, diet, exercise, hygiene, responsibility, and sharing" (Martin, quoted in Giorgianni, 2003, p. 6) that can profoundly affect family health now and in the future. Areas of focus include family consumption patterns, rest and sleep patterns, exercise and leisure activities, and safety practices.

FAMILY CONSUMPTION PATTERNS As we have seen in other chapters, a large percentage of Americans are obese or overweight. In other parts of the world, many people are malnourished. These dichotomous states of ill health are both related to family consumption patterns, either overconsumption or underconsumption of nutrients. For many Americans, family consumption patterns include excessive amounts of fat and calories but deficiencies in many vitamins and minerals due to low intake of fruits and vegetables. Healthy diets are difficult to achieve given the fast-paced nature of American family life. Family members often have little time to spend on food preparation and may rely heavily on fast foods rather than balanced family meals. Other families may have difficulty affording healthful foods.

Cultural patterns evident in food selection, preparation, and consumption may also influence family health status. For example, the excessive use of fried or high-fat foods sometimes seen among Latinos or families in the southern United States contributes to the increased incidence of atherosclerosis, heart disease, and stroke among members of these populations.

Other consumption patterns that affect family health status include the use of tobacco, alcohol, and illicit drugs. Approximately 25% of U.S. men and 20% of women are current smokers (Centers for Disease Control, 2005), and a significant number of U.S. children are exposed to cigarette smoke in the home. Drug and alcohol abuse by family members affects health in a number of ways. Substance abuse affects the personal physical and emotional health of the substance-abusing member and may result in the inability to carry out necessary family functions, adversely affecting the health status of other family members. In addition, substance abuse may contribute to family violence or neglect.

REST AND SLEEP Family rest and sleep patterns may also be a source of problems. For example, a new baby may sleep during the day and cry at night. This will adversely affect parents' rest and their subsequent performance the next day.

Another problem frequently encountered with respect to family sleep patterns is that of differing work schedules. If, for example, one parent works days and the other works nights, this situation may limit their opportunities to interact with each other and with their children. A parent's typical rest and sleep schedule may also require children to play at a neighbor's house during the day or find quiet pastimes at home.

EXERCISE AND LEISURE Regular exercise is necessary for good health. The earlier children are included in such activities, the more likely they are to build lifetime habits of exercise. Exercise and leisure activities that include the entire family also promote cohesion. At times, it is also helpful to plan leisure activities that are unique to certain members of the family. This allows for individuality among family members and promotes a balance between family togetherness and separateness that is needed for individual development.

The nurse can also help the family identify potential health risks involved in leisure activities. For example, are safety helmets worn by all family members on bike trips? What are the safety rules when the family goes swimming? Is a backyard pool covered when not in use to prevent a child from going in alone or falling in accidentally?

High costs and low income may limit the activities that families can do together, but should not eliminate them. The availability of low-cost recreational opportunities in the community is an area for assessment at the population level.

HOUSEHOLD AND OTHER SAFETY PRACTICES Safety practices such as the use of seat belts, infant safety seats, cribs with safe spacing between rails and proper mattress width, proper disposal of hazardous substances, and safety education for children are important considerations in family assessment. Are these behavioral safety factors evident in the household? Who is the person most attentive to family safety issues? What family behaviors contribute to health risks for members?

Health System Considerations

Factors related to the health system dimension also affect family health. Two major considerations for individual families are family attitudes to health and response to illness and family use of available services. Aggregate level considerations include the availability and effectiveness of health services provided to families in the population.

FAMILY ATTITUDES TOWARD HEALTH AND RESPONSE TO ILLNESS Culturally determined attitudes toward health and illness also influence family health status. Families as a whole may see health promotion and illness prevention as a priority, or these activities may be valued for some family members and not others. For example, parents may make an effort to meet the health promotion needs of their children, but neglect their own needs or those of older family members. Similarly, family members may only seek health care when their ability to perform their respective functions is impaired. In part, this may be the result of cultural definitions of health and illness, but may also arise from lack of access to affordable health care services.

Family response to illness is another important influence on family health. How do members deal with illness? Part of learning about this aspect of family life is determining who in the family decides when an ill family member should stay home from work or school and whether an ill member should receive health care. For example, in some families the mother decides who is ill and consults the father when she believes that the illness is severe enough to require the services of a health care provider. Family caregivers may themselves be in need of nursing intervention in order to function effectively in their caregiving role. As we saw earlier, family caregivers provide much of the care to ill family members. Unfortunately, they often receive little support from health care professionals in doing so. Too often, they are expected to accept responsibility for care without the required knowledge or abilities (Giorgianni, 2003). Community health nurses should assist family caregivers with the emotional as well as physical and cognitive challenges of caregiving.

USE OF HEALTH CARE SERVICES Family functions with respect to illness vary with the type of illness. For example, family functions in the case of acute illness include providing or obtaining health care, reassigning roles, and supporting the sick person. Additional functions in dealing with chronic illness include avoiding or coping with medical crises, preserving the family's quality of life, and arranging treatment modes and mechanisms. In the face of terminal illness, family functions also include dealing with shock and fear and minimizing pain and discomfort.

Do family members have a source of health care? Do they have health insurance? Often, there may be providers available for mothers and children because of federal and state programs. Fathers and other young adult males, however, are often excluded from these programs. The nurse may be asked to help families find health care for excluded family members who become ill.

Health care may be limited because of a lack of funds, language barriers, distance to health care facilities, transportation limitations, and many other problems. The nurse needs to determine these deterrents to access and find resources within the community to help families obtain health care. Occasionally, even when families have health insurance, members are not able to take full advantage of this resource because they do not understand what services are covered (or not covered). The nurse can help them understand insurance benefits or refer families to resources in the community who can explain insurance benefits and how to use them.

Assessing Family Health

Family health is an attribute of the family as a unit and encompasses more than the health status of individual family members (Soubhi & Potvin, 2000). Not all family–nurse interactions require a complete family assessment. The focused assessment below can identify situations in which a complete assessment is warranted.

Assessment of family health takes place with respect to individual families and the overall health of families within the population. A tool for assessing the health of individual families is found in the *Community Assessment Reference Guide* 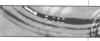 designed to accompany this text.

Family assessment begins with a determination of the health status of individual family members. This information may be available in a family record, or some data elements may have been provided by referring agencies. Most information on health and illness in family members, however, will come from interviews with individual members or from specific family informants (e.g., the mother regarding the health of children). Information on family composition by age, gender, and

---

FOCUSED ASSESSMENT

Indications for Family Assessment

- Difficulty achieving developmental milestones
- Problems considered by the family to be family issues
- A child or adolescent experiencing problems
- Issues affecting family relationships
- Psychiatric admission of a family member
- Hospital admission of a family member
- Family crisis situation

Data from: Wright, L. M., & Leahey, M. (2005). Nurses and families: A guide to family assessment and intervention (4th ed.). Philadelphia: F. A. Davis.

race/ethnicity can be obtained from the same sources. Interviews with family informants can also provide information on family history of conditions with a genetic predisposition as well as data regarding the immunization status of family members.

Information on the developmental status of each family member and the family unit as a whole is also obtained. The community health nurse may conduct developmental tests such as the Denver Developmental Screening Test (DDST) to determine the developmental status of young children. Interviews and observation will provide information regarding the developmental status of older family members and the family unit.

The community health nurse should also collect data regarding biophysical considerations at the aggregate level. For example, effective health care planning for families requires information about the proportion of elderly families and those with young children in the population and the number of families with disabled members or other individual health problems that may affect overall family health. A focused assessment related to the biophysical dimension of family health is presented below. The questions included in the focused assessment might be adapted in assessing families as an aggregate within the population.

The community health nurse assesses a variety of considerations in the psychological dimension at both the individual family level and the aggregate level. As noted earlier, elements for consideration in this dimension include communication among family members, family dynamics, coping strategies and emotional strengths, child-rearing practices, family goals, the presence or absence of mental health problems, and the existence of family crises.

Mealtime is a good time to assess family interaction. It is here that the nurse can determine whether meals are a time of light conversation or heated argument, whether all family members eat together, and whether mealtimes contribute to family solidarity. It is also important to assess the content of communications. Are they superficial

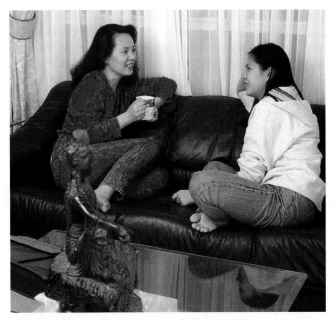

Effective communication is an important factor in family health. (© Bob Daemmrich/The Image Works)

or does the family engage in values clarification discussions? The type of statements made or questions asked tell the nurse a great deal about family interactions. For example, "You are wrong about that" and "Tell me more about your point of view" indicate different attitudes about interactions among family members. The latter, open-ended response facilitates communication, whereas the previous accusatory statement impedes it.

The nurse should ascertain what areas of communication are taboo (off limits) for family members. Typical areas include feelings, sexual issues, and religion. For example, in some families, members are not expected to express feelings of anger. Another example would be an expectation that family members do not discuss family problems with outsiders. If certain topics are found to be taboo, the nurse may need to alter his or her approach to data gathering. For example, if one of the areas closed to discussion involves feelings, the nurse might try engaging in self-disclosure, thus acting as a role model. Another way to alter the approach is to gather data by examining areas related to the taboo issue. This may also help the nurse to identify the reason for resistance to communication about a specific area.

In assessing family communication patterns, the nurse will also be gathering data related to family relationships and family dynamics. How does one assess relationships within the family? Initially, information regarding subgroups is compiled. For example, the nurse may notice that a mother–daughter subgroup has excluded the father from the decision-making process.

Communication within and between subgroups is then assessed in terms of both content (what is said) and process (who says it and how it is said). This is followed by identification of the relationship as supportive or

---

FOCUSED ASSESSMENT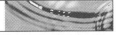

Biophysical Considerations in Family Assessment

- What is the age, gender, and racial/ethnic composition of the family?
- How adequately have individual family members accomplished age-appropriate developmental tasks?
- Do individual family members' developmental stages create stress in the family?
- What developmental stage is the family in? How well has the family achieved the tasks of this and previous developmental stages?
- Do family members have any existing physical health conditions that are affecting family function?
- Is there a family history of genetic predisposition to disease?
- What is the immunization status of family members?

close, demanding, maternal, and so on. Subgroups are described in terms of how they relate. For example, one may describe the sibling group as one that shares feelings and actions, or siblings may be described as alienated from each other. Positive self-image on the part of a family member is the result of daily family interactions that bolster the individual's feelings of self-worth. A child who is criticized too often may develop a poor self-image. The nurse can assess the self-esteem of family members by observing nonverbal behavior as well as their communication patterns with others.

Family dynamics are assessed by observing family leadership patterns. Who are the primary decision makers? Who controls conversations? Is there a leader in the family? What leadership style does the leader employ? Do family members respect the leader? Do they respect each other? Respect requires that children view parents as individuals as well as parents. Likewise, parents need to learn to respect their children as individuals.

The community health nurse can assess how the family copes by observing behavior during life change events or by obtaining information on how the family has dealt with a major move, job change, or loss of a family member in the past. Assessment of family resilience or hardiness can also be obtained by asking how the family has dealt with adverse circumstances in the past.

A family's emotional strengths or resilience become evident as the nurse observes interactions and communicates with family members over time. The nurse should look for evidence of family cohesion and the degree of sensitivity to others displayed by each family member. For example, the nurse might observe whether a mother anticipates her child's needs or whether there is a general feeling of warmth and caring. The nurse should also estimate the degree to which family members support and praise each other. The results of these observations help the nurse to estimate how well the family is meeting the emotional and psychological needs of its members.

The nurse should also explore child-rearing practices employed by the family and determine the type of discipline used, who administers it, and the types of behavior that elicit disciplinary action. The nurse would determine whether parents and other adults in the family support each other's decisions in matters of discipline. For example, if the child is punished by the mother, does the child attempt to avoid punishment by manipulating the father? If so, are the adults able to discuss and support a joint decision? Ultimately, parents need to teach self-discipline, so it is important to assess whether they provide adequate role models for children. A more detailed discussion of discipline is included in Chapter 16∞. Much of the information on child rearing and discipline obtained in a family health assessment is derived from observation of parent–child interactions and interviews with family informants.

Family goals, another element of the psychological dimension of family health, may be difficult to assess because families often are not consciously aware of them. The nurse, however, can be aware of and observe for evidence of family goals; these include producing children and ensuring their survival, exchanging love and emotional support, and providing for economic survival or affluence. Family members can also be asked to describe and prioritize family goals. At the aggregate level, knowledge of the cultural groups in the area and their perspectives on acceptable family goals also gives community health nurses some insight into possible family goals. Family members can also be asked to describe interactions with the outside world as a means of identifying conflicts between family and societal goals. For example, if the family has children in school, parents might be asked about the quality of their interactions with school personnel. Similarly, if local news stories highlight incidents of "police brutality," family members can be asked about their perceptions of local police activities and their effects on family life.

Community health nurses should also assess families for the presence of mental health problems. This information can be gleaned from observations of family interactions as well as interviews with family informants. Occasionally, the reason that families have been referred for community health nursing services is the existence of mental health problems in one or more family members. In such cases, some information about mental health status among family members should be available from the referring agency. Nurses working with families experiencing mental illness should assess the impact of the illness on family function and address the resulting health problems of both the individual and the family as a whole.

At the aggregate level, community health nurses can develop a picture of psychological dimension factors that have the potential for affecting the health of families within the population. The incidence and prevalence of family violence or suicide, for example, can suggest potential problems that may be faced by individual families as well as societal attitudes that may contribute to problems. Similarly, the extent of mental illness in the population may suggest psychological dimension factors impinging on family health.

Assessment of crisis situations for individual families involves first determining whether or not a crisis exists. If the family is experiencing a crisis, the nurse would then assess factors contributing to the crisis and family members' perceptions of the crisis situation. The nurse would also explore family responses to prior crises as well as family member's ideas for ways to deal with the crisis situation. A particularly important element of assessing a crisis situation is determining the level of risk for suicide or homicide by family members. Asking family members to describe the crisis as well as their feelings related to it will provide most of the data required for crisis assessment. The community health nurse may also explore with families the availability of internal and external resources that might help to resolve the crisis situation.

At the aggregate level, there are usually no statistical data available regarding the number of families that are experiencing crises. Community health nurses can, however, get some sense of the magnitude of family crises from interviews with family counselors. These providers should also have some insight into the types of crises most often experienced by families. Police data on the number of calls related to family altercations can also provide some indication of the level of family crises experienced in the community. Community health nurses can also gather data on social conditions that are likely to precipitate family crises. For example, unemployment and poverty levels in the community can provide information on some of the stresses experienced by families.

Potential questions for a focused assessment of psychological considerations in family assessment are presented below. The questions suggested can be modified to assess the needs of families in the overall population.

FOCUSED ASSESSMENT

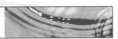

Psychological Considerations in Family Assessment

- What are the typical modes of family communication? How effective are family communication patterns? What areas are taboo in family communication?
- How cohesive is the family? Do family members exhibit close supportive relationships?
- How are decisions made in the family? By whom? Which family members have input into decisions? Who is responsible for carrying out family decisions?
- Who is the leader in the family? Does the leader use a leadership style appropriate to the age and abilities of other family members?
- Do family members express respect for each other?
- Is there evidence of violence within the family? What forms of discipline are used in the family? Is the discipline used appropriate?
- What emotional strengths does the family exhibit? How does the family deal with change?
- What coping strategies does the family use? How effective are these strategies?
- What are the family's goals? Do individual goals conflict with or complement family goals? What values are reflected in the family's goals?
- Is there evidence of mental illness in the family? What is the effect of mental illness on family relationships? On family function?
- How well does the family deal with crisis? Is there an existing crisis within the family? If so, what type of crisis is it?
- What are the perceptions of the family regarding the crisis situation?
- Is there potential for harm to family members as a result of the crisis (e.g., homicide or suicide)?
- What defense mechanisms and coping strategies has the family employed?
- What internal and external sources of support are available to deal with the crisis?
- What options for action are available to resolve the crisis situation? To what extent are family members aware of options? What are the advantages and disadvantages of the options available?

To assess a specific family's physical environment, it is important to describe the home and its condition. Information such as the address, whether the family owns or rents the home, whether the home is big enough for the family, the presence of safety hazards, and family plans for fire or other disasters are all relevant to the family's health status and can be derived from observations and interviews with family members. Potential hazards to be considered in assessing a family's physical environment include:

- Peeling paint (especially lead-based paint in older homes)
- Loose throw rugs, toys, or other safety hazards in walkways
- Broken furniture
- Broken stairs or stair railings (inside or outside the home)
- Broken porch floorboards or railings
- Hazardous materials within children's reach
- Plumbing that does not allow for sanitary disposal of human wastes
- Overcrowding
- Absence of fire alarms in the home
- Lack of a fire or other disaster plan
- Lack of a poison control plan (posted telephone numbers)
- Numerous house pets such as cats or dogs
- Close proximity to a heavily traveled highway
- Lack of a fenced-in yard for small children

Tools for assessing home safety for families with children and families with older members are included in the *Community Assessment Reference Guide* designed as a companion to this text.

The community health nurse should note if there are any air, water, or noise pollution problems in the external environment that would increase the family's risks of disability and illness. It is important to determine what the sources of pollution are and the effects of pollution on the family.

After making this assessment, the community health nurse may want to question family members about perceptions of their environment. Does the family feel safe in this neighborhood? What are the hazards they perceive? Do they have an emergency plan if their safety should be jeopardized? Is the family aware of any existing pollutants in their neighborhood? Questions for a focused assessment of physical environmental considerations in family health are presented on page 342.

At the aggregate level, the community health nurse would obtain similar information about environmental conditions within the community. What is the proportion of unsafe housing in the community? What sources of pollution are present? What is the disaster potential in the community and how might a disaster affect resident families? The answers to these and other questions will give the community health nurse some

FOCUSED ASSESSMENT

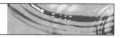

Physical Environmental Considerations in Family Assessment

- Where does the family live?
- What is the physical condition of the home? Are there safety hazards in the home?
- Is plumbing adequate? Is the amount of space available adequate for the number of persons in the family?
- Does the family have an emergency plan?
- How safe is the neighborhood? Are there environmental hazards in the neighborhood?
- Does the family have access to necessary goods and services (e.g., grocery stores)?

idea of the environmental conditions that may be faced by families in general as well as by specific families.

With respect to sociocultural dimension factors, the nurse assesses family roles and their effectiveness in meeting family needs. The nurse identifies the presence or absence of formal and informal roles, determines how well roles are performed, and examines their effects on family function and cohesiveness. Much of this information will be derived from observations of family interaction. The nurse will also want to assess for evidence of role conflict by asking family members about the roles they play and how those roles influence their physical and emotional well-being. The nurse can also assess the family's ability to adjust roles to the changing needs of its members and can provide anticipatory guidance about adjustments that will be needed. At the societal level, information on cultural expectations regarding family roles within the overall population or in ethnic subgroups can help the community health nurse identify the potential influence of family roles on health and illness. The nurse can compare individual family culture with that of the community in which they live and determine if there are differences present that may create problems for the family or the children of the family. Principles of cultural assessment, discussed in Chapter 9∞, are applicable to the assessment of the sociocultural dimension of families.

An individual family's social class and economic status can profoundly affect its health status. The community health nurse can assess these elements of the sociocultural dimension by observation of family living conditions and interviews with key family informants. At the aggregate level, data on the proportion of families living in poverty and the educational and economic levels of the population or subgroups in the population can provide information on the potential effects of social and economic factors on the health of individual families.

Families may also have other external resources available to them. To assist families in dealing with social environmental stressors, the community health nurse needs to identify the resources available to the family. External resources include those materials or sources of assistance available to the family from the community. The nurse's assessment of the family's external resources may suggest ways of dealing with identified health problems. Questions that elicit this information relate to neighborhood sources of financial assistance, transportation, housing, health care, and education. The nurse would gather data on the types of social services and social support systems available to families in need. For example, the nurse might examine local telephone or social service agency directories for the types of services available to address family needs. The nurse should also investigate relational support systems such as kin networks, friends, and neighbors in interviews with family members.

Community health nurses should be alert to the effects of both separation and reunification on refugee and immigrant families and assist them in dealing with the myriad problems that may result. Knowledge of the number of refugee families in the community and their countries of origin will assist the community health nurse in identifying some of the potential problems that these families may experience.

At the population level, the community health nurse should assess conditions that affect the social environment of families as well as the overall availability of social resources for families. What is the level of unemployment in the community? What is the availability of jobs, particularly for families with low education levels? What social and cultural attitudes prevalent in the population may affect family health and function? Similarly, the nurse would assess the resources available to families such as financial assistance, education for parenting, and so on. Potential questions for a focused assessment of sociocultural considerations in individual families are presented below. These questions may be adapted to assess factors impinging upon families at the population level.

FOCUSED ASSESSMENT

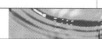

Sociocultural Considerations in Family Assessment

- What formal and informal roles are enacted by family members? How flexible and interchangeable are these roles?
- How congruent are family roles with those of the dominant culture?
- Is there evidence of role conflict? Role overload?
- How adequate are family role models?
- Are essential family roles being adequately performed?
- Are there expected changes in family roles? How will the family adapt to these changes?
- What cultural and religious factors influence family health status?
- What is the family's income? Is the income sufficient to meet the family's needs?
- Are family members employed? What are the occupations of family members? Do occupational roles conflict with family roles? Do occupational roles present health hazards for family members?
- Is this a refugee family? If so, how have they adapted to their changed environment?

Community health nurses also assess behavioral dimension factors and their effects on family health. A family's nutritional status can be assessed through physical assessment of each member and by observing the way in which the family selects, purchases, and prepares food. If any family members are nutritionally impaired, the nurse will need to determine the underlying causes. Is it lack of money to buy food? Does the person who prepares food lack information that would ensure good family nutrition? How is food prepared?

Other consumption patterns of interest to the nurse include the use of alcohol, drugs, medications, tobacco, and caffeine. Is the use of any of these substances causing a family member to be unable to carry out his or her role and functions within the family? Does the mother's smoking, for instance, aggravate her child's respiratory condition? Are prescription drugs being used as prescribed? Are any side effects evident from the use of prescription drugs? Are over-the-counter (OTC) products used appropriately? The answers to these and similar questions assist the nurse to identify problems arising from family consumption patterns. Similarly, aggregate-level data on consumption patterns, particularly those related to tobacco, drugs, and alcohol, can suggest problems that may be experienced by individual families.

Assessment of the type and frequency of physical activity by family members should also be addressed. Community health nurses can ask family members to describe physical and leisure-time activities. At the aggregate level, the nurse can obtain information on the types of leisure-time activities available to families in the community through examination of the telephone book, personal observation of the community, or interviews with staff at recreational facilities. With the individual family, the nurse would explore whether there are exercise or leisure activities that meet the needs of individual family members as well as activities that the family engages in together.

Family safety practices should be considered in assessing the behavioral dimension of family health. Areas to be addressed include seat belt and infant/child safety seat use, use of other safety devices (e.g., bicycle helmets), storage and disposal of hazardous substances, and safety education for children. Information in these areas can be obtained by observation or in interviews with family members. Family sexual practices can also be assessed in interviews with key family informants. These and other behavioral dimension considerations are included in the focused assessment questions provided at right. The questions provided reflect assessment of the individual family, but can be adapted to assess families at the aggregate level as well.

Health system considerations in family assessment include the family's attitudes toward health and response to illness and their use of health services. Community health nurses would gather information

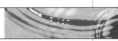

FOCUSED ASSESSMENT

Behavioral Considerations in Family Assessment

- What are the food preferences and consumption patterns of the family? How are foods usually prepared? By whom?
- Do family members smoke, or use or abuse alcohol or other substances?
- What medications are used by family members? Is medication use appropriate? Are medications stored safely?
- Do family members get adequate rest and exercise?
- What kinds of leisure activities do family members engage in? Do leisure activities pose any health hazards?
- Do family members engage in appropriate safety precautions in the following areas?
  - Consistent seat belt use
  - Use of safety equipment such as eye and ear protection
  - Use of infant safety seats
  - Cribs with safe spacing between rails and proper mattress width
  - Proper storage and disposal of hazardous substances
  - Safety education of children regarding not talking to or going with strangers, crossing the street safely, and using seat belts and safety equipment such as helmets, goggles, and ear protection
  - Safe use of appliances and craft equipment such as saws, glues, and drills
- Who in the family engages in sexual activity? Is there a need for contraceptives? What is the attitude of family members toward sexual activity?

on family perceptions of health and illness and the priority accorded to health promotion activities. Family members can be asked about their use of health services, including the type of services and when they are sought. The community health nurse should also explore families' practical responses to illness. In some families, home remedies or cultural health practices are used before a health care provider is consulted. The community health nurse needs to assess whether these practices are harmful to sick family members and whether to encourage the family to seek professional assistance. Chapter 9 ∞ addressed ways in which the nurse can determine which cultural health practices may be harmful and how to help families choose other modes of care.

It is important to learn where family members go for health care and whether their choice provides any preventive health services or dental care. Many private medical doctors provide only sickness care, and families may need information about where to go for preventive services such as immunizations, health teaching, and dental care.

At the aggregate level, the community health nurse should assess the availability of health services needed by families in the population. What illness-preventive and health-promotive services are available? Are they accessible to all families in the population or only to certain subgroups? What secondary and tertiary preventive services are available?

Aggregate-level assessment also focuses on the effectiveness of health services provided to families in the population and the extent to which those services are utilized. For example, are prenatal services available but underutilized by families in the community or by certain segments of the community? Local figures on the proportion of pregnancies for which no prenatal care is received is one measure of service utilization. Similarly, the nurse might obtain data on the number of nonemergent visits to emergency departments suggesting inappropriate use of emergency services for routine illness. Accessibility and affordability of services available to families in the community should also be assessed. Again, general information on the types of services available can be gleaned from the telephone directory. Information on costs and other accessibility issues (e.g., hours of operation, types of insurance taken) can best be obtained through interviews or surveys of local providers and health care agencies. Tips for a focused assessment of health system considerations related to family health are provided below. In addition, Appendix F on the Companion Website includes a tool for family assessment incorporating considerations in each of the six dimensions of health. The tool is also included in the *Community Assessment Reference Guide* designed to accompany this text to assist community health nurses to assess the health status of a specific family or families as an aggregate within the population.

Diagnostic Reasoning and Care of Families

The data obtained during family health assessment enable the nurse to make informed decisions about the health care needs of families. These needs are stated in the form of nursing diagnoses. The community health nurse may develop nursing diagnoses related to individual families or to families as a group within the larger population. For example, the nurse may diagnose "family exhibiting ineffective coping related to changes in roles and relationships in a newly constituted stepfamily as evidenced by conflict between stepmother and

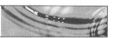

FOCUSED ASSESSMENT

Health System Considerations in Family Assessment

- How does the family define health and illness? How does the family prioritize health in relation to other family needs and goals?
- How do family members deal with illness?
- Who makes health-related decisions in the family? Who carries out those decisions?
- What health-related behaviors do family members exhibit?
- What is the family's usual source of health care?
- Is the family's use of health care services appropriate?
- Does the family have health insurance? If so, are all family members covered? What services are covered?
- How adequate are the primary, secondary, and tertiary prevention services available to families?
- How available, accessible, and affordable are health services for families in the community?

stepchildren." An example of an aggregate family nursing diagnosis might be "families with chronically ill children at risk for increased stress related to lack of adequate community support services."

Planning and Implementing Health Care for Families

Not all families will require community health nursing intervention. Some indications of the need for intervention, based on nursing diagnoses derived from the family health assessment, include:

- Illness in a family member with a detrimental effect on the family unit
- Family factors that contribute to ill health in a family member
- Recent diagnosis of serious illness in a family member
- Marked deterioration in the health status of a family member
- Hospital admission or discharge of a family member
- Missed or delayed developmental milestones
- Death of a family member
- Presence of psychological, environmental, sociocultural, behavioral, or health system factors detrimental to family health and function

When intervention is required, community health nurses plan nursing interventions to address identified needs. These interventions may be directed toward improving the health of specific families or of all families within a population and may take place at the primary, secondary, and tertiary levels of prevention. Population-level interventions will often involve the creation or expansion of an infrastructure that supports effective family function and provides services needed by families in the population.

Primary Prevention

Primary prevention for individual families may involve health promotion and protection or illness prevention. Community health nurses can educate family members regarding the need for adequate nutrition, rest, and physical activity to promote health. Safety education and advocating use of safety devices or equipment are some potential approaches to health protection with families. Similarly, the nurse may teach family members how to minimize lead exposure in residential areas with high levels of lead contamination in soil or water or advocate with landlords for removal of lead-based paint or other safety hazards in older housing. Illness prevention may include teaching effective hygiene, referring for immunization, or advocating for access to safe water and food supplies as well as other interventions.

At the aggregate level, primary preventive activities by community health nurses are likely to be directed toward advocacy for environmental protection and social justice or assuring the availability of health promotion and illness prevention services to families. For example, community health nurses may be actively involved in local initiatives to guarantee families a living wage or to assure that immunization and other health promotion and illness prevention services are available to low-income families.

Teaching coping skills and modeling effective communication strategies with adolescents are two interventions that community health nurses might employ to prevent family crises. The community health nurse may advocate for a balance between increasing independence and supervision of adolescents. Advocacy related to financial difficulties (e.g., linking families to available sources of financial support, employment assistance, and so on) may also help to alleviate factors that contribute to family crises. Primary prevention for family crisis also includes providing anticipatory guidance related to common crises of family life and assisting families to develop effective coping strategies to combat the stress of situational crises.

It may be impossible, and sometimes undesirable, to prevent a crisis situation from occurring; however, the nurse can assist the family to prepare for and cope with the event. For example, the birth of a child or change of employment may be a very desirable event. Such an event requires changes in lifestyle and family adaptation that might precipitate a crisis. The nurse can assist the family to explore areas in which change will be required, avenues for accomplishing these changes, and strategies for dealing with the anxiety related to change. Through primary prevention implemented via anticipatory guidance, potential crises may be averted even though stressful events occur.

Secondary Prevention

Secondary prevention activities with families may be aimed at assisting families to obtain needed care for existing health problems or helping families to deal with these problems. For example, the nurse might facilitate a family meeting to discuss role allocation in order to minimize role overload on a few family members. Similarly, the nurse might refer a family with a substance-abusing member to community resources to help them deal with the problem. In the advocacy role, the nurse may help families explore treatment options or obtain approval for substance abuse treatment coverage under their insurance plan. The community health nurse might even engage in advocacy with an employer to assure access to an available employee assistance program (EAP).

Community health nurses may also be instrumental in linking families with other services needed to resolve existing family health problems. For example, they may encourage a wife and mother to remove herself and her children from an abusive situation as well as provide information on where the woman can get help. In this instance, the community health nurse may need to advocate with local police or court officials for adequate protection for the woman and her children. At a more mundane level, the community health nurse may refer family members to sources of medical assis-

tance to deal with existing illnesses. For example, the nurse may refer a family to a community clinic for treatment of the grandmother's hypertension.

Crisis intervention is an important element of secondary prevention in the care of many families. Crisis intervention focuses on secondary prevention and is directed toward helping members to discuss and define the problem and to express their feelings concerning the crisis situation. The nurse is an active listener and participates attentively, but the family must do the work. The emphasis is on bringing feelings out into the open. The nurse must be truthful, honest, and forthright, and should not give false reassurance about the situation.

Exploration of coping mechanisms already used enables the nurse to help the family examine ways to cope. The nurse's involvement includes helping the family to explore other options for dealing with the situation. The pros and cons of each of these alternatives should be discussed with the family. At this stage, the nurse may need to be fairly directive in assisting family members to implement agreed-upon strategies for resolving the crisis. For example, if the family has decided to confront a substance-abusing member with the need for treatment, the nurse may need to assign specific tasks to certain family members to implement the confrontation.

Advocacy for secondary preventive services may be needed at the population level. The community health nurse may be actively involved in alerting health policy makers to the need for family services and in initiating plans for programs to meet those needs. For example, if the nurse's assessment indicates that most families in the population are dual-earner or single-parent families whose needs for childcare services are not being met, he or she may initiate community efforts to provide additional childcare resources. Similarly, knowledge of widespread violations of housing codes in rental housing for families seen by the nurse may lead to reports to the housing authority and advocacy activities on the part of the nurse to promote code enforcement.

Tertiary Prevention

With respect to tertiary prevention, community health nurses may assist families to cope with long-term health problems or to deal with the consequences of those problems. For example, a nurse might suggest home modifications that permit a disabled family member to be more functional within the family or help a family coping with Alzheimer's disease to locate respite care. Another example of tertiary prevention is assisting families to deal with the loss of a loved one, particularly during holidays and anniversaries (Klicker, 2002). Phone calls to caregivers of people with Alzheimer's disease have been found to be a helpful tertiary prevention measure for dealing with caregiver burden (Chang et al., 2004). Similarly, creative arts interventions have shown success in reducing stress and anxiety and improving emotions in caregivers of family members with cancer

MediaLink Case Study: Family Health

(Walsh, Martin, & Schmidt, 2004). After successful resolution of a crisis, tertiary prevention might involve following up with the family to help them recognize their use of the problem-solving process, identify how the crisis might have been averted if possible, and engage in activities that will prevent future crises from occurring.

Tertiary prevention activities may also occur at the aggregate level. For example, the community health nurse might advocate for the development of respite services for family caretakers or create support groups for crisis-prone families to help them avoid future crises.

Evaluating Health Care for Families

Evaluation of family care begins as the nurse examines the adequacy of the assessment database and continues as he or she evaluates alternative approaches to meeting families' health care needs. Post-intervention evaluation focuses on the achievement of objectives of family care and the processes and structures that promote accomplishment of these objectives.

Evaluation will occur at the level of individual families who receive care and at the population level. With respect to the care of individual families, the nurse would examine whether care has resulted in expected family outcomes. Is the family better able to cope with stress? Have communications between parents and adolescent children improved? The nurse would also assess the appropriateness of interventions employed and the quality of their implementation. Were the interventions appropriate to the family's cultural beliefs and practices? To the family's education level? Did the family experience frustration in following through on referrals because the nurse did not select appropriate resources or did not effectively prepare the family for acting on the referral?

At the aggregate level, evaluation will focus on outcomes and processes of care for groups of families rather than individual families. Is respite care readily available to families that need it? Is respite care provided in the most cost-effective manner? What are the effects of respite care on the level of stress experienced by families with disabled members? These and other questions can address outcome and process evaluation of programs designed to serve groups of families within the population.

Much of the work of community health nurses involves care of families in a variety of health care settings. Family care should be based on the principles presented in this chapter and should contribute to the improvement of the overall health status of the population in which the family lives. Use of the nursing process in the context of community-focused care permits community health nurses to meet the health needs of family clients as well as those of the larger community.

Case Study

A Family in Need

Alfinia Michaels is a 45-year-old single parent of two children, a boy of 8 years and a girl of 5. She has recently been diagnosed with breast cancer and is scheduled to have a lumpectomy and reconstruction of her right breast in 2 weeks. Ms. Michaels is divorced and is responsible for the care of her 79-year-old father, who has mild Alzheimer's disease. Her father is still capable of caring for himself during the day while she works, but cannot be left alone overnight and cannot care for the children. Ms. Michaels has one sister who lives approximately 150 miles away. She states that she and her sister have always been close. Ms. Michaels's former husband lives in the same community. He provides child support and health insurance for the children and takes them every other weekend. Ms. Michaels does not have health insurance because she works two part-time jobs, neither of which includes benefits. She tells the community health nurse she doesn't have any idea how she will pay for her surgery and the chemotherapy that will follow. She is worried about care of her father and her children during her hospitalization and afterwards.

1. What biophysical, psychological, physical environmental, sociocultural, behavioral, and health system factors are influencing this situation?
2. Is this a crisis situation? If so, what type of crisis would this be?
3. What nursing interventions might the community health nurse employ with this family?
4. How could the nurse evaluate the effectiveness of nursing intervention?
5. How might your interventions be different if you find that many families in the population are experiencing similar problems?

Test Your Understanding

1. List at least five different types of families. What are the characteristic features of each type? (pp. 318–321)

2. What are the basic components of family structure? What are the five major functions performed by families? Give some examples of how family structure might influence the ability to effectively perform family functions. (pp. 324–327)

3. What are the basic concepts of systems theory? How are these concepts applied to families? (pp. 321–323)

4. How do Duvall's and Carter and McGoldrick's stages of family development differ? How are they similar? (pp. 323–324)

5. Describe assessment considerations related to the biophysical, psychological, physical environmental, sociocultural, behav-

ioral, and health systems dimensions to be addressed in assessing a family. Give an example of how each might influence family health. (pp. 327–338)

6. How do formal family roles differ from informal roles? Give an example of each type of role. (p. 333)

7. How does a maturational crisis differ from a situational crisis? Give an example of each type of crisis. (p. 332)

8. Provide examples of family interventions at the primary, secondary, and tertiary level of prevention. Describe how you might evaluate the effectiveness of your interventions. (pp. 334–346)

EXPLORE MediaLink

http://www.prenhall.com/clark
Resources for this chapter can be found on the Companion Website.

Audio Glossary
Appendix F: Family Health Assessment and
    Intervention Guide
Exam Review Questions

Case Study: Family Health
MediaLink Application: Foster Parenting
    (video)
Media Links

Challenge Your Knowledge
Advocacy Interviews

References

Aldred, H., Gott, M., & Gariballa, S. (2005). Advanced heart failure: Impact on older patients and informal caregivers. *Journal of Advanced Nursing, 49,* 116–124.

American Association of Retired Persons (AARP). (2002). *Beyond 50: A report to the nation on trends in health security.* Washington, DC: Author.

Asahara, K., Momose, Y., Murashima, S., Okubo, N., & Magilvy, J. K. (2001). The relationship of social norms to use of services and care giver burden in Japan. *Journal of Nursing Scholarship, 33,* 375–380.

Cannuscio, C. C., Colditz, G. A., Rimm, E. B., Berkman, L. F., Jones, C. P., & Kawachi, I. (2004). Employment status, social ties, and caregivers' mental health. *Social Science & Medicine, 58,* 1247–1256.

Cannuscio, C. C., Jones, C., Kawachi, I., Colditz, G. A., Berkman, L., & Rimm, E. (2002). Reverberations of family illness: A longitudinal assessment of information caregiving and mental health in the nurses' health study. *American Journal of Public Health, 92,* 1305–1311.

Carter, B., & McGoldrick, M. (1999). Overview: The expanded family life cycle: Individual, family, and social perspectives. In B. Carter & M. McGoldrick (Eds.), *The expanded family life cycle: Individual, family and social perspectives* (3rd ed., pp. 1–26). Boston: Allyn & Bacon.

Casper, L. M., & Bianchi, S. M. (2002). *Continuity and change in the American family.* Thousand Oaks, CA: Sage.

Centers for Disease Control and Prevention. (2005). *Healthy people data.* Retrieved September 25, 2005, from http://wonder.cdc.gov/data 2010

Chang, B. L., Nitta, S., Carter, P. A., & Markham, Y. L. (2004). Perceived helpfulness of telephone calls: Providing support for caregivers of family members with dementia. *Journal of Gerontological Nursing, 30*(9), 14–21.

Chiu, L., Shyu, W-C., & Liu, Y-H. (2001). Comparisons of the cost-effectiveness among hospital chronic care, nursing home placement, home nursing care, and family care for severe stroke patients. *Journal of Advanced Nursing, 33,* 380–386.

Clark, P. C., Dunbar, S. B., Shields, C. G., Viswanathan, B., Aycock, D. M., & Wolf, S. L. (2004). Influence of stroke survivor characteristics and family conflict surrounding recovery on caregivers' mental and physical health. *Nursing Research, 53,* 406–431.

dos Rets, S., Zito, J. M., Safer, D. J., & Soeken, K. L. (2001). Mental health services for youths in foster care and disabled youths. *American Journal of Public Health, 91,* 1094–1099.

Duvall, E., & Miller, B. (1990). *Marriage and family development* (6th ed.). New York: Harper College.

Ellwood, D. T., & Jencks, C. (2004). The spread of single-parent families in the United States since 1960. In D. P. Moynihan, T. M. Smeeding, & L. Rainwater (Eds.), *The future of the family* (pp. 25–65). New York: Russell Sage Foundation.

Fellmeth, R. C. (2003). The child care system in the United States. In H. M. Wallace, G. Green, & K. J. Jaros (Eds.), *Health and welfare for families in the 21st century* (2nd ed., pp. 171–196). Sudbury, MA: Jones and Bartlett.

Flaskerud, J., & Lee, P. (2001). Vulnerability to health problems in female informal caregivers of persons with HIV/AIDS and age-related dementias. *Journal of Advanced Nursing, 33,* 60–68.

Friedman, M. M., Bowden, V. R., & Jones, E. (2003). *Family nursing: Research, theory, and practice* (5th ed.). Upper Saddle River, NJ: Prentice Hall.

Giorgianni, S. J. (Ed.). (2003). *How families matter in health: Challenges of the evolving 21st-century family.* New York: Impact Communications.

Goodman, J. H. (2004). Paternal postpartum depression, its relationship to maternal postpartum depression, and implications for family health. *Journal of Advanced Nursing, 45,* 26–35.

Han, H. R. (2003). Korean mothers' psychosocial adjustment to their children's cancer. *Journal of Advanced Nursing, 44,* 499–506.

Hofferth, S. L. (2003a). Did welfare reform work: Implications for 2002 and beyond. In H. M. Wallace, G. Green, & K. J. Jaros (Eds.), *Health and welfare for families in the 21st century* (2nd ed., pp. 138–148). Sudbury, MA: Jones and Bartlett.

Hofferth, S. L. (2003b). The American family: Changes and challenges for the 21st century. In H. M. Wallace, G. Green, & K. J. Jaros (Eds.), *Health and welfare for families in the 21st century* (2nd ed., pp. 71–79). Sudbury, MA: Jones and Bartlett.

Jungbauer, J., Stelling, K., Dietrich, S., & Angermeyer, M. C. (2004). Schizophrenia: Problems of separation in families. *Journal of Advanced Nursing, 47,* 605–613.

Kiernan, K. (2004). Unmarried cohabitation and parenthood: Here to stay? European perspectives. In D. P. Moynihan, T. M. Smeeding, & L. Rainwater (Eds.), *The future of the family* (pp. 66–95). New York: Russell Sage Foundation.

Klicker, R. L. (2002). *Guidelines: Grief and the holidays.* Madison, AL: Guideline Publications.

Lee, I., Lee, E.-O., Kim, H. S., Park, Y. S., Song, M., & Park, Y. H. (2005). Concept development of family resilience: A study of Korean families with a chronically ill child. *Journal of Clinical Nursing, 13,* 636–645.

Lyons, K. S., Stewart, B. J., Archbold, P., Carter, J. H., & Perrin, N. A. (2004). Pessimism and optimism as early warning signs for compromised health for caregivers of patients with Parkinson's disease. *Nursing Research, 53,* 354–362.

McCann, J. J., Herbert, L. E., Bienias, J. L., Morris, M. C., & Evans, D. A. (2004). Predictors of beginning and ending caregiving during a 3-year period in a biracial community population of older adults. *American Journal of Public Health, 94*, 1800–1806.

McCubbin, M. A., & McCubbin, H. I. (1993). Families coping with illness: The resiliency model of family stress, adjustment, and adaptation. In C. B. Danielson, B. Hamel-Bissell, & P. Winstead-Fry (Eds.), *Families, health and illness: Perspectives on coping and intervention* (pp. 21–63). St. Louis: Mosby.

McCubbin, H. I., Thompson, A. I., & McCubbin, M. A. (2001). *Family measures: Stress, coping, and resiliency—Inventories for research and practice.* Honolulu, HI: Kamehameha Schools.

Mjelde-Mossey, L. A., Barak, M. E. M., & Knight, B. G. (2004). Coping behaviors as predictors of drinking practices among primary in-home dementia caregivers. *Journal of Applied Gerontology, 23*, 295–308.

National Institute for Occupational Health and Safety. (2001). Occupational and take-home lead poisoning associated with restoring chemically stripped furniture—California, 1998. *Morbidity and Mortality Weekly Report, 50*, 246–248.

Navaie-Waliser, M., Feldman, P. H., Gould, D. A., Levine, C., Kuerbis, A. N., & Donelan, K. (2002). When the caregiver needs care: The plight of vulnerable caregivers. *American Journal of Public Health, 92*, 409–413.

Patterson, J. M. (2002). Integrating family resilience and family stress theory. *Journal of Marriage and Family, 64*, 349–360.

Polatnick, M. R. (2000). Working parents. *National Forum, 80*(6), 38–41.

Rainwater, L., & Smeeding, T. M. (2004). Single-parent poverty, inequality, and the welfare state. In D. P. Moynihan, T. M. Smeeding, & L. Rainwater (Eds.), *The future of the family* (pp. 96–115). New York: Russell Sage Foundation.

Ray, R. A., & Street, A. F. (2005). Ecomapping: An innovative research tool for nurses. *Journal of Advanced Nursing, 50*, 545–552.

Rosenbach, M., Lewis, K., & Quinn, B. (2003). Children in foster care: Challenges in meeting their health care needs through Medicaid. In H. M. Wallace, G. Green, & K. J. Jaros (Eds.), *Health and welfare for families in the 21st century* (2nd ed., pp. 197–205). Sudbury, MA: Jones and Bartlett.

Rousseau, C., Rufagari, M., Bagilishya, D., & Measham, T. (2004). Remaking family life: Strategies for re-establishing continuity among Congolese refugees during the family reunification process. *Social Science & Medicine, 59*, 1095–1108.

Saloviita, T., Italinna, M., & Leinonen, E. (2003). Explaining the parental stress of fathers and mothers caring for a child with intellectual disability: A double ABCX model. *Journal of Intellectual Disability Research, 47*, 300–312.

Sherman, P., & Redlener, I. (2003). Homeless women and their children in the 21st century. In H. M. Wallace, G. Green, & K. J. Jaros (Eds.), *Health and welfare for families in the 21st century* (2nd ed., pp. 469–480). Sudbury, MA: Jones and Bartlett.

Soubhi, H., & Potvin, L. (2000). Homes and families as health promotion settings. In B. D. Poland, L. W. Green, & I. Rootman (Eds.), *Settings for health promotion: Linking theory and practice* (pp. 44–67). Thousand Oaks, CA: Sage.

Strunnin, L., & Boden, L. I. (2004). Family consequences of chronic back pain. *Social Science & Medicine, 58*, 1385–1393.

Sullivan, M. T. (2004). Caregiver strain index. *Dermatology Nursing, 16*, 385–386.

Svavarsdottir, E. K., & Rayens, M. K. (2005). Hardiness in families of young children with asthma. *Journal of Advanced Nursing, 50*, 381–390.

Takeda, Y., Kawachi, I., Yamagata, Z., Hashimoto, S., Matsumura, Y., Oguri, S., et al. (2003). Multigenerational family structure in Japanese society: Impacts on stress and health behaviors among women and men. *Social Science & Medicine, 59*, 69–81.

U.S. Census Bureau. (2004). *Poverty: 2003 highlights.* Retrieved September 30, 2004, from http://www.census.gov

U.S. Census Bureau. (2005). *Statistical abstract of the United States: 2004–2005.* Retrieved April 12, 2005, from http://www.census.gov/prod/pubs/04statab

Usita, P. M., Hall, S. S., & Davis, J. C. (2004). Role ambiguity in family caregiving. *Journal of Applied Gerontology, 23*(1), 20–39.

Vellone, E., Sansoni, J., & Cohen, M. Z. (2002). The experience of Italians caring for family members with Alzheimer's disease. *Journal of Nursing Scholarship, 34*, 323–329.

von Bertalanffy, L. (1973). *General systems theory.* New York: George Braziller.

von Bertalanffy, L. (1981). *A systems view of man.* Boulder, CO: Westview.

Walsh, S. M., Martin, S. C., & Schmidt, L. A. (2004). Testing the efficacy of a creative-arts intervention with family caregivers of patients with cancer. *Journal of Nursing Scholarship, 36*, 214–219.

Wright, L. M., & Leahey, M. (2005). *Nurses and families: A guide to family assessment and intervention* (4th ed.). Philadelphia: F. A. Davis.

Yosef, A-R. (2004). Male Arab-Muslim's health and health promotion perceptions and practices. (Unpublished manuscript).

Zwelling, E., & Phillips, C. R. (2001). Family-centered maternity care in the new millennium. Is it real or is it imagined? *Journal of Perinatal and Neonatal Nursing, 15*(3), 1–12.

Care of Populations

CHAPTER OBJECTIVES

After reading this chapter, you should be able to:

1. Discuss the rationale for including members of the population in every phase of population health assessment and health program planning.
2. Describe factors in each of the six dimensions of health to be considered in assessing the health of a population.
3. Describe the components of a population nursing diagnosis.
4. Identify at least five tasks in planning health programs to meet the needs of populations.
5. Analyze the elements of a program theory or logic model and its usefulness in health program planning.
6. Describe four levels of acceptance of a health care program.
7. Describe three types of considerations in evaluating a health care program.

KEY TERMS

 MediaLink
http://www.prenhall.com/clark

Additional interactive resources for this chapter can be found on the Companion Website. Click on Chapter 15 and "Begin" to select the activities for this chapter.

Advocacy in Action

Community Nursing Guidance Clinics in Japan

Kenkounippon21 is a national mandate in Japan much like *Healthy People 2010* in the United States. As this mandate for health promotion through individual and social efforts was being developed, the Japanese Nursing Association was developing a new system of community nursing services that included the use of volunteer services. An assessment of community needs indicated a need for education and consultation services for clients with minor health problems. Based on this assessment, community health nursing faculty met with the local nursing association to propose a project to meet this need. They also visited the city office, met with the director of health promotion and local public health nurses, and visited a nursing alumni association and a medical association in the community. All of them agreed to collaborate in initiating a new voluntary nursing service. The local nursing association provided the funds; the city office provided the place; the nursing alumni association recruited volunteer nurses; and the medical association supported the new service. Nursing faculty members wrote grants to purchase equipment to measure bone mass, energy expenditure, blood pressure, and body mass index.

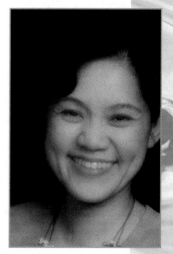

The nursing faculty group established a center to provide volunteer nursing services in May 2004. The center is open on Saturdays from 2 to 4 pm twice a month at a citizens' plaza. The location is easily accessible to community members, and they can choose among a variety of free services, including nursing guidance and education, health measurement, health diary, and information and referral services. Through their ability to network with multiple segments of society, these nurses have created a program that meets the needs of both individual clients and the community.

Ariko Noji

Niigata College of Nursing, Joetsu City, Niigata, Japan

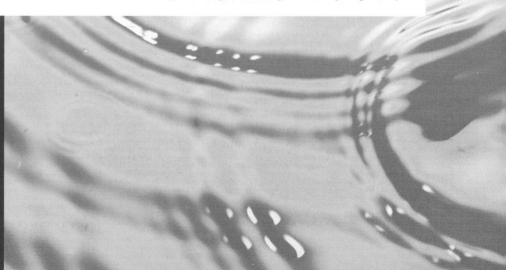

*N*owhere is the advocacy role of community health nurses more apparent than in the care of population groups. From the beginnings of community health nursing in the United States, community health nurses have been assessing the needs of population groups and planning and implementing programs to meet those needs. As noted several times in earlier chapters, the focus of community health nursing is on the health of population groups or aggregates. In many instances, this focus entails providing care to communities or to target groups within communities. Communities, as we saw in Chapter 2∞, are "groups composed of individuals, families, organizations, or businesses that share a common language, common values, a common history, or a common purpose" (Nardi, 2003a, p. 2). A target group is a subgroup within the community whose members exhibit particular health needs (such as victims of family violence) or are at particular risk for the development of problems (e.g., members of refugee groups).

This care of whole population groups is sometimes referred to as **population health management**, which is defined as "accountability and management of the health of an entire community regardless of system membership or insurance status" (Greene & Kelsey, as quoted in Robertson, 2004, p. 495). Population health management involves health promotion and illness prevention strategies at the community level designed to improve overall population health status.

Although community health nurses have long been involved in advocacy and program development to address the health needs of population groups, this focus was subsumed within care of individuals and families for many years. For example, a set of objectives for public health nursing developed by the National Organization for Public Health Nursing (NOPHN) in 1931 focused on the care of individuals and families, with community-level initiatives aimed at developing resources to meet their needs. By 1949, a new statement of *Public Health Nursing Responsibilities in a Community Health Program*, also by NOPHN, reflected an expanded focus for public health nursing in community program planning. According to this statement, community health nurses were expected not only to participate in planning nursing services but also to address social problems affecting health. Most recently, in 2003, the Quad Council, an association of nursing organizations with a focus on community health, developed a new set of competencies that maintains this focus on population health, with care of individuals and families within the context of population-level practice (Abrams, 2004). Today, skills in population assessment and program planning are expected of nurses prepared at the baccalaureate level (Clark & Buell, 2004).

Most population-based health care interventions are developed in collaboration with members of other professions and community residents rather than by

GLOBAL PERSPECTIVES

*C*ommunity health nurses in the United States have only recently begun to reclaim their role in the care of populations. Explore the international community health nursing literature to determine the extent to which community health nurses in other countries engage in population-based care.

community health nurses in isolation. In the past, interventions for population groups frequently entailed health professionals' identification of problems and development and implementation of programs to solve them with minimal input from group members. More recently, health professionals have advocated the involvement of members of the population at all stages of intervention, from participation in identifying community needs and capabilities to the development, implementation, and evaluation of programs that enhance local capacity to meet those needs.

THE EPIDEMIOLOGY OF POPULATION HEALTH

Factors that influence community health can be organized in various ways. For example, one might address the physical features of the community, availability of a healthy environment, health services provided, or sociocultural features of the population. The community's reputation might also have a bearing on factors that influence population health status (Macintyre & Ellaway, 2003). For example, an area with a reputation as being dangerous might hamper physical activity by community members. Factors influencing community health could also be examined in light of the leading health indicators delineated in *Healthy People 2010*◆ and discussed in Chapter 2∞. In this chapter, we will use the six dimensions of health to frame our discussion of factors affecting the health of population groups.

Biophysical Considerations

Human biological factors influencing a population's health reflect specific physical attributes of its members. The first of these attributes is age. Others reflect the genetic inheritance and physiologic function of community members.

The age composition of the population is an important indicator of probable health needs. Typically, there is a greater need for health services in areas with large numbers of the very young and the very old. Large numbers of women of childbearing age increase the need for prenatal and family planning services. Accident prevention is a major consideration in populations with large numbers of school-age and younger children.

Another population factor related to age composition is the annual birth rate, which provides information on the growth of the younger segments of the population. The annual birth rate is calculated on the basis of the number of live births during the year in relation to the total population of the community. Birth rates are calculated per 1,000 persons. Birth statistics are usually compiled by official local and state health agencies and can be obtained from these sources.

Age-specific death rates also provide valuable information regarding the health status of the population. An age-specific death rate is the number of deaths in a particular age group compared with the population within that group. Because of the relatively small number of deaths in some age groups, the multiplier used in calculating age-specific death rates is 100,000. Excess deaths (deaths over the number that would be expected for that age group in the general population) for any age group in the population would indicate the presence of health problems.

The average age at death also provides an indication of overall population health. If people in the community typically die at a relatively young age, this suggests the existence of health problems that are contributing to these early deaths. Native Americans, for example, have shorter expected life spans than the rest of the population because of the high incidence of such health problems as chronic disease and alcoholism and high rates of homicide.

One feature of the genetic inheritance of the population is its distribution by gender. Many health problems such as obesity, hypertension, and various forms of cancer are more prevalent in one gender than in the other. Knowing the gender distribution in the community sharpens the index of suspicion with regard to these problems. Knowing the composition of the population with respect to gender assists the assessment team to identify health needs and plan programs to meet them. For example, the knowledge that women constitute 79% of a community's population might suggest the need for easily accessible detection programs for cancer of the cervix and breast.

The racial or ethnic composition of a community is another important factor in assessment. Knowledge of the ethnicity and racial origin of the population helps to pinpoint health problems known to be prevalent in certain groups, such as sickle cell disease in African Americans and diabetes in some Native American tribes.

Information about physiologic function in a population is derived from morbidity and mortality data as well as other health status indicators such as immunization levels. Mortality rates of concern to the community health nurse include the crude death rate, cause-specific death rates, and death rates among specific segments of the population, such as the elderly, minority groups, and the homeless.

The crude death rate reflects all deaths in the population regardless of age or cause of death. The crude death rate presents a picture of the overall health status of the community, but it does not suggest the presence of specific health problems that may be contributing to deaths.

Cause-specific death rates, on the other hand, provide information about a population's specific health problems. Cause-specific death rates are the number of deaths in the population attributable to specific conditions such as diabetes, heart disease, or suicide. They are calculated in proportion to the total population using a multiplier of 100,000. When death rates due to specific causes are higher than those of populations with a comparable age composition, health care programs may be needed to deal with these causes of death.

The majority of health problems are nonfatal, and many existing health problems in the population are not brought to light by examining mortality statistics alone. For this reason, those conducting a community assessment must consider morbidity as well as mortality rates. Morbidity rates reflect the extent of illness present in the population. The two morbidity statistics of greatest significance in population health assessment are prevalence and incidence rates. Prevalence rates indicate the *total* number of cases of a particular condition at any given time. Incidence rates indicate the number of *new* cases of the condition identified over a period. For example, eight new cases of tuberculosis may have been diagnosed in Buffalo County last month (incidence), but 39 people in the county are currently under treatment for active tuberculosis (prevalence).

Immunity is the final consideration related to biophysical factors influencing community health. Immunization levels and the overall immune status of the population influence susceptibility to a variety of communicable diseases. Even when specific individuals do not have immunity to a particular disease, if immune levels in the community are high, their chances of being exposed to the disease are diminished. This protective element of general community immunization levels is referred to as "herd immunity."

Psychological Considerations

The psychological environment influences the health of the population by increasing or mediating exposure to stress and affects the ability of the population to function effectively. In addition, elements of the psychological dimension may enhance or impede community action to resolve identified health problems. Some of the areas to be considered in the psychological dimension of community health include the future prospects of the community, significant events in the population's history and the response to those events, communication networks existing within the population, and the adequacy of protective services. Other considerations in this area include evidence of psychological problems such as suicide and homicide rates and identifiable sources of stress within the population.

Learning about a community's prospects helps those conducting a population health assessment to gain a clearer picture of the psychological climate within the population. If a community is growing and productive, for example, apathy regarding community problems is less likely than might be the case if the community is economically depressed and faltering. A community that is in decline or has multiple problems is also more likely to have multiple sources of stress that affect the health of its residents.

Similarly, information about a population's history can provide insight into previous and current health problems and how the population has dealt with them. Historical information may also provide some clue as to how the community will deal with subsequent problems and where community strengths lie. For example, historical information on the cohesive response of community members to a past crisis suggests a strength that will enable the population to face future crises.

The psychological environment created by relationships between subgroups within the population should also be explored. Harmonious relations between groups indicate a psychological climate that is conducive to cooperative community action to resolve identified problems. Tension and distrust between groups, on the other hand, may make resolution of population health problems more difficult.

The adequacy of protective services provided by law enforcement, fire, and other emergency personnel can profoundly influence the psychological climate of an area. Adequate protective services help to create a psychological environment that enhances feelings of personal safety and security. Where these services are inadequate to meet residents' needs, stress and insecurity are created and can negatively influence the health of the population.

Communication is an important contributing factor in the psychological climate of a population, therefore, the adequacy of communication networks should also be explored. This includes the availability and accessibility of a telecommunication infrastructure in the community (Bingler, 2000). Communication in the community may be formal or informal. Formal channels include media such as radio, television, and newspapers, as well as the form that public announcements may take. Informal communications take place outside of these channels. For example, rumors about a particular religious or ethnic group may serve to exacerbate intergroup tension and strife. The degree of trust placed in official formal communications is another element of the psychological dimension that may enhance or detract from community health.

Other indicators of the psychological environment in a population include annual incidence rates for homicide and suicide. Rates for specific subgroups within the population should also be examined, for there is usually considerable variation among different racial and ethnic groups. For example, both suicide and homicide rates are frequently higher for minority group members than

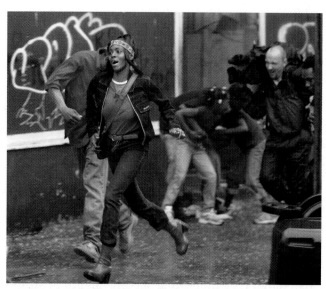

Conflict between groups in the population affects the overall health status of its members. (Getty)

for the general population in most communities. Examination of these figures and their distribution in the population may help to identify factors contributing to poor psychological health in certain subgroups or in the population in general.

Common sources of stress within the environment also influence community health. Widespread unemployment, lack of available housing, and crowded living conditions are sources of stress in a population. These and other sources of stress serve to create a psychological environment that is not conducive to health.

Physical Environmental Considerations

Physical environmental factors affecting a population include its location, its type (e.g., rural, urban, or suburban) and size, topographical features, and climate. Other physical factors to be assessed include the type and adequacy of housing and considerations related to water supply, nuisance factors, and potential for disaster.

The location, climate, and physical geography or topography of the community provide indications of some health problems likely to occur in the community. An area that is heavily wooded, for example, might increase the index of suspicion for problems such as Rocky Mountain spotted fever and Lyme disease. On the other hand, a dry, arid desert area would be more conducive to problems of heat exhaustion.

Size and population density, as well as the type of community, are other factors that influence the types of health problems encountered and resources available to the population. Certain health problems are more prevalent in urban areas than in rural ones and vice versa. Statistics indicate that suicide is more prevalent in urban communities, whereas one would expect a problem like rabies to occur more often in a rural area where wild animals are likely to be infected. Urban dwellers are less likely to encounter rabid animals because of regulations regarding vaccination of pets. Rural and urban areas also have unique strengths. For example, rural communities are often characterized by a tendency for neighbors to help each other, whereas urban areas generally have a greater variety of health care services within close proximity.

Housing is another important physical environmental factor. Inadequate, unsafe, or unsanitary housing conditions contribute to a variety of health problems including communicable diseases spread by poor sanitation, lead poisoning due to lead-based paint in older homes in poor repair, and unintentional injuries resulting from safety hazards. Overcrowding has been found to increase the incidence of a number of health concerns. Communicable diseases are spread more rapidly in crowded conditions, and the prevalence of stress-related conditions such as alcohol abuse, suicide, and other forms of violence increases with crowding as well.

The source of a population's water supply is another important physical environmental consideration. Are most residents supplied by local water systems or do they have independent wells? What is the level of *potability*, or drinkability, of the water? Is the population's water supply safe for drinking, or does it pose biological or chemical hazards to health? The presence or absence of fluoride in the water supply is a possible indicator of dental health.

Disposal of wastes is another area of consideration in the physical environmental dimension of population health. Disposal methods for various types of materials, particularly hazardous wastes, should be considered. Do disposal methods ensure adequate safeguards for the health of the public, or is there potential for environmental pollution as a result of waste disposal? Concerns about hazardous waste disposal were addressed in Chapter 10∞.

Physical environmental factors within the community may also contribute to accidental injuries. For example, particularly dangerous intersections may be the sites of frequent motor vehicle accidents, or large numbers of swimming pools in the area may contribute to the incidence of drowning.

Nuisance factors such as insects, noxious plants, and other substances may provide additional physical health hazards or prove offensive to the senses, thereby decreasing the quality of life for the population. Nearby dairy farms, for example, might provide insect breeding grounds that contribute to the incidence of insect-borne diseases, or there might be an airport that presents a noise hazard. Another consideration in terms of nuisances is the presence of various pollutants in the environment. The effects of pollution and the community health nurse's responsibility with regard to pollution were discussed in Chapter 10∞.

Finally, within the population's physical environment there may be the potential for either natural or human-caused disasters. Is the population situated on a major fault line and subject to earthquakes? Is there a chemical manufacturing plant close by that presents a potential hazard? Assessment of the potential for disaster and the community health nurse's role in planning for disaster response are addressed in more detail in Chapter 27∞.

Sociocultural Considerations

From the previous discussion it is clear that sociocultural and psychological dimensions are closely interrelated. Social and cultural factors influence the psychological dimension and have other effects on health as well. Considerations in assessing the sociocultural dimension include information about community government and leadership, language, income and education levels, employment levels and occupations, marital status and family composition, and religion. Other areas to be addressed include transportation and the availability of goods and services needed by residents.

A community's government and power structure are important considerations in terms of planning and implementing programs designed to solve population health problems and to make effective use of resources. Who holds the purse strings? How are decisions made? Who are the decision makers in the community? Community members conducting the health assessment should identify both formal and informal leaders. In one isolated community, for example, no program was successful unless it first received approval from one elderly matriarch. It was she who controlled the community despite the presence of elected officials.

Information on the population's official leadership can be obtained from the mayor's office or from other local governmental agencies. Informal leaders may be more difficult to identify, but, if they do not already know this information, assessment team members can ask key informants in the community (e.g., school principals, clergy, and official leaders) who the informal leaders are. Other health care providers and business leaders might also provide information on informal leadership within the community.

Language is another important sociocultural factor affecting the health of the population. Language influences interactions among community members as well as their ability to obtain needed goods and services. Closely related to language are the cultural affiliations within the population. Major cultural differences between racial and ethnic segments of the community can create stress and increase the potential for civil strife and discord. Information about cultural affiliations also provides insights into health-related attitudes and behaviors and directions for tailoring health service interventions to enhance their effectiveness.

The average income of community residents also has bearing on a population's health status. For example, a strong relationship exists between the economic status of the population and certain critical indicators of health. Economic status influences the ability of residents to provide for basic necessities and to gain access to health care services. In addition, the income of residents influences the tax base of the community and the types of services the community is able to provide. For example, when many residents are unemployed or have low incomes, they have less money to spend. Businesses take in less money and community revenues from sales and other taxes are decreased. Consequently, the community is less able to provide essential services for its citizens.

Income is closely related to education level. People who have received a lesser education may have lower-paying jobs. They also tend to have less health-related knowledge, and, consequently, lower levels of health. Both income and education levels are indicators of a population's standard of living and, indirectly, of its health status. The prevalence of several acute and chronic conditions in the population (e.g., tuberculosis, pneumonia, and heart disease) tends to decline as income and education levels rise.

Because large numbers of people within a population are usually employed, it is important to consider the types of occupations and possible health hazards involved. Persons in some occupational groups are at higher risk for certain health problems than those in other groups. For example, histoplasmosis occurs frequently among people who work with birds (e.g., poultry farmers), and black lung (pneumoconiosis) is prevalent among coal miners.

In addition to information about employment, the level of unemployment in the population provides an indication of possible health problems. Unemployment contributes to stress and to decreased income levels that affect access to health care as well as other necessary goods and services.

Religious affiliations within a population can either foster or impede health practices. Religious beliefs may affect health or influence the acceptability of health programs to community members. For example, some religious groups may be averse to the idea of providing on-site health care services in high schools because of the fear that contraceptive services will be provided. Similarly, local religious groups may provide significant community resources and should be included in assets assessment.

Marital status and family composition are social environmental factors that might influence the health of a population. Those conducting a population health assessment would consider the number of single-parent families and older persons living alone. Generally, married individuals have lower death and illness rates than those who are unmarried; therefore, information about marital status in the population can provide clues to overall health status.

Accessibility of transportation is an important factor related to the use of health services and is, therefore, a necessary component of the assessment. Transportation difficulties compound health problems where large numbers of people are poor or elderly, chronically ill or disabled, poorly motivated with respect to health, or who are mothers with small children.

Behavioral Considerations

Behavioral factors influence the health status of a population and its members. Areas to be considered in this dimension include consumption patterns, leisure pursuits, and other health-related behaviors.

Consumption patterns play a major part in the development of health or illness. In assessing consumption patterns in the community, the assessment team would examine dietary patterns and the use of potentially harmful substances.

Information is needed on the general nutritional level of the population and on specific dietary patterns. For example, information would be sought on the prevalence of overweight individuals in the population or the incidence of anemia in school-age children. Another area for consideration is any ethnic nutritional patterns that might influence health either positively or negatively. For example, movement away from traditional foods to typical American dietary practices has contributed to obesity and a variety of chronic diseases among many ethnic cultural groups.

The use of harmful substances is another area to explore. The level of alcohol consumption within the population should be examined, both for the population in general and for specific target groups. The extent of both legal and illegal drug use may also merit investigation, including the types of substances abused and the typical sources of abused substances. The extent of smoking and other forms of tobacco use in the population should also be considered.

Information about leisure activities prevalent in the population can also indicate the potential for certain kinds of health problems. For example, boating, waterskiing, and related recreational activities increase the risk of drowning and similar accidents. On the other hand, if watching television is the primary form of recreation, there may be increased potential for heart disease and other conditions associated with a sedentary lifestyle. The presence or absence of recreational opportunities available to the population may also affect the psychological environment and the ability of community members to deal with stress effectively.

Health System Considerations

Health care system factors can profoundly affect the health of a population. Assessment in this dimension involves identifying existing services, assessing their level of performance, and identifying areas in which services are lacking. Relevant information includes the types of health care services available to community residents and their effectiveness in addressing community health needs. What types of primary, secondary, and tertiary preventive services are available? How adequate are these services to meet the needs of the people? The availability and accessibility of specific types of services and how effectively they are used can influence population health. For example, the percentage of pregnant women in the community who receive prenatal care and the point in the pregnancy at which care usually begins affect maternal and infant health. The availability and adequacy of services provided by emergency medical personnel and by emergency rooms or trauma centers are other examples of factors in the health system dimension that influence community health. Other questions relate to the availability and accessibility of certain types of health care providers. For example, there may be several physicians in town, but none of them provide prenatal services because of malpractice concerns.

The extent to which available health services are overused or underused may also affect the health status of the community, and factors that contribute to overuse and to underuse would be considered. For example, emergency room services might be overused because many community members cannot afford a regular source of health care and seek care only in crisis situations. Conversely, the services of clinics and physicians might be underused because they are offered at inconvenient times or places, because people have no means of transportation to such services, or because residents may simply not be aware of the need for or availability of certain services.

Another area for consideration is the financing of health care. Considerations to be addressed include who pays for health care services, the adequacy of funding sources for meeting population health needs, the priority given to health-related concerns in planning budgetary allocations, the extent of health insurance coverage in the population, and the availability of funds to pay for care for the indigent (see Chapter 5∞). Financing of health care can also provide an indirect indication of prevailing attitudes toward health. Adequate health care budgeting indicates that health is considered a public priority.

Other considerations related to the health care system include community definitions of health and illness and the use of culturally prescribed health practices and practitioners. As we saw in Chapter 9∞, culturally determined health behaviors may have both positive and negative effects on a community's health status. For example, herbal remedies used by some cultural groups may have positive effects, but when used in combination with scientific medicine, may impede treatment or create adverse health effects.

ASSESSING POPULATION HEALTH

A population or **community assessment** is the process by which data are compiled regarding a community's health status and resources and from which nursing diagnoses are derived. An accurate assessment is the basis of any community health endeavor and is essential to planning any program designed to meet health-related needs. Assessment data provide the foundation for community health nursing advocacy to assure that identified needs are met. Population or community health assessment can be approached from two perspectives. A needs assessment approach focuses on community health problems. A population assessment, on the other hand, provides an overall picture of community health status, including community strengths and assets as well as needs or problems (Ervin, 2002). Population health assessments can serve a variety of functions, including identifying problems, risk factors, and needs as perceived by its members (Swinney, Anson-Wonkka, Maki, & Corneau, 2001); determining community interests and priorities related to health (Center for Health Improvement, 2004); describing population lifestyles; and delineating community strengths and resources. Population health assessment can also facilitate decision making, particularly with respect to resource allocation, provide skill training for residents, facilitate group mobilization, and enable consciousness raising (Hancock & Minkler, 2005; Plescia, Koontz, & Laurent, 2001).

Population health assessment should be based on several general principles, including the following:

- Multiple sources of information should be sought to provide an overall picture of community health rather than the view of one segment of the population.
- Assessment should address the needs of specific subgroups within the population (e.g., vulnerable populations such as the elderly or members of diverse cultural groups).
- Assessment should consider all potential stakeholders in the population. **Stakeholders** are those concerned with the outcomes of the assessment (e.g., community residents, officials, health care providers, funders).
- Assessment should identify population assets as well as needs or problems.
- Assessment should be conducted or directed by persons with experience in population health assessment. (Center for Health Improvement, 2004)

Incorporating Community Members in Population Health Assessment

Including members of the community in the population health assessment process is a form of community health nursing advocacy. It is only through their incorporation in assessment, planning, implementation, and evaluation processes that their voices are truly heard. Community participation in population health assessment facilitates development of an accurate and comprehensive picture of the health status of the population. The inclusion of grassroots community members may offset the adherence to organizational agendas that may be displayed by members of specific agencies and provides a more comprehensive and balanced picture of the population's health (Kone et al., 2000). Such inclusion may occur through the use of rapid participatory appraisal (RPA) (Lazenbatt, 2002) or participatory action research (PAR) (Severtson, Baumann, & Will, 2002). The approaches are similar in that they include community members in all phases of community assessment and action to address identified community needs. RPA involves collecting data at several levels. The first level addresses information about community structure, composition, interest, and capacity. At the second level, data are collected regarding community needs and assets. The third level of appraisal addresses services available to meet identified needs, and the fourth level considers social policy as it affects capacity to meet population health needs (Lazenbatt, 2002).

Participatory action research has been found to be particularly effective in assessing population groups subject to prior exploitation. Many population groups have been subjected to repeated assessment with little resulting benefit to the community (Clark & Buell, 2004). Because in PAR community members are involved in all stages of assessment, program planning, implementation, and evaluation, distrust of health care personnel and other authority figures may be diminished and health-related outcomes augmented. PAR has been described as occurring in three cycles, an education and analysis cycle, an investigation cycle, and an action cycle (Severtson et al., 2002). In the education cycle, community members are educated for participation and areas for assessment are identified, questions developed, and data collection mechanisms identified. In the investigation cycle, data are collected and analyzed and findings reported back to the community. In the action cycle, community members and others engage in collaborative efforts to address population health needs.

Community participation in population health assessment and planning requires community engagement. **Community engagement** has been defined as the "process of working collaboratively with and through groups of people affiliated by geographic proximity, special interest, or similar situations to address issues affecting the well-being of those people" (CDC/ATSDR Committee on Community Engagement, 1997, p. 9). A joint committee of the Centers for Disease Control and Prevention (CDC) and the Agency for Toxic Substances and Disease Registry (ATSDR) has developed several principles of community engagement. These principles include the following:

- Clarify the purpose and goals for engagement and the populations to be engaged.
- Learn about the community and their perceptions of those promoting engagement.

- Establish trusting and collaborative relationships in the community.
- Accept the need for community self-determination.
- Partner with the community to bring about change.
- Respect diversity within the population.
- Mobilize community assets and develop community capacities and resources to sustain community health endeavors.
- Cede control of actions and interventions to members of the population.
- Anticipate and plan for a long-term commitment to the population. (CDC/ATSDR Committee on Community Engagement, 2004)

Data Sources for Population Health Assessment

Usually, a wide variety of data are collected in a population assessment. The breadth and depth of data collected will vary somewhat depending on the scope of the assessment, but for a comprehensive assessment of population health status, data on all aspects of health and factors that affect health are required. Assessment data may be either quantitative or qualitative. *Quantitative* data reflect numbers of people, characteristics, or events within the population. Examples of quantitative data include the number of people in specific age or ethnic groups and the rates of specific diseases and causes of death within the population. *Qualitative* data focus on perceptions of health, attitudes, and health concerns as voiced by members of the population. For example, community members' identification of adolescent pregnancy, substance abuse, and lack of affordable housing as health-related problems in the community reflects qualitative data.

Population assessment data may be obtained in several ways including use of focus groups, key informant interviews, surveys of residents, secondary analysis of existing data, and use of data from geographic information systems (Nardi, 2003a). A focus group is "a group of people who have personal experience of a topic of interest and who meet to discuss their perceptions and perspectives on that topic" (Clark et al., 2003, p. 456). Perspectives may be formulated or changed in the context of group discussion (Webb, 2002), and the nature of the interaction among focus group participants is itself considered data (Owen, 2001).

Assessment team members might also interview members of the community and key informants. **Key informants** are people who, because of their position in the community, possess information and insights about the community. Key informants include both formal and informal community leaders. Examples of key informants include public officials, school and health care personnel, prominent businesspeople, and local clergy. Again, it is important not to restrict interviews to these sources, but also to interview typical residents of the community because of the possible differences in perceptions of the community's health needs. General surveys of members of the population may also be used to collect either quantitative or qualitative assessment data.

Community assessment data may already exist in other forms. For example, the local health department will have a variety of data on the incidence of specific communicable diseases and may also collect additional data on a routine basis. Data may also be obtained from the records of health care providers and institutions, community service agencies, civic organizations, and other groups. Data from other focused assessments may also be available. For example, a local agency may have collected data related to transportation needs among the elderly.

Asset mapping is another means of collecting data about a community, particularly regarding its resources. **Asset maps** are geographic maps of the community indicating the location of specific community assets. A community assessment may involve the development of several asset maps, each related to a different type of community resources. For example, one asset map might indicate the location and types of educational resources available in the community, whereas another identifies agencies and organizations providing health care services. In addition to asset maps, community members engaged in population assessment may conduct capacity inventories that catalog the skills, expertise, and capabilities of individual community members and community organizations (Sharpe, Greaney, Lee, & Royce, 2000).

Asset maps may make use of **geographic information systems (GISs)**, which are computerized databases that collect and store information and display it in the form of maps and geographic distributions of various factors. In a GIS, data are geocoded by census block to enable specific data to be located on a map of the area (Nardi, 2003a). Geographic information systems are useful for identifying areas or segments of the population at risk for specific health problems or targeting interventions to areas of greatest need (Riner, Cunningham, & Johnson, 2004).

Information on biophysical factors influencing health will come from a number of sources. For example, information on the age, gender, and racial/ethnic composition of the population can be obtained from census figures for the census tracts that make up the community. Data on gender and racial composition may also be available from state and local agencies. Birth and death statistics are usually compiled by official local and state health agencies and can be obtained from these sources. Information on mortality may also be available from other sources. For example, insurance companies or trauma centers might be able to provide information on motor vehicle fatalities, and homicide figures may be available from local law enforcement agencies. Information on age at death is compiled by local health agencies,

but may also be obtained by a review of death certificates or examination of obituaries published in local newspapers.

Local and state health departments also compile statistics on the incidence and prevalence of certain reportable health conditions. These conditions include many communicable diseases, but may also include other conditions for which special surveillance programs are in place. For example, in some areas information is compiled on newly diagnosed cases of hypertension. Another indicator of population morbidity is the *rate under treatment* or the number of people seeking assistance for specific health problems. For example, the number of people being treated for depression says a great deal about the mental health of the population and may be obtained from local treatment facilities. For other conditions, the assessment team may need to seek other sources of data. Cancer registries may be a source of information about the incidence and prevalence of certain forms of cancer, and local health care facilities and providers may have figures related to the incidence of other conditions. For example, the local hospital may have data on the number of clients hospitalized for diabetes, myocardial infarction, and other conditions.

Immunization levels within the population also provide information on the physiologic function of its members. Information on immunization levels is usually extrapolated from immunization figures derived from school records. In areas where a large number of school-age children are not immunized, there are probably also large numbers of unimmunized younger children, and overall immunization levels in the general population are also likely to be low. School immunization records, however, are not always an accurate indicator of high immunization levels. Because immunization is required for school entry in most places, school-age children may be immunized, while younger children remain unimmunized. For additional data on immunization levels, the assessment team might want to examine the records of public immunization clinics as well as those of private physicians who provide immunization services.

In addition to obtaining information regarding the population being assessed, the assessment team will also want to obtain similar figures for other populations in order to make comparisons. Comparison figures on morbidity and mortality at state and national levels can be obtained from state health departments and from various federal publications, respectively. One publication that contains a great deal of information on morbidity and mortality statistics is the *Morbidity and Mortality Weekly Report* published by the Centers for Disease Control and Prevention (CDC). Such data are also available online at the CDC Web site (*http://www.cdc.gov*). National morbidity and mortality data can also be obtained from health and life insurance companies as well as voluntary agencies concerned with specific

FOCUSED ASSESSMENT

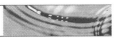

Biophysical Considerations in Population Health Assessment

- What is the age composition of the population? What is the annual birth rate? What are the age-specific death rates in the population? What is the average age at death of population members?
- What is the racial and ethnic composition of the population? What is the relative proportion of men and women? In specific age groups? What genetically determined illnesses, if any, are prevalent in the population?
- What are the cause-specific mortality rates for the population? What physiologic conditions are prevalent? What is the extent of disability within the population? How does the population of interest compare with state and national morbidity and mortality figures?
- What is the overall immunization level in the population?

FOCUSED ASSESSMENT

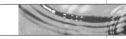

Psychological Considerations in Population Health Assessment

- What stressors affect the health of the population? How do members of the population usually deal with crises? What significant events have occurred in the history of the population? What was the response to those events? What are the population's prospects for the future?
- How cohesive is the population? Is there evidence of tension between groups in the population?
- How adequate are protective services?
- What are the formal communication channels in the population? The informal channels?
- What are the prevalence rates for mental illnesses in the population? What is the homicide rate? Suicide rate?
- What are the rates of crime in the population? What types of crimes are prevalent?

health problems, such as the American Cancer Society and the American Heart Association. Comparisons may also be made with prior data for the population being assessed. This trend data can indicate changes in community health problems over time. Tips for a focused assessment of biophysical considerations in population health are presented above.

Information on the psychological dimension of community health is obtained primarily through observation and through interviews with area residents. Again, it is important to get a broad representation of community membership among the people interviewed. The assessment team should be alert to unrest and conflict between groups within the population and the implications of such psychological tensions for the health of the population and its members. Information in this area may be derived from a review of local news articles or from police data regarding civil unrest.

Those assessing the health of a population would obtain information about the availability and quality of police and fire services, as well as information on the availability and adequacy of legal services, services for victims of abuse, and consumer protection services. Community residents can be surveyed to determine their perceptions of the quality of these services. Community insurance agencies might also have data on injuries related to violence or fires that would provide indirect evidence of protective services. Information on rates for fire insurance coverage in the community also reflects the quality of services. Data about the psychological environment of a population might be obtained using the focused assessment questions provided above right.

For the most part, the physical environmental characteristics of a community can be observed. For example, the nurse or other members of the assessment team might drive through the community assessing its geographic features, nuisance factors, and the general adequacy of housing. Information about pollution,

water supply, and waste disposal might be obtained from local government bureaus or the nearby public health agency. Data on population size and density are available from census figures or from local government agencies. This information, as well as information on the typical climate and geographic features, may also be available in local publications or from the chamber of commerce. A focused assessment for physical environmental conditions affecting a population's health is provided below.

In the sociocultural dimension, the nurse and others should assess the degree to which language presents a barrier to health education or to the provision of other health care services. Key informants in the population can provide information about languages spoken. Schoolteachers and principals, for example, are

FOCUSED ASSESSMENT

Physical Environmental Considerations in Population Health Assessment

- Where is the population located (urban, rural region)? How large is the area occupied by the population? How densely populated? What topographical features could influence the health of population members? What is the local climate like?
- What is the quality of housing in the population? Is affordable housing available? Are dwellings in good repair?
- What is the population's source of water? Is the water supply adequate to meet population needs? Is it safe for consumption? How is waste disposal handled?
- What plants and animals are common in the area?
- Is there evidence of environmental pollution that may affect health?
- Are there nuisance factors present in the area? If so, what are they? How do they affect health?
- Is there potential for disaster in the population? If so, what kind of disasters are likely? What is the extent of disaster preparation in the population?

knowledgeable about languages spoken by their students. Those conducting the community assessment may also derive this information from personal observation in the community. For example, they may spend time observing stores where large segments of the population shop or check for newspapers and radio and television broadcasts in languages other than English.

Another aspect of language to be assessed is the use of colloquialisms by local residents. Are there unique ways in which community members express themselves? Unfortunately, much of this information is gleaned by trial and error on the part of the nurse; however, the nurse can ask key informants about the use of colloquialisms and about their meaning.

Assessment team members also need to identify the host of cultural factors within the community that may affect its health status (see Chapter 9 ∞). Information on cultural groups in the population can be obtained from key informants and through observation. The presence of ethnic markets and restaurants, as well as non-English newspapers and radio stations can also provide information on the ethnic/cultural composition of the population.

Information on income and education levels, other important sociocultural influences on population health, can be obtained from census figures. This information may also be available from local government agencies or school districts. In addition to determining the education level of the population, education resources should be examined. This information enables the assessment team to make diagnoses regarding the adequacy of resources for meeting identified health needs. The telephone directory is a good starting place for obtaining information on education facilities in the area. Assessment team members can then interview administrators of those facilities or review their brochures and other publications to determine the types of education programs offered. Local school personnel can also provide information on education opportunities available to the population.

Information about community businesses and industries is available from the local chamber of commerce. The numbers of people employed in specific occupations can be obtained from major employers in the area. Questions should also be asked about health hazards presented by community occupations. The community assessment team would address the potential for exposure to hazardous substances (e.g., asbestos and chlorine gas), radiation, noise, or vibration, as well as the potential for injury due to falls or use of hazardous equipment. In addition to determining the potential for occupational injury or illness, the team would obtain figures on the extent to which such conditions occur. This type of information may be obtained from the illness and accident records of major employers or may be available from the state occupational health agency.

Unemployment figures can be obtained from state or local employment offices. Occupational data derived from a community assessment might be based on the focused assessment included on page 361.

Telephone directories and Internet data can provide a picture of the religious groups represented in the population. Membership rosters of specific houses of worship can provide information on the number of people affiliated with each religious group. The assessment team can also interview members of local religious groups to determine the extent of their influence on health and their level of involvement in health-related activities. For example, some congregations may organize periodic blood pressure screening events or provide health-related education programs for their members.

Information on marriage and family composition is available from census data for the area. Vital statistics collected by the local health department can also provide data on marriages and the frequency of divorce among community members.

With respect to transportation, the assessment team can obtain information on the number of families with cars from area census data. Information on other forms of transportation can be gleaned from the telephone directory or Internet and by contacting bus and taxi companies to determine routes and fares.

In addition, the assessment team members would obtain data on the types and adequacy of goods and services available to the population, including recreational programs, local shopping facilities, prices for goods and services, and social service programs. Much of this information can be obtained through participant observation. For example, the nurse might shop in local stores or look for recreational pursuits. Information about the number and types of stores and services is also available in the telephone directory and possibly on the Internet. Newspaper advertisements provide information on local prices. Finally, assessment team members can contact personnel at local social service agencies to obtain information about the services offered. Data related to a community's sociocultural environment might be obtained using the focused assessment questions provided on page 361.

Information on dietary patterns may be obtained by interviews and surveys of community residents as well as by observation of foods purchased in grocery stores. The assessment team would determine the number of residents who smoke and whether that number is increasing or decreasing. Indirect indicators of the use of alcohol, drugs, and tobacco include sales of these items. This information can be obtained from interviews with personnel in stores that sell these items or from information about the related taxes collected. Information on substance abuse may be reflected in law enforcement agencies' records of arrests or accidents related to drugs and alcohol. Information can also be obtained on the number of admissions to drug and alcohol treatment facilities.

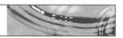

FOCUSED ASSESSMENT

Sociocultural Considerations in Population Health Assessment

- How are community decisions made? Who makes them? Who holds power in the population? How is that power exercised? What is the population's governance structure? How effective is governance? Who are the formal and informal leaders in the population?
- What cultural groups are represented in the population? What languages are spoken? What cultural beliefs and behaviors are prevalent in the population? What is the character of relationships between members of different cultural groups in the population?
- What religious affiliations are represented in the population? What effect do they have on community life and health?
- What is the general education level of the population? What educational resources and facilities are present?
- What is the income level and distribution within the population?
- What is the rate of unemployment in the population? Who are the major employers in the area? What kinds of occupations are represented? What occupational health hazards are present?
- How accessible is transportation in the community?
- What is the marital status of the population? What is the typical family structure in the population?
- How accessible are goods and services to members of the population?

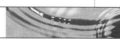

FOCUSED ASSESSMENT

Behavioral Considerations in Population Health Assessment

- What are the usual food preferences and consumption patterns in the population? What is the nutritional level in the population? What percentage of the population is overweight? Underweight?
- What is the extent of drug abuse in the population? How easy is it to obtain drugs?
- What is the extent of alcohol and tobacco sales in the population? What is the prevalence of arrests related to alcohol and other drugs? What is the extent of tobacco use in the population? What is the rate of hospital admissions for health problems related to alcohol, drug, and tobacco use?
- What exercise and leisure opportunities are available to the population? To what extent are they utilized? Do leisure activities pose any health or safety hazards?
- What is the attitude of the population toward sexual activity? Toward homosexuality? What is the prevalence of unsafe sexual practices in the population? What is the extent of contraceptive use in the population?
- To what extent do members of the population engage in safety practices (e.g., seat belt use)?

Community self-help groups, such as a local chapter of Alcoholics Anonymous, may also provide information on the extent of substance abuse problems. Data reflecting a community's consumption patterns would include information derived from the focused assessment above right.

Information on leisure-related exercise is usually obtained by means of interviews and surveys. To determine the extent of interest in various forms of exercise, assessment team members might also contact groups that offer exercise-related classes or businesses that sell related equipment. In addition, they can observe for joggers or other exercise enthusiasts as they move about the community. Information on recreational opportunities can be obtained from the telephone directory and the Internet, from direct observation, and from events publicized in the newspaper or other means of communication employed in the community.

Members of the population conducting the health assessment should also examine the prevalence of other health-related behaviors. For example, information would be obtained on the extent of seat belt use in passenger vehicles or the use of safety devices in certain occupational settings. Information on failure to use seat belts might be available from policy or insurance records of motor vehicle accidents, and failure to use occupational safety devices would be reflected in OSHA accident reports.

The assessment team would also be interested in such behaviors as the extent of heterosexual and homosexual activity and use of condoms and other forms of protection against conception and sexually transmitted diseases. Two negative indicators of contraceptive use are the proportion of births that are unintended and the local abortion rate. In areas with a high prevalence of injection drug use, assessment team members would also try to obtain information on the extent of needle sharing and other practices that contribute to the spread of HIV/AIDS infection and hepatitis C. Much of this information is available only through observation and through interviews of key informants. Assessment of behavioral factors related to population health is based on the focused assessment questions provided above.

In assessing factors in the health system dimension, community members would obtain information on the type of health services available to residents. Such information can be derived from a variety of sources, such as the telephone directory, the Internet, word-of-mouth, and personal observation. Referral services provided by professional organizations or agencies such as local senior citizens groups can also supply information on health care providers and facilities. Health care institutions are also a source of information on services provided and fees involved.

Utilization figures for health care services can be obtained from health care facilities and providers in the community. Information on health insurance coverage may be available from insurance agencies or major health care facilities in the area, or through community surveys. Health care facility records may also contain data on the percentage of the population without health insurance. Information about recipients of Medicaid and Medicare benefits is available from the agencies that

ETHICAL AWARENESS

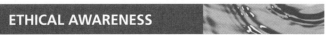

You have been working with a group of community residents to assess the health needs of the population. Part of the effort has involved focus-group sessions with several ethnic minority groups to elicit their perceptions of community health. Some of the comments made in the focus groups indicate dissatisfaction with the services of the major primary health care provider in the community. This provider is concerned about the effect these comments will have on his clientele and wants to have them eliminated from the assessment team's report. Other team members do not think this is appropriate. The provider is a member of the assessment team and has been one of the primary funders of the assessment. As leader of the assessment team, what would you do in this situation?

administer these programs. Information on other sources of funding for health care services can be solicited from public officials as well as local health care agencies and institutions.

The focused assessment questions provided below can help you assess health system factors affecting population health. A tool to guide a comprehensive assessment of health system considerations and considerations related to the other dimensions of health is included in Appendix G on the Companion Website and in the *Community Assessment Reference Guide* designed to accompany this text. Table 15-1◆ provides several sources of population assessment information and examples of data that might be obtained from each source.

In addition to determining appropriate data collection methods, the nurse and community members preparing to conduct a community assessment explore methods for organizing and analyzing the data obtained. When modes of data organization and analysis are identified as much as possible prior to data collection,

FOCUSED ASSESSMENT

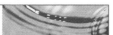

Health System Considerations in Population Health Assessment

■ What types of primary, secondary, and tertiary preventive services are available to the population? How accessible are these services? Are the types of services available adequate to meet population health needs? Are available services culturally relevant to members of the population?

■ To what extent are available health care services utilized? What barriers to service utilization exist in the population?

■ Are there alternative or complementary health services available to the population? To what extent do members of the population use alternative/complementary health services? What is the level and quality of interaction between alternative and scientific health care systems?

■ How are health care services financed? What proportion of the population has health insurance? What level of priority is given to health care services in budgeting local funds? What are community attitudes toward health care services and providers?

Type of Data	Source	Example
TABLE 15-1	**Sources of Population Assessment Data**	
Quantitative	Census figures	Age composition of population
		Racial composition of population
	Local agencies	Child abuse incidence figures from child protective services
		Diabetes admissions from hospitals
		Immunization levels from schools
	Community surveys	Frequency of health services use
		Common health problems
	Observation	Number and types of educational institutions
		Number and types of recreational opportunities
	Newspaper reports	Incidence of homicide
		Incidence of motor vehicle fatalities
	Telephone book	Number and types of health care providers
		Number and types of churches
Qualitative	Community surveys	Attitudes toward health
		Attitudes toward specific health issues
	Key informant interviews	Perceptions of community health needs
	Resident interviews	Perceptions of health needs
	Observation	Quality of housing
	Participant observation	Barriers to health care for handicapped individuals

interpretation of the masses of information obtained becomes much easier.

The Population Health Assessment Process

Nardi (2003b) has outlined a seven-step community or population assessment process that forms the acronym **PROCESS**. Steps as delineated include:

- **P**urpose: Identification of the purpose of the assessment or issue to be addressed.
- **R**efine: Refinement of the questions to be answered by means of the assessment.
- **O**rganize: Identification of data needs, collection methods, and organizing strategies to prepare data for analysis.
- **C**ompare: Comparison of data collected against *Healthy People 2010*◆ benchmarks or other standards.
- **E**valuate: Evaluation of existing programs and services against benchmarks.
- **S**ummary: Summarization of findings and recommendations.
- **S**ubmit: Submit a report of assessment findings to interested stakeholders.

As an example of this assessment process, we can examine a community assessment involving focus groups of community residents (Clark et al., 2003). The purpose of the assessment was to gain community members' perceptions about health assets and issues in the community. Input from segments of the community that are frequently silent and invisible was considered particularly important in creating an accurate picture of the health-related assets and needs of the community, so the assessment was specifically designed to include these segments of the population. A steering committee was formed that included community agency representatives and community residents to develop and refine the questions to be answered in the community assessment. These questions were pilot-tested at a community fair and revised based on responses obtained. The steering committee organized a series of focus groups with different segments of the community based on age, ethnicity, perspective (e.g., health providers, school parents and teachers, area businesspeople). Focus group findings were compared to prior community data as well as indicators of healthy communities, and the availability of existing mechanisms to address identified problems was evaluated. Findings were summarized in the context of the dimensions model of community health nursing and disseminated to a wider segment of the community in a community forum that included residents as well as local policy makers. As a result of the forum, working groups were formed to address the highest priority problems. As one problem is resolved, these working groups are reconfigured to address additional issues, and the work prompted by the initial assessment continues 5 years later.

DIAGNOSTIC REASONING AND POPULATION HEALTH

The collection of data on factors influencing the health status of a population or a community is the first step in identifying resources and health needs. To be of any value, the data must be interpreted and analyzed to derive nursing diagnoses. In other words, assessment data are used to identify health-related needs that are amenable to nursing action and the resources that will support action. Community or population nursing diagnoses should reflect existing, emerging, and potential threats to health, as well as strengths or competencies.

Diagnostic reasoning in the care of communities involves comparing population assessment data to identified standards to uncover health problems and identify assets. One type of standard that may be used in data analysis is the general health status of the state or the nation. For example, the community health nurse can compare data for the population with data for the state or the nation as a whole. In doing so, the nurse might ask the following questions: How does this group stand in relation to the larger population on a variety of measures of health status? Is the local birth rate higher or lower than that of the state or the nation? How do death rates compare? For example, the southern region of Georgia has been labeled the "stroke belt" because the death rate for cerebrovascular accidents far exceeds

that of the rest of the nation. Do morbidity rates for various illnesses exceed national and state rates? How do income and education levels compare?

Another standard with which to compare present data is found in the history of the community or target group. How do current rates compare with those of a year ago? Five years ago?

Members' perceptions of areas of need are a third type of standard with which to compare the data gathered. What health problems are mentioned in interviews with group members? What problems are perceived by other health care professionals and community leaders? What are the expectations of the population regarding these problems?

Diagnostic reasoning gives rise to "statements of risk, condition, trend, potential problem, strength, or latent situation about a community or population" (Ervin, 2002, p. 206). Population or community nursing diagnoses provide a comprehensive picture of the population's health. Diagnoses may be either positive or negative. Positive diagnoses reflect population strengths. Positive diagnoses may also indicate improvements in the population's health status. Components of a population nursing diagnosis include a potential adverse situation or risk, identification of the group or population subgroup at risk, group factors or characteristics contributing to the risk, and indicators that support the conclusion that an increased risk is present (Ervin, 2002). Inclusion of these four elements of the diagnosis provides information about the causative factors involved and provides direction for action as needed. Examples of positive and negative population nursing diagnoses are provided below. As indicated in the negative example, factors related to the risk may be related to an absence of relevant health-related services as well as to other factors or behaviors in the population.

SPECIAL CONSIDERATIONS

SAMPLE POSITIVE AND NEGATIVE POPULATION NURSING DIAGNOSES

Negative Nursing Diagnosis

Large adolescent population [population subgroup] at risk for sexually transmitted diseases (STDs) [risk situation] related to self-report of unprotected sexual activity by 75% of high school students, lack of knowledge related to STD transmission, and lack of access to condoms [population characteristics related to risk], as evidenced by: (a) gonorrhea incidence rate of 357 per 1,000 population, (b) 30% increase in number of cases of *Chlamydia trachomatis* infection in last year, and (c) 5% increase in sexually transmitted hepatitis B among adolescents [evidence of elevated risk].

Positive Nursing Diagnosis (Demonstrating Improvement)

Diminished risk of STDs [risk situation] for adolescents [population subgroup] related to older age at initiation of sexual activity and 50% increase in condom use by sexually active adolescents [population characteristics related to risk], as evidenced by 50% decrease in gonorrhea and chlamydia infection rates among adolescents [evidence of decreased risk].

PLANNING HEALTH CARE FOR POPULATIONS

Whenever a negative diagnosis is made, planning to address the unmet need or risk situation is warranted, and the community health nurse should engage community members in planning health care initiatives to meet the identified needs of the population. These initiatives may take the form of projects or programs (Longest, 2004). Projects and programs differ primarily in their anticipated time frame. Projects are time-limited, whereas programs are health care initiatives designed to occur over an extended period of time. In this chapter, we focus on the development of health care programs rather than short-term projects.

Planning is a collaborative and systematic process used to attain a goal. Planning is collaborative in the sense that persons who will be affected by the planned program need to be involved in its planning. It is systematic in that change is consciously and deliberately brought about.

Systematic planning is essential to effective health care programming and is based on three underlying premises (Gottlieb, as cited in Jonas, 2003):

- Effective health systems respond to the needs of the population and are accountable to members of the population.
- Resources are limited, so must be used to the population's greatest advantage.
- Health is a societal value that should outweigh other economic or social ends (although this may not always be apparent in today's political milieu).

The program planning process may incorporate a variety of steps depending on the planning model used. For our purposes, we will use a five-step model that includes defining and prioritizing the issue to be addressed, creating the planning group, analyzing the issue, developing the program, and setting the stage for evaluation.

Defining and Prioritizing Population Health Issues

A large-scale population health assessment will usually identify a number of health issues that could be addressed through health program planning. In some cases, several different issues may be addressed simultaneously through the development of several separate health care delivery programs. In others, several related issues may be combined and addressed by a single, more comprehensive program. In any event, it is unlikely that all of a population's health-related problems, issues, and needs can be addressed at once given the finite resources available. For this reason, it is necessary to examine the issues derived from the assessment, prioritize them, and define the issue or issues to be addressed in program planning.

The criteria used to prioritize population health needs are essentially the same as those used in working with individuals and families: (a) severity of the threat to the community's health, (b) degree of the community's concern about the need, and (c) extent to which meeting one need depends on meeting other needs. It is likely that the priorities of the population group involve needs that are easily perceived. Community participation in the assessment process helps community members to become aware of less obvious needs that might have greater priority than other more obvious ones.

The process of assigning priority to the health needs identified in a population health assessment involves developing criteria for decision making, establishing standards for minimally acceptable levels of the criteria, and assigning weights to the criteria. For example, a high-priority problem will usually meet criteria of severity, significant community concern, and high cost to society. A standard for severity might be that a minimum of 20% of the population be affected by the problem; whereas significant community concern would be evident if at least 30% of community members surveyed mentioned a particular problem as needing attention. Possible standards for cost to society might be the number of days of lost school or work attendance or the actual monetary cost for medical treatment for the problem. Each of these three criteria (and others developed) would be given a weight reflecting its relative importance in decisions about priorities. For example, high societal cost might be given greater value than the level of concern expressed about a given problem. All of the problems identified in the population health assessment would be evaluated in terms of the weighted criteria, and those with higher priority scores would be addressed first in efforts to resolve population health problems. At this point, community health nurses may need to advocate for giving community concerns a high priority, even when health care providers may see other problems as more important.

Once health-related issues have been prioritized, the community health nurse and other group members can define the specific problem or set of problems to be addressed by program planning. For example, the group may need to determine whether the issue to be addressed is obesity in the general population or obesity as it occurs in school-aged children. Depending on the way the issue is defined, approaches to its resolution may be quite different.

BUILDING OUR KNOWLEDGE BASE

Plescia, Koontz, and Laurent (2001) described the use of a community assessment by an integrated health care delivery system to design a primary care facility to meet population health care needs. Design a study to determine the extent to which managed care organizations in your area use community assessment findings to plan service delivery. What would you do with your findings?

Definition of the problem or issue to be addressed should also lead to establishment of specific goals for its resolution. Program goals are broad statements of desired outcomes that provide the general direction for program development, in contrast to objectives, which are measurable indicators of program accomplishments (Center for Health Improvement, 2004). A goal statement should speak to the resolution of the identified issue. For example, if the issue to be addressed is poor nutrition among older members of the population, the goal would be to improve the nutritional status of older persons.

Creating the Planning Group

The group of people who develop a health care program to meet an identified population health need may be the same as those who participated in the population health assessment. More than likely, however, there will be a need to include others in the planning process who have specific expertise or interest related to the issue to be addressed. The community health nurse may need to advocate for the inclusion of specific people in the planning body, particularly members of the target group. Because of their connections in the community, community health nurses are likely to know of community members who would be assets to the planning group.

For health program planning to be successful, it is important to determine who should be included in the planning group. Generally speaking, five categories of people should be included in the planning group: those in authority who must approve or fund the program, people with expertise related to the issue to be addressed, those who will implement the program, those who will benefit from it, and, finally, people who might resist the program. Those with authority to address the issue should be included because they usually control resources that will be required to implement the program and because they may resist the program if they see it as overlapping or competing with other existing programs. People with expertise related to the issue have knowledge of potential solutions to the problem that have been used elsewhere and may be effective with the population of interest. They are also usually in a position to identify alternatives that have been shown to be unsuccessful in the past.

Health care providers may fall into the expert category, but may also be implementers of the program. Implementers are in a position to implement a program as designed or to sabotage it and their buy-in is essential if the program is to be implemented effectively. Implementers may also have insights into what will and will not work in a given situation. Responsibility for ultimate acceptance and use of a program lies with those who are intended to benefit from it. Potential beneficiaries of a program should be involved in planning to ensure that the program planned meets their needs and is culturally acceptable to them.

It may seem contrary to common sense to include people who are likely to resist development and implementation of a program in planning. In reality, however, incorporating resisters into the planning group often converts them into supporters. Their presence during program planning permits incorporation of program elements that will defuse their resistance. When they are satisfied that the program planned is not a threat to their own interests or values, they will then act to convince other potential resisters of the benefits of the program. Special considerations in creating a planning group to address the health care needs of prison inmates are presented below. Given the particular issue to be addressed, there may be additional people who do not fall into any of these categories who should be included in the planning group. For example, if media advocacy will be needed to gain public acceptance of the program, members of the local media should be invited to join the planning group.

In addition to determining who should be involved, other tasks in creating the planning group include developing planning competence among group members and formulating a group philosophy. Group members should also engage in the tasks of group development discussed in Chapter 13 ∞.

Few health care professionals or consumers have any educational background or experience in program planning. For this reason, the community health nurse or other planning group leader may find it necessary to educate members of the planning group in regard to

---

Think Advocacy

Policy makers in your community have decided to conduct a comprehensive community assessment to determine what public health services should be expanded, what services can be eliminated, and what additional services are needed. You have been appointed to the committee planning the assessment. At the first meeting you notice that there are no community residents represented on the committee. How would you go about advocating for community participation in all facets of the assessment and subsequent decision making?

SPECIAL CONSIDERATIONS

CREATING A PLANNING GROUP TO ADDRESS THE HEALTH CARE NEEDS OF INMATES

Those in authority: Corrections officials, elected officials

Experts: Health care providers with experience in correctional settings, corrections experts, financial analysts to determine potential program costs

Implementers: Corrections personnel, health care personnel

Beneficiaries: Inmates and their families

Resisters: Corrections officials and personnel, taxpayers, elected officials

Others: Inmate advocates

planning processes and activities. It may also be necessary to prevent the group from engaging in activities for which an adequate foundation has yet to be provided. In doing so, the community health nurse needs to exercise well-developed skills in group dynamics addressed in Chapter 13∞. Other tasks to be accomplished at this stage of planning include establishing the organizational structure of the group and clarifying the roles and responsibilities of planning group members.

The next task in creating the planning group, formulating a philosophy, is not often carried out as a conscious activity, but is an assumption on the part of group members. For example, there must be some type of commitment to adequate health care for prison inmates before a group would even consider planning a program to meet prisoners' needs. It is, however, important that the philosophies of various members of the planning group be compatible. Therefore, group members should be encouraged to verbalize their philosophies and to identify and deal with areas of conflict between philosophies. The development of a joint philosophy is sometimes referred to as "visioning" and is a process in which group members develop a collective view of what they hope to accomplish (Sharpe et al., 2000).

Analyzing the Issue and Choosing an Intervention

The next task in program planning is to analyze the issue or problem, its contributing factors, and potential alternative solutions. Much of the data required for this analysis may already be available from the population health assessment, but the planning group may find that they need to collect additional information related to the issue. For example, the population health assessment may have identified problems related to adequate housing that include issues of safety, affordability, and landlord intimidation, but the committee may need more information on the kinds of safety risks present in local housing, the extent of those risks, who is affected by housing affordability issues and why, and which tenants are being intimidated by landlords and why. The planning group will then develop methods for collecting the additional information needed for effective planning to address the housing issue.

Analysis of the issue to be addressed also includes determining the level of prevention involved in its resolution. Is the issue one that requires a primary prevention intervention? Or does problem resolution require intervention at the secondary or tertiary prevention level?

Other information to be obtained and analyzed by the planning group may relate to potential solutions to problems identified (Easterling, Gallagher, & Lodwick, 2003a). What strategies have other communities used to address similar problems? How effective were those strategies? What features of those strategies might be appropriate to this population? Which of the strategies could be implemented in this population or how might the strategies need to be adapted to be appropriate to this population? Some potential solutions have greater research support for their effectiveness than others. The Task Force on Community Preventive Services (2005) has developed information on a variety of community-based interventions linked to achievement of *Healthy People 2010*◆ objectives. The task force has identified a number of interventions that have strong research support as well as many that have insufficient evidence of their effectiveness to warrant use in many population situations.

Information obtained should be analyzed by the planning group to gain a complete picture of factors contributing to the problem and to assist in identifying or developing a strategy to address those factors and resolve the problem. Usually such an analysis will lead to several alternative approaches to problem resolution that must themselves be analyzed in the light of criteria established by the planning group for acceptable solutions. Examples of critical criteria for solutions to population health problems might be that such solutions fit within available budgetary resources or that they be acceptable to ethnic or religious groups within the population.

Potential solutions to problems should always be evaluated in terms of cost, feasibility, acceptability, availability of necessary resources, efficiency, equity, political advantage, and identifiability of the target group. Generally speaking, an alternative that costs less will be viewed more favorably, other factors being equal, than one that costs more, or one alternative may be selected over another because its implementation is more feasible. For example, it is considerably easier to install a traffic light at an accident-prone intersection than to build a bridge to route one intersecting road over the other.

Potential solutions should also be evaluated in terms of their acceptability to policy makers, implementers, and the population. Policy makers are unlikely to approve an alternative that diminishes their power or authority, and implementers are certainly unlikely to accept a potential solution that requires them to work overtime or without pay if another alternative is available. Similarly, community members affected by the proposed program may find one alternative more acceptable than another for a variety of reasons.

Alternative solutions may also differ in terms of the resources needed to implement them. Generally speaking, an alternative that requires fewer resources or for which resources are already available is more likely to be endorsed than one that requires extensive or scarce resources. For example, a group seeking to improve the nutritional status of schoolchildren may select an alternative that makes use of existing facilities used to prepare meals for senior citizens rather than one that necessitates providing kitchen facilities in each school. Efficiency is a related criterion on which alternative solutions to a particular problem can be evaluated. An efficient alternative makes better use of available resources and is usually viewed more favorably than an inefficient one. An asset-oriented assessment can provide a picture of the resources already available within the population and can assist in assessing the relative resource needs of alternative solutions.

Questions of equity also arise in evaluating alternative solutions to a problem. Alternatives that unfairly discriminate against one segment of the population are usually rejected. For example, one alternative to the problem of dealing with teen pregnancy might be to provide contraceptive services in the larger high schools. If, however, these schools tend to serve the upper-middle-class segment of the population while lower-class students attend smaller schools, this alternative would discriminate against a segment of the population also needing service.

Political consequences also need to be considered. For instance, an alternative plan that provides services to a highly vocal voting bloc might be viewed more favorably by politicians than one that serves a less politically involved minority group. Evaluation of alternatives may also involve forecasting regarding the effects of other possible events on the problem or its solution. For example, if a vaccine for HIV infection is likely to be available in the near future, the community may not want to put a lot of resources into a condom promotion program.

Finally, alternative solutions should be evaluated in terms of the identifiability of the target group. One potential solution for preventing the spread of AIDS might be to screen all prostitutes in the population for HIV infection. It is somewhat difficult, however, to identify this group of people, as prostitution is an illegal activity in most places. It might be easier to screen everyone who requests contraceptive services because this group is both sexually active and identifiable.

Consideration of possible sources of opposition also contributes to selection of the most appropriate alternative. If it is known that members of the local PTA would vigorously oppose a "sex fair" as a means of educating adolescents on sexual issues, another less threatening alternative would be more appropriate.

Analysis of alternatives leads to selection of one or more choices judged to meet the criteria set for acceptable solutions. Once this selection has been made, the planning group can proceed to the tasks involved in developing the actual program.

Developing the Program

The four primary tasks involved in developing the program include identifying program objectives, delineating the program theory, delineating actions to achieve objectives, and identifying and obtaining resources. Each of these tasks will be briefly addressed here.

EVIDENCE-BASED PRACTICE

Lazenbatt (2002) described several attributes of evidence for *best practices*, including the following:

- Validity: Practice guidelines, if followed, actually lead to improved health.
- Replication: Other groups will identify a practice as "best" given similar evidence.
- Reliability: Health professionals apply the practice in the same way.
- Flexibility: The practice is able to accommodate the client into the decision-making process.
- Clarity: The definitions of the practice are clear and easily understood.
- Dissemination: The practice is widely disseminated.

Describe a practice considered *best practice* in community health practice (e.g., immunization for preventing immunizable diseases). How well does the practice exemplify these attributes?

Identifying Program Objectives

The first step in actually developing the program is to identify the objectives the program is intended to accomplish. Objectives are statements of specific outcomes expected to result from the program that contribute to the realization of the overall goal.

Program developers usually address two kinds of objectives, outcome objectives and process objectives. Outcome objectives reflect the expected results of the program for its intended beneficiaries and, in the case of population-level programming, for the overall population. An outcome for a smoking cessation program, for example, might be that 75% of program participants successfully quit smoking within 6 months of starting the program. An outcome objective at the population level might be a 50% reduction in the prevalence of smoking within the population in the year after program implementation.

Outcome objectives may be designed at multiple levels and may include immediate, intermediate, and ultimate outcomes (Grembowski, 2001). For instance, immediate objectives of a nutrition education program might be that people understand the new food pyramid and are able to use the pyramid to select an appropriate number of servings of each category of food. An intermediate objective might be that people change their dietary habits based on the education received. An ultimate or long-term objective might be a 30% decrease in the prevalence of obesity within the population.

Process objectives designate the level of expected performance of program staff in carrying out the program. Using our nutrition education program as an example, a process objective might be that the program is provided to 300 people over the course of a year. Another process objective might be that the program is provided in three different languages.

Effective program objectives reflect the following characteristics:

- **Measurable:** Achievement of the objective can be measured. Measurability involves specification of an expected level of achievement (e.g., 75% of smoking cessation program participants will stop smoking).
- **Precise:** The expected outcome is clear and precisely stated.
- **Time specific:** The objective includes a statement of the time within which it should be accomplished.
- **Reasonable or practical:** The objective is practical and able to be met with a reasonable amount of effort and using a reasonable level of available resources.
- **Within group capability:** The objective is within the competence of the planning group to accomplish, given members' expertise and authority.
- **Legal:** The objective can be achieved using legal activities.
- **Congruent with community morals and values:** The objective is consistent with the values and morals of implementers and members of the population or target group.
- **Carries minimal side effects:** The objective has minimal side effects, and these effects are acceptable to program beneficiaries.
- **Fits budgetary limitations:** The objective can be accomplished within existing budgetary constraints.

Using the ultimate outcome objective for our smoking cessation program as an example, the objective is both precise and measurable in that we expect a 50% (measurable) decrease in smoking behavior (not overall tobacco use) in the population. The objective is also time specific in that we expect it to be achieved within one year of program initiation. It is also legal, in that it is not illegal for people to stop smoking; however, it may not be reasonable to expect such a dramatic drop in the prevalence of smoking as a result of the program. If the population values health and does not attach some religious or cultural value to smoking, the objective is also congruent with population morals and values. Achieving the objective also carries minimal side effects for the beneficiaries (temporary irritability, potential weight gain), but these side effects are outweighed by the benefits of smoking cessation. At this point, we do not know for sure if the objective fits within the group's capabilities or if it fits budgetary limitations because we do not know what those capabilities or limitations are, but it is reasonable to suspect that the objective also meets these criteria.

Delineating the Program Theory

To develop effective health care programs for populations, it is helpful to know how the program is supposed to work. A **program theory** or logic model is an explanation of how elements of a program interact to produce the expected outcomes (Longest, 2004) or a conceptual model of the interventions planned and how they work to achieve program outcomes (Linnan & Steckler, 2002). Program theories are most often presented graphically showing the interrelationships among elements of the program and their relationship to expected outcomes.

Program theories usually consist of five interrelated elements: program inputs, processes, outputs, outcomes, and impact (Longest, 2004). In addition, program theories are actually a composite of two types of theory, a theory of cause and effect and a theory of implementation, both of which are required for program success (Grembowski, 2001). The theory of cause and effect links interventions with the outcomes they are designed to produce. The theory of implementation describes the strategies for implementing the program in a real-life situation.

In addition to describing how a program is expected to produce the desired results, program theories or logic models serve several other purposes. Obviously, they identify the theoretical framework underlying the program, but they also provide guidance for organizing program evaluation efforts and determine the program's readiness for evaluation. Finally, they enable program planners to assess the fidelity of the program in meeting its expected outcomes (Dykeman, MacIntosh, Seaman, & Davidson, 2003). Figure 15-1 presents a partial program theory for our smoking cessation program.

Rectangles in Figure 15-1 indicate the theory of cause and effect. The ovals contain elements of the theory of implementation and suggest intervention activities designed to bring about the desired outcome, smoking cessation for program participants. The theory of cause and effect suggests that although many smokers wish to stop smoking they are unable to do so because of the difficulties involved in stopping an addictive behavior. However, the theory also suggests that knowledge of addictive behaviors as well as one's own motivation for that behavior can help people quit smoking. Knowledge can also assist people to identify substitute behaviors that can achieve the same purpose as smoking. Development of this knowledge occurs through program activities such as education and keeping a log of one's smoking behavior. Since interpersonal support is also predicated to help people deal with addictive behaviors, another intervention to be included in the program is the formation of a support group for participants. No one will participate in the program, however, unless they are made aware of it, which suggests that another necessary activity involves recruiting participants through program marketing.

Delineating Actions to Accomplish Objectives

The next step in the planning process is delineating specific actions required to carry out the program. This is usually considered the "nitty-gritty" of planning, and many planning groups mistakenly jump immediately to

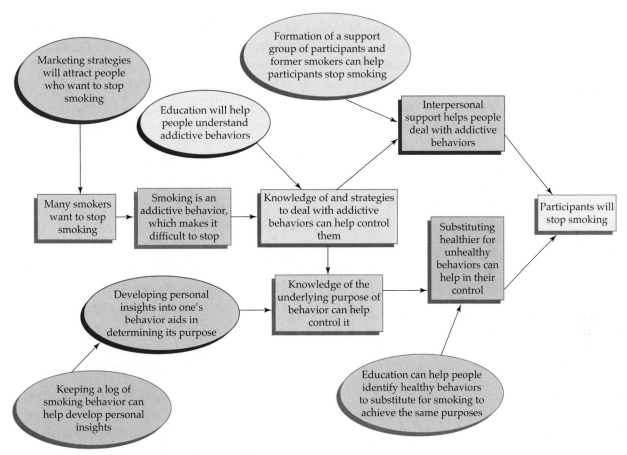

FIGURE 15-1 Partial Program Theory for a Smoking Cessation Program

this phase of activity. For planning to be effective, however, this step must be preceded by those discussed earlier. In this stage of program planning, the community health nurse may need to function as an advocate within the planning group for interventions that are evidence-based and logically connected to the desired outcomes. The community health nurse may also need to advocate for interventions that are culturally and linguistically appropriate to the target population and that consider the population's educational and economic assets.

In this phase of planning, the step-by-step details of the plan are developed. To a large extent, many of the major activities involved in carrying out the program have already been delineated in the development of the program theory. Using the smoking cessation program example, required activities will include developing the educational curriculum, designing a marketing strategy and materials, developing the organizational structure for the support group, and so on. Each of these activities has subactivities that need to be completed. For example, some of the activities related to marketing will include determining whether to employ a marketing firm, deciding on the message and what media will be used to disseminate it, determining how people should register for the program, and so on down to the last detail of how the marketing campaign will be carried out. Activities related to the educational component of

the program include determining when and where to hold group sessions, what content should be presented at each session, and what teaching-learning strategies will be used.

Identifying and Obtaining Resources

Once program activities have been delineated in detail, the resources needed to carry them out can be identified. Resources include personnel, money, materials, and time. To continue with the previous example of smoking cessation, a variety of resources will be needed to implement the program. Personnel resources may include people knowledgeable about smoking, its health effects, and addictive behaviors; people with marketing expertise; and artists and designers to develop attractive marketing and curricular materials. Funds will be needed to produce teaching and recruiting materials and to pay staff. Materials needed include curricular and recruiting materials as well as facilities and equipment for the educational sessions and support group meetings. Many of these resources may have been identified in the course of the asset-oriented population health assessment.

The planning group must not only decide what resources are required but also specify how these resources can be obtained. Will the group write a grant proposal or lobby the local government for funds for the program? Will they hire someone to create marketing materials or design them themselves? Can materials be printed at cost by a local printer? The final consideration with respect to resources is that of time. The time needed to put the program into operation must be determined and specific timelines for various components of program development set. Community health nurses as advocates may assist with grant writing to obtain resources needed for program implementation. They may also assist in linking communities to existing resources.

Setting the Stage for Evaluation

When the detailed plan has been constructed and specific activities delineated, the planning group should begin to set the stage for evaluation. At this point in the planning process, setting the stage for evaluation includes two aspects, evaluating the plan itself and planning for program evaluation. With respect to the plan, is it based on identified needs of the target group or population or is it unrelated to those needs? Is the plan flexible enough to adapt to changing circumstances in the foreseeable future? How efficient will the planned program be? Could program efficiency be improved by modification of the plan? Finally, how adequate is the plan? Have all constraints and contingencies been addressed? Answers to these and similar questions enable the planning group to evaluate the plan and to identify the need for any modifications before implementation. Again, the program theory or logic model can assist in evaluating the plan itself. Are the cause-and-effect relationships assumed in the model based on evidence? Are the links clear and direct, or have some necessary activities been forgotten? Have the elements of the theory of implementation been identified in sufficient detail to prevent any surprises during program implementation?

The second aspect in setting the stage for evaluation is beginning to plan for evaluation of program effectiveness. This may seem a bit premature because the program has not even started; however, it is essential. Unless planning for program evaluation is incorporated at this stage, the data needed for evaluating program outcomes and processes may not be available when the time arrives for actual evaluation.

Planning evaluation involves four considerations. The first of these is determining criteria on which the program should be evaluated. The second consideration is the types of data to be collected and the means used to collect the data. Determining the resources needed to carry out the evaluation is the third consideration. Finally, the planning group should determine who will evaluate the program. All of these considerations are addressed in greater detail in the section on evaluating population-based health care programs. At this juncture it is sufficient to reemphasize the point that planning for evaluation begins during program planning, not after the program has been implemented.

Effective health program planning involves all of the steps discussed here. When steps are ignored or bypassed, the program planned is likely to be less effective and its implementation may prove more difficult. The steps of program planning are summarized above.

IMPLEMENTING POPULATION HEALTH CARE

It is not enough for the planning group to plan for a health care program to meet identified population needs. The group must also ensure that the plan is implemented as designed. The goal of implementation is to integrate program activities into community networks in such a way that the program is sustained as long as the need for it continues. Implementing a health program involves several considerations. These include getting the plan accepted, performing the tasks involved in implementing the program, and using strategies that foster implementation of the program as planned.

Plan Acceptance

Acceptance of the planned program occurs at four levels. The first level is acceptance by community policy makers. If policy makers have been represented on the planning group, this level of acceptance should already have been achieved. If not, community health nurses can serve as advocates in presenting the plan to policy makers or in preparing community members to present the plan themselves. For example, a group of community health nursing students wanted to present information on STD prevention at their religious-sponsored university. A faculty member assisted the students to couch their prevention message in a way that would be acceptable to members of the campus community. She

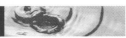

*R*ecent community health research has provided evidence of the effectiveness of using community workers drawn from the local population and from ethnic minority groups targeted by particular programs to assist with the implementation of population health programs (Farquhar, Michael, & Wiggins, 2005; Krieger, Takaro, Song, & Weaver, 2005). What advantages do you think using such workers might have? What challenges would their use entail? What do you think the effects of program involvement would be for these workers?

then met with the Vice President for Student Affairs to gain his support for the project.

The second level of acceptance involves convincing those who are to carry out the plan to implement it as designed. Again, if program implementers have been adequately represented in the planning effort, this level is already partially achieved. All that remains is for the implementers to convert the plan into an operational program.

Acceptance and participation in the planned program by members of the target group is the third level of acceptance. If, for example, the planned program involves providing contraceptive services to sexually active adolescents, the third level of acceptance involves adolescents' participation in the program. Acceptance at this third level may require marketing the program to the intended target population. Marketing involves the design and use of methods to influence people's choices of actions to be taken (Fos & Fine, 2000), in this case adolescents' choice to obtain contraceptive services.

The fourth level of acceptance involves potential resisters (Ervin, 2002). Resisters, particularly those with influence with any of the prior three groups, can make or break a program. They can influence policy makers to reject the program or withhold required funding. They

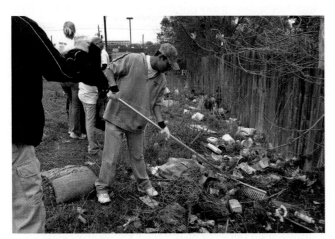

Community clean-up projects promote efforts for a clean environment. (©Bob Daemmrich/The Image Works)

may also influence participation in the program by members of the target population or convince implementers to sabotage the program. Once again, if potential resisters have been included effectively in the planning group, their influence on program implementation is more likely to be positive than negative. Using the STD example, the Vice President for Student Affairs was a potential resister. Because of the community health nursing faculty member's advocacy, he became a supporter of the program and helped to defuse other sources of resistance on campus.

Tasks of Implementation

Three basic tasks are involved in program implementation: activity delineation and sequencing, task allocation, and task performance. Necessary activities have been broadly outlined during the program planning phase. Now they must be specifically delineated and subactivities identified. This involves identifying needed categories of action and the skills required for their performance. At this point, implementers would determine the appropriate sequencing of activities and might establish a specific time frame for their accomplishment. Returning to the program theory in Figure 15-1, program implementation would entail determining the details of the marketing program and the activities needed to establish the smokers' support group.

Task allocation involves identifying the expertise of program implementers relative to the skills needed to effectively implement the program. Also at this point, responsibility is assigned for various activities delineated. Such assignments must be communicated to those involved, and they must be provided with whatever education or training is required to implement the program. Finally, the activities themselves are carried out and the planned program is put into operation.

Strategies for Implementation

Program implementation can be enhanced if several specific implementation strategies are employed. The first of these strategies is to assign responsibility for coordination of the total effort to one person. Identifying preparatory steps to each activity and listing them in sequence also fosters implementation of the program as planned.

Another strategy is periodic consultation with those implementing the program to address any difficulties that arise. Finally, the chances of implementing the program as planned are enhanced when everyone involved is clearly informed of expectations and the time frame for meeting expectations.

Members of the planning group, or designated others, must monitor implementation of the program to determine any barriers to implementation or any changes needed in the plan itself. Monitoring should address at least five areas: the adequacy of funds budgeted to carry

Advocacy in Action

Gaining Credibility

The U.S. Department of Housing and Urban Development (HUD) has a grant program called "Community Outreach Partnership Centers" (COPC) to assist universities to form partnerships with their local communities that address identified community needs. Nursing projects are often part of COPC initiatives. One such project was a health information and referral service (HIRS) designed to link community members to existing health and social services in the area. When the project was initiated, the community health nursing faculty member who wrote the grant anticipated considerable business from people needing help in finding a source of care. She and the nursing graduate hired to staff the center were somewhat surprised to find that, in spite of advertising their services to local churches and other agencies, they received few customers. Although the university had been located in the community for more than 30 years, it was not considered an integral part of the community, even though the School of Nursing had been periodically involved in some community activities.

The HIRS needed a way to gain credibility in the community. The community health nurses began by offering blood pressure screening in the context of other programs provided at the community center where the HIRS was located. When local residents came to a bread distribution program, the community health nurses were there to offer blood pressure screenings. They also did screenings during a senior lunch program and other regularly scheduled activities at the community center and other locations. The nurses provided health education as the opportunity arose in the context of the blood pressure screening activities. When the nurses became familiar to community residents, their help was sought for other health-related problems, and the original intent of the HIRS was realized. The whole process took nearly a year. Now, many years later, the HIRS is the only one of the COPC projects that remains operational because the School of Nursing and the community have written collaborative grants to continue a valued service.

---

out the program, the ability of personnel to address program needs, the adequacy of other program resources, the timing of actual activities versus the planned sequence of action, and the production of the expected output (Veney & Kaluzny, 2005). Again, using the smoking cessation example, the planning group might note whether the funds budgeted for the program are sufficient to cover program costs and whether the educators can develop a curriculum that motivates participants to stop smoking. Similarly, the group might note whether there is sufficient space for group sessions as well as the appropriateness of the planned activity sequence. Finally, the group would monitor the number of participants in the program and their response to program activities.

EVALUATING POPULATION-BASED HEALTH CARE PROGRAMS

Evaluating the effects of health-related programs is an essential feature in the care of populations. Program evaluation is needed for many of the same reasons that a systematic process is used in program planning. Health care providers recognize the limitation of available resources and must be accountable to the community members who use the program and, particularly, to the community members who pay for the program. They must be able to justify the program's existence and continuation. This can be done only by documenting the effectiveness of programs in solving the problems they were designed to address.

Evaluation of a particular program may be undertaken for a variety of reasons. Some of these include justifying program continuation or expansion, improving the quality of service provided, determining future courses of action, and determining the impact of the program. Other reasons for evaluation might be to call attention to the program, to assess personnel performance, or to assuage political expectations. The underlying purpose for program evaluation, however, is to make better programmatic decisions (Veney & Kaluzny, 2005). The importance of program evaluation is highlighted by the following comment, "Evaluation is an essential part of public health; without evaluation's close ties to program implementation, we are left with the unsatisfactory circumstance of either wasting resources on ineffective programs or, perhaps worse, continuing public health practices that do more harm than good" (Vaughan, 2004).

The Centers for Disease Control and Prevention have developed a *Framework for Program Evaluation in Public Health*. This framework poses a series of general questions that can guide program evaluation (Center for Health Improvement, 2004). These questions include the following:

- What will be evaluated?
- What aspects of the program will be considered in judging its performance?
- What standards will be used to judge the program's performance?

- What evidence will be used to compare program performance with the standards selected?
- What conclusions can be drawn from comparing program data with the standards selected?
- How will the evaluation information be used to improve program effectiveness?

The first four questions guide the development of the evaluation plan. The last two address analysis and use of evaluative data.

In addition to general questions that can be addressed by a program evaluation, there are several criteria that can be used to judge the worth or value of a health-related program. These criteria are presented in Table 15-2◆.

Considerations in Program Evaluation

There are a number of considerations to be made in designing a program evaluation. These include the purpose of the evaluation, who should conduct the evaluation, political considerations, ethical considerations, and considerations about the type of evaluation to be conducted.

Evaluation Purpose

The purpose of the evaluation influences all other aspects of the process. For example, if the purpose of the evaluation is to justify continuing a program, the evaluation will focus on determining whether the program has a beneficial effect on the health of the population group for which it is designed. On the other hand, if the purpose is to decide whether programs are under- or overused, evaluation will focus on the number of persons served. In other words, the purpose of the evaluation influences the types of data collected and how they are used.

Possible purposes for evaluation include deciding to continue or discontinue the program, improving the program, testing a new idea or approach, comparing two similar programs, making decisions to add or drop an element of a program, determining the feasibility of implementing the program elsewhere, and allocating resources among competing programs (Grembowski, 2001). Other potential purposes for program evaluation include justifying program expenditures, determining if the implementation timeline is on target, gaining support for program expansion, drawing attention to the program, and demonstrating the achievements of the program (Ervin, 2002).

Evaluator Considerations

Another consideration in planning for evaluation is the question of who will conduct the evaluation. Should the evaluators be people who implement the program? Program beneficiaries? Outside experts? Or someone else? Considerations in selecting who will evaluate the program include trust and credibility, access and cooperation, hidden agendas, and confidentiality. Who will have credibility in evaluating the program? An outside expert might have credibility with policy makers, but less with program participants or community members. Program implementers might be trusted by other staff and by program beneficiaries, but be somewhat biased in their approach to data analysis and conclusions drawn. Policy makers might also conduct the evaluation, but might have hidden agendas related to the program, as might program staff.

Program implementers will have access to much of the data needed for the evaluation and may have the cooperation of other staff members and beneficiaries. An outside expert is likely to be relatively objective in his or her evaluation, but is not as well acquainted with possible data sources and may not be trusted by program staff and beneficiaries, which might lead to decreased cooperation on their part. Outside evaluators also tend to be a rather expensive alternative.

Another possibility, and one that is in keeping with participatory research in community assessment, and community participation in program planning, is empowerment evaluation. **Empowerment evaluation** is defined as "an interactive and iterative process by which the community, in collaboration with the support team, identifies its own health issues, decides how to address them, monitors progress toward its goals and uses the information to adapt and sustain the initiative" (Fetterman, as quoted in Minkler & Wallerstein, 2005, p. 43).

Empowerment evaluation assists communities to develop the skills to assess and improve their own quality of life. In empowerment evaluation, the community health nurse evaluator serves as an educator, advocate, and facilitator, and community members determine the focus and methods for the evaluation and participate in data collection and analysis and use of the findings. If community members are to collect

TABLE 15-2	General Criteria for Program Evaluation
Criterion	Description
Relevance	The program is appropriate to meet the identified needs of the population
Adequacy	The program is able to address all aspects of the problem or issue
Progress	Program implementation is congruent with the program plan
Effectiveness	The program produces the anticipated intermediate outcomes
Impact	The program achieves ultimate outcomes as anticipated
Efficiency	There is a reasonable relationship between input and output; resource expenditure is reasonable in relation to program results
Sustainability	Both program effects and the program itself are capable of being sustained over time

Data from: Veney, J. E., & Kaluzny, A. D. (2005). Evaluation and decision making for health services (4th ed.). Chicago: Health Administration Press.

evaluation data, consideration should be given to confidentiality issues if client records are used as a data source. The evaluation team should consider all of these possibilities before determining who will conduct the evaluation.

Political Considerations

Program evaluation occurs within a political context, and so political factors should be considered in designing the evaluation. Evaluations, for example, may be undertaken purely for political reasons (Grembowski, 2001). One political purpose might be to delay decisions about the program. For example, some policy makers may be calling for the discontinuation of a program. Others who support the program, however, may propose an evaluation of program effects to delay any action taken with respect to the program. Policy makers may also choose to evaluate a program in order to escape pressure from competing interest groups. For example, different segments of the population may support different alternative solutions to an identified problem. In this instance, evaluation of programs based on the different alternatives may give policy makers support for choosing one alternative over another.

Program evaluation may also be conducted to provide legitimacy for prior decisions or to support program expansion. For example, data on the effectiveness of adapting a Parents as Teachers program (a national program to promote school readiness in children) specifically for Hmong families were used to support adaptation of the program to Hispanic families in the same community. Finally, program evaluation may be used to promote support for the program. In this instance, those proposing the evaluation may want to highlight only positive aspects of the program rather than conduct a comprehensive evaluation of program effects (Grembowski, 2001).

In addition, community health nurses and community members engaged in program evaluation may want to consider the political uses to which evaluation findings may be put. For example, positive evaluation findings may be used to support reelection of public officials who supported program initiation. Conversely, negative findings may be used to bolster the candidacy of a political opponent. Negative findings regarding program effectiveness may be used to close programs that provide other benefits for a community (e.g., visibility of cultural minority groups, employment opportunities for community members, and so on).

Ethical Considerations

Ethical conflicts must be anticipated in program evaluation. Participation in the evaluation should be voluntary for staff and clients alike. This poses some problems in that staff members are sometimes unwilling to reveal information that reflects poorly on them or on the program that employs them. To circumvent this reluctance, the evaluator needs to have a variety of sources of data that provide an overall picture of the program and its effects.

Confidentiality is another issue. Persons who provide data need to be assured that their individual responses will not be identifiable. There is also the question of who will have access to the findings of the evaluation. Should findings be shared only with those involved in the program? With their supervisors? With funding agencies or regulatory bodies? The use to which findings can be put is also of concern. Can the evaluator publish the information? Will it be used to fire personnel?

Finally, the evaluation team must consider the risks and benefits accruing from the evaluation. Is there potential for harm to the participants, either clients or staff? Do the anticipated benefits of the evaluation outweigh any possible risks?

Type of Evaluation

The last major consideration in evaluating a health care program is the type of evaluation to be conducted. Program evaluation may occur either prospectively or retrospectively (Grembowski, 2001). In a prospective evaluation, the evaluation is planned and evaluative criteria are determined prior to program implementation. Retrospective evaluation is designed after the program is completed or at least in the process of being implemented. Although prospective evaluation is the recommended approach, there are many occasions in which community health nurses may be involved in retrospective evaluation. For example, community health nurses may be asked to assist in the evaluation of existing programs for which evaluative mechanisms and criteria were not established during program planning. At times, community health nurses will be asked to evaluate programs that do not even have clear expected outcomes. In those instances, the first step in the evaluation process is to determine what the program is expected to achieve.

Whether the approach used in program evaluation is prospective or retrospective, there are three basic types of evaluation that can be conducted: implementation monitoring, process evaluation, and outcome evaluation. Many program evaluations incorporate more than one type of evaluation.

IMPLEMENTATION MONITORING Implementation monitoring involves examining the extent to which the program has been implemented as planned (Ervin, 2002; Lazenbatt, 2002). Has the organizational structure of the program been implemented as designed? Structure reflects the delivery system characteristics of the program including its organization, the types of personnel employed, types of clients served, and so on (Aday, Begley, Lairson, & Balkrishnan, 2004). Evaluative questions that might be asked in implementation monitoring include the following:

- Do program staff have the education and expertise to carry out the program and meet identified community needs?
- Is the program attracting the anticipated number and type of participants? Are there barriers to access to services for some segments of the community? If so, what are they and how can they be overcome?
- Are program activities being implemented as planned? If not, what factors are impeding planned implementation?
- Is program implementation proceeding along the anticipated time frame? If not, what factors are delaying implementation of various elements of the program?

PROCESS EVALUATION The second type of evaluation is process evaluation. Here, one is concerned with the quality of interactions between program staff and recipients (Aday et al., 2004). Process evaluation examines program performance and may take the perspective of quality assurance or quality improvement. The focus in quality assurance is on making sure that the processes by which care is provided meet certain established standards. If the standard has been met, no action is warranted and program operation continues unmodified. Quality improvement, on the other hand, focuses on continuing improvement in program performance. The philosophy behind quality improvement, also referred to as continuous quality improvement (CQI) or total quality management (TQM), is that clients' needs and expectations change over time and that an effective health care program is continually changing to better meet those needs. This can be achieved only if the processes of care are being continually examined and improved as needed. Quality improvement focuses on enhancing the processes of care to create more effective outcomes.

Process evaluation addresses questions of what is working (or not working) within the program and why (Anderson, Guthrie, & Schirle, 2002). Process evaluation also helps to determine why program objectives may not be met (Grembowski, 2001). In addition, process evaluation may be useful in implementing the program in other places (Billings, 2000). For example, information about processes that worked and did not work in one setting, may assist in developing more effective processes in other similar settings.

Process evaluation also examines the context in which the program operates (Linnan & Steckler, 2002). When the context changes, the program may also need to change to continue to be effective in achieving its outcomes. For example, an existing community immunization program may have been planned prior to the arrival of a large refugee population. Program processes will need to be changed to incorporate outreach activities,

informed consent, and education regarding side effects in other languages to accommodate the cultural background of this new group of beneficiaries.

Additional considerations that may be incorporated in process evaluation include issues of efficiency, cost, equity, adequacy, quality, timeliness, and satisfaction with care received. Efficiency evaluation addresses the use of resources in relation to the outcomes achieved by the program. Cost reflects the entire cost of the program and its acceptability to implementers, policy makers, and funding sources. Programs may be highly effective, but may be delivered at a cost too high to be supported. Equity concerns the extent to which the needs of the entire target population, rather than only certain segments, are met. Adequacy, on the other hand, addresses the extent to which all of the related needs of the target population are met by the program. Quality evaluation reflects whether the care provided by the program meets established standards. Evaluation of timeliness addresses whether services are provided within an anticipated time frame. Finally, satisfaction with program services is evaluated from the perspectives of the individuals who receive them, providers, and the community at large. Possible process evaluation criteria and potential evaluative questions are provided in Table 15-3◆. Evaluative questions are considered in the context of an immunization program for vaccine-preventable diseases.

Process evaluation may also address one or more of the qualities of successful health improvement programs. A given program can be evaluated in terms of how well it incorporates the following features:

- Incorporates intensive approaches to problem resolution
- Is based on community commitment to solving the problem
- Is multidisciplinary in nature and incorporates interagency alliances as needed
- Takes place in a variety of settings
- Is based on prior needs assessment
- Employs culturally sensitive interventions
- Uses a variety of implementers as appropriate (including community workers)
- Adequately trains program staff
- Uses effective support materials (e.g., appropriate literature)
- Addresses health needs holistically
- Promotes community empowerment
- Uses evidence-based interventions
- Employs systematic processes for evaluation (Lazenbatt, 2002)

For example, a part of the evaluation might focus on the appropriateness of marketing strategies and literature for a multiethnic population or for a specifically targeted ethnic group. Or the evaluation might focus on the relative effectiveness of different types of providers

TABLE 15-3	Process Evaluation Criteria and Related Evaluation Questions
Criterion	**Potential Evaluation Questions**
Context	▪ Has the context within which the program operates changed? (e.g., are community members able to get immunizations from other sources, or has there been a change in the population needing program services?) ▪ Is there still a need for the program given the altered program context? ▪ Are changes needed in the program to adapt to changes in the context? (e.g., does the immunization program need to adapt to provide services to non-English-speaking community members?)
Efficiency	▪ What is the cost of the program per unit accomplishment (e.g., what is the cost of an immunization program per child fully immunized?) ▪ Are resources (time, personnel, equipment and supplies, funding) being used as efficiently as possible? (e.g., would immunization services in the context of other services, such as WIC services, reach more clients?) ▪ How much waste occurs in the use of program resources? (e.g., how many doses of vaccine expire before they can be used?)
Cost	▪ What is the overall cost of the program? ▪ Is the cost of the program acceptable given the level of benefits achieved? ▪ What is the cost of the program in terms of lost opportunities? (e.g., what other programs might be funded with that money or implemented with staff time?)
Equity	▪ Are various segments of the target population benefiting equally from the program? If not, why? (e.g., are Hispanic clients less likely to take advantage of immunization services? If so, why?) ▪ Do some segments of the target population have difficulty obtaining program services? (e.g., does an immunization program provide services to children but not to adults?)
Adequacy	▪ Does the program address all of the target population's needs in the area to be addressed? (e.g., does an immunization program provide all the required immunizations for school entry or only some of them?)
Quality	▪ Do the services provided conform to recognized standards? (e.g., are parents given accurate information on which to give informed consent for immunizations? Are they informed of potential reactions and what to do about them?) ▪ Is the performance of staff monitored to determine the quality of services provided? If so, what do results indicate? (e.g., do staff use appropriate immunization techniques for people of different ages?) ▪ What indicators are used to measure quality in the services provided? Are these indicators valid and reliable? (e.g., how is the performance of staff in providing immunizations services evaluated?)
Timeliness	▪ Are program services received in a timely fashion and within an expected time frame? ▪ Are services available when requested, or do clients have to wait to obtain services? (e.g., can parents get their children immunized when needed, or do they have to wait for an appointment?) ▪ Are expected program results achieved within an expected time frame? (e.g., have community immunization levels increased to the expected level in the anticipated time from program initiation?)
Satisfaction	▪ What is the level of satisfaction with the program expressed by program beneficiaries? By service providers? By the community? ▪ What are areas of dissatisfaction, if any? What factors contribute to dissatisfaction with the program? ▪ Are program recipients satisfied with the services provided by the program? ▪ Are they satisfied with program outcomes? ▪ Are policy makers satisfied that the program is achieving its intended outcomes at a reasonable cost?

in achieving program goals (e.g., professional providers versus community workers).

OUTCOME EVALUATION Outcome evaluation focuses on the consequences of the program for the health and welfare of the population, irrespective of how well organized or efficient the program was. Outcome evaluation documents the effects of the program and justifies decisions to continue, modify, or eliminate it. The greatest difficulty in evaluating the effects of community health programs lies in the extended time between interventions and their effects (Easterling, Gallagher, & Lodwick, 2003b). For this reason, outcome evaluation may focus on immediate, intermediate, and ultimate outcomes or on *effect* and *impact*.

A program's effect is the degree to which specific outcome objectives were met. This addresses the achievement of immediate, and possibly intermediate, outcomes. Using the example of the health department

immunization program, the effect of the program is evaluated when one determines whether the *Healthy People 2010*◆ objectives of full immunization coverage for 90% of children aged 19 through 36 months and influenza vaccine coverage for 90% of noninstitutionalized adults over age 65 have been achieved. If the objectives have been achieved, the program can be considered effective. If not, the evaluator must determine to what degree the objective has been met and whether continuation of the program is warranted. For example, if vaccine coverage was achieved for 85% of young children in the community, extending the program would probably be considered. If, on the other hand, only 60% of the children in this age group are fully immunized, alternative approaches may need to be considered.

The impact of a program is how well it serves to attain overall goals. If the goal was to decrease the incidence of vaccine-preventable diseases, for example, the achievement of improved immunization rates should contribute to goal achievement. If, however, the goal was to reduce the incidence of communicable diseases in general, increasing immunization rates will only be partially successful, since some communicable disease cannot be prevented with immunization. In this instance, the program was effective in accomplishing its objective, but accomplishing the objective did not lead to achievement of the overall goal.

Valid impact evaluation is based on five common-sense criteria. First, the impact studied should be consistent with the program theory. In other words, based on the cause and effect relationships contained in the program theory, the intervention chosen should logically contribute to the outcome studied. Using our immunization program as an example, getting more people to accept immunizations should logically lead to increased immunization rates, which should, in turn, lead to decreased incidence of vaccine-preventable diseases. Second, the program should precede the outcome measured. Third, the evaluation should rule out other possible explanations for achievement of the outcome. Fourth, conclusions regarding a positive impact of the program should be based on the presence of statistically significant relationships. Finally, the measures used to assess outcomes should be both reliable and valid (Grembowski, 2001).

Health programs can have a number of outcomes. Often, the outcomes arise out of the program's stated objectives as in the examples above. Other outcomes may also be of interest. Usually, however, it is not feasible or even possible to examine all of a program's possible outcomes, so the evaluation team will need to decide which outcomes will be the focus of program evaluation. Several criteria have been suggested for making this decision. First, the outcomes studied should be valued by persons involved in the program—the recipients, the implementers, or the funders. Second, a multidimensional array of outcomes should be examined to provide information about the overall worth of the program. Third, outcomes should be selected for which objective and measurable data can be obtained. Fourth, the outcomes selected should be logically connected to the program and should be effects that can be attributed to the program rather than to other factors. Finally, both long-term and short-term outcomes of the program should be assessed whenever possible (Schalock, 2000).

For each outcome selected, the evaluation team will develop one or more outcome measures to assess that outcome. **Outcome measures** involve the assessment of one or more variables related to expected program results (Fos & Fine, 2000). Immunization rates and incidence rates for vaccine-preventable diseases might be outcome measures to evaluate an immunization program.

Community health programs may incorporate specific nursing-sensitive outcomes included in the Nursing Outcomes Classification (NOC) system. NOC is a taxonomy of outcomes that can be affected by nursing intervention, often in conjunction with other health

professionals and community residents and agents. Each NOC outcome includes a set of indicators that can be used to evaluate its achievement. In its second edition, NOC included six community-level outcomes that have been tested and found to be valid and sensitive to nursing intervention. These outcomes include (a) community competence, (b) community health status, (c) community health: immunity, (d) community risk control: chronic disease, (e) community risk control: communicable disease, (f) community risk control: lead exposure (Head et al., 2004). Indicators for the outcome of community risk control: communicable disease might be relevant to the evaluation of our immunization program.

In designing a program evaluation, the evaluation team needs to decide which types of evaluation are appropriate—implementation monitoring, process evaluation, or outcome evaluation. A particular program can be evaluated with respect to any one aspect or a combination of several. The aspects selected depend on the purposes of the evaluation and the time and other resources available. Most health program evaluations will incorporate several aspects of evaluation.

The Evaluation Process

Like any other systematic process, evaluation takes place in a series of specific steps. Some of these steps, such as planning the evaluation, have already been completed as part of the total planning process. Other steps include collecting data, interpreting data, and using evaluative findings. These steps have been likened to a three-act play (Grembowski, 2001). The first act involves asking the question; the second act involves answering it; and the third act involves using the data generated for program decisions.

Evaluation Planning

In asking the evaluation question, the evaluation team reviews the program theory, specifies program objectives (process and outcome) to be addressed, translates the program theory and objectives into evaluation questions, and selects the questions to be addressed in the evaluation process. Goals for the evaluation, evaluative criteria, types of data needed, and appropriate methods of data collection were established as part of the planning process. Evaluative criteria and type of evaluation are based on the purpose of the evaluation and the evaluation questions asked. If the intent of the evaluation is to determine the extent to which outcome objectives are met, evaluative criteria will be derived from those objectives. In the immunization program example, evaluative criteria related to outcome objectives would include immunization levels and disease incidence in the population. If the intent is to assess the efficiency of the program, evaluative criteria might include the number of immunizations given, the length of time people had to wait for immunizations, and the effectiveness of marketing strategies for reaching specific target populations.

Data needed to answer the evaluation questions are determined and data collection procedures established. Planning evaluation also involves determining the necessary equipment and supplies. If, for example, the evaluation team wanted to know if adequate levels of immunity had been achieved in those immunized, they would need supplies for drawing and testing blood samples. It is more likely, however, that evaluation of the program will involve collecting data on the percentage of the population immunized based on a survey of immunization records and the incidence of disease based on local surveillance strategies.

Collecting, Analyzing, and Interpreting Data

The evaluative criteria chosen influence the types of data collected and the manner in which they are collected. Data collection strategies may also need to take into consideration the language of program participants, their ability to read (in which case printed surveys would not be appropriate), or other elements of the program context. For the immunization program, records will need to be kept regarding the number and types of immunizations given, categories of persons to whom they were given (e.g., children, adults, members of ethnic groups). Data collection will also necessitate generating information on the existing immunization rates in the community if that has not already been obtained in the assessment that motivated program planning.

Once data have been collected, they must be analyzed and interpreted. Analysis may involve conducting statistical tests of relationships or identification of concepts and themes from qualitative information. The evaluation team should identify analysis strategies that are consistent with the evaluation questions to be asked.

The next step in the evaluation process is interpreting the findings. In this step, data are compared with the evaluative criteria. In evaluating the achievement of the outcome objectives of an immunization program, the evaluation team would compare the community immunization rates to those specified in the program objectives. If the program has achieved a 90% immunization rate for children 19 to 36 months of age and for noninstitutionalized persons over age 65, the program would be judged to be effective and would probably be continued. If the program has only achieved rates of 80% and 75%, respectively, but these rates are higher than those prior to the program, the program might be considered somewhat effective. The extent of improvement would need to be considered, however, in deciding whether to continue the program.

Data may also be used to assess the processes by which the program is carried out. For example, in the community focus group project described by Clark and associates (2003), one of the process objectives for the assessment was to include specific segments of the population in the assessment. When the assessment process was evaluated, the steering committee found that focus group participation mirrored community composition in terms of age, ethnicity, and the proportion of residents versus service providers in the community. Thus, the process objective was judged to be met.

In examining data related to the efficient use of supplies, an evaluation team might look at what percentage of vaccines purchased was used and what percentage was wasted. If the criterion derived from process objectives specified that less than 5% of vaccine supplies purchased be wasted and the team finds that closer to 10% was actually wasted, the program processes are not operating as efficiently as planned.

Disseminating and Using Evaluation Findings

Effective use of evaluation findings requires that they be communicated to those who need them. This includes those who will make decisions regarding the program as well as those who are contemplating similar programs. The task of the evaluation team, at this point, is to determine who should be told about the evaluation findings and conclusions and when and how communication of results will occur. Findings then need to be translated into language that will be understood by various stakeholder audiences and should be used to derive specific recommendations regarding the program. Finally, the team communicates the findings in appropriate forms to the stakeholder groups. In keeping with community empowerment strategies, members of the community should certainly comprise one stakeholder group to whom findings and recommendations are communicated.

The findings of the evaluation should be used as a basis for decisions about the program. Basically, three decisions can be made based on evaluative findings: to continue, to modify, or to discontinue the program. If the evaluation team finds that the program's objectives are being achieved, they may recommend continuing the program. If the team finds that only a few community members are participating in the program, they may recommend either stopping the program or taking steps to increase participation. For example, perhaps marketing strategies need to be changed to target specific ethnic groups with low immunization rates who are not taking advantage of the program. Looking at program efficiency, if the assessment team finds that 10% of the vaccines purchased are being wasted, various waste control practices may need to be instituted.

Factors in each of the six dimensions of health are considered by community health nurses in assessing the health needs of communities and other population groups. Planning to meet those needs then employs an organized and systematic process involving development of planning competence, developing goals and objectives based on program theory, and delineating resources and actions needed to accomplish goals and objectives. Implementation and evaluation of health care delivery programs are also systematic processes employed by community health nurses.

Case Study

Caring for Copper City

You are the community health nurse assigned to Copper City, a small town in New Mexico with a population of 3,000. You have just arrived in town and have been given the task of assisting community members to assess the health needs of the community and developing a plan to meet those needs. Your assessment committee consists of yourself, one of the local physicians, the elementary school principal, two teachers, the pastors of two local churches, the owner of one of the local copper mines, and five community residents.

During the assessment, the assessment team obtains the following information: Copper City is a small town run by a city council and a mayor. Most of these officials are administrators of the local copper mines or owners of large chicken farms in the area. The town is in a largely rural area, 50 miles from Tucumcari. The surrounding countryside is hot and arid.

The ethnic composition of the town is 80% Caucasian of European ancestry and 20% Latino, primarily of Mexican descent. Fifty percent of the town's population is under 8 years of age. There are very few elderly persons in the community, because Copper City is a relatively new town that grew up around copper mines discovered in the last 20 years. The birth rate is 30 per 1,000 population. Approximately 10% of all births are premature, and the neonatal death rate is 50 per 1,000 live births. Only about 10% of the women receive prenatal care during their pregnancies.

The major industries in the area are copper mines and chicken farms, which employ approximately 85% of the adult men and 50% of the women. The majority of the Latino population works on the chicken farms. The remaining 15% of the adult men and another 20% of the adult women are employed in offices and shops in the town. The unemployment level is 0.5%, far lower than that of the state and the nation.

The average annual family income is $8,000, and 75% of the population is below the poverty level. Nearly one third of those below the poverty level receive some form of aid such as Medicaid or Temporary Aid to Needy Families (TANF).

The predominant religion among the Caucasian population is Methodist, and among the Latino group it is Roman Catholic. There are two Methodist churches in town, one Catholic church, and a small Southern Baptist congregation.

Many of the Latino group subscribe to alternative health practices. They frequently seek health care from a local *yerbero* (herbalist). They may also drive to a nearby town to solicit the services of a *curandera* (faith healer). Close to one third of the Latino population speaks only Spanish.

The average education level for the community is tenth grade. For the Spanish-speaking group, however, it is only third grade.

Education facilities in the town include a grade school and a high school. The high school also offers adult education classes at night. There is a Head Start program that enrolls 50 children, but no other childcare facilities are available.

There is a high incidence of tuberculosis in the community, and anemia and pinworms are common problems among the preschool and school-age children. Several of the men have been disabled as a result of accidents in the mines.

The only transportation to Tucumcari is by car or by train, which comes through town morning and evening. About half of the families in town own cars.

There is one general practice physician and one dentist in the town. The nearest hospital is in Tucumcari, and the funeral home hearse is used as an ambulance for emergency transportation to the hospital. The driver and one attendant have had basic first aid training but have not been educated as emergency medical technicians. The county health department provides family planning, prenatal, well-child, and immunization services one day a week in the basement of the larger of the two Methodist churches. In addition to yourself, the staff consists of a physician, one licensed practical nurse, a master's-prepared family nurse practitioner, and a nutritionist. The well-child and immunization services are heavily used, and immunization levels in the community are high among both preschoolers and school-age youngsters.

1. What are the biophysical, psychological, physical environmental, sociocultural, behavioral, and health system factors influencing the health of this community?
2. What assets are present in this community that might assist with problem resolution?
3. What community nursing diagnoses might you derive from the assessment team's data?
4. What health problems are evident in the case study? Which do you think are the three most important problems for this community? Why have you given these problems priority over others? Do you think other members of the assessment team would prioritize them differently? Why or why not?
5. Select one of the three top-priority problems and design a health program to resolve it. Be sure to address the following:
   - Level of prevention involved
   - Who should be involved in the planning group, why, and how you would obtain community participation in planning
   - Additional information you would need, if any, and where you would obtain that information
   - Goals and objectives for the program
   - Resources needed to implement the program
6. How would you gain acceptance of your program?
7. How would you go about implementing the program?
8. How would you conduct outcome and process evaluation of the program?

Test Your Understanding

1. Why should community or target group members be incorporated into all phases of population health assessment and program planning and evaluation? (pp. 356–357)

2. What biophysical, psychological, physical environmental, sociocultural, behavioral, and health system factors should be addressed in a comprehensive population health assessment? (pp. 351–356)

3. What are the elements of a population nursing diagnosis? Give examples of positive and negative population nursing diagnoses. (p. 363)

4. Identify at least five tasks in planning a health program to meet the needs of populations. What would be the role of the community health nurse with respect to each task? (pp. 364–370)

5. Define program theory. How is program theory used to develop a health care program? Give an example of a program theory underlying a community health program with which you are familiar. (p. 368)

6. What are the four levels of acceptance of a health care program? How might community health nurses influence acceptance at each level? (pp. 370–371)

7. Discuss three of the five types of considerations in evaluating a health care program? How might each influence the program evaluation process? (pp. 373–377)

EXPLORE MediaLink

http://www.prenhall.com/clark
Resources for this chapter can be found on the Companion Website.

Audio Glossary
Appendix G: Community Health Assessment and Intervention Guide
Exam Review Questions

Case Study: Influencing the Health of a Community
MediaLink Application: Tobacco-Free Kids (video)

Media Links
Challenge Your Knowledge
Advocacy Interviews

References

Abrams, S. E. (2004). From function to competency in public health nursing, 1931 to 2003. *Public Health Nursing, 21,* 507–510.

Aday, L. A., Begley, C. E., Lairson, D. R., & Balkrishnan, R. (2004). *Evaluating the healthcare system: Effectiveness, efficiency, and equity* (3rd ed.). Chicago: Health Administration Press.

Anderson, D., Guthrie, T., & Schirle, R. (2002). A nursing model of community organization for change. *Public Health Nursing, 19,* 40–46.

Billings, J. R. (2000). Community development: A critical review of approaches to evaluation. *Journal of Advanced Nursing, 31,* 472–480.

Bingler, S. (2000). The school as the center of a healthy community. *Public Health Reports, 115,* 228–233.

Center for Health Improvement. (2004). *Health policy guide: Evidence-based policies to improve the public's health.* Retrieved August 25, 2004, from http://www.healthpolicycoach.org/advocacy.asp?id=23

Centers for Disease Control and Prevention/Agency for Toxic Substances and Disease Registry Committee on Community Engagement. (1997). *Principles of community engagement.* Washington, DC: Author.

Centers for Disease Control and Prevention/Agency for Toxic Substances and Disease Registry Committee on Community Engagement. (2004). *Principles of community engagement: Part 2.* Retrieved May 17, 2005, from http://www.phppo.cdc.gov/dphsdr/FaithBase/PCE/part2.asp

Clark, M. J., Cary, S., Diemert, G., Ceballos, R., Sifuentes, M., Atteberry, I., et al. (2003). Involving community in community assessment. *Public Health Nursing, 20,* 456–463.

Clark, N., & Buell, A. (2004). Community assessment: An innovative approach. *Nurse Educator, 29,* 203–207.

Dykeman, M., MacIntosh, J., Seaman, P., & Davidson, P. (2003). Development of a program logic model to measure the processes and outcomes of a nurse managed community health clinic. *Journal of Professional Nursing, 19,* 197–203.

Easterling, D. V., Gallagher, K. M., & Lodwick, D. G. (2003a). Practical lessons for promoting health at the community level? In D. V. Easterling, K. M. Gallagher, & D. G. Lodwick (Eds.), *Promoting health at the community level* (pp. 219–246). Thousand Oaks, CA: Sage.

Easterling, D. V., Gallagher, K. M., & Lodwick, D. G. (2003b). What do case studies say about community-based health promotion? In D. V. Easterling, K. M. Gallagher, & D. G. Lodwick (Eds.), *Promoting health at the community level* (pp. 195–218). Thousand Oaks, CA: Sage.

Ervin, N. (2002). *Advanced community health nursing practice: Population-focused care.* Upper Saddle River, NJ: Prentice Hall.

Farquhar, S. A., Michael, Y. L., & Wiggins, N. (2005). Building on leadership and social capital to create change in 2 urban communities. *American Journal of Public Health, 95,* 596–601.

Fos, P. J., & Fine, D. J. (2000). *Designing health care for populations: Applied epidemiology in health care administration.* San Francisco: Jossey-Bass.

Grembowski, D. (2001). *The practice of health program evaluation.* Thousand Oaks, CA: Sage.

Hancock, T., & Minkler, M. (2005). Community health assessment or healthy community assessment: Whose community? Whose health? Whose assessment? In M. Minkler (Ed.), *Community organizing and community building for health* (2nd ed., pp. 138–157). New Brunswick, NJ: Rutgers University Press.

Head, B. J., Aquilino, M. L., Johnson, M., Reed, D., Maas, M., & Moorhead, S. (2004). Content validity and nursing sensitivity of community-level outcomes from the Nursing Outcomes Classification (NOC). *Journal of Nursing Scholarship, 36,* 251–259.

Jonas, S. (2003). *An introduction to the U.S. health care system* (5th ed.). New York: Springer.

Kone, A., Sullivan, M., Senturia, K., Chrisman, N. J., Ciske, S. J., & Frieger, J. W. (2000). Improving collaboration between researchers and communities. *Public Health Reports, 115,* 243–248.

Krieger, J. W., Takaro, T. K., Song, L., & Weaver, M. (2005). The Seattle-King County Healthy Homes Project: A randomized, controlled trial of a community health worker intervention to decrease exposure to indoor asthma triggers. *American Journal of Public Health, 95,* 652–659.

Lazenbatt, A. (2002). *Evaluation handbook for health professionals.* London: Routledge.

Linnan, L., & Steckler, A. (2002). Process evaluation for public health interventions and research: An overview. In L. Linnan & S. Steckler (Eds.), *Process evaluation for public health interventions and research* (pp. 1–23). San Francisco: Jossey-Bass.

Longest, B. B. (2004). *Managing health programs and projects.* San Francisco, Jossey-Bass.

Macintyre, S., & Ellaway, A. (2003). Neighborhoods and health: An overview. In I. Kawachi & L. F. Berkman (Eds.), *Neighborhoods and health* (pp. 20–42). Oxford: Oxford University Press.

Minkler, M., & Wallerstein, N. (2005). Improving health through community organization and community building. In M. Minkler (Ed.), *Community organizing and community building for health* (2nd ed., pp. 26–50). New Brunswick, NJ: Rutgers University Press.

Nardi, D. A. (2003a). Introduction to health and wellness needs assessment. In D. A. Nardi & J. M. Petr (Eds.), *Community health and wellness needs assessment: A step-by-step guide* (pp. 1–22). Clifton Park, NY: Delmar Learning.

Nardi, D. A. (2003b). Steps of the community health and wellness assessment process. In D. A. Nardi & J. M. Petr (Eds.), *Community health and wellness needs assessment: A step-by-step guide* (pp. 23–45). Clifton Park, NY: Delmar Learning.

Owen, S. (2001). The practical methodology and ethical dilemmas of conducting focus groups with vulnerable clients. *Journal of Advanced Nursing, 36,* 652–658.

Plescia, M., Koontz, S., & Laurent, S. (2001). Community assessment in a vertically integrated health care system. *American Journal of Public Health, 91,* 811–814.

Riner, M., Cunningham, C., & Johnson, A. (2004). Public health education and practice using geographic information system technology. *Public Health Nursing, 21,* 57–65.

Robertson, J. F. (2004). Does advanced community/public health nursing practice have a future? *Public Health Nursing, 21,* 495–501.

Schalock, R. L. (2000). *Outcome-based evaluation* (2nd ed.). New York: Plenum Press.

Severtson, D., Baumann, L., & Will, J. (2002). A participatory assessment of environmental health concerns in an Ojibwa community. *Public Health Nursing, 19,* 47–58.

Sharpe, P. A., Greaney, M. L., Lee, P. R., & Royce, S. W. (2000). Assets-oriented community assessment. *Public Health Reports, 115,* 205–211.

Swinney, J., Anson-Wonkka, C., Maki, E., & Corneau, J. (2001). Community assessment: A church community and the parish nurse. *Public Health Nursing, 18,* 40–44.

Task Force on Community Preventive Services. (2005). *Guide to community preventive services: What works to promote health?* New York: Oxford University Press.

Vaughan, R. (2004). Evaluation and public health. *American Journal of Public Health, 94,* 360.

Veney, J. E., & Kaluzny, A. D. (2005). *Evaluation and decision making for health services* (4th ed.). Chicago: Health Administration Press.

Webb, B. (2002). Using focus groups as a research method: A personal experience. *Journal of Nursing Management, 10,* 27–35.

Advocacy in Action

The Power of Research and Publication

As part of a capstone public health nursing course, senior nursing students in a Middle Eastern country conducted telephone interviews about the use of child safety seats. The students interviewed parents of children aged 1 to 13 months who lived in a geographically defined community. The community had relatively high income and educational levels, and most families had telephones and private automobiles. Students found that only 20% of parents reported transporting their children in child safety seats during the child's last car ride. The remainder reported that the child was held in someone's arms or transported in a baby carrier. Based on the data, the students planned educational interventions to be integrated into well-child care for this population.

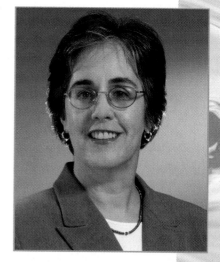

After the students graduated, the instructor thought that if wealthy and comparatively well-educated parents didn't transport their children in child safety seats, then the issue of safe transport of children would likely be an important one for the country at large. She urged the graduates to disseminate the findings of their study, but they were busy learning new skills and told the instructor to feel free to disseminate the findings herself. The instructor and a colleague developed a manuscript based on the students' findings that was published in a local nursing journal. This article was picked up by the local press, and multiple newspapers ran articles about the issue of safe transport of children in cars. The nursing instructor was interviewed by local media, helped legislators draft legislation requiring the use of safety seats, and testified before a legislative committee. Less than three years after the students completed their project, legislation was passed mandating the use of child safety seats in that country.

Derryl Block, PhD, MPH, RN

Professor and Chair Professional Program in Nursing

Director BSN-LINC

University of Wisconsin–Green Bay

16 CHAPTER

Meeting the Health Needs of Child and Adolescent Populations

CHAPTER OBJECTIVES

After reading this chapter, you should be able to:

1. Identify factors affecting the health of children and adolescents.
2. Describe at least five primary prevention measures appropriate to the care of children and adolescents and analyze the role of the community health nurse with respect to each.
3. Identify at least three approaches to providing secondary preventive care for children and adolescents and give examples of community health nursing interventions related to each.
4. Describe three tertiary preventive considerations in the care of children and adolescents and analyze the role of the community health nurse with respect to each.

KEY TERMS

anticipatory guidance **395**
attention deficit hyperactivity disorder (ADHD) **409**
Denver Developmental Screening Test (DDST) **384**
development **384**
developmental milestones **384**
fetal alcohol syndrome (FAS) **393**
growth **384**
herd immunity **387**
menarche **385**

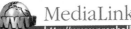

MediaLink
http://www.prenhall.com/clark

Additional interactive resources for this chapter can be found on the Companion Website. Click on Chapter 16 and "Begin" to select the activities for this chapter.

*A*ccording to the Federal Interagency Forum on Child Health and Family Statistics (2004), children under 18 years of age comprised 25% of the U.S. population. This figure encompassed nearly 73 million children and adolescents. By 2020, the proportion of the population under age 18 is expected to decrease slightly to 24%. Children and adolescents have specific health needs and problems that can be addressed by community health nurses. Community health nursing practice with children and adolescents involves assessing the health status and needs of these populations; deriving community health diagnoses; designing and implementing programs of care at primary, secondary, and tertiary levels of prevention to meet those needs; and evaluating the effectiveness of these programs.

THE EPIDEMIOLOGY OF CHILD AND ADOLESCENT HEALTH

Factors in each of the six dimensions of health influence the health of children and adolescents. We will briefly examine considerations related to the biophysical, psychological, physical environmental, sociocultural, behavioral, and health system dimensions as they affect the health of these populations.

Biophysical Considerations

Biophysical considerations related to the health of children and adolescents include the effects of maturation and aging and factors that affect both, genetic inheritance, and physiologic function. Factors contributing to health and illness among children and adolescents in each of these areas will be briefly addressed.

Age and Maturation

Areas to be assessed with respect to maturation and aging include growth and development. **Growth** is an increase in body size or change in the structure, function, and complexity of body cells until a point of maturity. Overweight and obesity are serious problems related to growth in the U.S. child and adolescent populations, whereas many children in other parts of the world are malnourished and exhibit growth retardation. In 2000, for example, 15% of 6- to 11-year olds and 16% of adolescents in the United States were overweight or

obese (National Center for Health Statistics [NCHS], 2005b). At the same time, 8% of low-income children under 5 years of age exhibited growth retardation (Centers for Disease Control and Prevention [CDC], 2005a). Similarly, news reports in 2005 indicated that as many as one third of poor children in China were malnourished. There may also be significant disparities among subgroups within the population with respect to growth parameters. For example, refugee children are often below their age mates for height and weight due to malnutrition in their countries of origin. Obesity is also more prevalent in some child and adolescent populations than in others. For example, in 2000, 24% of Mexican American school-aged children in the United States were obese or overweight compared to 15% of the general population (CDC, 2005a). When rates of obesity among children and adolescents in the population are high, community health nurses can identify contributing factors and advocate for programs to prevent or treat obesity. For example, a nurse might advocate for more physical activity and healthier meals in school settings or for the development of recreational opportunities that encourage physical activity among children and adolescents.

Development is a process of patterned, orderly, and lifelong change in structure, thought, or behavior that occurs as a result of physical or emotional maturation. With the individual child or adolescent, the community health nurse would assess the extent to which specific developmental milestones have been met. **Developmental milestones** are critical behaviors expected at specific ages, and their assessment can be accomplished using a variety of tools addressed in your basic pediatric nursing text. Development from birth to 6 years of age is often assessed by means of the **Denver Developmental Screening Test (DDST)**, a test of age-specific development in four areas: fine motor, gross motor, personal-social, and language development. Failure to develop normally may result from a number of causes. At the population level, the community health nurse would focus on the extent of developmental delay in the population. The most common cause of delayed development is mental retardation, which will be discussed in more detail later in this chapter. Other causes of developmental delays are acute and chronic illness and lack of an environment that fosters development. When the latter is the case, the community health nurse can advocate with parents and other caretakers for conditions that stimulate appropriate development. For example, in some families, younger children do not develop language skills appropriate to their ages because family members anticipate and address their needs without the child having to voice them in understandable language. In such a case, the community health nurse would encourage parents and older siblings not to meet the child's needs until the child has indicated them verbally. Similarly, community health nurses may need to

EVIDENCE-BASED PRACTICE

*E*vidence-based practice requires that research be conducted with the same types of people to whom findings will be applied. For this reason, the federal government has ruled that all research receiving federal support include children as subjects, if relevant to the study. Why is such a ruling appropriate? What ethical dilemmas might this policy pose? In what types of studies would inclusion of children as subjects not be appropriate?

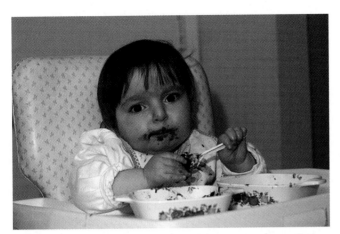

Children need opportunities to develop age-appropriate skills. (Molly Schlachter)

advocate for a balance between independence and supervision for adolescents so they gradually become independent from their parents. Nurses may also need to reassure parents that testing of family values is a normal part of adolescence, not evidence of rebellion.

Another maturational or developmental consideration for the adolescent population is the usual age at which adolescents become sexually mature, which may differ for different segments of the community. For example, African American adolescents may become sexually mature at an earlier age than their Caucasian or Asian counterparts.

Menarche, the first appearance of menstrual flow in the adolescent girl, usually occurs between 12 and 13 years of age. Menarche that occurs too early (age 8 or younger) is associated with precocious puberty, an anomaly of the endocrine system. Delayed menarche (after age 18) is also a signal that the endocrine system is not functioning properly. Either early or late onset of

menses is cause for referral for medical evaluation. Menarche may appear earlier or later than average in some ethnic populations, and the nurse should be familiar with population parameters for the onset of menstruation.

The physical and emotional changes that occur just prior to and with menarche have the potential to create physical or psychological problems for the adolescent girl. Assessment of preadolescent girls should include the extent of sexual changes, knowledge of menstruation, and preparation for the event. If menarche has occurred, other considerations related to menstruation may include menstrual regularity, extent and duration of flow, and the experience of dysmenorrhea, or painful menstruation. The nurse would also inquire about signs and symptoms of premenstrual distress (premenstrual syndrome) such as depression, irritability, nervousness, tension, inability to concentrate, breast tenderness, bloating, edema, fatigue, headache, and food cravings. Symptoms of premenstrual distress may be severe and require medical referral or may be less severe and respond to dietary changes and exercise. Menarche heralds the beginning potential for pregnancy, so the typical age of menarche in the population, or within certain subpopulations, can suggest the age at which sex education should be undertaken. Community health nurses also need to be aware of cultural attitudes to menarche within the population. Menarche in some societies is met with female genital mutilation, and community health nurses should be aware of the extent to which women in the community may have been subjected to this practice.

Physical sexual maturation in the male typically begins between ages 9.5 and 14 years and is completed between ages 14 and 18 years. Adolescent males are typically very concerned with sexual and physical development, often comparing themselves to other males and

Advocacy in Action

Developmental Delay

As both a pediatric nurse practitioner and a public health nurse working in a county health department, I had the opportunity to see clients in the child health clinic and to follow up with home visits as needed. One day in clinic I saw a 9-month-old child who was barely sitting and unable to accomplish most of the age-appropriate tasks of the Denver Developmental Screening Test (DDST). The child's mother seemed also to have a significant level of developmental delay, so I decided to make a home visit prior to making a referral for a complete diagnostic workup. When I arrived at the home, I discovered the mother had been leaving the baby in her crib in a back bedroom except when she had to feed, bathe, or change her. The mother obviously took good physical care of the child. She knew

enough to feed the baby and keep her clean and dry, but, given her own limited mental capabilities, she had no idea that a baby required stimulation. There were no toys or other objects to interest the child, and she was left consistently without stimulation of any kind.

The father of the child lived in the home, but worked two jobs. When he arrived home at night, the baby was usually in bed, and he had no idea that his wife was not interacting with the baby other than to meet her physical needs. I encouraged him to make time to play with the baby and taught the mother how to talk to and play with the child. Once the mother realized the importance of interaction with the child, she was happy to comply. After 6 months or so of appropriate stimulation, the child was on track developmentally.

many times experiencing anxiety about the possibility that their development is delayed or inadequate. In some cases, this anxiety can be sufficient to cause social impairment or serious emotional distress, and the community health nurse should make a special effort to be supportive and accepting. The community health nurse can also assist adolescent male clients by offering information and reassurance about the normal patterns and variations in growth and development. In the majority of adolescent males, a degree of transient gynecomastia (enlargement of the breasts) occurs. This is variable in degree, but can be a source of significant concern to the adolescent; again, reassurance, explanation, and acceptance are of benefit.

During this period, adolescents become increasingly concerned with the values of peers and are increasingly focused on achieving acceptance from the peer group. They are prone to value the opinions of peers over those of parents, and attitudes are more reflective of peers than of family. Adolescent males often experience identity uncertainty, and may engage in a variety of behaviors that, although perhaps disconcerting to family or other adults, are necessary experiments in determining their self-concepts. Hormonal changes result in increased growth and libido, confronting adolescent males with the possibility of new (and perhaps anxiety-provoking) roles; these changes are also mirrored in the behavior of peers, on which the teenager tends to model his own behaviors and choices.

Adolescent males may feel embarrassed about the physical and emotional changes they experience. For example, they may have spontaneous and ill-timed erections or nocturnal emissions. Physical development and social circumstances, coupled with peer pressure and a desire to conform, may lead to varying degrees of sexual activity, presenting the risks of unwanted pregnancy and sexually transmitted diseases. It is not unusual for some of the adolescent male's sexual exploration to involve sexual contact with other males; approximately 50% of all males have had such contact at some point, and there is no correlation between such sexual activity and later sexual orientation (though the adolescent may again experience significant anxiety, guilt, or shame about this experimental behavior). Other adolescent males may begin to discover a same-sex orientation during these years and should be supported as well.

Over time, the adolescent male's preoccupation with sexual performance and activity as the major parameters of a relationship are increasingly replaced by romantic attributes and genuine caring; initially, these romantic views are often stereotypical and exaggerated, but this also changes as he progresses through early adulthood. Again, the nurse's role involves assessing the young male's development relative to existing norms; providing education about growth, development, sexuality, and related risks and safety precautions; and

providing reassurance and guidance relative to the changes experienced. Community health nurses can also advocate for appropriate sexuality education for adolescents to help them deal with the many issues surrounding sexual maturation.

Genetic Inheritance

Genetic inheritance is another biophysical consideration in the assessment of child and adolescent populations. Gender and racial or ethnic background are two intrinsic genetic factors that influence the health of children and adolescents. Male and female children and children of different racial and ethnic groups tend to experience different types of health problems. For example, the nurse might identify the prevalence of urinary tract infections in school-age girls as a community problem because urinary tract infections occur more frequently in girls than in boys in this age group. Similarly, screening tests for sickle cell disease should be routinely conducted on African American children and others at risk.

Physiologic Function

Considerations related to physiologic function include the incidence and prevalence of specific physical health problems in the child and adolescent populations. Information on the leading causes of child and adolescent deaths in the population provides an overview of the health status of these two groups. According to the U.S. Census Bureau (2004b), the leading causes of death for children 1 to 4 years of age in 2001 in descending order were accidents (contributing to more than a third of all deaths in this age group), congenital malformations, neoplasms, assault/homicide (a staggering 8% of deaths), and diseases of the heart. Accidents remained the leading cause of death for children aged 5 to 14 years (40% of deaths) and adolescents and young adults from 15 to 24 years (45%), with neoplasms, congenital malformations, homicide (4.5%), heart disease, and suicide (2.6% of deaths) following for 5- to 14-year-olds. Among 15- to 24-year-olds, causes of death after first-ranked accidents included homicide (16%), suicide (12%), malignant neoplasms, and diseases of the heart. The community health nurse would explore relevant mortality figures for the child and adolescent populations in his or her community.

Not all illnesses result in death, and assessment of the child and adolescent population may reveal high prevalence rates of other acute and chronic illnesses. For example, 45,000 new cases of epilepsy are diagnosed each year in children under 15 years of age (Epilepsy Foundation, 2005). Another one in every 400 to 500 children and adolescents has type 1 diabetes (American Diabetes Association, n.d.). Other acute and chronic conditions may also be found in this population. If acute and chronic diseases are prevalent among the child and adolescent population in the community, community health nurses may need to advocate for effective illness prevention programs or services to deal with existing illness. For example, if a large proportion of the school population has asthma, the community health nurse may advocate for creation of school-based asthma management programs. Similarly, if the prevalence of childhood cancers is high, community health nurses may initiate investigation of environmental factors that may be contributing to high prevalence.

Another aspect of physiologic function that should be explored with respect to the child and adolescent populations is immunization. Maintenance of high rates of immunization among children not only protects individual children from disease, but also serves to protect other members of the population via herd immunity. **Herd immunity** is the level of protection provided to unimmunized people when immunization rates are high among the rest of the population. If most children, for example, are immunized against varicella (chickenpox), the chances of an adult without immunity being exposed to the disease are considerably reduced. Recommended immunizations for children and adolescents are summarized in Table 16-1◆. The immunization schedule is updated by the Advisory Committee on Immunization Practices (ACIP) each year and published in a January issue of *Morbidity and Mortality Weekly Report*. Up-to-date information on recommended immunizations is also available from the National Immunization Program Web site at http://www.cdc.gov/nip. When immunization levels within the population are low, community health nurses may need to advocate with parents for needed childhood immunizations for individual children or with health care delivery systems to make sure that immunizations are available. For example, the community health nurse might advocate for development of outreach immunization clinics for low-income families in underserved neighborhoods.

Psychological Considerations

A number of considerations related to the psychological dimension influence the health status of child and adolescent populations. These include family dynamics, parental coping and mental health, mental health problems in the child and adolescent population, and the potential for and extent of abuse.

Family Dynamics, Parental Expectations, and Discipline

Family dynamics affect the child's or adolescent's interactions with parents and other family members and influence the child's self-image and development of self-esteem. Children who are subjected to denigration, neglect, or harsh discipline may grow up considering themselves unworthy of love or esteem. Children may also internalize feelings and roles based on the dynamics of their families of origin. For example, children of divorced parents may experience feelings of guilt or emotional distress related to the dissolution of their family. Similarly, children in foster care have been shown to have twice the incidence of mental disorders as non-foster-care children receiving Supplemental Security Income through the Social Security program and 15 times the incidence among children receiving other forms of public aid (dos Rets, Zito, Safer, & Soeken, 2001). Research has also shown consistently that children exposed to hostility and aggressive behaviors by other family members are more likely to display these behaviors themselves.

TABLE 16-1	**Recommended Child and Adolescent Immunizations**									
Age	HBV	DTaP	Hib	IPV	PCV	MMR	Td	Var	Inf	MCV4
Birth	#1*									
1 month	#2*									
2 months		#1*	#1*	#1	#1					
4 months		#2	#2	#2	#2					
6 months	#3*	#3	#3	#3*	#3				✓*	
12 months			#4*		#4*	#1*		#1*	✓	
15 months		#4*								
24 months	†							†	✓	
4–6 years		#5		#4		#2*			✓	
11–12 years						#2†	#1		✓	#1
13–18 years							†		✓	

HBV, hepatitis B virus; DTaP, diphtheria and tetanus toxoids and acellular pertussis; Hib, *Hemophilus influenzae* type b; IPV, inactivated polio vaccine; PCV, pneumococcal conjugate vaccine; MMR, measles–mumps–rubella; Td, tetanus and diphtheria toxoids, adult type; Var, varicella; Inf, influenza (yearly), MCV4, meningococcal conjugate vaccine

* Indicates earliest acceptable time of dose; doses may be given within a window of time beginning at the time indicated
†Initiate series or give immunization if not given previously
✓ Given annually

Data from: Centers for Disease Control and Prevention. (2006). Recommended childhood and adolescent immunization schedule–United States, 2006. Morbidity and Mortality Weekly Report, 54(51–52), Q-1–Q-4.

Parental expectations of children shape children's expectations of themselves and others. Failure to meet parental expectations may contribute to guilt and depression, whereas unrealistic parental expectations may result in inappropriate discipline for behaviors that are normal for a child's or adolescent's developmental stage. For example, parents may expect a 3-year-old child to be toilet trained even at night and punish the child for bedwetting when this is still normal behavior at this age. Parental expectations may also stifle adolescent development. For example, in many Asian cultures, adolescents may be expected to choose an occupation that brings benefit or recognition to the family rather than one in which the adolescent may be personally interested. Such expectations may cause conflict within the family or psychological problems for the adolescent.

Parental Coping and Mental Health

Parental stress levels affect their ability to parent effectively. The number of women with small children in the population may provide indirect information on coping abilities, since child rearing has been found to contribute

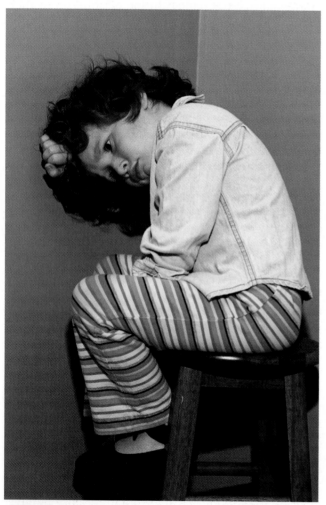

Discipline is frequently a thorny issue in raising children. (Molly Schlachter)

to cumulative stress, and the mental health of women with young children tends to be worse than those without children, particularly when accompanied by low resource levels (Jun, Subramanian, Gortmaker, & Kawachi, 2004). Similarly, the level of mental health problems in the adult population can affect parents' abilities to be effective in caring for their children.

Mental Health Problems Among Children and Adolescents

The frequency and types of mental health problems encountered in children and adolescents also provide information about the health status of these populations. According to the U.S. Department of Health and Human Services (2002), approximately 1 in 10 U.S. children and adolescents has some functional impairment due to mental illness. Only 20% of these children and adolescents receive needed mental health services, and many of them end up in jail. Depression is a significant problem, although depression may be difficult to diagnose in these age groups. Approximately 1 of every 33 children and 1 in 8 adolescents experience significant depression (Childers, 2004). High rates of mental illness in the child and adolescent population may necessitate community health nursing advocacy for effective treatment services. For example, a community health nurse may assist schoolteachers and counselors to set up a program that facilitates identification and referral of depressed students for treatment services.

Abuse

Physical, sexual, and psychological abuse and neglect are other problems that affect the psychological health of children and adolescents. The effects of childhood abuse are many and varied and may include future prostitution, drug and alcohol abuse, and more unprotected sexual activity (Dilorio, Hartwell, & Hansen, 2002). There were approximately 906,000 confirmed cases of child maltreatment in the United States in 2002. Most of these (61%) involved neglect, but physical, sexual, and psychological abuse were also reported. Abused children are at risk for adverse health effects as well as behavior problems as adults.

In 2002, there were 1,500 confirmed deaths due to abuse of U.S. children (National Center for Injury Prevention and Control, 2004a). The homicide rate in the first day of life is 10 times that of any other age period, and more than 9% of homicides occur in the first week of life (Epidemiology Program Office, 2002). Among adolescents 15 to 19 years of age, homicides account for 12.4% of all firearms-related deaths (Federal Interagency Forum on Child and Family Statistics, 2004). In addition, abuse of children and adolescents results in direct judicial, law enforcement, and medical costs of $24 billion a year in the United States. Indirect costs of abuse are estimated at $69 billion per year (National Center for Injury Prevention and Control, 2004a).

You have encountered a 6-year-old boy who you suspect is being physically abused by his father. The family has come to the United States illegally from Central America. You know that as a nurse you are required by law to report instances of child abuse. You are afraid if you report the abuse, however, that the family will be deported and the child will be blamed for this outcome. In that event, he is likely to be subjected to even more abuse. What would you do in this situation?

Abuse of children is not just a problem in the United States or even in the developed world, but is a worldwide problem. For example, according to the United Nations Population Fund (2003) as many as 20% to 30% of young girls are sexually abused in India, Jamaica, Mali, Tanzania, and Zimbabwe, and 30% of young women in South Africa report that their first sexual experience was forced. In addition, an estimated 700,000 to 4 million women and children are forced into the international sex trade every year in response to conditions of poverty, low social status of women, lax border surveillance, and police collusion. In India, approximately 40% of sex workers are children under the age of 18.

Risk factors and protective factors for abuse are summarized in Table 16-2◆. The problem of child abuse and potential nursing interventions are addressed in more detail in Chapter 32∞.

According to United Nations Population Fund (2003) figures, approximately 130 million girls and young women have been subjected to female genital cutting (FGC), also known as female genital mutilation (FGM) or female circumcision. FGC is a cultural practice in more than 28 countries throughout the world and is designed to control female sexuality. An estimated 6,000 incidents of FGC occur each day. Prevalence estimates range from 5% of young women in the Democratic Republic of Congo to 98% in Somalia. Figures for 1995 indicated that 97% of married women aged 15 to 49 years in Egypt had been subjected to FGC; 1998 figures for Mali were as high as 94%.

Although many countries have laws banning FGC, these laws are often poorly enforced. Recently several countries have begun initiatives to prevent FGC. For example, in Kenya, "circumcision with words" has been advocated. This program provides an alternative rite of passage that preserves positive elements of cultural practices but substitutes a week of seclusion, education, and counseling followed by a community celebration of girls' coming of age. Another program in Senegal, promoted by the organization Tostan, has resulted in agreements by 18% of registered villages to abandon FGC and early marriage.

What is the prevalence of FGC in your community? What cultural groups might promote FGC? What actions have been taken, if any, to prevent FGC? What additional actions are warranted and how could community health nurses be involved in these activities?

TABLE 16-2	Risk Factors and Protective Factors for Abuse of Children and Adolescents
Risk Factors	**Protective Factors**
▪ Disability or mental retardation among victims	▪ Supportive families
▪ Social isolation of families	▪ Nurturing parenting skills
▪ Parental lack of knowledge/understanding of child needs and development	▪ Stable family relationships
▪ Family history of domestic abuse	▪ Household rules and child monitoring
▪ Poverty/unemployment	▪ Employment
▪ Family disorganization/intimate partner violence	▪ Adequate housing
▪ Lack of family cohesion	▪ Access to health and social services
▪ Substance abuse	▪ Adequate role models outside the family
▪ Young single-parenthood	▪ Supportive communities
▪ Negative parent–child interactions	
▪ Parental stress or mental illness	
▪ Prevalence of community violence	

Data from: National Center for Injury Prevention and Control. (2004a). Child maltreatment: Fact sheet. Retrieved June 16, 2005, from http://www.cdc.gov/ncipc/factsheets/cmfacts.htm

Physical Environmental Considerations

Children are more susceptible than adults to a variety of environmental pollutants. For example, because their nervous systems are not yet fully developed, young children are more susceptible than adults or older children to the effects of lead poisoning. This may be even more apparent in some population groups. For instance, 30% of refugee children in one study developed elevated blood lead levels after resettlement due to living in older housing contaminated with lead-based paint and the effects of acute and chronic malnutrition due to economic conditions in their countries of origin (National Center for Environmental Health, 2005). Overall, however, the prevalence of elevated blood lead levels has declined significantly in recent years (Meyer et al., 2003).

Insecticide exposure and air pollution are other continuing problems for children and adolescents. From 1997 to 2000, for example, 52% of reported pesticide exposures in the United States occurred in children. An estimated 85% of families store and use pesticides with poisoning potential (Belson et al., 2003). In addition, more than one third of U.S. children in 2002 lived in areas that did not meet one or more National Ambient Air Quality Standards (Federal Interagency Forum on Child and Family Statistics, 2004). Community health nurses should be alert to the presence of environmental pollutants and other hazards and their effects on children.

Safety hazards are another major factor in the physical environment that influences the health of children of all ages. Safety concerns are related to children's physical surroundings and their ability to gain access to dangerous substances. Injuries accounted for 9% of all hospitalizations of children in 2000 (Wise, 2004), and the injury death rate among children aged 5 to 14 years was 17.3 per 100,000 population. Among 1- to 4-year-olds, the injury mortality rate was 33.3 per 100,000 children (Federal Interagency Forum on Child and Family Statistics, 2004). Motor vehicle accidents are, of course, the primary issue with respect to both child and adolescent safety. In 2003, for example, 6 children under 15 years of age were killed each day and 694 injured in motor vehicle accidents. In spite of evidence that use of seat-positioning booster seats results in a 59% decrease in the probability of injury of child passengers, only 22% of states and the District of Columbia have laws requiring booster seat use, and a recent telephone survey indicated that only 21% of 4- to 8-year-olds actually used booster seats (Centers for Disease Control and Prevention [CDC], 2005b). Approximately one fourth of motor vehicle accident deaths in children under 14 years of age involved alcohol use by the driver of the vehicle. In most cases, children riding with drivers who had been drinking were not restrained (Division of Unintentional Injury Prevention, 2004).

Young children are also injured as pedestrians and while riding on bicycles and tricycles. In 2003, for example, more than 7,000 children 1 to 14 years old were injured by a vehicle backing over them, and nearly half of deaths from back-over accidents in children occurred in their own driveways. Injury rates are six times higher for child pedestrians than for those riding bicycles and tricycles (National Center for Injury Prevention and Control, 2005).

Drowning is the second leading cause of death for children aged 1 to 14 years and the seventh cause of death for children of all ages (National Center for Injury Prevention and Control, 2004b). Children under 1 year of age most often drown in the bathtub, buckets, or toilet, whereas among children 1 to 4 years of age, residential swimming pools are the most common avenue for drowning deaths. Among adolescents, alcohol is involved in 25% to 50% of drownings. Approximately three times as many children and adolescents are seen in emergency departments for nonfatal submersion injuries as die (National Center for Injury Prevention and Control, n.d.d). Choking also accounts for significant morbidity in children. In 2001, more than 17,000 children were treated in emergency departments for choking incidents, and it is estimated that one death occurs for each 110 nonfatal episodes of choking (Division of Unintentional Injury Prevention, 2002). Advocacy for child and adolescent safety is an important aspect of community health nursing for this population. In carrying out this advocacy role, community health nurses might campaign for effective enforcement of seat belt legislation or for gun safety education for local families and youth.

Sociocultural Considerations

A variety of sociocultural factors affect the health of children and adolescents. As we saw earlier, a number of these factors have implications for children's psychological health. In addition, factors such as employment, family income, and education levels affect access to health care services and knowledge of health care needs. For example, in the United States income is strongly associated with infant mortality (Rodwin & Neuberg, 2005) as well as effective control of chronic illness. In 2003, 17.6% of U.S. children were living in poverty, an increase from 16.7% in 2002, and the proportion of those in poverty is higher than for any other age group (U.S. Census Bureau, 2004a). In addition, half of poor children are in families that are considered "severely poor," those with incomes below 50% of the federal poverty level (Wise, 2004). In 2002, 0.8% of children under 18 years of age lived in households that were food insecure, where both adults and children experienced actual hunger at some times. This figure rises to 2.4% of households in poverty (Federal Interagency Forum on Child and Family Statistics, 2004).

Although significant proportions of both elderly and children are affected by poverty, current U.S. policy requires these two groups to compete for resources, with children and adolescents often coming out the losers. For example, the income for elderly persons has risen in recent years, whereas that for families with children has remained flat. In 1967, 37% of social welfare expenditures were directed to services for children. This figure declined to 25% in 1986, and expenditures for the elderly increased from 21% to 33% in the same time period. Actual per capita spending has increased for both groups, but grew 191% for the elderly from 1965 to 1986 compared to only 107% for children and adolescents. Health care providers have voiced concerns regarding allocation decisions that are prompted by political and economic conditions rather than the needs of the groups involved (Newacheck & Benjamin, 2004).

In addition to affecting family income, parental employment may also have other effects on the health of children and adolescents. Although 72% of U.S. children were living in two-parent families in 2003, in many of these families as well as in single-parent families, parents work. In 2002, for example, 55% of women who had given birth to a child in the last year were in the work force (U.S. Census Bureau, 2004b). Working parents may have less time and energy to interact effectively with their children, and children and adolescents may be less effectively supervised by working parents. For instance, in 2001, nearly 3% of children in kindergarten to third grade cared for themselves for at least some portion of the day. Self-care increases with age, with 25% of fourth to eighth graders caring for themselves (Federal Interagency Forum on Child and Family Statistics, 2004).

Parental work schedules have also been shown to affect child and adolescent health and welfare (Strazdins, Korda, Lim, Broom, & D'Souza, 2004). Many parents work nonstandard schedules precisely to allow them to arrange favorable childcare; however, childcare may be less available at nonscheduled times (e.g., during evening and night shifts). Nonstandard work hours also limit parent availability to children when children are home from school and diminish family time. Parents may be prevented from attending many family and community events involving their children, and nonstandard schedules may affect parental sleep and parenting capabilities. In one study, nonstandard parental work schedules were associated with increased likelihood of one or more behavioral or emotional problems in children of all ages. Among 2- to 3-year-olds, children whose parents worked nonstandard hours were more likely to exhibit hyperactivity/inattention, physical aggression, and separation anxiety than those whose parents worked regular hours. Similarly, among 4- to 11-year-olds, children with parents on nonstandard work schedules were more likely to display hyperactivity/inattention and physical aggression, but were also more likely to exhibit conduct disorder and commit property offenses.

Parental education level affects income and knowledge of effective parenting. These effects are compounded when one or more parents do not speak the dominant language of the community. In 2003, 15% of U.S. children had a parent without a high school education, and 20% had at least one foreign-born parent. In 1999, nearly 17% of children and adolescents in the United States spoke a language other than English in their homes, and 5% had difficulty speaking or understanding English (Federal Interagency Forum on Child and Family Statistics, 2004).

Legislation and media are two other important sociocultural factors that influence the health of child and adolescent populations. Legislation may have positive or negative effects. For example, legislation mandating graduated driver licensing requirements for adolescents have been shown to result in stricter limits on driving privileges for adolescents and fewer accidents (Simons-Morton, Hartos, Leaf, & Preusser, 2005). Similarly, legislation regarding immunization of middle school students has been associated with increased immunity to measles, mumps, and rubella and hepatitis B (Averhoff et al., 2004).

Media coverage and role models are often associated with the assumption of risky behaviors such as smoking, drinking, and sexual activity by adolescents, but media may have beneficial effects as well. For instance, "truth" advertising campaigns that acquainted adolescents with tobacco company documents indicating specific plans to target adolescent markets were credited with a 22% decline in smoking prevalence among youth in one study (Farrelly, Davis, Haviland, Messeri, & Healton, 2005).

Prejudice in the social environment may also affect children. For instance, they may be subjected to ridicule by other children at school because of their dress, physical appearance, family culture, or religion. Family religious affiliation may provide social support, but can also lead to potential health problems. For example, children who receive exemption from immunization on the basis of religious beliefs are 22 times more likely to get measles and 6 times more likely to get pertussis than immunized children. When these children are in childcare or elementary school settings, their risk increases 62-fold and 16-fold, respectively (California Department of Health Services, 2001).

Behavioral Considerations

Several behavioral considerations also affect the health of children and adolescents. Behavioral considerations may relate to behaviors of children and adolescents themselves and those of their parents. Major areas for consideration in the behavioral dimension include nutrition, rest and exercise, and exposure to hazardous substances.

Nutrition

Earlier we noted the need for the community health nurse to assess the extent of poverty and hunger in the population. This is particularly important in developing countries, but should not be neglected in the United States and other areas of the developed world where poverty affects certain subgroups within the population. In the United States, however, nutritional deficits are more likely to reflect the lack of specific nutrients or caloric excess.

Community health nurses should be alert to child feeding practices in the community such as the extent to which newborns are breast-fed or bottle-fed, the availability of fast food in the community, and the extent to which families frequent fast food establishments. Exclusive breast-feeding for the first 6 months is the recommended dietary standard for infants. Based on data from the 1991–1994 National Health and Nutrition Examination Survey (NHANES), however, less than half of children (47%) were exclusively breast-fed at 7 days after birth. This figure declined to 10% at 6 months (Li, Ogden, Ballew, Gillespie, & Grummer-Strawn, 2002). Less exclusive breast-feeding has been associated with increased

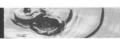

CULTURAL COMPETENCE

Child-rearing practices can vary significantly from one cultural group to another. Differences in child-rearing practices can create problems when cultures interact with each other or when members of ethnic cultural groups interact with health care professionals. What are some examples of these types of cross-cultural difficulties involving ethnic groups in your area? How might they be addressed?

asthma and atopic conditions (e.g., atopic dermatitis) in children as well as other adverse effects (Oddy et al., 2004). Breast-feeding is strongly influenced by cultural beliefs and practices and with a family's degree of acculturation. Cultural influences on breast-feeding were addressed in more detail in Chapter 9∞.

Dietary practices are also important among toddlers and older children and adolescents. Although the quality of diets improved slightly among preschool children in the United States from 1977 to 1998, there remains a need to increase consumption of fruits and vegetables and decrease total and saturated fat intake, juice, and sugar (Kranz, Siega-Riz, & Herring, 2004). In 1999–2000, approximately 20% of children aged 2 to 6 years consumed a healthy diet, compared to only 8% of those aged 7 to 12 years and 4% of adolescents. Conversely, 6%, 13%, and 19%, respectively, had poor diets. The vast majority of children at all age groups had diets that needed improvement in one or more areas (Federal Interagency Forum on Child and Family Statistics, 2004).

As we saw earlier, obesity is a common problem related to diet and nutrition in the United States and worldwide. According to NHANES data, the prevalence of obesity in 6- to 11-year-olds increased threefold from 1960 to 2000 (Thorpe et al., 2004). The focused assessment provided below can be used to assess the nutritional status of individual children or can be adapted for use with groups of children in specific age ranges.

Rest and Exercise

Problems of obesity can be combated by adequate exercise as well as healthier diets, yet few children and adolescents engage in recommended levels of physical activity. In 2002, for example, the Youth Media Campaign Longitudinal Survey (YMCLS) found that 61.5% of U.S. children aged 9 to 13 years did not participate in any organized physical activity outside of school, and 22.6% did not engage in any free-time physical activity (National Center for Chronic Disease Prevention and Health Promotion, 2003). Many public health professionals have called for an increase in physical education in schools to promote physical activity among school-age children and adolescents (Datar & Sturm, 2004). Special attention should be given to the activity needs of children with chronic illness and handicapping disabilities. For example, children with asthma were found in one study to have higher basal metabolic indices due to reduced activity as a result of their reactive airway disease (Oddy et al., 2004). Again, community health nurses can advocate for age-appropriate physical activities for children and adolescents.

Exposure to Hazardous Substances

Exposure of children and adolescents to hazardous substances (e.g., lead) in the physical environment was addressed earlier; however, children and adolescents are exposed to other hazardous substances through

---

FOCUSED ASSESSMENT

Assessing the Nutritional Status of Children and Adolescents

Infant (birth–1 year)

- Is the infant breast- or bottle-fed?
  - If breast-fed,
    - How often does the infant nurse?
    - How long does the infant nurse?
    - Does the mother alternate breasts?
    - Is the mother's nutritional intake adequate?
    - Does the infant seem satisfied?
  - If bottle-fed,
    - How often does the infant eat?
    - How much formula is consumed in 24 hours?
    - What type of formula is used? Is it iron fortified?
    - Do caretakers prepare formula correctly?
    - Do caretakers use appropriate feeding techniques (e.g., not propping the bottle)?
    - Does the infant tolerate the formula well?
- Is the infant gaining weight?
- At what point did parents introduce solids?
- How much solid food does the infant eat?
- Do parents use individual foods rather than less nutritious combination foods (such as vegetable and beef combinations)?
- Is one new food introduced at a time? Over several days?
- Has the 1-year-old started eating table food?
- Is the child weaned from the bottle by 1 year?

Toddler, preschool, and school-age child (2–10 years)

- What foods is the child eating?
- How much food is the child eating?
- Is the child's diet well-balanced?
- Is the child eating the recommended number of daily servings of fruits, vegetables, and grains?
- Is the child's diet low in saturated fat and sodium?
- Is the child's calcium and iron intake adequate?
- Are any snacks provided nutritious?
- Is the child's growth pattern normal for his or her age?

Additional questions for preadolescent and adolescent (11–18 years)

- Is protein and calcium intake adequate to accommodate growth spurts?
- Is iron intake sufficient to accommodate blood loss in menstruating girls?
- Is the preadolescent/adolescent overweight or underweight for his or her height?
- Does the preadolescent/adolescent engage in food fads?
- Does the preadolescent/adolescent engage in binge eating or purging?
- Is the preadolescent/adolescent excessively concerned about body size?

their own behavior or that of parents and other family members. For example, in 2002, more than 11% of women giving birth in the United States smoked during their pregnancies (Division of Reproductive Health, 2004a). Although this represents a decline in maternal smoking of 38% from 1990 to 2002, many infants continue to be adversely affected by maternal smoking during pregnancy. Smoking during pregnancy is associated with poor birth outcomes and health problems such as increased gastric reflux, colic, sudden infant death syndrome (SIDS), and lower respiratory tract infections (Gaffney, 2001) as well as more than 900 infant deaths per year from 1997 to 2001 (Office on Smoking and Health, 2005a). In addition to the physical effects of fetal exposure to tobacco smoke, maternal smoking during pregnancy has been associated with behavioral problems in children (Wakschlag, Pickett, Cook, Benowitz, & Leventhal, 2002).

Maternal smoking during pregnancy also has significant economic effects on families and on society. In 1996 alone, smoking-attributable neonatal expenditures amounted to $366 million, roughly $704 for every woman who smoked during pregnancy (Division of Reproductive Health, 2004b). Smoking also has preconceptual effects and has been associated with infertility and delay in conception (Division of Reproductive Health, 2004a). Maternal smoking during pregnancy decreases with increasing levels of education. For example, fewer than 3% of college-educated women smoked during pregnancy, compared to 27% of those without a high school diploma. Lower rates of smoking cessation and higher rates of relapse are also associated with lower education levels (Jun et al., 2004).

Children and adolescents are not just exposed to the effects of smoking in utero. An estimated 30% to 60% of U.S. children under 5 years of age are exposed to tobacco smoke in the home (Gaffney, 2001), and in 1999, 19% of children under 7 years of age lived in a home with a regular smoker (Federal Interagency Forum on Child and Family Statistics, 2004). In addition, children and adolescents themselves may smoke or use other forms of tobacco. In 2004, for example, nearly 12% of middle school children and 28% of high school students reported tobacco use (Office on Smoking and Health, 2005b). In 2003, 5% of eighth graders, 9% of tenth graders, and 16% of twelfth graders smoked daily, and although these figures are not good, they are the lowest recorded since children in these grade levels began to be surveyed (Federal Interagency Forum on Child and Family Statistics, 2004).

Children and adolescents may also be exposed to alcohol and other drugs. **Fetal alcohol syndrome (FAS)** is a condition resulting from maternal alcohol consumption during pregnancy and is characterized by growth retardation, facial malformations, and central nervous system dysfunctions that may include mental retardation. FAS is also associated with spontaneous abortion, ectopic pregnancy, stillbirth, fetal death, low birth weight, preterm delivery, and intrauterine growth retardation. Other potential effects of FAS include placenta previa, abruptio placenta, premature rupture of membranes, and increased risk of SIDS in the infant (Beck, Morrow, Lipscomb, & Johnson, 2002).

FAS is a growing problem in many areas of the world. For example, although the rate of FAS in the United States is relatively low (0.3 to 1.5 per 1,000 live births), it is as high as 40.5 to 46.4 per 1,000 births in South Africa (National Center on Birth Defects and Developmental Disabilities, 2003). Even though U.S. rates of FAS are relatively low, approximately 5,000 infants each year are affected (CDC, 2004a), and its prevalence is likely to be underestimated due to failure to diagnose affected infants (Division of Birth Defects and Developmental Disabilities, 2002). The prevalence of alcohol use during pregnancy actually increased from 12.4% of pregnant women in 1991 to 16.3% in 1995 before dropping back down to 12.8% in 1999 (National Center on Birth Defects and Developmental Disabilities, 2002). Exposure to other drugs (e.g., cocaine) or infectious agents, such as herpes or HIV, may also occur during pregnancy, putting infants at risk for a variety of serious health consequences.

Alcohol-related neurodevelopmental disorders (ARNDs) and alcohol-related birth defects (ARBDs) are three times more common than FAS. Immediate effects of these perinatal exposures to alcohol include poor intrauterine growth, small stature, facial abnormalities, poor coordination, hyperactivity, and sleep and suck problems in infancy. Long-term consequences may include learning disabilities, speech and language delays, difficulties performing activities of daily living, and poor judgment and reasoning abilities. Perinatal alcohol exposure also places those affected at higher risk for psychiatric problems, crime, unemployment, and school dropout. FAS and other effects can be prevented by encouraging pregnant women to refrain from alcohol and drug use during pregnancy. For those children affected, early enrollment in special education programs can help mitigate the long-term effects of perinatal alcohol exposure (National Center on Birth Defects and Developmental Disabilities, 2004d).

As with tobacco, children and adolescents may expose themselves to alcohol and other drugs. In 2002, for example, nearly 12% of 12- to 17-year-olds reported being current users of illicit drugs (U.S. Census Bureau, 2004b). In 2003, 10% of eighth graders, 20% of tenth graders, and 24% of twelfth graders reported illicit drug use. Again, these are some of the lowest figures reported since 1993. Similar figures were noted for heavy drinking among children and adolescents—12% of eighth graders, 22% of tenth graders, and 28% of twelfth graders (Federal Interagency Forum on Child and Family Statistics, 2004).

Sexual Activity

Adolescent sexual activity can have a profound influence on health in this population group, particularly in terms of unwanted pregnancy and sexually transmitted diseases (STDs). Adolescent boys generally initiate sexual activity earlier than girls, with an average age of initiation of sexual intercourse by boys at 16.9 years and girls at 17.4 years (Alan Guttmacher Institute, 2002). According to the 2001 Youth Risk Behavior Surveillance System (YRBSS), 45.6% of U.S. high school students reported engaging in sexual intercourse. Boys were more likely to report intercourse than girls (48.5% versus 42.9%). Black and Hispanic students were more likely than White students to have had intercourse. A small percentage (6.6%) of students initiated sexual activity prior to 13 years of age, and boys were more than twice as likely as girls to initiate early sexual activity. Among those students who were sexually active at the time of the survey, only 57.9% reported condom use during their last episode of intercourse, and only 18% of respondents or their partners used oral contraceptives. Black students were more likely than White and Hispanic students to report condom use, but White students were more likely to report use of oral contraceptives. One fourth of the sexually active students reported that alcohol or drug use preceded their last sexual intercourse (Grunbaum et al., 2002).

Nearly 5% of high school students in the 2001 YRBSS reported having been pregnant or gotten someone else pregnant. Pregnancy was more likely among minority adolescents than their White counterparts (Grunbaum et al., 2002). In 2001, 18% of legal abortions occurred among girls 19 years of age and under. This amounted to a total of 138,000 abortions, more than 4,700 of which occurred in girls under 15 years of age. Abortions were performed in approximately three fourths of pregnancies in girls under age 15 and two thirds in girls 19 years of age or younger (Strauss et al., 2004).

Although one usually thinks of adolescent pregnancy as primarily affecting girls, boys are also involved. Approximately 2% of U.S. births and 5% of abortions involve boys 15 to 17 years of age, and another 5% and 8%, respectively, involve young men 18 to 19 years of age (Alan Guttmacher Institute, 2002). Pregnancy poses significant health risks for adolescent girls and may delay or impede educational and vocational plans for both boys and girls. Community health nurses may need to advocate for effective sexuality education for boys and girls as well as for access to condoms and contraceptive services for those who are sexually active.

Violence

Earlier we discussed the effects of abuse on children and adolescents, but these population groups are exposed to and may participate in other forms of violence as well. For example, in 2003, 33% of high school students participating in the YRBSS reported being involved in a physical fight in the previous year. Boys were more likely than girls to report involvement in fighting (40.5% versus 25.1%). Fortunately, these figures have declined somewhat from 1991 reports (50.2% for boys and 34.4% for girls). Similarly, somewhat fewer students reported carrying weapons in 2003 (17%) than in 1991 (26%), but more students reported being threatened with a weapon in 2003 (9.2%) than in 1991 (7.3%), and more students did not attend school in 2003 than in 1991 because of safety concerns (5.4% versus 4.4%) (Division of Violence Prevention, 2004).

Health System Considerations

A number of factors in the health care delivery system influence the health of children and adolescents. Some of these factors include attitudes toward health and health care, usual sources of health care, and use of health care services. In 2002, only half of children with special health needs had a regular source of health care (Wise, 2004), and many well children do not have a regular source of care or a "medical home." A medical home is a regular source of health care that is characterized by access to preventive care, 24-hour availability of ambulatory and inpatient care, continuity, access to subspecialty referrals and interaction between providers and school and community agencies as needed, and maintenance of a central health record for the child.

Poor children, in particular, may lack a regular source of care, relying on emergency departments for care. This practice increases the costs of care and decreases opportunities for basic preventive and health-promotive services. Emergency departments have, however, been shown to be effective places for recruiting children who are eligible for the State Child Health Insurance Program (SCHIP) (Gordon, Emond, & Camargo, 2005). Having a regular source of care is impeded by reimbursement patterns of federal insurance programs for children. Welfare reform efforts have contributed to periods of uninsurance for low-income families including children (Holl, Slack, & Stevens, 2005).

In 2003, 8.4 million U.S. children (11.4%) had no health insurance coverage (U.S. Census Bureau, 2004a), another 5.8 million were enrolled in SCHIP, and slightly more than 17 million were insured by Medicaid (U.S. Census Bureau, 2004b). In 2002, Medicaid covered one fifth of all U.S. children and 40% of children in low-income families. In addition, Medicaid paid for the care of 70% of children with chronic disabilities (Klein, Stoll, & Bruce, 2004). By June 2004, SCHIP enrollment had declined to 3.7 million children due to state legislative changes limiting eligibility and enrollment and increasing premiums and cost-sharing provisions for children of low-income families (Blewett, Davern, & Rodin, 2004).

ASSESSING THE HEALTH STATUS OF CHILD AND ADOLESCENT POPULATIONS

Community health nurses provide services to individual children and adolescents and their families as well as to these populations as aggregates. Whether services are provided to individuals or population groups, community health nurses must first assess their health status and health needs. The focus of this chapter is on meeting the needs of children and adolescents as population groups. A tool for assessing the health of an individual child or adolescent is provided in Appendix H on the Companion Website and in the *Community Assessment Reference Guide* 📖 designed as a companion volume to this text. Here we will focus on the assessment of populations of children and adolescents using the dimensions of health as a framework.

In assessing the health of child and adolescent populations, the nurse would gather data on rates of growth and the prevalence of departures from normal growth. For example, the nurse might examine the records of school-aged children to determine the proportion of children above or below normal parameters for height and weight. The prevalence of obesity in these populations would also be determined. The incidence of maturational problems such as developmental retardation could be extrapolated from the number of children with these problems in schools or in interviews with physicians and others who provide health services to these children.

Information on sexual maturity, as well as on attitudes toward sexual maturity and sexual activity, has implications for the prevention of adolescent pregnancy and sexually transmitted diseases, and can be determined in interviews with community informants such as school officials and members of religious groups as well as in general community surveys. Community health nurses may also assess the knowledge of adults in the community with respect to normal maturation and development in children and adolescents. Armed with this information, community health nurses can design programs for parents that promote effective child and adolescent growth and development and provide anticipatory guidance for parents in dealing with developmental transitions experienced by their children. **Anticipatory guidance** involves providing information to parents and others regarding behavioral expectations of children and adolescents at a specific age, before they reach that age.

Community health nurses should also be familiar with the gender and ethnic composition of the child and adolescent populations in their communities. They would also obtain information on the prevalence of conditions with a tendency to genetic transmission (e.g., sickle cell disease or diabetes) in their communities in order to begin primary preventive services for condi-

tions with high prevalence during childhood. Gender, racial, and ethnic composition of the child and adolescent population is available from census figures. The prevalence of some genetically transmitted conditions may be calculated by local health authorities, but may also be available from voluntary organizations specializing in these diseases.

Child and adolescent mortality data can be obtained from the local health department, which may also provide information on the incidence and prevalence of certain conditions in these populations. For example, the incidence of gonorrhea in the adolescent population would be available from health department sources. Data on other forms of morbidity for which official figures are not collected may be available from voluntary organizations or health care providers in the community. For example, information on the incidence and prevalence of diabetes in children and adolescents may be available from the local chapter of the American Diabetes Association. Similarly, school systems may have data on the number of school absences related to childhood asthma. Local hospitals and other health care agencies may have figures on the numbers of children and adolescents seen with specific conditions.

Information on the level of child and adolescent immunization in the population may be obtained from local health departments, schools, preschools, or clinics and physicians' offices that provide primary care services. Conversely, incidence rates for immunizable childhood diseases are available from local and state health departments. Assessment of biophysical factors affecting the health of children and adolescents can be guided by the focused assessment questions provided below.

Psychological dimension factors would also be assessed in determining the health status of the child

MediaLink

Appendix H: Child and Adolescent Health Assessment

FOCUSED ASSESSMENT

Biophysical Considerations Influencing Child and Adolescent Health

- What is the age composition of the child and adolescent population?
- What is the gender composition of the child and adolescent population?
- What is the racial/ethnic composition of the child and adolescent population?
- What are the gender-specific attitudes and expectations regarding boys and girls in the population?
- What is the extent of growth retardation in the child and adolescent population?
- What is the extent of developmental delay in the child and adolescent population? What are the typical causes of delays?
- What are cause-specific child and adolescent mortality rates in the population?
- What are the rates of morbidity for specific acute and chronic health problems in the child and adolescent population?
- What is the level of immunization coverage in the child and adolescent population?

and adolescent populations. With the individual child or adolescent, the community health nurse would assess family dynamics as described in Chapter 14∞. When assessing the health of children and adolescents as a population group, however, similar kinds of information about family dynamics (e.g., role structure, communication patterns, authority) are often not available. The nurse can, however, obtain information related to the sociocultural dimension, such as the prevalence of divorce and single-parent families, that may provide some insights into family dynamics that contribute to mental health or illness in children and adolescents.

In a similar vein, there will probably be no specific aggregate data available regarding parental expectations and discipline as there would be if a community health nurse were assessing an individual child or adolescent. However, the nurse can extrapolate inferences about parental expectations and discipline from knowledge of cultural attitudes, beliefs, and behaviors toward parenthood and child rearing among cultural and ethnic groups in the community. How are children generally viewed within the cultures represented in the population? How is discipline typically handled? Do disciplinary practices or typical parental expectations of children have any implications for the health of the child and adolescent populations in the community? The answers to these and other similar questions are best derived from observations in the community and through interviews with knowledgeable community informants.

Aggregate information is also unlikely to be available regarding the extent of coping among parents of children and adolescents in the population. The community health nurse can, however, make inferences based on data regarding stressors encountered by parents. For example, family size, the extent of single-parenthood, and other sociocultural factors faced by parents contribute to stress, which may tax coping abilities.

Community health nurses could obtain information on the extent of mental health problems in the child and adolescent population from psychiatric facilities in the area as well as from interviews with school counselors and other mental health service providers. Similar information can also be obtained with respect to mental health problems among adults in the community since many of these adults will be the parents of the child and adolescent populations.

Community health nurses should examine the incidence and prevalence of abuse of children and adolescents in their jurisdictions. Data on abuse will be available from local child protective service agencies as well as from police files. In addition, nurses should be alert to the presence of factors in the population that promote child and adolescent abuse and those that are protective against abuse, as indicated in Table 16-2◆. The focused assessment provided above right includes questions that can guide assessment of psychological factors affecting the health of the child and adolescent population.

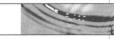

FOCUSED ASSESSMENT

Psychological Considerations Influencing Child and Adolescent Health

- What is the extent of mental illness in the child and adolescent population? Among parents?
- What are the cultural expectations of children and adolescents in the population? To what extent do these expectations create stress for children and adolescents?
- What is the suicide rate among children and adolescents in the population?
- What are the typical approaches to discipline in the population?
- What is the extent of abuse in the child and adolescent population? What forms of abuse are prevalent? What factors contribute to abuse of children and adolescents? What is the attitude of the population to abuse of children and adolescents?

With respect to the physical environmental dimension, community health nurses should assess both the presence of hazardous conditions in the environment and public knowledge of safety-related behaviors. A tool to assess safety hazards in the environment of individual children is provided in the *Community Assessment Reference Guide* designed to accompany this text.

Community health nurses should obtain information on the morbidity and mortality resulting from child and adolescent safety hazards as well as the types of injuries occurring in their communities. Mortality data will be available from the local health department as well as from insurance departments. Both mortality data and information on nonfatal injuries among children and adolescents may be obtained from local emergency departments, poison control centers, and health care providers. Information on safety hazards present in the community can be derived from observations by community health nurses or in community surveys. A focused assessment for the physical environmental dimension is included below.

Community health nurses assessing the health of the child and adolescent populations would also obtain information related to the sociocultural dimension such as local income, employment, and education levels. Much of this information is available in census data or from local social service agencies. Employment figures

FOCUSED ASSESSMENT

Physical Environmental Considerations Influencing Child and Adolescent Health

- What safety hazards are present in the community? How do they affect the health of the child and adolescent population?
- How adequate is family housing in the community?
- What environmental pollutants are present in the community? How do they affect the health of the child and adolescent population?

may also be available from local government offices or employment agencies.

Parental education levels have implications for health knowledge and behaviors as well as for child performance in school and later success as adults, and community health nurses should assess the extent to which these factors exist in their communities and the effects they have on the health of children and adolescents in the community. Community health nurses should also examine high school completion rates among adolescents as well as the percentage of younger children held back in one or more grades. Such information can be obtained from local school officials or from state boards of education.

Community health nurses can also observe the quality of health-related messages provided through advertising, news coverage, and other media. Driving through the community or perusing magazines and newspapers read by children and adolescents in the community can provide some sense of the kind and level of negative advertising to which they are exposed as well as the presence of positive health-related messages. An overview of local television programming can provide similar information.

Information related to intergroup conflicts and discriminatory practices in the community that may affect the health of children and adolescents can be derived from a review of local news articles. School officials may also provide insight into racial or ethnic group conflicts that may affect the health of children and adolescents. The prevalence of fighting and other forms of violence involving children or adolescents may also be determined from school informants or local police data. Information on religious affiliations in the community can be suggested by perusal of the telephone directory. Insights into religious attitudes and practices that may influence the health of children and adolescents is best derived from interviews and other interactions with knowledgeable members of local groups and congregations. Community health nurses should also be aware of the extent of religious exemptions related to immunization and the potential effects of such exemptions. Assessment of sociocultural factors influencing child and adolescent health can be guided by the focused assessment questions provided at right.

With respect to the behavioral dimension of health, community health nurses would assess the nutritional status of children and adolescents in the community. Knowledge of basic dietary patterns of cultural subgroups in the population may be obtained from observation or interviews with knowledgeable community informants. Nurses can also assess the nutritional content of school lunch menus or observe purchases made in local grocery stores. Community health nurses should also assess the extent of dietary problems among children and adolescents, such as obesity or malnutrition, as well as the factors that contribute to those

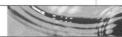

FOCUSED ASSESSMENT

Sociocultural Considerations Influencing Child and Adolescent Health

- What are the culturally defined roles for children and adolescents in the community? What effect do these roles have on health?
- How do social factors such as educational level, employment, and income affect the health of the child and adolescent population?
- What is the extent of parental employment outside the home? How does this affect child and adolescent health?
- What is the extent of employment among the child and adolescent population? What effect does employment have on health?
- What is the availability of childcare services in the community? How adequate are childcare services to meet the needs of working parents?
- How adequate are educational opportunities available to the child and adolescent population?
- How do legislative initiatives affect the health of the child and adolescent population?

problems. Height and weight screening of children and adolescents in school settings can provide some of this data. Community health nurses should also be knowledgeable regarding infant feeding practices prevalent in the community and promote breast-feeding whenever possible. Again, this type of information may vary among cultural groups in the community and can best be obtained through observation or interviews with members of different ethnic groups.

Community health nurses will also assess the opportunities provided in the community for physical activity by children and adolescents as well as the actual levels of activity exhibited. School curricula can be examined for their inclusion of physical activities. The extent of participation in sports activities can also be determined. Other information on opportunities for recreational activities can be obtained from the telephone book and from observations of children at play in parks and neighborhoods.

Assessment of the health status of child and adolescent populations would also include information related to the incidence of hazardous substance exposures discussed earlier as well as types of exposures and their effects on the health of children and adolescents. Tobacco use by adolescents can be determined by observation in areas where they "hang out." Community surveys may also be used to provide information on tobacco, drug, and alcohol use. Police records may contain information on the number of adolescents arrested for crimes involving alcohol or drug use.

Community health nurses working with adolescent populations would also assess the extent of sexual activity and unsafe sexual practices (e.g., failure to protect against STDs or pregnancy) within the population. In addition, they would determine the rate of adolescent pregnancy and the availability of health and other services needed to meet the needs of pregnant adolescents and those who are sexually active. Adolescent pregnancy rates would be available from the local health department or from labor and delivery units of area hospitals. Data related to sexual practices would best be obtained by surveys of adolescent populations.

Rates of violence among children and adolescents are another aspect of assessing the health of these populations. Community health nurses might obtain data from local school officials regarding the extent of physical fighting on campuses. Police records might also indicate the extent to which children and adolescents are perpetrators or victims of violence in the local community. Behavioral considerations in child and adolescent health can be explored using the focused assessment questions provided below.

Community health nurses assessing the health status of child and adolescent populations will obtain information on the relative percentage of children without health insurance as well as those who have public or private sources of insurance coverage. Community health nurses can also determine the number of children seen for nonemergency purposes in emergency departments. Information on the use of health-promotive and illness-preventive services (e.g., utilization of immunization services, dental services, etc.) by children and adolescents can also be obtained from agencies and facilities that provide these services. Local Medicaid offices would have information on the number of children and adolescents with Medicaid coverage, and health care providers and emergency departments

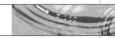

FOCUSED ASSESSMENT

Health System Considerations Influencing Child and Adolescent Health

- What percentage of the child and adolescent population has a regular source of health care?
- What is the extent of insurance coverage in the child and adolescent population?
- How adequate are available health services in meeting the needs of the child and adolescent population?
- To what extent do health care needs of the child and adolescent population go unmet?
- To what extent does the child and adolescent population make use of available health promotion and illness prevention services?

could provide information on the number of children seen who have no insurance coverage. The focused assessment provided above can guide the assessment of health system factors influencing child and adolescent health.

DIAGNOSTIC REASONING AND THE HEALTH OF CHILD AND ADOLESCENT POPULATIONS

Based on the data gathered in the assessment of the child or adolescent population, the community health nurse derives diagnoses or statements based on health status and health care needs. Both positive and problem-focused nursing diagnoses may be derived from the data obtained. Diagnoses may reflect the need for primary, secondary, or tertiary preventive measures. For example, a positive community nursing diagnosis related to primary prevention is "high immunization levels due to high parental motivation and access to immunization services." On the other hand, a problem-focused nursing diagnosis related to immunizations is "lack of appropriate immunizations for age due to lack of access to low-cost immunizations." Another problem-focused nursing diagnosis for the population related to primary prevention is "increased potential for child abuse due to widespread unemployment and increased community incidence of mental health problems."

Nursing diagnoses related to secondary prevention are necessarily problem focused because secondary prevention is warranted when actual health problems exist. An example of a nursing diagnosis for the child population might be "lack of services available in the community to meet the needs of children with developmental problems." For adolescents, a relevant nursing diagnosis might be "increased incidence of adolescent pregnancy due to widespread sexual activity, lack of effective sexuality education, and lack of access to contraceptive services." Nursing diagnoses at the population level might also reflect physical environmental, psychological, sociocultural, or behavioral

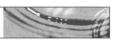

FOCUSED ASSESSMENT

Behavioral Considerations Influencing Child and Adolescent Health

- What are the dietary patterns typical of children and adolescents in the community?
- What are the physical activity patterns typical of children and adolescents in the community?
- What recreational activities are available to the child and adolescent population? What health benefits and hazards are posed by recreational activities?
- What are the effects of dietary and physical activity patterns on the health of the child and adolescent population?
- What is the extent of child and adolescent exposure to tobacco in the home? To use of other substances?
- What is the extent of tobacco, alcohol, and drug use among the child and adolescent population?
- What is the extent of sexual activity among children and adolescents?
- To what extent is safety instruction (including sexual safety) provided to children and adolescents?
- What is the extent, if any, of female genital mutilation among adolescent girls?
- To what extent do children and adolescents engage in effective safety practices (e.g., seat belt use, protective recreational equipment, condom use).

considerations affecting children's and adolescents' overall health status.

At the level of tertiary prevention, nursing diagnoses focus on the need to prevent complications of existing problems or to prevent the recurrence of problems. For example, the nurse might derive nursing diagnoses of "lack of respite for families of children with chronic health problems" or "barriers to effective participation in physical activity by children with handicapping conditions."

PLANNING AND IMPLEMENTING HEALTH CARE FOR CHILD AND ADOLESCENT POPULATIONS

Just as the nursing diagnoses derived from an assessment of child or adolescent health may reflect health problems at primary, secondary, and/or tertiary levels of prevention, interventions may be planned at each level to address identified health needs of children or adolescents.

Primary Prevention

A number of general interventions may be used to promote the health of children and adolescents or to prevent the development of health problems. These categories of intervention all reflect primary prevention and include assuring access to health care; preventing prematurity, low birth weight, and infant mortality; promoting growth and development; providing adequate nutrition; promoting physical activity; promoting safety; preventing communicable diseases; promoting dental care; supporting effective parenting; and other primary prevention activities.

Assuring Access to Health Care

One of the best means of promoting the health of children and adolescents is to ensure that they have access to needed health care services. Community health nurses can be instrumental in linking individual children and adolescents to needed services and in assuring that health services are available to these population groups. This can be accomplished by implementing several strategies that have been recommended for improving child health in general and reducing disparities in health status among subpopulations of children and adolescents. These strategies include the following:

- Assuring that all children and adolescents have a regular source of primary health care
- Eliminating copayments and cost sharing for primary care services
- Establishing disincentives for seeking health care directly from specialists
- Including assessment of the adequacy of primary care services in all quality assurance activities
- Supporting the education of primary care providers

- Developing information systems to monitor health activities and detect differences among subpopulations of children and adolescents (Starfield, 2004)

Implementing these strategies at the level of the individual child or adolescent will usually require referral to an effective source of primary health care. Implementation may also involve referral for public insurance programs such as SCHIP or Medicaid for those children and adolescents who are eligible for these programs. At the population level, implementing these strategies will most likely require community health nurses to be politically active in advocating and planning for services to meet identified child and adolescent health care needs.

Preventing Prematurity, Low Birth Weight, and Infant Mortality

Another approach to primary prevention with children and adolescents is action to reduce rates of prematurity, low birth weight, and infant mortality. Premature birth and low birth weight are two of the major contributors to infant mortality worldwide. In 2002, infant mortality was highest in Afghanistan at 189 deaths per 1,000 live births. Mortality among children under 5 years of age was greatest in Angola, with 262 deaths for every 1,000 live births (World Health Organization, 2004). In the United States, total infant mortality for that year was considerably lower, at 7 per 1,000 live births, but varied greatly among subpopulations. For example, the infant mortality rate was more than twice as high among non-Hispanic Blacks (13.9 per 1,000) as among non-Hispanic Whites (5.8 per 1,000). Higher rates were also seen among Hawaiian (9.6), Native American (8.6), and Puerto Rican infants (8.2). Lower infant mortality rates were noted among other ethnic populations, with the lowest seen among Chinese infants (3 per 1,000) (CDC, 2005b). In 2000, the United States ranked 25th among developed nations with respect to infant mortality and 33rd in relation to deaths among children under 5 years of age. The lower ratings of the United States when compared to other industrialized countries are thought to be a result of greater income disparities among U.S. families, the absence of universal health care, and the existence of policies inimical to effective primary health care (e.g., lack of regular source of care, frequent changes in insurance status among low-income families, etc.) (Starfield, 2004).

Although progress has been made in this area, with an 11% decrease in overall infant mortality in the United States from 1995 to 2001 (NCHS, 2005c), much remains to be done, both with respect to infant mortality and its primary underlying causes. In 2002, for example, low birth weight (LBW) babies accounted for 7.8% of all births in the United States. Adolescent mothers are more likely than older mothers to have a low birth weight baby. For example, in 2002, 13.8% of babies born to girls under 15 years of age and 9.9% of those born to girls aged 15 to 19 years were LBW compared to only 7.1% of mothers

MediaLink Case Study: Promoting Children's Health and Safety

25 to 29 years of age. Mothers who smoked during pregnancy also had a higher percentage of LBW babies than nonsmokers (12% vs. 7.5%). (U.S. Census Bureau, 2004b). Very low birth weight (VLBW) babies (those born weighing less than 3 pounds 4 ounces or 1,500 grams) have a 75% to 100% greater risk of death in the first month of life than normal weight babies (Regional Perinatal Programs of California, 2004). Although VLBW babies account for only 2% of all U.S. births, they contribute to 68% of neonatal deaths, and survivors have multiple problems throughout life (Wise, 2004).

Babies born prematurely are often of low or very low birth weight. In addition to contributing to death, prematurity and low birth weight start young children off at a disadvantage that may or may not be overcome in later years. For example, in one longitudinal study in New Zealand, babies born prior to 32 weeks gestation were found to make greater health care service demands and were six times more likely to be hospitalized in childhood than those born at term. In addition, 32% of these children required state-funded special education services (Olsen & Maslin-Prothero, 2001). In another study, extremely preterm infants had higher rates of cognitive impairment, mild to severe disability, and cerebral palsy than age mates born at full term (Marlow, Wolke, Bracewell, & Samara, 2005).

In spite of the overall decline in infant morality in the United States (45% from 1980 to 2000), the percentage of LBW babies has actually increased by nearly 12% and VLBW by more than 24% during the same period (Division of Reproductive Health, 2002). An estimated 200 VLBW babies are born each day in the United States (Nisbet, 2004). Both prematurity and low birth weight and subsequent infant mortality can be prevented by a group of community health nursing interventions including delayed pregnancy, early and effective prenatal care, adequate prenatal nutrition, and prevention of smoking during pregnancy. According to the Pregnancy Risk Assessment Monitoring System, in 1999 one third to one half of all pregnancies in the United States were unintended. These figures were even higher for women with lower educational levels. In 2002, 82% of

BUILDING OUR KNOWLEDGE BASE

A study by Koniak-Griffin, Anderson, Verzemnieks, and Brecht (2000) found that home visits by community health nurses to pregnant adolescents had no significant effects in terms of type of delivery (vaginal or caesarean) or birth weight among their infants, but did result in fewer days of birth-related hospitalizations and rehospitalizations for the infants. In addition, the group of adolescent mothers who were visited by community health nurses had better educational outcomes than those who were not visited. How might you replicate this study to provide sufficient evidence upon which to base routine community health nursing practice? Whom might you include as subjects? Would you want your subjects to be ethnically diverse or homogeneous? Why?

legal abortions occurred among unmarried women, and slightly more than 18% occurred in girls younger than 19 years of age (Strauss et al., 2004). Each year approximately half a million teenage girls give birth in the United States. The direct societal costs of adolescent pregnancies for welfare, Medicaid, and foster care services are estimated at $6.9 billion per year (Koniak-Griffin, Anderson, Verzemnieks, & Brecht, 2000). Community health nurses can educate the public, particularly adolescents, regarding sexuality and contraception to prevent unintended pregnancies. In addition, they can advocate for effective and accessible contraceptive services for adolescents and other women of childbearing age. They may also need to ensure that services are available to provide care to pregnant teens and to support them in their role as parents. Particular attention is needed to see that adolescent mothers continue to meet their own personal developmental tasks as well as meeting those of their children. This may necessitate advocacy on the part of community health nurses for educational assistance and other support services for adolescent parents.

For women who carry their pregnancies to term, approximately 16% to 30% receive late or no prenatal care (Beck et al., 2002). Community health nurses can refer individual clients to prenatal services and engage in political advocacy to make sure that such services are available to all women of childbearing age. They can also educate the public regarding the need for adequate prenatal care.

In addition to promoting prenatal care, community health nurses can educate pregnant women regarding the need for good nutrition during pregnancy and make referrals for supplemental nutrition programs such as the Supplemental Nutrition Program for Women, Infants, and Children (WIC). WIC participation among pregnant women has been associated with a decreased incidence of low birth weight (Kowaleski-Jones & Duncan, 2002).

Promoting Growth and Development

To develop properly, children need an environment conducive to growth and development. Community health nurses can assist parents and communities in creating such environments. They can educate both the general public and specific families regarding developmental milestones children and adolescents need to accomplish. They can alert parents to the challenges posed by these milestones through anticipatory guidance, discussed earlier. Community health nurses can also advocate for community programs and environmental conditions that promote growth and development within safe parameters. For example, they can promote sports appropriate to children's abilities and developmental levels and foster the use of effective safety equipment in such programs. In addition, nurses can advocate for humanistic educational programs that promote emotional and physical, as well as cognitive, development. A tool for assessing developmental levels in children and adolescents is provided in the *Community Assessment Reference Guide* 📋 designed to accompany this text.

Providing Adequate Nutrition

For infants, providing adequate nutrition can best be met by promoting breast-feeding. It is estimated that exclusive breast-feeding for the first 6 months could prevent 720 post-neonatal deaths (from 1 to 28 days of age) each year in the United States. Breast-fed infants have a 20% lower mortality risk than infants who are bottle-fed and also experience lower rates of infectious disease incidence (Regional Perinatal Programs of California, 2004). The effects of breast-feeding are also seen among VLBW infants, with one study indicating that exclusive breast-feeding saved $200 to $400 in health care costs per infant during the first year of life (Nisbet, 2004).

Good nutrition is also an issue for older children and adolescents. From 1999 to 2000, 15% of U.S. children were overweight, more than twice as many as in 1976 to 1980 (6%) (Federal Interagency Forum on Child and Family Statistics, 2004). Although children are overeating, they are not eating many of the nutrients needed for good physical health. For example, in one national survey, not quite 30% of girls and just over 45% of boys aged 11 to 18 years had diets that met the daily requirements for calcium intake. Similarly, the diets of large percentages of children and adolescents were deficient in fruits, vegetables, and grains, but overabundant with respect to fats (Neumark-Sztainer, Story, Hannan, & Croll, 2002).

Community health nurses can educate the public regarding the efficacy of breast-feeding and the need for and contents of an adequate diet for children and adolescents. In addition, they can advocate for nutritional supplementation programs and for adequate nutrition programs in schools and other institutional settings. Community health nurses can also promote policies that diminish access to "junk foods" for children and adolescents. For example, they can spearhead initiatives to remove candy and soft drink vending machines from schools and recreational areas and promote healthy fast food alternatives at popular chain restaurants. A tool for assessing the nutritional status of children and adolescents is provided in the *Community Assessment Reference Guide* 📋 designed as a companion volume for this text.

Promoting Physical Activity

Promoting physical activity among children and adolescents is another intervention aimed at promoting health and, in particular, preventing obesity. Based on 2003 data related to achievement of the *Healthy People 2010*◆ objectives for physical activity among high school students, much remains to be done in this area. For example, although the target is to increase the percentage of adolescents regularly engaged in moderate physical activity from a baseline of 27% in 1999 to 35% by 2010, current figures (25% in 2003) actually indicate movement away from the target. Similar findings are noted for objectives related to vigorous physical activity and daily participation in physical education activities at school. Only for the objective related to decreasing television viewing to less than 2 hours per day do data indicate movement toward the 2010 goal of 75%, increasing from 57% in 1999 to 62% in 2003 (CDC, 2005a). Community health nurses can help to educate children and adolescents on the need for increased physical activity and advocate for the inclusion of physical activity in school curricula. They can also advocate for neighborhood environments that promote physical activity (e.g., schools within walking or biking distance of homes, bicycle paths, and safe activity areas).

Promoting Safety

As we saw earlier, accidental injuries are a major cause of death and disability among children and adolescents, and community health nurses should be actively involved in promoting safety across the age spectrum. Again, parental and public education are the primary means for accomplishing this objective, but community health nurses can also campaign for safe conditions in play areas as well as the development and enforcement of safety regulations such as seat belt and helmet use, effective labeling and storage of household chemicals, and so on.

Community health nurses can promote the use of safety devices and equipment. For example, in 2003, 1,519 children under 14 years of age died in motor vehicle accidents and 220,000 were injured. This amounts to 4 deaths and 602 injuries per day. In half of the fatalities, children were riding in the car unrestrained. In one study, only 15% of child passengers were properly harnessed into correctly installed safety seats. Children are most often restrained when they are riding with a driver who also uses safety restraints. In fact, according to some figures, as many as 40% of children riding with unrestrained drivers did not use appropriate restraints

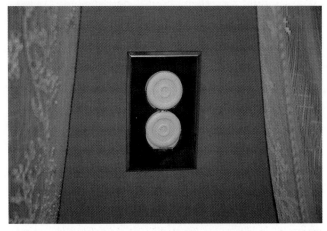

Child-proofing a home entails different strategies for children of different ages. (Patrick J. Watson)

(National Center for Injury Prevention and Control, n.d.a). Federal government figures indicate that use of appropriate child safety restraints decreases the risk of death by 50%, and placing children in the back seat of the vehicle reduces the risk of fatality by 30% (46% if the vehicle is equipped with front-seat air bags) (CDC, 2002a). Community health nurses educate individual families and their children, as well as the general public, regarding the need for effective restraint. In addition, they may campaign for strict enforcement of restraint legislation for all vehicle occupants.

Playground safety is another issue for children and adolescents. Each year, more than 205,000 preschool and elementary-age children are seen in emergency departments for injuries that occur on playgrounds (National Program for Playground Safety, 2005). In 1995, the treatment costs for these injuries amounted to $1.2 billion (National Center for Injury Prevention and Control, n.d.b). More than three fourths of these injuries (76%) occur on public play equipment, and nearly half (45%) occur at school. Although the majority of injuries occur in public settings, 70% of playground fatalities occur at home. The National Program for Playground Safety has developed recommendations for preventing playground injuries that can be used by community health nurses to educate parents and the general public regarding playground safety. These recommendations include:

- Adult supervision of children in play activities
- Choice of age- and developmentally appropriate play equipment
- Provision of safe surfacing below play equipment
- Regular maintenance of all equipment and play surfaces (National Program for Playground Safety, 2005)

Accidental and, among adolescents and preadolescents, intentional poisoning are other areas of concern for community health nurses caring for child and adolescent populations. More than 2.2 million poison

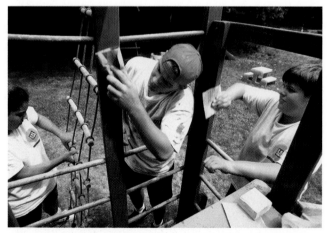

Playground safety is an important issue for child health. (Robert Harbison)

exposures were reported to poison control centers in the United States during 2000, nearly 53% involving children under 6 years of age (CDC, 2002c). Most of these incidents (90%) occurred in the home. Among adolescents, half of the poisoning incidents were intentional suicide attempts (National Center for Injury Prevention and Control, n.d.c). Community health nurses can actively promote safety education regarding the use and storage of poisonous materials among the general public. They may also be involved in efforts to promote effective labeling of hazardous substances and in suicide prevention activities with youth. These activities are discussed in more detail in Chapter 32∞. Selected elements of an educational program to promote child and adolescent safety in the community are included in Table 16-3◆. The *Community Assessment Reference Guide* 🗒 designed as a companion reference for this text contains an assessment tool that community health nurses can use to assess home safety for children and adolescents.

Preventing Communicable Diseases

The most effective means of preventing many communicable diseases among children and adolescents is, of course, immunization. Community health nurses may be actively involved in referring individual children and adolescents for immunizations and in assuring that immunization services are available to these populations. Community health nurses may also educate the public, particularly adolescents, regarding practices to prevent specific communicable diseases such as HIV/AIDS.

IMMUNIZATION Routine immunization of children has resulted in a 99% decline in the incidence of vaccine-preventable diseases (CDC, 2004b). Immunization is credited with preventing 10.5 million cases of disease and 33,000 deaths each year in the United States. In addition to the savings in lives and suffering, each dollar spent on immunizations saves an estimated $6.30 in direct medical expenses and $18.42 in indirect costs, for an annual savings to society of $42 billion (Trust for America's Health, 2004).

By 2 years of age, U.S. children should have received as many as 23 doses of vaccine to protect them against 12 communicable diseases. In 2003, 27.5% of children aged 19 to 35 months were deficient in one or more doses of the recommended vaccines (CDC, 2005c). By the end of 2004, immunization coverage in this age group for all vaccines except varicella had reached the *Healthy People 2010◆* goal of 80% (Immunization Services Division, 2005b). Because of state and local regulations, immunization coverage is usually somewhat higher among school-aged children. During the 2003–2004 school year, for example, the extent of coverage for seven major vaccines (polio, DTP, measles, mumps, rubella, hepatitis B, and varicella) ranged from 93.3% for varicella to 96% for

Age	Safety Education
TABLE 16-3	**Educational Elements to Promote Child and Adolescent Safety**
Infant (birth–1 year)	Not leaving child unattended on elevated surfaces or in bath Use of car seat restraint Use of safety straps in high chairs, strollers, swings, infant seats, etc. Use of flame-retardant sleepwear Crib safety: Narrow spaces between slats, bumper pads, no plastic coverings, nontoxic paint, no soft pillows Toy safety: No sharp edges or small parts, no long strings, siblings' toys out of reach
Toddler (2–3 years)	Not leaving child unattended in bath or pool Use of car seat restraint Adequate adult supervision Home safety: Outlet covers, sharp and poisonous objects locked away, medications out of reach, child-resistant containers, gated stairs, bathroom doors closed, no dangling electrical cords Play equipment: Age-appropriate and in good repair, on appropriate surface Toy safety: Age-appropriate toys, no small parts Fenced yard/swimming pool
Preschool child (4–6 years)	Use of booster seat in vehicle Adequate adult supervision Home safety: Outlet covers, sharp and poisonous objects locked away, medications out of reach, child-resistant containers, gated stairs, bathroom doors closed, no dangling electrical cords Play equipment: Age-appropriate and in good repair, on appropriate surface Toy safety: Age-appropriate toys, no small parts, adult supervision with potentially hazardous toys Safety practices: Education regarding interaction with strangers, crossing the street, fire safety, water safety
School-age child (6–12 years)	Use of booster seat/adult seat belt based on height and weight Sports safety: Age-appropriate sports, use of safety equipment, adequate adult supervision Firearms: Locked separately from ammunition Safety practices: Education regarding stranger interactions, caring for self at home, sports, bicycling and helmet use, water safety, use of medications, swimming instruction
Adolescent (13–18 years)	Safe driving Use of seat belts Sports safety: Age-appropriate sports, use of safety equipment, adequate adult supervision Safety practices: Education regarding use of firearms, caring for self and others at home, use of medications, dangerous situations (e.g., alcohol and driving, fighting), stranger interactions Sexuality: Abstinence, safe sexual practices Use of drugs and alcohol

mumps (National Immunization Program, 2004). Hepatitis A coverage, however, lags rather far behind the other vaccines, with 51% of children in high-risk states, 25% in states with moderately high incidence, and only 1.4% of children in low-risk states being immunized (National Immunization Program, 2005). Similarly, influenza immunization in children and adolescents at high risk for complications was less than 35% during the 2004–2005 influenza season (Division of Adult and Community Health, 2005), and only 36% of 6- to 23-month-old children received the recommended influenza vaccine (Immunization Services Division, 2004).

In addition to the vaccines required by most states and local jurisdictions, the Advisory Committee on Immunization Practices has recommended routine immunization for meningococcal disease for all adolescents before high school entry. The goal is to provide routine immunization for all children at 11 years of age by 2008. Meningococcal vaccine is also recommended for previously unimmunized college students living in dormitories, military recruits, and travelers to endemic areas (Bilukha & Rosenstein, 2005).

Despite the benefits of immunization, there are still children in the United States and worldwide who remain unimmunized for one or more immunizable diseases. Periodic outbreaks of disease may occur in these populations. From 2001 to 2003, for example, the incidence rate for pertussis was 55.2 per 100,000 infants under 1 year of age. Incidence was nearly eight times higher for children under 6 months of age than for those 6 months to 1 year of age. Incidence among adolescents aged 10 to 19 years nearly doubled in the same period, suggesting waning immunity among previously immunized children (Epidemiology and Surveillance Division, 2005). Factors in poor immunization coverage include cost, lack of health insurance, inability to get appointments, parental lack of knowledge regarding the need for immunizations, and missed opportunities for immunization on the part of health care providers (O'Connor, Maddocks, Modie, & Pierce, 2001). Religious beliefs also play a part in outbreaks among groups that do not approve of immunization.

A number of interventions by community health nurses can improve immunization rates among children and adolescents. As mentioned earlier, nurses can refer individual clients and their families for available immunization services and educate parents and the public regarding the need for immunizations. They can also help to educate other providers to prevent missed opportunities for immunization. For example, they might campaign for providing initial hepatitis B immunizations at birth, which has been shown to increase the probability that the entire immunization series will be completed (CDC, 2002b). Community health nurses can also promote provider and client participation in immunization registries. Immunization registries are central databases used to record immunizations for all children in a jurisdiction. When they are regional in nature, they relieve the difficulty of immunization records scattered among many different providers. Registries also permit notification of needed immunizations and have been shown to increase immunization rates in participating populations (Kempe et al., 2004). Registries with additional capabilities for managing vaccines, reporting adverse vaccine events, storing lifespan immunization histories, and interacting with electronic medical records are called immunization information systems (IISs). Unfortunately, as of December 2003, only 44% of children under 6 years of age were enrolled in an IIS (Immunization Services Division, 2005a).

PREVENTING OTHER COMMUNICABLE DISEASES Because many communicable diseases are not immunizable conditions, community health nurses must engage in other activities to prevent these conditions in children and adolescents. HIV/AIDS and other sexually transmitted diseases are areas of concern for community health nurses working with child and adolescent populations. In 2002, for example, an estimated 2,292 children under age 13 and 732 adolescents 13 and 14 years of age were living with AIDS in the United States (U.S. Census Bureau, 2004b). As we saw in Chapter 6∞, incidence rates are much higher for children in other parts of the world, particularly Africa. For most young children, HIV transmission occurs during pregnancy, the birth process, and via breast-feeding. Perinatal transmission of HIV infection, however, can be reduced from 25% to 2% with effective treatment of pregnant women (County of San Diego Health and Human Services Agency, 2004). Community health nurses can be actively involved in referring pregnant women for prenatal care and in promoting routine HIV screening during pregnancy. For those women who are infected, community health nurses can provide case management services for diagnosis and treatment as well as educating them and the general public about the dangers of breast-feeding in the presence of HIV infection. They can also arrange for screening of infants born to HIV-infected women and make referrals for treatment as needed. Prenatal treatment with zidovudine has been credited with a decrease in perinatal HIV transmission from 19% to 3% during 1993 to 2000 (National Center for HIV, STD, and TB Prevention, 2002). Prenatal care and screening can also help identify women with other sexually transmitted diseases (STDs) (e.g., syphilis, genital herpes, and hepatitis B) that can be transmitted perinatally to their infants.

Adolescents may also be at high risk for sexually transmitted diseases due to increased sexual activity. Community health nurses can educate this group regarding STD transmission and can promote use of condoms and safe sexual practices. In addition, community health nurses may need to advocate for condom availability to sexually active adolescents.

Hygiene and protection of food and water supplies are additional measures to prevent communicable diseases in children and adolescents, particularly in developing areas of the world. In the United States, acute gastroenteritis results in an estimated 300 deaths

per year in children under 5 years of age. Worldwide mortality from these diseases approaches 1.5 to 2.5 million deaths each year (King, Glass, Bresee, & Duggan, 2003). Community health nurses can educate the public regarding hygiene and preventing contamination of food and water supplies. They can also advocate for safe water and food supplies at the societal level.

Promoting Dental Care

Dental hygiene should begin as soon as the child's first tooth erupts. At this time parents can be encouraged to rub teeth briskly with a dry washcloth. Later, parents can begin to brush the child's teeth with a soft toothbrush. Older children can be taught to brush and floss their own teeth with adult supervision. Use of fluoridated toothpaste should be encouraged in areas with unfluoridated water; parents can give fluoride-containing vitamins to infants in such areas. In addition to instructing parents about the need for preventive dental care, community health nurses can be actively involved in promoting fluoridation of community drinking water.

Community health nurses can educate the public about the need to wean infants from the bottle before a year of age to prevent bottle-mouth syndrome. The use of sugarless snacks and rinsing the mouth after eating—when brushing is not possible—can also be encouraged. Finally, community health nurses should encourage parents to obtain regular dental checkups for children and to get prompt attention for dental problems. Financial assistance may be needed for such services for low-income families. In such cases, the community health nurse should make a referral for Medicaid in those areas where dental care is covered or work to promote the availability of such services in the population.

Supporting Effective Parenting

Parenting has been described as one of the hardest jobs in the world and the one for which we receive the least preparation. In one study, both mothers and fathers described their first year as parents as overwhelming, with problems related to lack of confidence in the parental role, the demands of being parents, time for oneself, and feeling drained and fatigued (Nystrom & Ohrling, 2004). Other studies have shown that the availability of social support contributes to parental efficacy, the ability to "organize and execute a set of tasks related to parenting a child" (de Montigny & Lacharite, 2005, p. 387). In a review of related literature, the authors found four factors that contributed to efficacy: positive mastery experiences in past care of infants, vicarious experience obtained through parent training programs, verbal persuasion by significant others of one's capabilities, and an appropriate physical and affective state (e.g., not being fatigued or under stress).

Other studies have noted that both structural and functional elements of social support influence parenting abilities. Structural elements include formal and informal social networks and the people who make up those networks. Informal networks are comprised of family members and friends, whereas formal networks include health care professionals. Functional elements of social support address the kinds of support available to the parent and usually include informational, instrumental, emotional, and appraisal support (Warren, 2005). Each of these types of support can be provided by community health nurses to the parents of children and adolescents. For example, they may provide informational support by educating families regarding the needs of children and adolescents, or emotional support in dealing with the frustrations of parenthood. They may also provide appraisal support by giving parents both positive and negative feedback on their performance as parents. Less often, community health nurses may provide instrumental support by actually caring for a child, arranging respite services for a parent, or advocating the presence of such services in the community.

Support for parenting for parents of young children may frequently address issues of discipline. Table 16-4◆ provides several general principles of child and adolescent discipline that community health nurses can use to educate community members. The converse of promoting effective discipline of children and adolescents is preventing abuse of children and adolescents by their parents and other adults or older siblings. In the United States, the role of the community health nurse in identifying and reporting child abuse is quite clear cut. Community health nurses are part of a group of professionals, including health care providers, teachers, and others, who are required by law to report any suspicion of abuse of a child or adolescent. The role of the nurse is not as clearly defined in other countries, however. For example, one study in Scotland found considerable confusion among community health nurses regarding their responsibility with respect to child protection issues as well as the extent of activity by community health nurses in detecting cases of abuse. Many nurses in the study perceived detection and reporting of abuse as in conflict with their traditional role of support to families (Crisp & Lister, 2004). Contrary to these perceptions, however, identification and reporting of child abuse can foster effective parenting because it gives parents an opportunity to learn more appropriate ways to interact with their children.

Other Primary Prevention Activities

Additional primary preventive measures may be warranted for children with specific illnesses. For example, parents of children with AIDS and other immunosuppressive conditions should be taught to minimize exposure to opportunistic infections. Special intervention may also be warranted to create a healthy self-image in children with chronic conditions or disabilities. For

TABLE 16-4	Principles of Effective Discipline and Related Considerations
Principle	**Disciplinary Consideration**
Importance	Employ discipline for important matters Do not automatically say "no" to everything Determine what is unacceptable behavior
Consistency	Maintain consistency in what is considered unacceptable behavior Maintain consistency between and among authority figures If a behavior is acceptable in some situations and not in others, make sure children understand the difference and why it is so
Calm	Never act in anger Employ a "cooling off" period, if needed, and make sure children understand the need to deal with anger appropriately
Time	Allow time for compliance with directions before taking disciplinary action
Limits	Set rules and limits for behavior ahead of time and make sure children are aware of them Make sure limits are within the child's age and developmental capacity to comply Give a warning for unanticipated unacceptable behaviors the first time
Understanding	Make sure children understand the rules and the reasons for them
Prevention	Prevent unacceptable behavior rather than punish it whenever possible Remove sources of temptation from younger children Provide adequate adult supervision of children
Investigation	Ascertain the facts of the situation before taking disciplinary action Ask for the child's explanation of the situation and his or her behavior When the behavior is unacceptable but the child's reasons are appropriate, make sure he or she understands why the behavior should not be repeated
Meaningfulness	Make sure children understand the reason for disciplinary action Explain how the child can improve his or her behavior Use a form of discipline appropriate to the child and the situation

example, the physically handicapped child can be helped to develop skills such as artistic ability that contribute to a positive self-image. Primary preventive interventions employed by community health nurses in caring for children are summarized in Table 16-5◆.

Secondary Prevention

Secondary prevention is geared toward resolution of health problems currently experienced by children and adolescents. Activities are directed toward screening for conditions, care of minor illness, care of children and adolescents with chronic conditions, and care of those with terminal illnesses.

TABLE 16-5 Primary Prevention Interventions for Child and Adolescent Populations

Focus	Interventions
Assuring access to health care	Making referrals to sources of health care Promoting a regular source of health care for all children and adolescents Advocating health insurance coverage for children and adolescents
Reducing prematurity, low birth weight, and infant mortality	Sexuality education Promoting effective contraception to prevent unplanned pregnancies Promoting effective prenatal care and advocating for low-cost pregnancy services Promoting supplemental nutrition programs for pregnant women and children and making referrals to existing programs Promoting smoking cessation and alcohol abstinence during pregnancy
Promoting growth and development	Educating parents and the public regarding normal growth and development Advocating environments that promote adequate growth and development of children and adolescents Promoting continued development of adolescent parents as well as their children
Providing adequate nutrition	Promoting breast-feeding Educating parents, children, and the public regarding nutritional needs of children and adolescents Advocating healthy nutrition in schools and day care centers Advocating for healthier food choices in restaurants and other venues
Promoting physical activity	Educating children and adolescents regarding the need for physical activity Advocating for physical activity in school curricula Advocating for environments conducive to physical activity
Promoting safety	Encouraging provision of adequate supervision of children and adolescents Advocating for strong legislation and strict enforcement to protect children and adolescents Promoting use of effective safety devices Teaching children and adolescents regarding safety issues Advocating elimination of safety hazards in the environment
Preventing communicable diseases	Promoting immunization and referring for immunization services Modifying immunization practices or schedules for children with special needs Promoting prenatal care and screening for HIV and other STDs in pregnant women Promoting condom use and safe sexual practices among adolescents Educating the public and families with respect to good hygiene and protection of food and water supplies Advocating for effective sanitation and safe food and water supplies
Promoting dental care	Promoting dental hygiene Advocating access to dental care services
Supporting effective parenting	Providing support for parents Educating parents for care of children and adolescents Advocating for respite care as needed Assisting parents with discipline issues Educating parents for realistic expectations of their children Taking action to minimize parental sources of stress
Other primary prevention activities	Meeting the primary prevention needs of children with special needs

Screening for Health Problems

Screening for conditions at birth is usually employed when treatment soon after birth leads to improved health outcomes. Each state determines the panel of required screenings for newborns born in that state. In 2004, required newborn screening panels ranged from 4 tests to 40. Criteria for the selection of mandatory screening tests include the prevalence of the condition; the cost, feasibility, and accuracy of screening tests; the effectiveness of early intervention; and the availability of treatment. CDC recommends that newborn screening programs include follow-up treatment systems, parental education, and primary provider information systems (Grosse et al., 2004).

Routine screening for existing conditions takes place at other ages as well as at birth. Table 16-6◆ provides information about routine screening procedures for selected age groups. Other screening procedures may be warranted for children and adolescents in certain circumstances. For example, children with a family history of diabetes may be screened for this condition. Similarly, children or adolescents who have been exposed to traumatic events (e.g., school violence, natural disaster) should be screened for depression and other mental health problems. Community health nurses may be actively involved in providing routine and specialized screening services or may need to advocate for access to these services for the child and adolescent populations.

Caring for Minor Illness

Each year approximately 12 million children under the age of 5 years die of treatable conditions, mostly as a result of pneumonia, diarrhea, malaria, measles, and

TABLE 16-6	Routine Screening Procedures for Children and Adolescents
Age	**Screening Procedure**
Birth	Phenylketonuria (PKU), hypothyroidism, hearing, hemoglobinopathies, sickle cell disease, galactosemia, maple syrup urine disease, homocystinuria, biodatinase, congenital adrenal hyperplasia, cystic fibrosis
1 month	Lead, Denver Developmental Screening Test (DDST)
1–2 months	Head and chest circumference, height and weight (and periodically thereafter)
3 months	Blood pressure (and periodically thereafter)
3–4 months	Vision (and periodically thereafter)
6 months	Hematocrit or hemoglobin
9 months	Tuberculin skin test
1 year	DDST
2 years	DDST
3 years	Dental (and periodically thereafter)
5 years	School readiness, immunization status
6–12 years	Hearing, vision, school performance
11–18 years	Use of tobacco and alcohol and sexual activity (and periodically thereafter), immunization status, scoliosis, STDs and Papanicolaou smear (if sexually active)

Think Advocacy

Rowe, Onikpo, Lama, Cokou, and Deming (2001) conducted a study to examine the extent to which community health workers (CHWs) implemented WHO strategies for Integrated Management of Childhood Illness for children under the age of 5 years. They found that a significant portion of the community health workers failed to correctly implement the guidelines. Major areas of deficit included incomplete assessment, incorrect diagnosis and treatment, inappropriate drug therapy, missed opportunities for immunizations, and failure to refer children for professional care when needed. Qualitative data obtained from CHWs indicated reasons for these deficits included conflicts among health workers, overload, failure to use knowledge acquired in training, low morale and motivation, poor time management, lack of equipment, and lack of fluency in the local language. Other reasons given for poor implementation of guidelines were impatient parents or other caregivers, caregiver demands for medications, CHW perceptions that caregivers would report all of a child's symptoms without questioning or prompting or would be alarmed if told of a child's diagnosis, and CHW unwillingness to use charts or other diagnostic and treatment aids for fear of being thought incompetent. How might you address the factors contributing to poor implementation of guidelines by CHWs so that all the children seen receive adequate treatment for their illnesses?

malnutrition. The World Health Organization has established strategies for the Integrated Management of Childhood Illness for children 1 month to 5 years of age. These strategies include guidelines for assessing, diagnosing, treating, and referring ill children, counseling their caregivers, and immunizing them as needed (Rowe, Onikpo, Lama, Cokou, & Deming, 2001). Community health nurses can educate the public regarding appropriate home treatment for minor illness and when professional care is required.

Many minor illnesses and health care problems can be addressed effectively if parents or other caregivers know how to deal with them. For other problems, or when home care does not resolve the problem, professional care is required. Appendix C∞ provides some guidelines that community health nurses can use to educate individual families and the general public regarding treatment of minor health problems in children and adolescents. Community health nurses can educate parents and the public on the signs of illness in children, appropriate measures to be taken at home, and when to seek medical intervention. Caretakers and the public should be acquainted with what is normal and what is abnormal, as well as what home remedies are appropriate and what might be harmful. In addition to providing such information, community health nurses frequently are called on to assess the health status of specific children and recommend appropriate interventions or make referrals for medical assistance.

Caring for Children and Adolescents with Chronic Illness

We most often think of chronic illness in the context of caring for elderly clients, but roughly 31% or 20 million U.S. children are affected in some way by chronic illness (Meleski, 2002). An estimated 400,000 of these children experience chronic, life-threatening conditions (Jennings, 2005). Chronic illness has been defined as "an incurable condition that interferes with long-term function and requires special assistance to manage" (Meleski, 2002, p. 48). Based on figures from the U.S. Federal Interagency Forum on Child and Family Statistics, 3% of children under 5 years of age and 7% of those aged 5 to 17 years have activity limitations due to chronic conditions. Approximately two thirds of these children experience only mild limitations, but 29% have moderate limitations and 5% are severely limited by their conditions (Meleski, 2002). The percentage of children who experience activity limitation due to chronic disease has more than tripled in the past four decades (Newacheck & Benjamin, 2004). Children with chronic conditions have three times as many physician contacts and hospitalizations and eight times as many hospital days as those without chronic illnesses. In fact, an estimated 80% of nontrauma spending in the care of children is allocated to chronic illness care (Wise, 2004). Chronic conditions may also affect children's performance or their interactions with others in the school setting. Problems posed by chronic illness in school settings are addressed in more detail in Chapter 23∞.

MediaLink Appendix C: Health Problems in Children

Parental uncertainty has been shown to be a key feature of parental response to diagnosis of serious illness in their children. Uncertainty has been defined as the "inability to determine the meaning of illness related events" as a result of the inability to categorize an event due to a lack of understandable cues (Mu, 2005, p. 368). Four dimensions have been noted in the literature with regard to parental uncertainty in the face of serious illness in a child: ambiguity regarding the illness state; lack of information regarding the illness, its management, and its effects; the complexity of information and care systems; and the unpredictability of the child's prognosis, quality of life, and functional ability (Santacroce, 2003).

Parents of children and adolescents with chronic health problems have reported ongoing personal trauma throughout periods of diagnosis, treatment, and survivorship. Some of the traumas reported include having to approve or give painful treatments, watching their child's condition deteriorate, and being constantly alert for recurrent or subsequent health problems (Santacroce, 2003). Trauma and disequilibrium seem to center around five specific periods of transition in chronic illness: initial diagnosis, symptom exacerbation, movement to a new care setting (e.g., hospitalization), periods of parental absence (e.g., divorce or separation), and times when the child would be expected to experience a normal developmental transition such as learning to walk or talk, school entry, puberty, or a 21st birthday (Meleski, 2002). The approach of adulthood may be a particularly stressful time for families, as they are faced with the possible need for residential placement if children are not capable of living independently (Green, S., 2004). Coming of age may also make children ineligible for previously covered services, and each year half a million adolescents reach the age when they are ineligible for continued services (Wise, 2004).

Another period when disequilibrium may be experienced occurs when treatment regimens change, even if the change is not in response to the child's deteriorating condition. For example, parents of children with diabetes who were switched to insulin pumps reported having to rethink their disease management strategies with the advent of this technology. Changes required greater vigilance and more frequent glucose monitoring than they were accustomed to doing (Sullivan-Bolyai, Knafl, Tamborlane, & Grey, 2004).

Two models have been used to explain parental reaction to the presence of serious disease in their children. The first is a time-bound model in which parents are believed to adapt over time to the presence of the disease. In the chronic sorrow model, on the other hand, parents adapt, but may never accept the illness and experience continuing sorrow that fades and burgeons based on circumstances in the life of the child and the family. Perhaps the most appropriate model is one that integrates both perspectives: parents and families do adapt, but are apt to experience periods in which adaptation is more or less difficult (Meleski, 2002). Factors that may affect adaptation include family coping abilities, the availability of social support and appropriate services, respite, and the level of stigma attached to the child's condition, which may be influenced by cultural norms (Mu, 2005).

Many children and adolescents and their families need to learn to cope with the effects of chronic illness on a daily basis. Coping has been defined as the "specific cognitive and behavioral efforts by which an individual and family attempt to reduce or manage the demands placed upon them" (Mu, 2005, p. 368). McCubbin found three patterns of family coping in the presence of cystic fibrosis in a child that may have application for families dealing with other chronic illnesses. The first coping pattern involved maintenance of family integration, optimism, and cooperation. The second pattern addressed maintenance of self-esteem of family members and mobilizing social and psychological sources of support. The third pattern was understanding the disease and its effects through interactions with providers and with other parents whose children also were affected (Mu, 2005).

Much intervention with families with children experiencing chronic illness has focused on development of family resilience or hardiness. Hardiness "refers to the internal strengths and durability of the family, and is characterized by a sense of control over outcomes of life, a view of change as growth-producing, and an active rather than passive orientation in adapting to stressful situations" (Svavarsdottir & Rayens, 2005, p. 382). There is some evidence to suggest, however, that resilience may be associated with greater internalization of feelings such that negative effects of illness are just less visible rather than less real.

Research on families dealing with children and adolescents with chronic illnesses has identified a number of common themes that are relevant to community health nursing care of these population groups. Some of these themes address family interactions, and some deal with interactions with health care providers and the health care system. Others reflect the economic burden experienced by families. Families describe the need to live as normal a life as possible but being challenged by the need to be constantly alert to crises and the shift in perception of the home as a place of safety and refuge to one of providing care. The presence of a chronic illness in a child results in changes in family relationships with the affected child and among other family members. Families may also be at higher risk for social isolation due to the inability to find adequate care for the affected child. Parents describe ambiguity in their parental role and role conflict between the parental and formal caregiver roles, and frequently experience adverse health effects themselves related to fatigue, depression, fear, and panic (Wang & Barnard, 2004). Parents may also feel burdened by the need to provide emotional support to the child with a chronic illness as well as to his or her siblings, with limited emotional support for themselves (Svavarsdottir, 2005).

Health system factors that affect family response to chronic illness include fragmentation of care and lack of social support for parental caregivers. Parents may find themselves engaged in frequent battles to obtain needed health and education services for their children, and support programs for families of children with chronic illnesses are usually severely underfunded, if they exist at all. Parents also describe being unprepared for the demands of their new caregiver role and may view the presence of a community health nurse as both helpful and disruptive of family routine and privacy (Wang & Barnard, 2004).

Children and adolescents experience a wide variety of chronic health problems. A few of the major problems affecting these age groups will be addressed here.

HIV INFECTION AND AIDS Prevalence and prevention of HIV/AIDS in children and adolescents was addressed earlier in this chapter. Here we will concentrate on the role of the community health nurse in caring for children and adolescents with HIV infection or active AIDS. The primary aspect of this role lies in management of the disease and prevention of opportunistic infections. Community health nurses may refer children for diagnosis and treatment services, and may be involved in long-term follow-up for children with HIV/AIDS. In addition to halting the progression of the disease, highly active antiretroviral therapy (HAART) has been shown to reduce the incidence of opportunistic infections (OI) in children with AIDS. HAART is the most effective means of combating OI, since many protozoan, fungal, and viral infections are not amenable to antibiotic therapy (Mofenson, Oleske, Serchuck, Van Dyke, & Wilfert, 2004). Community health nurses monitor HAART therapy in children and observe for treatment effects and medication side effects. They can also educate clients and family members in dealing with side effects. In addition, they would also be alert to signs of OI in HIV-infected children and adolescents and refer them for treatment in keeping with new treatment guidelines published by CDC in 2004 (Mofenson et al., 2004).

ATTENTION DEFICIT HYPERACTIVITY DISORDER Attention deficit hyperactivity disorder is one of the three most common conditions in children (with asthma and otitis media) (Leslie & Stein, 2003) and the most common psychiatric disorder in the United States (Singh, 2004). **Attention deficit hyperactivity disorder (ADHD)** is a chronic condition characterized by poor attention span, impulsive behavior, and hyperactivity. Attention deficit with associated hyperactivity is frustrating for the children affected and for everyone who interacts with them.

Prevalence estimates for ADHD in the general population range from 4% to 12% (Leslie & Stein, 2003) with a 7% prevalence among children 6 to 11 years of age. More than three fourths of those affected are boys (Singh, 2004). Children with ADHD usually exhibit poor school performance and poor peer relationships and often have problems with family relationships (Leslie & Stein, 2003). Twenty to thirty percent of children with ADHD also have specific learning disabilities, including reading and spelling disabilities (e.g., dyslexia) and writing and arithmetic disorders. Other conditions that may occur in conjunction with ADHD include Tourette syndrome (a neurological disorder characterized by nervous tics and uncontrollable swearing), oppositional defiant disorder (stubborn, defiant, belligerent behavior), conduct disorder, anxiety and depression, and bipolar disorder (National Institutes of Mental Health [NIMH], 2003). Children with ADHD have also been shown to be at higher risk for injury due primarily to lack of attention to risk situations (National Center on Birth Defects and Developmental Disabilities, 2004a).

An additional 8 million adults are also affected by ADHD, which affects education and employment in adult life. Adults with ADHD also have higher rates of divorce, lower life satisfaction, and higher risks for substance abuse. Failure to complete their education is another common problem. Even those who manage to complete high school earn an average of $10,791 a year less than their counterparts who are not affected by ADHD, and college graduates earn on average $4,334 less than their nonaffected counterparts. Roughly one third of adults with ADHD are not diagnosed until after 18 years of age. Approximately half of adults with ADHD go on to have a child with the disorder, suggesting a genetic component to the disease (American Medical Association, 2004). Overall estimates of ADHD in the U.S. population stand at 5 million, with approximately half of those cases undiagnosed (Federwisch, 2005).

Only approximately 3% of school-age children with ADHD are receiving methylphenidate (Ritalin) therapy, and the prevalence of therapy has increased sixfold in the last decade (Singh, 2004). Ritalin is one of several medications used for the treatment of ADHD. Ritalin has been approved for use in children 6 years of age and older, but other drugs (e.g., Adderall and dextrostat) may be used with children as young as 3 (NIMH, 2003). Despite some controversy regarding the number of children on medication for ADHD, a recent NIMH study indicated that children on medication fared better than those without, whether or not they received behavioral therapy (Federwisch, 2005). For some children, particularly those with anxiety, poor academic performance or social skills, poor parent–child interaction, or oppositional defiant disorder, a combination therapy including medication management and behavioral treatment was more effective than either therapy alone (NIMH, 2003).

Treatment goals for children and adolescents with ADHD include the following:

- Decreasing symptoms through medication management and behavior modification
- Addressing co-existing medical conditions through medical management
- Addressing co-existing mental health problems through pharmacologic and behavioral therapies
- Addressing co-existing learning disabilities through special education services
- Addressing environmental and family stressors
- Promoting adequate development
- Promoting child and family competence (Leslie & Stein, 2003)

Community health nurses can be particularly helpful in assisting families with medication management and behavioral modification. They can also advocate for environments that minimize symptoms. For example, children with more green play areas have been shown to exhibit fewer ADHD symptoms than those without green play areas (Kuo & Taylor, 2004). Similarly, regular routines and organizing strategies can help students maintain focus and improve performance (NIMH, 2003). For example, a written schedule posted on the refrigerator can include activities such as homework, chores, and specific play activities (e.g., computer games or outdoor play). Community health nurses can also advocate for the necessary special education services as well as refer individual children and adolescents for diagnostic and treatment services. School nurses may be particularly helpful as case managers for children and adolescents with ADHD.

Community health nurses should also attend to the needs of those who care for children and adolescents with ADHD. Mothers, in particular, have been shown to blame themselves and to be blamed by others for their children's hyperactivity (Singh, 2004). These families may require a great deal of emotional support by the community health nurse.

OTHER CHRONIC AND DISABLING CONDITIONS Children and adolescents experience a variety of other chronic physical and mental conditions. For example, asthma is the leading cause of hospitalizations and emergency department visits among children (Nicholas et al., 2005) and the leading cause of school absence (Navaie-Waliser, Misener, Mersman, & Lincoln, 2004). The incidence of asthma in U.S. children nearly tripled from 3.7% of children in 1980 to 12.7% twenty years later (Wise, 2004). In 2003, an estimated 9 million U.S. children and adolescents had been diagnosed with asthma (NCHS, 2005a). Asthma is also a growing problem worldwide, with prevalence ranging from 10% to 50% of children in some countries (Huey, 2001).

Environmental modification may help control airway reactivity in children and adolescents with asthma.

For example, in one study, community health workers' efforts to assess home environments and educate families regarding elimination of asthma triggers resulted in fewer asthma symptom days, fewer asthma triggers in the home, less urgent care use, and increased quality of life for caregivers (Krieger, Takaro, Song, & Weaver, 2005). Removing pets from the homes of children with asthma has proven particularly effective in controlling symptoms (Shirai, Matsui, Suzuki, & Chida, 2005).

Seizure disorders are another type of chronic condition that may affect the health of children and adolescents. According to the Epilepsy Foundation (2005), each year approximately 300,000 people experience a first convulsion. More than one third of them (120,000) are children under 18 years of age, and 75,000 to 100,000 are children under 5 years of age who experience febrile seizures. Many of those who experience a first seizure, however, go on to develop chronic seizure disorder without any known cause. Overall, approximately 326,000 children under 14 years of age have diagnosed epilepsy, and roughly 1% of the U.S. population can be expected to develop epilepsy before the age of 20.

Medication is highly effective in the treatment of epilepsy, with approximately 70% of those treated remaining seizure-free for 5 or more years, at which time three fourths of them can discontinue medication without a return of seizures. Unfortunately, 10% of those with seizure disorders will be unable to gain control of them despite treatment (Epilepsy Foundation, 2005).

Caring for children and adolescents with seizure disorders involves assisting them to cope with the perceived or real stigma attached to the disease as well as encouraging compliance with medical therapy. Adolescents, in particular, may need to be referred for counseling if their condition contributes to a poor self-image or difficulty with interpersonal interactions, especially in the school setting. For children and adolescents whose disease is uncontrolled by medication, community health nurses may need to provide assistance in dealing with the limitations imposed by their condition. For example, the nurse might educate them about the inadvisability of swimming alone or help adolescents cope with their inability to obtain a driver's license. Both children and parents may need to be helped to cope with the fear and uncertainty caused by uncontrolled seizures. School nurses, in particular, may be in a position to educate others about seizure disorder and advocate for fair treatment of those affected.

Growing numbers of children are also affected by diabetes. Although children are most likely to develop type 1 diabetes, there are indications of growing incidence of type 2 diabetes among children as well, particularly among Native American, African American, and Hispanic youth (American Diabetes Association, n.d.). Overall, an estimated 210,000 people under 20 years of age have diabetes (National Diabetes Information Clearinghouse, n.d.).

Care of children and adolescents with diabetes is centered around controlling the disease while maintaining as normal a lifestyle as possible. Community health nurses will educate children and their parents regarding the need for dietary control, use of medication, exercise, and the need to monitor illness and injury carefully to prevent diabetic complications. Again, the community health nurse may need to function as an advocate for children with diabetes, particularly in the school setting. For example, in addition to educating others about the disease, the nurse may need to see that the school meal programs contain foods appropriate to a diabetic diet. The nurse can also assist older children and adolescents in designing their diet, so they can participate in activities enjoyed by their peers (e.g., a class picnic or an occasional trip to the local fast food restaurant).

Obesity is another chronic condition with increasing prevalence among children and adolescents. In 2000, for example, 15.3% of children were obese, compared to only 5.7% in 1980 (Wise, 2004). Community health nurses can be particularly effective in addressing the problem of obesity by promoting healthy diets and physical activity. Nurses can advocate for healthy school meal programs as well as healthy diets in the home setting. In addition, many community health nurses have been actively involved in local initiatives to remove vending machines or discontinue the sale of junk food on school premises. They can also make referrals to weight control programs for overweight and obese children and adolescents or establish such programs within school or recreational settings (e.g., a local Boys and Girls Club). In addition, they can attempt to decrease the stigma attached to being overweight or refer children and youth for counseling to improve self-image if needed.

Many children also experience congenital heart disease, hearing loss, and a variety of developmental disorders. Approximately 8 of every 1,000 babies are born with congenital heart disease. Children with congenital heart disease often exhibit delayed growth compared to normal children and have been shown to have increased exercise intolerance and risks for depression and anxiety disorders as adults (Chen, Li, & Wang, 2004; Green, A., 2004). Another 1 to 3 children per 1,000 live births have congenital hearing loss, yet, in 2001, only 65% of infants were screened for hearing loss (Division of Human Development and Disability, 2003).

Developmental disabilities encompass a variety of conditions "that initially manifest in persons ≤ 18 years and result in impairment of physical health, mental health, cognition, speech, language, or selfcare" (National Center on Birth Defects and Developmental Disabilities, 2004c). Mental retardation is the most common of these disabilities and affects 1% of U.S. children 3 to 10 years of age. Mental retardation may be caused by injury, disease, brain abnormality, genetic disorder, or fetal alcohol syndrome. The average lifetime costs for mental retardation in 2003 dollars were more than $1 million per person, with 76% of these costs going toward indirect support costs (National Center on Birth Defects and Developmental Disabilities, 2004e).

Cerebral palsy (CP) and autism are other developmental disabilities that affect children and adolescents. The overall prevalence of CP is 2.8 per 1,000 children aged 3 to 10 years. Average lifetime costs for a single person with CP in 2003 were $921,000 (National Center on Birth Defects and Developmental Disabilities, 2004b; 2005). Autism occurs less often, with an estimated prevalence of 2 to 6 per 1,000 children aged 3 to 10 years, and more than 500,000 people aged 10 to 21 years affected (National Center on Birth Defects and Developmental Disabilities, 2005).

The conditions described above and other chronic illnesses may result in disability for those affected. In the last two decades, perspectives on disability have been changing. In 1980, the WHO International Classification of Impairment, Disability, and Handicap (ICIDH) differentiated among these three effects of chronic conditions. Impairment was defined as a "loss or abnormality of psychological, physiological, or anatomical structure or function" (Kearny & Pryor, 2004, p. 164). Disability was defined as "any restriction or lack (resulting from impairment) of ability to perform an activity in the manner or within the range considered normal for a human being" (p. 164). Finally, a handicap was defined as "a disadvantage for a given individual, resulting from impairment or disability, that limits or prevents the fulfillment of a role that is normal (depending on age, sex and social and cultural factors) for that individual" (p. 164).

In 2001, WHO replaced this classification with the International Classification of Functioning, Disability, and Health (ICF), shifting from a personal-tragedy or consequences-of-disease perspective to a social-components-of-health perspective. In the social model, disability is not a property of the individual, but is a "multidimensional phenomenon resulting from the interaction between people and their physical and social environment" (WHO as quoted in Kearny & Pryor, 2004, p. 166). From this new perspective, functional ability and disability are not inherent in the individual and his or her health status, but are the product of the interaction between health status and contextual factors in the individual's environment. This perspective highlights the need to modify contextual factors such that disability is minimized to the extent possible. For example, community health nurses may work to remove asthma triggers from home and school environments to minimize airway reactivity in children with asthma. Similarly, they may be actively involved in environmental modifications that promote free access to educational, recreational, and service settings for people in wheelchairs. Although these kinds of modifications are often taken for granted in the United States, where compliance with the Americans with Disabilities Act is mandated for all public buildings, there are no such efforts underway in many other countries.

The interaction between health status and environment may lead to the creation of special needs in children with serious chronic conditions. Children with special needs have been defined by the U.S. federal government as "those who have or are at risk for a chronic physical, developmental, behavioral, or emotional condition, and who also require health and related services of a type or amount beyond that required by children generally" (Maternal and Child Health Bureau [MCHB], 2001, p. 2).

The Maternal and Child Health Bureau (2001) has established a plan to address the health of children with special needs. The plan includes six goals to be met in the care of all children with special needs. A similar set of eight goals has been established by the U.S. Department of Health and Human Services (2002) for dealing with chronic mental health problems in children and adolescents. Both sets of goals are presented in Table 16-7◆.

Community health nurses can educate both caregivers and the public regarding the mental health needs of children and adolescents and those of children with special needs. In addition, they can recognize signs of mental illness or other chronic health problems in children and refer them for screening, diagnosis, and treatment as needed. Community health nurses can assist children and adolescents with chronic illnesses and their families to cope with the day-to-day challenges of their conditions through education and emotional support. For example, they can educate the public and families regarding asthma self-management or diabetes control. They can also refer families to needed sources of support and advocate for the availability and accessibility of support and care services for children and adolescents in need of them. Finally, they can work to minimize the stigma attached to chronic illness through public education.

Caring for Children and Adolescents with Terminal Illness

Nearly 53,000 children die each year, approximately half of them from chronic disorders, and another 400,000 have life-threatening illnesses (Childers, 2005). The two primary functions of community health nurses in the care of children and adolescents are palliative care and assisting families with grieving. The World Health Organization has defined palliative care for children as "total care of the child's mind, body, and spirit" (quoted in Childers, p. 25). The goal of palliative care is to enhance the quality of life of the child and his or her family through control of symptoms and alleviation of other conditions (e.g., loneliness, depression) that may diminish quality of life. Palliative care also seeks to ensure continued effective functioning of the family unit (Jennings, 2005). Community health nurses may be involved in the provision of palliative care for individual children or adolescents or refer clients for palliative care services. At the aggregate level, they can work to assure the availability of palliative care services in the community and their accessibility to all those in need of them.

Family communication is another issue that can be addressed through palliative care. One communication issue that challenges families is whether to discuss the impending death with the child and with his or her siblings. Research has shown that impending death is harder on the child when it is not acknowledged by his or her parents (Childers, 2005) and that parents who discussed death with their seriously ill child did not regret having done so. On the other hand, parents who did not discuss the impending death with their child did regret not having done so and experienced more continuing depression and anxiety afterwards than parents who discussed death with their child (Kreicbergs, Valdimarsdottir, Onelov, Henter, & Steineck, 2004).

Some providers have noted the fine line between hope and realism that must be maintained to assist

TABLE 16-7	Goals for Addressing the Health Needs of Children and Adolescents with Special Needs and Those with Mental Health Problems	
Children and Adolescents with Special Needs	**Children and Adolescents with Mental Health Problems**
▪ Provide coordinated, ongoing, comprehensive care for all children with special needs within a medical home	▪ Promote public awareness and reduce the stigma of mental illness
▪ Provide adequate public or private insurance to pay for needed services	▪ Study and promote effective treatment services
▪ Provide early and continuing screening for special needs for all children	▪ Improve recognition of mental health problems in children and adolescents
▪ Incorporate families of children with special needs in decision making to improve satisfaction with care	▪ Eliminate disparities in access to mental health care services
▪ Develop easily used community-based systems of care for children with special needs	▪ Improve the mental health care infrastructure
▪ Provide services needed to make transitions to all aspects of adult life (e.g., health care, employment, independent living)	▪ Increase access to and coordination of mental health services
	▪ Educate providers to recognize and manage mental health problems in children and adolescents
	▪ Monitor access to and coordinate mental health services

Data from: Maternal and Child Health Bureau, 2001; All aboard the 2010 express. Rockville, MD: Author; U.S. Department of Health and Human Services, 2002. Children's mental health is national priority. Prevention Report, 16 (2), 5–6.

families to deal with a terminal illness and the thought of the death of a child or adolescent. Providers may need to "plant the seeds of bereavement" even while parents are attempting every last effort to save their child. Providers may begin to discuss the possibility of death with the family when the child him- or herself expresses knowledge that something is very wrong, when parents begin to acknowledge the potential for death, or when siblings begin to question the possibility of death (Wolfe, 2004).

The grief of parents for a child may not follow the traditional pattern of grieving, which was based on research conducted with grieving widows or widowers. The death of an older person is considered a normal, albeit sad, event. The death of a child, however, is considered unnatural, at least in the developed world where child fatality rates are relatively low. Acceptance of death is more difficult since it is perceived as unnatural for parents to outlive their children. Unlike a dead spouse, who might eventually be replaced by a new love, a child is irreplaceable. Parents experience not only the loss of the child but also the loss of all of their hopes and dreams for that child. Traditional grief work usually involves the breaking of bonds with the deceased; however, research with bereaved parents has shown that they are often comforted by maintaining links with their deceased child through linking objects (e.g., a favorite toy), religious devotions, and rituals that evoke memories of the child. Parents often find that talking about the child with others who remember him or her helps, as does exploring the meaning of the child's life. On the other hand, parents may experience intense loneliness and difficulty discussing the child with others who have not experienced similar losses (Davies, 2004).

Community health nurses can assist dying children and their families to deal with their feelings about an impending death and can make referrals for counseling, respite, and other services as needed. They may also provide information about the condition and palliative activities, help families create lasting memories of the child, or hold memorial events for groups of parents who have lost children (Childers, 2005). At the population level, community health nurses can initiate bereavement groups and advocate for the availability of both palliative and bereavement services for terminally ill children and their families. They can also advocate insurance coverage for both palliative and bereavement services. Community health nursing foci and interventions related to secondary prevention for children and adolescents are presented in Table 16-8◆.

Tertiary Prevention

Tertiary prevention is geared toward the particular health problems experienced by children or adolescents. Generally, there are three aspects to tertiary prevention with children and adolescents: preventing recurrence of problems, preventing further consequences, and, in the case of chronic illness or disability, promoting adjustment.

Preventing Problem Recurrence

Community health nurses may educate parents and children to prevent the recurrence of many health problems experienced by children. For example, the parent

TABLE 16-8 Secondary Prevention Interventions for Child and Adolescent Populations	
Focus	**Interventions**
Screening for health problems	■ Providing routine screening services for children and adolescents ■ Interpreting screening test results for families and making referrals for follow-up diagnosis and treatment ■ Advocating for available and accessible screening services
Caring for minor illness	■ Educating families and the public to recognize signs of minor illness in children and adolescents ■ Educating families and the public regarding home care of minor illness and how to know when professional care is needed ■ Providing or referring for treatment for minor illness when needed ■ Advocating available and accessible services for minor illness care
Caring for children and adolescents with chronic illnesses	■ Educating families and the public regarding signs of chronic illness in children and adolescents ■ Referring individual children and adolescents for diagnosis and treatment of chronic illness ■ Providing case management services for children and adolescents with chronic illness ■ Assisting families to adapt to the care needs of a child or adolescent with chronic illness ■ Teaching children and adolescents and their families for self-management of chronic illness ■ Referring caretakers of children and adolescents with chronic illnesses for respite services ■ Promoting normal growth and development in children with chronic illness ■ Advocating environmental changes to minimize disabilities due to chronic illness ■ Advocating available and accessible diagnostic and treatment services for children and adolescents with chronic illness
Caring for children and adolescents with terminal illness	■ Providing or referring families for palliative care ■ Assisting families with the grief process ■ Referring children and adolescents and their families for support services as needed ■ Initiating bereavement care ■ Advocating available and accessible palliative and bereavement care for children and adolescents and their families

may need information on the relationship of bottle propping to otitis media to prevent subsequent infections. Similarly, education about the need to change diapers frequently, to wash the skin with each diaper change, and to refrain from using harsh soaps to wash diapers may help prevent continued diaper rash. Preventing recurrence of conditions like lead poisoning may require environmental changes and political activity to promote those changes. For adolescents, tertiary prevention may focus on promoting use of contraceptives to prevent subsequent pregnancies, or condom use to prevent recurrent STDs.

Preventing Consequences

Tertiary prevention related to preventing further consequences of health problems is most often employed with children and adolescents who have chronic conditions. For example, the child with diabetes requires attention to diet, exercise, and medication to control the diabetes and prevent physical consequences of the disease itself. At the same time, attention must be given to promoting the child's adjustment to the condition and normalizing his or her life as much as possible. Nursing interventions would be geared toward convincing the child to stick to his or her diet and promoting social interactions with peers.

The nurse might also need to intervene to prevent or minimize the consequences of a child's condition for the rest of the family. For example, the nurse might need to point out to parents that in their concern for the child with a chronic heart condition, they are neglecting the needs of siblings. Tertiary prevention for an infant with AIDS may entail educating parents on the disposal of bodily fluids and excreta to prevent infection of other family members. Tertiary prevention may entail a wide variety of activities on the part of the nurse, from education on how to deal with specific conditions to referral for assistance with major medical expenses. Nurses may also need to act as advocates for children with chronic conditions. The example that most readily comes to mind is the need for advocacy for children with AIDS who are still well enough to attend school.

Emotional support by the nurse is a very important part of tertiary prevention for children with chronic conditions. Parents' and children's feelings about the condition need to be acknowledged and addressed. The nurse can also reinforce positive activities on the part of parent or child. Again, this support may need to be extended as families go through the grieving process. Grieving will probably occur with most chronic illnesses, even those that are not terminal, and the nurse should be prepared to reassure families that their feelings of grief are normal and to support them through this process.

Promoting Adjustment

The community health nurse may also engage in activities that are designed to return the child and family to a relatively normal state of existence. For children or adolescents with chronic illnesses or disabilities, this means restoring function as much as possible, preventing further loss of function, and assisting the child and his or her family to adapt lifestyles and behaviors to the presence of a chronic condition. The community health nurse might accomplish this by encouraging the family to discuss problems posed by the child's condition and to view the condition in the most positive light possible. The nurse should also encourage the family to normalize family life as much as possible. For example, if the Little League activities of a sibling have been curtailed because of an exacerbation of the child's illness, parents should make an attempt to reinstitute those activities as soon as the youngster's condition is stable, or the family can be encouraged to call on members of their support network to take the sibling to baseball practice and games.

With the advent of information technology, adjustment may be fostered by computer-mediated parent support groups. Parents of children with special needs or specific chronic illnesses can find support from parents who experience similar problems. Computer-mediated support groups have been shown to assist parents to find needed assistance and to improve parent–child interactions. In addition, computer-mediated groups have the advantage of eliminating the problem of finding appropriate childcare for a child with special needs that exists with participation in face-to-face support groups (Baum, 2004). Interventions that might be used by community health nurses in tertiary prevention with children and adolescents and their families are presented in Table 16-9◆.

EVALUATING HEALTH CARE FOR CHILD AND ADOLESCENT POPULATIONS

The effectiveness of nursing interventions for the individual child or adolescent is assessed in the same manner that care of any specific client is evaluated. Has intervention fostered the child's growth and development? Is the child's nutrition adequate for normal needs? Is the child up to date on his or her immunizations? Have physical or psychological hazards been eliminated from the child's environment? Is the child receiving health care as needed? Have acute health care problems been resolved?

The community health nurse would also examine the extent to which care has contributed to the adjustment of the child and family to an existing chronic disease or disability. Are parents comfortable and adequately prepared to parent a child with special needs? Do they perform this role adequately? Have complications of the child's condition been prevented?

The community health nurse may also be involved in evaluating the effects of interventions at the aggregate level. This might entail evaluating the extent to

TABLE 16-9	Tertiary Prevention Interventions for Child and Adolescent Populations	
Focus	**Interventions**
Preventing recurrence	▩ Educating children, adolescents, their families, and the public to prevent recurrence of health problems ▩ Advocating societal and environmental changes needed to prevent recurrence of health problems
Preventing consequences	▩ Monitoring and promoting effective disease management for children and adolescents with chronic conditions ▩ Advocating for support services for children and adolescents with chronic conditions ▩ Promoting development of children and adolescents with chronic conditions ▩ Providing or referring for counseling for children and adolescents and their families as needed ▩ Providing emotional support for children, adolescents, and their families ▩ Referring caretakers for respite care as needed
Promoting adjustment	▩ Promoting lifestyle changes consistent with effective disease management ▩ Promoting normal family life as much as possible ▩ Promoting communication within the family and between the family and health care providers ▩ Initiating or referring families to existing support groups ▩ Advocating for societal and environmental changes necessary for effective adjustment to a chronic illness

which national objectives for the health of children and adolescents have been achieved. Evaluative data regarding the status of several of these objectives are summarized below. For the most part, data are derived from the *Healthy People 2010*◆ Web site. As can be seen from the table, a few of the objectives (e.g., those related to low birth weight, preterm birth, and visual impairment) are actually moving away from the targeted levels. Community health nurses might be involved in gathering data related to the status of these objectives in their own communities to evaluate the effectiveness of child and adolescent care.

Community health nursing services for children and adolescents are one of the most effective means of enhancing the health of the population. Community health nurses can educate the public, parents, and children on health-promoting behaviors and provide early intervention for existing health problems to minimize their effects on the health of individual children and on the population during childhood and adolescence and on into adulthood.

HEALTHY PEOPLE 2010

Goals for Population Health◆

OBJECTIVE	MOST RECENT BASELINE	DATA	TARGET
▩ 1-4b. Increase the proportion of children and youth aged 17 years and under who have a specific source of ongoing care	93%	94%	97%
▩ 1-9a. Reduce pediatric hospitalizations for asthma (per 100,000 children)	23.0	21.4	17.3
▩ 6-9. Increase inclusion of children with disabilities in regular education programs	45%	47%	60%
▩ 8-11. Eliminate elevated blood lead levels in children 1 to 5 years of age	4.4%	NDA	0
▩ 9-3. Increase the proportion of females at risk of unintended pregnancy who use contraceptives (age 15 to 19 years)	93%	NDA	100%
▩ 9-7. Reduce pregnancies among adolescent females (per 1,000 girls 15 to17 years of age)	68	NDA	43
▩ 9-10. Increase the proportion of sexually active girls who use effective barrier contraception	68%	NDA	75%
▩ 14-24. Increase the proportion of young children (19 to 35 months) who receive all vaccines that have been recommended for universal administration for at least five years	73%	80.9%	80%
▩ 14-26. Increase the proportion of children who participate in fully operational population-based immunization registers	21%	45%	95%
▩ 15-20. Increase use of child restraints	92%	95%	100%
▩ 15-33. Reduce maltreatment and maltreatment fatalities of children (per 1,000 children)	12.6	12.4	10.3
▩ 15-38. Reduce physical fighting among adolescents	36%	33%	32%
▩ 15-39. Reduce weapon carrying by adolescents on school property	6.9%	6.1%	4.9%
▩ 16-1c. Reduce infant deaths (per 1,000 live births)	7.2	7.0	4.5
▩ 16-2. Reduce child death rates (per 100,000 children)			
a. 1 to 4 years	34.1	31.2	18.6
b. 5 to 9 years	17.2	15.2	13.3

Continued on next page

HEALTHY PEOPLE 2010 *continued*

16-3. Reduce deaths of adolescents (per 100,000)			
a. 10 to 14 years	21.5	19.5	16.8
b. 15 to 19 years	69.5	67.8	39.8
16-10. Reduce			
a. low birth weight	7.6%	7.8%#	5%
b. very low birth weight	1.4%	1.5%#	0.9%
16-11. Reduce preterm births	11.6%	12.1%#	7.6%
16-17. Increase abstinence among pregnant women			
a. alcohol	86%	NDA	94%
b. cigarette smoking	87%	87%	98%
c. illicit drugs	98%	NDA	100%
16-19. Increase the proportion of mothers who breast-feed their babies (at 6 months)	29%	33%	50%
18-2. Reduce the rate of suicide attempts by adolescents (12-month average)	2.6%	2.9%#	1%
19-3. Reduce the proportion of children and adolescents who are overweight or obese (6 to 19 years)	11%	15%#	5%
19-4. Reduce growth retardation in low-income children	8%	8%#	5%
21-2. Reduce untreated dental decay in			
a. 2 to 4 years	16%	NDA	9%
b. 6 to 8 years	29%	NDA	21%
c. adolescents	20%	NDA	15%
22-6. Increase the proportion of physically active adolescents	27%	25%#	30%
26-9. Increase in high school seniors never using			
a. alcohol	19%	23%	29%
b. illicit drugs	46%	49%	56%
27-2. Reduce tobacco use by adolescents (past month)	40%	27%	21%
27-9. Reduce child tobacco exposure at home	20%	NDA	10%
28-4. Reduce blindness and visual impairment in children and adolescents (per 1,000 children)	24	25	20
28-12. Reduce otitis media in children and adolescents (visits per 1,000 children)	344.7	302.9	294

Objectives moving away from the 2010 target

NDA = *No data available for this objective*

Data from: *Centers for Disease Control and Prevention. (2005).* Healthy People Data 2010. *Retrieved August 3, 2005, from http://wonder.cdc.gov/data2010*

Case Study

Promoting Child Health

You have received a referral to visit Mrs. Kwon, a 24-year-old mother with a newborn baby. There is also another child in the family, Mandy, who is 3. Mrs. Kwon's pregnancy and delivery were uneventful, and mother and baby were discharged after 2 days in the hospital. When you make your home visit, Mrs. Kwon tells you that the baby is spitting up an ounce or so of formula after each feeding but had gained almost a pound at her 2-week visit to the pediatrician yesterday. Otherwise, the baby is doing well.

When you first arrive in the home, Mandy is sitting with her back to you watching cartoons on television. The TV is rather loud, and she does not seem to be aware that a visitor has arrived. While you are talking to Mrs. Kwon, Mandy turns around and sees you. She picks up her rag doll and comes to lean against her mother's knee with her thumb in her mouth. She seems to be rather pale compared with her mother's coloring.

Mandy pulls at her mother's sleeve to get her attention. When Mrs. Kwon continues to tell you about the baby spitting up, Mandy hits the infant with her doll. Mrs. Kwon scolds her and then tells you that Mandy used to be a very good girl, but ever since they brought the new baby home, she has been throwing tantrums and sucking her thumb.

1. What biophysical, psychological, sociocultural, behavioral, and health care system factors are influencing the health of these two children? Based on Mandy's pallor, what environmental factor may be present in this situation?
2. What screening tests and immunizations should these two children have had?

3. Based on the data presented above, what are your nursing diagnoses?

4. How could you involve members of the family in planning to resolve the problems identified?

5. What primary, secondary, and/or tertiary preventive measures might you employ with this family?

6. What community resources for child health would be helpful to this family? How would you go about locating them?

7. How would you go about evaluating the effectiveness of your nursing interventions?

Test Your Understanding

1. What is the difference between growth and development? How would you go about assessing each? (p. 384)

2. What are some safety considerations in the care of children and adolescents? (p. 390)

3. Describe at least five primary prevention measures appropriate to all children and adolescents. What modifications might be needed in these measures when caring for a child or adolescent with a chronic or terminal illness or a disability? (pp. 399–405)

4. What are four areas in providing secondary prevention services to children and adolescents? Give an example of a community health nursing intervention related to each. (pp. 405–413)

5. What are the three considerations in tertiary prevention for children and adolescents with existing health problems? Give an example of a community health nursing intervention related to each consideration. (pp. 413–414)

EXPLORE MediaLink

http://www.prenhall.com/clark
Resources for this chapter can be found on the Companion Website.

Audio Glossary
Appendix C: Nursing Interventions for Common Health Problems in Children
Appendix H: Child and Adolescent Health Assessment and Intervention Guide

Exam Review Questions
Case Study: Promoting Children's Health and Safety
MediaLink Application: Adolescent Risk-Taking (video)

Media Links
Challenge Your Knowledge
Update *Healthy People 2010*
Advocacy Interviews

References

Alan Guttmacher Institute. (2002). *Sexual and reproductive health: Women and men.* Retrieved September 18, 2005, from http://www.guttmacher.org/pubs/fb_10-02.html

American Diabetes Association. (n.d.). *National diabetes fact sheet.* Retrieved March 8, 2006, from http://www.diabetes.org/diabetes-statistics/national-diabetes-fact-sheet.jsp

American Medical Association. (2004). *Breaking news: The social and economic impact of ADHD.* Retrieved June 7, 2005, from http://www.ama-assn.org/ama/pub/category/print/12869.html

Averhoff, F., Linton, L., Peddlecord, K. M., Edwards, C., Wang, W., & Fishbein, D. (2004). A middle school immunization law rapidly and substantially increases immunization coverage among adolescents. *American Journal of Public Health, 94,* 978–984.

Baum, L. S. (2004). Internet support groups for primary caregivers of a child with special health care needs. *Pediatric Nursing, 30,* 381–390.

Beck, L. F., Morrow, B., Lipscomb, L. E., & Johnson, C. H. (2002). Prevalence of selected maternal behaviors and experiences, Pregnancy Risk Assessment Monitoring System (PRAMS), 1999. *Morbidity and Mortality Weekly Report, 51*(SS-2), 1–27.

Belson, M., Kieszak, S., Watson, W., Blindauer, K. M., Phan, K., Backer, L., et al. (2003). Childhood pesticide exposures on the Texas-Mexico border: Clinical manifestations and poison center use. *American Journal of Public Health, 93,* 1310–1315.

Bilukha, O., & Rosenstein, N. (2005). Prevention and control of meningococcal disease: Recommendations of the Advisory Committee on Immunization Practices. *Morbidity and Mortality Weekly Report, 54*(RR-7), 1–21.

Blewett, L. A., Davern, M., & Rodin, H. (2004). Covering kids: Variation in health insurance coverage trends by state, 1996–2002; Despite nationwide improvements, variation persists in levels of children's coverage among states. *Health Affairs, 23,* 170–180.

California Department of Health Services. (2001, February 14). *Miniupdate, 1.*

Centers for Disease Control and Prevention. (2002a). Child passenger safety week, February 10–16, 2002. *Morbidity and Mortality Report, 51,* 104.

Centers for Disease Control and Prevention. (2002b). Hepatitis B vaccine. *Morbidity and Mortality Weekly Report, 51,* 33.

Centers for Disease Control and Prevention. (2002c). National poison prevention week, March 17–23, 2002. *Morbidity and Mortality Weekly Report, 51,* 215.

Centers for Disease Control and Prevention. (2004a). Indicators for Chronic Disease Surveillance. *Morbidity and Mortality Weekly Report, 53*(RR-11), 1–114.

Centers for Disease Control and Prevention. (2004b). National Infant Immunization Week, April 25–May 1, 2004. *Morbidity and Mortality Weekly Report, 53,* 290.

Centers for Disease Control and Prevention. (2005a). *Healthy People Data 2010.* Retrieved

August 3, 2005, from http://wonder.cdc.gov/data2010

Centers for Disease Control and Prevention. (2005b). Infant mortality rates, by selected ethnic populations—United States, 2002. *Morbidity and Mortality Weekly Report, 54,* 126.

Centers for Disease Control and Prevention. (2005c). National Infant Immunization Week, April 24–30, 2005. *Morbidity and Mortality Weekly Report, 54,* 361–362.

Centers for Disease Control and Prevention. (2006). Recommended childhood and adolescent immunization schedule—United States, 2006. *Morbidity and Mortality Weekly Report, 54*(51–52), Q-1–Q-4.

Chen, C.-W., Li, C.-Y., & Wang, J.-K. (2004). Growth and development of children with congenital heart disease. *Journal of Advanced Nursing, 47,* 260–269.

Childers, L. (2004). Baby blues. *Nurseweek, 17*(21), 24.

Childers, L. (2005). Caring to the end. *Nurseweek, 18*(11), 14–15.

County of San Diego Health and Human Services Agency. (2004). *Standards of care for the prevention of perinatal HIV transmission in San Diego County.* San Diego: Author.

Crisp, B. R., & Lister, P. G. (2004). Child protection and public health: Nurses' responsibilities. *Journal of Advanced Nursing, 47,* 656–663.

Datar, A., & Sturm, R. (2004). Physical education in elementary school and body mass index: Evidence from the Early Childhood Longitudinal Study. *American Journal of Public Health, 94,* 1501–1506.

Davies, R. (2004). New understandings of parental grief: Literature review. *Journal of Advanced Nursing, 46,* 506–513.

de Montigny, F., & Lacharite, C. (2005). Perceived parental efficacy: Concept analysis. *Journal of Advanced Nursing, 49,* 387–396.

Dilorio, C., Hartwell, T., & Hansen, N. (2002). Childhood sexual abuse and risk behaviors among men at high risk for HIV infection. *American Journal of Public Health, 92,* 214–219.

Division of Adult and Community Health. (2005). Estimated influenza vaccination coverage among adults and children—United States, September 1, 2004–January 31, 2005. *Morbidity and Mortality Weekly Report, 54,* 304–307.

Division of Birth Defects and Developmental Disabilities. (2002). Fetal alcohol syndrome—Alaska, Arizona, Colorado, and New York, 1995–1997. *Morbidity and Mortality Weekly Report, 51,* 433–435.

Division of Human Development and Disability, National Center on Birth Defects and Developmental Disabilities. (2003). Infants tested for hearing loss—United States, 1999–2001. *Morbidity and Mortality Weekly Report, 52,* 981–984.

Division of Reproductive Health. (2002). Infant mortality and low birth weight among black and white infants—United States, 1980–2000. *Morbidity and Mortality Weekly Report, 51,* 589–592.

Division of Reproductive Health. (2004a). Smoking during pregnancy—United States, 1990–2002. *Morbidity and Mortality Weekly Report, 53,* 911–915.

Division of Reproductive Health. (2004b). State estimates of neonatal health-care costs associated with maternal smoking—United States, 1996. *Morbidity and Mortality Weekly Report, 53,* 915–917.

Division of Unintentional Injury Prevention, National Center for Injury Prevention and Control. (2002). Nonfatal choking-related episodes among children—United States, 2001. *Morbidity and Mortality Weekly Report, 51,* 945–948.

Division of Unintentional Injury Prevention, National Center for Injury Prevention and Control. (2004). Child passenger deaths involving drinking drivers—United States, 1997–2002. *Morbidity and Mortality Weekly Report, 53,* 77–79.

Division of Violence Prevention. (2004). Violence-related behaviors among high school students—United States, 1991–2003. *Morbidity and Mortality Weekly Report, 53,* 651–655.

dos Rets, S., Zito, J. M., Safer, D. J., & Soeken, K. L. (2001). Mental health services for youths in foster care and disabled youths. *American Journal of Public Health, 91,* 1094–1099.

Epidemiology and Surveillance Division, National Immunization Program. (2005). Pertussis—United States, 2002–2003. *Morbidity and Mortality Weekly Report, 54,* 1283–1286.

Epidemiology Program Office. (2002). Variation in homicide risk during infancy—United States, 1989–1998. *Morbidity and Mortality Weekly Report, 51,* 187–189.

Epilepsy Foundation. (2005). *Epilepsy and seizure statistics.* Retrieved March 8, 2006, from http://www.efa.org/answerplace/statistics.cfm

Farrelly, M. C., Davis, K. C., Haviland, L., Messeri, P., & Healton, C. G. (2005). Evidence of a dose-response relationship between "truth" antismoking ads and youth smoking prevalence. *American Journal of Public Health, 95,* 425–431.

Federal Interagency Forum on Child and Family Statistics. (2004). *America's Children 2004.* Retrieved June 16, 2005, from http://www.childstats.gov/ac2004

Federwisch, A. (2005). Paying attention: Helping families cope with ADHD. *Nurseweek, 18*(21), 10–12.

Gaffney, K. F. (2001). Infant exposure to environmental tobacco smoke. *Journal of Nursing Scholarship, 33,* 343–347.

Gordon, J. A., Emond, J. A., & Camargo, C. A. Jr. (2005). The State Children's Health Insurance Program: A multicenter trial of outreach through the emergency department. *American Journal of Public Health, 95,* 250–253.

Green, A. (2004). Outcomes of congenital heart disease: A review. *Pediatric Nursing, 30,* 280–284.

Green, S. (2004). The impact of stigma on maternal attitudes toward placement of children with disabilities in residential life care facilities. *Social Science & Medicine, 59,* 799–812.

Grosse, S. D., Boyle, C. A., Botkin, J. R., Comeau, A. M., Kharrazi, M., Rosenfeld, M., et al., (2004). Newborn screening for cystic fibrosis: Evaluation of benefits and risks and recommendations for state newborn screening programs. *Morbidity and Mortality Weekly Report, 53*(RR-13), 1–37.

Grunbaum, J. A., Kann, L., Kinchen, S. A., Williams, B., Ross, J. G., Lowry, R., et al. (2002). Youth Risk Behavior Surveillance—United States, 2001. *Morbidity and Mortality Weekly Report, 51*(SS-4), 1–62.

Holl, J. L., Slack, K. S., & Stevens, A. B. (2005). Welfare reform and health insurance: Consequences for parents. *American Journal of Public Health, 95,* 279–285.

Huey, F. L. (Ed.). (2001). *Global impact of innovations on chronic disease in the genomics era.* New York: Pfizer.

Immunization Services Division, National Immunization Program. (2004). Estimated influenza vaccination coverage among adults and children—United States, September 1–November 30, 2004. *Morbidity and Mortality Weekly Report, 53,* 1147–1153.

Immunization Services Division, National Immunization Program. (2005a). Immunization Information System progress—United States, 2003. *Morbidity and Mortality Weekly Report, 54,* 722–724.

Immunization Services Division, National Immunization Program. (2005b). National, state, and urban area vaccination coverage among children aged 19–35 months—United States, 2004. *Morbidity and Mortality Weekly Report, 54,* 717–721.

Jennings, P. D. (2005). Providing pediatric palliative care through a pediatric supportive care team. *Pediatric Nursing, 31,* 195–200.

Jun, H.-J., Subramanian, S. V., Gortmaker, S., & Kawachi, I. (2004). Socioeconomic disadvantage, parenting responsibility, and women's smoking in the United States. *American Journal of Public Health, 94,* 2170–2176.

Kearney, P. M., & Pryor, J. (2004). The International Classification of Functioning, Disability, and Health (ICF) and nursing. *Journal of Advanced Nursing, 46,* 162–170.

Kempe, A., Beaty, B. L., Steiner, J. F., Pearson, K. A., Lowery, N. D., Daley, M. F., et al. (2004). The regional immunization registry as a public health tool for improving clinical practice and guiding immunization delivery policy. *American Journal of Public Health, 94,* 967–972.

King, C. K., Glass, R., Bresee, J. S., & Duggan, C. (2003). Managing acute gastroenteritis among children: Oral rehydration, maintenance, and nutritional therapy. *Morbidity and Mortality Weekly Report, 52*(RR-16), 1–16.

Klein, R., Stoll, K., & Bruce, A. (2004). *Medicaid: Good medicine for state economies, 2004 update.* Retrieved August 30, 2004, from http://www.families.org

Koniak-Griffin, D., Anderson, N. L. R., Verzemnieks, I., & Brecht, M.-L. (2000). A public health nursing early intervention program for adolescent mothers: Outcomes from pregnancy through 6 weeks postpartum. *Nursing Research, 49,* 130–138.

Kowaleski-Jones, L., & Duncan, G. J. (2002). Effects of participation in the WIC program on birthweight: Evidence from the National Longitudinal Survey of Youth. *American Journal of Public Health, 92,* 799–804.

Kranz, S., Siega-Riz, A. M., & Herring, A. H. (2004). Changes in diet quality of American preschoolers between 1977 and 1998. *American Journal of Public Health, 94,* 1525–1530.

Kreicbergs, U., Valdimarsdottir, U., Onelov, E., Henter, J.-I., & Steineck, G. (2004). Talking about death with children who have severe malignant disease. *New England Journal of Medicine, 351,* 1175–1186.

Krieger, J. W., Takaro, T. K., Song, L., & Weaver, M. (2005). The Seattle-King County Healthy Homes project: A randomized, controlled trial of a community health worker intervention to decrease exposure to indoor asthma triggers. *American Journal of Public Health, 95,* 652–659.

Kuo, F. E., & Taylor, A. F. (2004). A potential natural treatment for attention-deficit/hyperactivity disorder: Evidence from a national study. *American Journal of Public Health, 94,* 1580–1586.

Leslie, L. K., & Stein, M. T. (2003). Attention-deficit hyperactivity disorder. In H. M. Wallace, G. Green, & K. J. Jaros (Eds.), *Health and welfare for families in the 21st century* (2nd ed., pp. 407–421). Sudbury, MA: Jones and Bartlett.

Li, R., Ogden, C., Ballew, C., Gillespie, C., & Grummer-Strawn, L. (2002). Prevalence of exclusive breastfeeding among US infants: The Third National Health and Nutrition Examination Survey (Phase II, 1991–1994). *American Journal of Public Health, 92,* 1107–1112.

Marlow, N., Wolke, D., Bracewell, M. A., & Samara, M. (2005). Neurological and developmental disability at six years of age after extremely preterm birth. *New England Journal of Medicine, 352,* 9–19.

Maternal and Child Health Bureau. (2001). *All aboard the 2010 express.* Rockville, MD: Author.

Meleski, D. D. (2002). Families with chronically ill children: A literature review examines approaches to helping them cope. *American Journal of Nursing, 102*(5), 47–54.

Meyer, P. A., Pivetz, T., Dignam, T. A., Homa, D. M., Schoonover, J., & Brody, D. (2003). Surveillance for elevated blood lead levels among children—United States, 1997–2001. *Morbidity and Mortality Weekly Report, 52*(SS-10), 1–21.

Mofenson, L. M., Oleske, J., Serchuck, L., Van Dyke, R., & Wilfert, C. (2004). Treating opportunistic infections among HIV-exposed and infected children: Recommendations from CDC, the National Institutes of Health, and the Infectious Diseases Society of America. *Morbidity and Mortality Weekly Report, 53*(RR-14), 1–92.

Mu, P.-F. (2005). Paternal reactions to a child with epilepsy: Uncertainty, coping strategies, and depression. *Journal of Advanced Nursing, 49,* 367–376.

National Center for Chronic Disease Prevention and Health Promotion. (2003). Physical activity levels among children aged 9–13 years—United States, 2002. *Morbidity and Mortality Weekly Report, 52,* 785–788.

National Center for Environmental Health. (2005). Elevated blood lead levels in refugee children—New Hampshire, 2003–2004. *Morbidity and Mortality Weekly Report, 54,* 42–46.

National Center for Health Statistics. (2005a). Percentage of children aged < 18 years who have ever had asthma diagnosed by age

group—United States, 2003. *Morbidity and Mortality Weekly Report, 54,* 312.

National Center for Health Statistics. (2005b). Prevalence of overweight among children and teenagers by age group and selected period—United States, 1963–2002. *Morbidity and Mortality Weekly Report, 54,* 203.

National Center for Health Statistics. (2005c). Racial/ethnic disparities in infant mortality—United States, 1995–2002. *Morbidity and Mortality Weekly Report, 54,* 553–556.

National Center for HIV, STD, and TB Prevention. (2002). Progress toward elimination of perinatal HIV infection—Michigan, 1993–2000. *Morbidity and Mortality Weekly Report, 51,* 93–97.

National Center for Injury Prevention and Control. (n.d.a). *Child passenger safety: Fact sheet.* Retrieved June 16, 2005, from http://www.cdc.gov/ncipc/factsheets/childpas.htm

National Center for Injury Prevention and Control. (n.d.b). *Playground injuries: Fact sheet.* Retrieved June 16, 2005, from http://www.cdc.gov/ncipc/factsheets/playgr.htm

National Center for Injury Prevention and Control. (n.d.c). *Poisonings: Fact sheet.* Retrieved June 16, 2005, from http://www.cdc.gov/ncipc/factsheets/poisoning.htm

National Center for Injury Prevention and Control. (n.d.d). *Water-related injuries: Fact sheet.* Retrieved June 16, 2005, from http://www.cdc.gov/ncipc/factsheets/drown.htm

National Center for Injury Prevention and Control. (2004a). *Child maltreatment: Fact sheet.* Retrieved June 16, 2005, from http://www.cdc.gov/ncipc/factsheets/cmfacts.htm

National Center for Injury Prevention and Control. (2004b). Nonfatal and fatal drownings in recreational water settings—United States, 2001–2002. *Morbidity and Mortality Weekly Report, 53,* 447–452.

National Center for Injury Prevention and Control. (2005). Nonfatal motor-vehicle-related backover injuries among children—United States, 2001–2003. *Morbidity and Mortality Weekly Report, 54,* 144–146.

National Center on Birth Defects and Developmental Disabilities. (2002). Alcohol use among women of childbearing age—United States, 1991–1999. *Morbidity and Mortality Weekly Report, 51,* 273–276.

National Center on Birth Defects and Developmental Disabilities. (2003). Fetal alcohol syndrome—South Africa, 2001. *Morbidity and Mortality Weekly Report, 52,* 660–662.

National Center on Birth Defects and Developmental Disabilities. (2004a). *ADHD: Attention-deficit/hyperactivity disorder.* Retrieved June 16, 2005, from http://www.cdc.gov/ncbddd/adhd/injury.htm

National Center on Birth Defects and Developmental Disabilities. (2004b). *Cerebral palsy.* Retrieved June 16, 2005, from http://www.cdc.gov/ncbddd/dd.ddcp.htm

National Center on Birth Defects and Developmental Disabilities. (2004c). Economic costs associated with mental retardation, cerebral palsy, hearing loss, and vision impairment—United States, 2003. *Morbidity and Mortality Weekly Report, 53,* 57–59.

National Center on Birth Defects and Developmental Disabilities. (2004d). *Fetal alcohol*

syndrome. Retrieved June 16, 2005, from http://www.cdc.gov/ncbddd/fas/fasask.htm

National Center on Birth Defects and Developmental Disabilities. (2004e). *Mental retardation.* Retrieved June 16, 2005, from http://www.cdc.gov/ncbddd/dd/ddmr.htm

National Center on Birth Defects and Developmental Disabilities. (2005). *Autism.* Retrieved June 16, 2005, from http://www.cdc.gov/ncbddd/autism/asd_common.htm

National Diabetes Information Clearinghouse. (n.d.) *National diabetes statistics.* Retrieved June 16, 2005, from http://diabetes.niddk.nih.gov/dm/pubs/statistics/index.htm

National Immunization Program. (2004). Vaccination coverage among children entering school—United States, 2003–2004 school year. *Morbidity and Mortality Weekly Report, 53,* 1041–1044.

National Immunization Program. (2005). Hepatitis A vaccination coverage among children aged 24–35 months—United States, 2003. *Morbidity and Mortality Weekly Report, 54,* 141–144.

National Institutes for Mental Health. (2003). *Attention deficit hyperactivity disorder.* Retrieved March 8, 2006, from http://www.nimh.nih.gov/publications/NIMHadhdpub.pdf

National Program for Playground Safety. (2005). *Playground-related statistics.* Retrieved June 16, 2005, from http://www.playgroundsafety.org/resources/statistics.htm

Navaie-Waliser, M., Misener, M., Mersman, C., & Lincoln, P. (2004). Evaluating the needs of children with asthma in home care: The vital role of nurses as caregivers and educators. *Public Health Nursing, 21,* 306–315.

Neumark-Sztainer, D., Story, M., Hannan, P. J., & Croll, J. (2002). Overweight status and eating patterns among adolescents: Where do youths stand in comparison with the *Healthy People 2010* objectives? *American Journal of Public Health, 92,* 844–851.

Newacheck, P. W., & Benjamin, A. E. (2004). Intergenerational equity and public spending; The United States should embrace a new doctrine of fairness to ensure that vulnerable populations are not forced to compete for resources. *Health Affairs, 23,* 142–146.

Nicholas, S. W., Jean-Louis, B., Ortiz, B., Northridge, M., Shoemaker, K., Vaughan, R., et al. (2005). Addressing the childhood asthma crisis in Harlem: The Harlem Children's Zone Asthma Initiative. *American Journal of Public Health, 95,* 245–249.

Nisbet, C. (2004, Summer). Human milk for the very low birthweight infant. *Perinatal Care Matters,* pp. 1–2.

Nystrom, K., & Ohrling, K. (2004). Parenthood experiences during the child's first year: Literature review. *Journal of Advanced Nursing, 46,* 319–330.

O'Connor, M. E., Maddocks, B., Modie, C., & Pierce, H. (2001). The effect of different definitions of a patient on immunization assessment. *American Journal of Public Health, 91,* 1273–1275.

Oddy, W. H., Sherriff, J. L., de Klerk, N. H., Kendall, G. E., Sly, P. D., Beilin, L. J., et al. (2004). The relation of breastfeeding and body mass index to asthma and atopy in children: A prospective cohort study to age 6 years. *American Journal of Public Health, 94*, 1531–1537.

Office on Smoking and Health, National Center for Health Promotion and Disease Prevention. (2005a). Annual smoking-attributable mortality, years of potential life lost, and productivity losses—United States, 1997–2002. *Morbidity and Mortality Weekly Report, 54*(RR-7), 1–21.

Office on Smoking and Health, National Center for Health Promotion and Disease Prevention. (2005b). Tobacco use, access, and exposure to tobacco in media among middle and high school students—United States, 2004. *Morbidity and Mortality Weekly Report, 54*, 297–301.

Olsen, R., & Maslin-Prothero, P. (2001). Dilemmas in the provision of own-home respite support for parents of young children with complex health care needs: Evidence from an evaluation. *Journal of Advanced Nursing, 34*, 603–610.

Regional Perinatal Programs of California. (2004, Summer). Breastfeeding decreases infant mortality. *Perinatal Care Matters*, p. 2.

Rodwin, V. G., & Neuberg, L. G. (2005). Infant mortality and income in 4 world cities: New York, London, Paris, and Tokyo. *American Journal of Public Health, 95*, 86–90.

Rowe, A. K., Onikpo, F., Lama, M., Cokou, F., & Deming, M. S. (2001). Management of childhood illness at health facilities in Benin: Problems and their causes. *American Journal of Public Health, 91*, 1625–1635.

Santacroce, S. J. (2003). Parental uncertainty and posttraumatic stress in serious childhood illness. *Journal of Nursing Scholarship, 35*, 45–51.

Shirai, T., Matsui, T., Suzuki, K., & Chida, K. (2005). Effect of pet removal on pet allergic asthma. *Chest, 127*, 1565–1571.

Simons-Morton, B. G., Hartos, J. L., Leaf, W. A., & Preusser, D. F. (2005). Persistence of effects of the checkpoints program on parental restrictions of teen driving privileges. *American Journal of Public Health, 95*, 447–452.

Singh, I. (2004). Doing their jobs: Mothering with Ritalin in a culture of mother-blame. *Social Science & Medicine, 59*, 1193–1205.

Starfield, B. (2004). U.S. child health: What's amiss, and what should be done about it?; A strong primary care infrastructure is key to improving and reducing disparities in children's health. *Health Affairs, 23*, 165–170.

Strauss, L. T., Herndon, J., Chang, J., Parker, W. Y., Bowens, S. V., Zane, S. B., et al. (2004). Abortion surveillance—United States, 2001. *Morbidity and Mortality Weekly Report, 53*(SS-9), 1–32.

Strazdins, L., Korda, R. J., Lim, L. L.-Y., Broom, D. H., & D'Souza, R. M. (2004). Around-the-clock: Parent work schedules and children's well-being in a 24-h economy. *Social Science & Medicine, 59*, 1517–1527.

Sullivan-Bolyai, S., Knafl, K., Tamborlane, W., & Grey, M. (2004). Parents' reflections on managing their children's diabetes with insulin pumps. *Journal of Nursing Scholarship, 36*, 316–323.

Svavarsdottir, E. K. (2005). Caring for a child with cancer. *Journal of Advanced Nursing, 50*, 153–161.

Svavarsdottir, E. K., & Rayens, M. K. (2005). Hardiness in families of young children with asthma. *Journal of Advanced Nursing, 50*, 381–390.

Thorpe, L. E., List, D. G., Marx, T., May, L., Helgerson, S. D., & Frieden, T. R. (2004). Childhood obesity in New York City elementary school students. *American Journal of Public Health, 94*, 1496–1500.

Trust for America's Health. (2004). *Closing the vaccination gap: A shot in the arm for childhood immunization programs*. Retrieved September 28, 2004, from http://www.healthyamericans.org

United Nations Population Fund. (2003). *State of world population 2003: Making 1 billion count: Investing in adolescents' health and rights*. Geneva, Switzerland: Author.

U.S. Census Bureau. (2004a). *Poverty: 2003 highlights*. Retrieved September 30, 2004, from http://www.census.gov

U.S. Census Bureau. (2004b). *Statistical abstract of the United States: 2004–2005*. Retrieved May 12, 2005, from http://www.census.gov/prod/2004pubs/04statab

U.S. Department of Health and Human Services. (2002). Children's mental health is national priority. *Prevention Report, 16*(2), 5–6.

Wakschlag, L. S., Pickett, K. E., Cook, E. Jr., Benowitz, N. L., & Leventhal, B. L. (2002). Maternal smoking during pregnancy and severe antisocial behavior in offspring: An overview. *American Journal of Public Health, 92*, 966–974.

Wang, K.-W. K, & Barnard, A. (2004). Technology-dependent children and their families: A review. *Journal of Advanced Nursing, 45*, 36–46.

Warren, P. L. (2005). First-time mothers: Social support and confidence in infant care. *Journal of Advanced Nursing, 50*, 479–488.

Wise, P. (2004). The transformation of child health in the United States; Social disparities in child health persist despite dramatic improvements in child health overall. *Health Affairs, 23*, 9–25.

Wolfe, L. (2004). Should parents speak with a dying child about impending death? *New England Journal of Medicine, 351*, 1251–1253.

World Health Organization. (2004). *The world health report*. Geneva, Switzerland: Author.

Meeting the Health Needs of Women

CHAPTER OBJECTIVES

After reading this chapter, you should be able to:

1. Identify at least two factors in each of the dimensions of health as they relate to the health of women.
2. Identify health problems common to women.
3. Describe at least three unique considerations in assessing the health needs of lesbian, bisexual, and transgender clients.
4. Identify concerns in primary prevention for women and analyze the role of the community health nurse with respect to each.
5. Describe areas of secondary prevention activity with women and design community health nursing interventions related to each.
6. Describe two elements of secondary prevention of physical abuse of women and analyze the role of the community health nurse in addressing abuse.
7. Describe at least two actions that the community health nurse can take to provide more sensitive and effective care to lesbian, bisexual, and transgender clients.

KEY TERMS

MediaLink

Additional interactive resources for this chapter can be found on the Companion Website. Click on Chapter 17 and "Begin" to select the activities for this chapter.

Advocacy in Action

Breast Cancer Screening among Older African Americans

A group of eight nursing students in a Midwestern city had their public health clinical experience in a high-rise apartment building for low-income disabled seniors, most of whom were African American. When they interviewed several female residents, the students found that many of the women had not had a mammogram in several years, and some had never had a mammogram. Most of these women were older and had limited mobility. Several of them were in wheelchairs, and most had difficulty finding affordable transportation.

The students decided that finding mammogram services for this population would be an appropriate intervention and began calling area hospitals to see if mammography services 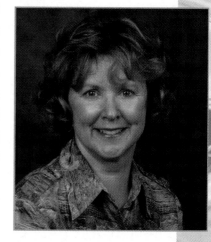 were wheelchair accessible and if transportation was available for clients. They found one hospital with wheelchair-accessible services, but no transportation. The students continued calling until they had reached every mammogram resource in the metropolitan area. Finally they located a wheelchair-accessible mammogram van that would come to the apartment building, but it was booked for the next three months. After conferring with leaders in the apartment community, they set a date for the mammogram van. The nurse manager of the mammogram van was delighted to provide services to a population that had been considered "hard to reach."

The students publicized the date of the mammogram van visit. They called on residents in their apartments to explain the procedure, teach self-breast examination, and preregister the women according to scheduled appointments. The students faxed registrations to the mammogram office and obtained missing information, such as Medicare and Medicaid numbers, and birth dates when needed. The semester was over by the date of the mammogram van's visit to the apartment complex. With cooperation from instructors in the two classes, the students incorporated this activity into a community health project class they took the subsequent semester. On the day the mammogram van was at the apartment, the students were present to assist residents in getting to the van and completing the procedure.

This work occurred in the spring of 2004. As a result of the students' advocacy, the mammogram van now visits the apartment complex yearly. The women living in the apartments are supporting the mammogram van and bring their female friends and family for testing.

Sheila Adams-Leander, RN, MSN

Doisy College of Health Sciences

School of Nursing, Saint Louis University

Women's health is defined as "health and illness issues that are unique to or more prevalent or serious in women, have causes or manifestations specific to women, and occur across the life span and within the context of women's lives" (U.S. Department of Health and Human Services [USD-HHS], n.d., pp. 1–2). The Department of Health and Human Services acknowledged the ongoing contribution of nursing to the health care of women in the following words: "Members of the nursing profession have a long tradition of providing health services to women. From the inception of modern nursing to the present, nurses have been concerned with promoting the health of women and their families" (p. 1).

Although nursing education has long prepared nurses to care for women and their health concerns, a study by the American Association of Colleges of Nursing identified several areas related to women's health that should receive greater attention in nursing curricula. These areas included cultural competence in communicating with women, lesbian issues, women with disabilities, and specific prevention of a variety of conditions that affect women (USDHHS, n.d.). Although many of these conditions also affect men, there is a need for interventions tailored to addressing these conditions in the context of women's lives. Specific recommendations for nursing curricula related to women's health included:

- Examination of gender-specific communication styles and cultural competence in communicating with women clients
- Attention to the health consequences of trauma experienced by women
- Gender-specific health care decision making
- Issues of physical activity and nutrition as they relate to women's health
- Sex and gender differences in the development, manifestation, and treatment of specific conditions
- Lesbian and gay health issues
- Health issues posed by disability in women (USDHHS, n.d.)

In 2003 there were more than 87 million women between 20 and 64 years of age in the United States, roughly 30% of the population (U.S. Census Bureau, 2005). By 2050 the number of women in this age group is expected to grow to 93.2 million, but the percentage of young and middle adult women is expected to remain about the same, while the percentage of older women will increase significantly. Women have unique health care needs, not only because of their anatomy and reproductive functions, but also because of their vulnerability within society. Women live longer than men and experience more chronic health problems. Women also tend to have fewer resources with which to address health care

problems than men. Community health nursing services to women can greatly improve the health of the overall population.

The importance of improving the health of women in the United States is reflected in the national health objectives for the year 2010. Multiple objectives specifically target the health needs of women (USDHHS, 2000). These objectives can be viewed by accessing the *Healthy People 2010*◆ Web site at http://www.healthypeople.gov. Selected objectives are included at the end of this chapter.

This chapter addresses care of young adult and middle adult women. The health needs of older women are the focus of Chapter 19∞.

THE EPIDEMIOLOGY OF WOMEN'S HEALTH

Factors influencing women's health status occur in each of the six dimensions of health. In this chapter, we will briefly examine factors in the biophysical, psychological, physical environmental, sociocultural, behavioral, and health system dimensions that contribute to health and illness among women.

Biophysical Considerations

Biophysical factors are of concern to the community health nurse working to improve the health of women in the community. Specific areas for consideration include genetic inheritance, maturation and aging, and physiologic function.

Genetic Inheritance

Women are prone to a number of genetically related or genetically linked conditions. For example, cancers of the breast have been shown to occur more frequently among women whose mothers, sisters, aunts, or grandmothers have had similar cancers. Similarly, diseases of the thyroid gland seem to occur more frequently among women than men, as do diabetes, asthma, various forms of dermatitis, and hay fever–type allergies, all of which may involve genetic predisposition to disease.

ETHICAL AWARENESS

Approximately one in every 2,000 babies born each year in the United States has both male and female physical or hormonal characteristics. Genital reassignment surgery is performed on 100 to 200 of these babies each year (Sember, 2000). Since parents do not know what gender identity the child will adopt in later life, do you think they should wait until the child is old enough to participate in the decision to have surgery performed? Why or why not? If surgery is performed in infancy, should the child be informed? Why or why not? If yes, when should the child be informed?

Maturation and Aging

In general, physical maturation of females follows the developmental schedule typical of children. Sexual maturation, however, follows a unique trajectory in women. Stages of sexual maturation and the relevant time periods are presented in Table 17-1◆. Menarche was addressed in Chapter 16∞. As noted in Chapter 16∞, menarche in some societies is met with female genital mutilation, and community health nurses should be aware of the extent to which women in the community may have been subjected to this practice.

Premenopause is the period of a woman's life in which she is most likely to become pregnant. These childbearing years generally last from menarche to age 40, when women enter the perimenopausal period. In 2003, approximately 72% of young and middle adult women, or 22% of the total U.S. population, were of childbearing age (U.S. Census Bureau, 2005).

Menstruation during premenopause is usually free of medical complications; however, 3% to 5% of women may be affected by **premenstrual dysphoric disorder (PMDD)**, a condition of depressed mood and irritability severe enough to interfere with interpersonal relationships and everyday activities. PMDD usually begins in late adolescence and may worsen with age (Eli Lilly and Company, 2004d).

Perimenopause is a transition period between premenopause and menopause, when the physical and hormonal changes that herald cessation of menstruation occur. Perimenopause may last from 3 to 9 years, but the average is 4 years. Anywhere from 20 to 50 million U.S. women will experience menopause in the next decade and are currently in the perimenopausal stage (Lewis, 2004; McGinley, 2004). Perimenopause is characterized by less predictability regarding menstrual cycles in terms of frequency, duration, and amount of bleeding. Perimenopause may also be associated with a variety of vasomotor symptoms, sleep disturbance, anxiety, and depression. The psychological distress that sometimes accompanies perimenopause is more common in the early perimenopausal period and diminishes after

menopause (Bromberger et al., 2001). Hormone replacement therapy may be effective in addressing the discomforts of the perimenopausal period. Some herbal preparations, such as black cohosh and plant phytogens, may also be used to deal with the symptoms associated with perimenopause, and community health nurses should be aware of the extent to which these preparations are used by women in the community, as well as their knowledge about potential adverse effects of use (American College of Obstetricians and Gynecologists, 2001; Wilson, 2004). There is some evidence to suggest that the discomforts experienced by some women during perimenopause are, at least in part, a function of cultural expectations. For this reason, community health nurses should also explore cultural beliefs, attitudes, and behaviors related to perimenopause and menopause among women in the community. The effects of perimenopause may also arise from socioeconomic factors in women's lives, but it is at present unknown how much psychological distress is the result of hormonal changes and how much derives from socioeconomic and cultural influences (Bromberger et al., 2001).

Menopause is the cessation of menstruation that occurs with advancing age. Menopause has occurred when the woman has been without menses for 12 months. The average age for menopause is 50 years, but normal menopause can occur as early as age 40. Some women experience menopause as a result of surgical interventions such as hysterectomy. Early menopause may be associated with increased health problems such as osteoporosis and increased mortality risk. In at least one study of African American women, early menopause has been associated with smoking, overweight, and oral contraceptive use (Palmer, Rosenberg, Wise, Horton, & Adams-Campbell, 2003).

Postmenopause extends from menopause until death and may cover as much as one third of women's lives (Lewis, 2004). Because of the hormonal changes that occur with menopause, the postmenopausal period is a time of increased risk for a number of health problems. Several of these, such as osteoporosis and heart disease, are discussed in the section addressing physiologic function. Community health nurses may engage in advocacy to change negative social attitudes toward perimenopausal and menopausal women. Conversely, they may assist women to deal effectively with the effects of these negative attitudes as well as the physical discomforts of menopause. Finally, community health nurses can be actively involved in educating women to minimize the negative effects of menopausal changes (e.g., bone loss) on their health.

Other areas for consideration with respect to maturation and aging include the effects of aging in general on health status (which will be addressed in Chapter 19∞) and women's emotional maturation.

TABLE 17-1	Stages of Sexual Maturation in Women
Stage	**Typical Time Frame**
Prepuberty	Birth to menarche
Menarche	Time of first menstruation (typically around age 13 years)
Premenopause	Reproductive years, potential for childbearing
Perimenopause	Transitional period 3 to 9 years prior to menopause (typically begins about age 40)
Menopause	Achieved after 12 consecutive months without menstruation (typically around age 50)
Postmenopause	Menopause to death (may be as much as a third of life)

Physiologic Function

Physiologic function is another biophysical consideration influencing the health of women as a population group. Specific considerations in this area include the incidence and prevalence of specific illnesses and functional limitations, reproductive issues of pregnancy and infertility, and immunization levels.

PHYSICAL ILLNESS AND DISABILITY Women are affected by a variety of acute and chronic illnesses that may not occur in men (e.g., uterine cancer), have different risk factors and manifestations than the same diseases in men, or may require different approaches to treatment than the same diseases in men. Women are more likely than men to experience multiple chronic diseases and to be disabled as a result of them. In addition, physiologic differences in drug metabolism between men and women lead to differences in treatment effects (Huey, 2001). Several conditions and their effects on women will be discussed here. In addition, women are more likely to experience disability with chronic conditions than men, so the prevalence and effects of disability in women are also examined.

The leading causes of mortality in U.S. women in 2002 were (a) heart disease, (b) cancer, (c) stroke, (d) chronic lower respiratory diseases, (e) Alzheimer's disease, (f) diabetes, (g) accidents, (h) pneumonia and influenza, (i) nephritis, nephrotic syndrome, and nephrosis, and (j) septicemia (Centers for Disease Control and Prevention [CDC], 2004a).

More than 356,000 deaths occurred among U.S. women in 2002 as a result of heart disease (CDC, 2004a). Women are more likely than men to die within one year of myocardial infarction (MI) and are more likely to have a second MI. In 2002, the age-adjusted rate for heart disease mortality among U.S. women was 197 per 100,000 women. Although this is a significant decrease from the 1950 rate of 484.7 per 100,000 women, considerable work remains to be done in preventing heart disease in women. The 2002 cerebrovascular mortality rate for women in the United States was 55.2 per 100,000 women compared to 175.8 per 100,000 in 1950 (CDC, 2004a). Although breast cancer is often considered the most serious illness for women, approximately half of women will eventually die as a result of heart disease or stroke compared to only 1 in 30 women who will die from breast cancer. An estimated 83% of women are considered at risk for heart disease, yet only 26% have been diagnosed as at risk or consider themselves at risk (Wilson, 2002). More than a third of women have multiple risk factors for heart disease and stroke (Division of Adult and Community Health, 2005b). Community health nurses can advocate for conditions that prevent premature mortality among women as well as for effective health care services to address the conditions that contribute to mortality.

Chronic Illness   Other conditions affecting women may not cause death but contribute to significant morbidity. Leading worldwide causes of physical morbidity in women include heart disease, HIV infection, osteoarthritis, cerebrovascular disease, diabetes, and rheumatoid arthritis. Some risk factors for heart disease include hypertension, elevated cholesterol levels, and obesity, all of which are present in significant numbers of women. From 1999 to 2002, for example, more than one fourth (25.7%) of U.S. women 20 to 74 years of age had hypertension, compared to only 20% in the 1988–1994 period. During the same period, 17% of women had high cholesterol levels. This latter figure, however, indicates some effect of public health interventions to lower cholesterol levels, being slightly less than half of the proportion of women affected in 1960 to 1962 (35.6%). The prevalence of overweight and obesity among women, however, is not as encouraging. Prevalence of overweight in women increased more than 50% from 40.2% in the 1960–1962 period to 61.7% in the 1999–2002 period. Obesity more than doubled in the same time period from 15.7% of U.S. women to 34% (National Center for Health Statistics [NCHS], 2005a). These and other risk factors for cardiovascular disease are discussed in more detail in Chapter 29 ∞.

Although breast and cervical cancer mortality has declined considerably in recent years, cancer remains a significant health problem for women. Approximately one third of women will receive a diagnosis of cancer at some time in their lives (CDC, 2004b). In 2002, the U.S. mortality rate for women for all cancers was 163.1 per 100,000 women. For breast cancer, the rate was 25.6 per 100,000 women, a decrease from 31.9 in 1950. Lung cancer deaths among women, on the other hand, have increased nearly eightfold since 1950, rising from 5.8 per 100,000 women to 41.6 in 2002 (CDC, 2004a). Uterine cancer remains the most common reproductive cancer in women, with differential mortality among some groups. For example, although the incidence of uterine cancer in Black women is 31% higher than in White women, mortality is 84% higher (Madison, Schottenfeld, James, Schwartz, & Gruber, 2004). More than 12,000 new diagnoses of cervical cancer are made each year, and cervical cancer results in 4,400 deaths per year. This is considerably lower than in the past due to widespread screening with Papanicolaou smears (CDC, 2004b). Community health nurses may be active advocates for the availability of cancer screening services for women, particularly among older women and those from ethnic minority groups. They may also educate women regarding the need for cancer screening.

Chronic pulmonary diseases, including asthma and its underlying conditions, are also major contributors to death and disability in women. In 2002, the age-adjusted mortality rate for chronic lower respiratory diseases was 37.4 per 100,000 women, more than two and a half times the 1980 rate of 14.9 per 100,000 women (CDC,

MediaLink   Case Study: Promoting Women's Health

2004a). In 2000, the prevalence of self-reported emphysema or chronic bronchitis among adult women was more than one and a half times that for men and had increased by nearly 36% from 1980. In addition, the rate of hospitalization for chronic obstructive pulmonary disease increased from 38.2 per 10,000 women in 1980 to 40.2 in 2000, an increase of 281,000 actual hospitalizations (Mannino, Homa, Akinbami, Ford, & Redd, 2002).

Nearly 6% of women in the United States have a diagnosis of diabetes, and another 2.3% have undiagnosed diabetes (CDC, 2004a). This amounts to a little over 9 million women. From 1990 to 2000, the prevalence of diabetes in women increased 50%, with rates among ethnic minority women twice those of White women (National Center for Chronic Disease Prevention and Health Promotion, 2002). Women represent slightly over half (52%) of all persons with diabetes in the United States (Division of Diabetes Translation, 2002).

Diabetes contributes to significant mortality and morbidity among women. For example, women aged 25 to 44 years with diabetes have three times the mortality of women without diabetes. Diabetes is also a significant contributing factor for cardiovascular disease, chronic renal failure, and blindness. Women with diabetes from 45 to 64 years of age have three times the risk for cardiovascular disease as those without diabetes, and diabetes more often leads to cardiovascular disease in women than men. Women with diabetes also have a worse prognosis in cardiovascular disease than men (National Center for Chronic Disease Prevention and Health Promotion, 2002).

Gestational diabetes mellitus (GDM) occurs in 2.5% to 4% of all pregnancies in the United States. GDM is reflected in abnormally high blood glucose levels as a result of pregnancy. Anywhere from 5% to 10% of women with gestational diabetes are diagnosed as having type 2 diabetes after delivery, and another 20% to 50% go on to develop type 2 diabetes in the next 5 to 10 years. Children born to mothers with gestational diabetes also have a greater risk than other children of developing type 2 diabetes later in life. Among women with diabetes at the time of pregnancy, poor disease control, particularly during the first trimester, leads to complications including spontaneous abortion and congenital abnormalities in the infant (National Center for Chronic Disease Prevention and Health Promotion, 2002).

Rheumatoid arthritis is the most common chronic condition in women, and women have a higher prevalence of arthritis than men. In 2002, arthritis affected nearly 28% of U.S. women and only 18% of men (Division of Adult and Community Health, 2005c). Approximately 23% of U.S. women over 40 years of age experience some activity limitation as a result of arthritis (National Women's Law Center et al., 2000).

Human immunodeficiency virus (HIV) infection and acquired immune deficiency syndrome (AIDS) are other diseases that affect large numbers of women. Although initially a disease of gay men, the percentage of women with active cases of AIDS has tripled in the last decade (National Women's Law Center et al., 2000), and women are the fastest-growing group with new HIV infections worldwide. In 1999, for example, 15,000 new infections occurred each day, 40% of which occurred in women (Maman et al., 2002). In 2002, the U.S. age-adjusted female mortality rate for AIDS was 2.5 per 100,000 women (down from 5.3 per 100,000 in 1995). HIV/AIDS mortality rates per 100,000 U.S. women ranged from 0.4 for those 15 to 24 years of age to 6.7 for women aged 35 to 44 years. In 2003, the incidence rate for new cases of AIDS was 9 per 100,000 women 13 years of age and older (CDC, 2004a), and women comprised 28% of people in the United States with HIV infection or AIDS (Division of HIV/AIDS Prevention, 2005). Advocacy by community health nurses is needed to increase efforts to protect women from HIV infection, particularly in cultural groups where women are not empowered to insist on condom use by their partners. Community health nurses may also advocate for available screening and treatment services for women.

Osteoporosis is another physiologic condition of concern for women during the perimenopausal and postmenopausal years. **Osteoporosis** is a common metabolic bone disease characterized by a loss of bone minerals that weakens bones so that fractures occur more easily. Approximately 8 million U.S. women and 2 million men have osteoporosis, and another 3 million are at high risk for the disease (Curry & Hogstel, 2002). Peak bone mass occurs at about 25 years of age, and loss of 0.5% to 1% of bone mass per year begins at about age 40. Osteoporosis has a variety of causes, including long-term use of certain medications (e.g., steroids, anticonvulsants), genetic disorders such as hemophilia and thalassemia, vitamin D deficiency, hypercalciuria, Cushing's syndrome, hyperthyroidism, type 1 diabetes, chronic liver disease, and Crohn's and celiac diseases. Other conditions that may lead to osteoporosis include gastrectomy, multiple myeloma, lymphoma and leukemia, anorexia nervosa, rheumatoid arthritis, and chronic renal failure (Shepherd, 2004). Chemotherapy for breast cancer, small frame, low body weight or increased height, family history of osteoporosis, and Caucasian or Asian ancestry are other risks for osteoporosis for some women (*Excellence in Clinical Practice*, 2000; McGinley, 2004; Shepherd, 2004).

For women, loss of bone mass is accelerated during and after menopause, and continuing loss may occur at rates of 2% to 4% per year after menopause (McGinley, 2004). As much as one third of bone mass may be lost in the first 6 years after menopause (Eli Lilly and Company, 2004c). Loss of bone mass may be influenced by lifestyle factors such as caffeine intake, use of long-acting sedatives, physical inactivity, smoking, and low calcium intake (McGinley, 2004; Shepherd, 2004). Prevalence of osteoporosis increases with age, with approximately half of women over age 45 years and 90% of those over 75 years affected (McGinley, 2004).

Osteoporosis is the leading cause of fractures in adult women. In the United States osteoporosis contributes to 1.5 million fractures each year. Similar figures for the United Kingdom stand at 200,000 osteoporotic fractures per year (Sandison, Gray, & Reid, 2004). Annual U.S. costs are estimated at $14 billion (McGinley, 2004), with estimated costs of £1.7 billion per year in the United Kingdom. Approximately 50% of women lose their independence following a hip fracture, and 20% die within 6 months (Sandison et al., 2004).

Disability in Women   In addition to causing mortality and morbidity in the population, many of the conditions discussed above, as well as others, contribute to disability among women. As we saw in Chapter 16 ∞, disability results from an interaction between a person's functional abilities and the environment. In 2002, 12.3% of U.S. women experienced some limitation of activity due to chronic conditions (U.S. Census Bureau, 2005). The prevalence of limitation increased with age, with only 6.3% of those 18 to 44 years of age affected, compared to 13.7% of women in the next decade of life, and 21.1% of those aged 55 to 64 years (CDC, 2004a). This amounts to approximately 30 million American women living with disabling conditions. These women have what has been described as a "thinner margin of health" because routine health problems may cause greater difficulty for them than for women without disability (Jones & Bell, 2004).

Studies of women with disability have found that they tend to define health in terms of functional capacity. In one study, personal factors contributing to impairment and stress included weakness, fatigue, recurring symptoms, memory problems, and aphasia. Environmental factors included the inability to care for children, insufficient help with personal care, income insufficient to address illness-related needs, and the need to live with one's parents. Lack of spontaneity was an additional effect of disability reported by women in the study because of the need to plan activities around the limitations imposed by their disability (Nosek et al., 2004).

A review of related literature indicated that women with disabilities tend to experience difficulties in five major areas: physical function, coping, self-care, roles and relationships, and sociocultural issues (O'Neill & Morrow, 2001). Women with disabilities report more symptoms, more chronic illnesses, and poorer perceptions of personal health than men. Physical functional ability and levels of fatigue are often used as a measure of health, and women often have inaccurate perceptions of symptoms and their meaning, leading them to engage in ineffective control of their physical disease.

Coping, in the context of chronic illness and disability, is defined as a "cognitive process whereby people learn to tolerate the effects of illness" (O'Neill & Morrow, 2001, p. 263). People with disabilities generally engage in two types of coping: problem-focused and emotion-focused. Problem-focused coping involves management or alteration of the source of stress, whereas emotion-focused coping involves managing one's emotional response to the stressor. Coping may also be characterized by active/confrontive or passive/avoidance strategies. In active/confrontive coping, one faces the problem and attempts to develop a viable solution. Some of the strategies used in active coping include positive reappraisal, distancing, seeking spiritual guidance, and exerting self-control. Passive or avoidance coping involves verbal expression of distress to reduce tension and may employ strategies such as denial, hoping for change, and hoping for a miracle. Avoidance coping has been linked to worse psychosocial adjustment in the face of disability. In general, women are more likely to use confrontive than passive strategies except in the face of severe functional disability or the presence of frightening symptoms. Whatever style of coping employed, women with disability tend to have more depression and lower quality of life scores than men, most likely because of differences in the availability of economic resources to deal with the consequences of disability (O'Neill & Morrow, 2001).

With respect to self-care, women often have difficulty managing chronic illness and disability. Strategies for self-care include both symptom control strategies and mechanisms for mobilizing resources. Women have been found to exhibit few behavioral strategies to control symptoms, but have wider social networks and more social support than men. Women with disabilities may have particular difficulty incorporating health promotion strategies into their disease management plan. For example, men with chronic conditions are twice as likely as women to engage in exercise (O'Neill & Morrow, 2001). In part this may be due to the reported failure of health care providers to discuss strategies for health promotion with women experiencing disabilities.

Interpersonal relationships appear to be more important to women than to men, and interpersonal conflict has more negative consequences in terms of disease control than for men. Women are more likely than men to seek assistance, but are also more likely to experience loss of independence related to chronic and disabling conditions. Disabilities may create restrictions that lead to loss of family roles, changes in living arrangements, disrupted social relationships, and potential social isolation (O'Neill & Morrow, 2001).

All of the relationship effects of chronic disability are compounded by sociocultural issues such as poverty and language barriers. Poverty requires a focus on economic survival rather than optimal control of one's chronic condition. This may be particularly true for immigrant women, who number among the poorest in the population. Immigrant women and others with low educational levels may be hampered by language barriers from interacting effectively with health care professionals to address their disabilities or from obtaining information related to their condition that would promote self-care (O'Neill & Morrow, 2001). Community health nurses may be able to join other activist groups to advocate for educational and economic opportunities for women. They may be particularly helpful in making a case for assistance for women who are caring for disabled family members or who are disabled themselves.

REPRODUCTIVE ISSUES Because of their sex, a variety of reproductive issues affect women that are not encountered by men. Earlier, we discussed menstrual difficulties that are experienced by a small number of women as well as some of the consequences of the maturational stage of menopause. Other reproductive issues (in addition to reproductive cancers discussed earlier) include contraception and infertility and pregnancy.

Contraception and Infertility As we saw in Chapter 16∞, approximately half of all pregnancies in the United States are unintended. Half of these pregnancies end in abortion and half in the birth of a live infant (Beck, Morrow, Lipscomb, & Johnson, 2002). The prevalence of unintended pregnancy suggests that women of childbearing age are not using contraceptives for a variety of reasons. Many women may have misconceptions regarding conception and pregnancy; for example, some folk beliefs hold that conception is most likely to occur during menstruation. Others, particularly adolescents, may not be knowledgeable about or have access to effective contraception. In 1995, for example, roughly 28% of women in the United States were surgically sterile, 40% used nonsurgical contraceptive methods, 4% were seeking pregnancy, and 5% were pregnant or had recently delivered a child, again suggesting a large number (33%) of sexually active women who were not using any form of contraceptive (U.S. Census Bureau, 2005).

Even for those using contraceptives, the method selected may have implications for health. For example, use of nonoxynol-9 spermicide preparations, while preventing pregnancy, may actually increase one's risk for HIV infection. Such products are also not protective against other sexually transmitted diseases (Division of Reproductive Health, 2002a). Similarly, use of oral contraceptives may give women a false sense of security and increase sexual activity because the fear of pregnancy is diminished. Use of condoms, on the other hand, not only is relatively effective in preventing pregnancy, but also prevents a wide array of sexually transmitted diseases (STDs).

The converse of unwanted pregnancy is infertility, which is experienced by a number of women throughout the world. In some cultures, failure to produce offspring devalues the woman as a person and leads to social stigma and stress for those affected (Hsu, Tseng, Banks, & Kuo, 2004). In the United States, use of assisted reproductive technology has increased. In fact, the number of procedures performed increased 18% just in the period from 1996 to 1998. Only about 25% of these procedures result in live births, and 56% of those result in

multiple births (compared to 3% of all pregnancies). Assisted reproductive technology is also associated with increased risk of complications of pregnancy, prematurity, low birth weight, and long-term disability in the infants (Division of Reproductive Health, 2002b). Community health nurses may need to advocate for the availability of fertility services, as well as for contraceptive services for clients who do not wish to become pregnant.

Pregnancy Although considered a natural condition rather than an illness, pregnancy may pose a variety of problems for women and their families. Each year, an estimated 4 million births occur in the United States. Anywhere from 15% to 25% of these pregnancies result in antepartum hospitalization for complications. In one study, 43% of women had some type of problem during their delivery hospitalization, and 31% had at least one obstetric complication or preexisting medical condition that created a high-risk situation (Daniel, Berg, Johnson, & Atrash, 2003).

Pregnancy-related mortality has decreased significantly in the United States, dropping from 73.7 per 100,000 live births in 1950 to 7.6 in 2002 (CDC, 2004a). In spite of this improvement, more than 4,200 pregnancy-related deaths occurred among U.S. women between 1991 and 1999 (Chang et al., 2003). Maternal mortality worldwide varies considerably, from zero per 100,000 live births in Iceland to 2,000 in Sierra Leone (World Health Organization [WHO], 2004).

Maternal deaths in the United States may be due to lack of prenatal care, presence of existing health conditions (e.g., diabetes or HIV infection) that complicate pregnancy, or advanced age at conception, as well as a variety of other factors. In 2002, for example, nearly 4% of pregnancies in the United States received late or no prenatal care (U.S. Census Bureau, 2005). Lack of prenatal care has been linked to adverse maternal and infant outcomes. Approximately 20% of all U.S. births occur to women born outside the United States (NCHS, 2002). Many of these women encounter language and economic barriers to prenatal care. Immigrant women in particular may be in poor health prior to pregnancy due to deprivation in their country of origin, placing them at increased risk for poor outcomes and making prenatal care imperative. Community health nurses can make referrals for prenatal care and other reproductive services for women and can work to make sure that such services are available to women of all ethnic groups and economic levels. They can also educate women regarding the need for prenatal care.

With the advent of highly active antiretroviral therapy (HAART), perinatal transmission of HIV infection has decreased from 25% to 2% in the United States. Not all HIV-infected women, however, have access to HAART, particularly in underdeveloped countries where HIV infection is endemic among women of childbearing age. Even for those who receive HAART, HIV infection increases maternal risks in pregnancy due to the need for cesarean section at 38 weeks gestation for women with an HIV RNA load above 1,000, as well as those with unknown viral loads or who have not been adequately treated (County of San Diego Health and Human Services Agency, 2004).

Advanced maternal age at conception also increases the potential for poor pregnancy outcomes for mother and baby. In 2000, more than 500,000 U.S. women over 35 years of age gave birth. Later pregnancy is a result of several social factors such as delayed marriage, childbearing in second marriages, pursuit of education and career opportunities, and expanded options for previously infertile women (Davis-Snavely, 2004).

Homicide is another cause of pregnancy-related fatality. In one major metropolitan hospital, homicide was the leading cause of death among women during pregnancy or within 90 days of delivery. A homicide rate of 1.7 deaths per 100,000 live births was noted, and higher rates of homicide with pregnant victims was associated with younger age (under 20 years), being Black, or having late or no prenatal care (Chang, Berg, Saltzman, & Herndon, 2005).

Some women must cope with fetal or infant death. As noted earlier, culture plays a significant role in the response to the death of an infant. For example, Taiwanese women who experience stillbirth report feelings of guilt, incompleteness, and personal failure. Fetal loss affects their maternal identity and their cultural role as women. In addition, cultural taboos against discussing death, participating in death-related events, and expressing one's grief in public limit their ability to grieve effectively and adapt to the loss (Hsu et al., 2004). Fetal loss also leads to depression and anxiety in subsequent pregnancies for both partners, but more so for women than men. The effects on subsequent pregnancies does not, however, seem to affect bonding with later infants (Armstrong, 2002). Community health nurses can assist women who have lost infants to cope with their grief. For example, nurses may link these women to support groups or counseling services. They may also need to advocate for time to grieve with family members or friends who expect the woman to "grieve, then get on with her life."

Even a pregnancy with a normal course and favorable outcome may result in problems for the mother. For example, some women may experience postpartum depression that has significant health effects for them and their children. Postpartum depression is characterized by dysphoric mood, feelings of inadequacy in the maternal role, poor sleep and appetite, and poor concentration (Hung, 2004). Postpartum depression in mothers has been associated with delayed language development and behavior problems in their children (Kahn, Zuckerman, Bauchner, Homer, & Wise, 2002). In addition, a depressed mother is less likely to be able to effectively care for and nurture her infant.

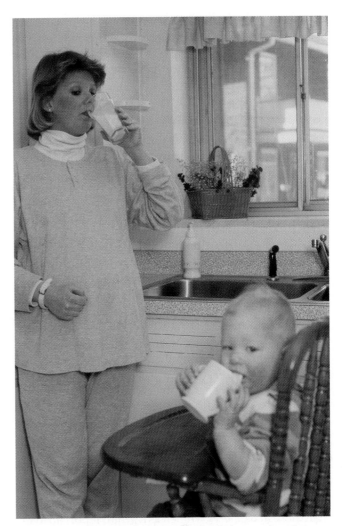

Women's health needs extend beyond those related to reproductive issues. (Patrick J. Watson)

Development of postpartum depression appears to be mediated by social support and cultural factors. The postpartum period is characterized by major changes and adjustments in women's lives. During this time women need to recover from the physical stresses of pregnancy and delivery, while meeting the needs of their newborn and often maintaining other responsibilities as well. Women in some cultures are less likely to experience postpartum depression than those in other cultural groups. The differences noted are believed to arise from the existence of cultural rituals in the postpartum period and social recognition of the mother's role transition in low-incidence cultures. In these cultures, new mothers are likely to receive more in the way of systematic instrumental support from extended family members and friends (Hung, 2004). Maternal role adaptation is also influenced by levels of perceived social support available, relationship with one's partner, and life satisfaction.

IMMUNITY Immunizations are the last aspect of physiologic function to be considered in relation to women's physiologic health status. Women's immunization rates, like those for all adults, are lower than recommended. Immunizations of particular concern for women include rubella and tetanus vaccine, but women should receive influenza and other immunizations as appropriate.

Psychological Considerations

Factors in the psychological dimension can have a profound effect on women's health. Areas of particular concern are stress and coping abilities, the psychological implications of sexual identity, and mental health and illness in the female population.

Stress and Coping

The first area for consideration related to the psychological dimension and its effect on women's health is the extent of women's exposure to stress and their abilities to cope with that stress. It is well known that stress contributes to a variety of illnesses in both men and women. For example, stress plays a part in the development of tuberculosis and hypertension. Severe life events and the stress that accompanies them have also been shown to be related to breast cancer in women. In one study, stress was found to interact with women's personal psychological traits to affect health. Women in this study who were subjected to medium to high levels of stress who were less assertive, less hardy, and less able to express themselves had more physical symptoms than women who scored favorably in these areas (Kenney & Bhattacharjee, 2000). Women, in general, have been found to be less happy and to experience more stress than men. In fact, U.S. women as a group report an average of 3.5 days per month when their mental health was not perceived as good (National Women's Law Center et al., 2000). Women were also more than one and a half times more likely to report serious psychological distress than men during the 2000–2001 period (CDC, 2004a). Although women tend to experience more stress than men, they often have better coping skills and are more likely than men to seek social support (Williams, 2003).

Sources of stress for women include stresses related to interpersonal relationships, financial status, children, and family health. Levels of stress also appear to be greater contributors to self-reported health, functional health, and chronic disease for women than men (Denton, Prus, & Walters, 2004). Women's coping ability is particularly affected by circumstances such as domestic violence, which leads to changes in the type of coping strategies employed. As noted earlier, women generally tend to use confrontive coping strategies. At least one study has shown, however, that higher levels of domestic violence are associated with avoidance coping. More severe violence has also been associated with enforced social isolation and avoidance by members of the social support network, further reducing abused women's abilities to cope with the situation (Waldrop & Resick, 2004).

Sexuality

Elements of both the psychological and social dimensions affect issues of sexuality in women, but because of the implications of sexuality for women's mental health, they will be addressed under the psychological dimension. Many women are embarrassed to discuss issues of sexuality, and teenagers, in particular, may have a number of fears and misconceptions. In assessing adolescent girls, the community health nurse obtains information related to attitudes and anxieties about menstruation as well as knowledge of menstrual physiology and hygiene. Social factors such as family and cultural attitudes and knowledge and parental education level may affect family willingness or ability to assist the young girl with the physical, emotional, and practical issues posed by menarche.

The nurse cannot assume that older women do not have some of the same concerns regarding menstruation and sexuality as teenagers. Women may have questions about their sexuality, guilt about sexual activity or possible infertility, and difficulty in developing healthy sexual identities. As we will see later in this chapter, these concerns are frequently magnified for the lesbian, bisexual, or transgender client. Community health nurses should assess women's comfort with sexuality and their sexual identity and assist them to voice concerns in these areas.

Sexual activity by women, especially teenagers, may have a variety of psychological precursors. For example, the adolescent may think that if she is still a virgin at age 15, there is something wrong with her. Or, if she perceives her mother as asexual or "Madonna-like," she may rebel and seek sexual outlets totally unlike those of her mother. The nurse assesses clients' knowledge and attitudes about sexual identity and sexual activity.

Menopause, at the other end of the reproductive spectrum, also has psychological implications. In U.S. society, menopausal women have not been held in high esteem. Society's lack of regard for the older woman adds to her emotional stress, thereby limiting her abilities to cope with physical and psychological changes occurring at this time.

Sexual identity and conformity to societal expectations with respect to one's sexual or gender role may also pose problems for both men and women. **Sexual identity** refers to one's perceptions of self as male or female. **Sexual orientation**, on the other hand, reflects one's attraction for members of the same sex (homosexual), opposite sex (heterosexual), or both (bisexual). Sexual identity and sexual orientation are not synonymous. One may identify as female and be attracted to either men or women or both. Nor is sexual identity synonymous with biological sex. **Transgender individuals** are those whose gender identity and expression contrast with their biological sex (Nemoto, Operario, Keatley, Nguyen, & Sugano, 2005) or who express

TABLE 17-2	Typology of Biological Sex, Sexual Identity, and Sexual Orientation		
Category	Biological Sex	Sexual Identity	Sexual Orientation
Heterosexual man	Male	Male	Attracted to women
Heterosexual woman	Female	Female	Attracted to men
Gay	Male	Male	Attracted to men
Lesbian	Female	Female	Attracted to women
Bisexual man	Male	Male	Attracted to both men and women
Bisexual woman	Female	Female	Attracted to both men and women
Transgendered man	Female	Male	Varies
Transgendered woman	Male	Female	Varies

discomfort with their biological gender and identify instead with members of the opposite sex (Nemoto, Operario, Keatley, Han, & Soma, 2004). Table 17-2◆ presents a typology of biological sex, sexual identity, and sexual orientation associated with commonly used terms. Sexual activity may or may not reflect either sexual identity or orientation, since more than attraction may affect sexual activity. For example, a heterosexual male may be sexually attracted to women but engage in sexual activity with other men based on circumstances (e.g., imprisonment or in sex-for-money or sex-for-drug exchanges).

Sexual identity, orientation, or activity that is not in conformity with one's biological sex can create a variety of psychological and social problems for both men and women. Such problems encountered by women are discussed in more detail in the section dealing with the health needs of lesbian, bisexual, and transgender women. Similar problems for men are addressed in Chapter 18∞.

Mental Health and Illness

Women more often internalize emotional stress, leading to internalized disorders such as depression and anxiety, whereas men exhibit more externalization of stress in outward behavior (Williams, 2003). It is estimated that 10% to 25% of women will experience clinical depression at some point in their lives (Matthews, Hughes, Johnson, Razzano, & Cassidy, 2002). Women experience depression at a rate twice that of men (Skarsater, Dencker, Bergbom, Haggstrom, & Fridlund, 2003) and also experience more symptoms at an earlier age than men (Huey, 2001). Depression is most common among women 18 to 44 years of age (Eli Lilly and Company, 2004b). General risk factors for depression include genetic predisposition, hormonal factors, previous episodes of depression, poor coping, poverty, negative life events and psychosocial stressors, and substance abuse. The presence of chronic illness, particularly cardiovascular disease, has also been linked to the incidence of depression, with more severe consequences among women who are already at higher risk for depression than men (Eli Lilly and Company, 2004a). Women also experience unique risks related to their social role and social and economic status, gender socialization, the presence of dependent children, and victimization (Matthews et al., 2002).

Women at all ages are less likely than men to commit suicide, but a significant number of women each year succumb to despair and end their lives. In 2002, the age-adjusted suicide mortality rate for women was 4.2 per 100,000 women, down from 6.8 per 100,000 women in 1970 (CDC, 2004a). Population estimates of depression in women as well as rates for attempted and completed suicide are important data for an aggregate assessment of women's health.

Other mental health problems that are prevalent among women include eating disorders, post-traumatic stress disorder (PTSD), and chronic fatigue syndrome. Women also experience schizophrenia, which tends to occur at a later age in women than in men. Peak incidence of schizophrenia in women occurs from ages 20 to 30 years, and symptoms rarely begin after age 45 (National Institute of Mental Health, 2005). An estimated 1% to 3% of U.S. women have bulimia nervosa, an eating disorder that impairs function and ultimately imperils life. Bulimia is characterized by recurrent episodes of binge eating followed by compensatory mechanisms, such as purging by means of self-induced vomiting or use of laxatives, diuretics, or emetics (Spearing, 2001). In one study, women with bulimia identified four major difficulties associated with the disease: self-isolation, fear, being at war with one's mind, and pacifying one's mind. Affected women tended to isolate themselves from others in order to disguise their pattern of binge eating and purging. They also reported living in fear of being judged by others, of gaining weight and "being fat," and of having to live without the bingeing and purging behaviors around which their lives revolved. Women also described a constant battle to rationalize their behavior as normal and feeling "possessed" by their cravings. Finally, they reported purging to deal with self-generated feelings of guilt about overeating or to relieve uncomfortable feelings of fullness (Broussard, 2005).

Anorexia nervosa is another eating disorder characterized by active resistance to maintaining a minimal body weight, an overwhelming fear of becoming fat, and disturbed perceptions of one's own body weight or shape. An estimated 0.5% to 3.7% of U.S. women suffer from anorexia. Anorexia results in mortality rates nearly 12 times higher than the annual death rate for all other causes among women 15 to 24 years of age. Other women (2% to 5% of the U.S. adult population) suffer from binge eating disorders in which they engage in uncontrollable eating at least 2 days a week in a 6-month period. Unlike women with bulimia, those with binge eating disorders do not engage in compensatory purging strategies (Spearing, 2001).

Although PTSD was first identified among men suffering from post-combat trauma, it is being identified in women more and more often. PTSD is a mental health condition characterized by flashbacks to the traumatizing event, anger, anxiety, depression, and isolation (Beck, 2004). PTSD most commonly arises as an aftermath of prior abuse, particularly sexual abuse, but may not exhibit all of the symptoms found in combat veterans with this disorder. PTSD after prior sexual abuse may surface during pregnancy and interfere with client–provider interactions in prenatal care, self-care during pregnancy, or maternal sensitivity to the needs of the child. Sexually abused women with PTSD have also been shown to be at high risk for revictimization, self-harm, substance abuse, and eating disorders (Seng, Low, Sparbel, & Killion, 2004).

Pregnancy and childbirth themselves may result in PTSD in some women. PTSD related to childbirth has been found in 1.5% to 6% of U.S. births (Beck, 2004). Similarly, female genital mutilation (FGM) has been found to result in PTSD in as many as 30% of victims in some studies (Behrendt & Moritz, 2005).

Chronic fatigue syndrome, which is characterized by severe fatigue with no identifiable physical cause, is another condition that affects women more often than men. Chronic fatigue may result in changes in self-concept, alienation, and decreased quality of interpersonal interactions. Women with chronic fatigue often report that their symptoms are disregarded and dismissed by health care providers. Although fatigue often correlates with depression and low perceived personal power, most typical treatment with antidepressants does not seem to result in long-term improvement (Dzurec, Hoover, & Fields, 2002).

Physical Environmental Considerations

Physical environmental factors also influence the health of women. They are exposed to physical environmental hazards both at home and in the work setting. In the home, environmental hazards include household chemicals used to clean, inhalants such as powders and sprays, and the potential for falls related to stools, stairs, and throw rugs. The effects of the workplace on women's health are covered later in this chapter during the discussion of the occupational component of the sociocultural dimension. Physical environmental dimension factors are particularly evident in rates for

accidental injuries. Although women have far lower injury rates than men, significant morbidity and mortality are related to unintentional injuries in women. Another area for consideration is the reproductive effects of environmental pollutants, and the community health nurse should be alert to connections between environmental conditions and adverse pregnancy outcomes in the population.

In addition, lack of exposure to sunlight in the physical environment may lead to vitamin D deficiency. Since vitamin D is required for calcium absorption, this physical environmental factor may increase the potential for osteoporosis and fracture injuries (Curry & Hogstel, 2002).

Sociocultural Considerations

Many sociocultural dimension factors affect the health status of women. Social determinants of health appear to be more relevant for women than men and appear to contribute significantly to disparities in health status, self-rated health, functional ability, and chronic conditions between men and women (Denton et al., 2004). Some of the more influential factors among these are societal pressures regarding roles and relationships, occupational and economic issues, and violence and abuse.

Roles and Relationships

Women often define themselves in terms of relationships with others. Women's roles in these relationships are culturally defined by the society in which they live. Society even specifies how women should look. U.S. entertainment media, in particular, promote a strong cultural value for thinness, often leading women to engage in poor health behaviors and resulting in eating disorders and depression. Research has indicated that these sociocultural effects can be mediated by women's internal feelings of self-confidence or self-criticism and by their relationships with significant others in their lives (Paquette & Raine, 2004). Many of women's relationships entail caregiving roles in which they have primary responsibility for the care of children, spouses, aging parents, and ill family members that compounds the stresses of daily life. In 2003, for example, 57% of U.S. women were married, and more than 20% were divorced or widowed. Eighty-one percent of single-parent households with children were headed by women (U.S. Census Bureau, 2005), and more than one fourth of these households (28%) had incomes below federal poverty levels (U.S. Census Bureau, 2004b).

Women are often responsible for caring for the home and children as well as older family members. In addition, women are often employed outside the home. For example, in 2002, 55% of U.S. women who had had a child in the previous year were employed in the workforce (U.S. Census Bureau, 2005), and as of 2004, only California had a paid family leave policy for care of a new child or ill family member (National Women's Law Center et al., 2004). Childcare responsibilities have been shown to pose a cumulative burden for women due to chronic strain that is exacerbated by low levels of resources and low socioeconomic status. Parenting stress contributes to lower levels of mental health in mothers of young children that is often compounded by problems with childcare and stressful working situations, but may be mitigated by social support from family and friends (Jun, Subramanian, Gortmaker, & Kawachi, 2004). Women's health and health-related behaviors have been shown to be negatively related to living with elderly family members, particularly for low-income workers and unemployed housewives (Artazcoz, Borrell, Benach, Cortes, & Rohlfs, 2004).

Women's roles and responsibilities are culturally defined, and may have differential impacts on women's health and well-being. In many cultural groups, women operate from a highly familial point of view, putting the needs of family members ahead of their own and thereby neglecting or jeopardizing their own health (Ro, 2002). For example, access to prenatal care in underdeveloped countries has been affected by such mundane considerations as the inability to spare time from meeting familial responsibilities for obtaining water (McCray, 2004). Cultural buffers may also serve to mediate the effects of trauma on women, as proposed in the indigenist model of coping discussed in the Cultural Competence box at right. Different cultures also value men and women differently within the societal framework, which may have implications for health and health care service access. For example, in India, boys are more highly valued than girls and are more likely to be immunized and to receive better nutrition than girls, contributing to health problems for women later in life (Borooah, 2004). These attitudes toward women also have other health and social implications with regard to educational opportunities, freedom of choice, and ability to negotiate safe sexual practices, to name a few areas of influence.

Cultural expectations also define communication patterns in terms of gender. Gender determines appropriate topics of conversation as well as the words and phrases that may appropriately be used. Gender differences lead to the lack of a common language between men and women and contribute to miscommunication, particularly in the area of sexuality, but also in other aspects of life. For example, Mexican men can discuss sex and initiate discussion of sex, but women are not expected to discuss this area. In the context of sexual communication, "no" may be difficult to interpret. Similarly, men are allowed to swear, but women are not. Women are more likely to ask questions, whereas men may try to fake knowledge. Women are more likely to discuss relationships and feelings than men. Even when similar words are used, interpretation may be different based on gender expectations within the culture (Marston, 2004).

CULTURAL COMPETENCE

Walters and Simoni (2002) have suggested an indigenist model of coping to examine cultural mediating factors in the effect of trauma on health and health-related behaviors. They noted that Native American women are located in a so-called fourth world, which the authors defined as "situations in which a minority indigenous population exists in a nation wherein institutionalized power and privilege are held by a colonizing subordinating majority" (p. 520). They suggested that the effects of trauma experienced by fourth world groups on health and health-related behaviors are mediated by cultural buffers that promote coping. Trauma may result from historical trauma (e.g., attempts to eliminate indigenous cultures), current experiences of discrimination, or traumatic life events (including physical or sexual abuse). Cultural mediating factors suggested for Native American women include positive identity attitudes (failure to internalize negative attitudes toward oneself or one's group), degree of enculturation (identification with one's traditional culture), spiritual coping, and use of traditional healing practices. The authors suggested that these cultural coping factors may have positive influences on health-related behaviors and health status. To what extent might a similar indigenist model apply to other minority populations? What aspects of the model might need to be adapted to the particular population? What cultural mediating factors may be operating in the selected population(s)?

Occupational and Economic Issues

Both occupational and economic issues can have direct and indirect effects on women's health. More than 12% of adult women in the United States live in poverty, and employed women earn less than three fourths of men's income for the same jobs (National Women's Law Center et al., 2004). In 2002, nearly twice as many women as men had annual incomes under $10,000 (U.S. Census Bureau, 2005). Divorced women, particularly those with children, are at special risk for the effects of poverty. Many of these women do not receive court-mandated child support payments from ex-spouses. Although state agencies are becoming more adept at recovering outstanding child support payments, with 12 states recovering nearly 60% of outstanding amounts, many states have policies that prevent families on Temporary Assistance for Needy Families (TANF) from receiving any part of the support payments recovered (National Women's Law Center et al., 2004).

Lower income is frequently associated with higher incidence of disability, chronic disease, and generally poor health, and women's health status has been shown to decline as their income declines. In one study, for example, people served by "safety net systems" designed to meet the health care needs of low-income families often delayed or did not receive care due to lack of insurance coverage and competing priorities for the monies available to them. Women in this study were found to be more likely to delay care than men. Additional reasons given for delaying care were inability to take time from work, care of children and others, lack of transportation, and being too sick to seek care (Diamant et al., 2004).

Employment and occupation are sociocultural dimension factors that have profound effects on the health of many women. In 2003, 60% of the adult female population in the United States was employed, and this figure is expected to climb to 61.6% by 2012 (U.S. Census Bureau, 2005). Women tend to receive less pay than men in their jobs. For example, in 2003, twice as many women as men were paid at hourly rates at or below minimum wage (2.3% versus 1.1%), and the median wage of hourly women workers was only $11.01 compared to $13.25 for men. Similarly, the median annual family income for families headed by single women in 2002 was $29,000, compared to $41,000 for families headed by single men (U.S. Census Bureau, 2005).

Many women in the paid labor force continue to work in traditional "women's jobs" such as nursing, teaching, the garment industry, and secretarial/clerical and service jobs. Although considered "women's work," these jobs are not without health risks. Physical risks arise from chemicals, radiation, infectious disease, noise, vibration, and repetitive movements. Employed women also have a higher incidence of musculoskeletal problems than men, possibly due to repetitive work, poor ergonomic work design, and reduced opportunity to rest and exercise at home as a result of family obligations outside of work (Strazdins & Bammer, 2004).

As more women enter the world of "men's work," such as heavy industry, construction, mining, and factory work, they face a different set of physical hazards. Health risks arise from heavy lifting, use of dangerous machinery, and tools that were designed for larger men rather than smaller women. Minority women are at higher risk than White women for job-related injury because they often take jobs that others will not. Their economic need prevents them from saying no or quitting. Women are also more likely than men to work in small companies that do not provide health insurance benefits (National Center for Chronic Disease Prevention and Health Promotion, 2002).

High-tech employment, once touted as safe, also entails health risks. The scrupulously clean area needed to produce a computer chip or to work with computers contains potential threats to human reproduction posed by radiofrequency or microwave radiation, video display terminal radiation, and arsine and chlorine gases. Working women today face essentially the same physical hazards as working men. They have the same risks for reproductive failure, respiratory ailments, skin disorders, and cancer. The health risks of the work setting are discussed in more detail in Chapter 24∞.

The psychological environment of the workplace can be as detrimental to women's health as its physical hazards. For example, studies have shown that it is not

GLOBAL PERSPECTIVES

The plight of women worldwide is a serious one that merits immediate and sustained global attention. In the course of 5 years, maternal deaths increased more than 100,000 and now occur at a rate of 600,000 deaths per year. Much of the burden of mortality in women is due to HIV/AIDS. In 2000, 1.3 million women died of AIDS and worldwide prevalence was an estimated 16.4 million women.

Women's poor health status is linked to a broad array of social, cultural, and economic factors. Based on the World Health Organization's gender:poverty ratio calculations, the poverty rate for women exceeds that for men in 12 of every 15 developing nations and in 5 of every 8 developed nations. Women often experience single parenthood or widowhood, both of which are related to greater poverty. Poverty results in both direct and indirect effects that influence women's health. In many groups, cultural norms favor entitlement for men over women, and the division of labor in many households worldwide remains very traditional, with women retaining responsibility for the home and children despite the fact that more women than ever before are in the workforce.

Labor force participation by women increases their access to both material and social support, but adds to the burden of their work when combined with family responsibilities. In addition, work increases the potential for toxic exposures and other occupational risks. Women, more often than men, are employed in low-income, high-risk jobs. Even women who work at home are exposed to more risks from the use of hazardous cooking fuels and pesticides (Doyal, 2004). Although the worldwide health status of women has improved in some respects in recent years, much remains to be accomplished.

the female administrator who suffers the most from stress and depression, but women in the more traditional positions of secretary and clerk. It is postulated that stress is intensified by the lack of freedom to control one's work that secretaries and clerks experience. The "dead-end" quality of these jobs with little possibility of advancement may decrease incentive. In addition, the low salaries available for secretaries and clerks add stresses related to financial insecurity.

Social factors in the work environment also affect women's health. The world of work for women differs from that for men in several ways. First, more jobs are open to men than to women. In addition, those jobs that are open to women often provide unequal pay and levels of benefits compared with similar jobs among men. Finally, until a 1991 Supreme Court ruling, women were more often barred from work based on reproductive capacities than were men. Childbearing has also been blamed for women's late entry into the workforce and women's lack of training and education.

There are no uniform policies for paid medical or family leave for U.S. women despite federal mandates for such leaves, and only three states have provisions for medical or family leave beyond the federal mandate as well as paid disability leave (National Women's Law

Center et al., 2000). Consequently, when a woman must have time off from work because of pregnancy or caring for ill or disabled family members, she must often take it without pay.

Childcare is another social environmental factor that creates problems for the working woman. Employer or community assistance with childcare is practically nonexistent. Invariably, women must find quality childcare on their own. If children are sick, it is usually the mother who stays home, often without pay, to care for them. Work may also interfere with childcare responsibilities in other ways. For example, although breastfeeding is encouraged by official Hong Kong health policy, fewer than three fourths of Hong Kong hospitals provided space for female employees to pump their breasts, and in only one quarter of these did the facilities provide privacy. In addition, only 11% of the institutions permitted specific time to pump breasts, with others requiring employees to use regular breaks or lunchtimes to do so (Dodgson, Chee, & Yap, 2004).

Disproportionate pay between traditional women's jobs and such "men's work" as road construction is a strong incentive for women to seek such jobs. Women who enter male-dominated jobs often feel pressure to prove they are equal to men in ability. They may not speak out against safety hazards because they do not want to appear weak or "unable to take it." Sexual harassment is another problem that may be encountered by women in the work setting. Although there are laws prohibiting such abuse, women may not complain because they need work so badly.

Minority women must contend with a higher degree of discrimination and lack of job opportunity than White women. They are particularly subject to dead-end and hazardous jobs with low pay and few benefits. Minority women are also less likely to finish high school, more likely to become the head of a single-parent household, and more likely to have job-related illnesses than their White counterparts.

Social factors related to approaching retirement may affect the health status of the middle-aged woman. The woman who is nearing retirement needs to be aware of and plan for the financial shortfalls that are likely to occur with retirement. Leaving the workforce means living in poverty for many older people. Retirement assets are usually tied to lifetime income. Women who worked for low pay and poor benefits will have neither pensions nor full Social Security benefits. A divorced woman may draw Social Security from her ex-husband's account if they were married at least 10 years, but widows face declining incomes following the death of a spouse.

Violence and Abuse

Abuse of women is the product of many psychological and sociocultural dimension factors, and it fosters a psychological environment detrimental to women's health.

Because it is primarily social and cultural conditions that allow abuse to occur, the issue is addressed here within the discussion of the sociocultural dimension. Psychological dimension factors contributing to abuse of women are also addressed.

An estimated 10% to 50% of women worldwide are assaulted by a male partner. Women's risk of violence is increased by financial dependence, their partners' association with other women, an inability to negotiate condom use, their partners' use of alcohol, and interactions with multiple partners. Additional risk factors include low educational level, short-term relationships, lower household income, drug use, and HIV infection. In one study, for example, HIV-infected women were 10 times more likely to report one or more episodes of violence in their lives than uninfected women. Violence may increase the risk for HIV infection through forced sexual activity or the inability to negotiate condom use (Maman et al., 2002).

Psychological dependence on males and poor self-esteem on the part of both the victim and the abuser are some of the psychological factors resulting in abuse. Feelings of shame and worthlessness may hamper the woman's ability to seek help while in an abusive situation. Societal attitudes toward abused women often compound the problems of abuse for victims.

Violence against women is a pervasive, underrecognized, and culturally condoned phenomenon in American society and in other cultural groups. An estimated 3% to 5% of adult intimate relationships involve intimate partner violence (IPV) (Murty et al., 2003), and nearly a third of women age 14 through college age experience some form of dating violence (Smith, White, & Holland, 2003). According to the Youth Behavioral Risk Surveillance System (YBRSS), nearly 10% of high school girls report being "beat up" by boyfriends, and 21% have been sexually assaulted. The lifetime risk of being physically hurt by a dating partner is over 15%, and the lifetime risk of rape among 9th to 12th grade girls is 9%. Women physically assaulted during high school have been found to be at higher risk for revictimization as college students than those assaulted in childhood (Smith et al., 2003). In 2002, the incidence rate for forcible rape was 64.8 per 100,000 U.S. women, down from 80.5 in 1990, but still twice as high as the rate for men. The incidence of any IPV in 2000 was six times higher among women than men (466.5 versus 75 per 100,000 population) (U.S. Census Bureau, 2005). In part, this difference is due to greater reluctance on the part of men to report being victims of IPV, but also reflects women's more vulnerable position in an intimate relationship.

In 2002, the age-adjusted female rate of death from homicide was 2.8 per 100,000 women, a decrease from 4.4 per 100,000 women in 1980 (CDC, 2004a). Adult women accounted for nearly 22% of U.S. homicide victims in 2002 (U.S. Census Bureau, 2005). In most cases homicide against women is perpetrated by a current or former intimate partner. Anywhere from 5% to 22% of women seen in primary care settings may be subject to IPV that may escalate to homicide. Advocacy groups recommend routine screening of all women in primary care settings for IPV, and in one study, inclusion of screening questions on multiple intake forms resulted in documented assessment for IPV in 72% of all women seen (Scholle et al., 2003). Risk of IPV may be even higher among some cultural groups. For example, immigrant Southeast Asian women have been found to be at higher risk for IPV than other groups due to family disruption and lack of extended family support, immigration-related social isolation, and lack of awareness of available help (Raj & Silverman, 2003).

Domestic violence such as spouse abuse is rarely a one-time event. By the time injuries are identifiable as inflicted by a batterer, a woman may have been abused for several years. If the woman does not ask for help or injuries are not discovered, battering usually increases in severity and frequency. Only four states have mandated assessment protocols, training, and screening for domestic violence and prohibit insurance companies from discriminating against victims of domestic violence (National Women's Law Center et al., 2000). Risk factors and prevention strategies for abuse of women are addressed in more detail in Chapter 32∞.

Behavioral Considerations

Behavioral dimension factors also affect the health of women clients. Areas of particular concern include dietary consumption patterns; tobacco, alcohol, and drug use; and physical activity and exercise. Unprotected sexual activity, another behavioral consideration, was addressed in the context of issues related to contraception earlier in the chapter. Dietary concerns may be particularly problematic among women, many of whom are obese or overweight or who engage in fad diets to attain or maintain a fashionably slim figure. Fad dieting is especially prevalent among adolescent females who also have high incidence rates for eating disorders such as bulimia and anorexia nervosa. In addition to the influence of obesity and overweight on heart disease and other chronic health conditions, research indicates that overweight and obese pregnant women have a significantly greater risk for gestational diabetes mellitus, eclampsia, cesarean section, and delivery of a macrosomic child (a child with an abnormally large body) (Baeten, Bukusi, & Lambe, 2001).

Overweight and obesity are endemic conditions among the U.S. population, particularly among women. In the period 1999–2002, for example, nearly two thirds (61.7%) of women 20 to 74 years of age were overweight, and more than a third (34%) were actually obese. The prevalence of obesity has more than doubled since the 1960–1962 time period (CDC, 2004a). Calcium intake is another dietary concern among women due to the

increased risk of osteoporosis. Conversely, a diet high in fruits, vegetables, potassium, and magnesium has a protective effect against osteoporosis (Shepherd, 2004).

Smoking is another consumption pattern that is problematic for women. Although the number of male smokers has declined rather dramatically in the last few years, the number of women who smoke has not declined as rapidly, leading to corresponding increases in lung cancer and heart disease among women. In addition to the negative effects of smoking with respect to cancer incidence and cardiovascular disease, smoking promotes urinary calcium excretion, increasing women's risks for osteoporosis (Curry & Hogstel, 2002).

In 2002, more than 20% of U.S. women over 18 years of age smoked. This is only a slight decline from 22.9% in 1990 (U.S. Census Bureau, 2005). Several factors contribute to the continued prevalence of smoking among women. These include attempts to control weight, perceptions that smoking controls negative mood, extensive targeting of women by tobacco company advertising, and the dependence of the media on tobacco revenue and sponsorship of women's fashions, athletics, and other events by tobacco companies that stifle media coverage of the negative effects of smoking (CDC, 2002). Women with disabilities who smoke are at even greater risk for these effects (Jones & Bell, 2004). Low socioeconomic status and parenting responsibility for young children are other factors associated with smoking among women (Jun et al., 2004).

Substance use and abuse among women is another area of concern related to consumption patterns. Although women still tend to abuse alcohol and drugs less often than men, the incidence of such problems among females is increasing. Overall, 17% of adult women in the United States reported binge drinking (CDC, 2004b). As noted earlier, a significant proportion of pregnant women use alcohol and 2% reported binge drinking in 2002, contributing to poor pregnancy outcomes and fetal alcohol syndrome in their offspring (National Center on Birth Defects and Developmental Disabilities, 2004). Problems of drug and alcohol abuse are addressed in Chapter 31∞. Both alcohol and caffeine consumption promote diuresis and calcium excretion, increasing one's risk for osteoporosis (Curry & Hogstel, 2002).

Another major behavioral consideration that influences women's health is physical activity and exercise.

BUILDING OUR KOWLEDGE BASE

Jones and Bell (2004) noted that there is little information on the extent of alcohol use among women with disabling conditions or on the effects of alcohol on their disabilities. How would you go about designing such a study? Would you focus on women with a specific disability, or those with any disabling condition? Why? What alcohol effects would you examine? How would you measure them?

An active lifestyle promotes overall health and is associated with a 50% reduction in the risk of hip fractures due to osteoporosis (Shepherd, 2004). In spite of the benefits of physical activity, however, over half of all U.S. women are sedentary, and CDC data indicate that less than 30% of minority women achieve even moderate levels of physical activity. In one study, although most of the older African American and Native American women surveyed believed that physical activity was important for health, few participated in any form of exercise or other physical activity. Participants in the study reported a number of constraints for physical activity, including job and family demands, fatigue, illness, and lack of facilities and opportunities for physical activity. Other barriers included economics, major life changes or traumas, safety concerns, weather, and the hassle associated with personal care (e.g., showering) after physical activity (Henderson & Ainsworth, 2003).

Sexual activity among women is another behavioral dimension consideration. The extent of sexual activity within the population influences the health of women in terms of the potential for pregnancy and exposure to STDs. Health-related practices associated with sexual activity also affect health. For example, failure to use barrier contraceptives increases one's risk of both pregnancy and STDs.

Health System Considerations

Lack of attention to women's health needs, lack of illness prevention and health promotion resources, health insurance discrimination, and lack of support for the informal caregiver in the home are health care system issues that adversely affect women. The medical system tends to focus on female reproductive problems, frequently to the exclusion of other health problems faced by women. Failure to recognize and deal with physical abuse is just one example of failure of the health care system to meet the needs of women. By and large, the health care system has only recently come to recognize the special health needs of the female client.

Services provided by the health care system tend to focus on secondary and tertiary prevention of injury and disease. Few efforts are made to provide preventive health care, particularly for women, and those preventive health services that are available are not always offered at a time when busy working women can take advantage of them. Compounding this problem is the lack of provision for childcare while women seek preventive health care services.

In a periodic review of state policies affecting women's health, the National Women's Law Center et al. (2004) found that only one policy issue was addressed by all 50 states and the District of Columbia in 2004. That policy dealt with Medicaid coverage of breast and cervical cancer care for women less than 65 years of age. Table 17-3◆ summarizes the extent to which some of the major policy goals for women's health have been met by the states.

The cost of health care is a barrier to health service utilization for women. Women are less likely than men to have employment-based health insurance, and they are more likely to work in part-time jobs or jobs that do not offer this benefit. Single women are also less likely to be able to pay the monthly insurance premiums. This situation is particularly hard on divorced and separated women with children who are already faced with financial difficulties. According to U.S. Census Bureau figures, in 2003, 59.5% of women had employment-based health insurance and another 28.4% were covered by Medicaid (13.4%) or Medicare (15%). The remaining 14.4% of women had no insurance coverage (U.S. Census Bureau, 2004a). In 2002, more than half (53.5%) of uninsured persons in the United States were women (U.S. Census Bureau, 2005).

Research indicates that, for all ethnic groups, having a regular source of health care is the greatest predictor of the use of preventive services (Cornelius, Smith, & Simpson, 2002), yet during 2001 and 2002, 11.4% of women had no regular source of care (CDC, 2004a). Discontinuous insurance coverage increases lack of access to care due to the inability to develop a relationship with a consistent health care provider. Many uninsured women rely on emergency departments or hospital clinics for care, thereby increasing societal expenses for care.

Even when women do have health insurance coverage, many essential services are not covered. For example, as indicated in Table 17-3◆, private insurance coverage for breast, cervical, and colorectal cancer and osteoporosis screening is not mandated by all states, and Medicaid programs in all 50 states and the District of Columbia have been expanded to cover only breast and cervical cancer screening. Many private insurance plans do not cover the cost of contraceptive services even though provision of contraceptives would be cost-effective in terms of preventing unintended pregnancies, pregnancy complications, and STDs (Kurth, Weaver, Lockart, & Bielinski, 2004). In fact, one state-funded program for contraceptive services in California was credited with preventing 108,000 unplanned pregnancies, 50,000 unintended births, and 41,000 induced abortions (Foster et al., 2004).

Another problem for working women attributable to the health care system is the lack of support for the informal caregiver. Women may be forced to quit their jobs to care for a sick child or elderly family member but cannot expect the financial support that might be available for institution-based care of the loved one. As noted in Table 17-3◆, only one state mandates paid employee leave to care for family members.

In addition to giving up employment to care for family members, women engaging in such care often receive little support from friends and family or respite services from the health care system. These circumstances often lead to excessive strain and diminished

TABLE 17-3   Selected Policy Goals for Women's Health and Their Achievement in the United States

Policy Area	Policy Goal	Level of Goal Achievement
Access to health insurance coverage	• Meet Healthy People goal for access to health insurance	• No state met goal
	• Presumptive eligibility for Medicaid by pregnant women	• Met by 31 states
	• Increase income eligibility for Medicaid for working parents	• Met by 5 states
	• Simplify Medicaid enrollment procedures	• Met by 25 states
	• Provide coverage for childless adults	• Met by 7 states (down from 8 in 2001)
	• Regulate access to private health insurance for people without employer-sponsored or public coverage	• Met by 5 states
Access to health care providers and services	• Provide Medicaid coverage for breast and cervical cancer care	• Met by all states (includes District of Columbia)
	• Provide adequate Medicaid pharmaceutical coverage	• Met by 12 states
	• Provide coverage for mental health services	• Met by 4 states
	• Mandate private insurance coverage of contraceptive services	• Met by 20 states
	• Provide access to emergency contraception services	• Met by 3 states
	• Eliminate parental consent requirements for abortion services	• Met by 16 states
	• Provide public funds for abortion services for women who cannot afford them	• Met by 17 states
	• Mandate managed care coverage of participation in clinical trials	• Met by 17 states
	• Mandate the right to external review of managed care plan decisions if desired	• Met by 44 states
	• Mandate provision of interpretation and translation services for clients with limited proficiency in English	• Met by 6 states
Availability of preventive and health-promotive services	• Improve mammography screening	• Met by 43 states
	• Improve Pap smear screening	• Met by 3 states
	• Improve colorectal screening	• Met by 19 states
	• Improve cholesterol screening	• Met by 10 states
	• Mandate mammography coverage by private insurance	• Met by 21 states
	• Mandate colorectal screening coverage by private insurance	• Met by 17 states
	• Mandate osteoporosis screening coverage by private insurance	• Met by 8 states
	• Mandate Pap smear screening coverage by private insurance	• Met by 25 states
	• Mandate Chlamydia screening coverage by private insurance	• Met by 2 states
	• Expand food stamp outreach programs	• Met by 24 states
	• Improve nutrition education	• Met by 50 states
	• Mandate smoking cessation coverage by private insurance	• No state met goal
	• Provide Medicaid coverage of smoking cessation services	• Met by 7 states
	• Provide direct access to OB/GYN services	• Met by 40 states
	• Provide access to diabetes-related services	• Met by 42 states
Reduce economic disparities	• Increase collection of outstanding child support payments	• Met by 12 states
	• Mandate paid leave for care of new child or ill family member	• Met by 1 state
	• Prohibit insurance discrimination for victims of domestic violence	• Met by 22 states
	• Prohibit employment discrimination based on sexual orientation	• Met by 15 states
	• Prohibit insurance discrimination based on genetic information	• Met by 28 states
	• Increase high school completion rates	• Met by 8 states

Data from: *National Women's Law Center & Oregon Health & Science University. (2004).* Making the grade on women's health: A national and state-by-state report card. *Retrieved August 13, 2005, from http://www.nwlc.org*

health for the caregiver. Common effects for these caregivers include depression, insomnia, functional limitations, and diminished health status as well as delay in seeking health care services for themselves (Lee, Colditz, Berkman, & Kawachi, 2003).

THE EPIDEMIOLOGY OF HEALTH FOR LESBIAN, BISEXUAL, AND TRANSGENDER WOMEN

Lesbians and bisexual and transgender women comprise a segment of the female population with whom the community health nurse will knowingly or unknowingly come in contact. According to U.S. Census Bureau (2005) figures, 5% of unmarried partner households consist of women living with a female partner. Although not all of these partnerships may include lesbian sexual orientation, an estimated 1% of the U.S. female population is lesbian, and an additional 7% are bisexual (Scheer et al., 2002). The proportion of the population that includes transgender individuals is not known. All of these subpopulations comprise the lesbian, gay, bisexual, and transgender (LGBT) community. Women in these subpopulations have many health needs in common with their heterosexual counterparts, but they also have unique needs that are not often known or acknowledged by health care providers. Most attention and research related to the LGBT community has focused on the psychological issues of "coming out" and the prevalence of STDs (Boehmer, 2002).

The American Psychiatric Association recognizes that homosexuality is neither a choice nor a psychiatric disorder; it is a normal variant and an inherent part of a person's identity. Sexual orientation is not chosen; it is discovered. Being a lesbian means that a woman's primary affectional and sexual preferences are for other women. Lesbians exist in all cultures, races, religions, and classes. They cannot be identified by appearance, assumed role, or mannerisms. Lesbians are at high risk for misunderstanding and discrimination because they share the homosexual label with men, yet they have much in common with heterosexual women.

In examining lesbianism and other sexual orientations from a dimensions-of-health perspective, the goal is for the nurse to become better able to meet clients' needs by gaining greater understanding and insight into the similarities and differences between these subgroups and the heterosexual population. Using this knowledge, the nurse is then able to formulate a more sensitive and effective plan of care for the client.

Biophysical Considerations

There are no differences in the maturational or aging processes between lesbian, bisexual, and transgender women and heterosexual women. Sexual identity formation is a similar process of confusion, self-awareness, and acceptance, but leads to different outcomes in each group. Although it is sometimes assumed that the needs of lesbians are similar to those of gay men, their needs are actually quite different and differ as well from those of bisexual and transgender women. There have been no medical problems identified that are specifically attributable to being lesbian or bisexual, but there are some potential differences in risk factors that may put these women at higher risk for certain diseases.

From a gynecologic viewpoint, women who engage in sexual activity exclusively with other women seem to be at lower risk for some sexually transmitted diseases (STDs) than their heterosexual counterparts. Human papillomavirus (HPV), candidiasis, *Trichomonas vaginalis*, herpes virus infection, HIV infection, and bacterial vaginoses, however, are transmissible between women and occur even in lesbians who have not had sex with male partners (Bauer & Welles, 2001; Hawke, 2002; Silenzio & White, 2000a). Unfortunately, less than one fourth of lesbian women in some studies voice concern regarding STD exposure, and few report being regularly tested for STDs. The probability of exposure to STD for women with only female partners increases with the number of partners (Bauer & Welles, 2001). Bisexual women have the same risk of STDs as heterosexual women and may serve as a reservoir of disease for other women (Scheer et al., 2002). Transgender

women have also been shown to be at increased risk for HIV infection (Nemoto et al., 2005). In fact, the prevalence of HIV infection ranges from 11% to 78% of male-to-female transgender persons in different locations in the United States (Nemoto et al., 2004). Complacency regarding risk for STDs should be discouraged, and lesbian, bisexual, and transgender women should be as selective in their sexual partners as possible.

Although actual disease figures have not demonstrated an increased incidence of breast cancer among lesbian women (possibly because of underreporting in this largely hidden group), there is a higher prevalence of certain risk factors for breast and endometrial cancer in this group (Meyer & Bowen, 2000). Nulliparity, late childbearing, low rates of oral contraceptive use, and high rates of smoking prevalence are all risk factors that are prevalent among lesbian women (Sandovsky, 2000).

Routine Pap smears are as important for the lesbian, bisexual, or transgender client as for heterosexual women. Studies have shown that lesbians have cervical dysplasia and carcinoma in situ. The incidence of these cervical disorders rises sharply in women who have had several sexual encounters with men, just as for their heterosexual counterparts. Because lesbian women typically do not use contraceptive services (a common route to health care services for heterosexual women), they may miss opportunities for routine breast and cervical cancer screening. Similarly, lack of regular health care may minimize opportunities for routine blood pressure checks and cholesterol testing, placing lesbian women at higher risk for cardiovascular disease. Increased risk for heart disease may also lie in the fact that lesbian and bisexual women smoke more than their heterosexual sisters and tend to have a higher body mass index (Silenzio & White, 2000b). Transgender women (male-to-female) may also continue to have as many risk factors for health problems as heterosexual men. For example, genital reassignment surgery does not usually entail removal of the prostate gland, so the potential for prostate cancer still exists (King County Public Health, 2005).

Psychological Considerations

Psychological factors affecting lesbian, bisexual, and transgender women are closely entwined with social factors. A woman who realizes that she has a same-sex orientation has three basic choices. She can live openly as a lesbian, thereby setting herself up for potential rejection by her family, loss of her job or professional reputation, and societal labeling and abuse. Second, she can deny her identity and put her energy into fulfilling the accepted female role. Third, she can live a lesbian life but maintain a heterosexual appearance. The second and third options are also those available to a biological male who perceives himself as a woman.

The lesbian, bisexual, or transgender woman who does not live her identity openly must deal, on a daily basis, with the fear that someone will discover who she really is. This involves the complex task of vigilance about how she looks and acts, where she is, who she is with, and what she says. This means that the lesbian or bisexual woman must constantly monitor her responses and change pronouns to misrepresent the identity of her partners. She must hide from coworkers, family, or friends important life events such as a new relationship or the breakup of an old one. Although lesbian women grieve such losses, their grief is not sanctioned by society and is another source of hidden stress. Transgender women also run the risk of rejection and physical assault if their biological maleness is discovered or, if they continue to maintain a male role in some venues, if their transgender activities are discovered. Recently, members of the LGBT community have also had to deal with increased fears of being "outed" by other, more militant individuals. *Outing* involves publicizing another's sexual orientation without their consent.

Coming out is an important emotional occurrence experienced by members of the LGBT community. A lifelong process, **coming out** can be generally defined as one's realization and admission to oneself and to others of a homosexual or bisexual orientation or nonbiological gender identity. Although the process of coming out usually occurs in the tumultuous years of the late teens and early twenties, it can happen at any time in life. Coming out frequently encompasses critical aspects of awareness of same-sex feelings and attractions, initial lesbian encounters or recognition of a different gender identity, participation in the LGBT subculture, labeling of self, and disclosure to significant others. Stages of coming out have been delineated by several authors, but stage models fail to acknowledge that coming out may be more of a continuous process with no specific end point. Lesbians may be "out" to some people in their lives, but not to others (McDonald, McIntyre, & Anderson, 2003). As noted by some authors,

> There are constant transitions in the self and social networks in coming out. Coming out is best understood in terms of the constant transitions that young men and women undertake. There is always someone else to "come out" to whenever new associations are made. For this reason, one can never be wholly "out" (Ridge, Hulme, & Peasley, 2003, p. 284).

The coming out process may encompass contradictory feelings of excitement and relief at having found an inner answer to guilt, sadness, and anger about what the person is losing or giving up. She must come to terms with any guilt she experiences for being different and for not fulfilling her role in the heterosexual lifestyle to which she has been socialized. She may also mourn the loss of her relationship with a spouse or lover, the fact that she may not fulfill parental expectations of a wedding and grandchildren, and the knowledge that she may never be totally socially acceptable. Additionally, many women go through the coming out process without the influence or support of the LGBT subculture, thereby adding isolation to the difficulty of the task. The coming out process may be even more difficult for those from minority cultures who already bear a certain amount of stigma due to membership in an ethnic minority group. These women may be marginalized by both the heterosexual ethnic community and the LGBT community since neither has a true picture of the difficulties they face.

From a mental health perspective, although mental health is of concern among lesbians and bisexual women, they are no more likely to be diagnosed with psychiatric disorders than heterosexual women. Their level of social and psychological functioning is indistinguishable from that of their heterosexual counterparts. The community health nurse must be aware, however, of the medical and psychological implications of the emotional stresses that arise from the moral and social

SPECIAL CONSIDERATIONS

COMING OUT AND SOCIAL SUPPORT FOR TRANSGENDER WOMEN

Sister of the Heart

I walked alone in darkness
Through the forest gloom of night
I longed to find the meadow
To feel the sun so bright

The forest was the people
The ones who couldn't see
The face I showed to them
Was not the real me

There was no way out
Of this prison made by man
The dictates of society
Kept me well in hand

I had heard of others
Who escaped out of the night
They found the path of freedom
That led them to the light

I could not take that path
I could not take that road
The demands of my existence

Were much too great a load

And then I met another
Whose sorrows, thoughts, and dreams
Though it was just online
Were so similar to mine

Although she did not take it
She knew where lay the path
She gave to me the courage
To face the world's wrath

Deserted by so many
Friends and family
She was always there
To set things right for me

She and others like her
Have become my family
She accepts me as I am
She knows the real me

I have yet to reach the meadow
Though I have made a start
When I do, I'll find her
My sister of the heart.

Source: Dummer, L. R. (2004). Unpublished poem. Reprinted with permission from L. R. Dummer.

stigma attached by much of society to a lesbian, bisexual, or transgender identity. As a result of these stresses, lesbian, bisexual, and transgender women may be at greater risk of mental distress, depression, substance abuse, and suicide (Meyer, Rothblum, & Bradford, 2000). Mental distress in transgender women may manifest in attempts at self-mutilation (Sember, 2000).

Some authors suggest that lesbian, bisexual, and transgender women may internalize negative social attitudes to their sexual identities, leading to greater risk of suicide. Whether this greater risk is an actual fact remains an area of controversy. One recent major study, the National Lesbian Health Care Survey, found no more depression in lesbians than in other women, but other studies have provided some evidence of increased risk for mental health problems (Matthews et al., 2002; Mays & Cochran, 2001; Meyer, Rothblum, & Bradford, 2000). There is also evidence, however, of greater risk of mental health problems and suicide attempts in LGBT adolescents than among their heterosexual counterparts (Cochran, Stewart, Ginzler, & Cauce, 2002; Pinhey & Millman, 2004). For example, approximately 30% of youth suicides occur among gay and lesbian youth, and in one study, gay and lesbian youth were two to three times more likely to attempt suicide than their heterosexual age mates. In addition, recent studies have indicated prevalence of suicidal ideation in 4% to 76% of gay and lesbian youth compared to 19% to 29% of the general adolescent population (Russell & Joyner, 2001). Same-sex attraction has also been found to be associated with increased depression, anxiety, conduct disorder, and other disorders in adolescents (Ridge et al., 2003).

Sociocultural Considerations

Elements of the sociocultural dimension create problems that lesbian, bisexual, and transgender women deal with on a daily basis. A woman cannot usually be included in one of these groups without experiencing social problems. The discrepancy between socially prescribed behaviors and sexual and affectional needs automatically sets up a conflict between these women and their environments. The routine conflict with the environment; homophobia; and religious, legal, familial, and economic constraints all combine to make life more difficult for these women.

Homophobia, an irrational fear, hatred, or intolerance of homosexuals, encompasses a belief system that is believed to justify discrimination against gays and lesbians. Transgender females may be stigmatized by the lesbian/bisexual group as well as by the heterosexual population (Meyer, Silenzio, Wolfe, & Dunn, 2000).

Homophobia is used to justify discrimination against and abuse of homosexuals. As of 2004, only 15 states had strong laws prohibiting employment discrimination based on sexual orientation (National Women's Law Center et al., 2004), and state and local laws supporting nondiscrimination are frequently overturned.

Homosexual activity is criminalized in 16 states (Meyer, Silenzio et al., 2000), and lesbians are subjected to many forms of legal discrimination in employment, promotion, and so on. Lesbians are also discriminated against in terms of benefits usually granted to heterosexual married couples. For example, lesbians are not able to receive their partners' Social Security benefits on their deaths (White, Bradford, Silenzio, & Wolfe, 2000), nor can they file a joint tax return, claim family or bereavement leave, or inherit their partners' property.

In addition to legal sanctions, lesbian, bisexual, and transgender women risk the loss of social support due to rejection by family and friends. Loss of traditional sources of support has led to the creation of LGBT communities that offer a variety of health and social services as well as companionship and emotional support. Some authors have noted, however, that the commercial LGBT scene (e.g., gay bars) may not be supportive, but may in fact be impersonal and alienating, particularly for younger people (Ridge et al., 2003). Some professional organizations have gay and lesbian interest groups, and some local governments have developed special offices to address the needs of gay and lesbian populations (Sell & Wolfe, 2000). Among the health professions, some authors have noted that there are fewer role models for non-heterosexually-oriented men and women than in the arts and other fields of science. Historically, many gay and lesbian health care providers drew on their own discriminatory experiences to fuel a personal commitment to caring for other vulnerable populations (Hansen, 2002).

Lesbian, bisexual, and transgender women are frequently subjected to social stigma, discrimination, rejection, and verbal and physical violence (Perkins, 2004). In 2002, for example, 1,464 hate crimes motivated by sexual orientation were committed in the United States (U.S. Census Bureau, 2005). Approximately one third to one half of lesbians have reported being the object of a verbal hate crime, and 5% to 10% have been assaulted. It is estimated that only 13% to 14% of violent episodes are reported for fear of further stigmatization. In fact, 16% to 30% of lesbian, gay, bisexual, or transgender victims report victimization by police personnel (Dean & Bradford, 2000). Another 5% report being hassled by police in general (Mays & Cochran, 2001). Lesbians may

Think Advocacy

How would you go about advocating for rights for LGBT couples equal to those afforded to heterosexual married couples in your state? What activities, if any, are already underway in this effort? Who is engaged in these advocacy activities? What sources of resistance would this kind of policy change encounter? How would you counteract that resistance? What groups or agencies might support your advocacy efforts?

also experience violence, called *horizontal violence*, from their partners. Figures for intimate partner violence among lesbian, bisexual, and transgender women are similar to those reported by heterosexual women, and the potential for domestic violence in same-sex couples should not be ignored. Lesbian, bisexual, and transgender women, as well as heterosexual women, should be assessed for evidence of abuse and the incidence and prevalence of domestic abuse in the community determined.

From a religious perspective, many Christian denominations advocate sexual activity only in the context of procreation. Most, especially fundamentalist denominations, consider homosexuality biologically unnatural, sinful, and condemned by the Bible, and religious traditions may cause a sense of shame in lesbian, bisexual, and transgender women affiliated with more conservative religions. In recent studies, many Americans considered homosexuality to be immoral, but others are more tolerant of nonheterosexuality than in the past. In a 1999 U.S. survey, only 13% of respondents believed that members of the LGBT community should not have equal rights, compared to 33% in 1977 (Casper & Bianchi, 2002). Similarly, public thinking about the causes of sexual orientation has changed, although perceptions of the general public do not parallel perceptions of those with nonheterosexual orientations. For example, approximately a third of the general public in one study believed that people are born with a particular sexual orientation, compared to three fourths of gay and lesbian individuals who held this belief. Similarly, 56% of the general public believed that one can change one's sexual orientation if one chooses to do so, whereas 90% of gay and lesbian respondents indicated that this is not possible (Casper & Bianchi, 2002).

Behaviors considered inappropriate, but tolerated, in the heterosexual population are sanctioned more heavily among nonheterosexuals. For example, cohabitation is less acceptable among same-sex couples than among heterosexual couples. Similarly, messages of support and health prevention for gay and lesbian youth may be construed as promoting gay lifestyles, whereas STD prevention messages for other sexually active youth are accepted (Ridge et al., 2003).

Many women realize and act on their same-sex preferences after they are married and have children; others choose to have children after coming out. It is estimated that there are 1 to 5 million lesbians raising 6 to 14 million children. Research consistently indicates no negative outcomes for these children, in particular that children of lesbians are no more likely than other children to be gay or lesbian. In spite of these findings, courts may deny custody of children to a lesbian parent purely on the basis of her lesbianism (Scout, 2000).

Lesbian parents also face other potential legal difficulties related to their families. Some states prohibit adoption by gay or lesbian couples. Some lesbian women may choose artificial insemination in order to become pregnant. Because lesbians may be denied service by traditional sperm banks, they may enter into dubious agreements with known donors that may not be supported later in a court of law (Scout, 2000). Similarly, if the biological parent should die, the partner may have difficulty retaining custody of children unless guardianship has been legally specified.

Economically, lesbians may have higher educational attainments and earn more than their heterosexual counterparts (Casper & Bianchi, 2002). Disclosure of lesbian, bisexual, or transgender sexual identity or orientation in the work setting, however, could lead to being passed over for promotion, subtle or overt harassment, or termination, particularly if these women work with children or young women. In one study, 39% of lesbian and bisexual women reported not being hired for a particular job, compared to only 16.9% of heterosexual women. Another 34% reported being passed over for promotion, compared to only 14% of their heterosexual counterparts (Mays & Cochran, 2001). As was noted under psychological factors, the ever-present fear of discovery adds immeasurable anxiety and tension to the inherent stress of work. Nevertheless, the economic and occupational achievements of lesbians are similar to those of their heterosexual counterparts.

EVIDENCE-BASED PRACTICE

James and Platzer (1999) presented several ethical considerations in conducting research with marginalized groups such as women with nonheterosexual orientations. These include issues of vulnerability, balancing researcher versus clinician roles, and the possibility of adding to negative stereotypes. Several of these issues are compounded when the researchers are members of the group studied. Marginalized groups may be vulnerable to bias and damage due to researchers' lack of familiarity with the culture and high levels of unmet needs. Confidentiality issues are particularly relevant when the group is characterized by social stigma. In addition, research with marginalized groups is frequently poorly funded, limiting the availability of support counseling when participation in the research causes adverse psychological effects. Researchers who are themselves members of the marginalized group create a potential for bias and also face the ethical dilemma of possibly adding to negative stereotypes of the group if unfavorable findings are discovered (e.g., if research should indicate that children of lesbian parents have higher rates of attempted suicide than other children—which is *not* the case).

- To what extent do you think these ethical issues apply to research with women in general as well as to research with lesbians or bisexual or transgender women?
- What actions might researchers take to minimize potentially harmful effects of these ethical issues?
- How should researchers address the issue of maintaining the rigor of the research study in the face of subjects' identified clinical needs?

Behavioral Considerations

Research suggests that lesbian, bisexual, and transgender women have higher rates of smoking than heterosexual women, and young lesbians have been shown to smoke more than young gay males (Silenzio & White, 2000b). Tobacco companies have targeted LGBT youth, and approximately 48% of lesbian women smoke, more than twice as many as their heterosexual counterparts. The average age for smoking initiation is younger for LGBT youth than for others, and they may have more difficulty with smoking cessation. Lesbian smokers have a risk of breast, colorectal, and other cancers five times higher than that of heterosexual women. Smoking triggers immune system changes that affect prognosis in hepatitis C and other STDs for which bisexual and transgender women are at particular risk (Washington, 2002).

Although lesbianism does not cause alcohol or substance abuse, there is a perception among researchers, clinicians, and lesbians themselves that such problems may be more prevalent and severe among lesbians than in the general population. In part, this is the result of earlier studies conducted on samples solicited in lesbian bars yielding biased samples. Among more recent studies, some researchers have found rates of alcohol and drug use comparable to those of heterosexual women, and some have found higher rates. There is some evidence, however, that younger lesbians have somewhat higher rates of tobacco, marijuana, and cocaine use than their heterosexual counterparts (Silenzio, White, & Wolfe, 2000). Both young boys with same-sex attraction and young girls with bisexual attraction have been found to be at higher risk for substance use and abuse than heterosexual adolescents. They also smoked more, got drunk or drank alone more often, and used more illicit drugs than other youth (Russell, Driscoll, & Truong, 2002). Homeless LGBT youth are at particular risk of starting or escalating substance use and abuse (Cochran et al., 2002).

Lesbian and bisexual women have been found, in some studies, to have higher rates of drug use, greater numbers of sexual partners, and more partners who have sex with prostitutes than strictly heterosexual women. Women who have sex with women comprise 20% to 30% of female intravenous drug users (IDUs) in the United States. Bisexual women are also more likely than other IDUs to engage in injection and sexual behaviors with men who have sex with men, increasing their risks for hepatitis B and HIV infection in high prevalence areas as well as other STDs (Friedman et al., 2003). Bisexual women have also been found to be more likely to have sex with HIV-infected men and engage in anal sex or sexual activity for money (Scheer et al., 2002).

Community health nurses can assist lesbian, bisexual, and transgender women clients by being alert to cues that would indicate patterns of substance abuse, by not assuming that the alcoholism is related to sexual preference, by respecting their reluctance to enter traditional treatment programs that are not designed to meet their needs, by being familiar with resources in the community to assist those women with substance abuse issues, and by involving their significant others in the treatment plan.

Health System Considerations

Beyond reproductive issues, many health needs of women have not been adequately addressed by the U.S. health care system. This propensity tends to be heightened when the woman is of color; a rape victim; addicted to drugs or alcohol; a lesbian, bisexual, or transgender female; or otherwise stigmatized. As noted by several authors, "our society is dominated by the rhetoric of heterosexism, in which 'heterosexuals occupy the position of privilege, and non-heterosexuals are considered other'" (Gray et al., as cited in McDonald et al., 2003, p. 706). Lesbian interactions with the health care system have been characterized by episodes of neglect, discrimination, and abuse.

Three general types of barriers to health care for lesbian, bisexual, and transgender women have been identified: structural barriers, financial barriers, and personal and cultural barriers. Structural barriers relate to the availability and organization of health care services. For example, the short office visits mandated by managed care plans may limit the ability of lesbian, bisexual, and transgender clients to develop the rapport with their providers required for optimal care. Similarly, lack of family insurance coverage may limit the ability of lesbian families to be cared for as a unit by providers who are familiar with the entire family. Finally, there is a systematic lack of recognition of the rights of partners in decision making, visiting, and so on (Solarz, 1999).

Financial barriers relate primarily to the lack of insurance coverage among lesbians. Because of their lack of legal status as a married couple, lesbian partners usually do not have access to spousal insurance benefits, and lesbian women are less likely than heterosexual women to be insured. Surveys of lesbians indicate that 12% to 27% of this population may be uninsured. In the National Lesbian Health Care Survey, 16% of lesbians indicated that they did not receive needed care because of costs (Solarz, 1999). Even for those with health insurance, many may choose not to seek care for fear of breach of confidentiality. This is particularly true of lesbians who are insured under an employer's self-insurance plan in which employers have access to employees' health records (White, Bradford, Silenzio, & Wolfe, 2000).

A variety of personal and cultural barriers also inhibit effective care for lesbian, bisexual, and transgender clients. Health care for women arises out of heterosexual assumptions, and, as noted earlier, contraceptive needs are often a mode of entry for women into the health care system. Because they typically do not have contraceptive needs, lesbian clients may miss opportunities for preventive health and screening services readily available to other women.

Lesbian, bisexual, and transgender clients may also not seek care because of negative provider attitudes or fears of violation of confidentiality (Ridge et al., 2003). Gender identity disorders are still classified as mental illness in the Diagnostic and Statistical Manual of the American Psychiatric Association (McLeer, 2004), and more lesbian and bisexual women (7%) report being denied or given inferior care than heterosexual women (3%) (Mays & Cochran, 2001). In some studies, 9% of lesbians reported that their partners were not allowed to accompany them to examinations and were not included in treatment discussions. Some gay and lesbian clients also reported rough or violent digital examinations after disclosure of their sexual orientation (White, Bradford, & Silenzio, 2000). A study of Swedish nurses revealed positive attitudes toward nonheterosexual clients among 62% of the nurses, but the authors concluded that nursing students needed more education regarding sexual orientation and homosexuality (Rondahl, Innala, & Carlsson, 2004). A few health care providers may even continue to advocate for reparative therapy. Reparative therapy is therapy designed to reverse a same-sex orientation (Meyer, Silenzio et al., 2000).

Counseling and preventive services often assume a heterosexual orientation, and intake forms and interview questions may make it difficult to alert providers to nonheterosexual orientations. Approximately 27% of lesbians in some studies have reported that their providers assumed that they were heterosexual, and 11% describe contraceptives being "forced" on them (Scout, 2000). Conversely, providers may fail to give counseling in areas where lesbian clients may be at risk (e.g., for STDs) (Hawke, 2002).

For effective care to occur, providers need to be aware of and knowledgeable regarding clients' sexual orientations, but the design of the health care system makes disclosure difficult and places the burden of disclosure on lesbian, bisexual, and transgender clients. The GLBT Health Access Project (n.d.) has developed standards of care for LGBT clients that address concerns related to health care personnel, clients' rights, intake and assessment procedures, service planning and delivery, confidentiality, and community outreach and health promotion. In addition, the King County Public Health Department (2005) has developed practice guidelines for use with this population. These standards and guidelines are summarized on page 445 as special considerations in the care of lesbian, bisexual, and transgender clients.

ASSESSING WOMEN'S HEALTH

Care of women as a population group begins with an assessment of health status. Community health nurses may assess the health status of individual women as well as the status of women as an aggregate within the population. In this chapter, we focus on women as a population group and provide focused assessment questions to guide data collection related to factors in each of the six dimensions of health. Appendix I on the Companion Website contains a generic tool for assessing the health status of adult clients that can be used to assess women's health. A tool for assessing the health status of individual heterosexual or nonheterosexual women can also be found in the *Community Assessment Reference Guide* designed as a companion volume to this text.

In assessing biophysical dimension factors influencing the health status of the female population, the community health nurse would examine the incidence of genetic predisposition of certain diseases in the population. For example, the nurse might collect data related to the prevalence of diabetes or heart disease in the overall population, since these are likely to affect women as well as other population groups in the community.

Nurses should assess the relative proportion of women at different ages and different stages of sexual maturation in the population. These data, available from census figures, will provide a picture of the health care needs of women as a subsegment of the population.

Assessment considerations related to the maturational stage of premenopause include pregnancy rates, the proportion of unintended pregnancies in the population, the extent of prenatal care, and information on pregnancy outcomes for women and children. All of this information is routinely collected by local health departments. Consideration should also be given to the availability and use of contraceptive methods by women who do not desire to become pregnant. This kind of information could be obtained by surveys of health agencies that provide contraceptive services. Community health nurses should be alert to increased incidence of PMDD in the community as well as knowledgeable regarding the availability of treatment for those affected.

Community health nurses should also explore with women's health care providers the age at which menopause typically occurs in the population, as well as the extent of factors that may contribute to early menopause and increased health risk. Age at menopause and factors affecting this stage of women's lives may vary among racial and ethnic groups in the community. Another assessment component related to maturation and aging includes the psychological and social effects of aging. Community health nurses can interview knowledgeable community informants regarding attitudes toward women in local community culture(s) as well as women's attitudes toward age and aging.

Assessment of physiologic function also includes the collection of data related to the presence or absence of physical illness in the population. Data on communicable disease incidence and other selected conditions among women may be available from local health authorities or from major providers (e.g., hospitals, clinics) in the area. Mortality data and causes of death for

SPECIAL CONSIDERATIONS

CARING FOR LGBT POPULATIONS

The following general principles are appropriate in providing care to LGBT populations:

- Identify personal beliefs, values, and attitudes toward caring for LGBT individuals.
- Recognize that sexual identity and sexual orientation are not the same thing.
- Recognize that sexual behavior is not synonymous with sexual orientation.
- Avoid assumptions regarding sexual orientation or identity.
- Revise intake and assessment forms and processes to include language appropriate to LGBT clients.
- Emphasize confidentiality and describe how it will be protected.
- Develop and implement specific procedures regarding confidentiality for LGBT clients.
- Be knowledgeable regarding LGBT issues and health concerns.
- Educate employees regarding the health needs of the LGBT population.
- Be knowledgeable regarding LGBT services in the community and facilitate referrals as appropriate.
- Ask for specific feedback regarding the cultural sensitivity of services.
- Develop and implement complaint procedures for discriminatory services.
- Respect partners as you would any other client's family members.
- Address issues of homophobia among staff members.
- Ask about social support and mental health issues.
- Don't assume that all health concerns are related to sexuality.
- Provide appropriate health promotion and illness prevention strategies (e.g., continued breast examinations for transgender men [female-to-male transition] and prostate examinations for transgender women [male-to-female transition], STD prevention for all sexually active clients).
- Provide support, particularly for youth who remain unsure about their sexual identity or orientation.
- Screen for domestic violence as with any other client.
- Promote employment and visibility of LGBT employees and board members.
- Fully include LGBT employees in benefits packages offered to other employees.
- Develop and implement explicit policies that prohibit discrimination in services to LGBT individuals.
- Develop partnerships with other organizations and agencies serving the needs of the LGBT population.

Data from: GLBT Health Access Project. (n.d.). Community standards of practice for provision of quality health care services for gay, lesbian, bisexual, and transgendered clients. *Retrieved August 14, 2005, from http://www.glbthealth.org; King County Public Health. (2005).* Gay, lesbian, bisexual, and transgender health: Culturally competent care for GLBT people: Recommendations for health care providers. *Retrieved August 14, 2005, from http://www.metrokc.gov/health/glbt/ providers.htm*

women are also available from these sources. Information related to other health conditions among women could be obtained from local providers or health care institutions or by means of community surveys. Similar types of information should be collected with respect to lesbian, bisexual, and transgender women. Data regarding the kinds of health problems experienced by these subgroups of women may be available from providers in the community who care for them or through surveys of members of these groups. Assessment of HIV status and prevalence of other STDs may be particularly warranted for bisexual and transgender women as well as for sexually active heterosexual women.

Community health nurses would also assess the extent and type of functional limitations posed by disabling conditions among women. This information is best derived from surveys of women in the community. Nurses could also assess environmental conditions contributing to disability by observation in the community and interviews with community informants. The availability of resources to assist women to deal with disabling conditions can be obtained by consulting the local telephone or social services directory or speaking to the staff of social service agencies that provide this assistance. At the level of the individual client, the nurse would assess factors contributing to disability as well as the effects of disability on all facets of women's lives.

The extent of infertility, another consideration in assessing the health of the female population, may be extrapolated from the number of couples that seek infertility services from providers in the community. Information on contraceptive use among women who do not desire to become pregnant is best derived from community surveys of women of childbearing age. Local prenatal clinics, family planning services, and labor and delivery units may have data on the extent of failed contraception or unintended pregnancy. Abortion data may also be available from these sources as well as from local health department figures on therapeutic and spontaneous abortions.

Community health nurses would also assess the immunization status of individual women clients as well as immunization levels in the population as a whole. These data may not be as readily available as data on childhood immunization levels and may need to be derived from provider records or community surveys. The focused assessment questions provided on page 446 can assist the community health nurse in examining biophysical factors influencing the health of women in the nurse's community.

With respect to the psychological dimension, community health nurses assessing the health of women would consider stress and coping abilities, sexuality, and the prevalence of mental health and illness among women in the population. It is unlikely that aggregate data on the levels of stress experienced by women or the adequacy of their coping skills will be readily available. Community health nurses will most probably need to obtain this information from community surveys or from indirect indicators such as the incidence and prevalence of depression and other mental health problems in the community. They may also be able to get some sense of the extent of these conditions from records of mental health professionals or agencies in the community.

Information on sexual identity within the female population is also difficult to obtain. Community health nurses can observe for elements of a lesbian, bisexual, or transgender culture in the community and speak to members of that culture to get some sense of the extent of these sexual identities in the community. Other data may come from counselors or other professionals sought by members of these groups to deal with the psychological and social ramifications of nonheterosexual identities. Community health nurses should assess for feelings of guilt, isolation, or depression among lesbian, bisexual, and transgender women who have come or are coming to grips with their identities.

Community health nurses assessing the health of the female population should explore the extent of mental health problems among women as well as the psychosocial factors that contribute to their incidence and prevalence. Information on the incidence and prevalence of conditions such as depression, schizophrenia, eating disorders, and so on may be available from local mental health providers. Community health nurses should be aware of social and cultural factors that promote unhealthy body images among women that lead to eating disorders. Data on the prevalence of mental health issues and suicide among lesbian, bisexual, and transgender women are also needed and can be obtained from providers who serve these groups for

FOCUSED ASSESSMENT

Psychological Considerations in Assessing Women's Health

- What are the sources of stress to which women in the population are exposed?
- What are the incidence and prevalence of mental illness in the female population? What specific mental health problems are prevalent in the population?
- What is the societal attitude toward women? Does this attitude contribute to stress for women in the population?
- What is the extent of nonheterosexual orientation in the female population? What are the societal attitudes toward nonheterosexual orientation? How does this affect the level of stress experienced by women in the population?

mental illness or from local mortality figures for suicide. Community surveys of these groups may also provide relevant data. The questions in the focused assessment below provide guidance for assessing factors in the psychological dimension influencing women's health.

The effect of physical environmental dimension factors on women's health can best be determined by observation. Community health nurses may also seek out incidence and prevalence figures on environmentally caused diseases in women from local health departments and from local employers. Information on environmental factors within the home that affect women's health status can be obtained through observation or community surveys. Focused assessment questions are provided below to direct examination of physical environmental factors influencing women's health.

One of the major sociocultural factors to be assessed in determining the health status of the female population is that of roles and relationships with others. Community health nurses should assess cultural definitions of women's roles and relationships within the population and the effects of those definitions on women's health and health-related behaviors. Nurses would also determine the proportion of women in the population who engage in family caregiver roles and the extent of support and respite services available to them. Much of

FOCUSED ASSESSMENT
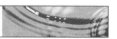

Biophysical Considerations in Assessing Women's Health

- What is the age composition of the female population?
- What is the racial/ethnic composition of the female population?
- What are the main causes of mortality in the female population?
- What acute and chronic illnesses are prevalent in the female population? What factors contribute to the prevalence of these conditions?
- What percentage of the female population are of childbearing age? What is the annual birth rate in the population? What is the fertility rate?
- What is the level of immunity to specific communicable diseases among the female population?

FOCUSED ASSESSMENT

Physical Environmental Considerations in Assessing Women's Health

- To what environmental health hazards are women in the population exposed?
- What environmental hazards are posed by occupational settings?
- Are women engaged in recreational pursuits that pose physical environmental hazards?
- To what extent does the physical environment promote or impede healthy behaviors by women (e.g., physical activity)?

this data can be obtained in interviews with community informants or by means of community surveys.

The proportion of women employed in the labor force is available from census data. Specific data on the types of jobs in which women are employed can be obtained from local businesses or business associations. The incidence of occupational injuries and illness among women can be derived from the same sources or from state OSHA data. Community health nurses assess individual women's occupational and economic status and the effects of these factors on their health. In addition, they obtain information about women's income levels, occupations, and other societal factors that may impinge on their ability to work or influence the economic and occupational effects on health for the population.

Domestic violence is another sociocultural factor that impinges heavily on the health of women. Assessment

at the aggregate level includes the prevalence of various forms of abuse of women as well as the presence of risk factors for abuse in the general population. Societal attitudes and responses to abuse are other important aspects of the assessment. Information on the incidence and prevalence of abuse can be derived from police records and from data kept by agencies that assist these women, but only capture a small segment of the abuse that probably occurs. Community surveys and data from emergency departments are other means of identifying the extent of abuse of women in the population.

In assessing a potentially abused woman, the nurse needs to ask the client about depression, the possibility of suicide, and her risk of being killed by her partner. Another important consideration is the woman's willingness to leave the situation. Many women in such situations continue to hope that their partner will change or are fearful

Advocacy in Action

Eva's Plight

The story begins on a Friday afternoon when I made an unscheduled visit to Eva, an 88-year-old woman I had visited earlier in the month. She had begun to show signs of declining health and I felt it wise to check on her. Eva, a widow, lived with her adopted son in the two-family brick home that she and her husband had purchased many years before. John was severely hearing impaired and had not worked for many years. There were no other children, and the only relatives were distant cousins who had limited contact with Eva and her son.

When I got there, I noted that Eva was not seated in her usual place on the living room couch. She was instead in her bed curled up in a fetal position, almost unresponsive to my voice. As I moved closer to her bed and called her name several times, she awoke. She nodded when I asked whether she was comfortable. When I asked if she had eaten, she shook her head.

I went to the kitchen, found a can of chicken soup, and opened it. As the soup was heating up, I decided to freshen Eva up a bit, and that was when I discovered the first problem: lack of water due to an unpaid water bill. Doing the best I could to straighten and freshen Eva, I asked her son to put her in her wheelchair. He did, but he was very rough, causing Eva to wince in pain as her tiny frame hit the hard plastic seat of the wheelchair. Problem number two identified: ineffective coping (son) related to anxiety or stress.

I left John to feed his mother and returned to my office at the parish where I began to make plans for dealing with this crisis. I first contacted the water department, explained the situation, and assured them that the bill would be negotiated early the following week. The water was turned on later that

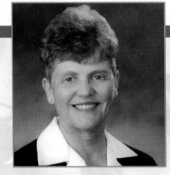

day. Next, I contacted a member of the parish who was a lawyer and friend of the family. He suggested the steps we should take to secure guardianship for Eva given that neither she nor her son could manage their personal or financial affairs. Because it was a weekend, nothing could be done until Monday morning, but plans were made to petition the court for a guardian. I arranged for members of the parish to provide food and companionship throughout the weekend.

Early Monday morning I signed the petition and the court formally began to process the paperwork. Two days later, a hearing was held regarding our petition for guardianship. As the parish nurse and petitioner, I was called before the judge, who asked a number of questions pertinent to Eva's well-being. So too was the guardian ad litem, who reported that since Eva's nutritional status had improved she was coherent and able to make her own decisions. However, based on my assessment and documentation of visits with Eva over the previous 3 years, the judge appointed a guardian for Eva.

My relationship with Eva continued after the appointment of the guardian. As the parish nurse and someone who knew Eva well, I was contacted by the guardian for suggestions on an extended care placement. Eva passed away three weeks later. Then problem three was identified: inability to cope (son) related to death of mother, initiating advocacy on John's behalf.

Judith Mouch, MSN, MA
University of Detroit Mercy

that the partner will hunt them down and further injure them if they try to leave. Another common fear is that the partner will attempt to win custody of the children if the woman leaves.

In assessing the health status of the lesbian, bisexual, and transgender populations, community health nurses should explore community attitudes toward LGBT lifestyles and their effects on members of these groups. They should also examine laws that support or discriminate against lesbian, bisexual, and transgender women. In addition, community health nurses should identify supports available for members of the LGBT community, their effects, and the extent to which they are utilized by this population. With respect to individual lesbian, bisexual, or transgender women, community health nurses should be sensitive to feelings of guilt, abandonment, or anger or suicidal tendencies experienced as a result of societal attitudes and values. Coming out to family members may be particularly difficult in the context of a conservative social or religious milieu. Community health nurses can also explore with lesbian mothers and providers of support services the use and availability of legal safeguards related to custody of children. Sociocultural factors influencing the health of the female population can be identified using the focused assessment questions provided above right.

With respect to behavioral dimension factors, community health nurses would gather data related to dietary consumption patterns, including cultural influences on diet and meal patterns. They would also determine the extent of obesity and other diet-related problems in the population. In addition, they would examine other consumption patterns, such as the extent of smoking, alcohol, and drug use, and the extent of and opportunities for physical activity among women. They would also explore social and cultural attitudes toward these health-related behaviors as well as toward behaviors such as seat belt use. In addition, community health nurses should examine the proportion of women in the population who are sexually active and their use of contraceptive measures and safe sexual practices. Much of this information is derived from observations, police records of alcohol and drug arrests, or community surveys. Similar data could be obtained with respect to the lesbian, bisexual, and transgender population, but would be derived primarily from community surveys or in interviews with knowledgeable informants or health care providers and counselors. The focused assessment provided at right can guide exploration of behavioral factors influencing the health of women in the population.

Assessment of health system factors influencing the health of women would address the proportion of women who have health insurance and the extent of conditions covered by various types of insurance. Community health nurses would also obtain information

FOCUSED ASSESSMENT

Sociocultural Considerations in Assessing Women's Health

- What are the social roles expected of women? What effects do these role expectations have on women's health?
- What opportunities for social interaction are available to women in the population?
- What is the extent of social support available to women in the population?
- What is the percentage of single-parent families headed by women in the population?
- What is the typical educational status of women in the population?
- What is the economic status of women in the population? Are women allowed to own property in their own names? Are they allowed to control money and other family resources?
- What transportation opportunities are available to women in the population?
- To what extent do women in the population function as caretakers for other family members? To what extent do these women experience caretaker burden?
- What percentage of women in the population is employed? What are the typical occupations for women in the population? What effects do occupation and employment setting have on women's health? What support do employers provide for women's other roles and responsibilities?
- What childcare services are available to working women? What is the cost of these services?
- What are the incidence and prevalence of abuse of women in the population? What are the societal attitudes toward abuse of women? What resources are available to abused women in the population?

on the use of services by uninsured women (e.g., use of emergency departments) and the extent to which women forgo health care services due to lack of access or affordability. Community health nurses should also examine the availability of services needed by women in the population. For example, are there sufficient providers of obstetrical and gynecological services

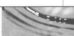

FOCUSED ASSESSMENT

Behavioral Considerations in Assessing Women's Health

- What are the dietary consumption patterns typical of women in the population?
- What is the prevalence of smoking among women in the population?
- What is the extent of alcohol and other drug use in the population?
- To what extent do women in the population engage in safety practices (e.g., seat belt use)?
- To what extent do women who are sexually active engage in safe sexual practices?
- What is the extent of contraceptive use in the population?
- To what extent do women engage in health screening practices such as mammography and so on?

in the community to meet the needs of the female population? Are contraceptive services available and affordable? Finally, community health nurses would be alert to the extent of use of available services by women and barriers to their use (e.g., language, lack of childcare, lack of hours outside women's work times). With respect to the lesbian, bisexual, and transgender population, community health nurses could gather data on their perceptions and use of health care services by means of community surveys. Information on provider attitudes toward and knowledge of the health needs of lesbian, bisexual, and transgender women can be derived from provider surveys or interviews with health care providers in the community. Community health nurses could also observe the extent to which provider offices and other facilities reflect the standards and guidelines for care of these population groups. Health system factors affecting the health status of women can be explored using the focused assessment questions provided below.

DIAGNOSTIC REASONING AND CARE OF WOMEN

Based on information obtained during assessment, community health nurses develop nursing diagnoses that direct further interventions. These diagnoses reflect both positive health states and potential or existing health problems and the factors contributing to them. Nursing diagnoses might relate to health problems experienced by an individual woman such as "role overload due to employment, single parenthood, and lack of a social support network." Or diagnoses may be made at the aggregate level regarding the health needs of groups of women. An example of a nursing diagnosis at this level might be a "need for adequate and inexpensive childcare due to the number of single-parent working women and a lack of affordable childcare."

FOCUSED ASSESSMENT

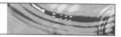

Health System Considerations in Assessing Women's Health

- What percentage of the female population has a regular source of health care?
- What are the attitudes of women toward health and health care services?
- What percentage of the female population has health insurance coverage?
- What health services are available to women in the population? Are health care services needed by women available to all segments of the population?
- What barriers to obtaining health care do women encounter?
- What are the attitudes of health care providers to care of women? To care of nonheterosexual women?

PLANNING AND IMPLEMENTING HEALTH CARE FOR WOMEN

In planning to meet the identified health needs of the female population, community health nurses incorporate the general principles of planning discussed in Chapter 15∞. It is important to keep in mind the unique needs of female clients. Participation by women in planning health care services is particularly important in view of the passive and dependent role expected of female clients by health care providers of the past. Women need to be encouraged to be active participants in health care decision making.

Planning and implementing care for groups of women also need to be based on women's unique circumstances. Services should be offered at times when women, especially working women, can take advantage of them. Provision for transportation and childcare services during appointments might also need to be considered. Financing of such programs can be problematic, given the lower earning capacity of many women, and political activity to ensure program funding may need to be part of the planning process. Planning to meet the health needs of female clients may involve developing primary, secondary, or tertiary preventive interventions.

Primary Prevention

Four goals for wellness direct primary preventive interventions for women:

- Maintaining balance, perspective, and priorities in life
- Developing and maintaining healthy relationships
- Developing and maintaining a healthy sense of self
- Developing and maintaining a physically healthy body and preventing acute and chronic illness (Olshansky, 2000)

An additional goal for some women is promoting healthy pregnancy outcomes. Primary preventive measures related to each of the goals will be briefly discussed.

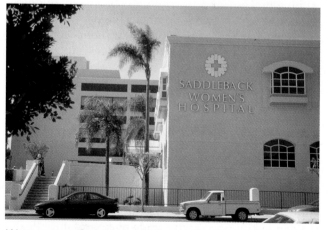

Women are often in need of specialized health care services. (Myrleen Ferguson)

Maintaining Balance, Perspective, and Priorities

Women may need assistance with a variety of conditions in their lives to help them achieve the first goal of wellness. For example, they may need referrals to existing social service programs for assistance in achieving economic balance. Similarly, they may need help in balancing multiple roles. Intervention in this area may be particularly important for single women with children who may be fulfilling both parental roles as well as the breadwinner role. Women caretakers may also need help in learning to balance personal needs with those of other family members or may need respite from continual demands on their time and energy. Community health nurses can also advocate for the availability of needed supports and services for women. For example, they might assist in the development of respite services for women who care for young children or disabled family members. Or they might advocate with the women themselves, encouraging them to take needed time for themselves and to delegate some of their responsibilities to others if possible.

For lesbian, bisexual, and transgender women, the aspects of life to be balanced may be even more complex, and community health nurses can assist them to find resources that help them to achieve the desired level of balance. For example, referrals may be needed to address legal problems of child custody or inclusion of partners in health-related decisions (e.g., drafting of a durable power of attorney).

There may also be a need to assist women to achieve balance in the work setting. The community health nurse may work to change the psychosocial environment of the work setting by means of several strategies. These strategies include educating and socializing women to expect wage equity and to believe that their work is as important as a man's, promoting legislation to prevent job discrimination, educating women about their rights, and encouraging women to challenge sexual harassment. Additional strategies include supporting women running for political office, influencing the legislative process, and promoting collective bargaining, mentoring, and networking among women. A final strategy is active participation in organizations working for changes to benefit women.

The community health nurse working in the occupational setting can provide primary preventive care for women by identifying and understanding stressors affecting women in the work setting, counseling regarding work options, encouraging women to report safety hazards (or the nurse can report them personally), encouraging organization of women in the work setting, fostering personal preventive measures such as the use of protective devices, and keeping a log of jobs and exposure to hazardous materials and health changes. Another major contribution can be made by community health nurses who have clients experiencing role proliferation. These nurses can assist clients to plan efficient use of

time, to use outside help when possible, and to let go of minor household duties that can wait. Single parents particularly need help in this area.

Primary prevention for female clients also involves assistance in the development of coping skills and assertiveness. Interventions can be designed to improve women's self-esteem and to teach them how to cope with life stress in effective ways. These kinds of interventions may be particularly important for lesbian, bisexual, and transgender women who are subjected to multiple stressors.

Developing and Maintaining Healthy Relationships

Development of coping skills and self-esteem not only assists women in maintaining balance in their lives, but also assists in the development of healthy relationships. Another critical intervention in this area is prevention of domestic abuse. Community health nurses can assist in the development of societal conditions that prohibit abuse (e.g., strong sanctions for abusers, assistance for women at risk for abuse, etc.). Primary prevention of abuse is addressed in more detail in Chapter 32∞.

Developing and Maintaining a Sense of Self

Interventions in this area are important for all women, but may be particularly critical for lesbian, bisexual, and transgender women who are experiencing the coming-out process or who are experiencing guilt over their sexual orientation. Abused women may also need to develop a strong sense of self to avoid blaming themselves for the abuse. Community health nurses can be active in the development of societal attitudes that value women and that promote the economic and social status of women.

Young girls approaching menarche, women experiencing perimenopause and menopause, and infertile women may also be in particular need of interventions to assist them to develop or maintain strong self-images. Working women who are entering retirement or mothers who are experiencing the departure of children from the home may need help coming to grips with changes in their roles without feeling devalued or useless. Similarly, women who have decided to leave an abusive situation or obtain a divorce may need assistance in dealing with feelings of guilt, loss, and depression. Community health nurses can provide anticipatory guidance regarding all of these changes and assist women to work through them effectively without diminished self-esteem. In addition, nurses can provide assistance with the practical aspects of change (e.g., menstrual education, referral for hormone replacement therapy [HRT], financial assistance, etc.).

Developing a Physically Healthy Body and Preventing Illness

A number of primary preventive interventions center on promotion of physical health and prevention of illness. General measures for promoting health in women are similar to those for all clients and include adequate nutrition, rest and exercise, immunization, and abstinence from unhealthy behaviors such as tobacco, alcohol, and drug use. Attention should also be given to healthy behaviors such as the use of seat belts and other safety devices and use of preventive health services (including contraceptive services as needed). With respect to physical activity, women should also be educated regarding prevention of exercise-related musculoskeletal injury and encouraged to be realistic in goal setting and injury prevention (Gilchrist, Jones, Sleet, & Kimsey, 2000).

One of several health promotion strategies specific to women is provision of prenatal care. Although some progress has been made in this area (83.7% of pregnant U.S. women in 2002 began prenatal care in the first trimester, compared to only 68% in 1970), 3.6% of women either delayed obtaining prenatal care until the third trimester of pregnancy or received no prenatal care at all (CDC, 2004a). Reasons given for delaying receipt of care were not knowing they were pregnant, inability to afford care, and inability to get an appointment. Community health nurses can assist in early case finding of pregnant women and referral for services. In addition, they can educate the public regarding the need for early prenatal care and advocate for access to prenatal care services for all segments of the population.

For those women who do not wish to become pregnant, community health nurses can provide information about contraceptive options and make referrals for contraceptive services. At the aggregate level, community health nurses may need to advocate for the availability of such services, particularly for adolescents or low-income women.

Health promotion is also needed by women in the perimenopausal and postmenopausal years. These women should be educated regarding the need for dietary supplementation with calcium and vitamin D and weight-bearing exercise to prevent osteoporosis. Long-term calcium supplementation has been shown to reduce the risk of fractures by 24% to 30% (Shepherd, 2004). Sun exposure on the face, hands, and arms for short periods without sunscreen and dietary vitamin D supplementation promote calcium absorption and should be encouraged in perimenopausal and postmenopausal women (Curry & Hogstel, 2002). Women should also be encouraged to limit alcohol intake and refrain from smoking since both increase calcium excretion. In spite of documented benefits from these lifestyle changes, only limited numbers of women engage in them, even after being identified as at risk for osteoporosis. In fact, in one study in Scotland, only 21% of women changed their dietary habits after being told of their risk for osteoporosis (Sandison et al., 2004).

There is some evidence to indicate that only current, not past, use of HRT is associated with decreased risk of hip fractures (Yates et al., 2004). Conversely, two major national studies on the effects of estrogen on postmenopausal women were discontinued due to increased risks for breast cancer, stroke, cardiovascular disease, and blood clots. The conclusion reached was that the potential for harm outweighed the possible benefits of HRT in the prevention of chronic diseases. Based on these findings, the U.S. Preventive Services Task Force (2005a) has recommended against the use of combined estrogen and progestin HRT in postmenopausal women despite the evidence of its effectiveness in preventing fractures and possible evidence of a preventive effect for colorectal cancer due to the increased potential for harm.

Because of concerns regarding the safety of HRT or because of perceptions of menopause as a natural phenomenon, a growing number of women are shifting to the use of botanical preparations for relief of menopause symptoms. Other women may employ acupuncture or other complementary or alternative therapies (National Center for Complementary and Alternative Medicine, 2005). Many of these remedies have limited evidence of effectiveness. For example, black cohosh has been shown to be somewhat effective in addressing dysmenorrhea and premenstrual syndrome and may provide short-term relief for hot flashes in menopause, but it is contraindicated in persons at risk for breast cancer and may contribute to endometrial cancer. Dong quai, often used as part of tailored herbal preparations, has no documented effect and is contraindicated for use with anticoagulants (Wilson, 2004). Controlled studies suggest that 20% to 30% of the response achieved with estrogen preparations may be explained by a placebo effect (National Center for Complementary and Alternative Medicine, 2005). Suggestions for educating clients regarding the use of botanicals are presented on page 452.

Given the confusing information regarding HRT or natural botanicals, community health nurses may need to assist clients to make informed decisions regarding osteoporosis prevention and dealing with menopausal symptoms. Some authors have suggested a tailored approach to assisting women with HRT decision making, taking into account the woman's personal risk of breast cancer and other possible adverse effects (McBride et al., 2002). For women whose risk of cancer or heart disease outweighs that of osteoporosis, HRT may not be appropriate.

Communicable disease prevention entails such interventions as immunization and safe sex activities. Tetanus–diphtheria immunization is recommended at 10-year intervals for all adults, including women, and women of childbearing age who are not immune to rubella should receive one dose of measles, mumps, and rubella (MMR) vaccine. Similarly, women who do not have documented immunity to chickenpox should receive varicella vaccine. Other immunizations recommended, particularly for elderly women or those with chronic diseases, include annual influenza vaccinations and one dose of pneumococcal vaccine. Standing orders for nurses and pharmacists to give immunizations as needed and provision of immunizations in pharmacies, community centers, workplaces, churches, and so on can enhance the immunization status of women as well as other groups (McKibben et al., 2000; Postema & Breiman, 2000). Community health nurses may be involved in giving immunizations, making referrals to immunization sources, or assuring the availability of immunization services to women clients.

Education on barrier contraceptive methods should be given to sexually active women who are not in exclusive monogamous relationships for both partners. This is a need for all women, whether heterosexual, lesbian, bisexual, or transgender, who are at risk for STDs. Emphases in primary prevention interventions for women's health are summarized in Table 17-4◆.

Promoting Healthy Pregnancy Outcomes

In spite of a general broadening of their focus to multiple types of health problems at the population level, community health nurses retain their traditional commitment to promoting healthy pregnancy outcomes for mother, infant, and other family members. Because of their presence in the community, community health nurses may become aware of women early in the course of their pregnancies, providing the opportunity for referral for early initiation of prenatal care. Many community health nurses also provide care during pregnancy and into the postpartum recovery period.

Early in the pregnancy, the community health nurse would educate the woman regarding appropriate

TABLE 17-4	Primary Prevention Emphases in the Care of Women
Primary Prevention Goal	**Foci**
Maintaining balance, perspective, and priorities	• Maintaining economic balance • Balancing multiple roles • Balancing personal needs and caretaking responsibilities • Coming to grips with one's sexual orientation • Balancing work and family responsibilities • Balancing work and life stress • Developing coping and assertiveness skills
Maintaining healthy relationships	• Preventing domestic violence • Promoting healthy communication styles
Maintaining a sense of self	• Developing and maintaining one's self-identity • Receiving anticipatory guidance for role changes
Maintaining physical health and preventing illness	• Obtaining adequate nutrition • Obtaining adequate rest and exercise and preventing injury • Staying current on immunizations • Abstaining from unhealthy behaviors (e.g., smoking, alcohol and drug use) • Using safety precautions • Obtaining prenatal care • Preventing osteoporosis • Practicing safe sex

---

CLIENT EDUCATION — **Use of Botanical Preparations**

- Use of herbal remedies and dietary supplements should be reported to one's primary health care provider.
- "Natural" products do not have guaranteed safety or efficacy.
- Interactions of botanicals with prescription drugs may be dangerous.
- Lack of production standardization may result in differences in content and efficacy of products from batch to batch or from manufacturer to manufacturer.
- Lack of quality control in production may result in contamination, adulteration, or misidentification of botanical sources.
- Compounding errors may result in toxicity in custom-blended botanical preparations.
- Botanicals should not be used by pregnant or lactating women or those planning to become pregnant.
- Botanicals should not be taken in doses larger than those recommended.
- Some botanicals are known to have adverse effects.
- A small positive response to use of botanicals could be a result of a placebo effect.

Data from: American College of Obstetricians and Gynecologists. (2001). Use of botanicals for management of menopause symptoms. ACOG Practice Bulletin: Clinical Management Guidelines for Obstetrician-Gynecologists, 28, 1–15. Retrieved August 13, 2005, from http://www.acog.org/from_home/ publications/misc/pb028.htm

nutrition, exercise, dental hygiene, sexual activity, signs and symptoms of complications, and fetal development. If the woman smokes or uses other drugs, the nurse would educate her on the potential harmful effects of these behaviors for the fetus and encourage quitting. The community health nurse also monitors the progress of the pregnancy and helps the woman deal with its discomforts (e.g., nausea, breast tenderness, back pain). In addition, the nurse monitors blood pressure and other signs of complications (e.g., edema, urinary protein). When signs of complications occur or the woman is at high risk for adverse pregnancy outcomes, the nurse can reinforce the need to seek medical attention. The community health nurse may also need to help the client deal with the interactive effects of pregnancy and other health conditions (e.g., asthma).

As the pregnancy progresses, the community health nurse monitors fundal height and weight gain, assesses for fetal heart tones, and continues to monitor blood pressure and other signs of complications. The nurse also assists the client to begin preparation for the infant's arrival. If there are other children in the home, the nurse might discuss the potential for sibling rivalry and ways to minimize siblings' negative reactions. The nurse may also assist the woman and other adults in the home to envision how roles and relationships will change with the advent of a child. At this time, the community health nurse may also begin educating the mother regarding signs and symptoms of labor and the labor process.

Closer to the time of delivery, the community health nurse may refer interested clients and their significant others for childbirth education classes, while continuing to monitor the status of the pregnancy. He or she may also begin to educate the family regarding childcare and safety issues as well as make sure that plans have been made for appropriate supplies for the infant or care of older children when the mother goes into labor. Plans for breast-feeding or bottle-feeding the infant and for returning to work can also be discussed. The nurse may also begin discussing contraceptive options with clients who desire to prevent or delay subsequent pregnancies and may make referrals for childcare services for women returning to work. Education at this time may also address the need for infant immunizations.

Throughout the pregnancy, the community health nurse should assess and help family members deal with emotional reactions to the pregnancy. The nurse should also be alert to potential signs of abuse of the pregnant woman and refer her for assistance and protective services if needed. The nurse may also engage in a variety of other referrals to assist the woman and family to deal with service and financial needs related to the pregnancy. For example, the nurse might refer a low-income woman to the supplemental nutrition program for Women, Infants, and Children (WIC). A checklist of recommended community health nursing interventions in the prenatal period is included in the *Community Assessment Reference Guide* ▢ designed to accompany this text.

After delivery, the nurse will assess the physiological status of both mother and newborn as well as the psychological response of the mother, maternal–infant bonding, and the responses of other family members. The community health nurse may need to advocate for changes in role expectations for the mother to accommodate the additional role demands of caring for the infant. The nurse may also encourage other family members to participate in the care of the infant or other home care responsibilities. Postpartum care should also be encouraged as well as follow-up on contraceptive care decisions. Finally, the nurse can assist the mother and other family members to deal with the exigencies of a newborn in the home. For example, the nurse may teach the mother how to bathe and dress the baby, how to correctly position the baby at breast, or how to deal with a reaction to first immunizations. The *Community Assessment Reference Guide* ▢ designed to accompany this text provides an inventory that can be used to guide care of mother and newborn in the postpartum period.

At the population level, community health nurses can advocate for the availability of prenatal care and can work to make sure that safe delivery options and adequate nutrition are available to all pregnant women. They can also promote self-help groups among women

or families with young infants or arrange for childbirth and childcare classes in local venues. Finally, they can advocate for the availability of contraceptive services for women who do not desire subsequent pregnancies.

Secondary Prevention

Secondary prevention focuses on screening and diagnosis and treatment for existing health problems.

Screening

Several organizations make recommendations for routine screening procedures among women. For example, the American Cancer Society has made recommendations for breast and cervical cancer screening in women. Similarly, the U.S. Preventive Services Task Force has examined evidence regarding the effectiveness of specific screening procedures in different population groups (e.g., men, women, children, adults, people with specific risk factors) and developed an extensive set of recommendations for routine screening practices. Routine screening procedures specifically recommended for women are summarized in Table 17-5◆. Individual women should, of course, also be screened for other health problems for which they may be at risk.

Many women do not receive recommended routine screening procedures. For example, in 2002, only 89% to 98% of women in various states had ever had a Papanicolaou smear and only 85% to 94% had ever received a mammogram (Balluz et al., 2004). Screening figures are even lower for minority women. Based on 2001–2002 data, 70% to 85% of minority women had had a mammogram in the previous 2 years, and 68% to 89% had received a Papanicolaou smear (Liao et al., 2004). Lower rates of screening are also associated with lack of health insurance, lower educational levels, and being foreign-born (Hewitt, Devesa, & Breen, 2002). Overall in 2000, 81% of all U.S. women over 18 years of age had had a Pap smear in the previous 2 years (CDC, 2004a), and in 2003, 70% of adult women in the United States had had a mammogram at some time in their lives (NCHS, 2005b). Women are slightly more likely than men to have had a cholesterol check in the last 5 years (Division of Adult and Community Health, 2005a).

Community health nurses can educate the public regarding the need for routine screening procedures and can advocate for the availability of screening services for all segments of the female population. Community health nurses may also be involved in case management for women whose screening tests are positive. These women may need assistance in accessing further diagnostic and treatment services (Lawson, Henson, Bobo, & Kaeser, 2000).

Diagnosing and Treating Existing Problems

Community health nurses refer women for medical or social assistance with any identified health problems. Problems unique to female clients for which secondary

TABLE 17-5   Routine Screening Recommendations for Women

Type of Screening	Recommendation
Asymptomatic bacteriuria	**U.S. Preventive Services Task Force:** All pregnant women at 12–26 weeks gestation
Cervical cancer (Papanicolaou smear)	**American Cancer Society**: All women 3 years after becoming sexually active and no later than age 21; every 2 to 3 years after age 30 with previous negative tests; not after age 70 with negative tests for the last 10 years; not after total hysterectomy
	U.S. Preventive Services Task Force: All sexually active women with a cervix; not after age 65 with previous negatives; not after total hysterectomy
Chlamydia trachomatis	**U.S. Preventive Services Task Force:** All sexually active women and pregnant women less than 25 years of age, other women at high risk
Clinical breast examination	**CDC:** Women aged 50–69 years
	U.S. Preventive Services Task Force: Insufficient evidence to recommend routine screening
Colorectal cancer	**U.S. Preventive Services Task Force:** Women over age 50 (fecal occult blood and/or sigmoidoscopy); no evidence of effectiveness of screening colonoscopy
Depression	**U.S. Preventive Services Task Force:** Adult women in practice settings where follow-up is available
Diabetes	**U.S. Preventive Services Task Force:** Adult women with hypertension or hyperlipidemia
Gonorrhea	**U.S. Preventive Services Task Force:** All sexually active and pregnant women with risk factors
Group B streptococcus	Vaginal and rectal screening for all pregnant women
Hepatitis B	**U.S. Preventive Services Task Force:** All pregnant women at first prenatal visit
Herpes simplex virus	**U.S. Preventive Services Task Force:** Not recommended for asymptomatic pregnant women
HIV infection	**U.S. Preventive Services Task Force:** All pregnant women; all adults and adolescents at risk
Intimate partner violence	**U.S. Preventive Services Task Force:** No evidence of screening effectiveness **Women's advocacy groups:** All primary care and emergency department interactions with women
Lipid disorders (total cholesterol and HDL-C)	**U.S. Preventive Services Task Force:** All women over age 45
Mammogram	**U.S. Preventive Services Task Force:** All women age 40 and over (every 1 to 2 years)
Obesity	**U.S. Preventive Services Task Force:** All adult women
Osteoporosis	**U.S. Preventive Services Task Force:** All women after age 65, women at high risk over age 60
Preeclampsia	**U.S. Preventive Services Task Force:** All pregnant women (via blood pressure) at first prenatal visit and periodically
Rh(D)	**U.S. Preventive Services Task Force:** All pregnant women at first prenatal visit and 24–28 weeks gestation unless the father is known to be Rh(D) negative
Rubella susceptibility	**U.S. Preventive Services Task Force:** All women of childbearing age at first clinical encounter (immunize if susceptible and not pregnant, immunize after delivery if pregnant)
Self-breast examination (SBE)	**U.S. Preventive Services Task Force:** Insufficient evidence to recommend routine screening
Sexually transmitted diseases	All sexually active women, including lesbian, bisexual, and transgender women
Syphilis	**U.S. Preventive Services Task Force:** All pregnant women and others at risk
Tobacco use	**U.S. Preventive Services Task Force:** All adult women and pregnant women

Data from: American Cancer Society, 2002; Bauer & Welles, 2001; CDC, 2004b; Division of STD/AIDS Prevention, 2002; Schrag, Gorwitz, Fultz-Butts, & Schuchat, 2002; U.S. Preventive Services Task Force, 1996a; 1996b; 2001a; 2001b; 2002a; 2002b; 2002c; 2002d; 2003a; 2003b; 2003c; 2003d; 2004a; 2004b; 2004c; 2004d; 2004e; 2005b; 2005c; 2005d. See references for full citations.

prevention may be required include infertility, fertility control, menopause, and physical abuse. Secondary prevention may also be required for existing acute and chronic health conditions.

Treatment for infertility generally requires referral to a fertility specialist. The role of the community health nurse with respect to infertility focuses on case finding, referral, and support during a fertility workup. The nurse can also assist the client and her significant other in considering alternative options such as adoption, artificial insemination, and in vitro fertilization. The nurse may also refer couples to self-help groups for assistance in dealing with psychological problems of infertility. In addition, the community health nurse may assist infertile women to deal with the psychological ramifications of their condition. This may be particularly needed for women from cultural groups in which a woman's identity or worth is based on her ability to have children. At the population level, community health nurses can work with other elements of the health and social systems to assure that infertility services are available to those who need them.

Helping women who are having difficulty using a contraceptive method is another aspect of nursing care at the level of secondary prevention. Some women discover that they cannot use the method they have chosen and just stop using it. This can lead to unwanted pregnancy. The nurse can counsel, teach, and refer as needed to help each woman or couple find the best way to control fertility or to plan for children. Occasionally, secondary prevention in this area may entail presenting the client with options for dealing with the problem of an unintended pregnancy.

During perimenopause, referral to a physician or nurse practitioner for estrogen replacement therapy can take place if the client expresses discomfort related to hot flashes or has risk factors predisposing her to osteoporosis. If the client decides to be evaluated for estrogen replacement therapy, the nurse should describe what to expect during the initial visit. Generally, this visit entails a complete history and physical and several laboratory tests including a fasting blood glucose, complete blood count, blood lipids, liver function tests, and Pap smear. Some physicians also do an endometrial biopsy to determine the potential for endometrial cancer. This procedure is painful for the client and should be discussed by the nurse to alleviate fear and assist the client to cope with the procedure. Community health nurses can also educate clients and the general public on lifestyle approaches to the treatment of osteoporosis (e.g., calcium and vitamin D supplementation and weight-bearing physical activity).

Menopause may cause vaginal dryness and discomfort during sexual intercourse. The nurse can counsel women concerning longer foreplay and the use of vaginal lubricants to relieve the problem.

Some women also experience decreased sexual desire. The community health nurse can help clients explore contributing factors in this experience such as depression, a feeling of being at the end of the reproductive years, and acceptance of a new phase of life. Self-help groups for women who are having similar problems are extremely beneficial during this stage of life. If there is no such group in the local community, the nurse might start one by inviting clients to meet and begin discussions.

Secondary prevention related to physical abuse of women has two dimensions. The first of these is dealing with the physical and psychological effects of physical abuse, and the second is dealing with the source of the problem itself. Recognizing the problem is a prerequisite to either dimension of treatment. Female clients should be asked in a caring and sensitive manner about any violence in their lives. Careful recording of the history and of information regarding old and new injuries is important in the diagnosis of abuse. Such a record may reveal a pattern the woman is unwilling or unable to admit to the nurse. If there is evidence of abuse, it is unethical for the nurse not to confirm this diagnosis with the client. Allowing the woman to describe what is happening to her through open-ended questions is therapeutic and can serve as the first step in stemming the cycle of abuse.

It is important that the nurse convey to the client that she does not deserve to be abused and that the nurse is concerned about her. These critical statements are needed to convey to the client that someone cares and that she is not worthless, helpless, or deserving of abuse.

It is not easy for a community health nurse to intervene in an abusive relationship. Inherent in such situations are reasons to fear that intervention will not be successful, that the woman may become depressed and suicidal or resent the nurse for interfering in a private family matter, or that the male abuser may punish the woman or the nurse. Such fears have kept health care professionals from pursuing evidence and attempting to help women in abusive situations.

When the nurse is able to work through and conquer personal fear and is able to identify a client in an abusive relationship, the nurse should encourage the client to discuss the circumstances of her abuse. It is important that the client realize the danger inherent in her situation.

Once the diagnosis of abuse is made, the primary goal is to assist the woman to reestablish a feeling of control and to empower her to change the situation. Supportive counseling and reassurance are essential. The nurse should let the woman work out her problems at her own pace. Each woman has the capacity to change when she is ready. The nurse must realize that the victim will feel ambivalence in the relationship she has with her partner. The nurse should support realistic ideas for change and assist the client in altering unrealistic ideas. The nurse should help the client to clarify her beliefs about the situation. The nurse should also help to identify myths about abuse that the client may have internalized. For example, if the victim believes that she deserves the beatings, the nurse can assure the client that her partner is totally responsible for his or her own actions.

The nurse can help the client explore alternative plans for solutions to her problem. What are her personal supports? Is there anyone to whom she can go for help? The client may want to go home. If the client can do this without risk of suicide or homicide, the nurse should help her plan strategies for managing at home and provide her with resources for assistance or escape should the need arise. If necessary, however, the community health nurse can also help the woman to plan a quick getaway. The client needs to accumulate extra money, collect necessary documents like birth certificates and immunization records for children, pack a change of clothing, and carry a few emergency supplies. If the client has children, she should take them with her if she leaves or risk losing them to the abuser if he or she should claim that the client abandoned them.

The nurse should avoid becoming another controller in the life of the client. The physically abused woman needs every opportunity to develop independence. Nurses tend to want to rescue victims to stop the violence, but they cannot make decisions for the woman. Although nurses can provide information on shelters and other resources, they must allow the woman to make her own decisions.

Nurses should be familiar with the resources they recommend. Are they reliable? Will they assist the woman to become independent while providing a safe haven for her and her children? If the client is a lesbian, bisexual, or transgender woman, will her needs be effectively met in the shelter? Or will she be subjected to hostility and further abuse?

Community health nurses can also provide assistance in referrals for medical care for injuries and for counseling to deal with contributing factors and psychological effects of abuse. Such services may be needed for children as well as the woman. The woman should also be cautioned that her children may resist being removed from their home and other family members. If this should be the case, the community health nurse can help the client cope with grief and hostility on the part of the children. The client may also need help in dealing with her own grief over the loss of a significant relationship.

When adequate treatment facilities to meet the secondary prevention needs of women are not available, community health nurses can become actively involved in advocating for these services and in developing and implementing them. Community health nurses may also need to advocate for the availability of services for certain specific segments of the population, for example, low-income women or lesbian women.

Tertiary Prevention

As with all clients, tertiary prevention in the care of women focuses on rehabilitation and preventing the recurrence of health problems. Areas in which tertiary prevention are particularly warranted for the female client include pregnancy, abuse, and STDs. Tertiary prevention may also be needed to deal with some of the effects of menopause or chronic illness.

Tertiary prevention with respect to pregnancy involves the use of an effective contraceptive to prevent subsequent pregnancies. Again, the nurse may be involved in education, counseling, and referral for contraceptive services.

In the case of abuse, tertiary prevention necessitates the rebuilding of the woman's life and that of her family. This may involve developing new financial resources as well as ways of coping with problems. The woman needs to become self-sufficient. Again, referrals to a variety of agencies to help with employment skills and provide counseling may be of assistance. Nurses may also need to collaborate with other segments of the community to assure enforcement of protections for abused women and availability of services to assist them in rebuilding their lives.

Women can also be helped to prevent recurrence of STDs or to cope with the life changes necessitated by a diagnosis of HIV/AIDS or chronic hepatitis B or C. Tertiary prevention related to STDs is discussed more fully in Chapter 28∞. Other tertiary prevention measures may be warranted for existing chronic health problems. For example, women may need to be assisted to adapt to lifestyle changes necessitated by chronic illness or to manage symptoms such as pain. Tertiary prevention for chronic physical and mental health conditions are addressed in Chapters 29 and 30∞.

EVALUATING HEALTH CARE FOR WOMEN

Health care provided to women should be evaluated using the evaluative process described in Chapter 15∞. Once more, it is important to evaluate both the quality of the care given and its outcomes. Because of the dependent role of many women, it is particularly important that they play an active role in evaluating the health care they are given. At the national level, the year 2010 objectives for the health of women can provide criteria for evaluating women's health care services◆. Evaluative information on selected national objectives related to women's health is presented on page 457. Information on other objectives that relate to women, as well as to other segments of the population, is included in relevant chapters.

Women's health care needs are many and varied and are often poorly addressed by existing health care systems. Community health nurses may provide health care for women at all three levels of prevention: primary, secondary, and tertiary. Care may also be provided to individual women or to groups of women within the population, and often involves advocacy for services to meet women's needs.

HEALTHY PEOPLE 2010
Goals for Population Health

OBJECTIVE	BASELINE	MOST RECENT DATA	TARGET
1-1. Increase the proportion of women with health insurance	84%	85%	100%
1-4c. Increase the proportion of women with an ongoing source of care	85%	86%	96%
2-9. Reduce the number of cases of osteoporosis	16%	NDA	8%
3-2. Reduce lung cancer deaths (per 100,000 women)	40.2	41.6	44.9*
3-3. Reduce breast cancer deaths (per 100,000 women)	26.6	25.6	22.3
3-4. Reduce cervical cancer deaths (per 100,000 women)	2.8	2.6	2.0
3-11a. Increase the proportion of women who have ever received a Pap test	92%	93%	97%
3-13. Increase the proportion of women aged 40 and over who have received a mammogram in the past 2 years	67%	70%	70%*
9-1. Increase the proportion of pregnancies that are intended	51%	NDA	70%
9-3. Increase contraceptive use among those who do not desire pregnancy	93%	NDA	100%
9-12. Reduce the proportion of married couples unable to conceive or maintain a pregnancy	13%	NDA	10%
9-13. Increase the proportion of health insurance policies that cover contraceptive services	NDA	NDA	NDA
15-34. Reduce the rate of physical assault by intimate partners (per 1,000 women)	4.4	2.6	3.3*
15-35. Reduce the rate of rape or attempted rape (per 1,000 women)	0.8	0.7	0.7*
16-4. Reduce maternal deaths (per 100,000 live births)	9.9	8.9	3.3
16-5. Reduce pregnancy complications (per 100 deliveries)	31.2	31.9	24#
16-6. Increase the proportion of pregnant women who receive early and adequate prenatal care	74%	75%	90%
16-17c. Increase abstinence from cigarette smoking by pregnant women	87%	89%	99%
19-2. Reduce the proportion of women who are obese	25%	33%	15%#
19-12c. Reduce iron deficiency anemia among females of childbearing age	11%	12%	7%#
22-1. Reduce the proportion of women with no leisure-time physical activity	43%	40%	20%
27-1. Reduce tobacco use by women	22%	20%	12%

NDA—No data available
* Objective has been met
# Objective moving away from target

Data from: Centers for Disease Control and Prevention. (2005). Healthy people data. Retrieved September 5, 2005, from http://wonder.cdc.gov/data2010

Case Study

Meeting a Woman's Health Needs

Susan is 25 years old, married, and the mother of two girls. She is pregnant for the third time. You have scheduled a home visit with her following a referral from the community clinic where she is receiving prenatal care. According to the referring agency, Susan does not always keep her appointments, and the baby is small for gestational age. The prenatal clinic requests that you teach nutrition and encourage her to keep her appointments.

When you arrive at the home, Susan is reluctant to allow you inside. She turns her face away and does not look at you as she answers your questions. Because you know that every woman has the potential for being a victim of physical abuse, you ask Susan if someone has hurt her. In a nonthreatening, caring, and sensitive manner you say, "I see many women in my practice who are in a relationship with a person who hits or abuses them. Did someone hurt you?" Susan begins to cry and says, "My husband hit me last night." She allows you to come in, and you observe that she has a black eye and a swollen jaw. Her two small children are thin and poorly clothed. The house, though neat, is sparsely furnished.

In speaking with Susan, you find out that her husband works in a local factory and has been denied a promotion and a raise in the last week. He seems to blame Susan for becoming pregnant again and causing more financial worries. Susan tells you that she has been missing appointments at the prenatal clinic because of her black eye and the lack of transportation when her husband is at work.

1. What are the biophysical, psychological, sociocultural, behavioral, and health system factors operating in this situation?
2. What are your nursing diagnoses in this situation?
3. How would you address the two aspects of secondary prevention of physical abuse of women in this case?
4. What other secondary preventive measures seem to be warranted in this situation?
5. What primary and tertiary preventive interventions might be appropriate in working with Susan?
6. How will you evaluate whether intervention has been successful?

Test Your Understanding

1. What are the major human biophysical, psychological, sociocultural, behavioral, and health system factors that influence the health status of women? (pp. 423–438)

2. What are some of the health problems common to women? Which of these problems also affect men's health status? How do these common problems differ between men and women? (pp. 425–429)

3. What are some of the considerations that are unique in assessing the health needs of lesbian, bisexual, and transgender women? (pp. 438–449)

4. What are the major concerns in primary prevention for women? What roles might a community health nurse play with respect to each? (pp. 449–453)

5. Describe areas for consideration in secondary preventive activities in the care of women. Give examples of nursing interventions in each of these areas. (pp. 453–456)

6. What are the two aspects of secondary prevention of physical abuse of women? What is the role of the community health nurse with respect to each? (pp. 455–456)

7. What actions can community health nurses take to provide more sensitive and effective care to lesbian, bisexual, or transgender women? (p. 445)

EXPLORE MediaLink

http://www.prenhall.com/clark
Resources for this chapter can be found on the companion Website.

Audio Glossary
Appendix I: Adult Health Assessment and Intervention Guide
Case Study: Promoting Women's Health

Exam Review Questions
MediaLink Application: Discussing Menopause (video)
Media Links

Challenge Your Knowledge
Update *Healthy People 2010*
Advocacy Interviews

References

American Cancer Society. (2002). New cervical cancer early detection guidelines released. Retrieved February 3, 2003, from http://www.cancer.org

American College of Obstetricians and Gynecologists. (2001). Use of botanicals for management of menopause symptoms. *ACOG Practice Bulletin: Clinical Management Guidelines for Obstetrician-Gynecologists, 28*, 1–15. Retrieved August 13, 2005, from http://www.acog.org/from_home/publications/misc/pb028.htm

Armstrong, D. S. (2002). Emotional distress and prenatal attachment in pregnancy after perinatal loss. *Journal of Nursing Scholarship, 34*, 339–345.

Artazcoz, L., Borrell, C., Benach, J., Cortes, I., & Rohlfs, I. (2004). Women, family demands, and health: The importance of employment status and socio-economic position. *Social Science & Medicine, 59*, 263–274.

Baeten, J. M., Bukusi, E. A., & Lambe, M. (2001). Pregnancy complications and outcomes among overweight and obese nulliparous women. *American Journal of Public Health, 91*, 436–440.

Balluz, L., Ahluwalia, I. B., Murphy, W., Mokdad, A., Giles, W., & Harris, V. B. (2004). Surveillance for certain health behaviors among selected local areas—United States, Behavioral Risk Factor Surveillance System, 2002. *Morbidity and Mortality Weekly Report, 53*(SS-5), 89–94.

Bauer, G. R., & Welles, S. L. (2001). Beyond assumptions of negligible risk: Sexually transmitted diseases and women who have sex with women. *American Journal of Public Health, 91*, 1282–1286.

Beck, C. T. (2004). Post-traumatic stress disorder due to childbirth. *Nursing Research, 53*, 216–224.

Beck, L. F., Morrow, B., Lipscomb, L. E., & Johnson. (2002). Prevalence of selected maternal behaviors and experiences, Pregnancy Risk Assessment Monitoring System (PRAMS), 1999. *Morbidity and Mortality Weekly Report, 51*(SS-2), 1–27.

Behrendt, A., & Moritz, S. (2005). Posttraumatic stress disorder and memory problems after female genital mutilation. *American Journal of Psychiatry, 162*, 1000–1002.

Boehmer, U. (2002). Twenty years of public health research: Inclusion of lesbian, gay, bisexual, and transgender populations. *American Journal of Public Health, 92*, 1125–1130.

Borooah, V. K. (2004). Gender bias among children in India in their diet and immunization against disease. *Social Science & Medicine, 58*, 1719–1731.

Bromberger, J. T., Meyer, P. M., Kravitz, H. M., Sommer, B., Cordal, A., Powell, L., et al. (2001). Psychologic distress and natural menopause: A multiethnic community study. *American Journal of Public Health, 91*, 1435–1442.

Broussard, B. B. (2005). Women's experience of bulimia nervosa. *Journal of Advanced Nursing, 49*, 43–50.

Casper, L. M., & Bianchi, S. M. (2002). *Continuity and change in the American family*. Thousand Oaks, CA: Sage.

Centers for Disease Control and Prevention. (2002). Women and smoking: A report of the Surgeon General, Executive Summary. *Morbidity and Mortality Weekly Report, 51*(RR-12), 1–13.

Centers for Disease Control and Prevention. (2004a). *Health United States, 2004 with chartbook on trends in the health of Americans*. Retrieved August 9, 2005, from http://www.cdc.gov/nchs/data/hus/hus04.pdf

Centers for Disease Control and Prevention. (2004b). Indicators for chronic disease surveillance. *Morbidity and Mortality Weekly Report, 53*(RR-11), 1–114.

Chang, J., Berg, C. J., Saltzman, L. E., & Herndon, J. (2005). Homicide: A leading cause of injury deaths among pregnant and postpartum women in the United States, 1991–1999. *American Journal of Public Health, 94*, 471–477.

Chang, J., Elam-Evans, L. D., Berg, C. J., Herndon, J., Flowers, L., Seed, K. A., et al. (2003). Pregnancy-related mortality surveillance—United States, 1991–1999. *Morbidity and Mortality Weekly Report, 52*(SS-2), 1–8.

Cochran, B. N., Stewart, A. J., Ginzler, J. A., & Cauce, A. M. (2002). Challenges faced by homeless sexual minorities: Comparison of gay, lesbian, bisexual, and transgender homeless adolescents with their heterosexual counterparts. *American Journal of Public Health, 92*, 773–777.

Cornelius, L. J., Smith, P. L., & Simpson, G. M. (2002). What factors hinder women of color from obtaining preventive health care? *American Journal of Public Health, 92*, 535–539.

County of San Diego Health and Human Services Agency. (2004). *Standards of care for the prevention of perinatal HIV transmission in San Diego County*. San Diego: Author.

Curry, L. C., & Hogstel, M. O. (2002). Osteoporosis. *American Journal of Nursing, 102*(1), 26–32.

Daniel, I., Berg, C., Johnson, C. H., & Atrash, H. (2003). Magnitude of maternal morbidity during labor and delivery: United States, 1993–1997. *American Journal of Public Health, 93*, 631–634.

Davis-Snavely. (2004, Summer). Advanced maternal age and increased-pregnancy-related morbidity and mortality. *Perinatal Care Matters*, p. 3.

Dean, L., & Bradford, J. (2000). Violence and sexual assault. In Gay and Lesbian Medical Association & Center for Lesbian, Gay, Bisexual, and Transgender Health (Eds.), *Lesbian, gay, bisexual, and transgender health: Findings and concerns* (pp. 29–32). New York: Author.

Denton, M., Prus, S., & Walters, V. (2004). Gender differences in health: A Canadian study of the psychosocial, structural, and behavioral determinants of health. *Social Science & Medicine, 58*, 2585–2600.

Diamant, A. L., Hays, R. D., Morales, L. S., Ford, W., Calmes, D., Asch, S., et al. (2004). Delays and unmet need for health care among adult primary care patients in a restructured urban public health system. *American Journal of Public Health, 94*, 783–789.

Division of Adult and Community Health. (2005a). Disparities in screening for and awareness of high blood cholesterol—United States, 1999–2002. *Morbidity and Mortality Weekly Report, 54*, 117–119.

Division of Adult and Community Health. (2005b). Racial/ethnic and socioeconomic disparities in multiple risk factors for heart disease and stroke—United States, 2003. *Morbidity and Mortality Weekly Report, 54*, 113–117.

Division of Adult and Community Health. (2005c). Racial/ethnic disparities in the prevalence and impact of doctor-diagnosed arthritis—United States, 2002. *Morbidity and Mortality Weekly Report, 54*, 119–123.

Division of Diabetes Translation. (2002). Socioeconomic status of women with diabetes—United States, 2000. *Morbidity and Mortality Weekly Report, 51*, 147–148, 159.

Division of HIV/AIDS Prevention. (2005). HIV transmission among black women—North Carolina, 2004. *Morbidity and Mortality Weekly Report, 54*, 89–94.

Division of Reproductive Health, National Center for Chronic Disease Prevention and Health Promotion. (2002a). Nonoxynol-9 spermicide contraceptive use—United States, 1999. *Morbidity and Mortality Weekly Report, 51*, 389–392.

Division of Reproductive Health, National Center for Chronic Disease Prevention and Health Promotion. (2002b). Use of assisted reproductive technology—United States, 1996 and 1998. *Morbidity and Mortality Weekly Report, 51*, 97–101.

Division of STD/AIDS Prevention. (2002). HIV testing among pregnant women—United States and Canada, 1998–2001. *Morbidity and Mortality Weekly Report, 51*, 1013–1016.

Dodgson, J. E., Chee, Y.-O., & Yap, T. S. (2004). Workplace breastfeeding support for hospital employees. *Journal of Advanced Nursing, 47*, 91–100.

Doyal, L. (2004). Putting gender into health and globalization debates: New perspectives and old challenges. In N. K. Poku & A. Whiteside (Eds.), *Global health and governance: HIV/AIDS* (pp. 43–60). New York: Palgrave Macmillan.

Dzurec, L. C., Hoover, P. M., & Fields, J. (2002). Acknowledging unexplained fatigue of tired women. *Journal of Nursing Scholarship, 34*, 41–46.

Eli Lilly and Company. (2004a). *Women's health: Cardiovascular mental health*. Retrieved August 13, 2005, from http://www.lilly.com/products/health_women/cardiovascular/mental_health.html

Eli Lilly and Company. (2004b). *Women's health: Depression facts and figures*. Retrieved August 13, 2005, from http://www.lilly.com/products/health_women/depression/facts_figures.html

Eli Lilly and Company. (2004c). *Women's health: Osteoporosis facts and figures*. Retrieved August 13, 2005, from http://www.lilly.com/products/health_women/osteoporosis/facts_figures.html

Eli Lilly and Company. (2004d). *Women's health: PMDD facts and figures*. Retrieved August 13, 2005, from http://www.lilly.com/products/health_women/pmdd/facts_figures.html

Excellence in Clinical Practice. (2000). Chemotherapy may cause bone loss in women. *1*(3), 4.

Foster, D. G., Klaisle, C. M., Blum, M., Bradsberry, M. E., Brindis, C. D., & Stewart, F. H. (2004). Expanded state-funded family planning services: Estimated pregnancies averted by the Family PACT program in California, 1997–1998. *American Journal of Public Health, 94*, 1341–1346.

Friedman, S. R., Ompad, D. C., Maslow, C., Young, R., Case, P. Hudson, S. M., et al. (2003). HIV prevalence, risk behaviors, and high-risk sexual and injection networks among young women injectors who have sex with women. *American Journal of Public Health, 93*, 902–906.

GLBT Health Access Project. (n.d.). *Community standards of practice for provision of quality health care services for gay, lesbian, bisexual, and transgendered clients*. Retrieved August 14, 2005, from http://www.glbthealth.org

Gilchrist, J., Jones, B. H., Sleet, D. A., & Kimsey, C. D. (2000). Exercise-related injuries among women: Strategies for prevention from civilian and military studies. *Morbidity and Mortality Weekly Report, 49*(RR-2), 15–33.

Hansen, B. (2002). Public careers and private sexuality: Some gay and lesbian lives in the history of medicine and public health. *American Journal of Public Health, 92*, 36–44.

Hawke, M. (2002). Just like everyone else. *Nursing Spectrum Western Edition, 3*(12), 20–21.

Henderson, K. A., & Ainsworth, B. E. (2003). A synthesis of perceptions about physical activity among older African American and American Indian Women. *American Journal of Public Health, 93*, 313–317.

Hewitt, M., Devesa, S., & Breen, N. (2002). Papanicolaou test use among reproductive-age women at high risk for cervical cancer: Analyses of the 1995 National Survey of Family Growth. *American Journal of Public Health, 92*, 666–669.

Hsu, M.-T., Tseng, Y.-F., Banks, J. M., & Kuo, L.-L. (2004). Interpretations of stillbirth. *Journal of Advanced Nursing, 47*, 408–416.

Huey, F. L. (2001). Global impact of innovations on chronic disease in the genomics era. *The Pfizer Journal, 11*(2), 13.

Hung, C.-H. (2004). Predictors of postpartum women's health status. *Journal of Nursing Scholarship, 36*, 345–351.

James, T., & Platzer, H. (1999). Ethical considerations in qualitative research with vulnerable groups: Exploring lesbians' and gay men's experiences with health care—A personal perspective. *Nursing Ethics, 6*(1), 73–81.

Jones, G. C., & Bell, K. (2004). Adverse health behaviors and chronic conditions in working-age women with disabilities. *Family and Community Health, 27*(1), 22–36.

Jun, H.-J., Subramanian, S.V., Gortmaker, S., & Kawachi, I. (2004). Socioeconomic disadvantage, parenting responsibility, and women's smoking in the United States. *American Journal of Public Health, 94*, 2170–2176.

Kahn, R. S., Zuckerman, B., Bauchner, H., Homer, C. J., & Wise, P. H. (2002). Women's health after pregnancy and child outcomes at age 3 years: A prospective cohort study. *American Journal of Public Health, 92*, 1312–1318.

Kenney, J. W., & Bhattacharjee, A. (2000). Interactive model of women's stressors, personality traits, and health problems. *Journal of Advanced Nursing, 32*, 249–258.

King County Public Health. (2005). *Gay, lesbian, bisexual, and transgender health: Culturally competent care for GLBT people: Recommendations for health care providers.* Retrieved August 14, 2005, from http://www.metrokc.gov/health/glbt/providers.htm

Kurth, A., Weaver, M., Lockart, D., & Bielinski, L. (2004). The benefit of health insurance coverage of contraceptives in a population-based sample. *American Journal of Public Health, 94*, 1130–1132.

Lawson, H. W., Henson, R., Bobo, J. K., & Kaeser, M. K. (2000). Implementing recommendations for the early detection of breast and cervical cancer among low-income women. *Morbidity and Mortality Weekly Report, 49*(RR-2), 37–55.

Lee, S., Colditz, G., Berkman, L., & Kawachi, I. (2003). Caregiving to children and grandchildren and risk of coronary heart disease among women. *American Journal of Public Health, 93*, 1939–1944.

Lewis, S. J. (2004, July). After menopause: Novel marker helps to identify women at risk for heart disease. *Journal of Family Practice (Supplement)*, S18-24.

Liao, Y., Tucker, P., Okoro, C. A., Giles, W. H., Mokdad, A. H., & Harris, V. B. (2004). REACH 2010 surveillance for health status in minority communities—United States, 2001–2002. *Morbidity and Mortality Weekly Report, 53*(SS-6), 1–35.

Madison, T., Schottenfeld, S., James, S. A., Schwartz, A. G., & Gruber, S. B. (2004). Endometrial cancer: Socioeconomic status and racial/ethnic differences in stage at diagnosis, treatment, and survival. *American Journal of Public Health, 94*, 2104–2111.

Maman, S., Mbwambo, J. K., Hogan, N. M., Kilonzo, G. P., Campbell, J. C., Weiss, E., et al. (2002). HIV-positive women report more lifetime partner violence: Findings from a voluntary counseling and testing clinic in Dar es Salaam, Tanzania. *American Journal of Public Health, 92*, 1331–1337.

Mannino, D. M., Homa, D. M., Akinbami, L. J., Ford, E. S., & Redd, S. C. (2002). Chronic obstructive pulmonary disease surveillance—United States, 1971–2000. *Morbidity and Mortality Weekly Report, 51*(SS-6), 1–16.

Marston, C. (2004). Gendered communication among young people in Mexico: Implications for sexual health interventions. *Social Science & Medicine, 59*, 445–456.

Matthews, A. K., Hughes, T. L., Johnson, T., Razzano, L. A., & Cassidy, R. (2002). Prediction of depressive distress in a community sample of women: The role of sexual orientation. *American Journal of Public Health, 92*, 1131–1139.

Mays, V. M., & Cochran, S. D. (2001). Mental health correlates of perceived discrimination among lesbian, gay, and bisexual adults in the United States. *American Journal of Public Health, 91*, 1869–1876.

McBride, C., M., Bastian, L. A., Halabi, S., Fish, L., Lipkus, I. M., Bosworth, H. B., et al. (2002). A tailored intervention to aid decisionmaking about hormone replacement therapy. *American Journal of Public Health, 92*, 1112–1113.

McCray, T. M. (2004). An issue of culture: The effects of daily activities on prenatal care utilization patterns in rural South Africa. *Social Science & Medicine, 59*, 1843–1855.

McDonald, C., McIntyre, M., & Anderson, B. (2003). The view from somewhere: Locating lesbian experience in women's health. *Health Care for Women International, 24*, 697–711.

McGinley, A. M. (2004). Health beliefs and women's use of hormone replacement therapy. *Holistic Nursing Practice, 18*(1), 18–25.

McKibben, L. J., Stange, P. V., Sneller, V., Strikas, R. A., Rodewald, L. E., & Briss, P. A. (2000). Use of standing orders programs to increase adult vaccination rates: Recommendations of the Advisory Committee on Immunization Practices. *Morbidity and Mortality Weekly Report, 49*(RR-1), 21–26.

McLeer, S. V. (2004). Mental health services. In H. S. Sultz & K. M. Young, *Health care USA: Understanding its organization and delivery* (4th ed., pp. 335–366). Sudbury, MA: Jones and Bartlett.

Meyer, I., & Bowen, D. (2000). Lesbian, gay and bisexual health concerns: Cancer. In Gay and Lesbian Medical Association & Center for Lesbian, Gay, Bisexual, and Transgender Health (Eds.), *Lesbian, gay, bisexual, and transgender health: Findings and concerns* (pp. 15–17). New York: Author.

Meyer, I., Rothblum, E., & Bradford, J. (2000), Mental health and mental disorders. In Gay and Lesbian Medical Association & Center for Lesbian, Gay, Bisexual, and Transgender Health (Eds.), *Lesbian, gay, bisexual, and transgender health: Findings and concerns* (pp. 21–26). New York: Author.

Meyer, I., Silenzio, V., Wolfe, D., & Dunn, P. (2000). Introduction/background. In Gay and Lesbian Medical Association & Center for Lesbian, Gay, Bisexual, and Transgender Health (Eds.), *Lesbian, gay, bisexual, and transgender health: Findings and concerns* (pp. 4–9). New York: Author.

Murty, S. A., Peek-Asa, C., Zwerling, C., Stromquist, A. M., Burmeister, L. F., & Merchant, J. A. (2003). Physical and emotional abuse reported by men and women in a rural community. *American Journal of Public Health, 93*, 1073–1075.

National Center for Complementary and Alternative Medicine. (2005). Alternative therapies for managing menopausal symptoms. Retrieved August 13, 2005, from http://nccam.nih.gov/health/alerts/menopause

National Center for Chronic Disease Prevention and Health Promotion. (2002). *Interim Report: Proposed recommendations for action—A national public health initiative on diabetes and women's health.* Retrieved October 2, 2002, from http://www.cdc.gov/diabetes/pubs/interim/summary.htm

National Center for Health Statistics. (2002). State-specific trends in U.S. live births to women born outside the 50 states and the District of Columbia — United States, 1990 and 2000. *Morbidity and Mortality Weekly Report, 52*, 1091–1095.

National Center for Health Statistics. (2005a). *Health, United States, 2005 with chartbook on trends in the health of Americans.* Retrieved December 23, 2005, from http://www.cdc.gov/nchs/data/hus/hus05.pdf

National Center for Health Statistics. (2005b). Percentage of women who reported ever having a mammogram. *Morbidity and Mortality Weekly Report, 54*, 18.

National Center on Birth Defects and Developmental Disabilities. (2004). Alcohol consumption among women who are pregnant or might become pregnant—United States, 2002. *Morbidity and Mortality Weekly Report, 53*, 1178–1181.

National Institute of Mental Health. (2005). *Schizophrenia.* Retrieved March 8, 2006, from http://nimh.nih.gov/publicat/schizoph.cfm

National Women's Law Center, Focus/University of Pennsylvania, & The Lewin Group. (2000). *Making the grade on women's health: A national and state by state report card.* Washington, DC: National Women's Law Center.

National Women's Law Center and Oregon Health & Science University. (2004). *Making the grade on women's health: A national and state-by-state report card.* Retrieved August 13, 2005, from http://www.nwlc.org

Nemoto, T., Operario, D., Keatley, J., Han, L., & Soma, T. (2004). HIV risk behaviors among male-to-female transgender persons of color in San Francisco. *American Journal of Public Health, 94*, 1193–1199.

Nemoto, T., Operario, D., Keatley, J., Nguyen, H., & Sugano, E. (2005). Promoting health for transgender women: Transgender resources and neighborhood space (TRANS) program in San Francisco. *American Journal of Public Health, 95*, 382–384.

Nosek, M. A., Hughes, R. B., Howland, C. A., Young, M. E., Mullen, P. D., & Shelton, M. L. (2004). The meaning of health for women with physical disabilities: A qualitative analysis. *Family and Community Health, 27*(1), 6–21.

Olshansky, E. (2000). Goals for women's wellness. In E. Olshansky (Ed.), *Integrated women's health: Holistic approaches for comprehensive care* (pp. 69–80). Gaithersburg, MD: Aspen.

O'Neill, E., & Morrow, L. (2001). The symptom experience of women with chronic illness. *Journal of Advanced Nursing, 33*, 257–268.

Palmer, J. R., Rosenberg, L., Wise, L. A., Horton, N. J., & Adams-Campbell, L. L. (2003). Onset of natural menopause in African American women. *American Journal of Public Health, 93*, 299–306.

Paquette, M.-C., & Raine, K. (2004). Sociocultural context of women's body image. *Social Science & Medicine, 59*, 1047–1058.

Perkins, R. (2004). Diversity in health care delivery. *Pfizer Journal, VIII*(2), 4–14.

Pinhey, T. K., & Millman, S. R. (2004). Asian/Pacific Islander adolescent sexual orientation and suicide risk in Guam. *American Journal of Public Health, 94*, 1204–1206.

Postema, A. S., & Breiman, R. F. (2000). Adult immunization programs in nontraditional settings: Quality standards and guidance for program evaluation. *Morbidity and Mortality Weekly Report, 49*(RR-1), 1–13.

Raj, A., & Silverman, J. G. (2003). Immigrant South Asian women at greater risk for injury from intimate partner violence. *American Journal of Public Health, 93*, 435–437.

Ridge, D., Hulme, A., & Peasley, D. (2003). Queering health: The health of young same-sex-attracted men and women. In P. Liamputtong & H. Gardner (Eds.), *Health, social change and communities* (pp. 282–305). Oxford: Oxford University Press.

Ro, M. (2002). Moving forward: Addressing the health of Asian American and Pacific Islander Women. *American Journal of Public Health, 92*, 516–519.

Rondahl, G., Innala, S., & Carlsson, M. (2004). Nurses' attitudes to lesbians and gay men. *Journal of Advanced Nursing, 47*, 386–392.

Russell, S. T., Driscoll, A. K., & Truong, N. (2002). Adolescent same-sex romantic attractions and relationships: Implications for substance use and abuse. *American Journal of Public Health, 92*, 198–202.

Russell, S. T., & Joyner, K. (2001). Adolescent sexual orientation and suicide risk: Evidence from a national study. *American Journal of Public Health, 91*, 1276–1281.

Sandison, R., Gray, M., & Reid, D. M. (2004). Lifestyle factors for promoting bone health in older women. *Journal of Advanced Nursing, 45*, 603–610.

Sandovsky, R. (2000). Sexual orientation and associated health care risks. *American Family Physician, 62*, 2685.

Scheer, S., Peterson, I., Page-Shafer, K., Delgado, V., Gleghorn, A., Ruiz, J., et al. (2002). Sexual and drug use behavior among women who have sex with both women and men: Results of a population-based study. *American Journal of Public Health, 92*, 1110–1112.

Scholle, S. H., Buranosky, R., Hanusa, B. H., Ranieri, L., Dowd, K., & Valappil, B. (2003). Routine screening for intimate partner violence in an obstetrics and gynecology clinic. *American Journal of Public Health, 93*, 1070–1072.

Schrag, S., Gorwitz, R., Fultz-Butts, K., & Schuchat, A. (2002). Prevention of perinatal group B streptococcal disease: Revised guidelines from CDC. *Morbidity and Mortality Weekly Report, 51*(RR-11), 1–22.

Scout. (2000). Family planning. In Gay and Lesbian Medical Association & Center for Lesbian, Gay, Bisexual, and Transgender Health (Eds.), *Lesbian, gay, bisexual, and transgender health: Findings and concerns* (pp. 17–18). New York: Author.

Sell, R., & Wolfe, D. (2000). Educational and community-based programs. In Gay and Lesbian Medical Association & Center for Lesbian, Gay, Bisexual, and Transgender Health (Eds.), *Lesbian, gay, bisexual, and transgender health: Findings and concerns* (pp. 13–15). New York: Author.

Sember, R. (2000). Transgender health concerns. In Gay and Lesbian Medical Association & Center for Lesbian, Gay, Bisexual, and Transgender Health (Eds.), *Lesbian, gay, bisexual, and transgender health: Findings and concerns* (pp. 32–43). New York: Author.

Seng, J. S., Low, L. K., Sparbel, K. H., & Killion, C. (2004). Abuse-related post-traumatic stress during the childbearing years. *Journal of Advanced Nursing, 46*, 604–613.

Shepherd, A. J. (2004). An overview of osteoporosis. *Alternative Therapies, 10*(2), 26–33.

Silenzio, I., & White, J. (2000a). Sexually transmitted diseases. In Gay and Lesbian Medical Association & Center for Lesbian, Gay, Bisexual, and Transgender Health (Eds.), *Lesbian, gay, bisexual, and transgender health: Findings and concerns* (pp. 26–27). New York: Author.

Silenzio, I., & White, J. (2000b). Tobacco use. In Gay and Lesbian Medical Association & Center for Lesbian, Gay, Bisexual, and Transgender Health (Eds.), *Lesbian, gay, bisexual, and transgender health: Findings and concerns* (p. 29). New York: Author.

Silenzio, I., White, J., & Wolfe, D. (2000). Substance abuse. In Gay and Lesbian Medical Association & Center for Lesbian, Gay, Bisexual, and Transgender Health (Eds.), *Lesbian, gay, bisexual, and transgender health: Findings and concerns* (pp. 27–29). New York: Author.

Skarsater, I., Dencker, K., Bergbom, I., Haggstrom, L., & Fridlund, B. (2003). Women's conceptions of coping with major depression in daily life: A qualitative, salutogenic approach. *Issues in Mental Health Nursing, 24*, 419–431.

Smith, P. H., White, J. W., & Holland, L. J. (2003). A longitudinal perspective on dating violence among adolescent and college-age women. *American Journal of Public Health, 93*, 1104–1109.

Solarz, A. L. (Ed.). (1999). *Lesbian health: Current assessment and directions for the future.* Washington, DC: National Academy Press.

Spearing, M. (2001). *Eating disorders: Facts about eating disorders and the search for solutions.* Retrieved March 8, 2006, from http://www.nimh.nih.gov/publicat/NIMHeatingdisorder.pdf

Strazdins, L., & Bammer, G. (2004). Women, work, and musculoskeletal health. *Social Science & Medicine, 58*, 997–1005.

U.S. Census Bureau. (2004a). *Historical health insurance tables.* Retrieved October 1, 2004, from http://www.census.gov

U.S. Census Bureau. (2004b). *Poverty: 2003 highlights.* Retrieved September 30, 2004, from http://www.census.gov

U.S. Census Bureau. (2005). *Statistical abstract of the United States: 2004–2005.* Retrieved May 12, 2005, from http://www.census.gov/prod/2004pubs/04statab

U.S. Department of Health and Human Services. (n.d.) *Women's health in the baccalaureate nursing school curriculum: Report of a survey and recommendations.* Washington, DC: Author.

U.S. Department of Health and Human Services. (2000). *Healthy People 2010* (Conference edition, in two volumes). Washington, DC: Author.

U.S. Preventive Services Task Force. (1996a). Screening: Preeclampsia. Retrieved August 13, 2005, from http://www.ahrq.gov/clinic/uspstf/uspspree.htm

U.S. Preventive Services Task Force. (1996b). Screening: Rubella. Retrieved August 13, 2005, from http://www.ahrq.gov/clinic/uspstf/uspsrubl.htm

U.S. Preventive Services Task Force. (2001a). Screening for chlamydial infection. Retrieved August 13, 2005, from http://www.ahrq.gov/clinic/uspstf/uspschlm.htm

U.S. Preventive Services Task Force. (2001b). Screening for lipid disorders in adults. Retrieved August 13, 2005, from http://www.ahrq.gov/clinic/uspstf/uspschol.htm

U.S. Preventive Services Task Force. (2002a). Osteoporosis—screening. Retrieved August 13, 2005, from http://www.ahrq.gov/clinic/uspstf/uspsoste.htm

U.S. Preventive Services Task Force. (2002b). Screening for breast cancer. Retrieved August 13, 2005, from http://www.ahrq.gov/clinic/uspstf/uspsbrca.htm

U.S. Preventive Services Task Force. (2002c). Screening for colorectal cancer. Retrieved August 13, 2005, from http://www.ahrq.gov/clinic/uspstf/uspscolo.htm

U.S. Preventive Services Task Force. (2002d). Screening for depression. Retrieved August 13, 2005, from http://www.ahrq.gov/clinic/uspstf/uspsdepr.htm

U.S. Preventive Services Task Force. (2003a). Screening for cervical cancer. Retrieved August 13, 2005, from http://www.ahrq.gov/clinic/uspstf/uspscerv.htm

U.S. Preventive Services Task Force. (2003b). Screening for diabetes mellitus, Adult type 2. Retrieved August 13, 2005, from http://www.ahrq.gov/clinic/uspstf/uspsdiab.htm

U.S. Preventive Services Task Force. (2003c). Screening for obesity in adults. Retrieved August 13, 2005, from http://www.ahrq.gov/clinic/uspstf/uspsobes.htm

U.S. Preventive Services Task Force. (2003d). Counseling: Tobacco use. Retrieved August 13, 2005, from http://www.ahrq.gov/clinic/uspstf/uspstbac.htm

U.S. Preventive Services Task Force. (2004a). Screening for asymptomatic bacteriuria. Retrieved August 13, 2005, from http://www.ahrq.gov/clinic/uspstf/uspsbact.htm

U.S. Preventive Services Task Force. (2004b). Screening for family and intimate partner violence. Retrieved August 13, 2005, from http://www.ahrq.gov/clinic/uspstf/uspsfamv.htm

U.S. Preventive Services Task Force. (2004c). Screening for hepatitis B virus infection. Retrieved August 13, 2005, from http://www.ahrq.gov/clinic/uspstf/uspshepb.htm

U.S. Preventive Services Task Force. (2004d). Screening for Rh (D) incompatibility. Retrieved August 13, 2005, from http://www.ahrq.gov/clinic/uspstf/uspsdrhi.htm

U.S. Preventive Services Task Force. (2004e). Screening for syphilis infection. Retrieved August 13, 2005, from http://www.ahrq.gov/clinic/uspstf/uspssyph.htm

U.S. Preventive Services Task Force. (2005a). Chemoprevention for hormone replacement therapy. Retrieved August 13, 2005, from http://www.ahrq.gov/clinic/uspstf/uspspmho.htm

U.S. Preventive Services Task Force. (2005b). Screening for genital herpes. Retrieved August 13, 2005, from http://www.ahrq.gov/clinic/uspstf/uspsherp.htm

U.S. Preventive Services Task Force. (2005c). Screening for gonorrhea. Retrieved August 13, 2005, from http://www.ahrq.gov/clinic/uspstf/uspsgono.htm

U.S. Preventive Services Task Force. (2005d). Screening for human immunodeficiency virus infection. Retrieved August 13, 2005, from http://www.ahrq.gov/clinic/uspstf/uspshivi.htm

Waldrop, A. E., & Resick, P. A. (2004). Coping among adult female victims of domestic violence. *Journal of Family Violence, 19*, 291–302.

Walters, K. L., & Simoni, J. M. (2002). Reconceptualizing native women's health: An "indigenist" stress-coping model. *American Journal of Public Health, 92*, 520–524.

Washington, H. (2002). Burning love: Big tobacco takes aim at LGBT youths. *American Journal of Public Health, 92*, 1086–1095.

White, J., Bradford, J., & Silenzio, V. (2000). Health communication. In Gay and Lesbian Medical Association & Center for Lesbian, Gay, Bisexual, and Transgender Health (Eds.), *Lesbian, gay, bisexual, and transgender health: Findings and concerns* (pp. 11–13). New York: Author.

White, J., Bradford, J., Silenzio, V., & Wolfe, D. (2000). Access to quality health services. In Gay and Lesbian Medical Association & Center for Lesbian, Gay, Bisexual, and Transgender Health (Eds.), *Lesbian, gay, bisexual, and transgender health: Findings and concerns* (pp. 10–12). New York: Author.

Williams, D. R. (2003). The health of men: Structured inequalities and opportunities. *American Journal of Public Health, 93*, 724–731.

Wilson, J. (2004). Botanicals' effect on menopausal symptoms. *Holistic Nursing Practice, 18*, 274–275.

Wilson, N. (2002). What women don't know can hurt them. *Nursing Spectrum MetroEdition, 3*(7), 16W–17W.

World Health Organization. (2004). *The world health report*. Geneva, Switzerland: Author.

Yates, J., Barret-Connor, E., Barlas, S., Chen, Y. T., Miller, P. D., & Siris, E. S. (2004). No long-term benefit shown for bones after HRT. *Journal of Family Practice, 53*, 444, 447.

Meeting the Health Needs of Men

CHAPTER OBJECTIVES

After reading this chapter, you should be able to:

1. Describe major considerations in assessing the biophysical, psychological, physical environmental, sociocultural, behavioral, and health care system factors affecting men's health.
2. Describe factors that contribute to adverse health effects for gay, bisexual, and transgender men.
3. Identify major considerations in primary prevention for men and analyze the role of the community health nurse with respect to each.
4. Describe secondary prevention considerations for men and related community health nursing roles.
5. Identify areas of emphasis in tertiary prevention for men and analyze the role of the community health nurse in each.

KEY TERMS

disclosure **480**
erectile dysfunction (ED) **467**
gender dysphoria **475**
heterosexism **476**
joblessness **471**
reframing **484**
unemployment **471**

MediaLink
http://www.prenhall.com/clark

Additional interactive resources for this chapter can be found on the Companion Website. Click on Chapter 18 and "Begin" to select the activities for this chapter.

Advocacy in Action

Juan

Juan was a Spanish-speaking man in his 70's who had recently moved to the area from Puerto Rico with his family. He had problems with high blood pressure, which we were treating at St. Agnes Nurses Center. Over the course of a couple of weeks, we noticed that Juan appeared depressed. After exploring this further, we discovered that he was unhappy because in his native land he was used to working to support his family and was very upset by his inability to work here.

The nurses put their heads together, and within a week or so I accompanied Juan to the local grocery store. I spoke with the manager about Juan and told Juan about the job opportunity that was available. After I helped Juan complete the application, he was hired.

I occasionally ran into Juan at the grocery store and was always greeted with a big smile as well as an exuberant "Hola, mi amiga!"

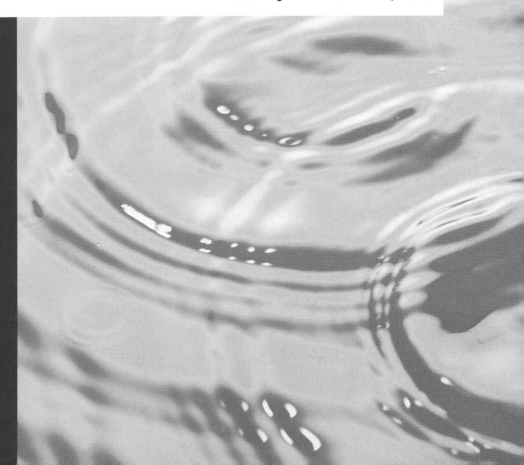

Vienna Tomesheski, BA, BSN, RN

Med-Surg Staff Nurse, Paoli Hospital, PA

*I*n 2003, men between the ages of 20 and 64 years constituted roughly 30% of the U.S. population. This amounted to 87.8 million men in age groups that are more likely than any other segment of the population to lack access to health care services. By 2030, although the proportion is expected to remain stable, the actual number of men in this age group is expected to increase by 4.3 million to more than 92 million men (U.S. Census Bureau, 2005). Although health care services have traditionally been built around men's health care needs, U.S. men die an average of 7 years earlier than women (Huey, 2001), and mortality rates for all but one of the top 15 causes of death are higher for men than women (Williams, 2003). Only since the late 1990s has men's health been considered a separate and specific area of health care endeavor (White & Banks, 2004).

Men differ from women in their patterns of physical health disorders and health-related needs. These differences are attributable to (a) physiologic differences between men and women, (b) differences in health-related habits and health-seeking behavior, and (c) differences in social roles, stress, and coping. A great deal of health-related literature has been written about specific problems that influence men's health status (e.g., cardiovascular disease, lung cancer, etc.). Very little, however, is written about the overall health needs of men. The health care of men has been fragmented, approached from an episodic perspective. Little effort has been made to provide comprehensive, holistic health services.

Lack of emphasis on holistic health for men is evident in previous versions of the national health objectives. Women, children, and the elderly are among the populations that have been specifically targeted in previous sets of objectives; men have not. Only in the most recent objectives is prostate cancer addressed (U.S. Department of Health and Human Services [USDHHS], 2000)◆. Many of the past and current objectives will benefit men. The lack of attention to the total health of men, however, is a justifiable concern of community health nurses. The focus of this chapter is on preparing community health nurses to provide holistic care to men as a population group.

THE EPIDEMIOLOGY OF MEN'S HEALTH

Factors in each of the six dimensions of health affect men's health status. We will briefly consider major factors in the biophysical, psychological, physical environmental, sociocultural, behavioral, and health system dimensions and their influence on the health of the male population.

Biophysical Considerations

Men experience a variety of physical health conditions, many of which can be prevented or their effects ameliorated by effective community health nursing interven-

tion. In 2002, the leading causes of death for men were (a) heart disease, (b) malignant neoplasms, (c) unintentional injuries, (d) cerebrovascular disease, (e) chronic lower respiratory diseases, (f) diabetes mellitus, (g) influenza and pneumonia, (h) suicide, (i) nephritis, nephrotic syndrome, and nephrosis, and (j) chronic liver disease and cirrhosis. The overall age-adjusted male mortality rate for 2002 was 1,013 deaths per 100,000 men, compared to only 715.2 per 100,000 women (Centers for Disease Control and Prevention [CDC], 2004a). Men are twice as likely as women to die from heart disease, bronchitis, and accidental injuries, and three times more likely to commit suicide (Donaldson, 2004). Table 18-1◆ provides a comparison of male and female mortality for selected causes of death in the United States. Worldwide, the most frequent cause of death in young and middle adult men is traffic accidents. Other significant causes of male mortality and morbidity in developing regions are depression and bipolar disorder, alcohol use, violence, tuberculosis, the effects of war, suicide, schizophrenia, and anemia (Huey, 2001).

Men also experience higher levels of morbidity for many health problems than do women (Table 18-2◆). For example, cancer diagnoses occur 1.3 times more often in men than women (Williams, 2003), and one half of men will have a diagnosis of cancer at some time in their lives compared to only one third of women (CDC, 2004b). Men are also more likely to die from cancers than women, primarily because the major site for cancer in men is the lung, with poor prognosis for recovery. Women, on the other hand, often have more highly detectable and treatable cancers (Division of Cancer Prevention and Control, 2004). Much of the difference in cancer mortality between men and women is attributable to malignant melanoma, one of the most virulent

TABLE 18-1	Age-adjusted Male and Female Mortality from Selected Causes, United States, 2002 (per 100,000 population)		
Cause of Mortality	Men	Women	Ratio Men to Women
Overall	1,013.7	715.2	1.4 to 1
Heart disease	297.4	197.2	1.5 to 1
Cerebrovascular disease	56.5	55.2	ca. 1 to 1
Malignant neoplasms	238.9	163.1	1.5 to 1
Cancer of lungs, trachea, bronchus	73.2	41.6	1.75 to 1
Lower respiratory diseases	53.5	37.4	1.4 to 1
HIV/AIDS	7.4	2.5	2.9 to 1
Homicide	9.4	2.8	3.4 to 1

Data from: Centers for Disease Control and Prevention. (2004). Health, United States, 2004. Retrieved August 9, 2005, from http://www.cdc.gov/ nchs/data/hus/hus04.pdf

TABLE 18-2	Age-adjusted Male and Female Morbidity from Selected Causes, United States, 2002		
Cause of Morbidity	Men	Women	Ratio Men to Women
AIDS (per 100,000 population)	27.4	9.0	3 to 1
Lung cancer (per 100,000 population)	73.6	46.4	1.6 to 1
Colorectal cancer (per 100,000 population)	59.5	44.1	1.3 to 1
Prostate cancer (per 100,000 population)	171.4	N/A	N/A
Cancer of oral cavity and pharynx (per 100,000 population)	14.6	6.2	2.3 to 1
Stomach cancer (per 100,000 population)	11.5	5.6	2 to 1
Pancreatic cancer (per 100,000 population)	12	9.2	1.3 to 1
Bladder cancer (per 100,000 population)	35.5	8.8	4 to 1
Arthritis	17.8%	23.7%	
Activity limitation due to chronic conditions	12.3%	12.3%	
Elevated blood cholesterol	16.9%	17%	
Hypertension	25.1%	25.7%	
Overweight	68.8%	61.7%	
Obesity	28.1%	34.0%	
Injury (per 100,000 population)	92.9	77.2	1.2 to 1

Data from: Centers for Disease Control and Prevention. (2004). Health, United States, 2004. Retrieved August 9, 2005, from http://www.cdc.gov/nchs/data/hus/hus04.pdf; Division of Adult and Community Health. (2005c). Racial/ethnic disparities in the prevalence and impact of doctor-diagnosed arthritis—United States, 2002. Morbidity and Mortality Weekly Report, 54, 119–123; U.S. Census Bureau. (2005). Statistical abstract of the United States: 2004–2005. Retrieved August 16, 2005, from http://www.census.gov/prod/2004pubs/04statab

forms of skin cancer. Melanoma mortality increased 66% among U.S. men from 1969 to 1999. It has subsequently declined in younger men due to earlier age at diagnosis, but continues to be high in men over 65 years of age (Culpepper & McKee, 2004). Differences in melanoma mortality between men and women most likely arise from differential exposure to sunlight in occupational and recreational activities.

Men develop heart disease at earlier ages and die earlier than women, and gender differences in traditional risk factors for heart disease have been found to explain only approximately 40% to 50% of the difference in mortality (Purcell, Daly, & Petersen, 2004; Weidner & Cain, 2003). On average, one in four men will die from myocardial infarction, compared to one in six women (Purcell et al., 2004).

Although the prevalence of self-reported emphysema or chronic bronchitis has been found to be lower in men than in women (45.5% and 73.2%) and women make slightly more total visits to providers for these conditions, the annual rate of visits per 1,000 men is higher than that for women (46.8 visits per 1,000 men and 43.4 for women). In addition, men are more likely to be hospitalized for chronic obstructive pulmonary disease (COPD) than women at 42.4 hospitalizations per 1,000 men compared to only 40.2 per 1,000 women. Men are also more likely than women to die as a result of COPD, with mortality rates of 82.6 per 100,000 for men in 2000 versus 56.7 per 100,000 for women (Mannino, Homa, Akinbami, Ford, & Redd, 2002).

Breast cancer and osteoporosis, often considered diseases of women, can also be found in men. In 2001, for example, an estimated 1,400 to 1,600 men received a diagnosis of breast cancer and an estimated 400 deaths occurred. Breast cancer incidence in the United States increased by 50% from 1995 to 2000. Risk factors for male breast cancer include a family history of the disease (in male or female relatives), age 50 to 60 years, Klinefelter's syndrome with its extra X chromosome, gynecomastia, a history of radiation therapy as a child, and cirrhosis or parasitic liver disease. Breast cancer diagnosis for a man brings feelings of isolation, embarrassment, and loss of self-image (Banks, 2002).

Osteoporosis, which is a frequent occurrence in postmenopausal women, also occurs in men. The World Health Organization has defined osteoporosis as a bone matter density 2.5 standard deviations below the mean for young adults (Lim & Fitzpatrick, 2004). As many as 2 million American men are affected by osteoporosis, with as many as 3 million more at risk for the disease (Curry & Hogstel, 2002). An estimated one in every eight men will experience an osteoporotic fracture at some point in their lives. Men account for approximately 30% of hip fractures and 20% of vertebral fractures due to osteoporosis (Lim & Fitzpatrick, 2004). Age-related bone loss begins for both men and women after age 40 and progresses at 0.5% to 1% loss in bone density per year. Although men do not experience the accelerated bone loss suffered by women at menopause, a 60-year-old man has a 25% chance of an osteoporotic fracture at some point in his life (Shepherd, 2004). Most risk factors for osteoporosis are similar for men and women, but men have higher levels of some risk factors (e.g., smoking, alcohol use) than women. Other predisposing factors include long-term corticosteroid use, hypogonadism, organ transplantation, gastrointestinal conditions such as celiac disease and pancreatic insufficiency, chronic liver disease, diabetes, and a variety of medications, such as anticonvulsants, psychotropic drugs, and immunosuppressants (Lim & Fitzpatrick, 2004).

Men also have higher rates of sexually transmitted diseases (STDs) than women. For example, the incidence of gonorrhea among men in their early 20s is 500 to 600 cases per 100,000 population. Similar incidence is also seen for *Chlamydia trachomatis*, a sexually transmitted disease often thought to occur primarily in women. In 2002, men had incidence rates for primary and secondary syphilis three times those for women (CDC, 2005). Men often have very little knowledge of STDs beyond HIV infection, gonorrhea, and syphilis and less knowledge of STD prevention (Alan Guttmacher Institute, 2004). Approximately 80% of U.S. adults with AIDS are men, and genital herpes affects one in every six men (Pinkelman, 2002a).

In addition to experiencing conditions that occur in women, but at frequently lower rates of incidence, men are subject to some unique biophysical conditions. Among these are prostate and testicular cancers and erectile dysfunction. An estimated 230,000 new cases of prostate cancer were expected to be diagnosed in U.S. men in 2004 (Johnson, 2004). Prostate cancer is the second leading cause of cancer deaths in men and contributes to 10% of all deaths in men. One in every six men will develop prostate cancer in his lifetime and one in 32 men will die of this disease despite increasing survival rates with treatment (Pinkelman, 2002b). Prostate cancer may result in feelings of inadequacy that lead to changes in relationships, feelings of lost manhood, and changes in sexual feelings, as well as to erectile dysfunction (Johnson, 2004). Although prostate cancer is frequently not life threatening, its implications for men's quality of life cannot be underestimated. Prostate cancer and benign prostatic hyperplasia (BPH) may both obstruct urinary flow, resulting in reduced urinary flow, increasing frequency, and nocturia. Approximately 43% of middle-aged and older men experience BPH (Kirby & Kirby, 2004). An additional 2% to 6% of men at any given time may experience prostatitis, an inflammation of the prostate gland and the most common urological diagnosis in men over age 50. Prostatitis may cause pain, difficulty voiding, and sexual dysfunction, all symptoms that can significantly alter quality of life (Nickel, 2004).

Testicular cancer is the most common cancer in men 15 to 44 years of age and causes 2% of all cancers in men. Overall incidence of testicular cancer in men under 50 years of age is 2 per 1,000 men. Men with a history of cryptorchism (an undescended testicle) account for 10% of testicular cancers, and the risk increases sixfold for testes that remain in the abdominal cavity. Even nor-

mally situated testes are affected in 20% of cases of one maldescended testicle. Surgical removal of the undescended testicle is recommended if the testicle cannot be effectively placed and maintained in the scrotal sac. Trauma is another contributing factor in testicular cancer, as is intrauterine exposure to hormones such as diethylstilbestrol or radiation (Hendry & Christmas, 2004).

In addition to its life-threatening potential, testicular cancer has profound psychological implications for men in terms of sexuality, self-identity, and fertility. Five-year survival rates for testicular cancer are high at 90%, but sexuality concerns may delay seeking treatment and contribute to greater potential for death. Anywhere from 15% to 30% of men with testicular cancer have long-term sexual dysfunction after treatment, and a diagnosis of testicular cancer may lead to feelings of inadequacy, hopelessness, and depression (Gurevich, Bishop, Bower, Malka, & Nyhof-Young, 2003).

Erectile dysfunction (ED), formerly called impotence, occurs when a man cannot achieve or maintain an erection sufficient for satisfactory sexual activity (Carson, 2004). The relatively high prevalence of ED was not recognized until a landmark study in Massachusetts in 1994 indicated that 52% of men between 40 and 60 years of age experienced some level of difficulty (Solomon & Jackson, 2004). Approximately 20% to 30% of U.S. men (approximately 30 million) have erectile dysfunction, but only 5% to 10% seek treatment for this problem (Chua & Bakris, 2004; Johnson, 2004). Worldwide prevalence of ED is estimated at more than 150 million men and is expected to double by 2025 (Kirby, 2004). The incidence of ED increases with age, with approximately 39% of men aged 40 to 50 years affected compared to 70% of those over age 70 (Johnson, 2004). Research has indicated that both age and atherosclerotic processes contribute to the development of ED, but that diminished blood flow due to atherosclerosis has a greater effect on its development than age (Solomon & Jackson, 2004).

An estimated 35% of men 40 to 70 years of age experience moderate to severe ED that may be due to a number of factors. Some of the common contributing factors are chronic diseases such as diabetes, hypertension, and arteriosclerosis; medications used to treat these and other conditions; and anxiety. For example, 39% to 64% of men with cardiovascular disease also experience ED, and the presence of erectile dysfunction may suggest coronary heart disease or a worsening of an existing cardiac condition. In addition, 44% to 64% of men who have had myocardial infarction develop ED. Similarly, more than 68% of men with hypertension develop ED, and the prevalence increases in men with both hypertension and diabetes. Over half of men with diabetes will experience erectile dysfunction at some point (Kirby, 2004), and men with diabetes are four times more likely than other men to experience complete ED (Solomon & Jackson, 2004).

Obesity has also been linked to erectile dysfunction; a man with a 42-inch waist is 50% more likely to have erectile difficulties than one with a 32-inch waist (Calandra, 2004). Renal failure and alcohol use are additional contributing factors in erectile dysfunction (Johnson, 2004). Smoking appears to be another risk factor, and pharmacologic treatment for many of the conditions that cause ED may also contribute to erectile dysfunction. For example, statin therapies for cardiovascular disease may exacerbate ED, and sexual dysfunction is a common side effect of many antihypertensive medications (Solomon & Jackson, 2004).

Infertility is another condition that poses significant threats to men's self-image. Male infertility is implicated in approximately half of couples unable to conceive, either independently or in conjunction with female fertility factors. Approximately 25% of male infertility arises from unknown causes. Possible causes of infertility include prior surgeries, pelvic trauma, sexually transmitted disease, genetic causes such as Klinefelter's syndrome, medication use, and toxic exposures. One relatively common and treatable cause of male infertility is varicocele, a dilatation of spermatic veins, which can be addressed with surgical intervention. Hormone therapies or in vitro fertilization may be effective for other forms of infertility (Alam, Niederberger, & Meacham, 2004).

Another area to be addressed in assessing men's physiologic function is the presence of adverse effects related to accidental injury. Males at all ages have higher rates of unintentional injuries than females. This is particularly true for motor vehicle accidents. In the 2001–2002 period, for example, men accounted for 17% more emergency department visits than women (CDC, 2004a). Unintentional firearms mortality among men from 1993 to 1998 was eight times higher than among women (Gotsch, Annest, Mercy, & Ryan, 2001). As we will see later in this chapter, many of these differences arise from risk behaviors engaged in by men. Other factors that may contribute to accidental injuries and should be assessed by the community health nurse are sensory impairments. These impairments, if undetected and uncorrected, may contribute to a variety of physical and psychological health problems.

The last aspect of physiologic function to be considered in assessing the health status of men is immunization levels. Men, as well as women, should be immunized against tetanus and diphtheria (Td), influenza, and pneumococcal disease, and susceptible men should also receive varicella vaccine. Although men are more likely than women to have received tetanus vaccines in the last 10 years, they are less likely to have received influenza vaccine in the past year or to ever have received pneumococcal vaccine (Singleton, Greby, Wooten, Walker, & Strikas, 2000).

GLOBAL PERSEPECTIVES

Around the world, men fare worse than women in many health-related venues. For example, in 2003, differences in life expectancy at birth varied from 2 years less for men than women in the African Region of the World Health Organization (WHO) to 9 years less in the European Region. Similarly, health life expectancy varied from 1 to 6 years, with men having a shorter expectation of a healthy life span. In fact, men in the African Region, on average, can expect only 40 years of healthy life before dying at the relatively young age of 46 years (WHO, 2005). In part, these differences are due to differences in disease and injury incidence and behavioral risk factors and would be even worse if not for the relatively high rates of maternal mortality in much of the developing world.

Mean systolic blood pressure is consistently higher among men than women in each of the six WHO regions. Similarly, tobacco use among adolescent boys is nearly twice that of girls in all WHO regions except the Americas (WHO, 2005). Men also have higher levels of alcohol consumption and greater risk of accidental injury than women. Poverty and poor employment opportunities can threaten men's mental and physical health status, particularly in areas where gender socialization casts men as the primary breadwinner in the family. In addition, growing urbanization and movement of young men to large cities to find employment separates them from the support of extended families, contributing to depression and substance abuse (Alan Guttmacher Institute, 2005a; Monts, 2002a).

What other factors may contribute to the global lower health status of men than women? To what extent do these factors contribute to differences in your own community?

Psychological Considerations

Several related elements of the psychological dimension are of concern to community health nurses caring for men. These elements include socialization, stress, and coping abilities, as well as suicide as an outcome of ineffective coping.

Men, like women, have several basic psychological needs. These include the needs to know and be known to others, to be mutually interdependent, to love and be loved, and to live meaningful lives. Society, however, has socialized both men and women to accept a stereotypical male role that makes it difficult to meet these needs. General dimensions of this stereotyped role include a need to actively differentiate oneself from women and refrain from behaviors ascribed to women (such as demonstrating affection or seeking help) and a need to see oneself as superior to others. Other dimensions include the need to be strong and self-reliant and to be more powerful than others, even if this means resorting to violence to demonstrate one's power.

Because of this stereotyped view of the masculine role, men experience social pressures to conform that sometimes conflict with health. Socialized to view the male role as strong or invulnerable, a man may have difficulty admitting health-related frailties to a community health nurse. Similarly, men who believe that taking physical risks is fundamental to their masculinity may experience more frequent health impairment from trauma. Pressure to assert one's manliness also contributes to early initiation of sexual activity by young men, putting them at risk for STDs and unintended fatherhood (Alan Guttmacher Institute, 2005a). In addition, internalization of the typical male gender role has been shown to be associated with less attention to routine screenings such as testicular self-examination (Gurevich et al., 2003). As can be seen in these examples, when societal messages about male roles are internalized by men, they become psychological factors influencing health-related behaviors.

Men may also have a stronger psychological need than women to see themselves as healthy and even invulnerable. Because men tend to value strength and endurance more than women, they are more likely to conceal or suppress pain and other perceived indicators of frailty. An example of this state of mind can be seen in the male post–myocardial infarction client who resumes shoveling snow against the recommendations of health care professionals and his family, and who continues the activity despite the return of the now-familiar angina. As a result of this need for strength in his self-image, the male client minimizes the importance of the problem. Consequently, when shoveling snow causes further angina, he may seek health care less readily and use it less effectively than would a female client in a similar situation.

Similar responses may occur with mental health problems. Traditional American culture prohibits men from expressing emotions other than anger and aggression, and men may be unable to express grief, sadness, or powerlessness, allowing these emotions to fester and contributing to depression (Calandra, 2004). Gendered communication styles are another aspect of gender socialization that may make it difficult for men to express needs and feelings (Marston, 2004).

Based on data from 1993 to 2001, men less frequently reported frequent mental distress than women (7.2% versus 10.3%) (National Center for Chronic Disease Prevention and Health Promotion, 2004). Men are also less likely than women to report depression, but still account for 20% of diagnoses of clinical depression. Physicians are also less likely to diagnose depression in men than women (Monts, 2002b). Men are less willing to acknowledge depression and deal with it less well than women, contributing to a variety of health problems (Weidner & Cain, 2003). For example, depression is more often associated with coronary heart disease in men than in women (Monts, 2002b).

Conversely, male values of strength and endurance do not always adversely affect a male client's health. Some men who value strength actually may be more motivated to exercise and maintain a higher level of general fitness and to seek preventive health care to preserve their sense of themselves as strong and invulnerable.

Another psychological barrier to men's health is the male client's conflicting response to feelings regarding a health problem. For example, a man who values strength may exercise regularly, but he may avoid having a swelling in his groin examined because he cannot cope effectively with the fear that the swelling may represent a threat to his sexuality. This is particularly true with respect to problems like testicular growths, because testicular integrity is closely linked to perceptions of manliness, sexual attractiveness, and desirability (Gurevich et al., 2003).

As we saw in Chapter 17∞, men and women are exposed to different types of stress and cope with stress in different ways. For example, men are more likely than women to engage in avoidant coping strategies (Weidner & Cain, 2003). Similarly, post-traumatic stress disorder (PTSD) arises from different types of events and manifests differently in men and women. One frequent cause of PTSD in men is combat exposure, which contributes to approximately 28% of PTSD in men. In one study, PTSD was found to contribute to 7.4% of depression, 8% of substance abuse disorder, 12% of job loss, 9% of current unemployment and divorce or separation, and 21% of partner or spouse abuse in combat veterans (Prigerson, Maciejewski, & Rosenheck, 2002).

PTSD and other mental health problems may contribute to suicide. Although women make more suicide attempts, rates of completed suicide are four times higher in U.S. men than women (Monts, 2002b). Suicide mortality is highest among White men, at 19.1 per 100,000 population, compared to 4.3 per 100,000 among White women. Similar gender differences are noted for Black men (10.0 per 100,000) and women (1.8 per 100,000) (U.S. Census Bureau, 2005).

Suicide claims more lives among men annually than many of the diseases that health care professionals combat so effectively. Because suicide is such a frequent cause of mortality for men, it is important that community health nurses assess the male population for the presence of suicide risk factors:

- Significant portions of the population 15 to 24 years of age or older than 65 years
- High rates of chronic physical or mental disorders (particularly those that are progressively debilitating or that lead to deterioration in function)
- High rates of depression
- High rates of substance abuse

Physical Environmental Considerations

With the exception of the occupational environment, which is addressed in the discussion of the sociocultural dimension, the effects of the physical environment on men's health are much the same as they are on women's health. Pollution, overcrowding, and safety hazards adversely affect both. Men, however, may have increased exposure to environmental hazards due to occupational and leisure activity choices.

Sociocultural Considerations

Many influences on men's health arise from the sociocultural dimension. We have already discussed the influences of gender socialization, a sociocultural factor, on men's psychological health. Other considerations in the sociocultural dimension affecting men's health include family interactions, economic and occupational issues, and issues related to violence.

Family Interactions

By far, the largest proportion of men live within a family situation, which may create both positive and negative health effects. Worldwide, most men are married by the time they are in their 30s, but delayed marriage is associated with higher educational levels. By their 40s to mid-50s, most men have been married, some of them several times (Alan Guttmacher Institute, 2005a). Approximately 27% of American men marry in their early 20s, and this figure doubles by the late 20s. White and Hispanic men tend to marry earlier than Black men. About 70% of men in their 30s are married and 80% of men in their 40s are married or cohabiting (Alan Guttmacher Institute, 2004). In 2003, 61% of adult men were married, 28% had never married, nearly 3% were widowed, and close to 9% were divorced (U.S. Census Bureau, 2005).

Marriage has been shown to have a protective health effect for men and less so for women; however, because of socialization to a stereotyped male role and gender communication styles discussed earlier, men may have difficulty interacting within the family in ways that effectively meet their psychological needs. Differing role expectations between husband and wife may lead to marital conflicts and, in some cases, spouse or child abuse. Family violence and its effects on health are discussed in more detail in Chapter 32∞. It is, however, important for the community health nurse dealing with male clients to assess the marital status of the male population.

Parenting is another aspect of family interaction that may affect men's health. Approximately one fourth of U.S. men have had a child by 20 years of age and 50% by age 30. Early parenthood is more likely among minority men and those with lower educational levels. Younger men are often involved in pregnancies that end in abortion. In fact, in the United States, 13% of pregnancies that result in abortion involve adolescent fathers, and 53% involve men in their 20s. Half of all live births in the U.S. involve men in their 20s (Alan Guttmacher Institute, 2002), and 80% of births involving men in their early 20s and 50% in the late 20s occur

outside of marriage. Thus, men may have children who do not live with them. Divorce may also separate many men from their children. Sixty-seven percent of U.S. men in their 30s and 85% of men in their 40s have one or more children who may or may not be living with them (Alan Guttmacher Institute, 2002). In fact, an estimated 11% of U.S. men in their 30s have biological children who do not live with them (Alan Guttmacher Institute, 2004).

Because of typical male socialization, many men have little or no childcare experience, yet the increase in the number of working women has led to greater assumption of childcare duties by men. Married women with children have been shown to spend 50% more time with them than their fathers do, although the amount of time men spend with their children increased about one hour per day between 1965 and 1995 (Alan Guttmacher Institute, 2002). Many men may find themselves single parents as a result of divorce or the death of their wives. Others may have partial custody of children as a result of divorce. In 2003, 19% of single-parent households were headed by men, an increase from 17% in 2000. Four percent of these single male-headed households included three or more children (U.S. Census Bureau, 2005).

Although stressful, parenthood, like marriage and particularly in the context of marriage, may have a protective health effect for men. In one study, for example, married men with children had lower overall mortality rates and lower rates of death due to ischemic heart disease, accidents, and addictions than single childless men and fathers who did not live with their children. Single parenthood by men was also associated with lower mortality rates than childlessness or noncustodial parenthood, but differences were not as great as for married men with children (Weitoft, Burstrom, & Rosen, 2004).

Divorce is one of the most significant stressors a person can experience, and it frequently has a profound effect on physical and psychological health. Divorced men, in particular, have been shown to experience increased morbidity and mortality as compared with married men. Men may respond to divorce or its

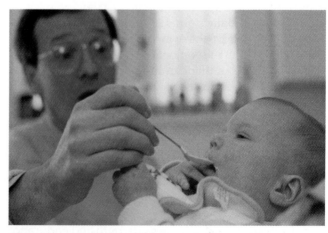

More men are raising children as single parents.
(Patrick J. Watson)

aftermath with intense anger, a profound sense of loss, or significant depression. Suicidal behavior occasionally occurs as the man reacts to the divorce as an assault against his self-image and self-worth, or homicidal behavior if he directs his anger toward his ex-spouse. Widowed men also fare less well than widowed women (Weitoft et al., 2004). Although women are more likely than men to experience divorce, separation, or widowhood in their 40s, men tend to have greater health effects due to the loss of a spouse (Alan Guttmacher Institute, 2002; Weitoft et al., 2004).

Economic and Occupational Issues

In most cultures, men are the primary breadwinners for the family, although more and more women throughout the world can be found in the workforce. Worldwide poverty and poor employment prospects undermine men's ability to fulfill their provider roles. Unemployment may be high in many developing countries and urbanization may lead young men to leave their families for extended periods of time to seek employment where it can be found (Alan Guttmacher Institute, 2005a). In the United States, men fare better than women in terms of their economic status, yet economic influences can have profound effects on their health status.

Economic status is closely linked to employment and unemployment. Some authors make a distinction between the societal experience of unemployment and the individual experience of "joblessness." From this perspective, **unemployment** is the proportion of the workforce that is not employed at a specific point in time and is a statistical measure reflecting the general state of the economy. **Joblessness**, on the other hand, is the personalized experience of being out of work when one desires employment. Joblessness can have significant implications for both physical and mental health among men since "most men in America gain at least part of their sense of manhood from their participation in the workforce" (Cooke, 2004, p. 156). Although joblessness affects the mental health of both men and women, its mental health effects seem to be worse for men than women (Artazcoz, Benach, Borrell, & Cortes, 2004).

In 2003, nearly 69% of U.S. men over 16 years of age were employed, and employment rates are expected to rise to 73% by 2012. Slightly more than 5% of employed men hold more than one job. Another 6% of men were unemployed in 2003, 62% of them due to job loss. The median hourly wage for all men was $13.25, but more than 1% of male workers over age 25 received minimum wage or less. Similarly, the median family income for families headed by a man without a spouse present was $41,711, but 483,000 of these families have annual incomes less than $15,000. Nearly 15 million men (11.2% of all U.S. men) had incomes below poverty level in 1999, only slightly less than women at 13.5% (U.S. Census Bureau, 2005). In 2003, 13.5% of male-headed households had incomes below poverty level (U.S. Census

Bureau, 2004b). Poverty is one of several reasons that men are more likely than women to be homeless. Despite the differences in the incidence of homelessness among men and women, homeless shelter systems are often better designed to meet the needs of women and children than those of men (Archambault, 2002). Issues related to homelessness will be addressed in more detail in Chapter 20∞.

Men are more likely than women to be employed in jobs that entail physical health risks. In 2002, for example, the rate of occupational injury deaths was nearly 10 times higher for men (6.8 per 100,000 employed workers) than women (0.7 per 100,000). The highest rates of death occurred in agriculture, forestry, fishing, mining, and construction, enterprises less likely to employ women (CDC, 2004a). In addition, a higher percentage of men (4%) than women (3.8%) have work-related disabilities (U.S. Census Bureau, 2005).

Economic status is also associated with educational levels. Men are more likely to drop out of high school than women and less likely to attend college. In 2002, for example, only 62% of men aged 16 to 24 years were enrolled in college, compared to 68% of women (U.S. Census Bureau, 2005).

Violence and Trauma

Earlier, we discussed the implications of PTSD for men's psychological health. PTSD and other health problems arise from exposure to a variety of forms of violence and trauma. Men are more likely than women to be exposed to societal violence in many forms. For example, in 2002 men constituted 78% of homicide victims over 18 years of age. In 2002, the homicide rate for men was 9.4 per 100,000 men, down from 13.6 in 1976, but still more than three times the rate for women (2.8 per 100,000) (CDC, 2004a; U.S. Census Bureau, 2005). Men are also exposed to higher rates of physical assault than women. In 2002, the assault victimization rate for men was 23.9 per 1,000 men compared to 19.8 for women (CDC, 2005).

Violence also occurs in families, and men, as well as women, are subjected to intimate partner violence (IPV). Men, however, are less likely to be injured as a result of IPV. In one study of IPV in rural settings, more men than women (4.7% versus 2.9%) reported being the victim of at least one episode of severe physical violence by their partner. Men were less likely than women, however, to report emotional abuse (30.2% and 46.7%, respectively). Interestingly, men engaged in farm work reported more physical abuse and controlling abuse than other men, possibly related to the greater stress and economic uncertainty experienced in agriculture than in other areas of employment (Murty et al., 2003). Overall, men report considerably less IPV than women, with rates of 4.2 per 1,000 women in 2000 compared with only 0.8 per 1,000 men (CDC, 2005). In part, however, these differences may be related to men's reluctance to report being victims of IPV because of threats to their self-image.

Trauma also results from unintentional injury. In 2002, men experienced six times as many firearms-related deaths as women and nearly twice as many deaths related to poisoning. The unintentional injury mortality rate for men was similarly nearly twice that for women. Men also experience high rates of injury requiring emergency department services. For example, the rate of emergency department visits for men in 2002 was 154 per 1,000 men compared to 123 per 1,000 women (CDC, 2005).

Behavioral Considerations

Behavioral factors seem to make a greater contribution to men's health status than to that of women, probably because men are generally more likely than women to engage in high-risk behaviors (Denton, Prus, & Walters, 2004). Because of their gender socialization, men are more inclined to engage in high-risk behaviors and less apt to perform healthful behaviors (Griffiths, 2004). Some behavioral considerations to be addressed in assessing men's health include consumption patterns, exercise and leisure, sexual activity, and other behavioral risk factors.

Consumption Patterns

Consumption patterns include diet as well as substance use and abuse. As we saw earlier, U.S. men are more likely than women to be overweight, but less likely to be obese. In the United Kingdom, 21% of men are considered obese and an additional 40% are overweight. Healthy weight involves 10% to 20% of body weight as fat. Less than 10% body fat is considered underweight and unhealthful, 20% to 25% is considered overweight, and greater than 25% is considered obese (Campbell, 2004). As of 2000, only 32% of U.S. men over 20 years of age had achieved a healthy diet, compared to 35% of women (CDC, 2005). With respect to specific nutrients, men are less likely than women to consume the recommended five or more servings of fruits and vegetables per day (CDC, 2004b), but more likely to eat six or more servings of grains. Based on baseline data for the *Healthy People 2010*◆ objectives, only 32% of men restricted their fat intake to less than 10% of their daily calories. Men were more likely than women (63% versus 39%) to have sufficient calcium in their diets, but women were five times more likely than men to restrict their sodium intake to recommended dietary limits (CDC, 2005).

With respect to substance use and abuse, men are involved in more than three times more alcohol-related motor vehicle accidents than women, and men are more likely to engage in binge drinking. For example, 51% of college-age men report binge drinking, compared to 33% of women, and similar differences occur with older age groups. In addition, men are twice as likely as women to die of cirrhosis, a major consequence of alcohol consumption, and nearly twice as likely to experience a drug-induced death (CDC, 2005). As we saw in

Chapter 17∞, men are more likely than women to smoke (25% and 20%, respectively), and women smokers are slightly more likely than men to attempt to quit smoking (CDC, 2005).

Exercise and Leisure

Men are more likely than women to engage in leisure-time physical activity, but in 2002, 35% of U.S. men did not engage in any leisure-time physical activity at all. Another 35% of men engaged in moderate physical activity and 27% in vigorous activity (CDC, 2005). Higher levels of physical activity have been shown to be associated with decreased risk of hip fracture (Mussolino, Looker, & Orwoll, 2001), as well as improved cardiovascular health.

Men and women increasingly share similar leisure patterns in American culture. Nevertheless, men still tend to be more active in competitive contact sports and, more often than women, to choose leisure activities involving some degree of physical risk (skydiving, white-water rafting, rock climbing). Participation in athletic sports is closely linked with images of masculinity and reinforces tendencies to aggressiveness and violence, increasing the potential for injury. Expectations of masculinity may also lead men to downplay the severity of injuries, delay treatment, and take insufficient time for healing. Men also tend to choose leisure activities associated with alcohol consumption. For these reasons, men experience relatively greater incidence of recreation-related trauma.

Sexual Activity

On average, men are sexually active for approximately 10 years prior to marriage, and the average age for initiating sexual activity in the United States is 16.9 years (Alan Guttmacher Institute, 2002; 2005b). Less than 10% of boys are sexually active at age 15, but approximately 90% have initiated sexual activity by age 20 (Pinkelman, 2002a). Worldwide, most men have initiated sexual activity prior to their 20th birthday. In various populations, anywhere from 15% to 65% of single men report more than one sexual partner, and 7% to 36% of married men report extramarital partners. More than twice as many men as women report multiple partners, although men may exaggerate the number of partners and women may underreport due to gender socialization expectations for male and female behavior (Nnko, Boerma, Urassa, Mwaluko, & Zaba, 2003). Men are often unaware of measures to prevent STDs, and knowledge of condom use to prevent STDs ranges from a low of 6% of men in Bangladesh to 82% of men in Brazil (Alan Guttmacher Institute, 2005a). Most men with multiple sexual partners do not use condoms, and those that do tend to use them for contraceptive purposes rather than STD prevention (Alan Guttmacher Institute, 2004; 2005a). In the United States, condom use is relatively high at first intercourse (close to two thirds) but declines with increased age, with only 16% of sexually active men using condoms by age 35 to 39 years (Alan Guttmacher Institute, 2002).

Other Behavioral Risk Factors

Use of seat belts and other safety devices is another behavior that can significantly affect men's health. Because of masculine socialization to risk as an element of manliness, men are less likely than women to engage in a variety of safety practices, including seat belt or helmet use. They are also more likely to engage in high-risk recreational activities, particularly in the context of alcohol or drug use.

Another relatively recent phenomenon that may affect men's health is the increase in genital piercing. Piercing is not a new phenomenon, and historical texts refer to various forms of piercing. Similarly, anthropologists have found evidence of genital piercing in some ancient cultures. In men, piercing may involve the pubis just above the penis, the glans, the foreskin, frenum, body of the penis, or the scrotum, as well as the nipples. Piercings may be singular or multiple. Piercing is not regulated in any way in most countries, and there are no data regarding complications resulting from piercing. There have been cases of hepatitis B and C and HIV transmission associated with piercing, but it is difficult to ascribe causality since many men who engage in piercing have other risk factors for these diseases. Localized bleeding, infection, and cellulitis are other possible complications. Urethral fistulas have also been noted in some cases. Allergic reactions to metal rings and studs and difficulty with hygiene have also been reported. Piercings have also occasionally proved hazardous to sexual partners in terms of injury and choking hazards (Anderson & Holmes, 2004). Community health nurses should be alert to the extent of a "piercing culture" among the male population and its possible implications for health.

Health System Considerations

Generally speaking, men define health as the ability to be employed and to be economically independent, and, in some cases, to have adequate sexual function (Hjelm, Bard, Nyberg, & Apelqvist, 2005). Despite unhealthy lifestyles and shorter lives than women, 70% of men consider themselves to be in good health. As noted earlier, on average, women live 7 years longer than men, and White women live an average of 14 years longer than Black men. Gender socialization leads men to "tough out" pain and not seek help until conditions interfere with their ability to work. In addition, media portrayals of men engaged in unhealthy behaviors contribute to risk taking and negative health effects in men (Monts & Smith, 2002).

All of these factors combine to make men less likely than women to seek health care services. Each year, men make 130 million fewer visits to health care providers than women, and in any given year, approximately 37 million men have not seen a provider in the last year (Monts & Smith, 2002). In addition, only 14% of men 15 to 49 years of age make reproductive health visits in any given year, and reproductive health needs of men are largely ignored (Alan Guttmacher Institute, 2004, 2005b). Even in the face of symptoms, men may delay seeking care. For example, men who perceive themselves to be in "good" health may wait as long as 3 years before seeking assistance for recognizable symptoms of testicular cancer. Physicians may also succumb to genderized perspectives in delaying referrals for specialist care. Young men are not supposed to present with possible life-threatening illness (Griffiths, 2004).

Factors other than gender socialization may also prohibit men from seeking health care. Some of these factors include lack of trust in providers, language barriers, lack of health insurance, financial difficulties, and difficulty relating to providers. Lack of health insurance is a particularly salient factor in men's failure to access health care services. In 2003, only 84% of U.S. men had health insurance, 61% through employment, 11% through Medicaid, and 12% under Medicare. Another 17% had no coverage at all (U.S. Census Bureau, 2004a). During the previous year, men constituted 53.5% of those who were without health insurance for the entire year (U.S. Census Bureau, 2005). Lack of health insurance is even more prevalent among young adult men; 40% of men 20 to 24 years of age are uninsured, compared to only 30% of women in the same age group (Alan Guttmacher Institute, 2002).

CULTURAL COMPETENCE

*I*n many cultural groups, men and women do not interact with or touch each other unless they are family members. This may make some men uncomfortable interacting with female nurses. In addition, in some cultural groups, women have lower social status than men, and men are the authority figures. These cultural perspectives may make men less willing to see female nurses as knowledgeable and make them hesitant to act on health-related information presented by women. How might you go about counteracting these cultural perspectives in planning health education offerings designed to improve men's health in the community?

U.S. men and women have similar levels of coverage under employment-based health insurance. Many government services, however, are designed to meet the needs of women and children rather than men, and women are more likely than men to have coverage under Medicaid (Alan Guttmacher Institute, 2002). It is often difficult for men to obtain Medicaid coverage, but a depressed economy leads to greater unemployment or employment in jobs that do not provide health insurance benefits and less employment-based coverage. Section 1115 of the Social Security Act permits states to request waivers to provide care to groups of people (including men) who would not ordinarily be eligible for Medicaid services. Unfortunately, few states have done so. A few programs have been developed to provide primary care services for nondisabled men 50 to 64 years of age with incomes at or below 50% of the federal poverty level. Even with these few programs, however, it is sometimes difficult to find providers willing to accept Medicaid reimbursement (Bufalini, 2002). A few additional programs have been set up to meet the needs of homeless clients, who are primarily men, and in 2002, 154 such Health Care for Homeless Centers existed throughout the United States (Archambault, 2002).

Another factor in men's failure to use health care services on a level commensurate with women is their perceived lack of a need for health care. Women routinely enter the health care system through services related to pregnancy, contraception, and routine screenings (e.g., Papanicolaou smears). These services serve as avenues for other health promotion activities as well as for detection of illness. Men do not routinely access any health-promotive services that would provide a similar door to other needed health care. Health care services are not crafted to target men, nor are many providers educated specifically to address the health care needs and motivations (or lack thereof) of men (White & Banks, 2004).

THE EPIDEMIOLOGY OF HEALTH FOR GAY, BISEXUAL, AND TRANSGENDER MEN

Homosexuality has been present throughout recorded human history, but, until recently, it has rarely been considered in terms of its effects on men's health status and health behaviors (Savage, Harley, & Nowak, 2005). An estimated 2.8% to 9% of U.S. men are believed to be homosexual in their sexual orientation (Meyer, Silenzio, Wolfe, & Dunn, 2000). This figure includes both gay men (those who have a primary sexual or affectional orientation to members of the same sex) and bisexual men (those who may interact sexually with both men and women). Transgenderism is relatively rare, occurring in approximately one in 30,000 U.S. men. Rates of transgenderism are somewhat higher in countries like the Netherlands with policies that support sexual

reassignment surgery or so-called sex change operations (Sember, 2000). Although no specific number of gay, bisexual, or transgender men is available, approximately 5% of unmarried partner households in United States in 2000 were comprised of two men (U.S. Census Bureau, 2005). Many other gay, bisexual, or transgender men may not live in partnered arrangements.

There is no general consensus on the use of the terms *heterosexual, homosexual,* and so on, primarily because the terms are defined differently by different groups. Homosexuality is culturally defined, and what is considered homosexual in one culture may not be in another, even if it involves same-sex sexual activity (Murray, 2000). For example, 24% of African American men and 15% of Latino men who had sex with other men identified themselves as heterosexual (Scout & Robinson, 2000). Similar lack of clarity occurs in definitions of bisexuality. For instance, in one study, 82% of men who self-identified as gay also had sexual interactions with women, yet did not consider themselves bisexual (Taylor, 1999). Definitions may incorporate one or more of three dimensions: one's sexual identity orientation, sexual behavior, and/or sexual attraction (Sell, 2000). For the purposes of this book, self-identification as a gay, bisexual, or transgender individual will be used as the primary means of distinguishing membership in these groups. Readers should be aware, however, that different definitions have been used in some of the research that will be reported here. Where relevant, the term "men who have sex with men" (MSM) will be used since it encompasses both gay and bisexual men as well as some men who self-identify as heterosexual despite occasional same-sex sexual activity.

Biophysical Considerations

Biophysical considerations related to gay, bisexual, and transgender men's health include maturation and aging and the presence of physical illnesses. Although gay culture emphasizes youth, there is a significant older population among both gays and lesbians. Gay men and lesbians are estimated to constitute approximately 6% of the older population of the United States (Heath, 2002), with 1 million to 3 million gay men over 65 years of age. This number is expected to rise to 4 million by 2030 (Hawke, 2002). An additional 545,000 to 872,000 lesbians and gay men over 65 are estimated in the United Kingdom (Price, 2005). Because of their marginal status in society, older gay men and lesbians may have more difficulty than others in obtaining assistance in old age (Hawke, 2002), creating a population of particular concern to community health nurses.

Gay, bisexual, and transgender men tend to be at greater risk for a number of physical health problems than their heterosexual counterparts. In part, this is due to the greater prevalence of high-risk behaviors in this population, as well as to their reluctance to seek medical care. Much of the attention given to health issues among gay, bisexual, and transgender men to date has focused on the extent of sexually transmitted diseases in this population. From 2000 to 2001, for example, the number of cases of syphilis in the United States increased by more than 15% in men; most of this increase occurred among men who have sex with men (Natinsky, 2002). Since 2001, approximately 60% of all cases of primary and secondary syphilis have occurred in MSM, and half of MSM with primary and secondary syphilis are co-infected with HIV (Division of STD Prevention, 2004b). MSM also contribute greatly to the incidence of HIV infection in cities considered "AIDS epicenters," U.S. cities with unusually high rates of HIV infection. HIV incidence ranged from 14% to 31% of MSM in Chicago, Los Angeles, San Francisco, and South Beach, Florida (Webster et al., 2005). Many MSM, particularly Black MSM, do not perceive themselves to be at risk for HIV infection. For example, in a 1994–1998 Young Men's Survey in six U.S. cities, 93% of HIV-infected Black MSM did not know they were infected and 71% stated that there was "no chance" or it was "very unlikely" that they were infected. Forty-two percent also perceived themselves at low risk of ever being infected (Division of HIV/AIDS Prevention–Intervention, Research, and Support, 2002).

MSM are also at risk for other STDs. For example, they are at increased risk for lymphogranuloma venereum (LGV), a sexually transmitted disease rarely seen in the general U.S. population. Risk of LGV is increased with sexual contact with European gay, bisexual, and transgender men. Because of the presence of ulcerative lesions, LGV increases one's susceptibility to HIV infection and other STDs (Division of STD Prevention, 2004a). Because of anal insertive sexual activity, many MSM are also at risk for sexual transmission of enteric diseases such as *Shigella flexneri, Entamoeba histolytica, Giardia lamblia, Campylobacter, Shigella*, and hepatitis A (Division of Bacterial and Mycotic Diseases, 2005). They may also be at increased risk for "gay bowel syndrome," an intestinal infection due to anal intercourse, as well as for anal carcinoma. Due to their frequent lack of interaction with health care providers, MSM may also have undetected prostate cancer. In addition, low levels of testosterone may lead to erectile dysfunction at higher rates than in the general population (Hawke, 2002).

There is some evidence to suggest that gay, bisexual, and transgender men may also be at increased risk for certain forms of cancer. In part, this increased risk may relate to the effects of stress on the immune system, with clients who don't disclose their sexual orientation at even higher risk than other gay, bisexual, and transgender men. Among gay and bisexual men with HIV infection, rates of Kaposi's sarcoma are thousands of times higher than in the general population. Incidence of Kaposi's sarcoma among gay and bisexual men has declined with the advent of more effective treatments for AIDS. The incidence of AIDS-related non-Hodgkin's lymphoma is also higher among MSM than among heterosexual groups. Gay and bisexual men also appear to be at increased risk for anal cancers, though not for cancers at other sites, than the heterosexual male population. This increased risk is thought to be due to the increased prevalence of human papillomavirus infection and smoking as risk factors among gay men. In addition, survival rates for gay men with cancer are lower than in the general population, probably due to HIV/AIDS comorbidity and delay in disease detection and treatment (Meyer & Bowen, 2000).

Immunity is another consideration in the biophysical dimension. In addition to routine immunizations suggested for adults, gay, bisexual, and transgender men should also receive immunization for hepatitis A and B. Unfortunately, figures indicate low immunization rates for these diseases among the homosexual population (3%) (Silenzio, 2000). Community health nurses should assess immunity among individual clients as well as levels of immunity in the gay, bisexual, and transgender population at large.

Homosexual males are also vulnerable to other physiologic conditions found among their heterosexual counterparts. Due to discriminatory attitudes among some health care professionals and prior unpleasant experiences with the health care system, however, many homosexuals may not volunteer information about health problems or seek assistance. These barriers to care help to explain the lower cancer survival rates among this population. For this reason, community health nurses should carefully assess homosexual clients for evidence of physical illness.

Psychological Considerations

Homosexuality was considered a psychiatric disease by the American Psychiatric Association until 1993 (Savage et al., 2005), and the "gender dysphoria" experienced by some transgender individuals is still considered a mental illness. **Gender dysphoria** is a sense of incongruity between one's physical gender and one's self-perceptions (Sember, 2000). The American Psychiatric Association has retained the diagnosis of gender identity disorder in its *Diagnostic and Statistical Manual of Mental Disorders IV-TR*, but is moving to a consideration of pathology only in those individuals who exhibit significant levels of distress over their transgender identity (McLeer, 2004; Meyer, Rothblum, & Bradford, 2000). These individuals may be at particular risk for suicide, auto-castration, or substance abuse. Psychological well-being seems to increase and gender dysphoria to disappear in most individuals who experience sexual reassignment surgery (Sember, 2000). In the interim, however, community health nurses may need to be particularly alert to suicidal ideation in these individuals.

Although gay, bisexual, and transgender men do not appear to be any more intrinsically susceptible to mental illness than their heterosexual counterparts, there is some evidence to suggest that they have a slightly higher prevalence of mental illness, possibly as a result of perceptions of discrimination (Mays & Cochran, 2001). MSM have been shown in some studies to have higher prevalences of substance abuse, partner violence, depression, and childhood sexual abuse than the heterosexual population. In addition, increased numbers of psychosocial problems have been linked to greater prevalence of high-risk sexual behaviors and HIV infection in MSM (Stall et al., 2003). Same-sex attraction has also been linked to the incidence of depression, anxiety, conduct disorder, suicide ideation and suicide attempts, and other disorders (Ridge, Hulme, & Peasley, 2003).

Suicide is a particular problem among gay, bisexual, and transgender men, particularly among youth, and the link between same-sex attraction and suicide attempts is stronger for boys than for girls, particularly when both partners were of the same ethnic group (Pinhey & Millman, 2004). The lifetime prevalence of suicide ideation for adult gay men and lesbians is estimated at 24% to 41%, with 7% to 20% of gay men and lesbians actually attempting suicide sometime in their lives. Among gay and lesbian youth, 20% to 40% attempt suicide. In one study, MSM attempted suicide over five times more often than men who had only female partners (Paul et al., 2002). Other studies have noted a link between sexual orientation and suicide mediated by depression, hopelessness, alcohol abuse, and victimization (Russell & Joyner, 2001).

Psychological factors also seem to influence sexual risk behaviors among MSM. For example, MSM who have been found to have high relationship needs are more likely than others to maintain steady partner relationships. Conversely, those whose sexual behavior is motivated by pleasure seeking are more likely to have a number of casual relationships; they are also more likely than those in steady relationships to engage in unprotected anal intercourse (UAI) (Craft, Smith, Serovich, & Bautista, 2005).

Sociocultural Considerations

Factors in the sociocultural dimension have a profound impact on the health status and health-related behaviors of gay, bisexual, and transgender men. Gay men and lesbians have been described as a "sociological minority," which is defined as "any segment of the population subjected to negative acts and behaviors inflicted by the rest of society" (Savage et al., 2005, p. 134). Discrimination against gay men and lesbians has been attributed to homophobia, a "fear of lesbian and gay male individuals or of homosexual feelings within oneself leading to hatred, loathing, prejudice, and possible discrimination toward individuals known or perceived to be lesbian or gay" (Savage et al., 2005, p. 135). Some authors note, however, that the use of the term *homophobia* restricts responses to gay men and lesbians to an individual phenomenon, when it is evident that it is in reality a societally constructed entity that influences many

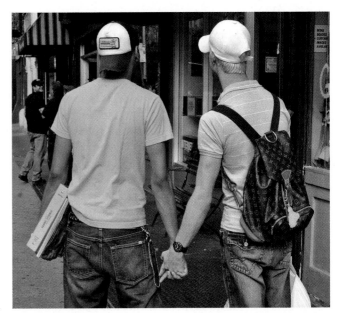

Gay men may experience discrimination in health care settings as well as in the wider society. (© Lee Snider/ The Image Works)

aspects of the sociocultural environment. For that reason, many authors prefer the term **heterosexism**, which is defined as an "ideological system that denies, denigrates, and stigmatizes any non-heterosexual form of behavior, identity, relationship, or community" (Herek, as quoted in Savage et al., 2005, p. 135).

Heterosexism results in oppression through force or imposition or by deprivation (Savage et al., 2005). Oppression by force is seen in physical abuse and victimization of MSM, whereas oppression by deprivation is reflected in failure to afford same-sex partners in long-term relationships the same benefits accorded to heterosexual married couples. Oppression may occur in a variety of forms, including language, assumptions of heterosexuality, simultaneous support and denial of civil rights, criminalization of same-sex sexual behavior, and failure to educate health care professionals and counselors regarding the health needs of nonheterosexual clients (Savage et al., 2005).

MSM who are members of cultural minority groups may be faced with even more conflict. For example, some authors have noted that Latino gay and bisexual men in Southern California are simultaneously exposed to more relaxed attitudes to homosexual behavior in the majority culture and strict cultural attitudes. Community programs, such as SOLAAR (Superacion, Orgullo y Lucha Atraves de Amor en Relaciones), are designed to enhance self-understanding within this cultural conflict and to promote long-term monogamous relationships among Latino MSM to reduce the risk of HIV exposure (Conner et al., 2005). This program employed social marketing strategies similar to those discussed in Chapter 11∞ to specifically target Latino gay and bisexual clients, and has been successful in recruiting participants from a wider geographic range than that achieved prior to the social marketing campaign.

Cultural conflicts similar to those experienced by Latino MSM may also be encountered by older gay men who developed their sexual identities in an age when it was more prudent to keep one's sexual orientation hidden. This group may be at particular disadvantage in dealing with the effects of societal heterosexualism. For example, in the United Kingdom, surviving partners of homosexual relationships cannot claim property, register the partner's death, or claim other social benefits available to heterosexual spouses. In addition, disability and lack of avenues for care may necessitate disclosure of previously unknown sexual orientation, leaving clients open to discrimination on the basis of both age and sexual orientation (Price, 2005).

Societal attitudes toward what many consider deviant behavior may lead to prejudice, discrimination, harassment, and victimization. For example, more than 50% of gay men reported experiencing discrimination in their lives, compared to only 34% of heterosexual men (Mays & Cochran, 2001), and associations have been found among psychosocial distress, perceptions of discrimination, and experiences of victimization in MSM. In some studies, 28% of gay men reported violence or criminal activity directed at them because of their sexual orientation. Gay, lesbian, and bisexual youth are more likely to be involved in physical fighting in school than other youth (25% to 38% of gay youth versus 7% to 19% of others) (Huebner, Rebchook, & Kegeles, 2004). Similarly, half of older gay men and lesbians report being physically abused, and three fourths report verbal abuse (Heath, 2002). In 2002, Federal Bureau of Investigation statistics indicated 1,464 hate crimes in the United States based on sexual orientation, 68% of which were directed at homosexual men (U.S. Census Bureau, 2005). Gay men have also been found to be disproportionately victimized by heterosexual men in prison settings. Most male-to-male sexual assaults involve unprotected anal intercourse, with the attendant risks of trauma and STD (Dean & Bradford, 2000).

Family interaction is another element of the sociocultural dimension that affects the health of gay, bisexual, and transgender men. Disclosure of homosexuality or transgenderism to family members and their response, homosexual relationships, and homosexual parenting are the three primary aspects of family interaction to be assessed by the community health nurse.

Two different themes occur in families' responses to disclosure of a family member's homosexuality: loving acceptance or conventionality, which results in rejection of the homosexual family member. All families who come to know of homosexual or transgender members need to deal with feelings of grief, guilt, and fear for their child or sibling.

For those families that are able to accept homosexuality or transgenderism in one of their members, acceptance appears to come about in stages similar to the stages of grief experienced with the loss of a loved one. The first stage is one of grief, followed by a period of denial during which parents may see their child's professed sexual identity as a "phase" that he or she will grow out of. This stage is followed successively by stages characterized by guilt and anger and, finally, acceptance (Barret & Robinson, 2000). Unfortunately, some families never achieve the stage of acceptance of their loved one's sexual orientation.

Parental response to the disclosure of homosexuality is strongly influenced by a variety of factors: the strength of traditional gender role conceptions, perceptions of the probable attitudes of significant others in the family's social network, and parental age and education level (younger and better educated parents tend to be more accepting). Affiliation with conservative religious ideologies and intolerance of other stigmatized groups are other factors that suggest a negative response to disclosure.

Gay males may face decisions about disclosure to wives as well as parents and siblings. Contrary to popular belief, many homosexual men are or have been married, and about half of these men have children. Some gay men do not become aware of their homosexuality until after marriage. Others marry in an attempt to deny or hide their sexual orientation. Responses of wives to the disclosure of homosexuality vary considerably and may include feelings of living with a "stranger," guilt, development of an asexual friendship or a semi-open relationship in which both husband and wife are free to take outside lovers, or a desire for divorce. Transgender identity changes can be particularly devastating to marital relationships, as the spouse questions not only the husband's sexual identity but her own as well (Sember, 2000). Community health nurses should assess the extent of clients' disclosure of their sexual identities and the effects of the responses received. Nurses should also assess the needs of family members for assistance in dealing with the disclosure.

Disclosure to family members is usually not a onetime event. As families grow and change, both the homosexual family member and others face decisions regarding disclosure to extended family members, to inlaws as siblings marry, and possibly to children and grandchildren (Barret & Robinson, 2000).

Parenting by gay, bisexual, and transgender men brings its own stresses, many of them similar to those experienced by lesbian parents. Gay or bisexual men may become fathers in a number of ways: in heterosexual relationships prior to coming out, as foster parents or through adoption, or in cooperation with a lesbian woman or surrogate mother. Gay fathers may be marginalized by both the heterosexual and homosexual communities, and partners may resent the intrusion of children into the relationship (Barret & Robinson, 2000). Gay fathers may also be forced to be less open about their sexual identities than they might otherwise be in order to prevent court actions and potential loss of custody. This often means that they cannot openly live with a same-sex partner and may be denied the companionship and support afforded to heterosexual and even lesbian couples (Lambert, 2005).

The mistaken societal view that homosexuality can be transmitted to children has motivated a great deal of research on the effects of homosexual parenting on children. Heteronormative family forms require such research to be defensive in nature, effectively proving that living in a homosexual household is not detrimental to children (Hicks, 2005). In actuality, gay fathers have been found to show greater warmth and responsiveness to children and to provide more limits to children's behavior than heterosexual fathers. Gay fathers are also more likely than lesbian mothers to encourage play with gender-specific toys. In general, parental sexual orientation has not been found to affect children's gender identity or sexual orientation. Children of gay and lesbian parents may be more open to early experimentation with same-sex behaviors than those of heterosexual parents, but no relationship has been shown to final gender identification or sexual orientation. Similarly, no effects have been noted for children's personal development, although younger children of homosexual parents may be somewhat more likely than others to be teased. This effect seems to dissipate as children get older, and children of homosexual parents develop normal peer relationships (Lambert, 2005).

Disclosure of one's sexual identity to children is another dilemma faced by gay, bisexual, and transgender men. Depending on when and how disclosure occurs, children may exhibit the same range of responses shown by other family members. Some considerations in disclosure of sexual identity to children are provided below.

SPECIAL CONSIDERATIONS

DISCLOSURE OF SEXUAL ORIENTATION OR IDENTITY TO CHILDREN

- Come to grips with your own sexual identity before trying to explain it to children.
- Children are never too young to be told, but explanations must be couched in terms the child can understand.
- Disclose to children before they suspect or are informed by others.
- Plan the disclosure; do not let it occur in an impromptu fashion.
- Make the disclosure in a private setting where interruptions are unlikely.
- Inform the child in an objective and straightforward manner; do not "confess."
- Stress that your relationship with the child will not change.
- Be prepared for questions and respond to them honestly.

Data from: Barret, R. L., & Robinson, B. E. (2000). Gay fathers: Encouraging the hearts of gay dads and their families. San Francisco: Jossey-Bass.

BUILDING OUR KNOWLEDGE BASE

Savin-Williams and Esterberg (as cited in Lambert, 2005) suggested several areas for research regarding parenting by gay and lesbian clients. These areas include:

- How is gay or lesbian parenthood viewed in the context of the current legal and social system in the United States?
- How do gay and lesbian parents construct identities as parents as well as homosexuals? How do their identities differ with their circumstances?
- How do gay and lesbian parents interact with social institutions related to parenting (e.g., schools)? What are the effects of this interaction on parents and social systems?
- How is the transition to parenthood for gay and lesbian parents similar to and different from that of their heterosexual counterparts?
- How does parenthood affect the character of gay and lesbian relationships?
- What support is available to gay and lesbian parents from their social networks (both traditional and within the gay and lesbian community)?

How might you design a study to address one or more of these questions? How might you include ethnic minority groups whose participation in research on homosexuality has been limited?

Gay men frequently establish long-term partnerships with same-sex partners, although cohabitation by same-sex couples is less socially acceptable than among heterosexual couples (Casper & Bianchi, 2002). Gay couples' relationships are subjected to the same kinds of stress as heterosexual relationships, but this stress may be exacerbated by the absence of social support for the marital role. Therapists who work with gay and lesbian couples have identified several additional issues that threaten the stability of their relationships. These issues include differences in the stages of coming out between partners, differences with respect to extended family involvement, inequalities of power, and financial conflict and disparity in income (Barret & Robinson, 2000). With the exception of the stage of coming out, these same issues may also affect the stability of relationships among heterosexual couples.

Gay, bisexual, and transgender men may experience violence and abuse in intimate relationships, just as partners in heterosexual relationships do. In one study of four U.S. cities, for example, 34% of MSM reported psychological or symbolic battering, 22% reported physical battering, and 5% reported sexual battering by their partners in the last 5 years. Battering was more likely to occur if the victim was younger, had a low educational level, or was HIV-infected (Greenwood et al., 2002).

The occupational risks and concerns experienced by gay men, another consideration in the social environment, relate primarily to avoiding discrimination and rejection in the workplace. For example, 22.5% of gay men report not being hired for a position versus 18.5% of heterosexual men. Similarly, gay men are more likely than heterosexual men to report being passed over for promotion (17% versus 13%) (Mays & Cochran, 2001). No clearly established occupational health risks pertain to gay or bisexual lifestyles. It should, however, be noted that in occupational settings where masculine roles are stereotypical and exaggerated (e.g., construction), there may be an increased incidence of acting out of homophobic thinking, resulting in an increased risk of assault. Nursing assessment should focus on such potential safety risks and should consider the possibility that gay men who are unable to accept their sexual orientation may themselves enact exaggerated masculine roles and experience the related safety risks these behaviors may entail.

Societal attitudes toward nonheterosexual orientations have changed somewhat in some segments of the American population and elsewhere in the world. For example, a 1999 survey indicated that only 13% of the U.S. population thought that gay men and lesbians should not have equal rights regarding employment, compared to 33% in 1977. Although many people continue to see homosexuality as a moral issue, others are more tolerant than was previously the case, and people who are personally acquainted with gay and lesbian individuals are more accepting of this population than those who are not (Casper & Bianchi, 2002). In spite of these changes, there is continuing evidence of discrimination and violence against gay, bisexual, and transgender men.

Gay, bisexual, and transgender men may participate in the "gay culture," although transgender men may be less likely to do so than others. Some authors have noted, however, that some elements of gay and lesbian networks (e.g., gay bars) are not supportive and may promote alcohol and drug use in MSM (Ridge et al., 2003; Thiede et al., 2003; Webster et al., 2005).

Behavioral Considerations

Behavioral factors are also important influences on the health of gay, bisexual, and transgender men. One study conducted in seven U.S. cities indicated drug use prevalence in 66% of gay men, and 28% of MSM reported using three or more drugs. In addition, 29% of study respondents used drugs frequently, and 4% were injection drug users. Drug use was found to be more common in bisexual men, those who self-identified as heterosexual, runaway youth, and those subjected to forced sexual intimacy (Thiede et al, 2003). Drug use may be higher among MSM in some parts of the country than others. For example, 37% of MSM in South Beach, Florida, reported using three or more recreational drugs in the previous year, compared to 18% in New York City, Chicago, San Francisco, and Los Angeles (Webster et al., 2005). Increased risk of HIV infection has been linked to methamphetamine and other "club" drug use among

EVIDENCE-BASED PRACTICE

Webster et al. (2005) described the use of a population-based survey of men who have sex with men (MSM) in the South Beach, Florida, area to tailor interventions to this subpopulation in preventing HIV infection. Community members responded to survey findings by creating a community-wide education effort to address the intertwined problems of recreational drug use, unprotected intercourse, and HIV infection. The survey highlighted differences in the extent of HIV infection in the local population of MSM and contributing factors from other high-incidence areas throughout the country. These differences permitted development of tailored interventions specific to the population at greatest risk. How might a similar approach be used to identify key factors and intervention strategies in your own area?

MSM. Methamphetamine use is also associated with higher-risk sexual behaviors (Boddiger, 2005). Bisexual men, in particular, have been shown to engage in a variety of high-risk behaviors (Russell, Driscoll, & Truong, 2002).

MSM are also more likely to smoke and to initiate smoking at an earlier age than their heterosexual counterparts; gay, lesbian, bisexual, and transgender youth have been particularly targeted by tobacco company marketing campaigns (Washington, 2002). In one study, 31.4% of MSM were smokers, compared to 24.7% of men in the general population (Greenwood et al., 2005). General figures for smoking prevalence lie at 46% for gay men. In addition to smoking more, gay men tend to find smoking cessation more difficult than their heterosexual counterparts, and gay youth who smoke are more likely than others to engage in other high-risk behaviors. Besides being damaging to health in terms of increased risk for lung and other cancers and heart disease, smoking triggers immune system changes that affect prognosis of hepatitis C and other STDs common among MSM (Washington, 2002).

In addition to smoking and drug use, many MSM engage in high-risk sexual behaviors such as "bare backing." *Bare backing* is the term for intentional unprotected anal intercourse (UAI) (Craft et al., 2005). In part, the move away from condom use to UAI is motivated by perceptions among gay, bisexual, and transgender men that HIV/AIDS is now "curable" with the advent of newer, more effective drugs (Hawke, 2002). Other reasons for UAI reported in the literature include general tendencies toward risk taking, identifying HIV infection with being gay or as a rite of passage, guilt about personal survival when others have died of the disease, a desire to be metaphorically "impregnated," and attempts to get attention due to illness (Ridge et al., 2003). Additional reasons for failing to use condoms include perceptions of their ineffectiveness in preventing HIV infection and associations with erectile dysfunction (Webster et al., 2005).

Unprotected receptive anal intercourse in the previous 6 months was reported by 48% of MSM in a study conducted in six U.S. cities, and 55% reported unprotected insertive anal intercourse (Koblin et al., 2003). Some MSM also engage in oral-anal sexual encounters that put them at increased risk of hepatitis A infection (Allard et al., 2001) and transmission of syphilis, particularly during the secondary stage of the disease. Oral lesions also increase the potential for HIV transmission (Division of STD Prevention, 2004b). In fact, MSM accounted for 40% of all cases of primary and secondary syphilis diagnosed in 2002, and diagnosis was strongly associated with HIV coinfection (Division of STD Prevention, 2003). From 1999 to 2002, MSM accounted for 60% of new diagnoses of HIV infection (Division of HIV/AIDS Prevention, 2003b). Hepatitis C, on the other hand, has not been shown to be transmitted by sexual activity among MSM except in the context of intravenous drug use (Alary et al., 2005).

Sexual motivation, quality of relationships, disclosure of sexual orientation and HIV status, and sex trading are some of the factors that influence UAI among MSM. Craft and associates (2005) found four types of needs that were satisfied by sexual encounters among MSM. Pleasure-focused motivations reflected perceptions of sexual intimacy as meeting personal physical, emotional, and sexual needs. Partner-focused motivations reflected sexual activity to meet the needs of the partner. MSM motivated by substitution needs used sexual intimacy to meet other personal needs, such as relief of depression, and so on. Sexual activity based on relationship needs was motivated by attempts to strengthen relationships with the sexual partner. MSM motivated by pleasure-focused and substitution needs were more likely than other MSM to engage in casual sexual interactions. Those motivated by relationship-focused needs were more likely to have a steady partner.

Relationships with steady or casual partners have also been shown to influence UAI, although the direction of influence is not consistent. In some studies, UAI is more likely to occur with steady than casual partners. For example, in Craft et al.'s (2005) study, 70% of UAI occurred among steady partners. In another study, 29% of those in steady partnerships with someone whose HIV status was negative or unknown engaged in UAI (Denning & Campsmith, 2005), and 25% of men with nonsteady partners who reported insertive anal intercourse engaged in UAI (Division of HIV/AIDS Prevention, 2004).

Many MSM do not disclose their sexual orientation and may self-identify as heterosexual. **Disclosure** is the term used to describe the explicit revealing of one's sexual orientation to others. Nondisclosure is prevalent among MSM who self-identify as heterosexual (Denning & Campsmith, 2005). These men are at particular risk for HIV infection (Division of HIV/AIDS Prevention, 2003a). Other gay, bisexual, and transgender men may

choose to disclose their sexual orientation to certain people and not to others. MSM may also fail to disclose HIV status. MSM with steady partners are more likely to disclose their HIV status to their "main partner." For example, only 19% of MSM in one study had not disclosed HIV status to their regular partner, but 43% failed to disclose their status to casual partners. HIV-positive MSM have been found to be more likely to disclose their status if the partner is known to also be HIV-positive and least likely to disclose if the partner's HIV status is unknown, possibly for fear of rejection (Poppen, Reisen, Zea, Bianchi, & Echeverry, 2005). Disclosure of HIV status influences condom use, with condoms more likely to be used when partners are "seroconcordant," either both positive or both negative.

Sex trading, or engaging in sexual activity in return for money, drugs, shelter, or food, also occurs among MSM, particularly those who do not self-identify as gay. In one study, sex trading occurred among 62.5% of MSM, and MSM who engaged in sex trading were more likely than other MSM to engage in unprotected sexual activity. Sex trading places the individual MSM at risk for STDs as well as endangering his non-sex-trade male and female sexual partners. Sex trading was associated with crack cocaine and injection drug use, childhood abuse, and homelessness (Newman, Rhodes, & Weiss, 2004). A higher percentage of transgender men than other MSM may engage in sex trading to pay for sexual reassignment surgery. Because transgender prostitutes are stigmatized by both heterosexual and gay and lesbian prostitutes, they are often forced to take the least desirable customers who are least likely to agree to condom use. In addition, transgender individuals may resort to self-injecting hormones and engage in needle sharing, which increases their risk of HIV infection and hepatitis B (Sember, 2000).

Health System Considerations

The final category to be addressed in the epidemiology of gay, bisexual, and transgender men's health is the health system dimension. Gay, bisexual, and transgender men may encounter homophobia and heterosexism among health care workers and care delivery systems. In addition, the perception of homophobia represents a significant barrier to health care. For example, gay men and lesbians have been found to be somewhat more likely to perceive that heterosexual individuals are made more uncomfortable by them than is actually the case (Casper & Bianchi, 2002).

Despite possible exaggerations of perceptions of discrimination, however, gay, bisexual, and transgender men are subjected to discrimination in some health care settings (Perkins, 2004). In a survey of members of the Gay and Lesbian Medical Association, 67% indicated seeing gay and lesbian clients receive substandard care based on their sexual orientation (White, Bradford, Silenzio, & Wolfe, 2000). In another study, 3.1% of gay and bisexual men reported being denied care or given inferior care (Mays & Cochran, 2001). Even when the health care provider, whether an individual or an institution, is devoid of homophobia, various circumstances may threaten the gay client and act as health barriers. For example, assessment questions about birth control practices, if answered truthfully, might have the effect of requiring that a client disclose his sexual identity. For the client who fears loss of health care benefits (due to assumed higher risk of AIDS for all gay men), this is a situation to be avoided. Confidentiality issues may also prevent gay and bisexual men at risk for HIV infection from being tested. An estimated half of gay men in the United Kingdom do not disclose their sexual orientation to their primary providers, and one third of them would be unhappy for their providers to have this information. Reasons given for nondisclosure include perceptions that the information is not relevant, fear of stigma or discrimination, and fear of release of information to insurance companies and others (Durham, 2004).

Another problem in the current health care system is the lack of providers who are knowledgeable regarding the health care needs of gay, bisexual, and transgender clients. This lack exists among providers of mental health and other services as well. Inability to communicate effectively with gay, bisexual, and transgender clients may lead to inaccurate diagnoses and inappropriate treatment plans as well as impaired compliance with health-related recommendations (White, Bradford, & Silenzio, 2000). In some reports as many as 50% of gay men and lesbians who seek counseling report dissatisfaction with the services received (Savage et al., 2005). Effective health care services for gay, bisexual, and transgender men display the same characteristics as those for lesbian women presented in Chapter 17∞.

The effects of the health care system on transgender men in the United States may be even more profound than for gay and bisexual men. Sexual reassignment surgery is covered under national health insurance in the Netherlands, Great Britain, and Australia. In the United States, requests for coverage under Medicaid are addressed on an individual basis and are frequently not decided in favor of the client. Availability of surgery is often dependent on the individual client's ability to pay for services out of pocket. The long-term effects of surgery have not been adequately studied, although immediate responses to surgery have been almost uniformly favorable. Hormone therapy does, however, have some adverse side effects, including a twentyfold increase in thromboembolism for men receiving estrogen, some reports of breast cancer, liver disease, increased risk for heart disease, increased blood pressure, sterility, mood changes, and a decreased sex drive, among others. For women receiving testosterone, side effects may include increased cholesterol and lipid levels, heart disease, mood changes, male pattern baldness, acne, and cessation of menses (Sember, 2000).

ASSESSING THE HEALTH OF THE MALE POPULATION

The first requisite for effectively meeting the health needs of men is an accurate assessment of their health status and health needs. Here we will focus on assessing the health of men as a segment of the population. A tool that can be adapted for use in assessing the health status and needs of individual male clients is included in Appendix I on the Companion Website. A tool specifically designed to assess men's health is included in the *Community Assessment Reference Guide* designed as a companion volume to this text 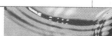.

In conducting an assessment of this population, the community health nurse would gather data related to factors in each of the six dimensions of health discussed earlier. Information related to the biophysical dimension would be primarily derived from local morbidity and mortality data. Mortality data and a great deal of morbidity information will be available from the local health department. Other morbidity data (e.g., the extent of hospitalizations for specific conditions such as diabetes, cardiovascular disease, or asthma among men) may be available from local hospitals. Other health care agencies (e.g., clinics, disease registries, or voluntary organizations) may also have relevant morbidity and mortality data for male clients. For example, local emergency departments may be able to provide statistics on accidental injuries among men. Similarly, local police departments may have data on accident-related calls and the injuries suffered. For other conditions, such as erectile dysfunction and immunization levels among men, there are often no statistical data available and information may be best obtained by means of community surveys. Community surveys or rehabilitation service data might address the extent of activity limitation in the male population. The focused assessment provided below can assist the community health nurse in determining biophysical factors that influence the health of the male population.

With respect to psychological dimension factors, local psychiatric units should be able to provide

FOCUSED ASSESSMENT

Biophysical Considerations in Assessing Men's Health

- What is the age composition of the male population?
- What is the racial/ethnic composition of the male population?
- What are the main causes of mortality in the male population?
- What acute and chronic illnesses are prevalent in the male population? What factors contribute to the prevalence of these conditions?
- What is the prevalence of sexual dysfunction in the male population?
- What is the level of immunity to specific communicable diseases among the male population?

information regarding hospitalizations for mental health problems. Again, police departments may have figures on arrests made for aberrant behavior, or clients taken to psychiatric facilities. Psychiatric service providers can also be interviewed to get an estimate of the numbers of men who seek care for mental health issues such as depression and PTSD. Data on the extent of suicide among men will be available from local mortality figures. Community surveys may be used to gain information regarding the levels of stress experienced by the male population, coping strategies used, and their effectiveness. Cultural immersion or interviews with persons knowledgeable regarding local cultures are effective means for determining male gender socialization and its effects on health status and health-related behaviors. Questions to guide the assessment of psychological factors affecting the health of men in the population are included in the focused assessment provided below.

General information related to the physical environment and its effects on the health of men would be similar to that gathered for a comprehensive community assessment as discussed in Chapter 15∞. In addition, the nurse would obtain information regarding occupational and recreational exposures to hazardous conditions. The local Chamber of Commerce or Business Association will probably have data on the types of business and industry present in the community. The telephone book may be a good source of information on recreational opportunities available to men in the community. In addition, direct observation by means of a "windshield survey" could provide information related to physical environmental conditions and their effects on men's health. Police departments may also have data on dangerous intersections or other road hazards that contribute to motor vehicle accidents. Assessment questions related to physical environmental factors influencing men's health are provided above right.

Community health nurses assessing the health of the male population would also obtain information

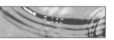

FOCUSED ASSESSMENT

Psychological Considerations in Assessing Men's Health

- What are the sources of stress to which men in the population are exposed?
- What are the incidence and prevalence of mental illness in the male population? What specific mental health problems are prevalent in the population?
- What is the rate of suicide in the male population?
- How are men socialized in the population? Does socialization contribute to health problems among men? How does male socialization affect coping abilities?
- What is the extent of nonheterosexual orientation in the population? How does this affect the level of stress experienced by men in the population?

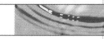

FOCUSED ASSESSMENT

Physical Environmental Considerations in Assessing Men's Health

- To what environmental health hazards are men in the population exposed?
- What environmental hazards are posed by occupational settings? By recreational pursuits among men?
- To what extent does the physical environment promote or impede healthy behaviors by men (e.g., physical activity)?

related to sociocultural dimension factors. Much of this data will be available from community census figures. For example, information regarding income, employment, educational levels, and single parenthood among men in the population is available through the census. Local government may also have figures on the extent of homelessness among men in the community. Interviews with local informants will provide information on typical family roles played by men and their gender socialization to these roles. Local authorities will also have some information on the extent to which men are perpetrators or victims of violence. General employment and unemployment figures are available from census data,

FOCUSED ASSESSMENT

Sociocultural Considerations in Assessing Men's Health

- What are the social roles expected of men? What effects do these role expectations have on men's health?
- What opportunities for social interaction are available to men in the population? How do men in the population typically interact with others?
- To what extent are men perpetrators or victims of violence? What are the health effects of exposure to violence?
- What is the extent of social support available to men in the population?
- What is the percentage of single-parent families headed by men in the population?
- What is the typical educational level of men in the population?
- What is the economic status of men in the population? What is the average income of men in the population?
- What effects do economic, educational, and employment levels have on men's health?
- What transportation opportunities are available to men in the population?
- To what extent do men in the population function as caretakers for other family members? To what extent do these men experience caretaker burden?
- What percentage of men in the population is employed? What are the typical occupations for men in the population? What effects do occupation and employment setting have on men's health? What support do employers provide for men's other roles and responsibilities?
- What childcare services are available to working single male parents? What is the cost of these services?

and current levels of employment can be obtained from local employment offices. Information on the types of employment available in the community can be obtained from local newspapers as well as the Chamber of Commerce or Business Association discussed earlier. Information on marriage and divorce among the male population is available from vital statistics collected by local government agencies. The focused assessment provided on page 482 includes questions for assessing the effects of sociocultural dimension factors on the health of the male population.

Most information regarding consumption patterns, exercise and leisure, sexual activity, and other behavioral dimension factors that influence health will be obtained primarily from community surveys. In some instances, indirect measures of behavior are available. For example, information regarding sales of tobacco and alcohol or arrests for illicit drug use would give some idea of the extent of these behaviors. Similarly, the prevalence of STDs in the population would suggest lack of condom use. Some information related to exercise and leisure activities can be obtained from observation or from interviews with owners of businesses that support these activities. For example, the nurse can observe the number of men who walk or jog in the park in the evening or speak with proprietors of exercise facilities regarding the extent of their use by men in the community. Assessment of behavioral considerations in men's health can be guided by the focused assessment questions included below.

Finally, the community health nurse would assess factors related to the health system dimension such as the extent to which men in the population use available health services. Such data can be obtained from the providers of health care services or from insurers who pay for them. In addition, the nurse would obtain information on the extent of health insurance coverage in the male population. In part, this information can be extrapolated from unemployment figures since the unemployed are unlikely to have health insurance. Local agencies may also have information regarding the extent of health insurance in the population. For example, a

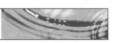

FOCUSED ASSESSMENT

Behavioral Considerations in Assessing Men's Health

- What are the dietary consumption patterns typical of men in the population?
- What is the prevalence of smoking among men in the population?
- What is the extent of alcohol and other drug use in the population?
- To what extent do men in the population engage in safety practices (e.g., seat belt use)?
- To what extent do men who are sexually active engage in safe sexual practices?
- To what extent do men engage in health screening practices such as testicular self-exam?

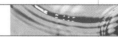

FOCUSED ASSESSMENT

Health System Considerations in Assessing Men's Health

- What percentage of the male population has a regular source of health care?
- What are the attitudes of men to health and health care services? How do they define health and illness?
- What percentage of the male population has health insurance coverage?
- What health services are available to men in the population? Are health care services needed by men available to all segments of the population?
- What barriers to obtaining health care do men encounter?
- What are the attitudes of health care providers to care of men? To care of nonheterosexual men? How do these attitudes affect health care utilization by men?

local hospital would have data on the number of male clients served who did not have health insurance coverage. Similarly, local businesses could provide data on the number of employees who receive employment-based health insurance benefits. Information on health insurance status can also be obtained through community surveys.

Similar types of information related to factors in each dimension of health would be obtained with respect to the gay, bisexual, and transgender population. Unfortunately, information may be more difficult to obtain for this population than for the general population of men, but a few data sources may exist. For example, mortality data for suicide may provide some indication of the number of suicidal men who were members of the gay, bisexual, or transgender community. For the most part, however, community surveys, interviews, and observation will be the most profitable means of obtaining information for these subgroups of men. The focused assessment included above can assist the community health nurse in gathering data related to health system factors affecting the health of men in the population.

DIAGNOSTIC REASONING IN THE CARE OF MEN

Community health nurses use data from their assessment of the male population to identify health needs and determine appropriate nursing diagnoses. Nursing diagnoses may reflect positive or negative health states or increased risk for disease. A positive diagnosis might be "High prevalence of adequate physical activity due to presence of multiple low-cost opportunities for exercise." An example of a negative diagnosis might be "increased risk of sexually transmitted diseases among young adult men due to unprotected sexual activity." Based on the diagnoses derived from the assessment of men's health status and health needs, the community health nurse would collaborate with other segments of the community to plan, implement, and evaluate health care delivery programs to meet the needs of this population.

PLANNING AND IMPLEMENTING HEALTH CARE FOR MEN

Interventions to improve the health status of men in the population may occur at primary, secondary, or tertiary levels of prevention. The level of prevention chosen for community health nursing interventions depends on the status of health problems to be addressed.

Primary Prevention

Although it is difficult to generalize about male clients' attitudes toward health promotion activities, there are some commonly encountered patterns of health behavior among men. One such behavior is a tendency to view exercise as sufficient to compensate for unhealthy behaviors such as a high intake of fats in the diet. Men also tend to attribute greater significance to health changes they can sense than to those they cannot (e.g., they can sense pain but not elevated blood pressure). Because men tend to rate their health as very good or excellent more often than women, they may feel they do not need to be actively involved in health promotion activities. They may also err in their health appraisal efforts, stemming from a tendency to believe that their past athletic or current work activities may provide for their present health needs ("When I was a teenager I would run all day." "I work hard all day in the fresh air. What could be healthier than that?"). Community health nurses may need to advocate among men for changing attitudes to health and health-related behaviors through health education initiatives and reframing approaches.

Reframing, which focuses on helping men to see the same situation in a different light, is one technique that can be used to promote positive behavioral change. A second technique for promoting change involves emphasizing alternate ways of coping with anxiety or fearfulness. Education, of course, is a crucial aspect of any primary prevention strategy. Education is perhaps most effective when teaching is initiated with school-age male youngsters, as this is the stage when lifelong health values and habits are forming. Health promotion by family members is known to be a significant motivator and predictor of client compliance and outcomes, and involvement of family members in educational efforts and treatment planning is usually of significant benefit.

General approaches to promoting health among men are included in the HEALTH program, a six-point program intended to facilitate creation of health care services that better meet the health promotion needs of men. HEALTH is an acronym that stands for **H**umanize, **E**ducate, **A**ssume, **L**ocate, **T**ailor, and **H**ighlight. Health services for men should humanize the experience of illness by emphasizing the normality of experiencing and

acknowledging pain, weakness, fear, and similar emotions to defuse the "macho" gender socialization to which men are subjected. Community health nurses can advocate for realistic health-related messages that emphasize the normality of these experiences and assist men to see them in the light of catalysts for health-related behaviors. Community health nurses working with men should educate them regarding the need for screening, primary prevention, and risk reduction. It may also be helpful in working with men to assume the worst and to overexaggerate risks to make the point of the need for change in health-related behaviors. Community health nurses and other health care providers should also locate support for men's health through follow-up telephone calls and return visits for health promotion purposes after acute care needs have been met. Health care services for men should also be tailored to their specific needs with input from those involved. Community health nurses, in particular, are in a position to advocate for the inclusion of men in planning health services relevant to their needs. For example, a community health nurse might identify men who are single parents and encourage them to be involved in the development of support services for men who are parenting alone. Finally, effective health care services for men highlight strengths and lay out the costs and benefits of health-promoting behaviors such as smoking cessation, hypertension control, and so on, in terms that are relevant to men (Monts & Smith, 2002). Community health nurses can help to draft health-related messages in language that is meaningful to men, addressing consequences and benefits in meaningful terms. For example, a community health nurse might approach the need for health promotion and illness prevention among men in terms of their continued ability to work or support their families, both elements of male gender socialization.

Primary prevention for health concerns specific to men focuses on increasing their use of health-promoting behaviors in the areas of chronic disease prevention, coping, immunization, safety practices, and elimination of high-risk behaviors. Chronic diseases in men can be prevented through adequate nutrition, physical activity, and weight control and elimination of behaviors such as smoking. Education for the prevention and control of other underlying diseases can also help to prevent chronic disease. For example, compliance with hypertension treatment can minimize the risk of developing cardiovascular disease. More information on primary prevention of chronic illnesses is provided in Chapter 29∞.

Environmental modification can also help to prevent chronic diseases and injuries. For example, community health nurses can be advocates for environments that promote physical activity among men and for the elimination of hazardous exposures in work and other settings that put men at risk for environmentally caused diseases.

Promoting coping strategies among men would focus primarily on moving men from a reliance on avoidant coping mechanisms to more confrontive types of coping. This may necessitate specific education for coping as early as grade school and continuing on throughout the educational process. Coping education can also be employed in settings where men experience considerable stress such as the workplace. Community health nurses can advocate for and develop coping skills training programs tailored to men in both school and work settings.

Immunizations for men should focus on prevention of diseases such as tetanus, hepatitis A and B, influenza, and pneumonia for those at highest risk of disease due to occupational exposure (e.g., working outdoors or around animals) or high-risk behaviors such as oral-anal intercourse or injection drug use. Gay, bisexual, and transgender men are at particular risk for hepatitis A in the context of oral-genital and oral-anal sexual encounters and should be immunized. Concerted immunization efforts in this population are particularly warranted in the event of outbreaks of hepatitis A (Allard et al., 2001). Men with chronic conditions, particularly chronic respiratory conditions, or who work with susceptible populations should routinely receive immunizations for influenza and pneumonia. Because most adult men are part of the workforce, community health nurses may need to advocate for immunization services at times and locations that fit busy schedules. In addition, they can advocate for workplace policies that promote immunization, particularly in settings where risk of infectious disease is high. For example, a community health nurse might promote development and enforcement of a policy mandating regular tetanus boosters among construction workers. The nurse working in this setting might also monitor immunization status among employees and provide tetanus immunizations as needed.

Health promotion related to safety issues for men would focus on both injury prevention and safe sexual practices. Because of men's socialization to accept personal risk and their tendency to engage in high-risk behaviors, injury prevention often depends on legislation and regulation. Community health nurses can advocate for the passage and enforcement of legislation related to use of seat belts and other protective devices. Community health nurses can also monitor and report occupational safety hazards that put men at risk for injury or toxic exposures. Legislative advocacy may also be required in this area. Groups of men can also be educated regarding the need for effective injury prevention and the possible long-term consequences of injury.

Education may also need to focus on safe sexual practices. The Alan Guttmacher Institute (2005a) has recommended an ABC approach for sexual health promotion for men: **A**bstinence, **B**eing faithful to one partner, and **C**ondom use. Specific services are needed for men's reproductive health needs as well as women's. For example, one hospital instituted a program for addressing the sexual needs of young men that resulted in 83% of young men participating reporting that they would be able to resist peer pressure for sexual activity and 94%

Think Advocacy

Howard, Davis, Evans-Ray, Mitchell, and Apomah (2004) described the establishment of a "teen-friendly" clinic for both male and female adolescents to meet the need for sexual clinical and education services for this age group. The clinic was established based on the evaluation of an educational program in which adolescent boys achieved gains in knowledge about and changes in attitudes toward sexual activity and indicated that they would use protection during sexual intercourse if available. Provision of such services is often resisted in many communities in the belief that it promotes sexual activity among adolescents. How would such a service be viewed in your community? Where might resistance to the program originate? How would you go about advocating for such a program?

reporting intentions to use STD protection during intercourse (Howard, Davis, Evans-Ray, Mitchell, & Apomah, 2004). Again, community health nursing advocacy may be required before such programs for men are developed.

The ABC approach would also be effective for promoting safe sexual activity among MSM. Additional preventive practices may also be warranted in this population. For example, the Division of Bacterial and Mycotic Diseases (2005) of the Centers for Disease Control and Prevention recommends that MSM who have diarrhea refrain from oral-genital or anal-genital activity, and that MSM wash their hands and genital areas with soap and water before and after sexual intercourse. Additional recommendations include the use of gloves during digital-anal contact, condoms for oral-genital or anal-genital sexual activity, and dental dams for oral-anal contact to prevent transmission of enteric pathogens. Programs to prevent UAI among men who have sex with men have yielded mixed results, however. In one study, for example, the prevalence of UAI among MSM exposed to an educational intervention decreased from 37% to 27%, whereas that for the control group increased. Unfortunately, although UAI reportedly decreased in the experimental group, 31% of the participants compared to only 21% of the controls developed at least one new STD during the study period (Imrie et al., 2001). The SOLAAR program discussed earlier has been somewhat more successful in promoting monogamous relationships and decreased risk of STD exposure in Latino MSM (Conner et al., 2005). Community health nurses can be actively involved in educating MSM for safer sexual practices and in advocating these practices in venues that reach MSM. For example, a community health nurse might advocate for a condom dispenser in a prominent location in a gay bar or convince gay publications to include articles advocating safer sexual practices. Nurses might even volunteer to write health-related articles for these publications.

Another approach to primary prevention in men is the elimination of high-risk behaviors. Elimination of high-risk sexual behaviors has already been addressed, but attention should also be given to smoking cessation and prevention or cessation of illicit drug use. Community health nurses can educate men about the need for smoking cessation and make referrals to smoking cessation services. They can also advocate for smoke-free workplace legislation to limit places where smoking is permitted or for coverage of smoking cessation assistance under health insurance plans. They can engage in similar interventions related to drug use, which is discussed in more detail in Chapter 31 ∞. Community health nurses may also need to advocate for the availability of such services and for their coverage under health insurance.

One additional primary preventive intervention for gay, bisexual, and transgender men is that of empowerment. There is a need for this population to "reconstruct their interpersonal and intrapersonal spheres to yield positive self-concepts and to diminish heterosexism" (Savage et al., 2005). Empowerment for this subset of men involves both psychological and community empowerment. Psychological empowerment occurs within the individual at three levels: intrapersonal, interactional, and behavioral. Intrapersonal empowerment entails constructing positive perceptions of self in the context of one's sexual orientation. Interactional empowerment reflects the individual's perceptions of the social environment, and behavioral empowerment involves action to influence one's social and political environments. Community empowerment occurs at the group level and entails efforts by the gay and lesbian community to address issues through political activity (Savage et al., 2005).

Community health nurses can work with individual gay, bisexual, and transgender men to promote psychological empowerment. They can also work at the societal level to promote community empowerment for this population. In part, they can accomplish community empowerment by working to eliminate heterosexism, particularly in health care settings, and by assisting groups of gay, bisexual, and transgender men to form coalitions with other marginalized groups and represent their position in a variety of social venues (Savage et al., 2005). Table 18-3◆ presents a summary of the major foci in primary prevention for men as well as examples of community health nursing interventions related to each focus.

Secondary Prevention

Secondary prevention involves the earliest possible detection of health needs through effective screening. It also encompasses the actual treatment of the health needs or disorders themselves.

Community health nurses may participate in health screening activities by providing or encouraging the client's use of such health measures as blood pressure screening and cardiovascular risk-assessment programs in public, educational, or occupational settings. Men are more likely than women to have multiple risk factors for heart disease and stroke (Division of Adult and Community Health, 2005b), and community health

TABLE 18-3	Primary Prevention Foci and Sample Interventions in the Care of Men
Focus	**Sample Interventions**
Reframing	• Creating health care systems tailored to address men's needs and health-related perceptions
Preventing chronic illnesses	• Promoting healthy diet • Promoting physical activity • Advocating for environmental modifications to promote health • Referring for treatment of underlying conditions that contribute to chronic illness (e.g., hypertension) • Advocating for available and accessible health preventive services
Enhancing coping	• Teaching confrontive coping strategies
Providing immunization	• Educating men on the need for immunizations • Providing immunization services • Advocating for availability and insurance coverage of adult immunization services
Promoting safety	• Educating men regarding the need to use safety devices • Educating men regarding safe sexual practices • Monitoring and eliminating environmental safety hazards • Advocating for safety legislation
Eliminating risk behaviors	• Educating men regarding smoking and drug use • Referring men for smoking and drug use cessation programs • Advocating for insurance coverage for smoking and drug use cessation services
Advocating empowerment	• Promoting personal psychological empowerment at all levels • Assisting the gay, bisexual, and transgender community with community empowerment activities

nurses can design, implement, and promote participation in risk assessments for the male population. Blood cholesterol screening is one example of such services. In 2003, nearly three fourths of U.S. men (71.8%) had received blood cholesterol screening services in the previous 5 years, slightly less than among women (74.4%). At that time, only two states had achieved the *Healthy People 2010*◆ objective of cholesterol screening in 80% of the U.S. adult population (Division for Heart Disease and Stroke Prevention, 2005). Men with elevated cholesterol levels, however, are twice as likely as women to have them controlled (Division of Adult and Community Health, 2005a).

Nurses can also facilitate the offering and use of screening examinations by other health care professionals within the community, such as rectal examinations and blood testing for prostate cancer and chest x-rays for lung cancer. Early detection of testicular cancer is an important area for secondary prevention by community health nurses.

One intervention that facilitates detection of testicular cancer is teaching the testicular self-examination

(TSE) technique. In one study, as many as 64% of men rarely or never engaged in TSE (Wynd, 2002). Because testicular cancer occurs primarily in young men, the community health nurse can often educate and motivate clients efficiently (and minimize individual embarrassment in the process) by working with groups of males in school or work settings.

Prostate cancer screening can employ a digital rectal examination or testing for prostate-specific antigen (PSA), although both are limited in their effectiveness in identifying disease. Because prostate cancer may not have adverse effects in many men, widespread screening programs are controversial. It is also unknown whether or not treatment increases survival rates, since the prognosis for 5-year survival is high even without treatment. In addition, treatment of prostate cancer may have a variety of adverse effects, including erectile dysfunction, urinary incontinence, depression, and hot flashes. The suggested approach to determining the need for screening and treatment for prostate cancer includes informing the client regarding the consequences of the disease and the potential benefits and disadvantages of available screening and treatment options, dealing with questions and concerns, discussing rationale for different choices, and coming to a joint decision with the client regarding the advisability of screening and/or treatment (Pinkelman, 2002b).

Routine screening procedures for men include tobacco use and alcohol misuse, colorectal cancer, hypertension, lipid disorders, and obesity. Other screening tests are recommended for men at particular risk for certain conditions. Recommendations of the U.S. Preventive Services Task Force (2005) for screening in men are presented in Table 18-4◆. Community health nurses may need to advocate for access to routine screening services, particularly among low-income men and those without health insurance.

Community health nurses may refer men with existing health problems for medical evaluation and treatment. They may also participate in the treatment of illnesses experienced by male clients. In the case of ischemic and certain other cardiac disorders, for example, stress has been shown to impact negatively on treatment outcomes, in some cases leading to a threefold increase in mortality (e.g., in post–myocardial infarction clients). Treatment programs that identify high-stress clients during hospitalization, that track and reduce their stress levels after discharge, and that provide prompt assistance from nurses in the community when episodes of increased stress occur can result in significant reduction of the stress-related mortality experienced by post–myocardial infarction clients. Again, advocacy may be required to assure access to diagnostic and treatment services for men. For example, a community health nurse might assist in the development of stress reduction programs in the workplace or in the development of coping skills training programs in school and work settings.

TABLE 18-4	Routine Screening Recommendations for Men
Type of Screening	**Recommendation**
Alcohol misuse	All adult men
Colorectal cancer	Men over 50 years of age (fecal occult blood &/or sigmoidoscopy); no evidence of effectiveness of screening colonoscopy
Depression	Adult men in practice settings where follow-up is available
Diabetes	Adult men with hypertension or hyperlipidemia
Hypertension	All men 18 years of age and older
HIV infection	All men at risk of infection
Lipid disorders (total cholesterol and HDL-C)	All men over 35 years of age; men under 35 years of age with risk factors
Obesity	All adult men
Syphilis	All men at risk
Tobacco use	All adult men

Data from: U.S. Preventive Services Task Force. (2005). The guide to clinical preventive services, 2005. Retrieved August 13, 2005, from http://www.ahrq.gov/clinic/pocketgd.pdf

A special treatment issue for transgender men involves counseling regarding their options. Not all transgender men (or women) are happy with the results of sexual reassignment surgery (SRS), and clients should be assisted to examine the benefits of treatment options. These options include hormone therapy, surgical intervention, and assistance with legal, emotional, and financial issues. There is also a need for social advocacy to promote options other than SRS as legitimate grounds for changing one's gender legally (Fee, Brown, & Laylor, 2003).

Tertiary Prevention

Tertiary prevention for men is directed at those disorders that influence men's health in some ongoing manner or that have a likelihood of recurrence. The goals of tertiary prevention are to assist men in coping with the continuing manifestations of illness and to reduce the likelihood of future episodes of an illness. To this end, it is useful to group tertiary prevention measures into care directed toward those disorders that affect men's sexual functioning or sexual identity or as they present a threat to notions about male strength. Tertiary prevention measures also would be directed at supporting compliance with long-term therapy.

One area for tertiary prevention measures by the community health nurse involves those disorders that affect the male client's sexual functioning or sexual identity, such as testicular cancer and erectile dysfunction. Male clients with testicular cancer may face significant emotional distress owing to the effects of treatment on their sexuality. Treatment for testicular cancer is surgical removal of the affected testes followed by hormonal therapy. These treatments, along with their side effects

MediaLink Case Study: Promoting Men's Health

Advocacy in Action

A Hypertensive Emergency

Every once in a while, a community health nurse finds him- or herself advocating for something with a client rather than on the client's behalf. This is what occurred when community health nurses working in an information and referral center encountered a client with a soaring blood pressure. The client, an African American gentleman in his late forties to early fifties, had a blood pressure of 210/170. This was his first visit to the nursing center, so the nurses had no previous blood pressure readings for him. He did not have a history of hypertension and was symptom free.

After allowing him to rest, we took several more blood pressure readings. They remained extremely high, and the nurses strongly suggested that he go immediately to the emergency department. Because the client did not feel ill and did not have health insurance or a regular provider, he was extremely reluctant to do so. The nurses finally talked him into going to the ED. Once there, he was admitted, and an emergency angioplasty was performed. When he subsequently returned to the center, his blood pressure had approximated normal levels, and he was recovering well from the angioplasty.

(loss of fertility, emasculation), can have a profound impact on the client's self-image and psychosocial functioning (Gurevich et al., 2003). Community health nurses may need to advocate for development of and access to services dealing with sexual dysfunction. They may also be instrumental in changing men's attitudes to sexual dysfunction and their willingness to seek help.

An important area of tertiary prevention in this regard involves encouraging men to join support groups. Interaction with other men who have experienced the same problems can be very effective in facilitating adjustment to treatments that so tangibly affect men's sense of masculinity. On a one-to-one basis, the nurse can be accepting, supportive, and facilitative of the male client's expression of his feeling of loss. Community health nurses may also be instrumental in initiating supportive groups for these men or in advocating their availability in the community.

Some disorders may affect men's sense of strength; this is particularly true of cardiovascular disorders. The heart is a symbol of masculine strength for some men. Consequently, cardiovascular disorders not only can leave residual symptoms and physiological impairment, but can also threaten a man's self-image. Men with cardiovascular disease often benefit from interventions that support their self-image as masculine and from discussing their feelings about their illness. As noted elsewhere, stress management training also can have a significant positive effect on outcomes for men who have cardiovascular disease. These interventions are essential to promote adjustment and compliance with treatment.

Of course, community health nurses should also support and reinforce men's positive responses to cardiac rehabilitation efforts initiated in other treatment settings. Foremost among these would be weight control, limited intake of saturated fats, regular exercise, compliance with follow-up examinations and medications, and control of other disorders that exacerbate cardiovascular disease (hypertension, diabetes).

In the case of some chronic disorders, especially those producing no overt symptoms, men tend to be lax about complying with long-term treatment recommendations. This is especially true for male clients with hypertension. Interventions that help men understand the importance of controlling this disorder and that build on their perceptions of masculinity are very helpful. Maintaining a regimen of antihypertensive medications may be especially difficult for men when side effects interfere with necessary masculine roles. Examples of such side effects could include impotence, dizziness, and decreased tolerance for physical activity. Nurses can assist the men by teaching ways to compensate for these side effects, thereby helping them to maintain a sense of control over circumstances. In cases in which the side effects are not manageable and are affecting clients' masculinity (impotence), collaborating with the client's physician or assisting the client to discuss the problem with the physician can lead to acceptance of the treatment for hypertension.

Preventing recidivism, or rehospitalization, in instances of substance abuse is a major tertiary intervention in working with men. Interventions that decrease the likelihood of recidivism include encouraging the use of therapeutic support groups (Alcoholics Anonymous) and education regarding factors that predispose one to continued substance abuse (poor coping skills, co-dependent relationships, maintaining social contacts with abusers). It is also important for the community health nurse to consider the client's family and significant others when caring for substance-abusing men. Families and significant others can be either enablers of substance abuse or corrective forces leading to its elimination. Education of family and support persons regarding behaviors that produce improvement and those that permit further substance abuse is essential, and referrals to family treatment and support services are also of value.

Two special considerations in tertiary prevention for men include assisting transgender men to adjust to the effects of sexual reassignment surgery and use of the Internet for disease self-management information. SRS may result in loss of sexual feeling and appetite. In addition, the continuation of male facial features may make male-to-female transgender persons less satisfied with the outcome of surgery than might otherwise be expected. Facial feminization surgery is possible, but usually at an additional cost of up to $30,000 (Fee et al., 2003). In addition, community health nurses must help monitor transgender individuals for effects related to hormone therapy such as increased risk of heart disease, stroke, and breast cancer.

The Internet may be a particularly valuable tool for educating men regarding tertiary prevention and self-management of chronic illnesses as well as for motivating primary prevention activities by men (Division of STD Prevention, 2003). More and more, the U.S. population is turning to the Internet as a source of information. Community health nurses can help to create Web sites to provide such information as well as monitor existing sites for their accuracy and credibility.

EVALUATING HEALTH CARE FOR MEN

As in working with other population groups, community health nursing plans and interventions are evaluated by determining the degree to which population health goals have been met. It is also important to determine whether interventions were efficient. Could the same results have been accomplished with less expense of time or other resources?

The effects of interventions for men at the aggregate level can be assessed in terms of the accomplishment of national health objectives. The current status of selected objectives related to men's health is presented below. Information about objectives related to men's health is available on the *Healthy People 2010*◆ Web site at http://wonder.cdc.gov/data 2010. As we can see in the table, many of the objectives are actually moving away from their 2010 targets, and only three objectives have actually been met. Even for most of the objectives that are actually progressing toward the established targets, progress is so slight as to suggest that target goals will not be met by 2010 without additional concerted efforts.

Men have a variety of health care needs that they may or may not acknowledge. Community health nurses can be actively involved in encouraging men to seek health care as needed. They may also provide direct services to male clients, particularly with respect to education for primary prevention. In addition, community health nurses may be involved in advocacy activities to assure the availability and accessibility of needed services to improve men's health status.

HEALTHY PEOPLE 2010

Goals for Population Health◆

OBJECTIVE	BASELINE	MOST RECENT DATA	TARGET
1-1. Increase the proportion of men with health insurance	81%	82%	100%
1-4. Increase the proportion of men with a source of ongoing care	84%	85%	96%
2-3. Reduce the proportion of men with chronic joint symptoms	1.6%	ND	1.2%
2-11. Reduce activity limitation due to chronic back pain (per 1,000 men)	31	29	25
3-1. Reduce cancer deaths (per 100,000 men)	251.9	238.9	159.9
3-2. Reduce lung cancer deaths (per 100,000 men)	76.9	73.2	44.9
3-7. Reduce prostate cancer deaths (per 100,000 men)	33.3	27.9	28.8*
3-8. Reduce melanoma cancer deaths (per 100,000 men)	2.6	2.6	2.5
5-2. Prevent new cases of diabetes (per 1,000 men)	5.5	6.7	2.5#
5-5. Reduce the diabetes death rate (per 100,000 men)	89	91	45#
12-1. Reduce coronary heart disease deaths (per 100,000 men)	260	180	166
12-7. Reduce stroke deaths (per 100,000 men)	63	57	48
12-9. Reduce the proportion of men with high blood pressure	30%	ND	16%
12-14. Reduce the proportion of men with high blood cholesterol levels	19%	ND	17%
12-15. Increase the proportion of men who have had their blood cholesterol checked in the last 5 years	64%	ND	80%
13-2. Reduce the number of AIDS cases among MSM	17,847	15,917	13,385
14-3f. Reduce the number of cases of hepatitis B in MSM	7,135	8,063	1,808#
14-6. Reduce new cases of hepatitis A (per 100,000 men)	12.7	3.7	4.5*
14-28b. Increase hepatitis B vaccine coverage among MSM	9%	ND	60%

Continued on next page

HEALTHY PEOPLE 2010 *continued*

15-2. Reduce hospitalization for nonfatal spinal cord injuries (per 100,000 men)	7.6	5.4	2.4
15-3. Reduce firearm-related deaths (per 100,000 men)	18.4	18.6	4.1#
15-12. Reduce emergency department visits due to injury (per 1,000 men)	146	154	126#
15-13. Reduce unintentional injury deaths (per 100,000 men)	49.8	51.5	17.5#
15-15. Reduce motor vehicle accident deaths (per 100,000 men)	20.4	21.3	0.2#
15-32. Reduce homicides (per 100,000 men)	9.1	9.4	3.0#
15-34. Reduce physical assault by intimate partners (per 100,000 men)	1.3	0.08	3.3*
15-37. Reduce physical assaults (per 1,000 men)	37.4	23.9	13.6
18-1. Reduce suicide deaths (per 100,000 men)	17.4	18.4	5#
19-2. Reduce the proportion of men who are obese	20%	28%	15%#
20-1. Reduce occupational injury deaths (per 100,000 men)	7.7	6.9	3.2
22-1. Reduce the proportion of men who engage in no leisure-time physical activity	36%	35%	20%
25-2. Reduce new cases of gonorrhea (per 100,000 men)	125	124	19
25-3. Reduce cases of primary and secondary syphilis	3.6	3.8	0.2#
26-1. Reduce deaths and injuries due to alcohol and drug-related motor vehicle accidents (per 100,000 men)	9.2	ND	4.0
26-3. Reduce drug-induced deaths (per 100,000 men)	9.4	11.7	1.0#
27-1. Reduce tobacco use by men	26%	25%	12%
27-5. Increase smoking cessation attempts by men who smoke	39%	42%	75%

NDA—No data available

* Objective has been met

 # Objective moving away from target

Data from: Centers for Disease Control and Prevention. (2005). Healthy people data. Retrieved September 5, 2005, from http://wonder.cdc.gov/data2010

Case Study

Promoting Sexual Health in Men

There is a high rate of sexually transmitted diseases among men in the community where you are employed as a community health nurse. Particularly high incidence rates are noted for *Chlamydia trachomatis* and gonorrhea. Significant disparities are noted in incidence rates among Caucasian, African American, and Latino men, with incidence higher among young African American and Latino men than among Caucasians, although incidence among all three groups is high. STD incidence does not seem to be associated with sexual orientation since high rates are noted for both exclusively heterosexual men and those who have sex with other men.

1. How might you address the problem of STD incidence at the population level?
2. What additional information might you need to determine appropriate interventions for the problem?
3. What other segments of the community would you involve in developing your interventions?

Test Your Understanding

1. What are the major factors in the biophysical, psychological, physical environmental, sociocultural, behavioral, and health system dimensions influencing men's health? (pp. 465–474)

2. What are some of the factors that contribute to adverse health effects for gay, bisexual, and transgender men? (pp. 474–481)

3. Identify at least four areas for primary prevention with men. How might the community health nurse be involved in each? (pp. 484–486)

4. What are the major secondary prevention considerations for men? Give an example of at least one community health nursing intervention related to each consideration. (pp. 486–487)

5. Identify areas of emphasis in tertiary prevention for men. How might the community health nurse be involved in each? In what kinds of situations might tertiary prevention be required? (pp. 487–489)

EXPLORE MediaLink

http://www.prenhall.com/clark
Resources for this chapter can be found on the Companion Website.

Audio Glossary
Appendix I: Adult Health Assessment and
   Intervention Guide
Exam Review Questions

Case Study: Promoting Men's Health
MediaLink Application: Prostate Cancer (video)
Media Links
Challenge Your Knowledge

Update *Healthy People 2010*
Advocacy Interviews

References

Alam, S., Niederberger, C. S., & Meacham, R. B. (2004). Evaluation and treatment of male infertility. In R. S. Kirby, C. C. Carson, M. G. Kirby, & R. N. Farah (Eds.), *Men's health* (2nd ed., pp. 261–266). London: Taylor & Francis.

Alan Guttmacher Institute. (2002). *Sexual and reproductive health: Women and men*. Retrieved September 18, 2005, from http://www.guttmacher.org/pubs/fb_10-02.html

Alan Guttmacher Institute. (2004). *In their own right: Addressing the sexual and reproductive health of American men*. Retrieved September 18, 2005, from http://www.guttmacher.org/pubs/summaries/exs_men.html

Alan Guttmacher Institute. (2005a). *In their own right: Addressing the sexual and reproductive health of men worldwide*. Retrieved September 18, 2005, from http://www.guttmacher.org/pubs/summaries/exs_itorintl.pdf

Alan Guttmacher Institute. (2005b). *Sexual and reproductive health information and services for men dangerously lacking*. Retrieved September 18, 2005, from http://www.guttmacher.org/media/presskits/2005/03/15/index.html

Alary, M., Joly, J. R., Vincelette, J., Lavoie, R., Turmel, B., & Remis, R. S. (2005). Lack of evidence of sexual transmission of hepatitis C virus in a prospective cohort of men who have sex with men. *American Journal of Public Health, 95*, 502–505.

Allard, R., Beauchemin, J., Bedard, L., Dion, R., Tremblay, M., & Carsley, J. (2001). Hepatitis A vaccination during an outbreak among gay men in Montreal, Canada, 1995–1997. *Journal of Epidemiology and Community Health, 55*, 251–256.

Anderson, W. R., & Holmes, S. A. (2004). Genital piercing. In R. S. Kirby, C. C. Carson, M. G. Kirby, & R. N. Farah (Eds.), *Men's health* (2nd ed., pp. 407–414). London: Taylor & Francis.

Archambault, D. (2002). The health needs of homeless men. *Community Health Forum, 3*(5), 37–39.

Artazcoz, L., Benach, J., Borrell, C., & Cortes, I. (2004). Unemployment and mental health: Understanding the interactions among gender, family roles, and social class. *American Journal of Public Health, 94*, 82–88.

Banks, M. (2002). Richard Roundtree's road to recovery from male breast cancer. *Community Health Forum, 3*(5), 22–25.

Barret, R. L., & Robinson, B. E. (2000). *Gay fathers: Encouraging the hearts of gay dads and their families*. San Francisco: Jossey-Bass.

Boddiger, D. (2005). Methamphetamine use linked to rising HIV transmission. *The Lancet, 365*, 1217–1218.

Bufalini, M. (2002). Barriers to state coverage for single males. *Community Health Forum, 3*(5), 46–48.

Calandra, J. (2004). Transition—Not "male menopause"—The norm for middle-aged men. *Nurseweek, 17*(26), 27–28.

Campbell, I. W. (2004). Obesity and men's health. In R. S. Kirby, C. C. Carson, M. G. Kirby, & R. N. Farah (Eds.), *Men's health* (2nd ed., pp. 55–62). London: Taylor & Francis.

Carson, C. (2004). Erectile dysfunction: Diagnosis and treatment. In R. S. Kirby, C. C. Carson, M. G. Kirby, & R. N. Farah (Eds.), *Men's health* (2nd ed., pp. 343–357). London: Taylor & Francis.

Casper, L. M., & Bianchi, S. M. (2002). *Continuity and change in the American family*. Thousand Oaks, CA: Sage.

Centers for Disease Control and Prevention. (2004a). *Health, United States, 2004*. Retrieved August 9, 2005, from http://www.cdc.gov/nchs/data/hus/hus04.pdf

Centers for Disease Control and Prevention. (2004b). Indicators for chronic disease surveillance. *Morbidity and Mortality Weekly Report, 53*(RR-11), 1–114.

Centers for Disease Control and Prevention. (2005). *Healthy people data*. Retrieved September 6, 2005, from http://wonder.cdc.gov/data2010

Chua, D., & Bakris, G. (2004). Hypertension. In R. S. Kirby, C. C. Carson, M. G. Kirby, & R. N. Farah (Eds.), *Men's health* (2nd ed., pp. 89–100). London: Taylor & Francis.

Conner, R. F., Takahashi, L., Ortiz, E., Archuleta, E., Muniz, J., & Rodriguez, J. (2005). The SOLAAR HIV prevention program for gay and bisexual Latino men: Using social marketing to build capacity for service provision and evaluation. *AIDS Education and Prevention, 17*, 361–374.

Cooke, C. L. (2004). Joblessness and homelessness as precursors of health problems in formerly incarcerated African American men. *Journal of Nursing Scholarship, 36*, 155–160.

Craft, S. M., Smith, S. A., Serovich, J. M., & Bautista, D. T. (2005). Need fulfillment in the sexual relationships of HIV-infected men who have sex with men. *AIDS Education and Prevention, 17*, 217–226.

Culpepper, K. S., & McKee, P. H. (2004). Cutaneous melanoma. In R. S. Kirby, C. C. Carson, M. G. Kirby, & R. N. Farah (Eds.), *Men's health* (2nd ed., pp. 171–183). London: Taylor & Francis.

Curry, L. C., & Hogstel, M. O. (2002). Osteoporosis. *American Journal of Nursing, 102*(1), 26–31.

Dean, L., & Bradford, J. (2000). Violence and sexual assault. In Gay and Lesbian Medical Association & Center for Lesbian, Gay, Bisexual, and Transgender Health (Eds.), *Lesbian, gay, bisexual, and transgender health: Findings and concerns* (pp. 29–32). New York: Author.

Denning, P. H., & Campsmith, M. L. (2005). Unprotected anal intercourse among HIV-positive men who have a steady male sex partner with negative or unknown HIV serostatus. *American Journal of Public Health, 95*, 152–158.

Denton, M., Prus, S., & Walters, V. (2004). Gender differences in health: A Canadian study of the psychosocial, structural, and behavioral determinants of health. *Social Science & Medicine, 58*, 2585–2600.

Division for Heart Disease and Stroke Prevention. (2005). Trends in cholesterol screening and awareness of high blood cholesterol—United States, 1991–2003. *Morbidity and Mortality Weekly Report, 54*, 865–870.

Division of Adult and Community Health. (2005a). Disparities in screening for and awareness of high blood cholesterol—United States, 1999–2002. *Morbidity and Mortality Weekly Report, 54*, 117–119.

Division of Adult and Community Health. (2005b). Racial/ethnic and socioeconomic disparities in multiple risk factors for heart disease and stroke—United States, 2003. *Morbidity and Mortality Weekly Report, 54*, 113–117.

Division of Adult and Community Health. (2005c). Racial/ethnic disparities in the prevalence and impact of doctor-diagnosed arthritis—United States, 2002. *Morbidity and Mortality Weekly Report, 54*, 119–123.

Division of Bacterial and Mycotic Diseases. (2005). *Shigella flexneri* type 3 infections among men who have sex with men—Chicago, Illinois, 2003–2004. *Morbidity and Mortality Weekly Report, 54,* 820–822.

Division of Cancer Prevention and Control, National Center for Chronic Disease Prevention and Health Promotion. (2004). Cancer survivorship—United States, 1971–2001. *Morbidity and Mortality Weekly Report, 53,* 526, 528–529.

Division of HIV/AIDS Prevention—Intervention, Research, and Support. (2002). Unrecognized HIV infection, risk behaviors, and perceptions of risk among young black men who have sex with men—Six U.S. cities, 1994–1998. *Morbidity and Mortality Weekly Report, 51,* 734–736.

Division of HIV/AIDS Prevention, National Center for HIV, STD, and TB Prevention. (2003a). HIV/STD risks in young men who have sex with men who do not disclose their sexual orientation—Six U.S. cities, 1994–2000. *Morbidity and Mortality Weekly Report, 52,* 81–68.

Division of HIV/AIDS Prevention, National Center for HIV, STD, and TB Prevention. (2003b). Increases in HIV diagnoses—29 states, 1999–2002. *Morbidity and Mortality Weekly Report, 52,* 1145–1148.

Division of HIV/AIDS Prevention. (2004). High-risk sexual behavior by HIV-positive men who have sex with men—16 sites, United States, 2000–2002. *Morbidity and Mortality Weekly Report, 53,* 891–894.

Division of STD Prevention, National Center for HIV, STD, and TB Prevention. (2003). Internet use and early syphilis infection among men who have sex with men—San Francisco, California, 1999–2003. *Morbidity and Mortality Weekly Report, 52,* 1229–1232.

Division of STD Prevention, National Center for HIV, STD, and TB Prevention. (2004a). Lymphogranuloma venereum among men who have sex with men—Netherlands, 2003–2004. *Morbidity and Mortality Weekly Report, 53,* 985–987.

Division of STD Prevention, National Center for HIV, STD, and TB Prevention. (2004b). Transmission of primary and secondary syphilis by oral sex—Chicago, Illinois, 1998–2002. *Morbidity and Mortality Weekly Report, 53,* 966–968.

Donaldson, S. L. (2004). Inequalities and men's health. In R. S. Kirby, C. C. Carson, M. G. Kirby, & R. N. Farah (Eds.), *Men's health* (2nd ed., pp. 8–14). London: Taylor & Francis.

Durham, N. (2004, August 30). Over half of gay men not out to GPs. *General Practitioner,* 17–18.

Fee, E., Brown, T. M., & Laylor, J. (2003). One size does not fit all in the transgender community. *American Journal of Public Health, 93,* 899–900.

Gotsch, K. E., Annest, J. L., Mercy, J. A., & Ryan, G. W. (2001). Surveillance for fatal and nonfatal firearm-related injuries—United States, 1993–1998. *Morbidity and Mortality Weekly Report, 50*(SS-2), 1–34.

Greenwood, G. L., Paul, J. P., Pollack, L. M., Binson, D., Catania, J. A., Chang, J., et al. (2005). Tobacco use and cessation among a household-based sample of US urban men who have sex with men. *American Journal of Public Health, 95,* 145–151.

Greenwood, G. L., Relf, M. V., Huang, B., Pollack, L. M., Canchola, J. A., & Catania, J. A. (2002). Battering victimization among a probability-based sample of men who have sex with men. *American Journal of Public Health, 92,* 1964–1969.

Griffiths, S. (2004). Men as risk takers. In R. S. Kirby, C. C. Carson, M. G. Kirby, & R. N. Farah (Eds.), *Men's health* (2nd ed., pp. 243–250). London: Taylor & Francis.

Gurevich, M., Bishop, S., Bower, J., Malka, M., & Nyhof-Young, J. (2003). (Dis)embodying gender and sexuality in testicular cancer. *Social Science & Medicine, 58,* 1597–1607.

Hawke, M. (2002). Just like everyone else. *Nursing Spectrum, Western Edition, 3*(12), 20–21.

Heath, H. (2002). Opening doors: Working with older lesbians and gay men. *Nursing Standard, 16*(48), 18–19.

Hendry, W. F., & Christmas, T. J. (2004). Testicular cancer. In R. S. Kirby, C. C. Carson, M. G. Kirby, & R. N. Farah (Eds.), *Men's health* (2nd ed., pp. 359–366). London: Taylor & Francis.

Hicks, S. (2005). Is gay parenting bad for kids? Responding to the "very idea of difference" in research on lesbian and gay parents. *Sexualities, 8,* 153–168.

Hjelm, K. G., Bard, K., Nyberg, P., & Apelqvist, J. (2005). Beliefs about health and diabetes in men of different ethnic origin. *Journal of Advanced Nursing, 50,* 47–59.

Howard, M., Davis, J., Evans-Ray, D., Mitchell, M., & Apomah, M. (2004). Young men's sexual education and health services. *American Journal of Public Health, 94,* 1332–1335.

Huebner, D. M., Rebchook, G. M., & Kegeles, S. M. (2004). Experiences of harassment, discrimination, and physical violence among young gay and bisexual men. *American Journal of Public Health, 94,* 1200–1203.

Huey, F. L. (2001). Global impact of innovations on chronic disease in the genomics era. *The Pfizer Journal, 11*(2), 13.

Imrie, J., Stephenson, J. M., Cowan, F. M., Wanigaratne, S., Billington, A. J. P., Copas, A. J., et al. (2001). A cognitive behavioral intervention to reduce sexually transmitted infections among gay men: Randomised trial. *British Medical Journal, 322,* 1451–1456.

Johnson, B. K. (2004). Prostate cancer and sexuality: Implications for nursing. *Geriatric Nursing, 25,* 341–347.

Kirby, M. (2004). Erectile dysfunction: Cardiovascular risk and the role of the primary care physician. In R. S. Kirby, C. C. Carson, M. G. Kirby, & R. N. Farah (Eds.), *Men's health* (2nd ed., pp. 145–157). London: Taylor & Francis.

Kirby, R. S., & Kirby, M. (2004). Benign and malignant diseases of the prostate. In R. S. Kirby, C. C. Carson, M. G. Kirby, & R. N. Farah (Eds.), *Men's health* (2nd ed., pp. 285–298). London: Taylor & Francis.

Koblin, B. A., Chesney, M. A., Husnik, M. J., Bozeman, S., Celum, C. L., Buchbinder, S., et al., (2003). High risk sexual behaviors among men who have sex with men in 6 US cities: Baseline data from the EXPLORE study. *American Journal of Public Health, 93,* 926–932.

Lambert, S. (2005). Gay and lesbian families: What we know and where to go from here. *The Family Journal: Counseling and Therapy for Couples and Families, 13*(1), 43–51.

Lim, L. S., & Fitzpatrick, L. A. (2004). Osteoporosis in men. In R. S. Kirby, C. C. Carson, M. G. Kirby, & R. N. Farah (Eds.), *Men's health* (2nd ed., pp. 203–221). London: Taylor & Francis.

Mannino, D. M., Homa, D. M., Akinbami, L. J., Ford, E. S., & Redd, S. C. (2002). Chronic obstructive pulmonary disease surveillance—United States, 1971–2000. *Morbidity and Mortality Weekly Report, 53*(SS-6), 1–16.

Marston, C. (2004). Gendered communication among young people in Mexico: Implications for sexual health interventions. *Social Science & Medicine, 59,* 445–456.

Mays, V. M., & Cochran, S. D. (2001). Mental health correlates of perceived discrimination among lesbian, gay, and bisexual adults in the United States. *American Journal of Public Health, 91,* 1869–1876.

McLeer, S. V. (2004). Mental health services. In H. S. Sultz & K. M. Young, *Health care USA: Understanding its organization and delivery* (4th ed., pp. 335–366). Sudbury, MA: Jones and Bartlett.

Meyer, I., & Bowen, D. (2000). Lesbian, gay and bisexual health concerns: Cancer. In Gay and Lesbian Medical Association & Center for Lesbian, Gay, Bisexual, and Transgender Health (Eds.), *Lesbian, gay, bisexual, and transgender health: Findings and concerns* (pp. 15–17). New York: Author.

Meyer, I., Rothblum, E., & Bradford, J. (2000). Mental health and mental disorders. In Gay and Lesbian Medical Association & Center for Lesbian, Gay, Bisexual, and Transgender Health (Eds.), *Lesbian, gay, bisexual, and transgender health: Findings and concerns* (pp. 21–26). New York: Author.

Meyer, I., Silenzio, V., Wolfe, D., & Dunn, P. (2000). Introduction/background. In Gay and Lesbian Medical Association & Center for Lesbian, Gay, Bisexual, and Transgender Health (Eds.), *Lesbian, gay, bisexual, and transgender health: Findings and concerns* (pp. 4–9). New York: Author.

Monts, R. (2002a). Depression among migrant farm workers. *Community Health Forum, 3*(5), 52–54.

Monts, R. (2002b). Men don't seek treatment for depression. *Community Health Forum, 3*(5), 53.

Monts, R., & Smith, S. (2002). Why don't men obtain preventive care? *Community Health Forum, 3*(5), 8–13.

Murray, S. O. (2000). *Homosexualities.* Chicago: University of Chicago Press.

Murty, S. A., Peek-Asa, C., Zwerling, C., Stromquist, A. M., Burmeister, L. F., & Merchant, J. A. (2003). Physical and emotional abuse reported by men and women in a rural community. *American Journal of Public Health, 93,* 1073–1075.

Mussolino, M. E., Looker, A. C., & Orwoll, E. S. (2001). Jogging and bone mineral density in men: Results from NHANES III. *American Journal of Public Health, 91,* 1056–1059.

Natinsky, P. (2002). The return of syphilis. *Community Health Forum, 3*(5), 30–31.

National Center for Chronic Disease Prevention and Health Promotion. (2004). Self-reported frequent mental distress among adults—United States, 1993–2001. *Morbidity and Mortality Weekly Report, 53*, 963–966.

Newman, P. A., Rhodes, F., & Weiss, R. (2004). Correlates of sex trading among drug-using men who have sex with men. *American Journal of Public Health, 94*, 1998–2003.

Nickel, J. C. (2004). Prostatitis. In R. S. Kirby, C. C. Carson, M. G. Kirby, & R. N. Farah (Eds.), *Men's health* (2nd ed., pp. 315–327). London: Taylor & Francis.

Nnko, S., Boerma, J. T., Urassa, M., Mwaluko, G., & Zaba, B. (2003). Secretive females or swaggering males? An assessment of the quality of sexual partnership reporting in rural Tanzania. *Social Science & Medicine, 59*, 299–310.

Paul, J. P., Catania, J., Pollack, L., Moskowitz, J., Canchola, J., Mills, T., et al. (2002). Suicide attempts among gay and bisexual men: Lifetime prevalence and antecedents. *American Journal of Public Health, 92*, 1338–1345.

Perkins, R. (2004). Diversity in Health Care Delivery. *Pfizer Journal, VIII*(2), 4–14.

Pinhey, T. K., & Millman, S. R. (2004). Asian/Pacific Islander adolescent sexual orientation and suicide risk in Guam. *American Journal of Public Health, 94*, 1204–1206.

Pinkelman, M. A. (2002a). In their own right: Men's sexual and reproductive health issues on the line. *Community Health Forum, 3*(5), 20.

Pinkelman, M. A. (2002b). Search for consensus: Prostate. *Community Health Forum, 3*(5), 17–19.

Poppen, P. J., Reisen, C. A., Zea, M. C., Bianchi, F. T., & Echeverry, J. J. (2005). Serostatus disclosure, seroconcordance, and unprotected anal intercourse among HIV-positive Latino men who have sex with men. *AIDS Education and Prevention, 17*, 227–237.

Price, E. (2005). All but invisible: Older gay men and lesbians. *Nursing Older People, 17*(4), 16–18.

Prigerson, H. G., Maciejewski, P. K., & Rosenheck, R. A. (2002). Population attributable fractions of psychiatric disorders and behavioral outcomes associated with combat exposure among US men. *American Journal of Public Health, 92*, 59–63.

Purcell, H., Daly, C., & Petersen, S. (2004). Coronary heart disease in men (reversing the "descent of man"). In R. S. Kirby, C. C. Carson, M. G. Kirby, & R. N. Farah (Eds.), *Men's health* (2nd ed., pp. 101–109). London: Taylor & Francis.

Ridge, D., Hulme, A., & Peasley, D. (2003). Queering health: The health of young same-sex-attracted men and women. In P. Liamputtong & H. Gardner (Eds.), *Health, social change and communities* (pp. 283–305). Oxford: Oxford University Press.

Russell, S. T., Driscoll, A. K., & Truong, N. (2002). Adolescent same-sex romantic attractions and relationships: Implications for substance use and abuse. *American Journal of Public Health, 92*, 198–202.

Russell, S. T., & Joyner, K. (2001). Adolescent sexual orientation and suicide risk: Evidence from a national study. *American Journal of Public Health, 91*, 1276–1281.

Savage, T. A., Harley, D. A., & Nowak, T. M. (2005). Applying social empowerment strategies as tools for self-advocacy in counseling lesbian and gay male clients. *Journal of Counseling & Development, 83*, 131–137.

Scout, & Robinson, K. (2000). HIV/AIDS. In Gay and Lesbian Medical Association & Center for Lesbian, Gay, Bisexual, and Transgender Health (Eds.), *Lesbian, gay, bisexual, and transgender health: Findings and concerns* (pp. 18–20). New York: Author.

Sell, R. (2000). Methodological challenges to studying lesbian, gay, bisexual, and transgender health. In Gay and Lesbian Medical Association & Center for Lesbian, Gay, Bisexual, and Transgender Health (Eds.), *Lesbian, gay, bisexual, and transgender health: Findings and concerns* (pp. 43–47). New York: Author.

Sember, R. (2000). Transgender health concerns. In Gay and Lesbian Medical Association & Center for Lesbian, Gay, Bisexual, and Transgender Health (Eds.), *Lesbian, gay, bisexual, and transgender health: Findings and concerns* (pp. 32–43). New York: Author.

Shepherd, A. J. (2004). An overview of osteoporosis. *Alternative Therapies, 10*(2), 26–33.

Silenzio, I. (2000). Immunization and infectious diseases. In Gay and Lesbian Medical Association & Center for Lesbian, Gay, Bisexual, and Transgender Health (Eds.), *Lesbian, gay, bisexual, and transgender health: Findings and concerns* (p. 21). New York: Author.

Singleton, J. A., Greby, S. M., Wooten, K. G., Walker, F. J., & Strikas, R. (2000). Influenza, pneumococcal, and tetanus toxoid vaccination of adults—United States, 1993–1997. *Morbidity and Mortality Weekly Report, 49*(SS-9), 39–62.

Solomon, H., & Jackson, G. (2004). Risk factors in men with erectile dysfunction. In R. S. Kirby, C. C. Carson, M. G. Kirby, & R. N. Farah (Eds.), *Men's health* (2nd ed., pp. 159–170). London: Taylor & Francis.

Stall, R., Mills, T. C., Williamson, J., Hart, T., Greenwood, G., Paul, J., et al. (2003). Association of co-occurring psychosocial health problems and increased vulnerability to HIV/AIDS among urban men who have sex with men. *American Journal of Public Health, 93*, 939–942.

Taylor, B. (1999). "Coming out" as a life transition: Homosexual identity formation and its implications for health care practice. *Journal of Advanced Nursing, 30*, 520–525.

Thiede, H., Valleroy, L. A., MacKellar, D. A., Celentano, D. D., Ford, W. L., Hagan, H., et al. (2003). Regional patterns and correlates of substance abuse among young men who have sex with men in 7 urban areas. *American Journal of Public Health, 93*, 1915–1921.

U.S. Census Bureau. (2004a). *Historical health insurance tables.* Retrieved October 1, 2004, from http://www.census.gov

U.S. Census Bureau. (2004b). *Poverty: 2003 highlights.* Retrieved September 30, 2004, from http://www.census.gov

U.S. Census Bureau. (2005). *Statistical abstract of the United States: 2004–2005.* Retrieved August 16, 2005, from http://www.census.gov/prod/2004pubs/04statab

U.S. Department of Health and Human Services. (2000). *Healthy people 2010* (Conference edition, in two volumes). Washington, DC: Author.

U.S. Preventive Services Task Force. (2005). *The guide to clinical preventive services, 2005.* Retrieved August 13, 2005, from http://www.ahrq.gov/clinic/pocketgd.pdf

Washington, H. (2002). Burning love: Big tobacco takes aim at LGBT youths. *American Journal of Public Health, 92*, 1086–1095.

Webster, R. D., Darrow, W. W., Paul, J. P., Roark, R. A., Taylor, R. A., & Stempel, R. R. (2005). Community planning, HIV prevention, and a needs assessment for men who have sex with men: The South Beach health survey. *Sexually Transmitted Diseases, 32*, 321–327.

Weidner, G., & Cain, V. S. (2003). The gender gap in heart disease: Lessons from Eastern Europe. *American Journal of Public Health, 93*, 768–770.

Weitoft, G. R., Burstrom, B., & Rosen, M. (2004). Premature mortality among lone fathers and childless men. *Social Science & Medicine, 59*, 1449–1459.

White, A. K., & Banks, I. (2004). Help seeking in men and the problems of late diagnosis. In R. S. Kirby, C. C. Carson, M. G. Kirby, & R. N. Farah (Eds.), *Men's health* (2nd ed., pp. 1–7). London: Taylor & Francis.

White, J., Bradford, J., & Silenzio, V. (2000). Health communication. In Gay and Lesbian Medical Association & Center for Lesbian, Gay, Bisexual, and Transgender Health (Eds.), *Lesbian, gay, bisexual, and transgender health: Findings and concerns* (pp. 11–13). New York: Author.

White, J., Bradford, J., Silenzio, V., & Wolfe, D. (2000). Access to quality health services. In Gay and Lesbian Medical Association & Center for Lesbian, Gay, Bisexual, and Transgender Health (Eds.), *Lesbian, gay, bisexual, and transgender health: Findings and concerns* (pp. 10–12). New York: Author.

Williams, D. R. (2003). The health of men: Structured inequalities and opportunities. *American Journal of Public Health, 93*, 724–731.

World Health Organization. (2005). *World health statistics 2005.* Retrieved September 21, 2005, from http://www.who.int/healthinfo/statistics/whostat2005en1.pdf

Wynd, C. A. (2002). Testicular self-examination in young adult men. *Journal of Nursing Scholarship, 34*, 251–255.

Advocacy in Action

The Credit Card

Mrs. A. is an 83-year-old widow who lives alone in a small four-plex that she owns. She has a son who lives in the area and stops by frequently to check on her. He has a learning disability and does not read, so he is not involved in her financial affairs, nor does she want him to be.

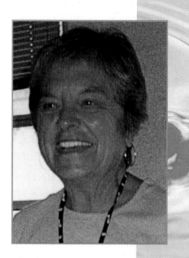

Because of problems with her teeth, including pain and not being able to chew, Mrs. A. went to a local dentist. While she was at the dentist's office having x-rays taken, a clerk came in and asked her to sign a paper without any explanation. Mrs. A. signed the paper but did not know why or ask any questions. Later she said she thought it was permission for them to do the dental work.

Six weeks later Mrs. A. received a bill from a credit card company for over $2,000, including finance charges. The bill was a prepayment for dental work that would be done over several office visits. This was the first she knew that she had signed for a credit card while at the dentist's office. Mrs. A. does not have any credit cards at present, and her only experience with a credit card was a bad one years ago. She had planned to pay for the dental work herself, as it was done, and had no desire to put the bill on credit. She called the credit card company but was unable to get a satisfactory answer. She also called the dentist's office, but they would only say that she signed for the card.

The community health nurse working with Mrs. A. called the credit card company and explained the situation. They were sympathetic and asked for a written synopsis of the details, but did not offer much hope. The next step was to contact the elder abuse division of the district attorney's office. Mrs. A. was advised to send a registered letter to the dentist. She received no response. The next week, Mrs. A. and the community health nurse met with the dentist. Mrs. A. indicated that she no longer wanted him as her dentist and that she would never have signed the credit card if she had known what it was. After a lengthy discussion and threats to report the dentist to the Better Business Bureau, he agreed to waive all credit card charges, including interest. The dentist wrote a check to the credit card company, and an agreement was signed.

Without the intervention of the community health nurse, Mrs. A. would have been faced with an extensive bill and finance charges for dental work that had not yet even been done.

Connie Curran, MSN, RN, PHN

Community Health Nurse

Bayside Community Center

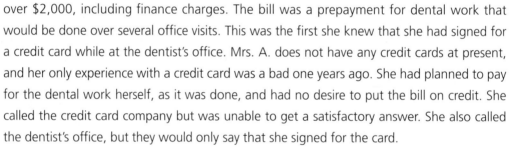

Meeting the Health Needs of Older Clients

CHAPTER OBJECTIVES

After reading this chapter, you should be able to:

1. Describe three categories of theories of aging.
2. Describe biophysical, psychological, physical environmental, sociocultural, behavioral, and health system factors influencing the health of the elderly population.
3. Identify major considerations in primary prevention in the care of older adults and analyze community health nursing roles related to each.
4. Describe secondary preventive measures for at least four health problems common among older clients.
5. Identify at least three foci for tertiary prevention with older clients and give examples of related community health nursing interventions.
6. Identify considerations that may influence the community health nurse's approach to health education for older clients.
7. Analyze the influence of factors unique to older clients on evaluation of nursing care.

KEY TERMS

advanced activities of daily living (AADLs) **502**
ageism **497**
aging **496**
basic activities of daily living (BADLs) **502**
comorbidity **498**
dementia **504**
elderly support ratio **511**
functional status **502**
instrumental activities of daily living (IADLs) **502**
life-sustaining treatment **535**
old-age dependency ratio **511**
palliative care **534**
respite **536**
senescence **496**
social network **509**
transnationalism **509**
validation therapy **531**

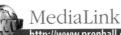

MediaLink
http://www.prenhall.com/clark

Additional interactive resources for this chapter can be found on the Companion Website. Click on Chapter 19 and "Begin" to select the activities for this chapter.

According to the Federal Interagency Forum on Aging-related Statistics (2004), the older population of the United States increased tenfold during the 20th century and is expected to increase to 87 million by 2050. Increased longevity and decreasing fertility are continuing to change the proportion of elderly people in relation to other age groups in the population. Life expectancy has increased by 2 years each decade over the last 50 years and is expected to increase by another 10 years worldwide by 2050 (Plese, 2005b). In the United States, although overall life expectancy at birth was 77.2 years, additional life expectancy for a person who was 65 years of age in 2001 was another 18.1 years (Centers for Disease Control and Prevention [CDC], 2004b). Worldwide, Japan has the highest life expectancy at birth at 82 years (World Health Organization [WHO], 2005).

By 2030, the elderly population throughout the world is expected to increase to 973 million people, and the number of older adults will more than triple in developing countries, which will account for 71% of the world's elderly population. In 2004, elderly persons already constituted more than 20% of the total population of 22 countries. Italy had the highest proportion of elderly residents at nearly a quarter of the population (24.5%) (World Health Organization, 2004), but China has the largest elderly population in the world in terms of actual numbers (You, Deans, Liu, Zhang, & Zhang, 2004). The number of centenarians (people over 100 years of age) is expected to increase fifteenfold by 2050 to 2.2 million persons worldwide, and in 2005 there were already 300 to 450 "super centenarians" (those more than 110 years of age) in the world (Plese, 2005b).

In the United States, the proportion of the population over 65 years of age is expected to increase from 12.4% in 2000 to 19.6% in 2030, and the actual number of elderly people will more than double from 35 million to 71 million. In addition, the number of people over 80 years of age in the United States is expected to increase from 9.3 million in 2000 to 19.5 million in 2030 (Division of Adult and Community Health, 2003c). Much of this increase will come in ethnic minority populations, with a decrease in the proportion of non-Hispanic White residents from 87% to 67% of the elderly population, an elevenfold increase in the Hispanic elderly population, and small increases in the proportion of elderly residents of other minority groups (Manly & Mayeux, 2004).

As the world's population ages, there will be a growing demand for health care services that improve the quality of life as well as longevity. This emphasis on quality of life can be seen in the national health objectives for 2010 addressing the health needs of the elderly. A major thread throughout these objectives is to reduce activity limitations that impair the quality of life for older persons (U.S. Department of Health and Human Services [USDHHS], 2000). These objectives can be viewed on the *Healthy People 2010*◆ Web site, which can be accessed at http://wonder.cdc.gov/data2010.

Concern for the health of the older population of the world also stems from a desire to minimize health care expenditures. Because of the prevalence of multiple chronic illnesses, the elderly account for a significant percentage of all health care expenditures worldwide. For example, in the United States, people over 65 years of age accounted for 45% of all days of hospital care and 38% of hospital discharges in 2003 (National Center for Health Statistics [NCHS], 2005d). Health care costs for people age 65 years and over in developed nations are three to five times those for younger people (Division of Adult and Community Health, 2003c). Improving the health of this population can decrease the societal burden of their care as well as promoting a better quality of life.

Nurses have long provided care to individual older clients and to the elderly as a population group. The American Association of Colleges of Nursing and the John A. Hartford Foundation Institute for Geriatric Nursing (2000) have developed a set of 30 competencies required of baccalaureate preparation for care of the elderly in the United States. These competencies primarily address knowledge required for care of individual elderly clients, but can be adapted to the care of the elderly as a vulnerable population. This latter application to the health of the elderly population is the thrust of this chapter.

THEORIES OF AGING

Aging is defined as "maturation and senescence of biological systems" (Albert, Im, & Raveis, 2002, p. 1214). Some authors prefer the term **senescence**, which is defined as "progressive deterioration of body systems that can increase the risk of mortality as an individual gets older" (Tabloski, 2006, p. 15). Aging or senescence involves a gradual and progressive loss of function over time that is not synonymous with an increase in disease (Malavolta, Mocchegiani, & Bertoni-Freddari, 2004), although the effects of aging may place older people at higher risk for disease.

A number of different theories have been advanced to explain how and why aging occurs. Generally speaking, these theories can be divided into three categories: biological theories, psychological theories, and sociological theories. Biological theories attempt to explain the biophysical changes that occur in aging and are of two basic types, programmed theories and error theories. Programmed aging theories propose that genetic codes regulate cell reproduction and death and that organ deterioration and eventual death are programmed in one's genetic makeup (Saxon & Etten, 2002). Specific programmed aging theories address longevity, declining endocrine function, and declining immune function. In error theories, hypothesized

TABLE 19-1	Stages and Foci of Erikson's and Peck's Developmental Theories	
Life Stage	Erikson's Stages	Focus
Infancy	Stage 1: Trust vs. mistrust	Erikson: Development of a sense of trust in self and others
Childhood	Stage 2: Autonomy vs. shame and doubt	Erikson: Development of the ability to express oneself and cooperate with others
Childhood	Stage 3: Initiative vs. guilt	Erikson: Development of purposeful behavior and the ability to evaluate one's own behavior
Childhood	Stage 4: Industry vs. inferiority	Erikson: Development of belief in one's own abilities
Adolescence	Stage 5: Identity vs. role confusion	Erikson: Development of a sense of self and plans to actualize one's potential
Adolescence/early adulthood	Stage 6: Intimacy vs. isolation	Erikson: Development of one's capacity for reciprocal relationships
Middle age	Stage 7: Generativity vs. stagnation	Erikson: Promotion of creativity and productivity and development of the capacity to care for others
		Peck: Development of the ability to value wisdom over physical competence
		Shifting relationships to emphasize friendship and companionship over sexual satisfaction
		Development of flexibility in roles and relationships
		Development of mental and intellectual flexibility
Late adulthood	Stage 8: Ego identity vs. despair	Erikson: Acceptance of one's life as unique and worthwhile
		Peck: Development of the ability to value one's self outside of work roles
		Development of abilities to adapt to physical changes and effects of aging
		Maintenance of an active interest in the external world

cumulative environmental assaults stretch the body's ability to respond and cause accumulation of metabolic toxins that impair normal function (Tabloski, 2006).

Psychological theories of aging focus on psychological changes that occur with age and propose that effective aging requires development of effective coping strategies over time. Major theories in this area include Jung's theory of individualism, in which the individual's mental focus changes from the external to the internal world, and the developmental theories (Tabloski, 2006). Erik Erikson's stage theory of development proposed eight stages of life in which the individual needed to accomplish specific developmental tasks that would facilitate task accomplishment in later stages. Peck took Erikson's last two stages, which encompass the last 40 to 50 years of life, and subdivided them into seven more discrete stages that cover middle age and older adult life (Saxon & Etten, 2002). In Peck's final stage, the individual engages in life review in preparation for death. Table 19-1◆ presents an overview of developmental theories and associated foci for task accomplishment.

Sociological theories of aging focus on changes in roles and relationships that occur with advancing age. Theories in this group tend to be mutually exclusive. For example, disengagement theory proposes that individuals disengage from life as a means of making way for a younger generation in preparation for death. The process may actually work in reverse, however, with society disengaging from and isolating older individuals as a result of **ageism**, which is prejudice or discrimination based on chronological age or appearance of age. In activity and continuity theories, however, older persons maintain their interest in life, but their specific interests change (Tabloski, 2006).

THE EPIDEMIOLOGY OF HEALTH FOR OLDER CLIENTS

Factors in each of the six dimensions of health influence the health of the older population, often with greater effects than on the health of people in younger age groups. Here we will examine some of the major

CULTURAL COMPETENCE

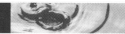

*D*ifferent cultural groups have differing attitudes toward the elderly and the conditions that often affect them. For example, in many cultures, the elderly are revered and respected for their wisdom, yet in these same cultures, stigma attached to certain conditions may make caring for older clients with these conditions difficult. Zhan (2004) described the additional burden on caregivers of family members with Alzheimer's disease (AD) due to perceived stigma among Chinese clients. In a qualitative study of Chinese caregivers for older clients with AD, she noted that diagnosis was often delayed because, even though family members recognized problems, they were ashamed to admit them to others, including health care providers. There were also differences in perceptions of the disease between caretakers, who saw AD as a brain dysfunction, and family members and others in the community, who ascribed AD to fate, wrongdoing, getting old and forgetful, worrying too much, being crazy, and bad *feng shui*. Some also thought AD was communicable and so shunned both client and family members to avoid contagion. Cultural factors, such as inability to speak English, also prevented clients and families from obtaining access to some services for persons with AD.

Cultural values did have one positive aspect, however. Because of the strong cultural value given to care of the elderly, caregivers felt satisfaction in their caregiving that allowed them to cope with the stresses of caregiving as well as the stigma in the community.

What are the responses of other cultural groups to diagnoses such as AD in the elderly? How do cultural factors influence the care of these older persons? How might community health nurses intervene in cultural groups that attach stigma to AD and similar diseases?

influences on the health of the older population in each dimension.

Biophysical Considerations

Major considerations related to the biophysical dimension of health include those related to maturation and aging and physiologic function, including immunization status.

Maturation and Aging

Whatever the ultimate causes of aging, aging has certain rather universal effects that result in a number of changes in both form and function. These changes may be the result of senescence or of cumulative exposures to risk factors over long periods of time (Albert et al., 2002). The major change involved in aging is loss of physical reserve capacity, which results in both cognitive and physical slowing, increased response to stress, a more easily disrupted equilibrium, and a need to pace oneself (Saxon & Etten, 2002). These effects are seen in slowed reaction times, decreased psychomotor and walking speed, loss of verbal memory, declining strength, decreased urine flow, and loss of skeletal muscle. The physiologic changes that occur with aging occur at different rates for different people and are normal effects. They may, however, increase the older client's

risk of developing illness and disability. Physical changes related to aging and their possible implications for health are summarized in Table 19-2♦.

Aging also results in changes in patterns of disease that may make diagnosis or treatment of illness more difficult. These changing disease patterns include comorbidity, differences in symptom experience, and perceptions of many symptoms of disease as a normal part of aging (Williams, 2005). **Comorbidity**, the coexistence of many chronic physical and/or mental illnesses in the same person at the same time, complicates both diagnosis and treatment of illness in older adults. For example, drug therapies for one condition may interact with treatment of another condition, interfering with therapeutic effects or causing adverse effects. In addition, older people may not present with classic symptoms of a given condition, making diagnosis more difficult. For example, many older people do not experience the chest pain typical of myocardial infarction. Finally, older clients, family members, and health care providers may inaccurately interpret abnormal symptoms as facets of normal aging (e.g., many people believe that pain and stiffness are normal concomitants of age).

The goal of community health nursing with respect to aging is to foster healthy aging and to promote active aging, defined by WHO as "the process of optimizing opportunities for health, participation, and security in order to enhance quality of life as people age" (quoted in Plese, 2005b, p. 5). Three requisites have been proposed for healthy aging: (a) accepting the limitations posed by bodily changes, (b) modifying one's lifestyle as needed to accommodate these changes, and (c) developing new personal standards of achievement and life goals consistent with the constraints imposed by the effects of aging (Saxon & Etten, 2002). The role of the community health nurse is to assist the elderly population to mitigate the adverse effects, prevent unnecessary deterioration in function, and promote quality of life for older clients.

Physiologic Function

Older populations experience increased mortality and morbidity rates relative to younger groups of people. They also experience higher rates of many other problems that affect their quality of life, such as pain and incontinence. A few of these physiologic effects will be discussed here. With respect to mortality, age-specific death rates increase with age for most diseases. For example, the mortality rate for heart disease in 2002 was 241.5 per 100,000 persons aged 55 to 64 years, but more than doubled for the next age group (615.9 per 100,000), then nearly tripled for those aged 75 to 84 years (1,677 per 100,000), then more than tripled again for those over age 85 (5,466 per 100,000). Similar escalation with age is noted in mortality rates for cerebrovascular disease, malignancies, chronic lower respiratory diseases, and other chronic illnesses (CDC, 2004a).

TABLE 19-2	Common Physical Changes of Aging and Their Implications for Health	
System	Changes Noted	Possible Health Implications
Integumentary		
Skin	Decreased turgor, sclerosis, and loss of subcutaneous fat, leading to wrinkles	Lowered self-esteem
	Increased pigmentation, cherry angiomas	
	Cool to touch, dry	Itching, risk of injury, insomnia
	Decreased perspiration	Hyperthermia, heatstroke
Hair	Thin, decreased pigmentation	Lowered self-esteem
Nails	Thickened, ridges, decreased rate of growth	Difficulty trimming nails, potential for injury
Cardiovascular	Less efficient pump action and lower cardiac reserves	Decreased physical ability, fatigue with exertion
	Thickening of vessel walls, replacement of muscle fiber with collagen	Elevated blood pressure, varicosities, venous stasis, pressure sores
	Pulse pressure up to 100	
	Arrhythmias and murmurs	
	Dilated abdominal aorta	
Respiratory	Decreased elasticity of alveolar sacs, skeletal changes of chest	Decreased gas exchange, decreased physical ability
	Slower mucus transport, decreased cough strength, dysphagia	Increased potential for infection or aspiration
	Postnasal drip	
Gastrointestinal	Wearing down of teeth	Difficulty chewing
	Decreased saliva production	Dry mouth, difficulty digesting starches
	Loss of taste buds	Decreased appetite, malnutrition
	Muscle atrophy of cheeks, tongue, etc.	Difficulty chewing, slower to eat
	Thinned esophageal wall	Feeling of fullness, heartburn after meals
	Decreased peristalsis	Constipation
	Decreased hydrochloric acid and stomach enzyme production	Pernicious anemia, frequent eructation
	Decreased lip size, sagging abdomen	Change in self-concept
	Atrophied gums	Poorly fitting dentures, difficulty chewing, potential for mouth ulcers, loss of remaining teeth
	Decreased bowel sounds	Potential for misdiagnosis
	Fissures in tongue	
	Increased or decreased liver size (2–3 cm below costal border)	Potential for misdiagnosis
Urinary	Decreased number of nephrons and decreased ability to concentrate urine	Nocturia, increased potential for falls
Reproductive		
Female	Atrophied ovaries, uterus	Ovarian cysts
	Atrophy of external genitalia, pendulous breasts, small flat nipple, decreased pubic hair	Lower self-esteem
	Scant vaginal secretions	Dyspareunia
	Vaginal mucosa thinned and friable	
Male	Decreased size of penis and testes, decreased pubic hair, pendulous scrotum	Lowered self-esteem
	Enlarged prostate	Difficulty urinating, incontinence

Continued on next page

TABLE 19-2	Common Physical Changes of Aging and Their Implications for Health *(continued)*	
Musculoskeletal	Decreased muscle size and tone	Decreased physical ability
	Decreased range of motion in joints, affecting gait, posture, balance, and flexibility	Increased risk of falls, decreased mobility
	Kyphosis	Lowered self-esteem
	Joint instability	Increased risk of falls, injury
	Straight thoracic spine	
	Breakdown of chondrocytes in joint cartilage	Osteoarthritis, joint pain, reduced abilities for activities of daily living
	Osteoporosis	Increased risk of fracture
Neurological	Diminished hearing, vision, touch, and increased reaction time	Increased risk for injury, social isolation
	Diminished pupil size, peripheral vision, adaptation, accommodation	
	Diminished sense of smell, taste	Decreased appetite, malnutrition
	Decreased balance	Increased risk of injury
	Decreased pain sensation	Increased risk of injury
	Decreased ability to problem-solve	Difficulty adjusting to new situations
	Diminished deep tendon reflexes	
	Decreased sphincter tone	Incontinence (fecal or urinary)
	Diminished short-term memory	Forgetfulness
Endocrine		
Thyroid	Irregular, fibrous changes	
Female	Decreased estrogen and progesterone production	Osteoporosis, menopause
Male	Decreased testosterone production	Fatigue, weight loss, decreased libido, impotence, lowered self-esteem, depression

Older populations are even more prone to morbidity from acute and chronic illness than to death, and the bulk of the burden of many of these conditions is borne by the older segments of the population.

ACUTE HEALTH CONDITIONS Because of decreased organ function and immune function that accompanies aging, older people are often at greater risk for acute illnesses and injuries as well as for developing serious complications of disease. Accidental injuries are acute conditions that significantly affect the health of the elderly. For example, in 2002, the rate of injury-related emergency department visits for older clients was 1,192.5 per 10,000 men and 1,369.4 per 10,000 women (CDC, 2004a). Accidental injuries are the seventh leading cause of death over age 65 years and the fifth leading cause for people over age 85 (Hurley et al., 2004). Most of these injuries are related to falls, with one third of older adults in the United States each year experiencing a fall (Huang & Acton, 2004). Mortality is 12% to 20% higher among older people experiencing a hip fracture as a result of a fall than among non-fallers. Annual costs for hip fractures resulting from falls in the United States amount to $6 billion (Yuan et al.,

2001). Injuries are addressed in more detail in the section on safety later in this chapter.

Influenza and pneumonia are two other acute health conditions that disproportionately affect the elderly. Influenza causes more than 36,000 deaths each year (Harper, Fukuda, Uyeki, Cox, & Bridges, 2005). From 1990 to 1999, more than 32,000 influenza-related deaths occurred each year among people over 65 years of age (Epidemiology and Surveillance Division, 2004). Similar patterns are evident for pneumococcal pneumonia, with hospitalizations among the elderly increasing by 93.5% from 1991 to 1998 (Baine, Yu, & Summe, 2001) and more than 3,000 deaths in people over 65 years of age in 1999 alone (CDC, 2004b). In 2001, influenza and pneumonia together constituted the fifth leading cause of death in people over 85 years of age (U.S. Census Bureau, 2005).

Although a smaller proportion of the population is affected than in other age groups, 10% of AIDS cases occur in people over 50 years of age in the United States. In addition, from 1991 to 1996, the incidence of AIDS increased more in the population over 50 years of age than in the 13- to 49-year-old group (Rose, 2004). In 2002, an estimated 8,900 people over 65 years of age in the United States were living with AIDS (U.S. Census

Bureau, 2005). In 2003, incidence rates for AIDS in people over 60 years of age were 6.3 per 100,000 men and 1.5 per 100,000 women (CDC, 2004a). Although these rates are less than a quarter of those for people aged 13 to 59 years, they are significant because many providers do not think of AIDS in the older population and because of the added complication posed by AIDS in the control of other health problems among the elderly. Community health nurses may need to advocate for treatment facilities that meet the specific needs of older clients with AIDS or for health education programs particularly targeted to this population.

CHRONIC DISEASE AND DISABILITY Both the incidence and prevalence of chronic illnesses increase with age. An estimated 84% of people over 65 years of age have at least one chronic illness, and 62% have two or more chronic conditions (Tanner, 2004). By age 80, three fourths of women have two or more chronic conditions, the major contributors to disease burden being arthritis, hypertension, heart disease, and hearing and vision problems (Yoon & Horne, 2004). Chronic illness contributes to an increasing number of days in bed. For example, in 2003, the average number of days in bed due to chronic disease was only 3.5 for people aged 18 to 44 years and 6 days for those aged 45 to 64 years, but increased with age to 6.6 days for those 65 to 74 years old and 9.4 days for those over 75 years of age (NCHS, 2005a).

Arthritis affects 60% of people over 65 years of age in the United States. The percentage of people affected by this disease is expected to remain relatively stable through 2030 (58% of the elderly population), but the actual number of people with arthritis or chronic joint symptoms is expected to double to 41.1 million (Division of Adult and Community Health, 2003b). Arthritis is the most frequent cause of disability in the United States. Arthritis pain limits movement, which leads to deconditioning of joints and muscles and greater pain with movement. Without treatment, arthritis leads to a continuous pain-movement cycle that limits function and increases the potential for disability (Davis, Hiemenz, & White, 2002).

Hypertension and consequent cardiovascular disease are other common chronic illnesses in older populations. From 1999 to 2002, for example, hypertension affected 59% of men aged 65 to 74 years and 68% of those over 75 years of age. The percentage of women in each age group is even higher, at 72.5% of those 65 to 74 years of age and 83% of those over age 75 (CDC, 2004a). Heart disease and stroke incidence also increase with increasing age. In 2001, for example, 50% to 74% of hospitalizations for cardiovascular disease, coronary heart disease, angina, or stroke occurred among people over 65 years of age, and people over 85 years of age constitute 84% of cardiovascular and coronary heart disease deaths (Johnson, 2004). As we saw in Chapter 17 ∞, the risk of cardiovascular disease increases substantially in women after menopause (Lewis, 2004).

The rate of hospitalization for stroke also increases with age. In 2001, for example, the rate of stroke hospitalization nearly doubled each decade after age 65 years, from 10.3 per 100,000 people aged 65 to 74 years to 20.5 per 100,000 of those 75 to 84 years of age, to 29.9 per 100,000 of those over age 85 years (Division of Adult and Community Health, 2003a).

Cardiovascular disease often leads to congestive heart failure (CHF), and 7% to 10% of people over age 80 have some degree of CHF. The incidence of CHF increases ninefold for men and elevenfold for women with every decade from age 50 to 80 years (Resnick, 2005).

Malignant neoplasms are the leading cause of death in people 65 to 74 years of age in the United States, at which point they are replaced by heart disease as the leading cause of death (U.S. Census Bureau, 2005). Approximately 60% of all new cancer diagnoses each year occur in people over 65 years of age, and people in this age group account for 61% of all cancer survivors (Division of Cancer Prevention and Control, 2004). Prostate cancer incidence in men increases with age; men aged 60 to 79 years have a twelvefold higher risk than younger men (Calabrese, 2004). An estimated 8% of men over age 80 have prostate cancer (Pinkelman, 2002). Breast cancer mortality in women also increases with age. For example, in 2002, mortality rates increased from 56.2 per 100,000 women aged 55 to 64 years to 191.5 per 100,000 women 85 years of age and over (CDC, 2004a).

Diabetes is another chronic illness that affects the health status of the elderly. From 1999 to 2000, for example, approximately 19% of people over 60 years of age had diabetes (CDC, 2004a). About 4.5 million women over age 60 years have diabetes, and nearly one fourth of them remain undiagnosed (National Center for Chronic Disease Prevention and Health Promotion, 2002a).

Chronic obstructive pulmonary disease (COPD) is a group of diseases that affect pulmonary function and includes chronic bronchitis, chronic obstructive bronchitis or emphysema, and combinations of these diseases. COPD is the fourth leading cause of death in the United States and is expected to become the third leading cause by 2020 (National Heart, Lung, and Blood Institute, 2003). In 2002, the latest year for which statistics are available, the overall age-adjusted U.S. mortality rate for lower respiratory diseases including COPD was 43.5 per 100,000 population. COPD death rates are far higher among the elderly, however, climbing to 163 per 100,000 among people age 65 to 74 and 637.6 among those 85 years of age and older (NCHS, 2005b). COPD may make even minimal exertion difficult for those affected and is a significant cause of disability among the elderly.

Even for chronic diseases that do not have a higher incidence among older adults, the effects of disease may be more pronounced with age. For example, only 45% of people with multiple sclerosis (MS) are over 55 years of age, but older persons with MS must deal with continuing deterioration as well as the usual effects of aging. In addition, older people with MS tend to display a more rapid rate of decline in function than those diagnosed at younger ages (Finlayson, Van Denend, & Hudson, 2004).

Chronic disease in the elderly often leads to functional limitations and disability. **Functional status** is the ability to perform tasks and fulfill expected social roles. Assessment of functional status includes exploration of abilities at three levels of task complexity: basic, intermediate or instrumental, and advanced activities of daily living. **Basic activities of daily living (BADLs)** are personal-care activities and include the ability to feed, bathe, and dress oneself, and toileting and transfer skills (getting in or out of a chair or bed). Intermediate or **instrumental activities of daily living (IADLs)** are tasks of moderate complexity, including household tasks such as shopping, laundry, cooking, and housekeeping, as well as abilities to take medications correctly, manage money, and use the telephone or public transportation. **Advanced activities of daily living (AADLs)** involve complex abilities to engage in voluntary social, occupational, or recreational activities.

Disability in the older population is defined as "difficulty with household and personal self-maintenance activities severe enough to threaten independent living" (Albert et al., 2002, p. 1215). Some authors propose three distinct pathways leading to disability in the elderly (Albert et al., 2002). In the first pathway, senescence, or the normal effects of aging, lead to frailty, which is seen as a preclinical stage to disability. Frailty is characterized by increasing weakness, slowness, and poor endurance, which make it difficult for the older person to engage in activities of daily living (ADLs). When these effects reach a threshold of "physical and cognitive capacity required for completion of daily tasks" (p. 1215), disability results.

The second pathway to disability reflects the direct effects of chronic diseases on stamina, strength, sensibility, dexterity, and the effect of pain and balance difficulties that decrease the capacity to perform ADLs. Albert

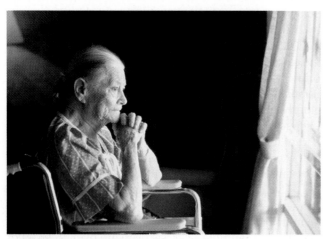

Disability may result in social isolation for many older clients. (Mark Richards)

and associates (2002) noted that senescence and disease can interact to contribute to disability. In the third pathway, environmental factors contribute to disability when difficulties in performing ADLs are compounded by lack of access to assistive and prosthetic devices or absent social and psychological resources to offset these difficulties. In one study, approximately 54% of disability in the elderly was attributed to the direct effects of chronic disease, 28% to frailty alone, and 18% was potentially related to environmental conditions (Albert et al., 2002). Other authors noted that more than 3 million people in Britain experienced locomotor disability, the inability to walk, climb stairs, or maintain balance. They found that personal difficulties arose primarily from the gap between the disability and environmental conditions that would allow people to function effectively in the face of the disability (Ebrahim, Papacosta, Wannamethee, & Adamson, 2004).

The extent of disability in the elderly population declined from 25% in 1984 to 20% in 1999. Despite the decrease in the percentage of the population affected, the actual number of older people experiencing disability increased due to the increasing size of this population (Federal Interagency Forum on Aging-related Statistics, 2004).

In 2002, an estimated 42% of people over 65 years of age in the United States experienced one or more disability. For 29% the disability was physical in nature; 14% experienced sensory limitations; 11% had mental disabilities of some kind; 9.5% experienced self-care limitations; and 20% were unable to go outside their homes without assistance. Just over 6% of people over age 65 experienced limitations in ADLs, and twice as many (12%) had difficulties with IADLs (U.S. Census Bureau, 2005).

Activity limitations vary with age and gender. In 2002, 25% of people aged 65 to 74 years experienced activity limitations, compared to 45% of those over age 75 (U.S. Census Bureau, 2005). The percentage of people aged 65 to 74 years with BADL limitations was 2.7%, whereas 9.6% of those over age 75 had BADL limitations. With respect to IADLs, the respective percentages were 6% and 18.9% (CDC, 2004a). The cause of disability may also vary with age. Between 65 and 84 years of age, disability is most often due to chronic physical conditions such as arthritis, hypertension, and heart disease. After age 85, disability due to cognitive and sensory problems, such as Alzheimer's and vision and hearing impairment, are more common (Huey, 2001). For example, memory impairment is found in approximately 5% of people aged 65 to 69 years, but 32% of those over 80 years of age (Federal Interagency Forum on Aging-related Statistics, 2004). Nearly 4% of women and 10% of men aged 65 to 74 years have hearing problems, and these figures increase to 13% of women and 18% of men who are 75 years of age or older (NCHS, 2005c). Approximately 18% of people over 70 years of age in the United States have visual difficulties, and 8.6% have both hearing and vision problems. People with both hearing and vision impairment were nearly three times more likely to consider themselves in poor health and were half as likely as those with neither impairment to report their health as excellent. Similarly, those with impairments in both senses were almost three times as likely as those with neither impairment to be depressed or confused and to have difficulty walking and were nearly four times more likely to have difficulty preparing meals. Those with vision problems were three times more likely to have difficulty going places and were more than twice as likely to have problems taking medications as people with neither hearing nor vision problems (Crews & Campbell, 2004).

The prevalence of disability in the older population also varies by gender. Although women have lower mortality rates than men and lower incidence and prevalence rates for some chronic illnesses, they tend to report lower quality of life and more disability and physical limitations than men. In general, about half of women over 65 years of age have some sort of functional disability (National Center on Birth Defects and Developmental Disabilities, 2005). In studies, 52% of older women report functional limitations compared to 37% of men. Women also report more limitations and greater disability than men do. Mobility limitations were reported by women one and a half times more often than men, and women were also more likely than men to report use of assistance in ADLs. In addition, women reported more pain and stiffness and greater fatigue related to chronic illness than men (Murtaugh & Hubert, 2004).

In addition to impaired quality of life for older people, disability presents significant costs to society. For example, in 1995 the estimated cost of older people transitioning from an independent to a dependent status due to disability amounted to a total of $26.1 billion. Average annual costs for people who developed a disability in a given year but remained in their home were $3,400. For those living at home who began and ended the year with a disability, average costs were doubled to $6,800. When disability resulted in nursing home placement, annual costs escalated to $21,000 per person (Guralnik, Alecxih, Branch, & Wiener, 2002).

PAIN Pain is a symptom that accompanies a wide variety of acute and chronic illnesses and is a common problem experienced by the older population. It is estimated that at least 70% of older adults experience chronic pain, most often as a result of arthritis and neuralgias (Davis et al., 2002). Unrelieved pain can diminish quality of life for the elderly through its functional, cognitive, emotional, and social effects. The normal effects of aging may lead to a slightly higher pain threshold for the elderly, such that older clients may not experience the pain typical of some conditions, making diagnosis more difficult. Pain is, however, prevalent and is often undertreated in older persons. The incidence of pain has been found to double

after the age of 60 years and increases each decade thereafter (Hanks-Bell, Halvey, & Paice, 2004).

Poor pain management in the elderly centers around client and provider decisions related to pain management. One study identified several barriers to arthritis pain management that are relevant to other causes of pain. These barriers included lack of access to care or treatment, an accelerating pain-movement cycle, lack of use of adaptive resources, emotional distress and its effects on pain and pain management, knowledge deficits regarding pain management, age-related perceptions by clients and providers that pain is normal in old age, and poor communication with providers (Davis et al., 2002).

INCONTINENCE Incontinence is another manageable physiologic condition that affects the quality of life of the elderly. Urinary incontinence has both psychological and social effects for older individuals, as well as economic consequences. For example, it is estimated that the 2002 cost of urinary incontinence was $2.2 billion (Phillips, 2004). Approximately 17 million people in the United States experience urinary incontinence or overactive bladder, but only about 15% of them seek help with the condition. Estimated prevalence in U.S. community-dwelling elders is 37% to 41%, with European studies suggesting that 20% of men and 24% of women are affected (Cooper & Kaplan, 2004; Heidrick & Wells, 2004).

Urinary incontinence may be of four general types: stress incontinence, overflow incontinence, urge incontinence, and functional incontinence (Dash, Foster, Smith, & Phillips, 2004). Stress incontinence occurs with movements that stress the urethral sphincter, such as coughing or sneezing. Overflow incontinence is due to residual urine remaining in the bladder from incomplete emptying. Urge incontinence is characterized by a sudden uncontrollable need to urinate, and functional incontinence is due to impaired mobility to reach the toilet in

ETHICAL AWARENESS

You are caring for an elderly gentleman with terminal lung cancer. He is experiencing considerable pain and has been given a prognosis of about 6 months' survival time. He tells you that he and his wife have been exploring the idea of assisted suicide and have found a physician who may be willing to help them. His wife experiences severe pain due to her arthritis and is never pain free, although pain medications decrease the level of pain to some extent. He had been doing most of the work in the home (cooking, washing, etc.) until recently. They have no family in the area and his wife's older brother lives in another state and is caring for his wife, who has Alzheimer's disease. Your client is afraid that when he dies, his wife will have no one to care for her and will suffer even more. He says they would "like to be together in death" just as they have been in life for over 50 years. Assisted suicide is illegal in your state. What will you do in this situation?

time or decreased manual dexterity in undressing. Incontinence in any given individual may combine several types (Teunissen, de Jonge, van Weel, & Lagro-Janssen, 2004). Incontinence may also be related to medications, such as anticholinergics, psychotropics, antidepressants, diuretics, sedatives, alpha-adrenergic blockers and agonists, calcium channel blockers, and muscle relaxants, or to alcohol or caffeine use (Dash et al., 2004).

Older clients may also experience fecal incontinence related to limited mobility and difficulty getting to the toilet and removing their clothing. Other causes of fecal incontinence include diarrhea caused by a variety of factors, constipation resulting in overflow incontinence, irritable bowel syndrome, incomplete evacuation, rectal neoplasms, neurological problems (e.g., stroke, multiple sclerosis, dementia), congenital malformations, accidental or surgical trauma, and pelvic floor denervation due to vaginal delivery, rectal prolapse, or chronic straining at stool (International Foundation for Functional Gastrointestinal Disorders, 2006a). Approximately 2.2% to 6.9% of the general population experiences fecal incontinence, but prevalence may be as high as 47% of elderly nursing home residents (International Foundation for Gastrointestinal Disorders, 2003). Although fecal incontinence is more common in older clients than in younger ones, it is not a normal part of aging (National Digestive Diseases Information Clearinghouse, 2004).

Both fecal and urinary incontinence are distressing to older clients because of the loss of control and feelings of reversion back to babyhood. Clients with incontinence may isolate themselves from others and become virtually housebound due to feelings of embarrassment and incompetence. They may also be reluctant to share problems of incontinence with health care providers. Community health nurses may need to advocate with older clients themselves to encourage them to seek treatment. They may also need to educate the public regarding incontinence and the potential for treatment.

Psychological Considerations

Psychological considerations that particularly influence the health of the older population include cognitive impairment, stress, and depression. Although cognitive impairment has a number of biophysical causes, it is addressed here because the majority of its effects are mental, with physiological effects arising from the mental deficits caused. Some other psychiatric illnesses will be noted in the elderly population, some of which may be superimposed on other physical illnesses or may result from physical illness. By 2030, 15 million older adults in the United States are expected to have some form of psychiatric illness, the most common of which will be dementia, depression, and anxiety disorders. Symptoms of schizophrenia seem to diminish with age, but older clients are at greater risk for extrapyramidal side effects of psychotropic medications than younger people. In addition, hearing and vision impairments that often accompany aging may increase the potential for confusion and delusions (Calandra, 2003).

Cognitive Impairment

Elements of cognitive function that may be impaired in the elderly include attention span, concentration, judgment, learning ability, memory, orientation, perception, problem solving, psychomotor ability, reaction time, and social intactness. Although slight decline in some of these areas (e.g., memory) or increased slowness in others (e.g., learning or reaction time) may be expected with age, marked changes are not consistent with the normal aging process. **Dementia** is a loss of intellectual function in multiple domains including memory, problem-solving ability, judgment, and others (Garand, Buckwalter, & Hall, 2000). *Dementia* is a general term used to encompass cognitive deficits that include progressive memory loss and at least one other symptom such as aphasia (difficulty with written or verbal communication), apraxia (inability to correctly use objects), or agnosia (loss of comprehension of auditory, visual, or tactile sensations) (Vogel, 2003). Dementia is found in 2% of people aged 65 to 70 years and 11% to 40% of those over 80 years of age (Chang, Nitta, Carter, & Markham, 2004).

Alzheimer's disease (AD) is the most common cause of dementia, affecting 3% of people over 65 years of age in the United States, and 20% of those over 85 years of age (Vogel, 2003). In the future as many as 47% of people over age 85 are expected to develop the disease. Similarly, the estimated prevalence of dementia in the United Kingdom is 4% to 6% (Minardi & Blanchard, 2004). During the 1990s, as many as 360,000 new cases were diagnosed each year in the United States, and this number is expected to climb to 959,000 per year by 2050 (Hurley et al., 2004; National Institute on Aging, 2002). There are currently 4 million Americans with Alzheimer's disease (Kolanowski, Fick, Waller, & Shea, 2004), and the number who will require care due to the effects of dementia is expected to increase by 350% before 2050 (Brown & Alligood, 2004). These figures may be even higher for ethnic minority groups who tend to have higher rates of cognitive impairment, dementia, and Alzheimer's disease than the non-Hispanic White population (Manly & Mayeux, 2004). Although Alzheimer's disease is the primary cause of dementia, it may also be caused by other conditions. For example, 20% to 60% of people with Parkinson's disease, especially severe disease, develop dementia. Other potential causes of dementia include Pick's disease (a rare degenerative neurological disease), Korsakov's syndrome (due to prolonged alcohol abuse), HIV infection, head trauma, and classic Creutzfeldt-Jakob disease (CDC, 2005a; Vogel, 2003). Circulatory deficiencies in chronic heart failure may also lead to cognitive deficits in memory, learning ability, executive function, and psychomotor speed. In fact, cognitive deficits may occur in as many as 30% to 80% of clients with congestive heart failure (Bennett, Suave, & Shaw, 2005).

Alzheimer's dementia usually progresses in stages characterized by progressive impairment. In the early stage, the client experiences mild cognitive impairment, increased difficulty learning and retaining new material, and difficulty with complex tasks that require reasoning, spatial orientation, and language. Additional characteristics of this stage include increasing difficulty with problem solving, managing finances, accomplishing routine tasks, and remembering specific words. People in middle-stage Alzheimer's disease exhibit inability to recognize family and friends not seen regularly, difficulty in completing simple tasks, wandering and becoming lost, mood changes, irritability, agitation, and sleep disturbance. Late Alzheimer's disease is characterized by a substantial decline in verbal, recognition, and comprehension skills; inability to comprehend language; gait disturbances and loss of the ability to walk; urinary incontinence; and loss of the ability to feed oneself and swallow, with consequent poor nutrition (Vogel, 2003).

The confusion experienced in Alzheimer's disease may be exacerbated by changes in one's surroundings, and maintenance of familiar surroundings may help clients remain comfortable and retain some functional abilities. This is due to the fact that priming or conditioning memory (habit) tends to be retained in many people with AD, in contrast to explicit memory (conscious, directed effort to recall information) and procedural memory related to learned skills such as feeding oneself (Son, Therrien, & Whall, 2002). The focused assessment below contains questions to guide assessment of cognitive function in older clients.

FOCUSED ASSESSMENT

Assessing Cognitive Function in Older Clients

Attention Span

- Does the client focus on a single activity to completion?
- Does the client move from activity to activity without completing any?

Concentration

- Is the client able to answer questions without wandering from the topic?
- Does the client ignore irrelevant stimuli while focusing on a task?
- Is the client easily distracted from a subject or task by external stimuli?

Intelligence

- Does the client understand directions and explanations given in everyday language?
- Is the client able to perform basic mathematical calculations?

Judgment

- Does the client engage in action appropriate to the situation?
- Are client behaviors based on an awareness of environmental conditions and possible consequences of action?
- Are the client's plans and goals realistic?
- Can the client effectively budget income?
- Is the client safe driving a car?

Learning Ability

- Is the client able to retain instructions for a new activity?
- Can the client recall information provided?
- Is the client able to correctly demonstrate new skills?

Memory

- Is the client able to remember and describe recent events in some detail?
- Is the client able to describe events from the past in some detail?

Orientation

- Can the client identify him- or herself by name?
- Is the client aware of where he or she is?
- Does the client recognize the identity and function of those around him or her?
- Does the client know what day and time it is?
- Is the client able to separate past, present, and future?

Perception

- Are the client's responses appropriate to the situation?
- Does the client exhibit evidence of hallucinations or illusions?
- Are explanations of events consistent with the events themselves?
- Can the client reproduce simple figures?

Problem Solving

- Is the client able to recognize problems that need resolution?
- Can the client envision alternative solutions to a given problem?
- Can the client weigh alternative solutions and select one appropriate to the situation?
- Can the client describe activities needed to implement the solution?

Psychomotor Ability

- Does the client exhibit repetitive movements that interfere with function?

Reaction Time

- Does the client take an unusually long time to respond to questions or perform motor activities?
- Does the client respond to questions before the question is completed?

Social Intactness

- Are the client's interactions with others appropriate to the situation?
- Is the client able to describe behaviors appropriate and inappropriate to a given situation?

Stress, Coping, and Depression

Like people in other age groups, older clients experience stress and have a broad range of abilities to cope with stress. Unlike others, however, older people may have fewer resources to allow them to cope effectively with stress. During 2001–2002, for example, 2.4% of the U.S. population over 65 years of age reported serious psychological distress (CDC, 2004a). Coping with the helplessness and loss of power often associated with chronic illness may be particularly difficult for older persons, who often need to achieve a balance between assistance and independence (Tanner, 2004). Studies of older people suggest that they prefer to manage stress themselves whenever possible. This has been found to be true in Asian populations, perhaps because of the cultural imperative to "save face" or in response to the absence of effective social support. Approaches to stress management found among older Asian clients include participation in enjoyable activities, having positive thoughts, and expressing thoughts and feelings to family and friends. Study subjects were less likely to seek professional help due to fear of stigma, cost, not wanting to worry others, difficulty communicating with providers, not knowing where to go, or perceptions that help would not be effective (Kwong & Kwan, 2004).

When older people cannot cope with the stress encountered in their lives, they may become depressed. Estimates of the overall prevalence of depression in the elderly vary from 2% (with 15% to 30% experiencing mild or "subsyndromal depression") (Antai-Otong, 2004) to 15% to 20% of the general elderly population (Loughlin, 2004; Weeks, McGann, Michaels, & Penninx, 2003) to 26% to 44% of the homebound elderly (Loughlin, 2004). According to the Federal Interagency Forum on Aging-related Statistics (2004), 11% of older men and 18% of women are clinically depressed. These figures may increase as "baby boomers" begin to age, because this group has higher rates of depression, suicide, anxiety, and substance abuse disorders than previous cohorts (McLeer, 2004).

Many older clients with depression have a previous personal history of depressive disorders; others develop depression for the first time late in life. Risk factors for late-onset depression include family history of depression, cognitive impairment, loss of interest in life, low socioeconomic status, inadequate support systems, negative life events such as retirement or loss, physical or mental comorbidity, and divorce, separation, or widowhood (Antai-Otong, 2004). Depression has also been linked to loneliness and decreased life satisfaction (Minardi & Blanchard, 2004).

In addition to diminished quality of life, depression in the elderly has been associated with diminished immunity and increased risk of substance abuse as a means of coping with depression (Calandra, 2003). Depression has also been linked to falls in the elderly, perhaps as a result of postural and gait changes that often occur in the context of depression. Conversely, antidepressant therapy may also predispose the elderly to falls (Turcu et al., 2004). Depression increases health care use and costs and may lead to functional decline and dependence (Weeks et al., 2003).

Depression may be difficult to diagnose in the elderly for several reasons. Comorbid depression is often missed in the presence of critical illness or undertreated when it is recognized (Weeks et al., 2003). Providers and family members may miss symptoms of depression, attributing them to aging. At the same time, older clients may feel shame related to their perceived inability to cope and not voice their feelings of depression, or may fail to recognize them for what they are (Calandra, 2003). Many medications used to treat chronic illness in the elderly may also contribute to feelings of depression. Some authors have voiced a need for standardized tools for screening for depression in the elderly that account for the many confounding factors (Weeks et al., 2003).

At its extreme, depression may lead to suicide, which is a significant problem among the elderly, particularly among older men. From 2000 to 2003, the average annual suicide rate for people over 65 years of age in the United States was 27.34 per 100,000 men and 4.43 per 100,000 women (National Center for Injury Prevention and Control, 2005a). Suicide rates increase with age for older men, but decrease slightly among women. In 2002, for example, suicide mortality affected 13.5 per 100,000 men aged 65 to 74 years, rose to 17.7 per 100,000 for 75- to 84-year-olds, and was highest among men 85 years or older. Comparable figures for women in these age groups were 4.1, 4.2, and 3.8 per 100,000 women (CDC, 2004a). White men over 85 years of age have the highest suicide rate of any age or racial group (American Association of Retired Persons [AARP], 2002).

Physical Environmental Considerations

Conditions in the physical environment also affect the health of older populations. For example, living in neighborhoods with problems of traffic, noise, crime, trash and litter, poor lighting, and inadequate public transportation has been associated with increased risk of functional loss among elderly residents. As the number of problems in the neighborhood increased, greater loss of physical function occurred. Neighborhood factors have also been

---

BUILDING OUR KNOWLEDGE BASE

Turcu et al. (2004) found that among patients who were admitted to a geriatric unit as a result of a fall, those who were depressed had lower motor ability scores than those who were not depressed. They noted, however, that their data did not suggest whether depression was a contributing factor in the falls or was a consequence of injury sustained in a fall. How might you design a study to address this issue?

linked to problems of social isolation, hearing impairment, cognitive impairment, and depression in the elderly (Balfour & Kaplan, 2002). Similar findings have been noted for functional deterioration in unsafe neighborhoods (Blazer, Sachs-Ericsson, & Hybels, 2005).

Physical environmental conditions may also have a direct effect on physical health status. For example, in 2002, 45% of older persons in the United States lived in counties with ozone levels above federal standards. This figure represented an increase from 26% in 2000. Another 19% lived in areas with excessive particulate matter (Federal Interagency Forum on Aging-related Statistics, 2004). Both ozone and particulate matter have an adverse effect on respiratory function, particularly in people with chronic respiratory diseases. In fact, a 4-year national study found that older people had higher rates of cardiovascular and respiratory diseases than younger people when exposed to fine particle pollution, and that disease rates increased with age even among the elderly (National Institute of Environmental Health Sciences, 2006).

Safety hazards are another major consideration with respect to the physical environment of the elderly. Older clients may live in older housing with multiple safety hazards. Or, given recent energy prices, older persons on fixed incomes may have significantly more difficulty heating or cooling their homes than in the past. Both heat and cold have more profound effects on elderly persons than on younger ones due to changes in heat-regulating mechanisms that occur with aging. For example, heat wave mortality has been associated with increasing age, particularly in the presence of lower socioeconomic status, poor housing quality, and lack of air conditioning (Center for Climatic Research, 2004). The companion *Community Assessment Reference Guide* 🖉 designed to accompany this text provides a tool for assessing home safety for older clients.

Conversely, older people may live in settings that promote health and independence. Residential areas that provide opportunities for safe exercise by the elderly or assist with accomplishment of routine tasks can delay functional deterioration. Unfortunately, in 2002, only 2% of the Medicare population lived in settings with at least one such service available (Federal Interagency Forum on Aging-related Statistics, 2004).

Sociocultural Considerations

Sociocultural considerations that have a major impact on the health of the elderly population include family roles and responsibilities, social support, and economic and employment factors. Abuse and violence are other sociocultural factors that have a profound influence on the health of this vulnerable population.

Family Roles and Responsibilities

Family configurations and the resulting roles and responsibilities change over time. Children grow up and marry or move away; spouses divorce or die. Older clients may need to adjust to a variety of changes in family roles and responsibilities, some of which are looked forward to and some of which are not. In 2003, 3% of people over 65 years of age in the United States had never married, 56.5% were married, 31.6% were widowed, and 8% were divorced (U.S. Census Bureau, 2005).

Living arrangements for older clients are many and varied. In 2003, people over 65 years of age constituted 36% of those living alone in the United States and constituted 26% of heads of households. Thirty one percent of people lived alone, 54% with spouses, and 15% with others (usually grown children) (U.S. Census Bureau, 2005). Women constitute 80% of older persons living alone, and older women are three times more likely than older men to be widowed (Callen, 2004). In fact, approximately 40% of all older women live alone, compared to 73% of older men who live with spouses (Leenerts, Teel, & Pendleton, 2002). Baby boomers are particularly likely to live alone as they age (Plese, 2002).

Older people are accepting greater responsibility for raising grandchildren than in the past. In 2000, for example, an estimated 42% of people over 65 years of age assumed at least partial responsibility for caring for their grandchildren (U.S. Census Bureau, 2005). In 2003, 14.5% of U.S. grandmothers had been caring for their grandchildren for 6 months or longer. These responsibilities

GLOBAL PERSPECTIVES

*I*n many cultural groups, care of aging parents is expected to be performed by children. Lee and Law (2004) noted that in Hong Kong, this traditional pattern of intergenerational care is rapidly changing due to societal changes. Some of these changes include the increasing economic pressure on women to be employed, career plans, smaller families with fewer children to share the burden of elder care, and weakening family bonds. Although the pattern of care is changing, most elderly residents in Hong Kong have engaged in little or no planning with respect to retirement. The authors make the case that advance planning with respect to financial, health, residential, and psychological issues is associated with better adjustment and quality of life among retirees. In their study, however, they found that most Hong Kong residents moving toward retirement age had engaged in only 3 of 19 retirement planning activities, if any retirement planning was done at all. More than half of the respondents (52%) had initiated financial savings for retirement, and 57% had begun to quit unhealthful behaviors such as smoking to enhance health status. An additional 51.5% had begun to exercise regularly to promote their health. Far fewer people had engaged in such activities as buying life or accident insurance, arranging for regular health care services, planning living arrangements, considering how to spend time after retirement, obtaining information about retirement from a variety of sources, or discussing retirement with family, friends, and others.

To what extent do you think these findings are typical of the U.S. pre-retirement population? Of people in other parts of the world? How might you go about obtaining information on retirement attitudes and planning practices in other cultural settings?

often devolved on grandparents when their adult children died, were divorced, were mentally ill, or were incarcerated. Caring for grandchildren has been linked to depression, insomnia, hypertension, diabetes, functional limitations, and poor self-reported health in caregivers. In fact, in one study, caring for grandchildren 21 hours a week or more increased coronary heart disease risk by 150% (Lee, Colditz, Berkman, & Kawachi, 2003).

Caregiving responsibilities may also be undertaken by older persons in the care of aging spouses. Societal policies to promote "aging in place," or allowing people to remain in their own homes as they grow older, will increase the requirements for assistance and caregiving by family members (Magnusson & Hanson, 2005). More than one fifth of U.S. households include someone who requires caregiving, and in 81% of these households the recipient of care is someone over 50 years of age (Plese, 2005a). More than half of the adult population in the United States (54%) have provided care to a family member in a given year; 44% of these caregivers are men. A surprising number of caregivers are young people, many of them young men. Studies indicate that anywhere from 12% to 18% of adult caregivers in the United States are between the ages of 18 and 25 years (Levine et al., 2005). A caregiver is defined as "an individual aged 16 or over who provides or intends to provide a substantial amount of care on a regular basis for another individual who is 18 or over" (Merrell, Kinsella, Murphy, Philpin, & Ali, 2005, p. 550).

Family caregivers have been described as an "unpaid extension of the health care system" (Hunt, quoted in Plese, 2005a, p. 5). The average family caregiver, for instance, provides nearly 18 hours of care per week, and 17% of caregivers provide more than 40 hours of care a week (Plese, 2005a). For women, in particular, caring may become their "life's work" by the time they have spent several years caring for children, then for aging parents, and later for aging spouses (Plese, 2002). Caregiver responsibilities range from personal physical care and assistance with activities of daily living to supervision to financial management and guardianship to complete care (Davis, Burgio, Buckwalter, & Weaver, 2004). Roughly one fourth of family caregivers provide assistance with three or more ADLs, and 80% assist with IADLs. Both men and women provide assistance with IADLs, but women are more likely than men to assist with personal care. The broad range of responsibilities required of caregivers necessitates expertise in many areas that some older clients do not have (Plese, 2005a).

Research has suggested that when caregiving is based on mutually agreed-upon rules for the relationship, there is less strain for both caregiver and recipient (Coeling, Biordi, & Theis, 2003). Unfortunately, such mutual decision making often cannot occur in the face of Alzheimer's disease and other forms of dementia. Studies of caregivers of older people with AD indicate a number of concerns and challenges. These include dealing with change, managing competing responsibilities, providing the broad spectrum of care discussed above, finding and using community resources, and dealing with physical and emotional responses to caregiving (Farran, Loukissa, Perraud, & Paun, 2004). More than half (57%) of those caring for elderly family members are employed, and an estimated 12% of the U.S. workforce provide care for elderly relatives, yet only 42% of large employers have programs in place to assist family caregivers, leaving caregivers to juggle work and caregiving responsibilities on their own (Plese, 2005a). Some states provide for family medical leave for care of ill family members. Unfortunately, although family medical leaves permit caretakers to keep their jobs, most such leaves are unpaid, and caretakers may not be able to afford to take advantage of them.

Frequently, even when resources are available from employers or others in the community, older caregivers are not aware of them or do not perceive themselves as caregivers eligible for assistance. Older caregivers have been found to be less likely to request assistance from either formal or informal support networks, since they may perceive their care as part of an ongoing relationship, rather than as caregiving per se (McGarry & Arthur, 2001). Changes in social structure related to smaller families, more women working, higher divorce rates, and an increasingly mobile population have diminished the social networks of many older people, often leaving them to deal with caregiving tasks in relative isolation (Hoskins, Coleman, & McNeely, 2005).

Most caregivers for people with Alzheimer's disease are aging spouses who have their own health problems that are compounded by the physical and psychological burdens of caregiving. The ability to initiate or continue caregiving activities is predicated on maintenance of the same level of health in both caregiver and recipient (McGarry & Arthur, 2001). Unfortunately, the stress of caregiving often leads to diminished health for caregivers. For example, spouses caring for persons with dementia have been found to have more anxiety disorders, falls, rheumatologic disease, and diabetes. Caregiver strain has also been associated with increased cardiovascular disease risk (Kolanowski et al., 2004). Women caregivers of aging spouses have been referred to as "hidden patients" because of the lack of attention to the physical and emotional effects of caregiving (Jansson, Nordberg, & Grafstrom, 2001). Older

Think Advocacy

What groups might be approached to form a coalition to advocate for support services for caretakers of older clients with Alzheimer's disease? Why would you include these specific groups in your coalition?

caregivers, in general, have poorer self-reported health status than their non-caregiving counterparts, and caregivers may not attend to their own health care needs. For example, 85% of older caregivers in one study reported previously engaging in a variety of health-promotive activities, but only 63% still performed these activities at the time of the study (Matthews, Dunbar-Jacob, Sereika, Schulz, & McDowell, 2004).

Caregiver strain is also heightened by changes in relationships, particularly in the face of dementia. Relationship changes occur with both the care recipient and other family members (Vellone, Sansoni, & Cohen, 2002). Loss of companionship of the care recipient and social isolation are two of the relationship changes that Alzheimer's caregivers have noted as creating strain (Hoskins et al., 2005). Caregivers may also experience loneliness, which has been found to be less frequent when caregiver and recipient live together. Cohabitation, however, may lead to greater social isolation when activities with others are constrained by caregiving responsibilities (Ekwall, Sivberg, & Hallberg, 2005). In some cultural groups, caregiving may also be accompanied by the stress of stigma. For example, Chinese caregivers for people with Alzheimer's disease face stigma related to cultural perceptions of AD as a result of fate, wrongdoing, worrying too much, craziness, bad feng shui, or contagion (Zhan, 2004).

Caregiving by older people also has financial burdens for both caregivers and for society. For example, approximately 60% of care costs for persons with dementia are paid out-of-pocket by caregivers (Kolanowski et al., 2004). Average monthly costs for caregiving for those with the highest care needs amount to $200 to $325 (Plese, 2005a).

Social Support

Social support is another major sociocultural influence on the health of the elderly population. Social support occurs at societal, neighborhood, and individual levels. At the societal level, social support is a function of the sense of solidarity felt by subsegments of the population with other segments. In many European countries, for example, there is greater solidarity in which younger people feel a greater responsibility for the welfare of older generations than is usually the case in the United States (Edwards, 2004). In stable neighborhoods, opportunities for social interaction increase social support available from neighbors who can be called upon at short notice because of their propinquity (McGarry & Arthur, 2001).

Social support may arise from either informal or formal social networks. A **social network** is the web of social relationships within which one interacts with other people and from which one receives social support. Social support includes emotional, instrumental, or financial assistance from the social network. The informal social network consists of friends, family members, and neighbors, whereas the formal network comprises health and social service providers. Religious affiliation may provide a form of social support that often bridges the formal and informal networks. For example, many congregations provide material and emotional support to their members. In addition, religious affiliation has been associated with greater use of preventive services (Benjamins & Brown, 2004).

Some authors have noted that examination of the health of elderly populations should include consideration both of the social support available and perceptions of its adequacy among recipients (Tanner, 2004). Most older persons seek social support most often from family members, particularly spouses. In one Japanese study, for example, for married older adults with spouses, the spouse was the most important source of social support, followed by adult children and others. For elders without spouses, adult children were the most important source of support (Okabayashi, Liang, Krause, Akiyama, & Sugisawa, 2004). The quality of support provided, however, is affected by several factors, including residential propinquity, co-residence, and past relationships (Davey, Janke, & Savla, 2005). Residential propinquity is associated with household assistance, but not financial assistance, and prior financial support from parents has been linked to later financial support of parents by their children. Co-residence may involve mutual support between generations or couples. For example, adult children may provide housing for their parents, who, in turn, provide assistance with childcare.

For immigrant families, intergenerational support may be transnational in nature, where some family members live in one country and some in another. **Transnationalism** is defined as "the process by which immigrants forge and sustain multistranded social relations that link together their societies of origin and resettlement" (Basch, Glick, Schiller, & Szanton Blanc, as quoted in Burholt & Wenger, 2005, p. 154). Transnational social support may be made more difficult by monetary exchanges, immigration laws, and other forces that regulate movement of people and objects across international borders. Some refugee immigrant families may not even have transnational support available. Many refugee families have been separated or have had family members killed. In addition, family members left in the country of origin may not have the freedom to contact immigrant members or may have little in the way of support to offer. Community health nurses can be actively involved in linking these clients to other sources of support (e.g., churches or other organizations). They may also advocate for the availability of necessary support services for these older clients.

Economic and Employment Factors

Although older people in the United States are somewhat better off financially as a total group than some other age groups, economic forces still have a significant impact on the health of the elderly. In 2002, for example, the median household income for people over 65 years of age was $23,152, up from $16,882 in 1974 (Federal Interagency Forum on Aging-related Statistics, 2004), compared to a median income of $42,409 for all U.S. households (U.S. Census Bureau, 2005). From 1984 to 2001, the median net worth of older households increased by 82% (Federal Interagency Forum on Aging-related Statistics, 2004), and older adults control 70% of U.S. wealth and 75% of the wealth of the United Kingdom (Plese, 2005b). Poverty among U.S. elderly declined from 25% in 1970 to 11% in 1996 (Imamura, 2002), and from 1965 to 1986 social welfare spending for the elderly in the United States increased from 21% of national expenditures to 33% (Newacheck & Benjamin, 2004). Despite these figures, approximately 10% of the U.S. elderly population in 2003 had an annual income below poverty level (U.S. Census Bureau, 2004b). Nearly a third (31%) of households headed by persons over 65 years of age had annual incomes below $15,000 in 2002, and the elderly comprised nearly 9% of food stamp recipients (U.S. Census Bureau, 2005). More than 20% of U.S. elderly fall into the lowest quartile for income, compared to only 6% in the Netherlands (Edwards, 2004), and older women are twice as likely as men to be poor (National Center for Chronic Disease Prevention and Health Promotion, 2002a).

Most of the income for this age group (39%) derives from Social Security payments, 25% from continued earnings, 19% from retirement pensions, and 14% from other asset income. For the lowest fifth of the population, 83% of annual income is derived from Social Security. Although many older people own their own homes, 40% of those in the lowest quintile for annual income spend 40% of their income on housing alone (Federal Interagency Forum on Aging-related Statistics, 2004).

Income levels influence access to health care as well as to other necessary goods and services. For example, in 2003, less than 54% of older adults with incomes below poverty level received influenza vaccinations, compared to 58% of the total Medicare population and 71% of those who could afford supplemental insurance in addition to Medicare (Immunization Services Division, 2005). Similarly, in 1999 1.2 million Medicare beneficiaries did not have a prescription filled, half of them due to the cost of the medication (AARP, 2002). In addition, in one study, socioeconomic status as measured by home and car ownership was associated with decreased risk of disability in older men (Ebrahim et al., 2004).

Employment and retirement are other factors that affect the health of older people indirectly through their effects on economic status as well as more directly. In 2003, 3.3% of the U.S. population over 65 years of age were employed, with approximately equal percentages among men and women (U.S. Census Bureau, 2005). Older workers are just as productive as younger ones,

but they do have increased health risks in some areas. For example, occupational injury rates in 2002 were nearly twice as high among those over age 65 as among other age groups (CDC, 2004a), and disability risk is higher in occupations involving manual labor than in other occupational groups (Ebrahim et al., 2004). As noted earlier, older workers are also at greater risk of disease and complications related to influenza, which is rapidly transmitted in workplace environments.

There is a great deal of concern lately about retirement funding. Much has been written in the United States about the Social Security and Medicare systems in particular. At present, most countries have set 65 years of age as the minimum age for drawing public pension benefits, and many employers have mandatory retirement at a specific age. Only Australia and the United States prohibit mandatory retirement except in certain age-dependent occupations (Edwards, 2004). Retirees throughout the world have been promised benefits of 37% to 70% of their earnings per year, with the United States about in the middle of this range at 45% (Plese, 2005b). Because of increased longevity,

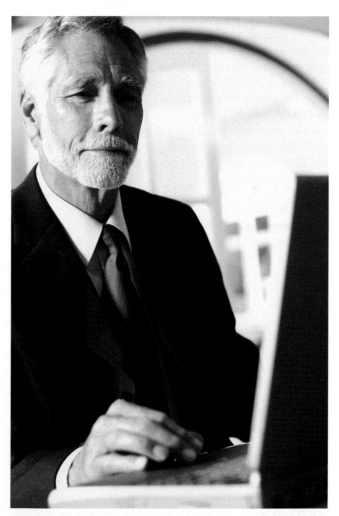

Older individuals may continue to be successfully employed beyond the typical retirement age. (Image Source)

many people can expect to spend a quarter of their lives in retirement (Lee & Law, 2004). The **old-age dependency ratio**, or the number of nonworking elders to workers, is expected to double in the developed world and triple in less developed nations from current figures of one elder per nine workers to one to four, or even one to two. Another related concept is the **elderly support ratio**, or the number of people over 65 years of age per 100 people aged 20 to 64 years (Division of Adult and Community Health, 2003c). Increases in these two ratios result in a declining tax base from which to fund services to the elderly as well as other segments of the population.

With the increasing numbers of elderly, the cost of public pension and health care benefits is expected to increase from 12% to 24% of the gross domestic product (GDP) by 2040. To stabilize expenditures at the current percentage of GDP, benefits would need to be cut by 30% to 60% (Plese, 2005b). With respect to health care services, however, reducing benefits would be a short-term solution at best. Reducing access to and payment for health care will only add to later societal costs for conditions that could have been prevented or treated in much less expensive fashion earlier.

In addition to the increased expenditures for elderly services, there will be a stagnation of markets with less money available for other forms of personal and government spending. More caregiving will be required of fewer young family members, resulting in what has been labeled the "4-2-1 phenomenon"—four aging grandparents and two aging parents to be cared for by one working adult (Plese, 2005b). Some countries such as China and Japan have already begun to experience this phenomenon.

Another result of the aging of the population is an aged workforce and employers losing skilled and experienced employees to retirement. Because of the smaller number of younger people in the workforce, employers will have difficulty replacing these people at all, much less with people of comparable levels of expertise. One solution proposed to address all of these concerns is that of "reinventing the last third of life as a time of continued productivity rather than retired leisure" (Plese, 2005, p. 8). Retaining older employees in the workforce would have benefits for employers as well as for the employees. Employers will continue to retain highly competent employees who will continue to be productive rather than a drain on society. Continued employment, whether paid or volunteer, full-time or part-time, has been found to have health benefits for older persons. Not working, on the other hand, has been linked to increased incidence of suicide and other health effects. In one study, for example, not working reduced longevity by as much as 14 years (Plese, 2005b). Retaining employees in the workforce might have the added benefit of improving the health of family members as well. For instance, news media recently addressed a new

phenomenon in Japan called "retired husband syndrome." This syndrome is experienced by wives of men who retire and expect their wives to meet their demands for service (N. A., 2005).

For older clients to continue to be productively employed, a number of changes will be required in the workplace and in society at large. Increased emphasis on health promotion in the workplace will be required to keep employees healthy and productive. Societal changes will be required to promote a move to an "age-neutral" society in which older workers are not seen as less creative or productive. Employers will also need to develop more flexible work patterns and schedules to accommodate employees who prefer part-time work and retraining programs to help older employees keep up with new skill needs. Finally, both local and societal action will be required to end age discrimination in and out of the workplace (Plese, 2005b).

Abuse and Violence

One final sociocultural consideration that affects the health of the older population is that of violence and abuse. The increase in the older population has been accompanied by a disproportionate increase in elder abuse or maltreatment. Between 1986 and 1996, reports of elder abuse increased by 150%, compared to only a 10% increase in the population. In part, this increase may be due to better reporting, but also probably stems from an actual increase in abusive events. Elder abuse is defined as "the mistreatment, neglect, or exploitation of an elderly person" (Orhon, 2002, p. 22).

From 3% to 6% of people over 65 years of age in the United States experience abuse or neglect each year (Meeks-Sjostrom, 2004). This amounts to 700,000 to 1.2 million cases of abuse per year (Fulmer, 2002). In 2001, more than 33,000 older adults were treated for assault-related injuries in U.S. emergency departments (National Center for Injury Prevention and Control, 2003). Elder abuse occurs throughout the world, with 27.5% of elders in Hong Kong reporting at least one incident of abuse by a caretaker in the past year and overall prevalence of abuse at 4.6% of elders in Australia and 15.5% in Greece. In Canada, the prevalence of abuse ranges from 1.1% for verbal abuse in some studies to 20% for financial abuse. In other studies in the United Kingdom, 45% of caregivers admitted to at least one form of abuse of an older person (Yan & Tang, 2004). The average U.S. homicide rate for people over 65 years of age from 2000 to 2003 was 2.3 per 100,000 population overall (CDC, 2004a), 2.8 per 100,000 men, and 1.38 per 100,000 women (National Center for Injury Prevention and Control, 2005a). Elder abuse may be physical, verbal or emotional, sexual, or financial, or involve neglect, abandonment, or self-neglect (Fulmer, 2002; Meeks-Sjostrom, 2004; Mouton et al., 2004), and its effects may be physical or psychological. Elder abuse is discussed in more detail in Chapter 32∞.

Behavioral Considerations

Research has indicated that sociocultural and behavioral lifestyle factors have greater effects on biological systems in the older population than aging itself (Williams, 2005). Behavioral factors, such as diet and other consumption patterns, physical activity, sexuality, and medication use, have important influences on the health of the older population. Factors in each of these areas will be briefly addressed.

Diet

Diet figures significantly in many health problems experienced by older clients. Conversely, health problems such as loss of teeth may affect dietary intake. Nearly 8% of the total U.S. population is edentulous (without any teeth), but this percentage increases to nearly 25% of those over 60 years of age (Beltran-Aguilar et al., 2005). Presence or absence of teeth, diminished gastric secretion and motility, and diminished sense of taste or smell may affect older clients' ability or desire to eat a nutritious diet.

Some of the nutrition-related problems experienced by the older population include malnutrition, obesity, elevated cholesterol levels, dehydration, and deficiencies in certain specific nutrients. Between 2% and 16% of the elderly population in the United States is malnourished. Annual hospitalization costs for malnourished elders are twice those of older people who are not malnourished, with an average length of stay 5.6 days longer. In one study of older clients admitted to an acute care setting, none of those assessed as malnourished perceived themselves to be so (Callen, 2004).

Another 30% of the elderly population is obese, and during the period of 1999 to 2002, 69% of all those over 65 years of age in the United States were overweight (Federal Interagency Forum on Aging-related Statistics, 2004). Older individuals with disabilities are even more likely to be obese. For example, a 1998–1999 survey in eight states and the District of Columbia found that, although obesity affected 14% of all those over 65 years of age, 24% of disabled elderly were obese (Division of Human Development and Disability, 2002). In addition, nearly 14% of men and 33% of women aged 65 to 74 years had elevated cholesterol levels. These figures decreased slightly in the population over 75 years of age to 10% and 26.5%, respectively (CDC, 2004a).

Interestingly, obesity in women over 70 years of age has been associated with the absence of health promotion measures. For example, obese older women were less likely than women of normal weight to receive influenza immunizations in one study (Østbye, Taylor, Yancy, & Krause, 2005). These women may choose not to seek care for routine health promotion due to embarrassment regarding their weight or fears that providers will chastise them for their obesity.

Chronic dehydration is another dietary problem that occurs frequently in older populations. In one study, as many as 48% of elderly clients seen in emergency departments suffered from chronic dehydration. Dehydration leads to loss of muscle function, depression, altered states of consciousness, and renal failure and contributes to increased potential for medication toxicity, hypo- or hyperthermia, and infection. Dehydration is often unrecognized in the elderly, and mortality may be as much as seven times higher in dehydrated elders than in the general elderly population. Annual costs of dehydration in the older population are estimated at more than $1 billion, but this may be an underestimate because of the tendency for this diagnosis to be missed in older clients (Bennett, Thomas, & Riegel, 2004).

Finally, older clients may be lacking in specific nutrients such as iron, protein, and calcium. Calcium, in particular, is needed to prevent or ameliorate the effects of osteoporosis. Many older women, however, do not know that they should continue calcium intake into their older years. In one study, even after an educational intervention related to the need for dietary calcium, many women most at risk for osteoporosis had not increased their calcium intake (Sandison, Gray, & Reid, 2004). Many older clients also take a variety of vitamins and food supplements. In fact, it is estimated that two thirds of people aged 60 to 100 years take vitamins and food supplements, and limit caffeine, sugar, and fat intake (Matthews et al., 2004).

Other Consumption Patterns

Other consumption patterns that affect the health status of the older adult population include alcohol and tobacco use. According to the Federal Interagency Forum on Aging-related Statistics (2004), 10% of older men and 9% of women smoked in 2002. Elderly smokers are more likely than their younger counterparts to have health-related effects due to diminished respiratory function as a result of aging. An estimated 70% of smokers want to quit the habit, and 46% of them make the attempt (Andrews, Heath, & Graham-Garcia, 2004).

Many older clients believe that smoking cessation will not make much difference with respect to their health. Smoking cessation at any age, however, can have beneficial effects. For example, smoking cessation at age 65 years has been found to add 1.4 to 2 years of life for men and 2.7 to 3.7 years for women (Taylor, Hasselblad, Henley, Thun, & Sloan, 2002).

Alcohol consumption may also affect the health of the older adult population. In one study, half of the men and women 55 to 65 years of age consumed alcohol three or more times a week, and 38% of women and 48% of men reported seven or more drinks per week (Moos, Brennan, Schutte, & Moos, 2004). Misuse of alcohol and other drugs (e.g., benzodiazepines) is relatively common, particularly among older women. An estimated 1.8 million women (7%) over 59 years of age abuse alcohol, and 2.8 million (11%) abuse psychotropic drugs. Approximately one third of women who misuse drugs and alcohol begin to do so after 60 years of age.

Aging diminishes the ability of the body to metabolize alcohol and other drugs. Increased body fat also results in slower excretion of alcohol, which is a water-soluble substance. These factors contribute to higher alcohol-related mortality among older women than men (50% to 100% higher) (Finfgeld-Connett, 2004). In addition to its direct effects on the body, alcohol-related disease increases the risk of hip fracture by more than twofold (Yuan et al., 2001).

Physical Activity

As with their perceptions of the need for continued calcium intake, many older people do not believe they need to engage in much physical activity. Exercise by older adults, however, has been shown to prevent disability and hospital admission, improve lipid profiles, reduce body fat, and prevent osteoporosis (Schneider, Mercer, Herning, Smith, & Prysak, 2004). In addition, exercise in the presence of congestive heart failure increases exercise capacity, decreases symptoms, and improves quality of life (Resnick, 2004).

Exercise provides both physical and psychological benefits for older clients. In the physical realm, exercise contributes to improved cardiovascular function, better control of hypertension and hyperlipidemia, cancer prevention, and prevention of gallstones as well as osteoporosis. Additional physical benefits include reduction in diabetes risk; increased muscle, bone, and joint strength; and decreased risk of falls (National Center for Chronic Disease Prevention and Health Promotion, 2002b). Psychologically, physical activity contributes to emotional well-being and improved self-assurance and self-concept and may be linked to improvements in cognition, at least to perceptions of improvement (Blumenthal & Gullette, 2002).

In spite of evidence regarding the benefits of physical activity, many older adults remain sedentary. About half of those who start an exercise program stop within 6 months. According to 2000 figures, fewer than a third of people aged 65 to 74 years engaged in 20 minutes of moderate physical activity three or more times a week (Schneider et al., 2004). These figures decrease with age, with only 9% of people over 85 years of age engaging in regular physical activity (Federal Interagency Forum on Aging-related Statistics, 2004). In the United States, less than 6% of older adults meet the national objectives for both physical activity and strength training (Division of Nutrition and Physical Activity, 2004).

Sexuality

Sexuality considerations related to the older population include knowledge, attitudes, values, and behaviors, as well as changes in anatomy and physiology due to the aging process (Johnson, 2004). Research indicates that primary health care providers assume that older clients are asexual and rarely discuss sexual issues with members of the older adult population. Evidence suggests that, despite these perceptions, sexuality continues to be

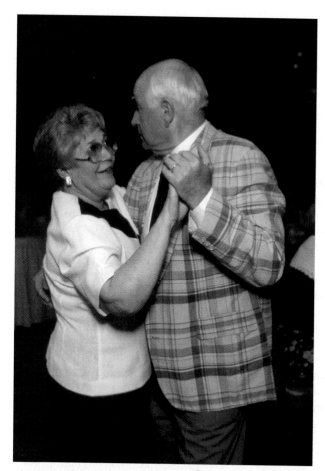

Physical activity is an important element of physical and mental health. (Patrick J. Watson)

an area of importance for many older people. In fact, in the United Kingdom, more than 16,000 people over 50 years of age are seen annually in genitourinary clinics, most of them for sexually transmitted diseases. Similarly, people over 50 years of age constitute 11% of those with AIDS in the UK, most of whom acquired their infection through sexual activity (Gott, Hinchliff, & Galena, 2004).

Older clients may also have concerns regarding sexual dysfunction. Because most older people grew up in an era when sexuality was not a topic for discussion, they may find it difficult to talk about such concerns with health care providers. As we saw in Chapter 18∞, many of the medications used to treat chronic diseases common in the elderly cause impotence in men. Similarly, aging may decrease vaginal secretions, making intercourse painful for older women. Both older men and women may experience diminished sexual interest, which may interfere with marital intimacy.

Medication Use

Medication use and misuse are significant factors in the health of the older adult population. Medication use is increasing among the elderly. For example, according to the Federal Interagency Forum on Aging-related

Statistics (2004), older persons in the United States filled an average of 18 prescriptions per year in 1992; by 2000 this figure had increased to 30 prescriptions per person per year. Approximately 94% of women over 65 years of age take at least one prescription medication, 57% take five or more, and 12% take ten or more medications. Among older men, 91% take at least one medication, 44% take five or more, and 12% take ten or more prescription drugs (Logue, 2002). Approximately 40% of all U.S. prescriptions are written for people over 65 years of age (Edlund, 2004). On average, older persons take three times as many prescription medications as younger ones, and the incidence of drug reactions and interactions is two to three times higher than in younger people (Yoon & Horne, 2001).

In addition to taking multiple prescription medications, older adults may also use a variety of over-the-counter (OTC) medications and herbal therapies, compounding the potential for drug interactions and adverse reactions. An estimated 90% of older adults use OTC medications in addition to prescription drugs (Edlund, 2004). In one study, nearly 36% of rural elderly women used some type of self-directed complementary therapy, primarily herbal preparations used for health promotion purposes (Shreffler-Grant, Weinert, Nichols, & Ide, 2005). In another study, 43% of older women used herbal preparations, for an average of 2.5 preparations used per woman. In addition, the women in the study used an average of 3.2 prescription drugs each, and 3.8 nonprescription medications (Yoon & Horne, 2001). A subsequent study by the same authors found that the herbal products most often used were ginger, garlic, glucosamine, ginkgo, and aloe, and that older women frequently used complementary therapies in conjunction with prescription medications (Yoon & Horne, 2004). It is estimated that as many as 3 million U.S. elders may be at risk for herb/vitamin/prescription drug interactions (Edlund, 2004).

In addition to the combination of multiple drugs, OTC medications, and herbal remedies, medication use in the elderly is complicated by the effects of aging. As age increases, lipid compartments increase from 14% of body weight to 30%, which has implications for drug absorption and metabolism (Williams, 2005). These changes in drug metabolism increase the risk of adverse reactions as drug excretion slows and the potential for overdose increases (Caterino, Emond, & Camargo, 2004).

Older clients may also have difficulty taking medications as recommended. An estimated 50% of the elderly have difficulty adhering to medication regimens. Medication misuse and nonadherence have been linked to more than 11% of hospital admissions and 10.5% of emergency department visits by older clients. Overall nonadherence has been found to range from 14% to 77% among older populations, depending on the method used to measure nonadherence. Using electronic monitors, one study found that 43% of clients underdosed,

overdosed, or missed a dose for more than 20% of their medications (Schlenk, Dunbar-Jacob, & Engberg, 2004).

Factors that contribute to medication nonadherence include drug regimen characteristics, health beliefs, side effects, extent of social support, depression, and cognitive function (Schlenk et al., 2004). Drug regimens may be complicated or burdensome in terms of the number of medications, the number and timing of doses, and the number of providers prescribing different medications. In one study, for example, 54% of older clients had more than one prescribing physician, and 36% used more than one pharmacy (Safran et al., 2005). Health beliefs regarding personal self-efficacy or medication efficacy may also affect adherence, as does the occurrence of annoying side effects. In fact, in one study, 57% of older people discontinued prescription medications on their own initiative, 92% of those in response to side effects (Schlenk et al., 2004).

The availability of social support has also been linked to medication adherence. For example, adherence has been found to increase in the presence of assistance with ADLs and to decrease for persons living alone. Depression is also a contributing factor. In one study, depressed clients were nonadherent with medications on 55% of days, whereas nondepressed clients were only nonadherent 31% of days (Schlenk et al., 2004). Cognitive functional ability also affects medication adherence in terms of forgetting to take medications or inability to understand the regimen in terms of dose, timing, route of administration, and other instructions.

Cost of medications is another significant factor in nonadherence. Average annual drug costs per Medicare enrollee in 2000 were $1,340. In a 2003 study conducted by the Kaiser Family Foundation, average annual drug costs per Medicare enrollee had increased to $2,322, and 40% of enrollees had annual drug costs over $2,000 (Brinckerhoff & Coleman, 2005). In another 2003 study, 27% of all seniors studied lacked prescription drug coverage under their health insurance. This figure increased to a third of poor and near-poor elderly. Approximately 26% of participants reported forgoing at least one prescription in the previous year due to cost, and another 12% reported cutting back on basic needs to be able to afford medications. One third of participants reported $100 or more out-of-pocket expenses for medications each month (Safran et al., 2005), and 95% of the U.S. population over 65 years of age had out-of-pocket expenses (Federal Interagency Forum on Aging-related Statistics, 2004). In 2002, out-of-pocket drug costs for older Americans amounted to $87 billion, and this figure was expected to rise to $120 billion by 2005 (Brinckerhoff & Coleman, 2005). Cost may also figure into fears of running out of medications and spacing doses at wider intervals than ordered to conserve medication (Alemagno, Niles, & Treiber, 2004).

During the late 1990s, spending on prescription drugs increased 15% per year for several years. From

1997 to 2001, Medicare expenditures for drugs increased 71.6% more than inflation rates, and this was prior to the advent of Medicare prescription drug coverage. These increasing costs have been the result of a 10% increase in the number of elderly using prescriptions, a 24% increase in the number of prescriptions per person, and a 26% increase in the actual cost of prescription drugs. Using cardiovascular drugs as an example, there has been a 55% increase in spending despite increased use of generic drugs to fill many prescriptions. Similarly, total spending for hormones and psychotherapeutic agents doubled, and spending for analgesics increased by 125%. This latter increase was primarily due to increased use of cyclooxygenase and decreased use of NSAIDS due to safety concerns (Moeller, Miller, & Banthin, 2004).

Inappropriate medication use among the elderly is compounded for cultural minority groups. Cultural factors such as language difficulties, values, and economic status may interfere with medication adherence, as does cultural stereotyping by providers. One study identified four factors influencing medication compliance in ethnic minority groups: difficulty with English, cultural barriers in the health system, lack of health insurance, and failure to consult providers regarding medication discontinuation or use of ancillary therapies (Zhan & Chen, 2004). Inappropriate medication use among older clients, including members of ethnic minority groups, may also be related to deteriorating vision and inability to read prescription labels. The focused assessment provided below can guide evaluation of medication use in elderly clients.

Health System Considerations

The demand for health care services increases sevenfold after 70 years of age compared to that among people under age 60. Most of this increase is due to greater use of expensive technology, but a significant portion of the increase is due to the multiple chronic illnesses experienced by older adults. For these reasons early diagnosis and effective treatment of chronic illness can help to decrease the societal burden of care for the elderly.

The concept of aging in place was conceived as a way of improving the quality of life for older adults and of decreasing the cost burden of their care by maintaining older individuals in their homes whenever possible and providing care in the least expensive setting. Two perspectives are taken on aging in place. In the first, aging in place is conceived as case management to permit provision of care at a consistent level (e.g., with the older adult continuing to reside in their own home). The second perspective views aging in place as provision of a full continuum of services, delivery methods, and policy directions in a system that helps older people successfully navigate various levels of care as they are needed (Bertsch & Taylor-Moore, 2005). Unfortunately, however, a number of health system factors impede effective aging in place. Three of those factors will be addressed here: access to care, prescription drug coverage, and interactions with health care providers.

Health Care Access

Access to health care services for older Americans has improved significantly since the advent of Medicare in the 1960s. In 2003, Medicare provided health insurance coverage for 13.7% of the total U.S. population. Forty-one million Medicare recipients were 65 years of age or over, and another 35 million were disabled. Although only 0.8% of the elderly did not receive Medicare, this still amounted to 286,000 older adults without health insurance coverage (U.S. Census Bureau, 2004a, 2005).

The costs of health care to those without insurance can be prohibitive. For example, hospitalization rates among the elderly in the United States increased by 23% from 1970 to 2000, and the average length of stay in the hospital for people over 65 years of age was 6 days in 2000. Hospitalization costs in 1999 averaged $2,546 for all Medicare beneficiaries, but rose to an average of $7,222 per person for those with Alzheimer's disease (Rosenfeld & Harrington, 2003). Older persons without health insurance cannot afford care at these rates. In some locales, primary health care services may be available from free clinics. Unfortunately, free clinics do not exist in many areas, and, even where they occur, they may not be able to meet the care needs of the uninsured. Similarly, "charity care" or uncompensated care provided by some hospitals may not meet the local needs for care among the elderly. In addition, uncompensated care may threaten the fiscal viability of health care organizations and force their closure, further diminishing access to care for older clients (Pricewaterhousecooper Health Research Institute, 2005). The effects of uncompensated care are discussed in more detail in Chapter 8∞.

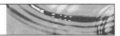

FOCUSED ASSESSMENT

Assessing Medication Use in Older Clients

- Is the client taking prescribed medications?
- Is the client taking over-the-counter (OTC) medications?
- Are any of the client's medications contraindicated by existing health conditions?
- Do OTC medications potentiate or counteract prescription medications?
- Do prescription medications potentiate or counteract each other?
- Does the client take prescription and OTC medications as directed (e.g., correct dose, route, time)?
- Does the client comply with other directions regarding medications (e.g., not taking with dairy products)?
- Is the client aware of potential food–drug interactions or drug–drug interactions?
- Are medications achieving the desired effects?
- Is the client experiencing any medication side effects?
- What is the client doing about medication side effects, if any?
- Is the client exhibiting symptoms of any adverse medication effects?

Advocacy in Action

Getting into the System

Students working in a student-faculty "miniclinic" held weekly in a local church identified an elderly woman with a blood pressure of 212/184. The woman was uninsured and did not have a regular health care provider. She refused to go to the emergency room even though the students and their instructor strongly urged her to do so. Failing that, the students and faculty member tried to get her an appointment with a physician. Without insurance, however, no one would see her.

The client was eligible for Medicaid. At first she assured the students that she would go to the Medicaid office to apply, but when she was seen week after week with the same high blood pressure and no progress on her Medicaid application, the problem of transportation surfaced. She had no means of transportation herself, and her son, a construction worker, could not—or would not—take time from work to help his mother apply. After many phone calls, the students were able to arrange for an intake worker to come to the woman's home and complete the Medicaid application. The application was approved, and the students found a physician who would care for the woman. She was started on antihypertensive medications and her blood pressure returned to normal.

Even for those with Medicare, access to care may be limited. Medicare pays only 54% of the health care costs for the elderly in the United States. Medicaid pays another 10%, and 15% of costs are covered by private insurance. The remaining 21% of costs are paid for out-of-pocket by the elderly themselves, and the percentage of people with out-of-pocket costs has increased from 83% in 1977 to 95% in 2000 (Federal Interagency Forum on Aging-related Statistics, 2004). Approximately half of the out-of-pocket expenses incurred by Medicare recipients are for Part B premiums. By 2050, Medicare beneficiaries can be expected to spend 30% of their income on health care (AARP, 2002).

In 2002, 40.1 million Americans had Medicare Part A coverage for hospitalization, but only 38 million had Part B coverage for provider fees, outpatient costs, and other costs. Sixty percent of the population also had supplemental insurance through private insurance providers (CDC, 2004a). Many older clients cannot afford either Part B coverage under Medicare or private supplemental insurance due to the cost of premiums. For 6 million of the poorest elderly, Medicaid covers the cost of Medicare Part B premiums as well as prescription drugs and some other expenses not covered under Medicare (Klein, Stoll, & Bruce, 2004), but for others the cost of premiums is prohibitive. Similarly, many older clients cannot afford private supplemental insurance for expenditures not covered under Medicare. Private health insurance coverage may be as much as two to four times more expensive for people aged 50 to 60 years than for the typical 25-year-old, and the extent of supplemental coverage has actually declined from 90% in 1998 to 60% in 2002 (American Association of Retired Persons, 2002; CDC, 2004a). Ethnic minority groups may have particular difficulty obtaining supplemental insurance due to small fixed incomes (Angel, Angel, & Markides, 2002). Lack of supplemental insurance coverage may also affect receipt of health promotion and illness prevention services. For example, in 2003, only 58% of older persons with Medicare coverage alone received influenza immunizations, compared to 71% of those with supplemental insurance coverage (Immunization Services Division, 2005).

In 2000, 5% of Americans over 65 years of age reported delaying needed care because of costs. Although this figure is down from 10% in 1992, it still represents a large segment of the older population who are not receiving appropriate care (Federal Interagency Forum on Aging-related Statistics, 2004).

Cost is not the only factor that may impede access to health care services for older clients. In one study, for example, 12% of older clients reported at least one of several barriers to obtaining care. The most commonly reported barrier was lack of responsiveness on the part of physicians, followed by medical bills, lack of transportation, unsafe streets and neighborhoods, and fear of serious diagnoses or unwanted tests. Some respondents also cited lack of a regular provider as a barrier to care, although 93% of the sample reported seeing the same provider on each visit. Finally, older clients also cited responsibilities for the care of others and work responsibilities as barriers to care (Fitzpatrick, Powe, Cooper, Ives, & Robbins, 2004). Other authors have noted that the health care system is often unresponsive to the needs of older clients as a result of inconvenient office locations, lack of parking, and short encounters that do not allow clients time to voice their concerns (Williams, 2005).

Older clients may also lack access to specific kinds of services. For example, most older clients do not have long-term-care insurance. Currently, Medicaid pays for 46% of nursing home costs in the United States, but many older clients are not eligible for Medicaid (Federal Interagency Forum on Aging-related Statistics, 2004). Medicare pays for short stays in long-term-care facilities, but 25% of nursing home and home health care costs are paid out-of-pocket. Public financing of long-term care is expected to increase 20% to 21% in the United States and the United Kingdom between 2000 and 2020. In the interim, however, many older people are not able to access needed long-term-care services. Due to their emphasis on care of the elderly, Japan's public contribution to long-term care is expected to increase by 102% in the same time period (Division of Adult and Community Health, 2003c).

Older clients may also lack access to care for problems related to substance abuse. In one study, 37% of physicians reported that they do not have time to discuss substance abuse with older clients. Similarly, 20% reported that managed care plans do not cover treatment for alcohol abuse. Medicare coverage for substance abuse treatment is limited to hospital detoxification and 50% of the costs of outpatient care. In addition, providers often lack the knowledge to intervene effectively or are uncomfortable discussing substance abuse with older clients. Finally, few treatment programs are designed to meet the needs of older adults. The author concluded that only 1% of older women in need of treatment for alcohol abuse actually receive the needed services (Finfgeld-Connett, 2004).

Prescription Drugs

Two elements of the health care system related to prescription drugs affect the health of older populations. The first is prescription of inappropriate drugs, and the second is the cost of medications.

In approximately 13% of emergency visits from 1992 to 2000, older clients were given inappropriate medications. This amounted to more than 16 million inappropriate prescriptions provided in emergency departments alone. Six drugs were found to account for 70% of the inappropriate prescriptions: promethazine, meperidine, propoxyphene, hydroxyzine, diphenhydramine, and diazepam. Study findings indicated that as the number of drugs prescribed increased, the number of inappropriate drugs also increased. Many inappropriate drugs are also prescribed in primary care settings when providers do not attend to the altered risk-benefit ratio for many drugs when taken by the elderly. Certain drugs should not be prescribed for older clients, and others should not be given in specific doses, for extended periods of time, or in the presence of specific comorbid conditions (Caterino et al., 2004). Table 19-3◆ provides information on selected drugs that are not appropriate for administration to older clients.

As we noted earlier, the cost of prescription drugs is one of the impediments to medication compliance among the elderly. Overall spending on drugs in the United States increased by more than 15% in 2002. A third of this increase was attributed to increased prices of medications rather than increased numbers of prescriptions. Over a 3-year period, the prices of the 30 name-brand drugs most often prescribed for older clients increased 22%, at 4.3 times the rate of inflation from January 2003 to January 2004, and 3.6 times the inflation rate over the previous 3 years (Mahan, 2004).

Prior to initiation of Medicare Part D, an estimated 65 million Americans, including 30% of Medicare beneficiaries, had no insurance coverage for prescription drugs. Some elderly had medication coverage under Medicaid, but this program has increased the amount paid out-of-pocket by recipients. Similarly, employers and private insurance plans that cover prescription drugs have increased copayments or reduced the level of prescription drug benefits. Approximately 28% of Medicare recipients rely on retirement benefits for prescription drug coverage, but many employers have recently eliminated or reduced coverage. For example, in 2003, 57% of firms with retiree coverage increased out-of-pocket costs for recipients, and in 2002, 40% fewer firms offered drug coverage than in 1994 (Mahan, 2004).

Medicare Part D, or the Medicare Prescription Drug, Improvement, and Modernization Act of 1993,

TABLE 19-3	Hazardous Medications for Elderly Clients	
Drug Classification	**Specific Medications**	**Potential Hazard**
Analgesics	Meperidine, pentazocine, propoxyphene	Confusion, hallucinations
Anticholinergics/antihistamines	Chlorpheniramine, diphenhydramine, hydroxyzine, cyproheptadine, promethazine, tripelennamine, dexchlorpheniramine	Confusion, blurred vision, constipation, dry mouth, lightheadedness, urinary difficulty or incontinence
Antidepressants	Amitriptyline, chlordiazepoxide-amitriptyline, perphenazine-amitriptyline, doxepin	Severe anticholinergic effects, sedation
Barbiturates	All except phenobarbital	Addiction potential
Benzodiazepines, long-acting	Chlordiazepoxide, clindinium-chlordiazepoxide, diazepam, quazepam, halazepam, chlorazepate	Sedation, increased fall risk
GI antispasmodics	Dicyclomine, hyoscyamine, propantheline, belladonna alkaloids	Anticholinergic effects
Muscle relaxants and antispasmodics	Carisoprodol, chlorzoxazone, cyclobenzaprine, metaxalone, methocarbamol, oxybutynin	Anticholinergic effects, sedation, weakness
Nonsteroidal anti-inflammatory drugs (NSAIDS)	Naproxen, oxaprozin, piroxicam	GI bleeding, renal failure, high blood pressure, heart failure

Data from: Wooten, J., & Galavis, J. (2005). Polypharmacy: Keeping the elderly safe. RN, 68(8), 44–50.

was intended to help meet the need for prescription drug coverage for older Americans. When the act is fully implemented in 2006, beneficiaries may choose to enroll in the program with a monthly premium cost of $35. After client payment of an annual deductible of $250 (which will increase to $445 in 2013), Medicare will pay 75% of annual prescription drug costs up to $2,250, with the client responsible for the remaining 25% out-of-pocket or through supplemental insurance. Recipients are responsible for paying 100% of annual drug costs in the "doughnut hole" from $2,250 to $5,100, after which Medicare will pay 95% with a 5% copayment by the recipient (Henley, 2004, Miller, 2004a). Excluding premiums, total out-of-pocket costs for prescription drugs for people with drug use over $5,100 will be $3,600. This figure will rise to $6,400 in 2013 (Henley, 2004). In other nations—the Netherlands, for example—the elderly have extended prescription drug coverage with few copayments (Edwards, 2004). The new law specifically prohibits Medicare from negotiating for blanket drug discounts as other federal health care systems, such as the Veterans Administration, currently do (Mahan, 2004). This means that older clients, as well as the general population, will bear the primary burden for escalating drug costs.

Some local and state jurisdictions have begun contracting with Canadian pharmacies in an effort to control drug costs. For example, a city program in Burlington, Vermont, saved $54,000 in a single year purchasing drugs for employees and retirees from Canada. Similarly, Montgomery, Alabama, saved so much money in purchasing Canadian drugs that they waived copayments for covered citizens. Drug import programs tend to focus on medications used for chronic conditions so prevalent among the elderly. Unfortunately, many of these programs have been threatened with sanctions for violating the Federal Food and Drug Act. Some question has been raised regarding the safety of drugs imported internationally, but many of these drugs are manufactured in the United States and then sold overseas. They can often be resold at lower costs than in the United States because of government regulation of drug prices (Wiebe, 2004).

Client–Provider Interactions

The third major health system consideration that affects the health of older populations is the quality of interactions with health care providers. These interactions are shaped by knowledge and attitudes on the part of providers as well as clients. As reflected in the discussion of inappropriate prescriptions given to older adults, some providers do not have the knowledge or expertise to provide effective care to this population. In one study, for example, nurses had less accurate knowledge of aging and its effects than members of other professions and more anxiety about working with aging clients, and they voiced perceptions that care of the elderly has lower prestige value than work with other populations. The

authors also found that nurses have more positive attitudes toward working with older populations when they work directly for a specific service provider rather than through a "temp" agency, when they had specific geriatric content in their educational programs, and when they worked outside of geriatric residential settings (Wells, Foreman, Gething, & Petralia, 2004).

Difficulties in provider–client interactions may also arise from communication barriers and lack of empowerment of older persons. Guinn (2004) identified three requisites for empowering older clients in health interactions. First, older clients must actively participate in the encounter and in the identification of problems to be addressed. Second, they must contribute to identification of health care goals. A third strategy for empowerment is rehearsal, in which older clients rehearse questions and other forms of input prior to interactions with health care professionals.

Barriers to effective communication between older clients and health care providers may stem from client attitudes and abilities or from provider characteristics. Client attributes that may impede communication include diminished communication abilities due to declining hearing, vision, or cognitive ability; diminished self-worth; and lack of knowledge about health-related issues. Provider-related barriers may include ageist attitudes and discrimination, as well as lack of knowledge and expertise regarding the needs of and interventions appropriate to older clients (Guinn, 2004).

Differences may also arise from the primary foci of providers and clients. According to the National Institute on Aging (2004), providers, especially physicians, focus on disease and its treatment, whereas the primary focus of many older clients is on quality of life. The Institute highlights the need for effective communication to achieve four specific outcomes: preventing errors, strengthening the provider–client relationship and promoting compliance, making efficient use of the time of both, and achieving better client outcomes.

An additional barrier to communication between health care providers and older clients is a phenomenon called "elder speak." Elder speak is an approach to communication with the elderly that conveys a message of incompetence and control and may take one of two forms: excessively nurturing communication and controlling communication. Elder speak may be characterized by a slow rate of speech, exaggerated intonation, elevated pitch and volume, frequent repetition, and the use of simple vocabulary and grammar. Other characteristics may include use of inappropriate terms of endearment (e.g., "honey" or "sweetie"), use of the plural pronoun "we," and use of questions that prompt a specific answer (e.g., "you want to wear this pretty blue sweater, don't you?") such as one might use with a child. An estimated 20% of communication occurring in nursing home settings involves elder speak, and as many as 40% of older clients in both institutional and home settings report caregivers who use speech that they perceive as demeaning, patronizing, or implying their own incompetence (Williams, Kemper, & Hummert, 2004).

Even when providers think they may be communicating effectively, this may not be the case. For example, in one study of primary care physicians caring for clients with Alzheimer's disease and their families, physicians reported providing a variety of information and support that family members reported not receiving. For instance, 80% of the providers believed that Alzheimer's disease can be stabilized, at least temporarily, but only 32% of the caregivers reported having been given this information. Similarly, 74% of the physicians reported that they always provided referrals to community support groups for caregivers, yet only 24% of caregivers said that the providers actually did so (Alzheimer's Association, 2001).

Providers have also been found to neglect to address health promotion activities with older client populations. For example, according to the National Center for Chronic Disease Prevention and Health Promotion (2002b), only 52% of health care providers ask older clients about their activity levels. In the same vein, as we saw earlier, few providers are willing to address issues of substance abuse or sexuality with their older clients.

ASSESSING THE HEALTH OF THE OLDER POPULATION

In the preceding discussion, we have identified a number of factors that influence the health of elderly populations. The task of a given community health nurse working with a given population of elderly individuals is to assess the extent to which these factors are influencing the health of the specific population and the effects of these factors. Here we will focus on assessing the health of older clients as a population group. A tool that can be adapted for use in assessing the health of individual older adults is included in Appendix I on the Companion Website. The *Community Assessment Reference Guide* deigned to accompany this text contains an assessment tool specific to the health status and needs of older clients.

Basic information about the relative proportion of older individuals in the population can be obtained from census figures or other local population figures. Similarly, information on communicable diseases among the elderly will be available from local health department statistics. Health department statistics will also provide information on mortality due to both acute and chronic health conditions. Morbidity data, on the other hand, may be more difficult to obtain. Local acute-care institutions may have data on the number of older persons admitted for specific conditions, or registries may exist for certain selected illnesses (e.g., some forms of cancer). A local Office of Aging and Independence Services may also have figures related to the incidence and prevalence of specific conditions or disabilities.

Such information may also be derived indirectly from the number and type of requests for home care assistance, although these figures are likely to underestimate the true need, since many elders may not request assistance even when it is needed. The focused assessment on page 520 provides guidance for assessing the extent of functional limitations and disabilities in the elderly population. The data included in the assessment will be collected primarily through community surveys.

Churches and other religious groups may also be able to provide some sense of the extent of disability within the congregation or the number of requests for assistance by older members. Community surveys of the older population may also provide information on the extent of acute and chronic illness as well as disability, immunization status, use of health care services, and so on. The effectiveness of pain control or the prevalence of incontinence are other factors that are best assessed in community surveys, as are data on stress, coping, depression, and other psychological factors. Questions for assessing biophysical factors affecting the health of the older population are included on page 520. Some data on rates of treatment for psychiatric disorders may be available from local primary care providers and specific psychiatric services. Emergency department statistics may also provide insights into the kind and frequency of health problems experienced by older adults in the population. Additional areas for consideration in the psychological dimension are reflected in the focused assessment questions provided on page 520.

Much of the information related to physical environmental factors affecting health will be obtained by direct observation and through community surveys. Considerations related to physical environmental influences on the health of older clients are included in the focused assessment questions provided on page 521. Information on many sociocultural factors may also be derived from community surveys, but local social service agencies may also have information related to income levels among the elderly, formal social support available in the community, and so on. Figures related to income, poverty, educational levels, and so on are also available from census data. Information regarding the participation of older clients in the workforce may be available from local employers as well as from census data. Aggregate data regarding family roles and responsibilities among the older population are best derived from community surveys, but local social service agencies may have some data on these factors within segments of the population. Information on elder abuse and violence will most likely be available from local police departments and protective service agencies, although local emergency departments can provide data on the frequency with which older clients are seen for injuries resulting from violence. The focused assessment questions included on page 521 can guide community health nurses' exploration of sociocultural factors influencing the health of the older population.

MediaLink

Appendix I: Adult Health Assessment

FOCUSED ASSESSMENT

Assessing Disability in the Elderly Population

Basic Activities of Daily Living

What proportion of the population over 65 years of age has difficulty with

- Feeding (feeding self, chewing, or swallowing)?
- Bathing (getting into or out of a bathtub or shower, manipulating soap or washcloth, washing hair, effectively drying all body parts)?
- Dressing (remembering the order in which clothes are put on, dressing self, bending to put on shoes and socks, manipulating fasteners, putting on and removing sleeves, combing hair, applying makeup)?
- Toileting (ambulating to the bathroom, urinary urgency, removing clothing, positioning self on toilet, lifting from a sitting position on toilet, cleaning self after urination or defecation, replacing clothing)?
- Transfer (getting from lying to sitting position, standing from a sitting position, lying or sitting down)?

Instrumental Activities of Daily Living

What proportion of the population over 65 years of age has difficulty with

- Shopping (transporting self to shopping facilities, navigating within shopping facilities, lifting products from shelves, handling money, carrying purchases to and from car, storing purchases)?
- Laundry (collecting dirty clothing, sorting clothes to be washed or dry-cleaned, accessing laundry facilities, manipulating containers of soap, etc., lifting wet clothing into dryer, hanging or folding clean clothes, putting clean clothing away)?
- Cooking (planning well-balanced meals, safely operating kitchen appliances and utensils, reaching dishes and pots and pans, cleaning and chopping foods, carrying food to the table)?
- Housekeeping (identifying the need for housecleaning, light housekeeping, doing heavy chores, doing yard maintenance)?
- Taking medication (remembering medications, opening medication bottles, swallowing medications, giving injections, etc.)?
- Managing money (budgeting effectively, writing checks, balancing checking account, remembering to pay, and recording payment of bills)?

Advanced Activities of Daily Living

What proportion of the population over 65 years of age has difficulty with

- Social activity (maintaining a group of people with whom to socialize, transporting self to social events, seeing and hearing well enough to interact with others, tiring easily, being fearful of incontinence or embarrassed over financial difficulties)?
- Occupation (carrying out occupational responsibilities, if any)?
- Recreation (having the physical strength and mobility to engage in desired recreational activities, maintaining a group of people with whom to pursue recreation, transporting self to recreational activities)?

Most information on behavioral considerations affecting the health status of the older population will be derived from community surveys. Some data may also be available from local police records of arrests for substance abuse–related crimes by older individuals or from local mental health facilities regarding the frequency of hospitalizations for substance abuse among the elderly. Again, however, these data are likely to reflect only the "tip of the iceberg" since many substance abusers in all age groups do not seek treatment. Emergency department data on older clients seen for malnutrition, dehydration, and substance abuse–related health problems may also help to clarify the extent of behavioral factors affecting the older population. Issues related to sexuality, on the other hand, are best addressed with community surveys. Some data related to physical activity by older clients may be derived from observations of physical activity in and around the community, but community surveys may also serve to elicit these data.

Information on medication use among older clients in the community can be derived in a variety of ways. Health care providers may have a sense of the extent of medication noncompliance within this population in their practices. Similarly, pharmacies may provide anecdotal evidence of prescription refills that do not jibe with the dose and frequency of medication prescribed. Some agencies may also use electronic monitors or other devices to monitor medication compliance in individual clients, and some agencies may aggregate

FOCUSED ASSESSMENT
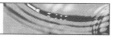

Assessing Biophysical Factors Influencing Older Clients' Health

- What is the age composition of the elderly population?
- What are the primary causes of death in the elderly population?
- What is the incidence and prevalence of acute and chronic disease in the elderly population?
- What is the extent of disability in the elderly population? What types of disability are prevalent?
- What is the immune status of the elderly population? What proportion of the elderly population has received pneumonia vaccine? What proportion has received recent influenza and tetanus immunizations? What is the extent of immunity to other diseases in the elderly population (e.g., pertussis, diphtheria)?

FOCUSED ASSESSMENT
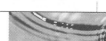

Assessing Psychological Factors Influencing Older Clients' Health

- What sources of stress is the elderly population exposed to? What is the extent of coping abilities in the elderly population?
- What is the prevalence of cognitive impairment in the elderly population? What levels of cognitive impairment are represented in the population (e.g., mild confusion, vegetative states)?
- What is the extent of mental illness in the elderly population? What mental illnesses are prevalent in the population? What are the rates of suicide and attempted suicide in the elderly population?

FOCUSED ASSESSMENT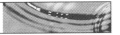

Assessing Physical Environmental Factors Influencing Older Clients' Health

- How adequate is housing available to the elderly population? What is the extent of home ownership in this population? What safety hazards are presented by housing for the elderly? Are rentals and taxes within the budgetary limitations of most of the elderly population?
- Does the physical environment of the community promote or impede physical activity in the elderly population?
- What health effects does environmental pollution have for the elderly population?

this data at the population level. Considerations in assessing behavioral factors influencing the health of the elderly population are reflected in the focused assessment provided at right.

Information on access to health care as well as use of health care services can be obtained from local providers as well as community surveys of the elderly population. The local Social Security and Medicaid offices should have data on the number of older persons enrolled in these

FOCUSED ASSESSMENT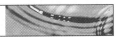

Assessing Sociocultural Factors Influencing Older Clients' Health

- What are societal attitudes toward the elderly? To what extent does the society provide support services for its older members?
- What is the ethnic composition of the elderly population? What languages are spoken among the elderly population? How does culture influence the health of the elderly population?
- What religious affiliations are represented among the elderly population? What health and social services are provided to the elderly population by religious organizations in the community?
- What is the level of economic support available to the elderly population? What is the income distribution within the elderly population? What are the typical sources of income for members of the elderly population? What is the proportion of elderly living in poverty or near poverty?
- What is the typical education level in the elderly population? How does education level influence health?
- What proportion of the elderly population is working? What are the occupations typical of elderly members of the population?
- What retirement planning and assistance are available to older members of the population?
- What proportion of the older population is engaged in caretaking for other family members? What is the effect of caretaking on their health?
- What transportation resources are available to the elderly population? Are they accessible to older clients with mobility limitations? Are they affordable?
- What shopping facilities and other services are available to older members of the population? Are they accessible and affordable?
- What is the extent of social isolation in the elderly population? What resources are available in the community to limit social isolation?

FOCUSED ASSESSMENT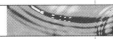

Assessing Behavioral Factors Influencing Older Clients' Health

- What are the typical dietary patterns among the elderly in the population? What is the extent of obesity in the elderly population? What nutritional deficits are prevalent in the elderly population?
- What is the extent of smoking, alcohol, and drug use in the elderly population? What are the treatment rates for alcohol and drug abuse?
- To what extent do members of the elderly population engage in health-related behaviors such as testicular self-examination, mammography, and so on?
- To what extent do members of the elderly population employ safety precautions such as seat belt use?
- What proportion of the elderly population drives? What is the incidence of motor vehicle accidents among this population?
- What prescription and over-the-counter medications are typically taken by elderly clients? What is the incidence of adverse events due to inappropriate medication use in the population?

programs in the local population as well as data on expenditures and types of services for which reimbursement is provided. Finally, community surveys and health institutions can provide information on the extent or lack of health care insurance in the older population. The quality of interactions between providers and older clients, however, is likely to be available only through community surveys or small-scale qualitative studies involving participant observation. Focused assessment questions related to the health system dimension are provided below.

DIAGNOSTIC REASONING AND CARE OF OLDER POPULATIONS

Once the community health nurse has determined the extent to which factors in each of the dimensions of health are affecting the health of the older population and determined what those effects are, he or she would

FOCUSED ASSESSMENT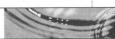

Assessing Health System Factors Influencing Older Clients' Health

- What proportion of the elderly population has a regular source of health care?
- What is the level of insurance coverage among the elderly population (e.g., Medicare A and B, supplementary insurance)?
- To what extent are medication needs covered by insurance plans among the elderly population?
- What preventive and restorative health care services are available to members of the elderly population? To what extent are these services used by the population? How adequate are these services in meeting the needs of the elderly population?
- To what extent are palliative services, end-of-life care, and hospice services available and accessible to the elderly population?

derive community nursing diagnoses related to the population's health status. These diagnoses would reflect the problems identified in the elderly population as well as the availability of resources within the community to address these problems.

Nursing diagnoses may be either positive or negative. An example of a positive diagnosis might be "continued maintenance of older clients in their own homes due to the availability and accessibility of assistance with ADLs." Positive diagnoses usually indicate that no further nursing intervention is needed, but that the health status of the population in this area should continue to be monitored. A negative diagnosis might be "lack of assistance with ADLs for older persons with functional disabilities." In this instance, the diagnosis would indicate the need for intervention by nurses and others in the community to resolve the identified problem.

PLANNING HEALTH CARE FOR OLDER POPULATIONS

Planning to meet the health care needs of older clients may take place at the primary, secondary, and tertiary levels of prevention. Major emphases in planning health care for older clients should be on successful aging and promotion of self-care. As noted earlier, aging can result in loss of functional abilities, stamina, and so on, but these losses can be balanced to achieve successful aging. Health care for older clients should be based on the standards for gerontological nursing practice developed by the American Nurses Association (2001). These standards are included in the Special Considerations Box below.

Primary Prevention

Primary prevention among the elderly is imperative for several reasons. First, they are the fastest-growing segment of the population. In addition, they exhibit the

SPECIAL CONSIDERATIONS

SCOPE AND STANDARDS OF GERONTOLOGICAL NURSING PRACTICE

Standard I. Assessment: The gerontological nurse collects patient health data.

Standard II. Diagnosis: The gerontological nurse analyzes the assessment data in determining diagnosis.

Standard III. Outcomes identification: The gerontological nurse identifies expected outcomes individualized to the older client.

Standard IV. Planning: The gerontological nurse develops a plan of care that prescribes interventions to attain expected outcomes.

Standard V. Implementation: The gerontological nurse implements the interventions identified in the plan of care.

Standard VI. Evaluation: The gerontological nurse evaluates the older adult's progress toward attainment of expected outcomes.

highest prevalence of chronic illness, and finally, they use the majority of health care services (Wang, 2001). Increasing longevity necessitates a primary prevention focus on health promotion and illness prevention. As noted by members of a global summit on aging, "Because we will be in real trouble if these extra years are not accompanied by more vigor and less disability, we need health policies that support the social, economic, and environmental conditions that promote active aging and give everyone—young and old—access to the best medical and nonmedical resources" (Telling, as quoted in Plese, 2005b, p. 5). The need for prevention among the older population was highlighted in the following comment from the same international forum:

> The short-term thinking about prevention is the most costly policy mistake being made . . . Frailty must be addressed before it happens. Technology is only part of the solution. The solution for polio was not better iron lungs. The solution for healthy aging is not better long-term care institutions; it is prevention, better care early in the disease process, and investment in innovation. (Telling, as quoted in Plese, 2005b, p. 19)

Community health nurses may need to actively advocate for the availability of preventive services to older clients. They may also need to advocate among the elderly population for use of these services.

The Centers for Disease Control and Prevention has identified five roles for which it should be responsible in promoting the health of the older population. These roles are also the responsibility of other jurisdictions (e.g., state and local government), but at a more circumscribed level. These roles and responsibilities are as follows:

- Provide high-quality information and resources to health care providers and members of the general public regarding health promotion activities
- Support prevention activities by local providers and organizations
- Integrate public health prevention expertise with networks of services for the older population
- Identify and implement effective prevention efforts
- Monitor changes in the health status of the older adult population (Division of Adult and Community Health, 2003c)

Primary prevention of disability in the older population requires interruption of the three pathways to disability discussed earlier in this chapter: prevention or delay of fragility; prevention, recognition, and treatment of conditions that contribute to disability; and alteration of the environment to promote independence and prevent disability even in the face of diminished health (Albert et al., 2002). Unfortunately, health promotion and illness prevention are often neglected in the elderly population. For example, Medicare's emphasis on health promotion and illness prevention is piecemeal at best, and Medicare funding only covers a portion of the clinical preventive services recommended for older adults. The Partnership for Prevention (2003) suggested two possible avenues for increasing the focus on promotion and prevention for Medicare beneficiaries. The first is an incremental approach that involves adding coverage for specific services or groups of services. The second approach is to provide a comprehensive examination at age 65 (or when people become eligible for Medicare benefits) that would address existing conditions and provide basic health promotion and illness prevention services and education. This second approach would not, however, address the needs of this population for continuing health promotion and illness prevention services such as annual influenza immunization or continued monitoring of diet, exercise, and other health promotion activities.

Both health promotion and illness prevention in the care of older populations may involve an emphasis on self-care. Leenerts and associates (2002) identified five dimensions of self-care for health promotion in the elderly. The first dimension incorporates the internal and external environment in which self-care occurs. The internal environment includes factors internal to the client him- or herself, such as motivation, self-concept, physical health status, and emotional health. The external environment encompasses the physical, social, and cultural contexts in which self-care takes place. Community health nurses may need to advocate for changes in the external environment that support self-care by older clients. For example, a community health nurse might assist a community to develop a program of assistance with shopping and heavy household chores, allowing frail older clients to remain in their own homes. The second dimension is self-care ability, which involves both knowledge of needed self-care and the physical ability to carry it out. The third dimension, education, provides the link between self-care ability and self-care activity, the fourth dimension of self-care in health promotion. Community health nurses may be particularly helpful in providing older clients with the knowledge required for effective self-care. Self-care activity includes the client's repertoire of activities needed for self-care. The fifth and final dimension is the outcome of self-care, hopefully improved health status.

Health promotion and illness prevention often depend on changes in health-related behaviors. Although we often think about behavioral change as occurring at the individual client level, behavior-related interventions should actually occur at three levels: individual, community, and national (Cutler, 2004). Community health nurses can be particularly active in promoting activity at each of these levels. At the individual level, community health nurses can educate clients to take steps to modify factors that place them at risk for disease and injury. At the community level, initiatives can be undertaken to change environmental factors that influence health-related behaviors. These initiatives may include public policy interventions such as designing communities to promote safe opportunities for exercise by all age groups, but particularly for the elderly. At the national level, comprehensive campaigns can be undertaken to address widespread behavior change among either clients (e.g., the recent campaign on weight control and physical activity) or health care providers (e.g., the development of national guidelines for preventive activities). In the next few sections, we will examine some of the major considerations in primary prevention among older adults.

Nutrition

Adequate nutrition is important for the older population to maintain health, prevent disease, and prevent further effects of existing chronic conditions. Adequate nutrition for health promotion frequently entails a reduction in caloric intake. For example, caloric needs decrease roughly 7% for each decade after 30 years of age for men and 10% for women. Specific caloric needs vary from person to person: older persons engaged in physical activity and resistance training do not experience such a marked reduction in caloric needs (Tabloski, 2006).

Despite reduced caloric needs, older adults continue to require a balance of all other nutrients. Nutritional deficits are most frequently noted for calcium; iron; vitamins A, D, and C; the B vitamins riboflavin and thiamine; and dietary fiber. Care should be taken, however, in the use of fat-soluble vitamins A, D, E, and K, which are stored in the body more readily than water-soluble vitamins and may lead to vitamin toxicity in the older population due to diminished metabolism (Tabloski, 2006). Community health nurses can promote the health of older clients by educating this population regarding their nutritional requirements.

Other, more general interventions may also be needed to improve older clients' nutritional status by eliminating impediments to good nutrition. For example, social isolation may need to be addressed because people tend to eat better in company with others. Older clients can be referred to senior nutrition centers, or family members can be encouraged to drop by at mealtimes to eat with older clients who live alone. Interventions may also be required to deal with nausea, poorly fitting dentures, or other factors that may impede good nutrition. Community health nurses may also need to be active in the development and implementation of programs to meet the nutritional needs of the older population where these services do not already exist, or in increasing access to existing services for underserved segments of the population.

Safety

Safety is an area of significant concern in the care of the older population. Injuries are the eighth leading cause of death in people over 65 years of age in the United States (Division of Unintentional Injury Prevention, 2003), and the fifth leading cause in countries such as Finland (Kannus, Parkkari, Niemi, & Palvanen, 2005) and China

(You et al., 2004). The majority of these deaths are related to falls resulting in hip fractures. An estimated 16% of White U.S. women will experience a hip fracture sometime in their lives. Seventeen percent of these women will die within one year, and half will never regain their independence. Hip fracture incidence has actually been found to be increasing with recent birth cohorts (Samelson, Zhang, Kiel, Hannan, & Felson, 2002). Risk factors for falls in the elderly include arthritis, problems with gait or balance, poor muscle strength, and vision problems. The risk of falls also increases with the number of medications taken. On average, 3,000 falls among the elderly each year in the United States require hospitalization for traumatic brain injury, with an annual cost of $50 million (Division of Surveillance and Informatics, 2003). Cognitive ability also affects falls and fracture mortality (Williams & Jester, 2005). In fact, therapeutic interventions in dementia may actually increase the potential for falls. For example, hypnotics used for agitation may increase gait disturbances or drowsiness, leading to falls and other accidental injuries (Hurley et al., 2004).

Exercise by older adults can reduce the risk of falling by as much as 15% (Division of Unintentional Injury Prevention, 2003). In one study, for example, biweekly exercise sessions in community settings combined with at-home exercise significantly improved balance and mobility in elderly clients (Robitaille et al., 2005). Interventions may also be aimed at reducing environmental risks for falls and effective medication management. Individualized risk assessments have been shown to increase self-efficacy related to falls, environmental safety, and knowledge of medication safety (Huang & Acton, 2004).

Another area of concern is that of driving by older clients with sensory impairments or diminished reaction times. From 1990 to 1997, the number of motor vehicle deaths among older clients increased 14%, and nonfatal motor vehicle injuries increased by 19% (National Center for Injury Prevention and Control, 2005b). Drivers over 65 years of age have threefold higher crash rates per mile driven than any other group except teenagers. Because they drive fewer miles, however, motor vehicle accident rates per number of drivers are comparable. Men over 65 years of age drive an average of 10,000 miles per year (a 74% increase in the last 30 years), and women average 5,000 miles per year (a 31% increase). Most older drivers decide for themselves when it is appropriate to stop driving, although women are 78% more likely to stop than men. Each year more than 600,000 older drivers decide to stop driving, and this decision is often associated with depression and social isolation. Based on longevity projections, older men can anticipate 7 years of needing other sources of transportation and women 10 years (Foley, Heimovitz, Guralnik, & Brock, 2002). Unfortunately, transportation services for the elderly are often lacking, leaving older populations with decreased mobility and diminished opportunities for social interaction.

Motor vehicles are also problematic when older people are pedestrians. In many areas, the bulk of pedestrian fatalities occur among elderly individuals. In areas where there are large numbers of elderly, nurses can campaign for traffic signals at heavily used crossings, strict enforcement of speed limits, and public awareness of the presence of older adults.

Community health nurses can initiate and participate in education campaigns related to safety issues for the older population. In addition, they can support initiatives that promote safe environments for the elderly. Finally, they may need to engage in activity to promote access to public transportation to meet the needs of the elderly, particularly those with disabilities that may limit their ability to use existing public transportation systems.

Home and neighborhood safety and prevention of elder abuse are two other safety concerns with older populations. Community health nurses can be active in promoting police activity to make neighborhoods safe for older clients to move about in them. They may also be involved in the development of neighborhood watch programs and in programs to alert public safety officials that older clients are residing in particular places. This is particularly important for older disabled individuals in the community. For example, nurses can participate in the development of programs to identify homes with older residents so fire and police personnel can meet their special needs in the event of an emergency.

The last area of concern in promoting the safety of older clients is preventing abuse and neglect. Elder abuse and neglect frequently occur when those caring for elderly clients are unable to cope with the resulting stress. Providing support for these caretakers, teaching positive coping skills, and providing periodic respite care may help to prevent abuse. Assisting older clients to maintain their independence may also help prevent the development of a potentially abusive situation. Specific interventions for preventing abuse are discussed in more detail in Chapter 32∞.

Immunization

The Advisory Committee on Immunization Practices (ACIP) (2004) recommends tetanus and diphtheria immunization every 10 years, annual influenza immunization, and one dose of pneumococcal vaccine for all older adults in the United States. Additional recommendations for older adults at particular risk of disease include three doses of hepatitis A, two doses of hepatitis B, and two doses of varicella vaccine for susceptible persons of all ages. In addition, adults with medical or exposure indications should receive meningococcal vaccine. It is estimated that for every million persons who receive influenza vaccine, 900 deaths and 1,300 hospitalizations are prevented (Centers for Medicare and Medicaid Services [CMS], 2004). Similar, but less pronounced, effects are noted for other immunizations.

Unfortunately, immunization is an often neglected intervention among older clients. For example, only 40% of people over 65 years of age have had a tetanus booster in the last 10 years (Matthews et al., 2004). Similarly, as of 2003, only 55% of this population had received pneumococcal vaccine (Centers for Disease Control and Prevention, 2003). During the 2004–2005 influenza season, only 63% of people over age 65 received influenza vaccine (Division of Adult and Community Health, 2005). Immunization levels are often lower in certain subsegments of the elderly population. For example, in 2003, only 54% of older people with incomes below poverty level received influenza immunizations, compared to 58% of the total Medicare population and 71% of those with both Medicare coverage and supplemental health insurance (Immunization Services Division, 2005). The three reasons most often given for not receiving influenza immunizations, which also have relevance for failure to receive other recommended immunizations, are lack of knowledge of the need for immunization, concerns regarding potential side effects, and lack of vaccine availability (CMS, 2004).

Community health nurses can be active in providing immunization services for older adults as well as in educating the older population regarding the need for immunizations. Nurses may also be involved in the design of programs and services to meet the immunization needs of the older population, making sure that all segments of the population have access to services. In 2003, ACIP recommended that nurses and pharmacists be allowed to provide influenza and pneumonia immunizations under standing orders without a physician's signature. CMS also published rules removing the requirement for a physician's signature for immunizations as part of the Conditions of Participation for hospitals, nursing homes, and home health agencies receiving Medicare and Medicaid funding (Centers for Disease Control and Prevention, 2003).

Rest and Exercise

Many people believe that the need for exercise decreases with age; however, older people need exercise as much as their younger counterparts. Thirty minutes of aerobic exercise 5 days a week is recommended for older adults (Resnick, 2005). Exercise sessions should also include 10 to 15 minutes of warm-up exercises and a 10- to 15-minute cool-down period (Resnick, 2004). The American College of Sports Medicine also recommends strength training at least twice a week as part of a comprehensive physical activity program. Strength training has been associated with improved health and fitness, increased muscle strength and endurance, increased bone density, improved insulin sensitivity and glucose metabolism, decreased fall risk, and continued independent living (Division of Nutrition and Physical Activity, 2004). Unfortunately, members of the older adult population often fail to engage in recommended physical activity. Barriers to physical activity among the elderly include lack of time, pain, boredom, fatigue, unsafe environments, fear of injury, lack of awareness of the need to exercise, environments not conducive to physical activity, and failure to set reasonable exercise goals (Resnick, 2005). Community health nurses can help design and provide physical activity programs for older adults that address these barriers. As we saw earlier, community-based exercise programs can have positive effects on physical activity among older clients. Similarly, a cognitive behavioral intervention designed to promote exercise in this age group was found to result in moderately increased overall exercise behavior in experimental subjects as compared to a control group (Schneider et al., 2004).

The quality of rest is another consideration in caring for the older adult population. Many older adults experience insomnia that may be due to underlying disease states, medications, or use of alcohol, tobacco, or caffeine. Interventions that may assist clients with insomnia include treating underlying diseases, keeping a sleep log to determine possible triggers to wakefulness, adjusting medication regimens as needed, and promoting good sleep hygiene. The last can be accomplished by promoting exercise (particularly outdoor activity); increasing exposure to light; avoiding alcohol, tobacco, and caffeine after midafternoon; napping for 30 minutes or less, if at all, during the day; and not working or reading in bed. Other possible interventions include developing a relaxing bedtime routine, promoting pain control, and keeping the environment bright during the day and dark at night (Williams, 2004). Community health nurses can educate clients with sleep problems regarding these strategies. They may also refer them for medical care of underlying diseases or for changes in medications that may be contributing to wakefulness.

Smoking Cessation

Smoking cessation is another primary prevention activity that may be beneficial for the older population in preventing smoking-attributable health problems. As we saw earlier, it is never too late to stop smoking. In addition to the obvious cardiovascular and respiratory effects, not smoking has been associated with decreased risk for colorectal cancer (Kather, 2005). A five As model has been developed to assist with smoking cessation in older adults. Elements of this model are:

- **A**sking about smoking behaviors
- **A**dvising clients regarding the need to stop smoking
- **A**ssessing clients' willingness to stop smoking
- **A**ssisting them with smoking cessation strategies or referral to smoking cessation programs
- **A**rranging for follow-up to support smoking cessation and monitor its effectiveness (Andrews et al., 2004)

Community health nurses can refer older clients who smoke to smoking cessation programs. They can also campaign for access to such programs and coverage of smoking cessation under health insurance plans.

Maintaining Independence

Because of physical and economic limitations, it is sometimes difficult for older persons to maintain their independence. Decreased income and physical inability to care for themselves sometimes force older clients to give up their own residence and live with family members. Whatever the living arrangements of the older client, community health nurses should assist them to maintain the highest degree of independence possible. Some older clients may be able to continue to live alone if referred to supportive services such as homemaker aides, transportation services, and Meals-on-Wheels. When older persons are living with family members, the nurse can encourage family members to foster independence in the client. This may mean encouraging families to assign specific roles within the household to the older family member. Community health nurses can also be actively involved in designing and implementing programs intended to assist older clients to age in place.

Life Resolution

Creating meaning for one's life is one of the developmental tasks to be accomplished by older adults. This entails developing a personal set of goals and the ability to view one's life as having been productive. Reminiscence is one way of accomplishing life resolution and achieving positive feelings about one's own life. The community health nurse must recognize and foster older clients' need to reminisce and should encourage family members to do so as well. This is sometimes difficult given the nurse's busy schedule and the number of clients who need to be seen; however, nurses should be able to find some time during interactions with older clients to listen to these reminiscences and to help clients reflect on their lives. In spite of cognitive losses, reminiscence or "life review" has also been shown to be effective with some clients with Alzheimer's disease (Haight, 2001). Primary preventive interventions for older adult populations are summarized in Table 19-4◆.

Secondary Prevention

As with other population groups, secondary prevention with older adults focuses on screening and treatment of disease. Because of the prevalence of chronic illness, self-management of disease is another important area of emphasis in secondary prevention.

Screening

Screening for older clients is another aspect of care that is often neglected. Many people believe that it is not necessary to engage in early detection of disease because the benefits of treatment are minimal among the elderly.

TABLE 19-4 Primary Prevention Strategies for Older Adult Populations	
Area of Concern	Primary Prevention Strategies
Diet and nutrition	Educate public regarding nutritional needs of older adults.
	Assure access to nutritional foods.
	Eliminate social and environmental barriers to good nutrition.
Safety	Educate public regarding safety issues for older adults.
	Promote exercise to strengthen muscles, bones, and joints.
	Eliminate environmental safety hazards.
	Educate older drivers regarding the hazards of driving.
	Promote alternative forms of transportation for older adults.
	Initiate or promote programs to alert fire and police personnel to older clients in specific residences.
	Promote family coping abilities and relieve stress to prevent abuse of older persons.
Immunization	Educate older populations regarding the need for immunizations.
	Provide immunization services and assure their accessibility to all segments of the older population.
	Develop immunization programs in places where older clients are frequently found.
Rest and exercise	Educate the older population on the need for exercise.
	Participate in the development of physical activity programs that address the most common barriers to exercise among older clients.
	Develop programs to deal with insomnia in the elderly.
Smoking cessation	Assist in the development of programs to assist older clients with smoking cessation.
	Educate the older population on the need for and benefits of smoking cessation.
Maintaining independence	Participate in the development of services that allow clients to live independently as long as possible.
	Promote environments that support independent living by the older population.
Life resolution	Encourage reminiscence.

A number of disease conditions can still be effectively treated in the older population, however, if found early enough. For example, older adults are perceived to have a poor prognosis for colorectal cancer, yet surgery is quite effective following early detection of disease. An estimated third of deaths due to colorectal cancer could be prevented with screening in persons over the age of 50 (Kather, 2005). Unfortunately, in 2001, 69% of people in this age group had not had a test for fecal occult blood in the previous 2 years (CDC, 2004b), and only 34% of adults over age 50 have ever had a sigmoidoscopy (Matthews et al., 2004). Similarly, risk reduction for breast cancer fatality is greatest among women over 50 years of age, and early detection can reduce mortality by 25% to 30% (CDC, 2004b), yet from 2000 to 2002, 16% of women between 65 and 74 years of age and 23% of those 75 years of age and older had not had a mammogram in the previous 2 years (Division of Cancer Prevention and Control, 2005).

A number of routine screening procedures are recommended for the older adult population. These procedures are summarized in Table 19-5◆. As noted in the table, general recommendations are to discontinue annual Papanicolaou smears at age 65 or 70 years. Some authors, however, note a need to continue this screening test in older women who are sexually active due to the potential for human papilloma virus (HPV) infection (Neher, 2004). As noted above, many of the recommended screening practices are not provided to older clients.

Community health nurses can educate older clients regarding the need for routine screening and refer them for screening services. Clients with particular risk factors or symptoms of possible disease should also be referred for screening and diagnostic services as appropriate. For example, a community health nurse might refer an older immigrant woman with a persistent productive cough for tuberculosis screening or refer a client with an elevated blood pressure for possible diagnosis and treatment of hypertension. Community health nurses may also need to advocate for access to screening services for older clients. For example, a nurse might advocate expanding breast cancer education and screening programs to target older women.

TABLE 19-5 Routine Screening Recommendations for Older Adult Populations

Type of Screening	Recommendation
Abdominal aortic aneurysm	**U.S. Preventive Services Task Force:** One-time screening in male smokers aged 65 to 75 years; recommend against routine screening in older women
Colorectal cancer	**U.S. Preventive Services Task Force:** All adults over age 50 (fecal occult blood and/or sigmoidoscopy); no evidence of effectiveness of screening colonoscopy
Depression	**U.S. Preventive Services Task Force:** Older adults in practice settings where follow-up is available
Elder abuse	**U.S. Preventive Services Task Force:** Insufficient evidence for effectiveness of routine screening
Hearing impairment	**U.S. Preventive Services Task Force:** All older adults
Hypertension	**U.S. Preventive Services Task Force:** All older adults
Lipid disorders (total cholesterol and HDL-C)	**U.S. Preventive Services Task Force:** All adults over age 45 (total cholesterol and HDL-C)
Mammogram	**U.S. Preventive Services Task Force:** Women over age 40 (with or without clinical breast examination)
Osteoporosis	**U.S. Preventive Services Task Force:** All adults over age 65 (over age 60 for those with risk factors) **Scientific Advisory Council of the Osteoporosis Society of Canada:** All women over age 65
Papanicolaou smear	**American Cancer Society:** Not recommended for women over age 70 with three consecutive normal smears **American College of Obstetricians and Gynecologists:** An individual decision between provider and client **Canadian Task Force on Preventive Health Care:** Not recommended for women over age 70 with four consecutive normal smears **U.S. Preventive Services Task Force:** Not recommended for women over age 65 with previous normal smears
HIV infection	All men at risk of infection
Obesity	All adult men
Syphilis	All men at risk
Tobacco use	All adult men

Data from: Curran, D. R. (2004). Should we discontinue Pap smear screening in women aged > 65 years? Journal of Family Practice, 53, 308–309; Shepherd, A. J. (2004). An overview of osteoporosis. Alternative Therapies, 10(2), 26–33; U.S. Preventive Services Task Force. (2005). The guide to clinical preventive services, 2005. Retrieved August 13, 2005, from http://www.ahrq.gov/clinic/pocketguide.htm; U.S. Preventive Services Task Force. (2005). Screening for abdominal aortic aneurysm. Retrieved August 13, 2005, from http://www.ahrq.gov/clinic/uspsaneu.htm

Disease Self-management

Effective chronic disease control requires a combination of supportive care, self-management, maintenance of function, and prevention of further disability. Over time, chronic illness requires an increasing burden of self-management. The ability to cope with the demands of self-management are complicated by three features of chronic illness: interference with functional abilities, limited effectiveness of treatment modalities, and disruption of one's daily routine. As noted by one author, life is often "consumed with the demands imposed by the coping strategies expected" in dealing with chronic illness (Tanner, 2004, p. 313). One's ability to cope with chronic illness is based on perceptions of four factors: the severity of the condition, one's personal responsibility for dealing with it, the controllability of its effects, and the changeability of the situation.

Tanner (2004) described three requisites for self-management of chronic disease. The first requisite is the presence of physical, environmental, mental, and socio-economic factors that promote effective disease management. For example, one must have the cognitive ability, economic resources, and knowledge of and access to a variety of community services needed to manage the chronic condition. Depression is an emotional factor that may preclude an environment conducive to self-management of disease.

The second requisite for effective self-management of disease is the knowledge and skills required to discontinue unhealthy behaviors, learn and execute replacement behaviors, and learn and execute related behaviors. The final, and perhaps most critical, requisite is the desire to cope with one's illness and take action.

Self-management of chronic disease involves a number of activities, including symptom response and monitoring, compliance with complicated medical and lifestyle regimens, and developing the skills needed for self-management. Steps that can promote self-management of disease among older clients mirror the nursing process and include establishing treatment goals, identifying alternative methods to achieve these goals, planning short-term interventions to achieve goals, implementing the plan, and evaluating and revising the plan (Tanner, 2004).

Managing medications is an important element of self-management of chronic illness. Community health nurses may assist with this task by encouraging providers to simplify medication regimens as much as possible for older adults. Targeted interventions that assist older adults with medication compliance may also be helpful. Technological interventions such as prompting devices, electronic dispensers, monitoring devices, and data management systems may be effective for clients who can afford them, but research is needed to test their effectiveness in practice (Logue, 2002). In one study, electronic monitors increased medication compliance among older women from various ethnic backgrounds.

Other research has indicated that expanded instructions in simple language also improves adherence (Robbins, Rausch, Garcia, & Prestwood, 2004). Results of another study indicated that the MD.2® automated medication dispensing system resulted in decreased time spent in nursing visits on medication review as well as fewer missed doses, lower hospitalization rates and fewer emergency department visits, and a decrease in the overall number of prescription medicines required (possibly due to better compliance and, therefore, increased effectiveness) (Buckwalter, Wakefield, Hanna, & Lehmann, 2004). Unfortunately, many elderly clients cannot afford these technological advances. Other, less expensive, strategies include pill organizers (Alemagno et al., 2004; Miller, 2004b) and telephone reminders (Buckwalter et al., 2004), and community health nurses can advocate the use of such strategies with low-income clients. Some automated reminder or dispensing systems are available via the Internet (http://www.epill.com, http://www. ontimrx.com, http://www.medpromot. com) (Miller, 2004b).

With increasing drug advertising, clients may request specific drugs, and community health nurses need to be knowledgeable in answering clients' questions about drugs for their conditions. Community health nurses can also refer clients to Web sites that provide comparisons of the effectiveness of specific medications. Effectiveness comparisons for multiple categories of drugs are available from the Drug Effectiveness Review Project (2005) or from AARP (2005) (http://www.ohsu.edu/drugeffectiveness/reports/final. cfm, http://www.aarp.org/health/comparedrugs).

Clients may also have questions about Medicare part D prescription drug coverage benefits, and community health nurses can either educate clients themselves

---

EVIDENCE-BASED PRACTICE

Logue (2002) described a variety of technology-based devices that may help improve medication compliance among older clients. She also noted a lack of evidence on the effectiveness of such devices for promoting compliance and suggested a number of self-medication outcomes that could be used in such research. These included (a) objective symptom measurement and physical examination (e.g., blood pressure monitoring), (b) direct indicators (e.g., blood glucose levels, or blood serum levels of medications), (c) indirect indicators (e.g., pill counts, prescription refills, pill diaries), subjective report of clients and families, and the frequency of visits to primary care providers and emergency departments.

Examine the health care literature. To what extent have these outcome measures been used to evaluate the effectiveness of technology-based interventions in promoting medication compliance among the elderly? What conclusion can be drawn from these studies? What other factors related to their effectiveness in the general population have not been addressed (e.g., the cost of technology for some segments of the population)? How might research be designed to address these additional factors?

or refer them to other sources of information. Community health nurses may also need to advocate for effective drug coverage for older clients and assist them to select prescription drug plans that best meet their personal needs. For example, during the transition to Medicare part D, many community health nurses found themselves battling drug plans to assure that clients' needs for medications were met. This was particularly true for clients with dual eligibility for Medicare and Medicaid who were used to having prescription drugs covered by Medicaid at low copayment rates. Following initiation of Medicare part D, some clients found that higher copayments were required or that some previously covered drugs were not covered under specific plans. Community health nurses worked with the Social Security Administration, local offices of Aging and Independent Services, prescription drug plans, and local pharmacies to assure continued medication access for these clients. At the aggregate level, community health nurses also need to advocate coverage of a set of drugs most commonly used by older clients under all Medicare-approved prescription drug plans. The provisions of Medicare part D are discussed in more detail in Chapter 8∞.

The effectiveness of self-management of chronic illness may be evaluated based on symptom assessment and physical examination, direct indicators of disease processes (e.g., blood glucose levels), or indirect indicators of medication compliance (e.g., pill counts, prescription refills). Additional measures of effectiveness include subjective reports of clients or family members or the frequency of visits to primary health care providers or emergency departments (Logue, 2002).

Dealing with Common Health Problems

As noted earlier, older clients experience a variety of health problems related to the effects of aging. They are also subject to problems stemming from chronic and communicable diseases. Secondary prevention for communicable diseases and chronic conditions is addressed in detail in Chapters 28 and 29∞. Here we will address interventions for some of the health problems commonly found in older populations. Community health nurses can assist individual clients in dealing with these problems or educate the older population in general. Some of the common problems encountered in caring for older clients include skin breakdown, constipation, urinary and fecal incontinence, sensory loss, mobility limitations, pain, and cognitive impairment. Additional problems that may be encountered by community health nurses working with this population include depression, social isolation, abuse and neglect, and substance abuse. Inadequate financial resources and the need for advocacy at individual and population levels are also areas that may be addressed by means of community health nursing interventions.

Some problems, like fecal and urinary incontinence, chronic pain, and cognitive impairment, are particularly distressing to clients and their caregivers and warrant specific consideration here. Urinary incontinence occurs in approximately 15% of older men and 30% of older women (National Institute on Aging, 2004). Generally speaking, behavioral approaches have proven more effective than medication in reducing urinary incontinence (Teunissen et al., 2004). Recommended interventions include decreasing fluid intake after the evening meal, urinating every 2 to 3 hours during the day, Kegel exercises, and eliminating constipation. Additional approaches may include treatment of underlying physical causes, use of prescription drugs, or modification of existing drug regimens (Dash et al., 2004).

Treatment of fecal incontinence may also employ a variety of strategies depending on its cause and severity. Community health nurses should encourage clients with incontinence to be examined by their primary care provider to identify any underlying medical conditions. In addition, community health nurses can suggest several dietary changes that may improve continence. For example, if incontinence is due to watery stools or to constipation, increasing bulk in the diet may contribute to stools that are more formed and easier to control. Conversely, for some people, high-fiber diets may have a laxative effect, increasing the problem of incontinence. Specific foods that relax the internal anal sphincter (e.g., caffeine-containing beverages and foods such as coffee, tea, and chocolate) may need to be avoided. Other foods that may contribute to fecal incontinence include cured meats, spicy foods, alcohol, dairy products, fruits (e.g., peaches and pears), fatty foods, and artificial sweeteners (National Digestive Diseases Information Clearinghouse, 2004).

Keeping a food diary may allow the client to identify other foods that cause problems. Community health nurses can educate clients about other dietary strategies that may help, including:

- Eating smaller, more frequent meals
- Eating food and drinking liquids at different times
- Eating an appropriate amount of fiber and focusing on foods with soluble fiber (e.g., bananas, rice, bread, potatoes, applesauce, cheese, smooth peanut butter, yogurt, pasta, oatmeal)
- Drinking sufficient fluids (64 ounces per day unless fluids are otherwise contraindicated) (National Digestive Diseases Information Clearinghouse, 2004)

Medications may also be used in the control of fecal incontinence, but clients should be encouraged to consult their primary care providers rather than use over-the-counter remedies. Bowel training using Kegel exercises or developing regular bowel patterns has also been found to be helpful in dealing with fecal incontinence (International Foundation for Functional Gastrointestinal Disorders, 2006b).

Community health nurses can also assist older clients with fecal or urinary incontinence to address the psychological effects of these problems. Some easy suggestions are to carry a backpack with cleanup supplies and a change of clothing whenever one leaves the house, locate restrooms before they are needed, use the toilet before leaving home, wear disposable undergarments or sanitary pads if needed, or use oral fecal deodorants for frequent episodes of incontinence.

Chronic pain in the elderly is often overlooked or undertreated. As we saw earlier, a significant proportion of older clients experience ongoing pain that is perceived by them and by their providers and caretakers to be a normal part of aging. Others experience pain as a result of a variety of chronic illnesses. A number of barriers exist to effective pain control in the older population. These barriers may relate to providers, to clients and/or their families, or to the health system in general (Hanks-Bell et al., 2004). Provider-related barriers include lack of expertise in pain assessment and management with older clients, concerns related to regulatory scrutiny in the prescription of pain medication, fear of opioid side effects, inability to assess pain in clients with cognitive impairment, and the previously mentioned perception that pain is normal in the aged. Client/family barriers include fear of medication side effects and addiction, reluctance to be considered a "bad patient," and, again, the fatalism exemplified in the belief that pain is part of aging, to be accepted. Health system barriers include the cost of pain medication, insufficient time to adequately assess pain and its management during client encounters, and cultural biases in the health professions against opioid use. Community health nurses can help educate the general public, as well as health care providers, regarding the need for appropriate pain control in the elderly. In addition, they can assist in the development of alternative options for pain control (e.g., development of and insurance coverage for acupuncture, guided imagery, and other pain relief services). Community health nursing advocacy may be required with health care providers, with family members, or within the health system to develop attitudes and services that support effective pain control for older clients. For example, the community health nurse might educate family members, or even clients themselves, regarding the improbability of addiction. Or, the nurse may need to advocate for access to pain-control services for low-income elderly clients.

The shortness of breath characteristic of advanced COPD can also be very disabling for older clients. In addition to referring clients for medical evaluation and possible therapy with bronchodilators, steroids, and oxygen, community health nurses can assist clients with COPD in implementing a variety of strategies that may improve lung function and limit disability. The primary intervention among smokers is, of course, smoking cessation. Clients with COPD who stop smoking have slower progression of disease than those who do not (Rennard, 2005). Community health nurses can refer clients who smoke to smoking cessation programs. They

may need to advocate with insurance plans for coverage of such services as necessary therapy for COPD.

Community health nurses can also suggest that clients refrain from excessive use of cough medicines to control the chronic cough characteristic of COPD because they decrease clearance of secretions, making clients more susceptible to respiratory infection. The nurse can also refer clients for pneumonia vaccine as well as annual influenza immunization to prevent infection. Nutrition is another important aspect of COPD control; more than 30% of patients with severe COPD exhibit malnutrition (Rennard, 2005). Suggestions for improving the nutritional status of clients with COPD include the following:

- Clearing airways and resting before eating
- Eating slowly and taking small bites that are chewed thoroughly
- Choosing foods that are easy to prepare and to chew
- Asking family members to help with meal preparation
- Eating smaller, more frequent meals
- Drinking fluids at the end of the meal instead of before or with food
- Sitting up straight while eating and using pursed-lip breathing during the meal
- Obtaining meals from a local Meals-on-Wheels program
- Eating the main meal early in the day to provide energy for the rest of the day (Cleveland Clinic, 2005c)

Pulmonary rehabilitation is another approach to controlling the debilitating effects of COPD. Comprehensive pulmonary rehabilitation may include education, exercise, psychosocial support, and the use of specific breathing techniques such as pursed-lip breathing, diaphragmatic breathing, and controlled coughing (Cleveland Clinic, 2005a, 2005b, 2005d). Easy-to-follow client instructions for these breathing techniques are available at the Web site of the Cleveland Clinic at http://www.clevelandclinic.org/health. Community health nurses can teach these strategies to clients with COPD as well as advocate for access to necessary diagnostic and treatment services.

As we saw earlier, the number of older adults with cognitive impairment is expected to increase significantly in the next few decades. In older clients, it is particularly important to distinguish among depression, dementia, and delirium, as each of these conditions may produce similar effects. Depression, as we will see in Chapter 30∞, can be effectively treated in most older clients. Treatment goals for depression in the elderly include reduction of suicide risk, improved level of function, and improved quality of life. Older antidepressant medications (e.g., tricyclic antidepressants, or TCAs) are cardiotoxic and may be less well tolerated in the elderly than newer drugs, leading to increased risk of overdose and mortality. For this reason, these drugs should not be routinely used to treat depression in older clients. Instead, "novel antidepressants" (e.g., selective serotonin reuptake inhibitors,

SSRIs) are recommended with close monitoring of treatment and adverse effects. Older clients are also more likely than younger ones to experience "discontinuation syndrome," a temporary condition that may include severe cognitive impairment, so they should be cautioned against abruptly stopping their medications (Antai-Otong, 2004). Community health nurses may advocate with health care providers for recognition and treatment of depression in elderly clients. They may also engage in political advocacy to assure access to treatment services for the older population. The principles of political advocacy were discussed in Chapter 7∞.

Delirium is usually characterized by a sudden onset and is generally reversible if the underlying cause is identified and treated. Some possible causes of delirium in the elderly include drug toxicity, infectious diseases, problems with elimination, exacerbation of chronic illness, or development of new disease processes. Other potential causes of delirium include changes in the psychosocial context such as a recent loss, a move to a new residence, or hospitalization. Dementia, on the other hand, is characterized by a gradual onset, progressive decline, and irreversibility (Henry, 2002; Naylor, 2003).

Recently, there has been progress in the development of drug therapies to retard the progression of Alzheimer's disease. Until a truly effective treatment is found, however, early detection and advance planning for progressive decline are the best modes of control for this condition (National Institute on Aging, 2002). The most effective approaches to care of individual clients with Alzheimer's disease combine medication, lifestyle changes, and supportive services for both clients and their families (Alzheimer's Association, 2001).

The goal of treatment in the face of cognitive impairment is to maintain the client's quality of life as much as possible. Specific medications such as donepezil, galantamine, and rivastigmine may be helpful in slowing cognitive decline in clients with Alzheimer's disease, particularly when initiated early in the disease process. Antidepressants, mood stabilizers, and antipsychotics may also be warranted for some clients (Vogel, 2003), although, as we saw earlier, use of these medications may lead to accidental injury in some clients. Activities that enhance memory capabilities may also be of some help. Similarly, exercise, hand massage, and therapeutic touch have been shown to be of some benefit (Bates, Boote, & Beverly, 2004; Vogel, 2003). Consistent routines, reduction of environmental stimulation and triggers for agitated or aggressive behavior, and adequate rest are other interventions that may assist the cognitively impaired client (Vogel, 2003).

In the past, reality orientation was recommended as a strategy for dealing with confusion in older people, particularly those with dementia. Reality orientation was a practice of reminding the client of "reality" when they strayed too far from it. For example, the nurse might persistently inform a client with dementia that

her husband would not be coming to visit her because he died 3 years ago or that she cannot find the closet because she is no longer living in her old home. Research has indicated, however, that the effect of reality orientation was not to reorient the client to the present but to create anxiety and distress (Allen, 2000).

A more recent approach is termed **validation therapy**, a therapeutic approach to dealing with dementia by *validating* and accepting what the client perceives as reality. Validation therapy is based on the theory that people attempt to resolve unfinished life issues and that retreat into a specific *unreality* is an attempt to do that. It also presupposes that there is a reason for the behavior exhibited. Validation classifies dementia behaviors into four progressive stages: malorientation, time confusion, repetitive motion, and vegetation (Validation Training Institute, 2003). In the malorientation stage, the client expresses past conflicts in "disguised forms." For example, a client may believe that her daughter is her mother and reenact conflicts from the past. In the time confusion stage, the client retreats inward and may not be in touch with reality, but still attempts to resolve old life issues. In the repetitive motion stage, movements replace words in the attempt to resolve past conflicts, and finally, in the vegetation stage, the client gives up trying to resolve life issues and retreats from the world. In the validation approach, the caregiver (nurse or family member) accepts what the client perceives as reality and tries to redirect them without engaging in confrontations aimed at orienting them to reality. For example, a confused client may be asking when her dead husband will arrive. Rather than reminding her that he will never arrive because he is dead, the caretaker might just say, "Oh, not for a while yet, let's have lunch while we wait," redirecting the client's attention to a positive activity without causing distress.

Although validation therapy was developed between 1963 and 1980, there is limited research examining its effectiveness in addressing the problems of dementia. A recent meta analysis of research in this area found only three studies that met inclusion criteria. Based on the results of the analysis, the author concluded that there was "insufficient evidence from randomized trials to allow any conclusion about the efficacy of validation therapy for people with dementia or cognitive impairment" (Briggs, 2006, p. 3).

Advocacy may be required to be sure that treatment and supportive services are available in the community for older clients with impaired cognitive function and their families. Advocacy for respite care for caregivers is particularly important, and community health nurses may even advocate with caregivers themselves to take advantage of such services. Finally, advocacy is needed to support continuing research on the effectiveness of therapeutic approaches in dealing with the issues of dementia and cognitive impairment in the elderly. Secondary prevention interventions for these and other problems common among older clients are presented in Table 19-6◆.

TABLE 19-6 Secondary Prevention Strategies for Common Problems in the Older Population

Client Problem	Secondary Prevention Strategies
Skin breakdown	Inspect extremities regularly for lesions.
	Keep lesions clean and dry.
	Eliminate pressure by frequent changes of position.
	Refer for treatment as needed.
Constipation	Encourage fluid and fiber intake.
	Discourage ignoring urge to defecate.
	Encourage regular exercise.
	Encourage regular bowel habits.
	Use mild laxatives as needed, but discourage overuse.
	Administer enemas as needed; discourage overuse.
	Administer bulk products or stool softeners as indicated.
Urinary incontinence	Refer for urological consult or treatment of underlying physical causes.
	Refer for modification of medication regimen as needed.
	Encourage frequent voiding.
	Teach Kegel exercises.
	Decrease fluids after the evening meal.
	Assist with bladder training.
	Encourage use of sanitary pads, panty liners, etc., with frequent changes of such aids.
	Keep skin clean and dry; change clothing and bed linen as needed.
	Offer bedpan or urinal frequently or assist to bedside commode at frequent intervals.
Fecal incontinence	Refer for medical treatment of underlying causes as needed.
	Educate for dietary changes to address contributing factors.
	Encourage avoidance of caffeinated beverages and chocolate.
	Suggest smaller, more frequent meals.
	Suggest eating and drinking at different times.
	Encourage consumption of soluble fiber.
	Encourage sufficient fluid intake.
	Teach Kegel exercises or bowel training.
	Suggest strategies to decrease embarrassment.
Sensory loss	Provide adequate lighting.
	Keep eyeglasses clean and hearing aids functional.
	Eliminate safety hazards.
	Use large-print books or materials.
	Use multisensory approaches to communication and teaching.
	Avoid using colors that make discrimination difficult.
	Speak clearly and slowly, at a lower pitch.
	Eliminate background noise.
	Assist clients to obtain voice enhancers for phone.
	Use additional herbs and spices, but use with discretion.
	Purchase small amounts of perishable foods.
	Check pilot lights on gas appliances frequently.
	Encourage the use of smoke detectors.
Mobility limitation	Provide assistance with ambulation, transfer, etc.
	Assist clients to obtain equipment such as walkers and wheelchairs.
	Install ramps, tub rails, etc., as needed.
	Promote access to public facilities for older persons.

Continued on next page

TABLE 19-6	Secondary Prevention Strategies for Common Problems in the Older Population *(continued)*
	Assist clients to find alternative sources of transportation.
	Make referrals for assistance with personal care or instrumental activities as needed.
Pain	Plan activities for times when pain is controlled.
	Encourage warm soaks.
	Encourage adequate rest and exercise to prevent mobility limitations.
	Encourage effective use of analgesics.
	Refer for assistance with alternative pain control measures.
COPD (shortness of breath)	Refer for medical therapy (e.g., bronchodilators, steroids, oxygen), as needed.
	Educate regarding safety precautions with oxygen therapy.
	Encourage smoking cessation, as needed.
	Advocate for coverage of smoking cessation under health insurance plans.
	Encourage and refer for pneumonia and influenza immunization.
	Promote adequate nutrition.
	Encourage small, easily prepared and eaten meals or ask for assistance in meal preparation from family members.
	Discourage use of cough suppressants.
	Suggest taking fluids at the end of the meal rather than before or with foods.
	Refer to Meals-on-Wheels, if appropriate.
	Suggest sitting upright to eat.
	Educate client for pursed-lip breathing, diaphragmatic breathing, and controlled coughing.
	Promote physical activity as tolerated.
	Advocate for access to necessary diagnostic and treatment services.
Cognitive impairment	Apply principles of validation therapy, if helpful.
	Refer for Alzheimer's drug therapy as indicated.
	Refer for antidepressant, mood-stabilizing, or antipsychotic medications as needed.
	Promote exercise (register wanderers with national registry if appropriate).
	Promote activities to enhance memory (e.g., discussion of current events, games, puzzles, etc.).
	Educate families and caregivers regarding the progression of disease.
	Provide hand massage or therapeutic touch services or teach these interventions to caregivers.
	Establish consistent daily routines.
	Reduce environmental stimulation and triggers for aberrant behavior.
	Provide adequate rest.
Depression	Accept feelings and reflect on their normality; encourage client to ventilate feelings.
	Refer for counseling or medications as needed.
Social isolation	Compensate for sensory loss; enhance communication abilities.
	Improve mobility; provide access to transportation.
	Assist client to obtain adequate financial resources.
	Refer client to new support systems.
	Assist client to deal with grief over loss of loved ones.
Abuse or neglect	Assist caretakers to develop positive coping strategies.
	Assist families to obtain respite care or day care for older members.
	Refer families for counseling as needed.
	Arrange placement in temporary shelter.
	Assist families in making other arrangements for safe care of older clients.
	Advocate for laws and protective services systems that protect older clients from abuse.
Substance abuse	Identify problem drinking by older clients.
	Refer for therapy, Alcoholics Anonymous, or Al-Anon as appropriate.

Continued on next page

TABLE 19-6	Secondary Prevention Strategies for Common Problems in the Older Population *(continued)*	
	Observe for toxic effects of alcohol ingestion.	
	Maintain hydration and nutrition.	
Inadequate financial resources	Refer for financial assistance.	
	Assist with budgeting and priority allocation.	
	Educate for less expensive means of meeting needs.	
	Function as an advocate as needed.	

Tertiary Prevention

Tertiary preventive activities for older clients focus on preventing complications of existing conditions and preventing their recurrence. Tertiary prevention for the individual client depends on the problems experienced by the client. For example, tertiary prevention for an abused older client may include long-term counseling for family members, whereas prevention related to financial inadequacies may involve assistance with budgeting. Four specific areas of tertiary prevention in the care of older populations will be addressed here. These include monitoring health status, palliative care, end-of-life care, and caring for caregivers.

Monitoring Health Status

As we saw earlier, the majority of older clients will experience one or more chronic health conditions, and the prevalence of these conditions increases with increasing age. Community health nurses can be actively involved in monitoring the continuing health status of individual older clients and in the development and implementation of programs to monitor the effectiveness of provider intervention and self-management. For example, community health nurses may advocate for the initiation of community programs to support the needs of clients with diabetes or pain control for populations with arthritis. Monitoring of hypertension is another important role for community health nurses. In one study, older clients perceived ongoing blood pressure monitoring as reassuring and contributing to effective decisions regarding self-management. Monitoring provided opportunities to educate clients regarding their conditions and treatment regimens, as well as ensuring regular social contact and demonstration of concern (Vivarai-Dresler & Bakker, 2004). Community health nurses should advocate for, and in some cases provide, disease management and monitoring services available to all segments of the older population, particularly low-income older clients.

Palliative Care

Palliative care is another important consideration in tertiary prevention with the older adult population. Because of the incurability of many chronic conditions, the only avenue open for intervention is symptom management. **Palliative care** is care that addresses pain and symptom relief without attempting to cure the underlying disease process. The intent of palliative care is to decrease suffering and improve quality of life for both clients and families (Zerwekh, 2006). Although often viewed in the context of end-of-life care, as indicated in this definition, palliative care is also warranted when symptom control is the primary goal of care. Important features of palliative care include relief of pain and other symptoms, effective communication with health care providers, and achievement of a sense of completion. Goals for palliative care include the following:

- Sustained relationships with client and family
- Continued independence and function as long as desired by the client
- Aggressive symptom relief
- Physical, psychosocial, and spiritual support
- Attention to client needs in the context of the family and community
- Family involvement in care
- Incorporation of cultural and spiritual perspectives in care
- Determination of goals based on client and family values and choices
- Care provided through a multidisciplinary approach
- Acknowledgment and relief of caregiver burden
- Development of support systems in home and community (Zerwekh, 2006)

Palliative care often takes place in hospice settings. Unfortunately, Medicare's requirement for hospice care includes forgoing all further curative measures and a projected life expectancy of less than 6 months, leading to initiation of hospice care too late in the trajectory of disease (Matesa, 2002). Some hospices, particularly those in managed care systems, are now instituting separate palliative services that may be initiated prior to actual hospice care. In 2002, however, only 26% of hospitals provided palliative care programs, primarily due to lack of insurance coverage for such programs (Plese, 2002). Some managed care organizations cover the cost of palliative care, but costs are often borne as out-of-pocket expenses by older clients or their families.

Last Acts (2002), an advocacy group for end-of-life care, identified five principles of palliative care:

- Respect for the goals, likes, and choices of clients
- Attention to the medical, emotional, social, and spiritual needs of clients
- Support for family members

- Promotion of access to necessary health care providers and settings
- Promotion of excellent end-of-life care through support and assistance to caregivers

Community health nurses may be involved in providing palliative care to older clients and others with incurable conditions. Such care presents a number of challenges, including provision of pain relief and holistic care and dealing with symptoms such as fatigue and breathlessness, among others. In one study, community health nurses reported being unprepared to discuss death with clients' families or to deal with other areas of communication. For example, community health nurses experienced difficulty regarding disclosure of the client's condition or prognosis to the client or to family members. Community health nurses also reported being unprepared to deal with the emotional reactions of family members (particularly anger) and with their own personal emotional reactions to caring for these clients (Dunne, Sullivan, & Kernohan, 2005). In addition to providing care to individual clients, community health nurses may be actively involved in developing palliative care services and in advocating coverage of these services under both public and private health insurance programs.

End-of-life Care

Three specific considerations must be addressed in providing effective end-of-life care to older clients. These include formulation of advance directives, personal preparation for death, and actual care of the dying client.

In 1990, the Patient Self-determination Act required hospitals, nursing homes, hospices, managed care organizations, and other agencies receiving Medicare and Medicaid funds to inform clients of their right to refuse treatment and formulate advance care directives (Kleespies, 2004). Advance care planning is defined as "a process of discussion between professionals, families, and patients aimed at quality of care at the end of life" (Laakkonen, Pitkala, Strandberg, Berglind, & Tilvis, 2004, p. 247). Advance care planning may result in specific documents such as living wills or health-related powers of attorney. These documents specify circumstances in which life-sustaining treatment is or is not to be provided and appoint a surrogate to make decisions regarding life-sustaining treatments in the event of the client's incapacitation (Last Acts, 2002). **Life-sustaining treatment** is defined as "any medical intervention that would have little or no effect on the underlying disease, injury, or condition, but is administered to forestall the time of death or to reinstate life when death can be regarded as having occurred" (Kleespies, 2004, p. 57).

Three assumptions form the underlying premise for advance care directives: (a) people complete them, (b) the treatment preferences expressed are accurate and current, and (c) surrogate decision makers are able to interpret advance directives in light of the circumstances of a given situation. Unfortunately, research suggests that none of these assumptions is consistently met (Kleespies, 2004). For example, in one study in Finland, only 12% of the population studied had executed a living will. Among those who had a living will, 46% indicated that they would want to have cardiopulmonary resuscitation performed if needed, in contrast to the declarations in their living will documents (Laakkonen et al., 2004). In another study, subjects perceived both advantages and disadvantages to advance directives. Advantages included protection of personal integrity and support for family decision making; however, participants also saw advance directives as opening the possibility of euthanasia. They also voiced concerns that changes in perspective after executing an advance directive would not be taken into consideration and 57% of them indicated that they might not want to adhere to advance directives during dying (Seymour, Gott, Bellamy, Ahmedzai, & Clark, 2004). Studies of clients with cancer in intensive care units have also indicated that the presence of advance directives did not influence whether or not life-support interventions were initiated (Last Acts, 2002).

To be effective, advance care planning documents must be supported by state policies, usually legislation, that promote their implementation. Last Acts (2002) has identified six criteria for such state-level policies. The first criterion is that policies recommend one advance directive to address foreseeable circumstances. Second, states should avoid mandating a specific format for advance directives. The third criterion is that state policy gives precedence to the designated surrogate decision maker that overrides the written document or to the most recent directive. Fourth, state policies should authorize specific default surrogate decision makers in the event that none have been named. Fifth, close friends, as well as family members, should be recognized as possible surrogates. Finally, states should establish a statewide do-not-resuscitate (DNR) order for emergency medical services in the state. Unfortunately, by 2002, only seven states had laws related to advance directives that addressed all criteria (Last Acts, 2002).

Based on the difficulties noted with formal documents, some authors suggest that, in advance care planning, it "now seems more important to investigate the process of advance care planning in the doctor-patient relationship and to explore the poorly understood values and motives behind the expressed preferences" (Laakkonen et al., 2004, p. 248). The same need for exploration of desires and the values underlying them would seem to exist for families as well, and community health nurses may need to advocate for such discussions. They may also need to advocate compliance with advance directives by family members or health care providers when these directives have been written.

Preparation for death usually also entails a number of practical activities involved in getting one's affairs in order. Older clients may need to make decisions about funeral arrangements or the disposition of their belongings. Both nurses and family members should be encouraged to listen to clients in their reflections on such matters, rather than put them off with assurances that they "won't die for a long time yet." Community health nurses may need to advocate with family members to encourage them to address older clients' concerns about dying. Nurses may also need to refer clients for legal assistance with wills, burial plans, and other financial arrangements. Many communities have low-cost legal aid services available to elderly clients. Community health nurses should keep in mind, however, the cultural differences in preparation for death that clients may exhibit (Mitty, 2001). For example, in many cultures, such decisions are believed to be the responsibility of children, and the dying client should not be bothered. In others, discussion of death is believed to hasten its occurrence, so clients are not willing to explore plans related to their deaths.

"End-of-life care begins the moment there is a shift from trying to challenge the illness to trying to challenge the suffering of the human who is experiencing serious life-threatening illness" (Plese, 2002, p. 7). End-of-life care includes five essential services: assessment of the living situation, management of symptoms and promotion of quality of life, promotion of advance care planning, counseling for client and family, and provision of continuity, communication, and coordination of care. The Palliative Care Task Force (Henderson, 2004) has identified five principles of end-of-life care. These principles are as follows:

- Respect for client and family goals, preferences, and choices
- Provision of comprehensive care
- Use of interdisciplinary expertise
- Attention to caregiver concerns
- Use of systems and mechanisms that support dying clients and their families

At present, more than half of older Americans die in hospitals, although 70% express the desire to die at home. Approximately half of dying clients do so in pain, and only 42% of U.S. hospitals have formal pain management programs and 23% provide hospice services. Only seven states have high-quality pain management policies. In addition, no state has more than 1% of primary care providers who are certified in palliative care, and only 15 states have more than 1% of full-time-equivalent registered nurses with certification (Last Acts, 2002). Community health nurses can be active in promoting effective end-of-life policies through legislative advocacy. Locally, they can help to ensure that advance directives will be implemented and support clients and family members in their execution.

End-of-life care also includes care for family members of the dying client. Community health nurses can assist families with both anticipatory grief and grief after the death of a loved one. In addition, they can advocate for effective services that assist with the management of grief. As many as 35% of bereaved family members have been found to meet the criteria for major depression, yet their depression is often unrecognized and few services are available to them. Anticipatory grief is defined as "any grief occurring prior to a loss, as distinguished from the grief that occurs at or after a loss" (Aldrich, as quoted in Lewis & McBride, 2004, p. 45). Anticipatory grief is experienced in response to an impending loss, and may be characterized by withdrawal, detachment, or caring and love. Community health nurses can assist families to share information and feelings and to resolve unfinished business in either practical or relational realms. Community health nurses may also need to help families adjust to changes in roles, particularly in cultural groups in which loss of people in specific designated roles may have a greater impact on the family (Lewis & McBride, 2004).

Caring for Caregivers

The last major consideration in tertiary prevention with the older population is caring for those who provide care to this group. The National Family Caregiver Support Program (NFCSP) has identified five core services needed by caregivers. These include information, referral to needed assistance, counseling, respite, and help with supplies, assistive devices, and so on (Plese, 2005a). Caregivers need information regarding the older client's condition and treatment regimen as well as the availability of services in the local community and how to obtain them. Information may also be needed on managing life changes and on dealing with financial and legal issues, particularly in the face of increasing cognitive impairment in the recipient of care (Alzheimer's Association, 2001). Many caregivers lack information about resources available to them. In some instances, services may be perceived as unable to meet the religious and cultural needs of some segments of the population (Merrell et al., 2005). Caregivers may also benefit from counseling services that help them to cope with the physical and emotional burdens of caregiving. Counseling may prevent caregivers from being "engulfed" by their caregiving role (Brown & Alligood, 2004). **Respite**, the provision of temporary relief from caregiving responsibilities, is often lacking for many caregivers who have 24-hour, 7-day-a-week responsibilities for the care of their aging family members. When available, respite may be provided by informal (other family members and friends) or formal support networks. Finally, caregivers may need help with obtaining needed supplies and assistive devices or in dealing with the financial burden of caregiving.

Both health care systems and caregivers themselves give rise to barriers to caregiver empowerment. Caregiver-related barriers may include an absence of focus on self, reluctance to share caregiving duties with

TABLE 19-7 Tertiary Prevention Strategies in the Care of Older Populations

Focus	Tertiary Prevention Strategies
Monitoring health status	Monitor health status and treatment effects for individual older clients.
	Design and implement programs to monitor health status in older client.
Palliative care	Provide palliative care or refer individual clients for palliative care services.
	Advocate for accessible palliative care services for population groups.
End-of-life care	Assist individual clients and families with advance care planning.
	Advocate for adherence to advance directives within health care systems.
	Advocate for effective state and national policies related to advance directives.
	Provide culturally sensitive and appropriate end-of-life care to individual clients.
	Advocate for access to hospice and other end-of-life services.
	Advocate for changes in reimbursement for end-of-life services.
Caregiver support	Provide support to individual caregivers, including referral to available support services.
	Educate the public and caregivers regarding their own needs.
	Promote caregiver empowerment.
	Advocate for support services for caregivers.
	Advocate for insurance coverage of supportive services needed by caregivers.

others, reluctance to consider or discuss the effects of caregiving on their own health, and lack of awareness of caregiver support services (Plese, 2005a). Caregivers may focus on the needs of the care recipient to the exclusion of their own needs. They may also feel a duty and responsibility for caregiving as part of their relationship with the recipient. In addition, as we saw earlier, many caregivers do not perceive themselves as such and do not realize that they are eligible for whatever supportive services may exist. Barriers related to the health system include a lack of attention to the needs of caregivers and lack of availability of and funding for caregiver support services. Specific services that may be needed to support caregivers include domiciliary assistance with personal care, social work services to maintain clients in home settings without undue burden on caregivers, respite care, support groups, and interactions with multidisciplinary teams that can address the multiple needs of clients and their caregivers (Hoskins et al., 2005). Community health nurses can be actively involved in supporting individual caregivers and referring them for needed assistance, including respite services and counseling. They can also function as advocates to assure that such services are provided and that caregivers in all segments of the population have access to culturally sensitive and appropriate support. Selected strategies for tertiary prevention in the care of older populations are presented in Table 19-7◆.

IMPLEMENTING CARE FOR OLDER POPULATIONS

Two major considerations in implementing care for older populations are health education directed at this group and political advocacy. Information sources for educating clients and the general public on health issues of concern to older populations are presented on page 538. Health education initiatives are based on the general principles of teaching and learning discussed in Chapter 11∞, but there are also some unique considerations in implementing education programs for the older adult population.

Older adults may exhibit some decline in linguistic skills with age. Auditory communication may be too fast-paced for comprehension or contain too much information to be easily comprehensible (Qualls, Harris, & Rogers, 2002). Sensory losses also need to be considered when teaching the older client population. Strategies to circumvent hearing loss include using a lower-pitched voice; facing the listener while speaking; employing nonverbal teaching techniques; using clear, concise terminology; and having the client use a hearing aid if needed. The effects of hearing loss can also be minimized by limiting background noise, reemphasizing important points, and supplementing verbal with written materials.

The use of glasses, a magnifying glass, and large print may help to minimize visual deficits. Learning can also be enhanced by visual materials using black lettering on white or yellow paper, providing adequate lighting, and eliminating glare in the learning environment.

In implementing health education plans for older adults, the nurse may need to repeat material more frequently. Because of decreases in short-term memory, it may take longer for some older clients to learn new material. Once material is learned, however, older clients retain it as well as younger ones. Multisensorial presentation, multiple repetitions, reinforcement of verbal content with written materials, and use of memory aids (e.g., a calendar for taking medications) may also assist learning in older clients.

Because response times are longer for older people than for their younger counterparts, lessons should proceed at a slower pace, and the nurse should allow more time for responses on the part of the client. Self-paced

CLIENT EDUCATION   Information Resources for Older Clients

Information Category	Agency/Organization	Information Category	Agency/Organization
Abuse	National Center on Elder Abuse	Exercise and nutrition (cont.)	Healthy Aging Campaign
	http://www.elderabusecenter.org		http://www.healthyaging.net
Advanced care directives	Aging with Dignity		National Institute on Aging
	http://www.agingwithdignity.com		http://www.niapublications.org
	Partnership for Caring		http://www.nia.nih.gov/exercisebook
	http://www.partnershipforcaring.org		National Policy and Resource Center on Nutrition and Aging
Alzheimer's disease	Alzheimer's Association		http://www.fiu.edu
	http://www.alz.org		USDA Food and Nutrition Information Center
	Alzheimer's Disease Education and Referral Center (ADEAR)		http://www.nal.usda.gov/fnic
	http://www.alzheimers.org	Financial barriers to care	Medicare Rights Center
Caregiving	American Association of Retired Persons (AARP)		http://www.medicarerights.org
	http://www.aarp.org/life/caregiving		National Council on Aging
	Family Caregiver Alliance		http://www.benefitscheckup.org
	http://www.caregiver.org		Pharmaceutical Research and Manufacturers of America
	National Alliance for Caregiving		http://www.helpingpatients.org
	http://www.caregiving.org	Immunization	National Immunization Program
	National Family Caregivers Association		http://www.cdc.gov/nip/recs/adult-schedule.htm
	http://www.nfcacares.org	Mental health/ substance abuse	American Association for Geriatric Psychiatry
Cultural competence	National Council on Interpreting in Health Care		http://www.aagponline.org
	http://www.ncihc.org/index.htm		National Clearinghouse for Alcohol and Drug Information (NCADI)
	National Institutes of Health (NIH)		http://www.health.org
	http://www.salud.nih.gov		National Institute of Mental Health (NIMH)
	U.S. Office of Minority Health		http://www.nimh.nih.gov
	http://www.omhrc.gov	Sexuality	Sexuality Information and Education Council of the United States
Driving/safety	American Association of Retired Persons (AARP)		http://www.siecus.org/pubs/biblio/bibs0012.html
	http://www.aarp.org/drive	Social services	Eldercare Locator
	Getting Around Safe & Sound and Granddriver		http://www.eldercare.gov
	http://www.aamva.org/drivers/drv_AgingDrivers.asp	Urinary incontinence	American Foundation for Urological Diseases
	http://www.granddriver.info		http://www.afud.org
End-of-life care	National Hospice and Palliative Care Organization		National Institute of Diabetes and Digestive and Kidney Disorders (NIDDK)
	http://www.nhpco.org		http://www.niddk.nih.gov
Exercise and nutrition	Centers for Disease Control and Prevention		The Simon Foundation for Continence
	http://www.cdc.gov/agomg/index.htm		http://www.simonfoundation.org/html
	http://www.cdc.gov/nccdphp/dnpa/index.htm		
	http://www.cdc.gov/nccdphp/dnpa/physical/growing_stronger/growing_stronger.pdf		

instruction is helpful. Motivation to learn can be heightened by increasing client participation in the lesson and by setting easily attainable, progressive goals that enhance success and satisfaction. Irrelevant material can confuse clients and should be eliminated from the presentation.

Endurance may be somewhat limited in older clients, so teaching sessions should be kept short (10 to 15 minutes per session). Lessons should be scheduled at times of the day when learners are rested and comfortable. Health education for older clients should not be time limited, as they may need more or less time to learn specific material. Again, learning should be broken down into small, progressive steps so that periodic success will continue to motivate older learners.

The teaching-learning process should also allow for rest periods as needed.

Political advocacy may be needed to implement primary, secondary, and tertiary prevention strategies with older populations. Political advocacy is based on the general principles discussed in Chapter 7∞ but may require more effort than advocacy for other population groups in countries like the United States that are affected by pervasive ageism. Advocacy efforts may need to start at local levels, with research that documents the cost savings of health promotion strategies and effective end-of life care. For example, it has been demonstrated that every Medicare dollar spent on hospice services actually saves $1.52 in hospitalization costs and that expenditures for hospice clients in the last month of life are two thirds lower than those for clients who do not receive hospice services (Plese, 2002). Similarly, the cost savings associated with family caregiving versus formal care can be used as justification for services to support caregivers.

EVALUATING HEALTH CARE FOR OLDER POPULATIONS

Evaluating the effectiveness of health care for older members of the population can occur at the individual or aggregate level. At the individual level, the community health nurse would assess the client's health status and the effects of primary, secondary, and tertiary interventions in improving health status. On occasion, the effectiveness of care would be measured in terms of a peaceful death and the physical and emotional health of family members and caregivers.

At the aggregate level, evaluation of the effects of care on the health of the elderly can be measured, in part, by the level of accomplishment of relevant national health objectives. The status of selected national objectives for the year 2010 related to the health of older clients is reflected below. As we can see, only one of the objectives for this age group has been met, and four objectives are actually moving away from their targets. These data indicate that more effort is required to promote the health of the older U.S. population.

Because older clients frequently have multiple health problems, many people consider care for older individuals as incongruent with the population-focused health promotion emphasis of community health nursing. Primary, secondary, and tertiary prevention efforts by community health nurses, however, can decrease the burden of illness experienced by older clients themselves as well as by society.

HEALTHY PEOPLE 2010
Goals for Population Health◆

OBJECTIVE	BASELINE	MOST RECENT DATA	TARGET
▓ 1-9c. Reduce hospitalization rates for immunization-preventable pneumonia (per 10,000 persons over 65)	10.6	11.2	8#
▓ 2-9. Reduce cases of osteoporosis in adults 50 years of age and older	10%	NDA	8%
▓ 2-10. Reduce hospitalization for vertebral fractures due to osteoporosis (per 10,000 persons over 65)	17.5	14.1	14.0
▓ 3-12. Increase colorectal cancer screening with fecal occult blood in persons 50 years of age and older	35%	33%	50%#
▓ 12-6. Reduce hospitalization for heart failure in:			
a. Adults 65 to 74 years of age (per 1,000 people)	13.2	12.3	6.5
b. Adults 75 to 84 years of age (per 1,000 people)	26.7	27.1	13.5#
c. Adults 85 years and older (per 1,000 people)	52.7	50.4	26.5
▓ 14-5. Reduce invasive pneumococcal infections (per 100,000 people)	62	51	42
▓ 14-29. Increase immunization among those 65 years of age and older for:			
a. Influenza	64%	66%	90%
b. Pneumococcal disease	46%	56%	90%
▓ 15-15. Reduce motor vehicle crash deaths (per 100,000 people over 70 years of age)	23.7	23.1	9.2
▓ 15-16. Reduce pedestrian deaths (per 100,000 people over 70 years of age)	3.9	2.7	1
▓ 15-28. Reduce hip fractures (per 100,000 people over 65 years of age			
a. Females	1,055.8	1029.2	416.0
b. Males	592.7	484.2	474.0
▓ 19-1. Increase the proportion of people over 60 years of age at healthy weight	36%	28%	60%#
▓ 21-4. Reduce the proportion of older adults who have lost all of their teeth	26%	24%	20%

Continued on next page

HEALTHY PEOPLE 2010 *continued*

■ 22-1. Reduce the proportion of adults with no leisure-time physical activity as follows:			
a. 65 to 74 years of age	51%	47%	20%
b. Over 75 years of age	64%	61%	20%
■ 24-4. Reduce hospitalizations for asthma (per 10,000 people over 65 years of age)	17.7	21.4	11#
■ 24-10. Reduce activity limitation due to COPD in:			
a. Men over 65 years of age	4.4%	4.4%	1.5%
b. Women over 65 years of age	3.3%	3.2%	1.5%
■ 27-1. Reduce tobacco use (older adults)	11%	9%	12%*

NDA—No data available

* Objective has been met

 # Objective moving away from target

Data from: *Centers for Disease Control and Prevention. (2005).* **Healthy people data.** *Retrieved September 5, 2005, from http://wonder.cdc.gov/data2010*

Case Study

Caring for an Elderly Woman

Henrietta Walker is a 68-year-old African American woman who has been referred for community health nursing services following her discharge from the hospital. She was hospitalized after being found unconscious in her room by her 50-year-old daughter. A diagnosis of diabetes mellitus was made, and Mrs. Walker was placed on 15 units of NPH insulin daily. She and her daughter were instructed on injection technique and a diabetic diet at the hospital.

Mrs. Walker lives with her daughter and son-in-law and their three teenage boys (ages 18, 15, and 13). They live in a lower-class neighborhood, and the son-in-law works at the local textile plant. His income is barely enough for the family to live on. Mrs. Walker does not know how she will pay her hospital bill. She has Medicare, Part A, and a small Social Security income, but she does not have any supplemental health insurance.

Mrs. Walker's vision is failing, probably as a result of undiagnosed diabetes of long standing. She hears well but is 80 pounds overweight, so is unsteady on her feet. The family lives in a second-floor apartment, and there is no handrail on the stairs outside the apartment. Mrs. Walker tries to help out around the house because her daughter works. She says she does not want to be a burden to her daughter and her son-in-law. Mrs. Walker's husband died of a heart attack 8 months ago, and that was when she came to live with her daughter. Mrs. Walker's daughter says that her mother's presence has caused some friction among the boys because the two younger ones now have to share a room.

1. What are the biophysical, psychological, physical environmental, sociocultural, behavioral, and health system factors influencing Mrs. Walker's health?
2. What nursing diagnoses can be derived from the information presented in the case study? Be sure to include the etiology of Mrs. Walker's problems where appropriate.
3. How would you prioritize these diagnoses? Why?
4. How would you go about incorporating client participation in planning interventions for Mrs. Walker's health problems?
5. List at least three client care objectives that you would like to accomplish with Mrs. Walker.
6. Describe some of the primary, secondary, and tertiary prevention strategies that would be appropriate in resolving Mrs. Walker's health problems. Why would they be appropriate?
7. How would you evaluate your nursing intervention? What criteria would you use to evaluate care?

Test Your Understanding

1. What are the three categories of theories of aging? What theories fit within each category? (pp. 496–497)

2. What are some of the biophysical, psychological, physical environmental, sociocultural, behavioral, and health system factors that affect the health of older clients? (pp. 497–519)

3. What are the major emphases in primary prevention in the care of older clients? Give examples of community health nursing interventions related to each. (pp. 522–526)

4. Describe at least one secondary preventive measure in each of four common health problems encountered among older clients. (pp. 526–534)

5. Identify at least one tertiary prevention measure in each of the four emphasis areas discussed in this chapter. (pp. 534–537).

6. What are two major considerations in implementing health-related interventions with older adults? In what ways are these considerations similar to and different from care of other age groups? (pp. 537–539)

EXPLORE MediaLink

 http://www.prenhall.com/clark
Resources for this chapter can be found on the Companion Website.

Audio Glossary
Appendix I: Adult Health Assessment and
  Intervention Guide
Exam Review Questions

Case Study: Caring for the Aged
MediaLink Application: Defying
  Ageism (video)
Media Links

Challenge Your Knowledge
Update *Healthy People 2010*
Advocacy Interviews

References

Advisory Committee on Immunization Practices. (2004). Recommended adult immunization schedule—United States, October 2004–September 2005. *Morbidity and Mortality Weekly Report, 53,* Q1–Q4.

Albert, S. M., Im, A., & Raveis, V. H. (2002). Public health and the second 50 years of life. *American Journal of Public Health, 92,* 1214–1216.

Alemagno, S. A., Niles, S. A., & Treiber, E. A. (2004). Using computers to reduce medication misuse of community-based seniors: Results of a pilot intervention program. *Geriatric Nursing, 25,* 281–285.

Allen, J. (2000). *Using validation therapy to manage difficult behaviors.* Retrieved March 16, 2006, from http://www.ec-online.net/Community/Activists/difficultbehaviors.htm

Alzheimer's Association. (2001). *The Alzheimer's disease study: Communication gaps between primary care physicians and caregivers.* Retrieved December 20, 2001, from http://www.alz.org

American Association of Colleges of Nursing & the John A. Hartford Foundation Institute for Geriatric Nursing. (2000). *Older adults: Recommended baccalaureate competencies and curricular guidelines for geriatric nursing care.* Washington, DC: American Association of Colleges of Nursing.

American Association of Retired Persons. (2002). *Beyond 50.02: A report to the nation on trends in health security.* Washington, DC: Author.

American Association of Retired Persons. (2005). Effective and safe prescription drugs. Retrieved October 18, 2005, from http://www.aarp.org/health/comparedrugs

American Nurses Association. (2001). *Scope and standards of gerontological nursing practice* (2nd ed.). Washington, DC: American Nurses Publishing.

Andrews, J. O., Heath, J., & Graham-Garcia, J. (2004). Management of tobacco dependence in older adults. *Journal of Gerontological Nursing, 30*(12), 13–24.

Angel, R. J., Angel, J. L., & Markides, K. S. (2002). Stability and change in health insurance among older Mexican Americans: Longitudinal evidence from the Hispanic Established Populations for Epidemiologic Study of the Elderly. *American Journal of Public Health, 92,* 1264–1271.

Antai-Otong, D. (2004). Antidepressants and older adults. *Advance for Nurses, 1*(7), 15–17.

Baine, W. B., Yu, W., & Summe, J. P. (2001). Epidemiologic trends in the hospitalization of elderly Medicare patients for pneumonia, 1991–1998. *American Journal of Public Health, 91,* 1121–1123.

Balfour, J., & Kaplan, G. (2002). Neighborhood environment and loss of physical function in older adults: Evidence from the Alameda County study. *American Journal of Epidemiology, 155,* 507–515.

Bates, J., Boote, J., & Beverly, C. (2004). Psychosocial interventions for people with a milder dementing illness: A systematic review. *Journal of Advanced Nursing, 45,* 644–658.

Beltran-Aguilar, E. D., Barker, L., K., Canto, M. T., Dye, B. A., Gooch, B. F., Griffin, S. O., et al. (2005). Surveillance for dental caries, dental sealants, tooth retention, edentulism, and enamel fluorosis—United States, 1988–1994 and 1999–2002. *Morbidity and Mortality Weekly Report, 53*(SS-3), 1–43.

Benjamins, M. R., & Brown, C. (2004). Religion and preventative health care utilization among the elderly. *Social Science & Medicine, 58,* 109–118.

Bennett, J. A., Thomas, V., & Riegel, B. (2004). Unrecognized chronic dehydration in older adults: Examining prevalence rates and risk factors. *Journal of Gerontological Nursing, 30*(11), 22–28.

Bennett, S. J., Suave, M. J., & Shaw, R. M. (2005). A conceptual model of cognitive deficits in chronic heart failure. *Journal of Nursing Scholarship, 37,* 222–228.

Bertsch, D. K., & Taylor-Moore, P. C. (2005). Elderly want to "age in place." *NurseWeek, 18*(14), 17–18.

Blazer, D. G., Sachs-Ericsson, N., & Hybels, C. F. (2005). Perception of unmet basic needs as a predictor of mortality among community-dwelling older adults. *American Journal of Public Health, 95,* 299–304.

Blumenthal, J. A., & Gullette, E. C. D. (2002). Exercise interventions and aging: Psychological and physical benefits in older adults. In K. W. Schaie, H. Leventhal, & S. L. Willis (Eds.), *Effective health behavior in older adults* (pp. 157–177). New York: Springer.

Briggs, N. M. (2006). *Validation therapy for dementia.* Retrieved March 16, 2006, from http://www.cochrane.org/reviews/en/ab001394.html

Brinckerhoff, J., & Coleman, E. A. (2005). What you need to know about the Medicare

Prescription Drug Act. *Family Practice Management, 12*(3), 49–52.

Brown, J. W., & Alligood, M. R. (2004). Realizing wrongness: Stories of older wife caregivers. *Journal of Applied Gerontology, 23,* 104–119,

Buckwalter, K. C., Wakefield, B. J., Hanna, B., & Lehmann, J. (2004). New technology for medication adherence: Electronically managed medication dispensing system. *Journal of Gerontological Nursing, 30*(7), 5–8.

Burholt, V., & Wenger, G. C. (2005). Migration from South Asia to the United Kingdom and the maintenance of transnational intergenerational relationships. In M. Silverstein & K. W. Schaie (Eds.), *Annual review of gerontology and geriatrics (Vol. 24), Focus on intergenerational relations across time and space* (pp. 153–176). New York: Springer.

Calabrese, D. A. (2004). Prostate cancer in older men. *Urologic Nursing, 24,* 258–269.

Calandra, J. (2003). Mental health & older adults: Mental illness in later life. *NurseWeek, 16*(25), 21–22.

Callen, B. (2004). Understanding nutritional health in older adults: A pilot study. *Journal of Gerontological Nursing, 30*(1), 36–43.

Caterino, J. M., Emond, J. A., & Camargo, C. A. (2004). Inappropriate medication administration to the acutely ill elderly: A nationwide emergency department study. *Journal of the American Geriatric Society, 52,* 1847–1855.

Center for Climatic Research, University of Delaware. (2004). Impact of heat waves on mortality—Rome, Italy, June–August, 2003. *Morbidity and Mortality Weekly Report, 53,* 369–371.

Centers for Disease Control and Prevention. (2003). Facilitating influenza and pneumococcal vaccination through standing orders programs. *Morbidity and Mortality Weekly Report, 52,* 68–69.

Centers for Disease Control and Prevention. (2004a). *Health United States, 2004 with chartbook on trends in the health of Americans.* Retrieved August 9, 2005, from http://www.cdc.giv/nchs/data/hus/hus04.pdf

Centers for Disease Control and Prevention. (2004b). Indicators for chronic disease surveillance. *Morbidity and Mortality Weekly Report, 53*(RR-11), 1–114.

Centers for Disease Control and Prevention. (2005a). *CJD (Creutzfeldt-Jakob disease, classic).* Retrieved March 16, 2006, from http://www.cdc.gov/ncidod/dvrd/cjd/index.htm

Centers for Disease Control and Prevention. (2005b). *Healthy people data*. Retrieved September 5, 2005, from http://wonder.cdc.gov/data2010

Centers for Medicare & Medicaid Services. (2004). Influenza vaccination and self-reported reasons for not receiving influenza vaccination among Medicare beneficiaries > 65 years—United States, 1991–2002. *Morbidity and Mortality Weekly Report, 53,* 1012–1015.

Chang, B. L., Nitta, S., Carter, P., & Markham, Y. K. (2004). Perceived helpfulness of telephone calls: Providing support for caregivers of family members with dementia. *Journal of Gerontological Nursing, 30*(9), 14–21.

Cleveland Clinic. (2005a). *Controlled coughing.* Retrieved March 16, 2006, from http://www.clevelandclinic.org/health/health-info/docs/2400/2413.asp?index=8697

Cleveland Clinic. (2005b). *Diaphragmatic breathing.* Retrieved March 16, 2006, from http://www.clevelandclinic.org/health/health-info/docs/2400/2409.asp?index=9445

Cleveland Clinic. (2005c). *Nutritional guidelines for people with COPD.* Retrieved March 16, 2006, from http://www.clevelandclinic.org/health/health-info/docs/2400/2411.asp?index=9451

Cleveland Clinic. (2005d). *Pursed-lip breathing.* Retrieved March 16, 2006, from http://www.clevelandclinic.org/health/health-info/docs/2400/2408.asp?index=9443

Coeling, H. V., Biordi, D. L., & Theis, S. L. (2003). Negotiating dyadic identity between caregivers and care receivers. *Journal of Nursing Scholarship, 35,* 21–25.

Cooper, K. L., & Kaplan, S. A. (2004). The overactive bladder and incontinence. In R. S. Kirby, C. C. Carson, M. G. Kirby, & R. N. Farah (Eds.), *Men's health* (2nd ed., pp. 417–430). London: Taylor & Francis.

Crews, J. E., & Campbell, V. A. (2004). Vision impairment and hearing loss among community-dwelling older Americans: Implications for health and functioning. *American Journal of Public Health, 94,* 823–829.

Curran, D. R. (2004). Should we discontinue Pap smear screening in women aged > 65 years? *Journal of Family Practice, 53,* 308–309.

Cutler, D. M. (2004). Behavioral health interventions: What works and why? In N. B. Anderson, R. A. Bulatao, & B. Cohen (Eds.), *Critical perspectives on racial and ethnic differences in health in late life* (pp. 643–674). Washington, DC: National Academies Press.

Dash, M. E., Foster, E. B., Smith, D. M., & Phillips, S. L. (2004). Urinary incontinence: The Social Health Maintenance Organization's approach. *Geriatric Nursing, 25,* 81–87.

Davey, A., Janke, M., & Savla, J. (2005). Antecedents of intergenerational support: Families in context and families as context. In M. Silverstein & K. W. Schaie (Eds.), *Annual review of gerontology and geriatrics* (Vol. 24), *Focus on intergenerational relations across time and space* (pp. 29–54). New York: Springer.

Davis, G. C., Hiemenz, M. L., & White, T. L. (2002). Barriers to managing chronic pain of older adults with arthritis. *Journal of Nursing Scholarship, 34,* 121–126.

Davis, L. L., Burgio, L. D., Buckwalter, K. C., & Weaver, M. A. (2004). Comparison of in-home and telephone-based skill training interventions with caregivers of persons with dementia. *Journal of Mental Health, 10,* 31–44.

Division of Adult and Community Health. (2003a). Hospitalizations for stroke among adults aged >65 years—United States, 2000. *Morbidity and Mortality Weekly Report, 52,* 586–589.

Division of Adult and Community Health. (2003b). Projected prevalence of self-reported arthritis or chronic joint symptoms among persons aged >65 years—United States, 2005–2030. *Morbidity and Mortality Weekly Report, 52,* 489–491.

Division of Adult and Community Health. (2003c). Trends in aging—United States and worldwide. *Morbidity and Mortality Weekly Report, 52,* 101–106.

Division of Adult and Community Health. (2005). Estimated influenza vaccination coverage among adults and children—United States, September 1, 2004–January 31, 2005. *Morbidity and Mortality Weekly Report, 54,* 304–307.

Division of Cancer Prevention and Control, National Center for Chronic Disease Prevention and Health Promotion. (2004). Cancer survivorship—United States, 1971–2001. *Morbidity and Mortality Weekly Report, 53,* 526, 528–529.

Division of Cancer Prevention and Control, National Center for Chronic Disease Prevention and Health Promotion. (2005). Breast cancer screening and socioeconomic status—35 metropolitan areas, 2000 and 2002. *Morbidity and Mortality Weekly Report, 54,* 981–985.

Division of Human Development and Disability. (2002). State-specific prevalence of obesity among adults with disabilities—Eight states and the District of Columbia, 1998–1999. *Morbidity and Mortality Weekly Report, 51,* 805–808.

Division of Nutrition and Physical Activity, National Center for Chronic Disease Prevention and Health Promotion. (2004). Strength training among adults >65 years—United States, 2001. *Morbidity and Mortality Weekly Report, 53,* 25–28.

Division of Surveillance and Informatics. (2003). Non-fatal fall-related traumatic brain injury among older adults—California, 1996–1999. *Morbidity and Mortality Weekly Report, 52,* 276–278.

Division of Unintentional Injury Prevention. (2003). Nonfatal injuries among older adults treated in hospital emergency departments—United States, 2001. *Morbidity and Mortality Weekly Report, 52,* 1019–1022.

Drug Effectiveness Review Project. (2005). *Drug effectiveness review project reports.* Retrieved October 17, 2005, from http://www.ohsu.edu/drugeffectiveness/reports/final.cfm

Dunne, K., Sullivan, K., & Kernohan, G. (2005). Palliative care for patients with cancer: District nurses' experiences. *Journal of Advanced Nursing, 50,* 372–380.

Ebrahim, S., Papacosta, O., Wannamethee, G., & Adamson, J. (2004). Social inequalities and disability in older men: Prospective findings from the British regional heart study. *Social Science & Medicine, 59,* 2109–2120.

Edlund, B. J. (2004). Medication use and misuse. *Journal of Gerontological Nursing, 30*(7), 4.

Edwards, M. (2004). As good as it gets. *AARP Magazine, 47*(6A), 42–49, 90.

Ekwall, A. K., Sivberg, B., & Hallberg, I. R. (2005). Loneliness as a predictor of quality of life among older caregivers. *Journal of Advanced Nursing, 49,* 23–32.

Epidemiology and Surveillance Division. (2004). Influenza and pneumococcal vaccination coverage among persons aged >65 years and persons aged 16–64 years with diabetes or asthma—United States, 2003. *Morbidity and Mortality Weekly Report, 53,* 1007–1012.

Farran, C. J., Loukissa, D., Perraud, S., & Paun, O. (2004). Alzheimer's disease caregiving information and skills. Part II: Family caregiver issues and concerns. *Research in Nursing & Health, 27,* 40–51.

Federal Interagency Forum on Aging-related Statistics. (2004). *Older Americans 2004: Key indicators of well-being.* Washington, DC: Author.

Finfgeld-Connett, D. L. (2004). Treatment of substance misuse in older women: Using a brief intervention model. *Journal of Gerontological Nursing, 30*(8), 30–37.

Finlayson, M., Van Denend, T., & Hudson, E. (2004). Aging with multiple sclerosis. *Journal of Neuroscience Nursing, 36,* 245–251.

Fitzpatrick, A. L., Powe, N. R., Cooper, L. S., Ives, D. G., & Robbins, J. A. (2004). Barriers to health care access and who perceives them. *American Journal of Public Health, 94,* 1788–1794.

Foley, D. J., Heimovitz, H. K., Guralnik, J. M., & Brock, D. B. (2002). Driving life expectancy of persons aged 70 years and older in the United States. *American Journal of Public Health, 92,* 1284–1289.

Fulmer, T. (2002). Elder abuse and neglect assessment. *Try this: Best practices in nursing care to older adults.* New York: Hartford Geriatric Institute for Nursing.

Garand, L., Buckwalter, K. C., & Hall, G. R. (2000). The biological basis of behavioral symptoms in dementia. *Issues in Mental Health Nursing, 21,* 91–107.

Gott, M., Hinchliff, S., & Galena, E. (2004). General practitioner attitudes to discussing sexual health issues with older people. *Social Science & Medicine, 58,* 2093–2103.

Guinn, M. J. (2004). A daughter's journey promoting geriatric self-care: Promoting positive health care interactions. *Geriatric Nursing, 25,* 267–271.

Guralnik, J. M., Alecxih, L., Branch, L. G., & Wiener, J. M. (2002). Medical and long-term care costs when older persons become more dependent. *American Journal of Public Health, 92,* 1244–1245.

Haight, B. K. (2001). Life reviews: Helping Alzheimer's patients reclaim a fading past. *Reflections on Nursing Leadership, 27*(1), 20–22.

Hanks-Bell, M., Halvey, K., & Paice, J. A. (2004). Pain assessment and management in aging. *Online Journal of Issues in Nursing.* Retrieved September 2, 2004, from http://www.nursingworld.org/ojin/topic21/tpc21_6.htm

Harper, S. A., Fukuda, K., Uyeki, T. M., Cox, N. J., & Bridges, C. B. (2005). Prevention and control of influenza: Recommendations of the Advisory Committee on Immunization Practices (ACIP). *Morbidity and Mortality Weekly Report, 54*(RR-8), 1–41.

Heidrick, S. M., & Wells, T. J. (2004). Effects of urinary incontinence: Psychological well-being and distress in older community-dwelling women. *Journal of Gerontological Nursing, 30*(4), 47–54.

Henderson, M. L. (2004). Gerontological advance practice nurses as end-of-life care facilitators. *Geriatric Nursing, 25,* 233–237.

Henley, E. (2004). What the new Medicare prescription drug bill may mean for providers and patients. *Journal of Family Practice, 53,* 389–392.

Henry, M. (2002). Descending into delirium. *American Journal of Nursing, 102*(3), 49–56.

Hoskins, S., Coleman, M., & McNeely, D. (2005). Stress in carers of individuals with dementia and community mental health teams: An uncontrolled evaluation study. *Journal of Advanced Nursing, 50,* 372–380.

Huang, T.-T., & Acton, G. J. (2004). Effectiveness of home visit falls prevention strategy for Taiwanese community-dwelling elders: Randomized trial. *Public Health Nursing, 21,* 247–256.

Huey, F. L. (Ed.). (2001). Global impact of innovations on chronic disease in the genomics era. *The Pfizer Journal* (Global ed.), *11*(2), 1–36.

Hurley, A. C., Gauthier, M. A., Horvath, K. J., Harvey, R., Smith, S. J., Trudeau, S., et al. (2004). Promoting safer home environments for persons with Alzheimer's disease: The home safety/injury model. *Journal of Gerontological Nursing, 30*(6), 43–51.

Imamura, E. (2002). Amy's chat room: Health promotion programmes for community dwelling elderly. *International Journal of Nursing Practice, 8,* 61–64.

Immunization Services Division, National Immunization Program. (2005). Influenza vaccination levels among persons aged > 65 years and among persons aged 18–64 years with high-risk conditions—United States, 2003. *Morbidity and Mortality Weekly Report, 54,* 1045–1049.

International Foundation for Functional Gastrointestinal Disorders. (2003). *Prevalence of bowel incontinence.* Retrieved March 15, 2006, from http://www.aboutincontinence.org/prevalence.html

International Foundation for Functional Gastrointestinal Disorders. (2006a). *Common causes of bowel incontinence.* Retrieved March 15, 2006, from http://www.aboutincontinence.org/causes.html

International Foundation for Functional Gastrointestinal Disorders. (2006b). *Treatment for bowel incontinence.* Retrieved March 15, 2006, from http://www.aboutincontinence.org/treatment.html

Jansson, W., Nordberg, G., & Grafstrom, M. (2001). Patterns of elderly spousal caregiving in dementia care: An observational study. *Journal of Advanced Nursing, 34,* 804–812.

Johnson, B. K. (2004). Sexuality and heart disease: Implications for nursing. *Geriatric Nursing, 25,* 224–226.

Kannus, P., Parkkari, J., Niemi, S., & Palvanen, M. (2005). Fall-induced deaths among elderly people. *American Journal of Public Health, 95,* 422–424.

Kather, T. A. (2005). Colorectal cancer: Guidelines for prevention, screening and treatment. *Advance for Nurses, 20*(5), 15–17.

Kleespies, P. M. (2004). *Life and death decisions: Psychological and ethical considerations in end-of-life care.* Washington, DC: American Psychological Association.

Klein, R., Stoll, K., & Bruce, A. (2004). *Medicaid: Good medicine for state economies, 2004 update.* Retrieved August 30, 2004, from http://www.familiesusa.org

Kolanowski, A. M., Fick, D., Waller, J. L., & Shea, D. (2004). Spouses of persons with dementia: Their healthcare problems, utilization, and costs. *Research in Nursing & Health, 27,* 296–306.

Kwong, E. W.-Y., & Kwan, A. Y.-H. (2004). Stress management methods of the community-dwelling elderly in Hong Kong: Implications for tailoring a stress-reduction program. *Geriatric Nursing, 25,* 102–106.

Laakkonen, M.-L., Pitkala, K. H., Strandberg, T. E., Berglind, S., & Tilvis, R. S. (2004). Living will, resuscitation preferences, and attitudes towards life in an aged population. *Gerontology, 50,* 247–254.

Last Acts. (2002). *Means to a better end.* Retrieved January 29, 2003, from http://www.lastacts.org/files/misc/meansfull.pdf

Lee, S., Colditz, G., Berkman, L., & Kawachi, I. (2003). Caregiving to children and grandchildren and risk of coronary heart disease among women. *American Journal of Public Health, 93,* 1939–1944.

Lee, W. K. M., & Law, K., W.-K. (2004). Retirement planning and retirement satisfaction: The need for a national retirement program and policy in Hong Kong. *Journal of Applied Gerontology, 23,* 212–233.

Leenerts, M. H., Teel, C. S., & Pendleton, M. K. (2002). Building a model of self-care for health promotion in aging. *Journal of Nursing Scholarship, 34,* 355–361.

Levine, C., Hunt, G. G., Halper, D., Hart, A. Y., Lautz, J., & Gould, D. A. (2005). Young adult caregivers: A first look at an unstudied population. *American Journal of Public Health, 95,* 2071–2075.

Lewis, I. D., & McBride, M. (2004). Anticipatory grief and chronicity: Elders and families in racial/ethnic minority groups. *Geriatric Nursing, 25,* 44–47.

Lewis, S. J. (2004, July, Supplement). After menopause: Novel marker helps to identify women at risk for heart disease. *Journal of Family Practice,* S18–S24.

Logue, R. M. (2002). Self-medication and the elderly: How technology can help. *American Journal of Nursing, 102*(7), 51–55.

Loughlin, A. (2004). Depression and social support: Effective treatments for homebound elderly adults. *Journal of Gerontological Nursing, 20*(5), 11–15.

Magnusson, L., & Hanson, E. (2005). Supporting frail older people and their family carers at home using information and communication technology: Cost analysis. *Journal of Advanced Nursing, 51,* 645–657.

Mahan, D. (2004). *Sticker shock: Rising prescription drug prices for seniors.* Retrieved August 30, 2004, from http://www.familiesusa.org

Malavolta, M., Mocchegiani, E., & Bertoni-Freddari, C. (2004). New trends in biomedical aging research. *Gerontology, 50,* 420–424.

Manly, J. J., & Mayeux, R. (2004). Ethnic differences in dementia and Alzheimer's disease. In N. B. Anderson, R. A. Bulatao, & B. Cohen (Eds.), *Critical perspectives on racial and ethnic differences in health in late life* (pp. 95–141). Washington, DC: National Academies Press.

Matesa, J. (2002, November). Barriers to hospice care and some proposed policy solutions. *State Initiatives in End-of-life Care, 17,* 1–8.

Matthews, J. T., Dunbar-Jacob, J., Sereika, S., Schulz, R., & McDowell, B. J. (2004). Preventive health practices: Comparison of family caregivers 50 and older. *Journal of Gerontological Nursing, 30*(2), 46–54.

McGarry, J., & Arthur, A. (2001). Informal caring in late life: A qualitative study of the experiences of older carers. *Journal of Advanced Nursing, 33,* 182–189.

McLeer, S. V. (2004). Mental health services. In H. S. Sultz & K. M. Young, *Health care USA: Understanding its organization and delivery* (4th ed., pp. 335–366). Sudbury, MA: Jones and Bartlett.

Meeks-Sjostrom, D. (2004). A comparison of three measures of elder abuse. *Journal of Nursing Scholarship, 36,* 247–250.

Merrell, J., Kinsella, F., Murphy, F., Philpin, S., & Ali, A. (2005). Support needs of carers of dependent adults from a Bangladeshi community. *Journal of Advanced Nursing, 51,* 549–557.

Miller, C. A. (2004a). Getting older adults through the maze of Medicare prescription drug benefits. *Geriatric Nursing, 25,* 190–191.

Miller, C. A. (2004b). Teaching older adults medication self-care. *Geriatric Nursing, 25,* 318–319.

Minardi, H. A., & Blanchard, M. (2004). Older people with depression: A pilot study. *Journal of Advanced Nursing, 46,* 23–32.

Mitty, E. L. (2001). Ethnicity and end-of-life decision-making. *Reflections in Nursing Leadership, 27*(1), 28–31.

Moeller, J. F., Miller, G. E., & Banthin, J. S. (2004). Looking inside the nation's medicine cabinet: Trends in outpatient drug spending by Medicare beneficiaries, 1997 and 2001; Costly new drugs do have an impact on overall drug spending. *Health Affairs, 23,* 217–225.

Moos, R. H., Brennan, P. L., Schutte, K. K., & Moos, B. S. (2004). High-risk alcohol consumption and late-life alcohol use problems. *American Journal of Public Health, 94,* 1985–1991.

Mouton, C. P., Rodabough, R. J., Rovi, S. L. D., Hunt, J. L., Talamantes, M. A., Brzyski, R. G., et al. (2004). Prevalence and 3-year incidence of abuse among postmenopausal women. *American Journal of Public Health, 94,* 605–612.

Murtaugh, K. N., & Hubert, H. B. (2004). Gender differences in physical disability among an elderly cohort. *American Journal of Public Health, 94,* 1406–1411.

N. A. (2005). Husband fatigue. *The Week, 5*(231), 11.

National Center for Chronic Disease Prevention and Health Promotion. (2002a). *A national public health initiative on diabetes and women's health.* Retrieved October 2, 2002, from http://www.cdc.gov/diabetes/pubs/interim/background.htm

National Center for Chronic Disease Prevention and Health Promotion. (2002b). Prevalence of health-care providers asking older adults about their physical activity levels—United States, 1998. *Morbidity and Mortality Weekly Report, 51,* 412–414.

National Center for Health Statistics. (2005a). Average number of bed days during the preceding 12 months among persons aged >18 years, by age group—United States, 2003. *Morbidity and Mortality Weekly Report, 54,* 803.

National Center for Health Statistics. (2005b). *Health, United States, 2005 with chartbook on trends in the health of Americans.* Retrieved December 23, 2005, from http://www.cdc.gov/nchs/data/hus/hus05.pdf

National Center for Health Statistics. (2005c). Percentage of adults who reported being deaf or having a lot of trouble hearing without a hearing aid, by sex and age group—United States, 2003. *Morbidity and Mortality Weekly Report, 54,* 635.

National Center for Health Statistics. (2005d). Percentage of hospital discharges and days of care, by age group—United States, 2003. *Morbidity and Mortality Weekly Report, 54,* 584.

National Center for Injury Prevention and Control. (2003). Nonfatal physical assault-related injuries among persons aged >60 years treated in hospital emergency departments—United States, 2001. *Morbidity and Mortality Weekly Report, 52,* 812–816.

National Center for Injury Prevention and Control. (2005a). Homicide and suicide rates—National Violent Death Reporting System, six states, 2003. *Morbidity and Mortality Weekly Report, 54,* 377–380.

National Center for Injury Prevention and Control. (2005b). *Older adult drivers: Fact sheet.* Retrieved June 9, 2005, from http://www.cdc.gov/ncipc/factsheets/older.htm

National Center on Birth Defects and Developmental Disabilities. (2005). *Women with disabilities.* Retrieved June 6, 2005, from http://www.cdc.gov/ncbddd/wwomen/default.htm

National Digestive Diseases Information Clearinghouse. (2004). *Fecal incontinence.* Retrieved March 15, 2006, from http://digestive.niddk.nih.gov/ddiseases/pubs/fecalincontinence/

National Heart, Lung, and Blood Institute. (2003). *Chronic obstructive pulmonary disease.* Retrieved March 16, 2006, from http://www.nhbli.nih.gov/public/lung/other/COPD-fact.pdf

National Institute on Aging. (2002). *Alzheimer's disease: Unraveling the mystery.* Washington, DC: U.S. Department of Health and Human Services.

National Institute on Aging. (2004). *Working with your older patient: A clinician's handbook.* Bethesda, MD: Author.

National Institute for Environmental Health Sciences. (2006). *Elderly have higher risk for cardiovascular, respiratory disease from fine particle pollution.* Retrieved March 16, 2006, from http://www.nih.gov/news/pr/mar2006/niehs-08.htm

Naylor, M. (2003). Delirium, depression often overlooked. *American Journal of Nursing, 103*(5), 116.

Neher, J. O. (2004). Clinical commentary. *Journal of Family Practice, 53,* 310.

Newacheck, P. W., & Benjamin, A. E. (2004). Intergenerational equity and public spending; The United States should embrace a new doctrine of fairness to ensure that vulnerable populations are not forced to compete for resources. *Health Affairs, 23,* 142–146.

Okabayashi, H., Liang, J., Krause, N., Akiyama, H., & Sugisawa, H. (2004). Mental health among older adults in Japan: Do sources of social support and negative interaction make a difference? *Social Science & Medicine, 59,* 2259–2270.

Orhon, A. (2002). Elder abuse: Mistreatment of older Americans on the rise. *NurseWeek, 15*(23), 22–23.

Østbye, T., Taylor, D. H. Jr., Yancy, W. S. Jr., & Krause, K. M. (2005). Associations between obesity and receipt of screening mammography, Papanicolaou tests, and influenza vaccination: Results from the Health and Retirement Study (HRS) and the Asset and Health Dynamics Among the Oldest Old (Ahead) study. *American Journal of Public Health, 95,* 1623–1630.

Partnership for Prevention. (2003). *A better Medicare for healthier seniors: Recommendations to modernize Medicare's prevention policies.* Retrieved July 25, 2003, from http://www.prevent.org

Phillips, B. B. (2004). Skip to the loo, my darlin': Urinary incontinence 1850–present. *Geriatric Nursing, 25,* 74–80.

Pinkelman, M. A. (2002). Search for consensus: Prostate. *Community Health Forum, 3*(5), 17–19.

Plese, N. K. (Ed.). (2002). At peace with dying: A healthy approach to the end of life. *The Pfizer Journal, 6*(2), 1–36.

Plese, N. K. (Ed.). (2005a). A profile of caregiving in America (2nd ed.) *The Pfizer Journal, IX*(4), 1–40.

Plese, N. K. (Ed.). (2005b). Global summit on the aging workforce. *The Pfizer Journal, IX*(3), 1–40.

Pricewaterhousecooper's Health Research Institute. (2005). *Acts of charity: Charity care strategies for hospitals in a changing landscape.* Retrieved December 27, 2005, from http://healthcare.pwc.com/cgi-local/hcregister.cgi?link=reg/charitycare.pdf&update=true

Qualls, C. D., Harris, J. L., & Rogers, W. A. (2002). Cognitive-linguistic aging: Considerations for home health care environments. In W. A. Rogers & A. D. Fisk (Eds.), *Human factors interventions for the health care of older adults* (pp. 47–67). Mahwah, NJ: Lawrence Erlbaum Associates.

Rennard, S. I. (2005). *Patient information: Overview of the management of COPD.* Retrieved March 16, 2006, from http:patients.uptodate.com/print.asp?print=true&file=lung_dis/4567

Resnick, B. (2004). Encouraging exercise in older adults with congestive heart failure. *Geriatric Nursing, 25,* 204–211.

Resnick, B. (2005). Exercise for older adults. *Advance for Nurses, 2*(4), 19–21.

Robbins, R., Rausch, K. J., Garcia, R. I., & Prestwood, K. M. (2004). Multicultural medication

adherence: A comparative study. *Journal of Gerontological Nursing, 30*(7), 25–32.

Robitaille, Y., Laforest, S., Fournier, M., Gauvin, L., Parisien, M., Corriveau, H., et al. (2005). Moving forward in fall prevention: An intervention to improve balance among older adults in real-world settings. *American Journal of Public Health, 95,* 2049–2056.

Rose, M. A. (2004). Planning HIV education programs for older adults: Cultural implications. *Journal of Gerontological Nursing, 30*(3), 34–39.

Rosenfeld, P., & Harrington, C. (2003). Hospital care for the elderly. *American Journal of Nursing, 103*(5), 115.

Safran, D. G., Neuman, T., Schoen, C., Kitchman, M. S., Wilson, I., Cooper, B., et al. (2005). *Prescription drug coverage and seniors: Findings from a 2003 national survey.* Retrieved August 13, 2005, from http://www.cmwf.org/publications/publications_show.htm?doc_id=273944

Samelson, E. J., Zhang, Y., Kiel, D. P., Hannan, M. T., & Felson, D. T. (2002). Effect of birth cohort on risk of hip fracture: Age-specific incidence rates in the Framingham study. *American Journal of Public Health, 92,* 858–862.

Sandison, R., Gray, M., & Reid, D. (2004). Lifestyle factors for promoting bone health in older women. *Journal of Advanced Nursing, 45,* 603–610.

Saxon, S. V., & Etten, M. J. (2002). *Physical change & aging: A guide for the helping professions* (4th ed.). New York: Tiresias Press.

Schlenk, E. A., Dunbar-Jacob, J., & Engberg, S. (2004). Medication non-adherence among older adults: A review of strategies and interventions for improvement. *Journal of Gerontological Nursing, 30*(7), 33–43.

Schneider, J. K., Mercer, G. T., Herning, M., Smith, C. A., & Prysak, M. D. (2004). Promoting exercise behavior in older adults: Using a cognitive behavioral intervention. *Journal of Gerontological Nursing, 30*(4), 45–53.

Seymour, J., Gott, M., Bellamy, G., Ahmedzai, S. H., & Clark, D. (2004). Planning for the end of life: The views of older people about advance care statements. *Social Science & Medicine, 59,* 57–68.

Shepherd, A. J. (2004). An overview of osteoporosis. *Alternative Therapies, 10*(2), 26–33.

Shreffler-Grant, J., Weinert, C., Nichols, E., & Ide, B. (2005). Complementary therapy use among older rural adults. *Public Health Nursing, 22,* 323–331.

Son, G.-R., Therrien, B., & Whall, A. (2002). Implicit memory and familiarity among elders with dementia. *Journal of Nursing Scholarship, 34,* 263–267.

Tabloski, P. A. (2006). *Gerontological nursing.* Upper Saddle River, NJ: Pearson.

Tanner, E. (2004). Chronic illness demands for self-management in older adults. *Geriatric Nursing, 25,* 313–317.

Taylor, D. H. Jr., Hasselblad, V., Henley, S. J., Thun, M. J., & Sloan, F. A. (2002). Benefits of smoking cessation for longevity. *American Journal of Public Health, 92,* 990–996.

Teunissen, T. A. M., de Jonge, A., van Weel, C., & Lagro-Janssen, A. L. M. (2004). Treating urinary incontinence in the elderly—Conservative measures that work: A systematic review. *Journal of Family Practice, 53,* 25–32.

Turcu, A., Toubin, S., Mourey, F., D'Athis, P., Manckoundia, P., & Pfitzenmeyer, P. (2004). Falls and depression in older people. *Gerontology, 50,* 303–308.

U.S. Census Bureau. (2004a). *Health insurance coverage: 2003.* Retrieved September 30, 2004, from http://www.census.gov

U.S. Census Bureau. (2004b). *Poverty: 2003 highlights.* Retrieved September 30, 2004, from http://www.census.gov

U.S. Census Bureau. (2005). *Statistical abstract of the United States, 2004–2005.* Retrieved May 5, 2005, from http://www.census.gov/prod/2004pubs/04statab

U.S. Department of Health and Human Services. (2000). *Healthy people 2010* (Conference edition, in two volumes). Washington, DC: Author.

U.S. Preventive Services Task Force. (2005a). *The guide to clinical preventive services, 2005.* Retrieved August 13, 2005, from http://www.ahrq.gov/clinic/pocketguide.htm

U.S. Preventive Services Task Force. (2005b). *Screening for abdominal aortic aneurysm.* Retrieved August 13, 2005, from http://www.ahrq.gov/clinic/uspstf/uspsaneu.htm

Validation Training Institute. (2003). *What is validation?* Retrieved March 16, 2006, from http://www.vfvalidation.org/whatis.html

Vellone, E., Sansoni, J., & Cohen, M. Z. (2002). The experience of Italians caring for family members with Alzheimer's disease. *Journal of Nursing Scholarship, 34,* 323–329.

Vivarai-Dresler, G., & Bakker, D. A. (2004). Blood pressure monitoring: Older adults' perceptions. *Journal of Gerontological Nursing, 30*(1), 44–52.

Vogel, C. (2003). Dementia: Prompt detection, family education make the difference. *NurseWeek, 16*(8), 21–22.

Wang, H.-H. (2001). A comparison of two models of health-promoting lifestyle in rural elderly Taiwanese women. *Public Health Nursing, 18,* 204–211.

Weeks, S. K., McGann, P. E., Michaels, T. K., & Penninx, B. W. J. H. (2003). Comparing various short-form geriatric depression scales leads to the GDS-5/15. *Journal of Nursing Scholarship, 35,* 133–137.

Wells, Y., Foreman, P., Gething, L., & Petralia, W. (2004). Nurses' attitudes toward aging and older adults: Examining attitudes and practices among health services providers in Australia. *Journal of Gerontological Nursing, 30*(9), 5–13.

Wiebe, C. (2004). Drug import programs defy federal warnings, reap benefits. *Medscape Business of Medicine, 5*(2). Retrieved October 13, 2005, from http://www.medscape.com/viewarticle/490299

Williams, A., & Jester, R. (2005). Delayed surgical fixation of fractured hips in older people: Impact on mortality. *Journal of Advanced Nursing, 52,* 63–69.

Williams, J. R. (2004). Gerontological nurse practitioner care guidelines: Sleep management in elderly patients. *Geriatric Nursing, 25,* 310–312.

Williams, K., Kemper, S., & Hummert, M. L. (2004). Enhancing communication with older adults: Overcoming elderspeak. *Journal of Gerontological Nursing, 30*(10), 17–25.

Williams, M. E. (2005). *Physical diagnosis in elderly people.* Retrieved April 24, 2005, from http://www.medscape.com/viewprogram/3955_pnt

Wooten, J., & Galavis, J. (2005). Polypharmacy: Keeping the elderly safe. *RN, 68*(8), 44–50.

World Health Organization. (2004). *The world health report 2004.* Geneva, Switzerland: Author.

World Health Organization. (2005). *World health report 2005: Make every mother and child count.* Retrieved December 16, 2005, from http://www.who.int/why/2005/annexesen.pdf

Yan, E. C.-W., & Tang, C. S.-K. (2004). Elder abuse by caregivers: A study of prevalence and risk factors in Hong Kong Chinese families. *Journal of Family Violence, 19,* 269–277.

Yoon, S.-J. L, & Horne, C. (2001). Herbal products and conventional medicines used by community-residing older women. *Journal of Advanced Nursing, 33,* 51–59.

Yoon, S. L., & Horne, C. (2004). Perceived health promotion practices by older women: Use of herbal products. *Journal of Gerontological Nursing, 30*(7), 9–15.

You, L., Deans, C., Liu, K., Zhang, M. F., & Zhang, J. (2004). Rising awareness of fall risk among Chinese older adults: Use of the home fall hazards assessment tool. *Journal of Gerontological Nursing, 30*(6), 35–42.

Yuan, Z., Dawson, N., Cooper, G. S., Einstadter, S., Cebul, R., & Rimm, A. A. (2001). Effects of alcohol-related disease on hip fracture and mortality: A retrospective cohort study of hospitalized Medicare beneficiaries. *American Journal of Public Health, 91,* 1089–1093.

Zerwekh, J. V. (2006). *Nursing care at the end of life: Palliative care for patients and families.* Philadelphia: F. A. Davis.

Zhan, L. (2004). Caring for family members with Alzheimer's disease. *Journal of Gerontological Nursing, 30*(8), 19–29.

Zhan, L., & Chen, J. (2004). Medication practices among Chinese American older adults: A study of cultural influences. *Journal of Gerontological Nursing, 30*(4), 24–33.

Advocacy in Action

Safe at Home

Homeless women and children face a variety of challenges in their lives and do not need to experience any further risks to their health. However, students working in a group of homes for homeless women and their children noted a number of safety hazards that put the children, in particular, at risk of injury. Each of the homes had been a single-family dwelling but now housed three or four homeless women and many young children.

Most of the women were attempting to escape abusive situations and often did not have the knowledge or energy to engage in childproofing the homes. In addition, the staff was not always aware of structural safety hazards present in the homes. The students decided that safety was a significant issue that they could address. They began by assessing the safety hazards in the seven homes. All the homes had fenced play areas for the children, but in some of them the surface below the play areas was hard and in others play equipment was in poor repair and presented several safety hazards. Inside the homes, there were a number of other safety hazards. The women frequently left medications and sharp utensils within easy reach of small children. Cleansers and other toxic materials were in easy reach, and there were no outlet covers or latches on the cabinet doors. Most of the mothers had little knowledge of home safety or potential hazards.

Based on their assessment, the students undertook a number of initiatives. They created a home safety training manual for each house and conducted safety education classes for the mothers living there. In addition, they obtained donations of outlet covers and cabinet latches from local merchants that they installed in each house. They also alerted the agency responsible for the homes regarding the play area and equipment hazards, and the administrator was able to get a local construction company to redesign the outdoor areas, put in safe play surfaces, and construct safe play equipment. With the safety training manual, agency staff were able to orient subsequent residents to safety issues in the homes, and the project took on a life of its own.

Meeting the Needs of Poor and Homeless Populations

CHAPTER OBJECTIVES

After reading this chapter, you should be able to:

1. Analyze the effects of factors contributing to poverty and homelessness.
2. Identify biophysical, psychological, physical environmental, sociocultural, behavioral, and health system factors that influence the health of poor and homeless clients.
3. Describe approaches to primary prevention of homelessness and analyze related roles of community health nurses with respect to each.
4. Identify major areas of emphasis in primary prevention of health problems in poor and homeless clients.
5. Identify areas in which secondary preventive interventions may be required in the care of poor and homeless individuals and analyze the role of the community health nurse in these interventions.
6. Identify strategies for tertiary prevention of poverty and homelessness at the aggregate level.
7. Describe considerations in implementing care for poor and homeless individuals.
8. Identify the primary focus of evaluation for care of poor and homeless clients.

KEY TERMS

MediaLink

http://www.prenhall.com/clark

Additional interactive resources for this chapter can be found on the Companion Website. Click on Chapter 20 and "Begin" to select the activities for this chapter.

As we have seen in several previous chapters, sociocultural factors play a significant role in determining the health status of population groups. The health-related effects and community health nursing roles with respect to two interrelated sociocultural factors, poverty and homelessness, are explored in detail in this chapter.

OVERVIEW OF POVERTY AND HOMELESSNESS

In 1948, the United Nations General Assembly adopted the Universal Declaration of Human Rights, which stated that "everyone has the right to a standard of living adequate for the health and well-being of himself and his family, including food, clothing, housing, and medical care social services, and to the right to security in the event of unemployment, sickness, disability, widowhood, old age, or other lack of livelihood in circumstances beyond his control" (cited in Thiele, 2002, p. 712). The following year, in the United States, the Housing Act of 1949 proposed "the realization as soon as feasible of the goal of a decent home and suitable living environment for every American family" (cited in Freeman, 2002, p. 709). To further the objectives of these two pieces of legislation, the World Health Organization developed six *Health Principles of Housing* as follows. Healthful housing:

- protects against communicable diseases through access to a safe water supply, sanitary disposal of excreta and solid wastes, drainage of surface water, support for personal and domestic hygiene, safe food protection, and structural safeguards against disease transmission
- protects against injury, chronic disease, and poisoning by means of safe construction materials, structural safety, ventilation and light, and absence of exposure to hazardous conditions or substances
- reduces psychological and social stress
- provides an improved housing environment
- supports informed use of housing
- protects populations at risk (Thiele, 2002)

The responsibility of governments with respect to housing were further delineated in the core principles of housing justice emphasized by the National Coalition for the Homeless (2005n). These principles include the right of every person to basic economic rights, including housing; the responsibility of society to meet housing needs; the need for economic and social support for adequate housing; the right of homeless individuals to services and programs provided to housed individuals; the need for tailored services and programs to meet the needs of people without adequate housing; and the right to equal access to housing regardless of one's life circumstances. The final principle of the Coalition is that provision of universal access to adequate housing is a measure of an effective society.

Unfortunately, many of the world's societies do not achieve these principles of housing justice. Worldwide, more than 1 billion people live in inadequate housing in urban areas alone (Population Information Program, 2003), and many more are literally or virtually homeless. Adequate housing is a community health concern because of its effects on the health of the population. These effects occur in three ways: through poor physical conditions of housing, through the absence of affordable housing, and through location of housing in unhealthy places (Freeman, 2002).

Defining Poverty and Homelessness

Both poverty and homelessness are defined in multiple ways. **Poverty** is "having insufficient money, goods, or means of support" (Wilton, 2004, p. 26), but what is considered *sufficient* may vary from one definition to the next. The most common definition of poverty in the United States is an income lower than the federally identified poverty level. In 2005, the poverty threshold for a family of four was an annual income less than $19,350 (Center for Medicaid and State Operations, 2005). The "near poor" have incomes 100% to 199% above the federal poverty level (National Center for Health Statistics, 2003). In Canada, poverty is determined by *low-income cut-offs* identified by Statistics Canada (Wilton, 2004).

Poverty may also be defined in terms of the percent of one's income spent on essential goods and services (e.g., food, shelter, clothing) or one's income relative to the median income in the local area. In Canada, for example, the poor generally spend more than 56.2% of their income on essentials (Wilton, 2004). In the context of the U.S. Rural Rental Housing Loan Program, very low income is defined as an income 50% below the area median income (AMI), and low-income households are below 50% to 80% of the AMI (National Coalition for the Homeless, 2005f). Measurable definitions of poverty are important because they often determine clients' eligibility for assistance programs. For example, eligibility may be restricted to individuals or families with incomes at or below the defined poverty level. In some programs, eligibility may be set at 100% or 150% above poverty level.

Homelessness also has multiple definitions, depending on the purpose of the definition. One of the most commonly used definitions is that posed by the Stewart B. McKinney Homeless Assistance Act of 1987, the first federal legislation in the United States dealing with the problem of homelessness. In the McKinney Act, a **homeless individual** is defined as a person who "lacks a fixed, regular, and adequate nighttime residence; and . . . has a primary residence that is: (a) a supervised publicly or privately operated shelter designed to provide temporary accommodations . . . (b) an institution that provides a temporary residence for individuals intended to be institutionalized, or (c) a public or private place not

GLOBAL PERSPECTIVES

The World Health Organization Regional Office for Europe has described homelessness as "a complex concept embracing states of rooflessness, houselessness, living in insecure accommodation, or living in inadequate accommodation" (Wright & Tompkins, 2005, p. 2). The *roofless* include people without shelter, newly arrived immigrants, and those displaced by disaster or violence. Those who are *houseless* are living in temporary shelter, but also include those who are released from prisons, hospitals, or foster homes with nowhere to go. Those *living in insecure accommodation* include those doubled up with friends and family, as well as those who are in the process of being evicted and "squatters" who take up residence in areas not designed for human habitation (e.g., warehouses and city parks). Those who are *living in inadequate accommodation* include people living in overcrowded or substandard housing. Having a home is defined as "having an adequate dwelling (or space) over which a person and his/her family can exercise exclusive possession, being able to maintain privacy and enjoy social relations, and having a legal title to occupy" (p. 2).

Compare the WHO definition of homelessness to that used in the McKinney Act in the United States. What are the implications for determining the extent of homelessness? For determining eligibility for services designed to address the needs of homeless populations? How does the definition of having a home relate to the criminalization of homelessness seen in many jurisdictions in the United States?

designed for, or ordinarily used as, a regular sleeping accommodation for human beings" (National Coalition for the Homeless, 2005t, p. 1). Being homeless has also been defined as "having spent more than seven consecutive nights in a shelter or other non-dwelling" (Swigart & Kolb, 2004, p. 162). Unfortunately, these definitions fail to recognize the large segment of the population who are virtually homeless but are living doubled and tripled up with friends or family or who are living in substandard housing (National Coalition for the Homeless, 2005s). In various studies, anywhere from 46% to 82% of homeless families had been living with others just prior to becoming homeless, and a typical family may spend as long as 4 years doubled up with friends or family members (Bolland & McCallum, 2002).

A more inclusive definition that does include these populations as well as others (e.g., those living in hotels) is provided in the definition of homeless children and youth in the McKinney-Vento Act dealing with the education of homeless children and youth. In this legislation, homeless children and youth are

(a) individuals who lack a fixed, regular, and adequate nighttime residence . . . and (b) include (i) children and youth who are sharing the housing of other persons due to loss of housing, economic hardship, or a similar reason; are living in motels, hotels, trailer parks, or camping grounds due to lack of alternative adequate accommodations; are living in emergency or transitional shelters; are abandoned in hospitals; or are awaiting foster care placement; (ii) children and youth who have

a primary nighttime residence that is a public or private place not designed for or ordinarily used as a regular sleeping accommodation for human beings . . . (iii) children and youth who are living in cars, parks, public spaces, abandoned buildings, substandard housing, bus or train stations, or similar settings, and (iv) migratory children who qualify as homeless for purposes of this subtitle because the children are living in circumstances described in clauses (i) through (iii). (National Coalition for the Homeless, 2005t)

The Magnitude of Poverty and Homelessness

There are no exact figures on the number of poor or homeless persons in the United States. In 2003, 12.5% of all persons in the United States had incomes below poverty level, an increase from 12.1% in 2002. This amounts to 35.9 million people (U.S. Census Bureau, 2005). From 1982 to 1998, the income of the wealthiest 1% of the American population increased by 42%, whereas that for the poorest 40% decreased by 76% (Wise, 2004). Despite these figures, the median per capita income is highest in the Americas, at $15,850 per year. The poorest region is Africa, where the per capita income is only $560. Fewer than 5% of the population of the European Region lives in poverty, compared to 39% in the African Region. An estimated 70% of the world's extremely poor population is women (World Health Organization [WHO], 2003, 2005).

The relationship between poverty and homelessness is well established and is best conveyed by the following statement: "Being poor can mean that one is an illness, an accident, or a paycheck away from homelessness" (Bringing America Home, 2005e, p. 1). As with poverty, the exact number of homeless persons is unknown and, in fact, varies from one day to the next. The best estimate is that approximately 3.5 million people, including 1.35 million children, are homeless in the United States in any given year. These figures include approximately 1% of the total U.S. population (National Coalition for the Homeless, 2005o) and 6.3% of those in poverty (Milby, Schumacher, Wallace, Freedman, & Vuchinich, 2005). Approximately one tenth of these people are chronically homeless (Caton et al., 2005). The number of homeless people may be largely underestimated due to the failure to include those who are homeless for short periods of time, those who are housed with others, or those who are just invisible to officials (National Coalition for the Homeless, 2005s; Sherman & Redlener, 2003, p. 1).

Worldwide, 20 to 40 million urban families are homeless and many others live in temporary structures. Each year several million of the world's families are forcibly evicted from the places where they are living (Population Information Program, 2003). U.S. homelessness rates tripled between 1987 and 1997, and even though the number of shelter beds doubled in many locations and tripled in others, the need for shelter remains largely unmet (National Coalition for the Homeless, 2005o). In 2004, requests for shelter in 27 U.S. cities increased by 7%, and 32% of requests were denied due to lack of resources (National Coalition for the Homeless, 2005k).

An estimated 6.5% of all adults in the United States, or 12 million people, have been literally homeless at some time in their lives (Anderson & Rayens, 2004), and on any given night 500,000 to 700,000 persons may be homeless (Swigart & Kolb, 2004). Who are these homeless individuals? In 2003, 39% of the homeless were children under 18 years of age (National Coalition for the Homeless, 2005t). Approximately 42% of these children were under 6 years of age, and 20% were over 11 years of age. Half of these children have been homeless more than once, and 23% have been homeless three or more times (Clement, 2003). About 5% of the homeless are *unaccompanied youth*, "individuals under the age of eighteen who lack parental, foster, or institutional care" (National Coalition for the Homeless, 2005, p. 1). Between 500,000 and 1 million young people run away from home each year, and 200,000 may be on the streets at any one time (Clement, 2003).

Families are the fastest-growing segment of the homeless population, accounting for 40% of the urban homeless population in 2004 and a larger proportion of the homeless in rural areas (National Coalition for the Homeless, 2005k). The number of families represented among the urban homeless increased by 5% in only 2 years, and in rural areas, single mothers with children make up the bulk of the homeless population (Bringing America Home, 2005b). As noted by the National Coalition for the Homeless, "Homelessness is a devastating experience for families. It disrupts virtually every aspect of family life, damaging the physical and emotional health of family members, interfering with children's education and development, and frequently resulting in separation of family members" (2005k, p. 1). Members

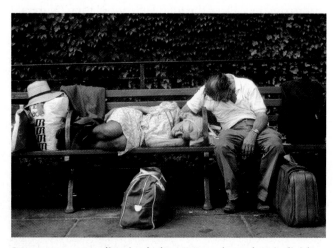

Due to overcrowding in shelters, many homeless individuals have no choice but to sleep outside. (© Andrew Holbrooke/The Image Works)

of ethnic minority groups are more likely to experience poverty and homelessness in urban areas than is the Caucasian population. Overall, African Americans comprise 49% of the homeless population, 35% are Caucasian, 13% Hispanic, 2% Native American, and 1% Asian. In a study in Philadelphia, 20% of African American women had been homeless sometime in the prior 7 years, compared to 4.8% of Hispanic women, 1.2% of Caucasian women, and 0.9% of Asian women (Webb, Culhane, Metraux, Robbins, & Culhane, 2003). In rural areas, on the other hand, homeless individuals and families are more likely to be Caucasian (National Coalition for the Homeless, 2005t). Homelessness in minority populations has been found to be more often due to external socioeconomic factors (e.g., poverty and unemployment) than to internal factors such as substance abuse (Cooke, 2004).

Another rapidly increasing segment of the homeless population is the elderly. For example, there was a 60% increase in the number of people over 55 years of age in Massachusetts shelters from 1999 to 2002. There is some debate regarding the age at which a homeless person should be considered elderly. Generally, however, 50 years of age is used as a cut-off because homeless people tend to age faster than the general population and a 50-year-old homeless individual may have a health status similar to that of a 70-year-old in the general population (National Coalition for the Homeless, 2005m). The increase in homelessness among the elderly is due, in large part, to the loss of affordable housing in the context of fixed incomes.

Older householders have approximately one chance in three of experiencing *worst-case housing*. **Worst-case housing** is defined as having an income below 50% of the area median income, being involuntarily displaced from housing, paying more than half of one's income for rent and utilities, or living in substandard housing (National Coalition for the Homeless, 2005k). Only 37% of very-low-income elderly receive federal housing assistance, and current Supplemental Security Income (SSI) benefits (an additional Social Security benefit for low-income elderly individuals) fall well below poverty level, and pay less than half of the fair market rent (FMR) in even the most generous states (National Coalition for the Homeless, 2005m).

Older homeless individuals are also less likely than others to request shelter due to fears of victimization. In one study, half of the older homeless persons responding had been robbed and one fourth had been assaulted in the previous year. Older homeless persons, like most elderly people, also tend to have more health problems than their younger counterparts and are less likely to be aware of eligibility for benefits and more likely to need assistance in navigating the social services system (National Coalition for the Homeless, 2005m).

U.S. veterans are another group that experience homelessness, accounting for roughly 23% of the total homeless population and 33% of homeless men.

According to Veterans Administration (VA) estimates, as many as 200,000 veterans may be homeless on any given night, and 529,000 to 840,000 veterans are homeless at some time during the year (National Coalition for Homeless Veterans, n.d.). Veterans have been found to be as much as three times more likely to become homeless than the general population (Nyamathi et al., 2004). Somewhat surprisingly, homelessness among veterans has not been linked to combat experience, but is associated with high rates of mental illness and addictive disorders. Approximately half of homeless veterans experience problems with substance abuse, and an estimated 45% experience mental illness (National Coalition for Homeless Veterans, n.d.). Homeless female veterans have been found to be even more likely than male veterans to have serious psychiatric disorders and less likely to be employed or to have addictive disorders (National Coalition for the Homeless, 2005l). Although the Veterans Administration provides services to more than 100,000 homeless veterans each year, at least 80% of the homeless veteran population is not served by the VA. A portion of this population is served by the more than 200 community-based veterans organizations across the country (National Coalition for Homeless Veterans, n.d.).

Epidemiologic Factors Affecting the Health of Poor and Homeless Populations

The epidemiology of poverty and homelessness has two aspects, factors that contribute to these conditions and factors that influence their effects on the health status of poor and homeless populations. Here we will examine both aspects in light of considerations in each of the dimensions of health.

Biophysical Considerations

Biophysical factors, in conjunction with factors in other dimensions, may lead to poverty and homelessness. Conversely, poverty and homelessness have serious consequences for biophysical health that vary with age and prior health status.

Certain health conditions may contribute to poverty and homelessness due to limited ability to work (Nielsen, Juon, & Ensminger, 2004). For example, people with HIV/AIDS are at greater risk for homelessness than the general population for a number of reasons. Hospitalization and excessive fatigue may interrupt employment, leading to loss of income and consequent inability to pay for housing. They may also experience discrimination and job loss due to their condition. In one study conducted in several cities, 44% to 50% of housed clients with HIV/AIDS feared becoming homeless due to inability to afford housing. In another study, 40% of 12,000 people with HIV/AIDS surveyed had been homeless at least once (National Coalition for the Homeless, 2005j).

Homeless individuals, particularly homeless youth, may also be at greater risk for HIV infection as a result of sexual abuse and exploitation and the practice of engaging in sex for money (Robertson et al., 2004). The median prevalence of HIV/AIDS in the homeless population is three times that in the general population, but may be as high as 62% in some subpopulations of the homeless. Homeless individuals with HIV/AIDS also tend to be sicker and have higher mortality rates than those with housing because of the additional stress of being homeless (National Coalition for the Homeless, 2005j). Homelessness, particularly among those with HIV/AIDS, also increases the risk of tuberculosis (TB), due to crowded conditions in shelters, and homeless individuals with TB usually have more advanced disease than their housed counterparts (National Coalition for the Homeless, 2005j).

Poverty has long been linked to ill health. One measure of this link is the number of days of activity limitation experienced due to illness. From 1993 to 2001, 15% of Americans with annual incomes under $15,000 experienced 14 or more days of activity limitation, compared to only 6.2% of those with incomes over $50,000 (Zahran et al., 2005).

The health effects of poverty and homelessness are exacerbated for both the young and the elderly. For example, homeless children are twice as likely as other children to report fair or poor health and four times more likely to experience developmental delays (Bringing America Home, 2005d). In addition, homeless children are two to six times more likely than other children to have asthma and twice as likely to experience lead poisoning. They also have a higher incidence of dental problems, poor nutrition, anemia, ear infection, upper respiratory infection and bronchitis, diarrhea, skin conditions, accidental injuries, obesity, and failure to thrive (Clement, 2003; Sherman & Redlener, 2003). Homeless children are also less likely to be up to date on immunizations. For example, in one study, only 11% of sheltered adolescents were adequately immunized (Ensign, 2001). Homeless adolescents often experience sexually transmitted diseases (STDs) and pregnancy. Approximately 80% of homeless youth are sexually active before 15 years of age. They have incidence rates for HIV infection two to ten times higher than other teenagers and are also at risk for hepatitis B. Other health problems common in this

EVIDENCE-BASED PRACTICE

Characteristics of homeless populations and the factors contributing to their homelessness vary from one geographic locale to the next. Solutions to the problem of homelessness must be based on causes specific to the local area. How might you go about determining the extent and causes of homelessness in your own area? Who comprises the homeless population in your area and what are their health needs? What needs for primary, secondary, and tertiary prevention are evident in your local homeless population?

population include skin conditions, injuries, dental problems, and poor nutrition (Clement, 2003).

Health problems common among homeless adults include asthma, bronchitis, hypertension, heart disease, peptic ulcer, cancer, arthritis, diabetes, and STDs (Wilson, 2004). Other frequently noted problems include malnutrition and TB and other respiratory diseases, due to the lack of housing and overcrowding in shelters (Krieger & Higgins, 2002). Homeless individuals tend to experience higher mortality from most causes than does the housed population (Wilde, Albanese, Rennells, & Bullock, 2004). Additional problems include frostbite, leg ulcers, liver disease, peripheral vascular disease, hepatitis C, vision problems, skin conditions, and trauma due to accidental injury and assault (Kushel, Perry, Bangsberg, Clark, & Moss, 2002; National Coalition for the Homeless, 2005h; Swigart & Kolb, 2004). As we can see from this list of common conditions, homeless persons often suffer multiple acute and chronic conditions that require long-term treatment and monitoring that is difficult in circumstances of homelessness (National Coalition for the Homeless, 2005h). Inadequate diet and lack of access to medications and health care supplies make disease management difficult. In addition, survival stress experienced by many homeless persons may lead them to put health needs at a lower priority than basic survival needs (Archambault, 2002).

The elderly are at particular risk of health problems stemming from homelessness. All of the usual problems of the elderly discussed in Chapter 19∞ are intensified by homelessness. The homeless elderly are particularly susceptible to the effects of communicable diseases, exposure, burns, and trauma due to alcohol use, physical or mental impairment, or assault. The elderly homeless population is also more likely than younger groups to experience chronic disability due to physical, mental, or emotional impairment.

Psychological Considerations

Psychological factors can lead to homelessness when people are unable to cope with the demands of daily life and have limited support systems. Family dynamics in the family of origin have been linked to homelessness in adulthood. In one study, for example, homeless women were less likely to have good support networks, were less likely to call on existing networks for assistance, and had networks that were less functional than stably housed women. Women who were unable to engage in reciprocal relationships or who reported conflictive relationships in childhood were at greater risk of homelessness. The authors noted the "significance of families of origin and learning how to develop and utilize support systems in preventing or reducing homelessness" and attributed increased vulnerability to homelessness as adults to the absence or inhibited development of abilities to interact effectively with support systems (Anderson & Rayens, 2004).

Mental illness is another psychological factor that contributes to homelessness. Estimates of the extent of psychiatric illness in the homeless population vary, but best estimates suggest that 20% to 25% of the homeless population experiences severe mental illness (National Coalition for the Homeless, 2005r), and 45% of homeless veterans have psychiatric diagnoses (Nyamathi et al., 2004). Some authors note that these figures only take into account homeless individuals with serious diagnoses and fail to account for many other mental health problems experienced by this population (Archambault, 2002). Others caution that the prevalence of mental illness in a specific homeless population changes over time and that intervention strategies need to address these changes (North, Eyrich, Pollio, & Spitznagel, 2004).

Mental illness interferes with one's ability to perform instrumental activities of daily living that permit one to remain adequately housed. In one study, 86% of the homeless individuals surveyed had a history of drug or alcohol problems or mental illness, and 30% experienced all three at some point in their lives (Wilde et al., 2004). Homeless clients with psychiatric illness are often noncompliant with therapeutic recommendations, exhibit more symptoms, and have higher rates of hospitalization for mental illness than housed persons with mental health problems (Caton et al., 2000).

Many authors cite the move to deinstitutionalize the mentally ill in the 1950s and 1960s as the cause of increasing homelessness among this population (Bohrer & Faulkner, 2004; McLeer, 2004). **Deinstitutionalization** was the process of discharging large numbers of mentally ill persons from mental institutions in an attempt to enable them to live in the least restrictive environment possible. This move was prompted by recognition of the appalling conditions prevalent in many institutions for the mentally ill. Although the intent of deinstitutionalization was laudable, the results were not. Unfortunately, there was no concurrent move to provide the community services needed for the mentally ill to live in noninstitutional settings, leaving them to fend for themselves. Other authors, however, point out that the increase in homeless mentally ill persons did not actually occur until the 1980s, when income and housing assistance programs for this population were withdrawn (National Coalition for the Homeless, 2005r). Loss of these socioeconomic supports prevented many mentally ill clients, prohibited from working by their disabilities, from being able to pay rent and resulted in their homelessness. In addition, the stigma of mental illness, combined with the stigma of homelessness, makes it more difficult for these individuals to obtain needed services (Bohrer & Faulkner, 2004).

Some homeless persons without preexisting mental illness exhibit psychological problems as a result of their homelessness. For example, data indicate that one third of homeless women have attempted suicide, compared to only one fourth of housed women (National Coalition for the Homeless, 2005k). Similarly, in one study, more than half of homeless adolescents had considered suicide (Clement, 2003). Homeless youth have also been found to have high rates of depression and conduct disorder, and rates of post-traumatic stress disorder (PTSD) are three times higher in this population than among adolescents in general (National Coalition for the Homeless, 2005p). Younger children's mental health is also affected by homelessness, and homeless children are more likely than their housed age mates to experience anxiety, depression, and withdrawal (Bringing America Home, 2005d). In addition, homelessness has been linked to child behavior problems, and fear of homelessness may lead to mental health problems in children (Krieger & Higgins, 2002).

Mental illness may also affect one's ability to escape homelessness. Homeless mentally ill individuals have been found to be homeless for longer periods of time than other homeless persons and to have less family contact, more barriers to employment, and more contact with the criminal justice system (National Coalition for the Homeless, 2005r). Conversely, good mental health, as evidenced in effective coping skills, has been linked to shorter episodes of homelessness (Caton et al., 2005).

Physical Environmental Considerations

Physical environmental factors also contribute to the effects of homelessness on health. Exposure to cold, even in the mildest climates, can lead to hypothermia (Clement, 2003). This is particularly true when people are lying on concrete or are clothed in wet garments. Overcrowding and poor sanitary conditions in shelters contribute to the spread of communicable diseases among a population that is already debilitated by exposure and poor nutritional status. As noted earlier, TB is rapidly spread in overcrowded shelter environments (Division of Applied Public Health Training, 2003).

Unsafe physical environments also present health hazards for young children. In addition to the potential for physical injury, the restrictions placed by parents on children's activities in unsafe surroundings may result in developmental delays.

Rural environments also pose physical environmental hazards for the poor and homeless due to the lack of available shelters and lack of access to assistance services. Rural poor and homeless individuals are more likely than members of the urban homeless population to live in a car, camper, or severely deteriorated housing (National Coalition for the Homeless, 2005s).

Sociocultural Considerations

Sociocultural dimension factors play a major role in the development of poverty and homelessness and in their effects on health. Lack of affordable housing, inadequate social support and welfare reform, mobility, and employment are some of the societal conditions that contribute to conditions of poverty and homelessness.

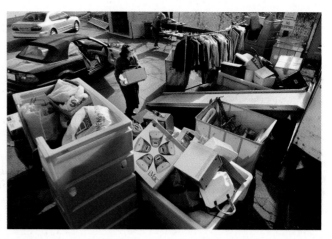

Thrift stores help the poor and the homeless to stretch their resources, but still may not meet all their needs. (Chip Somodevilla/Getty)

Other considerations to be addressed in this dimension include school attendance for homeless children and youth and considerations related to criminal justice, civil rights, and violence.

LACK OF AFFORDABLE HOUSING In addition to poverty, lack of affordable housing is the primary cause of homelessness in the United States. From 1973 to 1993, more than 2 million low-rental housing units disappeared from the housing market. Some were abandoned due to poor condition, others were demolished in the process of gentrification, and still others became unaffordable due to increases in rents. During the same period the number of households needing low-income housing increased significantly. From 1995 to 1997, the number of housing units renting for less than $300 per month declined by 19%, and between 1991 and 1995, the median rent for low-income housing increased by 21% (Bringing America Home, 2005b). Currently there is a gap of 4.4 million units between the available housing supply and the need for low-rent housing (National Coalition for the Homeless, 2005k), and it is estimated that an increase of 250,000 low-rent units would be needed each year for the next 20 years to meet the demand (Bringing America Home, 2005b).

Part of the loss of affordable housing stems from **gentrification**, which is defined as the displacement of low-income housing by higher-income space use such as luxury apartments, condominiums, or office buildings. Another aspect of the problem is the loss of many

BUILDING OUR KNOWLEDGE BASE

Lack of affordable housing is one of the primary factors contributing to homelessness in many areas of the United States. What strategies would you use to determine the availability of low-income housing in your area? How do housing costs compare to local wages for different subgroups in the community?

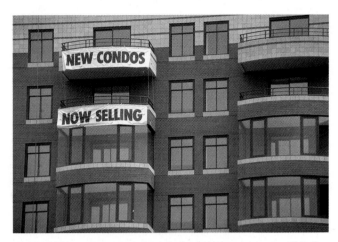

Single-room-occupancy hotels (SROs) that once provided low-cost shelter in many inner-city neighborhoods are being replaced by high-rent condominiums and luxury apartments. (© Rachel Epstein/The Image Works)

single-room occupancy (SRO) units in inner city areas. From 1970 to the mid-1980s, more than 1 million SROs were lost, many to the gentrification process in city center areas in large metropolitan settings. During this period, New York City lost an estimated 87% of downtown SRO units, Chicago lost all of its SROs, Los Angeles lost half, and San Francisco lost 43% (National Coalition for the Homeless, 2005a).

In rural areas homelessness is often precipitated by the occurrence of major structural or physical problems that make houses unsafe for human habitation. Approximately 30% of rural households in the United States, or 6.2 million households, have at least one major problem with housing. Housing availability in rural areas is also complicated by long distances to workplaces, lack of transportation, and insecure tenancy due to changes in local real estate markets (e.g., trailer park displacement by high-income single-family dwellings). Interestingly, many rural areas that are experiencing economic growth have the worst levels of low-income housing availability. When industry moves into an area, property values increase and so do rents, pricing out low-income residents (National Coalition for the Homeless, 2005s).

Worldwide, millions of people cannot afford housing that meets regulatory code standards. In addition, regulatory constraints control land acquisition and construction and do not foster development of low-income housing. In many parts of the world, it would take low-income families 15 to 30 years to be able to afford legal housing by saving 30% to 50% of their annual income (Population Information Program, 2003). Unfortunately, many people's incomes do not cover the basic necessities of life, much less allow for this level of savings.

POVERTY, SOCIAL SUPPORT, AND WELFARE REFORM The percentage of poor people in the U.S. population increased from 11.3% in 2000 to 12.1% in 2002, and the actual number of poor people increased by 4.3 million.

Increases in poverty stem from both declining wages and changes in public assistance programs. Since the 1980s income growth has not kept pace with rising housing costs. Family and individual incomes have declined while housing costs increased (National Coalition for the Homeless, 2005e; 2005o).

The American economy is increasingly divided into a highly paid skilled labor sector and a low-paid service sector (Freeman, 2002). In 1967, someone earning minimum wage could expect to support a family of three above poverty level. From 1981 to the 1990s, the federal minimum wage remained at $3.15 per hour, then increased in 1996 to $5.15 per hour. No increase in the minimum wage has been legislated at the federal level in the intervening years. Legislation in some states has increased the mandated minimum wage slightly beyond the federal minimum. Because of high rates of inflation, the real purchasing power of the minimum wage has decreased by 26% since 1979, and a full-time year-round employee receiving a federally defined minimum wage actually receives $1,778 less a year than the identified poverty level for a family of two. In no state, even those with the most generous minimum wage legislation, could one afford the fair market rent for a two-bedroom apartment. In fact, at the median state minimum wage, someone would need to work 87 hours per week to afford such an apartment at a cost of 30% of their monthly income, the federal definition of affordable housing (National Coalition for the Homeless, 2005e).

Many people, however, pay far more than 30% of their income for housing costs. In fact, 4.9 million households experience worst-case housing, paying more than 50% of their income for housing costs and having an income below 50% of the median for their geographic area. It is estimated that a minimum wage of $14.66 per hour would be required to enable a family to afford a two-bedroom home. This amount is nearly three times the current federal minimum wage and twice the minimum wage of any state (Bringing America Home, 2005e).

Changes in government programs to assist the poor have contributed to increased poverty and homelessness in two ways. First, the level of assistance provided has not kept pace with the rate of inflation. Consequently, individuals and families receiving aid fall deeper into poverty. Second, budgetary cutbacks have actually reduced benefits in some instances and stiffened eligibility requirements so that fewer of the working poor are eligible for aid. At the same time, taxes paid by the poor have increased. Some authors have noted a shift from welfare to "workfare" programs in the United States as well as in the United Kingdom and Canada (Wilton, 2004).

In 1996, the U.S. Congress passed the Personal Responsibility and Work Reconciliation Act, replacing the Aid to Families with Dependent Children (AFDC) program with the Temporary Aid to Needy Families (TANF) program, placing lifetime limits on receipt of

MediaLink Lenny Kravitz on Poverty (video)

ETHICAL AWARENESS

You are visiting a formerly homeless client, a single mother with three children under 8 years of age. She has been in subsidized housing for only 3 months. She is now working, and you discover that she is making about $50 more than the maximum that allows her to qualify for her housing subsidy. You know that there is a long list of people who are waiting to obtain subsidized housing, many of whom are in worse straits than this mother. Will you report her increased income to the housing authorities? Why or why not?

women previously on AFDC had chronic disabilities that limited their ability to work (Nielsen et al., 2004). Current and former welfare recipients have lower health status than the general population on several indicators, including glycosylated hemoglobin, blood pressure, body mass index, physical function, and smoking (Kaplan et al., 2005). Neither the health status nor the employability of many former AFDC recipients was considered in the design of welfare reforms.

Other federal programs that provided low-rent housing or housing subsidies to low-income individuals and families have also been cut. The U.S. federal government has ceased to build affordable housing and has actually demolished many older structures, replacing previous federal housing with housing vouchers intended to bridge the difference between an individual's or family's income and the cost of private rental (so called "section 8") housing. The point has been made, however, that housing vouchers may not be of much assistance in areas where low-income housing is scarce (Freeman, 2002). The average wait for section 8 housing is 24 months, but may be as long as 8 to 10 years in some areas (Sherman & Redlener, 2003).

Only about a third of poor renter households actually receive housing subsidies, and the availability of assistance is declining. For example, in 1976, 400,000 section 8 vouchers were authorized, but that number was reduced to 34,000 in 2003 (Bringing America Home, 2005b). Overall, federal housing support declined by 49% from 1980 to 2003 (National Coalition for the Homeless, 2005k). In addition, U.S. housing policies benefit the wealthy through mortgage interest tax deductions, reducing tax revenues that could help subsidize housing for the poor. It is estimated that the federal government loses $4 in income tax revenues for every $1 spent on housing assistance for the poor and homeless (Bringing America Home, 2005b). Federal housing assistance programs are summarized in Table 20-1◆.

benefits, and requiring recipients to be employed within 2 years of receiving benefits. The change also divorced Medicaid benefits from cash assistance programs. The intent of the legislation was to move recipients off the welfare rolls and to obtain gainful employment for them. TANF benefits and food stamps together, however, do not exceed the poverty level income in any state (National Coalition for the Homeless, 2005k). From 2000 to 2003, the number of poor children increased by 11%, yet the number of people receiving TANF benefits decreased by 9% (National Coalition for the Homeless, 2005k). Unfortunately, although many TANF recipients are finding employment, it is usually in low-paying jobs without benefits or sick leave, making it difficult for homeless women with children to provide adequately for their children. The federal legislation did not mandate support for childcare for working mothers, and although some states provide this assistance, many do not, making it even more difficult for low-income women to adequately care for dependent children.

Women on welfare are also more likely to have physical health problems than other women, and in 1997, as a result of welfare reforms, 675,000 people (including 400,000 children) lost access to federally funded health insurance (National Coalition for the Homeless, 2005h). In some studies, as many as 20% of

TABLE 20-1	Federal Housing Assistance Programs	
Program	Focus	Eligibility/Requirements
Section 811. Supportive Housing for Persons with Disabilities Program	• Small group homes, independent living projects, multifamily housing developments	• Very-low-income persons with disabilities over 18 years of age • Families with at least one disabled member
Section 202. Supportive Housing for the Elderly Program	• Construction, rehabilitation, or acquisition of structures to serve as supportive housing • Provision of support activities • Rental assistance to cover difference between costs and income	• Very-low-income persons age 62 years and older
Section 8. Housing Choice Voucher Program	• Rental assistance through a voucher system that permits renters access to privately owned housing	• Very-low-income families, elderly and disabled individuals • Income cannot exceed 50% of median income of area

Continued on next page

TABLE 20-1   Federal Housing Assistance Programs *(continued)*

		• Renters pay 30% of monthly income for rent and utilities
Section 8. Single-Room Occupancy	• Rehabilitation of existing structures to provide SRO units • Rental assistance to meet difference between cost and 30% of income • Rental assistance provided for 10-year period • May involve provision of some support services	• Very-low-income homeless individuals • Renters pay approximately 30% of income for rent • Rent must be equal to or less than 75% of HUD-established fair market rent (FMR) for an efficiency/studio unit
HOPE VI	• Destruction and replacement of public housing units or dramatic rehabilitation of existing units • Integration of low-income renters in middle-income areas • Provision of support services	• Intensive screening • Agreement to counseling and employment services
Public Housing	• Provision of rental housing to low-income families and individuals	• Low-income family, elderly, or disabled individual • U.S. citizen or eligible immigrant • Renters pay highest of (a) 30% of income, (b) 10% of monthly gross income, (c) shelter allowance, (d) locally determined minimum up to $50
Home Investment Partnerships Program	• Funding grants to states or communities to build, buy, or rehabilitate housing units for rental or ownership • Provision of rental assistance for occupants	• Local jurisdictions must contribute 25% match for funds • Income below 80% of area median
Section 502. Rural Home Ownership Direct Loan Program	• Loans to build, repair, renovate, or relocate houses (including mobile/manufactured homes) • Assistance with site purchase and water and sewage disposal arrangements	• Low- and very-low-income rural families without adequate housing • Able to afford mortgage payments, taxes, and insurance • 40% of funds must be used to serve families with incomes less than 50% of area median income
Section 515. Rural Rental Housing Loans	• Competitive mortgage loans to provide affordable rental housing • Provision of funds to buy and improve land and water and waste disposal systems	• Very-low-, low-, and moderate-income families, elderly, and disabled individuals • Renters pay higher of 30% of income or basic rent
Section 514/516. Farm Labor Housing Loans and Grants	• Loans and grants to buy, improve, or repair housing for farm laborers and those involved in aquaculture or on-farm processing	• U.S. citizens or permanent legal residents (temporary laborers, even if legally admitted, are not eligible) • Retired or disabled farm laborers living in such housing may remain there after retirement or disability

Data from: National Coalition for the Homeless. (2005). Federal housing assistance programs. Retrieved November 29, 2005, from http://www.nationalhomeless.org/publications/facts

MOBILITY Residential instability and population mobility are additional sociocultural factors that contribute to poverty and homelessness and to the lack of available social support systems. With the increasing mobility of the population, extended family members are often less available to help with material assistance. As we saw in Chapter 19∞, extended family support may be hampered by international mobility as well as movement within states and nations.

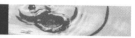

CULTURAL COMPETENCE

*H*omelessness is much less prevalent among some cultural groups than others (e.g., Muslims). Why do you think this might be the case? What other cultural groups do you think might exhibit similar protective factors for homelessness? How would you go about determining whether your assumption is correct?

Some homeless families and individuals may move to another location in an attempt to find work or housing. Approximately 70% of homeless families remain in the same general area, but the other 30% move (Clement, 2003). Loss of affordable housing may also mean moving to an area where shelter is available or moving from one shelter setting to another. As we will see later, this mobility poses difficulties in educating homeless children and youth.

A history of residential instability and mobility in childhood has also been linked to adult homelessness. Residential stability in childhood has been associated with both physical and mental health in middle adulthood. It has been hypothesized that residential stability permits the development of social capital and the ability to make social network connections that protect against homelessness later in life (Bures, 2003).

EMPLOYMENT Unemployment and underemployment are other major social factors contributing to homelessness. Although many people remain employed, there has been a shift in the job market from relatively well-paid manufacturing jobs to lower-paid employment in service industries (e.g., janitorial work). This phenomenon is referred to as **structural unemployment** or **deindustrialization** because it arises from changes in the nation's economic and occupational structure, such as the shifts from heavy to light industry and from manufacturing to technological occupations (Hirsch, Kett, & Trefil, 2002). In structural unemployment, jobs may be available, but those who are unemployed do not have the skills needed to qualify for them (Unemployment types, 2006). The emergence of high-technology occupations requires new sets of skills that many displaced workers do not have. Such changes in the structure of the job market have resulted in a situation in which 8.7 million people were unemployed in 2003 (U.S. Census Bureau, 2005).

The percentage of homeless people who are jobless varies from group to group. Overall, 42% of the homeless are employed, but many homeless individuals work at low-paying jobs that do not provide sufficient income to meet basic survival needs. An estimated 46% of jobs with the most growth from 1994 to 2005 provide incomes of less than $16,000 a year (Bringing America Home, 2005e). Many poor and homeless individuals are underemployed, a measure of those who are unemployed plus those who desire full-time work, but can only find part-time employment. Using this measure, in 2004, 9.9% of the U.S. population was underemployed, compared to an unemployment rate of 5.5%. In addition to declining real wages noted earlier, job security and stability have also declined, and displaced workers may have difficulty finding another job. Even when they do find work, however, many take jobs that pay an average of 13% less than former salaries. These workers also often find themselves in jobs that do not provide the benefits available from previous employment (National Coalition for the Homeless, 2005e).

Finding employment is difficult for most homeless individuals. Those with mental illness find it hard to maintain a job, if they can get one, because of their instability. Homeless single women with children, who account for almost half of homeless families, have problems of childcare while they work. In one study, for example, 30% of former welfare recipients reported having to leave work due to caregiving responsibilities (Kneipp, Castleman, & Gailor, 2004).

Even homeless persons with employable skills in areas where jobs are available may have difficulty negotiating the employment process. Lack of transportation may make it difficult to go to an interview or to get to work when a job is found. In addition, job application and interviews take time, which may prevent the individual from securing food or shelter for the night when these are obtained only after long waits in line in competition with many other homeless persons. Moreover, the homeless person may also find that he or she is penalized for working by reduction or even loss of assistance benefits and publicly financed health care coverage. Homeless individuals who cannot find regular work may engage in day labor or "shadow work." Shadow work may involve selling junk, personal possessions, or plasma; begging or panhandling; scavenging for food, salable goods, or money; and theft, all of which may carry criminal penalties in some jurisdictions (National Coalition for the Homeless, 2005q).

SCHOOL ATTENDANCE School attendance and its effects on school performance are other considerations affecting poor and homeless populations. In 2000, more than 930,000 children in kindergarten through 12th grade were homeless (Bringing America Home, 2005c). Frequent moves by homeless families result in frequent changes of school. Approximately 60% of U.S. children make an unscheduled school change between grades 1 and 12 (Kogut, 2004), often as a result of residential instability. It is estimated that every change results in the loss of 3 to 6 months of education. This affects school performance, and 23% of homeless children have repeated one or more grades (National Coalition for the Homeless, 2005d). In addition, homeless children and youth are four times more likely than their housed age mates to be below the 10th percentile in vocabulary and reading skills (Clement, 2003).

As noted by the National Coalition for the Homeless (2005d, p. 3), "School is one of the few stable, secure places in the lives of homeless children and youth—a place where they can acquire the skills needed to help them escape poverty." Unfortunately, the stability of the school environment is complicated by residency requirements, delay in the transfer of records, lack of transportation, and, often, lack of immunization records. Additional problems lie in getting children and youth assessed for special education needs, providing counseling, and promoting participation in before- and after-school activities. Unaccompanied youth also face problems with guardianship and liability. Approximately 87% of homeless children and youth are enrolled in school, but only 77% attend on a regular basis (National Coalition for the Homeless, 2005d).

The McKinney Act of 1987 attempted to fund states to provide educational services to homeless children and youth. The McKinney-Vento Act further requires school districts to maintain children in their prior schools whenever possible, to provide transportation as needed, and to provide immediate enrollment when a child moves to a new school regardless of prior receipt of official documents. Unfortunately, funds to provide these services are generally lacking. In 1990, Congress authorized $50 million for Education for Homeless Children and Youth (EHCY) programs, but the funds were never appropriated (National Coalition for the Homeless, 2005d). The 2003 EHCY budget was funded at $55 million, $15 million less than the amount authorized. The two McKinney Acts are also intended to fund preschool services for homeless preschoolers, yet only 15% of homeless preschool-age children were enrolled in preschool programs in 2000 (Bringing America Home, 2005c), partly because of long waiting times (30 days to 12 months) for public preschool programs (National Coalition for the Homeless, 2005d). As we will see in Chapter 23∞, school may be the only place that many poor children receive any health care. Difficulties with school attendance not only impair educational performance, but may also detract from the health status of these children.

CRIMINAL JUSTICE, CIVIL RIGHTS, AND VIOLENCE Homelessness and lack of basic necessities to support life may lead to crime, as well as prostitution, to obtain money. More often, however, homeless individuals are arrested for actions that, if conducted in private, would be perfectly acceptable. The homeless are overrepresented in jail, and recently released prisoners are at high risk of homelessness due to disruption of family and community ties. Mentally ill inmates have an even more difficult time reintegrating into society and have an even higher risk of homelessness (Kushel, Hahn, Evans, Bangsberg, & Moss, 2005). Approximately 54% of homeless men have a history of incarceration at some time in their lives (Cooke, 2004). A history of arrest has also

been found to be predictive of longer periods of homelessness than those experienced by persons without criminal records (Caton et al., 2005).

Many cities criminalize activities of homeless persons in an effort to render them invisible to the general public through incarceration "under the guise of assumed threats to public safety" (National Coalition for the Homeless, 2005q, p. 3). **Criminalization** is defined as "the process of legislating penalties for the performance of life-sustaining functions in public" (National Coalition for the Homeless, 2005q, p. 4). As noted by one author, "Homeless people are in a double bind. For them socially legitimated space does not exist, and so they are denied access to public space and public activity by laws of a capitalist society that is anchored in private property and privacy" (Mitchell, 2003, p. 135). This concept is further highlighted in statements by the National Coalition for the Homeless (2005q) that "because people without homes have no option but to perform necessary functions in public, they are vulnerable to judgment, harassment, and arrest for committing 'nuisance' violations in public" (p. 4) and that "cities have turned to the criminal justice system for housing, treatment, and even as a means of 'disappearing' homeless people" (p. 9).

Earlier, we saw that the number of available shelter beds is insufficient to meet the need in many jurisdictions. Another barrier to shelter that keeps people on the street and vulnerable to arrest for *nuisance* crimes is the cost of shelter, which may be as high as $5 to $10 per night and thus beyond the means of the most destitute homeless (National Coalition for the Homeless, 2005q). Fines imposed for *illegal* activities further deplete the money available to homeless individuals for obtaining housing. In addition, mental health and drug courts may also reserve shelter beds for sentencing purposes, further restricting the availability of shelter for many homeless individuals (Bringing America Home, 2005f).

In surveys conducted throughout the nation, 80% of communities have laws against camping or sleeping in public areas, yet 100% of these communities lack sufficient shelter beds to meet local needs. Police often conduct sweeps of areas where homeless people congregate prior to major political, entertainment, or sports events, and homeless people are banned outright from some high-income residential and tourist areas. In many places, public parks have been designated as "family" parks, making them off-limits for people without children. Similarly, bars have been placed in the center of public benches to prevent people from lying down on them. Increased policing of gentrified areas and tourist centers effectively removes the homeless from the sight of the more affluent members of society (Bringing America Home, 2005f).

Existing laws are selectively enforced, with homeless people, particularly members of ethnic minority groups, more often being arrested for nuisance activities than housed individuals (Bringing America Home,

2005f). The criminalization of activities by the homeless is costly to society and uses money that could be better spent in more positive initiatives to end homelessness. In fact, the cost of jailing a homeless offender, excluding the cost of police activity, is estimated to range from $40 to $140 per day. This is in excess of the cost of providing housing and other services, estimated at $30 per day (National Coalition for the Homeless, 2005q). The cost of criminalization is also higher than the cost of creating new affordable housing. In addition to the societal cost, criminalization also increases barriers to housing and other services for people who now have criminal records (Bringing America Home, 2005f).

Discrimination in terms of civil rights violations is not the only form of discrimination encountered by homeless individuals and families. In some cases, discrimination in housing markets may actually cause homelessness. Despite legislation to the contrary, Black individuals and families, elderly poor, people with HIV/AIDS, and those with psychiatric disorders frequently encounter discrimination in their efforts to obtain housing (Northridge, Stover, Rosenthal, & Sherard, 2003). In addition, exclusionary zoning ordinances prohibit construction of multifamily units or high-density housing in many high-income neighborhoods. Requirements for significant acreage upon which to build further restrict development of affordable housing and increase the price of what housing is available (Freeman, 2002).

Discrimination against the poor and homeless, at its extreme, results in violence and victimization. The National Coalition for the Homeless (2005g) identifies three types of perpetrators of *hate crimes*: mission offenders, scapegoat offenders, and thrill seekers. Mission offenders perceive themselves to be on a mission to cleanse the world of certain types of undesirable people. Scapegoat offenders engage in violence in response to feelings of frustration with circumstances (e.g., unemployment) that they attribute to members of a particular group. Thrill seekers act violently to derive pleasure from hurting others. The Coalition noted that most violence against homeless persons is committed by thrill seekers; however, they also state that the frequency of violence against the homeless rises with increased police action against this group and with negative city responses or portrayals of the homeless as responsible for societal ills.

From 1999 to 2004, a total of 386 violent acts against homeless individuals, resulting in 156 deaths, were reported. Victims ranged in age from 4 months to 74 years, and the perpetrators were as young as 11 years and as old as 65. In 2004 alone, 105 events were reported and 25 deaths occurred, with perpetrators ranging from 12 to 45 years of age (National Coalition for the Homeless, 2005g).

Violence may also be a cause of homelessness. For example, studies of homeless women indicate that 25% to 50% of them were abused in the year prior to becoming homeless. In one study, 46% of the women had remained in an abusive situation because of lack of other options. Loss of cash assistance programs may further limit the options for escape available to abused women and children (National Coalition for the Homeless, 2005c). Homeless youth may also be prior victims of abuse. Approximately 46% of runaway youth have been physically abused and 17% have been sexually abused (National Coalition for the Homeless, 2005p). Homeless youth are also at greater risk for violence and victimization on the street than adults. For example, in one study, 85% of homeless youth had witnessed a stabbing or shooting (Clement, 2003).

Behavioral Considerations

Behavioral considerations that are particularly relevant to the poor and homeless populations include diet and nutrition, rest, substance abuse, and sexual activity. Inadequate nutrition among poor and homeless individuals is a lifestyle factor leading to ill health. As housing and heating costs increase for poor families, food expenditures tend to decrease. In higher-income families, on the other hand, exceptionally cold weather and increased heating costs tend to be associated with increased food expenditures (Bhattacharya, DeLeire, Haider, & Currie, 2003). One million U.S. households are considered food insecure, and 3 million people experience hunger (Wehler et al., 2004).

The homeless, even those housed in shelters, rarely have access to kitchen facilities. Some shelters do provide meals, but they are rarely adequate to meet the nutritional needs of those served. This is particularly true in the case of homeless children, who frequently exhibit anemia or serious growth failure, and who go hungry twice as often as housed children (Bringing America Home, 2005d). In one survey, 20% of homeless individuals reported one or fewer meals a day; 39% reported hunger and the inability to afford food; and 40% had gone without food for one or more days (Clement, 2003). The homeless may also have difficulty meeting special dietary needs posed by chronic illness and pregnancy.

Homeless individuals may also have difficulty obtaining adequate rest. Because of increased crime and victimization at night, many homeless individuals may attempt to sleep in the daytime when they are less

---

Think Advocacy

The Bringing America Home Act (Bringing America Home, 2005a) is an ambitious piece of legislation aimed at addressing the multiple factors that contribute to homelessness in the United States. Access the Web site at http://www.bringingamericahome.org to see what organizations have endorsed this legislation. What organizations in your area might endorse the Act? How might you organize a campaign to support this piece of legislation?

vulnerable to attack. This further limits their ability to obtain many services that are offered only during the day. The inability to rest frequently places homeless individuals at greater risk for a variety of health problems and worsens existing health conditions. For example, the inability to lie down to rest may lead to venous stasis and contribute to leg and foot ulcers. These adverse effects on circulation are made worse if the homeless individual smokes. Smoking also intensifies the effects of respiratory infections contracted from others in crowded shelters.

Substance abuse is a behavioral factor that may contribute to homelessness when the abuser is unable, because of his or her addiction, to meet, or even care about, needs for shelter. Substance abuse may also lead to expenditure of money for alcohol or drugs that could be used for shelter. On the other hand, homelessness may lead to use and abuse of alcohol and drugs as a form of escape, or alcohol or drugs may be used to relieve symptoms of psychiatric illness. The precise connection between homelessness and substance abuse, however, is unclear. Competition for scarce housing resources may put those with drug and alcohol abuse problems at a disadvantage relative to other homeless individuals. Findings of studies showing a consistent link between addiction and homelessness have been called into question because of the preponderance of long-term shelter users and single homeless men in these studies (National Coalition for the Homeless, 2005a).

Changes in disability benefits have also made individuals with addictive disorders more vulnerable to homelessness. The Clinton administration eliminated eligibility for SSI and Social Security Disability Insurance (SSDI) for people whose disability is related to substance abuse (National Coalition for the Homeless, 2005a). In one study, 3% of homeless individuals had recently lost SSI or SSDI benefits, leaving them unable to support prior rents.

Nonheterosexual sexual orientation may be a precursor to homelessness, particularly among young people. In one study, for example, 35% of homeless youth reported homosexual or bisexual orientation as their reason for leaving home (Rew, Fouladi, & Yockey, 2002). Sex trading, or the exchange of sex for money or food, is a lifestyle that may arise as a result of homelessness. Sex trading is particularly prevalent among adolescent runaways who find no other way to earn enough money to support themselves (Clement, 2003). Homelessness has also been linked to sex trading among men who have sex with men (MSM) (Newman, Rhodes, & Weiss, 2004). Sex trading and injection drug use among some members of the homeless population place this group at risk for communicable diseases such as HIV infection and hepatitis B and C. Homelessness and poverty may also affect other health-related behaviors. For example, women with a history of adverse socioeconomic

circumstances at some point in their lives have been shown to be less likely to use hormone replacement therapy (Lawlor, Smith, & Ebrahim, 2004). Poverty and homelessness may also make it more difficult for people to engage in health-promoting and illness-preventing activities. We have already seen that homelessness is associated with decreased immunization levels among children. On a more positive note, some research has indicated that homeless individuals, particularly women, are open to healthy lifestyle behaviors when they are able to engage in them. For example, homeless women have been found to engage in behaviors related to physical activity, diet, and stress management (Wilson, 2004).

Health System Considerations

Health system factors may contribute to homelessness or limit access to care for poor and homeless persons. For example, medical bills for catastrophic illness, particularly for those who do not have health insurance, may catapult individuals and families into homelessness. As we saw earlier, thousands of people lost insurance coverage in 1997 as a result of changes in welfare benefits; another 725,000 individuals who were laid off lost employment-based health insurance (National Coalition for the Homeless, 2005k). In 2003, 16.5% of the U.S. population under 65 years of age had no health insurance (National Center for Health Statistics, 2005). Catastrophic illness in this population could easily lead to depletion of any existing savings, inability to pay rent, and eventually homelessness.

Noninstitutionalization of the mentally ill is another health system factor that may contribute to homelessness. **Noninstitutionalization** refers to a lack of hospitalization of persons with mental problems who are in need of care. Often, particularly in urban areas, people with mental illness are not hospitalized until they have deteriorated to the point where they are a danger to themselves or others. Such tolerance of deviant behavior prevents mentally ill individuals from obtaining help when they need it and when they could most easily benefit from it. In other situations, long waits for treatment may prevent individuals with mental illness or substance abuse disorders from obtaining help in a timely fashion and may lead to subsequent homelessness as they become less and less able to cope with life. Even when treatment becomes available, homeless individuals with no contact address cannot be reached and may be dropped from long waiting lists (National Coalition for the Homeless, 2005a).

More often than causing homelessness, however, health care system factors make it more difficult for homeless individuals to obtain health care and to prevent or resolve health problems. Financial costs are one barrier to health care for the homeless. Approximately 55% of the homeless population lacks health insurance (Wilde et al., 2004). Lacking regular health care providers, homeless individuals and families have rates of emergency department (ED) use three times those of the general population. For example, 40% of homeless individuals in one study made one or more ED visits in the previous year, and 8% had made three or more visits (Kushel et al., 2002). Many homeless individuals do not receive any care. Ten percent of homeless parents indicated that their children needed health care but did not receive it due to costs (Clement, 2003). Similarly, 13% of sheltered adolescents delayed getting recommended care due to costs (Ensign, 2001). Homeless veterans, on the other hand, may be slightly more likely to have a regular source of health care and receive needed care (Nyamathi et al., 2004). Some assistance is provided to help homeless individuals and families obtain needed health care. In 1987, the McKinney Act authorized creation of the Health Care for the Homeless (HCH) program. The program, which was reauthorized in 1996 under the Health Centers Consolidation Act and in 2002 under the Health Care Safety Net Amendments Act, provides grants to community-based organizations to support primary care services for homeless individuals (National Coalition for the Homeless, 2005h, 2005i). Some homeless individuals, particularly children, may also be eligible for Medicaid; however, the National Women's Law Center (2004) has noted that even eligible persons may not enroll in the Medicaid program because of the complexity of the enrollment process.

Cost is not the only barrier to health care access. Other problems include lack of transportation, long waits for service (which may mean missing a meal at the soup kitchen or being unable to obtain shelter for the night), fragmentation of services due to lack of case management, and billing practices that result in attaching the wages of those who earn next to nothing. Lack of childcare for other children may also prevent homeless parents from obtaining care for themselves or their children. Provider barriers include insensitivity to the needs and circumstances of the homeless and unwillingness to provide care to those with no means of payment.

Personal barriers posed by homeless persons themselves include priority placed on survival over health needs, denial of illness, fears of loss of personal control, lack of money, and embarrassment over personal appearance and hygiene. Homeless individuals and families may also lack the expertise or the energy to complete the processes involved in registration or application for services.

Lack of preventive care is a common problem among this population. Few pregnant homeless women receive prenatal care. These women and their offspring are at higher risk for complications of pregnancy than is the general population. Homeless women are also less likely to receive preventive services. Preventive care is also lacking for young children.

Think Advocacy

Wilde, Albanese, Rennells, and Bullock (2004) described the development of a nursing clinic for homeless men by nursing faculty and students. Based on the success of the clinic, shelter staff are more knowledgeable regarding the health needs of the homeless population and better able to meet those needs. How might you and your classmates establish such a service to serve the local homeless population? What services would be needed? Which of these services could be provided by nurses? By other health care and social service professionals? How might you go about obtaining these other services?

Compliance with treatment recommendations may also be difficult. Homeless clients may be unable to afford prescribed medications or may not have a watch to time doses correctly. They may not have access to water to take oral medications, and syringes for insulin may be lost or stolen. Other difficulties include retaining potency in medications exposed to frequent temperature changes and obtaining prescription refills. Treatment for HIV/AIDS is particularly difficulty among the homeless due to the complexity of most treatment regimens (National Coalition for the Homeless, 2005j).

Mental health services for poor and homeless populations are also lacking. Some observers have noted a mismatch between traditional community mental health services and the needs of the homeless population. Comprehensive services are seldom offered at one location, and mental health services seldom address the social factors contributing to homelessness.

COMMUNITY HEALTH NURSING AND CARE OF POOR AND HOMELESS POPULATIONS

Community health nurses may encounter homeless clients in a number of venues. They may work in or with shelters for homeless people. Or they may encounter virtually homeless people during home visits to other clients with whom homeless individuals may be staying. Community health nurses may also encounter homeless clients who seek to obtain services from other agencies where nurses are employed. Finally, homeless clients may be referred to community health nurses by other agencies and providers.

Homeless individuals may be reluctant to admit to their homelessness for a variety of reasons. They may feel embarrassed about their condition or may want to forestall intrusion into what they may feel is their own affair. Community health nurses should be alert to indicators of possible homelessness in clients they encounter. For example, a community health

Advocacy in Action

Interpreting for the Homeless

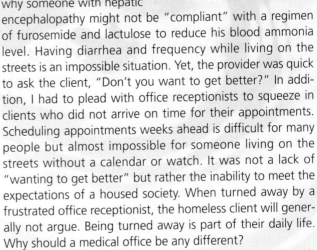

As an outreach nurse with Health Care for the Homeless in Phoenix, Arizona, I was constantly advocating for the homeless clients I served. Many individuals who are homeless have histories of mental illness, substance abuse, and physical abuse. They often do not trust the health care system and have generally had less than satisfying encounters with health care providers who could only identify the negative effects of their lifestyle rather than attempt to understand how to deliver culturally appropriate care to this vulnerable population.

As an outreach nurse, I was responsible for locating homeless individuals who were at risk, engaging them in services, and coordinating their health care. The locating wasn't difficult, but engaging and coordinating care proved to be. As clients came to trust me, I was able to schedule them for medical appointments and assured them that I would provide transportation and, more importantly, accompany them to appointments when possible.

Homeless people can be uncomfortable with meeting new people and having to sit in a waiting room full of people who may not appreciate their presence. They are concerned that the appointment may affect their ability to work that day. Picking up cans and panhandling do not allow for sick time. Many of my clients lived outside and did not have access to clean clothes or showers. I was prepared for the attitudes of the public, but not the attitude of the providers. The providers were quick to identify clients' negative health behaviors regardless of the reason they were seeking treatment. Rather than provide positive reinforcement for making and keeping an appointment, providers admonished clients for not coming in sooner. There was no consideration for their lifestyle in developing treatment plans. Clients who lived on the street would be told to go home, elevate the broken extremity, put ice on it, and call their orthopedic surgeon—none of which is possible for people living under a bridge or in a shelter.

Countless times I acted as an "interpreter" for my clients. I had to explain why someone with hepatic encephalopathy might not be "compliant" with a regimen of furosemide and lactulose to reduce his blood ammonia level. Having diarrhea and frequency while living on the streets is an impossible situation. Yet, the provider was quick to ask the client, "Don't you want to get better?" In addition, I had to plead with office receptionists to squeeze in clients who did not arrive on time for their appointments. Scheduling appointments weeks ahead is difficult for many people but almost impossible for someone living on the streets without a calendar or watch. It was not a lack of "wanting to get better" but rather the inability to meet the expectations of a housed society. When turned away by a frustrated office receptionist, the homeless client will generally not argue. Being turned away is part of their daily life. Why should a medical office be any different?

I am an advocate for a marginalized population that is unable to demand the medical care it deserves. I explain to providers how best to meet the needs of people who are homeless. I assist clients in navigating a health care system that has little understanding of the unique characteristics of people who are homeless. As an assistant clinical professor at ASU College of Nursing, I am educating new client advocates. During the senior year in community health nursing, I supervise students at a local shelter where they provide care to over 400 homeless residents. As a result of this clinical experience, the population welcomes over 60 new advocates each year.

Kay Jarrell, MS, RN
Clinical Assistant Professor
Arizona State University College of Nursing

---

nurse may note that a client has not taken a shower or washed his or her clothes in some time. Or the client may be hesitant when asked for a home address or may give the address of a known homeless shelter. Clients who report living with other family members or friends may also be virtually homeless. When faced with these indicators, the community health nurse can tactfully explore if the client is indeed homeless and if assistance is desired.

In other instances, clues may be more subtle. For example, in a hearing related to a college academic integrity violation related to plagiarism, the student explained his purchase of a paper from an Internet source as a result of not being able to work in his dorm room because his roommate was using drugs and he was afraid to be associated with him. When a community health nurse faculty member, who happened to be a member of the hearing committee, asked where the student was staying if he was not living in the dorm, he reported that he was living in one of the student lounges on campus. In addition to dealing with the academic integrity violation, the committee took immediate steps to obtain adequate housing for the student. However, his homeless plight would not have been identified if the community health nurse had not caught the cue buried in his defense of plagiarism.

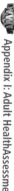

Assessing the Health of Poor and Homeless Populations

The first step in the care of poor and homeless segments of the population is assessing their health status and identifying the factors that influence their health. The community health nurse examines factors that contribute to homelessness in the population as well as the effects of homelessness on health. The focused assessment below provides some questions that can be used in assessing the health of the homeless population. The assessment tool included in Appendix I on the Companion Website can be used to assess the health of homeless clients.

Assessment data for poor and homeless populations may be somewhat more difficult to obtain than data about other, more easily observed populations.

Community health nurses working with homeless individuals or groups of homeless persons would be particularly alert for commonly encountered health problems. In addition, they would assess individual clients for the presence of any other chronic or communicable diseases, as well as for high prevalence rates for these conditions in the homeless population. Information regarding prevalent conditions can be sought from health professionals and agencies that care for homeless people. Some data on the age, gender, and ethnic composition of the homeless population may be available from shelter sites and social service agencies. Local churches may also have a sense of the number and types of homeless people served. Local government agencies may also have data on the extent of the homeless population and its composition.

FOCUSED ASSESSMENT

Assessing the Homeless Population

Biophysical Considerations

- What is the age composition of the homeless population? The ethnic and gender composition?
- What developmental effects has homelessness had? What acute and chronic health problems are prevalent? What is the prevalence of pregnancy?
- What is the immunization status of the homeless population (particularly children)?

Psychological Considerations

- What is the extent of mental illness in the homeless population? What is the extent of depression, anxiety, and suicide?
- What stresses are experienced by this population? How does the homeless population cope with stress?
- What are individual and group responses to being homeless? To seeking help?

Physical Environmental Considerations

- What are the effects of climatic conditions on the homeless population?
- Where do homeless individuals in the community seek shelter? How adequate are shelter facilities? What hygiene facilities are available to homeless persons?
- Do environmental conditions pose other health hazards for homeless individuals (e.g., flooding under bridges used for shelter)?

Sociocultural Considerations

- What is the community attitude to homelessness? To homeless individuals?
- What is the extent of family support available to the homeless individual? What is the extent of community support available to the homeless population?
- To what extent does family violence contribute to homelessness in the community?
- What effects do education, economic, and employment factors have on homelessness in the community? What proportion of the eligible homeless population is receiving financial assistance? What proportion of the homeless is employed? In what kind of work?

- What childcare resources are available to homeless women with children?
- What education programs are available for homeless children?
- What transportation resources are available to the homeless population?
- What is the availability of low-cost housing in the community? What is the availability of shelter for homeless persons? For individuals with special needs?
- What proportion of the homeless population consists of families? What proportion of homeless families are headed by women?
- What is the extent of crime victimization among homeless individuals?

Behavioral Considerations

- What food resources are available in the community for homeless individuals? What nutritional deficits do homeless individuals exhibit? What is the nutritional value of food available to homeless individuals and families?
- What is the extent of drug and alcohol abuse in the homeless population?
- What is the prevalence of smoking in the homeless population?
- Are there facilities available in the community for homeless individuals to rest during the day? What health effects does lack of rest have on the homeless individual?
- What is the extent of prescription medication use among the homeless population? Do homeless individuals have access to resources to help with medication expenses?
- What is the extent of sex trading and unsafe sexual activity in the population?

Health System Considerations

- What health care services are available to homeless persons in the community? To what extent are these services integrated with other services needed by the homeless population? What is the availability of mental health services for homeless individuals? Drug and alcohol treatment services? To what extent are preventive health services available to and utilized by the homeless population?
- Where do homeless persons usually obtain health care? What are the attitudes of health care providers toward homeless individuals?
- How is health care for homeless persons financed?

Information on the prevalence of specific conditions and immunization status can be obtained in surveys of the homeless population. Surveys of homeless individuals will need to be conducted in places where they congregate. For example, a community health nurse might survey individuals living in a shelter or those who take advantage of community meal programs. Because of the time needed to complete surveys, the lack of resources available to them (e.g., pens or pencils for completing written surveys), and varied levels of education among the homeless population, surveys will be most effective if conducted verbally in the context of other services. For example, the nurse might survey clients as they wait in line at a local soup kitchen or approach them for a few minutes of their time after they finish a meal. Privacy is often lacking in the lives of homeless individuals, and community health nurses should refrain from asking for highly personal information in public settings. Homeless individuals with substance abuse problems may also be wary of admitting these and other illicit behaviors (e.g., theft of food) unless assured of confidentiality. Community health nurses should endeavor to ask survey questions in language appropriate to the client's understanding and in ways that do not imply value judgments. Homeless individuals themselves may be involved in the development of survey tools that address their perceived needs in a sensitive and culturally appropriate manner. Community health nurses can also advocate for the involvement of homeless individuals in data collection and analysis and payment for temporary employment in these activities.

Surveys can also be a mechanism for collecting information on the extent of mental illness and the level of coping skills in the population. Psychiatric treatment facilities may also have data on the number of homeless individuals served and the types of diagnoses seen.

Environmental conditions and their effects on the homeless are often best assessed through observation. What is the local weather and how does it affect the homeless population? The adequacy of shelter facilities can be observed by visits to existing shelters. Other places where homeless people congregate can also be observed. At the same time, observations in public places can provide some information on the attitude of others toward obviously homeless individuals as well as on the extent of police activities related to the homeless. Local police records can also provide information on arrests for nuisance crimes.

The extent of family violence as a precursor to homelessness can best be determined by surveys of homeless individuals, particularly women and youth. Police and other protective services agencies are another source of information on family violence. These agencies may also provide information on the availability of shelters for victims of abuse. Shelter personnel can likewise be a source of information on the homeless population.

Educational and employment information can be obtained in a similar manner. Local social service agencies or employment offices may have information on places where homeless individuals may go to seek day labor. Observation and questioning of people in these locations can provide information on the kinds of jobs available and wages paid, as well as potential job hazards faced by the homeless population. Perusal of the local newspaper can also provide a sense of the job opportunities that may be available to homeless individuals. General community employment and economic data may be available from local chambers of commerce or government employment offices. Census data also include this information but may be outdated, depending on the recency of data collection.

Social service agencies and telephone books are potential sources of data regarding childcare availability. In addition, the community health nurse can contact local childcare providers to determine the availability of care for children in low-income families. Similarly, school districts can provide information on the availability of public preschool programs. School districts can also provide information on the number of homeless children enrolled in local schools, as well as the services available to meet their needs.

Information on shelter availability would most likely be obtained from social service agencies, local churches, or local government offices. These organizations may also have information regarding food resources and other services available to poor and homeless populations. Information on specific nutritive intake, however, is best obtained by observation in shelters or surveys of homeless individuals. Surveys could also be used to determine the extent of health-related behaviors such as smoking, alcohol and drug use, and sex trading, as well as the use of prescription medications. Crime victimization data would be available from local police departments.

General information on the availability of health services can be obtained from telephone directories, and specific agencies can be contacted to determine the type and extent of services provided to homeless individuals. Emergency departments, in particular, may have information on the frequency with which homeless individuals use ED services as a substitute for primary care. Local officials and health care agencies can also be contacted to determine how health care services for poor and homeless individuals are funded.

Diagnostic Reasoning and Care of Poor and Homeless Populations

Based on the assessment of the health status of poor and homeless clients and factors contributing to that status, nursing diagnoses may be derived at any of several levels. At the individual client level, the community health nurse may make diagnoses related to the existence of homelessness. As discussed before, the diagnostic statement includes underlying factors if identifiable, for example, "homelessness due to inability to pay for shelter" or "homelessness due to mental illness and inability to care for self."

Other kinds of diagnoses made at the individual or family level might relate to specific health problems resulting from or intensified by homelessness. As an example, the nurse might make a diagnosis of "stasis ulcers due to excessive walking and standing and inability to lie down at night" or "malnutrition due to inability to afford food and lack of access to cooking facilities."

Nursing diagnoses may also be made at the group or community level. For example, the community health nurse may diagnose a significant problem of homelessness in the community. Such diagnoses might be stated as "an increase in the homeless population due to recent closure of major community employer" or "an increase in the number of homeless families due to unemployment and reductions in public assistance programs." Diagnoses may also be made at the aggregate level relative to specific problems engendered by homelessness, for example, "increased prevalence of tuberculosis due to malnutrition and crowding in shelters for the homeless" or "increased incidence of anemia among homeless children due to poor nutrition."

Planning and Implementing Health Care for Poor and Homeless Populations

Planning to meet the needs of homeless clients should focus on long-term as well as short-term solutions to problems. Planning should also reflect the factors contributing to the needs of the homeless in a particular locale. For example, if most of the homelessness in one community is due to unemployment, long-term interventions would most likely be directed toward improving employment opportunities in the area or increasing the employability of those involved. If, on the other hand, a significant portion of homelessness in the area is due to mental illness and inability to care for self, attention would be given to providing supportive services for the mentally ill.

Planning should address the underlying factors contributing to homelessness as well as its health consequences. For example, providing shelter on a nightly basis may decrease the risk of exposure to cold for homeless persons but does nothing to relieve homelessness. In planning to meet the health needs of homeless clients, community health nurses may work independently or in conjunction with other health care and social service providers. When planning to address factors contributing to homelessness, however, the community health nurse frequently is part of a group of government officials and concerned citizens who have assumed responsibility for dealing with the overall problem of homelessness. The principles of coalition building, discussed in Chapters 7 and 13∞, will be helpful to community health nurses working with others to address problems of homelessness and poverty in the community.

Efforts to alleviate homelessness and its consequences may take place at the primary, secondary, or tertiary level of prevention. Community health nurses may be involved in activities at any or all three levels. As is true in caring for any client, planning care for a homeless client or population begins with prioritizing health needs. In many instances, the first priority would be obtaining shelter, a secondary preventive measure. Other health needs could then be addressed in terms of their priority. For each of the health care needs identified for the homeless client or population, the community health nurse would develop specific outcome objectives and design interventions at the primary, secondary, or tertiary level of prevention. Planning efforts should be a joint function of the community health nurse, homeless clients, who best know their situation and the kinds of interventions that are likely to be successful in that situation, and other concerned individuals.

Primary Prevention

Primary prevention may be directed at either preventing homelessness or preventing its health consequences. Primary prevention can occur at the individual or family level or at community levels. Community health nurses can help prevent individuals and families from becoming homeless by assisting them to eliminate factors that may contribute to homelessness. For example, if a family is threatened with eviction because of a parent's unemployment, the nurse can assist family members to obtain emergency rent funds from local social service agencies. The nurse can also encourage the family to apply for ongoing financial aid programs or assist the parent to find work.

As noted earlier, some people become homeless because of underlying psychiatric illness and an inability to deal with the requirements for maintaining shelter. Severely disturbed people may just wander away from home and take up residence on the streets. Homelessness in this group can be prevented by referrals for psychiatric therapy and counseling. Case management in the transition from hospital or prison to community may help to prevent homelessness in mentally ill or inmate populations. Nurses may also provide support services to families caring for mentally ill members to prevent these persons from becoming part of the homeless population. Placement in a sheltered home might also be an approach to preventing homelessness in the mentally disturbed person when family members either cannot or do not wish to care for the client. In addition, the community health nurse can monitor the effectiveness of therapy and watch for signs of increasing agitation or disorientation that may precede wandering. The nurse can also assist the disturbed person by giving concrete direction in such tasks as paying rent.

Runaway children and teenagers are another segment of the homeless population for whom homelessness may be prevented through primary preventive interventions. Efforts of community health nurses to promote effective communication in families and enhance parenting skills may prevent young people from feeling a need to run away. Similarly, efforts to prevent or deal with child abuse may prevent runaways.

Primary prevention at the community level to reduce the incidence of poverty and homelessness requires major changes in societal structure and thinking. Some suggested avenues for intervention include federal support for low-cost housing, increases in the minimum wage, and access to supportive services for the mentally and physically disabled to allow them to function effectively in society. Another suggestion aimed at reducing the incidence of poverty in families with children to prevent their homelessness is to provide childcare assistance and paid parental occupational leaves as needed.

Creating employment opportunities and programs to train people in employable skills is another possible primary preventive measure for both poverty and homelessness. Current public job training programs, however, have been criticized for their failure to facilitate job placement for those who complete the programs. Job training programs directed specifically toward the local job market have been suggested as more appropriate approaches to unemployment. Another societal intervention could be to provide a guaranteed annual income to all citizens. Such an approach is exemplified in part by social insurance programs such as Social Security and unemployment insurance that are not restricted to the poor but available to all eligible participants. Other social programs that may help to prevent homelessness include legal assistance to prevent evictions as well as increased housing subsidies (Caton et al., 2000). Changes in housing codes and tax laws to prevent loss of welfare benefits or allowing tax credits in shared housing situations may also be helpful. There is also a need for "discharge planning" for housing assistance for people displaced by building condemnation or renovation or release from prisons and other institutions.

Community health nursing involvement in such activities occurs primarily through advocacy and political action. As advocates, community health nurses can make policy makers aware of the needs of the homeless and can contribute to efforts to plan programs that prevent homelessness. Nurses can also engage in political activities such as those described in Chapter 7∞ to influence policies that help to eliminate these conditions. Comprehensive legislation was introduced before the U.S. Congress in November 2005 as part of the Bringing America Home Act (H.R. 4347). At that time, the bill was assigned to the House Ways and Means Committee. In March 2006, it was referred to the Subcommittee on Health, where it remains at this writing (Library of Congress, 2006). This legislation is a broad-based initiative acknowledging housing as a basic right for all and making provisions for a living wage, universal health care, dramatic services expansion for homeless individuals, and protection for temporary workers similar to that enjoyed by full-time employees. The Act also addresses civil rights protection for the homeless and the construction of new housing or rehabilitation of existing low-income housing (Bringing America Home, 2005a; National Coalition for the Homeless, 2005b). Community health nurses can be actively involved in promoting passage of this and similar legislation.

Community health nurses can also work to promote adoption of sound housing policies. Criteria for such policies include the creation of a social contract for decent housing funded at the federal level, redistribution of federally funded housing benefits (e.g., giving priority to localities with the greatest need), federal funding at levels needed to assure housing access, and policies that are sensitive to local housing market conditions (e.g., increasing subsidies in high-cost communities or building more housing in areas where housing is scarce) (Freeman, 2002).

Primary prevention may also be undertaken with respect to specific health problems experienced by homeless persons. Here, community health nurses may work with individuals, families, or groups of people. For example, community health nurses working with homeless substance abusers might advocate a program providing clean syringes to injection drug users. Failing that, the nurse might provide a simple bleach solution for injection equipment to minimize the risk of bloodborne diseases such as hepatitis and AIDS. Similarly, nurses may provide assistance to families with budgeting and meal planning to provide nutritious meals on limited incomes.

Community-based avenues for preventing homelessness among the mentally ill include providing access to services within the community that enable these persons to care for themselves adequately without institutionalization. Efforts may also be needed to ensure hospitalization for those persons who cannot be adequately maintained in the community. Treatment for substance abuse and secure places for convalescence after hospital discharge might also serve to prevent homelessness in this subgroup.

Also at the group level, nurses may engage in primary prevention for specific problems by encouraging community groups to provide shelters for homeless individuals. Nurses may also provide basic health care for the homeless, focusing particularly on primary preventive measures such as influenza vaccine and routine immunizations for children. For example, immunization services may be provided in nontraditional settings such as soup kitchens, shelters, and so on (Postema & Breiman, 2000). Adequate ventilation, reduced crowding, and use of ultraviolet lights in shelters may also help to prevent the spread of communicable disease.

Another area for primary prevention of the health consequences of homelessness is adequate nutrition. Community health nurses can advocate for food programs for the needy, including the homeless. They can also serve as consultants to existing food programs to ensure that meals are nutritionally adequate to meet the needs of the population served. Community health nursing activities in this area may also include attempts to arrange diets for homeless clients with special needs (e.g., assisting a diabetic client to select foods from those prepared in a shelter that approximate a diabetic diet as closely as possible).

Community health nurses can also work with other concerned citizens to initiate programs to provide adequate clothing and shoes for homeless clients. Efforts may also be needed to arrange for the homeless to bathe and wash their clothing. In some cities, day shelters that do not provide sleeping accommodations often provide homeless individuals an opportunity to shower and wash their clothing. These shelters may also provide a clean change of clothing on a periodic basis.

Another aggregate approach to preventing specific health problems among the homeless is providing universal access to health care through national health insurance or similar programs at the state level. Nurses can promote such programs through political activity and advocacy and may also be involved in implementing them by providing direct services to the homeless.

Secondary Prevention

Secondary prevention is designed to alleviate existing homelessness and its health effects. Community health nurses working with homeless individuals must first address their priority concerns for shelter and basic necessities before other health needs can be addressed (Drennan & Joseph, 2005). At the individual level, secondary interventions may include referral for financial assistance via "means-tested income transfers." **Means-tested income transfers** involve the distribution of cash or noncash assistance to individuals and families on the basis of income. As noted earlier, such programs frequently serve only the poorest of the poor and may necessitate loss of all resources before eligibility can be confirmed. Community health nurses may need to function as advocates to assist clients through the bureaucratic process frequently involved. This is particularly true for elderly clients and those with mental health problems. At the community level, nurses can advocate a review of eligibility criteria for means-tested income transfer programs so that a greater proportion of the homeless population is served.

Shelter is an immediate need for homeless individuals. The community health nurse can assist the homeless client to locate temporary shelter. This may be accomplished by means of referrals to existing shelters. If the nurse is not aware of homeless shelters provided in the community, he or she can contact a local YMCA or YWCA, a Salvation Army service center, or local churches for information on shelter availability. When organized shelter facilities are not available, the nurse may try contacting local houses of worship to see if members of religious congregations can provide shelter for a homeless person on a short-term basis. In making a referral for emergency shelter, the community health nurse would consider the needs of the particular client. Ideally, for example, the elderly and women and children would be referred to shelters where they are protected from victimization. Similarly, homeless persons with chronic health problems should be referred to shelters where health services are available and their conditions can be monitored on an ongoing basis.

At the aggregate level, community health nurses can work with government officials and other concerned citizens to develop shelter programs for homeless individuals or families. Avenues that might be pursued include school gymnasiums, churches, and public buildings. Many cities have used these and other buildings as temporary nighttime shelters for the homeless during cold weather. Plans might also be developed for more adequate shelters that provide other services as well as a place to sleep. In designing a shelter program, the community health nurse and other concerned individuals would employ the principles of program planning presented in Chapter 15∞.

For homeless persons with significant mental health problems, it may be necessary to create specialized shelters called **safe havens**, which are secure, stable places of residence that place few demands on those receiving help. Many mentally ill homeless individuals are not able to deal with the behavioral restrictions and other policies imposed by many typical homeless shelters. They need a place with limited restrictions that offers the same bed each night, a place to stay during the day, and a place to store their belongings. Because of the special needs of this segment of the homeless population, safe havens do not limit the length of stay for those served. Safe havens then become a stage in clients' progressive movement toward permanent housing in which they can learn to trust and relearn skills needed to maintain a permanent residence while unlearning the distrust required for survival on the streets.

Homeless persons with mental illness also require services tailored to meet their needs. Several authors note that the constant search for shelter, food, and other necessities interferes with treatment for mental illness and substance abuse problems. It is therefore helpful to combine treatment services with shelter and other services needed by the mentally ill and substance-abusing segments of the homeless population (Milby et al., 2005). Although this population has been characterized as generally noncompliant with treatment recommendations, pilot projects that involve outreach, available—but not mandatory—group therapy, and case management services have been shown to be effective in ensuring housing stability in this population (Shern et al., 2000). The provision of abstinence-only shelter for substance abusers is somewhat controversial. On one hand, abstinence-contingent shelter has been found to be useful in promoting treatment (Milby et al., 2005). On the other hand, the National Coalition for the Homeless (2005a) has noted that complete abstinence may not be a realistic goal for this population and that programs are needed that recognize and address the probability of relapse. Provision of housing assistance seems to be the key factor in helping this and other segments of the homeless population to remain housed. One study in New York, for example, demonstrated that 80% of those who received subsidized housing remained housed irrespective of the presence of mental and social disorders. Conversely, only 18% of those who did not receive housing subsidies were able to maintain a stable residence (National Coalition for the Homeless, 2005k).

Shelters are an emergency resource, not a solution to the problem of homelessness. Community health nurses should help homeless clients find ways to meet long-term shelter needs. For individual clients, this may mean referrals for employment assistance or other services to eliminate factors that resulted in homelessness. At the community level, nurses can participate in planning long-term solutions to the problems of homelessness. Unfortunately, such planning has not often been the focus of community attempts to deal with the problem. Community health nurses can advocate and participate in planning efforts to provide low-cost housing, employment assistance, job training, and other services needed to resolve community problems of homelessness. Initiating these planning activities may require political activity on the part of the community health nurse.

Planning for long-term resolution of the problem of homelessness for runaways involves a different set of strategies. The community health nurse can explore with the youngster his or her reasons for running away from home. Nursing interventions are then directed toward modifying factors that led the child to run away. For example, if the child was abused, the nurse can institute measures to prevent further abuse if the youngster returns to the home, or foster home placement can be arranged. If problems stem from poor family communication, the nurse can make a referral for family counseling or other therapeutic services. The nurse can also serve as a liaison between the child and his or her family, negotiating for changes that make the child's return possible.

Particular care should be taken to involve the child in planning interventions to resolve his or her situation. A child returned to his or her family unwillingly will probably run away again. In addition, such actions on the part of the community health nurse may also destroy any faith the child may have had in health care providers as a source of assistance.

At the aggregate level, community health nurses should alert community policy makers to the need for coordinated services for the homeless offered in a single location to meet the health and social needs of homeless clients (Rosenbaum & Zuvekas, 2000). They should also make sure that planning groups in which they participate plan services to address the needs of the homeless for housing, food, clothing, employment, childcare services for working parents, and adequate preventive and therapeutic health care services. Planning should also include avenues for outreach and follow-up services, particularly for the homeless who may be lost to service. Such comprehensive programs require changes in health care and social systems that may necessitate legislation and public policy formation that can be guided by nursing input.

Community health nurses can also provide curative services for a variety of health problems experienced by the homeless. For example, they may make referrals for food supplement programs or provide treatment for skin conditions or parasitic infestations. They will also be actively involved in educating clients for self-care. Homeless clients may have difficulty with simple aspects of treatment regimens. For example, if the homeless client does not have access to a clock or watch, it may be difficult to take medications as directed. Nurses can suggest the use of medications that can be taken in conjunction with set activities, such as on arising or at bedtime.

The special needs of homeless children and older persons require particular attention. One suggestion is age-segregated shelters or services specifically designed for older persons and families with children to prevent their victimization by other subgroups within the homeless population. Special attention also needs to be given to meeting the nutritional needs of these vulnerable groups as well as those of pregnant women.

Tertiary Prevention

Tertiary prevention may be aimed at preventing a recurrence of poverty and homelessness for individuals, families, or groups of people affected. Conversely, the emphasis may be placed on preventing the recurrence of health and social problems that result from conditions of poverty and homelessness.

Community health nursing involvement in tertiary prevention may entail political activity to ensure the provision of services to relieve poverty and homelessness on a long-term basis. This means involvement by nurses in efforts to raise minimum wages or to design programs to educate the homeless for employment in today's society. Advocacy and political activity may also be needed to ensure the adequacy of community services for the mentally ill to allow them to care for themselves or to support their families as caregivers.

At the individual or family level, community health nurses may be involved in referral for employment assistance or for educational programs that allow homeless clients to eliminate the underlying factors involved in their homelessness. Moreover, nurses might assist clients to budget their incomes more effectively or engage in cooperative buying efforts to limit family expenses. Community health nurses may also be actively involved in monitoring the status of mentally ill clients in the home and in assisting families of these clients to obtain respite care and other supportive services needed to prevent the mentally ill client from returning to a state of homelessness. In such cases, nurses also monitor medication use and encourage clients to receive counseling and other rehabilitative services.

Another avenue for tertiary prevention that may be employed at either the individual or group level is advocacy to prevent the criminalization of normal activities of life for homeless people. The National Coalition for the Homeless (2005q) has developed several recommendations that community health nurses and other advocates of homeless populations can implement. These include:

- Monitoring and documenting local arrests, fines, and harassment of homeless persons
- Empowering and organizing the homeless to advocate for themselves
- Providing legal advocacy for homeless individuals and advocating legislation to prevent criminalization
- Controlling and monitoring the activities of private security guards
- Mustering public and professional support for the Bringing America Home Act

Evaluating Care for Poor and Homeless Populations

Evaluating the effects of nursing interventions with poor and homeless clients can take place at two levels: the individual level and the population level. At the individual level, evaluation of the effectiveness of interventions reflects the client care objectives developed by the nurse and client in planning care. For example, if an objective for a homeless family was to provide them with an income sufficient to meet survival needs, the nurse and family would determine whether this objective has been achieved. Does the family now have sufficient income to provide adequate housing, appropriate nutrition, and other needs? If the objective was to find employment for the mother or father, has this been accomplished?

Evaluation of aggregate-level interventions must also be undertaken. For example, nurses and other concerned individuals will want to determine whether shelter programs are sufficient to meet the needs of the homeless population. Evaluation of tertiary prevention programs focuses on the extent to which interventions prevent people from returning to poverty and again becoming homeless. Are job training programs effective in increasing the income of participants above the poverty level? Criticism of current welfare programs seems to indicate that such programs do not effectively relieve the problems of the poor and homeless. If current programs are not effectively alleviating the problem, other solutions must be sought; community health nurses must be actively involved in developing those solutions.

The Working Group on Homeless Health Outcomes (1996) of the Bureau of Primary Health Care suggested that evaluation of programs for the homeless address both systems-level and client-level outcomes. Systems-level outcomes to be considered include ease of access to programs; the comprehensiveness of services offered; continuity of care, including appropriate referrals, follow-up, and case management; the degree to which an integrated set of services is provided; cost-effectiveness; focus on prevention; and client involvement in the design and implementation of services. Client-level outcomes include client involvement in and commitment to treatment, improved health status, improved functional status, effective disease self-management, improved quality of life, client choice of providers, and client satisfaction.

An additional focus for evaluation is the achievement of those national health objectives that relate to low-income individuals and families. The current status of some of these objectives is presented on page 570. Targets for achievement of other national objectives among the poor and near poor have also been developed, and the degree of success in achieving these targets can be assessed by visiting the *Healthy People 2010*◆ data Web site at http://wonder.cdc.gov/data2010. As we can see from the data, none of the objectives have reached the targets and little progress has been made with respect to most of them. Two of the objectives are actually moving away from the target, indicating that considerable work yet remains to protect the health of the poor, and particularly the homeless, population.

Poverty and homelessness are growing problems in the United States and throughout the world, and community health nurses may encounter poor and homeless individuals and families in a variety of settings. Community health nurses can provide direct health care services to these clients. They may also be actively involved in identifying and planning to deal with factors that contribute to poverty and homelessness.

HEALTHY PEOPLE 2010

Goals for Population Health◆

OBJECTIVE	BASELINE	MOST RECENT DATA	TARGET
■ 1-1. Increase the proportion of poor people with health insurance	65%	69%	100%
■ 1-4. Increase the proportion of poor people with a regular source of health care	79%	80%	96%
■ 1-6. Reduce the proportion of poor families with difficulty or delay in getting care	17%	NDA	7%
■ 8-22. Increase the proportion of poor families living in pre-1950s housing that has been tested for the presence of lead-based paint	18%	22%	50%
■ 8-23. Reduce the proportion of occupied housing units that are substandard	6.2%	NDA	3%
■ 11-1. Increase the proportion of poor households that have access to the Internet at home	NDA	NDA	80%
■ 14-24. Increase receipt of all immunizations among poor children	70%	68%	80%#
■ 19-4. Reduce growth retardation in low-income children	8%	8%	5%
■ 19-18. Increase food security and reduce hunger	69%	NDA	94%
■ 28-4. Reduce blindness and visual impairment in poor children and adolescents	34%	35%	20%#

NDA—No data available

Objective moving away from target

Data from: Centers for Disease Control and Prevention (2005). Healthy people data. Retrieved September 5, 2005, from http://wonder.cdc.gov/data2010

Case Study

A Homeless Family

Crystal is a 16-year-old girl with a 3-month-old baby boy. She has been referred for community health nursing services by her teacher at a special program for adolescents with children. In this program, the girls attend school while childcare services are provided for the children. During the day, the girls participate in the care of their infants and learn about childcare as well as the usual high school subject material. Crystal has been referred because she has not been coming to school and her teacher is concerned. The school does not have a home address or phone number for Crystal, but the teacher gives you the phone number of Crystal's grandmother. After several attempts, you finally contact the grandmother, who agrees to give Crystal a message to get in touch with you. The grandmother says that Crystal does not live with her and that she sees her only occasionally.

The following week you receive a call from Crystal. She is reluctant to give you an address but agrees to come to the health department with the baby. When she arrives, she tells you that she has not been going to school because the baby was ill and cannot return to the childcare center without a doctor's note that the baby is well. Crystal says she cannot afford to see a doctor. She has no health insurance and no money for health care. She began the application process for Medicaid but never followed through because it was "too much hassle." She lives with her mother and stepfather in a camper shell at a construction site where her stepfather is temporarily employed. She refuses to give you the location of this construction site, saying that they will probably move to a new site soon. Crystal says her parents provide her with food and formula for the baby, who appears clean and well nourished. The baby has not begun his immunizations, again because of lack of funds for health services.

Crystal says she is in good health but has not had a postpartum checkup. Although not currently sexually active, she has a steady boyfriend and is contemplating sexual intimacy with him. She asks about various types of contraceptives.

The father of her baby is no longer in the area and is not aware that Crystal had a baby. Crystal's own father is also removed from the picture and Crystal does not know where he is. When asked about her grandmother, Crystal says that they do not get along well and that her grandmother hardly speaks to her since she got pregnant.

Crystal is anxious to complete high school and enroll in a program to become a beautician. She tried recently to get a part-time job in a fast-food restaurant, but was told they wanted someone with experience. She socializes somewhat with the girls at school and goes with several of them to take their babies to the park and similar outings.

1. What health problems are evident in this situation? What are the biophysical, psychological, physical environmental, sociocultural, behavioral, and health system factors influencing these problems?

2. What primary prevention measures would you undertake with Crystal and her son?

3. What secondary prevention measures would be warranted to deal with existing health problems? Describe specific actions you would take to resolve these problems.

4. What could be done in terms of tertiary prevention to prevent further consequences or recurrence of health problems in this situation?

5. How would you evaluate the effectiveness of your interventions with Crystal? Describe the specific evaluative criteria you would use and how you would obtain the evaluative data needed.

Test Your Understanding

1. What are some of the biophysical, psychological, physical environmental, sociocultural, behavioral, and health system considerations that contribute to poverty and homelessness or affect the health of poor or homeless people? (pp. 551–562)

2. Describe at least three approaches to primary prevention of homelessness. How might community health nurses be involved in each approach? (pp. 565–567)

3. What are the major areas of emphasis in primary prevention of health problems among homeless clients? (pp. 565–567)

4. What are three areas in which secondary preventive activities may be appropriate in the care of poor and homeless

clients? What kinds of secondary preventive measures might a community health nurse employ in these areas? (pp. 567–568)

5. Identify at least two strategies for tertiary prevention of homelessness at the aggregate level. How might community health nurses be involved in implementing these strategies? (pp. 568–569)

6. What is the primary focus in evaluating care for homeless clients? Is this focus the same for evaluating care for individuals and families and care for groups of homeless people? (p. 569)

EXPLORE MediaLink

http://www.prenhall.com/clark
Resources for this chapter can be found on the Companion Website

Audio Glossary
Appendix I: Adult Health Assessment and Intervention Guide
Exam Review Questions

Case Study: Promoting the Health of the Homeless
MediaLink Application: Lenny Kravitz on Poverty (video)

Media Links
Challenge Your Knowledge
Update *Healthy People 2010*
Advocacy Interviews

References

Anderson, D. G., & Rayens, M. K. (2004). Factors influencing homelessness in women. *Public Health Nursing, 21,* 12–23.

Archambault, D. (2002). The health needs of homeless men. *Community Health Forum, 3*(5), 37–39.

Bhattacharya, J., DeLeire, T., Haider, S., & Currie, J. (2003). Heat or eat? Cold-weather shocks and nutrition in poor American families. *American Journal of Public Health, 93,* 1149–1154.

Bohrer, G. J., & Faulkner, P. (2004, October 4). Beyond standardized care for the homeless mentally ill. *NurseWeek,* pp. 31–33.

Bolland, J. M., & McCallum, D. M. (2002). Touched by homelessness: An examination of hospitality for the down and out. *American Journal of Public Health, 92,* 116–118.

Bringing America Home. (2005a). *Bringing America home: The campaign.* Retrieved November 29, 2005, from http://www.bringingamericahome.org

Bringing America Home. (2005b). *People need affordable housing.* Retrieved November 29, 2005, from http://www.bringingamericahome.org

Bringing America Home. (2005c). *People need education.* Retrieved November 29, 2005, from http://www.bringingamericahome.org

Bringing America Home. (2005d). *People need health care.* Retrieved November 29, 2005, from http://www.bringingamericahome.org

Bringing America Home. (2005e). *People need livable incomes.* Retrieved November 29, 2005, from http://www.bringingamericahome.org

Bringing America Home. (2005f). *People need their civil rights protected.* Retrieved November 29, 2005, from http://www.bringingamericahome.org

Bures, R. M. (2003). Childhood residential stability and health at midlife. *American Journal of Public Health, 93,* 1144–1148.

Caton, C. L. M., Dominguez, B., Schanzer, B., Hasin, D. S., Shrout, P. E., Felix, A., et al. (2005). Risk factors for long-term homelessness: Findings from a longitudinal study of first-time homeless single adults. *American Journal of Public Health, 95,* 1753–1759.

Caton, C. L. M., Hasin, D., Shrout, P. E., Opler, L. A., Hirschfield, S., Dominguez, B., et al. (2000). Risk factors for homelessness among indigent urban adults with no history of psychotic illness: A case-control study. *American Journal of Public Health, 90,* 258–263.

Center for Medicaid and State Operations. (2005). Medicaid at a glance, 2005. Retrieved December 21, 2005, from http://www.cms.hhs.gov/Medicaideligibility/downloads/MedGlance05.pdf

Centers for Disease Control and Prevention. (2005). *Healthy people data.* Retrieved September 5, 2005, from http://wonder.cdc.gov/data2010

Clement, M. S. (2003). *Children at health risk.* Malden, MA: Blackwell.

Cooke, C. L. (2004). Joblessness and homelessness as precursors of health problems in formerly incarcerated African American men. *Journal of Nursing Scholarship, 36,* 155–160.

Division of Applied Public Health Training, Epidemiology Program Office. (2003). Tuberculosis outbreak in a homeless population—Portland, Maine, 2002–2003. *Morbidity and Mortality Weekly Report, 52,* 1184–1185.

Drennan, V. M., & Joseph, J. (2005). Health visiting and refugee families: Issues in professional practice. *Journal of Advanced Nursing, 49,* 155–163.

Ensign, J. (2001). The health of shelter-based foster youth. *Public Health Nursing, 18,* 19–23.

Freeman, L. (2002). America's affordable housing crisis: A contract unfulfilled. *American Journal of Public Health, 92,* 709–712.

Hirsh, E. D., Jr., Kett, J. F., & Trefil, J. (Eds.), (2002). Structural unemployment. In *The new dictionary of cultural literacy* (3rd ed.). Retrieved March 19, 2006, from http://www.bartleby.com/59/18/structuralun.html

Kaplan, G. A., Siefert, K., Ranjit, N., Raghunathan, T. E., Young, E. A., Tran, D., et al. (2005). The health of poor women under welfare reform. *American Journal of Public Health, 95,* 1252–1258.

Kneipp, S. M., Castleman, J. B., & Gailor, N. (2004). Informal caregiving burden: An overlooked aspect of the lives and health of women transitioning from welfare to employment? *Public Health Nursing, 21*, 24–31.

Kogut, B. H. (2004). Why adult literacy matters. *Phi Kappa Phi Forum, 84*(2), 26–28.

Krieger, J., & Higgins, D. L. (2002). Housing and health: Time again for public health action. *American Journal of Public Health, 92*, 758–768.

Kushel, M. B., Hahn, J. A., Evans, J. L., Bangsberg, D. R., & Moss, A. R. (2005). Revolving doors: Imprisonment among the homeless and marginally housed population. *American Journal of Public Health, 95*, 1747–1752.

Kushel, M. B., Perry, S., Bangsberg, D., Clark, R., & Moss, A. R. (2002). Emergency department use among the homeless and marginally housed: Results from a community-based study. *American Journal of Public Health, 92*, 778–784.

Lawlor, D. A., Smith, G. D., & Ebrahim, S. (2004). Socioeconomic position and hormone replacement therapy use: Explaining the discrepancy in evidence from observational and randomized controlled studies. *American Journal of Public Health, 94*, 2149–2154.

Library of Congress. *H.R. 4347*. Retrieved March 19, 2006, from http://thomas.loc.gov/cgi-bin/bdquery/z?d109:h4347

McLeer, S. V. (2004). Mental health services. In H. S. Sultz & K. M. Young (Eds.), *Health care USA: Understanding its organization and delivery* (4th ed., pp. 335–366). Sudbury, MA: Jones and Bartlett.

Milby, J. B., Schumacher, J. E., Wallace, D., Freedman, M. D., & Vuchinich, R. E. (2005). To house or not to house: The effects of providing housing to homeless substance abusers in treatment. *American Journal of Public Health, 95*, 1259–1265.

Mitchell, D. (2003). *The right to the city: Social justice and the fight for public space*. New York: Guilford Press.

National Center for Health Statistics. (2003). *Health United States, 2003: Chartbook on trends in the health of Americans*. Washington, DC: Author.

National Center for Health Statistics. (2005). Percentage of persons aged <65 years without health insurance, by age group and number of uninsured months—United States, 2003. *Morbidity and Mortality Weekly Report, 54*, 385.

National Coalition for Homeless Veterans. (n.d.). *Facts and media: Background and statistics*. Retrieved March 19, 2006, from http://www.nchv.org/background.cfm

National Coalition for the Homeless. (2005a). *Addiction disorders and homelessness*. Retrieved November 29, 2005, from http://www.nationalhomeless.org/publications/facts

National Coalition for the Homeless. (2005b). *Bill to end homelessness in America introduced in Congress*. Retrieved November 29, 2005, from http://www.nationalhomeless.org/publications/facts

National Coalition for the Homeless. (2005c). *Domestic violence and homelessness*. Retrieved November 29, 2005, from http://www.nationalhomeless.org/publications/facts

National Coalition for the Homeless. (2005d). *Education of homelessness children and youth*. Retrieved November 29, 2005, from http://www.nationalhomeless.org/publications/facts

National Coalition for the Homeless. (2005e). *Employment and homelessness*. Retrieved November 29, 2005, from http://www.nationalhomeless.org/publications/facts

National Coalition for the Homeless. (2005f). *Federal housing assistance programs*. Retrieved November 29, 2005, from http://www.nationalhomeless.org/publications/facts

National Coalition for the Homeless. (2005g). *Hate, violence, and death on Main Street, USA, June 2005*. Retrieved November 29, 2005, from http://www.nationalhomeless.org/publications/facts

National Coalition for the Homeless. (2005h). *Health care and homelessness*. Retrieved November 29, 2005, from http://www.nationalhomeless.org/publications/facts

National Coalition for the Homeless. (2005i). *Health care for the homelessness program*. Retrieved November 29, 2005, from http://www.nationalhomeless.org/publications/facts

National Coalition for the Homeless. (2005j). *HIV/AIDS and homelessness*. Retrieved November 29, 2005, from http://www.nationalhomeless.org/publications/facts

National Coalition for the Homeless. (2005k). *Homeless families with children*. Retrieved November 29, 2005, from http://www.nationalhomeless.org/publications/facts

National Coalition for the Homeless. (2005l). *Homeless veterans*. Retrieved November 29, 2005, from http://www.nationalhomeless.org/publications/facts

National Coalition for the Homeless. (2005m). *Homelessness among elderly persons*. Retrieved November 29, 2005, from http://www.nationalhomeless.org/publications/facts

National Coalition for the Homeless. (2005n). *Housing justice*. Retrieved November 29, 2005, from http://www.nationalhomeless.org/publications/facts

National Coalition for the Homeless. (2005o). *How many people experience homelessness?* Retrieved November 29, 2005, from http://www.nationalhomeless.org/publications/facts

National Coalition for the Homeless. (2005p). *Homeless youth*. Retrieved November 29, 2005, from http://www.nationalhomeless.org/publications/facts

National Coalition for the Homeless. (2005q). *Illegal to be homeless, 2004 report*. Retrieved November 29, 2005, from http://www.nationalhomeless.org/publications/facts

National Coalition for the Homeless. (2005r). *Mental illness and homelessness*. Retrieved November 29, 2005, from http://www.nationalhomeless.org/publications/facts

National Coalition for the Homeless. (2005s). *Rural homelessness*. Retrieved November 29, 2005, from http://www.nationalhomeless.org/publications/facts

National Coalition for the Homeless. (2005t). *Who is homeless?* Retrieved November 29, 2005, from http://www.nationalhomeless.org/publications/facts

National Women's Law Center. (2004). *Making the grade on women's health*. Retrieved August 13, 2005, from http://www.nwlc.org/pdf/HR04findings_and_titlepage.pdf

Newman, P. A., Rhodes, F., & Weiss, R. (2004). Correlates of sex trading among drug-using men who have sex with men. *American Journal of Public Health, 94*, 1998–2003.

Nielsen, M. J., Juon, H.-S., & Ensminger, M. (2004). Preventing long-term welfare receipt: The theoretical relationship between health and poverty over the early life course. *Social Science & Medicine, 58*, 2285–2301.

North, C. S., Eyrich, K. M., Pollio, D. E., & Spitznagel, E. L. (2004). Are rates of psychiatric disorders in the homeless population changing? *American Journal of Public Health, 94*, 103–108.

Northridge, M. E., Stover, G. N., Rosenthal, J. E., & Sherard, D. (2003). Environmental equity and health: Understanding complexity and moving forward. *American Journal of Public Health, 93*, 209–214.

Nyamathi, A., Sands, H., Pattatucci-Aragon, A., Berg, J., Leake, B., Hahn, J. E., et al. (2004). Perception of health status by homeless US veterans. *Family and Community Health, 27*(1), 65–74.

Population Information Program, Center for Communication Programs. (2003). *Population reports: Meeting the urban challenge*. Retrieved July 25, 2003, from http://www.jhucpp.org

Postema, A. S., & Breiman, R. F. (2000). Adult immunization programs in nontraditional settings: Quality standards and guidance for program evaluation. *Morbidity and Mortality Weekly Report, 49*(RR-1), 1–13.

Rew, L., Fouladi, R. T., & Yockey, R. D. (2002). Sexual health practices of homeless youth. *Journal of Nursing Scholarship, 34*, 139–145.

Robertson, M. J., Clark, R. A., Charlebois, E. D., Tulsky, J., Long, H. L., Bangsberg, D. R., et al. (2004). HIV seroprevalence among homeless and marginally housed adults in San Francisco. *American Journal of Public Health, 94*, 1207–1217.

Rosenbaum, S., & Zuvekas, A. (2000). Health care use by homeless persons: Implications for public policy. *Health Services Research, 34*, 1303–1304.

Sherman, P., & Redlener, I. (2003). Homeless women and their children in the 21st century. In H. M. Wallace, G. Green, & K. J. Jaros (Eds.), *Health and welfare for families in the 21st century* (2nd ed., pp. 469–480). Sudbury, MA: Jones and Bartlett.

Shern, D. L., Tsemberis, S., Anthony, W., Lovell, A. M., Richmond, L., Felton, C., et al. (2000). Serving street-dwelling individuals with psychiatric disabilities: Outcomes of a psychiatric rehabilitation clinical trial. *American Journal of Public Health, 90*, 1873–1878.

Swigart, V., & Kolb, R. (2004). Homeless persons' decisions to accept or reject public health disease-detection services. *Public Health Nursing, 21*, 162–170.

Thiele, B. (2002). The human right to adequate housing: A tool for promoting and protecting individual and community health. *American Journal of Public Health, 92*, 712–715.

Unemployment types. (2006). *Wikipedia*. Retrieved March 19, 2006, from http://

en.wikipedia.org/wiki/Unemployment_types

U.S. Census Bureau. (2005). *Statistical abstract of the United States: 2004–2005*. Retrieved August 16, 2005, from http://www.census.gov/prod/2004pubs/04statab

Webb, D. A., Culhane, J., Metraux, S., Robbins, J. M., & Culhane, D. (2003). Prevalence of episodic homelessness among adult child-bearing women in Philadelphia, PA. *American Journal of Public Health, 93*, 1895–1896.

Wehler, C., Weinreb, L. F., Huntington, N., Scott, R., Hosmer, D., Fletcher, K., et al. (2004). Risk and protective factors for adult and child hunger among low-income housed and homeless female-headed households. *American Journal of Public Health, 94*, 109–115.

Wilde, M. H., Albanese, E. P., Rennells, R., & Bullock, Q. (2004). Development of a student nurses' clinic for homeless men. *Public Health Nursing, 21*, 354–360.

Wilson, M. (2004). Health-promoting behaviors of sheltered homeless women. *Family and Community Health, 28*(1), 51–63.

Wilton, R. (2004). Putting policy into practice? Poverty and people with serious mental illness. *Social Science & Medicine, 58*, 25–39.

Wise, P. (2004). The transformation of child health in the United States; Social disparities in child health persist despite dramatic improvements in child health overall. *Health Affairs, 23*, 9–25.

Working Group on Homeless Health Outcomes, Bureau of Primary Health Care. (1996). *Meeting proceedings*. Rockville, MD: Health Resources and Services Administration.

World Health Organization. (2003). *Right to water*. Geneva, Switzerland: Author.

World Health Organization. (2005). *World health statistics 2005*. Retrieved September 21, 2005, from http://www.who.int/health-info/statistics/whostat2005en1.pdf

Wright, N. M. J., & Tompkins, C. N. E. (2005). *How can health care systems effectively deal with the major health care needs of homeless people?* Retrieved December 12, 2005, from http://www.euro.who.int/HEN/Syntheses/homeless/ 20050124_11

Zahran, H. S., Kobau, R., Moriarty, D. G., Zack, M. M., Holt, J., & Donehoo, R. (2005). Health-related quality of life surveillance—United States 1993–2002. *Morbidity and Mortality Weekly Report, 54*(SS-4), 1–35.

IV Unit

Care of Populations in Specialized Settings

21 CHAPTER

Care of Clients in the Home Setting

CHAPTER OBJECTIVES

After reading this chapter, you should be able to:

1. Describe the advantages of a home visit as a means of providing nursing care.
2. Analyze challenges encountered by community health nurses making home visits.
3. Identify the major purposes of home visiting programs.
4. Describe major considerations in planning a home visit.
5. Identify tasks involved in implementing a home visit.
6. Analyze the effects of potential distractions during a home visit.
7. Discuss the need for both long-term and short-term evaluative criteria for the effectiveness of a home visit.
8. Describe the relationship between home health nursing and community health nursing.
9. Discuss the need for collaboration in home health and hospice nursing.
10. Discuss funding sources for home health and hospice care.
11. Apply evaluative criteria for home health and hospice care services.

KEY TERMS

certificate of need **597**
certification **596**
Health Plan Employer Data and Information Set (HEDIS) **599**
home health care **594**
home health resource group (HHRG) **597**
home visit **577**
hospice care **594**
Outcome and Assessment Information Set (OASIS) **596**
Outcome-Based Quality Improvement (OBQI) **599**
Outcome-Based Quality Monitoring (OBQM) **599**
proprietary agencies **594**

MediaLink
http://www.prenhall.com/clark

Additional interactive resources for this chapter can be found on the Companion Website. Click on Chapter 21 and "Begin" to select the activities for this chapter.

Advocacy in Action

Pain Control

As a home health care nurse, I am on the front lines of the community health care delivery team. I independently assess, monitor patients, and take a holistic approach to determine what my patients need in order to attain, improve, and preserve their health. Not only do I provide bedside nursing care in the home, I also act as my patient's advocate, which is one of the most important roles I have as a nurse—to protect the interests of my patients when they themselves cannot because of illness or insufficient knowledge.

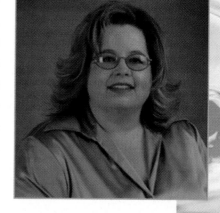

Pain control is a hot topic in nursing care. Home health care nurses deal with pain control issues daily. One 23-year-old client had been diagnosed with juvenile arthritis at age 13. By the ripe old age of 23, he had become so debilitated he required the use of a wheelchair. His vascular system had also been affected, and he had developed ulcerations on his lower extremities. The client subsequently had to be hospitalized due to developing osteomyelitis, which required IV antibiotic therapy through my home care agency. Upon admission, I noted that this client had been taking MS Contin and Oxycontin routinely for pain for several years. On one particular visit, the client indicated that he was almost out of his pain medication and asked if I would call and make an appointment for him at the local pain clinic where he had been treated for years. I called and they explained to me that his surgeon (who had seen him while he was hospitalized) needed to handle his pain medications. I then called the surgeon, who instructed me to call his family physician. I called the family physician, who in turn directed me back to the surgeon who had discharged him from the hospital.

My patient was obviously in pain, had been receiving routine pain meds for years, and I could not get a physician to prescribe pain medication before he began withdrawal symptoms. When I called the surgeon back, emphasizing that my patient needed to be seen within the next two days, I finally convinced him to see the patient. Had I not persisted, how long would it have taken for my patient to get his prescriptions?

Kim Clevenger, MSN, RN, C
Morehead State University

*H*istorical photographs of community health nurses often show them caring for clients in their homes. Indeed, home care was the initial focus of community health nursing. Home visiting by professional nurses in the United States began in 1877 with the work of the women's branch of the New York City Mission in the homes of the poor (Kendra & George, 2001). The home was where most clients were to be found and where community health nurses had to go to reach them. Today, the home is only one setting where community health nurses care for their clients. Despite the broadening of community health nursing over the years to encompass many other places and settings, the home visit remains a strategic tool for health care delivery. A home visit by a nurse is different from a social visit that might be made by friends or relatives. Home visitation has been defined as "a service delivery strategy that provides resources to people in their homes" (Miller, Kobayashi, & Hill, 2003, p. 174). A **home visit**, as conceptualized in community health nursing, is a formal call by a nurse on a client at the client's residence to provide nursing care.

Home visits are widely used by community health nurses as an intervention to achieve a number of purposes. Home visiting programs might be intended to address health promotion and health education needs of families in the general population or they may be targeted to individuals and families with specific needs. Home visiting, however, is not synonymous with home health nursing, which is usually directed to addressing specific physical health needs in a home setting. In this chapter, we will first address the general concept of the home visit as a nursing intervention and then consider the more specialized areas of home health and hospice nursing, both of which employ home visits as an intervention strategy.

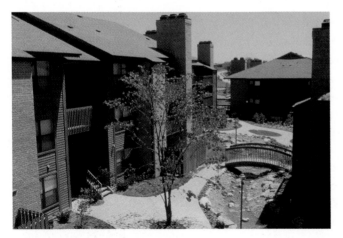

Community health nurses make visits to a variety of homes. (Patrick J. Watson)

PURPOSES OF HOME VISITING PROGRAMS

An array of health-related agencies conducts home visits, either as the major component of service or in addition to other services. Each agency has its own goals for the home visit program, but generally the purposes of visits can be grouped into four categories: case finding and referral; health promotion and illness prevention; care of the sick, which includes health restoration and maintenance; and care of the dying. Any given agency may incorporate several purposes within a home visiting program, but will usually emphasize one purpose over the others.

Case Finding and Referral

Some agencies engage in home visiting primarily to identify clients in need of additional services. These clients are then referred to appropriate sources of services to meet those needs. In this type of program, a minimum number of visits is usually required. In fact, the nurse frequently makes only a single visit to identify and deal with clients' needs. In other cases, the nurse might return to the home to follow up on referrals made. For example, a community with older housing initiated a lead abatement program. During the case finding stage of the program, nurses and outreach workers went from door to door to identify homes that had lead contamination. Identified families were then referred for blood lead levels and treatment if needed as well as to an abatement team to decrease lead in the home.

Health Promotion and Illness Prevention

Health promotion and illness prevention are the primary focus of many visits made by community health nurses, particularly those employed by official public health agencies. For example, in many jurisdictions, community health nurses routinely make home visits to new mothers. Community health nurses working in special projects that focus on prenatal and child health also emphasize health promotion and illness prevention in their visits. For instance, special prenatal health projects frequently employ home visits as well as regular clinic appointments as a means of promoting maternal and child health. Similarly, home visiting programs to enhance child development focus on health promotion and prevention of health problems. An example of a health promotion program was initiated with a large Hmong population. In the program, a community health nurse visited families with children from birth to age 3 and worked with them intensively to assist parents in promoting their children's development.

Care of the Sick

Specific "home health" agencies are primarily geared to meeting the needs of the sick in their homes. Home health care, in this context, refers to the delivery of

MediaLink Visiting Nurse Services, NYC (videos)

services in the home for the purpose of restoring or maintaining the health of clients. The great majority of clients who receive home health services are elderly persons (70.5% of care recipients in 2000) who have a variety of chronic illnesses. Common diagnoses among clients who receive home health services include circulatory problems (24%); musculoskeletal problems (10%, including 3.5% with osteoarthritis); respiratory problems (7%); endocrine, nutritional, metabolic, and immune disorders (9.5%, including 8% for diabetes); fracture (4%); malignant neoplasms (5%); and mental disorders (4%) (National Center for Health Statistics [NCHS], 2004a). The presence of multiple diagnoses and difficulties with functional abilities are other indicators of the need for home health services (Lee & Mills, 2000).

Indicators of potential needs for home health care services are summarized in Table 21-1◆.

Care of the Dying

Specialized home visiting services are provided to people with terminal illness by hospice agencies. In addition to home visits by nurses, hospices also provide a variety of other services, including visits by volunteers, caretaker respite, physical therapy, medications, durable medical equipment, counseling, and other spiritual care for clients and families. At the time of the 2000 National Home Health and Hospice Care Survey, more than 105,500 clients were receiving hospice services in the United States, and many thousands of clients had been discharged from services. Again, the majority of

TABLE 21-1	Clients Who Might Benefit From a Home Visit
Indication	Type of Client
Physical needs and conditions	Pregnant clients
	Ill, disabled, or frail elderly clients living alone or with others whose health is impaired
	Clients with physical or emotional problems that make it difficult to carry out activities of daily living
	Clients discharged from hospitals or nursing homes with continuing health needs
	Clients who need special procedures that family members cannot perform or need help in performing
	Clients who require periodic monitoring of chronic conditions
	Terminally ill clients and their families
	Clients with certain communicable diseases (e.g., HIV/AIDS, hepatitis, tuberculosis) that require care over time
	Clients who need rehabilitation services
	Clients who are recovering from work-related injuries
	Postpartum clients who experienced perinatal difficulties
Emotional needs	Clients with chronic mental health conditions
	Clients who are anxious about their condition or their ability for self-care
	Families undergoing crises
	Clients who have experienced the death of a child
	Clients who are at risk for suicide or who have experienced a recent suicide in the family
Family role changes	Adolescent parents
	First-time parents and their newborns
	Caretakers who need assistance or reassurance
	Caretakers who miss work frequently to provide care to family members
	Families with multiply handicapped children
	Families in which caretakers are experiencing stress
Health education needs	Clients who have significant knowledge deficits regarding health promotion, an existing condition, or its treatment
Psychosocial needs	Clients who live in unsafe physical environments
	Children who are experiencing difficulty in school
	Clients who have no regular source of health care
Other needs	Clients who are noncompliant with health recommendations
	Clients who need periodic review of medications
	Clients who are at risk for abuse or who have experienced abuse
	Children with a history of fetal drug exposure
	Children with attention deficit disorder or developmental delay

GLOBAL PERSPECTIVES

*H*ome health services originated and are organized differently in different countries. In the United States, there is no universal provision for home visits to any segment of the population. Home visitation services are based on need.

Home health care nursing in Japan began with voluntary visits by hospital nurses in the 1970s. In 1983, insurance reimbursement for home care was initiated under the Health and Medical Service Law for the Elderly, but the home was not recognized as an appropriate setting for care until legislative revisions in medical law in 1992. That legislation led to the establishment of a system of visiting nurse service stations (VNSSs), with nurses assuming executive leadership of stations (all prior services in hospitals and clinics had been under the direction of a physician) (Murashima, Nagata, Magilvy, Fukui, & Kayama, 2002). Originally established to provide home services to the elderly, the system was expanded to all age groups in 1994 (Ogata et al., 2004). Today home health care services in Japan are provided by VNSSs, hospitals, public municipalities, or private companies. Home care in Japan focuses on four areas: elder care, high-tech care, care for those with terminal illness (hospice care), and care of clients with mental illness.

In Canada, home care services have increased, but funding has not matched the need for services. Home care systems vary across provinces and may be based on one of four models: (a) all services from public employees, (b) professional services by public employees and personal care and homemaking services from private agencies, (c) case management by public employees and actual services from either public or private agencies, and (d) public payer contracts with both profit and non-profit agencies to provide services (Woodward et al., 2004).

Home visitation for the elderly has been a part of the national health systems in the United Kingdom (UK) since 1990 and in Australia since 1999, and all Danish municipalities must offer two preventive home visits a year to people over 75 years of age (Vass et al., 2004). Home visiting in the UK is believed to have started in 1867, when the Ladies Sanitary Reform Association promoted door-to-door services to the poor to provide education and assistance (Elkan, Robinson, Williams, & Blair, 2001). Early health visiting has been described as "a means of monitoring and encouraging socially acceptable norms for family health" among the laboring poor (Smith, 2004). Home visiting services shifted from a focus on the needs of the poor to a universally provided service in the early 20th century. In the 1990s, government policy emphasized services targeted specifically to persons at risk or in need. Debate continues as to the advisability of continuing universal services as opposed to targeted services (Bryans, 2004; Elkan et al., 2001). Home visiting in the UK is also attempting to make a shift from family-focused care to a more population-focused perspective, with greater attention to physical environmental and social conditions as well as education related to personal health behaviors (Smith, 2004).

In Poland, the Ministry of Health and Social Welfare published *The Outline of Community/Family Nurse Competence* in 1995. This document outlined basic family nursing services related to health promotion and illness prevention and provided for independent nursing services to families. In 1998, most home visiting services were provided by family nurses employed by primary practice physicians. By 2002, most visits were provided by nurses in independent practice who contracted with the National Health Fund to provide services. Studies of the effects of services before and after this change indicated that the number of visits had increased significantly, as had the degree of client satisfaction with care (Marcinowicz & Chlabicz, 2004).

---

these clients (81%) were over 65 years of age, but just under one fifth were younger (NCHS, 2004b).

Nurses employed by home health care agencies may also care for dying clients and their families. Family members, as well as dying clients, need information and support from nurses and others involved in home health and hospice care. Several aspects of the care of dying clients and their families were presented in Chapter 19∞. Both hospice and home health services are discussed in more detail later in this chapter.

THE HOME VISIT PROCESS

Although home visits have some distinct advantages over care provided in other settings, to be effective, home visits must be focused, purposeful events. Like any other nursing intervention, the home visit should be a planned event with specified goals and objectives. The nursing process provides a framework for systematically organizing the home visit to make it an effective nursing intervention.

Initiating the Home Visit

Home visits by community health nurses are initiated for a variety of reasons. Often the nurse receives a request for a visit from another health care provider or agency. Reasons for such requests include health care needs related to specific health problems or needs for health-promotive services. For example, many hospital obstetrics units refer all first-time mothers for home visits by community health nurses to provide assistance in parenting and to promote a successful postpartum course and adjustment to parenthood. Similarly, a physician might request a home visit to educate a hypertensive client about prescribed medications. In many countries outside the United States, home visits are universally available to mothers and children and to the elderly.

Referrals are an important source of information about clients needing home visits. For home visits to be initiated effectively, there must be regular processes for referrals from acute care settings, clinics, and other providers. In addition, good relationships between home visiting agencies and referral sources are critical to identifying those people most in need of visits (Wager, Lee, Bradford, Jones, & Kilpatrick, 2004).

Clients themselves might also initiate home visits. For example, a mother concerned about her child's recurrent nightmares may call and request a home visit by a community health nurse. Friends and family might also initiate a home visit. A neighbor might inform the nurse that he or she thinks the children next door are being abused, or a mother may request a home visit to help her daughter deal with the loss of a child. Finally, the community health nurse may initiate a home visit. The nurse might note that a child seen in the well-child clinic is developmentally delayed and decide to visit the home to see if environmental factors are contributing to the delayed development.

Other important aspects of initiating a home visit are communicating the reason for the home visit, creating appropriate expectations for the visit on the part of both client and nurse, overcoming fear, and building rapport with the client. As noted earlier, many clients are fearful and feel vulnerable about having a stranger in their homes. These feelings of vulnerability can be overcome by recognizing and addressing clients' fears, by building trust, and by promoting mutuality (Jack, DiCenso, & Lohfeld, 2005). Mutuality encompasses mutual understanding between client and nurse, sharing of personal information and experiences, respect, and provision of opportunities for client input in regard to the visit.

Conducting a Preliminary Health Assessment

Before the home visit, the nurse conducts a preliminary assessment to review existing information about the client and his or her situation. Previously acquired client data should be reviewed and factors influencing client health status identified. If the client is already known to the nurse or the agency, a certain amount of data is available in agency records, notes from previous visits, and other material. Such data can be used by the nurse to refresh his or her memory regarding the client's health status.

If the client is new to an agency, available data will probably be limited to that received with the request for services. In such a case, the nurse needs to look for general cues that suggest client strengths and potential problems. For example, if the home visit is requested for follow-up on a newborn and his adolescent mother, the nurse knows that infant feeding, sleep patterns, maternal knowledge of childcare, bonding, involution, maternal coping abilities, and family planning are areas that may need to be addressed with this family. Similarly, if the referral is for an elderly woman with uncontrolled hypertension, the nurse will identify areas related to diet, medication, safety, and exercise for investigation during the visit.

All aspects of the client's life should be reviewed to detect strengths, existing problems, and potential problems that may need to be addressed during the visit. Using the dimensions of health as a framework, the nurse reviews available information on biophysical, psychological, physical environmental, sociocultural, behavioral, and health system factors that influence the client's health status. By assessing client factors in each of these areas, the nurse enters the client's residence

better prepared to deal with the wide variety of client needs likely to be encountered.

Biophysical Considerations

In the biophysical dimension, the nurse would consider the effects of age and client developmental level on health status. For example, if the family includes adolescent children, the nurse might focus on sexuality issues, whereas home safety might be more relevant to a family with small children. The nurse would also obtain information on existing physical health problems and the presence of disability in clients as well as immunization status and other physiologic factors that influence health.

Psychological Considerations

Considerations related to psychological factors include evidence of family stress and coping. Nurses making home visits may often find themselves called upon to provide emotional support to individual clients or families in crisis, particularly until other services (e.g., counseling) can be obtained. The client with a terminal illness and his or her family are particularly in need of emotional support by the nurse.

Physical Environmental Considerations

In the physical environmental dimension, the nurse obtains information about the home environment with particular attention to home safety needs, based on the client's age, health status, and functional ability. Two home safety assessment tools, included in the *Community Assessment Reference Guide* 🔖 designed to accompany this text, may be of help to the nurse in this aspect of the assessment.

Other environmental safety conditions may relate to the client's condition or to therapeutic regimens to be implemented in the home. Continuous chemotherapy infusions, for example, are successfully administered in homes, but they present unique safety hazards. For example, some agents are extremely toxic to skin tissue. Needles and other equipment used to administer these agents also present contamination and injury hazards.

Infection control is another safety issue related to the provision of health care in the physical environment of the home. Infection control in the home has a dual focus: protecting the client and family and protecting the nurse. The nurse should adhere to the agency's standards of practice, incorporate universal precautions for preventing the spread of bloodborne diseases, and educate clients and family members in infection control measures, including universal precautions.

Community health nurses change dressings for infected wounds, change intravenous sites, provide central line care, transfuse clients, and work with clients diagnosed with many communicable diseases. Continuous assessment of the environment for established infection control standards and outcome criteria is a necessary function of the community health nurse in the home setting. In the preliminary assessment, the community health nurse is alert to the potential for problems related to infection control within the client's home environment.

Infection control procedures in the home are similar to those employed in other health care settings, but may require more creativity on the part of the nurse. For example, one community health nurse made an early morning visit to change the indwelling urinary catheter of a client in a remote rural area 60 miles from the health department. Because the nurse knew he would be visiting the client before going to the public health center, he put the necessary supplies in his car the day before. Unfortunately, the temperature dropped during the night, and when the nurse tried to inflate the bulb to keep the new catheter in place, the fluid was frozen in the syringe. The nurse did not have another catheterization set and could not return to the health department to get one, so he used the warmth of his sterile-gloved hand to thaw the syringe while maintaining a sterile field and keeping the catheter in place in the client's urethra.

The primary infection control measure in any setting is adequate handwashing before and after giving any direct care to clients. Hands should be thoroughly washed with soap and running water. Again, this may require some creativity on the part of nurses or family members in homes without running water. For example, the nurse may wet his or her hands, apply soap, and lather thoroughly, then ask a family member to pour clean water over the hands to rinse them. The nurse can also make a habit of carrying paper towels on home visits to avoid using family towels that were used previously. Many nurses now carry waterless hand cleansing agents with them on home visits. The nurse may also identify a need to instruct family members in the importance of handwashing in the care of the client and as a general measure for preventing the spread of disease.

Infection control in the home, as in other settings, involves the use of sterile precautions in any invasive procedures, appropriate disposal of bodily secretions and excretions, and isolation precautions as warranted by the client's condition. Nurses working in the home with clients who have bloodborne diseases such as AIDS and hepatitis should use universal blood and body fluid precautions. These precautions apply to any body fluids, including blood, semen, vaginal secretions, cerebrospinal fluid, synovial fluid, pleural fluid, peritoneal fluid, pericardial fluid, and amniotic fluid, and feces, nasal secretions, sputum, sweat, urine, and vomitus that contains visible blood. Identification of the possible need for universal precautions and other infection control measures during the preliminary assessment allows the community health nurse to plan effectively to promote personal safety and that of the client and family. Universal precautions to be taken by the nurse to prevent the spread of bloodborne disease are summarized above right.

Care should also be taken in the disposal of secretions and excretions of clients with other conditions. For example, sputum from clients with active tuberculosis

| HIGHLIGHTS | Universal Precautions for Preventing the Spread of Bloodborne Diseases |

- Use appropriate barrier precautions (e.g., gloves) to prevent skin and mucous membrane exposure when contact with human blood or other body fluids is anticipated.
- Wash hands and other skin surfaces immediately after contamination with blood or other body fluids.
- Take precautions to prevent injuries stemming from needles and other sharp instruments during or after procedures, when disposing of used equipment or needles, or when cleaning used equipment.
- Do not recap, bend, or break used needles; place them in a punctureproof container for disposal.
- Keep mouthpieces, resuscitation bags, or other ventilation devices at hand when the need for resuscitation is predictable.
- Use gloves in the direct care of clients and in handling client equipment when you have exudative skin lesions or weeping dermatitis.
- Use masks and protective eyewear during procedures that are likely to generate droplets of blood or other body fluids requiring universal precautions.
- Use gowns or aprons during procedures likely to generate splashes of blood or body fluids requiring universal precautions.
- Use gloves for digital examination of mucous membranes and endotracheal suctioning.
- Implement these precautions with all clients, not just those known to be infected with bloodborne diseases.

Data from: Division of Healthcare Quality Promotion (DHQP). (2005). Universal precautions for prevention of transmission of HIV and other bloodborne infections. Retrieved January 9, 2006, from http:www.cdc.gov/ncidod.dhqp/ bp_universal_precautions.html

should be handled with care, and the feces of chronic typhoid carriers should be disposed of in a municipal sewer system.

Sociocultural Considerations

Sociocultural dimension factors to be considered include the client's or family's economic status, interactions with the outside world, and occupational or employment considerations. The nurse would also obtain information on cultural or religious factors that influence the client's health as well as the extent of the client's social support

Think Advocacy

Berg, Hines, and Allen (2002) found that only 4% of homes of clients who used wheelchairs had received all five recommended structural modifications designed to address clients' functional limitations. Lack of modifications led to a higher incidence of falls with injuries. In part, modifications were not made because they were not covered by either private or government insurance programs. The authors suggested that "home environments that facilitate independence and that make it easier to move around should be considered a basic need for disabled persons" (p. 48). How might community health nurses advocate for this basic right? What might nurses and others do to get home modifications covered by health insurance plans?

CULTURAL COMPETENCE

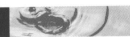

You are visiting the home of an elderly German American woman to check her blood sugar. Her home is quite rundown and in need of repairs. You notice that several of the window screens have holes and there are numerous flies in the home. Your client offers you a piece of coffee cake that a neighbor has brought her. Several of what appear, at first glance, to be raisins in the coffee cake are actually dead flies. Because of your client's diabetes and consequent retinopathy, she cannot see the flies. You know that among many German Americans hospitality is very important and your client will be insulted if you decline the offer. What will you do?

affect the plan of care for a young child. For instance, in some cultural groups even very young children may make independent decisions about taking medications or adhering to other elements of a treatment plan. If this is the case, the nurse will need to work with both parent and child to ensure compliance.

Behavioral Considerations

Behavioral dimension considerations would include information about the client's consumption patterns and nutritional needs based on age or health status. Information regarding substance use or abuse would also be relevant to the planning of effective nursing interventions.

Health System Considerations

The effects of the health system on the client are also an area to be addressed in the preliminary assessment. What is the source of payment for home health services? Does the client have access to other health promotion and health restoration services? Are these services effectively utilized by the client? The focused assessment below provides tips for assessing each of the six dimensions of health in a preliminary assessment in preparation for a home visit.

system. Client–family interactions are another feature of the sociocultural dimension that may influence the client's health. The nurse would also be alert to information about family caretaker responsibilities and how these might affect the health of both the client and the caretaker.

Cultural factors should also be considered. For example, the client's cultural food preferences or modes of preparation should be considered in planning to meet nutritional needs. Similarly, child-rearing practices may

FOCUSED ASSESSMENT

Assessing the Home Visit Situation

Biophysical Considerations

- What are the ages of persons in the home? Do the age and developmental level of persons in the home give rise to specific health needs?
- Do any persons in the home have existing physical health problems?
- Does anyone in the home have difficulty performing activities of daily living?
- Do persons in the home exhibit other physiologic states that necessitate health care (e.g., pregnancy)?

Psychological Considerations

- What is the emotional status of persons living in the home? How effective are the coping strategies used by persons living in the home? Is there a need for respite for family caregivers?
- Is there a history of mental illness in anyone living in the home?
- Do persons in the home interact effectively with one another? What effects do interpersonal interactions have on health? What is the potential for domestic violence in the home?

Physical Environmental Considerations

- Where is the home located? Is the neighborhood safe? Are there environmental conditions in the neighborhood that adversely affect health?
- Are there safety hazards in the home? Does the home environment accommodate the age-related safety needs of persons living there?
- Is the home in good repair? Does it have the usual amenities (e.g., running water, heat, electricity, refrigeration, cooking facilities)?

- Is the home equipped to meet special needs of persons living there (e.g., safe administration of oxygen, mobility aids)?
- Does the home situation pose an infection risk for persons living there?

Sociocultural Considerations

- What are the education and economic levels of persons living in the home? How do they affect health status?
- What is the extent of social support available to those living in the home? Do they make use of available social support?
- Are persons living in the home employed? How does employment affect health status and health care needs?
- Are there religious or cultural practices in the home that influence health?
- Is there sufficient provision for personal privacy in the home?

Behavioral Considerations

- Does anyone living in the home have special dietary needs? Are those needs being met?
- Does anyone living in the home smoke? What are the potential health effects of smoking on persons living in the home?
- Is there evidence of substance abuse in the home?
- Do any of those living in the home use medications on a regular basis? If so, are they used and stored appropriately?

Health System Considerations

- Is health care utilization by persons living in the home appropriate?
- Are there barriers to access to health care services for persons living in the home?
- How are home care services reimbursed?

Diagnostic Reasoning and the Home Visit

The diagnostic reasoning process is used to derive nursing diagnoses. The nurse examines available data and then develops diagnostic hypotheses that seem to explain the data. Hypothesis evaluation takes place when the nurse actually makes the home visit and obtains additional data to confirm or disconfirm the diagnostic hypotheses. The diagnostic hypotheses generated from the preliminary assessment, however, give the nurse some direction for planning nursing interventions to be performed during the home visit. Based on the data available in the preliminary assessment, the nurse makes nursing diagnoses related to health conditions to be addressed during the home visit. These diagnoses may be positive diagnoses, problem-focused nursing diagnoses, or health-promotive diagnoses.

Positive nursing diagnoses reflect client strengths evidenced in the preliminary assessment. For example, available data may indicate "effective coping with the demands imposed by a handicapped child due to a strong family support system." This diagnosis suggests that the nurse will reinforce family support as a factor contributing to effective coping.

Problem-focused nursing diagnoses may reflect potential problems or actual problems for which there is evidence in the preliminary assessment data. For example, an existing problem of "ineffective contraceptive use due to inadequate knowledge of contraceptive methods" may have been documented on a previous home visit. Unless there is also an indication that this problem has been resolved, the nurse will probably address it during the subsequent home visit. Preliminary assessment data may suggest potential problems as well. For example, the request for services might indicate that the client's husband is in the Navy and is due to leave on extended sea duty. This information would suggest a nursing diagnosis of "potential for ineffective coping due to loss of spousal assistance."

Nursing diagnoses might also reflect the need for health-promotive services. For example, there will soon be a "need for routine immunizations" for a newborn child. Similarly, the mother has a "need for postpartum follow-up due to recent delivery."

Planning the Home Visit

Based on the preliminary assessment, the community health nurse makes plans for a home visit to address the health needs most likely to be present in the situation. Tasks to be accomplished in planning the visit include reviewing previous interventions, prioritizing client needs, developing goals and objectives for care, and considering client acceptance and timing. Other tasks of this stage include delineating activities needed to meet client needs, obtaining needed materials, and planning evaluation.

Reviewing Previous Interventions

The first step in planning is to review any previous interventions related to client health needs and the efficacy of those interventions. This information allows the nurse to eliminate interventions that have been unsuccessful in the past and to identify interventions that have worked.

Prioritizing Client Needs

The next task is to give priority to identified client needs. Client care needs may be prioritized on the basis of their potential to threaten the client's health, the degree to which they concern the client, or their ease of solution. It is often impossible to address all of the client's health problems in a single visit, so the nurse must decide which needs require immediate attention. For example, if the wife has been admitted to an alcohol treatment center and there is no one to care for the children while the father works, provision of childcare and dealing with the children's feelings about their mother's absence may be the only things that can be accomplished on the initial visit. Other problems, such as poor nutritional habits and the need for immunizations for the toddler, can be deferred until a later visit.

Developing Goals and Objectives

After determining which client needs will be addressed in the forthcoming visit, the nurse develops goals and objectives related to each area of need. Goals are generally stated expectations, whereas objectives are more specific. In the previous example, the nurse's goal might be to enable the family to function adequately in the mother's absence. In this instance, an outcome objective might be that adequate childcare will be obtained so the father can return to work.

The health care needs that will be addressed during a home visit may reflect the primary, secondary, and tertiary levels of prevention. When health care needs occur in the realm of primary prevention, goals and outcome objectives reflect positive health states or the absence of specific health problems as expected outcomes of care. For example, a goal for primary prevention might be "development of effective parenting skills." A related outcome objective might be that the client "will display effective communication skills in relating to children."

Goals and objectives related to needs for secondary prevention focus on alleviation of specific problems. For example, a goal for a client with hypertension might be "effective control of elevated blood pressure" and the related outcome objective might be a blood pressure that is "consistently below 140/90." Similarly, goals and objectives for tertiary prevention reflect client achievement of a prior level of function or the prevention of recurrence of a health problem.

Considering Acceptance and Timing

In planning a home visit, the nurse should consider the client's readiness to accept intervention as well as the timing of the visit and the introduction of intervention. The nurse may find, for example, that a relatively minor problem with which the client is preoccupied must be addressed before the client is willing to deal with other health needs. As we saw earlier, clients may be fearful of home visits, particularly if they are viewed as evidence of poor performance on their part. For this reason the community health nurse may need to put considerable effort in a first contact into building a level of trust and rapport with the client.

Timing is another important consideration in planning an effective home visit. If the visit interferes with other activities important to the client, the client may not be as open to the visit as would otherwise be the case. Other activities that compete with a home visit for the client's attention might be the visit of a friend, an upcoming doctor's appointment, getting the children ready for an outing, or even something as mundane as a favorite soap opera. Prescheduling or rescheduling home visits can make the visit a more effective intervention if something else is interfering. In one study, consistent timing of visits was one of the factors that clients viewed as important in continuity of care. Clients were concerned about their inability to plan other aspects of their lives when the timing of home visits was inconsistent from one visit to the next (Woodward, Abelson, Tedford, & Hitchison, 2004).

Timing also relates to the degree of rapport established between client and nurse. Clients need time to develop trust in the nurse before intimate issues can be addressed. For example, a pregnant adolescent may feel too uncomfortable and threatened by the nurse during early visits to admit to prior drug use and ask about its effects on the baby. The nurse should judge the appropriateness of the timing in bringing up intimate issues for discussion and wait, if possible, until rapport is established with the client. Efforts at cost containment have often limited the number of visits that can be made to a particular client, so community health nurses must work to develop trust and rapport early in their interactions with clients.

Delineating Nursing Activities

The next aspect of planning the home visit is the planning of specific nursing activities for each nursing diagnosis to be addressed. Planned interventions should be based on evidence of their effectiveness and may incorporate practice guidelines, agency procedures and protocols, or elements of clinical pathways. The federal Agency for Healthcare Research and Quality (AHRQ) (formerly the Agency for Health Care Policy and Research [AHCPR]) has developed practice guidelines for several problems relevant to home health nursing. Current guidelines include those related to pressure ulcer prevention and treatment and cardiac rehabilitation. Prior guidelines include those for acute pain management, urinary incontinence, cataracts, depression, sickle cell disease, early HIV infection, benign prostatic hypertrophy, cancer pain management, unstable angina, heart failure, otitis media

with effusion, quality mammography, acute low back pain, poststroke rehabilitation, smoking cessation, and early Alzheimer's disease (AHRQ, 2001). Because of recent developments in treatment, these prior guidelines are no longer considered current, but may be of interest to home health nurses anyway. Current and prior guidelines may be accessed through the AHRQ Web page at http://www.ahrq.gov.

Agency procedures and protocols and clinical pathways may also be used as guides for planning nursing interventions during a home visit. Clinical pathways were addressed in detail in Chapter 12∞. Clinical pathways may differ from agency to agency and should be tailored to the goals and resources of the particular agency.

The activities planned reflect the nurse's assessment of health care needs and the factors influencing them. In the previous example, referral to a Head Start program may provide assistance with childcare, but only if the children involved are of the right ages. If the youngsters are of school age, the appropriate nursing intervention might be to help the father explore the possibility of an after-school program, if one is available, or have the children go home with the parents of a friend until the father can pick them up after work.

Nursing activities can focus on both health promotion and the resolution of health-related problems. For example, the community health nurse might provide the parents of a toddler with anticipatory guidance regarding toilet training or assist parents to discuss sexuality with their preteen daughter. Other positive interventions might focus on providing adequate nutrition for a young child or promoting a healthy pregnancy for a pregnant woman.

Specific interventions employed by the nurse might include referral, education, and technical procedures. For example, the nurse might refer a family to social services for financial assistance, teach a mother about appropriate nutrition for the family, or check a hypertensive client's blood pressure. The actions selected should be directed toward achieving the goals and objectives established while taking into account the constraints and supports in the individual client situation.

Obtaining Necessary Materials

One aspect of planning the home visit is obtaining materials and supplies that may be needed to implement planned interventions. Because the visit takes place in the client's home, the nurse cannot assume that necessary supplies will be available there. If the nurse plans to engage in nutrition education, he or she might want to leave a selection of pamphlets with the client to reinforce teaching. If planned activities involve weighing a premature infant, the nurse will want to take along a scale.

Equipment and supplies may also be needed for other procedures such as dressing changes, catheterizations, injections, and blood pressure checks. Because the nurse frequently does a physical assessment of one or

BUILDING OUR KNOWLEDGE BASE

Miller, Kobayashi, and Hill (2003) described the development of learning groups that included home visiting staff from several agencies. The purpose of the groups was to bring health care professionals together to discuss common concerns in the area of home visitation and to share information on strategies to address those concerns with an eye toward developing best practices in home health. The groups were intended to promote organizational change to improve services to at-risk families with young children.

What might be the relative advantages and disadvantages of such groups for the agencies participating? How might you conduct research to determine *best practices* based on group input?

more clients, additional equipment such as a stethoscope, percussion hammer, tongue blade, flashlight, and otophthalmoscope will need to be obtained prior to setting out for the visit.

Planning for Evaluation

As with every other process employed by community health nurses, the planning phase of the home visit process concludes with plans for evaluation. The nurse determines criteria to be used to evaluate the effectiveness of the home visit. Criteria for evaluating client outcomes are derived from the outcome objectives developed for the visit. Because the outcome of nursing interventions undertaken during a home visit may not be immediately apparent, the nurse needs to develop both long-term and short-term evaluative criteria. Short-term criteria are likely to be based on client response to interventions. For example, the nurse makes a referral for immunizations, but the mother cannot follow through on the referral and receive immunizations on the spot. The nurse, however, can evaluate the mother's response to the referral. Does the mother seem interested? Does she indicate that she will follow through on the referral? On subsequent visits, the nurse would employ long-term outcome criteria to evaluate the effects of interventions. In this instance, criteria would include whether the client had her child immunized.

Outcome evaluation addresses the level of prevention of the nursing interventions employed. Evaluative criteria for primary preventive measures, for example, reflect health promotion or the absence of specific health problems. For example, criteria for interventions to foster immunity to childhood diseases would include whether immunizations were obtained and the presence or absence of immunizable diseases such as measles. If the client develops measles, primary prevention of this disease obviously was not effective.

Evaluation of secondary preventive measures focuses on the degree to which an existing problem has been resolved. For example, a client's hypertension may have been uncontrolled because of poor medication compliance. Evaluative criteria in this instance would include

the degree of compliance achieved and the client's blood pressure measurements. Criteria to evaluate tertiary preventive measures reflect the degree to which a client has regained a prior level of health or prevented recurrent health problems. For example, have passive range-of-motion exercises helped a client recovering from a broken arm to regain strength and mobility? Or has parenting education by the nurse prevented further episodes of child abuse in an abusive family?

The nurse also develops criteria to evaluate implementation of the planned home visit. These criteria are derived from process objectives developed for the visit. For example, was the nurse adequately prepared to address the health care needs encountered during the visit? Were the appropriate supplies available for implementing planned interventions?

Implementing the Planned Visit

The next step in the home visit process is conducting the visit itself. Several tasks are involved in implementing the planned visit. These include validating the health needs and diagnoses identified in the preliminary assessment, identifying additional needs, modifying the intervention plan as needed, performing nursing interventions, and dealing with distractions.

Validating Assessment and Diagnoses

The first task in implementing the home visit is to validate the accuracy of the preliminary assessment. Problems identified from the available data may or may not exist when the nurse actually enters the home. For example, the nurse may find that the family's poor diet is not the result of lack of knowledge about nutrition, but stems from a lack of money to purchase nutritious foods. Or the nurse may find that what appeared to nurses on the postpartum unit to be poor maternal–infant bonding was not actually the case. Similarly, the nurse may discover that expected strengths or positive nursing diagnoses do not accurately reflect the client's actual health status. For example, a mother who appeared to be coping effectively with her child's handicap may really have been exhibiting denial of the condition. It is particularly important that the nurse involve the client in a reassessment of his or her needs and to modify the plan of care as needed, also in conjunction with the client.

Identifying Additional Needs

During the visit, the nurse collects additional data related to biophysical, psychological, physical environmental, sociocultural, behavioral, and health system factors to identify additional health care needs. For example, when the nurse arrives to visit a new mother and her infant son, the nurse may find that the client's father has recently had a heart attack and been taken to the hospital. The client may be much more in need of assistance in finding childcare for her new baby so she can spend time at the hospital than in discussing immunization and

MediaLink Case Study: Home Health Nursing

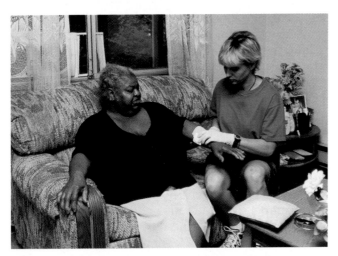

Community health nurses assess clients' physical health status.

postpartum concerns. Or the nurse may find that, in addition to having a new baby, the client's husband is out of work and the 12-year-old has been skipping school. Again, clients need to be actively involved in determining needs and prioritizing them if nurses are to avoid imposing their preconceived agenda for the visit.

Modifying the Plan of Care

Based on what the nurse finds in the course of the home visit and on input from the client or family, the initial plan of care may need to be modified. The nurse shares with the client the initial goals established for addressing health needs identified in the preliminary assessment, as well as additional problems identified, and together they set or revise goals. In doing this, the nurse may need to restructure priorities based on new data and client input. For instance, if the 2-year-old has cut her arm and is bleeding profusely when the nurse arrives, this problem takes precedence over the nurse's plan to discuss with the mother the potential for sibling rivalry. In other words, the nurse can either implement interventions as planned or modify the plan as the client's situation and desires dictate.

Performing Nursing Interventions

Only after the plan of care has been modified as needed does the nurse perform whatever nursing interventions are warranted by the client situation. As noted earlier, these activities may include primary, secondary, and tertiary preventive measures. For example, the nurse working with a new mother might discuss parenting skills as a means of preventing child abuse (primary prevention), give the mother suggestions for dealing with the infant's spitting up (secondary prevention), and discuss options for contraception to prevent a subsequent pregnancy (tertiary prevention).

Any or all of the three levels can be emphasized, depending on the situation encountered. For example, if the mother is inexperienced and concerned about childcare skills in feeding, bathing, and parenting, the emphasis would be on primary prevention. Conversely, if the nurse arrives to find a baby screaming with gas pains, emphasis is placed on making the infant more comfortable and relieving the mother's anxiety (secondary prevention). Once this has been accomplished, the nurse can focus on suggestions to prevent a recurrence of the problem (tertiary prevention).

Dealing with Distractions

One important consideration in implementing a home visit is dealing with distractions. Distractions are generally of three types: environmental, behavioral, and nurse-initiated. Environmental distractions arise from both the physical and social environments and may include background noise, crowded surroundings, and interruptions by other family members or outsiders. The occurrence of such distractions during the home visit can give the nurse a clear picture of the client's environment and the way in which the client and family interact among themselves and with others. For example, if mother and child are continually yelling at one another during the visit, this suggests the existence of family communication problems. On the other hand, positive interactions between a mother and her young child provide evidence of effective parenting skills.

Despite the information that can be gleaned from these distractions, their negative effects on the interaction between client and nurse need to be minimized. Requesting that the television be turned off during the visit or moving the client to a more private area can minimize some distractions. Or the nurse may ask an intrusive younger child to draw a picture to allow parent and nurse to talk with fewer interruptions. If there are too many distractions that cannot be eliminated or overcome, the nurse can ask the client if there is a better time for the visit, when fewer interruptions will occur, and reschedule the visit for a later date. For example, subsequent visits might be planned to coincide with the toddler's nap.

Behavioral distractions consist of behaviors employed by the client to distract the nurse from the purpose of the visit. Again, the use of such distractions can be a cue for the nurse that certain topics are uncomfortable for the client or that the client does not quite trust the nurse or may feel guilty about something. The nurse can benefit from the distraction by exploring the reasons for the client's behaviors and working to establish trust with the client.

The last category of distractions originates with the nurse. These distractions create barriers to relationships with clients. Fears, role preoccupation, and personal reactions to different lifestyles can distract the nurse from the purpose of the home visit. Nurses may fear bodily harm, rejection by the client, or the lack of control that is implicit in a home visit. In today's violent society, fear of bodily harm is understandable and nurses making home visits should employ the personal safety precautions addressed later in this chapter.

Community health nurses may also create distractions by being so preoccupied with their original purpose that they fail to see the need to modify the planned home visit. No planned intervention is so important that it cannot be postponed if more important needs intervene. Nurses who continue to pursue predetermined goals in the light of other client needs reduce their credibility with clients and create barriers to effective intervention. For example, the nurse who insists on talking about infant feeding when the client just had an argument with her husband and fears he will leave her is not meeting the client's needs.

Finally, community health nurses may be put off by the contrast between their own lifestyle and that of the clients they are visiting. In dealing with feelings engendered by such differences, it is helpful to understand that one's own attitudes are the product of one's upbringing and culture and that clients derive their attitudes in the same way. In dealing with lifestyle differences, the nurse must be aware of personal feelings and their impact on nursing effectiveness. The nurse must also determine what aspects of the client's lifestyle may be detrimental to health and focus on those, while accepting other differences in attitude or behavior as hallmarks of the client's uniqueness. Being thoroughly informed about cultural and ethnic differences also minimizes negative reactions by the nurse to such differences. Some of these differences are discussed in Chapter 9∞.

Evaluating the Home Visit

Before concluding the visit, the nurse evaluates the effectiveness of interventions in terms of their appropriateness to the situation and the client's response. This evaluation is conducted using criteria established in planning the visit. It may not be possible, at this point, to determine the eventual outcome of nursing care. The nurse can, however, examine the client's initial response to interventions. Was the mother interested in obtaining contraceptives? Is it likely that she will follow through on a referral to the immunization clinic? Did the client voice an intention to reduce fat intake? Could the client accurately demonstrate the correct technique for bottle-feeding the infant?

Evaluating the ultimate outcome of interventions may occur at subsequent visits. For example, on the next visit, the nurse might determine whether the mother obtained contraceptives. If she called but was not able to get an appointment, the nurse would determine the reason. Based on information obtained, there may be a need for advocacy on the part of the nurse. If the client did not seek contraceptive services, the nurse should determine the reason for her behavior. Was the client distracted by crises that occurred in the meantime, but plans to call for an appointment next week? Did she not have transportation to the clinic? Or maybe she does not really want contraceptives. If the client lacks transportation, the nurse might help her explore ways of getting transportation. If the client does not really want contraceptives, the nurse can either explore why or accept the client's wishes.

As noted earlier, evaluation of nursing interventions during a home visit should reflect the level of prevention involved. The nurse examines both the short-term and long-term effects of interventions at the primary, secondary, and tertiary levels of prevention, as appropriate. For example, if the home visit focused on secondary prevention, evaluation will also be focused at this level. If several levels were addressed during the visit, evaluation will focus on the effects of interventions at each level.

The nurse also evaluates his or her use of the home visit process. Was the preliminary assessment adequate? Was information available that the nurse neglected to review, resulting in unexpected problems during the visit itself? For example, did the nurse ask about the husband's reaction to the new baby when the record indicates the client is not married? Did the nurse miss cues to additional problems during the visit? Was the nurse able to plan interventions consistent with client needs, attitudes, and desires? Was the nurse able to deal effectively with distractions? If not, why not? Answers to these and similar questions allow the nurse to improve his or her use of the home visit process in subsequent client encounters.

Home visitation programs can also be evaluated in terms of their processes and outcomes. Home visits, although less expensive than hospitalization or some other means of service delivery, are not without cost, and the effects of such programs should be evaluated. Many home visiting programs have been found to be highly effective in achieving specific outcomes, but others have not shown any benefit. For example, some studies have indicated that home visits resulted in maintaining infant breast-feeding (AHRQ, 2003; Coutino, Cabral de Lira, Lima, & Ashworth, 2005), but a similar study in Italy showed no difference in the initiation or duration of breast-feeding (Di Napoli et al., 2004). Two longitudinal studies by Olds and associates have demonstrated significant effects of home visits on children and mothers in high-risk situations (Olds, Kitzman et al., 2004; Olds, Robinson et al., 2004). Other studies have demonstrated positive effects in pregnancy (Fetrick, Christensen, & Mitchell, 2003; Nguyen, Carson, Parris, & Place, 2003) and for chronic disease management related to stroke (Boter, Rinkel, & de Haan, 2004) and diabetes (Huang, Wu, Jeng, & Lin, 2004), but not for chronic lung disease (Kwok et al., 2004). A study by Paul, Phillips, Widome, and Hollenbeak (2004) found that newborns who received home visits had fewer hospital readmissions for jaundice and dehydration in the first 10 days of life than those who were not visited. Similarly, home visits to children with nutritional or psychosocial risk factors resulted in positive health effects compared to those who did not receive visits

(Worobey, Pisuk, & Decker, 2004), but did not appear to reduce risk for maternal or child abuse (Hahn et al., 2003). An overall review of 13 studies on the effects of home visiting on maternal and child clients found that about half were effective in achieving their targeted outcomes (McNaughton, 2004).

Some studies have found differential effects for home visiting programs for different populations. For example, Norr et al. (2003) found that a home visit program had greater effects on child health for African American mothers than for Hispanic mothers. Similarly, home visits have been found to be effective in improving functional status in women, but less so in men (Vass et al., 2004).

Documenting Home Visits

The last step in conducting a home visit is documenting what took place. As we will see later in this chapter, accurate documentation is particularly important in ensuring appropriate reimbursement for services. Several aspects of the visit should be documented. The nurse should document the actual (not preliminary) assessment of client health status and the health needs identified as well as the interventions employed to address these needs. Clients' responses to interventions should also be documented, as well as the long- and short-term outcomes of interventions. At the end of each visit, the nurse should also document future plans for care. Finally, at the end of services, the nurse should write a discharge summary of the interventions employed and the client's

health status at the close of care. If referrals have been made for continued care from other agencies, these should also be documented. The components of the home visit process are summarized in Table 21-2◆.

EVIDENCE-BASED PRACTICE

McNaughton (2004) conducted a review of 13 studies of the effects of nursing home visits to maternal child clients. She found that a wide range of problems was addressed by the nurses in the visits and that about half of the interventions were effective in accomplishing desired outcomes. McNaughton identified questions that had not yet been addressed in the literature related to nursing home visits. These questions included the types of problems for which home visiting is an effective intervention, and the "minimum dose" (number of home visits) needed to achieve desired outcomes. Another question that remains unanswered is the relative effectiveness of home visits conducted by community health nurses as compared to those by other professional and nonprofessional persons.

- Select a particular type of home visiting program, target population, or home-based practice (e.g., safety assessment) and examine the relevant literature. Have there been any reviews of studies examining the effectiveness of home visits for the type of problem, population, or practice you selected? If so, what were the findings regarding effectiveness?
- Do the reviews, if any, address the questions posed by McNaughton?
- If no published reviews are available, what conclusions can you draw from your own review of literature related to the program, population, or practice you selected?

TABLE 21-2	Elements of the Home Visit Process
Preliminary assessment	Review available client data to determine health care needs related to biophysical, psychological, physical environmental, sociocultural, behavioral, and health system dimensions.
Diagnosis	Develop diagnostic hypotheses based on preliminary assessment.
Planning	Review previous interventions and their effects.
	Prioritize client needs and identify those to be addressed during the visit.
	Develop goals and objectives for visit and identify levels of prevention involved.
	Consider client acceptance and timing of visit.
	Specify activities needed to accomplish goals and objectives.
	Obtain needed supplies and equipment.
	Plan for evaluation of the home visit.
Implementation	Validate preliminary assessment and nursing diagnostic hypotheses.
	Identify other client needs.
	Incorporate client into modification of plan of care to meet identified needs.
	Modify plan of care as needed.
	Carry out nursing interventions.
	Deal with distractions.
Evaluation	Evaluate client response to interventions.
	Evaluate long-term and short-term outcomes of intervention.
	Evaluate the quality of implementation in the home visit.
	Evaluate outcomes and quality of care at the aggregate as well as individual level.

Continued on next page

TABLE 21-2	**Elements of the Home Visit Process** *(continued)*
Documentation	Document client assessment and health needs identified.
	Document interventions.
	Document client response to interventions.
	Document outcome of interventions.
	Document future plan of care.
	Document client health status at discharge.

ADVANTAGES OF HOME VISITS

Why do community health nurses make home visits? It would seem to be more cost-effective for clients to come to the nurse. More clients might be seen in a given period if the nurse did not have to consider travel time or time wasted being lost in unfamiliar areas. What is there about a home visit that outweighs these obvious disadvantages?

The advantages of home visits can be viewed in terms of six major aspects: convenience, access, information, relationship, cost, and outcomes. With respect to convenience, many clients would prefer to be seen in their homes rather than clinics or other health care settings. Home visits permit health care services to be integrated into the client's usual routine. Moreover, clients are not subjected to the need to find transportation or to the long waits for service that frequently occur in other settings.

The access aspect of home visiting has two elements. First, clients who are immobile or lack transportation and cannot reach other care settings have access to care that might otherwise be unavailable to them. Similarly, community health nurses may gain access to clients who would not present themselves, for whatever reasons, for services provided in other settings. Second, home visits provide community health nurses with opportunities to identify other clients in need of services.

In the information aspect, the nurse making a home visit has opportunities to obtain a variety of information that is less easily obtained in other settings. The nurse gets a complete picture of the client, whether individual or family, and of his or her environment. The nurse can see firsthand the effects of physical environmental, psychological, and sociocultural factors on a client's health status. A home visit provides the nurse with information about possible resources and hazards that can influence a client's health. The interaction of family members during the visit might suggest the extent of a client's support network and the ability of family members to provide care. Similarly, detecting potential health hazards in a home, such as loose throw rugs in the home of an older client, can provide the stimulus for health education to promote physical safety.

In the home, the nurse can better assess the client's ability to perform activities of daily living (ADLs). Periodic contact in the client's home may permit the nurse to identify minor health changes for which clients would not seek help. The nurse may then act to prevent major problems.

Because the community health nurse has a more complete picture of a client as a result of a home visit, he or she has a better understanding of the client's needs and can better design interventions. Finally, during a home visit, the nurse is better able to monitor and evaluate the effects of interventions. For example, the client may tell the nurse in the clinic that he or she is adhering to a low-sodium diet as planned. If the nurse visits at home, however, and finds the client munching potato chips, it is readily apparent that dietary instruction has not been as effective as desired.

Ideally, the relationship aspect of home visiting has the advantage that the client is exercising autonomy and control. In the client's home the nurse is a guest; the client controls the situation. Unfortunately, this is not always as true as one might hope. Research, for example, has identified the tendency of community health nurses and other home visitors to dominate interaction in the home, allowing little opportunity for client input in the course of the visit. In part this may be the result of specific program foci for most home visitation programs that require the accomplishment of specific program-related tasks (Baggens, 2004; Bryans, 2004).

Effective community health nurses promote the aspect of control to foster clients' sense of empowerment. The nurse also acts as an enabler, assisting clients to find resources to take action on their own, and as an enhancer, helping clients build on personal strengths. Ideally, actions by the nurse lead to a collaborative atmosphere in which the client is fully involved in planning interventions, which in turn enhances the probability of successful implementation.

Another advantage to the relationship aspect of a home visit is the privacy and sense of intimacy created. Clients often feel freer to raise sensitive issues in the privacy of their own homes than in more alien health care settings. Thus, the community health nurse may gain more private insights into the client's situation.

The last element of the relationship aspect that frequently operates during a home visit is the continuity of the relationship itself. Often, community health nurses make several visits to an individual or family. This continuity intensifies the effects of the information dimension and other aspects of the relationship dimension, particularly intimacy. Continuity in the relationship may also permit services to others in the client's environment. For example, the nurse may provide education and referrals to enhance the health status of family care-givers. On occasion, however, the long-term nature of many home visiting relationships may contribute to challenges that we will address later.

Continuity in service provision in the home has been an important element identified by care providers, physicians, and clients and their caretakers. Continuity in care has been defined as "care that is experienced as running smoothly, that responds to clients' needs, and requires no special efforts for clients to maintain" (Woodward et al., 2004, p. 177). Research has suggested two aspects of continuity that are important, care management and actual service provision. Care management is more apparent as a requisite to physicians and case managers than it is to clients and their caretakers. Care management reflects planning, monitoring, and periodic review and modification of the plan of care and coordination of services. Clients and family caretakers, on the other hand, voiced more concern over continuity in direct service provision, particularly in terms of consistency in the knowledge and skills of providers, trusting relationships between provider and client/caretaker, and consistent timing of visits. Continuity was found to be facilitated by effective communication between provider and client and among providers and by consistency in providers (Woodward et al., 2004).

The cost aspect of home visiting is one reason this mode of delivering health care services has experienced a resurgence. Home care is less expensive than hospitalization or long-term facility placement. When clients can be maintained in good health in their homes, the overall cost of their care to society is reduced.

The final aspect of a home visit that contributes to its value is client outcomes. As we saw in the discussion of home visit evaluation, home visitation programs have been shown to achieve a variety of health-related outcomes for different population groups.

CHALLENGES OF HOME VISITING

Despite the many advantages of home visits, this mode of health care delivery is not without challenges. Some of these challenges arise out of the diversity of clients and the multiplicity of their problems. Clients differ in age, ethnic background, culture, health status, and attitudes toward health and health providers. They do not usually experience isolated problems but are faced with multiple problems that impinge on their health. The diversity of clients and the problems encountered in home visiting require the community health nurse to have a broad knowledge base to understand and deal with the variety of factors that may influence clients' health. The multiplicity of problems coupled with the diversity of clientele creates a variety of service demands that can seem overwhelming and lead to a great deal of stress for the visiting nurse.

Other challenges in home visiting derive from the community health nurse's need to maintain balance in his or her interactions with clients. Areas in which a delicate balance is required are depicted in Figure 21-1 and include a balance between intimacy and professional distance, assisting and devaluing clients, dependence and independence, altruism and realism, creativity and inadequacy, risk and safety, cost containment and quality, and, in some cases, health restoration and health promotion services. An additional area in which balance is needed is that of balance between task orientation and meeting the unique needs of clients and their families.

As noted earlier, home visits create a sense of intimacy between nurse and client that is not found in other health care settings. This intimacy, while advantageous in some respects, can make it difficult for nurses to maintain an appropriate professional distance in order to be most therapeutic. Although the home visit is not a social visit, a certain amount of socialization is necessary to establish rapport with clients. Nurses making home visits may disclose more about themselves than they would in other settings. Such self-disclosure can help establish rapport and a collaborative relationship with clients and help to equalize the balance of power between nurse and client, but the nurse must be careful to determine what level of self-disclosure is appropriate to the situation. In addition, the nurse will sometimes have to make difficult decisions about accepting hospitality or gifts. The client's offer may have cultural overtones, and refusal to accept may damage the nurse–client relationship. Often, the nurse may feel that the client cannot afford to give what is being offered. In each situation, the nurse must judge the potential effects of accepting or rejecting hospitality and gifts. When refusal to accept small gifts might be interpreted by the client as rejection, the nurse should gracefully accept. If more expensive gifts are offered, the nurse should decline tactfully. He or she might also indicate willingness to accept something of minimal monetary value. For example, the nurse might say, "I couldn't possibly accept that lovely vase, but I would love to have some of your delicious cookies" or anything else that seems appropriate. Such a response indicates acceptance of the client's generosity but not of an expensive item.

Another challenge arises out of the need to assist clients without conveying that clients are inadequate, that is, without devaluing them. Too often, when people are required to accept the help of others, they begin to perceive themselves as inadequate. This is where a collaborative relationship can be very beneficial. In a collaborative relationship, nurse and client work together to resolve problems, and the input of both is valued. Within this relationship, the nurse should convey a sense of self-efficacy that prevents clients from feeling inadequate to meet difficulties on their own.

The balance between assisting and devaluing clients affects self-determination. Clients have the right to determine for themselves whether they are going to act on health providers' suggestions. Because of the relationship engendered in the home visit situation, nurses may feel

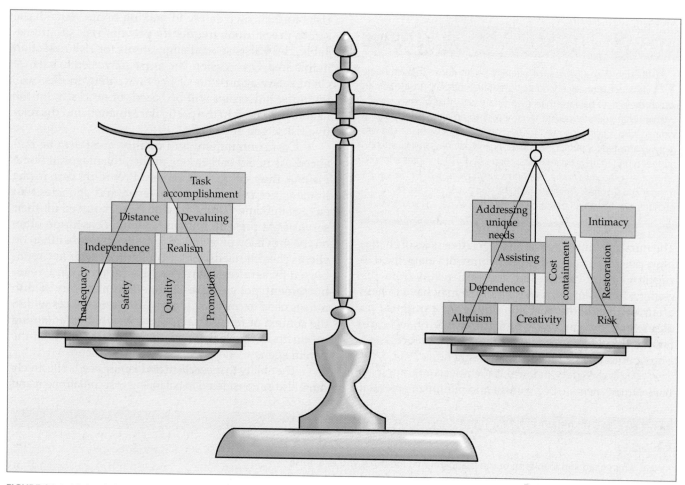

FIGURE 21-1 Maintaining Balance in Home Visiting

tempted to trade on the relationship to subtly coerce clients into actions that are "in their best interest." In a truly collaborative relationship, however, client and nurse together determine goals and the actions to achieve them. The nurse must always keep in mind that veto power lies with the client.

Another area in which balance is required is the level of dependence or independence of client function. The goal of a home visit is to promote client and family self-sufficiency; however, many clients may not reach this level until well into a series of home visits. Again, a collaborative relationship conveys the expectation that clients will do what they can, with assistance from the nurse as needed.

Because of the sometimes overwhelming nature of clients' problems, community health nurses making home visits must also maintain a balance between altruism and realism. The nurse cannot solve all of the client's problems and must focus on those problems that are amenable to nursing intervention. Nurses must also recognize that they will not be completely successful with all clients. The nurse, therefore, must learn to be satisfied with incremental progress rather than the dramatic improvements in clients' health status that may be seen in other health care settings. Having a realistic sense of what can be accomplished, given the resources available

to client and nurse, will diminish the stress of insurmountable client problems.

Balance is also required between creativity and inadequacy. In the home situation, community health nurses frequently have to deal with a lack of materials and resources that would be taken for granted in other settings. Community health nurses have thus learned to exercise their creativity and "make do" with whatever resources are available. For example, the nurse might suggest to a mother with limited income that she use simple homemade toys to stimulate an infant's development, or the nurse might arrange for support services from friends and neighbors to assist a client on a short-term basis. The nurse, however, must recognize when "making do" is no longer feasible but, rather, is contributing to inadequate care. In this situation, the nurse must seek other avenues to obtain the resources necessary to provide adequate client care. For example, the amount of assistance needed may tax the resources of the client's friends and family, and professional care must be sought.

The need for balance in the area of risk and safety affects both nurse and client. The nurse must decide what level of risk is acceptable without unduly jeopardizing the safety of the client or the nurse's own safety.

ETHICAL AWARENESS

*A*lthough it is quite rare, community health nurses making home visits occasionally encounter situations that are unsafe and in which they must balance their own safety with that of their clients. Imagine that you are making a home visit to an elderly homebound woman who is being followed for hypertension. The woman's son was recently arrested for producing and selling methamphetamines after his mother reported his activities to the police. About 10 minutes after you arrive, the son comes home. He is obviously intoxicated. He yells at his mother and says he is "going to beat the crap out of her." He says if you do not leave, he will do the same thing to you. What will you do?

The nurse may need to weigh the relative risks of changing a potentially hazardous environment versus the disruption to the client's life that will result from the change. For example, a visiting nurse may have to help a family decide the best alternative for caring for an older family member no longer capable of self-care. Should the older person live with family members, seek a companion, or be placed in a nursing home?

The risk–safety balance issue affects the nurse as well. Nurses need to be aware of and minimize potential risks to their own safety in making home visits. Basic safety precautions frequently prevent risk situations. Table 21-3◆ lists several suggestions for risk reduction in this area. On occasion, the nurse may need to balance client safety against his or her own safety. In this case, the nurse's decision will be based, of necessity, on the factors operating in the particular situation and the relative risk to self and client.

Cost containment and quality must also be balanced. As noted earlier, one of the advantages of home visits is their cost-effectiveness. Providing care in the home is not inexpensive, however, and agencies that engage in home visiting need to be reimbursed for their services. At present, reimbursement is based too often on the provision of technical care services rather than on clients' health needs. Frequently, nurses are not reimbursed for services such as health education. Until reimbursement policies are changed, community health nurses need to continue to provide these services within the context of reimbursable services while maintaining productivity levels that ensure the fiscal viability of the parent agency.

The ability to meet client and family needs effectively must also be considered in balancing cost containment and

---

TABLE 21-3 Personal Safety Considerations in Home Visiting

Appearance

- Wear a name tag and a uniform or other apparel that identifies you as a nurse.
- Do not carry a purse or wear expensive jewelry.
- Leave any valuables at home or lock them in the trunk of the car before leaving the office.

Transportation

- Keep your car in good repair and with a full tank of gas.
- Carry emergency supplies such as a flashlight and blanket.
- Always lock your car and carry keys in hand when leaving the client's home.
- Park near the client's home with your car in view of the home whenever possible.
- Avoid the use of public transportation if possible.
- Get complete and accurate directions to the home.

The Situation

- Call ahead to alert the client that you will be coming.
- Ask the client to secure pets before your visit.
- Walk directly to the client's home, without detours to local shops or other places.
- Keep one arm free while walking to the client's home.
- Avoid isolated areas, especially late in the day or at night.
- Knock before entering the client's home, even if the door is open.
- Make joint visits in dangerous neighborhoods or situations or employ an escort service if needed.
- Listen to the client's messages regarding potential safety hazards.
- Make home visits at times when illicit activity (such as drug transactions) is less likely to occur or when potentially dangerous family members will not be present.
- Carry a whistle that is easily accessible.
- Become familiar with personal defense techniques.
- Leave any situation that appears to hold a risk of personal danger.
- Stay alert and observe your surroundings.

quality. Sometimes the question is one of "cost containment for whom?" For example, it may cost society less to provide care in the home, but it may cost the family more. Family costs may include higher out-of-pocket costs for items not covered in the home setting by health insurance or lost wages if a family member needs to stay home to provide care.

Another area of balance related to cost containment versus quality is the balance between the provision of illness-related health restoration care and health-promotive care, the true focus of community health nursing. Health-promotive services are frequently not reimbursable in many home visit programs (particularly home health programs). Again, community health nurses may need to incorporate these kinds of services into the provision of reimbursable acute care services. Nurses must also be able to provide needed services to family members and caretakers that generate revenue.

The final area of balance of concern to community health nurses is that of task accomplishment versus consideration of unique needs of clients and families. As we saw earlier, community health nurses may be constrained by the need to accomplish specific purposes in a home visit. This may lead to an overemphasis on task accomplishment rather than meeting the specific needs of an individual client or family. For example, analysis of home visit interactions in one study identified a tendency on the part of nurses to address a preprogrammed agenda without assessing the need of the family for certain information or assistance. In fact, in some instances, nurses did not even listen to clients' expression of their needs but proceeded with what have been called "authoritative health persuasion techniques" geared to disseminating standard health information (Baggens, 2004).

Effective community health nurses are able to maintain balance in each of the areas addressed here. In maintaining that balance, nurses provide effective holistic care and yet maintain their own integrity and sanity.

Other challenges may arise in home visiting. The first may be getting clients' permission to visit in the first place. Because of increases in violent crime, families may be reluctant to admit strangers into their homes. In addition, clients are often unaware of referrals to community health nurses or may perceive them as unwarranted or intrusive. Moreover, some families may interpret being identified as being in need of home visits as "evidence of poor performance." In Great Britain, where home visiting is a routine health care service available to all families, this perception of labeling does not occur. In the United States, however, a home visit may be seen as evidence of inadequacy (Kearney, York, & Deatrick, 2000). In one study, mothers receiving home visits expressed feelings of vulnerability and powerlessness in the encounter (Jack et al., 2005). Because of this, community health nurses may be faced with the challenge of building rapport in an initial contact to permit a therapeutic interaction among nurse, client, and family. This task may be particularly difficult when clients do not have the option of refusing services, as in the case of suspected or confirmed child abuse.

Another challenge in home visiting is the ambiguity of the client situation. Visiting nurses repeatedly refer to the need to shift gears or move from a preconceived agenda to address more pressing needs identified in the family. Frequently, the nurse needs to accomplish this shift within the relatively restrictive service parameters of a given agency. Community health nurses may also be challenged by the need to avoid client abandonment when services continue to be needed but funding sources have been exhausted. Avoiding abandonment may require very creative problem solving by nurse and client to ensure receipt of needed services. Finally, program attrition is another challenge that may limit the effect of home visit programs, with an estimated 50% to 60% attrition from some programs (Navaie-Waliser et al., 2000).

HOME HEALTH AND HOSPICE CARE

A number of authors distinguish between home health care and community health nursing. The distinction arose from the early split between personal health care services and public health services when official health agencies began to emphasize population-based screening and health promotion services. Authors who make this distinction base it on the fact that home health nursing is primarily illness-focused and that it deals with individuals rather than population groups. Other authors, however, point out that home health nurses do deal with aggregate needs. From this perspective, home health nurses identify populations at risk and in need of home health services and define the role of home health nursing in meeting the needs of individual clients and the larger community. The community focus in home health comes in the planning of systems of care based on an assessment of community needs, characteristics, and resources.

Still other authors suggest that illness is both an individual or family problem and a community experience. This was the perspective of early community health nurses who provided personal health services in clients' homes and simultaneously campaigned to improve social conditions. These nurses and their supporters believed that the conditions of the sick in their homes influenced the health of society in general.

Although today home health nurses work primarily with ill individuals, they continue to employ knowledge of environmental, social, and personal health factors. That knowledge is a combination of public health science and nursing practice and is the hallmark of community health nursing. It would seem, then, that the distinction between community health nursing and home health nursing is an artificial one and that home health is actually a subspecialty within community health nursing in which the primary but not sole focus is health restoration. Effective home health nurses who provide holistic nursing care employ principles of community health nursing within the segment of the population that is ill. This perspective is supported by the *Scope and Standards of Home Health Nursing Practice* (American Nurses Association, 1999), which states:

> Home health nursing is a specialized area of nursing practice with its roots firmly placed in community health nursing. By definition, community health nursing practice includes nursing care directed toward individuals, families and groups with the predominant responsibility for care being to the population as a whole. The health care needs of the client determine the appropriate augmentation of home health nursing skills with community health nursing practice. (p. 3)

Home health nursing is characterized by holism, care management, resource coordination, collaboration, and both autonomous and interdependent practice. Interdependent practice involves collaboration with members of other health care disciplines, both professional (e.g., physicians, physical therapists) and nonprofessional (e.g., home health aides), as well as the client and family members.

Home health nurses, like other community health nurses, practice autonomously and are responsible for the achievement of designated outcomes of care. Home health nurses may also specialize in the care of terminally ill clients through the provision of hospice services. Home health care is defined as a "cadre of services for patients who are disabled, chronically or terminally ill, or are recovering from an acute illness" (Gaskell, 2003, p. 11). The official definition of **home health care** used by the federal government is care "provided to individuals and families in their place of residence for the purpose of promoting, maintaining, or restoring health or for maximizing the level of independence while minimizing the effects of disability and illness, including terminal illness" (NCHS, 2004f). Home care services are usually provided under the aegis of a home health agency, and may include a range of care from skilled nursing and therapy services to personal care and homemaking assistance (Qualls, Harris, & Rogers, 2002).

Hospice care is defined as "a program of palliative and supportive care services providing physical, psychological, social, and spiritual care for dying persons, their families, and other loved ones" (NCHS, 2004g). Hospice care may be provided in both home and in-patient settings, but we are concerned here only with home hospice services. Hospice care involves not only care for the terminally ill client, but also bereavement services and counseling for family members and others.

Home health care, as we know it today, originated in the work of voluntary agencies such as the Visiting Nurse Associations (VNAs), the first of which was established in 1886 as the Instructive Nursing Association. This association, established within the Boston Dispensary, later became the Boston VNA, an agency that is still in operation. The Metropolitan Life Insurance Company

home visiting program, discussed in Chapter 3∞, was established to provide home nursing services to policy holders with tuberculosis to limit fatality rates and insurance payouts (Gaskell, 2003). Home health care today continues to be focused on the resolution of specific health problems rather than on health promotion. Although health promotion may take place in home health care visits, it is not the initial purpose for the visit as it might be in other types of home visiting programs. The goal of home health care is to provide the services needed to restore the person to an optimal level of function given the constraints of chronic conditions, or in the case of hospice care, to provide for symptom amelioration until death.

From the 1930s to the 1950s the availability of hospital care decreased the need for home health care for the sick. Then, as hospital costs increased, home care was seen as an effective way to minimize the costs of providing care. In 1965, the Medicare home health benefit was established to provide home care to the elderly and others who qualified for Medicare. This led to the development of many proprietary home care agencies. **Proprietary agencies** are independent home health agencies owned by individuals or corporations that operate on a for-profit basis. The number of home health agencies peaked in 1996 at approximately 10,000 but declined by 30% from 1996 to 2000 (NCHS, 2004e). In 2000, there were more than 11,400 home health and hospice care agencies in the United States that were currently providing care to 1.46 million clients at the time of the National Home Health and Hospice Care survey and had recorded 7.8 million discharges (episodes of care) in a randomly selected single month prior to the survey (NCHS, 2004d).

These figures suggest the enormous amount of health care provided by home health and hospice agencies in the United States. In 2003, home health care accounted for 2.4% of all national health care expenditures ($40 billion), representing growth from 0.2% ($0.1 billion) in 1960 (NCHS, 2004b). It is likely that the need for home health services will increase in the future for several reasons. First, acute care settings will continue to attempt to reduce costs by shortening the length of hospital stays. Second, there are usually long waits for available beds in long-term-care facilities, necessitating maintenance at home for some clients who need long-term-care placement. Third, advances in technology make provision of highly technical care possible in the home setting, and finally, an aging population with multiple care needs will require greater levels of care (Ellenbecker, 2004; Fraser & Strang, 2004).

Home Care and Hospice Clients and Services

Most home health clients, as noted earlier, are elderly individuals. In fact, the rate of care per 10,000 population increases significantly with increasing age. In 2000, for example, 16.4 of every 10,000 people under 65 years of age were currently receiving home care services at the time of the national survey. For all people over 65 years of age, the rate increased to 277 per 10,000 population, and for those 85 years of age and over, the rate was more than twice as high, at 694.1 per 10,000 population. Three fourths of these clients received skilled nursing services, and 44% received personal care services. Physical therapy was provided to 27% of clients, occupational therapy to 8%, and dietary and nutritional services or intravenous services to 4%. In addition, 8% of home care clients received durable medical equipment, 6.5% received medications, and 8.6% received social services. Respite care was provided for 1.2%, referral to other sources of care to 2.5%, and transportation assistance to 1.8% of current clients (NCHS, 2004a).

Many clients had relatively short episodes of care by home health agencies, with an overall mean length of service of 41 days in the period from 1999 to 2000 (NCHS, 2005a), but some diagnostic categories required extensive length of service. For example, in 2000, clients with paralytic syndromes had a mean length of service of 414 days, those with Alzheimer's disease 368 days, and those with mental health problems 329 days. Length of stay for a pathological fracture averaged 255 days, whereas other chronic conditions had shorter length of stay in service (e.g., diabetes, 112 days; hypertension, 108 days; anemia, 123 days; and chronic obstructive pulmonary disease, 107 days) (NCHS, 2004a).

Like home health clients in general, hospice clients tended to be older, with 81% of current hospice clients in 2000 over 65 years of age. The rate of hospice care also increased with age, with 8 per 10,000 population under 65 years of age receiving hospice services, compared to 249.1 per 10,000 over 65 years and 673.3 per 10,000 people 85 years of age and over (NCHS, 2004b).

Home health agencies generally provide a typical set of services and have been found to have several common components, based on findings of the 3M Expert Design Project (Gaskell, 2003). These common elements include marketing strategies to increase referrals, intake processes in which client eligibility for services is determined and initial information is obtained, a financial division to handle billing, a medical records division, a quality assurance or quality improvement component, information systems, and a human resources division. Common services in the clinical services component include skilled nursing, dietetics, speech and language pathology services, medical social work services, homemaker and personal care services, and physical, occupational, and respiratory therapy services.

Collaboration in Home Health and Hospice Care

Clients' needs for home health or hospice services must be certified by a primary care provider before reimbursement for services will be forthcoming. Individual clients or families may contract independently for home health services, but unless the need for services is validated by the primary provider, payment will need to be made out of pocket. In other types of home visitation services, on the other hand, clients may self-refer or community health nurses may identify people in need of services while providing other services. In those types of home visiting programs, the decision of whether or not to provide services lies with the nurse and the client, not with a third party.

Because home health services are provided under the auspices of the primary care provider, there is a particular need for close collaboration among client, nurse, and primary provider. In addition, home health clients often need services provided by other health care professionals, such as physical therapists, dieticians, and so on. Again, it is extremely important for all those participating in the care of the client to be kept informed of the client's health status and to engage in collaborative care planning. A similar need also occurs in the case of hospice care. Physicians or nurse practitioners may need to be actively involved to ensure effective pain management. Similarly, spiritual care advisors and volunteers may be helpful in assisting the client and family members to adjust to the eventuality of death. For both home health and hospice care clients, there may be a need for durable medical equipment (DME) provided by outside vendors, and community health nurses often serve as liaisons to DME vendors, assisting clients to get the best possible care. Like other community health nurses, home health and hospice nurses may also make referrals for additional services to meet identified client needs. Referrals would be made using the process discussed in Chapter 12∞.

Technology and Home Care Services

Another area in which home health care differs from general community health nursing home visitation is that of care involving technology. Basic community health nursing is generally very low-tech care. Home health care, on the other hand, may rely on very sophisticated technology used in the home setting. Many services and procedures that were once only available in the hospital or outpatient setting are now being provided in homes. This requires that home health nurses be knowledgeable about high-tech equipment and procedures to a greater extent than is required of most community health nurses. Some of the more common concerns, such as safety considerations in the use of oxygen in the home and the need for universal precautions in dealing with blood and body fluids, are familiar to community health nurses in general.

Disposal of hazardous wastes in the home setting is another aspect of home care that is different from that in hospital settings. For example, clients who use lancets to check daily blood sugar levels should be educated on their appropriate disposal. Other more specialized equipment, such as infusion pumps or sophisticated monitors, may be less familiar and nurses who encounter clients using these technologies will need to be familiar with them. There is also a movement toward telemedicine with extremely sophisticated monitoring capabilities that will allow more in-depth follow-up for home health clients than currently exists.

Funding Home Health and Hospice Services

Home health and hospice services may be provided by a variety of different types of agencies. The major categories of agencies are for-profit or proprietary agencies, voluntary nonprofit agencies, and government and other agencies. As noted earlier, proprietary agencies provide home health and hospice services in order to generate revenue. Nonprofit agencies may be operated by church groups or other voluntary organizations (e.g., VNAs) and are supported by philanthropic donations as well as third-party payment from insurance or government sources. Some government agencies also provide home health services (e.g., the Veteran's Administration), and services may also be reimbursed under the auspices of pension plans or other organizations. In 2000, 34% of current home care clients received care from proprietary agencies, 57% from nonprofit agencies, and 9% from government-sponsored or other agencies (NCHS, 2004a). Among hospice clients in 2000, 22% were served by proprietary agencies, 73% by nonprofit agencies, and 4.5% by government or other agencies (NCHS, 2004b).

Whatever the type of home care or hospice agency, funding for services may be derived from private health insurance, government funding through Medicare or Medicaid, or, in some cases, personal out-of-pocket payment. Most home care and hospice agencies derive their funding from all of these sources. To receive reimbursement for services under Medicare or Medicaid, however, agencies must be certified. **Certification** is a process by which an agency is judged to meet specific conditions for participation in the Medicare or Medicaid programs. For Medicare these conditions are found in the *Home Health Conditions of Participation* (Gaskell, 2003). Similar conditions must be met for Medicaid certification. Agencies must be certified separately for participation in each program, although many home health and hospice agencies are certified by both programs. Many private insurance companies also require home health and hospice agencies to meet the Medicare and Medicaid certification requirements to be eligible for reimbursement for services provided (Gaskell, 2003).

Medicare was the source of payment for services to 52% of current home health clients in 2000, and Medicaid paid for services to another 20% of clients. Another 17% of home health services were provided under private insurance funding, and 10% under other sources of funding (NCHS, 2004a). Medicare was also the primary

source of funding for 80% of hospice clients, with private insurance covering 9% of clients, Medicaid 7%, and other sources 4% (NCHS, 2004b). Other sources of funding include religious organizations, foundations, Veterans Administration contracts, pension funds, and free care (NCHS, 2004f).

From 1990 to 2001, U.S. nursing home and home care expenditures doubled, with government funds footing most of the bill. Public financing of such care in the United States and the United Kingdom is expected to increase by 20% to 21% between 2000 and 2020 and by as much as 102% in countries like Japan (Division of Adult and Community Health, 2003). Home health care expenditures by Medicare increased three times faster than all other Medicare expenditures between 1990 and 1997 and are expected to increase an average of 7.3% per year from 2001 to 2012 (Ellenbecker, 2004). In 2004, home health care accounted for 3.4% of all Medicare Part A expenditures ($5.8 billion) and 4.2% of Part B expenditures ($5.9 billion). In the same year, Medicare expenditures for hospice care accounted for 4.4% of Part A costs, for a total of $7.6 billion (NCHS, 2005b).

The Medicare home health benefit was intended to be a short-term benefit for clients in a post-acute stage of illness. Now it is being used more and more often for long-term chronic care, which necessitates more intensive care of longer duration at higher cost (Keepnews, Capitman, & Rosati, 2004).

Medicare originally funded home care services on a fee-for-service, per-visit basis. In September 2000, however, Medicare shifted home health care to a prospective payment system (PPS) based on episodic payment at predetermined rates (Anderson, Clarke, Helms, & Foreman, 2005). An episode of care includes all care provided within a 60-day period. An episode begins with the first day of care and ends with the 60th day. If care is continued for longer than 60 days, this constitutes a separate episode of care and another payment is made (Gaskell, 2003). The home health agency receives 60% of the payment at the beginning of the episode and 40% at the end. If an episode of care involves fewer than five visits, however, the agency is not given the full payment, but is given a "low utilization payment" of approximately 11% of the scheduled amount. PPS permits 10 nursing visits as well as visits by physical, occupational, speech, and respiratory therapists (Anderson et al., 2005).

The rate of payment is dependent on three variables related to the client: clinical severity (C) of the client's condition, functional status (F), and anticipated service (S) utilization. Each client is scored on these three variables at the start of care on the basis of 23 questions included in the Start of Care OASIS assessment form. OASIS stands for **Outcome and Assessment Information Set**, a system of assessment and documentation developed by the Center for Health Care Policy and Research for use in Medicare home care agencies (Gaskell, 2003). Based on the composite CSF score, the client is placed in a **home health resource group (HHRG)**, a category similar to the diagnosis-related groups (DRGs) for Medicare hospitalization reimbursement. HHRGs are used to determine the rate of pay for an episode of home health care. Within the HHRG payment, the agency must provide all needed nursing and home care visits, disposable supplies (even those not related to the home health plan of care), and any needed outpatient services provided during the episode of care. Additional payments may be made for "therapy add-ons" or physical, occupational, or speech therapy services needed by the client. Medicare may also authorize outlier payments for clients with catastrophic care needs. These payments are intended to offset the losses encountered by the agency in serving these clients, but not to pay the entire cost of their care (Gaskell, 2003).

The HHRG payment may be changed if warranted by changes in the client's condition during an episode of care. Significant changes need to be documented on the Significant Change in Condition (SCIC) assessment form and must be accompanied by appropriate changes in the physician-ordered plan of care (Gaskell, 2003).

Home health care provided under private insurance may be funded on a fee-for-service, per-visit basis or under capitation arrangements, discussed in Chapter 8∞. Managed care organizations, on the other hand, tend to fund home care services on a prospective flat-rate basis similar to Medicare (Gaskell, 2003).

In addition to the requirements for agency certification, clients who receive services reimbursed under Medicare must meet certain eligibility requirements in addition to being eligible for Social Security benefits (Gaskell, 2003). These requirements include certification of the need for care and a care plan developed by the client's physician. Periodically, this plan of care must be reviewed and updated with recertification of the need for services. In addition, eligible clients must be homebound and need at least one of the following services: intermittent skilled nursing care; physical, speech, or occupational therapy; skilled observation and assessment; and case management and evaluation. Generally speaking, clients are considered homebound if they cannot leave their homes, except for health provider visits, without great difficulty. Medicaid home care eligibility criteria vary from state to state and usually require clients to "spend down" their assets to become financially eligible for care.

Licensing of Home Health and Hospice Services

Licensure of home health and hospice agencies is state or locally controlled, depending on where the agency is located. In California, for example, licensing is a state regulatory function. Some areas require a certificate of need prior to licensing a home health agency. A **certificate of need** is a statement providing evidence of the need for home health services in that area that are not being met by existing agencies. The trend appears to be toward increasing regulation of licensure for home health agencies; thus, the reader is encouraged to seek out licensing requirements for agencies in his or her own area.

In addition to state licensure, home health agencies may choose to be accredited by the Joint Commission on Accreditation of Healthcare Organizations (JCAHO) or the Community Health Accreditation Program (CHAP). Accreditation involves meeting more rigorous standards for quality of care and performance than the minimum standards set by state and federal governments.

Standards for Home Health and Hospice Nursing

Individual home health nurses, as well as agencies, should meet established standards. The standards for home health nursing have been established by the American Nurses Association (ANA) (1999) and reflect standards of care for individual clients and standards of performance. The standards of care relate to assessment, diagnosis, outcome identification, planning, implementation, and evaluation—in other words, the use of the nursing process in the care of clients. Standards of practice relate to quality of care, performance appraisal, education, collegiality, ethics, collaboration, research, and resource utilization. Each of the standards is accompanied by designated measurement criteria. The standards for home health nursing practice are summarized on page 598. A similar set of standards for hospice and palliative nursing practice was developed by the ANA and the Hospice and Palliative Nurses Association (2002).

Terminating Home Health and Hospice Services

The community health nurse may terminate home visiting services to a particular client when the goals and objectives established for care have been accomplished, when the duration of services surpasses allowable limits, when clients refuse continued services, or when a client dies. Other possible reasons for terminating services include safety concerns for the client or nurse, noncompliance with the treatment plan, needs that go beyond the capability of the agency to meet them, institutionalization, and repeated failure to find the client at home. In many of these instances, however, services should not be terminated until reasonable efforts have been made (e.g., to promote compliance or locate the client).

Obviously, it is less stressful for the nurse to terminate services to clients who no longer require them. Even then, the intimacy of the nurse–client relationship developed over a series of encounters may make it difficult for both nurse and client to "let go." In the case of agency moratoria on additional visits, clients with yet unmet needs may feel abandoned unless the nurse has made

Standards of Care

Assessment: The home health nurse collects client health data.

Diagnosis: The home health nurse analyzes the assessment data in determining diagnoses.

Outcome identification: The home health nurse identifies expected outcomes to the client and the client's environment.

Planning: The home health nurse develops a plan of care that prescribes intervention to attain expected outcomes.

Implementation: The home health nurse implements the interventions identified in the plan of care.

Evaluation: The home health nurse evaluates the client's progress toward attainment of outcomes.

Standards of Professional Performance

Quality of care: The home health nurse systematically evaluates the quality and effectiveness of nursing practice.

Performance appraisal: The home health nurse evaluates his or her own nursing practice in relation to professional practice standards, scientific evidence, and relevant statutes and regulations.

Education: The home health nurse acquires and maintains current knowledge and competency in nursing practice.

Collegiality: The home health nurse interacts with and contributes to the professional development of peers and other health care practitioners as colleagues.

Ethics: The home health nurse's decisions and actions on behalf of clients are determined in an ethical manner.

Collaboration: The home health nurse collaborates with the client, family, and other health care practitioners in providing client care.

Research: The home health nurse uses research findings in practice.

Resource utilization: The home health nurse assists the client or family in becoming informed consumers about the risks, benefits, and cost of planning and delivering client care.

careful preparation for termination. Client refusal of services may be perceived by the nurse as a personal rejection, and the nurse will need to work through feelings of frustration and come to an acceptance of the client's decision without loss of self-esteem. Even in the case of a client's death, the nurse may find it difficult to terminate relationships developed with the client's family.

True abandonment of clients is grounds for legal action. Clients who claim abandonment, however, must be able to prove that the provider unilaterally terminated the relationship without reasonable notice when the client required further care to prevent harm. Repeated failure of the client to be home for scheduled visits can be construed as termination of the provider–client relationship by the client rather than the provider. The precise number of missed visits that constitutes termination of the relationship should be determined on the basis of consistent agency policy. In the face of repeated failures to keep appointments, the agency must notify the client of the

possible consequences of this behavior and that he or she is perceived as having terminated the relationship. In the case of exhaustion of payment limits, clients can be offered the option of continuing services on a fee-for-service basis. If the client declines services on this basis, he or she is again perceived as terminating the relationship and cannot make a claim of abandonment against the agency (Hogue, 1998). Needless to say, all of these activities by the nurse and the client's response must be accurately documented to prevent a claim of abandonment. In such cases, the legal responsibility for care of the client has been met; the nurse will need to determine whether moral and ethical responsibilities have been met prior to deciding to terminate services to a client.

Effective termination actually begins with the initial home visit. The nurse should recognize and make clients aware that the relationship is necessarily time limited. It may be helpful at the outset of the relationship to specify a predetermined period during which services will be provided. The period designated may be mandated by agency policy or by mutually determined estimates of the time needed to accomplish established goals and objectives. As time passes, the nurse may need to remind the client that the time for termination is drawing near. When the time for termination actually arrives, the nurse and client can review goal accomplishment and the nurse can provide clients with continuing needs or surviving family members of deceased clients with referrals for sources of continued assistance.

Based on 2000 data, the most recent data available at the national level, a large majority of clients receiving home health services (71.5%) were discharged into the community with their problems resolved or under control. Roughly one fifth (20.5%) of home health discharges occurred when clients were transferred to another setting, such as a hospital (13.7%) or nursing home (2.6%). A small percentage of clients (2.3%) were discharged from services because they no longer met eligibility criteria (NCHS, 2004c). Not surprisingly, 85.5% of hospice clients were discharged due to death, but 3% were discharged due to hospitalization. Another 8% of hospice clients were discharged to the community either because their conditions were stable or their care was resumed by family members (NCHS, 2004h).

Evaluating Home Health and Hospice Services

Evaluation of home visiting services must be undertaken at both aggregate and individual levels. At the individual level, evaluation would be similar to the evaluation of all home visits discussed earlier. The OASIS system promotes documentation that supports assessment of care outcomes at both individual and aggregate levels (Keepnews et al., 2004). The OASIS documentation suite includes several documents that are required of home health agencies that receive

Medicare reimbursement. Components of the suite include (a) the Start of Care OASIS, a standardized assessment form used at the initiation of care, (b) a reassessment conducted after the 55th day of care and before the 60th day if care continues into another episode, and (c) the Discharge OASIS, completed at the close of care. The Discharge OASIS documents change in the client's health status at the end of care and must be completed within 48 hours of the last visit. Three types of outcomes are possible in assessing the client's health status including improvement in aspects of their condition, a decline in status or functional ability, or stabilization at a steady state with prevention of further decline (Gaskell, 2003).

One of the functions of the OASIS documentation suite is to permit home care agencies to assess their care relative to that provided by other home care agencies. This is facilitated by several reports that are generated by the OASIS system. The first type of report is the **Outcome-Based Quality Monitoring (OBQM)** report, also known as the Adverse Event Outcome report, which provides information on the types and frequency of adverse events experienced by clients (e.g., falls, medication errors). The second type of report is the **Outcome-Based Quality Improvement (OBQI)** report, or Risk-Adjusted Patient Outcome report (Gaskell, 2003). The OBQI report permits agencies to assess the outcomes of care across clients using specific health indicators (e.g., functional status, mental and emotional health, and medical condition) and compare outcomes to those achieved by other home health agencies. Data related to several of the outcome measures (e.g., improved ambulation, medication management, pain management, and others) are available to the general public to permit them to select an effective home health care agency (Keepnews et al., 2004).

The final type of report generated by the OASIS system is the Case Mix report, which provides information on the types of clients served by the agency. The financial viability of an agency depends on maintaining an appropriate case mix of clients with extensive service needs balanced by clients with less extensive needs (Gaskell, 2003). The Case Mix report allows the agency to examine the types of clients served and to target marketing efforts to recruiting clients to achieve a more balanced case mix if needed.

Home health agencies may also choose to use the Health Plan Employer Data and Information Set as a means of evaluating care given to clients as a whole. The **Health Plan Employer Data and Information Set (HEDIS)** is another data set developed by the nonprofit National Committee for Quality Assurance (NCQA, 2005) to rate managed care organizations and to provide prospective purchasers (usually employers) with information needed to select a health care plan. HEDIS collects data on several standardized performance measures and creates a "score card" that measures eight dimensions of the organization: effectiveness of care, access/availability of care, satisfaction with care, health plan stability, use of services, cost, consumer choice, and specific health plan descriptive information. Home health organizations can use HEDIS score card information as a marketing tool if they compare favorably with other home care agencies, or they can use HEDIS information to make informed decisions about the feasibility of contracting to provide home care services to specific managed care organizations.

In addition to evaluative data provided by OASIS and HEDIS, home health agencies should also attend to clients' level of satisfaction with the care provided. Both clients and their caretakers have identified indicators of good-quality and poor-quality care. In one study, good-quality care assisted clients to maintain independence and preserved their dignity. From the perspective of caretakers, good-quality care provided respite from the burden of caregiving, decreased emotional stress, provided social support, facilitated the learning of new skills, and helped them to navigate a complex health care system. Poor-quality care, on the other hand, increased caretaker stress and prevented desired respite. Poor-quality care was the result of one of three factors: incompetence of home care providers, unreliability, and personality conflicts between provider and client (Piercy & Dunkley, 2004).

Home visits, as a form of nursing intervention, have been used by community health nurses since the early days of their practice, and home visits remain a viable alternative to other health care delivery settings. The nursing process provides a context for structuring home visits to provide health care to individuals and their families. Home visits are used as a mechanism for service delivery in home health care and in providing some hospice services.

Case Study

The Home Visit

You are a community health nurse working for the Hastings City Health Department. Your supervisor took the following request for nursing services by phone and passed it on to you because the address is part of your district. You know that this address is in an older residential area with a large Hispanic population.

Hastings City Health Department

Request for Nursing Services

Source of Request: *La Paloma Hospital Maternity Unit*

Date of Request: *7-12-06*

Client: *Maria Flores*   Date of Birth: *10-21-86*

Address: *8359 Marlboro Way, Marquette, AR 36019*

Head of Household: *Juan Flores (client's father)*

Reason for Referral: *Delivered 5 lb. 7 oz. baby boy on 7-5-06. Gestational age 32 weeks. Baby remains in NICU with RDS. Prognosis good. Client had no prenatal care. Lives with parents and 2 younger sisters (ages 8 and 13). Both parents work, but family income insufficient to pay hospital bill. Family does not have insurance. Immigration status unknown. Request home assessment prior to anticipated discharge 8-1-06.*

1. Based on the information you have, what health care needs related to the biophysical, psychological, physical environmental, sociocultural, behavioral, and health system dimensions would you identify in your preliminary assessment? List your diagnostic hypotheses.

2. What nursing interventions would you plan for the health needs you are likely to encounter in a visit to this client? Identify your planned interventions as primary, secondary, or tertiary prevention measures.

3. What supplies and materials might you need on this home visit?

4. How would you go about validating your preliminary assessment and diagnostic hypotheses? How would you include Maria in planning for the interaction? Would you include other family members? Why or why not? Would you collaborate with other health care professionals or make any referrals in meeting Maria's needs? If so, with whom would you collaborate? What referrals would you make, and why?

5. What additional assessment data would you want to obtain during your visit?

6. What evaluative criteria would you use to conduct outcome and process evaluation of care provided to this client and her family?

7. On what basis would you make the determination to terminate services to Maria?

Test Your Understanding

1. Identify the major purposes of home visiting programs. How might programs differ with respect to purpose? (pp. 577–579)

2. Identify the major emphases in planning for a home visit. Give an example of each. (pp. 583–585)

3. What are the major tasks in implementing a home visit? Give an example of the performance of each task. (pp. 585–587)

4. What are some of the distractions that may occur during a home visit? What effect(s) might these distractions have on visit outcomes? Give an example of each and describe actions by the nurse that might eliminate the distraction. (pp. 586–587)

5. Why is there a need for both long-term and short-term criteria for evaluating the effectiveness of a home visit? Give examples of the use of both types of criteria. (pp. 585, 587)

6. Describe at least three advantages of home visits as a means of providing nursing care. (pp. 589–590)

7. What are some of the challenges faced by community health nurses making home visits? What community health nursing actions might be taken to address these challenges? (pp. 590–593)

8. What is the relationship between community health nursing and home health nursing? (pp. 593–594)

9. What are some of the types of home health agencies? In what ways do they differ? (p. 594)

10. Why is collaboration particularly important in home health and hospice nursing? (p. 595)

11. How are home health services funded? (pp. 596–597)

12. What are some evaluative criteria that could be used to assess home health and hospice care at the aggregate level? Give examples of the use of these criteria. (pp. 598–599)

EXPLORE MediaLink

http://www.prenhall.com/clark

Resources for this chapter can be found on the Companion Website.

Audio Glossary

Exam Review Questions

Case Study: Home Health Nursing

MediaLink Application: Visiting Nurse Services, NYC (2 videos)

Media Links

Challenge Your Knowledge

Advocacy Interviews

References

Agency for Healthcare Research and Quality. (2001). Clinical practice guidelines online. Retrieved May 18, 2001, from http://www.ahrq.gov

Agency for Healthcare Research and Quality. (2003, May). With outpatient breast-feeding support and a home visitor program, early postpartum discharge doesn't reduce breastfeeding. *Research Activities AHRQ, 273*, p. 8.

American Nurses Association. (1999). *Scope and standards of home health nursing practice.* Silver Spring, MD: nursesbooks.org

American Nurses Association and Hospice and Palliative Nurses Association. (2002). *Scope and standards of hospice and palliative nursing practice.* Silver Spring, MD: nursesbooks.org

Anderson, M. A., Clarke, M. M., Helms, L. B., & Foreman, M. D. (2005). Hospital readmission from home health care before and after prospective payment. *Journal of Nursing Scholarship, 37*, 73–79.

Baggens, C. A. L. (2004). The institution enters the family home: Home visits in Sweden to new parents by the child health care nurse. *Journal of Community Health Nursing, 21*, 15–27.

Berg, K., Hines, M., & Allen, S. (2002). Wheelchair users at home: Few home modifications and many injurious falls. *American Journal of Public Health, 92*, 48.

Boter, H., Rinkel, G. J. E., & de Haan, R. J. (2004). Outreach nurses support after stroke: A descriptive study on patients' and carers' needs and applied nursing interventions. *Clinical Rehabilitation, 18*, 156–163.

Bryans, A. N. (2004). Examining health visiting expertise: Combining simulation, interview, and observation. *Journal of Advanced Nursing, 47*, 623–630.

Coutino, S. B., Cabral de Lira, P. I., Lima, M. D. C., & Ashworth, A. (2005). Comparison of the effect of two systems for the promotion of exclusive breastfeeding. *The Lancet, 366*, 1094–1100.

Di Napoli, A., Di Lallo, D., Fortes, C., Franceschelli, C., Armeni, E., & Guasticchi, G. (2004). Home breast-feeding support by health professionals: Findings of a randomized controlled trial in a population of Italian women. *Acta Paediatrica, 93*, 1108–1114.

Division of Adult and Community Health. (2003). Trends in aging—United States and worldwide. *Morbidity and Mortality Weekly Report, 52*, 101–106.

Division of Healthcare Quality Promotion (DHQP). (2005). *Universal precautions for prevention of transmission of HIV and other blood-borne infections.* Retrieved January 9, 2006, from http://www.cdc.gov/ncidod.dhqp/bp_universal_precautions.html

Elkan, R., Robinson, J., Williams, D., & Blair, M. (2001). Universal vs. selective services: The case of British health visiting. *Journal of Advanced Nursing, 33*, 113–119.

Ellenbecker, C. H. (2004). A theoretical model of job retention for home health care nurses. *Journal of Advanced Nursing, 47*, 303–310.

Fetrick, A., Christensen, M., & Mitchell, C. (2003). Does public health nursing home visitation make a difference in the health outcomes of pregnant clients and their offspring? *Public Health Nursing, 20*, 184–189.

Fraser, K. D., & Strang, V. (2004). Decision-making and nurse case management. *Advances in Nursing Science, 27*(1), 32–43.

Gaskell, S. M. (2003). *Home health nursing: A comprehensive review of practical and professional issues.* Brockton, MA: Western Schools.

Hahn, R. A., Biluka, O. O., Crosby, A., Fullilove, M. T., Liberman, A., Moscicki, E. K., et al. (2003). First reports evaluating the effectiveness of strategies for preventing violence: Early childhood home visitation: Findings from the Task Force on Community Preventive Services. *Morbidity and Mortality Weekly Report, 52*(RR-14), 1–9.

Hogue, E. E. (1998). Avoiding legal liability for abandonment in the environment of health care reform. In M. McHann (Ed.), *What every home health nurse needs to know 2* (pp. 125–129). Memphis: Consultants in Care.

Huang, C.-L., Wu, S.-C., Jeng, C.-Y., & Lin, L.-C. (2004). The efficacy of a home-based nursing program in diabetic control of elderly people with diabetes mellitus living alone. *Public Health Nursing, 21*, 49–56.

Jack, S. M., DiCenso, A., & Lohfeld, L. (2005). A theory of maternal engagement with public health nurses and family visitors. *Journal of Advanced Nursing, 49*, 182–190.

Kearney, M. H., York, R., & Deatrick, J. A. (2000). Effects of home visits to vulnerable young families. *Journal of Nursing Scholarship, 32*, 369–376.

Keepnews, D., Capitman, J. A., & Rosati, R. J. (2004). Measuring patient-level clinical outcomes of home health care. *Journal of Nursing Scholarship, 36*, 79–85.

Kendra, M. A., & George, V. D. (2001). Defining risk in home visiting. *Public Health Nursing, 18*, 128–137.

Kwok, T., Lum, C. M., Chan, H. S., Ma, H. M., Lee, D., & Woo, J. (2004). A randomized, controlled trial of an intensive community nurse-supported discharge program in preventing hospital readmissions of older patients with chronic lung disease. *Journal of the American Geriatrics Society, 52*, 1240–1246.

Lee, T. T., & Mills, M. E. (2000). Analysis of patient profile in predicting home care resource utilization and outcomes. *Journal of Nursing Administration, 32*(2), 67–75.

Marcinowicz, L., & Chlabicz, S. (2004). Functioning of family nursing in transition: An example of a small town in Poland. Are there any benefits for patients? *Health Expectations, 7*, 203–208.

McNaughton, D. B. (2004). Nurse home visits to maternal-child clients: A review of intervention research. *Public Health Nursing, 21*, 207–219.

Miller, T. I., Kobayashi, M. M., & Hill, P. L. (2003). Home visitation learning groups: Community based professionals discovering best practices. In D. V. Easterling, K. M. Gallagher, & D. G. Lodwick (Eds.), *Promoting health at the community level* (pp. 173–194). Thousand Oaks, CA: Sage.

Murashima, S., Nagata, S., Magilvy, J. K., Fukui, S., & Kayama, M. (2002). Home care nursing in Japan: A challenge for providing good care at home. *Public Health Nursing, 19*, 94–103.

National Center for Health Statistics. (2004a). *Current home health care patients, 2000.* Retrieved January 6, 2005, from http://www.cdc.gov/nchs/data/nhhcsd/curhomecare00.pdf

National Center for Health Statistics. (2004b). *Current hospice care patients, 2000.* Retrieved January 6, 2005, from http://www.cdc.gov/nchs/data/nhhcsd/curhospicecare00.pdf

National Center for Health Statistics. (2004c). *Home health care discharges, 2000.* Retrieved January 6, 2005, from http://www.cdc.gov/nchs/data/nhhcsd/homecaredischarges00.pdf

National Center for Health Statistics. (2004d). *Home health and hospice care data.* Retrieved January 6, 2005, from ftp://ftp.cdc.gov/pub/Health_Statistics/NCHS/Datasets/Trends/Table1HH2000.pdf

National Center for Health Statistics. (2004e). *Home health care patients: Data from the 2000 National Home and Hospice Care Survey.* Retrieved January 6, 2005, from http://www.cdc.gov/nchs/pressroom/04facts/patients.htm

National Center for Health Statistics. (2004f). *Home health definitions of terms.* Retrieved January 6, 2005, from http://www.cdc.gov/nchs/about/major/nhhcsd/nhhcsdefhome-health.htm

National Center for Health Statistics. (2004g). *Hospice care definitions of terms.* Retrieved January 9, 2006, from http://www.cdc.gov/nchs/about/major/nhhcsd/nhhcsdefhos-picecare.htm

National Center for Health Statistics. (2004h). *Hospice care discharges, 2000.* Retrieved January 6, 2005, from http://www.cdc.gov/nchs/data/nhhcsd/hospicecaredischarges00.pdf

National Center for Health Statistics. (2005a). Average length of service provided to U.S. home health-care patients by selected period—United States, 1991–2000. *Morbidity and Mortality Report, 54*, 253.

National Center for Health Statistics. (2005b). *Health, United States, 2005 with chartbook on trends in the health of Americans.* Retrieved December 23, 2005, from http://www.cdc.gov/nchs/data/hus/hus05.pdf

National Committee for Quality Assurance. (2005). *The Health Plan Employer Data and Information Set (HEDIS).* Retrieved January 10, 2006, from http://ncqa.org/Programs/HEDIS

Navaie-Waliser, M., Martin, S., Campbell, M. K., Tessaro, I., Kotelchuck, M., & Cross, A. W. (2000). Factors predicting completion of a home visitation program by high-risk pregnant women: The North Carolina Maternal Outreach Worker Program. *American Journal of Public Health, 90*, 121–124.

Nguyen, J. D., Carson, M. L., Parris, K. M., & Place, P. (2003). A comparison pilot study of public health field nursing home visitation program interventions for pregnant Hispanic adolescents. *Public Health Nursing, 20,* 412–418.

Norr, K. F., Crittenden, K. S., Lehrer, E. L., Reyes, O., Boyd, C. B., Nacion, K. W., et al. (2003). Maternal and infant outcomes at one year for a nurse-health advocate home visiting program serving African Americans and Mexican Americans. *Public Health Nursing, 30,* 190–203.

Ogata, Y., Kobayashi, Y., Fukuda, T., Mori, K., Hashimoto, M., & Otosaka, K. (2004). Measuring relative work values for home care nursing services in Japan. *Nursing Research, 53,* 145–153.

Olds, D. L., Kitzman, H., Cole, R., Robinson, J., Sidora, K., Luckey, D. W., et al. (2004). Effects of nurse home-visiting on maternal life course and child development: Age 6 follow-up results of a randomized trial. *Pediatrics, 114,* 1550–1559.

Olds, D. L., Robinson, J., Pettitt, L., Luckey, D. W., Holmberg, J., Ng, R. K., et al. (2004). Effects of home visits by paraprofessionals and by nurses: Age 4 follow-up results of a randomized trial. *Pediatrics, 114,* 1560–1568.

Paul, I. M., Phillips, T. A., Widome, M. D., & Hollenbeak, C. S. (2004). Cost-effectiveness of postnatal home nursing visits for prevention of hospital care for jaundice and dehydration. *Pediatrics, 114,* 1015–1022.

Piercy, K. W., & Dunkley, G. J. (2004). What quality paid home care means to family caregivers. *Journal of Applied Gerontology, 23,* 175–192.

Qualls, C. D., Harris, J. L., & Rogers, W. A. (2002). Cognitive-linguistic aging: Considerations for home health care environments. In W. A. Rogers & A. D. Fisk (Eds.), *Human factors interventions for the health care of older adults* (pp. 47–67). Mahwah, NJ: Lawrence Erlbaum Associates.

Smith, M. (2004). Health visiting: The public health role. *Journal of Advanced Nursing, 45,* 17–25.

Vass, M., Avlund, K., Kvist, K., Hendriksen, C., Andersen, C. K., & Keiding, N. (2004). Structured home visits to older people. Are they only of benefit for women? A randomized controlled trial. *Scandinavian Journal of Primary Health Care, 22,* 106–111.

Wager, K. A., Lee, F. W., Bradford, W. D., Jones, W., & Kilpatrick, A. O. (2004). Qualitative evaluation of South Carolina's postpartum/infant home visit program. *Public Health Nursing, 21,* 541–546.

Woodward, C. A., Abelson, J., Tedford, S., & Hutchison, B. (2004). What is important to continuity in home care? *Social Science & Medicine, 58,* 177–192.

Worobey, J., Pisuk, J., & Decker, K. (2004). Diet and behavior in at-risk children: Evaluation of an early intervention program. *Public Health Nursing, 21,* 122–127.

Care of Clients in Official and Voluntary Health Agencies

CHAPTER OBJECTIVES

After reading this chapter, you should be able to:

1. Discuss the legal and regulatory parameters of nursing in official health agencies.
2. Describe the core functions and essential services of local health departments.
3. Discuss educational preparation for nursing in official health agencies.
4. Analyze the core competencies of the public health workforce as they relate to nursing in official health agencies.
5. Analyze community nursing diagnoses as they relate to nursing in official health agencies.
6. Analyze the role of the community health nurse in carrying out the core functions and essential services in local health departments.
7. Define faith community nursing.
8. Describe the philosophy of nursing in a faith-based community.
9. Describe the scope and standards of nursing in a faith-based community.
10. Differentiate among models for nursing in a faith-based community.
11. Describe the roles and functions of community health nurses in a faith-based community.

KEY TERMS

faith community **616**
faith community nurses **617**
health ministry **616**
parish nursing **617**
public health nurse (PHN) **608**
whole person health **616**

MediaLink
http://www.prenhall.com/clark

Additional interactive resources for this chapter can be found on the Companion Website. Click on Chapter 22 and "Begin" to select the activities for this chapter.

Advocacy in Action

Connie's Dilemma

Connie, a 40-year-old recovering drug abuser, called me one day with a request. She and her fiancé, also a recovering drug abuser and the father of her baby, had been looking for a Narcotics Anonymous meeting and had been unable to find one they could attend at a convenient time for both of them. She asked if I, as parish nurse, would approach the Parish Council and present her request to start up a Narcotics Anonymous meeting on Saturday evenings in the parish hall.

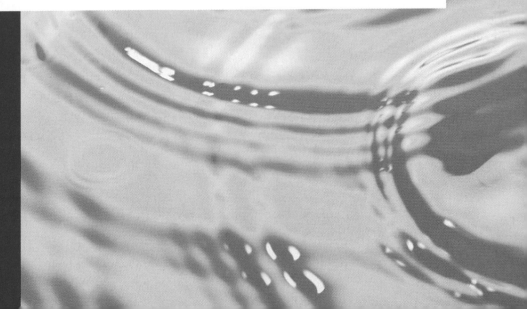

Realizing that Connie could not make the request herself and remain anonymous, I agreed to do so. However, I also realized that because of a past experience with the Youth Group, when some teens had used the parish hall for meetings that included the use of marijuana, the Parish Council would be reluctant to grant permission.

After investigating the experience of other churches that provided space, exploring the liability of the parish, and testing out the request among several members of the Parish Council, I presented Connie's request. In making the presentation, I emphasized the mission of the parish, which was to "raise the dead in spirit," provided the testimony of other pastors of churches that had Narc Anon meetings, and addressed the issue of the parish's liability. Connie's request was granted unanimously. The first Narc Anon meeting was held within a month, with 10 persons in attendance. Six months later, the number had grown to 40. Now, 8 years later, the Narc Anon meetings continue with an average attendance of 80 members. Truly, the spirits of those Narcotics Anonymous members have been raised.

Judith Mouch, MSN, MA

University of Detroit Mercy

hroughout this book, the point has been made that community health nursing focuses on the health of population groups, and that this focus, rather than the practice setting, is the core of community health nursing. In Chapter 5∞, we saw that the U.S. health care delivery system is composed of official and voluntary health agencies, both of which provide settings for the practice of community health nursing. In this chapter, we will explore exemplars of official and voluntary health agencies, the local health department and faith-based organizations, as settings for community health nursing practice. Local and state health departments and federal public health agencies are the official government agencies responsible for the overall health of the population. As we saw in Chapter 5∞, however, they are assisted in performing this responsibility by a wide variety of private-sector, nonprofit voluntary agencies and organizations. Faith communities that choose to engage in health-related ministries are a relatively new type of voluntary organization that engages in community health nursing activities.

COMMUNITY HEALTH NURSING IN AN OFFICIAL AGENCY: THE LOCAL HEALTH DEPARTMENT

Many community health nurses are employed in official health agencies, often at the local health department level. Although community health roles and functions in local health departments may vary somewhat from one jurisdiction to another, there are usually many similarities encountered in practice in these settings. In this chapter, we will examine some of those commonalities as well as some of the differences between the community health nursing role in official agencies and in voluntary organizations as exemplified by a faith-based health ministry.

Community health nursing in the United States originated in voluntary activities by nurses who were known as "public health nurses" because of their focus on the health of populations as well as of the individuals and families who comprised that population. The title *public health nurse*, or PHN, however, is now most commonly reserved for nurses who engage in public health practice within official public health agencies. This use of the title *public health nurse* is also true in other places, such as the United Kingdom (Carr & Davidson, 2004) and Ontario, Canada (Fliesser, Schofield, & Yandreski, 2003). Not all nurses who work in official public health agencies are public health nurses. Public health nurses generally have a specifically defined role related to the health of the whole population even though they may provide services to individuals and families within the population. For example, some local health departments employ public health nurses and another category of

nurses who may be called registered general nurses or clinic nurses, who may be responsible for the care of specific individuals. In Ireland, for example, public health nurses have a population focus with an emphasis on health promotion, and registered general nurses are responsible for secondary and tertiary prevention with individual clients (Clarke, 2004). Similar differentiation among nursing staff occurs in some health departments in the United States as well. For these reasons, we will use the term *public health nurse* in this chapter when referring to those community health nurses working in official health agencies whose focus of practice is the health of the entire population.

Legal and Regulatory Parameters of Public Health Nursing

Official health agencies are the only setting where community health nurses work in which many of their activities are derived from federal or state legislative mandates or local ordinances. Official agencies are charged by the particular level of government with protecting the health of the public, and public health nurses working in these agencies are actively involved in carrying out that mandate. For example, one of the functions of official public health agencies is to protect the public from communicable diseases. Under this mandate, public health nurses may investigate reports of communicable diseases. For instance, a public health nurse might conduct a followup interview of a community resident for whom a primary care provider has made a diagnosis of hepatitis A. In addition to obtaining information on the possible source of the client's infection and educating the client and family members to prevent the spread of disease, the public health nurse may be responsible for assuring that a close contact who prepares food in a local restaurant is removed from work until he or she has received hepatitis A vaccine and/or immune globulin and is determined

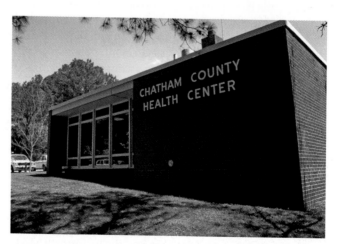

Public health nurses most often practice in official health agencies such as county health departments. (Billy E. Barnes/PhotoEdit)

to be free of disease. Similarly, public health nurses may be responsible for assuring that a chronic typhoid carrier does not work as a food handler or even provide food to groups of people (e.g., church members) on a volunteer basis.

Public health nurses are also charged with making sure that other health-related regulations are adhered to. For example, in the event of an influenza pandemic, quarantine measures may be instituted, and public health nurses may be responsible for assuring that those affected abide by quarantine restrictions. Similarly, clients with communicable tuberculosis (TB) who refuse treatment may be placed on home isolation under a judicial order. In this instance, it is often the public health nurse who makes sure that the client remains in his or her home and that only persons who have received chemoprophylaxis for TB are allowed to visit the home. Although clients must consent to treatment by public health nurses or official agencies, because of the legal mandate to protect the health of the public, failure to accept treatment for a communicable disease can result in restrictions of liberty when the appropriate court proceedings are implemented.

Public Health Functions and Essential Services in Local Health Departments

Local health department jurisdictions may include a city, a county, or a group of counties. For example, public health services for most of Los Angeles County are provided by the county department of health, but Pasadena and Long Beach, two cities within the county, have their own independent health departments. In some largely rural areas, on the other hand, one health department may provide services in several counties.

Many of the functions and activities of local health departments are mandated by state law or local ordinances. In addition to legislated functions, local health departments have primary responsibility for performance of the core functions and essential services of public health at the local level. The core functions of public health, as described in Chapter 5∞, are assessment, policy development, and assurance. These core functions were identified by the Institute of Medicine in its 1988 report, *The Future of Public Health*.

In 1994, in the context of health care reform legislation proposed by then President Clinton, a Public Health Functions Steering Committee was formed to develop a consensus on the essential elements of population-based health services. The committee was composed of representatives of the American Public Health Association (APHA), the Association of Schools of Public Health, the Association of State and Territorial Health Officials, the Environmental Council of the States, the Institute of Medicine, the National Association of County and City Health Officials, the National Association of State Alcohol and Drug Abuse Directors, the National Association of State

Mental Health Program Directors, the Public Health Foundation, and the U.S. Public Health Service. The committee identified the basic obligations of official health agencies and a set of essential services required to fulfill those obligations and accomplish the core functions of public health. The obligations identified included:

- Preventing epidemics and the spread of disease
- Protecting the public against environmental hazards
- Preventing injuries
- Promoting healthy behaviors and mental health
- Responding to disasters and aiding communities to recover from their effects
- Assuring the quality and accessibility of health services in the area (American Public Health Association, n.d.)

In meeting these obligations, official health agencies are responsible for the performance of certain essential services (National Public Health Performance Standards Program, n.d.). The core functions of public health and related essential services are presented in Table 22-1◆. The role of the public health nurse in providing these essential services is addressed later in this chapter.

Many local health departments have begun to redesign services to better address the core functions and essential services. Until recently, services were determined, in large part, by funding sources rather than the needs of the public (Avila & Smith, 2003). For example, Los Angeles County Department of Health Services has restructured its services around the essential services. The intent of the program is to protect and improve the health of the entire population while continuing to function as a safety net agency, providing services for those with no other source of care (Fielding, Luck, & Tye, 2003).

Some local health departments have used the 10 essential services to derive a system of indicators to assess the effectiveness of system performance. These indicators can be grouped as structural, process, and outcome indicators. Structural indicators address the infrastructure of the system and assess areas such as the adequacy of personnel to meet the needs of the population. Process indicators examine the ways in which services are provided, efficiency, and use of resources. Outcome indicators may address either intermediate or ultimate program outcomes. An example of an intermediate outcome might be increased immunization rates, whereas a related ultimate outcome might be decreased incidence of vaccine-preventable diseases (Derose, Asch, Fielding, & Schuster, 2003).

At the national level, the 10 essential public health services have been used to develop National Public Health Performance Standards for services provided by national, state, and local health systems (National Public Health Performance Standards Program, 2001). The performance standards include specific indicators related to each of the essential services. Local health departments may perform essential services themselves or

TABLE 22-1	Core Functions and Related Public Health Services
Core Function	**Essential Services**
Assessment	• Monitor health status to identify community health problems.
	• Diagnose and investigate health problems and health hazards in the community.
Policy development	• Inform, educate, and empower people regarding health issues.
	• Mobilize community partnerships to identify and solve health problems.
	• Develop policies and plans that support individual and community health efforts.
Assurance	• Enforce laws and regulations that protect health and ensure safety.
	• Link people to needed health care services and assure the provision of health care when otherwise unavailable.
	• Assure a competent public health and personal health workforce.
	• Evaluate effectiveness, accessibility, and quality of personal and population-based health services.
	• Research for new insights and innovative solutions to health problems.

Data from: National Public Health Performance Standards Program. (n.d.). The essential public health services. Retrieved January 16, 2006, from http://www.cdc.gov/od/nphpsp/EssentialPHServices.htm

assure that they are performed by some group or agency in the local jurisdiction (Beaulieu & Schutchfield, 2002).

Public Health Personnel

Community health nurses working in official public health agencies collaborate with a variety of people from other health-related and non-health-related disciplines. The Public Health Functions Project of the U.S. Department of Health and Human Services has recommended several specific occupational categories for public health practice. The breadth of disciplines represented will depend on the size of the public health agency, but community health nurses may encounter some or all of the disciplines included in Table 22-2◆. As noted earlier, local health departments may also employ nurses who are not public health nurses to provide care to individual clients and families that is not population-based. These nurses were not included in the occupational categories identified by the Public Health Functions project because their focus is not on the health of the overall population. For example, registered nurses, vocational nurses, or assistive personnel may work in STD clinics or in family planning, prenatal, or well-child clinics, providing services to specific clients in need of them. Health departments may also employ nurse practitioners to provide primary care services. Public health nurses may provide direct services within clinics, but they also have a broader practice mandate for addressing the overall health of the population. Public health nurses may also be responsible for supervising the practice of other nursing personnel.

Lay outreach workers or community health workers (CHWs) and volunteers are other categories of personnel that may be supervised by public health nurses. The role of community health workers in official health agencies is similar to that described in other settings in Chapter 13∞. Community health workers may be used in outreach, screening and case finding,

and health education activities. They may also assist with translation services for professional staff. Volunteers serve many of the same functions as CHWs except they are not paid personnel. For example, either CHWs or community volunteers may participate in house-to-house screening for lead exposure or to identify uninsured residents, providing them with referrals to services as needed.

In addition to supervising the activities of other nursing personnel, CHWs, and volunteers, public health nurses collaborate with other members of the public health team as well as other segments of society (e.g., residents, teachers, protective services personnel, government officials) to accomplish the core functions of public health. For example, a public health nurse might collaborate with teachers, school administrators, and health department substance abuse counselors and health educators to design a program to prevent substance use and abuse by local high school students. Local police and businesspeople who sell alcoholic beverages might also be involved in the collaborative effort. As another example, the nurse might refer a family with a rodent infestation to an environmental specialist for assistance or refer clients in need of specific services to a public health dentist or physician.

Public Health Nursing in a Local Health Department

Public health nurses are responsible for a large proportion of the essential services provided by local health departments. In the remainder of our discussion of the public health nursing role in the local official health agency, we will explore educational preparation for public health nursing, the use of nursing diagnoses in public health nursing, public health nursing as it relates to the core functions and essential services of public health agencies, and specific public health nursing roles in a local health department.

TABLE 22-2 Frequently Encountered Public Health Personnel

Occupational Category	Description
Alcohol/substance abuse counselor	Assesses and treats persons with alcohol or drug dependency problems; may engage in prevention programs
Biostatistician	Analyzes and interprets community health data
Epidemiologist	Investigates the determinants and distribution of disease, disability, and other health outcomes and develops means for prevention and control
Environmental engineer	Applies engineering principles to control, eliminate, ameliorate, and/or prevent environmental health hazards (assisted by environmental engineering technicians or technologists)
Environmental scientist/specialist	Applies biological, chemical, and public health principles to control, eliminate, ameliorate, and/or prevent environmental health hazards (assisted by environmental science technicians or technologists)
Health educator	Designs, organizes, implements, communicates advice on, and evaluates the effect of educational programs and strategies to support and modify health-related behaviors of individuals, families, organizations, and communities
Health information system specialist	Develops and maintains computer data and information systems
Health services manager/administrator	Plans, organizes, directs, controls, and/or coordinates health services, education, or policy
Mental health/substance abuse social worker	Provides services for persons having mental, emotional, or substance abuse problems
Mental health counselor	Emphasizes prevention and works with individuals and groups to promote optimal mental health; may help individuals deal with existing mental health problems
Occupational safety and health specialist	Collects data on workplace environments and exposures, implements and evaluates programs to limit chemical, physical, biological, and ergonomic risks to workers
Psychologist/mental health provider	Diagnoses and treats mental disorders by using individual, child, family, and group therapies
Public health social worker	Identifies, plans, develops, implements, and/or evaluates programs to address the social and interpersonal needs of populations
Public health attorney/ hearing officer	Advises on legal issues in enforcement of health regulations; may prosecute violation of public health regulations
Public health dentist	Provides preventive and curative dental services (assisted by public health dental workers such as dental hygienists and assistants)
Public health laboratory scientist	Develops, coordinates, and provides laboratory services; may provide oversight for regulation of laboratory practices and procedures (assisted by public health laboratory technicians or technologists)
Public health nurse	Provides nursing services to population groups, individuals, and families
Public health pharmacist	Develops and implements public policy for pharmaceuticals; may dispense pharmaceutical preparations
Public health physician	Provides preventive and curative physical health services
Public health policy analyst	Analyzes needs and plans for development of health programs, facilities, and resources; analyzes and evaluates the implications of alternative policies
Public health veterinarian	Provides preventive and curative services related to animals and control of animal diseases transmissible to people
Public health/public relations/ information/health communications/media specialist	Assists in the development and implementation of programs to communicate health-related messages

Data from: *Public Health Functions Project. (2000).* The public health workforce: An agenda for the 21st century. *Retrieved May 19, 2001, from* http://web.health.gov/phfunctions

Preparation for Public Health Nursing

When Florence Nightingale initiated the concept of public health nursing, she made it clear that this area of specialty practice required educational preparation beyond basic nursing preparation (Buhler-Wilkerson, 2001; McDonald, 2000). A similar need for postgraduate preparation for public health nursing was perceived in the United States.

Today, in some jurisdictions (e.g., California), **public health nurse (PHN)** is a legal term that designates a registered nurse who meets specific educational requirements for state certification for aggregate-level practice (including a minimum of a baccalaureate degree in nursing) (Board of Registered Nursing, 2004). Required educational preparation for PHN certification in California includes content in physical, mental, and developmental assessment; surveillance and epidemiology related to chronic and communicable diseases; health promotion and disease prevention; multicultural health care; research methodology and statistics; health education; and population-based practice. Other content requirements include legal and health care financing issues, family violence, case management, and emergency preparedness and response. In addition, public health nurses must complete a supervised clinical learning experience in public settings working with individuals, families, and communities (State of California, n.d.). Nurses with public health nurse certification in California are not restricted to employment in official public health agencies, nor do all nurses working in public health agencies have state PHN certification, as noted earlier.

Educational preparation beyond basic nursing education is required for public health nursing in other countries as well. For example, in Ireland, public health nurses must have educational preparation in general nursing, midwifery, and public health nursing and must be registered in all three areas (Clarke, 2004). Irish public health nurses must also have a minimum of 2 years of clinical nursing practice (Hanafin, Houston, & Cowley, 2002). Similarly, public health nursing practice in Finland requires a year of advanced studies in health promotion beyond the required 3 years of general nursing education (Jakonen, Tossavainen, Tupala, & Turunen, 2002). In Japan, public health nurses hold a different license from other nurses that is based on additional educational preparation and passing a national specialty examination (Yamashita, Miyaki, & Akimoto, 2005). Advanced educational preparation is also required for public health nursing in the United Kingdom (Nursing & Midwifery Council, 2004) and Manitoba, Canada (Manitoba Health, 1998).

Standards and Competencies for Public Health Nursing

Public health nurses working in local health departments should conform to the general standards and principles of community/public health nursing presented in Chapter 1∞. The standards reflect the use of the nursing process in population-based practice and are related to assessment of community health problems; diagnosis and priority setting; outcomes identification; planning, implementation, and coordination of programs and services. The standards also address the nurse's role in health education and health promotion, consultation, regulatory activities, and population health status evaluation. Additional areas of professional performance addressed by the standards include quality of practice, education, professional practice evaluation, collegiality and professional relationships, collaboration, ethics, research, resource

utilization, leadership, and advocacy on the part of community health nurses (American Nurses Association, 2007). Similar sets of standards for public and community health nursing practices have been created in other countries such as the United Kingdom (Nursing & Midwifery Council, 2004) and Canada (Community Health Nurses Association of Canada, 2003). These sets of standards have a more distinct population focus than U.S. standards and may be obtained at http://www.nmc-uk.org/AFrameDisplay.aspx?DocumentID=234 and http://www.communityhealthnursescanada.org/Standards/STandards%20Practice%20jun04.pdf, respectively.

To carry out the core functions of public health and provide the essential public health services, public health personnel, including nurses, must possess a basic set of skills. Requisite skills include research and analytic skills to collect, analyze, and interpret community health data; communication skills related to presentation, advocacy, and leadership; policy development and program planning skills; and skills derived from the basic public health sciences such as biostatistics and epidemiology. Additional skills required of those employed in public health agencies include cultural skills related to cultural competence and cultural sensitivity; financial planning and management skills such as contract negotiation and financial and organizational management skills; and skills in teaching (Public Health Functions Project, 2000). As we saw in Chapter 1∞, these basic competencies have been adapted to public health nursing in the Public Health Nursing Competencies developed by the Quad Council of Public Health Nursing Organizations (2004) and included in Appendix A∞.

Organizational Structures for Public Health Nursing

In addition to the overall redesign of health care delivery programs, some local health departments are returning public health nursing to the primary public health mission—improving the health of the entire population, with health department nurses providing primary care only as safety net agencies. For example, the Los Angeles County Department of Health Services has redesigned the public health nurse role in the agency, identifying two categories of public health nurses: district nurses and specialty program nurses. District nurses are so called because each nurse is responsible for addressing the health needs of all who reside in his or her district or assigned geographic area. District nurses are generalists educated to address a wide range of health needs across the age spectrum. Specialty program nurses, on the other hand, have special preparation in particular program areas such as tuberculosis control, maternal–child health, sexually transmitted disease control, and so on (Avila & Smith, 2003).

The intent in redesigning the public health nursing role was to accomplish three objectives:

- Movement away from a categorical focus on specific diseases and conditions to a more holistic approach

- Provision of consultation services to the community (either individuals or groups) with respect to health issues
- Participation as a service planning area team member addressing the broad spectrum of needs in the area

To this end, the district nurses have begun to conduct annual community assessments of their districts based on the 10 leading health indicators developed for the *Healthy People 2010*◆ objectives and other local health needs.

These assessments are intended to identify community assets as well as problems and provide the foundation for area health care planning (Avila & Smith, 2003). Community assessment by nurses in official public health agencies might be conducted in light of the focused assessment provided below. A complete tool to guide community assessment is included in Appendix G on the Companion Website and in the *Community Assessment Reference Guide* designed to accompany this text.

FOCUSED ASSESSMENT

Assessing Communities Using the Leading Health Indicators

Physical Activity

- What is the extent of physical activity in the community?
- What are community attitudes toward physical activity?
- What opportunities for physical activity are available for various age groups in the population?
- To what extent does the prevalence of physical disability or illness among community members influence physical activity?
- What physical environmental, socioeconomic, or cultural factors discourage physical activity in the community?
- What health effects related to lack of physical activity are prevalent in the community?

Overweight and Obesity

- What is the prevalence of overweight/obesity in the community?
- What cultural and socioeconomic factors contribute to overweight/obesity in the community?
- What resources exist for dealing with problems of overweight and obesity in the community?
- What health effects related to overweight and obesity are prevalent in the community?

Tobacco Use

- What is the extent of tobacco use in the community?
- Is tobacco advertising targeted to specific subsegments of the community?
- What legislative and regulatory factors influence tobacco use and sales in the community?
- What is the availability of tobacco use cessation assistance for people who want to quit?
- What health effects related to tobacco use are prevalent in the community?

Substance Abuse

- What is the extent of substance abuse in the community?
- In what subsegments of the population is substance abuse typically found?
- What substances are typically abused? By which subsegments of the population?
- What psychological, cultural, and socioeconomic factors influence substance abuse in the community?
- What is the availability of substance abuse treatment in the community?
- What harm-reduction strategies, if any, are in use in the community?
- What health effects related to substance abuse are prevalent in the community?

Responsible Sexual Behavior

- What is the extent of unprotected sexual activity in the community?
- What is the incidence of unwanted pregnancy in the community?
- What are the incidence and prevalence of sexually transmitted diseases (STDs) in the community?
- What is the extent of sexual activity by adolescents in the community?
- To what extent do members of the community engage in sexual activity with multiple sexual partners?
- To what extent is sexual activity by community members influenced by drug and alcohol use?
- What health services are available in the community to address pregnancy and STDs?

Mental Health

- What is the extent of mental illness in the community?
- What types of mental illness are prevalent?
- What are community attitudes toward mental health problems?
- What health services are available in the community to address mental health problems? How accessible are they to members of the population?

Injury and Violence

- What is the incidence of unintentional injury in the community? What types of injuries typically occur? What are the factors that influence the occurrence of unintentional injuries?
- What is the incidence of intentional injury resulting from violence? What types of violence are particularly prevalent in the community?
- What is the prevalence of disability as a result of accidental or intentional injury?
- What is the community attitude toward violence? What strategies are employed in the community to prevent violence?
- What services are available to address the needs of victims of intentional or unintentional injury?
- What services are available to address the needs of perpetrators of violence?

Environmental Quality

- What environmental pollutants are present in the community? What is the source of pollutants?
- What legal and regulatory factors influence environmental quality in the community?
- What health effects related to poor environmental quality are prevalent in the community?
- What other effects, if any, does the physical environment have on community health (e.g., opportunities for physical activity, safety concerns)?

Continued on next page

FOCUSED ASSESSMENT (Continued)

Immunization

- What are community immunization levels?
- What are community attitudes toward and levels of knowledge about immunizations?
- What socioeconomic or cultural factors impede immunizations?
- How available and accessible are immunization services to community members?
- What are the incidence and prevalence of immunizable diseases in the community?

Access to Care

- What proportion of the population is covered by health insurance?
- What proportion of the population has a regular source of health care?

- What is the extent of nonemergent care provided in local emergency departments?
- What proportion of the population receives preventive health services?
- To what extent do members of the population forgo health care for economic or other reasons (e.g., lack of knowledge, transportation to services, etc.)?

Other Indicators

- What other health problems are prevalent in the community (e.g., heart disease, hypertension, cancer, diabetes)?
- To what extent are these problems controlled in affected members of the community?
- What preventive activities are undertaken in the community with respect to these problems?

In the Irish public health nursing service and the British National Health System, distinctions are made between public health nurses, who have a population focus to their practice, and community health nurses, who provide more services on an individual client/family level. District nurses in Sweden are similar to those in Los Angeles County, and a similar approach is used in Finland, where public health nursing services may be based on sectoral or population-based models or a combination of both. Sectoral practice reflects a focus on a particular age group or health problem, similar to that of specialty program nurses in Los Angeles County, whereas population-based practice is similar to district nursing practice, described above (Jakonen et al., 2002). Some countries and U.S. health departments have separated services provided to specific population groups. Other countries, such as Australia, have begun to reunite functions under a generalist public health nurse role (Hanafin et al., 2002). Public health nurses working in specific jurisdictions need to become familiar with the organizational structure of public health nursing services and identify their particular role within that structure.

Nursing Diagnoses, Intervention Outcomes, and Public Health Nursing

As indicated throughout this book, community health nurses engage in the diagnostic reasoning process to develop community nursing diagnoses that are designed to direct intervention to achieve specific designated outcomes. One study of field records in one county health department found that 65 nursing diagnoses among those developed by the North American Nursing Diagnosis Association (NANDA) and 128 nursing interventions identified in the Nursing Interventions Classification (NIC) were used by public health nurses (Rivera & Parris, 2002).

Similarly, six population-based community nursing outcomes developed as part of the Nursing Outcomes Classification (NOC) have been tested for their applicability to nursing practice by public health nurses in official health agencies. The six diagnoses were (a) community competence, (b) community health status, (c) community health: immunity, (d) community risk control: chronic disease, (e) community risk control: communicable disease, and (f) community risk control: lead exposure. All of the outcomes were rated by practicing public health nurses as important and all of the outcome indicators were found to be important in assessing the achievement of outcomes. In addition, 45% of the indicators were felt to be capable of being influenced by nursing interventions, suggesting that community-level diagnoses may be useful in identifying and improving the health status of population groups (Head et al., 2004).

Public Health Nursing and Public Health Functions and Services

The efforts of public health nurses in local health departments are directed toward the accomplishment of the core public health functions and provision of the essential services outlined earlier. These efforts may be undertaken with individual clients and families as well as with population groups. With respect to the core function of assessment, for example, the public health nurse in a local health department may assess the health status of populations, target groups, families, or individuals. Similarly, he or she may recommend policy and program development to meet the needs of entire populations or subgroups of individuals and families within the population. The policy development function may also involve activities to develop standards of practice and criteria for service delivery. Finally, in relation to the assurance function, public health nurses may provide direct services to individuals and families, or evaluate the quality and effectiveness of health care services. Public health nursing roles and functions may also be examined in relation to the essential services provided by public health agencies as depicted in Table 22-3◆.

TABLE 22-3 Essential Public Health Services and Related Community Health Nursing Functions

Essential Service	Community Health Nurse Function
Monitor health status to identify community health problems.	• Conduct community assessments. • Collect data to monitor status of identified community health problems.
Diagnose and investigate health problems and health hazards in the community.	• Identify community assets and needs. • Identify factors contributing to community health problems. • Identify community health hazards and alert appropriate authorities.
Inform, educate, and empower people regarding health issues.	• Plan and implement health education programs. • Develop and disseminate health-related messages to the public. • Assist with community organization and empowerment.
Mobilize community partnerships to identify and solve health problems.	• Identify key community members. • Assist community members to articulate needs and plan to address them. • Identify potential coalition members to address particular health issues.
Develop policies and plans that support individual and community health efforts.	• Participate in community health program planning based on identified needs. • Advocate for relevant and culturally sensitive health care programs. • Advocate for involvement of community members in health program planning, implementation, and evaluation.
Enforce laws and regulations that protect health and ensure safety.	• Identify violations of health-related regulations and inform appropriate authorities. • Educate the public regarding health-related regulations.
Link people to needed health care services and assure the provision of health care when otherwise unavailable.	• Make referrals for health care services as needed. • Provide direct health care services as appropriate.
Assure a competent public health and personal health workforce.	• Assist in the education of community health nurses and other health care professionals.
Evaluate effectiveness, accessibility, and quality of personal and population-based health services.	• Participate in the planning and conduct of program evaluations to determine effectiveness, accessibility, and quality of services. • Use evaluative data to improve health care delivery.
Research for new insights and innovative solutions to health problems.	• Identify relevant research questions and participate in designing and conducting studies to answer them. • Test innovative practice models and delivery systems.

Several of the national health objectives for 2010 address the infrastructure and functions of local public health agencies (Centers for Disease Control and Prevention [CDC], 2005). These objectives can be viewed on the *Healthy People 2010*◆ Web site at http://wonder.cdc.gov/data2010. The targets for selected objectives are presented on page 613. Public health nurses may be actively involved in the accomplishment of these objectives. For example, public health nurses are the health care professionals most likely to develop and implement culturally and linguistically appropriate health promotion and disease prevention programs related to many of the health problems addressed in the objectives. Similarly, public health nurses may help to inform information systems personnel of the types of data needed in geographic information systems or assist local health authorities to develop health improvement plans that address state and national priorities.

Public Health Nursing Roles in a Local Health Department

Public health nurses working in local health departments also perform the community health nursing roles discussed in Chapter 1∞. The extent to which they engage in any one particular role, however, will depend on the focus and organizational structure of the particular health department. By virtue of their population health focus, public health nurses engage in all of the population-oriented roles. For example, community health nurses engage in the case-finding role in the context of other responsibilities. For example, a public health nurse working in a family planning clinic or making a home visit for child health may identify a woman who shows signs of intimate partner violence or notice a visitor to the home who has symptoms of tuberculosis. Similarly, public health nurses perform the leadership role in assisting community members to take action regarding a community health problem such as adolescent pregnancy or a high incidence of bicycle accidents among school-aged children. One population-oriented role that public health nurses may or may not be actively involved in is the researcher role. Even if public health nurses are not actively involved in conducting research, they will endeavor to incorporate research findings into their practice.

Delivery-oriented roles are performed by public health nurses primarily in the context of population-based delivery systems. For example, public health nurses may help develop systems that coordinate care for groups of clients with specific kinds of health problems

HEALTHY PEOPLE 2010
Goals for Population Health

OBJECTIVE	BASELINE	TARGET
7-11. Increase the number of health departments that provide access to culturally and linguistically competent health promotion and disease prevention programs related to:		
c. Cancer	30%	50%
g. Educational and community-based programs	33%	50%
h. Environmental health	22%	50%
i. Family planning	42%	50%
m. Heart disease and stroke	28%	50%
n. HIV	45%	50%
o. Immunizations and infectious diseases	48%	50%
q. Maternal and child health	47%	50%
r. Mental health	18%	50%
s. Nutrition and overweight	44%	50%
t. Occupational safety and health	13%	50%
u. Oral health	25%	50%
v. Physical activity and fitness	21%	50%
y. Sexually transmitted diseases	41%	50%
z. Substance abuse	26%	50%
aa. Tobacco use	24%	50%
23-3. Increase the proportion of local health data systems that use geocoding to promote use of geographic information systems	45%	90%
23-12. Increase the proportion of local jurisdictions that have a health improvement plan linked with their state plan	32%	80%

Data from: Centers for Disease Control and Prevention. (2005). Healthy people data. Retrieved September 6, 2005, from http://wonder/cdc.gov/data2010

Think Advocacy

Esperanza Gutierrez is a public health nurse working for the Jackson County Health Department. She is responsible for a low-income area in which many Latino clients live. Many of her clients live in apartment complexes owned by a few absentee Caucasian landlords. On several of her visits, Esperanza has noticed that the apartments are in need of repair and many are lacking smoke detectors, although they are required in rental units by state law. Others have bars on the windows that would prevent escape in case of fire. Her clients tell her that they have spoken to their landlords about repairs, but have received no response or are told to call a repairman and pay for the repairs themselves. Many of her clients speak no English and are afraid to report the safety hazards to the local housing authority for fear they will be evicted in retaliation. There are not enough rental units to meet the housing demand in the area, and apartments are often rented within a day of vacancy.

- What factors are influencing this situation?
- What action might Esperanza take to remedy the situation?
- What other segments of the county government might she involve in her efforts? What other community agencies might she involve? How might she go about obtaining their involvement?
- How might residents of the apartment complexes become involved?

requiring assistance from several health and social service sectors (e.g., those with HIV infection or pregnant adolescents). Similarly, public health nurses engage in collaboration with a wide variety of others in developing services and programs to meet the needs of population groups. They may also collaborate with others and coordinate care for individual and family clients. In the liaison role, public health nurses may serve as liaisons between community residents and other health care providers or with public officials. They may also serve a liaison function with individual clients and their families.

Some public health nurses may be involved in client-oriented community health nursing roles. Although the provision of direct care to individuals and families is receiving less emphasis in public health nursing than at some times in the past, many public health nurses still achieve population-level health outcomes in part through direct care to members of the population (Abrams, 2004). Almost all public health nurses are engaged in some manner in the educator function, and they often serve as referral resources for clients or communities in need of specific services. Many public health nurses also engage in case management for clients with long-term conditions (e.g., pregnancy, chronic illness). Table 22-4◆ compares

TABLE 22-4	Client-oriented, Delivery-oriented, and Population-oriented Community Health Nursing Roles as Performed by Public Health Nurses and Faith Community Nurses	
Role	Public Health Nurse	Faith Community Nurse
Caregiver	• Plan, implement, and evaluate care delivery systems based on assessed population needs • Sometimes provide direct care to individuals and families	• Provide direct care to individuals and families in the congregation based on needs • Sometimes plan, implement, and evaluate population-based programs to address identified needs
Educator	• Plan population-based health education programs • Occasionally provide health education to individuals and families	• Provide health education to individuals and families or groups within the congregation
Counselor	• Serve as a consultant to communities in addressing health care needs	• Assist members of the congregation with health-related decision making
Referral resource	• Refer individuals, families, and population groups to needed resources	• Refer individuals and families in the congregation to needed health and other services
Role model	• Role-model population-based practice for other health professionals and health profession students, including nursing students	• Role-model health-related behaviors for members of the congregation
Case manager	• Develop case management systems for specific groups within the population	• Provide case management services for members of the congregation
Coordinator	• Coordinate the provision of care by multiple agencies, health and social services providers, and other segments of the community	• Coordinate the activities of the faith community health ministry • Coordinate the health-related activities of volunteer members of the congregation
Collaborator	• Collaborate with broad segments of the community in developing, implementing, and evaluating health care programs based on identified population health needs	• Collaborate with other members of the ministerial team • Collaborate with health and social service providers in the community to meet the needs of specific clients
Liaison	• Assist population groups to connect with needed resources • Present the health-related needs of community members to policy makers	• Assist members of the congregation to obtain needed health care services
Case finder	• Identify trends in diseases and health problems occurring within the population	• Identify members of the congregation with specific health problems
Leader	• Assist communities in taking action to meet identified health needs	• Assist members of the congregation in taking action to meet identified health needs
Change agent	• Motivate and engineer change in health-related policies and health care delivery systems	• Assist members of the congregation to change health-related behaviors
Community mobilizer	• Organize community members to take action to address health-related concerns	• Organize members of the congregation to undertake health-related action
Coalition builder	• Develop associations with other community agencies and individuals to address identified population health needs	• Develop associations between the faith community and other community agencies and individuals to address the identified health needs of the congregation
Policy advocate	• Assist in the development of health-related policy to improve population health	• Assist in the development of health-related policies within the congregation (e.g., a ban on smoking in faith community facilities)
Social marketer	• Participate in the development of social marketing campaigns to change population health-related behaviors or attitudes or health-related policy	• Develop social marketing campaigns to change health-related behaviors or attitudes among members of the congregation
Researcher	• Possibly conduct research related to factors that influence population health or interventions that improve population health • Apply research findings to population-focused practice	• Possibly conduct research related to faith community nursing and its effectiveness • Apply research findings to faith community nursing practice

client-oriented, delivery-oriented, and population-oriented community health nursing roles as they might be executed by a public health nurse and a community health nurse employed in a faith community setting. As can be seen in the table, both public health nurses and faith community nurses are involved in similar roles and functions, but the level at which the roles are executed are quite different, with public health nurses performing roles at a broader population-based level.

The roles of public health nurses may also be examined in terms of the interventions wheel model discussed in Chapter 4∞. The 17 interventions included in the wheel can be implemented at individual-focused, community-focused, and systems-focused levels. At the individual level, the focus is on care provided to individuals and families within the population. At the community level, interventions center on changes in community norms, awareness, attitudes, and behaviors. Systems-level interventions focus on changes in organizations and health care delivery systems and structures (Keller, Strohschein, Schaffer, & Lia-Hoagberg, 2004). The utility of the interventions wheel has been tested in a health-department-based Medicaid Managed Care system. Specific interventions found to be useful in the program were outreach, individual health assessment, screening and surveillance, health education, case management, referral and follow-up, consultation, collaboration, and advocacy (Kaiser, Barry, & Kaiser, 2002). The interventions have also been successfully implemented to direct systems-level, community-level, and individual-level care in other state and local health departments (Keller et al., 2004).

Another role that is relatively unique to public health nurses in official health agencies is the development of community bioterrorism response plans. Although community health nurses in other settings are likely to be involved in developing response plans for their agencies, public health nurses are the ones most likely to participate in the development of response plans for local health departments. Bioterrorism preparedness roles for advanced-practice public health nurses could be adapted to respond to most disasters and include assessment to identify suspected bioterrorism, surveillance for bioterrorism effects, identification of desired response outcomes to a bioterrorist event, participation in the development of policies and response plans, dissemination of information to the public, referral for needed assistance in the event of bioterrorist exposures, and participation in evaluation of the effectiveness of response to a specific bioterrorist incident (Mondy, Cardenas, & Avila, 2003).

The overarching role of the public health nurse, of course, is advocating for the health of the public. Nursing advocacy in a public health setting may be somewhat more difficult than in other community health settings because nurses are functioning in a medically dominated and highly political bureaucracy in which activities are frequently mandated in response to changing political interests. In one study of a large public health agency, for example, public health nurses rated themselves as more influential in controlling their own practice than community members, but less influential than any other group of players (Falk-Rafael, 2005a). In other settings, public health nurses have been constrained by organizational structure or roles from engaging in population-based care and advocacy (Falk-Rafael, 2005b). For example, some authors have contended that failure to fund public health nursing positions on the basis of population needs rather than size has hampered the ability of public health nurses to engage in true population-based practice (Hanafin et al., 2002). Others have noted that the development of other nursing roles in public health departments that do not have a population focus has limited investment in public health nursing (Clarke, 2004). In some cases, public health nurses have themselves been reluctant to assume responsibility for population-based practice and advocacy (Carr & Davidson, 2004). Some research has found that work overload and expectations with respect to the primary care of individuals and families and lack of support has limited public health nurses' abilities to engage in population-level practice and advocacy even when these are organizational expectations. Public health nurses in one study engaged in population-based health projects on their own time and often provided for project needs from their own resources (McMurray & Cheater, 2004).

Public health nurses may need to advocate for their own ability to serve as community advocates and to protect and enhance their role in this area. They may also need to resist pressure to move away from a population focus on health promotion and illness prevention to address more categorically focused health needs (e.g., bioterrorism preparedness and disease prevention) (Falk-Rafael, 2005a). As noted by one author, "Nurses who practice at the intersection of public policy and personal lives are, therefore, ideally situated and morally obligated to include political advocacy and efforts to influence health public policy in their practice" (Falk-Rafael, 2005b, p. 212). This may mean advocating for sufficient funds to support public health nursing activity in official health agencies as well as advocacy for policies that directly affect the health of the population.

Advocacy for population health may involve empowering the communities with which public health nurses work. Community empowerment entails use of the strategies described in Chapter 13∞. One study of public health nurses in rural and urban health departments found that the nurses conceptualized empowerment as "an active, internal process of growth . . . toward actualizing one's full potential" that "occurred within the context of a nurturing nurse-client relationship" (Falk-Rafael, 2001, p. 4). The nurses also described three levels of awareness that related to empowerment of individual, family, or community clients. The first level was an awareness of one's own strengths and limitations. The second was an awareness of the right to have control over health issues and to participate in health-related decisions. The third level involved an awareness of political factors and their influence on health and health care services (Falk-Rafael, 2001). Public health nurses can work to create these levels of awareness in community members to empower them to take action with respect to community health issues.

Public health nurses may also engage in population health advocacy and community empowerment through the development of connections among three interacting levels of community: local communities, created communities, and communities of resources (Schulte, 2000). The local community is the geographic divisions of a public health jurisdiction. Created communities are groups of individuals and families connected by blood, marriage, or intended affiliations. The community of resources includes organizations developed to provide goods and services to residents in need of them. Public health nurses work to purposefully develop connections between these levels of

community. For example, they may link individual clients or families to service organizations, or coordinate the activities of several service organizations to meet the needs of the population. They may also connect several created communities to interact with service providers to design services appropriate to the needs of the population.

COMMUNITY HEALTH NURSING IN A VOLUNTARY AGENCY: A FAITH-BASED ORGANIZATION

As noted earlier, community health nursing may occur in official and voluntary agencies. According to the Public Health Nursing Section of the American Public Health Association (1996), nursing in voluntary agencies constitutes community health nursing when the focus is on the health of population groups that include both those persons who present for services and those who do not.

Health-related organizations within faith communities are a special type of voluntary health agency that present a relatively new practice setting for community health nursing. A **faith community** is "an organization of families and individuals who share common values, beliefs, religious doctrine, and faith practices that influence their lives" (Smith, 2003b). Faith communities may engage in **health ministry**, which is purposeful activity designed to help people in the congregation and surrounding community to achieve an optimal level of "whole person health" (Bay Area Health Ministries, 2001). **Whole person health** is a holistic concept that conceives of health as an integration of physical, psychological, social, and spiritual well-being (Story, 2003).

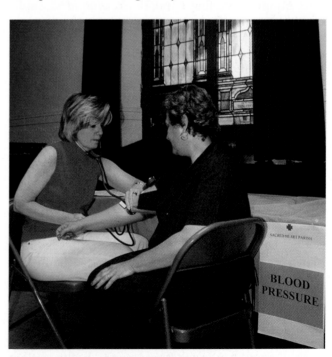

Some faith community nurses provide care to community residents as well as members of the congregation.

EVIDENCE-BASED PRACTICE

*E*vidence to support the effectiveness of public health nursing interventions is often lacking, but the Effective Public Health Practice Project of the Ontario, Canada, Ministry of Health has developed a process for systematic research reviews by which public health departments and public health nurses can create an evidence base for their practice. Elements of the process include the following:

- Formulating the question for the evidence review: Identification of the topic on which the review will center. Questions include identification of the population of interest (e.g., clients with HIV infection), an intervention (e.g., home visits), and an outcome (e.g., effects on medication compliance or symptom relief).
- Searching and retrieving relevant literature
- Establishing criteria for relevance of literature retrieved (e.g., specific types of study design, subject populations, etc.)
- Assessing the quality of relevant studies as strong, moderate, or weak, in terms of selection bias, design, control of confounding variables, blinding of participants and outcomes assessors, validity and reliability of data collection methods, and subject retention rates
- Retrieving data related to funding source, number of participants/dropouts, a description of the target populations, the intervention employed, outcomes, and the length of follow-up from studies judged to be of strong or moderate quality
- Writing a report that synthesizes the information retrieved for all studies reviewed
- Disseminating results of the review to policy makers and other appropriate personnel (Thomas, Ciliska, Dobbins, & Micucci, 2004)

Similar reviews have been undertaken by public health nursing administrators in Scotland (Elliott, Crombie, Irvine, Cantrell, & Taylor, 2004).

Identify a topic for a review of evidence that would be relevant to public health nursing practice in your own local health department. Who else might be involved in identifying appropriate topics and questions for systematic reviews?

Faith communities can provide a significant avenue for influencing the health of populations. In the United States alone, there are 265,000 to 350,000 congregations and 2,000 organized systems of religion. In addition, faith communities influence health and health care through interfaith and ecumenical systems, health institutions owned and operated by religious groups, and institutions that are strongly influenced by religious values and principles, as well as through the everyday activities of members of individual faith communities (Gunderson, 2000). For example, faith communities influence personality development and the development of health-related perspectives, motivate change in unhealthy behaviors, and convey messages of hope in adversity, promoting coping. Faith communities also influence perceptions of pain and disability, encourage caregiving and altruism, and provide a framework that gives meaning to life. Faith communities can influence health by virtue of their stability in the community and in the lives of their members, the respect with which they are viewed, their focus on respect for life and care of others, and their usual receptivity to health promotion interventions (Buijs & Olson, 2001). Faith communities may influence health through their involvement at any of three levels of health-related interventions:

- A recruitment venue for health-related activities provided by secular (nonreligious) sources
- A place for delivering health care services provided by secular agencies (by professionals or lay persons)
- Incorporation of a religious or spiritual focus into health care delivery programs (Holt, Kyles, Wiehagen, & Casey, 2003)

Many faith communities are becoming more actively involved in promoting the health of their members and engaging in activities related to this third level of involvement in health care interventions. These health promotion efforts have been found to be facilitated by the use of "parish" or faith community nurses who can integrate, coordinate, and institutionalize aspects of the faith community's health ministry in a way that is visible both to members of the congregation and to outsiders (Pattillo, Chesley, Castles, & Sutter, 2002). Multiple titles have been advanced for nurses working in this specialty area. The initial terminology, *parish nurse*, has been rejected by many people because many faith-based congregations are not organized as parishes and the term was believed to be too closely tied to certain faith traditions. Other titles used include *congregational nurse, health ministry nurse,* and *faith community nurse* (Pattillo et al., 2002). Because of its global nature and applicability to a broad array of faith traditions, the term *faith community nurse* is used in this book. Faith community nurses practice a newly recognized nursing specialty known as parish or faith community nursing. Faith community or **parish nursing** has been defined as "a health promotion, disease prevention role based on the care of the whole person . . . it is a professional model of health ministry

using a registered nurse" (Solari-Twadell, as cited in O'Brien, 2003, p. 51). Parish or **faith community nurses** are "registered nurses (RNs) with a significant personal religious history who join a church staff, either as volunteers or in paid positions, full- or part-time, and provide services that focus on the intersection of health, faith, and spirituality" (Vandecreek & Mooney, 2002, p. xviii). Faith community nurses focus on the promotion of health in the context of the faith community, building on the strengths of the congregation and providing services that are not otherwise available. They represent the concern of the congregation for members, and sometimes outsiders, who are experiencing health-related problems (Vandecreek & Mooney, 2002).

The number of nurses who function in this capacity is unknown, although the number is increasing. In one study, 57% of U.S. faith-based congregations engaged in some sort of social service programs, including those related to health. Most of these activities centered on primary prevention and health maintenance as well as specific health issues (e.g., smoking cessation, cardiovascular health, nutrition). Nearly one fourth of the programs provided services to members of the surrounding community in addition to members of the congregation (DeHaven, Hunter, Wilder, Walton, & Berry, 2004). Many of the health-related programs provided by U.S. faith communities are supported by the efforts of faith community nurses. Although the criteria for faith community nurses vary somewhat from congregation to congregation, Via Christi Regional Medical Center (n.d.) has identified some criteria that may be useful to congregations seeking to initiate a faith community nursing program. These criteria include the following:

- A registered nurse with a current license
- Willingness to participate in continuing education related to faith community nursing
- Previous clinical experience (preferably in community health, medical-surgical, emergency department, or outpatient department nursing)
- Belief in and willingness to support the healing ministry of the faith community
- Active participation in the faith community
- A holistic philosophy of health
- Expertise in communication and teaching
- Knowledge of health promotion and lifestyle modification strategies
- Familiarity with nursing and health-related issues
- Awareness of and compliance with the state nurse practice act and the nursing code of ethics
- An emphasis on confidentiality
- Ability to collaborate with the pastoral team

Historical Foundations of Nursing in a Faith-based Community

As we saw in Chapter 3∞, the early history of nursing included healthcare services provided by many religious groups. Faith community nursing traces its roots in the Christian tradition to the deaconesses of the early Christian church. The diaconal role in the early church included not only care for the sick but also the dispensing of alms, teaching, and assistance with liturgical ceremonies and is closely aligned with the modern role of the faith community nurse. The Kaiserswerth Deaconess program, established in 1836 by Theodor Fliedner and his wife Frederika Munster, was a faith-based program that significantly influenced Florence Nightingale in her contributions to modern nursing and community health nursing. The prominence of faith in health work was also seen in the writings of early nurses in the United States (O'Brien, 2003). The roots of care of the sick in parishes in the Roman Catholic tradition lie in the work of the Daughters of Charity, initiated by Vincent de Paul in 1629. The "rules" laid down for the sisters have relevance to modern faith community nursing and include the following:

- The need to be virtuous
- The need to maintain a professional relationship with the spiritual director and to avoid inappropriate relationships in an often intimate situation
- The need to be honest and direct with clients while avoiding incessant preaching
- The need to serve the whole person "so that those who die will leave the world better prepared" and to "assist those you serve to die well and those who recover to lead better lives" (Leonard, quoted in Solari-Twadell & Egenes, 2006, p. 13)
- The need to appropriately manage the nurse's time and to recruit and delegate to volunteers as appropriate
- The need for personal spiritual growth
- The need to care for family members as well as the sick individual, particularly children
- The need to recognize and adhere to the boundaries of practice
- The need to be aware of and set aside personal feelings
- The need to reject monetary gain for one's services

This last rule was not intended to imply that faith community nurses should not be paid for their services if they are employees of the congregation, but that they should direct any gifts in gratitude for services to the congregation (Solari-Twadell & Egenes, 2006).

Throughout history, there have been times of closer relationships between organized religion and public health efforts. For example, the control of tuberculosis at the close of the 19th century relied heavily on the promotion of public health messages of hygiene and sanitation by churches. Women's charitable organizations, many of them church based, supported many of the early health care services for the poor and indigent, and women as well as clergy were actively involved in campaigning for social conditions that would promote health. As public health became more of a scientific discipline dominated by physicians, however, women and the clergy were less involved in public health efforts.

Today, however, the ills that plague society are once again of interest to faith-based groups (e.g., adolescent pregnancy, substance abuse, violence), and faith communities have become more active in promoting healthy behaviors among their members (Gunderson, 2000). Public health agencies have also become more aware of the usefulness of congregations as a source of outreach and access to underserved populations (Holt et al., 2003).

The Reverend Granger W. Westberg saw congregations as playing a key role in illness prevention and in promoting whole-person health and initiated a health focus in the education of those in seminary training. He later implemented training for medical students in the connection of faith and health. In the 1960s, Rev. Granger implemented "holistic health centers," volunteer physician offices housed in church facilities that incorporated the services of a three-member team—pastor, physician, and nurse (Westberg, J., 2006).

The centers proved too costly to maintain, but they had demonstrated that the central feature in their effectiveness was the presence of nurses who spoke both the language of science and the language of faith and could translate between them (Patterson, 2003). Westberg engineered a partnership between Lutheran General Hospital and six Chicago-area churches, each with a faith community nurse, to provide health promotion services to their congregations (Palmer, 2001).

As noted earlier, the concept of faith community nursing has grown since its inception. Although begun in Christian denominations, the concept of faith community nurses has spread to Jewish and Muslim faith communities as well (Fitzgerald, 2000). In 1986, the International Parish Nurse Resource Center was established (O'Brien, 2003), and in 1992, the Interfaith Health Program of the Carter Center was initiated to help encourage best practices in faith community nursing and health ministries. Since then, a number of other organizations have been established to provide resources related to faith community nursing. In 1997, the American Nurses Association recognized faith community nursing as a distinct practice specialty (Fitzgerald, 2000), and began work with the Health Ministries Association to develop a set of standards for practice in the specialty. These standards will be addressed later in this chapter.

Philosophy of Nursing in a Faith-based Community

Faith community nursing focuses on the relationship between mind, body, and spirit in health, illness, and death. In this relationship, spirituality is recognized as a "dynamic force that nurtures and celebrates wholeness" (Swinney, Anson-Wonkka, Maki, & Corneau, 2001, p. 41) and contributes to health and a peaceful death. In the context of faith community nursing, illness is defined as "the experience of 'brokenness,' that is, the disintegration of body, mind, spirit; and disharmony with others, the environment, and God" (American Nurses Association and the Health Ministry Association, as quoted in Pattillo et al., 2002, p. 43). Faith community nursing focuses on total health and healing within the context of spiritual beliefs and values (Dryden, 2004).

The goals of faith community nursing are derived from this philosophical stance and include providing holistic care to members of the congregation and sometimes the larger community, preventing illness, and helping people obtain needed health care services. The faith community health ministry is intended to complement the health care delivery system in the larger community rather than to duplicate services (Swinney et al., 2001).

A health ministry presupposes belief that health is determined by four groups of factors—physical, mental, social, and spiritual—all of which can be modified by intervention. Four areas of interrelationship between faith and health have been identified. The first is the link between personal spirituality and healing. Scientific medicine is just beginning to explore the effect of faith on health and health outcomes. The second relationship is the link between faith structures or communities and public health, a link that is strengthened by the relationship-building efforts of faith community nurses. The third relationship deals with the changing roles and responsibilities for health activities assumed by public, private, nonprofit, and voluntary organizations. The last focus of activity lies in the changing vitality of faith structures, with greater assumption of responsibility for health ministries. This focus is exemplified by the fact that 10% to 15% of religious congregations ground their life in service to and fostering change in communities (Gunderson, 2000). Faith community nurses must themselves have an active spiritual life and must be able to incorporate spiritual interventions into their practice. Helping ability in the spiritual realm is characterized by the ability to access one's own spirituality, respect for spirituality in others, and the ability to offer spiritual as well as material resources to clients in need (Olson & Clark, 2000).

The need for spiritual care is particularly evident in times of transition. Like the types of crises discussed in Chapter 14 ∞, transitions may be developmental or situational in nature (Clark, 2000) and may give rise to a need for spiritual care as well as other interventions. Developmental transitions are expected and arise from normal growth, maturation, and change. They may be

experienced by individual members or families within the congregation or by the congregation as a whole. Marriage, death, or the birth of a child are expected transitions for individuals and families. The replacement of a pastor, priest, imam, or rabbi is an example of a developmental transition for the congregation. Situational transitions, on the other hand, are not expected and usually involve some aspect of loss. Unemployment is an example of a situational transition for an individual member of a congregation, whereas destruction of the church, synagogue, temple, or mosque imposes a situational transition on the congregation as a whole.

The foregoing underpinnings of faith community nursing can be summarized in four philosophical statements derived from the Statement of Philosophy for Parish Nursing endorsed at the First Invitational Educational Colloquium sponsored by the International Parish Nurse Resource Center (Solari-Twadell, 1999). These statements can be summarized as follows.

- Faith community nursing emphasizes the spiritual dimension but also addresses physical, psychological, sociocultural, and environmental dimensions of health.
- Faith community nursing integrates science with theology, and combines service with worship and nursing with pastoral care.
- The faith community nurse facilitates involvement of the faith community in health and healing.
- Spiritual health is central to well-being and may coexist with illness. Similarly, healing may occur in the absence of cure.

Standards and Competencies for Nursing in a Faith-based Community

As in other specialty areas of nursing practice, faith community nursing should be based on specific standards that promote effective, caring practice. The standards of practice for parish nursing summarized below were first published by the Health Ministries Association in conjunction with the American Nurses Association (ANA) in 1998. The standards of care reflect the nursing process and address assessment, diagnosis, outcome identification, planning, implementation, and evaluation. The standards of professional performance address quality of practice, education for competent practice, practice evaluation, collegiality, collaboration, ethics, research, resource utilization, and leadership similar to those put forth for community/public health nursing in general (ANA & Health Ministries Association, 2005). The standards are presented on page 620.

Competencies required of faith community nurses include the general competencies defined by the Institute of Medicine for health care professionals. These competencies include the ability to provide client-centered care, work effectively in interdisciplinary teams, engage in evidence-based practice, foster quality improvement, and effectively use information

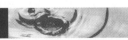

CULTURAL COMPETENCE

*R*eligious rituals are part of the cultural heritage of many faith communities. What are some of the religious rituals of your own faith community or one with which you are familiar? How might these rituals influence health? How do they differ from those of other faith communities? What role might a faith community nurse play in relation to these rituals?

SPECIAL CONSIDERATIONS

FAITH COMMUNITY NURSING: SCOPE AND STANDARDS OF PRACTICE

Standards of Practice for Faith Community Nursing

Standard 1. Assessment: The faith community nurse collects comprehensive data pertinent to the patient's wholistic health or the situation.

Standard 2. Diagnosis: The faith community nurse analyzes the wholistic assessment data to determine the diagnoses or issues.

Standard 3. Outcomes Identification: The faith community nurse identifies expected outcomes for a plan individualized to the patient or the situation.

Standard 4. Planning: The faith community nurse develops a plan that prescribes strategies and alternatives to attain expected outcomes for individuals, groups, or the faith community as a whole.

Standard 5. Implementation: The faith community nurse implements the specified plan.

> *Standard 5A. Coordination of Care:* The faith community nurse coordinates care delivery.
>
> *Standard 5B. Health Teaching and Health Promotion:* The faith community nurse employs strategies to promote wholistic health, wellness, and a safe environment.
>
> *Standard 5C. Consultation:* The faith community nurse provides consultation to facilitate understanding and influence the specified plan of care, enhance the abilities of others, and effect change.
>
> *Standard 5D. Prescriptive Authority and Treatment (Optional for appropriately prepared APRN):* The advanced practice registered nurse, faith community nurse uses prescriptive authority, procedures, referrals, treatments, and therapies in accordance with state and federal laws and regulations.

Standard 6. Evaluation: The faith community nurse evaluates progress toward attainment of outcomes.

Standards of Professional Performance for Faith Community Nursing

Standard 7. Quality of Practice: The faith community nurse systematically enhances the quality and effectiveness of faith community nursing practice.

Standard 8. Education: The faith community nurse attains knowledge and competency that reflects current nursing practice.

Standard 9. Professional Practice Evaluation: The faith community nurse evaluates one's own nursing practice in relation to professional practice standards and guidelines, relevant statutes, rules, and regulations.

Standard 10. Collegiality: The faith community nurse interacts with and contributes to the professional development of peers and colleagues.

Standard 11. Collaboration: The faith community nurse collaborates with the patient, spiritual leaders, members of the faith community, and others in the conduct of this specialized nursing practice.

Standard 12. Ethics: The faith community nurse integrates ethical provisions in all areas of practice.

Standard 13. Research: The faith community nurse integrates research findings into practice.

Standard 14. Resource Utilization: The faith community nurse considers factors related to safety, effectiveness, cost, and impact on practice in the planning and delivery of nursing services.

Standard 15. Leadership: The faith community nurse provides leadership in the professional practice setting and the profession.

Reprinted with permission from American Nurses Association & Health Ministries Association, Faith Community Nursing: Scope and Standards of Practice, © 2005. Silver Spring, MD: nursesbooks.org.

technology. Specific competencies required for faith community nursing will vary from one position to another depending on the needs of the faith community, but will generally include core competencies specific to the job description, competencies needed to address specific health issues in the congregation, age-specific competencies, and cultural competency. In addition, faith community nurses require competencies that allow them to intervene effectively in holistic care of body, mind, and spirit (Britt, 2006).

Models for Nursing in a Faith-based Community

Faith community nursing services vary greatly among faith communities, but can generally be grouped into one of several types of models or a blend of several models. The first distinction is between programs in which the faith community nurse is paid and those in which the nurse is an unpaid volunteer. In the paid model, the nurse is paid by either the faith community or by a health care organization that provides services to a faith

community. The paid employee model has the advantages of highlighting the professional nature of the health ministry and providing for a specific designated amount of time during which the faith community nurse is available. Paid professionals may also be perceived by members of the congregation as providing more confidential services than volunteer staff. In addition, employing a salaried nurse increases the potential pool of applicants for the position, allowing the congregation some choice in the selection of the nurse. Finally, having a paid position increases the visibility of the health ministry within the congregation (Patterson, 2003).

The use of volunteer faith community nurses, on the other hand, highlights the overall caregiving role of members of the congregation and usually leads to long-term commitment on the part of the nurse who is a member of the congregation. The volunteer faith community nurse is usually already known to and trusted by members of the congregation. Finally, the use of volunteers makes it easier to initiate a health ministry and results in lower costs to the faith community (Patterson, 2003). Despite these advantages, some authors have noted that the best outcomes are usually achieved with paid personnel (Dryden, 2004).

A second approach to differentiating among faith community nursing programs lies in the focus of services. This approach categorizes programs in three models: the mission-ministry model, the marketplace model, and the access model. In the mission-ministry model, the focus is on a ministry of reconciliation, health, healing, wholeness, and discipleship. The faith community nurse in this model is usually a member of the congregation. The role and scope of the nurse's practice is determined by the congregation and may encompass care to members alone or include services to the surrounding community (Smith, 2002, 2003a).

In a marketplace model, services are provided to members of a faith community by professional employees of a health care agency or organization who may or may not be members of the congregation (Smith, 2002). The role and scope of the faith community nurse are defined by the employing agency and often focus on interventions related to specific problems or issues (e.g., cardiovascular disease, smoking cessation). In this model, care is driven by economic values rather than by a value of stewardship as in the mission-ministry model (Smith, 2003a).

Access models are political in nature and focus on advocacy for underserved populations. In this model, the faith community nurse serves as a catalyst and social change agent to promote access to needed health care services either within the congregation or in the larger community (Smith, 2003a). Access models are primarily advocacy models in which the nurse functions as an advocate for the oppressed (Smith, 2002).

Faith community nurses functioning in programs based on the mission-ministry or access models may be either paid staff or volunteers. Those involved in a marketplace model are paid employees of the health system providing services.

Challenges of Nursing in a Faith-based Community

Nursing within a faith community has both advantages and disadvantages. The primary advantage lies in the congruence in belief systems of nurse and clients based on a shared faith. Faith communities also provide easy access to clients with whom the nurse may engage in health-promoting and illness-preventive behaviors. Because the nurse comes into contact with members of the faith community in realms other than those related to health, he or she has the opportunity for case finding and health promotion among people who might otherwise not encounter a health care provider. In addition, this forum for multiple interaction allows members of the congregation to get to know the nurse and develop trust in him or her.

Knowledge of members of the congregation outside the usual defined parameters of health care activities also poses some challenges in faith community nursing. For example, the nurse may have intimate knowledge of clients beyond what he or she might have in a more traditional setting. The intimacy of interaction in multiple spheres of clients' lives may make maintaining confidentiality more difficult. Members of the congregation may fear violation of confidentiality or the loss of the respect of the nurse if they disclose conditions or activities that would be frowned on by other members of the group. For example, an adolescent who believes himself to be gay may hesitate to consult the nurse if he fears her reaction based on the religious beliefs of the group.

An additional challenge in faith community nursing may involve setting parameters, particularly when the needs of the congregation exceed the time available or the role and abilities of the nurse (Carson & Koenig, 2002). Much like community health nurses in rural settings, nurses in faith communities may have difficulty maintaining boundaries and may find themselves "on call" at all times of the day or night. This may be resolved by having several nurses in the congregation who can assume responsibility for addressing members' needs, preventing overload of any one nurse.

Although most faith community nurses share the beliefs and values of the groups they serve, there may be some potential for conflict. The nurse's vision of his or her role may be different from that of the congregation or the pastoral team (Carson & Koenig, 2002). In addition, faith community nurses may find themselves in conflict with doctrinal issues that they believe are interfering with what is best for a given client. Conversely, nurses may find themselves in a position in which a particular client's actions or desires may conflict with the beliefs of the nurse and the religious group. Nurses working in faith community settings must have a highly developed personal code of ethics that will allow them to successfully resolve such conflicts. Faith community nurses may also encounter expectations from the external health care system that do not acknowledge the body-mind-spirit interface and expect the nurse to function as any other community health nurse (Carson & Koenig, 2002). Development of role clarity and clear communication of the role to others within and outside of the faith community can help the nurse to address these challenges (Solari-Twadell & McDermott, 2006a).

Faith community nurses may also encounter initial resistance to the concept of a health ministry on the part of the congregation if this is not part of their previous tradition. There may also be some feelings of jealousy on the part of other congregational staff members that requires the ability to partner without assuming responsibility for the work of others (Solari-Twadell & McDermott, 2006b). Respect for others' areas of responsibility and candid discussion of role overlap and boundaries can assist faith community nurses to deal with these responses (Hahn, Radde, & Fellers, 2002).

ETHICAL AWARENESS

You are covering the practice of a faith community nurse while she is on vacation. You are of a different religious faith than the congregation you are covering. An adolescent girl and her mother seek you out because the girl has been raped by her mother's boyfriend and is pregnant. The mother assures you she has initiated legal proceedings against the boyfriend and seems very supportive of her daughter. They are requesting a referral for abortion services. Your faith holds that abortion is never allowable, even in cases of rape. When you seek guidance from the pastor of this congregation, she suggests that abortion is probably the best option for this girl and would be supported by the tenets of their faith. What will you do?

Other challenges encountered by faith community nurses include allocating limited resources, developing and sustaining relationships with the congregation as well as with other members of the pastoral team, and accepting theological and personal differences while working collaboratively to address health problems. Developing indicators for effective practice is another challenge in faith community nursing. As with much of community health nursing focused on health promotion and illness prevention, it is difficult to document the effects of interventions. Assessing the outcomes of faith community nursing will be addressed in more detail later in this chapter. Finally, because they usually function alone within a congregation, faith community nurses may feel a sense of professional isolation (Carson & Koenig, 2002), which can be addressed by developing and sustaining a network of faith community nurses as well as by participating in organizations devoted to health ministries.

Preparation for Nursing in a Faith-based Community

As a new specialty in nursing practice, educational preparation for faith community nursing is less standardized than for other specialty areas. For example, most faith community nurses take continuing education programs of 30 or more hours related to the specialty (Dryden, 2004). As this specialty grows, education programs are likely to become more standardized. The International Parish Nurse Resource Center has developed a standardized curriculum that is used by many faith community nurse preparation programs. In 1994, the Center initiated a self-regulatory process for educational programs, developed a philosophy of parish or faith community nursing, and differentiated between basic orientation for the role and site-specific orientation to a particular faith community nurse position (McDermott & Solari-Twadell, 2006). The basic faith community nursing education program is intended to provide nurses with an understanding of the integration of faith and health, provide the knowledge and skills required for

beginning practice in this area, provide a peer support network, identify a support network for growth in the practice of faith community nursing, and foster commitment among the nurses to their own continued spiritual growth (Patterson, 2003).

In 2006, Health Ministries USA listed 20 educational programs that prepare faith community nurses. There have been some proposed curriculum changes for multiphase educational programs in this area, with phase one addressing basic role preparation, the context of faith community nursing, organization and administration of programs, and processes involved in faith community nursing. Phase two will address instruction on specific topical areas such as end-of-life care, screening, family and caregiver support, and the consultation process. Phase two will be followed by advanced workshops in areas such as teaching/learning, nutrition counseling, forgiveness facilitation, values clarification, and so on (McDermott & Solari-Twadell, 2006).

There is also movement to educate faith community nurses at the master's level in higher education institutions in nursing. The 2001 *Peterson's Guide to Nursing Programs* (Thomson Learning & American Association of Colleges of Nursing, 2001) did not list parish or faith community nursing or health ministry as an area of specialty practice within any existing graduate nursing programs. By 2006, however, a search for programs with these titles revealed eight programs in seven states and one Web-based program (All Nursing Schools, 2006).

Roles and Functions of Community Health Nurses in a Faith-based Community

The role of the faith community nurse has been described more as one of "being with" clients than of providing direct hands-on care (Carson & Koenig, 2002). The specific roles and functions of particular faith community nurses are dictated by the needs of the faith communities they serve. Because faith community nursing is an innovative field and the faith community nurse is often the only health professional present in the setting, he or she may have more latitude in defining the role than is permitted in more fully developed practice settings. In the first few years of his pilot faith community nursing project, Westberg identified five initial roles for faith community nurses: health educator, personal health counselor, referral agent, coordinator of volunteers, and developer of support groups (Westberg, G., 2006). Most authors consistently add two additional roles: integrator of faith and health and health advocate (Patterson, 2003). Solari-Twadell (2006) conducted a study of interventions from the Nursing Interventions Classification (NIC) system most commonly used by faith community nurses and found that they generally fell into six categories: basic physiologic care (e.g., exercise promotion), behavioral care (e.g., smoking cessation), safety (e.g., risk management and screening for health risks), family care (e.g., family and caregiver support), health system-related care (e.g., referral, consultation), and community care (e.g., health program development). She found that faith community nursing practice did not include hands-on care, medication management, laboratory testing, and similar interventions.

Most of the identified roles for faith community nurses are very similar to those of other community health nurses, so we will focus on a few specific elements of the role. The role of integrating faith and health is unique to faith community nursing and involves recognizing and making others aware of the connection between physical and emotional health and spiritual health (Patterson, 2003). The faith community nurse improves both physical and emotional health by intervening in the spiritual realm as well as with more mundane health care interventions. For example, the nurse might engage in prayer or other rituals as part of the healing function. In addition, faith community nurses model the integration of faith with health beliefs and behaviors.

Although the health educator role of the faith community nurse is very similar to that of all community health nurses, it may have the added feature of writing health messages for church bulletins and other publications (Dryden, 2004). Collaboration is another familiar community health nursing role that has special applications in faith community nursing. Components of the collaborative role for the faith community nurse are similar to those for all nurses: communicating effectively, developing and sustaining connections with clients and other providers, and cooperatively setting goals. The difference arises out of the number and variety of collaborative relationships in which faith community nurses engage. First and foremost, the nurse enters into a collaborative relationship with God. In addition, the nurse collaborates with a variety of individuals within and outside of the congregation. Within the congregation, the nurse must learn to collaborate effectively with pastoral staff, members of the congregation, and existing ministries, as well as with individuals and families to whom care is provided. Collaboration may also be required either within or outside the congregation with coordinators or directors of faith community nursing and with other faith community nurses. Similarly, collaboration with physicians may occur within or outside of the faith community. In addition, the faith community nurse will most likely collaborate with community agencies and possibly with schools of nursing. Finally, faith community health nurses must collaborate in larger world movements that affect the health of members of the congregation and the community at large (Blanchfield & McLaughlin, 2006). Faith community nurses may also be involved in coordination of care for individuals and families with complex needs (Dyess, 2002).

Another role function that deserves special emphasis in faith community nursing is that of working with volunteers. Health needs in all population groups, including faith communities, are usually beyond the capacity of a single person to address. Effective faith community nurses will make appropriate use of volunteer members of the congregation, but this requires skill and planning. The nurse may need to organize volunteer efforts or coordinate, and possibly redirect, existing volunteer programs to achieve desired health outcomes. Working with volunteers may require orienting them to the concept of a health ministry and training them to perform needed functions. Other components of successful volunteer programs include providing volunteers with meaningful work, sharing and confirming them in their faith, and respecting and valuing them for their contribution to the health ministry and as members of the faith community. On a more practical note, the nurse may need to ensure the availability of space for volunteer work and ceremonies that recognize their contributions (O'Brien, 2003).

Faith community nurses have a particularly important role in end-of-life care. Required competencies in this role include the ability to provide physical, emotional, and spiritual comfort; the ability to deal with one's own feelings and attitudes toward death; and the ability to assist the client, family members, colleagues, and oneself to cope with suffering, grief, loss, and bereavement. Faith community nurses working with dying clients assume the role of palliative caregivers, defined by the World Health Organization as persons who:

- Affirm life and accept death as a normal part of life
- Neither hasten nor postpone death
- Provide relief of pain and other symptoms
- Integrate psychological and spiritual care with physical care
- Support clients in their efforts to live as normally as possible for as long as possible
- Support families and others during illness and bereavement (Timms, 2003)

Because of the congruence of beliefs about death between the faith community nurse and clients and their families, faith community nurses can help to promote faith and reduce fears related to death. Because of their connections to the larger community, they can also refer clients and their families to sources of needed services in this critical time.

A final role that may be played by some faith community nurses is that of grant writing. As noted earlier, one of the challenges of faith community nursing is dealing with usually limited resources. Grant writing is one way to increase the resources available for elements of health ministries. Faith community nurses who are writing grant proposals, particularly to government agencies, should be careful, however, to assure that the requested funds are to be used for health-related purposes that do not have religious connotations. Only when the proposed use of funds does not violate the First Amendment provisions for separation of church and state can grant proposals be funded by official government agencies (Zimmerman, 2006).

Developing Faith Community Nursing Programs

Developing a faith community nursing program in a congregation would employ the principles of health program planning discussed in Chapter 15∞. Program development begins with an assessment of the health needs and resources available to the congregation. A congregational health needs assessment is also a way to introduce members of the congregation to the concept of faith community nursing and health ministry. An assessment of a faith community would employ the principles of community assessment discussed in Chapter 15∞ and might make use of the community assessment tool included in Appendix G on the Companion Website and in the *Community Assessment Reference Guide* 📄 designed to accompany this book. Some of the specific steps in initiating a program include identifying the theological foundation for a health ministry and developing an organizational structure and supervision mechanisms. The nurse and others involved in program development should delineate the long- and short-term goals of the health ministry and describe the role of the faith community nurse. Activities and qualifications of volunteer health ministers should also be identified. Practical issues in program development include finding space and funds for the program, defining lines of accountability, and dealing with possible liability issues. Finally, the planning group should develop a plan for evaluating the effectiveness of the health ministry. The focused assessment provided at right addresses some of the questions that might be asked in planning to develop a faith community nursing program.

Assessing the Outcomes of Nursing in a Faith-based Community

As with every other area of nursing practice, it is essential to evaluate the effectiveness of faith community nursing interventions. Specific outcomes to be assessed will depend on the health needs of the faith community. Possible outcomes might reflect primary, secondary, and tertiary prevention. For example, outcomes at the primary prevention level might address health risk modification (e.g., the extent of smoking cessation, improvements in home safety) or health promotion objectives (e.g., exercise participation among congregation members). Secondary prevention activities might be evaluated based on the level of control achieved in chronic diseases (e.g., hypertension control, reduced hospitalizations among diabetic members of the congregation,

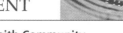

FOCUSED ASSESSMENT

Considerations in Developing a Faith Community Nursing Program

- What are the health needs of the congregation?
- What is the level of health knowledge among members of the congregation? Are there areas where health education is particularly needed?
- What are the attitudes of members of the congregation regarding health and health care services?
- Who will be the focus of care for the faith community nursing program? Members of the congregation? Others in the community? Both?
- What is the theological foundation for the faith community nursing program?
- Should the faith community nursing program employ paid staff or rely on volunteers? What qualifications should staff/volunteers have?
- What organizational structure should the program have? What should the lines of accountability and authority be?
- What are the long-term and short-term goals of the program? What kinds of services will be provided?
- Where will the program be housed? How will it be financed?
- What health-related resources are available to the faith community (e.g., expertise of members of the congregation, collaborative associations with other agencies)?
- How will the faith community deal with issues of professional liability?
- What criteria will be used to evaluate program effectiveness and how will effectiveness evaluation be conducted?

increased breast cancer screening participation), care coordination (e.g., transportation or childcare services provided), crisis intervention outcomes, and reconciliation outcomes. At the level of tertiary prevention, the effectiveness of care might be assessed in terms of improved functional status, spiritual well-being and acceptance of illness, caregiver well-being, or preparation for death. One meta analysis of studies of the effectiveness of faith-based health activities found that programs achieved a variety of significant health effects, including decreased cholesterol levels, decreased blood pressure, decreased weight, improved disease and symptom control, and increased participation in breast cancer screening activities (DeHaven et al., 2004).

BUILDING OUR KNOWLEDGE BASE

*I*n its modern form, faith community nursing is a relatively new phenomenon, and little research has been done regarding its effectiveness. How would you go about designing a study of the effectiveness of a specific faith community nursing program? Would your study be developed differently if you were looking at faith community nursing in general rather than a specific program? If so, how would it be different? What variables might you examine that would cut across faith community programs, and how would you measure them?

PUBLIC AGENCY/FAITH COMMUNITY COLLABORATION

As noted earlier, faith communities are beginning to be seen as important partners with official public health agencies in achieving core functions and essential public health services. Specific collaborative programs between faith communities and local health departments and other agencies are being developed to better meet the health care needs of the diverse populations served by each. Such collaborations can include state and local health departments, local health organizations, and colleges and universities, as well as faith communities (Pattillo et al., 2002). In 2005, U.S. President Bush established the White House Faith-based and Community Initiatives (2005) to support the work of faith-based and community organizations (FBCOs). Goals of the initiative include:

- Identifying and eliminating barriers to FBCO participation in federal grants
- Encouraging corporate and philanthropic support for social programs initiated by FBCOs
- Modifying legislation to permit charitable choice provisions that protect freedom of religion and preserve hiring rights by faith-based charities

Collaborative efforts between faith-based and official health organizations have a number of advantages, including the development of culturally specific interventions and capitalization on the strength of spiritual orientations. Such collaborations are often called faith-based initiatives and differ from faith community nursing in that they bring together faith-based communities and government agencies and funding sources and may include people of several different faiths (Kotecki, 2002).

Authors with experience in public/faith-based collaboration suggest several general considerations. The first of these is the need for a formalized structure for the initiative that includes a mission statement, goals, a statement of values, objectives, and specific activities to be undertaken to achieve the objectives (Pattillo et al., 2002). The formalized structure is best developed in written form when there are employment arrangements or liability considerations involved, when money will change hands, and when the responsibilities of collaborating partners need to be delineated. A written agreement is also beneficial when trust between collaborating partners is in the early stages of development (Zimmerman, 2006).

Other considerations in developing collaborative initiatives between faith communities and official health agencies include identifying groups and organizations that could be a part of the collaborative effort and "going where one is invited," honoring the priorities of the entities involved, finding a common language, promoting buy-in by officials and members of the faith community, addressing the concerns of the larger community in planning, supporting faith communities as co-owners of the program, and employing culturally sensitive staff (DiLeo, Graham, & Solari-Twadell, 2006). Additional recommendations include viewing the collaboration as an element of ministry in and of itself (Pattillo et al., 2002) and incorporating plans for the evaluation of the ministry with its development (DiLeo et al., 2006). One example of a collaborative effort resulted in the recruitment of more faith community nurses and increased competency among existing nurses, increased effectiveness of community resources, increased participation of academic institutions in both research and the education of faith community nurses, and increased visibility of faith community nursing programs (Pattillo et al., 2002).

In the two diverse settings presented here, the local health department and a faith community, community health nurses engage in a variety of similar tasks and functions. In the health department setting, these activities are directed toward accomplishing the three core public health functions—assessment, policy development, and assurance—as well as providing essential public health services. In the faith community setting, activities are determined by the needs of the congregation, but still encompass the aggregate focus on health and health promotion, assessing the needs of the congregation, developing policies and programs to address those needs, and assuring the provision of services through incorporation of the assets of the faith community and existing community services.

GLOBAL PERSPECTIVES

Faith community nursing in this century originated primarily as a North American innovation in nursing practice. How might this area of practice differ if carried out in another country? What effects might the presence of a national health care system have on the role of faith community nurses? How might faith community nursing differ in developed and developing nations?

Case Study

A Public Health/Faith Community Collaboration

You are a faith community nurse who has been approached by the nursing director of the local health department to solicit the participation of the faith community in an initiative to increase physical activity among youth in the larger community.

1. Is this an initiative that is likely to be congruent with the faith community's health ministry? Why or why not?
2. How might the faith community promote achievement of the objectives of the initiative?
3. What role might you, as the faith community nurse, play in this collaborative effort?
4. What criteria might be used to evaluate the effectiveness of the collaboration?

Test Your Understanding

1. How do the legal and regulatory parameters of public health nursing differ from those of community health nursing in other settings? (pp. 605–606)

2. What are the core functions and related essential public health services of official health agencies? How might public health nurses be involved in providing these essential services? (pp. 606–607, 611–616)

3. What are the core competencies of the public health workforce? How do these core competencies relate to public health nursing practice? (p. 609)

4. What are the roles and functions of public health nurses in carrying out the core functions and essential services in a local health department? (pp. 611–616)

5. What similarities and differences exist between community health nursing roles as performed in public health nursing and faith community nursing? (p. 614)

6. What are the basic philosophical tenets of faith community nursing? (pp. 618–619)

7. What is faith community nursing? How does it differ from other community health nursing practice settings? (pp. 616–617)

8. Describe the standards and competencies for faith community nursing practice. (pp. 619–620)

9. What features differentiate among the models of faith community nursing? (pp. 620–621)

10. What are the key functions of faith community nurses? Give an example of each. (pp. 622–624)

EXPLORE MediaLink

http://www.prenhall.com/clark
Resources for this chapter can be found on the Companion Website.

Audio Glossary
Appendix G: Community Health Assessment and Intervention Guide
Exam Review Questions

Case Study: A Nursing Experience in a Faith-Based Community
MediaLink Application: Nurse-Managed Services (video)

Media Links
Challenge Your Knowledge
Update Healthy People 2010
Advocacy Interviews

References

Abrams, S. E. (2004). From function to competency in public health nursing, 1931 to 2003. *Public Health Nursing, 21*, 507–510.

All Nursing Schools. (2006). *Search results for parish nursing*. Retrieved January 22, 2006, from http://allnursingschools.com

American Nurses Association. (2007). *Public health nursing: Scope and standards of practice*. Silver Spring, MD: nursesbooks.org.

American Nurses Association & Health Ministries Association. (2005). *Faith community nursing: Scope and standards of practice*. Silver Spring, MD: nursesbooks.org

American Public Health Association. (n.d.). *The essential services of public health*. Retrieved June 29, 2006, from http://www.apha.org/ppp/science/10ES.htm

Avila, M., & Smith, K. (2003). The reinvigoration of public health nursing: Methods and innovations. *Journal of Public Health Management, 9*(1), 16–24.

Bay Area Health Ministries. (2001). Promoting health and wellness in congregation and community. Retrieved May 19, 2001, from http://www.bahm.org

Beaulieu, J., & Schutchfield, D. (2002). Assessment of the validity of the National Public Health Performance Standards: The Local Public Health Performance Assessment Instrument. *Public Health Reports, 117*, 28–36.

Blanchfield, K. C., & McLaughlin, E. (2006). Parish nursing: A collaborative ministry. In P. A. Solari-Twadell & M. A. McDermott (Eds.), *Parish nursing: Development, education, and administration* (pp. 65–81). St. Louis: Mosby.

Board of Registered Nursing, State of California. (2004). *Instructions for applying for certification as a public health nurse in California*. Retrieved June 29, 2006, from http://www.rn.ca.gov/pdf/phn-app.pdf

Britt, J. (2006). Competencies for parish nursing practice. In P. A. Solari-Twadell & M. A. McDermott (Eds.), *Parish nursing: Development, education, and administration* (pp. 145–154). St. Louis: Mosby.

Buhler-Wilkerson, K. (2001). *No place like home: A history of nursing and home care in the United States*. Baltimore: Johns Hopkins University.

Buijs, R., & Olson, J. (2001). Parish nurses influencing determinants of health. *Journal of Community Health Nursing, 18*(1), 13–23.

Carr, S., & Davidson, A. (2004). Public health nursing: Developing practice. *Practice Development in Health Care, 3*, 101–112.

Carson, V. B., & Koenig, H. G. (2002). *Parish nursing: Stories of service and care*. Philadelphia: Templeton Foundation Press.

Centers for Disease Control and Prevention. (2005). *Healthy people data*. Retrieved September 6, 2005, from http://wonder/cdc.gov/data2010

Clark, M. B. (2000). Types of transitions in the lives of faith community members. In M. B. Clark & J. K. Olson (Eds.), *Nursing within a faith community: Promoting health in times of transition* (pp. 203–221). Thousand Oaks, CA: Sage.

Clarke, J. (2004). Public health in Ireland: A critical overview. *Public Health Nursing, 21*, 191–198.

Community Health Nurses Association of Canada. (2003). *Canadian community health nursing standards of practice*. Retrieved July 1, 2006, from http://www.communityhealthnurses canada.org/Standards/Standards%20Practice %20jun04.pdf

DeHaven, M. J., Hunter, I. B., Wilder, L., Walton, J. W., & Berry, J. (2004). Health programs in faith-based organizations: Are they effective? *American Journal of Public Health, 94,* 1030–1036.

Derose, S. F., Asch, S. M., Fielding, J. E., & Schuster, M. A. (2003). Developing quality indicators for local health departments. *American Journal of Preventive Medicine, 25,* 347–357.

DiLeo, J. W., Graham, C. S., & Solari-Twadell, P. A. (2006). Working with underserved congregations: A case study. In P. A. Solari-Twadell & M. A. McDermott (Eds.), *Parish nursing: Development, education, and administration* (pp. 297–304). St. Louis: Mosby.

Dryden, P. (2004). Heaven sent—Parish nurses are making a difference. Retrieved May 11, 2004, from http://www.medscape.com/viewarticle/474866

Dyess, S. M. (2002). Parish nursing. In C. C. Clark (Ed.), *Health promotion in communities: Holistic and wellness approaches* (pp. 409–417). New York: Springer.

Elliott, L., Crombie, I. K., Irvine, L., Cantrell, J., & Taylor, J. (2004). The effectiveness of public health nursing: The problems and solutions in carrying out a review of systematic reviews. *Journal of Advanced Nursing, 45,* 117–125.

Falk-Rafael, A. (2001). Empowerment as a process of evolving consciousness: A model of empowered caring. *Advances in Nursing Science, 24,* 1–16.

Falk-Rafael, A. (2005a). Advancing nursing theory through theory-guided practice: The emergency of a critical caring perspective. *Advances in Nursing Science, 28,* 38–49.

Falk-Rafael, A. (2005b). Speaking truth to power: Nursing's legacy and moral imperative. *Advances in Nursing Science, 28,* 212–223.

Fielding, J. E., Luck, J., & Tye, G. (2003). Reinvigorating public health core functions: Restructuring Los Angeles County's Public Health System. *Journal of Public Health Management, 9*(1), 7–15.

Fitzgerald, T. (2000). Body, mind, and soul: RNs reach out to the congregation through parish nursing programs. *NurseWeek, 13*(26), 16.

Fliesser, Y. L., Schofield, R., & Yandreski, C. (2003). Public health nursing: Nursing practice in a diverse environment. *RNAO Practice Page, 3*(2), 1–3.

Gunderson, G. R. (2000). Backing onto sacred ground. *Public Health Reports, 115,* 257–261.

Hahn, K., Radde, J. M., & Fellers, J. E. (2002). Spiritual care: Bridging the disciplines in congregational health ministries. In L. Vandecreek & S. Mooney (Eds.), *Parish nurses, health care chaplains, and community clergy: Navigating the maze of professional relationships* (pp. 130–141). New York: Haworth Press.

Hanafin, S., Houston, A. M., & Cowley, S. (2002). Vertical equity in service provision: A model for the Irish public health nursing service. *Journal of Advanced Nursing, 39,* 68–76.

Head, B., Aquilino, M. L., Johnson, M., Reed, D., Maas, M., & Moorhead, S. (2004). Content validity and nursing sensitivity of community-level outcomes from the nursing outcomes classification (NOC). *Journal of Nursing Scholarship, 36,* 251–259.

Health Ministries USA. (2006). *Training program resource list for parish nurses.* Retrieved January 22, 2006, from http://www.pcusa.org/health/usa/parishnursing/training.htm

Holt, C. L., Kyles, A., Wiehagen, T., & Casey, C. (2003). Development of a spiritually based breast cancer education booklet for African American Women. *Cancer Control, 10*(5), 37–44.

Institute of Medicine. (1988). *The Future of Public Health.* Washington, DC: National Academy Press.

Jakonen, S., Tossavainen, K., Tupala, M., & Turunen, H. (2002). Health and society in Finland: Public health nurses' daily practice. *British Journal of Community Nursing, 7,* 265–272.

Kaiser, M. M., Barry, T. L., & Kaiser, L. L. (2002). Using focus groups to evaluate and strengthen public health nursing population-focused interventions. *Journal of Transcultural Nursing, 13,* 303–310.

Keller, L. O., Strohschein, S., Schaffer, M. A., & Lia-Hoagberg, B. (2004). Population-based public health interventions: Innovations in practice, teaching, and management. Part II. *Public Health Nursing, 21,* 469–487.

Kotecki, C. N. (2002). Developing a health promotion program in faith-based communities. *Holistic Nursing Practice, 16*(3), 61–69.

Manitoba Health. (1998). *The role of the public health nurse within the Regional Health Authority.* Retrieved July 1, 2006, from http://www/gov/mb.ca/health/rha/rolerha.pdf

McDermott, M. A., & Solari-Twadell, P. A. (2006). Parish nursing curricula. In P. A. Solari-Twadell & M. A. McDermott (Eds.), *Parish nursing: Development, education, and administration* (pp. 121–131). St. Louis: Mosby.

McDonald, L. (2000). Florence Nightingale and the foundations of public health care, as seen through her collected works. Retrieved July 18, 2002, from http://www.sociology.uoguelph.ca/fnightingale/online_papers/dalpaper.htm

McMurray, R., & Cheater, R. (2004). Vision, permission and action: A bottom up perspective on the management of public health nursing. *Journal of Nursing Management, 12,* 43–50.

Mondy, C., Cardenas, D., & Avila, M. (2003). The role of an advanced practice public health nurse in bioterrorism preparedness. *Public Health Nursing, 20,* 422–431.

National Public Health Performance Standards Program. (n.d.). *The essential public health services.* Retrieved January 16, 2006, from http://www.cdc.gov/od/nphpsp/EssentialPHServices.htm

National Public Health Performance Standards Program. (2001). *Local public health performance standards.* Retrieved January 16, 2006, from http://www.cdc.gov/od/nphpsp/Documents/LocalModelStandardsOnly.pdf

Nursing & Midwifery Council. (2004). *Standards of proficiency for specialist community public health nurses.* Retrieved July 1, 2006, from http://www.nmc-uk.org/aFrameDisplay.aspx?DocumentID=234

O'Brien, M. E. (2003). *Parish nursing: Healthcare ministry within the church.* Sudbury, MA: Jones and Bartlett.

Olson, J. K., & Clark, M. B. (2000). Characteristics of faith community nurses. In M. B. Clark & J. K. Olson (Eds.), *Nursing within a faith community: Promoting health in times of transition* (pp. 122–140). Thousand Oaks, CA: Sage.

Palmer, J. (2001). Nursing's faith community: Parish nursing, connecting faith and health. *Reflections on Nursing LEADERSHIP, 27*(1), 17–19.

Patterson, D. L. (2003). *The essential parish nurse: ABCs for congregational health ministry.* Cleveland: Pilgrim Press.

Pattillo, M. M., Chesley, D., Castles, P., & Sutter, R. (2002). Faith community nursing: Parish nursing/health ministry collaboration model in Central Texas. *Family and Community Health, 25*(3), 41–51.

Public Health Functions Project. (2000). *The public health workforce: An agenda for the 21st century.* Retrieved May 19, 2001, from http://web.health.gov/phfunctions

Public Health Nursing Section, American Public Health Association. (1996). *The definition and role of public health nursing.* Washington, DC: Author.

Quad Council of Public Health Nursing Organizations. (2004). Public health nursing competencies. *Public Health Nursing, 21,* 443–452.

Rivera, J. C., & Parris, K. M. (2002). Use of nursing diagnoses and interventions in public health nursing practice. *Nursing Diagnosis, 13*(1), 15–22.

Schulte, J. (2000). Finding ways to create connections among communities: Partial results of an ethnography of urban public health nurses. *Public Health Nursing, 17,* 3–10.

Smith, S. D. (2002). Theoretical models of interdisciplinary relationships. In L. Vandecreek & S. Mooney (Eds.), *Parish nurses, health care chaplains, and community clergy: Navigating the maze of professional relationships* (pp. 217–226). New York: Haworth.

Smith, S. D. (2003a). Models for congregational and parish nursing programs. In S. D. Smith (Ed.), *Parish nursing: A handbook for the new millennium* (pp. 79–91). New York: Haworth Pastoral Press.

Smith, S. D. (2003b). Overview of parish nursing. In S. D. Smith (Ed.), *Parish nursing: A handbook for the new millennium* (pp. 25–35). New York: Haworth Pastoral Press.

Solari-Twadell, P. A. (1999). The emerging practice of parish nursing. In P. A. Solari-Twadell & M. A. McDermott (Eds.), *Parish nursing: Promoting whole person health within faith communities* (pp. 3–24). Thousand Oaks, CA: Sage.

Solari-Twadell, P. A. (2006). Uncovering the intricacies of the ministry of parish nursing practice through research. In P. A. Solari-Twadell & M. A. McDermott (Eds.), *Parish nursing: Development, education, and administration* (pp. 17–35). St. Louis: Mosby.

Solari-Twadell, P. A., & Egenes, K. (2006). A historical perspective of parish nursing: Rules for the sisters of the parishes. In P. A. Solari-Twadell & M. A. McDermott (Eds.), *Parish nursing: Development, education, and administration* (pp. 11–16). St. Louis: Mosby.

Solari-Twadell, P. A., & McDermott, M. A. (2006a). Challenges to the administration of the ministry of parish nursing practice. In

P. A. Solari-Twadell & M. A. McDermott (Eds.), *Parish nursing: Development, education, and administration* (pp. 227–331). St. Louis: Mosby.

Solari-Twadell, P. A., & McDermott, M. A. (2006b). Challenges to the ministry of parish nursing practice. In P. A. Solari-Twadell & M. A. McDermott (Eds.), *Parish nursing: Development, education, and administration* (pp. 103–107). St. Louis: Mosby.

State of California. (n.d.). *Title 16. California code of regulations, Division 14. Board of Registered Nursing, Article 9. Public health nurse.* Retrieved June 29, 2006, from http://www.rn.ca.gov/leg/pdf/approvedregs.pdf

Story, C. (2003). Barriers, difficulties, and challenges. In S. D. Smith (Ed.), *Parish nursing: A handbook for the new millennium* (pp. 113–128). New York: Haworth Pastoral Press.

Swinney, J., Anson-Wonkka, C., Maki, E., & Corneau, J. (2001). Community assessment: A church community and the parish nurse. *Public Health Nursing, 18,* 40–44.

Thomas, B. H., Ciliska, D., Dobbins, M., & Micucci, S. (2004). A process for systematically reviewing the literature: Providing research evidence for public health nursing interventions. *Worldviews on Evidence-based Nursing, 1,* 176–184.

Thomson Learning & American Association of Colleges of Nursing. (2001). *Peterson's guide to nursing programs* (7th ed.). Lawrenceville, NJ: Thomson Learning.

Timms, J. (2003). A role for parish nursing in end-of-life care. In S. D. Smith (Ed.), *Parish nursing: A handbook for the new millennium* (pp. 205–216). New York: Haworth Pastoral Press.

Vandecreek, L., & Mooney, S. (Eds.). (2002). *Parish nurses, health care chaplains, and community clergy: Navigating the maze of professional relationships.* New York: Haworth Press.

Via Christi Regional Medical Center, Center for Congregational Health Ministry. (n.d.). *The parish nurse.* Retrieved January 3, 2002, from http://www.via-christi.org/cchmweb... e1cd28625663900615e93!OpenDocument

Westberg, G. (2006). A personal historical perspective of whole person health and the congregation. In P. A. Solari-Twadell & M. A. McDermott (Eds.), *Parish nursing: Development, education, and administration* (pp. 5–10). St. Louis: Mosby.

Westberg, J. (2006). Introduction to: A personal historical perspective of whole person health and the congregation. In P. A. Solari-Twadell & M. A. McDermott (Eds.), *Parish nursing: Development, education, and administration* (pp. 3–5). St. Louis: Mosby.

White House Faith-based and Community Initiatives. (2005). *President Bush's faith-based and community initiative.* Retrieved January 22, 2006, from http://www.whitehouse.gov/government/fbci/overview2005.pdf

Yamashita, M., Miyaki, F., & Akimoto, R. (2005). The public health nursing role in rural Japan. *Public Health Nursing, 22,* 156–165.

Zimmerman, W. (2006). The public-private partnership: Expansion of the ministry. In P. A. Solari-Twadell & M. A. McDermott (Eds.), *Parish nursing: Development, education, and administration* (pp. 83–92). St. Louis: Mosby.

CHAPTER 23

Care of Clients in the School Setting

CHAPTER OBJECTIVES

After reading this chapter, you should be able to:

1. Identify the overall goal of a school health program.
2. Describe the components of a coordinated school health program.
3. Describe considerations in assessing biophysical, psychological, physical environmental, sociocultural, behavioral, and health system factors influencing the health of the school population.
4. Identify areas of emphasis in primary prevention in the school setting and analyze the role of the community health nurse in each.
5. Describe the facets of secondary prevention in the school setting and analyze related community health nursing roles.
6. Describe areas of emphasis in tertiary prevention in the school setting and analyze the role of the community health nurse with respect to each.

KEY TERMS

MediaLink
http://www.prenhall.com/clark

Additional interactive resources for this chapter can be found on the Companion Website. Click on Chapter 23 and "Begin" to select the activities for this chapter.

Advocacy in Action

The Missed Appointments

School-based health centers have become a common site for undergraduate public health nursing experiences. A group of students in a Midwestern city were assigned to a school-based health center to learn about population assessment and delivery of a range of health services to schoolchildren and their families. Two of the students selected children who were receiving special education as their population. Their first step was to check indicators of program success: school attendance and completed reports of special education team staffing sessions. *Staffing* refers to the collaboration of the special education team, including the parent, child, school nurse, psychologist, social worker, teacher, and other persons designated as appro-

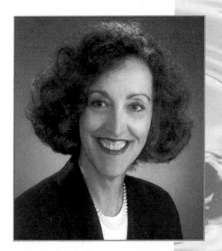

priate to meet a particular child's needs. Records of one sixth-grade child leaped out. The child had missed 16 days of school in 2 months, for an attendance rate of only 59%. On the staffing report, the nursing students noted that the mother had missed four scheduled appointments to meet with the special education team. They noted that multiple phone calls were made, but there was no answer, and finally, a note was made the week before that the phone was disconnected. A copy of a letter to the mother was enclosed, stating that the child's lack of attendance warranted a referral to the Department of Children and Family Services (DCFS).

The nursing students noted that the child's address was across the street from the school. They conferred with their clinical instructor and decided to make a home visit. The child answered the door reluctantly and, after a few moments, opened the door and showed them to a darkened bedroom. The nursing students discovered that the mother was undergoing chemotherapy, and the child was accompanying her to the hospital and then staying with her during episodes of nausea and vomiting. The mother reported that she was divorced and her two younger children were staying with relatives in another neighborhood during her treatment, but that she needed her daughter to help her manage public transportation and post-chemotherapy care.

The students reported their findings to the special education team and their instructor. After several phone calls, the students identified a local homemaker service for cancer patients and transportation services to the hospital. In addition, the special education director notified DCFS of the problem and a DCFS caseworker visited the mother to develop a plan for child-care coverage.

Without the nursing students' advocacy, expensive resources might have been spent to show that the procedure for working with families of children with special education needs was not personalized enough to "diagnose" staffing difficulties. Further, the label of "uncooperative" would have been applied to the mother.

Julia Muennich Cowell, PhD, RNC, FAAN

Professor and Chair, Community and Mental Health Nursing

Rush University Medical Center

*I*n 2003, there were more than 45 million children in elementary and secondary schools in the United States (Jones, Brenner, & McManus, 2003). This figure represents 95% of U.S. children 5 to 17 years of age (U.S. Department of Health and Human Services [USDHHS], 2003). By 2009, school enrollment in kindergarten through 12th grade is expected to increase to more than 54 million (Jones et al., 2003). These children spend a minimum of 6 hours a day in school settings year in and year out, making the school an obvious place to educate people for healthier lives (World Health Organization [WHO], 2002).

The relationship between health and education was aptly described by former U.S. Surgeon General Jocelyn Elders, who noted that "You can't educate a child who isn't healthy and you can't keep a child healthy who isn't educated" (quoted in Xu, Crane, & Ryan, 2002, p. 188). Health factors influence one's ability to learn. Education affects one's ability to engage in healthful behaviors. Schools with effective health programs can capitalize on existing resources to improve the health of the community, and school curricula, policies, and environments can promote healthy behaviors and attitudes for later life (Katz et al., 2005).

In a 2003 position statement, the National Association of School Nurses (NASN, 2003c) estimated that approximately 60,000 registered nurses provided care to more than 52 million students in public school systems. Most of these school nurses are community health nurses practicing in a specialized setting. Given their community health preparation, school nurses retain their concern for the health of the community and apply the principles of community health nursing to the needs of the overall community as well as to the needs of the school population. This multilevel focus of school nursing is reflected in the continuum of school nursing services described by Croghan, Johnson, and Aveyard (2004). The first level of services involves health promotion and illness prevention with individual students. At the second level, the nurse works with groups of students. The third level includes activities designed to affect the health of the whole school and the community, and at the fourth level, school nurses engage in public health programs related to the entire community.

The importance of the school health program as an avenue for improving the health of the population is evident in the number of national health objectives for the year 2010 that reflect health measures in schools. Of the 467 *Healthy People 2010* objectives, 107 are directed toward improving the health of young people and 21 are identified as critical (USDHHS, 2003). Several of these objectives are addressed later in this chapter, and the status of the full set of *Healthy People 2010* objectives can be reviewed at the Healthy People data site, http://wonder.cdc.gov/data2010◆. The importance of achieving these objectives is also seen in the four strategies adopted by the Division of Adolescent and School Health of the Centers for Disease Control and Prevention. These strategies include:

- Identifying and monitoring six critical risk behaviors (alcohol and drug use, injury and violence, tobacco use, nutrition, physical activity, and sexual behavior), school health policies, and programs
- Synthesizing and applying research findings to identify effective policies and procedures for promoting health in schools
- Funding programs to enable schools to implement comprehensive school health programs
- Providing technical assistance in evaluating school health programs (National Center for Chronic Disease Prevention and Health Promotion [NCCDPHP], 2005a, 2005c)

HISTORICAL PERSPECTIVES

School nursing is one of several traditional roles for community health nurses. It originated in the United States with compulsory school attendance and a concern for the number of children being excluded from school because of communicable diseases (Guttu, Engelke, & Swanson, 2004). Initial health activities in schools consisted of cursory physical inspections by physicians in New York City. Children who were found to have communicable diseases or parasitic infestations such as head lice were sent home. Because they received no treatment for their conditions, these children were excluded from school for extended periods of time and continued to serve as reservoirs of infection for friends and family members still in school. In response to this problem, Lillian Wald assigned nurses from the Henry Street Settlement to four New York City schools in a pilot project in school nursing in 1902. During that first year, the number of school exclusions declined 90%. Because of the success of the project, the New York City Board of Health hired additional nurses to continue this type of work (Kronenfeld, 2000).

School nursing in the United Kingdom actually predated development of the specialty in the United States and began in London in 1893. The focus of care, however, was essentially the same—preventing the spread of communicable diseases, improving hygiene, and decreasing truancy (Wolfe & Selekman, 2002). In 1907, the Education (Administrative Provision) Act provided a basis for disease surveillance in schools, and 1944 amendments to this British legislation mandated provision of school health services to all children. This mandate was followed in 1945 by regulations related to handicapped students. The establishment of the National Health Service (NHS) led to the separation of school health from other services and placed it under the jurisdiction of local education authorities. In 1977, however, the NHS Reorganization Act transferred responsibility for school health activities back to the NHS (Croghan et al., 2004).

The potential of schools as avenues for promoting health and dealing with social ills was recognized considerably earlier than the advent of specific health-related services in the school setting. For example, Benjamin Franklin advocated physical exercise as part of the school curriculum, and the report of the Massachusetts Sanitary Commission emphasized the importance of health education and the place of schools in providing it. In 1870, smallpox vaccination was required for school entry as a means of increasing immunization levels in the population, and in 1899 Connecticut made vision screening of schoolchildren mandatory.

In 1915, schoolchildren were enlisted as "modern health crusaders" by the National Tuberculosis Association to sell Christmas seals. This program also encouraged personal health behaviors by requiring participating children to keep a daily diary of 11 "health chores" (e.g., brushing one's teeth). Health education in schools arose from the temperance movement, which viewed schools as a vehicle for inculcating values antithetical to the use of alcohol, tobacco, and narcotics. These early attempts at promoting health education led to legislation mandating health education in schools in many states, and in 1928 the recommended health curriculum in the Sixth Yearbook of the Department of Superintendents of the National Education Association included topics such as mental, home, and sex hygiene; bodily functions as a basis for good health habits; causes of disease; nutrition; and posture (Allensworth, Lawson, Nicholson, & Wyche, 1997).

Early school nursing focused on preventing the spread of communicable disease and treating ailments related to compulsory school attendance. By the 1930s, however, the focus had shifted to preventive and promotive activities, including case finding, integration of health concepts into school curricula, and maintenance of a healthful school environment. Treatment of any health problems by the nurse was strongly discouraged to prevent infringement on the private medical sector.

School health nurses, dissatisfied with such a minimal role, continued to provide clandestine diagnostic services and treatment of minor ailments in addition to engaging in classroom teaching related to health. More recently, school nurses have begun to return to activities related to the diagnosis and treatment of health problems. Several factors account for current changes in the school nurse role. Among these is the number of families of school-age children in which both parents work. In these families, neither parent may have time to deal with their children's routine health problems. Other factors include increasing student diversity, higher incidence of mental health problems in school-aged children, lack of access to care, homelessness, and increasing use of foster care.

Mainstreaming is another major influence on the current role of school nurses in the United States.

Mainstreaming is the practice of placing children with serious illnesses or handicapping conditions in regular school settings and classrooms. The Rehabilitation Act of 1973 prohibited discrimination on the basis of disability and mandated access to public school education for children with disabilities. This requirement was expanded by the Education for All Handicapped Children Act of 1975 (PL 94–142), which mandated free and appropriate access to public education in the least restrictive environment possible, and the Individuals with Disabilities Act of 1997, which mandated access to educational opportunities for children with disabilities equal to those afforded their nondisabled age mates. A 1999 court decision further specified that school districts were responsible for providing nursing and other health services required to enable children with disabilities to effectively access educational programs (Wolfe & Selekman, 2002). Mainstreaming has created some difficulties for school health nurses. They now spend a considerable portion of their time caring for children with special needs, which may decrease the time available to meet the needs of other children in the school setting. Community health nurses in school settings may need to advocate for a balance between caring for the special-needs population and other children. They may also need to advocate for effective funding, personnel, facilities, and equipment to provide health care for children with special needs.

THE SCHOOL HEALTH PROGRAM

Health care is provided in schools for a number of reasons: the school environment itself may create hazards from which students must be protected; children need to be healthy to learn effectively; maintaining the health of children today produces healthier adults in years to come; and finally, there is a need to protect and enhance the health of the overall community. The national health objectives for 2010 reflect these points.

The overall goal of a school health program is to "ensure children reach their full academic and health potential through health promotion, protection, and surveillance activities" (Croghan & Johnson, 2004). This goal was traditionally achieved through three basic components of a school health program: health services, health instruction, and a healthy environment. More recently, other aspects of school life have also been considered integral features of a comprehensive school health program. According to the American School Health Association (2005, p. 1), a **school health program** is defined as "all the strategies, activities, and services offered by, in, or in association with schools that are designed to promote students' physical, emotional, and social development." A *coordinated school health program* incorporates the efforts of students, families, and communities to provide these strategies, activities, and services. Components of a coordinated school health program include the traditional elements of health services, health education, and a healthy environment, as well as physical education activities; nutrition services; staff health promotion; counseling and psychological services; and parent and community involvement (NCCDPHP, 2005b). Components of a coordinated school health program are depicted in Figure 23-1.

The health services component of a school health program should provide a wide variety of health care services. Health services are designed to meet the following goals:

- Appraisal, protection, and promotion of health
- Provision of access or referral to primary care services, including referral to a medical home
- Promotion of the use of primary care services
- Prevention and control of communicable diseases and other health problems
- Provision of screening and monitoring services
- Identification and resolution of student health problems
- Provision of emergency care and care in medical crises
- Promotion of sanitation and safety
- Provision of education and counseling to meet the health needs of individuals, families, and communities (American Academy of Pediatrics [AAP], 2001a; NCCDPHP, 2005b)

Broadly categorized, health services activities include assessment and screening, case finding, counseling, health promotion and illness prevention, case management, remedial or rehabilitation services, specific nursing procedures, and emergency care. Examples of activities in each of these categories are presented in Table 23-1◆.

The focus of the health education component of the school health program is educating students for health awareness and healthful behavior. Health education in the school setting focuses on both cognitive and affective learning. **Cognitive learning** involves acquisition of facts and information related to health and healthy behavior. **Affective learning**, on the other hand, refers to developing attitudes toward health and health behaviors that foster a healthy lifestyle. In the past, content areas for school-based health education included topics such as community health, consumer health, environmental health, family life, growth and development, nutrition, personal health, disease prevention and control, safety and accident prevention, and substance use and abuse. More recently, priority has been given to the six critical health behaviors identified earlier and other topics such as asthma, obesity, crisis preparedness and response, food safety, mental health, and skin cancer (NCCDPHP, 2005c).

The environmental component of the school health program includes activities directed toward improving

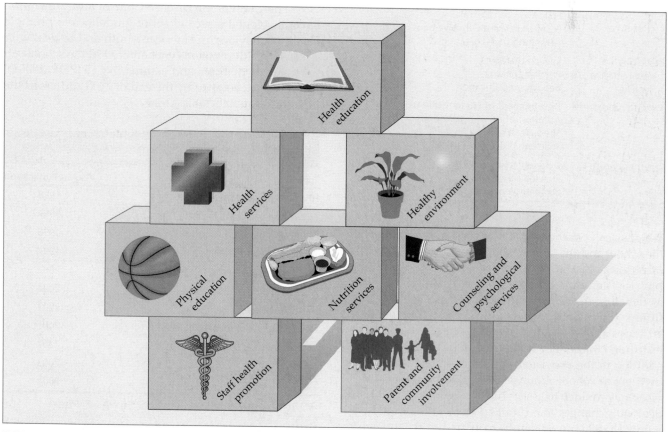

FIGURE 23-1 Components of the School Health Program

TABLE 23-1 Sample Activities Related to School Health Service Categories

School Health Service Category	Related Activities
Assessment and screening	Preschool entry assessments Transfer student health assessments Special appraisals for high-risk students or students referred by other school personnel Routine screening Home visiting for comprehensive assessment Monitoring chronic conditions and treatment effects
Case finding	Identification of communicable diseases Identification of chronic diseases Referral for diagnostic and treatment services Immunization surveillance Surveillance for selected health events
Counseling	Counseling to decrease health risks Counseling regarding existing health problems Anticipatory counseling for students, parents, staff
Health promotion/ illness prevention	Exclusion of students with communicable diseases Immunization of unimmunized students/ staff Health teaching in and outside of classrooms Health promotion activities for students/ staff (e.g., smoking cessation, weight control)
Case management	Liaison with community services Referral to outside services as needed Follow-up on referrals Fostering parental involvement Arranging transportation
Remedial/ rehabilitative services	Speech therapy Physical therapy Behavior modification
Nursing procedures	Development of student care plans Administration of medications Specialized nursing procedures Teaching procedures to other staff
Emergency care	Development of emergency protocols First aid services Postemergency assessment

The employee health component provides similar types of services for school employees in addition to assistance with physical health problems. Services to school employees serve several purposes, including reduction in illness and absenteeism, enhancement of interest in health issues and willingness to address them with students, and role-modeling healthy behaviors. The final component of the school health program is directed toward fostering partnerships among school, family, and community that enhance the health of the overall community.

STANDARDS AND GUIDELINES FOR SCHOOL HEALTH SERVICES

Three sets of standards and guidelines are helpful in planning and implementing school health services. The first set of guidelines was developed by a national task force incorporating input from several organizations concerned with the welfare of schoolchildren. This task force was spearheaded by the National Association of School Nurses and the American Academy of Pediatrics. The task force created a series of guidelines for school health services and policies linked to the *Healthy People 2010* objectives and organized around the components of a coordinated school health program (Robinson, Taras, Luckenbill, & Wheeler, 2000; Taras et al., 2004). A list of topics covered by the guidelines is available at http://www.nationalguidelines.org/toc.cfm.

The Centers for Disease Control and Prevention have developed a second set of guidelines to promote healthy behaviors in American youth and to deal with selected health problems encountered in the school setting such as diabetes and asthma (NCCDPHP, 2005d). Guidelines developed by the end of 2005 addressed the topics indicated in Table 23-2◆.

TABLE 23-2 CDC Guidelines and Strategies to Promote Healthy Behavior Among Young People

Topical Area	Year of Publication
HIV/AIDS prevention	1988
Promotion of physical activity	1997
Promotion of healthy eating	1996
Tobacco use and addiction prevention	1994
Skin cancer prevention	2002
Health, mental health, and safety	2004
Diabetes care	2003
Unintentional injury and violence prevention	2001
Asthma care	2002
Food safety	2003
Staff professional development	2002

Data from: National Center for Chronic Disease Prevention and Health Promotion. (2005). Healthy youth! School health guidelines and strategies. Retrieved February 8, 2006, from http://www.cdc.gov/HealthyYouth/ publications/guidelines.htm

the physical, psychological, and social environments of the school and the surrounding community. In the area of physical education, the emphasis is on promoting physical activity among school-age children as well as developing positive attitudes toward exercise and fitness that will continue throughout life. Positive attitudes and good food habits are also a focus of the nutrition component of the school health program in addition to the provision of healthful diets while children are at school. Counseling and psychological services are provided to assist students and their families to deal with changes and problem areas in their environments that may contribute to poor health and poor school performance.

The third set of standards relates specifically to nursing in the school setting and is contained in *School Nursing: Scope and Standards of Practice* (American Nurses Association [ANA] & NASN, 2005). The first national Standards for School Nursing Practice were published in 1983 by the American Nurses Association, the National Association of School Nurses, and the National Association of State School Nurse Consultants. The current standards for school health nursing were published in 2005 and are summarized in the Special Considerations box below. The standards for school nursing practice, like the standards for nursing practice in other specialty areas, reflect the use of the nursing process.

EDUCATIONAL PREPARATION FOR SCHOOL NURSING

Depending on the requirements of the particular jurisdiction, nurses working in school settings may have varying levels of education. In some parts of the country—for example, the Southeast—a person designated a "school nurse" may not even be a registered nurse. Because of the autonomy of nursing practice in the school setting and the complexity of the health problems addressed,

ideally the school nurse should be prepared at least at the baccalaureate level. This level of educational preparation guarantees that the nurse has the community health nursing background to deal effectively with the health needs of the school population.

In some states, employment as a school nurse requires advanced preparation beyond a baccalaureate degree in nursing. In California, for example, school nurses must complete a state-approved **school nurse credential program**. This is a nondegree program offered in an institution of higher learning that meets state requirements for educating school nurses. NASN and ANA (2001), the *Health, Mental Health and Safety Guidelines for Schools* (Taras et al., 2004), and the AAP (2001a) recommend post-baccalaureate preparation for school nursing.

Other school nurses may be prepared at the master's level in nursing. These nurses frequently function as nurse practitioners, promoting health and diagnosing and treating minor illnesses. Some, however, have advanced preparation in community health nursing and are involved in program planning rather than primary care of minor illnesses. National certification for school nursing practice is available from the National Board for the Certification of School Nurses (Taras et al., 2004).

SPECIAL CONSIDERATIONS

SCHOOL NURSING: SCOPE AND STANDARDS OF PRACTICE
Standards of Practice for School Nursing

Standard 1. Assessment: The school nurse collects comprehensive data pertinent to the client's health or the situation.

Standard 2. Diagnosis: The school nurse analyzes the assessment data to determine the diagnoses or issues.

Standard 3. Outcomes Identification: The school nurse identifies expected outcomes for a plan individualized to the client or the situation.

Standard 4. Planning: The school nurse develops a plan that prescribes strategies and alternatives to attain expected outcomes.

Standard 5. Implementation: The school nurse implements the identified plan.

> *Standard 5A. Coordination of Care:* The school nurse coordinates care delivery.

> *Standard 5B. Health Teaching and Health Promotion:* The school nurse provides health education and employs strategies to promote health and a safe environment.

> *Standard 5C. Consultation:* The school nurse provides consultation to influence the identified plan, enhance the abilities of others, and effect change.

> *Standard 5D. Prescriptive Authority and Treatment:* The advanced practice registered nurse uses prescriptive authority, procedures, referrals, treatments, and therapies in accordance with state and federal laws and regulations.

Standard 6. Evaluation: The school nurse evaluates progress towards attainment of outcomes.

Standards of Professional Performance for School Nursing

Standard 7. Quality of Practice: The school nurse systematically enhances the quality and effectiveness of nursing practice.

Standard 8. Education: The school nurse attains knowledge and competency that reflects current school nursing practice.

Standard 9. Professional Practice Evaluation: The school nurse evaluates one's own nursing practice in relation to professional practice standards and guidelines, relevant statutes, rules, and regulations.

Standard 10. Collegiality: The school nurse interacts with, and contributes to the professional development of, peers and school personnel as colleagues.

Standard 11. Collaboration: The school nurse collaborates with the client, the family, school staff, and others in the conduct of school nursing practice.

Standard 12. Ethics: The school nurse integrates ethical provisions in all areas of practice.

Standard 13. Research: The school nurse integrates research findings into practice.

Standard 14. Resource Utilization: The school nurse considers factors related to safety, effectiveness, cost, and impact on practice in the planning and delivery of school nursing services.

Standard 15. Leadership: The school nurse provides leadership in the professional practice setting and the profession.

Standard 16. Program Management: The school nurse manages school health services.

In 2003, the NASN adopted a resolution that every school district should have a full-time registered nurse in every school every day (NASN, 2003c). This recommendation is supported in the *Health, Mental Health and Safety Guidelines for Schools* and by the AAP (2001a). The *Healthy People 2010* goal is one nurse for every 750 students, but the NASN has recommended ratios of one nurse to 225 students when students with special needs are mainstreamed and one nurse to 125 severely chronically ill or disabled students (Taras et al., 2004). Unfortunately, these ratios are rarely met. In 2001, for example, 12 states mandated the presence of school nurses in public schools, but ratios ranged from one nurse to 3,000 students to one nurse per school (Domrose, 2003).

School nurses require a complex set of knowledge and skills to deal with the multiple health problems encountered in school settings. Required knowledge includes an understanding of the relationship between health and education, knowledge of normal growth and development, awareness of the standards for school nursing, and knowledge of legal issues in school health, particularly with respect to children with disabilities. Required skills include the ability to work independently in an educational setting and communicate with others as a representative of the school; case management abilities; skill in educating students, parents, and staff; skills related to complex medical and nursing procedures; and home visiting expertise (Taras et al., 2004).

THE SCHOOL HEALTH TEAM

Health problems identified in individual children or in the community served by the school are frequently beyond the capabilities of the community health nurse acting independently. To meet the needs of the school population and the community, the school health nurse often needs to participate as a member of a team.

Because identified health problems may be the consequence of factors beyond the control of health care professionals, the school health team often consists of a variety of individuals, not all of whom have a health or medical background. The team acts to design a school health program that meets the health needs of students and of the larger community.

The school health team should use the strategies discussed in Chapter 13 ∞ to create an effective team that can address the health needs of the population. One of the critical features of group development for the school health team is negotiating member roles. Group members should clarify for themselves the roles that each will play, so that infringement on anyone's professional territory is avoided.

Specific members of the team will vary with the identified needs of the population, but some of those who may be involved, in addition to the nurse, are parents, teachers, administrators, counselors, psychologists, social workers, physicians and dentists, a health coordinator, food service personnel, janitorial and secretarial staffs, public health officials and other public officials, and students. Additional team members in some school settings include nurse practitioners; unlicensed assistive personnel (UAPs); physical, occupational, and respiratory therapists; and speech pathologists. If unlicensed assistive personnel provide health services in the school setting (e.g., to assist in the care of students with special needs), the school nurse is responsible for delegating appropriate activities and supervising their performance. The school nurse may also assist in educating UAPs for activities as warranted. For example, the nurse may educate a parent volunteer about positioning a child with limited mobility to prevent pressure ulcers or suctioning a child with a tracheostomy. In educating UAPs, the school nurse would be sure to emphasize when the nurse or other provider needs to be notified of changes in a child's condition. The nurse may also educate other school personnel or volunteers in routine first aid and other simple health-related procedures (e.g., taking a temperature, assisting with height and weight screening).

Parents, of course, have the primary responsibility for the health of their children. With respect to the school health program, parents have a responsibility to reinforce health teaching at home and to follow up on referrals for assistance with health problems identified in their children. They should also provide input into the planning and evaluation of the school health program. Parents may also provide volunteer services for first aid or "sick room duty" when there is not a nurse employed full time. Community health nurses working in school settings may need to advocate for parent involvement in the development and design of school health services as well as evaluation of their effectiveness.

Teachers have a variety of responsibilities for the health of their students, such as motivating students in the development of good health habits, encouraging student responsibility for health, and observing students for signs of health problems. Teachers also have a responsibility to model healthy behavior and provide health instruction. Other responsibilities include assisting with screening efforts and measures to control the spread of disease and helping to identify factors in the physical, psychological, and social environments that are detrimental to the health status of students and coworkers. In addition, teachers may counsel students with health problems and may make referrals for assistance as appropriate.

School administrators include principals, district superintendents, and school board members. Administrators are responsible for the implementation of the school health program and should provide both material and nonmaterial support. They also function as liaisons between the school and the larger community. In collaboration with other team members, administrators participate in planning and evaluating the school health program. Other administrative responsibilities include hiring and evaluating health service employees and fostering collegial relationships among school health team members. Finally, administrators have the ultimate responsibility for the creation of a healthy and safe environment.

Some schools employ counselors, psychologists, or social workers or contract for their services as consultants. Counselors may provide emotional counseling or assistance to students in career decisions. Psychologists may also be involved in counseling for emotional problems. In addition, they may conduct psychological testing on selected youngsters to identify emotional problems or learning disabilities, or they may be called on to administer tests of school readiness to incoming children. Social workers may likewise counsel students regarding problems and may provide referrals for students and families to assist with socioeconomic problems. When the services of these specialists are not available in a particular school setting, many of these functions may be assumed by the school nurse, if he or she is educationally prepared to carry them out, or the nurse might make a referral to an outside source of assistance.

Physicians and dentists usually are not employed by a school system, but they may provide services on a contract or referral basis. Under a contractual arrangement, physicians and dentists may spend a certain amount of time in the school assessing health and dental needs or making treatment recommendations. In other instances, students may be referred to their own physicians or dentists for follow-up treatment of identified health problems. Physical, occupational, or respiratory therapists may be employed in some school systems that provide comprehensive health services or may serve as outside consultants in the care of individual children. School systems may also have similar kinds of interactions with speech pathologists.

The school nurse may function as the school's health coordinator, or the school health team may include a health coordinator who is not a nurse. The health coordinator may be a parent, teacher, or other person with some health-related preparation. Responsibilities of the health coordinator include serving as a liaison with families and with the community, arranging in-service education for staff, facilitating team relationships, and coordinating the health instruction program. Other areas of responsibility include planning for speakers on health topics, arranging health-related learning experiences such as field trips or health fairs, and reviewing materials for use in health education.

In schools where meals are provided, food service personnel are responsible for preparing and serving nutritious meals. They may also be responsible for planning menus, depending on their background and knowledge of the nutritional needs of school-age children. The school nurse may provide consultation on healthy diets appropriate to the age of children in a particular school. They may also need to advocate for the availability of foods to meet special dietary needs of children with specific health conditions (e.g., diabetes, difficulty swallowing).

The janitorial staff is usually responsible for maintenance of the physical environment. Remediation of physical health hazards usually comes under their jurisdiction as well. They also ensure the cleanliness of kitchen and sanitary facilities to prevent the transmission of disease.

Clerical personnel are responsible for maintaining student records and for processing family notification of screening test results and recommendations. They may also be responsible for notifying families in the case of student injury or illness.

Public health officials are not employed by the school, but still form part of the school health team in that they are responsible for inspection of school sanitation, cooking facilities, and immunization status. They also act to establish local health policy related to schools and other institutions and to safeguard the health of the overall community. Other public officials may also be involved in planning a school health program to meet the needs of the school's population. Fire or police personnel might be involved, for example, in designing safety education programs for children and their parents.

In older age groups, students within the school may also be part of the school health team. Student responsibilities include helping to maintain a healthful and safe environment and providing input regarding student health needs and planning to meet those needs. Older students should also be involved in evaluating the effectiveness of the school health program.

NURSING IN SCHOOL SETTINGS

NASN and ANA (2001) have defined **school nursing** as "a specialized practice of professional nursing that advances the well-being, academic success, and lifelong achievement of students" (p. 1). Depending on the needs of the school, school district, and community, the roles of community health nurses serving in schools may vary widely. Studies in the United Kingdom have noted a move away from screening and surveillance activities to a broader focus on health promotion, and have identified several common areas of practice. These include promoting a healthy lifestyle, addressing mental health needs, dealing with chronic health problems, and meeting the needs of particularly vulnerable children (Humphries, 2002). In other studies, school nurses in the UK have been found to be involved primarily in health needs assessment, sexual health activities, and parental support (Croghan et al., 2004).

Australian school nurses were found to engage in four primary roles: individual and group support for health decisions and ethical and moral choices, referral to other services as needed, marketing of health-promoting behaviors, and schoolwide health promotion initiatives (Barnes, Courtney, Pratt, & Walsh, 2004). Studies in New Zealand have suggested that advanced practice nurses should have roles related to chronic disease management, parenting education, and the needs of refugee and immigrant populations through health education and information services, health assessment, and referral (Clendon & White, 2001).

A joint statement of the NASN and the AAP indicated that school nurses provide acute, chronic, episodic, and emergency care, health education, and counseling services. They also advocate for children with disabilities. Specific roles identified for the school nurse included helping students and parents to locate a medical home, coordinating the school health services team, supervising unlicensed assistive personnel, assessing student health status and identifying problems, and developing individual health plans, particularly for students with special health needs (AAP, 2001a).

Community health nurses working in school settings apply the nursing process to the care of individual students and their families, to the school population, and to the larger community. In the remainder of this chapter we will explore the application of the nursing process to nursing care in school settings.

Assessing Health in School Settings

Use of the nursing process in the school setting begins with an assessment of health needs. The school nurse may assess the health status and needs of individual students or of the school population. In this chapter, we focus on assessing the health needs of the school population and identifying the factors influencing those

needs. Areas for consideration include the biophysical, psychological, physical environmental, sociocultural, behavioral, and health system dimensions of health.

Biophysical Considerations

Areas for consideration related to the biophysical dimension include maturation and aging as they affect health and health behaviors, genetic inheritance, and physiologic function.

MATURATION AND AGING School nurses work with students in preschool, elementary school, junior high and high school, and college and university settings. Consequently, the age of the client population influences the types of health problems that may be present. For example, prevention of childhood communicable diseases would receive greater emphasis in the preschool population, and sexuality issues and substance abuse would be of greater concern with adolescent populations. For college students, substance abuse and sexuality issues are also pertinent, as are stress-related problems stemming from academic pressures and being away from home.

Client maturation also influences the content and process of the health education component of the school health program. Basic hygiene conveyed via cartoon films is appropriate to the preschool or early elementary-age child; a frank discussion of sexuality and sexually transmitted diseases is appropriate with older groups of schoolchildren.

GENETIC INHERITANCE Aspects of genetic inheritance of particular interest to the school nurse are the gender and racial composition of the population. A predominance of females in a preschool or an elementary school increases the frequency with which the nurse will encounter students with symptoms of urinary tract infection as these are more common in girls than boys in all age groups except infants. In adolescent girls, there is increased risk of unwanted pregnancy, and sexually transmitted diseases are common among both girls and boys. Boys of all ages tend to have more sports-related injuries with which the nurse must deal (Chen, Smith, Deng, Hostetler, & Xiang, 2005).

The racial composition of the school population also influences the types of health problems encountered. For example, in schools with large African American populations, sickle cell screening might be included as a routine part of the school health program. The nurse must also be alert to the prevalence of other diseases that exhibit genetic predispositions, such as thalassemia and diabetes.

PHYSIOLOGIC FUNCTION An important aspect of the human biological component of the assessment is the physiologic function of the school population. School nurses may encounter students or staff with self-limiting health problems or chronic conditions that affect their abilities to function effectively in the school setting.

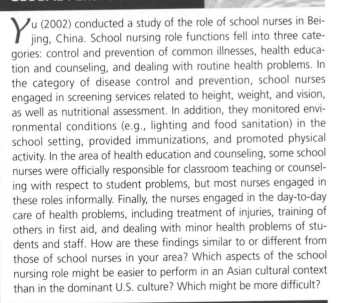

GLOBAL PERSPECTIVES

Yu (2002) conducted a study of the role of school nurses in Beijing, China. School nursing role functions fell into three categories: control and prevention of common illnesses, health education and counseling, and dealing with routine health problems. In the category of disease control and prevention, school nurses engaged in screening services related to height, weight, and vision, as well as nutritional assessment. In addition, they monitored environmental conditions (e.g., lighting and food sanitation) in the school setting, provided immunizations, and promoted physical activity. In the area of health education and counseling, some school nurses were officially responsible for classroom teaching or counseling with respect to student problems, but most nurses engaged in these roles informally. Finally, the nurses engaged in the day-to-day care of health problems, including treatment of injuries, training of others in first aid, and dealing with minor health problems of students and staff. How are these findings similar to or different from those of school nurses in your area? Which aspects of the school nursing role might be easier to perform in an Asian cultural context than in the dominant U.S. culture? Which might be more difficult?

Examples of self-limiting conditions include communicable diseases such as the common cold, influenza, and chickenpox and injuries such as a fractured arm or leg. Diabetes, seizure disorders, and minor visual or hearing problems are examples of chronic conditions that may have health and educational implications. Many of these conditions can be controlled if properly diagnosed and treated and do not necessarily interfere with the child's ability to function in school. Other chronic and handicapping conditions do interfere with school function. Examples are blindness, deafness, mental retardation, attention deficit hyperactivity disorder (ADHD), and long-term effects of fetal drug exposure. Conditions related to environmental or psychological stress may or may not affect physiologic function, although they may affect the child's ability to function effectively in the school situation.

The kinds of physical health problems seen by school nurses among students and staff are many and varied. Acute and chronic conditions commonly encountered in the school setting are listed in Table 23-3◆. Acute conditions include a variety of communicable diseases and injuries. For example, adolescents account for half of the 19 million STD diagnoses that occur each year (NCCDPHP, 2005c), and 80% of schoolchildren in one study visited the nurse for an injury of some sort and account for 4 million injuries a year (Barrios et al., 2001). From 10% to 31% of these injuries occur at school (Guttu et al., 2004), and 6% of all emergency medical service (EMS) dispatches are to schools. Serious injuries are more likely to occur among middle school and high school students than those in elementary schools. Falls and sports injuries are the cause of 77% of school injuries resulting in hospitalization (Barrios et al., 2001). Another commonly occurring acute problem in schoolchildren today is *backpack syndrome*, back pain due to

carrying heavy backpacks throughout the school day (Lewis & Bear, 2002). At the college and university level, new concerns for localized infection, hepatitis B, and HIV/AIDS center on the prevalence of tattoos and piercings (Williams, 2005).

Chronic health problems are encountered with greater frequency in today's schools than in the past. In part this is the effect of mainstreaming children with disabilities and in part an actual increase in chronic disease incidence in children. An estimated 15% of school-aged youth has some sort of chronic condition (Guttu et al., 2004). More than 5% of children experience school-related disability due to their conditions, and another 2% experience non–school-related activity limitations (Xiang, Stallones, Chen, Hostetler, & Kelleher, 2005). In 2002, 5.4 million U.S. children received special education services (Lewis & Bear, 2002). School nurses need to be conversant not only with care of minor illness and injury but also with the complex care of children with special needs.

Asthma and overweight are two of the most common chronic problems seen by today's school nurses. An estimated 6 million children under 18 years of age have asthma. Asthma in children is often poorly controlled, and 1.4% of U.S. children experience some level of limitation due to asthma. Asthma results in 14 million lost school days each year and $726.1 million in lost work time for their caretakers (Jones & Wheeler, 2004). According to the 2003 Youth Risk Behavior Survey (YRBS), nearly 19% of high school students had a diagnosis of asthma and nearly 38% of these students reported at least one attack at school during the previous year (Division of Environmental Hazards and Health Effects, 2005).

Obesity is another significant problem among school-aged children. The prevalence of overweight has tripled in this population in the last 20 years, and more

TABLE 23-3	Acute and Chronic Physical Health Problems Encountered in the School Setting	
Organ System Affected	**Conditions Encountered**
Cardiovascular system	Heart murmurs, hypertension
Central nervous system	Mental retardation, blindness, deafness, attention deficit hyperactivity disorder, learning disability, seizure disorder, meningitis, cerebral palsy
Endocrine system	Diabetes mellitus, thyroid disorders
Gastrointestinal system	Encopresis, hepatitis, diarrhea, dental caries, constipation, peptic and duodenal ulcer
Genitourinary/reproductive system	Sexually transmitted diseases, urinary tract infection, enuresis, dysmenorrhea, pregnancy
Hematopoietic system	Anemia, hemophilia, leukemia, sickle cell disease, lead poisoning
Immunologic system	AIDS and related opportunistic infections
Integumentary system	Acne, eczema, impetigo, lice, scabies, dermatitis, tinea corporis
Musculoskeletal system	Arthritis, sprains, fractures, scoliosis, Legg–Calvé–Perthes disease
Respiratory system	Upper and lower respiratory infections, strep throat, influenza, asthma, hay fever, pertussis, diphtheria, pneumonia
Other diseases	Measles, mumps, rubella, scarlet fever, chickenpox, infectious mononucleosis, otitis media, otitis externa, conjunctivitis, Lyme disease, cancer, hepatitis

than 9 million children aged 6 to 19 years (over 16%) are overweight (Katz et al., 2005; NCCDPHP, 2005c).

Immunity is another important consideration related to physiologic function in the school population. The community health nurse working in the school setting monitors the immunization status of students and school employees. For example, maintenance personnel are at risk for tetanus because of the potential for dirty injuries, and their immunization status should be monitored. For female teachers and other school personnel of childbearing age, the risk of rubella during pregnancy is increased by working with children, and they should also be adequately immunized.

A final health problem frequently encountered in the school population that may have a physiologic basis is attention deficit hyperactivity disorder (ADHD). ADHD was discussed in Chapter 16∞.

In addition to assessing the physiologic health status of the school population as a whole, the community health nurse working in a school setting will also assess the health status and needs of individual children. The AAP (2000c) has developed a policy for assessment in the school setting that includes both entry and periodic assessments that may be performed by school nurses. At entry into the school system, all children should receive a comprehensive medical history and assessment of preschool experiences; language, motor, social, and adaptive development; and immunization status, as well as a complete physical examination.

Periodic assessments should be based on age-appropriate guidelines and individual needs and should address new problems, medications, changes in status, and school progress. Assessment should also include screening at appropriate ages for vision, hearing, and dental problems, as well as emotional maturity, language, and motor skills. Assessments for sports participation should also include endurance and muscle strength assessment. All assessments performed in the school setting should include anticipatory guidance for children and/or parents and problem identification and referral as needed. Biophysical considerations in the school health setting are included in the focused assessment below.

FOCUSED ASSESSMENT

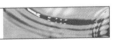

Biophysical Considerations in the School Setting

- What is the age composition of the school population (staff and students)? Do any of the students exhibit developmental delays? Are there specific developmental issues related to the age of the student population (e.g., sexual development)?
- What is the relative proportion of males and females in the school population? What is the racial/ethnic composition of the school population?
- What chronic or communicable conditions are prevalent in the school population?
- What are the immunization levels in the school population?

Psychological Considerations

The psychological environment of the school can either foster good health or undermine it. Aspects of the psychological dimension to be assessed include the nature of relationships among students and school staff members and between school and family, discipline, grading practices, parent–school relationships, and the presence of mental illness.

RELATIONSHIPS Jozefowicz-Simbeni and Allen-Meares (2002) described the structure of a school's ecological system as consisting of several system levels: microsystem, mesosystem, exosystem, macrosystem, and chronosystem. The microsystem consists of the family, school, and peer group. The mesosystem involves interrelationships among school, peer groups, and families. Community environments and social systems comprise the exosystem, and opportunity structures, resources, and cultural factors comprise the macrosystem. The chronosystem encompasses change in these systems over the course of one's lifetime.

Relationships in each of these systems can have profound effects on the health of students, staff, and community members. In the following paragraphs we will examine relationships among peers, student–teacher relationships, teacher–teacher relationships, and parent–school relationships. Although these relationships, in and of themselves, are part of the sociocultural dimension of the school setting, they are addressed here because of their profound psychological implications.

Peer Relationships The relationships of a student with his or her peers can create a psychological environment that is either conducive or detrimental to mental and physical health. The community health nurse can assess the extent to which students who have difficulties with peer relationships are encouraged to participate in group activities. Is there adequate adult supervision of student activities to moderate unhealthy peer relationships? If school personnel see that particular children are unable to participate or are even victimized, do they act to stop such behaviors? Are opportunities provided within the school setting and the curriculum for values clarification and learning about healthy interpersonal interactions?

Research has indicated that a sense of connectedness to one's school is associated with better achievement and less risk-taking behavior among young people (AAP, 2004). For example, connectedness has been negatively associated with substance abuse, delinquency, gang membership, violence, academic problems, and sexual activity in adolescents. School connectedness or bonding appears to have two independent components, attachment and commitment. Attachment involves close affective relationships with others in the school setting (either peers or adults), and commitment reflects a psychological investment in the school and its values and in doing well in school. Connectedness can be fostered through development of interpersonal problem-solving skills in students, development of refusal skills, and special programs to foster social skills (Catalano, Haggerty, Oesterle, Fleming, & Hawkins, 2004).

Conversely, students who have difficulty in relationships with their peers or who are harassed or bullied by others due to their looks or performance (either high-level or low-level performance) tend to withdraw from hurtful interactions and from participation in class or other activities. Popular students have been found to be role models for the behavior of other students, and when popular students harass others, other students frequently imitate their behavior. Research indicates that insults from high-status, popular students are even more hurtful than insults in general. In one study, students experienced an average of 34 insults per person per year (Bishop et al., 2004). In some instances, harassment goes beyond insults to physical victimization, and in the 2003 YRBS, more than 5% of high school students reported not attending school at least once in the previous month due to fear (Grunbaum et al., 2004). Bullying is one of several forms of societal violence addressed in more detail in Chapter 32∞.

Teacher–Student Relationships   Teacher–student relationships also affect the psychological climate of the school. Attachment to adults in the school setting has been found to foster a sense of connectedness and to benefit students in the development of resilience in the face of adversity. Teachers and other adults in the school setting, including the school nurse, can foster connectedness by engaging in proactive classroom management that provides for clear expectations and consistent routines, rewards desirable behaviors, and minimizes classroom disruption. Teachers can also make use of interactive teaching modalities to engage the interest of students and motivate their performance and can promote cooperative learning (Catalano et al., 2004).

The nurse assesses the quality of student–teacher relationships within the school in general and also between specific teachers and their students. Ideally, teachers are people who listen, reward appropriate behavior, maximize student assets, allow personal expression, and foster responsibility. Teachers who foster good student relationships tend to be enthusiastic and have a way of making learning fun. They exhibit a sincere concern for students and respect, accept, and trust them. They get to know their students well, encourage participation and curiosity, foster healthy competition, and encourage students to perform to their best potential. They also refrain from harsh or sarcastic comments, and they discipline students appropriately.

Unfortunately, not all teachers fit this picture. In assessing teacher–student relationships, the nurse identifies any tendencies on the part of teachers to use undue punishment or to make demands that students are incapable of meeting. Inconsistent demands or conflicting

expectations on the part of a teacher can also create stress in students and lead to physical and mental health problems. Nurses might note that certain children are singled out for punishment by a particular teacher and may need to function as advocates. School nurses should also be alert to the potential for emotional, physical, or sexual abuse of students by teachers (and, on occasion, of teachers by students).

Teacher–Teacher Relationships   The relationships among teachers in a school and between teachers and other school personnel also influence the psychological environment of students. The nurse should assess the extent to which healthy teacher relationships—those that are supportive, encourage creativity and freedom, and foster cooperation—exist within the school. Effective relationships among teachers foster sharing and self-confidence, recognize achievements, and provide guidance for teacher development. In schools where teacher–teacher relationships are strained, students may get caught in the middle between teachers, or student morale may be undermined by the stress created by strife among teachers. For example, if the basketball coach and a particular high school English teacher do not get along well, the coach may demand that basketball players cut English class for an extra practice before a championship game, and the English teacher may threaten to fail any player that cuts class. In this instance, the students cannot win. If they cut class, they may fail English. Conversely, if they miss the practice, they may be dropped from the team.

Parent–School Relationships   Another area for assessment is the quality of relationships between school personnel and parents, which can have a strong influence on the psychological climate of the school setting. When this relationship is cooperative, students do not receive conflicting messages about what is expected of them. On the other hand, when relationships between parents and school personnel are adversarial, students may again be caught in the middle of a power struggle, or students may attempt to exploit the situation by manipulating both parents and teachers to their own advantage.

School connectedness among students is promoted by collaborative parent–school relationships and can be further supported by behavior management training for parents. Parents can also assist their children through academic support skills and the development of a home environment conducive to school success (Catalano et al., 2004).

DISCIPLINE   In discussing the characteristics of supportive teachers, the issue of discipline was alluded to. In addition to looking at disciplinary measures employed by individual teachers, school nurses should assess the school's philosophy regarding discipline. Discipline should be used for inappropriate behavior and should not be unduly harsh. It is estimated that 1 to 2 million instances of corporal punishment occur in U.S. schools each year, and the AAP (2000a) has called for efforts to prohibit corporal punishment in all states. According to the Academy, school behavior/discipline plans should be schoolwide and should be consistent and clear with respect to behavioral expectations and consequences. Policies and plans should also include staff education relative to developing an environment that supports expected behaviors, basic behavior management strategies, and early recognition of mental health problems that contribute to inappropriate behavior (AAP, 2004).

In another policy statement, the AAP (2003) has noted the frequent inappropriateness of out-of-school suspensions and expulsions. The Academy noted that those children most likely to be suspended or expelled are also those most likely to lack home supervision, or to be abused, depressed, or mentally ill. In addition, suspension or expulsion is likely to exacerbate school problems and lead to crime, delinquency, and substance abuse as well as suicide. For these reasons, they recommend that suspension or expulsion be used only as a last-resort disciplinary measure and that school systems incorporate the following recommendations into their disciplinary plans:

- Early referral of students with discipline problems
- Encouragement of access to health care
- Notification of, and referral of students with discipline problems to, primary care providers for assessment
- Consultation with parents as soon as possible
- Consultation from primary health care providers in disciplinary actions

They also suggest that primary health care providers advocate for individual students and for sound school- and districtwide disciplinary policies and procedures. Finally, the policy statement suggests that effective social, emotional, and mental support for students experiencing problems may help to reduce the need for out-of-school suspension or expulsion.

In assessing the psychological dimension of the school setting, the school nurse determines whether rules of behavior are clearly communicated to students and whether expectations are realistic. The nurse should also assess whether discipline, when warranted, is administered fairly and in a manner that does not diminish the student's self-respect.

GRADING PRACTICES School and teacher grading policies should be clearly understood and fairly implemented. Particular grading practices are usually the province of the individual teacher, but the community health nurse can assess whether grading standards are consistent and grades are communicated to students privately to avoid humiliation. These kinds of concerns will most likely surface in interviews with children who are having difficulty in school or who are developing somatic complaints related to stress and perceived pressure. If graded

work is displayed, the nurse can examine the extent to which it is exhibited in ways so all students are made to feel good about some of their abilities. This is particularly important in elementary grades, when children incorporate perceptions of their school performance into either positive or negative self-images. If grading inequities are identified, the community health nurse can discuss them with the teacher or with school administrators.

MENTAL ILLNESS AND THE SCHOOL SETTING Approximately 20% of U.S. school-age children have mental health problems (an increase from 7% twenty years ago), and 5% of children develop severe disabling conditions due to mental health problems (AAP, 2004; Leighton, Worraker, & Nolan, 2003). In the United Kingdom, roughly 14% of children exhibit signs of mental health problems at any given time. The growing prevalence of mental illness in the school population is influenced by changes in family structure, family unemployment, loss of traditional community environments and social supports, and increases in disabling physical conditions. An estimated 80% of school staff in frequent contact with students (teachers, nurses, and social workers) has limited training in addressing child and adolescent mental health issues. In one study in the United Kingdom, mental health problems seen in schools stemmed from five general sources: problems at home, relational or performance problems at school, behavior problems (including substance abuse), emotional problems (e.g., poor self-esteem, anxiety, or depression), or major mental illness (e.g., schizophrenia, eating disorders, or drug-induced psychoses) (Leighton et al., 2003). Mental health problems commonly seen on college and university campuses include depression, anxiety, self-mutilation, eating disorders, and psychoses. In 2000, 17% of students seen in college health settings took some type of psychotropic medication, an 89% increase from 1994 (Williams, 2005).

It is not only students' mental health problems that affect their performance and level of achievement in school. Children whose parents have addictive disorders have been found to have higher incidence of asthma, hypertension, abdominal pain, headaches, gastrointestinal disorders, and allergies. They are more apt to be late to school, have a higher incidence of learning disability, and receive less assistance with homework than other children. In addition, these children are more likely to experience interpersonal difficulties, social isolation, school performance problems, low self-esteem, depression, anxiety, and phobias and to engage in antisocial behavior, delinquency, and substance abuse. Children with parents who have addictive disorders are at two to four times the risk of adolescent psychiatric disorders as other children and are more likely to be abused. In addition, they are four to six times more likely to develop drinking problems (Gance-Cleveland,

2004). School nurses should be alert to children whose parents have addictive behaviors and should endeavor to provide them with the psychological and social assistance needed to circumvent the effects of parental disability on health and school performance. The focused assessment below lists areas for consideration in assessing the psychological dimension of health in the school setting.

Physical Environmental Considerations

The average U.S. school building is 42 years old, and more than 75% of schools were built before 1970. An estimated one third of schools are in need of extensive repair or replacement of one or more buildings. In one national study, half of schools reported one or more "unsatisfactory environmental condition" such as poor ventilation, heating, lighting, or physical security. These environmental conditions were found to be worse in urban than rural or suburban schools. Nearly all schools provided access to indoor or outdoor facilities for physical activity. Regular inspections for physical safety hazards occurred in 80% to 90% of schools, depending on the focus of the inspection, and only 85% of schools were equipped with smoke detectors. Less than half of the elementary schools used the Consumer Product Safety Commission checklist to assess playground safety (Jones et al., 2003). The aging of school buildings provides an opportunity to redesign schools in a way that better promotes the health of students, staff, and the community (Bingler, 2000).

Another aspect of the physical environment of the school is the community in which the school is located. Distance and unsafe physical conditions interfere with students' ability to walk or bicycle to school (Division of Unintentional Injury Prevention, 2002; Sirard, Ainsworth, McIver, & Pate, 2005). Similarly, the number of fast food restaurants in close proximity to schools may influence dietary patterns. In one Chicago study, 78% of schools had at least one fast food restaurant within 800 meters of school property. Geographic positioning indicated that fast food restaurants seemed to be clustered around schools in greater numbers than would result from random placement in the community (Austin et al., 2005).

The nurse assesses both the internal and external physical environment of the school. The external environment includes the area surrounding the school. Assessment considerations here include traffic patterns, water hazards, use of pesticides, and rodent control in the area. The proximity of hazardous waste dumps or nuclear power plants, industrial hazards, and the presence of various forms of pollution are other environmental concerns in school settings. (See Chapter 10∞ for a discussion of environmental health issues.)

Several aspects of the school's internal environment, such as fire hazards and sanitation, are the responsibility of official agencies such as the fire department and health department; however, other aspects of the physical environment are rarely adequately assessed. The school health nurse needs to be alert to other hazards to physical safety that may be present in the school setting. Examples of these hazards are toxic art supplies, scientific equipment in laboratories, kitchen appliances in home economics classrooms, and chemical substances used either in chemistry labs or by maintenance and janitorial staffs. Animals in classrooms may also present safety hazards in terms of the potential for scratches and bites or disease transmission. Other conditions that may jeopardize safety include asbestos used in building materials, inadequate maintenance of fire hoses and extinguishers, and inoperable communications systems in the event of an emergency.

Other areas of concern are the safety of industrial arts classrooms, the gymnasium, and play areas. As noted in Chapter 16∞, the safety of outdoor play equipment should be inspected on a regular basis and repairs made as needed. A similar need exists for periodic assessment of sports equipment and practices. Other hazards associated with play areas include broken glass and other refuse on the playground. Hard surfaces below play equipment increase the potential for injuries stemming from falls.

Other assessment considerations with respect to the school's internal physical environment include noise levels within and outside of classrooms and the adequacy of lighting, ventilation, heating, and cooling. Food sanitation should also be assessed. If hot meals are provided at school, cooking facilities should be inspected regularly. Such inspections are usually the

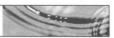

FOCUSED ASSESSMENT

Psychological Considerations in the School Setting

- What is the extent of connectedness to the school exhibited by students?
- How do peer relationships within the school affect health? Are there students who are harassed by others? What is the effect of this harassment?
- What is the overall character of teacher–student relationships within the school? Do these relationships support connectedness? Do they promote or impede student mental health?
- What is the character of relationships among teachers and between teachers and other school staff? What effect, if any, do these relationships have on the health of students? Of staff?
- What is the character of relationships between the school and parents? Between the school and the larger community? How do these relationships affect the health of the school population?
- What are the discipline policies and procedures in the school setting? Are they implemented fairly? What health effects do discipline policies have on students?
- What are the grading policies of the school? Are they implemented fairly?
- What is the extent of mental illness in the school population? To what extent does mental illness in family members affect the health of students?

official responsibility of the local health department, but the community health nurse should also assess these facilities periodically. If students bring their lunches, the potential for food poisoning from spoiled foods should be appraised.

Assessing sanitary facilities in the school is another area for consideration. Here, the nurse would examine the adequacy of toilet facilities for the size of the school population. The nurse would also periodically inspect sanitary facilities to make sure they are in good working order and do not pose hazards for the transmission of communicable diseases. Again, this area is usually the responsibility of health department personnel, but official inspections may occur only at lengthy intervals and the nurse should be aware of hazards that might arise in the interim.

Another area of concern with respect to sanitation is the use and cleaning of shower facilities. The nurse should assess that showers are adequately cleaned to prevent transmission of communicable conditions such as tinea pedis (athlete's foot).

Physical facilities for preventing the spread of disease by infected children should also be assessed. Are there places within the school where youngsters with infectious conditions can be isolated? All too often, these children are merely kept in the nurse's office until a parent can come for them. This presents opportunities for exposure of all those who visit the nurse while the child is there.

Special consideration should be given to the physical environment as it relates to handicapped children. Many physical barriers may exist, particularly in older schools, which limit the ability of handicapped youngsters to benefit from the education setting. Areas of concern include the presence of ramps, easily opened doors and windows, nonslip flooring, elevators, and curb modifications to eliminate the need to step up. Another consideration is access to toileting facilities by handicapped children. Are toilets accessible to wheelchairs? Are sinks placed so that a wheelchair can be maneuvered beneath them? The placement and height of mirrors, drinking fountains, and telephones is also of concern. Other considerations with respect to the environment of handicapped children are the adequacy of storage for wheelchairs and other special equipment, wheelchair space in classrooms and auditoriums, modification of laboratory and library carrels for wheelchair use, and the adequacy of evacuation plans for the handicapped in case of emergency. The intent is to create a school that is barrier-free so that all students, staff, and community members who may use the premises after school hours have access to facilities and equipment. Community health nurses may need to actively advocate for modifications in the school setting that address the needs of children (or employees) with disabilities.

Finally, the school nurse should assess the level of preparation in the school setting for disaster events or terrorist activities. Elements of an effective disaster response plan include personnel organization, forms, specific considerations, and the role of the nurse. Effective personnel organization usually includes an incident commander (usually an administrator) who coordinates the work of response teams and communications within and outside the school, and accounts for the welfare of all members of the school community. Other elements of the response organization include student management teams (usually teachers) who account for all students and staff, a first aid or health team, and search and rescue teams. Security teams should also be designated to secure the school site, control ingress and egress, direct traffic, and shut off electricity, gas, and water supplies as needed. A reunion team would be responsible for reuniting students with their parents, and a public information officer would supply needed information to the incident commander (Lewis & Bear, 2002).

Forms required in the event of a disaster include emergency information for all students and teachers, documentation forms for recording treatments and students released to parents, and site maps indicating the operations center, assembly and first aid areas, a reunion area, and a morgue, as well as the location of emergency supplies and shutoff valves. Other considerations in the school disaster response plan include water purification methods, first aid supplies, and supplies to meet the needs of disabled students. Schools, particularly those with younger children, may also stock "comfort packs" for each student to include pictures of family members and a 3-day supply of medications for students in need of them (Lewis & Bear, 2002).

The role of the school nurse with respect to disaster events or terrorist activities includes participation in developing the disaster plan. In the event of an actual disaster, the nurse assists in maintaining calm, triages injuries, and addresses the physical and psychological effects of the disaster. After a disaster event, the nurse helps to address the fears and grief of students and other staff members. In addition to meeting ongoing health care needs, the nurse should provide realistic and reliable information, facilitate referrals for support, and educate staff regarding the psychological effects of such events (Lewis & Bear, 2002). Disaster response will be addressed in more detail in Chapter 27∞. Elements of a focused assessment of physical environmental considerations in the school setting are summarized on page 645.

Sociocultural Considerations

The sociocultural dimension also plays a part in influencing the health status of members of the school community. Areas to be addressed in this dimension include culture and ethnicity, economic resources, legislation, abuse and violence, and the potential for terrorism.

FOCUSED ASSESSMENT

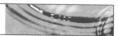

**Physical Environmental Considerations
in the School Setting**

- Are there health hazards present in the school or the surrounding neighborhood?
- Are food sanitation practices adequate to prevent communicable diseases, vermin infestation, etc.?
- Are school facilities adequate and in good repair? Are there adequate facilities for handicapped students or staff?
- What is the character of the environment surrounding the school? What health effects, if any, does the external environment have on the school population?
- What is the potential for disaster within the school setting? Is the school adequately prepared to respond to a disaster event?

CULTURE AND ETHNICITY Cultural factors in the school setting may affect educational priorities as well as health-related behaviors. What is the racial or ethnic composition of the school population? Are racial tensions present? Do religious beliefs influence the health of the school population? For example, if there are large numbers of children whose parents object to immunization on religious grounds, the nurse needs to be particularly alert to signs of outbreaks of childhood diseases such as measles, rubella, and diphtheria.

Another area for consideration is the cultural backgrounds of students and school personnel. Are they similar? Do cultural practices influence students' health? Do differences in cultural practices create tension among students or between students and staff? Cultural factors may also lead to inappropriate diagnoses of ADHD for behavior considered perfectly normal in the child's culture or child abuse in the face of cultural health practices such as dermabrasion or cupping. (See Chapter 9∞ for a discussion of these practices.) Children whose primary language is not English may also have difficulties in school, and the nurse should work to achieve culturally appropriate education for these children. Similarly, children of migrant families of whatever cultural or ethnic background may have their education disrupted by frequent moves.

CULTURAL COMPETENCE

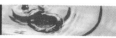

A large percentage of the children in your school are Mexican Americans or Mexicans whose families have come to the United States for work. Most of the families are here legally, but some are not. Several teachers have referred some of these children to you because of frequent absences (often of 3 days to a week) that are interfering with their achievement in school. When you contact the families to determine the reasons for children's absences, you discover that the families are making frequent trips to Mexico for a variety of family events and celebrations. What will you do about this situation?

ECONOMIC RESOURCES The level of resources available to the school is one element in assessing the sociocultural dimension of the school setting. The nurse also needs to assess the community's attitudes toward education because these attitudes determine the allocation of funds for both school and health programs. What level of priority is given to school funding in the community? Do community members support bond issues for school renovation or specific school-based programs? School districts with lower levels of financial resources have been found to be less likely to recognize students with health problems such as autism (Palmer, Blanchard, Jean, & Mandell, 2005). Community health nurses may need to advocate with school boards and other local officials for sufficient funding for school health services. Political advocacy may also be needed at state and national levels to assure adequate funding for education, particularly for school-based health services.

The economic levels of individual students and their families also influence the health status of the school population. Homelessness is an extreme socioeconomic factor that can have a profound effect on the health of school-age children. Homeless children often perform poorly in school or fall behind because of frequent moves. As a result of the McKinney Homeless Assistance Act, homeless children are guaranteed access to free and public education. Under this act, homeless children may be eligible for other services that must be provided by schools receiving assistance funds. These services may include clothing, a place to bathe and change clothes, free or reduced-cost meals, school supplies, tutorial assistance, and access to medical care. The problems of homelessness and its effects on children's health were addressed in Chapter 20∞.

Homelessness is often the result of divorce or violence within families. Children may be homeless because their mothers are fleeing an abusive situation. In such circumstances and in disputes over child custody, the school system needs to be alert to the potential for abduction of schoolchildren by the other parent. Similarly, abduction and mistreatment by strangers is an area of concern, and the school nurse should assess school policies designed to prevent such occurrences for their adequacy and the extent to which they are enforced.

Another factor closely related to family economic status is the prevalence of families in which both parents work. Unfortunately, children in dual wage-earner families are often sent to school when they are ill because there is no one at home to care for them. The nurse should assess the number of students who come to school ill and explore with parents their reasons for sending sick children to school. It may be a lack of awareness on the part of parents of the signs and symptoms of illness or the absence of other options.

The nurse should also assess before- and after-school care of children whose parents work. Many so-called *latchkey* children stay at home alone before and after school until parents return from work. Community health nurses can assess the availability of programs for children who are not mature enough to stay home alone and make referrals to these programs if they do not already exist within the school. In addition, nurses can assist parents to determine children's readiness to stay home alone and help to educate both parents and children on conditions that promote the safety of latchkey children.

LEGISLATION Legislation is another important sociocultural factor that influences health in the school setting. As we saw earlier, legislation related to education for children with disabilities has profoundly influenced the role of school nurses in caring for these children, many of whom have multiple health care needs. Public Law 94–142 mandated "free and appropriate public education" for all children aged 5 to 21 years. In 1990, this mandate was expanded to include children from 3 to 5 years of age in the Individuals with Disabilities Education Act (IDEA). Revisions to IDEA in 1997 defined 13 disabling conditions covered under the law and expanded coverage to children from birth to 21 years of age. Provisions of IDEA include:

- Education in the least restrictive environment possible
- Provision of multiple program options (regular classroom, supplemental services, designated services, special classes, special schools, and education in special settings such as the home or hospital)
- Classroom placement decisions based on evaluation by a designated multidisciplinary team that includes parents
- Development of an annual individual education plan (IEP) for each disabled child
- Definition of parent and student rights
- Provisions for confidentiality of information
- Designated instruction and services (e.g., speech, psychological, physical, and occupational therapy, and other health and educational services)
- Provisions for the application of school disciplinary rules to students with disabilities (Lewis & Bear, 2002)

Other legislative initiatives may also influence school health. For example, municipalities that place a high priority on tobacco control in general are more likely to have schools with smoke-free policies that prohibit school staff (as well as students) from smoking anywhere on campus (Kayaba, Wakabayashi, Kunisawa, Shinmura, & Yanagawa, 2005).

ABUSE, VIOLENCE, AND EXPLOITATION A particular need in today's society is to prevent violence in and around the school setting. From 1992 to 1994, 105 violent deaths were school-associated. Eighty-five incidents involved homicide and 20 were suicides (Barrios et al., 2001). In addition, the *Safe School Initiative* study found a total of 37 incidents of "targeted violence" on school campuses between December 1974 and May 2000 (Fein et al.,

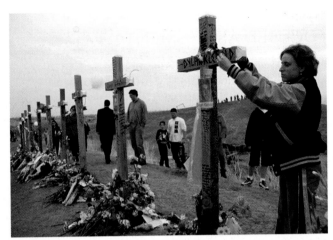

Community health nurses in schools may have to deal with the aftermath of school violence. (Steve Liss/Getty)

2002). Targeted violence is defined as "any incident of violence where a known or knowable attacker selects a particular target prior to their violent act" (Vossekuil, Fein, Reddy, Borum, & Modzeleski, 2002).

Violence within the school environment can be addressed by explicit codes of conduct that are clearly communicated to students and consistently and uniformly enforced. Weapons should be strictly banned from school campuses and the ban stringently enforced. Despite such bans, however, Youth Risk Behavior Surveillance data for 1999 indicated that more than 70 incidents of weapons carrying occurred per 100 students. These incidents involved slightly more than 17% of students nationwide (Kann et al., 2000). Peer counseling and off-campus counseling sites to address interpersonal problems have been effective means of reducing violence. The community health nurse in the school setting can assess the level of violence on campus as well as the effectiveness of steps taken to prevent violence. The nurse can also examine the inclusion of conflict resolution strategies and content on interpersonal relations in the school's health education curriculum.

Schoolchildren may also be subjected to violence and abuse outside of the school setting. In 2002, for example, 2.6 million referrals involving 5 million children were made to U.S. Child Protective Services (CPS), and 903,000 resulted in confirmed cases of neglect and physical, sexual, and emotional abuse. Children with disabilities are nearly twice as likely to be abused as other children, and, although boys and girls are abused with equal frequency, girls are four times more likely to experience sexual abuse (Massey-Stokes & Lanning, 2004).

The extent of crime in the school neighborhood is another aspect of the social environment to be assessed. Is violence a problem for children going to and from school? Is drug dealing going on in the area, and will youngsters be pressured to experiment with drugs? Questions for a focused assessment of sociocultural dimension considerations in the school setting are presented below.

Behavioral Considerations

Enrollment in school is itself a lifestyle factor that influences health. School attendance increases one's risk of exposure to a variety of communicable diseases. Children generally experience an increase in the number of acute illnesses during the first few years of school, whether at the day care/preschool level or with admission to elementary school.

The rigidity of the school day may also affect the health status of students. The nurse determines whether the organization of the school day is conducive to health. Assessment areas to be addressed include the extent to which periods of strenuous physical activity are alternated with periods of quiet study and the extent of opportunities for developing a variety of psychomotor as well as academic skills. The nurse also assesses whether mealtimes are arranged so that students have the energy reserves to handle the tasks of the school day. For younger children, this usually means providing a snack time. Another area for assessment is the scheduling of time for toileting activities. The nurse should determine whether children are given time to go to the lavatory or permitted to go when necessary to prevent chronic constipation or urinary tract infection. There should also be opportunities for children to obtain drinks of water. Such opportunities should increase in frequency with hot weather. Other areas to be addressed in the behavioral dimension include physical activity, diet and nutrition, substance use and abuse, safety practices, and gambling.

PHYSICAL ACTIVITY With the advent of television and computer game systems, children are much less physically active than they were a generation or two ago.

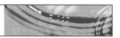

FOCUSED ASSESSMENT

Sociocultural Considerations in the School Setting

- What is the ethnic and cultural composition of the school population? How do ethnicity and culture affect the health of members of the school population?
- What are the community attitudes toward education? Toward the school? To what extent does the community support the school program?
- What economic resources are available to the school?
- What is the economic status of members of the school population? How does economic status affect access to health care?
- How do legislative initiatives affect the school and the health of the school population?
- What is the extent of violence in the school population? What are the factors underlying episodes of violence? What are the school's policies with respect to violence?
- To what extent are members of the school population subjected to violence and abuse outside the school setting?
- What is the potential for Internet exploitation of students?

According to *Healthy People 2010* tracking data, only 63% of high school students engaged in vigorous physical activity at least 3 days a week, and only 39% participated in daily physical activity in physical education classes. Conversely, 38% of students watched television for 2 or more hours a day (Centers for Disease Control and Prevention, 2005).

As noted earlier, many factors prevent students from walking or bicycling to school. This "active commuting" would provide opportunities for physical activity. On average, however, only 13% of U.S. schoolchildren engage in such active commuting to school, and in some studies only 5% of students do so (Sirard et al., 2005). Factors that deter these forms of physical activity include distance, traffic patterns, poor weather, crime, and school policies against walking or biking to school. Children who do not experience any of these barriers have been found to be six times more likely to walk or bike to school than those who do (Division of Unintentional Injury Prevention, 2002).

The American Academy of Pediatrics (2000b) has made several recommendations to promote physical activity in schools. These include policies that promote life-long physical activity, daily physical education involving physical activity, comprehensive health education including information about the need for and health effects of physical activity, adequate school resources for physical activity, and appropriately trained coaches and health education teachers. Additional recommendations include provision of physical activity instruction and programs and extracurricular activities that meet the needs and interests of all students (including those with disabilities), provision of safe environments for physical activity, including parents whenever possible in physical activity and education initiatives, and educating personnel to promote life-long enjoyable physical activity. Finally, the AAP recommended regular evaluation of physical activity programs and the establishment of relationships between schools and local recreation and sports programs.

Recreational activities should also be assessed. The need to examine recreational and sports equipment for safety hazards has already been touched on, but the nurse should also be aware of the types of recreational and competitive activities engaged in by students. Is there ample opportunity for physical activity? Is it adequately supervised? Are sports and recreational programs appropriate to children's ages and developmental levels? For example, contact sports are not appropriate for children in lower elementary grades because of the increased risk of injury. Another question is whether recreational activities are suited to children's interests. Are various opportunities available, or must all children engage in the same activity, whether they choose to or not? Is a gender bias evident in the recreational opportunities provided? For example, is soccer restricted to boys whereas girls are expected to play hopscotch or jump rope? Attention should also be given to the recreational needs of teachers. Are teachers given a break from classroom and playground duties?

The physical education curriculum of the school will also influence students' exercise behaviors. Many schools do not include the exposure to physical education activities required to meet the national health objectives. Research has indicated that features of the school environment such as physical improvements and supervision influence physical activity by students before and after school and at lunch. For example, the presence of permanent grounds improvements such as the installation of basketball and tennis courts and football and soccer goals increases the extent of physical activity by students. Similarly, adequate adult supervision also increases physical activity (Sallis et al., 2001). The school nurse should assess the extent to which the school physical education curriculum and the physical and social environments of the school promote physical activity.

DIET AND NUTRITION Nutrition is another behavioral dimension factor that should be assessed in the school population. The adequacy of lunches brought from home should be examined, as should evidence of poor nutrition of meals eaten at home. For example, the nurse would assess children for evidence of anemia or poor growth and development. In schools without a dietary consultant, the nurse should appraise the nutritional quality of school lunch and/or breakfast programs. Too often, food for such programs is purchased with an eye toward economy rather than nutritional value. School nurses may also encounter students who exhibit eating disorders and can assist with referrals for diagnostic and treatment services for these children. The type and prevalence of any food allergies among either students or staff is another consideration for assessment in this area. Community health nurses may need to educate food service personnel regarding food allergies and the need to avoid particularly allergenic foods (e.g., peanuts or use of peanut products in other foods) as a routine precaution.

The type and quality of food served in the school setting is important in determining food choices by members of the school population. In one study, although 89% of elementary, 92% of middle, and 94% of high schools had a cafeteria, fewer than 61% of elementary schools, 34% of middle schools, and 6% of high schools had policies restricting the availability of junk foods (Jones et al., 2003). In part, this is the result of the National School Lunch Act of 1946 that requires school lunch programs to be revenue-neutral, leading schools to plan cafeteria selections to meet the fast food preferences of children, contract with fast food companies to supply lunches, and provide vending machines that dispense junk food items (Richardson, 2004). In one study, for example, 90% of schools had a la carte menus, and 76% of high schools, 55% of middle schools, and 15% of elementary schools provided vending machines (Kubik, Lytle, Hannan, Perry, & Story, 2003).

SUBSTANCE USE AND ABUSE Other lifestyle behaviors should also be assessed, particularly among older students. The extent of tobacco use or use of alcohol or other drugs by students or staff should be explored, as should the extent of sexual activity among preadolescent and adolescent students. Approximately half of all adolescents aged 15 to 19 years are sexually active (Kann et al., 2000), and the nurse should assess the extent of sexual activity in the school population. More than 900,000 adolescents become pregnant each year (USDHHS, 2003), and school nurses must be alert to signs of pregnancy and sexually transmitted diseases as well as being aware of the potential for sexual assault in the school population. Similar assessments are needed with respect to substance use and abuse. In spite of the fact that 99% of school health education programs address problems of alcohol and drug use (Grunbaum et al., 2000) and that schools nationwide have policies prohibiting the use of tobacco, alcohol, and other drugs, use of these substances among preadolescents and adolescents remains high. In fact, in 2003, 8% of students reported using cigarettes on campus, and more than 5% reported use of alcohol at school. Nearly 6% of students reported marijuana use, and more than 28% of students reported being offered illegal drugs at school (Grunbaum et al., 2004). An estimated 4,000 children aged 12 to 17 years start smoking each day, and 14% report frequent smoking (AAP, 2004; NCCDPHP, 2005c). The school nurse should assess the extent of substance use and abuse in the school population, ease of access to these substances in the community, and the adequacy and enforcement of school policies regarding their use. The nurse should also be alert to signs of substance use and abuse in individual students and school personnel.

SAFETY PRACTICES Safety practices should also be assessed in the school setting. Approximately 8 million U.S. school children are engaged in sports activities, resulting in 1 million serious injuries each year in the 10- to 17-year-old group. Risk behaviors associated with injury include failure to use protective gear or seat belts, alcohol use, and access to weapons (Barrios et al., 2001). In one study, for example, only one third of high school athletes used discretionary protective equipment (Yang et al., 2005). Another safety practice that should be considered is the use of condoms by sexually active adolescents.

GAMBLING One final behavioral consideration that is increasingly of concern on school campuses is gambling. In one study, 76% to 91% of high school seniors reported gambling at some time. Approximately 4% to 6% of adolescents who gamble go on to become pathological gamblers, compared to only 1% to 3% of adults. Gambling among students often occurs on the Internet, and gambling is the fastest growing form of addiction among high school and college-age students (Lewis & Bear, 2002). The focused assessment below provides questions for assessing behavioral considerations in school health assessment.

Health System Considerations

The health of the school population is assessed at both the individual and community levels. At the individual level, the community health nurse assesses the usual source of health care for individual children and their families. Do children have a regular source of health care? Do they make use of health-promotive and illness-preventive services as well as curative services? Or is health care for children crisis oriented, focusing only on the treatment of acute conditions? Do children have unmet health needs because their families cannot afford care?

At the community level, the nurse assesses the availability of health care services to meet the needs of the school-age population. Are health-promotive and illness-preventive services easily accessible in the community? Are services available for youngsters with special health needs (e.g., handicapped children)? Are specific pediatric or adolescent services available? Is there access to contraceptive services or treatment of sexually transmitted diseases for the adolescent population? Is community attention to possible child abuse adequate?

FOCUSED ASSESSMENT

Behavioral Considerations in the School Setting

- What is the extent of physical activity in the school population? Does the school setting provide opportunities for safe physical activities to meet the needs and interests of all members of the school population?
- To what extent do students walk or bike to school? What factors support or impede "active commuting"?
- What recreational opportunities are available to the school population? Do recreational activities pose health hazards? Are appropriate safety equipment and devices used (e.g., in sports)?
- What are the dietary practices of the school population? To what extent do school food choices support or deter good nutrition?
- What is the prevalence of food allergies among the school population? What types of food allergies are represented? Do school food services avoid particularly allergenic foods?
- What is the extent of substance use and abuse in the school population? What are the school policies with respect to substance use (e.g., tobacco, alcohol)?
- Do any members of the school population use prescription medications on a regular basis? Are medications used, stored, and dispensed as directed?
- To what extent do members of the school population engage in other health and safety-related practices (e.g., seat belt use, condom use)?
- What is the extent of gambling among the school population?
- What is the extent of piercing and tattooing among the school population? To what extent do these practices influence health?

The nurse also assesses the relationship between the school and the health care community. Are private physicians conversant with regulations for excluding children with communicable conditions from school? Do physicians and other health care providers work cooperatively with school personnel to meet the health care needs of individual youngsters? Do health care providers in the community offer services within the school on either a paid or a voluntary basis?

Another consideration is the organizational structure for delivering health services in the school setting. Models of health care delivery in the schools include school-based health centers and school-linked health services and their natural extension, family health centers located in or near schools. A **school-based health center (SBHC)** is a program of health and social services provided in a school setting and designed to ensure access to necessary services. **School-linked health services** are "an innovative system of delivering services in which community agencies and school collaborate to provide a variety of health and social services to children and their families at or near school sites" (Jozefowicz-Simbeni & Allen-Meares, 2002). Another term for school-linked health services is *integrated school health services*. School-linked health services are coordinated by the school, but services may be provided at other locations in the community, whereas school-based health services are provided on campus (AAP, 2001b). Neither school-based nor school-linked services are intended to replace primary health care services provided by health professionals in the community, but both have been found to be economical ways to meet the needs of students who are not being served by existing community health services (Swider & Valukas, 2004). The AAP (2000c) has suggested that one aim of school health services should be to locate a medical home for all students and coordinate care provided with that of the primary care provider. Advantages of school-based and school-linked services include improved access to services, less educational time lost to health-related appointments, better compliance with follow-up recommendations, greater acceptability to students and families, opportunities to educate families regarding the use of primary care services, and better monitoring of behavioral and treatment effects (AAP, 2001b)

Both SBHCs and school-linked health services are efforts to provide accessible services to children who attend school. Family health centers extend these services to family members as well. Because of their centrality to community life, school-based clinics have been found to be a viable means of health care delivery. By 2003, more than 1,500 SBHCs in 45 states met the needs of more than 2 million school students (Wells, 2003; Williams, 2005). In addition to providing direct health care services to students and school staff, clinic personnel may be involved in health fairs; crisis intervention teams; classroom, parent, and teacher education; student health clubs; and other health promotion activities. School-based or school-linked health services may already exist in a particular system, or the community health nurse can assess the potential for their successful development.

Another innovative possibility links school health services and those provided by managed care organizations (MCOs) in areas of high managed care penetration or in schools that enroll large numbers of children who are involved in Medicaid managed care programs. In these programs, school nurses carry out many of the routine screening and health promotion activities among enrolled MCO clients. For example, they can increase the percentage of tuberculin skin tests that are read by saving parents a second trip to the provider's office for reading. School nurses also participate in multidisciplinary review of complex cases to prevent unwarranted referrals and increased costs for the MCO.

The nurse assessing a school system would also examine the availability of mental health services. Many children with recognizable mental health problems do not receive necessary services. Barriers to obtaining services include lack of transportation, cost, the absence of mental health professionals with expertise in treating children and youth, and stigma. These barriers also help to explain why 40% to 60% of children and families who begin therapy discontinue treatment prematurely (AAP, 2004).

The AAP (2004) recommended provision of school-based mental health services in three tiers. The first tier focuses on preventive mental health programs and curricula provided to all students. The second tier of services meets the needs of students who have mental health needs, but are basically able to function effectively in the school setting. The third tier involves services to students with severe mental health diagnoses.

Mental health service delivery may occur in one of three models: a school-supported model, a community connections model, or a comprehensive integrated model. In the school-supported model, mental health staff are employed by the school system. There may or may not be a separate mental health unit in the school system, and the school nurse serves as the entry point for services. In the community connections model, services are provided by outside agencies. Services may be provided on campus, within a school-based health center or through after-school programs, or by means of formal links to off-site service agencies. A comprehensive integrated model provides direct services on site at all three tiers, and mental health services are an integral part of the SBHC (AAP, 2004). Community health nurses in school settings should assess the availability of mental health services to the school population as well as the organization and quality of those services.

Tips for assessing health system considerations in a school setting are provided in the focused assessment at right. The community assessment guide included in

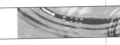

FOCUSED ASSESSMENT

Health System Considerations in the School Setting

- What health services are offered in the school setting? How are school health services funded? Is funding adequate to meet health needs?
- How are school health services organized?
- What is the availability of mental health services in the school setting? Are referrals made to outside sources of care as needed?
- How accessible are needed health services in the community? To what extent does the school population use available health services?
- To what extent are school health services coordinated with primary providers and community health services?

Appendix G on the Companion Website can be used to assess a school population. A specific guideline for conducting a population-based health assessment in the school setting is available in the *Community Assessment Reference Guide* designed to accompany this book.

Diagnostic Reasoning and Care of Clients in School Settings

The second aspect of the use of the nursing process in the school setting is deriving nursing diagnoses from assessment data. Diagnoses can be derived at two levels, in relation to individual students and in relation to the school population. Examples of diagnoses related to an individual student are "inability to participate in vigorous physical exercise due to exercise-induced asthma" and "need for referral to child protective services due to suspected physical abuse by father." Diagnoses related to a population group might be "safety hazard due to placement of play equipment on asphalt surface" and "need for drug abuse education due to high prevalence of drug abuse in the surrounding community."

Each of the sample diagnoses provided above contains a statement of the probable underlying cause of the problem. Such a statement provides direction for efforts to resolve the problem. With the individual examples, measures might be taken to provide less strenuous forms of exercise for the asthmatic child or to make a referral for child protective services in the abuse situation. One approach to the playground safety hazard might be to relocate play equipment to a sandy area.

Planning to Meet Health Needs in School Settings

Planning to meet health needs identified in the school setting takes place at two levels: the macrolevel, at which the general approach to providing health services in the school is planned, and the microlevel, at which plans are made to meet specific health needs of members of the school population. The community health nurse working in the school setting participates in planning efforts at both levels.

Macrolevel Planning

Health services are provided in keeping with an overall school health plan. The plan should specify the population to be served and the services to be provided. Typical categories of services include assessment of health status, problem management services, acute care services, and other preventive services such as immunizations and safety education. An additional component of the health services plan is specification of the personnel involved and of the resources needed to implement the program.

The health services plan should also address the nature of records to be kept. Categories to be addressed include clinical records related to the health of particular children or staff members, administrative records, and evaluative records. Planning for program evaluation should also be included in the plan. Finally, the plan should specify budgetary considerations related to salaries, facilities, and other expenses. Specific elements of the plan in each of these areas are listed in Table 23-4◆.

TABLE 23-4	Elements of the School Health Plan and Related Considerations
Health Plan Element	**Related Considerations**
Population served	Ages and grades of students involved Extent of service to be given to staff
Services provided	Assessment/screening services First aid Acute care services Problem management services Immunizations Safety education Health education Counseling services
Personnel	Categories of health personnel Qualifications of health personnel Functions and responsibilities Staff development needs
Resources	Facilities Equipment Supplies/postage Health records Telephone
Record system	Clinical records for individuals seen Administrative records Immunization records Absenteeism records Program evaluation records
Program evaluation	Focus of evaluation Data collection procedures Data analysis procedures
Budgetary considerations	Salaries Facility construction and maintenance Equipment and supply costs Record-keeping costs Staff development costs

Initial development of a health services plan in the school setting would entail use of the program planning process described in Chapter 15∞, and community health nurses working in the school setting should be involved in the development and periodic review and revision of the plan.

Microlevel Planning

The school health program includes microlevel planning for specific activities or programs at all three levels of prevention: primary, secondary, and tertiary.

PRIMARY PREVENTION Primary prevention in the school setting involves many of the same planning considerations as those used with children in general. Areas of emphasis in planning primary preventive measures in the school setting are immunization, safety, exclusion from school, health education, diet and nutrition, and exercise. Other concerns in primary prevention include developing a strong self-image, positive coping skills, and good interpersonal skills in students.

Immunization Young children are at particular risk for a variety of communicable diseases for which immunization is possible. Immunizations against measles, mumps, rubella, diphtheria, pertussis, tetanus, and polio are required for school entry. In many states immunization for *Haemophilus influenzae* B, varicella, and hepatitis B are also required. Immunizations are also available for hepatitis A and influenza. These diseases are discussed in more detail in Chapter 28∞ and Appendix E on the Companion Website.

The school nurse may be involved in referring individuals who are not immunized for appropriate services or may provide immunizations in the school setting. In addition to providing for routine immunizations, school nurses may also suggest other immunizations in the event of exposure to certain diseases, such as hepatitis A. Community health nurses may need to keep local school boards up to date on recommended immunizations and advocate for changes in immunization requirements to accommodate new national guidelines. Political advocacy may also be needed at the state level to change immunization requirements. At the same time, nurses may need to advocate for immunization waivers for specific children on the basis of religious beliefs or medical contraindications.

Injury/Violence Prevention and Safety Part of the school nurse's responsibility is to identify safety hazards and report them to those responsible for eliminating them. Safety education may also be the responsibility of the school nurse. In addition, the nurse might collaborate with others within and outside the school setting to reduce safety hazards in the surrounding area. Moreover, the nurse and other school personnel might become involved in cooperative efforts with local police to reduce drug traffic in the neighborhood.

MediaLink Appendix E: Communicable Diseases

The Centers for Disease Control and Prevention have identified eight guidelines for injury control and violence prevention in the school setting:

- Establishing a social environment that promotes safety
- Providing a safe physical environment
- Including safety in health education curricula and instruction
- Providing safe physical education, sports, and recreational activities
- Providing health, counseling, psychological, and social services for students in need
- Engaging in effective crisis and emergency response
- Involving families and communities in violence and injury prevention initiatives
- Educating school personnel on injury and violence prevention (Barrios et al., 2001)

Specific strategies for preventing violence and bullying in school settings include fostering a culture of respect for all, creating connections between students and adults in the school setting, and breaking the code of silence among students with respect to plans for school violence. Tasks involved in creating a safe, connected school environment where violence is prevented include assessing the school's emotional climate, emphasizing the need to listen to others, adopting a strong but caring stance against the code of silence, and preventing or intervening in bullying. Other tasks include involving members of the school population, parents, and the community in developing a culture of respect and safety, developing trusting relationships between students and at least one adult in the school setting, and creating mechanisms for sustaining safe schools (Fein et al., 2002).

Schools are also in a position to identify abuse and to engage in educational programs to prevent abuse. Students can be taught personal safety, coping and resiliency skills, decision making, impulse control, and anger management. Other curricular topics include conflict resolution and stress management. Parenting education can also be provided for parents to prevent abuse. Health services should also be provided for children who have been abused, and counseling and psychological and social services provided to address underlying factors. School personnel, including school nurses, are mandated by state law in all states to report suspected abuse to the appropriate authorities. Finally, schools can participate in community-wide efforts to prevent abuse (Massey-Stokes & Lanning, 2004).

Exclusion from School One of the earliest responsibilities of the school nurse was to determine when children should be excluded from school because they had communicable illnesses. Children were also excluded from school as part of an effort to stop the spread of scabies, lice, and other parasites among a highly susceptible

population. This responsibility still requires the school nurse to be knowledgeable of the signs and symptoms of communicable disease and infestation and to be aware of state and local regulations regarding school exclusion. Several conditions that usually warrant exclusion and guidelines for readmission are listed in Table 23-5◆.

The responsibility of the nurse does not stop with excluding the affected child from school. The nurse should also educate parents and children regarding the need to stay home from school when they are ill and about care during illness. The nurse may also make referrals for medical care as needed. In addition, the nurse follows up on children excluded from school to

TABLE 23-5	Conditions Typically Warranting Exclusion from School and Guidelines for Readmission
Condition	**Readmission Guidelines**
Bacterial conjunctivitis	After acute symptoms subside
Chickenpox	5 days after eruption of the first vesicles or after lesions are dried
Diphtheria	When negative cultures of nose and throat are obtained at least 24 hours after discontinuing antibiotics
Hepatitis A	One week after onset of jaundice
Impetigo (staphylococcal)	24 hours after treatment is initiated
Influenza	After acute symptoms subside
Measles	4 days after onset of the rash
Meningococcal meningitis	24 hours after chemotherapy is initiated or when the child is sufficiently recovered
Mononucleosis, infectious	After acute symptoms subside. Delay resumption of strenuous physical activity until spleen is nonpalpable.
Mumps	9 days after onset of swelling
Pediculosis	24 hours after application of an effective pediculocide
Pneumonia, pneumococcal and *Mycoplasma*	48 hours after initiation of antibiotics or when child is sufficiently recovered
Pertussis	After 5 days of antibiotic therapy or when child is sufficiently recovered
Respiratory disease (viral) and upper respiratory infection	After acute symptoms subside
Rubella	7 days after onset of the rash
Scabies	24 hours after treatment
Streptococcus (strep throat, scarlet fever, impetigo)	24 hours after treatment is initiated or when child is sufficiently recovered
Tinea corporis	Excluded only from gym, swimming pool, or other activities where exposure of other individuals may occur; activities resume after treatment is completed

make sure that they are receiving appropriate care and that they are able to return to school when there is no longer any danger of exposure to others.

Health Education   Health education in the school setting provides a foundation for healthy behaviors in adulthood. Most states and school districts require some form of health education at the elementary and junior and senior high school level. At the elementary level, health education is most likely to be incorporated into the total curriculum. Separate health courses are more likely at the junior and senior high level (Grunbaum et al., 2000).

The principles of health education discussed in Chapter 11∞ are particularly relevant to community health nursing in the school setting. The nurse may either serve as a resource for teachers on health content, provide health education classes, or both. The school nurse is also involved in the development of the health education curriculum. Activities involved in curriculum development in which the nurse may engage include the assessment of needs and resources, review of health curricula from other school systems, development of goals and objectives, and design of specific learning activities. In addition, the nurse may be involved in preparing teachers to participate in the health education program. Finally, the nurse participates in the implementation and evaluation of the program.

School nurses may also be involved in the provision of health education to school staff. School staff may also require education to enable them to promote their own health.

Diet and Nutrition   Nutrition is another important aspect of health promotion with the school population. As noted earlier, when this function is not performed by a dietitian or nutritionist, school nurses assess the nutritional status of children and monitor the nutritional value of school lunches. When nutritional offerings are inadequate, the nurse works with school administrators and food service personnel to improve the nutritional quality of meals served. The nurse may also educate children and their parents regarding nutrition and good dietary habits.

School nutrition services should be part of an integrated program of nutrition education. Research has indicated that students in schools with coordinated nutrition programs that incorporate recommendations for healthy eating experience less obesity and overweight, eat healthier diets, and engage in more physical activity than students in schools without such programs (Veugelers & Fitzgerald, 2005).

Exercise and Physical Activity   Exercise and physical activity are another important area for primary prevention in the school setting. The school health program must be designed to assure physical activity while students are in school and to promote continued activity throughout life.

EVIDENCE-BASED PRACTICE

*T*he Task Force on Community Preventive Services (Katz et al., 2005) determined that there was insufficient evidence for the effectiveness of any school-based intervention to prevent overweight and obesity. In large part, the reason for this determination was the lack of studies of outcomes related to weight control interventions. The task force members noted, in particular, that no studies were found examining the effects of such interventions among college students. They suggested research on the effectiveness of college- and university-based interventions to address this lack. How might you design an intervention to prevent overweight and obesity on your campus? Could similar studies be done on other college campuses to build an evidence base for college health practice? Why or why not?

Community health nurses working in school settings can be actively involved in developing physical education and activity programs appropriate to students' ages and interests. They may also be involved in integrating education on the need for physical activity into school curricula. Coordinated school-based interventions have been shown to increase physical activity in students (Pate et al., 2005).

Illness Prevention   Primary prevention in school settings involves preventing physical and emotional health problems. Obesity prevention is addressed with the primary prevention foci on physical activity and nutrition discussed above. Prevention of communicable diseases is addressed by immunization as well as by education regarding hygiene, safe sexual practices, and so on. Other recent foci in illness prevention in school settings include cancer prevention and prevention of mental health problems.

The American Cancer Society has made recommendations for coordinated school health programs related to cancer prevention to be achieved by 2005 and 2015. The 2005 recommendations included:

- Establishment of comprehensive education programs for cancer prevention in 20% of schools
- Establishment of health councils to direct school health efforts in 50% of school districts
- Employment of trained school health coordinators in 50% of school districts

The single 2015 goal is establishment of comprehensive school health education programs related to cancer prevention in 50% of all school districts (Winnail, Stevenson, & Dorman, 2004). No evaluation has yet been done to determine whether the 2005 goals were met.

Recommendations have also been made for school-based strategies to prevent skin cancer in particular. These recommendations include adoption of policies to minimize ultraviolet exposure in school settings, provision of an environment conducive to sun-safety practices, and health education on skin cancer prevention. Other activities related to skin cancer prevention include family involvement in prevention efforts, staff education regarding prevention, a focus on prevention in health services activities, and periodic evaluation of the effectiveness of prevention efforts (Glanz, Saraiya, & Wechsler, 2002).

According to the AAP (2004), prevention of mental health problems should incorporate development of personal assets and resilience in students, establishment of consistent behavioral expectations and discipline plans, and inclusion of mental health education in the school curriculum. The mental health education curriculum should address, at a minimum, self-image development, coping skills, and interpersonal skills.

Sound mental health is promoted by a strong self-image developed throughout childhood. Health promotion in the school setting should focus on the development of a healthy self-image as well as a healthy physical self. School nurses can foster self-image development by serving as role models in their dealings with children. They can also suggest to teachers learning activities that enhance development of a positive self-image.

On occasion, school nurses may need to function as advocates for children who do not have a strong self-image or for those who may be emotionally (or physically) abused by family members, peers, or even teachers. As noted earlier, the nurse should be aware of disciplinary measures used in the school and be alert to forms of discipline or unfair exercise of authority that are harmful to a child's self-image. When such circumstances are identified, the nurse might discuss his or her observations with teachers or other personnel involved and suggest other avenues for achieving the goals of disciplinary action. When corrective actions do not result from these interventions, the nurse may need to bring the problem to the attention of the appropriate authorities such as the school principal or members of the school board.

Occasionally, this requires filing a report of child abuse. In addition to reporting the situation, however, the nurse has a responsibility to provide counseling or referral for assistance to those involved and to serve as a support person for both victim and abuser. In such cases, referrals may also be needed to address socioeconomic problems that may be contributing to the situation.

Another aspect of primary prevention that should be fostered in schools is the development of coping skills. Students and personnel can be assisted to develop active problem-solving strategies that promote their abilities to cope with adverse circumstances. School health nurses can serve as role models in this respect and can also provide counseling that assists students and their families or staff to engage in positive problem solving. Nurses can also reinforce evidence of positive coping by making others aware of their abilities to cope.

In addition, the nurse can present information on stress and offer strategies for dealing with stress that enhance the development of sound coping skills.

The ability to interact effectively with others is essential to civilized society. Such abilities are not innate and must be learned. Education for effective interpersonal skills is another aspect of primary prevention with the school population. Again, the nurse can serve as a role model for effective interpersonal skills and can educate students, parents, and staff regarding interpersonal interactions and the development of communication skills. The nurse can also provide information on group dynamics and communication skills that can enhance interpersonal skills within groups. For example, the nurse might promote role-play in a class to which a handicapped child will soon be admitted or help youngsters learn how to express anger at a teacher in an appropriate manner. Aspects of primary prevention in the school setting and related community health nursing responsibilities are summarized in Table 23-6◆.

SECONDARY PREVENTION Secondary prevention deals with existing problems that require intervention. Generally speaking, secondary prevention involves screening for existing health conditions, referral, counseling, and treatment.

Screening Screening is a major facet of most school health programs and an important responsibility of the school nurse. The goals of screening programs within the school setting include the obvious goal of detecting disease as well as identifying children with special needs that require adjustment of the education program, promoting the importance of primary preventive measures, and evaluating the effectiveness of current measures. Screening can be used to detect health conditions that are amenable to treatment and that can be resolved with appropriate therapy. For example, vision screening is used to identify children with visual problems, the majority of whom can benefit from corrective lenses. Screening may also help to identify children with particular needs that necessitate adjustments in the education program. For example, developmental screening may help to identify youngsters with learning disabilities who will benefit from special education programs.

A screening program also provides an opportunity to stress the importance of primary prevention. Dental screening, for example, provides an excellent opportunity to educate students on the need for good dental hygiene (Cappelli & Brown, 2002). Finally, screening efforts provide one measure of the effectiveness of current preventive efforts. For example, hematocrit screening can provide evidence of one aspect of the efficacy of a school lunch program or nutrition education program in promoting good nutrition.

Screening is a cost-effective approach to the identification of health problems. Typical costs of a screening program include those of the screening procedure itself

TABLE 23-6	Areas of Emphasis in Primary Prevention in the School Setting and Related Community Health Nursing Responsibilities	
Area of Emphasis	**Community Health Nursing Responsibilities**
Immunization	Refer for immunization services as needed. Provide routine immunizations. Suggest additional immunizations as warranted by circumstances (e.g., an epidemic of hepatitis A).
Injury and violence prevention/ safety	Report safety hazards to appropriate authorities. Provide safety education. Collaborate in the development of school policies that promote safety. Collaborate with others to eliminate safety hazards in the community. Assess the emotional climate of the school and the potential for violence. Assist in creating a culture of respect for all members of the population. Identify and intervene in episodes of bullying. Foster effective relationships among students. Foster effective relationships between students and adults in the school setting. Identify and report child abuse. Provide health, psychological, and social services to address the effects of abuse and prevent subsequent abuse.
School exclusion	Determine need for exclusion from school. Explain need for exclusion to parents. Refer child for treatment of condition if needed. Educate children and parents on preventing the spread of communicable diseases. Follow up on children excluded from school to ensure appropriate care.
Health education	Participate in designing health education curricula. Provide consultation to teachers on health education topics. Provide in-service for teachers related to health education. Teach health education in the classroom. Arrange for other health education experiences (e.g., field trips or guest speakers). Arrange or provide health education for staff and/or families.
Food and nutrition	Provide consultation on menu planning. Educate children and families regarding nutrition.
Illness prevention	Teach hygiene and other measures for preventing communicable diseases. Assist in teaching about cancer prevention. Assist in development of policies to limit ultraviolet exposure. Promote development of strong self-image by providing a role model for teachers and others in positive interactions with children. Provide consultation to teachers on activities to enhance children's self-esteem. Function as an advocate for children who have poor self-esteem. Provide a role model for students and staff for effective coping and problem-solving skills. Provide counseling regarding coping and problem-solving skills. Reinforce use of appropriate coping skills. Educate students and staff on stress management and coping. Provide a role model for students and staff for effective interpersonal skills. Educate students, staff, and parents on group dynamics and communication skills.

and of retesting those with positive results, time spent by the nurse in referral, costs of diagnostic and treatment services, special education costs, and costs of corrective maintenance (e.g., for hearing aids or replacing eyeglasses). These costs tend to be far lower than the costs incurred when diagnoses are made later, after problems become more pronounced.

Screening programs typically undertaken in the school setting include screening of vision and hearing, dental screening, height and weight measurements, and screening for scoliosis. Other screening tests may also be employed, depending on the needs of the population served by the school. For example, tuberculosis, lead, sickle cell, and diabetes screening may be conducted in communities with high prevalences of these conditions.

The community health nurse in the school setting may perform a variety of roles with respect to screening programs. The nurse might arrange for the screening to be done, conduct the screening tests, or train volunteers to perform certain screening procedures. Moreover, the nurse is usually responsible for informing students and

ETHICAL AWARENESS

*K*atz et al. (2005) noted that the stigma attached to being overweight among school-aged children raises some ethical concerns regarding weight assessment in the school setting. They suggested interventions aimed at addressing both nutrition and physical activity as one means of dealing with the issue of labeling or stigmatization. Suggested interventions included combining nutrition and physical activity, providing additional time for physical activity in the school day, incorporating noncompetitive sports such as dance, and reducing sedentary activities, particularly television viewing.

parents of the results of screening tests and for interpreting those results. The nurse may also need to make referrals for follow-up diagnostic or treatment services. In addition, the nurse follows up on these referrals to make sure that students are receiving appropriate health care services.

Referral School health nurses make a number of referrals. In addition to referrals for following up on positive screening test results, the nurse may make referrals for a variety of other services. For example, the nurse might refer children who are not immunized to the local health department for immunizations, or a referral for counseling might be needed for a child with behavior problems. School personnel may also be referred for health problems that require medical attention. In making these and other referrals, the school nurse uses the principles of referral discussed in Chapter 12∞. If services to which children have been referred involve costs to the family, the nurse may need to assist the family to find sources of funding for these services.

Counseling Another important role for the school nurse in secondary prevention is that of counseling. As noted in Chapter 1∞, counseling involves assisting clients to make informed health decisions. Nurses may counsel individual students regarding personal problems, or they may assist students, families, and staff to engage in problem solving.

Treatment School nurses may also be involved in the actual treatment of existing health conditions. Treatment can involve emergency care in the event of illness or injury. School nurse practitioners might even engage in medical management of minor illnesses such as antibiotic treatment of otitis media.

Nurses may also be involved in providing specific treatments designed to minimize the effects of acute and chronic conditions. For example, the nurse may need to dispense prescribed medications or engage in specific technical procedures. The need for expertise in the use of medical technology in the school setting has increased dramatically and derives from the inclusion of children with a variety of physical, mental, and emotional health problems in the school population. The school nurse may also be involved in assisting students and staff with chronic illnesses such as diabetes or asthma to effectively manage their conditions.

School nurses may assist with physical therapy or perform procedures such as tracheostomy suctioning or catheterization. They may also be involved in programs for bowel or bladder training. Community health nurses working with handicapped children in the school setting may also find it necessary to educate other school personnel in procedures required and deal with the fears experienced by school staff regarding the child's condition.

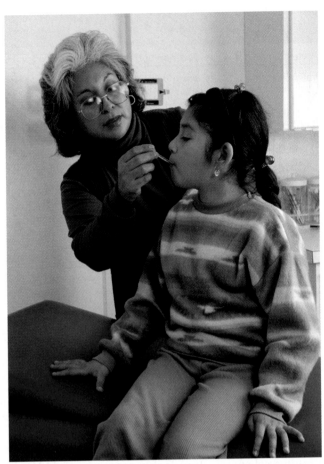

School health services may be some students' only source of health care. (Getty Images)

Caring for children with special health needs in the school setting entails the development of an Individualized Healthcare Plan (IHP). Components of the IHP include a health history, identification of special care needs (e.g., required procedures), an overview of the child's basic health status, and information about medications, including who dispenses them, timing, dosages, routes of administration, and so on. Additional elements of the plan include special dietary or nutritional needs, transportation needs, requirements for specialized equipment, identification of possible problems and strategies to solve them, and a plan for emergency action and transportation. Finally, the IHP should indicate review by the nurse, physician, parent, and school administrator and be incorporated in an easily retrievable location in the student's record. According to the NASN (2003a), IHPs should be developed for students who have multiple health needs, require lengthy care or multiple health care contacts, have daily health care needs, or have health care needs identified in the IEP.

In addition to planning care for students with special needs, the community health nurse monitors the therapeutic effects and side effects of medications and other treatments. Treatment may also involve monitoring self-medication by students. For conditions such as

TABLE 23-7	Considerations in Self-Medication Decisions in School Settings
Category	**Considerations**
Student-related considerations	▪ Disease severity and immediate need for medication ▪ Knowledge and skills related to self-medication ▪ History of disease episodes at school ▪ Adherence to relevant policies and procedures ▪ Experience of self-medication in other settings
Family-related considerations	▪ Desire for child to self-medicate ▪ Permission for sharing of information between school and primary provider
School-related considerations	▪ Health staff availability ▪ Distance to health area and medication storage ▪ Presence of episode triggers in school setting ▪ Availability of emergency services
Provider-related considerations	▪ Written disease management plan that includes self-medication ▪ Education of child in self-medication ▪ Assessment of child's medication administration technique

Data from: Jones, S. E., & Wheeler, L. (2004). Asthma inhalers in schools: Right of students with asthma to a free appropriate education. American Journal of Public Health, 94, 1102–1107.

asthma, the ability to self-medicate may mean a difference between adequately controlled and uncontrolled disease. Unfortunately, many schools have policies that prohibit self-medication by students. As of 2004, 38 states permitted self-medication by school students (Jones & Wheeler, 2004). Four categories of considerations have been suggested that influence asthma self-medication decisions in the school setting (Jones & Wheeler, 2004). These considerations can be adapted to other self-medication situations, and are summarized in Table 23-7◆.

Nurses who dispense medications in the school setting should follow similar guidelines, including obtaining a written order from the primary provider and written authorization from parents for medication administration, storage of medications in a secure area, and complete and accurate documentation of medication administration (Nurses Service Organization, 2004). According to NASN (2003b), medication management in school settings involves consideration of several issues: safe administration of medications; adherence to safe nursing practice and applicable law and regulations; monitoring of effects, side effects, and adverse reactions; effective communication with students, parents, school personnel, and health care providers; and proper documentation. Additional considerations include the use of alternative remedies and over-the-counter medications as well as prescription drugs, delegation of medication administration to unlicensed personnel, and confidentiality. Emphases in secondary prevention in the school setting and related community health nursing responsibilities are summarized in Table 23-8◆.

Think Advocacy

The local elementary school where you work has a policy that students may not self-medicate, including the use of inhalers by students with asthma. The reasoning of the administration is that students may overuse medications or share medications with classmates. According to school policy, students are to give their inhalers to the school nurse and come to the nursing office when they need to use them. You are present at this school only two and a half days a week. In your absence, the principal's secretary is supposed to unlock the nursing office and provide students with access to their inhalers. Each week, you have 10 to 12 students visiting the nursing office during the hours you are there to use inhalers. Because the campus is quite large, students may be coming from quite a distance and their asthma symptoms may be quite pronounced before they reach the nursing office. How would you go about advocating for a change in this policy? Would you advocate a change in policy for all children (K–6) or only for selected students? Why? What support might you try to draw on from other elements of the school population or from the outside community?

TABLE 23-8	Areas of Emphasis in Secondary Prevention in the School Setting and Related Community Health Nursing Responsibilities
Area of Emphasis	**Related Community Health Nursing Responsibilities**
Screening	Conduct screening tests or arrange for screening by others. Train volunteers in screening procedures. Interpret screening test results. Notify parents of screening test results. Make referrals for further tests or treatments as needed. Follow up on referrals to determine outcomes and to ensure appropriate care for identified conditions.
Referral	Refer children and families for health care and other services as needed. Refer other school personnel for needed services.
Counseling	Assist students, staff, or families to make informed health decisions. Counsel students, staff, or families regarding personal problems. Assist students, staff, or families to engage in problem solving.
Treatment	Provide first aid for illness or injury. Dispense medications prescribed for acute or chronic illnesses. Monitor self-medication by students. Develop the IHP for care of children with special health needs. Perform special treatments or procedures warranted by identified conditions. Teach others to perform special treatments or procedures. Monitor therapeutic effects and side effects of medications and other treatments.

TERTIARY PREVENTION Tertiary prevention is undertaken to prevent the recurrence of a problem or to minimize the effects of an existing one. To a large extent, tertiary preventive measures depend on the problems experienced by the student or staff member. Generally speaking, however, there are five aspects of tertiary prevention with which the school nurse is concerned: preventing the recurrence of acute problems, preventing complications, fostering adjustment to chronic illness and handicapping conditions, dealing with learning disabilities, and sustaining school-based health services.

Acute Conditions Preventing the recurrence of acute health problems depends on adequate treatment for existing problems and elimination of conditions that might lead to recurrence. For example, the school nurse might need to educate parents and children regarding the need to complete the course of therapy for otitis media, or education might be needed related to toileting hygiene (e.g., wiping from front to back) to prevent a recurrent urinary tract infection. The nurse might also engage in efforts to help an abusive parent or unduly harsh teacher find other ways to vent frustrations, or might make a referral to help alleviate financial difficulties that are taxing coping abilities.

Complications Tertiary prevention is also directed toward preventing complications of either acute or chronic health problems. For example, the school nurse might encourage parents of a child with strep throat to complete a course of antibiotics to prevent cardiac and urinary complications. Similarly, the nurse might suggest a cushion and frequent changes of position to prevent pressure sores in a student confined to a wheelchair.

Chronic Illness and Handicapping Conditions Tertiary prevention for children with chronic or handicapping conditions involves assisting them to adjust to their condition and preventing complications. Specific measures depend on the condition involved. For example, special arrangements for physical education might be needed to prevent recurrent attacks of exercise-induced asthma, and special attention to diet might be required for the diabetic child or staff member.

Major considerations in dealing with children with chronic illness in the school setting involve money, transportation and facilities, and equipment. Additional considerations include nutrition and psychological well-being. The school nurse may need to refer students and parents to sources of financial assistance as a way to deal with the long-term care requirements of chronic and handicapping conditions.

Transportation and facility considerations in the school setting include issues of physical access to facilities discussed earlier in this chapter. Another area for consideration is transportation to and from school and on field trips. The nurse identifies barriers to access in the school setting and serves as an advocate for the removal of those barriers. Likewise, the nurse attempts to arrange transportation and other circumstances so that students with chronic or handicapping conditions can participate in as many regular school activities, including field trips, as possible. Advocacy in this area might also be needed with parents of handicapped children who may have a tendency to overprotect them.

There may also be a need for special equipment to be used either at home or at school. The school nurse makes referrals to obtain such equipment or sees that it is provided by the school itself.

Nutrition may be particularly problematic for schoolchildren with chronic diseases or handicapping conditions. Youngsters with diabetes, for example, may need assistance in adapting a school lunch program to a diabetic diet. Severely handicapped children may need assistance with eating or may need to be fed. The school nurse assesses the special nutritional needs of children with these and similar conditions and then assists the child, family, and other school personnel to meet those needs. Again, advocacy may be required to assure the availability of special diets for children with particular nutritional needs.

The final consideration with children who have chronic illnesses or handicapping conditions is their psychological well-being. These children should be helped to adjust to their conditions and to participate as normally as possible in the school routine. Parents, teachers, and other children may need to be discouraged from undermining the child's independence by "doing for" them. Values clarification exercises can help other children understand the problems of handicapped or chronically ill children rather than make fun of them or pity them.

Psychological health may be particularly fragile among children with AIDS. There is a need to provide emotional support for these children as they deal with a stigmatized illness that may cause others to withdraw from them in fear. Again, the community health nurse in the school setting may need to function as an advocate to prevent social isolation of these and other children with chronic or handicapping conditions. Other concerns about the child with AIDS are the need to protect the child from infection and the use of universal precautions when dealing with blood and body fluids; both of these concerns may heighten the child's sense of isolation and alienation.

Learning Disability Because there does not seem to be any form of primary or secondary prevention available for learning disability, the focus in working with learning-disabled children is on minimizing the effects of their disability. Some of the interventions that may be planned to assist learning-disabled children are learning by activity, involving multiple senses in learning activities, using repetition, providing direction in small steps, and giving directions without irrelevant detail. Teaching at the appropriate level, a level that creates a challenge but does not lead to frustration, may also be helpful. Other useful strategies include avoiding drastic changes in activities, limiting distractions, and creating a climate in which success is ensured and reinforced as often as possible.

The nurse is involved in development of individualized education plans (IEPs) that allow children with learning disabilities, as well as those with other chronic or handicapping conditions, to learn as easily as possible. Again, attention must be given to the psychological effects of being tagged *learning disabled*. The nurse may need to function as an advocate with parents, teachers, and other children to avoid the application of labels that undermine the child's self-esteem. The nurse can also function as a role model in providing positive reinforcement for the child's strengths and accomplishments, however small.

Sustained School-based Services   Another tertiary prevention intervention directed toward the population level is activity to sustain school-based health services through continued funding. One suggestion for sustaining services involves converting school-based health centers to federally qualified health centers (FQHCs). FQHCs are designated health centers run by public or nonprofit private organizations that provide services in medically underserved areas. FQHCs are required to provide services to all ages and all populations regardless of ability to pay, to have a governing board that includes consumers as 51% of the board, to incorporate a sliding fee scale, and to provide directly or by referral diagnostic, preventive, treatment, and case management services. Other requirements are that the center must be open at least 32 hours per week, implement annual audit and third-party billing systems, produce revenues to cover at least 90% of its operating expenses, and develop a quality improvement program (Swider & Valukas, 2004).

Application for status as a FQHC involves both advantages and disadvantages for the school health system. On the plus side, health services are able to obtain cost-based reimbursement per visit and to increase their revenues by billing for third-party reimbursement from Medicaid and other insurance programs. FQHCs also get first access to new federal programs and access to drug pricing programs, as well as discounts for medical malpractice insurance for staff. Disadvantages include the need to provide services to all, developing accounting systems and coding for the cost of services in a market-based manner, and the loss of the ability to accept in-kind service donations. With respect to the last disadvantage, prospective donors (e.g., providers of health services) must donate funds to the FQHC, which are then used to purchase services they would previously have provided at no cost. Other options for sustaining funding for school-based health services are private foundation grants, state funding, other federal funding sources, and partnerships with community health organizations and agencies (Swider & Valukas, 2004). Considerations related to tertiary prevention in the school setting and related community health nursing responsibilities are summarized in Table 23-9◆.

Implementing Health Care in School Settings

Implementing health care for individuals or groups in the school setting frequently involves collaboration between the nurse and other members of the school health team. At the individual level, for example, the community health nurse may need to contact the private physician of a child with a chronic illness with information about adverse effects of medications or to request a change in the medical treatment plan based on

TABLE 23-9	Areas of Emphasis in Tertiary Prevention in the School Setting and Related Community Health Nursing Responsibilities	
Area of Emphasis	**Related Community Health Nursing Responsibilities**
Preventing recurrence of acute conditions	Eliminate risk factors for the condition. Teach students, staff, or parents how to prevent recurrence of problems. Make referrals that can assist in eliminating risk factors.
Preventing complications of and promoting adjustment to chronic and handicapping conditions	Assist parents with finding sources of financial aid to deal with chronic and handicapping conditions. Facilitate meeting special nutritional needs. Assist with meeting special needs for transportation and facilities. Provide for special equipment needs. Promote psychological well-being. Assist students, families, and staff to deal with the eventuality of death in terminal illnesses. Refer for counseling as needed. Function as an advocate as needed.
Preventing adverse effects of learning disabilities	Provide consultation for teachers in dealing with children's learning disabilities. Participate in the design of IEPs for children with disabilities. Function as an advocate for the learning-disabled child as needed. Serve as a role model in positively reinforcing the child's accomplishments.
Sustaining school-based health services	Assist with identification of mechanisms for continued funding of school-based health services. Assist with the development of plans to apply for FQHC status if warranted. Conduct research to document the outcomes of school-based health care services.

changes in the child's condition. The nurse also needs to solicit the cooperation of parents in following through on a referral for medical services, testing, counseling, or other services needed by their child.

Implementing care for groups within the school setting also requires collaboration between the nurse and others. For example, the nurse may invite local police personnel to participate in a drug education program to be presented in the school, or the nurse might work with teachers, media specialists, food service personnel, and others to implement an educational program on basic nutrition for elementary schoolchildren. Parental permission may be required in certain school-based health programs. For example, parents need to grant permission for screening procedures such as hematocrit testing. The nurse may also need to recruit parent or community volunteers to assist with screening programs or with other health-related programs such as a health fair.

Evaluating Health Care in School Settings

Evaluating the effectiveness of care in the school setting focuses on the outcomes of that care. Evaluation can occur at two levels, the individual child or the total school health program. Evaluative criteria for the care of the individual child reflect the effects of nursing care on the youngster's health status. For example, if a child is no longer abused by his parent, no longer has recurrent ear infections, or is now able to interact effectively with peers, the interventions of the nurse have probably been effective.

Evaluation of the overall school health program focuses on indicators of the health status of the total population. For instance, absentee rates might indicate how effective the program has been in preventing disease. Student screening test results may also provide information on the effectiveness of primary preventive efforts.

Changes in the prevalence of certain health problems within the school population may also indicate the efficacy of secondary preventive measures. For example, if alcohol abuse has been a problem among the student population, a declining prevalence of alcohol abuse would indicate that secondary measures are having an effect. Similarly, a decline in the teenage pregnancy rate would indicate that a sex education program is effective.

The processes used in evaluating the school health program are those discussed in Chapter 15∞. The school nurse collaborates with other members of the school health team in designing and implementing an evaluation of the program. Moreover, the nurse may also be involved in data collection related to the evaluation and in interpreting those data. Finally, the nurse should be actively involved in decisions made on the basis of evaluative data.

At the national level, national objectives for the year 2010 related to school health can provide additional evaluative criteria. Information on the current status of some of these objectives is presented on page 661◆. Another

Information on the current status of some of these objectives is presented on page 661◆.

BUILDING OUR KNOWLEDGE BASE

*I*n 1994, the Institute of Medicine committee studying comprehensive school health programs put forth recommendations for planned and continuously monitored school health services as part of public health and primary care systems and research on school-based services. In 1996, the American School Health Association (ASHA) and the National Association of School Nurses (NASN) collaborated to establish five priorities for research related to school health services:

- Research that is practice-based and relevant to school nursing practice
- The need for standardized research
- The need for school nurses to be educated to conduct and document research
- The need for funding to support research
- The need to include school nursing research in graduate-degree education requirements

Based on these priorities, Edwards (2002) conducted a Delphi study to identify specific topics for school nursing research. The topics identified included the following:

- The impact of school nursing services on student health
- The relationship between school nurse practice and educational outcomes
- The benefits and cost-effectiveness of school health services
- The value of school health services to the educational system
- Predictors of outcomes for student health, particularly for special needs students
- Nursing interventions for mental health promotion
- Characteristics of successful nursing interventions
- Prevention/intervention for children with chronic illnesses
- Core elements of school nursing practice
- Nursing interventions related to violence and substance abuse prevention

Select one of these topics and discuss with your classmates and instructors how you might design a study to address the topic. Where might you implement your study? What variables would you include? What type of design would you use?

mechanism for evaluating school health services is the School Health Index (SHI) developed by the National Center for Chronic Disease Prevention and Health Promotion (2005e) Division of Child and Adolescent Health. SHI is an assessment and planning guide that provides a series of self-assessment modules addressing the eight components of a school health program and five critical health topics as of 2005. Additional modules assessing other specific topics will be added as they are developed. Use of SHI creates a scorecard for each module that is then used to complete a planning questionnaire to guide program improvement.

Community health nursing in schools provides an opportunity for promoting health and preventing illness in children and their families. Community health nurses working in school settings at all levels can also assist students and staff with existing health problems, as well as designing school health programs that promote the health of the general public.

HEALTHY PEOPLE 2010

Goals for Population Health

OBJECTIVE	BASELINE	MOST RECENT DATA	TARGET
7-2. Increase the proportion of middle, junior, and senior high schools that provide comprehensive school health education related to:			
b. Unintentional injury	66%	68%	90%
c. Violence	58%	73%	80%
d. Suicide	58%	59%	80%
e. Tobacco use and addiction	86%	88%	95%
f. Alcohol and other drug use	90%	89%	95%#
g. Unintended pregnancy, HIV/AIDS, and STD	65%	62%	90%#
h. Unhealthy dietary patterns	84%	84%	95%
i. Inadequate physical activity	78%	76%	90%#
j. Environmental health	60%	60%	80%
7-3. Increase the proportion of college students who receive information on six priority health risks	6%	NDA	25%
7-4. Increase the proportion of elementary, middle, junior high, and senior high schools that have a nurse-to-student ratio of at least 1:750	28%	53%	50%*
6-9. Increase the proportion of children and youth who spend at least 80% of their time in regular education programs	46%	NDA	60%
22-8. Increase the proportion of schools that require daily physical education for all students			
a. Middle and junior high	6.4%	NDA	25%
b. Senior high	5.8%	NDA	5%*
22-9. Increase the proportion of adolescents who participate in daily school physical education	27%	28%	50%
22-10. Increase the proportion of adolescents who spend at least 50% of time in physical education classes being physically active	38%	39%	50%
27-11. Increase smoke-free and tobacco-free environments in schools (including all school facilities, property, vehicles, and events)	37%	45%	100%

NDA—No data available

* Objective has been met

Objective moving away from target

Data from: Centers for Disease Control and Prevention. (2005). Healthy People Data. Retrieved September 6, 2005, from http://wonder.cdc.gov/data2010

Case Study

Nursing in the School Setting

Brandon is a third grader in the school where you work as a school nurse. He comes to see you because he "has a stomachache." This is his third visit to your office in as many days. Each day, you have seen him for a similar complaint but have found no physical evidence of illness. According to his teacher, his appetite has been good at lunch, although his lunches are large and not particularly nutritious. Brandon says he is not constipated and has not had any diarrhea or vomiting. His abdominal pain usually disappears after he lies down in your office for about 20 minutes.

When you talk to the teacher, she tells you that lately the other children have been making fun of Brandon because he always comes in last in running games and can't run very fast during PE. Brandon is about 35 pounds overweight for his height and becomes short of breath with strenuous physical exercise. Brandon has two younger brothers who are both slender and have no difficulties with physical activity.

The teacher also mentions that Brandon has been talking during class and disturbing the other children. She has tried to take him aside and explain why he should not talk in class, but he continues. His grades are not the best in the world (they're not the worst either), but he has been discouraged lately because he is having trouble mastering long division.

1. What biophysical, psychological, sociocultural, behavioral, and health system factors are operating in this situation?
2. What nursing diagnoses would you derive from the information provided above? How would you prioritize Brandon's problems? Why?

3. Who else should be involved in developing a plan of care for Brandon?
4. Write at least two outcome objectives for Brandon's care.
5. What advocacy challenges might arise in meeting Brandon's needs?

6. What primary, secondary, and tertiary prevention measures would be appropriate in this case?
7. How would you evaluate the effectiveness of your interventions with Brandon? Be specific.

Test Your Understanding

1. What is the overall goal of a school health program? (p. 632)

2. What are the basic components of a school health program? (pp. 632–634)

3. What biophysical, psychological, physical environmental, sociocultural, behavioral, and health system factors may influence the health of the school population? (pp. 638–650)

4. What are the major areas of emphasis in primary prevention in the school setting? Describe at least two nursing activities related to each area. (pp. 651–654)

5. What are the facets of secondary prevention in the school setting? Identify at least two community health nursing responsibilities related to each facet. (pp. 654–657)

6. What are the major areas of emphasis in tertiary prevention in the school setting? How might the community health nurse be involved in each of these areas? (pp. 658–659).

EXPLORE MediaLink

http://www.prenhall.com/clark
Resources for this chapter can be found on the Companion Website.

Audio Glossary
Appendix E: Information on Selected Communicable Diseases
Appendix G: Community Health Assessment and Intervention Guide

Exam Review Questions
Case Study: Safety at School
MediaLink Applications: High School Stress (video)
Media Links

Challenge Your Knowledge
Update *Healthy People 2010*
Advocacy Interviews

References

Allensworth, D., Lawson, E., Nicholson, L., & Wyche, J. (Eds.). (1997). *Schools and health: Our nation's investment.* Washington, DC: National Academy Press.

American Academy of Pediatrics. (2000a). Policy statement: Corporal punishment in schools. *Pediatrics, 106,* 343.

American Academy of Pediatrics. (2000b). Policy statement: Physical fitness and activity in schools. *Pediatrics, 105,* 1156–1157.

American Academy of Pediatrics. (2000c). Policy statement: School health assessments. *Pediatrics, 105,* 875–877.

American Academy of Pediatrics. (2001a). Policy statement: The role of the school nurse in providing school health services. *Pediatrics, 108,* 1231–1232.

American Academy of Pediatrics. (2001b). Policy statement: School health centers and other integrated school health services. *Pediatrics, 107,* 198–201.

American Academy of Pediatrics. (2003). Policy statement: Out-of-school suspension and expulsion. *Pediatrics, 112,* 1206–1209.

American Academy of Pediatrics. (2004). Policy statement: School-based mental health services. *Pediatrics, 113,* 1839–1845.

American Nurses Association & National Association of School Nurses. (2005). *School nursing: Scope and standards of practice.* Silver Spring. MD: nursesbooks.org

American School Health Association. (2005). *What is school health?* Retrieved February 11, 2006, from http://www.ashaweb.org/whatis/html

Austin, S. B., Melly, S. J., Sanchez, B. N., Patel, A., Buka, S., & Gortmaker, S. L. (2005). Clustering of fast-food restaurants around schools: A novel application of spatial statistics to the study of food environments. *American Journal of Public Health, 95,* 1575–1581.

Barnes, M., Courtney, M. D., Pratt, J., & Walsh, A. M. (2004). School-based youth health nurses: Roles, responsibilities, challenges, and rewards. *Public Health Nursing, 21,* 316–322.

Barrios, L. C., Davis, M. K., Kann, L., Desai, S., Mercy, J. A., Reese, L. E., et al. (2001). School

health guidelines to prevent unintentional injuries and violence. *Morbidity and Mortality Weekly Report, 50*(RR-22), 1–73.

Bingler, S. (2000). The school as the center of a healthy community. *Public Health Reports, 115,* 228–233.

Bishop, J. H., Bishop, M., Bishop, M., Gelbwasser, L., Green, S., Peterson, E., et al., 2004. Why we harass nerds and freaks: A formal theory of student culture and norms. *Journal of School Health, 74,* 235–251.

Cappelli, D., & Brown, J. P. (2002). Validation of school nurses to identify gingivitis in adolescents. *American Journal of Public Health, 92,* 946–948.

Catalano, R. F., Haggerty, K. P., Oesterle, S., Fleming, C. B., & Hawkins, J. D. (2004). The importance of bonding to school for healthy development: Findings from the Social Development Research Group. *Journal of School Health, 74,* 252–261.

Centers for Disease Control and Prevention. (2005). *Healthy People Data.* Retrieved September 6, 2005, from http://wonder.cdc.gov/data2010

Chen, G., Smith, G. A., Deng, S., Hostetler, S. G., & Xiang, H. (2005). Nonfatal injuries among middle-school and high-school students in Guangxi, China. *American Journal of Public Health, 95*, 1989–1995.

Clendon, J., & White, G. (2001). The feasibility of a nurse practitioner-led primary health care clinic in a school setting: A community needs analysis. *Journal of Advanced Nursing, 34*, 171–178.

Croghan, E., & Johnson, C. (2004). Occupational health and school health: A natural alliance. *Journal of Advanced Nursing, 45*, 155–161.

Croghan, E., Johnson, C., & Aveyard, P. (2004). School nurses: Policies, working practices, roles, and value perceptions. *Journal of Advanced Nursing, 47*, 377–385.

Division of Environmental Hazards and Health Effects. (2005). Self-reported asthma among high school students—United States, 2003. *Morbidity and Mortality Weekly Report, 54*, 765–767.

Division of Unintentional Injury Prevention. (2002). Barriers to children walking and biking to school—United States, 1999. *Morbidity and Mortality Weekly Report, 51*, 701–704.

Domrose, C. (2003). Unkindest cuts. *NurseWeek, 16*(16), 11–14.

Edwards, L. H. (2002). Research priorities in school nursing: A Delphi process. *Journal of School Health, 72*, 173–177.

Fein, R. A., Vossekuil, B., Pollack, W. S., Borum, R., Modzeleski, W., & Reddy, M. (2002). *Threat assessment in schools: A guide to managing threatening situations and to creating safe school climates.* Washington, DC: U.S. Department of Education.

Gance-Cleveland, B. (2004). Qualitative evaluation of a school-based support group for adolescents with an addicted parent. *Nursing Research, 53*, 379–386.

Glanz, K., Saraiya, M., & Wechsler, H. (2002). Guidelines for school programs to prevent skin cancer. *Morbidity and Mortality Weekly Report, 51*(RR-4), 1–18.

Grunbaum, J. A., Kann, L., Kinchen, S., Ross, J., Hawkins, J., Lowry, R., et al. (2004). Youth risk behavior surveillance—United States, 2003. *Morbidity and Mortality Weekly Report, 53*(SS-2), 1–96.

Grunbaum, J. A., Kann, L., Williams, B. I., Collins, J. L., Kolbe, L. J., Williams, B. I., et al. (2000). Surveillance for characteristics of health education among secondary schools—School health education profiles, 1998. *Morbidity and Mortality Weekly Report, 49*(SS-8), 1–41.

Guttu, M., Engelke, M. K., & Swanson, M. (2004). Does the school nurse-to-student ratio make a difference? *Journal of School Health, 74*, 6–9.

Humphries, J. (2002). School nursing. In J. Canham & J. Bennett (Eds.), *Mentorship in community nursing: Challenges and opportunities* (pp. 166–172). London: Blackwell Science.

Jones, S. E., Brenner, N. D., & McManus, T. (2003). Prevalence of school policies, programs, and facilities that promote a healthy physical school environment. *American Journal of Public Health, 93*, 1570–1575.

Jones, S. E., & Wheeler, L. (2004). Asthma inhalers in schools: Right of students with asthma to a free appropriate education. *American Journal of Public Health, 94*, 1102–1107.

Jozefowicz-Simbeni, D. M. H., & Allen-Meares, P. (2002). Poverty and schools: Intervention and resources building through school-linked services. *Children & Schools, 24*, 123–136.

Kann, L., Kinchen, S. A., Williams, B. I., Ross, J. G., Lowry, R., Grunbaum, J. A., et al. (2000). Youth Risk Behavior Surveillance—United States, 1999. *Morbidity and Mortality Weekly Report, 49*(SS-5), 1–94.

Katz, D. L., O'Connell, M., Yeh, M.-C., Nawaz, H., Njike, V., Anderson, L. M., et al. (2005). Public health strategies for preventing and controlling overweight and obesity in school and worksite settings: A report on recommendations of the Task Force on Community Preventive Services. *Morbidity and Mortality Weekly Report, 54*(RR-10), 1–12.

Kayaba, K., Wakabayashi, C., Kunisawa, N., Shinmura, H., & Yanagawa, H. (2005). Implementation of a smoke-free policy on school premises and tobacco control as a priority among municipal health promotion activities: Nationwide survey in Japan. *American Journal of Public Health, 95*, 420–422.

Kronenfeld, J. J. (2000). *Schools and the health of children: Protecting our future.* Thousand Oaks, CA: Sage.

Kubik, M. Y., Lytle, L. A., Hannan, O. J., Perry, C. L., & Story, M. (2003). The association of the school food environment with dietary behaviors of young adolescents. *American Journal of Public Health, 93*, 1168–1173.

Leighton, S., Worraker, A., & Nolan, P. (2003). School nurses and mental health: Part 1. *Mental Health Practice, 7*(4), 14–16.

Lewis, K. D., & Bear, B. J. (2002). *Manual of school health* (2nd ed.). Philadelphia: Saunders.

Massey-Stokes, M., & Lanning, B. (2004). The role of CSHPs in preventing child abuse and neglect. *Journal of School Health, 74*, 193–194.

National Association of School Nurses. (2003a). *Position statement: Individualized health care plans.* Retrieved February 11, 2006, from http://www.nasn.org/Portals/0/positions/2003psindividualized.pdf

National Association of School Nurses. (2003b). *Position statement: Medication administration in the school setting.* Retrieved February 11, 2006, from http://www.nasn.org/Portals/0/positions/2003psmedication.pdf

National Association of School Nurses. (2003c). *Resolution: Access to a school nurse.* Retrieved February 11, 2006, from http://www.nasn.org/Portals/0/statements/resolutionaccess.pdf

National Center for Chronic Disease Prevention and Health Promotion. (2005a). *Healthy youth! About us: Our mission: Four strategies to promote national school health.* Retrieved February 8, 2006, from http://www.cdc.gov/HealthyYouth/about/mission.htm

National Center for Chronic Disease Prevention and Health Promotion. (2005b). *Healthy youth! Coordinated school health program.* Retrieved February 8, 2006, from http://www.cdc.gov/HealthyYouth/CSHP

National Center for Chronic Disease Prevention and Health Promotion. (2005c). *Healthy youth! Health topics.* Retrieved February 8, 2006, from http://www.cdc.gov/HealthyYouth/healthtopics/index/htm

National Center for Chronic Disease Prevention and Health Promotion. (2005d). *Healthy youth! School health guidelines and strategies.* Retrieved February 8, 2006, from http://www.cdc.gov/HealthyYouth/publications/guidelines.htm

National Center for Chronic Disease Prevention and Health Promotion. (2005e). *Healthy youth! School Health Index (SHI): Introduction.* Retrieved February 8, 2006, from http://www.cdc.gov/SHI/Static/Introduction.aspx

Nurses Service Organization (2004). Giving medications in daycare or school. *NSO Risk Advisor, 12*, 7.

Palmer, R. F., Blanchard, S., Jean, C. R., & Mandell, D. S. (2005). School district resources and identification of children with autistic disorder. *American Journal of Public Health, 95*, 125–130.

Pate, R. R., Ward, D. S., Saunders, R. P., Felton, G., Dishman, R. K., & Dowda, M. (2005). Promotion of physical activity among high-school girls: A randomized controlled trial. *American Journal of Public Health, 95*, 1582–1587.

Richardson, K. (2004). Highlights of obesity and the built environment: Improving public health through community design. Retrieved August 31, 2004, from http://www.medscape.com/viewarticle/487906

Robinson, J., & Taras, H., Luckenbill, D., & Wheeler, L. (2000). *Guidelines for school health programs to be developed.* Retrieved September 17, 2001, from http://www.schoolhealth.org/hmhs.htm

Sallis, J. F., Conway, T. L., Prochaska, J. J., McKenzie, T. L., Marshall, S. J., & Brown, M. (2001). The association of school environments with youth physical activity. *American Journal of Public Health, 91*, 618–620.

Sirard, J. R., Ainsworth, B. E., McIver, K. L., & Pate, R. R. (2005). Prevalence of active commuting at urban and suburban elementary schools in Columbia, SC. *American Journal of Public Health, 95*, 236–237.

Swider, S. M., & Valukas, A. (2004). Options for sustaining school-based health centers. *Journal of School Health, 74*, 115–118.

Taras, H., Duncan, P., Luckenbill, D., Robinson, J., Wheeler, L., & Wooley, S. (2004). *Health, mental health, and safety guidelines for schools.* Retrieved February 8, 2006, from http://www.nationalguidelines.org

U.S. Department of Health and Human Services. (2003). *Steps to a healthier US: A program and policy perspective. Prevention strategies that work.* Retrieved July 25, 2003, from http://www.healthierus.gov/steps

Veugelers, P. J., & Fitzgerald, A. L. (2005). Effectiveness of school programs in preventing childhood obesity: A multilevel comparison. *American Journal of Public Health, 95*, 432–435.

Vossekuil, B., Fein, R. A., Reddy, M., Borum, R., & Modzeleski, W. (2002). *Final report and findings of the safe school initiative.* Washington, DC: U.S. Department of Education.

Wells, J. (2003). Safety net. *NurseWeek, 16*(21), 18–19.

Williams, S. (2005). College infirmaries: From depression to tattoos. *NurseWeek, 18*(23), 26–27.

Winnail, S., Stevenson, B., & Dorman, S. (2004). New directions: A coordinated school health approach to cancer control. *Journal of School Health, 74,* 76–78.

Wolfe, L. C., & Selekman, J. (2002). School nurses: What it was and what it is. *Pediatric Nursing, 28,* 403–407.

World Health Organization. (2002). *Scaling up the response to infectious diseases.* Retrieved April 2, 2002, from http://www.who. infectious-disease-report/2002/framesintro. html

Xiang, H., Stallones, L., Chen, G., Hostetler, S. G., & Kelleher, K. (2005). Nonfatal injuries among US children with disabling conditions. *American Journal of Public Health, 95,* 1970–1975.

Xu, Y., Crane, P., & Ryan, R. (2002). School nursing in an underserved multiethnic Asian community: Experiences and outcomes. *Journal of Community Health Nursing, 19,* 187–198.

Yang, J., Bowling, M., Lewis, M. A., Marshall, S. W., Runyan, C. W., & Mueller, F. O. (2005). Use of discretionary protective equipment in high school athletes: Prevalence and determinants. *American Journal of Public Health, 95,* 1996–2002.

Yu, X. (2002). The role of school nurses in Beijing, China. *Journal of School Health, 72,* 168–170.

Care of Clients in Work Settings

CHAPTER OBJECTIVES

After reading this chapter, you should be able to:

1. Describe advantages of providing health care in work settings.
2. Identify types of health and safety hazards encountered in work settings.
3. Identify biophysical, psychological, physical environmental, sociocultural, behavioral, and health system factors that influence health in work settings.
4. Analyze spheres of social influence and their effect on the health of employees.
5. Describe types of health care programs in work settings.
6. Describe areas of emphasis in primary prevention in work settings and analyze the role of the community health nurse with respect to each.
7. Describe major considerations in secondary prevention in work settings and analyze the contribution of community health nursing in each.
8. Describe emphases in tertiary prevention in work settings and analyze the role of the community health nurse with respect to each.

KEY TERMS

company wellness policies **681**
emotional labor **674**
employee assistance program (EAP) **692**
ergonomics **682**
job strain **673**
occupational health nursing **668**
paraoccupational exposure **680**
postexposure prophylaxis (PEP) **688**
presenteeism **684**
screening **690**
work movement index **673**

MediaLink
http://www.prenhall.com/clark

Additional interactive resources for this chapter can be found on the Companion Website. Click on Chapter 24 and "Begin" to select the activities for this chapter.

Advocacy in Action

Stop Smoking

A public health nurse in Taichung County, Taiwan, assessed the community and found a high prevalence of smoking in local factories. Taiwanese workers like to make friends by giving cigarettes to each other and enjoy smoking together. Although Taiwan has legislation to promote smoking cessation and health education about smoking has been provided in schools, hospitals, restaurants, and public districts, factories are often resistant to smoking control. Employers do not perceive smoking to be a problem, and often think that cigarette smoking can improve worker effectiveness.

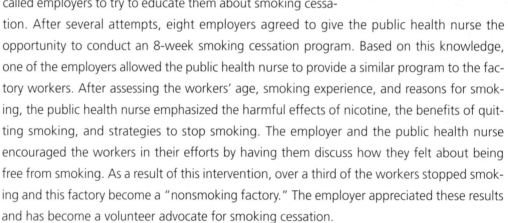

To create a "nonsmoking factory," the public health nurse called employers to try to educate them about smoking cessation. After several attempts, eight employers agreed to give the public health nurse the opportunity to conduct an 8-week smoking cessation program. Based on this knowledge, one of the employers allowed the public health nurse to provide a similar program to the factory workers. After assessing the workers' age, smoking experience, and reasons for smoking, the public health nurse emphasized the harmful effects of nicotine, the benefits of quitting smoking, and strategies to stop smoking. The employer and the public health nurse encouraged the workers in their efforts by having them discuss how they felt about being free from smoking. As a result of this intervention, over a third of the workers stopped smoking and this factory become a "nonsmoking factory." The employer appreciated these results and has become a volunteer advocate for smoking cessation.

The public health nurse reported the results of the intervention to the Health Bureau, and the Health Bureau and the nurse have developed guidelines to promote smoking cessation in occupational health settings. Because of the activities of the public health nurse and the volunteer employer, other factories have begun to provide smoking cessation programs for their workers.

Tzu-Chuan Chien Chen

Assistant Professor, Community Health, Hongkung University

*B*ecause nearly two thirds of the U.S. population over 16 years of age are employed, the work setting is an important place for promoting the health of the general population (Katz et al., 2005). Although the work environment contributes to a wide variety of health problems, it also provides opportunities to influence a major segment of the population regarding personal health behaviors.

The effects of work on health were noted by Bernardino Ramazzini, considered the father of occupational medicine, as early as 1700 (Franco, 2001). In 1713, Ramazzini wrote about the occupational effects on musculoskeletal health and the effects of the sedentary nature of some occupations (Ramazzini, 2001). Similarly, cutaneous anthrax was first associated with the handling of wool in 1837, although the disease itself was not diagnosed until 1880 (Bell, 2002). Henry Bell, a British physician who attended a man dying of anthrax sent the death certificate to the police maintaining that the employer had caused the death due to his failure to disinfect the wool the deceased was working with. Bell's actions led to an inquiry and the institution of voluntary guidelines for the wool industry that were in effect until 1899. In the early 20th century, Germany instituted *krankenhaussen*, sickness insurance funds for the working class, which prompted U.S. sociologists to promote occupational disease surveys. The first such survey was conducted in 1910 and focused on "occupational poisons," specifically occupational lead exposure (Hamilton, 2001). Despite this long history of knowledge of the effects of working conditions on health, thousands of workers are injured or develop occupational illnesses every year.

Over the years, however, employers have come to better appreciate that healthy employees are more productive and that it is in the employer's interest to promote and maintain employee health. Moreover, the escalating cost of health insurance makes health promotion increasingly cost-effective. One way that some companies have chosen to decrease health-related costs is to provide on-site health care for employees.

The importance of health care in the occupational setting can be seen in the national health objectives for the year 2010. In fact, one entire section of the objectives deals with health and safety in occupational settings (U.S. Department of Health and Human Services [USDHHS], 2000b). The status of selected objectives is addressed later in this chapter. The complete set of objectives and their current status can be reviewed on the *Healthy People 2010*◆ Web site, http://wonder.cdc.gov/data2010.

ADVANTAGES OF PROVIDING HEALTH CARE IN WORK SETTINGS

From a community health nursing perspective, there are a number of advantages to providing health care in work settings. They include the substantial amount of time that people spend in this setting and the fact that this time is spent on a regular basis. In addition, when employees are present, they are essentially a "captive audience," subject to powerful pressures from peers and employers to engage in healthy behaviors. For example, nonsmoking peers may object to smoking in their work or recreation areas, or employers may provide financial or nonfinancial incentives for healthy behavior. Another advantage is that the workforce frequently consists of people who may be at risk for a variety of health problems or who may be motivated to maintain their health to ensure their continued ability to work. Because health care personnel are frequently in the setting and mechanisms are in place for communicating health messages, health promotion in work settings is efficient and cost-effective. More and more companies are acknowledging the advantages of providing health care in the occupational setting.

Failure to address occupational health issues leads to a variety of consequences and costs for businesses themselves, as well as for society as a whole. Employers currently pay for a significant proportion of U.S. health care expenditures through employment-based health insurance premiums. In addition to health insurance costs, health issues present other visible and hidden costs in the work environment. Visible costs include those related to sickness, absenteeism, and employee turnover. Hidden costs may include low productivity, poor-quality work, poor customer service, accidents, and legal claims arising from illness and injuries due to the work environment.

OCCUPATIONAL HEALTH SERVICES

The goal of occupational health services is to "ensure that working adults reach and maintain their full working potential through health promotion, protection, and surveillance activities" (Croghan & Johnson, 2004, p. 158) or to "secure a safe and healthy environment and enhance the employees' ability to work" (Naumanen-Tuomela, 2001b, p. 108). The client for occupational health services may be the individual worker, the work community, or the organization.

Some authors have noted that occupational health services have focused, until recently, on individual employee risk behaviors and less on the public health context of occupational health. They identify a need to reconnect occupational health services with a public health perspective and suggest the use of one of four models for doing so. The ecosocial model integrates social and biological factors in exploring the influences of the work setting on health. The integrated workplace intervention model addresses both behavioral and environmental risks that influence worker health. The third model, a life course approach, views health as resulting from the cumulative effects of events over the course of a lifetime in which one's employment is one of many events. Finally, a sustainable production model focuses on primary prevention of occupational and environmental hazards as a mechanism for improving the health of employees as well as of the general public (Quinn, 2003).

When occupational health services have a public health focus, they occur at three levels: individual, community, and system (Naumanen-Tuomela, 2001a). Services provided to individual workers are aimed at affecting health knowledge and skills as well as individual health status. At the community level, services focus on the development of community norms, awareness, attitudes, practices, and behaviors that support health. At the systems level, services result in changes in organizations and social structures that benefit both individuals and the larger community.

Research in Finland identified four approaches to the provision of occupational health services that are comparable to possible arrangements for services in the United States. In the first approach, the business creates its own in-house health services to deal with the majority of health-related problems experienced by employees. Many companies that employ large numbers of workers provide in-house services. Smaller employers may choose to join with other organizations to establish health services then utilized by all. A third approach is to contract for services from municipal health care centers. For example, in the United States, companies may contract with organizations such as the American Cancer Society for smoking cessation programs offered in the work setting. Finally, the organization may purchase health care services from private medical facilities. For example, an employer may contract for health services for employees from a local hospital or clinic (Naumanen-Tuomela, 2001b).

When companies provide their own on-site services, community health nurses working in occupational health settings may be part of an occupational health team. In some small companies, the nurse is the only health care professional employed by the company. In such instances, other health care professionals interact with the nurse on a consultant basis. For example, the community health nurse might collaborate with an employee's primary health care provider to plan for the employee's return to work after an illness or injury. In other instances, the company may contract with outside providers for consultation services related to employee health needs.

Other companies have a well-developed occupational health team present within the facility. In addition to the community health nurse, such teams may include other nurses, physicians, safety engineers, industrial hygienists, counselors, ancillary nursing personnel (e.g., licensed practical nurses), toxicologists, emergency medical technicians, physicians' assistants, epidemiologists, laboratory and x-ray technicians, safety coordinators, and nurse practitioners. The functions and roles of most

of these individuals are already familiar to the reader. A few, however, may be unfamiliar. A safety engineer, for example, is responsible for monitoring the safety of the physical environment in the work setting, and an industrial hygienist has similar responsibilities for identifying and controlling physical, biological, and chemical hazards in the work setting. Toxicologists may be involved in research on the toxic effects of chemical exposures in the work setting, as well as in contributing to plans for the control and treatment of such exposures.

OCCUPATIONAL HEALTH NURSING

Not all nurses who practice in occupational settings are community health nurses. The community health nurse, however, is uniquely prepared to meet the health needs of the working population because of his or her knowledge of community health principles. Occupational health nursing is not a new role for the community health nurse. Nurses may have been employed in work settings as early as 1888 and certainly by 1895, when the Vermont Marble Company employed Ada M. Stewart (Parrish & Alfred, 1995). In 1943, a U.S. Public Health Service study recommended one nurse for every 300 employees to provide health services and advocacy in factories (Anglin, 1990). Since that time, the role of the occupational health nurse has been expanded along with other nursing roles. Several years ago, the U.S. Department of Labor defined occupational health nursing as "giving nursing service under general medical direction to ill or injured employees or other persons who become ill or suffer an accident on the premises of a factory or other establishment" (Hughes, 1979).

This definition does not, however, fully describe today's community health nursing role in work settings. It concentrates on the treatment aspects of care and the nurse's dependent functions and does not acknowledge the promotional and preventive aspects that are paramount in this practice setting. In the 2004 *Standards of Occupational and Environmental Health Nursing*, the American Association of Occupational Health Nurses (AAOHN, 2004b) defined **occupational health nursing** as

> the specialty practice that focuses on promotion, protection, and restoration of health within the context of a safe and healthy work environment. It includes the prevention of adverse health effects from occupational and environmental hazards. It provides for and delivers occupational and environmental health and safety programs and services to clients. (p. 270)

Educational Preparation for Occupational Health Nursing

Several types of nursing personnel may be found in occupational settings, including registered nurses prepared in associate degree and diploma programs in nursing as well as in baccalaureate degree programs; licensed practical nurses; and nurses prepared at the master's level. Because of the need to apply principles of community health nursing, nurses who engage in the full scope of the occupational health nurse's role should be prepared at least at the baccalaureate level in nursing. Advanced preparation in occupational health nursing may result in certification by AAOHN. Nurses working in occupational settings might also hold master's degrees in nursing. Educational preparation at this level might be in occupational health nursing, in community health nursing, or as a nurse practitioner.

Nurses in other settings may also be involved in providing care for health conditions related to work. This fact suggests that nurse practitioners working in ambulatory care settings where occupational conditions may be seen should have a basic grounding in the principles of occupational health.

Standards and Competencies for Occupational Health Nursing

Like other nursing specialties, occupational health nursing should be practiced in accordance with established standards. The AAOHN (2004b) has established 11 standards for competent occupational and environmental health nursing practice. These standards are summarized below.

In addition, AAOHN has developed a code of ethics for nursing practice in occupational health settings. According to the code of ethics, occupational health nurses

- Promote interdisciplinary collaboration with clients, other providers, and community agencies
- Safeguard employees' rights to privacy
- Safeguard employees from unethical and illegal actions
- Accept their obligation to society as licensed professionals

- Maintain personal competence and comply with applicable laws and regulations
- Promote the development of a professional body of knowledge while protecting employees' rights (AAOHN, 2004a)

Occupational Health Nursing Roles

The specific role functions of an occupational health nurse may vary somewhat from setting to setting, but there are some general commonalities among settings. These functions may generally be grouped as employee-centered functions, workplace and work community-centered functions, collaborative functions, administrative functions, and other functions (Naumanen-Tuomela, 2001b). Employee-centered functions include health promotion, protection, and illness prevention activities; primary care for health-related conditions; crisis care; rehabilitation; and counseling. Another function in this area might be the adaptation of work to the capabilities of workers based on their health status (Rose, 2002). Workplace and work community-centered functions include workplace surveillance and hazard detection, as well as communicating risk information to employees and employers (McPhaul & Lipscomb, 2004). Maintaining the first aid skills of employees is another community-centered function that may be performed by the occupational health nurse (Naumanen-Tuomela, 2001b).

The collaborative functions of occupational health nurses are carried out in cooperation with other members of the occupational health team and include identifying health and safety needs, prioritizing interventions, developing and implementing interventions and health care delivery programs, and evaluating the outcomes of care and the quality of service delivery (AAOHN,

SPECIAL CONSIDERATIONS

STANDARDS FOR OCCUPATIONAL AND ENVIRONMENTAL HEALTH NURSING

Standard 1. Assessment: The occupational and environmental health nurse systematically assesses the health status of the client(s).

Standard 2. Diagnosis: The occupational and environmental health nurse analyzes assessment data to formulate diagnoses.

Standard 3. Outcome Identification: The occupational and environmental health nurse identifies outcomes specific to the client(s).

Standard 4. Planning: The occupational and environmental health nurse develops a goal-directed plan that is comprehensive and formulates interventions to attain expected outcomes.

Standard 5. Implementation: The occupational and environmental health nurse implements interventions to attain desired outcomes identified in the plan.

Standard 6. Evaluation: The occupational and environmental health nurse systematically and continuously evaluates responses to interventions and progress toward the achievement of desired outcomes.

Standard 7. Resource Management: The occupational and environmental health nurse secures and manages the resources that support occupational health and safety programs and services.

Standard 8. Professional Development: The occupational and environmental health nurse assumes accountability for professional development to enhance professional growth and maintain competency.

Standard 9. Collaboration: The occupational and environmental health nurse collaborates with the client(s) for the promotion, prevention, and restoration of health within the context of a safe and healthy environment.

Standard 10. Research: The occupational and environmental health nurse uses resource findings in practice and contributes to the scientific base in occupational and environmental health nursing to improve practice and advance the profession.

Standard 11. Ethics: The occupational and environmental health nurse uses an ethical framework for decision-making in practice.

Data from: American Association of Occupational Health Nurses. (2004). Standards of Occupational and Environmental Health Nursing. AAOHN Journal, 52, 270–273. Reprinted by permission of American Association of Occupational Health Nurses.

2004b). Administrative functions may include tracking workers' compensation cases and cost-benefit analyses (Naumanen-Tuomela, 2001b).

CARE OF CLIENTS IN WORK SETTINGS

Nursing care in work settings is based on the use of the nursing process and includes assessment of the health of the population; development of nursing diagnoses; and planning, implementation, and evaluation of interventions to promote, protect, and restore health.

Assessing Health in Work Settings

Assessment of employee health status and health needs is undertaken from the perspective of biophysical, psychological, physical environmental, sociocultural, behavioral, and health system factors that influence health and illness in the working population.

Biophysical Considerations

Human biological factors to be addressed in assessing employee health status include those related to maturation and aging, genetic inheritance, and physiologic function.

MATURATION AND AGING The age composition of a company's workforce affects its health status. If employees are primarily young adults or adolescents, health conditions that may be noted with some frequency include sexually transmitted diseases, hepatitis, and pregnancy. Younger employees may also be at increased risk of injury due to limited job training and skills. In January 2006, U.S. Department of Labor (2006b) statistics indicated that 4% of the U.S. workforce was 16 to 19 years of age. Other data indicate that the United States employs more youth than any other developed country. As many as 5 million children and adolescents are legally employed and as many as 1 to 2 million more might be employed illegally without benefit of the health and safety standards applied to adult employment. Approximately half of 16- and 17-year-olds may be employed at least part of the time (Barrios et al., 2001), and in one study 56% of middle-school students worked for pay, 12% of them for 11 or more hours per week (Miller, 2004).

Younger workers are more likely to be injured on the job than older ones. In fact, youth in general are twice as likely as adults to be injured at work, and an average of 70 deaths occur each year among employees less than 18 years of age. Figures are even higher for agricultural workers, with youth being two to four times more likely to die of injuries as adults (Miller, 2004). In addition, younger agricultural workers are at greater risk of pesticide poisoning than older workers (Calvert et al., 2003). Overall, approximately 230,000 young people are injured at work each year, and roughly one third of them require care in an emergency department (Miller, 2004).

The health needs of older employees should also be considered. Because of prohibitions on forced retirement at specific ages, many employees are continuing in the workforce beyond the time when they would have retired. Economic need and a desire for continued productivity are two factors that may influence this trend. In January 2006, 17% of the U.S. workforce was over 55 years of age (U.S. Department of Labor, 2006b). By 2020, an estimated 80% of U.S. employees will be over 50 years of age (Plese, 2005b).

Musculoskeletal capacity diminishes and sensory impairments increase with age, placing older employees at higher risk for occupational injury. Although younger workers experience a higher rate of injury, older workers are at greater risk for occupational death. The occupational death rate for persons over 65 years of age is more than twice that of employees in other age groups (Division of Safety Research, 2001). In addition to the risk for injury and death, older workers planning to retire in the near future may need assistance with retirement planning and in dealing with retirement issues (see Chapter 19∞ for a discussion of these issues).

Older workers may also face discrimination in the workplace due to "stereotypes of disability, cognitive decline, inability to learn, and depression" (Plese, 2005b, p. 25). Many of these stereotypes are based on myths about older workers that include the following:

- Older workers are less creative than younger workers.
- Older workers are less productive than younger workers.
- Older workers value leisure time over employment.
- Older workers are more expensive to employ than younger workers.
- Older workers will become disabled or will be sick too often to be productive.
- Older workers are not as cognitively sharp as younger workers.
- It is too expensive to accommodate the needs of older workers.
- Additional training of older workers does not pay off.
- Older workers' best days are behind them. (Plese, 2005b)

Older workers will become a definite asset in many businesses and industries where there is a lack of younger workers to replace those who retire. In addition, older workers often possess experience and skills lacking in younger employees. Many older workers would remain in the work setting if their needs and preferences were accommodated. In fact, an estimated 13% of those who retired from jobs in the 1990s would have stayed on the job at least part-time if more flexible work schedules had been offered (Plese, 2005b).

Community health nurses working in occupational settings may find themselves advocating for the special needs of both younger and older workers. For example, they may need to encourage employers to arrange schedules to accommodate school schedules for younger employees. Similarly, they may need to advocate for equipment to assist with heavy lifting or other strenuous activities for older workers.

GENETIC INHERITANCE Genetic inheritance factors likely to be of greatest importance in the workforce are those related to race and gender. For example, in a largely African American labor force, hypertension may be prevalent. In an Asian population, particularly if large numbers are refugees, communicable diseases such as tuberculosis and parasitic diseases may be common.

In January 2006, 52% of the total U.S. workforce was women (U.S. Department of Labor, 2006b). The gender composition of the employee population affects the types of health conditions seen. For example, if large numbers of employees are women of childbearing age, there may be a need to provide prenatal or contraceptive services. There would also be a need to monitor more closely environmental conditions that may cause genetic changes or damage to an embryo. Occupational reproductive effects to be monitored include infertility, spontaneous abortion, low birth weight, pre- and postmaturity, birth defects, chromosomal abnormalities, preeclampsia, and an increased incidence of childhood cancers.

PHYSIOLOGIC FUNCTION Elements of physiologic function to be addressed in assessing the health of employees are the extent of injury and illness suffered by the population as well as immunization levels. In 2004, 4.3 million nonfatal injuries and illnesses occurred in the private employment sector. More than 2 million of these events required time away from work, job transfer, or restriction of job activities. This amounted to 2.5 cases per 100 full-time-equivalent (FTE) employees (U.S. Department of Labor, 2005b). Community health nurses in occupational settings must be prepared to recognize and deal with the multitude of illnesses and injuries likely to be encountered in the workplace.

Occupational illnesses include acute and chronic conditions that may affect an employee's ability to work as well as his or her quality of life. In 2004, 249,000 occupational illnesses were diagnosed. Although this figure reflects an 8% decrease from 2003 (U.S. Department of Labor, 2005b), it still represents an enormous burden in lost productivity as well as human suffering.

Illnesses experienced by employees may be acquired as a result of exposure to factors in the work setting. For example, workers in the adult film industry are at high risk for HIV infection, as well as for hepatitis B and other STDs (Division of STD Prevention, 2005). Similarly, miners frequently develop pneumoconiosis as a result of inhaling coal mine dust (Division of Respiratory Disease Studies, 2003), and employees who work with birds are at increased risk for histoplasmosis (Division of Bacterial and Mycotic Diseases, 2004). Highway repair poses an increased threat of silicosis (Valiante,

Schill, Rosenman, & Socie, 2004), and agricultural workers are at risk for pesticide poisoning (Reed, 2004).

The health care industry poses particular risks for occupational illness. In 2004, for example, 3 of the 14 industries with more than 100,000 new occupational illnesses were health-related settings. Hospitals contributed the most illnesses in this group, followed by nursing and residential facilities and primary care services (U.S. Department of Labor, 2005b). The overall illness rate in private industry in 2004 was 27.9 cases per 100 full-time-equivalent workers. In the health care and social assistance category of occupations, the rate was 41.7 per 100 FTE, but in the hospital sector, the rate of illness rose to 72.9 per 100 FTE (U.S. Department of Labor, 2005b, 2006a).

A large proportion of cancer deaths each year in the United States are attributable to workplace exposures. These include deaths from lung cancer, bladder cancer, and mesotheliomas (USDHHS, 2000a). Other cancers that may result from occupational exposures include those of the blood, bone, larynx, liver, nasal cavity and sinuses, peritoneum, pharynx, pleura, and skin (including scrotal malignancies).

Knowledge of the risk for and frequency of occupational illnesses in a particular work setting allows the community health nurse to advocate for appropriate worker protection systems and to effectively educate employees to minimize risks.

Other illnesses are not acquired as a result of working in a specific setting. These illnesses include a wide variety of chronic, and sometimes disabling, conditions that may affect employees' ability to work and their productivity while at work. These conditions may also be exacerbated by working conditions. Approximately 90 million people in the United States suffer from some type of chronic illness, and a significant number of them are included in the workforce (Sitzman, 2004a). One of the *Healthy People 2010*◆ objectives (objective 6.8) addresses the need to eliminate disparities in employment rates among adults with disabilities and those without disability. Another objective (2.5) focuses specifically on increasing the percentage of adults with arthritis who are employed (U.S. Department of Health and Human Services, 2000b).

Work-related asthma is a growing concern in occupational settings. Approximately 14 to 15 million Americans have asthma, and an additional 35 million have hay fever–type allergies that may be affected by their working conditions. In one survey of U.S. employees, 20% of respondents either suffered from asthma themselves or had a dependent with asthma. Approximately 9% of those surveyed had missed an average of 2.5 days of work in the last month due to allergies, and 6% missed an average of 3 days due to asthma. Another 19% lost partial days of work due to allergy and 11% due to asthma. Even when workers are not absent due to these conditions, their productivity is diminished (Putnam & McKibbin, 2004).

For the most part, cardiovascular diseases are influenced by personal risk factors of employees; however, evidence suggests that occupational factors may also contribute to the incidence of cardiovascular diseases. Some of these factors are exposure to metals, dust, and chemical inhalants, noise exposure, and psychological stress. Carbon disulfide, ethylene compounds, halogenated hydrocarbons, nitroglycerine, and nitrate exposures have also been associated with cardiovascular disease. The extent of one's control over one's job has also been shown to influence cardiovascular mortality. People with greater control tend to have lower mortality rates (Elovainio, Kivimaki, Steen, & Vahtera, 2004).

With greater numbers of women working today, there is growing concern regarding the reproductive and social effects of working conditions. Thus far, 1,000 occupational chemicals have been associated with reproductive effects in animals, but their human effects have not been assessed. Other working conditions, such as heat and radiation, also have reproductive effects. Although the primary concern is the impact on the female reproductive system, evidence indicates that exposure to some of these conditions (e.g., heat) can also affect the reproductive capabilities of men.

Neurotoxic conditions are another concern in occupational health. Some of the conditions encountered include heavy metal poisoning, behavior changes related to chemical exposure, and difficulty concentrating and performing one's job. Specific neurodegenerative disorders, such as presenile dementia, Alzheimer's disease, Parkinson's disease, and motor neuron disease, have also been associated with occupational factors. High prevalence of each of these conditions has been found among teachers, medical personnel, machinists and machine operators, scientists, writers, entertainers, and clerical workers. Selected conditions are also noted with some frequency among workers exposed to pesticides, solvents, and electromagnetic fields.

Noise-induced hearing loss and infectious diseases are other biophysical considerations in occupational settings. For example, first responders (fire fighters, emergency medical technicians) and health care personnel are at increased risk of bloodborne diseases (National Center for Infectious Diseases, 2000), whereas employees in manufacturing, construction, and other high-noise occupations are at greater risk for hearing loss.

With respect to dermatologic conditions arising from occupational factors, occupational health nurses are again in a position to assess the health status of employees. As with other types of health problems, the nurse should be aware of outbreaks of dermatologic conditions that indicate the presence of hazards in the environment and a need for control measures. Conditions encountered include a variety of rashes, pruritus, chemical burns, and desquamation.

Work-related injuries are another source of adverse effects on biophysical health. Each day approximately 11,000 workers are seen in emergency departments for injuries occurring on the job. Two hundred of these workers are hospitalized and 15 die of their injuries (Centers for Disease Control and Prevention [CDC], 2005b). Approximately 29% of all medically treated injuries in adults each year are work-related, and this figure climbs to almost half in some age groups (Smith et al., 2005). In 2004, the overall injury rate for private industry was 4.5 per 100 FTE, for a total of more than 4 million injuries (U.S. Department of Labor, 2006a). More than 5,700 of these injuries resulted in death, with nearly half of the deaths (43%) resulting from transportation accidents related to work. Other major causes of occupational fatalities included contact with objects or equipment (17.6%), falls (14%), assault and violence (14%), exposure to harmful substances or environments (8%), and fires or explosions (3%) (U.S. Department of Labor, 2005a). Occupational mortality rates increase with age, from 1.2 deaths per 100,000 workers aged 16 to 17 years to 11.3 per 100,000 employees over 65 years of age (National Center for Health Statistics, 2005).

Certain categories of industry account for a significant percentage of the occupational injuries and fatalities that occur each year. For example, in 2003, the rate of injury in the transportation and warehousing industries was 7.3 per 100 FTE, 6.6 per 100 FTE in manufacturing, and 3.8 in mining. Fourteen specific industries accounted for 46% of all injuries, with more than 100,000 cases each. This list was topped by hospitals, followed by nursing and residential care facilities. In fact, the combined

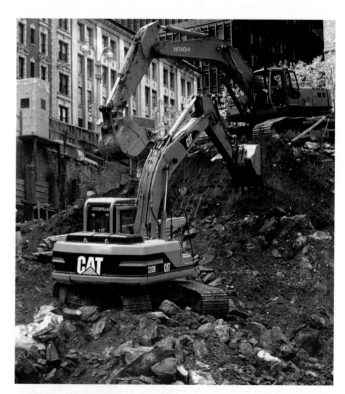

A variety of injuries may occur as a result of heavy equipment operation. (© Michael J. Doolittle/The Image Works)

health care and social assistance category accounts for 6.3% of all occupational injuries (U.S. Department of Labor, 2005b; 2006a).

Musculoskeletal injuries are the leading cause of lost workdays and workers' compensation claims among U.S. employees (Trinkhoff, Johantgen, Muntaner, & Le, 2005) and include injuries due to the cumulative trauma of repetitive activities as well as acute trauma. Causes of repeated trauma injury have increased fourteenfold in the last 20 years (Hopp, Lee, & Gest, 2004). Approximately 1.8 million U.S. workers each year experience musculoskeletal disorders such as carpal tunnel syndrome and back injuries, and these injuries lead to 600,000 work absences. The annual cost of musculoskeletal workplace injuries is $9 billion (Fee & Brown, 2001). The causes of carpal tunnel syndrome and other cumulative trauma disorders (CTDs) include repetitive motions, high-force actions, mechanical pressure, awkward posture, and vibration. Carpal tunnel syndrome results in a median loss of 30 days of work per injured employee, and back injury causes a loss of approximately 18 days per employee affected (Hopp et al., 2004). Although repetitive stress injuries have been commonly associated with computer use, they may also result from the repetitive motion of wrists, elbows, and shoulders involved in such occupations as laboratory work. In particular, pipetting requires high precision and increased muscle tension, resulting in damage to thumb and wrist (Andersen, 2004).

Nursing has the highest prevalence of back injuries of any occupational group throughout the world (O'Brien-Pallas et al., 2004). Risks for occupational back pain include overexertion, vibration, and increased body mass index. An increased **work movement index**, or the extent of bending, stooping, twisting, and extended reach involved in a job, is also associated with increased risk of back injury (Division of Surveillance, Hazard Evaluations, and Field Studies, 1999).

Occupational injuries and illnesses do not occur only among people who work for pay. Volunteer workers are also subject to occupational risks. An estimated 59,000 people in the United States volunteer a median of 52 hours per person per year. From 1993 to 2002, a total of 501 identifiable deaths occurred among volunteer workers (Division of Safety Research, 2005). Community health nurses, armed with knowledge of injury risks and rates among both employed and volunteer workers, can advocate for safer work environments. They can also educate both employees and volunteers to minimize injury risks.

The occupational health problems discussed here are only a few of the many physical health problems likely to be encountered by community health nurses working in occupational settings. Each occupational setting contains factors unique to that setting that influence the health of employees. The nurse should be cognizant of the factors operating in any given place, their effects,

and the appropriate measures of control. Occupational health nurses may be in a position to advocate for safe work environments or for policies and procedures that promote health and safety in the workplace.

Immunization is the final physiologic consideration in assessing health needs in the workplace. The nurse assesses the immunization status of employees, with special emphasis on groups of employees who may be at increased risk for certain diseases preventable by immunization. For example, employees who may be at risk for dirty injuries should be assessed for immunity to tetanus, whereas women of childbearing age should be assessed for immunity to rubella. Health care workers, on the other hand, should be particularly assessed for immunity to hepatitis B. Elements to be considered in an assessment of biophysical factors influencing health in the work setting are included in the focused assessment questions provided below.

Psychological Considerations

Assessment of psychological considerations in the work setting involves examination of two major areas, stressful working conditions that affect health and the presence of mental illness and its effects in the workplace.

STRESS IN THE WORKPLACE Two models are suggested for exploring the relationship of psychological factors that create stress and health effects in work settings. The first model is the job strain or demand-control-support model. **Job strain** is the result of high job demands coupled with low ability to control demands and low levels of social support (Niedhammer, Tek, Starke, & Siegrist, 2004). In this model, the psychological effects of work stress result from perceptions of high job demands over which the employee has little control (Godin & Kittel, 2004). *Decision latitude* is the term used for the extent of one's control over one's job and job performance (Vézina, Derriennic, & Monfort, 2004). Job decision latitude consists

FOCUSED ASSESSMENT

Biophysical Considerations in the Work Setting

- What are the age, gender, and ethnic composition of the employee population? What effects do these factors have on health in the work setting?
- What is the extent of injury in the population? What types of injuries are incurred? What factors contribute to injuries in the employee population?
- What occupation-related illnesses are common in the population?
- What other illnesses are experienced by the employee population? What is the level of disability in the population? What types of limitations are caused by disability?
- What is the effect of chronic illness or disability on the ability of employees to function effectively in the work setting? Do employees have preexisting health conditions that put them at greater risk for the toxic effects of workplace exposures?
- What are the immunization levels in the employee population?

of two components: decision authority and opportunities to participate in decisions affecting one's work and skill discretion, which is the opportunity to effectively employ personal skills and knowledge performing one's job (Elovainio et al., 2004). Low decision latitude has been linked to social isolation of employees and to increased risk of cardiovascular mortality, absences, poor self-reported health, and job strain (Vézina et al., 2004; Elovainio et al., 2004).

The second model relating psychological factors in the work setting to employee health is the effort-reward imbalance (ERI) model, in which job stress results from an imbalance between one's perceived work effort and the rewards received (Godin & Kittel, 2004). Like low job decision latitude, effort-reward imbalance has been shown to be associated with cardiovascular disease, risk factors for disease such as hypertension, elevated lipid levels, absence, and physiologic symptoms associated with stress (Niedhammer et al., 2004). Other potential effects of perceived imbalance include poor self-rated health, depression, anxiety, fatigue, and somatization (Godin & Kittel, 2004). Among nurses, occupational stress has been associated with poor health, lack of constructive thinking, and job dissatisfaction (Stacciarini & Troccoli, 2004). In other studies, the effort-reward ratio has been closely linked to depression among workers in three Eastern and Central European countries (Pikhart et al., 2004).

Perceptions of organizational justice have also been shown to be associated with job stress. Organizational justice refers to perceptions of fair treatment in the organizational setting. There are two components to organizational justice. The first component is procedural justice and reflects perceptions of the fairness of procedures employed in the work setting. The second component addresses relational justice, which involves perceptions of the quality of interpersonal treatment in making decisions. Relational justice reflects the degree of consideration and courtesy with which employees are treated in the work setting. Low perceived organizational justice may give rise to negative emotional reactions to perceptions of unfair treatment. Perceptions of organizational justice have been linked in some studies to the extent of worker absences (Elovainio et al., 2004).

Another relatively recent factor that contributes to stress in the workforce is what has been referred to as "emotional labor." **Emotional labor** has been defined as "the management of feeling to create a publicly observable facial and bodily display" (de Castro, Agnew, & Fitzgerald, 2004, p. 109) or as "the act of displaying the appropriate emotion" (Ashforth & Humphrey, as quoted in de Castro et al., 2004, p. 110). Emotional labor occurs in the context of service occupations when the employee cannot afford to display his or her true emotions for fear of alienating a client or customer. Jobs that require emotional labor are characterized by contact with the public, the necessity for producing a favorable

emotional state in the customer, and the opportunity for employers to control the emotional activities of their employees.

Research has indicated that employees may take one of two approaches to emotional labor. In the first approach, called "surface acting," the employee pretends to emotions that he or she does not feel. In "deep acting," the second approach, the employee actually changes his or her emotions to conform to those required for the job. For example, employees may take satisfaction in always being cheerful rather than resent the fact that they need to display a cheerful disposition. Emotional labor creates occupational stress when surface acting is used due to the dissonance between real emotions and those displayed. Deep acting, on the other hand, does not appear to increase occupational stress because it decreases dissonance (de Castro et al., 2004). Nursing as an occupation can be seen to require a significant amount of emotional labor, the stress of which may contribute to professional burnout.

Other psychological factors may contribute to stress in the workplace. For example, job barriers due to time pressures and poor technical or organizational designs that require additional steps to perform one's job have been shown to contribute to increased risk of hypertension in bus drivers (Greiner, Krause, Ragland, & Fisher, 2004). Similarly, intragroup conflict may diminish employee morale and productivity in any occupational setting. Some occupations may pose particular psychological risks. For example, the emotional stress and exhaustion characteristic of caring for dying clients contribute to burnout among hospice nurses (Payne, 2001).

Because of the position of trust that occupational health nurses usually have with employees, they may be among the first to recognize symptoms of stress in individual employees or the work group. With this knowledge, nurses can explore the sources of stress and advocate for improvements in working conditions. Even when the stress might be the result of misperceptions among employees (e.g., rumors that massive layoffs will take place or that the company is being sold), the effects on employee health and work ability can be significant. Community health nurses can help to identify these sources of stress and motivate employers to make changes to reduce stress levels.

MENTAL HEALTH AND ILLNESS IN THE WORKPLACE

Community health nurses are also in a position to identify employees with mental health problems or to recognize a high prevalence of these problems in the workforce. The sources of workplace stress discussed above may contribute to the development of actual psychiatric diagnoses, or employees may enter the workforce with one or more psychiatric illnesses. Depression, in particular, is a growing problem in the work setting and is the chronic illness most likely to lead to work absences (Zimmerman, Christakis, & Stoep, 2004). Approximately

5% of workers suffer from depression at any given time (Putnam & McKibbin, 2004). Estimated annual occupational costs for bipolar disease amount to more than $45 million (Matza, de Lissovoy, Sasane, Pesa, & Maus, 2004). A variety of stresses contribute to depression in the work setting. For example, lack of job control or job security, job-related conflict, high physical demands or physically uncomfortable work, and hazardous work environments have all been linked to employee depression. Conversely, higher job status has been associated with decreased risk of depression (Zimmerman et al., 2004).

Depression leads to a number of health-related consequences. For example, depression is a major risk factor for heart disease, high cholesterol, and elevated blood pressure, and depressed employees contribute to health care costs roughly twice those of nondepressed employees. Approximately 15% of people with major depression commit suicide. Depression also affects the morale and productivity of coworkers, and the costs to employers due to reduced productivity is estimated to be $33 million a year (Putnam & McKibbin, 2004).

Despite the prevalence of depression in the work setting, its preventability, and its costly consequences, few worksites have programs to address depression in employees. In surveys, only 12% of companies reported programs related to employee depression, and only 5% have developed comprehensive approaches to dealing with depression in the workforce. Because of the lack of attention to this problem, less than one third of those suffering from depression receive the care needed (Putnam & McKibbin, 2004).

Community health nurses may also encounter other psychiatric illnesses in the employee population, although usually with less frequency than depression. Schizophrenia and substance abuse are two of the additional diagnoses that may be encountered. Community health nurses should keep in mind several legal parameters related to psychiatric illness in the work setting. Employers are not permitted to ask about psychiatric illness in hiring decisions, and employees are not required to disclose such diagnoses unless they are requesting accommodations. Employers are also required by the Americans with Disabilities Act to make reasonable accommodations for employees with psychiatric disorders, particularly depression. Community health nurses working with employees with mental health problems may need to ensure access to needed treatment and advocate for accommodations in the work setting. They may also be involved in coordinating care, evaluating the functional ability of employees, and monitoring their use of psychotropic medications (Putnam & McKibbin, 2004).

In assessing psychological dimension factors influencing the health of clients in work settings, community health nurses identify psychological health problems prevalent in the population and assess factors contributing to psychological problems. The nurse can assess individual clients or the work group for the following indicators of psychological health problems:

- Increased absenteeism (especially on Mondays, Fridays, and the day after payday)
- Mood changes or changes in relationships with others (especially with health care providers)
- Increased incidence of minor accidents on and off the job
- Complaints of fatigue, weakness, or a general decrease in energy
- Sudden weight loss or gain
- Increased blood pressure
- Frequent stress-related illnesses
- Bloodshot or bleary eyes
- Facial petechiae (especially over the nose)

The focused assessment below provides guidelines for assessing psychological factors affecting health in the work setting.

Physical Environmental Considerations

Physical environmental factors contribute to a variety of health problems encountered in work settings. For example, in some studies, physical working conditions account for 42% of all work absences for musculoskeletal problems among women and 13% among men (Melchior et al., 2005). Rural workers are more likely to experience traumatic occupational fatalities than those in urban areas, particularly in certain industries. For instance, the mining industry contributes to 10,000 disabling injuries per year and agriculture to 150,000 injuries per year (10% of the entire agricultural workforce). In addition to the increased prevalence of injury, employees in these settings often have less access to injury compensation (Peek-Asa, Zwerling, & Stallones, 2004). In urban settings, urban sprawl contributes to a variety of respiratory infections, asthma, and injuries in workers due to extended commutes. Urban sprawl and age segregation in residential areas have also been found to contribute to decreased ability to work with others and increased work conflict and stress (Pohanka & Fitzgerald, 2004). For

FOCUSED ASSESSMENT

Psychological Considerations in the Work Setting

- To what extent does the work environment contribute to stress? What are the sources of stress in the work environment?
- How do employees cope with stress in the work environment?
- Does the work setting require emotional labor? How do employees in the setting approach emotional labor?
- Do employees encounter role conflicts between work and home? What are the sources of these conflicts? How do employees deal with them?
- What is the prevalence of mental illness among employees? How does the presence of mental illness affect employees' ability to work?

example, in areas where older people are primarily in senior residential settings, young people may not be exposed to the beliefs and values of an older generation and may be less able to understand the concerns of older people in the work setting. Of course, the reverse is also true, older people who do not interact with young people regularly may perceive their ways as strange and unfathomable. Urban sprawl tends to lend itself to segregation of residential areas by age more than rural or inner-city areas.

An estimated 89% of the U.S. workforce is employed in indoor work settings that have their own risks for disease and injury. Indoor environments are associated with increased respiratory diseases that result in impaired performance and decreased productivity, much of which is due to building characteristics. It is estimated that building improvements could lead to economic benefits ranging from $5 billion to $75 billion per year for the industries involved (Mendell et al., 2002).

Categories of health hazards in the physical environment include chemical hazards, physical hazards (radiation, noise, vibration, and exposure to heat and cold), electrical and magnetic field hazards, fire, heavy lifting and uncomfortable working positions, and potential for falls. Additional hazards that may be present in the workplace include exposure to metallic compounds and allergens and molds (Friis & Sellers, 2004).

Poor lighting and high noise levels may adversely affect vision and hearing, respectively. In addition, exposure to artificial light during the hours when melatonin production is affected has been linked to increased breast cancer incidence in nurses who work rotating night shifts, and the more years spent on night shift, the greater the increase in breast cancer incidence (Davis, Mirick, & Stevens, 2001; Schernhammer et al., 2001).

Night shift work has also been related to increased risk of coronary heart disease (Schernhammer et al., 2001).

Each year, more than 30 million workers are exposed to excessive noise levels, and noise-induced hearing loss is the second most common occupational health problem in the United States. Exposure to noise may also contribute to increased blood pressure, although research in this area to date has not provided any conclusive results (Penney & Earl, 2004). Heavy objects that must be moved may cause musculoskeletal injuries. In addition, there is the potential for falls or exposure to excessive heat or cold in many workplaces. All of these physical environmental factors contribute to the risk of occupational injury.

The use of toxic substances in work performance is another source of possible health problems related to the physical environment. Toxic substances may be encountered as solids, liquids, gases, vapors, dust, fumes, fibers, or mists. As noted earlier, a great number of toxic substances are present in the work environment that may result in respiratory, dermatologic, and other health problems. Of particular concern in this area is exposure to heavy metals (Table 24-1◆). The adverse effects of occupational exposure to lead, for example, have been known for more than 2,000 years. Despite this knowledge and efforts to minimize occupational exposure to lead and other heavy metals, significant numbers of workers in the United States have the potential for work-related lead exposure, and in many industries no mechanism is in place for biological monitoring of lead levels in employees with potential for exposure. Other metals of concern include mercury, arsenic, and cadmium. Exposure to lead and other metals occurs in a variety of occupations, including those listed in Table 24-1◆. Areas to be assessed relative to the potential for toxic exposures in the workplace include substances used in

TABLE 24-1 Occupational Sources and Health Effects of Heavy Metal Exposures

Metal	Occupational Sources	Health Effects
Antimony	Iron works, red dye manufacture	Irritation, cardiovascular and lung effects
Arsenic	Photographic equipment and supplies	Lung and lymphatic cancer, dermatitis
Cadmium	Soldering, battery manufacture, fuses, paint manufacture and painting, nuclear reactors	Lung cancer, prostatic cancer, renal system effects
Chromium	Steel manufacture, chrome plating, dye and paint manufacture, leather tanning	Lung cancer, skin ulcers, lung irradiation
Lead	Soldering; dispensing leaded gas; cable cutting and splicing; painting, casting, or melting lead; radiator repair; welding, grinding, or sanding lead-painted surfaces; battery manufacture; construction; paper hanging; foundries; plumbing	Kidney, blood, and nervous system effects
Mercury	Metal foil and leaf application, industrial measurement instruments, gold and silver refining	Central nervous system and mental effects
Nickel	Nickel plating, steel manufacture, heating coils, hydrogenation processes	Lung and nasal cancer, skin effects
Tungsten	Steel manufacture, x-ray tubes	Lung and skin effects
Zinc oxide	White paint manufacture	Metal fume fever

the setting and their level of demonstrated toxicity, portals of entry into the human body, established legal exposure limits, extent of exposure, potential for interactive exposures, and the presence of existing employee health conditions that put the individuals affected at greater risk for exposure-related illnesses. The nurse and other personnel would also assess the extent and adequacy of controls to prevent or limit exposures and the availability of and compliance with recommended screening and surveillance procedures.

For some people, seemingly innocuous substances may have toxic effects. For example, health care providers may be allergic to the latex gloves used in many settings. Similarly, the presence of food allergens in meals prepared in the work setting can have severe consequences for those with allergies. Community health nurses can be alert to the presence of people with specific allergies in the work setting and assist the company to eliminate the most common allergens. For example, the nurse might work with staff in an employee dining room to eliminate recipes that use peanuts or peanut oil. Similarly, the nurse can advocate for the use of nonlatex gloves in health care settings and other workplaces where gloves are used (e.g., by hotel cleaning staff members).

Equipment may also constitute an occupational health hazard. The use of heavy equipment or sharp tools can result in injury. There is also the potential for hand–arm vibration syndrome in the use of tools that vibrate or visual disturbance related to the use of computer display terminals. Another relatively recent physical hazard generated by widespread computer use is the potential for tendonitis and other similar conditions. Extreme or awkward postures have been associated with low back problems and repetitive or high-force

movements with carpal tunnel syndrome. The nurse in the occupational setting identifies the presence of any hazards in the physical environment that contribute to health problems. In addition, the nurse monitors the status of known hazards and their effects on the health of employees. The presence of modifiable hazards should lead to advocacy on the part of the nurse to change the physical work environment to eliminate or reduce the potential for exposure to these hazards. Some potential questions for evaluating hazardous conditions in work settings are included in the focused assessment presented below.

Sociocultural Considerations

The social environment of the work setting can influence employee health status either positively or negatively. The quality of social interactions among employees, attitudes toward work and health, and the presence or absence of racial or other tensions can all affect health status as well as employee productivity.

Assessment of sociocultural considerations affecting health in work settings focuses on four major areas. These include the effects of policy and legislation, the interactive effects of work and family life, workplace violence, and other sociocultural factors in the workplace.

POLICY AND LEGISLATION In the United States, health-related policy and legislation have a significant impact on the workforce. The three most influential pieces of legislation are the Occupational Safety and Health Act of 1970 (OSHA), workers' compensation, and the Americans with Disabilities Act. Other local and business-specific policies and regulations also affect the health of employees. OSHA was intended to develop and enforce safety standards in work settings. In addition, the legislation

FOCUSED ASSESSMENT

Physical Environmental Considerations in the Work Setting

- Does the physical environment of the work setting pose any health hazards?
- What potentially hazardous substances or conditions are associated with production processes (e.g., toxic chemicals, heat)?
- What potentially hazardous substances or conditions are associated with clerical processes (e.g., repetitive movements)? With other office processes (e.g., cleaning products, pesticides)?
- What is the typical extent and duration of exposure to hazardous substances or conditions?
- What are the designated exposure limits for substances and conditions in the work setting?
- What research evidence is there for adverse human health effects (e.g., toxicity, teratogenicity, potential for injury) associated with substances used or conditions existing in the work setting?
- Do low levels of exposure have a cumulative effect?
- What is the usual portal of entry or mechanism of exposure for a specific toxic agent or condition?

- What organ systems are typically affected by specific toxic agents or hazardous conditions?
- What are the usual signs and symptoms of toxicity/health effects?
- Are there synergistic effects among substances or between substances and other conditions (e.g., heat)?
- What are the recommended control practices to prevent or minimize potential for exposure?
- Are the recommended practices in place in a given occupational setting (e.g., ventilation, other engineering controls)?
- What are the recommended surveillance practices for monitoring environmental conditions and hazardous exposures? Are there surveillance systems in place for monitoring the presence or extent of hazardous conditions in the environment?
- Are food sanitation practices adequate to prevent communicable diseases, vermin infestation, etc.?
- Are there adequate facilities for handicapped employees?
- Are workstations designed to prevent injury and fatigue?
- Is there potential for a disaster in the work setting? Is there a disaster plan in place?

established the National Institute for Occupational Safety and Health (NIOSH) to conduct occupational research and provide for training and assistance to employers in safeguarding employee health. As of 2004, NIOSH has been relocated to the CDC Coordinating Center for Environmental Health, Injury Prevention, and Occupational Health (Fell-Carlson, 2004).

OSHA covers all private-sector employees except those who are self-employed, family employees on farms, and workers who are covered under other regulatory agencies (e.g., the Nuclear Regulatory Commission). Most agricultural workers are not covered unless a farming operation includes a migrant labor camp or employs more than 10 nonfamily employees (Fleming, 2004). The only public employees covered under OSHA are federal employees who were covered as a result of a Presidential Executive Order; however, many state occupational and safety plans cover both private- and public-sector employees (Fell-Carlson, 2004).

OSHA promulgates two types of occupation health and safety standards: horizontal standards and vertical standards (Fell-Carlson, 2004). Horizontal standards are general and cover all industries that fall under the auspices of OSHA. Vertical standards are specific to a given industry, such as the textile and sawmill standards developed specifically for those industries. All of the standards contain specific components, including required program elements, the need for a written program and parameters related to the standard, training requirements related to the standard, required hazard controls, exposure limits and medical surveillance requirements, and documentation requirements. Requirements for documentation and reporting apply only to injuries and illnesses that are work-related.

OSHA is charged with performing periodic inspections of worksites to determine whether standards are being enforced. Inspections may be conducted on a routine basis or may be triggered by certain specific events such as an employee death, hospitalization of three or more employees for work-related occurrences, employee complaints, or referrals from the media or other individuals. Inspections may also be conducted in the event of an imminent danger situation (e.g., possible rupture of a holding tank for hazardous materials) (Fell-Carlson, 2004). Unfortunately, the number and frequency of OSHA inspections and penalties for violation of standards have been steadily decreasing. In addition, OSHA has been criticized for the excessive length of time required to develop new exposure standards for hazardous substances, which may take as long as 5 to 10 years from proposal to enactment (Lurie, Long, & Wolfe, 1999). Finally, the U.S. Congress has periodically overturned OSHA regulations or blocked their timely implementation. For example, in 2001, Congress overturned the ergonomics standards just published the previous November (Fee & Brown, 2001). Community health nurses working in occupational settings may occasionally find themselves in the position of needing to report

GLOBAL PERSPECTIVES

Nuwayhid (2004) observed that the findings of occupational health research in the United States and other developed nations can be translated into practice with relative ease due to the existence of "political mechanisms to translate scientific findings into effective policies" (p. 1916). He pointed out, however, that these mechanisms are lacking in developing countries and that occupational health research should focus less on the "internal domain" of workplace hazards, work organization, exposure, and the effectiveness of occupational health services and programs and more on the "external-contextual domain." This latter domain consists of factors related to global, regional, and national policies and regulations; movement of populations and hazards; occupational mobility, unemployment, and retirement; disability and its economic and social burden; and vulnerable populations in the workforce (e.g., children, women, people with disabilities). He noted that developing nations need to address more pressing social and health issues before they can turn to issues related specifically to occupational health and illness and recommended that occupational health research in the developing world "should focus on the social and political issues and then move inward to address the peculiarities of the workplace" (p. 1918).

OSHA violations in order to protect employee health and safety. In addition, they may need to advocate for federal and state enforcement of health and safety regulations.

Workers' compensation legislation was passed in the United States in 1911 as the first instance of no-fault insurance in the nation (Hancock, 2004). Prior to establishment of the workers' compensation system, employees were required to prove employer responsibility for an illness or injury before they could claim recompense for lost wages or the cost of medical care. Workers' compensation provides protection for both employee and employer. Under the program, employees are guaranteed wage replacement and medical care costs if they are injured on the job. The system also protects employers from lawsuits by employees to recover lost wages or health care costs. Occupational health nurses are often responsible for tracking and administering workers' compensation for injured employees. They may also need to assist employees to obtain workers' compensation benefits.

The third piece of legislation that affects the workplace is the Americans with Disabilities Act (ADA). The implications of the act for the school setting were discussed in Chapter 23 ∞ and are similar for occupational settings. ADA was designed to ensure equitable occupational opportunity for those with disabilities. ADA provisions may be in conflict with OSHA regulations designed to limit risks to which employees are exposed (Daniels, 2003). Recent Supreme Court rulings have favored the right of employers to prevent people from working when a particular job would place the person him- or herself at risk due to limitations imposed by a disability. This particular ruling runs contrary to prior decisions that only possible danger to others justified employer decisions not to employ someone in a particular capacity (Barnes, Cleaveland, & Florencio, 2003; Daniels, 2003). Community health nurses may need to advocate for disabled workers when such decisions are made in the workplace.

Legislation regarding workplace issues is often influenced by union activity (Stern, 2003). For example, unions have been involved in the development of the workers' compensation program and in the tax deduction approved for employee health benefits. More recently, U.S. labor unions have been actively involved in the push to initiate national health insurance. Labor unions have also been influential in policy development in other, more authoritarian environments. For example, the input of trade unions and the Staff and Workers' Representative Congress has had an impact on the development of occupational health and safety policy in China (Chen & Chan, 2004). Community health nurses can also influence these policies by educating employers and employees alike and by advocating for policy change at local, state, and federal levels.

Local policies within specific business organizations have also been found to influence health and safety. For example, in early 2005, seven states had mandatory smoke-free workplace policies that covered 24% of the U.S. workforce (Bauer, Hyland, Li, Steger, & Cummings, 2005), including those working in bars and restaurants. Research has indicated that employees working in organizations with smoke-free worksite policies are almost twice as likely to quit smoking as those who work in organizations without such policies. Even those employees who do not quit smoking are likely to decrease their cigarette consumption (Bauer et al., 2005). Permissive workplace policies, on the other hand, may increase the risk for injury and illness. For example, people who work in settings where guns are permitted have a risk of homicide victimization five times higher than do people in settings where guns are prohibited (Loomis, Marshall, & Ta, 2005).

WORK AND FAMILY Although employees spend considerable time in the work setting, they do have lives outside of work. Interrelationships between work and family may support or impede employee and/or family health. For example, children of parents who work nonstandard work schedules (e.g., nights or evenings) have been found to have a greater risk for emotional and behavior problems than those whose parents work standard hours (Strazdins, Korda, Lim, Broom, & D'Souza, 2004). Nonstandard hours also prevent parental participation in many child-related activities and diminish the amount of time parents have available to interact with their children. Children in the 2- to 3-year-old age range may exhibit hyperactivity and inattention, physical aggression, and separation anxiety, whereas those aged 4 to 11 years may have a greater tendency to conduct disorders and property offenses (Strazdins et al., 2004). Nor are the effects of shift work confined to children. The adjustment and coping ability of workers on rotating shifts also appear to be affected by partners' perceptions of the degree of disruption caused by the changes (Newey & Hood, 2004).

Women may be more directly influenced by the interrelationships between work and family than men. For example, women have been found to have more musculoskeletal disorders than men, due in part to the limited time available to them for rest between work and family responsibilities (Strazdins & Bammer, 2004). Similarly, the self-perceived health status of Korean working women has been found to be strongly influenced by the extent of social support and work- and family-related stress (Kim, Cho, Lee, Marion, & Kim, 2005).

Employees, many of them women, also may be juggling care for someone with chronic illness with the

ETHICAL AWARENESS

*I*n 2002, the U.S. Supreme Court upheld employers' rights to make employment decisions for persons with disabilities based on the probable extent of risk to the employee's own personal health and safety. Previously, employers could only curtail employee's activity based on the presence of a threat to the safety or health of others (Barnes, Cleaveland, & Florencio, 2003). This decision rejected the position of advocates of the Americans with Disabilities Act that workers with disabilities should be able to determine for themselves the risks they are willing to take rather than have them determined for them (Daniels, 2003). What are the ethical implications of this decision? How might they affect people's employability? To what extent do you agree or disagree that an employer can take action to protect an employee from the consequences of employment on his or her own health status? What is the rationale for your position on this issue?

CULTURAL COMPETENCE

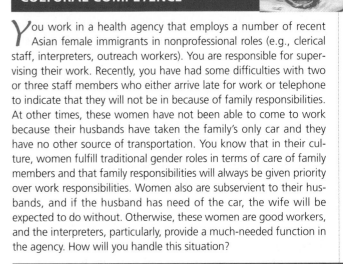

*Y*ou work in a health agency that employs a number of recent Asian female immigrants in nonprofessional roles (e.g., clerical staff, interpreters, outreach workers). You are responsible for supervising their work. Recently, you have had some difficulties with two or three staff members who either arrive late for work or telephone to indicate that they will not be in because of family responsibilities. At other times, these women have not been able to come to work because their husbands have taken the family's only car and they have no other source of transportation. You know that in their culture, women fulfill traditional gender roles in terms of care of family members and that family responsibilities will always be given priority over work responsibilities. Women also are subservient to their husbands, and if the husband has need of the car, the wife will be expected to do without. Otherwise, these women are good workers, and the interpreters, particularly, provide a much-needed function in the agency. How will you handle this situation?

routine duties of work and family. An estimated 12% of the workforce is caregivers for elderly parents, and the requirements of caregiving may cost employees more than $11 billion a year. Unfortunately, only 42% of large employers have any sort of assistance available for employees engaged in caregiving activities (Plese, 2005a). In 2003, for example, only 5% of employees received employer assistance with on-site or off-site childcare, and only 10% received assistance in locating childcare resources. Similarly, only 4% of the U.S. workforce had flexible work schedules that permitted them to work at home at times (U.S. Census Bureau, 2005).

The relationship between work and family life is a reciprocal one. Family and work relationships have been shown to affect recovery from carpal tunnel syndrome (Hopp et al., 2004). Conversely, occupational injuries and illnesses affect the family as well as the employee. For example, chronic back pain due to occupational injury affects one's ability to carry out family and social roles as well as work responsibilities (Strunin & Boden, 2004). In 2003, a disabling injury resulted in a 10-year loss of earnings ranging from $42,100 to $68,000 in five states even after compensation reimbursement. This amounts to 16% to 26% of earnings if the employee had not been injured. Workers' compensation reimburses only 32% to 41% of the loss incurred, leaving families with considerably less disposable income. In addition, disabling injuries may affect the employee's ability to carry out family roles, requiring other family members to take over these roles or even to take on additional caretaking roles for the injured family member (Boden, 2005).

A final aspect of the relationship between work and family relates to paraoccupational exposure to hazardous substances. **Paraoccupational exposure** occurs when employees are exposed to hazardous substances and in turn expose their families (usually via contaminated clothing). These exposures may involve metals, chemicals, or biological agents. For example, paraoccupational exposure to lead frequently occurs via contaminated clothing (Division of Surveillance, Hazard Evaluations, and Field Studies, 2001). Health care workers, on the other hand, may expose their families to infectious disease agents. Occupational health nurses can be particularly influential in teaching employees how to minimize paraoccupational exposures and in advocating employment policies that minimize the potential for exposure (e.g., through providing protective clothing and changing areas for employees working with hazardous materials).

WORKPLACE VIOLENCE Workplace violence is another sociocultural factor that can profoundly affect health and safety in the occupational setting. In 2004, 14% of workplace fatalities were the result of assault or violence (U.S. Department of Labor, 2005a). An estimated 20 workers are murdered each week in the United States, and another 19,231 are assaulted (Anderson, 2004; Ruff, Gerding, & Hong, 2004). Workplace violence has been defined by NIOSH as "violent acts, including physical assaults and threats of assault directed toward individuals at work or on duty" (quoted in Anderson, 2004, p. 24). Workplace violence may include either physical or verbal aggression against employees in the work setting (Ruff et al., 2004).

Four types of workplace violence have been identified. Criminal intent violence occurs in the context of commission of a crime. For instance, a store clerk may be injured during a robbery. The second type of violence is customer related, in which a client or customer becomes violent and injures an employee who is attempting to provide service. An example of this is a violent client in an emergency department who injures a health care provider. Worker-on-worker violence is the third type of violence, in which one employee is injured by another or by a former employee of the organization. The much-publicized murders of postal employees by other employees are an example of this type of violence. The fourth type of violence involves acts committed against an employee by someone who has a personal relationship with the employee outside of the work setting (e.g., a spouse). Roughly 17% of female homicides that occur in the work setting are perpetrated by husbands or boyfriends (Anderson, 2004).

Workplace violence may also include bullying or harassment. Harassment has been defined as the "creation of a hostile environment through unwelcome words, actions, and physical contacts that do not result in physical harm" (Anderson, 2004, p. 24). Both men and women are equally likely to bully others, but women are three times more likely than men to be the victims of workplace bullying. In approximately 81% of instances, the bully is in a superior position to the victim. Unfortunately, workplace bullying is not prohibited by law unless the harassment is linked to discrimination (Sitzman, 2004b).

Occupational health nurses may be faced with evidence of workplace violence or bullying and may be forced to advocate for clients. When the perpetrator is also the nurse's supervisor, this may place the nurse in an awkward position. When harassment is based on discrimination because of an employee's gender, ethnicity, or membership in another protected category, someone who reports harassment is protected from employer

ETHICAL AWARENESS

A pregnant female employee comes to see you because she is experiencing vaginal bleeding. During her visit, you notice bruises on her hips and abdomen. Eventually, she admits that her husband, who works for the same company, hit her several times last night. The employee begs you not to say anything or to write anything about the abuse in her record because they can't afford for her husband to lose his job, particularly with a first baby on the way. Your state does not have legislation mandating a report of spousal violence. What will you do?

retaliation. Unfortunately, however, this is not the case when the harassment cannot be linked to discrimination. Despite this disadvantage and the potential for retribution, nurses who are aware of bullying are ethically obliged to report it to the appropriate person or group and to advocate for the safety and security of the employee or employees affected.

OTHER SOCIOCULTURAL FACTORS A number of other sociocultural factors influence health in occupational settings. Such influence may occur in one of four spheres within the workplace social environment. The first sphere of influence involves the health-related behaviors of employees themselves and is addressed in the discussion of behavioral factors affecting health. The other three spheres are more directly related to the social environment of work settings.

The second sphere of influence on health in the workplace occurs among groups of coworkers, and the community health nurse should assess the influence of coworker groups on the health of individual employees and on the group as a whole. For example, a group of coworkers may decide that they do not wish to be exposed to smoke in their work area. This decision can lead to formal or informal bans on smoking in certain areas. Formal bans may occur when groups of employees request no-smoking policies from company management. When this is not the case, work groups may enforce the decision informally by exerting peer pressure on the smokers in the group. In other words, they can make life unpleasant for those who wish to smoke by ostracizing them or using other social sanctions. Another example of this sphere of social influence lies in the influence that more experienced employees have on the use of safety precautions by younger, less experienced workers who may imitate their behaviors. If older workers effectively use safety practices, younger workers are likely to do so as well; if they do not, younger workers are likely to imitate this behavior and increase their risk of injury.

The third sphere of influence is the management sphere. The nurse assesses management's attitudes toward health and health-related policies and the effects of these policies (or lack of them) on employee health. For example, management may decide on and enforce a no-smoking policy throughout the company, whether or not employees favor such a policy. As we saw earlier, smoke-free workplace policies are credited with decreasing annual cigarette consumption even among employees who continue to smoke.

Management also makes other kinds of policy decisions that affect employee health. For example, the type of health care coverage provided to employees is a management decision. A policy that provides "well leave" or extra vacation for those who have not taken sick leave may prompt employee efforts to promote health and prevent illness.

For employees to value wellness and health-promotive efforts, they must perceive them to be valued by employers. This means that wellness programs and other aspects of occupational health must receive the same degree of emphasis as other areas of business. It has been suggested that companies develop **company wellness policies**, statements of administrative commitment to employee health, and expectations of employees related to health promotion and maintenance, to convey the importance given to health issues. These companies must be seen to abide by, as well as create, such policies.

The last sphere of influence involves legal, social, and political action that influences the health of employees. A prime example of this is the regulation of conditions in work settings by agencies such as the Occupational Safety and Health Administration (OSHA) discussed earlier. Through legislation, society can mandate that business and industry create specific conditions that enhance the health of employees.

Additional sociocultural factors that may affect health in the work setting include languages spoken and cultural beliefs and behaviors. For example, employers may provide the traditional Western or Christian holidays but give no provision for important occasions in other cultural groups. Ethnic and cultural factors may also be the basis for discrimination in the work setting. For example, employees may be harassed by colleagues because of an accent, or employers may prohibit the wearing of culturally prescribed clothing, such as head scarves, in some employment settings. In other settings, such as India and Italy, businesses may close during the hottest part of the day, but stay open late into the evening.

The social capital available to employees in the work setting may also influence their health. In some studies, the security of employment and level of coworker trust, both elements of social capital, have been linked to self-reported health among employees (Liukkonen, Virtanen, Kivimaki, Pentti, & Vahtera, 2004). Social capital may also include job status. According to some studies, a move to a higher status job has been associated with decreased mortality among men. Conversely, movement to a lower-status job increases men's risk of death (Cambois, 2004).

Immigration status is another sociocultural factor that may influence the health of some segments of the working population. Immigrants and members of ethnic minority groups often have limited occupational choices available to them and frequently work in less safe and less desirable jobs (Richardson, Loomis, Bena, & Bailer, 2004). They tend to have higher rates of occupational injury and illness, but are often less eligible than other workers for compensation. They may also experience higher levels of unemployment and underemployment than the general working population. In one study, immigrant women voiced concerns about the high demands of their work and health issues related to physically demanding jobs, exposure to toxins and infectious disease, the psychological stress of work overload, financial strain, their immigration status, and the quality of relationships with their employers (Tsai, 2004). Guidelines for assessing sociocultural factors in occupational settings are presented in the focused assessment provided below.

Behavioral Considerations

As noted above, behavioral factors exemplified in individual decisions about health-related actions constitute the first sphere of social influence on employee health. Behavioral factors to be considered here include the type of work performed, consumption patterns, patterns of rest and exercise, use of safety devices, and working while ill.

TYPE OF WORK PERFORMED The type of work performed by an individual within a company can significantly influence the employee's health. The type of work performed determines the risk of exposure to various physical hazards and level of stress experienced. For example, factory workers in industries using lead may run the risk of lead poisoning, whereas executives in the same companies may be exposed to more stress. Approximately 58% of elevated blood lead levels resulting from occupational exposure occur in manufacturing settings, and 22% occur in construction (Division of Surveillance, Hazard Evaluations, and Field Studies, 2004). Another example of the effects of type of work performed and the related safety hazards is the increased risk of motor vehicle fatality among emergency medical services personnel. This increased risk is primarily due to failure to use safety restraints in the patient compartment

of the vehicle because of the need to be able to reach the client and needed supplies rapidly (Division of Safety Research, 2003).

The type of work done also influences the extent of exercise that employees obtain. Construction workers, for example, have ample opportunities for physical activity but also risk serious injury in the use of heavy equipment. Bank tellers, on the other hand, are at risk for cardiovascular and other diseases related to a sedentary lifestyle.

The community health nurse in an occupational setting should be conversant with the variety of jobs performed in that setting. The nurse should also be aware of the health hazards posed by each type of work performed and be alert to signs of health problems deriving from the work itself.

Another aspect of the type of work performed is that of **ergonomics**, the degree of fit between the employee and the job performed. The nurse should assess the degree to which employees are qualified to perform their particular job function and their interest in that job. Employees who work at jobs that do not interest them, that are beyond their capabilities, or that do not provide sufficient challenge may be at greater risk for both emotional and physical health problems than those who are better suited to their jobs. Ergonomics also reflects the design of workstations and their effects on health. For example, the height of a computer keyboard may influence the development of neck and shoulder problems. As noted earlier, the ergonomics standards established by OSHA were overturned by the U.S. Congress, leaving millions of employees at risk for fatigue and injury (Fee & Brown, 2001).

Community health nurses working in occupational health settings may be responsible for assessing the ergonomic features of a setting or a particular job. Ergonomic evaluation is commonly done when several employees develop work-related musculoskeletal disorders, but could be employed in a general assessment of the workplace to prevent musculoskeletal injuries. The purpose of an evaluation is to identify and correct factors contributing to injuries (Grayson, Dale, Bohr, Wolf, & Evanoff, 2005). In an evaluation, the employee is questioned about aspects of the work that are stressful, restrictions imposed by injury, and any accommodations attempted and their effectiveness. When possible, employees are observed performing their usual job duties. The evaluator also asks injured employees to identify tasks that are most difficult to accomplish as a result of injury. The difficult tasks frequently lead to the identification of specific factors that promote injury and that are amenable to change. In addition to changing features of the job or work environment, ergonomic analysis may lead to employee education in better work techniques to prevent injury (Grayson et al., 2005).

Another aspect of ergonomic evaluation is an assessment of tools and equipment used in the job and

FOCUSED ASSESSMENT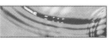

Sociocultural Considerations in the Work Setting

- Do OSHA regulations apply to the work setting? Are there other regulations that apply to the setting? If so, what are they and how do they affect employee health or the role of the occupational health nurse?
- What is the extent of workers' compensation claims in the work group? For what types of problems is compensation provided?
- How do provisions of the Americans with Disabilities Act affect the work setting?
- What effects, if any, does work in this setting have on family relationships? Do employees work nonstandard hours?
- What assistance, if any, is provided to employees relative to child-care or care of other family members?
- What is the educational, economic, and cultural background of employees? What languages are spoken by the employee population? How do cultural factors affect work, if at all?
- Does the work pose a high risk for crime victimization?
- Are there intergroup conflicts in the employee population? What is the potential for violence in the work setting?
- What is the extent of social support among employees? To what extent do coworkers support healthful behaviors?

their potential for injury. This may include both power equipment and hand tools and mechanical processes. A checklist was developed by one group of authors for assessing the ergonomic aspects of a variety of hand tools including snips, saws, hammers, screwdrivers, hammer, and caulking guns. Based on the evaluation checklist, most of the tools evaluated were lacking in a number of important ergonomic features increasing the potential for musculoskeletal injury (Dababneh, Lowe, Krieg, Kong, & Waters, 2004).

Some devices intended to ease work and prevent strain have even been found to promote injury. For example, one study that examined the use of a sling to assist nurses with lifting and transferring patients in acute care settings found that the sling actually increased back strain and exertion. The authors found that both the ergonomic properties of the sling itself and the postures assumed by nurses in its use affected back muscle strain indicating a need for further ergonomic evaluation of this and other devices used by nurses (Kothiyal & Yuen, 2004).

Another factor is the extent of multiple jobs held by employees, each of which presents its own unique risks and hazards. In addition, multiple-job holders have less time to rest and recover from the physical demands of the job as well as less time for family interactions. In January 2006, 5.3% of the U.S. labor force held multiple jobs. More than half of these individuals (53%) held one full-time and one part-time job, and 4% held two full-time jobs (U.S. Department of Labor, 2006b).

CONSUMPTION PATTERNS Consumption patterns of interest to the occupational health nurse include those related to food and nutrition, smoking, and drug and alcohol use. The influence of nutrition on health is well established, and the occupational health nurse assesses the nutritional patterns of employees with whom he or she works. In addition, the nurse assesses how the work environment affects eating habits. For example, sufficient opportunity may not be provided for employees to eat despite OSHA regulations regarding time and place for breaks and meals.

The nurse also determines whether food service is available to employees. If there is an employee cafeteria, the nurse may need to assess the nutritional quality of the food provided. If no food services are available in the workplace, the nurse would determine whether they are available nearby, or whether adequate storage facilities exist for employees who bring meals from home.

The prevalence of eating disorders in the workforce is another consideration related to dietary consumption. Occupational health nurses may identify employees (primarily, but not exclusively, young women) who have eating disorders. A number of screening tools are available to assist in identifying people with eating disorders, although some authors caution that many of the tools have not been adequately tested for their validity and that a sequential process should be used in which those

identified through screening as being at risk for an eating disorder receive more specific diagnostic tests to confirm the diagnosis (Jacobi, Abascal, & Taylor, 2004). One simple screening tool that has shown promise is the SCOFF questionnaire, which consists of five questions that address making oneself sick by overeating, worry about a loss of control over one's eating, a perception of oneself as fat in spite of others' assurances to the contrary, loss of more than 14 pounds over a 3-month period, and a dominance of food in one's life (Parker, Lyons, & Bonner, 2005). Occupational health nurses who identify employees with eating disorders would usually make a referral for diagnostic confirmation and treatment. Eating disorders are addressed in more detail in Chapter 30∞.

Smoking is another consumption pattern of concern to the occupational health nurse. Smoking is harmful to health in and of itself. In addition, smoking may increase the adverse effects of other environmental hazards in the work setting, particularly those that affect respiration. Many employers have recently begun to prohibit smoking except in carefully controlled areas in the workplace and have been active in promoting programs to help employees quit smoking. In addition to the health implications, such efforts cut employer expenses. The nurse assesses the extent of smoking in the employee population as well as the specific implications of smoking in that particular environment.

Employees may have problems with substance abuse. The prevalence of these problems should be monitored and the nurse should be alert to signs and symptoms of substance abuse in the employee population. Overindulgence in other substances, such as caffeine, may also pose a health hazard to employees. Worksite interventions have been shown to be successful in decreasing smoking and other drug use and in reducing fat intake and increasing consumption of fruits, vegetables, and fiber.

REST AND EXERCISE Work places many physical and psychological demands on people. Sometimes these demands result in inadequate rest and recreation, as with the executive who works constantly or the blue-collar worker who holds two jobs in an attempt to make ends meet. Conversely, work may also lead to too much sitting and too little exercise. Lack of rest may increase risk for injury or errors. For example, part-time farmers who have a second job have an increased risk of job injury when they use sleeping aids or experience sleep apnea problems (Spengler, Browning, & Reed, 2004). Similarly, there is an association between shift work and drug administration errors among nurses (Suzuki, Ohida, Kaneita, Yokoyama, & Uchiyama, 2005). Problems encountered in the work setting may also interfere with employees' ability to rest off the job. For example, one study of Japanese workers found that high levels of group conflict, job dissatisfaction, and depression were associated with increased risk of insomnia. Insomnia was also found to be linked to the physical work environment and low levels of coworker support (Nakata et al., 2004).

The nurse in the work setting assesses the amount of activity engaged in by employees and the balance between rest and exercise. He or she also obtains information on the types of recreation used by employees and any potential health hazards posed by recreational choices.

Many companies are recognizing the benefits of exercise in terms of both the physical and psychological health of employees. These companies are promoting physical exercise and may even provide facilities for exercise and recreation in the workplace. If this is the case, the nurse should be alert to potential health hazards and the potential for too much exercise. For example, if there is a company pool, an employee with epilepsy who swims to relieve tension should be cautioned against swimming alone. Similarly, an overweight executive should engage in physical activity cautiously to lessen the risk of heart attack or injury.

USE OF SAFETY DEVICES Another behavioral factor that is particularly relevant to health in the occupational setting is the use or nonuse of safety devices. Hazards present in the workplace frequently can be mitigated by the use of appropriate safety devices; however, this can occur only if employees use these devices consistently and appropriately.

The community health nurse identifies the need for safety devices and also monitors the extent to which they are used. For example, do individuals working in high-noise areas wear earplugs? Are those earplugs correctly fitted? Do people involved in heavy lifting wear weight belts, or do they ignore the potential for injury? Are heavy shoes or gloves worn in areas with dangerous equipment? Again, the attitude of management toward health promotion and illness prevention strongly influences employee behaviors. When administrators, for example, fail to use hearing protection in high-noise areas, they convey an attitude of disinterest in health, which frequently filters down to employees.

WORKING WHILE ILL A final behavioral factor that influences the health of employees in the work setting is working while ill, also called sickness **presenteeism** (Putnam & McKibbin, 2004). It is estimated that lost workdays and decreased productivity due to presenteeism cost U.S. employers more than $1.4 million each month or more than $17 million annually (Institute for Health and Productivity Management, 2002).

In addition to the lost productivity from employees whose performance is impaired by symptoms of illness, presenteeism is harmful to the ill employee as well as to others in the work setting. When an employee has a communicable disease, for example, coming to work while ill increases the risk of exposure for coworkers and clients. In addition, presenteeism may increase

overall risk of premature mortality. For example, in one study those workers who had taken no absences related to illness over a 3-year period had twice the risk for serious coronary events as those who had moderate levels of sickness absenteeism (Kivimaki et al., 2005).

Community health nurses working in occupational settings assess behaviors affecting the health of individual employees in the work setting as well as the prevalence of harmful behaviors in the work group. The focused assessment below provides some guidelines for assessing this aspect of health in the work setting.

Health System Considerations

Health system factors influencing employee health relate to both external and internal health care systems. The external system reflects the availability and accessibility of health care services outside the workplace, whereas the internal system consists of those services offered within the workplace.

THE EXTERNAL SYSTEM In assessing employee health status, the community health nurse in the occupational setting gathers information about the use of health services in the community at large. The nurse examines the type of services used and the reasons for and appropriateness of their use. The nurse also assesses the availability of services needed by company employees in the external health care system.

One of the work-related factors influencing use of outside health services is the availability of insurance coverage. Health insurance is an employment benefit for many, but large segments of the working population do not have health insurance coverage. Many of these

---

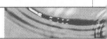

FOCUSED ASSESSMENT

Behavioral Considerations in the Work Setting

- What types of work are performed? Does the type of work pose health hazards?
- What behavioral factors influence health in the work setting?
- Do any members of the employee population use prescription medications on a regular basis? Are medications used, stored, and dispensed as directed?
- Are safety policies and procedures in place in the work setting? Are they enforced? Do employees use appropriate safety equipment and procedures?
- Do employees engage in other behaviors (e.g., smoking) that increase their risk of toxic effects from workplace exposures?
- Do employees get sufficient rest and exercise to promote their health? What opportunities are provided for physical activity in the work setting?
- What is the nutritional status of the employee population? What foods are available in the work setting? Does food availability promote good nutrition in the employee population?
- To what extent does sickness presenteeism occur in the employee population? What are the effects of presenteeism for the sick employee, for coworkers, and for the organization?

uninsured workers do not have sufficient income to afford health insurance themselves or out-of-pocket health care expenses. For example, in 2003, 56% of full-time U.S. employees and 9% of part-time employees were covered by an employer- or union-provided group health insurance plan (U.S. Census Bureau, 2005). Some of those not covered by employer-provided policies had health insurance from other sources (e.g., private or spousal coverage), but others had no insurance at all.

Even for insured employees, medical benefits have steadily declined due to high insurance costs. Copayments and deductibles have increased at the same time, further limiting access to care for some employees and their families. In 2005, for example, health insurance premiums accounted for 10.2% of public employees' salary and benefits, compared to only 6.9% in 1991. In private industry, the percentage of total compensation paid for health insurance did not increase as much during this time period, rising only from 6% to 6.8% of an employee's salary and benefits. From 1990 to 1996 alone, the percentage of employees required to contribute to the cost of employment-based health insurance rose from 42% to 51%, and the percentage of employees required to contribute to family coverage increased from 68% to 70%. During that same period, the average monthly contribution of the individual employee in a small business for personal health insurance coverage increased from $25 to $43. Monthly contributions for family coverage increased from $109 to $182. Overall, in 2003, employee contributions accounted for 35% of the premiums for work-based health insurance coverage (National Center for Health Statistics, 2005).

The occupational health nurse should become familiar with the insurance status of employees in the company and with the kinds of benefits covered under group policies, where they exist. Occupational health nurses may also need to advocate for affordable personal and family health insurance coverage for employees in the work setting.

THE INTERNAL SYSTEM The internal health care system consists of those health services and programs provided to employees in the work setting. In 2003, the cost of these in-house services amounted to $4.9 billion. Three general types of occupational health programs can be found in business and industry: programs aimed at controlling exposure to hazardous conditions; those emphasizing health promotion in the workplace; and comprehensive programs that attempt to meet a variety of employee health needs (Polanyi, Frank, Shannon, Sullivan, & Lavis, 2000). A few employers offer a fourth type of program that addresses the health needs of families as well as employees.

Programs to Control Toxic Exposures Programs to control or eliminate toxic substances and other hazardous conditions in the workplace usually occur in response to OSHA regulations. Control programs may involve engineering controls, controlled work practices, use of safety equipment or devices, or elimination of toxic substances from the work environment. In industries with this type of program, the community health nurse should assess the efficacy of these control measures and the extent to which they are adhered to in the setting. As noted earlier, the nurse may need to play an advocacy role to make sure that the organization complies with OSHA regulations.

Health Promotion Programs The second type of program involves both the development of organizational policies related to health promotion and the provision of health promotion programs. Policies seek to limit hospitalization and expenses for acute care services by promoting the health of the employee population and by encouraging a less expensive approach to providing services. For example, employers may have policies related to the need for a second opinion before covering employee expenses for elective surgery or encouraging home care rather than hospitalization whenever possible, or a company may initiate a no-smoking policy to promote smoking cessation or decrease the amount of tobacco use by employees.

The company may also provide health promotion programs aimed at fostering health-related behaviors among employees. Generally, a specific program focuses on one aspect of health care rather than taking a comprehensive approach to health promotion. These programs may be illness oriented rather than focusing on the promotion of overall health. For example, there may be emphasis on education for good body mechanics to prevent injuries or first aid for injuries, but little attention to overall health promotion. These programs also tend to focus on the individual employee's responsibility for his or her health and may neglect conditions within the work setting that create health problems. In this type of system, the community health nurse identifies the types of health promotion programs provided and the extent to which they meet employees' identified health needs. The nurse also reviews health-related policies and attempts to assure that they are beneficial to, rather than destructive of, employee health.

Comprehensive Programs The third type of occupational health program is a comprehensive approach to wellness that incorporates three aspects: awareness, lifestyle change, and change in environmental conditions to better promote health. These programs educate employees so as to promote health and prevent illness, but they also emphasize organizational programs, policies, and environmental changes that are conducive to health. For example, a company with a comprehensive health care approach might provide educational sessions on stress management and engage in organizational changes aimed at reducing the amount of stress engendered by the work setting, or the employer might provide on-site assistance with weight reduction or time and facilities for meditation, yoga, or massage. Again, the nurse assessing the influence of health care system factors on employees' health determines the extent to which the designated program meets employees' health needs.

Family Care In some work settings, comprehensive health care programs go beyond the provision of care to employees to include some form of direct care for family members. Employees who are concerned about their families may be less productive than they would be were their family situation less stressful. As more and more families are supported by two wage earners, employment of both spouses has implications for the life of the family and the well-being of children. Community health nurses who care for clients in work settings should be aware of the stresses involved in dual-career (or single-parent) families and how work schedules and conditions may affect the health of the family. Work schedules that allow for outside responsibilities and family life are very helpful, and the nurse may be able to influence management in the creation of flexible scheduling systems. The nurse may also be of assistance in helping employees deal with the stress of role overload.

Some companies are becoming more aware of the interplay of family influences and occupational factors in employee performance and are establishing systems designed to assist families. One effort is the establishment of childcare centers on company premises. Some centers provide care whether the child is well or ill. In such cases, the community health nurse working in this setting may assume responsibilities relative to the health of the children in the centers. These nurses need to be versed in pediatric as well as adult health care. Elder care services are also provided in a few occupational settings.

Even in occupational settings where there are no child or elder care facilities, nurses are asked for assistance in dealing with health problems of family members. The nurse may counsel the employee regarding resolution of family problems or may provide referrals to outside sources of assistance.

Nurses who have knowledge of problems experienced by members of employees' families are in a position to recognize paraoccupational exposure and to take action to correct such exposure. Nurses should be aware of the potential for such exposure and should make it a practice to ask employees questions designed to elicit information about family exposure to hazardous substances.

A focused assessment addressing health system considerations in the work setting is presented at right. The community assessment guide included in Appendix G on the Companion Website can be used to assess an employee population, and a specific tool for assessing health in work settings can be found in the

Community Assessment Reference Guide 🖵 designed to accompany this text.

Diagnostic Reasoning and Care of Clients in Work Settings

Community health nurses working in occupational settings derive nursing diagnoses from assessment information related to individuals or groups of employees. For example, the nurse might diagnose "inability to sleep due to work pressures" for a company executive or "poor employee morale due to increased tension and stress in the work setting." Other nursing diagnoses related to individual employees are a "need for referral for counseling due to heavy drinking" and "moderate hearing loss due to failure to use hearing protection in high-noise areas." Nursing diagnoses at the group level are a "potential for exposure to hepatitis B due to frequent contact with blood" for a group of laboratory technicians in a hospital, and the "potential for falls due to work in elevated areas" for a group of construction workers.

Planning Nursing Care in Work Settings

Interventions may be developed by the occupational health nurse alone or in conjunction with others in the work setting to address the health needs identified. In the case of individual clients, interventions would be tailored to individual needs and circumstances. When identified health problems affect groups of employees, planned interventions are likely to be more complex. Planning to meet the needs of groups in the workplace will employ the principles of health programming discussed in Chapter 15∞. Whether the client is an individual, a group of employees, or the total population in the work setting, interventions may be planned at primary, secondary, and tertiary levels of prevention.

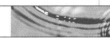

FOCUSED ASSESSMENT

Health System Considerations in the Work Setting

- What health services are offered in the work setting? How are health care services funded? Is funding adequate to meet health needs?
- How accessible are needed health services in the community? To what extent does the employee population use available health services?
- What is the extent of health insurance coverage in the employee population?
- What is the quality of interaction between internal and external health care services?
- To what extent are health promotion and illness/injury prevention emphasized in the work setting?
- What systems are in place to control and monitor toxic exposures in the work setting?
- Are surveillance procedures implemented in a systematic way to periodically assess all employees at risk for exposure?

Primary Prevention

Primary prevention in the occupational setting is directed toward promoting health and well-being and preventing illness, injury, and violence.

HEALTH PROMOTION Community health nurses in occupational settings educate employees to lead healthier lives. They also advocate for company policies that promote health. Baseline data for the *Healthy People 2010*◆ objectives indicated that 33% to 50% of worksites offer comprehensive health promotion programs to their employees, with larger companies more likely to provide such programs than small companies. The 2010 target is 75% of all worksites (CDC, 2005a). Workplace health promotion programs may focus on increasing awareness of the ill effects of unhealthy behaviors and encouraging behavior change among employees or on changing policies and conditions in the work setting to better promote health. In the latter focus, programs may be intended to alter the organizational culture of the work setting to reinforce the importance of health. Actions in these types of programs are directed at both the individual and the organization. For instance, the organization may strive to find effective ways to reduce stress in the work environment while incorporating a health behavior review as part of regular performance appraisals for employees.

An organizational culture that supports health conveys to employees that their health is a priority for the company. This message must be supported by company efforts to promote health within the organization. For example, some companies may promote exercise among employees, but an organizational culture that truly supports physical activity may allow time for exercise during the workday or provide facilities (e.g., weight rooms, walking paths) that actually promote physical activity. Similarly, an organizational culture that supports health will take steps to ban all forms of tobacco use in the work setting and will provide tobacco use cessation assistance for those employees who use tobacco. Another feature of an organizational culture that supports health is positive attitudes toward health-promoting behaviors among employees. For example, in such a culture employees who engage in physical activity are the norm, and those who do not are in the minority. Employees support each other in positive health-related behaviors. Community health nurses can be instrumental in promoting an organizational culture that supports health by convincing employers of the value of health promotion in terms of increased productivity, better morale, and reduced absenteeism. They can also help to develop positive attitudes to health promotion among employees by making health-promotion activities relevant to the goals and motivations of the employee group. For example, they might approach smoking cessation from the perspective of the benefits for employees' children if that is a strong motivator for members of the work group. Or they might plan physical activities that fit easily into the workday.

Health promotion programs in the occupational setting can be highly successful. For example, the Task Force on Community Preventive Services has recommended workplace interventions to address nutrition and increased physical activity. In fact, it is estimated that it would cost less than $1 per employee to provide on-site weight control programs for employee populations at risk for overweight and obesity (Katz et al., 2005). Similarly, stress management and other similar programs have also been shown to increase productivity and psychological health among employees as well as promote more healthful behaviors (van der Klink, Blonk, Schene, & van Dijk, 2001). Programs on how to improve one's commute to work are another opportunity for workplace health promotion programs (Pohanka & Fitzgerald, 2004). Community health nurses can be actively involved in designing and implementing these and other health promotion programs.

Further research is needed to document the long-term effects and costs of health promotion programs; however, research has indicated that the approach taken to health promotion initiatives can make a difference in outcomes. In a meta analysis of 95 quasi-experimental studies of workplace health promotion interventions, Burke and associates (2006) found that interventions that actively engaged participants (e.g., through hands-on learning or behavioral modeling) were consistently more effective in promoting health and safety behaviors than less engaging interventions (e.g., pamphlets, lectures, and video presentations).

Another avenue for health promotion is providing prenatal care to pregnant workers. This could involve referral for prenatal care if this service is not provided by the company health facility. The nurse might also monitor female employees for signs and symptoms of complications of pregnancy. The nurse may find it necessary to function as an advocate for an employee who needs to be relieved of some of her duties as the pregnancy progresses. For example, it may be necessary to move the employee to another position that does not require heavy lifting. The nurse may also be involved in childbirth education for pregnant employees or male employees and their spouses.

ILLNESS PREVENTION Preventing illness is the second aspect of primary prevention in the workplace. Illness prevention can involve either employee education or

---

EVIDENCE-BASED PRACTICE

*T*he Task Force for Community Preventive Services (Katz et al., 2005) has indicated that there is little evidence for the effectiveness of single-component interventions for reducing the prevalence of overweight and obesity in occupational settings. This lack of evidence is primarily due to the absence of studies of the effectiveness of such programs. How might you design a series of studies that address the effectiveness of single-focus intervention programs in work settings?

prevention of specific illnesses through immunization. For example, some industries routinely offer employees influenza immunization to cut down on illness-related absenteeism.

Another aspect of illness prevention involves modifying risk factors. Risk factors are personal or group characteristics that predispose one to develop a specific health problem. For example, it is well known that smoking increases one's risk of developing heart disease and lung cancer, so smoking is a risk factor for both of these problems.

Some risk factors can be modified or eliminated, thus decreasing one's chances of developing specific health problems. Again, using smoking as an example, people who quit smoking lower their risk of developing lung cancer. Occupational health nurses can be instrumental in assisting employees to modify risk factors, thereby helping them to prevent health problems. Some risk factors that receive particular attention in the occupational setting are smoking, elevated blood pressure, sedentary lifestyle, stress, and overweight.

Occupational health nurses can work on risk factor modification with individuals or groups of employees. They can also engage in risk factor modification efforts at the company level. One example of this would be efforts to convince company policy makers that a no-smoking policy should be instituted and enforced within the workplace. Nurses can also develop weight standards for job categories in which being overweight is particularly hazardous, or the nurse can recommend the use of safer products in place of toxic substances whenever possible.

At the individual level, the nurse can counsel employees regarding the hazards of smoking, particularly in conjunction with occupational exposure to respiratory irritants. They can also provide assistance to individuals who wish to quit smoking.

Other interventions may be used to prevent illness in specific occupational settings. For example, condom use and periodic screening have been recommended as mechanisms for preventing HIV infection and other STDs in the adult film industry (Division of STD Prevention, 2005). Similarly, adequate infection control procedures and engineering controls that provide adequate ventilation in areas where aerosols are generated can help to protect health care workers from tuberculosis (Division of Tuberculosis Elimination, 2004).

Specific illness prevention may also entail postexposure prophylaxis. **Postexposure prophylaxis (PEP)** is treatment for a communicable disease following a potential occupational exposure to the infectious agent. For example, health care providers caring for clients with known cases of hepatitis B or C or HIV infection may receive prophylactic treatment to prevent them from developing the disease (Beltrami et al., 2001; Panlilio, Cardo, Grohskopf, Heneine, & Ross, 2005). Occupational health nurses may be involved in actually providing employees with prophylactic treatment or in referring them for needed services. Prophylaxis will be addressed in more detail in Chapter 28∞.

Restructuring the work environment can help in minimizing occupational stress as a risk factor for health problems. Efforts in this direction include developing flexible schedules to minimize conflicts with employees' outside responsibilities. The nurse can also facilitate employee input into work-related decisions and strive to minimize role overload and role ambiguity. The nurse can also promote opportunity for social interaction, job security, and career development.

As is obvious, many of these efforts must be undertaken by management, but the nurse can provide management with evidence of related research and can provide the impetus for change in these areas. At the individual level, the occupational health nurse can be aware of the stressors experienced by employees in various jobs in the work setting. The nurse is also in a position to monitor the effects of stress on the individual employee and to counsel employees in stress management.

INJURY AND VIOLENCE PREVENTION Injury prevention in the work setting may entail employee education in a variety of areas. Employees need to be acquainted with safety procedures to prevent accidents. For example, there is a need to prevent needlesticks in health care settings, and staff may need to be educated regarding the appropriate disposal of sharps. Similarly, periodic reminders regarding good body mechanics in lifting patients may be needed in the health care setting. There may also be a need to educate employees in the correct use of safety equipment. For example, individuals working in some areas should wear protective clothing or use breathing apparatus. As noted earlier, safety education should be provided to both paid and volunteer employees. The nurse should explain the need for safety equipment and be responsible for monitoring its use. This may entail planning periodic visits to certain areas of the workplace to determine whether employees are indeed using safety equipment as directed.

Employees may also be in need of education in other areas related to injury prevention. Handling of hazardous substances, proper use of machinery, need for fluid replacement in high-heat areas, and good body mechanics are all educational topics that may be appropriate in certain industrial settings. Nurses may also provide education on first aid and cardiopulmonary resuscitation.

Another aspect of injury prevention in which the nurse may be involved is monitoring hazardous conditions in the workplace. The nurse should be aware of potential hazards and their appropriate management. In the absence of an industrial hygienist, the nurse may plan and conduct environmental testing to detect hazardous levels of chemicals, heat, or noise. Hazardous working conditions may reflect more than the physical

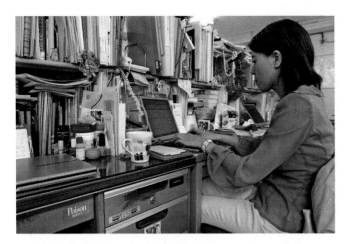

Injury prevention is important in office employment as well as in heavy industry. (© Zoriah/The Image Works)

work environment. For example, inadequate staffing has resulted in increased back injuries among nursing personnel. In fact, every 9% decrease in staffing levels has been shown to lead to a 65% increase in work-related injuries among nurses (Lipscomb, Trinkhoff, Brady, & Geiger-Brown, 2004). Similarly, low staffing ratios and poor unit organization have been linked to increased needlestick injuries in nursing settings (Clarke, Sloane, & Aiken, 2002).

The nurse may need to acquaint management with the occurrence of injuries due to hazardous conditions and advocate changes designed to protect employees from injuries. Recommendations for dealing with the problem of noise-induced hearing loss, for example, include engineering efforts to minimize noise production, use of properly fitted hearing protection devices, education of employees and managers in the use of protective

BUILDING OUR KNOWLEDGE BASE

LaMontagne, Oakes, and Turley (2004) indicated two major thrusts for occupational health research: intervention research and surveillance. Intervention research focuses on the effectiveness of a variety of interventions in preventing occupational injury and illness or in dealing with their consequences. Surveillance research, on the other hand, is directed toward identifying the frequency with which certain events occur in the work setting. Surveillance may take one of two forms, surveillance for health effects of occupational health conditions (e.g., the number of workers who develop carpal tunnel syndrome and the contributing factors) and surveillance for exposures (e.g., examination of exposures to pesticides among agricultural workers). Both forms of surveillance research are intended to identify health-related problems in occupational settings and their underlying factors as precursors to the design of interventions that would then be tested for their effectiveness using intervention research approaches. What are some potential research studies that might be conducted in community health nursing work settings? Which of these studies would be surveillance studies? Which would be intervention studies? What might be the implications of study findings for community health nursing practice?

devices and their importance, and periodic audiometric screening. The occupational health nurse may be actively involved in planning and executing the majority of these recommended activities, particularly in screening for hearing loss, fitting protective devices, and educating employees and supervisors. Control of noise-related hearing loss requires commitment on the part of employees and management to the proper use of protective devices. Motivating employees to use these devices and monitoring their use are crucial functions of the occupational health nurse.

Specific interventions may be required for specific types of injuries prevalent in a given work setting. For example, NIOSH (2004) has recommended the following elements of workplace safety policies related to motor vehicle accident injuries:

- Authorization of management to enforce driver safety policies and procedures
- Mandatory seat belt use for all occupants in all vehicles
- Use of vehicles with good safety ratings
- Maintenance and review of employee driving records
- Policies against distractions (e.g., use of cell phones) while driving
- Adequate licensing and qualifications for vehicles used
- Effective vehicle maintenance programs that include periodic comprehensive inspections, removal from service of any defective vehicles, and mandatory pre-trip sight inspections

Specific violence prevention programs may also be necessary in occupational settings with a high prevalence or risk for workplace violence. Some elements of workplace violence prevention might include adequate administrative support for violence prevention, assessment of the company history and rates of violence, determination of patterns of violence and contributing factors, and identification of workplace hazards that promote violence. An example of the latter might be poorly lighted or limited-visibility workstations or the known presence of significant amounts of money in the work setting. Other elements of workplace violence prevention include development of policies and procedures for reporting violence or potential violence and disciplinary consequences for violent behaviors in the work setting. Installation of security devices such as surveillance cameras and metal detectors may be appropriate in some settings. In other settings, visitor sign-in procedures may be appropriate. Additional interventions may include programs for dealing with aggressive behavior, anger management programs, and training for recognition of potentially violent situations (Ruff et al., 2004). Interventions related to primary prevention in the work setting, including violence prevention strategies, are summarized in Table 24-2◆.

TABLE 24-2 Primary Prevention Emphases and Interventions in Work Settings

Primary Prevention Emphasis	Interventions
Health promotion	• Education of employees for healthy behaviors
	• Assistance with elimination of unhealthy behaviors (e.g., smoking cessation)
	• Development of worksite policies that promote health (e.g., smoke-free workplace policies)
	• Development of work environments that promote health
Illness prevention	• Immunization
	• Postexposure prophylaxis for communicable disease exposures
	• Modification or elimination of risk factors in the work environment
	• Stress reduction/management education for employees
Injury prevention	• Safety education for employees (e.g., body mechanics, universal precautions for bloodborne pathogens)
	• Provision of adequate safety equipment
	• Monitoring effective use of safety equipment
	• Development of policies and procedures that prevent injury (e.g., comprehensive driver safety policies)
	• Modification or elimination of injury risk factors in the work setting
	• Development of adequate management support for injury prevention policies and procedures
Violence prevention	• Modification of worksite environments that promote violence
	• Installation of security devices if appropriate
	• Development of processes and procedures for handling workplace violence or potential for violence
	• Development of reporting procedures
	• Development of disciplinary sanctions for violent behavior in the work setting
	• Employee education on violence prevention, anger management, recognition of potentially violent situations

Secondary Prevention

Secondary prevention in work settings is aimed at recognizing and resolving existing health problems. General areas of involvement for occupational health nurses include screening and surveillance, treatment for existing conditions, and emergency care.

SCREENING AND SURVEILLANCE Screening activities can take any of three directions. Screening efforts begin with preemployment assessment of potential employees. Screening may also be conducted at periodic intervals to monitor employee health status. Finally, the work environment may be screened periodically for the presence or absence of hazardous conditions. The community health nurse would be involved in planning and implementing screening efforts at all three levels. **Screening** involves testing individual employees for indicators of disease or for risk factors that increase the potential for disease. Surveillance, on the other hand, involves the analysis of group data to identify trends and problems in the work setting rather than in individual employees (Rogers & Livsey, 2000).

Preemployment Screening For many employees, their first interaction with an occupational health nurse is the preemployment screening examination. The purpose of this initial screening is to facilitate employee selection and placement. Hiring an employee for a particular job is in part dependent on his or her physical, mental, and emotional capabilities for performing that job. A similar process may be needed when considering an employee for a change of job. These capabilities can be determined in an initial screening examination. At this time, the nurse usually obtains a complete health history from the employee and conducts a battery of routine screening tests. Nurse practitioners in the occupational setting may also conduct the physical examination.

For certain categories of jobs, preemployment screening may entail criminal background checks and/or drug screening. For example, a security guard who works for a firm that designs and builds equipment for use by the armed services would probably need to have a security clearance. Similarly, a school teacher may be required to undergo a criminal background check related to child abuse or molestation. Occupational health nurses will probably not be involved in a security check for a prospective employee, but they may be responsible for collecting specimens for drug screening tests. They may also be subject to screening themselves as health care institutions and other employers become more careful regarding the background of their employees.

Based on the information derived from the screening, the nurse may make determinations regarding the person's employability in a particular capacity. To make such determinations, the nurse must be familiar with the types of activities involved and stressors encountered in a particular job. The preemployment screening also

Advocacy in Action

Getting a Job

Jerry's prospective employer would not hire him because he had malignant hypertension. The occupational health agency that contracted with the employer for employment physicals was able to diagnose the HTN but offered no treatment options. Because Jerry was uninsured, he was cared for at the St. Agnes Nurses Center by one of the nurse practitioners. After a couple of months, Jerry's blood pressure was under control and he began working. Within a few months of beginning his job, he was promoted to store manager. We continue to care for Jerry, who will soon have health benefits through his employer.

We do countless physical exams required by individuals who are applying for employment. Without the physical they cannot get the job, and without a salary they cannot afford a physical—a definite catch 22.

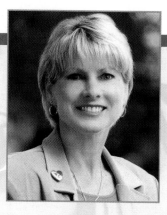

Maryann Lieb, RN, MSN
BSN Express Program Coordinator
College of Nursing, Villanova University

provides baseline data for determining the effects of working conditions on the health of employees. The questions included in the focused assessment provided below are designed to help determine an employee's fitness for a specific job. A work fitness inventory is also available in the *Community Assessment Reference Guide* designed to accompany this text.

FOCUSED ASSESSMENT

Evaluating Fitness for Work

Physical Health Considerations

- Does the employee have the physical stamina required?
- Does the employee have any mobility limitations that would interfere with performance?
- Does the employee have sufficient joint mobility to do the job?
- Does the employee have any postural limitations that would interfere with performance?
- Does the employee have the required strength for the job?
- Does the employee have the level of coordination required?
- Does the employee have problems with balance that would interfere with performance?
- Does the employee have any cardiorespiratory limitations?
- Is there a possibility for unconsciousness that would create a safety hazard?
- Does the employee have the required level of visual and auditory acuity?
- Does the employee have communication and speech capabilities required by the job?

Mental and Emotional Health Considerations

- Does the employee have the requisite level of cognitive function (e.g., memory, critical thinking)?
- Will the employee's mental or emotional state (e.g., depression) interfere with performance?
- Does the employee have the required motivational level?
- Does the employee have a substance abuse problem that would interfere with performance?

- Does the employee have effective stress management skills?
- Is there any possibility that the employee might endanger self or others?

Health Care Considerations

- Are there treatment effects that will interfere with performance (e.g., drowsiness from medications)?
- Will subsequent treatment plans interfere with performance (e.g., nausea due to future chemotherapy)?
- What is the employee's prognosis? Will existing conditions improve or deteriorate further?
- Does the employee have any special health needs to be met in the work setting (e.g., diabetic diet)?
- Are any assistive aids or appliances required? Will work processes or setting need to be adapted to accommodate these aids (e.g., space for a wheelchair)?

Task/Setting Considerations

- Are there risk factors in the work setting that would adversely affect the employee?
- What is the level of stress involved in the job?
- Will the employee be working with others or alone? What health effects might this have?
- What are the temporal aspects of the job and how will they affect health (e.g., shift work, early morning or late evening work, length of shift)?
- Is there travel involved in the job? How will this affect employee health?

Data from: Cox, R. A. F., & Edwards, F. C. (2000). Introduction. In R. A. F. Cox, F. C. Edwards, & K. Palmer (Eds.), Fitness for work: The medical aspects (3rd ed., pp. 1–24). Oxford: Oxford University Press.

Periodic Screening The nurse in the occupational setting also plans periodic screening activities to monitor employees' continuing health status. This is particularly true of employees working under hazardous conditions. For example, monitoring devices are used by personnel working with radiation and are periodically checked for exposure limits. Likewise, blood chemistries may be done at periodic intervals to test for exposure to toxic substances. Periodic blood pressure screenings and pulmonary function tests may also be warranted. In some occupational groups, such as the armed forces, employees are routinely screened for overweight and for physical capacity.

The types of screening done depend on the type of job performed, the risks involved, and the capabilities required. Some screenings are routinely performed on all employees in a particular setting. For example, employees may receive a routine physical examination at periodic intervals. Other screening tests are performed only on specific employees. For example, lead screening may be done routinely on individuals who work on a plant assembly line, but not on clerical personnel.

Nurses may also be actively involved in providing or promoting routine health screenings that are not related to employees' jobs. For example, the nurse may educate older male employees regarding the need for screening for prostate cancer, or teach men of all ages how to perform testicular self-examination. Similarly, nurses may encourage women to obtain regular Papanicolaou tests and mammography. In one study, for example, an occupational intervention consisting of education, group discussion, and outreach was successful in increasing the extent of cervical cancer screening among women employees. No effect was noted, however, in the rate of breast cancer screening between experimental and control groups (Allen, Stoddard, Mays, & Sorensen, 2001).

Occupational health nurses are frequently responsible for conducting these and other screening tests on employees. They may also interpret test results, explain them to employees, and take action when warranted by positive test results.

Environmental Screening Periodic screening of the environment may also be warranted, and, in the absence of industrial hygienists or safety engineers, the nurse may be responsible for planning and conducting environmental screenings. For example, the nurse may measure noise levels in various work areas at specific intervals to determine areas in which hearing protection is required. Similarly, measurements of volatile chemicals or radiation might be done in high-risk areas.

TREATMENT OF EXISTING CONDITIONS The second aspect of secondary prevention in the work setting is the diagnosis and treatment of existing health problems. Community health nurses are actively involved in planning health interventions for individual employees and should also participate in planning health programs to meet the needs of groups of clients.

Many industries go beyond treating only job-related illnesses and conditions to treating a variety of major and minor conditions. The rationale for the extension of services to non-job-related conditions is that any health problem, physical or emotional, can serve to impair the employee's performance. Also, treatment of these conditions within the work setting limits time lost in pursuing outside treatment, saving the company money in the long run.

Depending on the capabilities of the occupational health unit, employees with existing health problems may be referred to the external health care system for problem resolution, or treatment may be provided within the workplace itself. Those occupational health nurses who are nurse practitioners may treat illness in the work setting. Even nurses who are not nurse practitioners may treat minor conditions on the basis of protocols established in conjunction with medical consultation.

Occupational health nurses also need to plan to monitor the effectiveness of therapy, whether or not that therapy is provided by the occupational health unit. For example, an employee with hypertension might be followed by his or her primary care provider, but the occupational health nurse will monitor medication compliance and effects on the employee's blood pressure. In addition, the nurse will educate the employee regarding the condition and its treatment.

In the case of employees with problems related to substance abuse or stress, the community health nurse usually plans a referral to an appropriate source of assistance. The nurse may also need to function as an advocate for impaired employees, encouraging employers to provide coverage for treatment of psychological as well as physical illness. Nurses may also find it necessary to report substance abuse to supervisory personnel when either the health or the safety of other employees is threatened.

Community health nurses in occupational settings may also be involved in planning and implementing employee assistance programs for employees with psychological problems. An **employee assistance program (EAP)** is a program within the occupational setting designed to counsel employees with psychological problems and assist them in dealing with those problems. EAPs usually focus on motivating individuals to seek help and referring them for needed services. Substance abuse disorders and eating disorders are two types of problems addressed by EAPs. Generally, the occupational health nurse refers an employee to another source of services rather than providing care for these problems within the work setting. However, the nurse may be involved in the development and support of self-help groups within the employment setting to assist employees with these and other problems. For example, guided self-help and cognitive behavioral group therapy have both been found to be of help in treating bulimia nervosa, one of a group of eating disorders (Bailer et al., 2004; Pritchard, Bergin, & Wade, 2004). Similarly, an occupational health nurse might help to establish a bereavement group to assist employees who have experienced significant losses.

EMERGENCY RESPONSE Another aspect of secondary prevention in work settings is response to emergency situations. Nurses may find themselves dealing with both physical and psychological emergencies and should have a basic plan for dealing with various types of emergencies that may arise. Physical emergencies may result from serious accidents or from physical conditions such as heart attack, stroke, seizure disorder, and insulin reaction. Treatment for these emergencies is usually based on established protocols.

With respect to emergencies due to illness, it is helpful if the nurse has prior information related to the employee's condition. For example, if the nurse has prior knowledge that the client is diabetic, the diagnosis of hypoglycemic reaction will be reached and treatment initiated more rapidly than would otherwise be the case. For this reason, occupational health nurses should be well acquainted with employees' health histories.

Psychological emergencies may result in homicide, suicide, or both. Although businesses may have generalized protocols for dealing with such emergencies as threatened homicide or suicide, the nurse faced with such situations will probably need to exercise a great deal of creativity in planning to address a psychological emergency. General considerations include remaining calm and removing others from the immediate vicinity. The nurse *should not* plan any heroic measures that may endanger him- or herself, the employee, or others. Additional interventions are dictated by the situation. Again, prior identification of employees under excessive stress may help to prevent psychiatric emergencies.

Another psychological emergency with which occupational health nurses may need to deal is sexual assault. Most victims of sexual assault in the workplace are women, and most assaults occur at night when women are working in isolation from coworkers or the public. The nurse who encounters a female employee who has been sexually assaulted should address immediate physical and psychological needs, assess the client for suicidal tendencies, and refer her for counseling. The nurse may also need to act as an advocate with the legal and criminal justice systems and provide emotional support.

One further type of emergency that requires an occupational health nursing response is the emergency that affects large numbers of people. Examples of mass emergencies are fires or explosions, radiation exposure, and hazardous substance leaks. In addition to providing treatment for those injured in such emergencies, the nurse may be responsible for assisting in evaluating affected areas and in organizing to provide needed care. Occupational health nurses should be involved in planning the overall company response to such situations as well as in planning health care in such an eventuality. The role of the nurse in disaster preparedness is discussed in greater detail in Chapter 27∞. Major emphases in secondary prevention in work settings are summarized in Table 24-3◆.

TABLE 24-3 Secondary Prevention Emphases and Interventions in Work Settings

Secondary Prevention Emphasis	Interventions
Screening	• Preemployment screening
	• Determination of work capacity
	• Recommendations regarding work conditions or accommodations
	• Periodic employee screening
	• Periodic environmental screening
	• Reporting and interpreting screening findings and making referrals for care or environmental modification as needed
Treatment of existing conditions	• Treatment of work-related illness or injury
	• Provision of immediate first aid
	• Referral for outside medical assistance as needed
	• Development of health care delivery programs to address high prevalence problems in the occupational setting
	• Advocacy for adequate employee health insurance coverage
	• Advocacy for accessible internal or external health care services to meet employee health needs
Emergency response	• Assisting in the development of individual and disaster emergency response plans for the work setting
	• Responding to individual physical or emotional emergencies
	• Referral for continued treatment as needed
	• Responding to care needs in an occupational disaster
	• Evaluation of the health effects of occupational disasters

Tertiary Prevention

Tertiary prevention in work settings is directed toward preventing a recurrence of health problems and limiting their consequences. The types of tertiary intervention measures employed depend on the problems to be prevented. In many instances, primary prevention measures, which would be used to prevent a problem from occurring in the first place, can also be used as tertiary prevention to prevent its recurrence. For example, engineering measures may be used to prevent leakage of a toxic chemical or to prevent subsequent leaks if one has already occurred.

Generally speaking, tertiary prevention is geared toward preventing the spread of communicable diseases, preventing recurrence of other acute conditions, and preventing complications of chronic conditions. Sick-leave policies and employee immunization are examples of tertiary preventive measures that might be taken to stop the spread of influenza in the employee population. By encouraging employees to take advantage of sick-leave benefits when they or family members are ill, the nurse can minimize exposure of others in the occupational setting to communicable diseases and can control the spread of disease. Safety education might prevent a recurrence of accidental injuries due to hazardous equipment, and use of hearing protection might prevent further deterioration of an employee's hearing after noise exposure has already caused some damage. Similarly, treatment of an employee's hypertension can prevent further health problems.

Another aspect of tertiary prevention may be assessing an employee's fitness to return to work after an illness or injury. Assessment considerations in this case would be similar to those in preemployment assessment. Tertiary prevention interventions by occupational health nurses may also involve assisting employees to adapt to chronic illness or monitoring the status of workers' compensation claims. Dealing with chronic illness or disability in the work setting may be facilitated by the development of worksite disability management programs. Such programs provide disease management services in the work setting and have been shown to result in 10% to 15% cost savings for the organization by preventing days lost to work or follow-up appointments in the external health care system (Curtis & Scott, 2004).

Occupational health nurses may assist individual employees to cope with chronic illness in a number of ways. They may educate the client to enhance personal coping ability (e.g., through medication management, self-monitoring skills, etc.) or advocate with management or coworkers for support for self-care. For example, the nurse might arrange for flexible break or meal times to permit employees with diabetes to better manage their diets. Nurses may also advocate for working conditions that accommodate limitations or prevent further deterioration. For example, they may see that

the workstation for an employee with chronic back pain is ergonomically evaluated and any needed accommodations made. Occupational health nurses may also connect employees to sources of support, such as self-help groups, outside of the work setting. Finally, they may advocate for adequate health care provider support and insurance coverage to address the costs of needed care (Sitzman, 2004a). Tertiary prevention emphases in occupational settings are summarized in Table 24-4◆.

Implementing Health Care in Work Settings

Implementing nursing interventions in work settings frequently involves collaboration with others. Most often, collaboration occurs between the nurse and the employee. In other instances, the nurse may collaborate with health care providers and others within or outside of the occupational setting. For example, the nurse might collaborate with a pregnant employee's primary health care provider to monitor her progress throughout the pregnancy. Implementing the plan of care for an employee with carpal tunnel syndrome might involve collaboration with the primary care provider and with a supervisor to facilitate movement to a job that does not necessitate repetitive wrist movements.

When health problems affect groups of employees, implementing the plan of care might involve collaboration with other health care providers and with company management and other personnel. For example, the nurse who has documented an increased incidence of respiratory conditions due to aerosol exposures will advocate plans to resolve the problem. These plans need to be approved by management and implemented by engineering personnel, if engineering controls are required, or by company purchasing agents, if special respiratory protective devices are needed. In the latter instance, the nurse may be involved in determining the

TABLE 24-4 Tertiary Prevention Emphases and Interventions in Work Settings

Tertiary Prevention Emphasis	Interventions
Preventing the spread of communicable diseases	• Provide employee immunization • Educate on infection control procedures
Preventing the recurrence of other acute conditions	• Educate employees to prevent recurrent health problems • Advocate for environmental modifications to prevent recurrent problems
Preventing complications of chronic conditions	• Monitor treatment effects and disease status • Educate employees for disease self-management • Modify the work environment to accommodate limitations due to disability
Assessing fitness to return to work	• Follow up on workers' compensation claims • Assess recovery status • Modify work environment as needed to promote return to work

types of protective devices needed and recommending their purchase to management.

Evaluating Health Care in Work Settings

As in all other settings for nursing practice, the effectiveness of health care in work settings must be evaluated. Evaluation can focus on the outcomes of care either for the individual employee or for the total employee population. Evaluation is conducted on the basis of principles discussed in Chapter 15∞ and focuses on the achievement of expected outcomes and the processes used to achieve those outcomes. For example, the occupational health nurse may evaluate the effectiveness of body mechanics education in decreasing the incidence of back injuries. At the individual level, evaluation might focus on the impact of no-smoking education on an individual employee's smoking behavior.

Selected aspects of occupational health and safety programs can also be evaluated using a set of health and exposure surveillance indicators developed by the Council of State and Territorial Epidemiologists (2004). These indicators include 12 health effects indicators, 1 exposure indicator (for occupational lead exposures), 3 hazardous conditions indicators, 2 interventions indicators, and 1 socioeconomic impact indicator to assess the economic impact of work-related illness and injury. The indicators also include a user-friendly how-to guide on where to obtain relevant information related to each indicator and how to calculate the indicators for a specific occupational setting. The focus of each of the 19 indicators and relevant data sources are presented in Table 24-5◆.

Achievement of national objectives related to occupational health can be used to evaluate efforts in the local occupational setting or at regional, state, and national levels. The status of selected national objectives is presented on page 697.

Occupational settings contribute to a wide variety of health problems in individuals and in population groups, yet they also provide an ideal setting for influencing health-related behaviors and environmental conditions. Community health nurses employed in occupational settings can do much to promote the health of individual employees, work groups, and the general public.

TABLE 24-5 Occupational Health and Exposure Indicators and Relevant Data Sources

Indicator	Focus	Data Sources
Profile	Employment demographics	Current Population Statistics http://www.bls.gov/opub/gp/laugp/htm FERRET http://ferret.bls.census.gov/cgi-bin/ferret
1	Nonfatal work-related injuries and illnesses reported by employers	Occupational Safety and Health, Profile CD-ROM (available from Bureau of Labor Statistics) Survey of Occupational Injuries and Illnesses http://www.bls.gov/iff/home
2	Work-related hospitalization	Current Population Statistics http://www.bls.gov/opub/gp/laugp.htm
3	Fatal work-related injuries	Occupational Safety and Health, Census of Fatal Occupational Injuries CD-ROM (available from Bureau of Labor Statistics) http://www.bls.gov/iff/home

Continued on next page

TABLE 24-5   Occupational Health and Exposure Indicators and Relevant Data Sources *(continued)*

		Current Population Statistics http://www.bls.gov/opub/gp/laugp.htm
4	Work-related amputations with injuries with days away from work reported by employers	Occupational Safety and Health Profile, CD-ROM (available from Bureau of Labor Statistics)
5	Amputations filed with the State Workers' Compensation System	National Academy of Social Insurance http://www.nasi.org State Workers' Compensation System Data
6	Hospitalization for work-related burns	Current Population Statistics http://www.bls.gov/opub/gp/laugp.htm National Hospital Discharge and Ambulatory Surgery Data http://www.cdc.gov/nchs/about/major/hdasd.ncds.htm
7	Work-related musculoskeletal disorders with days away from work reported by employers	ftp://ftp.bls.gov/pub/special.request/ocwc/osh
8	Carpal tunnel syndrome cases filed with the State Workers' Compensation System	National Academy of Social Insurance http://www.nasi.org State Workers' Compensation System Data
9	Hospitalization from or with pneumoconiosis	http://quickfacts.census.gov National Hospital Discharge and Ambulatory Surgery Data http://www.cdc.gov/nchs/about/major/hdasd.ncds.htm
10	Mortality from or with pneumoconiosis	http://quickfacts.census.gov National Vital Statistics System http://www.cdc.gov/nchs/nvss.htm
11	Acute work-related pesticide-associated illness and injury reported to poison control centers	Current Population Statistics http://www.bls.gov/opub/gp/laugp.htm http://www.cste.org
12	Incidence of malignant mesothelioma	National Program of Cancer Registries http://www.cdc.gov/npcr National Hospital Discharge and Ambulatory Surgery Data http://www.cdc.gov/nchs/about/major/hdasd.ncds.htm
13	Elevated blood lead levels among adults	Current Population Statistics http://www.bls.gov/opub/gp/laugp.htm Adult Blood Lead Epidemiology Surveillance (ABLES) http://www.cdc.gov/niosh/topics/ABLES/ables.html
14	Percentage of workers employed in industries at high risk for occupational morbidity	Current Population Statistics http://www.bls.gov/opub/gp/laugp.htm County Business Patterns http://censtats.census.gov/cbpnaic
15	Percentage of workers employed in occupations at high risk for occupational morbidity	FERRET http://ferret.bls.census.gov/cgi-bin/ferret
16	Percentage of workers employed in industries and occupations at high risk for occupational mortality	FERRET http://ferret.bls.census.gov/cgi-bin/ferret
17	Occupational safety and health professionals	Council of State and Territorial Epidemiologists http://www.cste.org (requires membership to access)
18	OSHA enforcement activities	OSHA INSP-5 and INSP-9 Reports (State OSHA inspection reports) http://www.bls.gov/cew/home.htm
19	Workers' compensation awards	National Academy of Social Insurance http://www.nasi.org

Data from: Council of State and Territorial Epidemiologists. (2004). Occupational health effect and biological exposure indicators. Retrieved September 11, 2004, from http://www.cste.org/occupationalhealth.htm

HEALTHY PEOPLE 2010
Goals For Population Health

OBJECTIVE	BASELINE	MOST RECENT DATA	TARGET
7-5. Increase the proportion of worksites that offer a comprehensive employee health promotion program	33–50%	NDA	75%
7-6. Increase the proportion of employees that participate in employer-sponsored health promotion activities	67%	59%	75%#
14-3g. Reduce hepatitis B among occupationally exposed workers (per 100,000)	239	145	62
14-28c. Increase hepatitis B vaccine coverage among occupationally exposed workers	67%	NDA	98%
20-1. Reduce deaths from work-related injuries (per 100,000 workers)	4.5	4.0	3.2
20-2. Reduce work-related injuries resulting in medical treatment, lost work time, or restricted work activity (per 100 full-time workers)	6.2	5.0	4.3
20-3. Reduce the rate of injury and illness due to over-exertion or repetitive motion (per 100,000 workers)	675	497	338
20-5. Reduce deaths from work-related homicides (per 100,000 workers)	0.5	0.4	0.4*
20-6. Reduce work-related assault (per 100 workers)	0.85	0.87	0.60#
20-7. Reduce the number of persons who have elevated blood lead levels from work exposures (per 100,000 workers)	13.6	10.1	0
20-8. Reduce occupational skin diseases (new cases per 100,000 workers)	67	51	47
20-9. Increase the proportion of worksites that provide programs to prevent or reduce stress	37%	NDA	50%
20-10. Reduce occupational needlestick injuries among health care workers	600,000	NDA	420,000
27-12. Increase the proportion of worksites with formal smoking policies	79%	NDA	100%

NDA—No data available
* Objective has been met
 # Objective moving away from target
Data from: Centers for Disease Control and Prevention. (2005). Healthy people data. Retrieved September 5, 2005, from http://wonder.cdc.gov/data2010

Case Study

Nursing in the Work Setting

You are a community health nurse employed by a large manufacturing plant. On Wednesday you see several employees complaining of abdominal cramping and diarrhea. They all state that their symptoms started at home during the night. You get word from one of the plant supervisors that several of her employees called in sick this morning because of similar symptoms. In checking with other departments, you find that there are a number of absences throughout the plant. Two of the older employees and one who you know has AIDS have been hospitalized with severe dehydration. All of the people with cramps and diarrhea eat regularly in the cafeteria.

1. What are the biophysical, psychological, physical environmental, sociocultural, behavioral, and health system factors operating in this situation?
2. What are your nursing diagnoses?
3. What outcome objectives do you hope to achieve through intervention?
4. What secondary prevention measures will you employ in relation to your diagnoses? Why? What primary preventive measures might have prevented the occurrence of these problems? What tertiary prevention measures are warranted to prevent the recurrence of problems or complications?
5. How will you evaluate the effectiveness of your interventions?

Test Your Understanding

1. What are some of the advantages of providing health care in work settings? (p. 667)

2. What types of health and safety hazards are encountered in work settings? Describe at least one potential control measure for each type of hazard. (pp. 671–677)

3. What are some of the biophysical, psychological, physical environmental, sociocultural, behavioral, and health system factors that influence health in work settings? (pp. 670–686)

4. What are the spheres of social influence on the health of employees? (p. 681)

5. What types of health care programs may be found in work settings? What is the community health nurse's focus in each? (pp. 685–686)

6. What are the main areas of emphasis in primary prevention in work settings? Give an example of a community health nursing intervention related to each area. (pp. 687–690)

7. Describe the major considerations in secondary prevention in work settings. What activities might a community health nurse be involved in with respect to each? (pp. 690–693)

8. What are the areas of emphasis in tertiary prevention in work settings? Describe at least one community health nursing responsibility related to each area of emphasis. (p. 694)

EXPLORE MediaLink

http://www.prehall.com/clark
Resources for this chapter can be found on the Companion Website.

Audio Glossary
Appendix G: Community Health Assessment and Intervention Guide
Exam Review Questions

Case Study: Health Promotion at the Work Site
MediaLink Application: The City Health Inspector (video)

Media Links
Challenge Your Knowledge
Update *Healthy People 2010*
Advocacy Interviews

References

Allen, J. D., Stoddard, A. M., Mays, J., & Sorensen, G. (2001). Promoting breast and cervical cancer screening at the workplace: Results from the Woman to Woman study. *American Journal of Public Health, 91*, 584–590.

American Association of Occupational Health Nurses. (2004a). AAOHN code of ethics and interpretive statements. *AAOHN Journal, 52*, 140–142.

American Association of Occupational Health Nurses. (2004b). Standards of Occupational and Environmental Health Nursing. *AAOHN Journal, 52*, 270–273.

Andersen, E. (2004). Laboratory workers and musculoskeletal disorders—Examining ergonomic risk factors and solutions. *AAOHN Journal, 52*, 366–367.

Anderson, D. G. (2004). Workplace violence in long haul trucking. *AAOHN Journal, 52*, 23–27.

Anglin, L. T. (1990). *The roles of nurses: A history, 1900 to 1988.* Unpublished doctoral dissertation, Illinois State University.

Bailer, U., de Zwaan, M., Leisch, F., Strnad, A., Lennkh-Wolfsberg, C., El-Giamal, N., et al. (2004). Guided self-help versus cognitive-behavioral group therapy in the treatment of bulimia nervosa. *International Journal of Eating Disorders, 35*, 522–537.

Barnes, M., Cleaveland, K. A., & Florencio, P. S. (2003). *Chevron vs Echazabal*: Public health issues raised by the "threat-to-self" defense to adverse employment actions. *American Journal of Public Health, 93*, 536–540.

Barrios, L. C., Davis, M. K., Kann, L., Desai, S., Mercy, J. A., Reese, L. E., et al. (2001). School health guidelines to prevent unintentional injuries and violence. *Morbidity and Mortality Weekly Report, 50*(RR-22), 1–73.

Bauer, J. E., Hyland, A., Li, Q., Steger, C., & Cummings, K. M. (2005). A longitudinal assessment of the impact of smoke-free worksite policies on tobacco use. *American Journal of Public Health, 95*, 1024–1029.

Bell, J. H. (2002). Anthrax and the wool trade. *American Journal of Public Health, 92*, 754–757. (Reprinted from J. H. Bell, Anthrax: It's relation to the wool industry. In *Dangerous trades: The historical, social, and legal aspects of industrial occupations as affecting health, by a number of experts*, pp. 634–643, by T. Oliver, Ed., 1902, London: John Murray).

Beltrami, E. M., Alvarado-Ramy, F., Critchley, S. E., Panlilio, A. L., Cardo, D. M., Bower, W. A., et al., (2001). Updated U.S. Public Health Services guidelines for the management of occupational exposures to HBV, HCV, and HIV and recommendations for postexposure prophylaxis. *Morbidity and Mortality Weekly Report, 50*(RR-11), 1–52.

Boden, L. I. (2005). Running on empty: Families, time, and workplace injuries. *American Journal of Public Health, 95*, 1894–1897.

Burke, M. J., Sarpy, S. A., Smith-Crowe, K., Chan-Serafin, S., Salvador, R. O., & Islam, G. (2006). Relative effectiveness of worker safety and health training methods. *American Journal of Public Health, 96*, 315–324.

Calvert, G. M., Mehler, L. N., Rosales, R., Baum, L., Thompson, C., Male, D., et al. (2003). Acute pesticide-related illnesses among working youths, 1988–1999. *American Journal of Public Health, 93*, 605–610.

Cambois, E. (2004). Careers and mortality in France: Evidence on how far occupational mobility predicts differentiated risks. *Social Science & Medicine, 58*, 2545–2558.

Centers for Disease Control and Prevention. (2005a). *Healthy people data.* Retrieved September 6, 2005, from http:wonder.cdc.gov/data2010

Centers for Disease Control and Prevention. (2005b). Workers' Memorial Day—April 28, 2005. *Morbidity and Mortality Weekly Report, 54*, 401.

Chen, M.-S., & Chan, A. (2004). Employee and union inputs into occupational health and safety measures in Chinese factories. *Social Science & Medicine, 58*, 1231–1245.

Clarke, S. P., Sloane, D. M., & Aiken, L. H. (2002). Effects of hospital staffing and organizational climate on needlestick injuries to nurses. *American Journal of Public Health, 92*, 1115–1119.

Council of State and Territorial Epidemiologists. (2004). *Occupational health effect and biological exposure indicators.* Retrieved September 11, 2004, from http://www.cste.org/occupationalhealth.htm

Cox, R. A. F., & Edwards, F. C. (2000). Introduction. In R. A. F. Cox, F. C. Edwards, & K. Palmer (Eds.), *Fitness for work: The medical aspects* (3rd ed., pp. 1–24). Oxford: Oxford University Press.

Croghan, E., & Johnson, C. (2004). Occupational health and school health: A natural alliance. *Journal of Advanced Nursing, 45*, 155–161.

Curtis, J., & Scott, L. R. (2004). Integrating disability management plans into strategic decisions. *AAOHN Journal, 52*, 298–301.

Dababneh, A., Lowe, B., Krieg, E., Kong, Y.-K., & Waters, T. (2004). Ergonomics: A checklist for the ergonomic evaluation of nonpowered hand tools. *Journal of Occupational and Environmental Hygiene, 1*, D135–D145.

Daniels, N. (2003). *Chevron v Echazabal*: Protection, opportunity, and paternalism. *American Journal of Public Health, 93*, 545–548.

Davis, S., Mirick, D. K., & Stevens, R. G. (2001). Night shift work, light at night, and risk of breast cancer. *Journal of the National Cancer Institute, 93*, 1557–1562.

de Castro, A. B., Agnew, J., & Fitzgerald, S. T. (2004). Emotional labor: Relevant theory for occupational health practice in post-industrial America. *AAOHN Journal, 52*, 109–115.

Division of Bacterial and Mycotic Diseases, National Center for Infectious Diseases. (2004). Outbreak of histoplasmosis among industrial plant workers—Nebraska, 2004. *Morbidity and Mortality Weekly Report, 53*, 1020–1023.

Division of Respiratory Disease Studies. (2003). Pneumoconiosis prevalence among working coal miners examined in federal chest radiograph surveillance program—United States, 1996–2002. *Morbidity and Mortality Weekly Report, 52*, 336–340.

Division of Safety Research, National Institute of Occupational Safety and Health. (2001). Fatal occupational injuries—United States, 1980–1997. *Morbidity and Mortality Weekly Report, 50*, 317–320.

Division of Safety Research, National Institute for Occupational Safety and Health. (2003). Ambulance crash-related injuries among emergency medical services workers—United States, 1991–2002. *Morbidity and Mortality Weekly Report, 52*, 154–156.

Division of Safety Research, National Institute for Occupational Safety and Health. (2005). Fatal injuries among volunteer workers—United States, 1993–2002. *Morbidity and Mortality Weekly Report, 54*, 744–747.

Division of STD Prevention. (2005). HIV transmission in the adult film industry—Los Angeles, California, 2004. *Morbidity and Mortality Weekly Report, 54*, 923–926.

Division of Surveillance, Hazard Evaluations, and Field Studies, National Institute of Occupational Safety and Health. (1999). Back pain among persons working on small or family farms—Eight Colorado Counties, 1993–1996. *Morbidity and Mortality Weekly Report, 48*, 301–304.

Division of Surveillance, Hazard Evaluations, and Field Studies, National Institute of Occupational Safety and Health. (2001). Occupational and take-home lead poisoning associated with restoring chemically stripped furniture—California, 1998. *Morbidity and Mortality Weekly Report, 50*, 246–248.

Division of Surveillance, Hazard Evaluations, and Field Studies, National Institute for Occupational Safety and Health. (2004). Adult blood lead epidemiology and surveillance—United States, 2002. *Morbidity and Mortality Weekly Report, 53*, 579–582.

Division of Tuberculosis Elimination, National Center for HIV, STD, and TB Prevention. (2004). Nosocomial transmission of *Mycobacterium tuberculosis* found through screening for Severe Acute Respiratory Syndrome—Taipei, Taiwan, 2003. *Morbidity and Mortality Weekly Report, 53*, 321–323.

Elovainio, M., Kivimaki, M., Steen, N., & Vahtera, J. (2004). Job decision latitude, organizational justice and health: Multilevel covariance structure analysis. *Social Science & Medicine, 58*, 1659–1669.

Fee, E., & Brown, T. M. (2001). Editor's note. *American Journal of Public Health, 91*, 1381.

Fee, E., & Brown, T. M. (2002). John Henry Bell: Occupational anthrax pioneer. *American Journal of Public Health, 92*, 756–757.

Fell-Carlson, D. (2004). OSHA 101: An introduction to OSHA for the occupational health nurse. *AAOHN Journal, 52*, 442–449.

Fleming, M. J. (2004). Agricultural health: A new field of occupational health nursing. *AAOHN Journal, 52*, 391–396.

Franco, G. (2001). Bernadino Ramazzini: The father of occupational medicine. *American Journal of Public Health, 91*, 1382.

Friis, R. H., & Sellers, T. A. (2004). *Epidemiology for public health practice* (3rd ed.). Boston: Jones & Bartlett.

Godin, I., & Kittel, F. (2004). Differential economic stability and psychosocial stress at work: Associations with psychosomatic complaints and absenteeism. *Social Science & Medicine, 58*, 1543–1553.

Grayson, D., Dale, A. M., Bohr, P., Wolf, L., & Evanoff, B. (2005). Ergonomic evaluation: Part of a treatment protocol for musculoskeletal injuries. *AAOHN Journal, 53*, 450–457.

Greiner, B. A., Krause, N., Ragland, D., & Fisher, J. M. (2004). Occupational stressors and hypertension: A multi-method study using observer-based job analysis and self-reports in urban transit operators. *Social Science & Medicine, 59*, 1081–1894.

Hamilton, A. (2001). The health of immigrants. *American Journal of Public Health, 91*, 1765–1767. (Reprinted from *Exploring the dangerous trades: The autobiography of Alice Hamilton, MD*, by A. Hamilton, 1943, Boston: Little, Brown.)

Hancock, J. (2004). Making the transition to workers' comp case management. *NurseWeek, 17*(16), 22–24.

Hopp, P. T., Lee, K. E., & Gest, S. A. (2004). Carpal tunnel syndrome—The role of psychosocial factors in recovery. *AAOHN Journal, 52*, 458–460.

Hughes, H. V. (1979). A view from the top: Today's needs in occupational health service. *Occupational Health Nurse, 27*(2), 13–15.

Institute for Health and Productivity Management. (2002, January). Allergy and Asthma in the Workplace study reveals major work impact findings. *NEWS-line for Nurses, 12*.

Jacobi, C., Abascal, L., & Taylor, C. B. (2004). Screening for eating disorders and high-risk behavior: Caution. *International Journal of Eating Disorders, 35*, 280–295.

Katz, D. L., O'Connell, M., Yeh, M.-C., Nawaz, H., Njike, V., Anderson, L. M., et al. (2005). Public health strategies for preventing and controlling overweight and obesity in school and worksite settings: A report on the recommendations of the Task Force on Community Preventive Services. *Morbidity and Mortality Weekly Report, 54*(RR-10), 1–12.

Kim, G. W., Cho, W. J., Lee, C. Y., Marion, L. N., & Kim, M. J. (2005). The relationship of work stress and family stress to the self-rated health of women employed in the industrial sector in Korea. *Public Health Nursing, 22*, 389–397.

Kivimaki, M., Head, J., Ferrie, J. E., Hemingway, H., Shipley, M. J., Vahtera, J., et al. (2005). Working while ill as a risk factor for serious coronary events: The Whitehall II study. *American Journal of Public Health, 95*, 98–102.

Kothiyal, K., & Yuen, T. W. (2004). Muscle strain and perceived exertion in patient handling with and without a transferring aid. *Occupational Ergonomics, 4*, 185–197.

LaMontagne, A. D., Oakes, J. M., & Turley, R. N. L. (2004). *American Journal of Public Health, 94*, 1614–1619.

Lipscomb, J., Trinkhoff, A., Brady, B., & Geiger-Brown, J. (2004). Health care system changes and reported musculoskeletal disorders among registered nurses. *American Journal of Public Health, 94*, 1431–1435.

Liukkonen, V., Virtanen, P., Kivimaki, M., Pentti, J., & Vahtera, J. (2004). Social capital in working life and the health of employees. *Social Science & Medicine, 59*, 2447–2458.

Loomis, D., Marshall, S. W., & Ta, M. L. (2005). Employer policies toward guns and the risk of homicide in the workplace. *American Journal of Public Health, 95*, 830–832.

Lurie, P., Long, M., & Wolfe, S. M. (1999). *Report detailing Occupational Safety and Health Administration enforcement actions from 1972 through 1998* (HRG Publication #1494). Retrieved March 20, 2003, from http://www.citizen.org/publications/release.cfm?ID=6693

Matza, L., de Lissovoy, G., Sasane, R., Pesa, J., & Maus, J. (2004). The impact of bipolar disorder on work loss. *Drug Benefit Trends, 16*, 476–481.

McPhaul, K. M., & Lipscomb, J. A. (2004). Incorporating environmental health into practice: The expanded role of the occupational health nurse. *AAOHN Journal, 52*, 31–36.

Melchior, M., Krieger, N., Kawachi, I., Berkman, L., Niedhammer, I., & Goldberg, M. (2005). Work factors and occupational class disparities in sickness absence: Findings from the GAZEL cohort study. *American Journal of Public Health, 95*, 1206–1212.

Mendell, M. J., Fisk, W. J., Kreiss, K., Levin, H., Alexander, D., Cain, W. S., et al. (2002). Improving the health of workers in indoor environments: Research priority needs for an occupational research agenda. *American Journal of Public Health, 92*, 1430–1440.

Miller, M. E. (2004). Young adolescents in the workforce—A population at risk. *AAOHN Journal, 52*, 461–464.

Nakata, A., Haratani, T., Takahashi, M., Kawakami, N., Arito, H., Kobayashi, F., et al. (2004). Job stress, social support, and insomnia in a population of Japanese daytime workers. *Social Science & Medicine, 59*, 1719–1730.

National Center for Health Statistics. (2005). *Health, United States, 2005, with chartbook on trends in the health of Americans*. Retrieved December 23, 2005, from http://www.cdc.gov/nchs/data/hus/hus05.pdf

National Center for Infectious Diseases. (2000). Hepatitis C virus infection among firefighters, emergency medical technicians, and paramedics—Selected locations, United States, 1991–2000. *Morbidity and Mortality Weekly Report, 49*, 660–664.

National Institute for Occupational Safety and Health. (2004). Work-related roadway crashes—United States, 1992–2002. *Morbidity and Mortality Weekly Report, 53*, 260–264.

Naumanen-Tuomela, P. (2001a). Finnish occupational health nurses' work and expertise: The clients' perspective. *Journal of Advanced Nursing, 34*, 538–544.

Naumanen-Tuomela, P. (2001b). Occupational health nurses' work and expertise in Finland: Occupational health nurses perspectives. *Public Health Nursing, 18*, 108–115.

Newey, C. A., & Hood, B. M. (2004). Determinants of shift work adjustment for nursing staff: The critical experience of partners. *Journal of Professional Nursing, 20*, 187–195.

Niedhammer, I., Tek, M.-L., Starke, D., & Siegrist, J. (2004). Effort-reward imbalance model and self-reported health: Cross-sectional and prospective findings from the GAZEL cohort. *Social Science & Medicine, 58*, 1531–1541.

Nuwayhid, I. A. (2004). Occupational health research in developing countries: A partner for social justice. *American Journal of Public Health, 94*, 1916–1921.

O'Brien-Pallas, L., Shamian, J., Thomson, D., Alksnis, C., Koehoorn, M., Kerr, M., et al. (2004). Work-related disability in Canadian nurses. *Journal of Nursing Scholarship, 36*, 352–357.

Panlilio, A. L., Cardo, D. M., Grohskopf, L. A., Heneine, W., & Ross, C. S. (2005). Updated U.S. Public Health Services guidelines for the management of occupational exposures to HIV and recommendations for postexposure prophylaxis. *Morbidity and Mortality Weekly Report, 54*(RR-9), 1–17.

Parker, S. C., Lyons, J., & Bonner, J. (2005). Eating disorders in graduate students: Exploring the SCOFF questionnaire as a simple screening tool. *Journal of American College Health, 54*, 103–107.

Parrish, R. S., & Alfred, R. H. (1995). Theories and trends in occupational health nursing: Prevention and social change. *AAOHN Journal, 43*, 514–521.

Payne, N. (2001). Occupational stressors and coping as determinants of burnout in female hospice nurses. *Journal of Advanced Nursing, 33*, 396–405.

Peek-Asa, C., Zwerling, C., & Stallones, L. (2004). Acute traumatic injuries in rural populations. *American Journal of Public Health, 94*, 1689–1693.

Penney, P. J., & Earl, C. E. (2004). Occupational noise and effects on blood pressure: Exploring the relationship of hypertension and noise exposure in workers. *AAOHN Journal, 52*, 476–480.

Pikhart, H., Bobak, M., Pajak, A., Malyutina, S., Kubinova, R., Topor, R., et al. (2004). Psychosocial factors at work and depression in three countries of Central and Eastern Europe. *Social Science & Medicine, 58*, 1475–1482.

Plese, N. K. (Ed.). (2005a). A profile of caregiving in America (2nd ed.). *The Pfizer Journal, IX*(4), 1–40.

Plese, N. K. (Ed.). (2005b). Global summit on the aging workforce. *The Pfizer Journal, IX*(3), 1–40.

Pohanka, M., & Fitzgerald, S. (2004). Urban sprawl and you: How sprawl adversely affects worker health. *AAOHN Journal, 52*, 242–246.

Polanyi, M. F. D., Frank, J. W., Shannon, H. S., Sullivan, T. J., & Lavis, J. N. (2000). Promoting the determinants of good health in the workplace. In B. D. Poland, L. W. Green, & I. Rootman (Eds.), *Settings for health promotion: Linking theory and practice* (pp. 138–160). Thousand Oaks, CA: Sage.

Pritchard, B. J., Bergin, J. L., & Wade, T. D. (2004). A case series evaluation of guided self-help for bulimia nervosa using a cognitive manual. *International Journal of Eating Disorders, 36*, 144–156.

Putnam, K., & McKibbin, L. (2004). Managing workplace depression: An untapped opportunity for occupational health professionals. *AAOHN Journal, 52*, 122–129.

Quinn, M. M. (2003). Occupational health, public health, worker health. *American Journal of Public Health, 93*, 526.

Ramazzini, B. (2001). De morbis artificum diatriba [Diseases of workers]. *American Journal of Public Health, 91*, 1380–1382. (Reprinted from *De morbis artificum diatribe* Latin text of 1713, revised, with translation and notes by W. C. Wright, 1940, Chicago: University of Chicago.)

Reed, D. B. (2004). The risky business of production agriculture: Health and safety for farm workers. *AAOHN Journal, 52*, 401–409.

Richardson, D. B., Loomis, D., Bena, J., & Bailer, A. J. (2004). Fatal occupational injury rates in Southern and non-Southern states, by race and Hispanic ethnicity. *American Journal of Public Health, 94*, 1756–1761.

Rogers, B., & Livsey, K. (2000). Occupational health surveillance, screening, and prevention activities in occupational health nursing practice. *AAOHN Journal, 48*(2), 92–99.

Rose, J. (2002). Occupational health nursing. In J. Canham & J. Bennett (Eds.), *Mentorship in community nursing: Challenges and opportunities* (pp. 151–158). London: Blackwell Science.

Ruff, J. M., Gerding, G., & Hong, O. (2004). Workplace violence against K–12 teachers. *AAOHN Journal, 52*, 204–209.

Schernhammer, E. S., Laden, F., Speizer, F. E., Willett, W. C., Hunter, D. J., Kawachi, I., et al. (2001). Rotating night shifts and risk of breast cancer in women participating in the nurses' health study. *Journal of the National Cancer Institute, 93*, 1563–1568.

Sitzman, K. (2004a). Coping with chronic illness at work. *AAOHN Journal, 52*, 264.

Sitzman, K. (2004b). Workplace bullying. *AAOHN Journal, 52*, 220.

Smith, G. S., Wellman, H. M., Sorock, G. S., Warner, M., Courtney, T., Pransky, G. S., et al. (2005). Injuries at work in the US adult population: Contributions to the total injury burden. *American Journal of Public Health, 95*, 1213–1219.

Spengler, S. E., Browning, S. R., & Reed, D. B. (2004). Sleep deprivation and injuries in part-time Kentucky farmers. *AAOHN Journal, 52*, 373–382.

Stacciarini, J.-M., & Troccoli, B. T. (2004). Occupational stress and constructive thinking: Health and job satisfaction. *Journal of Advanced Nursing, 46*, 480–487.

Stern, A. L. (2003). Labor rekindles reform. *American Journal of Public Health, 93*, 95–98.

Strazdins, L., & Bammer, G. (2004). Women, work, and musculoskeletal health. *Social Science & Medicine, 58*, 997–1005.

Strazdins, L., Korda, R. J., Lim, L. L.-Y., Broom, D. H., & D'Souza, R. M. (2004). Around-the-clock: Parent work schedules and children's well-being in a 24-h economy. *Social Science & Medicine, 59*, 1517–1527.

Strunin, L., & Boden, L. I. (2004). Family consequences of chronic back pain. *Social Science & Medicine, 58*, 1385–1393.

Suzuki, K., Ohida, T., Kaneita, Y., Yokoyama, E., Uchiyama, M. (2005). Daytime sleepiness, sleep habits, and occupational accidents among hospital nurses. *Journal of Advanced Nursing, 52*, 445–453.

Trinkhoff, A. M., Johantgen, M., Muntaner, C., & Le, R. (2005). Staffing and worker injury in nursing homes. *American Journal of Public Health, 95*, 1220–1225.

Tsai, J. H.-C. (2004). Promoting immigrants' health—Relevance to occupational health nursing, *AAOHN Journal, 52*, 94–96.

U.S. Census Bureau. (2005). *Statistical abstract of the United States.* Retrieved May 12, 2005, from http://www.census.gov/prod/2004 pubs/04statab

U.S. Department of Health and Human Services. (2000a). *Health, United States, 2000.* Washington, DC: Author.

U.S. Department of Health and Human Services. (2000b). *Healthy people 2010* (Conference edition, in two volumes). Washington, DC: Author.

U.S. Department of Labor. (2005a). *Census of fatal occupational injuries (CFOI): Current and revised data.* Retrieved February 17, 2006, from http://www.bls.gov/iff/oshwc/cfoi/cftb02020.pdf

U.S. Department of Labor. (2005b). *Workplace injuries and illnesses in 2004.* Retrieved February 17, 2006, from http://www.bls.gov/iff/home.htm

U.S. Department of Labor. (2006a). *Table 3. Number and rate of nonfatal occupational injuries and illnesses by selected industry, all U.S., private industry, 2004.* Retrieved February 17, 2006, from http://www.bls.gov/GQT/servlet/RequestData

U.S. Department of Labor. (2006b). *The employment situation: January 2006.* Retrieved February 17, 2006, from http://www.bls.gov/news.release/pdf.empsit.pdf

Valiante, D. J., Schill, D. P., Rosenman, K. D., & Socie, E. (2004). Highway repair: A new silicosis threat. *American Journal of Public Health, 94*, 876–880.

van der Klink, J. J., Blonk, R. W., Schene, A. H., & van Dijk, F. J. H. (2001). The benefits of interventions for work-related stress. *American Journal of Public Health, 91*, 270–276.

Vézina, M., Derriennic, F., & Monfort, C. (2004). The impact of job strain on social isolation: A longitudinal analysis of French workers. *Social Science & Medicine, 59*, 29–38.

Zimmerman, F. J., Christakis, D. A., & Stoep, A. V. (2004). Tinker, tailor, soldier, patient: Work attributes and depression disparities among young adults. *Social Science & Medicine, 58*, 1543–1553.

25 CHAPTER

Care of Clients in Urban and Rural Settings

CHAPTER OBJECTIVES

After reading this chapter, you should be able to:

1. Describe various approaches to defining *rural* and *urban*.
2. Analyze barriers to effective health care in urban and rural areas.
3. Identify differences in biophysical, psychological, physical environmental, sociocultural, behavioral, and health system factors as they affect health in urban and rural areas.
4. Analyze differential effects of government policy on urban and rural community health.
5. Discuss assessment of health needs in urban and rural settings.
6. Describe goals for intervention in urban and rural settings.
7. Analyze approaches to evaluating the effectiveness of health care in rural and urban settings.

KEY TERMS

economies of proximity **712**
frontier areas **716**
health disparity population **705**
health professional shortage area (HPSA) **714**
medically underserved area (MUA) **714**
medically underserved populations (MUPs) **714**
metropolitan statistical area (MSA) **703**
organized indigenous caregiving (OIC) **716**
urbanization **703**

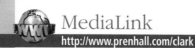

MediaLink

Advocacy in Action

Advocacy in a Rural Nurse-managed Clinic

A rural nurse-managed clinic that received initial funding from the state department of health was required to show proof of local financial support during the second year of the renewal funding application process. The community health nurse appeared before the county commissioners to make a request for funding and was denied because the commissioners understood neither the client population nor the need for the clinic in the community. The commissioners expressed the perception that the clients were unwilling to work and verbalized a negative "welfare stigma" regarding the clients. Their perceptions persisted even after the nurse informed them that the county was designated a medically underserved area 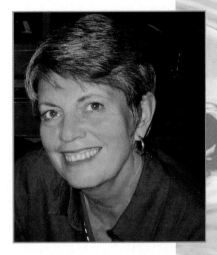 (MUA) and a health professional shortage area (HPSA), and explained that only county residents who lacked access to health care by virtue of being uninsured and who met the 200% level of the federal poverty guidelines could be seen at the clinic.

The community health nurse presented the problem to the clinic's Community Advisory Board, which included client and community representation. After strategizing with the board, the nurse arranged a meeting between the commissioners and some clients. She worked with the clients beforehand to help them advocate for themselves and tell their own stories. The clinic is situated in a community whose primary income base is tourism. The majority of clinic clients work in small shops and restaurants that do not provide health insurance to their employees. The commissioners were surprised to hear the real-life stories of the clients and to learn that they were in fact hardworking, productive community citizens who often held two or more jobs but still lacked access to health care. The advocacy of the clinic community health nurse was instrumental in securing funding from the commissioners, which has been sustained over the past 5 years. The financial support of the local community led in turn to increased funding from the state department of health.

Joyce Splann Krothe, DNS, RN

Associate Professor and Assistant Dean

Indiana University School of Nursing

hroughout the world people live in different kinds of environments, from crowded and deteriorating inner cities to planned suburban communities to isolated rural areas. Factors in each of these settings influence health in different ways, some positively and others negatively. Prior to the 20th century, people living in rural areas had generally better health and longer life expectancies than those in cities due to the crowding and poor sanitation that were characteristic of urban life. In large part, advances in public health have been spurred by a focus on the adverse health conditions present in urban areas (Knowlton, 2001), and as we saw in Chapter 3∞ early community health nursing in the United States was aimed at improving the health of impoverished immigrant populations in urban areas. More recently, however, people in urban areas in developed countries have had access to better health care services and better knowledge of health promotion and illness prevention than those in rural settings (Population Information Program, 2002). Changes in rural and urban environments have resulted in changes in factors that influence health in those settings. Much of the literature cited in other chapters in this book is specific to community health nursing in urban settings; less attention has been given to community health in rural settings. In this chapter, we compare and contrast factors that influence health in rural and urban settings and their implications for community health nursing as practiced in those settings.

WHAT IS URBAN? WHAT IS RURAL?

Although an estimated half of the world's population lives in cities, there is no clear definition of what *urban* means. **Urbanization** has been loosely defined by the

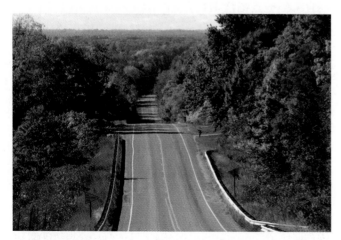

Great distances on poor roads may prevent rural residents from obtaining optimal health care. (©Jeff Greenberg/The Image Works)

National Center for Health Statistics (NCHS) (2005) as "the degree of urban (city-like) character of a particular geographic area" (p. 505). At the international level, the term *urban* can be applied to settlements of all sizes, but is generally reserved for settlements with populations of 20,000 or more people. *City* is a term often used in the international community to indicate "urban centers with large populations" (Population Information Program, 2002, p. 3). *Rural* is frequently defined as "not urban," but the National Rural Health Association maintains that the designation used for rural or urban residence should depend on the purpose for the designation and may legitimately vary from one program to another even in the same area, depending on the purpose of the program (National Rural Health Association, n.d.a).

The U.S. federal government has changed the definitions of urban and rural frequently, and different definitions are used by different agencies within the federal government, making comparisons between rural and urban areas over time and with respect to different aspects difficult. Commonly used definitions of rural and urban have been developed by the U.S. Census Bureau, the Office of Management and Budget (OMB), and the U.S. Department of Agriculture. Several of the approaches to defining urban and rural are summarized in Table 25-1◆.

The U.S. Census Bureau categorizes geographic areas as urbanized, urban clusters, or rural. Urbanized areas have central cores with populations of 50,000 or more. Urban clusters have core populations of 2,500 to 49,999 people. All other areas are considered rural. In 2000, 21% of the U.S. population lived in areas considered rural by the Census Bureau definition (Hart, Larson, & Lishner, 2005).

The OMB system classifies counties in terms of their metropolitan or nonmetropolitan character and their inclusion of a metropolitan statistical area. A **metropolitan statistical area (MSA)** is "a county or group of contiguous counties that contain at least one urbanized area of 50,000 or more population" (NCHS, 2005, p. 505). In the OMB system, metropolitan counties are classified as large, medium, or small. Large counties are those in an MSA with a million or more people; medium counties are included in MSAs with populations of 250,000 to 1 million people; and small counties are those in MSAs with less then 250,000 population. Nonmetropolitan counties are classified as micropolitan, nonmetropolitan counties or groups of counties that contain an urban cluster of 10,000 to 49,999 people, or nonmicropolitan, counties that do not contain an urban cluster of at least 10,000 people (NCHS, 2005).

A set of 10 rural–urban continuum codes used by the U.S. Department of Agriculture differentiates between metropolitan and nonmetropolitan counties based on the degree of urbanization and nearness to central metropolitan areas (Singh & Siahpush, 2002).

TABLE 25-1	Approaches to Defining Urban and Rural	
Approach	**Urban**	**Rural**
National Rural Health Association		Designation should depend on the purposes of the programs in which it is used.
U.S. Census Bureau	• Urbanized: Having a central core population of 50,000 or more • Urban clusters: Having a core population of 2,500 to 49,999 people	Areas with fewer than 2,500 people
Office of Management and Budget	• Metropolitan counties: Large: Include an MSA with 1 million or more people • Medium: Counties with MSAs of 250,000 to 1 million people • Small: Counties with MSAs of 50,000 to 250,000 people	• Nonmetropolitan counties: Micropolitan: Counties with an urban cluster of 10,000 to 49,999 people Nonmicropolitan: Counties with no urban cluster of at least 10,000 people
U.S. Department of Agriculture	• Metropolitan counties: Central counties with populations of 1 million or more people Counties on the fringe of central counties with populations of 1 million or more people Counties with populations of 250,000 to 1 million people Counties in metropolitan areas with populations less than 250,000 people	• Nonmetropolitan counties: Urban populations of 20,000 or more people adjacent to a metropolitan area Urban populations of 20,000 or more people not adjacent to a metropolitan area Urban populations of 2,500 to 19,999 people adjacent to a metropolitan area Urban populations of 2,500 to 19,999 people not adjacent to a metropolitan area Completely rural areas or areas with populations of fewer than 2,500 people adjacent to a metropolitan area Completely rural areas or areas with populations of fewer than 2,500 people not adjacent to a metropolitan area
Montana State Rurality Index	An index for an individual resident based on the population density of the county and the distance to the nearest emergency services	An index for an individual resident based on the population density of the county and the distance to the nearest emergency services

Data from: Hart, Larson, & Lishner, 2005; NCHS, 2005; Singh & Siahpush, 2002; Weinert & Boik, 1998. See references for full citations.

These codes are based on the OMB categories and are summarized in Table 25-1◆.

The Montana State University (MSU) rurality index is another approach to defining rurality. Rather than being county based, this index is person based and categorizes individual residents on the basis of their degree of rurality. The advantage of a resident-based index is that it allows comparisons of people within a county who differ from other people in the same county in terms of their rurality. This index allows comparisons between rural and urban populations within the same county. The index for a given individual is derived by creating a weighted score based on the population density of the county and the distance to the nearest emergency services. In the case of persons within a single county, the index is based on distance to emergency services alone (Weinert & Boik, 1998). Table 25-1◆ summarizes the features of various approaches to defining rural and urban communities.

For the most part, in this chapter, we will be using the term *rural* to describe groups with very low population densities (fewer than 2,500 people), which includes people in small rural communities, and the term *urban*, or metropolitan, to indicate central metropolitan areas.

URBAN AND RURAL POPULATIONS

Half of the world's present population lives in urban areas, and this is expected to increase to 60% by 2030, with more than 5 billion urban residents throughout the world. In 2000, 388 cities throughout the world had populations greater than 1 million, and the number of cities with populations over a million is expected to increase to 554 by 2015 (Population Information Program, 2002).

In the United States, 30% of the population lived in cities with populations of 5 million people or more at the time of the 2000 census (Knowlton, 2001). In 2004, 83% of the U.S. population lived in urban areas, an increase of roughly 1% since 2000 (Economic Research Service, 2005). The degree of urbanization of the population varies from one area to another. For example, 100% of the Washington, DC, area is considered urban, whereas only 38% of Vermont's population lives in urban areas. States such as California and New Jersey are more than

GLOBAL PERSPECTIVES

*T*he world's population is becoming increasing urbanized. In 1975, only 27% of the population in developing countries lived in urban areas. By 2000, the percentage had grown to 40%, and by 2030 an estimated 56% of the population in developing countries will be urbanized. In developed countries, 75% of the population were already living in urban areas by 2000. The United Nations anticipates that by 2015, there will be 21 "megacities," each with a population in excess of 10 million people, and 17 of these metropolises will be located in developing countries (Population Information Program, 2002).

Many urban areas throughout the world already lack the infrastructure to support existing population levels, with inadequate housing resources and services to meet human needs. An estimated 30% of the world's poor are concentrated in urban areas, and this figure is expected to climb to 50% by 2030. Many of the urban poor live in inadequate housing without access to potable (drinkable) water or sanitation. They also lack access to health care.

Some of the suggested strategies for dealing with the problems of increasing urbanization include the following:

- Improving local governance and shifting decision authority to municipal governments
- Engaging in urban planning to address land use, water, sanitation, waste management, and transportation issues
- Promoting planned industrial and economic development that considers environmental impact
- Upgrading housing stock in slum areas
- Developing and implementing plans for water conservation and managing the demand for water through economic constraints on use
- Developing efficient transportation systems with minimal reliance on private vehicles and cleaner technology to minimize environmental impacts
- Developing and implementing waste recycling programs (Population Information Program, 2002)

Many of these strategies are also appropriate to rural areas. To what extent are these strategies being implemented in your area? What would be required to implement these strategies? How might these requirements be met in developing areas of the world?

94% urban (U.S. Census Bureau, 2005b). Similar variation is noted worldwide. In the World Health Organization (WHO) European region, for example, 70% of the population lived in urban settings in 2005 compared with only 31% of the population in the Southeast African region (WHO, 2005).

Despite the imbalance between rural and urban populations in various parts of the world, and even in the United States, urban populations are growing, whereas rural ones are shrinking. In 1990, 78% of the U.S. population was considered urban, a figure that had increased to 79% by the next census (U.S. Census Bureau, 2005b). Similar rural-to-urban population shifts are occurring elsewhere in the world. Rapid growth in urban populations throughout the world is the result of three primary factors: migration from rural to urban areas, natural population

increase in urban populations, and reclassification of formerly rural areas as they have been built up (Population Information Program, 2002). Migration may occur because of declining agricultural employment or perceptions of better jobs, service access, or higher standards of living in urban areas. Natural population increases occur when births in the population outnumber deaths.

THE EPIDEMIOLOGY OF HEALTH AND ILLNESS IN URBAN AND RURAL POPULATIONS

Factors influencing the health status of rural and urban populations can be categorized into two types, compositional factors and contextual factors (Phillips & McLeroy, 2004). Compositional factors arise from the characteristics of the people who compose the population in a given area (e.g., proportion of the elderly in the population, presence of ethnic minority group members). Contextual factors are derived from characteristics unique to the setting itself, unique features of rural or urban environments. Both categories of factors may give rise to *health disparity populations*. A **health disparity population** has been defined by the National Institutes of Health as "a population where there is a significant disparity in the overall rate of disease incidence, prevalence, morbidity, mortality, or survival rates in the population as compared to the health status of the general population" (as quoted in Hartley, 2004, p. 1676).

Factors that arise in the biophysical, psychological, physical environmental, sociocultural, behavioral, and health system dimensions of health contribute to compositional and contextual factors influencing the health of both rural and urban populations. The types of factors present in each dimension, however, may differ considerably.

Biophysical Considerations

Biophysical considerations influencing the health of urban and rural populations include age and aging and the extent of physical illness in the population.

Age and Aging

Rural and urban populations differ considerably in their composition, with rural populations including more elderly individuals (Phillips & McLeroy, 2004). In fact, approximately 15% of the 61 million rural residents in the United States are over age 65 (Carty, Al-Zayyer, Arietti, & Lester, 2004). In 2000, 7.4% of the population in isolated rural areas were over 75 years of age, compared to 5.6% of urban populations (Phillips, Holan, Sherman, Williams, & Hawes, 2004). The percentage of elderly people in some rural areas is increasing faster than that in many urban centers as a result of three factors. The

MediaLink

Choosing a Career in Rural Health (video)

first and most obvious factor is aging in place—people already living in rural areas are growing older. The second is a decades-long pattern of movement of younger people out of rural areas. The third factor is the more recent phenomenon of older urban dwellers retiring to rural areas (Institute of Medicine, 2005; Rogers, 2002). Persons over age 60 living in nonmetropolitan areas are more likely than their urban counterparts to live alone, to have a high school education or less, and to report worse health. Rural elderly are also more likely than urban elderly to have incomes below poverty level (13.1% vs. 9.3%) and to own their own homes (Rogers, 2002). Community health nurses may need to advocate for income assistance or other services for the unmet needs of both rural and urban elderly poor.

More than 80% of U.S. children live in urban areas. Urban children in the 50 largest U.S. cities are more likely than their rural counterparts to have family incomes below poverty level (26% vs. 20%), to live with a single parent (37% vs. 25%), and to live in families in which no parent has full-time year-round employment (45% vs. 33%). In addition, urban children are more likely to live in a household headed by a high school dropout or to include an adolescent who has dropped out of school. Finally, children in large cities are more than four times as likely to live in a family without a vehicle (21% vs. 5%) (Annie E. Casey Foundation, 2004). This latter figure may be offset by the availability of public transportation in large cities.

Of the 20% of U.S. children who live in rural areas, approximately 1.3 million work and play in farm settings. Another half million nonfarm children work on farms, contributing to a high incidence of injuries to child farmworkers each year (Reed, 2004a). Community health nursing advocacy may be particularly warranted to promote farm safety for both children and adults in rural areas. Nurses may also need to advocate for safe environments in urban areas that are affected by high crime rates or pollution.

Urban and rural populations also display different patterns of disease prevalence with respect to age composition. When five major chronic disease categories are compared (heart disease, hypertension, diabetes, emphysema, and cancer), rural populations have higher percentages of younger people (under age 65) reporting these conditions. Surprisingly, after 65 years of age, self-reported prevalence of many of these conditions is higher in urban populations. This is particularly true of persons over 80 years of age, with the urban elderly having higher reported prevalence of all except diabetes (Wallace, Grindeanu, & Cirillo, 2004). Community health nurses may be active in advocating for preventive services for the physical health conditions that affect rural and urban populations as well as for curative and restorative services for those with existing disease. The types of services needed will be dictated by the kinds of conditions prevalent in any given area.

BUILDING OUR KNOWLEDGE BASE

*R*ural health care providers have identified a set of research priorities to be addressed with respect to the health of rural elderly populations and health care delivery in rural settings (Averill, 2003). Most of these priorities can be applied to the general population in rural areas and include:

- Identification of demographic patterns and trends, health service needs, and existing methods of service delivery
- Examination of systems of care delivery for effectiveness and efficiency
- Tracking of health care delivery outcomes for specific client populations and delivery systems
- Identification of needs of families and caregivers for elderly family members
- Perceptions of elders regarding access to care and the effectiveness of care received

Describe a study that might be designed to address one of these priorities. Would the study need to be modified if it was to be conducted in an urban, rather than rural, setting? Why or why not?

Physical Health Status

Differences between mortality rates in urban and rural areas are difficult to determine given the differing definitions of rural and urban that are used in many studies. For some conditions, rates for the most urban and rural areas are similar, but vary greatly from those encountered in suburban and "near rural" areas (Eberhardt & Pamuk, 2004). *Health United States, 2001, Urban and Rural Health Chartbook*, the rural counterpart of *Health, United States*, gave poorer ratings to rural than urban areas for 21 of 23 health indicators that addressed both physical and behavioral health (Hartley, 2004).

Generally speaking, rural areas have higher rates of premature mortality (before 75 years of age) than urban areas. Infant mortality is lowest in suburban communities, followed by urban areas, then rural areas, and mortality among people 1 to 24 years of age is 31% higher in the most rural counties than in the most urban areas and 65% higher than in suburban areas. Similarly, mortality rates among the 25- to 64-year-old group is 32% higher in rural than urban areas, but mortality in people over age 65 is only 7% higher in rural than urban populations (Eberhardt & Pamuk, 2004). Community health nurse advocacy for adequate prenatal care and education may help to offset differences in infant mortality. Advocacy for other health services in both rural and urban areas will depend on specific causes of morbidity and mortality.

COPD mortality is 32% higher for rural U.S. men than for their most urban counterparts (Eberhardt & Pamuk, 2004), and incidence of cancer is higher. Higher rural cancer mortality may be a result of later stage at diagnosis, particularly among rural ethnic minorities (Gamm, Hutchison, Dabney, & Dorsey, 2003). Rural accident mortality rates are twice as high as those for urban areas (Peek-Asa, Zwerling, & Stallones, 2004). One third of U.S. motor vehicle accidents occur in rural areas, yet rural populations account for two thirds of all motor vehicle accident fatalities (Gamm et al., 2003). Nonfatal injuries in rural areas occur at a rate almost 30 times higher than that seen in urban areas, with the exception of fracture and hip fracture rates, which are lower in rural than urban populations (Peek-Asa et al., 2004). Injuries are particularly prevalent among the farm population due to exposure to hazardous working conditions and work with heavy equipment and fractious animals (Spengler, Browning, & Reed, 2004).

Other nonfatal conditions, such as arthritis, have been found to be more prevalent in rural than urban populations, and rural adults are more likely to experience activity limitation due to chronic illness than urban elders (18% vs. 13%). Edentulism (loss of all teeth) is also more common among the rural elderly (38%) than among their urban counterparts (27%) (Eberhardt & Pamuk, 2004). Diabetes, dental caries, and obesity are also more common conditions in rural than urban populations (Gamm et al., 2003).

Rural–urban mortality differences also vary by gender. For example, heart disease mortality for women is highest in the urban north, followed by the rural south. For men, heart disease mortality is highest in the rural south. In general, however, heart disease, cerebrovascular disease, and hypertension are more prevalent in rural than in urban populations (Gamm et al., 2003).

Worldwide, the health of urban dwellers also tends to be better than that of their rural counterparts due to better access to health care and healthier living conditions. This is not true, however, for the urban poor, who may face more health risks due to inadequate housing, poor sanitation, and lack of other basic necessities in overcrowded urban settlements (Population Information Program, 2002). Community health nurses may be actively involved in advocating for provision of basic health care and health education services to improve the health of both urban and rural populations throughout the world. For example, they may advocate increased humanitarian aid from developed countries or they may be involved in the design of international health care systems that address urban and rural health care needs in developing nations.

A process similar to that used to develop the *Healthy People 2010* national health objectives was used among rural health care agencies and providers to identify an initial set of 10 top priorities for improving the health of rural populations. This initial set of priorities included heart disease and stroke, diabetes, mental health and mental disorders, oral health, tobacco use, substance abuse, maternal/child/infant health, nutrition and overweight, and cancer (Gamm et al., 2003). Additional priority issues that have been added since

then include injury and violence prevention, immunization and infectious diseases, public health infrastructure development, health education and community-based programming, and long-term care and rehabilitation (Gamm & Hutchison, 2004). Similar sets of priorities have been developed for specific subpopulations in rural settings. For example, priority diseases for rural American Indian/Alaskan Native populations include cardiovascular disease, cancer, diabetes, HIV/AIDS, sexually transmitted diseases (STDs), respiratory diseases, communicable diseases, malaria, and diarrhea. Other priority health concerns identified for this rural subpopulation included mental health and violence, child and adolescent health, women's health, tobacco use, maternal health and safety, emergency preparedness and response, immunization, nutrition, and safety of food and blood supplies (Baldwin et al., 2002). Community health nurses can be actively involved in advocacy efforts to address these rural health priorities at both state and local levels. For example, they may campaign for equitable allocation of state funds for health care services, particularly preventive services, in rural areas.

Psychological Considerations

In assessing an urban or rural population, the community health nurse will examine factors in the psychological dimension that influence population health. Actual rural and urban prevalences of mental health problems are probably similar, although rural men may have slightly higher prevalence of negative mood (Eberhardt & Pamuk, 2004). Migrant workers also display a higher incidence of depression than other rural residents. They, and members of other ethnic groups, are also less likely to seek treatment (Gamm et al., 2003; Monts, 2002). Community health nurses in areas that employ significant numbers of migrant workers are often those most likely to identify evidence of mental health problems in this population. Their advocacy may be required to assure access to care for mental illness among the migrant population.

Residents in both urban and rural areas are subjected to considerable levels of stress. For example, the rural farm population is faced with financial uncertainty, intense time pressures at certain seasons, uncertain weather, and intergenerational conflict that may lead to problems in interpersonal relationships, substance abuse, family violence, and suicide. Conversely, it is hypothesized that stressful conditions in urban areas, such as increased noise levels, sensory stimulation and overload, interpersonal conflict, and the vigilance needed regarding crime victimization and accidents, may also contribute to mental health problems (House et al., 2000). In fact, research has indicated that higher crime rates in urban areas are associated with increased incidence of asthma symptoms. Individuals

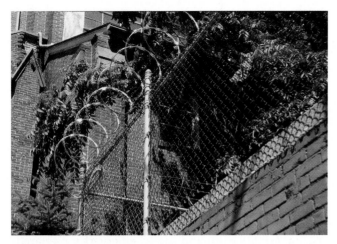

Unsafe neighborhoods with high crime rates create stress and poor health conditions.

with asthma who live in high-crime areas have greater symptom frequency than those who live in low-crime areas (Wright et al., 2004).

Areas in which differences do exist include the adequacy of mental health services and suicide rates. Rural mental health services are far less adequate than those available in urban areas. For example, 95% of metropolitan counties have available mental health services compared to only 80% of nonmetropolitan counties. Similarly, 87% of federally designated mental health professional shortage areas are in rural portions of the country. Three fourths of small rural counties lack the services of a psychiatrist and 95% have no access to child psychiatric services (Gamm et al., 2003).

Finally, rural areas have higher suicide mortality rates than urban settings. Rural counties have firearm-related suicide rates 1.5 times those of urban counties (Branas, Nance, Elliott, Richmond, & Schwab, 2004). For most age groups, rural men have suicide rates twice those among urban men. Rural suicide rates are 85% higher than those in urban areas for young women and 22% higher for working women (Singh & Siahpush, 2002). Reasons given for differences in rural and urban suicide rates include a rural cultural value on self-reliance, travel distance to and availability of mental health services, and greater social stigma attached to mental illness in rural cultures (Eberhardt & Pamuk, 2004; Gessert, 2003). Social stigma and the lack of anonymity in rural areas have even been suggested as reasons for purposeful underdiagnosis of mental health problems by health care providers, as well as for failure to seek assistance (Gamm et al., 2003). Community health nurses can advocate with providers to increase diagnosis and effective treatment of mental illness in rural, as well as urban, areas. They may also need to educate rural populations regarding mental illness in order to decrease the stigma that may prevent residents from seeking care for mental health problems. For both rural and urban dwellers, community health nurses

may need to actively advocate for access to affordable mental health services. For example, they may be active in political campaigns to increase coverage of mental illness and substance abuse under state Medicaid programs or to support the availability of tax-funded treatment services in both rural and urban areas of need. In Tennessee, for example, the Rural Health Association of Tennessee (2005), which includes rural nurses as well as other health professionals, was instrumental in negotiating the use of tobacco settlement funds for health and agricultural priorities.

Physical Environmental Considerations

As we saw in Chapter 10∞, both the built and natural environments affect health status. The built environment consists of buildings, spaces, and products created or modified significantly from their natural state by people, and the natural environment involves natural features of the area, including plant and animal life, terrain, and so on. The community health nurse assessing the health status of a particular rural or urban population would consider the effects of both the built and natural environments and interactions between them on the health of the population.

Differences between the built and natural environments are perhaps the most obvious differences between rural and urban settings. Elements of the built environment are probably more significant influences on health than those of the natural environment in urban settings. Health risks in the urban environment include noise exposure, crowding, and increased potential for environmental pollutants such as air pollution and heavy metals (Perdue, Stone, & Gostin, 2003). For example, approximately half of U.S. urban dwellers are exposed to excessive ozone levels, and many U.S. cities have particulate-matter air pollution levels one and a half to two times the national standard (Population Information Program, 2002). Central urban areas, however, have the advantage of being more energy efficient than rural or suburban areas. In fact, "suburban sprawl" has been described as being wasteful of both space needed for agricultural purposes and energy used to commute between widely separated residential, commercial, and industrial centers. Energy use increases threefold with movement from center city to suburban fringe areas as a result of greater motor vehicle use, and traffic congestion in small urban and rural areas is growing by 11% per year, twice the rate of increase in urban areas (Sierra Club, n.d., 2001). Urban areas have also been touted as safer in terms of accidents since the accident fatality rate involved for public transit is one twentieth the rate associated with personal automobile use (Hancock, 2000). Unfortunately, more than 140 million people in the United States live more than a quarter mile from a transit stop, and 41% of populations in small urban and rural areas do not have any access to public transit (Sierra Club, n.d.). Motor vehicle accident fatalities in rural areas are, in part, due to narrow two-lane roads that lack crash reduction features such as controlled entrances and exits, wide divided lanes, and traffic control devices. High speeds typical of travel on rural roads are also a factor (Peek-Asa et al., 2004). In addition, urban centers encourage exercise when destinations are within walking distance and contribute to less social isolation than more sparsely settled areas. As noted in Chapter 10∞, community health nurses can be active advocates for planned urban development that promotes physical activity. They can also advocate for changes in rural environments that increase access to needed transportation services or that promote safety (e.g., divided roads). For example, community health nurses may help to organize transportation cooperatives that improve access to goods and services for isolated rural residents.

In rural settings, the natural environment contributes to a variety of health risks. The presence of plants and wild and domesticated animals in the rural environment contributes to the potential for plant and animal allergens and zoonoses (diseases transmitted from animals to people) (National Center for Infectious Diseases, 2001). Dust and extreme weather conditions are other significant aspects of the natural environment in the rural setting that have health consequences. For example, weather conditions have been shown not only to decrease access to health care facilities, but also to impede home care in rural areas (Gallagher, Alcock, Diem, Angus, & Medves, 2002).

As noted in Chapter 20∞, deteriorated housing and lack of affordable housing may affect the health of urban residents, contributing to high levels of homelessness. In rural areas, this component is more apt to reflect the effects of substandard housing that is in poor repair, particularly among the elderly (National Coalition for the Homeless, 2005). Higher rates of fire-related mortality

Think Advocacy

Millersville is a small town of 3,000 people in rural Arizona. The main street of town is part of a four-lane undivided highway to Phoenix. The part of town traversed by the highway comprises about 20 blocks, four of which are lined by local stores and diagonal parking on either side. Except when it is raining, which is infrequent, most of the town's children ride their bicycles to the local elementary school, which is located on the highway three blocks south of the main shopping area. In the past 2 years, three children have been killed and seven others injured by cars speeding through town on the highway. There is a stop sign in the middle of town, but it does not seem to have reduced speeds or accidents. Research suggests that bicycle lanes divided from motor vehicle traffic by concrete barriers reduce child bicycle injuries. Although you have suggested creation of bicycle lanes on the section of the highway that bisects the town, the idea has been resisted by local merchants who do not want to give up the parking in front of their stores. They are afraid that if people from the outlying ranches have to park elsewhere and walk to the stores, they will take their business to the city 40 miles away. How would you go about advocating for a bicycle lane in town?

in rural areas have been associated with older homes and use of high-risk heating mechanisms. In addition, rural homes are less likely to have functioning smoke detectors (86%) than urban residences (93%) (Peek-Asa et al., 2004). An estimated 30% of rural homes have at least one major problem (National Coalition for the Homeless, 2005). In 2003, for example, 30% or more of households in 300 nonmetropolitan counties lacked adequate kitchen or bathroom facilities (U.S. Department of Agriculture [USDA], 2005). Safety education is one important form of community health nurse advocacy in both rural and urban areas. The types of issues addressed, however, are likely to differ, with rural safety focusing on issues of farm and traffic safety. Elimination of safety hazards in the home and use of smoke detectors will be relevant in both settings.

In the United States, rural housing issues are particularly serious for migrant and seasonal farmworkers who generally live in "camps," which often consist of temporary shelters erected for short periods of time. Although migrant camps are supposed to meet OSHA standards for housing and plumbing facilities, a survey by the Housing Assistance Council found that 52% of farmworker housing was crowded and 53% was deficient in bathtub/shower and laundry facilities. In addition, the lack of adequate sanitary facilities for workers in the fields promotes the spread of disease. Workers are often required to pay for the inadequate housing provided in camps, thus decreasing the funds available for food, health care, and other basic necessities (Culp & Umbarger, 2004). Community health nurses working with migrant workers can advocate for adequate housing.

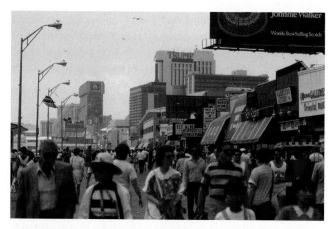

Crowding in urban areas can increase stress, leading to a variety of health effects. (Patrick J. Watson)

For example, they may report OSHA violations by farms that employ large numbers of migrant workers and do not provide adequate living facilities.

Worldwide, both urban and rural areas present physical environmental hazards to health. According to the World Health Organization (WHO, 2003), 600 million urban and 1 billion rural residents live in inadequate housing. Approximately one fourth of urban housing in developing countries is temporary in nature, and one third of it does not meet local housing codes. In some areas, such as sub-Saharan Africa, as much as 60% of urban housing is temporary quarters, and half of it does not meet building safety codes. Such temporary housing is often built in areas prone to natural disaster or with other unhealthy attributes. Legal housing is often too expensive for the urban poor to afford or not available at all. It is estimated that low-income households in many countries would need to save 30% to 50% of their income for 15 to 30 years to be able to afford legal housing that meets minimum safety standards (Population Information Program, 2002). Community health nurses can advocate for construction of safe housing units as well as for reasonable safety codes that do not price housing beyond the affordable range for most residents.

Although 100% of both urban and rural residents in the United States and other developed nations have access to improved water sources and sanitation, the same is not true for many developing countries. In many of these countries rural residents have far lower rates of access to these basic necessities than urban dwellers, and the greatest difference is noted in such countries as Papua New Guinea, where 88% of urban dwellers and 32% of rural residents have access to improved water, and Niger, where 79% of the urban population but only 4% of rural residents have adequate sanitation (WHO, 2004). Community health nurses can advocate development of safe water systems in both rural and urban areas. As indicated in Chapter 10∞, they can also educate rural and urban dwellers regarding inexpensive water purification methods and help to assure that the necessary supplies are available to and affordable for even the most needy. In the United States, many rural residents rely on wells as their primary source of drinking water, and many wells are contaminated with a variety of pollutants, particularly with agricultural runoff that includes pesticides and other hazardous substances.

The built environment also contributes to health risks in rural areas in the use of pesticides and other chemicals used in agriculture. For instance, in 2002, more than 483 million pounds of pesticides were applied to U.S. crops (U.S. Census Bureau, 2005b). Improper use of such chemicals and failure to follow safety instructions have resulted in human exposures to toxic and carcinogenic substances. In addition, 85% of fruits and vegetables are picked by hand, increasing the risk of toxic exposures for farmworkers (Culp & Umbarger, 2004). These exposures are compounded by lack of adequate shower and laundry facilities to wash away pesticide accumulations on skin or clothing. Exposure to high noise levels also occurs as a result of some aspects of the built rural environment (e.g., operation of farm machinery) (Reed, 2004b).

Finally, the built and natural elements combine to create sources of water pollution in rural areas. As noted in Chapter 10∞, agricultural runoff contaminated with chemical pesticides and heavy metals pollutes drinking water sources as well as local lakes and rivers. According to the Environmental Protection Agency, 91% of drinking water violations involve small water systems serving 25 to 3,300 people, many of which are in rural areas (U.S. Department of Health and Human Services [USDHHS], 2001). Urban sprawl also increases water runoff and potential contamination of water sources. Runoff is an increasing problem with the development of impervious surfaces in urban and suburban areas. Runoff is actually one and a half to four times higher in suburban than rural areas (Gaffield, Goo, Richards, & Jackson, 2003).

Sociocultural Considerations

Differences in sociocultural dimension factors between rural and urban settings, although not as immediately obvious as physical environmental factors, are nevertheless quite influential in their effects on population health status. Areas to be considered in assessing rural and urban populations include social values and conditions, economic issues, cultural factors, occupational factors, and factors related to health knowledge and values.

Rural cultures have been described as high-context cultures in which people experience sustained interactions with others (Phillips & McLeroy, 2004). Urban cultures, on the other hand, tend to be low-context cultures in which individuals are more socially isolated and experience greater mobility and frequent changes in relationships. Urban and rural areas also differ in terms of the potential number of social ties, which are likely to be more numerous in urban areas due to population density and greater opportunity to interact with others (Leyden, 2003).

Despite the enduring nature of interpersonal relationships in rural settings, long distances and lack of public transportation may lead to social isolation, particularly among the elderly. Social isolation may be particularly prevalent among migrant farmworkers from outside the United States. Many migrant workers are not able to return home to visit with families due to fears of being unable to return to the United States. In the past, most migrant workers would return home approximately every 9 months; now many are away from families for up to 4 years at a time (Monts, 2002).

Rural residents are more likely than urban dwellers to be married and tend to adhere to traditional gender roles. People in urban and rural settings also differ in terms of the likelihood of exposure to strangers and to unconventional norms, including gender norms. Urban areas are more heterogeneous in their population and residents are more likely to be exposed to attitudes and values different from their own (Fitzpatrick, 2000). Depending on the context of these encounters, they may lead to greater tolerance of differences or exhibitions of prejudice and discrimination. Rural areas are experiencing a growth in the diversity of their populations that may lead to tensions among racial and ethnic groups. Community health nurses may need to be actively involved in promoting cultural competence among residents. For example, they may advocate for cultural sensitivity training for employers of migrant workers or in rural and urban school settings.

Sustained interpersonal relationships in rural settings lead to the development of trust and informal support networks. These relationships may also result in the lack of anonymity and privacy discussed earlier and lead to less help-seeking for problems one does not want known by one's neighbors (Gamm et al., 2003). Urban society, on the other hand, may be characterized by stimulus overload and increasing complexity of interpersonal interactions that may result in a sense of "diffused responsibility" or failure to respond in the face of another's obvious need. Urban residents are twice as likely as rural dwellers to be victims of violence, and firearms-related homicide rates are three times higher in urban than rural areas (Branas et al., 2004). Gun safety education and advocacy are important aspects of health education by community health nurses.

Poverty affects health in both urban and rural settings, but those in rural areas are more likely to be poor than their urban counterparts. Per capita income for rural residents is nearly $10,000 less than among urban dwellers, and rural poverty rates are higher than those in urban areas (13.9% vs. 12.2%) (Economic Research Service, 2005). Within metropolitan areas, however, central-city populations are more likely to be poor (17.5%) than those living in non-central-city areas (9.1%) (U.S. Census Bureau, 2005a). Rural poverty is particularly prevalent among ethnic minorities and migrant or seasonal workers. Rural Black and Native American residents are three times as likely and rural Hispanics twice as likely to be poor as their rural White counterparts (Probst, Moore, Glover, & Samuels, 2004). Community health nurses may advocate for assistance to individual poor rural or urban families. They may also advocate for economic changes that will benefit the poor in either setting. For example, they may campaign for state legislation or local ordinances increasing the minimum wage to a living wage.

Each year, U.S. produce growers employ 750,000 to 5 million migrant and seasonal workers (Gamm et al., 2003). The 1983 Migrant and Seasonal Agricultural Worker Protection Act (AWPA) defined a seasonal worker as "a person employed in agricultural work of a seasonal or other temporary nature who is not required to be absent overnight from his or her permanent place of residence" (as quoted in Culp & Umbarger, 2004, p. 384). A migrant agricultural worker, on the other hand, was defined as "a person employed in agricultural work who is required to be absent overnight from his or her permanent place of residence, except for immediate family members of an agricultural employer or a farm labor contractor" (as quoted in Culp & Umbarger, 2004, p. 384). Under these definitions, then, adolescents who work on a farm during the summer months but return to their homes in town each night would be considered seasonal workers. People who move to an agricultural area for several months but have a home base elsewhere are considered migrant workers. For example, some migrant workers live in the Southwest, but travel to Midwestern states during peak planting and harvesting periods.

Migrant and seasonal workers are less likely than others in rural areas to be highly educated and more likely to live in poverty. In 2003, for example, 81% of 753,000 hired farmworkers had a twelfth-grade education or less. Nearly 83% of this population worked full-time, but the median weekly earnings were only $373 (U.S. Census Bureau, 2005b).

Poverty is also more prevalent among rural than urban elderly populations. In 2000, for example, more than 13% of people over 60 years of age living in non-metropolitan areas had incomes below poverty level, compared to just over 9% of the urban elderly (Rogers, 2002).

Worldwide, 70% of poor people live in rural areas, but urban poverty may have more severe consequences than rural poverty due to the dependence on cash income for goods and services in urban areas. Many rural families raise at least a portion of their food, and

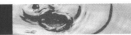

CULTURAL COMPETENCE

Traditionally, refugee and immigrant families enter the United States through major metropolitan areas, and the large majority of them remain in these or similar urban centers throughout the country. More recently, however, some refugee groups have begun to relocate to more rural areas. For example, many Laotian Hmong families have moved from San Diego to areas of North Carolina.

■ What do you think might be some of the reasons for this migration?
■ What are the social implications of an in-migration of a unique cultural group such as the Hmong into the rural culture of the Southeast?
■ What are the implications for community health systems in the North Carolina area?

urban residents throughout the world pay about 30% more for food than rural residents (Population Information Program, 2002). Other goods and services may be less expensive in urban areas due to **economies of proximity**, in which the cost of public services is decreased in areas of greater population density (Awofeso, 2003).

According to World Bank estimates, 330 million urban poor in the developing world earned less than US$1 per day in 1988. By 2000, this number had increased to 495 million. Approximately 20% of urban residents in half of the world's developing nations have incomes below the defined poverty level for their countries, and this figure rises to 50% in some countries (Population Information Program, 2002). Again, community health nurses may advocate for international aid or for economic changes within developing nations to offset poverty.

The economic situation of migrant workers in the United States is further complicated by political inequities. For example, although migrant workers are covered by minimum wage provisions of the 1966 Fair Labor Standards Act, they are specifically excluded from overtime compensation requirements. In addition, agricultural employers with fewer than 7 employees or 500 worker days of labor are exempted even from the minimum wage requirements. The Act also permits children as young as 10 to work in the fields. Because this legislation is often not enforced and migrant families may not have access to childcare, children may be working beside their parents at much earlier ages (Culp & Umbarger, 2004).

Again, community health nurses may advocate for public assistance for low-income families or for measures like the living wage that enable urban and rural families to afford basic necessities of life. Such advocacy may be particularly needed for migrant populations who may not advocate for themselves due to language barriers or fear of deportation or other retaliation. For example, community health nurses may work to see that the provisions of minimum wage legislation are upheld for migrant workers as well as for other employees. They may also work to change legislation so migrant workers are eligible for overtime pay.

Political inequities also occur for other segments of the rural population. For example, rural populations received approximately $261 less per capita in federal funding in 2000 than urban populations. Farming-dependent counties, however, receive slightly higher per capita rates of federal funding, primarily due to higher levels of loan funding (Reeder & Calhoun, 2002).

Rural populations are also less highly educated than urban dwellers. For example, in the 2000 census, nearly 60% of rural residents age 25 and older had a high school education or less, compared to 46% of the urban population. Conversely, more than a quarter of urban residents (26.4%) had completed college versus 15% of the rural population (Economic Research Service, 2005). Lack of education is more prevalent among some segments of the rural population than others.

As described in Chapter 20∞, significant poverty also exists in urban settings, and urban poor families are more likely to be headed by single parents than those in rural areas. Rates of homelessness due to poverty and other factors are higher in urban than in rural areas, but the number of homeless people in rural settings is increasing. Rural homeless are apt to be less visible because of the lack of social services and shelters where they might congregate. The rural homeless are also more likely than their urban counterparts to double or triple up in housing with family or friends, increasing their virtual invisibility (National Coalition for the Homeless, 2005).

Urban settings are more culturally diverse than rural settings, which can be both an advantage and a disadvantage depending on the character of relationships among population groups. Foreign-born persons are more likely to reside in urban than rural settings, but a significant proportion of this population is now migrating to rural areas (USDA, 2005). Because these immigrants tend to have more health-related needs than their U.S.-born counterparts, they are placing considerable strain on rural health care systems that are already overburdened. Movement of U.S.-born retirees with existing chronic illnesses and health care needs to rural areas has a similar effect on the social and health care infrastructures in rural settings (Phillips & McLeroy, 2004).

Occupational issues in urban settings are similar to those discussed in Chapter 24∞. Primary occupations in rural areas include agriculture, mining and other extractive industries, and manufacturing. Agricultural occupations are of two types: agricultural production and agricultural services. Agricultural production encompasses general farming and ranching; agricultural services occupations include custom crop and animal care, horticulture, and landscaping.

The primary differences between agricultural occupations and other rural and urban occupations is the absence of regulatory efforts. The Occupational Health and Safety Act of 1970 excluded agricultural workplaces, and this exclusion led to great differences in federal spending for health and safety in rural and urban settings. Exclusion from OSHA also means that occupational health and safety regulations are unenforceable on the 90% of U.S. farms that are family-owned or employ few paid workers (U.S. Census Bureau, 2005b). In addition, children engaged in work on family farms are not covered by the Fair Labor Standards Act, which leaves them at risk for hazardous working conditions and injury. Approximately 12,000 injuries occur to child farmworkers each year as a result of heavy machinery, work with animals, and other hazardous activities performed with little experience or training. Children are also more prone to agricultural injury than adults because of their limited strength and flexibility (Reed, 2004a). Another disparity lies in the fact that workers' compensation programs do not apply to rural workers in many states. Community health nurses can join other advocacy groups to address this inequity by reformulating workers' compensation legislation in their states.

Family violence and abuse are another consideration in examining the epidemiology of health and illness in urban and rural populations. Intimate partner violence may be more prevalent in rural areas due to isolation, lack of available services, and cultural differences in societal attitudes and norms. In one study, nearly 3% of rural women and nearly 5% of men reported at least one incident of severe physical abuse by an intimate partner. In addition, nearly 48% of rural women and 30% of men reported being victims of emotional abuse. Both physical and emotional abuse were found to be more common among young and unmarried couples. Interestingly, men engaged in farmwork reported more physical abuse and controlling abuse directed at them than other rural men, possibly due to the greater stress and economic insecurity of farmwork. Farm women, on the other hand, reported less abuse than nonfarm rural women (Murty et al., 2003).

The last sociocultural dimension factor to be considered in assessing factors influencing health in rural and urban settings lies in differences in the definitions of health and illness accepted by rural and urban residents. Definitions of health and illness differ widely in urban groups due to the greater heterogeneity of the population as well as greater cultural diversity. Rural definitions tend to be more homogeneous, reflecting a perception that health is synonymous with the ability to work (Gessert, 2003). This definition may lead rural residents to give work needs a higher priority than health needs and to put off seeking health care until conditions become severe. The self-reliance characteristic of rural culture, although often a strength, may also lead to rejection of needed health care services. Rural residents also tend to get fewer preventive health services than urban residents. Community health nursing advocacy may be required to assure provision of adequate health care services for both urban and rural populations. Advocacy may also be required among members of the population, particularly in rural areas, to change attitudes to health and health care.

Behavioral Considerations

Rural and urban populations also differ with respect to elements of the behavioral dimension as they affect health status. Areas for the community health nurse to consider in assessing a specific rural or urban population include diet, use of tobacco, use of alcohol and other drugs, physical activity, sexual activity, and health-related behaviors.

With respect to diet, rural residents are more likely than their urban counterparts to be overweight, and rural diets tend to contain more fat and calories than those of more urban populations. Rural populations also have little access to nutritionists and fewer weight control programs available to them (Gamm et al., 2003). Rural and urban populations may also differ in terms of meal patterns, particularly in the case of rural farm families who may plan meals in the traditional pattern connected with the workday, with the heaviest meal at noon. Urban families and nonfarm rural families are more likely to eat their largest meal in the evening.

Adequate nutrition may be particularly problematic for migrant farmworkers, who may rely on convenience foods while working and who have limited budgets for providing adequate diets. In addition, English language difficulties may force many families to rely on children to read labels and make food choices, with children selecting foods with high sugar content and few vegetables and fruits. The absence of transportation, adequate refrigeration, and cooking facilities may further hamper efforts to provide adequate family nutrition. Community health nurses may need to advocate for access to affordable healthful food sources for this population. For example, a nurse might organize transportation for a weekly shopping trip to a grocery store with reasonable prices for migrant farm families or encourage cooperative buying to achieve some economy of scale.

Tobacco use rates tend to be higher in rural populations than in urban settings. For example, cigarette smoking rates are 19% higher among rural than suburban youth and 32% higher among adults (Eberhardt & Pamuk, 2004). Rural youth are also more likely than their urban counterparts to use smokeless tobacco, and pregnant women in rural areas are less likely to refrain from smoking (Gamm et al., 2003).

Alcohol and tobacco are the most likely substances to be abused in rural areas. For example, more rural residents report five or more drinks on a single occasion than urban dwellers (Gamm et al., 2003), and prevalence of abuse may be as high as 29% among migrant

ETHICAL AWARENESS

*R*esearch has indicated that operation of heavy farm machinery—particularly tractors—by children is a serious risk factor for fatal injury. In your rural community, you are aware of several farm families whose use of children in this capacity places them at very high risk. This occurs primarily on small family farms where much of the machinery in use is aging and is not equipped with more modern safety devices, such as rollover protection on tractors. Would you become involved in political activity to ban operation of farm machinery by children less than 16 years of age? Why or why not? If not, what other action might you take to protect these children?

farmworkers, possibly as a result of social isolation and depression (Monts, 2002). Illicit drug use among adults, on the other hand, tends to be higher in large metropolitan areas. Among youth, however, rural adolescents have a higher prevalence of illicit drug use (14%) than youth in small and large metropolitan areas (10% each). Drug and alcohol abuse may have more severe consequences in rural areas due to lack of access to adequate treatment and the greater stigma attached to substance abuse (Gamm et al., 2003). Community health nursing advocacy can help to assure that treatment facilities are available and that substance abuse treatment is covered by health insurance. Nurses may also need to advocate among members of rural populations to change the perceptions of stigma attached to substance abuse diagnoses.

Lack of exercise is another common feature of rural residence. For example, lack of leisure-time physical activity has been found to be 50% higher in rural than suburban areas (Eberhardt & Pamuk, 2004), and rural schools are less likely than their urban counterparts to include physical education in the curriculum or to have exercise facilities (Gamm et al., 2003). Community health nurses can advocate inclusion of physical education in school curricula as well as the availability of low-cost avenues for physical activity. For example, a nurse might help to create an exercise club in a rural church or school or promote "mall walking" in an urban area.

Health-related behaviors are the final behavioral consideration in assessing the health of rural or urban populations. As noted earlier, rural residents tend not to receive preventive health care. In part, this is the result of lack of access to convenient services, but also reflects the definition of health as the ability to work. Rural residents have also been shown to be less likely than their urban counterparts to engage in health-promotive behaviors. Older persons in rural settings are less likely to receive influenza and pneumonia immunizations than those in urban areas, and older rural women are less likely than their urban counterparts to receive mammograms or Papanicolaou smears (Slifkin, Goldsmith, & Ricketts, 2000). Younger rural women, particularly those in ethnic minority groups, may also be less likely to obtain prenatal care or more likely to obtain care late in their pregnancies than those in urban areas (Baldwin et al., 2002; Gamm et al., 2003).

Rural residents may also be somewhat less likely than their urban counterparts to engage in the use of complementary or alternative medicines (CAM). For example, in one study, only 58% of rural residents reported use of CAM for pain relief compared to 77% of urban and 82% of suburban residents (Vallerand, Fouladbakhsh, & Templin, 2003). In another study, 17.5% of rural elders sought care from complementary providers, primarily for chronic health problems. Another 36% reported using self-directed CAM therapies

for health promotion purposes (Shreffler-Grant, Weinert, Nichols, & Ide, 2005).

Health System Considerations

Significant differences in health care systems in rural and urban areas influence the health of populations in these settings. Areas for consideration in assessing this dimension of health include the availability of and access to health care services, barriers to service use, and the influence of health policies and delivery systems on population health.

Health care services for many rural residents are less accessible, more costly to deliver, narrower in range and scope, and fewer in number than those available to their urban counterparts. This is true for most professional services, including those of physicians, dentists, nurses, and social workers, and is particularly true of services for the elderly in rural areas.

Nearly three fourths (70%) of federally designated health professional shortage areas in the United States are rural (National Rural Health Association, n.d.b). A **health professional shortage area (HPSA)** is defined as "a geographic area, population group, or medical facility that has been designated by the Secretary of the Department of Health and Human Services as having a shortage of health professionals" (National Health Service Corps, 2005, p. 1). HPSA designations may be made for shortages related to primary care, dental care, and mental health. Designation as a HPSA is based on one of two criteria: a ratio of population to full-time-equivalent primary care providers greater than 3,500:1 or a ratio between 3,500:1 and 3,000:1 and "an unusually high need for primary care services or insufficient capacity of existing primary care providers" (Center for Rural Health, n.d., p. 2).

Another designation for populations lacking access to health care services is that of a medically underserved area or population. A **medically underserved area (MUA)** is "a county or group of contiguous counties, a group of county or civil divisions or a group of urban census tracts in which residents have a shortage of personal health services." **Medically underserved populations (MUPs)** are "groups of people who face economic, cultural, or linguistic barriers to health care" (Bureau of Health Professions, n.d., p. 1). A given population may have a sufficient number of providers, therefore not qualifying for designation as a HPSA, and still contain MUPs. For example, if a significant group of Hispanics in the population cannot get adequate health care due to language barriers, the community may be designated a MUP even though it may have large numbers of health care providers overall. HPSAs, MUAs, and MUPs all exist in both rural and urban settings, but tend to be more common in rural communities.

There is a severe shortage of health care providers in many rural areas that does not occur in many urban populations. For example, the physician-to-population ratio is 139% higher for urban than rural counties. The ratio is 150% higher for dentists in urban counties and 130% higher for hospital-based registered nurses. From 1990 to 2000, nearly one fourth of nonmetropolitan counties lost primary care physicians, compared to only 7% of metropolitan counties. Although the number of physicians per population decreased in both rural and urban counties, the decrease in rural areas (37%) was more than twice that for urban populations (15%) (Ricketts, 2005). Approximately 65% of all rural counties are part of HPSAs, and this figure increases in counties with large ethnic minority populations (e.g., 81% of rural counties with large Hispanic populations, 83% of counties with primarily African American residents, and 92% of counties with populations consisting primarily of American Indians/Native Alaskans) (Probst et al., 2004).

Although 17% of the U.S. population lives in rural areas, fewer than 9% of all physicians and 14% of primary care physicians practice there. Rural and urban populations seem to fare equally well with respect to having a regular source of health care, but rural residents are less likely than their urban counterparts to have access to a regular source of care at night or on weekends. Approximately 30% to 40% of rural residents rely on care from a physician outside of their own local area. Factors contributing to the difficulty of attracting providers to rural areas include lack of sufficient population density to support specialty practices, differences between general practice and specialty reimbursement rates, professional isolation, and heavy workloads for the few providers in the area (Gamm et al., 2003).

The lack of specialty providers and rural cultural values of loyalty to local providers may influence primary care practice patterns, forcing providers to take on roles for which they are not prepared. This increases the risk for litigation for rural health care providers, particularly rural mental health nurses (Gibb, Livesey, & Zyla, 2003). These factors, as well as low population density, make it difficult for managed care organizations (MCOs) to maintain fiscal viability in rural areas (Waitzkin et al., 2002; Weeks et al., 2004). In addition, rural providers may find it difficult to participate in MCOs due to their lack of familiarity with managed care, lack of expertise in negotiating contracts, absence of alternative revenue sources, and increased use of mid-level providers (e.g., nurse practitioners) that may not be recognized for reimbursement by some MCOs. Many rural providers also lack the information systems capabilities needed for participation in an MCO (Waitzkin et al., 2002). Lack of providers is particularly noticeable with respect to specialty care.

As we saw earlier, similar disparities between urban and rural settings are noted with respect to the availability of mental health services. For example, the percentage of rural hospitals that have substance abuse treatment facilities in rural areas (10.7%) is less than half that of urban areas (26.5%). Likewise, the ratio of dentists to population is twice as high in large urban areas (60 per 100,000 people) as rural ones (30 per 100,000). In part, the lack of providers in rural areas is offset by the use of nonphysician primary care providers such as nurse practitioners, nurse midwives, and physician's assistants, and rural areas have slightly higher provider-to-population ratios for these categories of providers than urban areas (Gamm et al., 2003). The U.S. federal government also allows foreign physicians who do not meet licensure requirements to practice in HPSAs and provides Medicare bonus payments for physicians in these areas (Ricketts, 2005).

In addition to the shortage of physician providers faced by rural residents in general, members of minority populations in rural settings frequently do not have access to providers who understand their cultures and backgrounds. The problems of recruiting Caucasian providers to rural areas are compounded for ethnic minority providers, who may be faced with lack of acceptance and an even greater perception of being "outsiders."

Rural areas may fare slightly better than urban areas with respect to the public health workforce. For example, in one study of three states with large rural populations, rural health departments reported professional full-time-equivalent employees at a rate of 32.2 per 100,000 population, compared to only 29.2 per 100,000 in urban areas in those states. Rural health departments in these states reported almost twice as many nurses per 100,000 population as their urban counterparts (20.8 vs. 11.2). Unfortunately, nurses in rural health departments were more likely than those in urban areas to lack public health training or related clinical learning experiences, and many were employed only part-time. Rural health departments employed nearly twice as many nurse practitioners per 100,000 population as those in urban areas (1.7 vs. 1.1) (Rosenblatt, Casey, & Richardson, 2002).

Rural health departments may engage in a broader array of services than their urban counterparts, meeting needs that are not addressed by the private sector. For example, rural health departments provide 81% of all immunizations for children and adults in their jurisdictions. Urban health departments, on the other hand, provide only 64% of child and 65% of adult immunization services. Rural health departments also provide more personal care services with less privatization of services, do more community assessments, and provide more community outreach and education than urban departments. Only 7% of rural health departments, however, provide comprehensive primary care services versus 15% of urban health departments. Despite their generally broader array of services, rural health departments had lower funding levels, fewer medical specialists, less access to grant funding, and more difficulty recruiting personnel than urban health departments. Rural health departments also tended to be handicapped by lack of information technology, inadequate laboratory facilities, larger service areas with limited transportation availability, smaller hospitals for acute care needs, and greater fragmentation of resources (Berkowitz, 2004).

The bulk of services provided in rural U.S. health departments were provided by public health nurses (Berkowitz, 2004). This pattern is similar throughout the world, where the most frequent providers of health services in rural areas are nurses. In one study, for example, 84% of the systems responding employed nurses, 56% used physicians, 44% employed nurse practitioners, and 46% used nurse midwives. An additional 11% of systems employed lay health care workers and 10% employed traditional healers (Carty et al., 2004).

Generally speaking, rural areas worldwide have fewer health care providers than urban areas. According to WHO (2002) data, for example, the provider-to-population ratio in Cameroon is 1:400 in urban areas, but 10 times that in rural areas (1:4,000). Similarly, 85% of the population of Cambodia lives in rural settings, yet only 13% of health care workers are employed there. In Angola, 65% of the population is rural, but only 15% of health care workers are stationed in rural areas. The use of **organized indigenous caregiving (OIC)** strategies, which involves the training of local lay people for specific provider extender roles, has been advocated as a means of meeting rural service needs in the United States as well as overseas (May, Phillips, Ferketich, & Verran, 2003).

Emergency medical services (EMS) are another area in which rural populations may experience a deficit. Longer waits for emergency response, longer transport distances to hospitals, and lack of sophisticated emergency departments in rural hospitals increase the risk of trauma-related deaths. In fact, a 30-minute wait for EMS response has been found to increase the risk of death sevenfold. The average EMS response time in the rural United States is 18 minutes, more than eight times the response time in urban areas (Gamm et al., 2003). In addition, EMS personnel in rural areas are more likely than their urban counterparts to be volunteers and to lack adequate protocols for triage and transfer decisions (Peek-Asa et al., 2004). For example, 90% of EMS teams in rural **frontier areas** (those with a population density of fewer than seven people per square mile) are volunteers with only basic training (Gamm et al., 2003).

Health care in rural areas is also influenced by the relatively great distances to facilities and the lack of specialized facilities to meet particular needs (e.g., facilities for cancer therapy). Furthermore, small rural hospitals are at risk for low patient census and closure, further reducing availability of services. From 1990 to 2000, for example, 208 rural hospitals closed, and 29% of the rural

elderly must travel 21 to 30 miles to obtain acute care services. An additional 5% of this population travel more than 30 miles for acute care (Sanford & Townsend-Rocchiccioli, 2004).

Even when health facilities and providers are available, people in rural areas may have more difficulty making use of them than those in urban settings. Distance has already been mentioned as a barrier to health care. Other barriers that are relevant to both urban and rural residents, but are often more prevalent in rural areas, include cost and inconvenience. Rural residents are less likely than their urban counterparts to be insured. In 2003, nearly 19% of the rural population was uninsured, compared to 16% of people living in metropolitan statistical areas (NCHS, 2005). Poor and near-poor residents of rural areas are less likely to have Medicaid coverage (21%) than their urban counterparts (30%), and fewer rural residents receive health insurance benefits from employers (62% vs. 75%) (Eberhardt & Pamuk, 2004). Rural elderly are also less likely than older urban residents to have supplemental insurance in addition to Medicare coverage (Probst et al., 2004).

Many rural workers, especially those involved in agriculture, do not have "sick days" and may be unable to take time from work to obtain health care during the hours when facilities are typically open.

Community health nurses can advocate for the establishment of health care services that meet the needs of the population, particularly in rural areas. For example, a community health nurse may assist a rural community designated as a MUA to apply for federal funding for a rural health clinic (RHC) under the Rural Health Services Clinic Act. Both rural and urban populations may be assisted by community health nurses to obtain funds for community health centers (CHCs) or federally qualified health centers (FQHCs). Community health nurses might also assist local residents living in HPSAs and interested in health professional careers to apply for National Health Service Corps Scholarship and Loan Repayment programs with the understanding that they would practice in their own or another underserved area (Indiana State Department of Health, n.d.).

URBAN AND RURAL COMMUNITY HEALTH NURSING

Rural nursing has been defined as "the provision of health care by professional nurses to persons living in sparsely populated areas" (Long & Weinert, 1998, p. 4). Rural community health nursing originated in 1896, when Ellen M. Wood established an initial rural nursing service in Westchester County, New York. In 1911, Lydia Holman established an independent nursing service in Appalachia (Griffin, 1999), and in 1912, the American Red Cross founded the Rural Nursing Service, which later became the Town and Country Nursing Service. This organization was credited with decreasing infant and overall mortality and improving sanitation, hygiene, and nutrition in rural populations. The Town and Country Nursing Service continued until 1947, when it was disbanded due to the rise of official nursing agencies in state and local health departments. Other rural nursing services were provided by organizations such as the Frontier Nursing Service established by Mary Breckenridge in 1928 (Kalisch & Kalisch, 2004). More recent developments in rural nursing include the Migrant Health Act of 1962, which established the Migrant Health Program (Goldberg & Napolitano, 2001), and the passage of the Rural Health Clinic Service Act in 1977 (Oregon Health & Science University, 2006). Both of these pieces of legislation provided funding for health care services in rural areas that have addressed some of the health needs of the rural population and increased the use of nurse practitioners as providers of care. The Rural Health Clinic Service Act, in particular, mandated the use of mid-level practitioners such as nurse practitioners in underserved rural areas (Aday, Quill, & Reyes-Gibby, 2001).

As noted in Chapter 3∞, urban community health nursing in the United States began primarily with the efforts of Lillian Wald and others in the late 19th century. Occupational health nursing, which was primarily focused on urban manufacturing, also began about this time. Although occupational health risks related to agriculture were recognized as early as 1555, when the effects of breathing grain dust on the lungs of threshers were noted, little attention has been given to occupational health in rural areas until relatively recently. One other exception was the identification of anthrax among sheep handlers in the 1800s (Bell, 2002), discussed in Chapter 24∞. Thackrah's 1832 report on The Effects of Arts, Trades, and Professions addressed the effects of occupational postures on the health of the working poor, but there was no mention of agricultural occupations—in which bending, twisting, and heavy lifting are common occurrences—as contributing factors (Schenker, 1995).

Recent concerns about health influences in rural areas have led to the development of beginning theory related to rural nursing. Key concepts of rural nursing theory include work beliefs and health beliefs, isolation and distance, self-reliance, lack of anonymity, insider/outsider, and old-timer/newcomer (Long & Weinert, 1998). These key concepts and their relationships are summarized at right and discussed where relevant throughout the remainder of this chapter. No comparable theory of urban nursing has been noted in the literature.

Rural nurses tend to be generalists who may be required to deal with any type of health problem that arises. They are expected to be competent in multiple areas and expert in a few. Rural community health nurses should have generalized expertise related to childbearing, child health, injury prevention, health education, and so on. Urban nurses, on the other hand,

SPECIAL CONSIDERATIONS

KEY CONCEPTS AND RELATIONSHIPS IN A THEORY OF RURAL NURSING

- **Work beliefs and health beliefs:** Work and health are related. Work is of primary importance, and health is assessed in relation to the ability to work. Health needs are often secondary to work needs.
- **Isolation and distance:** Rural residents often live great distances from health care and other services. Despite these differences, however, they do not generally see themselves as isolated.
- **Self-reliance:** Rural residents are characterized by a strong desire to do and care for themselves. This may result in reluctance to seek help from others, reliance on informal support networks when care is sought, and resistance to seeking care from "outsiders."
- **Lack of anonymity:** Rural communities are close-knit and rural residents may feel a lack of privacy. For rural nurses, this means multiple different relationships with clients that are interrelated. For example, the nurse's credibility as a professional may be linked to perceptions of her performance as a wife and mother as well as to evidence of professional competence. The role diffusion caused by multiple roles within the community may lead to a broader diversity of tasks expected of rural nurses, including expansion into the practice realm of other disciplines.
- **Insider/outsider:** Rural residents prefer to receive services from people well known to them. Rural nurses must become actively involved within their communities in other than professional roles. This may be uncomfortable for nurses who try to maintain a clear separation between their personal and professional lives.
- **Old-timer/newcomer:** Rural residents may continue to perceive people who have lived in the area for several years as "newcomers," and rural nurses new to the area should expect a long period of being considered a newcomer before they are completely accepted by the population.

Data from: Long, K. A., & Weinert, C. (1998). Rural nursing: Developing the theory base. In H. J. Lee (Ed.), Conceptual basis for rural nursing (pp. 3–18). New York: Springer.

may have more opportunity for specialization because of the array of other providers available to fulfill other needs in urban areas.

Rural and urban nursing may also differ in the scope of practice. Because of the dearth of health professionals in many rural areas, rural community health nurses may be the only source of health care for many clients. Again, this demands a generalist perspective, but may also mean that the boundaries between nursing and medicine are less distinct than in urban settings. Rural nurses may often be required to engage in what would elsewhere be considered medical practice until a physician arrives, particularly in emergency situations (Gamm et al., 2003).

Care of population groups in both urban and rural settings relies on the nursing process as an organizational framework. However, the factors assessed as

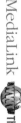

MediaLink The Urban HealthInstitute (video)

influencing health, the health problems identified, and intervention approaches may often differ.

Assessing Factors Influencing Health in Urban and Rural Populations

The first step in meeting the health care needs of urban and rural populations is to identify those needs through population health assessment. Such an assessment would be conducted using the principles discussed in Chapter 15∞. The focused assessments included in that chapter can be used to assess the health of either urban or rural populations. In addition, a community assessment tool that would be appropriate in the assessment of either rural or urban populations is provided in Appendix G on the Companion Website and in the Community Assessment Reference Guide 📄 designed to accompany this text.

Information about population composition, morbidity, and mortality for both rural and urban populations may be obtained from state agencies (e.g., departments of vital statistics or state health departments). Rural statistics may also be available from local, state, national, and international agencies dealing with rural concerns and issues. At the federal level, for example, the Office of Rural Health Policy of the Health Resources and Services Administration (HRSA) and the USDA provide a wide array of information about rural populations. Many states also have rural policy agencies (e.g., the California Rural Health Policy Council). Local governments in largely rural areas also collect population data. Generally these local agencies would be county health departments or other agencies. Finally, several voluntary organizations, such as the National Rural Health Association, collect information on rural populations. Similar organizations, such as the International Council of Nurses' (2005) Rural and Remote Nursing Network, the Rural Health Association of Tennessee (2005), the Australian Rural Nurses, Inc. (2003), and the Rural Nurse Organization (n.d.) may be found at U.S. state or national levels, in other countries, or internationally.

With respect to urban populations, city or county governments or other local agencies (e.g., Chambers of Commerce) collect a variety of data, and state and national data can be found by urban census tract or other designation (e.g., MSA). In addition, national and international voluntary agencies, such as the Urban Health Institute and the International Society for Urban Health, may provide a wealth of data on national or worldwide urban populations. The World Health Organization also collects data related to both urban and rural populations.

Other types of information included in an assessment of an urban or rural population may be derived from service agencies operating in the area. For example, crime statistics might be available from an urban police department, county sheriff's department, or state police agency. Similarly, information regarding morbidity and mortality as well as the extent of health insurance coverage might be obtained from local health care organizations.

Community health nurses might obtain still other forms of data from surveys of area residents. For example, the extent of depression in a rural or urban community can only be partially determined from treatment records because many people do not seek help for depression. Surveys of urban or rural dwellers would be apt to give a clearer picture of the extent of depression in the population. Finally, some information is best obtained through actual observation (e.g., housing conditions in the area, traffic hazards, and so on).

Diagnostic Reasoning and Care of Urban and Rural Populations

In rural areas, the etiology of nursing diagnoses is frequently related to a lack of resources and limited access to health care in the community. A nursing diagnosis of "potential for poor infant outcome due to extended travel time to nearest maternity delivery service" is common in today's rural health system and requires that the rural nurse providing prenatal care be most astute in assessing this client during her pregnancy. A second nursing diagnosis might be "increased suicide risk due to lack of access to and use of mental health services." This diagnosis may be attributable to limited access to health care as well as to perceptions of stigma frequently attached to mental illness among rural populations.

Nursing diagnoses developed for urban populations might also reflect unique factors affecting health in that setting. As an example, the nurse might make a diagnosis of "lack of physical activity due to fear of walking in high-crime neighborhoods." Another diagnosis related to urban populations might be "potential for hearing loss among children in schools adjacent to airport."

EVISDENCE-BASED PRACTICE

*H*uttlinger, Schaller-Ayers, and Lawson (2004) have advocated a population-based approach to health care delivery in rural areas. Population health is defined as "an approach [that] focuses on interrelated conditions and factors that influence the health of populations over the life course, identifies systematic variations in the patterns of occurrence, and applies the resulting knowledge to develop and implement policies and actions to improve the health and well-being of those populations" (Kindig & Stoddart, as quoted in Hartley, 2004, p. 1675). A population-based approach would work equally well to address health needs in urban settings. Population-based health care planning, however, must be based on an understanding of the health care needs of the particular population. Select an urban or rural population with which you are familiar. Then examine the literature for any information regarding the health problems and care needs of that population. Is there sufficient evidence on which to base health system planning? If not, how might that evidence base be developed?

MediaLink Case Study: Community Health Care in a Rural Area

Planning and Implementing Care for Urban and Rural Populations

Nursing interventions in rural and urban settings can be directed toward meeting the needs of individual clients, families, or population groups. Community health nurses play pivotal roles in planning intervention strategies for urban and rural populations. A key feature of planning interventions to address the health needs of either urban or rural populations would be the development of partnerships with community members and other groups and organizations in the setting. The development of such partnerships would employ the principles of coalition building discussed in Chapter 7∞ and the strategies for empowering communities presented in Chapter 13∞.

Overall goals for care in urban and rural settings are similar and include:

- Increasing access to health care services and decreasing barriers to their use
- Eliminating or modifying environmental risk factors
- Modifying social conditions that adversely affect health
- Increasing clients' abilities to make informed health decisions
- Developing systems of care that are population appropriate
- Developing equitable health care policies that address the diverse needs of urban and rural populations

Although the goals of care are similar for rural and urban populations, the means by which they are accomplished may be quite different. For example, increasing access to health care in rural settings may revolve primarily around increasing the number and variety of available providers or changing reimbursement rates and other characteristics of practice to attract providers to rural areas. In both urban and rural settings, increasing access may involve dealing with problems of cost, increasing insurance coverage, and developing systems that provide low-cost quality health care to these populations.

Interventions designed to decrease barriers to use of health care services may also differ significantly between urban and rural settings. For example, in urban settings, actions may be needed to increase the ability of providers to communicate with clients from multiple ethnic groups and cultures. With the movement of immigrants to rural areas, some actions along this line will be needed in rural settings as well, but providers are unlikely to be called on to communicate in multiple different languages and with multiple ethnic groups as occurs in urban areas. Decreasing barriers to care in rural settings may involve providing access to transportation services, changing times when services are provided, or finding creative ways to deliver services at great distances in cost-effective ways.

Activities to eliminate or modify environmental risks will also differ greatly between rural and urban settings. For example, skin cancer prevention education should be a high-priority focus among agricultural workers, whereas interventions to address high urban noise levels or reduce violent crime and gang activity may be more appropriate to urban settings.

In urban settings, action to modify social factors that adversely affect health may involve assisting clients to develop support systems or linking them to available health and social services. Community health nurses may also be involved in activities to promote the availability of affordable housing or to decrease unemployment levels. In rural settings, more focus is needed on providing support and respite for members of informal care networks and changing attitudes to the need for and use of health care services, particularly preventive services.

Increasing clients' abilities to make informed health decisions usually focuses on the type of decisions to be made and the health problems prevalent in the setting. For example, a rural community health nurse may focus on assisting clients with farm safety issues or use of preventive services. In the urban setting, on the other hand, community assessment data may suggest a need to focus on personal safety and crime prevention.

As noted earlier, the urban model of managed care may not be appropriate to meeting the needs of rural populations, and modified delivery systems may be required. Nurses may be involved in the development and implementation of creative modes of health care delivery in either urban or rural settings. For example, school-based clinics may be an effective mode of providing care in the urban environment. When children travel long distances to consolidated schools, however, the concept of the school as a central community structure that can support health services becomes less meaningful. It may be that faith community nursing or some other form of locally based nursing services may be a more appropriate vehicle for delivering nursing services in rural areas.

Finally, community health nurses should be actively involved in developing and promoting national and state health care policies that are equitable and address the diverse needs of both urban and rural populations. For example, nurses may advocate for higher reimbursement rates for providers in rural settings or for other incentives that attract and retain providers in rural communities, or community health nurses might become involved in revisions to policies that prevent both rural and urban immigrants from having access to certain health and social services.

Evaluating Health Care for Urban and Rural Populations

Nurses providing services in rural and urban settings must evaluate the outcomes of care as well as its cost-effectiveness. Outcomes of care in rural and urban settings may also be evaluated in terms of the accomplishment of the national health objectives. Several of the *Healthy People 2010* objectives deal with disparities in health care and

HEALTHY PEOPLE 2010

Goals for Population Health

OBJECTIVE	BASELINE	MOST RECENT DATA	TARGET
■ 1-1. Increase the proportion of people with health insurance:			
Metropolitan statistical areas (MSAs)	83%	84%	100%
Non-MSAs	80%	81%	100%
■ 1-5. Increase the proportion of people with a usual primary care provider:			
MSAs	77%	78%	85%
Non-MSAs	78%	80%	85%
■ 1-6. Reduce the proportion of families with difficulty in getting care:			
MSAs	12%	10%	7%
Non-MSAs	12%	12%	7%
■ 7-6. Increase the proportion of employees who participate in employer-sponsored health promotion:			
MSAs	66%	59%	75%#
Non-MSAs	73%	62%	75%#
■ 11-1. Increase the proportion of people with Internet at home:			
MSAs	26%	51%	80%
Non-MSAs	22%	49%	80%
■ 20-2d. Reduce injuries in agriculture, forestry, and fishing (per 100 full-time workers over age 16)	7.6	6	5.3
■ 22-1. Reduce the proportion of people with no leisure-time physical activity:			
MSAs	39%	37%	20%
Non-MSAs	43%	41%	20%

Objective moving away from target

Data from: Centers for Disease Control and Prevention. (2005). Healthy people data. Retrieved September 5, 2005, from http://wonder.cdc.gov/data2010

health care outcomes between rural and urban populations. These objectives and their current status may be viewed on the *Healthy People 2010* Web site, which may be accessed at http://wonder.cdc.gov/ data2010. Data regarding the status of some of these objectives are presented above. Similarly, the priority areas for rural health identified in *Rural Healthy People 2010* can be used as the basis for evaluating the effectiveness of rural health care.

Community health nursing in urban and rural settings displays some similarities but many differences. Effective community health nurses will be aware of these similarities and differences and will develop health care interventions accordingly. They will recognize that, although a particular intervention has demonstrated effectiveness in one setting, that effectiveness may not translate to other settings.

Case Study

Nursing in a Rural Setting

You are a rural community health nurse assigned to the county health department mobile van visiting a large migrant community at a local farm. Mr. Robert Kelbert is a 64-year-old African American migrant worker who comes into the mobile unit to have his blood pressure medication refilled. He will be in the county for the next 3 to 4 weeks to harvest the soybean crop. He usually attends a rural health clinic in the northern part of the state where he has been receiving his care and medications free.

Today, his blood pressure is 154/98, pulse 88, height 69 inches, and weight 198 pounds. He states he is "worn out" from the heat. He chews tobacco and drinks alcohol "some." He travels and stays with his son and family. His daughter-in-law does the cooking. During your interview, Mr. Kelbert tells you he is worried because two of the migrant workers have been given medicine for lung congestion and one of them has been coughing up blood.

1. In what ways is Mr. Kelbert's situation typical of that of rural clients in general? Of migrant farmworkers? In what ways is it different?

2. What are some of the biophysical, psychological, physical environmental, sociocultural, behavioral, and health system factors operating in this situation?

3. List three nursing diagnoses that you would identify for Mr. Kelbert.

4. What are your objectives for today's client visit?

5. How might your care for Mr. Kelbert differ from that provided to a client you see regularly at the rural health department?

6. What primary, secondary, and tertiary prevention measures are appropriate for Mr. Kelbert?

7. How will you follow up on this visit?

Test Your Understanding

1. Discuss differences in the definitions of *rural* and *urban*. What implications do these definitions have for health care policy? For research? (pp. 703–704)

2. What are some of the differences in factors that affect health in rural and urban settings? (pp. 705–718)

3. In what ways do policy inequities influence health in urban and rural settings? (pp. 712–713)

4. How might you go about assessing factors influencing health in urban and rural settings? (p. 718)

5. What are the primary goals for nursing intervention in urban and rural settings? How might accomplishment of these goals differ between settings? (p. 719)

6. How would you go about evaluating the effectiveness of nursing interventions in a rural setting? Would your approach to evaluation differ in an urban setting? (pp. 719–720)

EXPLORE MediaLink

http://www.prenhall.com/clark
Resources for this chapter can be found on the Companion Website.

Audio Glossary
Appendix G: Community Health Assessment and Intervention Guide
Exam Review Questions
Case Study: Community Health Care in a Rural Area

MediaLink Application: Choosing a Career in Rural Health (video)
MediaLink Application: The Urban Health Initiative (video)
Media Links

Challenge Your Knowledge
Update *Healthy People 2010*
Advocacy Interviews

References

Aday, L. A., Quill, B. E., & Reyes-Gibby, C. C. (2001). Equity in rural health and health care. In S. Loue & B. E. Quill (Eds.), *Handbook of rural health* (pp. 45–72). New York: Kluwer Academic/Plenum.

Annie E. Casey Foundation. (2004). *City & rural kids count data book*. Retrieved March 25, 2006, from http://www.aecf.org/publications/data/city_rural_databook.pdf

Australian Rural Nurses, Inc. (2003). *Mission and objectives*. Retrieved July 8, 2006, from http://www.aarn.au/about/mission.htm

Averill, J. (2003). Keys to the puzzle: Recognizing strengths in a rural community. *Public Health Nursing, 20,* 449–455.

Awofeso, N. (2003). The healthy cities approach—reflections on a framework for improving global health. *Bulletin of the World Health Organization, 81,* 222–223.

Baldwin, L.-M., Grossman, D. C., Casey, S., Hollow, W., Sugarman, J. R., Freeman, W. L., et al. (2002). Perinatal and infant health among rural and urban American Indians/Alaska Natives. *American Journal of Public Health, 92,* 1491–1497.

Bell, J. H. (2002). Anthrax and the wool trade. *American Journal of Public Health, 92,* 754–757.

(Reprinted from J. H. Bell, Anthrax: Its relation to the wool industry. In *Dangerous trades: The historical, social, and legal aspects of industrial occupations as affecting health, by a number of experts,* pp. 634–643, by T. Oliver, Ed., 1902, London: John Murray.)

Berkowitz, B. (2004). Rural public health service delivery: Promising new directions. *American Journal of Public Health, 94,* 1678–1681.

Branas, C. C., Nance, M. L., Elliott, M. R., Richmond, T. S., & Schwab, C. W. (2004). Urban–rural shifts in intentional firearm death: Different causes, same results. *American Journal of Public Health, 94,* 1750–1755.

Bureau of Health Professions. (n.d.). *Shortage designation*. Retrieved March 26, 2006, from http://bhpr.hrsa.gov/shortage

Carty, R. M., Al-Zayyer, W., Arietti, L. L., & Lester, A. S. (2004). International rural health needs and services research: A nursing and midwifery response. *Journal of Professional Nursing, 20,* 251–259.

Center for Rural Health, University of North Dakota. (n.d.). *Health professional shortage areas (HPSAs) and Medically underserved areas (MUAs)*. Retrieved March 26, 2006, from

http://www.med.und.nodak.edu/depts/rural/pdf/hpsa.pdf

Centers for Disease Control and Prevention. (2005). *Healthy people data*. Retrieved September 5, 2005, from http://wonder.cdc.gov/data2010

Culp, K., & Umbarger, M. (2004). Seasonal and migrant agricultural workers. *AAOHN Journal, 52,* 383–390.

Eberhardt, M. S., & Pamuk, E. R. (2004). The importance of place of residence: Examining health in rural and nonrural areas. *American Journal of Public Health, 94,* 1682–1686.

Economic Research Service. (2005). *Data fact sheets: United States*. Retrieved March 25, 2006, from http://www.res.usda.gov/StateFacts/US.htm

Fitzpatrick, K. M. (2000). *Unhealthy places*. New York: Routledge.

Gaffield, S. J., Goo, R. L., Richards, L. A., & Jackson, R. J. (2003). Public health effects of inadequately managed stormwater runoff. *American Journal of Public Health, 93,* 1527–1533.

Gallagher, E., Alcock, D., Diem, E., Angus, D., & Medves, J. (2002). Ethical dilemmas in home care case management. *Journal of Healthcare Management, 47*(2), 85–97.

Gamm, L., & Hutchison, L. (2004). *Rural Healthy People 2010—Evolving Interactive Practice. American Journal of Public Health, 94,* 1711–1712.

Gamm, L., Hutchison, L., Dabney, B., & Dorsey, A. (Eds.). (2003). *Rural healthy people 2010: A companion document to healthy people 2010* (vol. 1). College Station, TX: Texas A&M University System Health Science Center, School of Rural Public Health, Southwest Rural Health Research Center.

Gessert, C. E. (2003). Rurality and suicide. *American Journal of Public Health, 93,* 698.

Gibb, H., Livesey, L., & Zyla, W. (2003). At 3 am who the hell do you call? Case management issues in sole practice as a rural community mental health nurse. *Australasian Psychiatry, 11*(Suppl.), S127–S129.

Goldberg, B. W., & Napolitano, M. (2001). The health of migrant and seasonal farmworkers. In S. Loue & B. E. Quill (Eds.), *Handbook of rural health* (pp. 103–117). New York: Kluwer Academic/Plenum.

Griffin, J. (1999). Parish nursing in rural communities. In P. A. Solari–Twadell & M. A. McDermott (Eds.), *Parish nursing: Promoting whole person health within faith communities* (pp. 75–82). Thousand Oaks, CA: Sage.

Hancock, T. (2000). Healthy communities must also be sustainable communities. *Public Health Reports, 115,* 151–156.

Hart, L. G., Larson, E. H., & Lishner, D. M. (2005). Rural definitions for health policy and research. *American Journal of Public Health, 95,* 1149–1155.

Hartley, D. (2004). Rural health disparities, population health, and rural culture. *American Journal of Public Health, 94,* 1675–1678.

House, J. S., Lepkowski, J. M., Williams, D. R., Mero, R. P., Lanz, P. M., Robert, S. A., et al. (2000). Excess mortality among urban residents: How much, for whom, and why? *American Journal of Public Health, 90,* 1898–1904.

Huttlinger, K., Schaller-Ayers, J., & Lawson, T. (2004). Health care in Appalachia: A population-based approach. *Public Health Nursing, 21,* 103–110.

Indiana State Department of Health, Local Liaison Office. (n.d.). *Health professional shortage area and medically underserved area designations.* Retrieved March 26, 2006, from http://www.in.gov/isdh/publications/llo/shortages/shortage.htm

Institute of Medicine. (2005). *Quality through collaboration: The future of rural health.* Washington, DC: National Academies Press.

International Council of Nurses. (2005). *Rural and Remote Nursing Network (ICN-RRNN).* Retrieved December 15, 2005, from http://www.icn.ch/rrn_network.htm

Kalisch, P. A., & Kalisch, B. J. (2004). *American nursing: A history.* Philadelphia: Lippincott Williams & Wilkins.

Knowlton, K. (2001). Urban history, urban health. *American Journal of Public Health, 91,* 1494–1496.

Leyden, K. M. (2003). Social capital and the built environment: The importance of walkable neighborhoods. *American Journal of Public Health, 93,* 1546–1551.

Long, K. A., & Weinert, C. (1998). Rural nursing: Developing the theory base. In H. J. Lee (Ed.), *Conceptual basis for rural nursing* (pp. 3–18). New York: Springer.

May, K. M., Phillips, L. R., Ferketich, S. L., & Verran, J. A. (2003). Public health nursing: The generalist in a specialized environment. *Public Health Nursing, 20,* 252–259.

Monts, R. (2002). Depression among migrant farm workers. *Community Health Forum, 3*(5), 52–54.

Murty, S. A., Peek-Asa, C., Zwerling, C., Stromquist, A. M., Burmeister, L. F., & Merchant, J. A. (2003). Physical and emotional abuse reported by men and women in a rural community. *American Journal of Public Health, 93,* 1073–1075.

National Center for Health Statistics. (2005). *Health, United States, 2005 with chartbook on trends in the health of Americans.* Retrieved December 23, 2005, from http://www.cdc.gov/nchs/data/hus/hus05.pdf

National Center for Infectious Diseases. (2001). Outbreaks of *Escherichia coli* O157:H7 infections among children associated with farm visits—Pennsylvania and Washington, 2000. *Morbidity and Mortality Weekly Report, 50,* 293–297.

National Coalition for the Homeless. (2005). *Rural homelessness.* Retrieved November 29, 2005, from http://www.nationalhomeless.org/publications/facts

National Health Service Corps. (2005). *Health professional shortage areas.* Retrieved March 26, 2006, from http://nchs.bhpr.hrsa.gov

National Rural Health Association. (n.d.a). *How is rural defined?* Retrieved July 8, 2006, from http://www.nrharural.org/about/sub/ruraldef.html

National Rural Health Association. (n.d.b). *What's different about rural health?* Retrieved March 26, 2006, from http://www.nrharural.org/about/sub/different.html

Oregon Health & Science University. (2006). *Oregon Office of Rural Health: Rural health clinics.* Retrieved October 6, 2006, from http://www.ohsu.edu/oregonruralhealth/rclinpg.html

Peek-Asa, C., Zwerling, C., & Stallones, L. (2004). Acute traumatic injuries in rural populations. *American Journal of Public Health, 94,* 1686–1693.

Perdue, W. C., Stone, L. A., & Gostin, L. O. (2003). The built environment and its relationship to the public's health: The legal framework. *American Journal of Public Health, 93,* 1390–1394.

Phillips, C. D., Holan, S., Sherman, M., Williams, M. L., & Hawes, C. (2004). Rurality and nursing home quality: Results from a national sample of nursing home admissions. *American Journal of Public Health, 94,* 1717–1722.

Phillips, C. D., & McLeroy, K. R. (2004). Health in rural America: Remembering the importance of place. *American Journal of Public Health, 94,* 1661–1663.

Population Information Program, Center for Communication Programs. (2002). Retrieved July 25, 2003, from http://www.jhucpp.org

Probst, J. S., Moore, C. G., Glover, S. H., & Samuels, M. E. (2004). Person and place: The compounding effects of race/ethnicity and rurality on health. *American Journal of Public Health, 94,* 1695–1703.

Reed, D. B. (2004a). Collaboration between nurses and agricultural teachers to prevent adolescent agricultural injuries: The Agricultural Disability Awareness and Risk Education Model. *Public Health Nursing, 21,* 323–330.

Reed, D. B. (2004b). The risky business of production agriculture: Health and safety for farm workers. *AAOHN Journal, 52,* 401–409.

Reeder, R. J., & Calhoun, S. D. (2002). Federal funds in rural America: Payments vary by region and type of county. *Rural America, 17*(3), 74–76.

Ricketts, T. C. (2005). Workforce issues in rural areas: A focus on policy equity. *American Journal of Public Health, 95,* 42–48.

Rogers, C. C. (2002). The older population in 21st century rural America. *Rural America, 17*(3), 2–10.

Rosenblatt, R. A., Casey, S., & Richardson, M. (2002). Rural–urban differences in the public health workforce: Local health departments in 3 rural western states. *American Journal of Public Health, 92,* 1102–1105.

Rural Health Association of Tennessee. (2005). *About us.* Retrieved July 8, 2006, from http://www.rhat.org/About-Us.php

Rural Nurse Organization. (n.d.). *The history of RNO.* Retrieved July 8, 2006, from http://www.rno.org/about.htm

Sanford, J. T., & Townsend-Rocchiccioli, J. (2004). The perceived health of rural caregivers. *Geriatric Nursing, 25,* 145–148.

Schenker, M. B. (1995). Preventive medicine and health promotion are overdue in the agricultural workplace. *Wellness Lecture Series.* Davis, CA: University of California.

Shreffler-Grant, J., Weinert, C., Nichols, E., & Ide, B. (2005). Complementary therapy use among older rural adults. *Public Health Nursing, 22,* 323–331.

Sierra Club. (n.d.). *America needs more transit.* Retrieved March 1, 2006, from http://www.sierraclub.org/sprawl/reports/transit_fact_sheet.pdf

Sierra Club. (2001). *Clearing the air with transit spending.* Retrieved March 4, 2002, from http://www.sierraclub.org

Singh, G. K., & Siahpush, M. (2002). Increasing rural–urban gradients in US suicide mortality, 1990–1997. *American Journal of Public Health, 92,* 1161–1167.

Slifkin, R. T., Goldsmith, L. J., & Ricketts, T. C. III. (2000). *Race and place: Urban–rural differences in health for racial and ethnic minorities.* Chapel Hill, NC: North Carolina Rural Health Research Program.

Spengler, S. E., Browning, S. R., & Reed, D. B. (2004). Sleep deprivation and injuries in part-time Kentucky farmers. *AAOHN Journal, 52,* 373–383.

U.S. Census Bureau. (2005a). *Poverty: Historical poverty tables.* Retrieved March 22, 2006, from http://www.census.gov/hhes/www/poverty/histpov/histpov8/html

U.S. Census Bureau. (2005b). *Statistical Abstract of the United States: 2004–2005.* Retrieved May 12, 2005, from http://www.census.gov/prod/2004pubs/04statab

U.S. Department of Agriculture. (2005). *Rural America at a glance.* Retrieved March 25,

2006, from http://www.ers.usda.gov/publications/EIB4

U.S. Department of Health and Human Services. (2001). Health equity benefits everyone. *Prevention Report, 15*(2), 1–2.

Vallerand, A. H., Fouladbakhsh, J. M., & Templin, T. (2003). The use of complementary/alternative medicine therapies for the self-treatment of pain among residents of urban, suburban, and rural communities. *American Journal of Public Health, 93*, 923–925.

Waitzkin, H., Williams, R. L., Bock, J. A., McCloskey, J., Willging, C., & Wagner, W. (2002). Safety-net institutions buffer the impact of Medicaid managed care: A multi-method assessment in a rural state. *American Journal of Public Health, 92*, 598–610.

Wallace, B. R., Grindeanu, L. A., & Cirillo, D. J. (2004). Rural/urban contrasts in population morbidity status. In N. Glasgow, L. W. Morton, & N. E. Johnson (Eds.), *Critical issues in rural health* (pp. 15–26). Ames, IA: Blackwell.

Weeks, W. B., Kasiz, L. E., Shen, Y., Cong. Z., Ren, X., Miller, D., et al. (2004). Differences in health-related quality of life in rural and urban veterans. *American Journal of Public Health, 94*, 1762–1767.

Weinert, C., & Boik, R. J. (1998). MSU rurality index: Development and evaluation. In H. J. Lee (Ed.), *Conceptual basis for rural nursing* (pp. 449–471). New York: Springer.

World Health Organization. (2002). *Scaling up the response to infectious diseases.* Retrieved April 2, 2002, from http://www.who.int/infectious-disease-report/2002/investigating health.html

World Health Organization. (2003). *Right to water.* Geneva, Switzerland: Author.

World Health Organization. (2004). *World health report, 2004: Changing history.* Retrieved November 23, 2004, from http://www.who.int/whr/2004/annex/en

World Health Organization. (2005). *World Health Statistics, 2005.* Retrieved September 21, 2005, from http://www.who/int/healthinfo/statistics/whostat2005en1.pdf

Wright, R. J., Mitchell, H., Visness, C. M., Cohen, S., Stout, J., Evans, R., et al. (2004). Community violence and asthma mortality: An inner-city asthma study. *American Journal of Public Health, 94*, 625–632.

Advocacy in Action

Facilitating Reentry

Women who have been incarcerated are often at a loss when they are released from a correctional facility. They have often exhausted their social support networks and don't know where to turn for assistance with issues of housing, employment, and ongoing physical and mental health care. Welcome Home Ministries (WHM) is an organization started by a nurse/minister that attempts to assist women with the reentry process. Working one-to-one with women was effective in helping them to address their needs, but there was a need for basic information on services available to these women that could be provided to a wider audience, not just those who sought services at WHM.

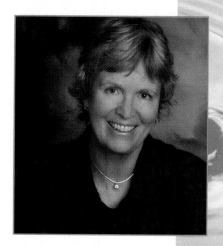

Community health nursing students of a local university undertook a project to identify services for which women were eligible and to produce a directory that could be distributed to women being released from the local jail and state prison. The students began by identifying categories of resources that women in reentry would need. They obtained this information in consultation with several recently released women who described their needs. The students explored services available in the community in each of the categories identified. They then interviewed staff at each of the agencies to get information on services provided, eligibility requirements, and how to obtain services. They were particularly careful to identify services for which previously incarcerated women would be eligible and that were in geographic areas that were easily accessible to the women.

Based on the information collected, the students created a services directory. WHM had a small grant that paid to print the directory. The directory was disseminated through WHM, as well as by the local sheriff's department and county jail personnel to women being released back into the community. With the students' assistance these women had a better chance of successfully reintegrating themselves into the community.

Diane Hatton, DNSc, RN

Professor, Hahn School of Nursing and Health Science

University of San Diego

26
CHAPTER

Care of Clients in Correctional Settings

CHAPTER OBJECTIVES

After reading this chapter, you should be able to:

1. Discuss the impetus for providing health care in correctional settings.
2. Differentiate between basic and advanced nursing practice in correctional settings.
3. Describe biophysical, psychological, physical environmental, sociocultural, behavioral, and health system factors that influence health in correctional settings.
4. Identify major aspects of primary prevention in correctional settings and analyze the role of the community health nurse in each.
5. Describe approaches to secondary prevention in correctional settings and analyze community health nursing roles with respect to each.
6. Discuss considerations in tertiary prevention in correctional settings and analyze related community health nursing roles.

KEY TERMS

detainees **726**
diversion **751**
forensic nurses **740**
jails **726**
juvenile detention facilities **726**
lockdown **749**
lockup **734**
medical parole **754**
parolee **752**
prisons **726**
probationer **752**
recidivism **751**
reentry **753**
search and seizure **749**
TB prophylaxis **746**

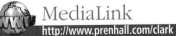

MediaLink
http://www.prenhall.com/clark

Additional interactive resources for this chapter can be found on the Companion Website. Click on Chapter 26 and "Begin" to select the activities for this chapter.

*T*he concept of prisons as a place to contain wrongdoers began as early as the 1600s with workhouses that were used to punish people who violated the law. Unfortunately, workhouses were also used to confine family members who were likely to impugn the family's honor through their activities, whether or not those activities were actually criminal in nature (Fagan, 2003). As we saw in Chapter 20∞, criminalization still occurs within populations that society would prefer to ignore, such as the homeless.

Correctional populations may be particularly vulnerable to a variety of health problems. In many instances, members of this population have not had access to effective health care services. In other cases, they have not seen health as a priority and frequently do not engage in practices that are conducive to good health. In addition, drug and alcohol use, which may result in incarceration, have both physical and psychological consequences for health. Incarceration, in and of itself, may have adverse health consequences.

Because of the great potential for coercion, correctional populations are also considered highly vulnerable to exploitation as research subjects. In addition to active coercion for participation, other more subtle forms of coercion may be employed. For example, inmates may agree to participate in research studies in order to obtain special privileges or gain additional time outside of cellblocks. For all these reasons, community health nurses working in correctional settings may be called on to engage in even greater advocacy efforts than might be required in other settings.

Correctional facilities provide a relatively new practice setting for community health nursing compared to the settings discussed in previous chapters. Correctional nursing, however, is congruent with the primary focus of community health nursing—the health of groups of people and the general public (Norman & Parrish, 2000). Corrections nursing frequently involves challenges not encountered in other community health nursing settings. Practice in a correctional setting requires autonomy and excellent assessment skills. Nurses are often responsible for triaging inmates during sick call and identifying those who need to be seen by physicians, nurse practitioners, or other providers. Nurses may also provide routine treatments, including medication, under agency protocols. Nursing in correctional settings operates within the constraints of the security system, which may contribute to increased job stress and frustration. Another source of stress is the fear of litigation by a population that is prone to threats of lawsuits (Morgan, 2003). Although there is some risk to the nurse's physical safety, many correctional nurses feel safer than they would in other settings such as emergency departments.

Another source of stress in the correctional setting is the potential for conflict between nursing values and

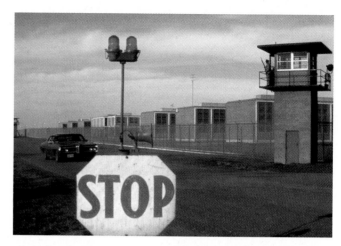

Providing health care to inmates of correctional settings presents multiple challenges. (John Bryson/Getty)

those of corrections personnel. Differences in values frequently give rise to the need for community health nursing advocacy in correctional settings to ensure that health care needs are balanced with custodial and security needs. For example, the primary concerns of the nurse are health care and meeting the health needs of inmates. For custodial personnel, however, the primary concern must be security. The priority placed on security may often make it difficult for the nurse to meet inmates' needs. For instance, giving medications such as insulin in a timely fashion may be impeded by security measures like lockdowns, when nurses are not ordinarily allowed into the areas where inmates are housed. Similarly, nurses may be expected to share information obtained while taking a health history (e.g., past drug use) with custodial or law enforcement personnel, when confidentiality and privacy are primary values of the nursing profession.

Correctional nursing takes place in three general types of facilities: prisons, jails, and juvenile detention facilities. **Prisons** are state and federal facilities that house persons convicted of crimes, usually those sentenced for longer than one year (Wolfe et al., 2001). Municipal or county facilities are usually called **jails** and house both convicted inmates and detainees. Convicted inmates in jails are usually serving sentences under a year in length. **Detainees** are people who have not yet been convicted of a crime. They are being detained pending a trial either because they cannot pay the set bail or because no bail has been set. They may also have violated the terms of probation or parole (National Center for HIV, STD, and TB Prevention, 2005). **Juvenile detention facilities** house children and adolescents convicted of crimes and those who are awaiting trial but who cannot be released in the custody of a responsible adult. Jails and juvenile detention facilities tend to be smaller and house fewer inmates than prisons.

Whatever the size of the facility or the terminology used, nurses working in correctional facilities must be committed to the belief that inmates retain their individual rights as human beings despite incarceration and that they have the same rights to health care as any other individual. Society does not categorically deprive any other group of individuals of access to adequate health care. In fact, there are carefully monitored standards of health care in such institutions as nursing homes, mental health facilities, and orphanages. It has only been as recently as 1979, however, that a program for accrediting health services in prisons was developed by the American Medical Association. Development of accreditation standards occurred at the request of the U.S. Department of Justice following a landmark court decision that depriving inmates of access to health care violated their civil rights (Stringer, 2001). Only since 1985 have published standards for nursing practice in such settings been available (American Nurses Association, 1985).

THE CORRECTIONAL POPULATION

On any given day, more than 2 million people are housed in U.S. correctional institutions, but as many as 10 million people may pass through the local, state, and federal correctional systems each year (Paris, 2005). At midyear 2004, there were 2.1 million inmates in U.S. prisons and jails, with approximately two thirds of this number housed in state and federal prisons and one third in local jails (Bureau of Justice Statistics [BJS], 2005d).

Incarceration rates have increased dramatically in the United States. From 1925 to 1973, rates remained relatively stable at 110 per 100,000 population (Travis, Solomon, & Waul, 2001). By the end of 2004, this figure had risen to 486 per 100,000 population or one of every 138 Americans (BJS, 2005e, 2005f; Golembeski & Fullilove, 2005), and if current rates of incarceration continue, 6.6% of all people born in the United States in 2001 will spend some time in prison during their lives (BJS, 2003a). Despite increases in bed capacity, local jails are operating at 94% of their capacity (BJS, 2005c). Federal and state facilities are over capacity with many facilities engaging in "double celling," a practice of placing more inmates in cells than are allowed based on national standards (Restum, 2005).

There are several reasons for this marked increase in correctional populations. First, there have been significant changes in sentencing guidelines, with mandatory sentences for specific crimes. In addition, criminal justice agencies have taken a more punitive approach to crime reduction, incarcerating more first-time offenders than in the past (Golembeski & Fullilove, 2005). Other reasons for the increase include longer sentences and less opportunity for discretionary release by parole boards, resulting in more inmates serving their entire sentences than in the past (BJS, 2003b). As a result, the United States now has the dubious distinction of having the highest rate of incarceration in the developed world (Restum, 2005).

From 1994 to 2004, the rate of incarceration for violent crime decreased significantly, with more convictions for drug and property offenses than for violent crimes (BJS, 2005a). Based on 2004 figures, incidence rates for rape were 1 per 1,000 population, and for assault with injury and robbery 2 per 1,000. Murder rates were 6 per 100,000 population in 2003 (BJS, 2005b).

THE NEED FOR HEALTH CARE IN CORRECTIONAL SETTINGS

Health care in correctional facilities is an appropriate endeavor for several reasons. First, the right to adequate health care is a constitutionally recognized right arising from the Eighth Amendment, which prohibits "cruel and unusual punishment" of those convicted of crimes. Detainees also have a constitutional right to health care under the Fifth and Fourteenth Amendments, which prohibit punishment of any kind without "due process" (e.g., conviction through the normal legal processes of the nation). In 1976, the U.S. Supreme Court handed down a decision that failure to provide adequate health care to correctional populations constituted unusual punishment and violated their constitutional rights (Weiskopf, 2005).

In addition to the constitutional right to health care, correctional care is good common sense for a variety of other reasons. Because of poverty, lower education levels, and unhealthy lifestyles that frequently involve substance abuse, inmates may enter a correctional facility with significant health problems. Because many of these individuals cannot afford to pay for care on the outside, the cost of care will be borne by society. Societal costs for this care will be lower if interventions occur in a timely fashion, before health problems become severe. Provision of care within the correctional facility also saves taxpayers the cost of personnel and vehicles to transport inmates to other health care facilities. Primary prevention in correctional settings is also cost-effective.

Another possible societal cost of failure to provide adequate health care to inmates lies in the potential for the spread of communicable disease from correctional facilities to the community (Inmate Infections Spread, 2005). Environmental conditions and behaviors within correctional facilities lend themselves to the transmission of communicable diseases such as tuberculosis. When inmates are released back into society, they may constitute a source of infection for the rest of the population.

Finally, correctional settings have been described as "inherently unhealthy environments" (Brodie, 2000, p. 15) and may themselves give rise to a variety of health problems. Correctional environments limit inmate autonomy;

MediaLink Interview with Author of *Acres of Skin* (video)

promote social isolation and communicable diseases; limit exercise; and foster boredom, stress, hostility, and depression. Services are needed to deal with these effects of incarceration as well as the myriad health problems inmates bring with them to correctional settings.

THE EPIDEMIOLOGY OF HEALTH AND ILLNESS IN CORRECTIONAL SETTINGS

Factors in each of the six dimensions of health influence the health status of clients and staff in correctional settings. The nurse assesses factors related to the biophysical, psychological, physical environmental, sociocultural, behavioral, and health system dimensions to identify health problems and to direct interventions to resolve those problems.

Biophysical Considerations

In the biophysical dimension, the nurse in the correctional setting needs to assess individual clients for existing physical health problems. He or she also needs to identify problems that have a high incidence and prevalence in the overall institutional population. Particular areas to be considered include the age, gender, and ethnic composition of the population and evidence of existing physical health problems as well as the population's immune status.

Age and Aging

Correctional populations vary greatly in their composition. The age group most likely to have ever been incarcerated is people aged 35 to 39 years (BJS, 2003a). Despite this majority, however, there are growing numbers of youth and the elderly in U.S. correctional facilities. In 2003, 2.2 million juveniles were arrested and 1.1 million cases were referred to juvenile courts. At any given time, more than 104,000 youth are incarcerated in juvenile correctional facilities (Teplin, Abram, McClelland, Washburn, & Pikus, 2005). Children and adolescents account for 17% of all arrests and 15% of arrests for violent crimes in the United States. Although these figures may seem high, the number of juvenile arrests for violent crimes actually decreased 47% from 1994 to 2002. In contrast, arrests for driving while under the influence of alcohol or drugs (DUI) increased 46% from 1993 to 2002, and drug abuse violations increased by 59% (Snyder, 2004). At midyear 2004, more than 7,000 youth were being held in local jails, and 2,477 state prisoners were under 18 years of age (BJS, 2005d). Juveniles are more apt to commit crimes in groups rather than alone and are more likely than adults to be arrested for violations (Snyder, 2004).

Juvenile inmates tend to have higher prevalence rates of a variety of physical and mental health conditions than their counterparts in the general population and usually have less access to care prior to incarceration. In one study, for example, 43% of juveniles

in detention centers had no previous health care provider and reported high rates of sexual abuse and sexual activity. Asthma was noted in 27% of the population, dental caries in 19%, sexually transmitted diseases in 12%, and scrotal masses were found in 11% of the youth (National Commission on Correctional Health Care [NCCHC], 2001b). Other studies have noted high incidence and prevalence rates for fractures, injuries, and chlamydial infection (Head, Kelly, Bair, Baillargeon, & German, 2000), as well as menstrual disorders, pregnancy, somatic complaints, and skin problems (American Academy of Pediatrics [AAP], 2001).

Incarcerated youth also display significant levels of mental illness and substance abuse. An estimated 15% of juvenile inmates display major mental disorders with functional impairment, but only about 15% of these receive treatment while incarcerated (Teplin et al., 2005). Identifying and treating mental health problems in juveniles in correctional settings may be complicated by their tendencies to minimize or exaggerate or fabricate symptoms. Many juvenile offenders may minimize mental health problems out of fear of being victimized if they are seen as weak or "crazy" or a desire to avoid administrative measures such as increased surveillance. Conversely, some youth may fabricate mental illness to receive psychotropic drugs or to induce peers to avoid them (Boesky, 2003).

Because of the move to try more juveniles as adults, particularly for violent crimes, the number of youth incarcerated in adult correctional facilities is growing. Because of the potential for victimization by older and stronger inmates, younger inmates should be in areas segregated both visually and auditorily (Shimkus, 2004b).

Incarcerated youth have different needs than adult inmates. For example, they have greater nutritional needs than adults (Shimkus, 2004b). In addition, correctional protocols are often based on the needs of adult inmates. For example, juvenile suicide prevention plans and staff training are often modeled on information from adult prisoners or from youth in the community and may not be effective with incarcerated youth (Hayes, 2004). Because of these differences, the National Commission on Correctional Health Care (NCCHC) (1999) has developed standards for juvenile detention facilities separate from those for adult facilities. Elements of these standards are presented as special considerations on page 729. In addition, the standards for adult correctional facilities include an appendix addressing the special needs of youth incarcerated in adult facilities (Shimkus, 2004b). The American Academy of Pediatrics (2001) has adopted a statement on care of juvenile offenders that includes the following recommendations:

- Incarcerated youth should receive care in keeping with AAP general guidelines for health supervision of children and adolescents, including immunization, care for psychosocial issues, and development of a "medical home."

- All youth should receive regular preventive services during incarceration.
- Incarcerated youth should receive prenatal services, parenting classes, and tobacco, alcohol, and other drug cessation services as needed.
- Pediatricians should be involved in policy development for incarcerated youth.
- Correctional personnel dealing with juvenile offenders should be specifically trained to address their needs.
- Youth incarcerated in adult settings should be segregated from the adult population by both sight and sound and should receive developmentally appropriate services.

Community health nurses may need to advocate for the application of these sets of standards and recommendations in the care of the juvenile correctional population.

The fastest-growing segment of corrections populations is the elderly, primarily because of extended sentences, with a large proportion of the population growing old in the correctional setting (Hills, Siegfried, &

SPECIAL CONSIDERATIONS

AREAS ADDRESSED BY NCCHC STANDARDS FOR JUVENILE CORRECTIONAL FACILITIES

- Access to care
- Communication and confidentiality
- Continuity of care
- Credentialing and orientation of staff
- Diet
- Emergency plans and procedures
- Employment of juvenile workers
- Environmental health and safety
- Exercise
- Grievances
- Hygiene
- Infection control
- Informed consent
- Kitchen sanitation
- Pharmaceuticals and medication administration
- Policies and procedures
- Research
- Reporting and notification
- Services (assessment, screening, diagnosis, treatment, oral health, mental health, health education and promotion, family planning, emergency, special needs)
- Staffing levels
- Sexual assault
- Substance abuse
- Suicide prevention
- Therapeutic restraint

Data from: National Commission on Correctional Health Care. (1999). A summary guide to revisions in the 1999 Standards for Health Services in Juvenile Detention and Confinement Facilities. Correct Care, 13(2), 18–19.

Ickowitz, 2004). The number of elderly inmates in state prisons increased more than 200% over a 10-year period (Richardson, 2003). People over 50 years of age are considered "old" in correctional systems due to the accelerated aging that occurs in correctional populations. In fact, the biological age of inmates over age 50 is, on average, 11.5 years more than their chronological age. This accelerated aging process is due to life histories that often include substance abuse and withdrawal, poor health care, and high-risk behaviors as well as the stress of incarceration (Shimkus, 2004a).

In 2004, people over 55 years of age constituted 5% of the state and federal prison population (BJS, 2005f) and nearly 4% of persons held in local jails (BJS, 2005d). Both medical and mental health problems increase in older clients. For example, approximately 40% of inmates over age 45 have been found to have medical problems, compared to 12% of those under age 24 years. Similarly, the incidence of mental health problems in inmates over 45 years of age was 48%, compared to 24% in the younger group (Maruschak & Beck, 2001). Common problems include incontinence, sensory impairments, limited mobility, respiratory disease, cardiovascular disease, and cancer. Other conditions experienced by this group are similar to those found in older populations in the community and include arthritis, hypertension, ulcers, and prostate disease (Shimkus, 2004a). Correctional facilities are often unprepared to address the health care needs of older inmates, nor are budgets designed to accommodate these needs. For example, it is estimated that health care costs for elderly inmates are approximately three times those for younger age groups (Hills et al., 2004) and may rise to as much as $60,000 to $70,000 per person per year (Shimkus, 2004a). Community health nurses may need to be actively involved in assuring that facilities and services are available to meet the needs of elderly inmates as well as to protect them from victimization by younger inmates.

Gender and Ethnicity

In 2004, women constituted 10% of the state and federal correctional population and 12% of the local jail population, but the rate of incarceration for women is growing faster than that for men. For example, the rate of incarceration among women has increased by 5% per year since 1995, compared to a 3.3% increase among men. The rate of incarceration among U.S. women in 2004 was 123 per 100,000 women; the rate for men was 1,348 per 100,000 (BJS, 2005d). Overall, there was a 313% increase in incarceration among women from 1981, compared to a 182% increase for men.

Similar differences are noted among incarcerated youth, with boys accounting for 71% and girls for 29% of juvenile arrests, but arrest rates are increasing faster for female juveniles than males. For example, DUI arrests from 1993 to 2002 rose 94% for girls versus 37% for boys. Similarly, drug abuse violations increased 120% for girls and only 51% for boys, and aggravated assault arrests increased 7% among adolescent girls, but decreased by 29% among boys in the same time period (Snyder, 2004). Women tend to be arrested more often for minor property crimes and drug offenses than violent crimes (Braithwaite, Treadwell, & Arriola, 2005).

Women inmates often have high rates of physical and mental health problems such as histories of physical and sexual abuse and early initiation of sexual intercourse and drug and alcohol use. Incarcerated women also have more unplanned and frequent pregnancies than women in the community and higher rates of STD, depression, suicide attempts, and dental problems (Newkirk, 2003). Female prisoners have twice the rates of mental illness as males, and in approximately one fourth of women, alcohol or drug use was associated with the offense for which they were arrested (Wagaman, 2003).

Incarcerated women are more likely to be unmarried, divorced, or separated than their community-dwelling counterparts, and have lower educational and economic levels than male inmates. Approximately 65% of women inmates are parents of minor children (Wagaman, 2003), and an estimated 1.3 million U.S. children have a mother who has been incarcerated. As many as 5% to 10% of women enter correctional systems pregnant, but few of them have received prenatal care prior to incarceration (Braithwaite et al., 2005). Prenatal services while incarcerated may be inadequate, with little prenatal education or availability of abortion or contraceptive services if desired. Conversely, some pregnant inmates report pressure to have an abortion when it is not desired. Women inmates have higher rates of low-birth-weight (LBW) babies than the general population, but the incidence of LBW among this population is similar to that of other high-risk populations (Mertens, 2001).

Women inmates have special needs not experienced by men. For example, they require both routine and nonroutine gynecologic care and have more difficulty with sleep disturbances due to anxiety and apprehension than men. In addition, their nutritional needs differ, and women tend to gain weight in correctional settings because the typical correctional diet is designed for more active men. Similarly, pain management needs may be influenced by higher levels of depression. Women's substance abuse treatment needs also differ from men's, and treatment often must address their histories of trauma and abuse (Wagaman, 2003). Women are more likely to request health care and mental health services than men, so staff levels in these areas may need to be higher than in facilities for men (Newkirk, 2003). Unfortunately, because they are fewer in number, incarcerated women are less visible than men (Braithwaite et al., 2005) and services may be less available. Because of gender socialization, women inmates may also be less able to articulate and advocate for themselves (Hills et al.,

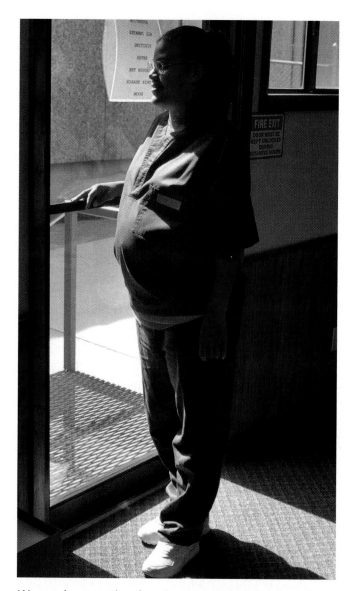

Women in correctional settings may have special needs, including care during pregnancy. (© Sean Cayton/The Image Works)

2004), leading to a need for community health nursing advocacy to assure that their health and social service needs are met.

Men and women also respond differently to the experience of being incarcerated. Men have been found to be most distressed by the loss of freedom, social rejection and loss of social status, autonomy, and self-control. Women, on the other hand, have similar concerns, but consider separation from family to be the most difficult aspect of incarceration. Other areas of concern for women include the constant stress of living in close proximity to others and lack of privacy with respect to personal property, modesty, and invasion of personal space. Men tend to view incarceration as an interruption in their lives, which will proceed normally on their release. Women are more likely to view incarceration as a significant change in their lives (Wagaman, 2003). Women, in particular, need support in dealing with family separation and in maintaining family relationships. Unfortunately, because of fewer numbers, women's correctional facilities are less likely to be located close to their place of residence than men's facilities (Braithwaite et al., 2005).

Another issue related to gender in correctional settings is the presence of transgendered individuals in the population. Concerns around transgendered individuals include housing decisions, safety, mental health issues, and maintenance of hormone therapy (American Public Health Association [APHA], 2003). Decisions need to be made whether to place these inmates in male or female housing. It is recommended that they be housed in the general correctional population if possible, with attention given to privacy for hygiene, appropriate clothing, and protection from assault by other inmates (Fry, 2003). These decisions will best be made in light of where the inmate is in the process of transition. Mental health services may also be needed to address issues of gender dysphoria or stigma (APHA, 2003).

Members of ethnic minority groups are disproportionately represented in correctional settings. Approximately 70% of the U.S. correctional population is comprised of minority group members (Paris, 2005), and one fourth of those housed in correctional facilities are African American. Black men are incarcerated at a rate seven times that of White men, and an estimated one in three African American men is under correctional supervision at any point in time (Cooke, 2004). In 2004, for example, 8.4% of all Black males age 24 to 29 were in prison (BJS, 2005f). The 2004 incarceration rate for Black men was 3,218 per 100,000 population compared to 1,220 per 100,000 and 463 per 100,000 for Hispanic and White men, respectively (BJS, 2005e). Similarly, two thirds of incarcerated women are members of ethnic minorities (Braithwaite et al., 2005). These and other similar figures have prompted concerns for inequities and prejudice within the justice system. Whether this is indeed the case, the fact remains that correctional populations are ethnically diverse, which may result in racial tensions within facilities as well as the need for culturally sensitive health care. Community health nurses may need to actively advocate for correctional health care services that meet the needs of a culturally and linguistically diverse population as well as advocate for fair treatment for all inmates regardless of ethnicity.

Physiologic Function

Environmental conditions and behavioral patterns in correctional settings foster the spread of communicable diseases. Although many communicable diseases are found in this population, four of particular concern are tuberculosis (TB), HIV infection and AIDS, hepatitis, and other sexually transmitted diseases (STDs). Nearly 4% of all TB diagnosed in the United States occurs among correctional inmates. Overall TB incidence is 5 times higher in state and federal prisons than in the general public (MacNeil, Lobato, & Moore, 2005), and may be as much as 6 to 15 times higher in some states (Francis J. Curry National Tuberculosis Center, 2003). Overcrowding and generally poor health status are two of the factors that promote the spread of tuberculosis (TB) in inmate populations. Moreover, co-infection with both TB and HIV is occurring in large segments of some correctional populations (Francis J. Curry National Tuberculosis Center, 2003). Additional complicating factors in the problem of tuberculosis in correctional facilities are the prevalence of multi-drug-resistant (MDR) tuberculosis and the tendency of inmates not to complete a full course of treatment. In some studies, for example, the rate of treatment completion among inmates is 59%, compared to 73% in the general population (MacNeil et al., 2005).

A large portion of all persons with tuberculosis will enter a correctional facility at some point. For example, in one year 40% of all persons with TB were admitted to a correctional facility during that year (Hammett, Harmon, & Rhodes, 2002). This makes correctional facilities ideal settings for minimizing the spread of TB in the general population. Community health nurses working in correctional settings should assess inmates for signs of tuberculosis as well as provide routine screenings for TB according to agency policy. Tuberculin skin test screening in jails may be inappropriate for many inmates who stay only one or two days, so the nurse should ask about TB symptomatology and history of exposure during the intake assessment to isolate potentially infectious inmates.

HIV infection and confirmed cases of AIDS are another growing problem in correctional facilities. Many inmates are at increased risk of infection because of injection drug use, and the potential for exposure during incarceration via continued drug use and homosexual activity is high. HIV prevalence peaked at rates 13 times those of the general population (Golembeski & Fullilove, 2005), but current rates are approximately five times those of the general population (Heines, 2005). Overall, rates for confirmed cases of AIDS are four times higher in correctional populations than on the outside (Braithwaite & Arriola, 2003). HIV infection rates are higher among incarcerated women than among men (Bauserman et al., 2003). For example, 3.4% of female prisoners in state correctional facilities in 2001 were HIV positive, compared to 2.2% of men (Bauserman, Ward, Eldred, & Swetz, 2001). Like TB, approximately 40% of people with HIV infection pass through correctional systems each year (Paris, 2005), making this setting a good place to identify them and initiate treatment.

Rates of HIV infection and AIDS diagnoses vary from one area of the country to another, and nurses should be aware of the overall prevalence of infection in their jurisdictions. Corrections nurses should assess all inmates for a history of HIV infection, high-risk behaviors, and a history or symptoms of possible opportunistic infections. In addition, community health nurses should advocate for effective treatment for HIV-infected inmates during incarceration and following their release into the community.

Drug use behaviors contribute to the increased incidence of tuberculosis and HIV infection in inmates. Such behaviors also place inmates at risk for other STDs and hepatitis B (HBV) and C (HCV). In addition to drug use, sexual activity and tattooing are other risk factors for HBV and HCV common in correctional populations. The prevalence of HBV infection in adult inmates ranges from 13% to 47% in different populations. As many as 1% to 3.7% of inmates may develop chronic HBV infection, a rate two to six times that of the general population. The incidence of new HBV infections in correctional settings may be as high as 3.8% per year, arguing for spread of disease during incarceration (Division of Viral Hepatitis, 2004c). Hepatitis C infection rates are nine to ten times higher in correctional populations than in the general public (Heines, 2005; Travis et al., 2001). In one study, prevalence rates for HIV, HBV, and HCV infection in a correctional population were 1.8%, 20.2%, and 23.1%, respectively (Macalino et al., 2004). In assessing individual inmates for health problems, the nurse should ask about a history of STDs and hepatitis B and C and should be alert to the presence of physical signs and symptoms of these diseases.

Other communicable diseases are also prevalent in correctional populations. For example, methicillin-resistant *Staphylococcus aureus* (MRSA) is a common occurrence in institutional settings, including jails and prisons (Tobin-D'Angelo et al., 2003). Similarly, *Chlamydia trachomatis* infection has been found in 22% of girls and 9% of boys admitted to juvenile detention facilities (Head et al., 2000). Higher syphilis rates are also found in correctional settings than in the general population (Wolfe et al., 2001).

Chronic illnesses of particular concern in correctional settings include diabetes, hypertension, heart disease, and chronic lung conditions such as asthma. Seizure disorders are also common, and inmates may also exhibit seizure activity during withdrawal from drugs and alcohol. Diabetes may be particularly difficult to control given the rigid structure of the correctional routine and the need to time hypoglycemic medications, meals, and exercise periods appropriately. The availability of vending machines and the use of commissary privileges as a reward may also complicate dietary control for inmates with diabetes. Many inmates with chronic conditions, particularly those with substance abuse problems, enter the correctional facility after prolonged periods without medications or may not know what medications they have been taking. In many instances, the nurse has to exert considerable ingenuity

to obtain an accurate health history from clients, family members, and health care providers in the community. Because of poor overall health status, inmates may also be especially susceptible to exacerbations of chronic conditions. The nurse should assess individual inmates for existing chronic conditions and should also identify problems with high incidence and prevalence in the correctional population with whom he or she works.

Injury is another area of physiologic function that should be assessed by the nurse. Injury may result from activities preceding arrest, from actions taken by arresting officers, or from accidents or assaults occurring during incarceration. The nurse should be aware of the potential for internal as well as visible injuries and should assess inmates for signs of trauma. Slightly more than one fourth of state and federal inmates reported injuries that occurred during their incarceration. Approximately two thirds of injuries were due to accidents, and the balance were related to fighting (Maruschak & Beck, 2001).

Dental health problems are also common among inmates. One particular problem that nurses in correction settings may encounter is a condition called "meth mouth." Meth mouth is characterized by severe erosion and decay of teeth and usually requires emergency dental services. Meth mouth results from several factors associated with methamphetamine use including gnashing of the teeth, poor oral hygiene, and dry mouth, which increases the acidic effects of methamphetamine. Methamphetamine use also leads to cravings for high-caffeine, high-sugar soft drinks that further contribute to tooth decay. In some correctional systems, meth mouth has been credited with doubling correctional health care costs over a 4-year period. The high demand for emergency dental services has also resulted in long waits for routine services by other inmates (Brunswick, 2005).

Pregnancy is the final biophysical consideration in assessing the health of correctional populations. As noted earlier, the number of female inmates increases annually. Because of prior drug use and poor health care, pregnant women in correctional settings may be at higher risk for poor pregnancy outcomes than women in the general population. Conversely, incarceration may improve pregnancy outcomes because it interrupts drug use and provides access to prenatal care that the women might not otherwise have. Care of pregnant women in correctional settings, however, is often hampered by lack of special diets to support pregnancy, lack of exercise, and inappropriate work assignments. Fetal health may also be compromised by problems encountered in drug and alcohol withdrawal in the correctional setting. Finally, the timely transfer of women in labor to obstetrical facilities is often hampered by the security constraints of the correctional facility (Fulco, 2001).

In assessing female inmates, the nurse should ask about the last menstrual period and solicit any symptoms of possible pregnancy. Because drug use can interfere with menses, menstrual history is not always reliable for indicating pregnancy or for suggesting length of gestation when pregnancy is confirmed. The nurse should also ask about high-risk behavior that may affect the fetus such as smoking, drug and alcohol use, and so on. The pregnant inmate's nutritional status should also be assessed. Other physical problems common in this population that may affect pregnancy outcomes include urinary tract infections and STDs, and the nurse should assess for symptoms of these conditions. Depression and anxiety are also common phenomena among these women. Advocacy may be required to assure adequate prenatal and perinatal care for pregnant inmates. For example, community health nurses may need to convince correctional personnel of the necessity of keeping outside appointments for high-risk pregnancy care, even when these require pulling security personnel away from the correctional facility.

Psychological Considerations

Psychological dimension factors can have a profound influence on health in correctional settings. The presence of mental illness in the correctional population is one of the major psychological factors influencing the health of this population. An estimated 16% of state prison inmates have serious mental illness or have been previously hospitalized for a psychiatric condition, and another 15% to 20% require some mental health care. Mentally ill inmates are often significantly disabled by their conditions and have a more difficult time adjusting to prison life than other inmates. Inmates are nearly four times more likely than the general population to experience schizophrenia, and approximately 6% of inmates have bipolar disorder. Major depression is present in approximately 9% of inmates and general anxiety disorders (including post-traumatic stress disorder [PTSD]) in 6%. Psychiatric disorders are more common in women inmates than men, with 34% of women experiencing PTSD and 17% experiencing major depression. Overall, as much as 80% of women inmates may have a lifetime history of one or more psychiatric disorders (Hills et al., 2004).

Juvenile inmates also experience high rates of mental illness, including attention deficit hyperactivity disorder (ADHD), conduct disorder, oppositional-defiant disorder, depression, and PTSD. Oppositional-defiant disorder is characterized by a consistent pattern of negative, hostile, and defiant behavior, whereas conduct disorder is the result of a basic disregard for rules and norms of behavior and for the rights of others (Boesky, 2003). Attempted suicide is a particularly prevalent problem among incarcerated youth, and as noted earlier, suicide prevention programs may not be designed to effectively address the needs of young inmates.

The high rates of PTSD in women and youth can be explained, in part, by past history of abuse. Approximately 25% to 31% of incarcerated youth have a history of abuse and neglect (American Academy of Pediatrics, 2001), and 50% to 80% of women inmates have been abused at some point in their lives (Wagaman, 2003).

Another 7% to 15% of young offenders may be mentally retarded, and an additional 17% to 53% may experience learning disabilities and other developmental disorders (American Academy of Pediatrics, 2001). The prevalence of mental retardation in correctional settings is two to three times that of the general population (Hills et al., 2004). Mentally retarded individuals, particularly youth, may be persuaded to participate in group crimes in order to be accepted by their peers without fully realizing the consequences of their actions. Developmentally disabled inmates may display deficits in both cognitive/intellectual function and adaptive capabilities, leading to greater difficulty adjusting to life in a correctional facility (Richardson, 2003). Because of their diminished mental capabilities, this group of inmates may have difficulty understanding instructions and display impulsivity and low frustration tolerance, earning them frequent punishment for infractions in the correctional setting (Hills et al., 2004). Mentally retarded inmates may be a subgroup in the correctional setting that requires particular advocacy on the part of community health nurses to assist them in their adjustment and to help correctional personnel recognize their limitations.

The increasing proportion of mentally ill persons in correctional institutions has several explanations (Broner, Borum, & Gawley, 2002; Fagan, 2003). "Get tough" philosophies and public initiatives that target nuisance crimes lead to more incarcerations, including among those with mental illness. Deinstitutionalization and the resulting closure of many locked psychiatric wards shifted mentally ill persons who could not cope with community living to jails and prisons. It is proposed by some that there may be as many as three times the number of mentally ill individuals in correctional settings as in mental hospitals (Bell, 2005). Some authors have described correctional institutions as a "safety net" for the care of the mentally ill (Cutler, Bigelow, Collins, Jackson, & Field, 2002). In addition, the federal "war on drugs" and the extent of co-occurring mental illness and substance abuse disorder put many mentally ill persons at increased risk of incarceration for drug offenses. Approximately 70% of mentally ill inmates also abuse alcohol and other drugs (Bell, 2005). Homelessness among the mentally ill and inability to compete for existing low-income housing also leads to their arrest and conviction, often for minimal crimes. Some studies have indicated that the mentally ill are more likely to be incarcerated than non-mentally ill offenders (Heines, 2005). Finally, the mentally ill have few legitimate economic opportunities, putting them at risk for criminal behavior to survive. In fact, in one study, 64% of persons discharged from mental hospitals were involved in some sort of criminal activity shortly after their discharge (Cutler et al., 2002).

By law, inmates are entitled to mental health services as well as medical treatment. Mental health services, however, may be lacking in some correctional systems, or the need for these services may go unrecognized. This is particularly true among women inmates, the elderly, and youth. An estimated 75% to 85% of state prisons provide mental health screening, assessment, and treatment services with medication management (Bell, 2005).

Incarceration itself is stressful and can lead to psychological effects, including depression and suicide. Incarceration also exacerbates existing mental illness. Correctional nurses should be alert to signs of depression and other mental or emotional distress in inmates, and assessment of suicide potential is a critical part of every intake interview. Suicide is the leading cause of death in jails and "lockups," and is the cause of nearly 100% of deaths among incarcerated juveniles. A **lockup** is a temporary holding facility in which inmates are placed prior to transportation to a jail or other facility. Suicide rates in prisons, on the other hand, are more or less comparable to those in the general population.

Finally, state and federal prison systems may house a number of inmates who have been sentenced to death, creating a need for emotional and psychological support. Corrections nurses working in systems with "death-row" inmates should assess them for evidence of psychological problems and refer them for counseling as appropriate.

Because of the increasing age of corrections populations, nurses may also encounter clients with terminal conditions in the correctional setting. These clients have the same end-of-life care needs as people in the general population. End-of-life care for terminally ill inmates is discussed in more detail later in this chapter.

Mental health challenges in dealing with correctional populations are many and varied. Some of these challenges include determining who has mental health problems and how they should be treated, managing behavior and symptoms associated with psychiatric illness, and recognizing and dealing with the negative mental health effects of incarceration. Other challenges include understanding the difficulty adjusting to incarceration that might be experienced by inmates with mental illness and determining the need for and providing specialized services (Hills et al., 2004). For example, few correctional settings deal effectively with the mental health needs of older inmates. Similarly, women and youth exposed to psychological trauma need therapy to deal with issues of abuse as well as co-occurring substance abuse. Community health nurses in correctional settings can engage in advocacy to assure that appropriate services are provided to these vulnerable population groups.

Physical Environmental Considerations

Factors in the physical environmental dimension also influence the health of correctional populations. The physical environment of the correctional setting is constrained by the need for security. Inmates may be relegated to specific spaces at specific times of the day. Because of the tremendous growth in the incarcerated population, jails and prisons are extremely overcrowded and few jurisdictions are not in violation of space standards for inmates. For example, at the end of 2003, local jails were at 94% of their capacity. State prisons were at capacity to 16% over capacity, and federal prisons were 39% over capacity (BJS, 2005d). Other physical environmental problems common in correctional settings include poor ventilation, lack of temperature control, and unsanitary conditions. Lack of funds for maintenance may lead to buildings in poor repair, creating safety hazards for both inmates and staff. Other areas that should be assessed by the nurse include the safety of recreational areas, fire protection, lighting, plumbing, solid waste disposal, and safety of the water supply. Additional considerations include vermin control, noise control, and the presence of high levels of radiation.

Because correctional facilities are often situated in areas away from the general population, they may be located in sites with disaster potential such as flooding, earthquake, and so on. The nurse should assess the potential for such disasters as well as the adequacy of the facility's disaster response plan. Disaster potential may also arise from prison industries. Inmate occupations may also present other physical hazards for individual clients that need to be assessed.

Sociocultural Considerations

A wide variety of sociocultural dimension factors influence the health status of correctional populations. An estimated 80% of law enforcement activity addresses social problems, yet police personnel are often ill-equipped to deal with them because of lack of understanding of the underlying dynamics of social problems. Like health care providers in correctional settings, law enforcement personnel may experience conflict between their law enforcement role and a role in resolving social problems. In addition, social problems that lead to criminal activity are given low priority at the societal level (Patterson, 2002). For example, the estimated cost of adequate treatment for persons with mental illness is one third to one half of the cost of incarceration for mentally ill offenders (Meyer, 2003). Sociocultural factors contribute to incarceration, and correctional systems have sociocultural effects on inmates and on the general society.

Particular elements of the sociocultural dimension that influence health in correctional settings include socioeconomic and cultural factors that lead to incarceration, family relationships, the correctional culture, and the potential for violence in the setting.

Socioeconomic and Cultural Influences

To a large extent, correctional populations tend to be at the low end of economic and educational spectrums. It is estimated that every 10% decrease in income is associated with a 10% to 20% greater likelihood of criminal activity and incarceration (Travis et al., 2001). Women offenders, in particular, often come from poverty-stricken neighborhoods with low levels of social capital (Reisig, Holtfreter, & Morash, 2002). Lower socioeconomic status is also associated with worse health status among inmates. For example, unmarried and homeless inmates and those of lower socioeconomic levels have been found to be at higher risk of TB infection than other inmates (Kim & Crittenden, 2005).

Housing is another socioeconomic issue that may contribute to incarceration. As we saw in Chapter 20∞, many activities performed by homeless individuals in ensuring their survival have been criminalized, with the result that they are often arrested for activities that would be tolerated in other members of society. The homeless are overrepresented in correctional populations, and recently released prisoners often become homeless due to poor reentry planning. Incarceration may also lead to homelessness due to the disruption of family and community ties and decreased employment and housing opportunities associated with the stigma of incarceration. In one study, one fourth of homeless individuals had a history of imprisonment, and homeless people who had been incarcerated had higher levels of health risk than other homeless individuals (Kushel, Hahn, Evans, Bangsberg, & Moss, 2005).

As we saw earlier, correctional populations include many minority group members who are frequently culturally and linguistically, as well as economically and educationally, disadvantaged (Paris, 2005). Many more inmates are being incarcerated as a result of immigration offenses than in the past. In fact, from 1995 to 2003 there was a 394% increase in federal incarcerations for immigration offenses, comprising 10% of all federal convictions in 2003 (BJS, 2005f). At midyear 2004, 20% of federal prisoners in the United States were non-citizens (BJS, 2005d).

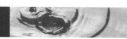
Family Relationships

Concerns for children can be a source of stress for many inmates. Approximately 75% of women inmates have children under 18 years of age (Hills et al., 2004), and the percentage of inmates with minor children increased by 55% over an 8-year period (Thigpen, Hunter, & Watson, 2002). As we saw earlier, separation from families was the most difficult aspect of incarceration for women, yet only slightly more than half of correctional systems consider place of residence and distance from families in placement decisions within the system. Approximately one third of institutions provide family visitation assistance, including help with lodging or transportation. Visitation assistance is more apt to be available in facilities that house men than in those that house women, although women's facilities are more likely to provide special family visitation space (Thigpen et al., 2002).

Women's facilities are twice as likely as men's to provide parenting education, but most such programs are provided without children present, prohibiting inmates from modeling learned skills with their own children (Thigpen et al., 2002). In one study, one third of children with mothers in state prison systems lived with their fathers during their mothers' incarceration; the rest lived with other family members or were placed in foster care. To date little research has been done on the effect of parental incarceration on children (Travis et al., 2001).

Problems caused by separation of children from their mothers have led some correctional facilities to allow young children, particularly newborns, to remain with their mothers in custody. According to a Bureau of Justice report (Thigpen et al., 2002), one fifth of state and large metropolitan departments of corrections house infants and small children with their incarcerated mothers, but only 17% are able to provide outside housing for pregnant women. Areas for concern in these types of programs that need to be addressed by correctional nurses and other correctional personnel include the security of children, liability issues, costs and mechanisms for providing health care and other services for children, the effects of incarceration on child development, charges of discrimination if pregnant and recently delivered inmates receive special consideration, and lack of interest in parenting by some incarcerated women (Fulco, 2001).

Family dynamics may also lead to incarceration, either directly or indirectly. For example, 15% of state prison inmates have been convicted of a violent crime against a family member (Durose et al., 2005). Family violence may also contribute to other criminal activity. In one study, for instance, South African men who observed abuse of their mothers during childhood were more likely to be arrested for physical violence against their partners as adults and for illegal firearms possession (Abrahams & Jewkes, 2005).

The Correctional Culture

The primary purpose of correctional institutions is custody and punishment, not health care. This custodial culture may pose considerable challenges to health care providers who must balance their health care and advocacy roles against security concerns and create a therapeutic environment without being perceived as a "soft touch" by either inmates or corrections personnel (Norman & Parrish, 2000).

Security concerns may also hamper provision of health care. In some institutions, nurses do not have immediate access to inmates unless security personnel are present. In other instances, transportation of inmates for outside services may be postponed if there are insufficient security personnel available to accompany them. There is also the potential for violence against health care providers and their use as hostages.

The nurse should be alert to the use of excessive force or punitive conditions to which inmates may be subjected. Correctional nurses will also assess the extent of social support available to inmates. Social support may arise from interactions and programs available within the correctional system or from continued interactions with persons or agencies outside the system (e.g., family). Development of social support systems may be particularly important for clients about to be released from the facility.

Some correctional facilities have assets that promote rehabilitation and permit inmates to earn some money. In some states, there are even provisions for inmates to work to repay the victims of their crimes. Such opportunities are less readily available to women inmates than men and are rarely adequate to meet the rehabilitation needs of all inmates. The presence of occupational opportunities, however, may contribute to a variety of occupational risks to health that should be assessed by nurses in correctional facilities. Occupational hazards for correctional facility staff, as well as those for inmates, should be considered. Corrections personnel, for example, are at higher risk for infectious disease exposure, with an estimated 3,000 blood-borne disease exposures among corrections personnel each year (Gershon, 2002). Physical and psychological safety considerations also present the need for constant vigilance among health care and other personnel in correctional settings (Weiskopf, 2005).

Violence and Abuse

As noted earlier, violence may lead to incarceration. Similarly, exposure to violence and abuse in one's past may increase the risk of incarceration, particularly among women and youth. Violence also occurs within correctional settings. Younger, smaller inmates or those with nonheterosexual orientations may be subjected to abuse by other inmates or by correctional personnel. Rates of sexual abuse of homosexual inmates may be as high as 41%, approximately four times that of the general inmate population (Coolman & Eisenman, 2003). Elderly, mentally ill, and mentally retarded inmates are also vulnerable to abuse within correctional settings. Inmates subjected to violence may need to be segregated from other inmates to ensure their safety, but isolation may result in creation or exacerbation of poor psychological response to incarceration. Community health nurses can be advocates for protection of these inmates in ways that promote rather than impair their mental health.

Inmates may also be abused by correctional staff (Braithwaite et al., 2005), and community health nurses working in correctional settings should be alert to signs of abuse. Women inmates in particular may be coerced to provide sexual favors in return for privileges (Coolman & Eisenman, 2003).

Behavioral Considerations

Behavioral dimension factors that influence the health of inmates and staff in correctional settings include diet, substance abuse, smoking, opportunities for exercise and recreation, and sexual activity. Inmates are more likely than the general public to engage in tobacco use and alcohol and drug use and abuse. With little to occupy their time, inmates may find themselves smoking more after incarceration than before. Smoking coupled with overcrowding, lack of exercise, and inadequate diet may increase inmates' risk of both communicable and chronic diseases. Access to tobacco is also a traditional reward for compliant behavior in correctional settings. Approximately 75% of all inmates smoke, far higher than the 23% of the general population, and only a few correctional facilities have or enforce smoking bans or promote smoke-free environments. Even when such bans do exist, 79% of them involve tobacco use only by inmates and do not include staff. Health care providers tend to see other addictive behaviors as having higher priority than smoking cessation, and 80% of corrections systems surveyed in one study do not provide smoking cessation programs or cessation aids (e.g., nicotine patches) (Porter, 2005). In 2004, California banned smoking, chewing tobacco, and snuff by inmates and staff in all state prisons and youth correctional facilities (NCCHC, 2004b).

Alcohol and other substance abuse is also common among correctional populations. One fourth of state prison inmates have been incarcerated for drug-related offenses (Brunswick, 2005), and 80% of the state correctional population has a history of drug and alcohol use, half of them at the time of commission of the crime for which they were incarcerated (Travis et al., 2001). Similarly, drug offenses accounted for 55% of federal convictions in 2003 (BJS, 2005f). In 2004, in 30% of all victimizations involving violent crimes, the perpetrator was using alcohol, and two thirds of intimate partner violence involves alcohol. In 20% of these crimes other drug use was also implicated (BJS, 2005a). An estimated 12% of all arrestees are alcohol dependent and as many as 4% may be addicted to opiates, yet only 28% of U.S. jail administrators surveyed reported detoxification of arrestees (Fiscella, Pless, Meldrum, & Fiscella, 2004).

The correctional nurse should assess substance use and abuse in individual clients as well as in the inmate population as a whole. The nurse should also assess nutritional status and particular dietary needs for individual inmates (e.g., those with diabetes). Nurses may need to advocate for special diets to accommodate medical or religious needs. Types of diets that may be needed include kosher diets, low-salt diets, diabetic diets, consistency-modified diets, allergy diets, bland diets, and diets to address specific renal problems or gastric reflux. Recently, there has been a trend toward the use of heart-healthy diets for the general inmate population as well (Wakeen & Roper, 2002), and community health nurses can advocate for such general dietary changes in correctional settings.

Sexual behaviors prior to and during incarceration can also influence inmate health status. Early initiation of sexual activity is common among inmate populations (e.g., before age 13) (Head et al., 2000), and 85% of infections such as HIV, HBV, and HCV are associated with preincarceration behaviors including sexual behavior and injection drug use (IDU) (Macalino et al., 2004). Among incarcerated youth, 90% of males in one study were sexually active, and more than 60% reported multiple sexual partners. Boys were more likely than girls to engage in high-risk sexual behaviors, but overall 95% of the study population engaged in three or more high-risk behaviors and 65% engaged in 10 or more such behaviors (Teplin, Mericle, McClelland, & Abram, 2003).

Sexual activity also occurs within the correctional setting. Such behavior may be consensual or nonconsensual, and high-risk behaviors such as anal intercourse are common (Restum, 2005). As many as 33% of inmates may be sexually assaulted while incarcerated (Macalino et al., 2004). Some authors note that "same-sex encounters during incarceration are defined as situational in nature and therefore not an individual or sustained sexual orientation" (Braithwaite & Arriola, 2003), so prevention messages targeted toward the gay and bisexual population may not be perceived as relevant to the general inmate population. Lack of access to condoms and the prevalence of STDs in correctional populations promotes

the spread of disease to others in the setting. For example, a 3.6% rate of new cases of HBV in one correctional study provides strong evidence for in-house transmission of disease (Kahn et al., 2005). The nurse should assess the extent of sexual activity among the correctional population and the availability and use of condoms within correctional systems. Nurses may also need to advocate for provision of condoms to sexually active inmates.

Other behavioral dimension factors that should be assessed include opportunities for and participation in exercise and recreational activities. Potential safety hazards posed by exercise and recreation activities should also be assessed.

Health System Considerations

Factors in the health system dimension also influence the health status of correctional populations. Correctional facilities are the only settings in which people have a constitutional right to health care (Treadwell & Ro, 2002). Because many inmates enter the correctional setting with multiple health problems, the adequacy of the correctional health care system has a significant influence on the health status of the population. Depending on several factors, including size and financial capabilities, correctional facilities may take one of two approaches to the provision of health care services for inmates. Services may be provided in-house by staff employed by the facility, or the agency may contract with other provider agencies for needed services. In many institutions, a combination of both approaches is used.

Whatever the approach used, a public health model of correctional health services would address assessment and early detection of health problems, treatment for existing conditions, prevention, health education, and continuity of care (Conklin, Lincoln, Wilson, & Gramarossa, 2003). Table 26-1◆ presents emphases related to each of these areas.

Specific areas to be addressed in the correctional health care system include health promotion and illness prevention services, medical and dental services, mental health services, and emergency response capabilities. Health promotion services will be discussed in more detail in the section on primary prevention in correctional settings. Minimum medical services should include screening, diagnostic, treatment, and follow-up services. Services begin with an initial health screening on admission to the facility. This initial screening is a brief immediate evaluation of whether it is safe to admit the inmate to the facility given his or her current health status. The initial screening also facilitates correct placement of the inmate within the facility, initiates planning to meet identified health needs, and provides aggregate data for use in overall program planning. Areas to be addressed in this screening include, at a minimum, evidence of infectious disease, existing health problems,

TABLE 26-1 Components and Emphases in the Public Health Model for Correctional Health Care

Component	Emphases	Component	Emphases
Detection and assessment	• Initial booking assessment • Dental health assessment • Mental health assessment • Information on accessing services in correctional system	Prevention (cont.)	• Immunization • Cessation counseling and relapse prevention to prevent long-term consequences of tobacco and other substance use • Dental health education • Prenatal care for pregnant inmates • Occupational health and safety for inmate workers and staff • Facility-wide smoking ban • Suicide prevention training for staff • Exercise and nutrition education for inmates and staff
Treatment	• Individualized treatment plan for identified health needs • Provision of pharmacy medications • Daily "sick call" triage system for new problems • Nursing clinic and treatment teams • Disease-specific education programs (group and individual) • On-site substance abuse and mental health treatment • Emergency services (on-site or contracted with local hospitals) for medical, psychiatric, and dental emergencies • Contracted surgical services at local hospitals		
		Health education	• Chronic disease management • HIV/AIDS education • Inmate wellness education programs
		Continuity of care	• Discharge planning beginning at admission • Collaboration between case manager and discharge planner • Planning to meet medical and social needs (e.g., housing, job training/placement, family reintegration, financial assistance) • Establishment of "medical home"
Prevention	• Communicable disease prevention education • Chronic disease screening and management to prevent complications		

Data from: Conklin, T., Lincoln, T., Wilson, R., & Gramarossa, G. (2003). Innovative model puts public health services into practice. Correct Care, 17(3), 1, 14–15.

current medications, evidence of disability or activity limitation, suicide risk, and other special needs (e.g., dietary restrictions, pregnancy, need for dialysis).

The correctional health care system should also make adequate provision for diagnostic and treatment services with access to health personnel evaluation in a timely fashion. In some situations, this may mean curtailing the discretion of corrections personnel in determining whether an inmate should be brought to the attention of health care providers. If necessary diagnostic and treatment services are not available within the facility, arrangements should be in place for securing these services elsewhere. The need for diagnostic and treatment services extends to dental health and mental health needs as well as to physical health problems.

Mental health services are also an important component of correctional health. Elements of effective mental health programming include the following:

• A correctional environment that supports program goals and provides a social climate and staff that promote mental health
• A view of mental health programming as congruent with institutional mission and values
• Service providers with appropriate background and training
• Program goals that address attitudes, associations, and behaviors that contribute to criminal activity
• Emphasis on the development of cognitive-behavioral problem-solving skills that relate actions to consequences

• Provision of post-program support within the correctional setting and at release into the community (Fagan, 2003)

Mental health services in correctional settings may occur at three levels: basic mental health services available to all inmates, services targeted to specific groups of inmates with similar problems or mental health treatment needs (e.g., youth, the elderly, inmates with substance abuse), and institutional-level services. Basic mental health services should include an initial intake assessment, crisis intervention, brief counseling, individual therapy, detention or segregation review, and record maintenance (Fagan, 2003). The initial intake assessment should address the risk or presence of mental illness, suicide risk, and potential danger to others. Crisis intervention activities may be required for inmates who are suicidal, the seriously mentally ill, victims of assault, mentally retarded inmates who are having difficulty adjusting to the correctional setting, or inmates experiencing other crisis events (Morgan, 2003).

The primary goal of counseling and therapeutic services in correctional settings is to stabilize the inmate and promote adaptation to the correctional setting, rather than to cure their mental illness. Therapeutic services may be individual or group oriented. Individual therapy tends to be provided for seriously disturbed inmates, whereas group therapies tend to be more problem focused (e.g., anger management, substance abuse) (Morgan, 2003).

Detention and segregation evaluations are part of the administrative support provided by mental health professionals in correctional settings. For example, mental health providers might evaluate an inmate for placement in the general housing population or recommend segregated housing. Another example of care at this level is evaluation of the suitability of parole (Morgan, 2003).

Record maintenance is a critical component of mental (and other) health services in correctional settings for several reasons. First, accurate documentation may help to prevent or at least minimize the consequences of litigation by inmates. Second, effective documentation promotes continuity of care for inmates who may be seen by multiple providers or be transferred among multiple correctional settings. Finally, documentation of treatment effects can help to demonstrate the worth of mental health services to system administrators (Morgan, 2003).

Level-two mental health services include specific treatment programs for particular subsegments of the correctional population. For example, services may be provided to women substance abusers who have a history of physical or sexual abuse. Other examples are treatment programs for inmates convicted of family violence crimes, counseling for "death row" inmates, and integrated treatment programs for inmates with dual diagnoses of mental illness and substance abuse. Mental health services for correctional personnel might also be included in this level of services (Fagan, 2003).

Institutional-level services would include consultations regarding system development or research. For example, mental health providers might assist in the development of initial assessment protocols or suicide prevention plans or the design of conflict management training for personnel.

A 3-year study by the National Commission on Correctional Health Care, entitled *The Health Status of Soon-to-be-released Inmates*, prompted a series of recommendations to the U.S. Congress related to correctional health care systems. These recommendations included the following:

- Surveillance for selected communicable and chronic diseases and mental illnesses in correctional populations
- Use of nationally accepted evidence-based clinical practice guidelines
- Establishment of a national vaccine program for incarcerated inmates
- Development and maintenance of a national literature database on correctional health care
- Initiation of a national ethical advisory panel for correctional health care
- Elimination of barriers to public health practice in correctional settings, including reducing barriers to the implementation of in-house public health programs, maintaining Medicaid enrollment during incarceration, mandating immediate Medicaid eligibility on release, supporting correctional system research, promoting improvement in inmate health care, and

encouraging primary and secondary prevention in correctional settings
- Promotion of prerelease planning to address needs for continuing health care services on release from correctional facilities (NCCHC, 2003)

Correctional health services tend to be chronically underfunded, and some authors have suggested Medicaid as a source of payment for services for eligible inmates (Conklin, 2004). At present, federal law prohibits people in correctional and mental institutions from obtaining care under Medicaid or Medicare, and most states terminate Medicaid benefits when someone is incarcerated. In 2004, however, the Center for Medicare and Medicaid Services (CMS) requested states to suspend, rather than terminate, Medicaid enrollment for those in correctional institutions (NCCHC, 2004a). Such a policy would make it easier for newly released inmates to obtain needed health services and maintain continuity of care (Cuellar, Kelleher, Rolls, & Pajer, 2005).

To offset some of the costs of health care, some correctional systems have instituted copayments for medical and dental services provided. The intent of this practice is to decrease service utilization rates and generate funds. The courts have upheld the initiation of small fees for care, ruling that although government has an obligation to provide care to inmates in correctional settings, there is no obligation to provide free care. In 1996, the National Commission for Correctional Health Care drafted a statement on the appropriate use of copayments for correctional health services. Some of the elements of that statement include the following:

- Copayments should be required only for services requested or initiated by the inmate.
- Copayments should not be assessed for screening, follow-up care for problems identified in screening, emergency services, hospitalization, infirmary care, laboratory or diagnostic services, pharmaceuticals, or mental health services.
- Copayments should be assessed only after services have been provided, not as a prerequisite for services.
- Copayments should be small and should not be cumulative in nature.
- Failure to pay a copayment should not be used as a reason to deny subsequent care.
- Inmates should be provided with a minimum balance in personal accounts to permit purchase of necessary hygiene items and over-the-counter medications, and copayments should not be deducted from this minimum.
- There should be a grievance system in place to address copayment grievances.
- Continuation of a copayment system should be contingent on evidence that it does not impede access to needed care (Vogt, 2002).

Copayments may deter inmates from obtaining needed health care and contribute to the spread of communicable diseases as well as increased costs for care of chronic conditions allowed to deteriorate. Correctional nurses may need to be actively involved in evaluating the effect of copayment systems on the health of inmates and the implications for the health of the general public if legitimate needs for services are not being addressed. They may also need to advocate for elimination of copayments if they are found to impede access to care.

The extent of emergency response capabilities (including suicide prevention programs) is another important aspect of the correctional health system. Emergencies may be inmate-specific or general. Examples of inmate-specific emergencies are medical emergencies (e.g., diabetic coma), psychiatric emergencies (e.g., suicide attempt), or traumatic injury. Systemwide emergencies could include inmate-generated emergencies (e.g., riots) or natural or human-caused disasters affecting the correctional setting. Community health nurses should advocate for and be involved in disaster planning for correctional settings. Disaster planning may include plans for evacuation of inmates as well as staff. For example, in 2005, Hurricane Rita forced the evacuation of more than 10,000 inmates from 10 prison facilities. In addition to plans for safe evacuation and provision for the health and survival needs of inmates and staff, correctional disaster plans must address public safety issues and prevent escape during evacuation (Murray, 2006). Disaster planning will be dealt with in more detail in Chapter 27∞.

The health care system within a correctional setting should also make adequate provision for efforts to control communicable diseases. This means screening programs, isolation of infectious inmates, and follow-up on contacts both within and outside the correctional system.

For health care services to be adequate to meet clients' needs, health care personnel must be available in adequate numbers and with adequate preparation for practice in correctional settings.

Another consideration related to the health system dimension is inmates' use of health care services prior to their incarceration. For example, the nurse might ask the female inmate when she had her last Pap smear or mammogram. The nurse would also want to explore prior interactions with health care providers related to existing health problems. For example, was the client being seen for hypertension or other health problems? Or has the client not been taking antihypertensive medications because he or she did not have the prescription renewed?

COMMUNITY HEALTH NURSING IN CORRECTIONAL SETTINGS

Correctional or "forensic" nursing is a specialized area of community health nursing with a special target population. **Forensic nurses** are "professional nurses who deliver health care to institutionalized populations in prisons, or to forensic patients in psychiatric facilities" (Weiskopf, 2005, p. 336). Work in correctional settings requires nurses to function within specific security parameters (Stanley, 2004a) and to understand both the legal and public health implications of care in this setting. Correctional settings place constraints on how nurses may care for clients, and nurses must often balance custodial and care functions. Studies of correctional nurses indicated that they are actively involved in advocacy and often take professional risks within the setting to meet inmates' needs or initiate changes in the system (Weiskopf, 2005). Nursing in correctional settings also requires superlative interpersonal skills and skills in collaborating with corrections personnel who often have a philosophical perspective far different from that of the nurse (Stanley, 2004b).

Standards for Correctional Health Care

Standards have been established for both correctional health care systems and for nursing practice within those systems. The American Public Health Association (APHA) (2003) has developed a set of principles that serve as a basis for health care services in correctional settings. Criteria for judging compliance with each of the principles have also been developed. Areas of focus and related considerations are presented in Table 26-2◆. In addition, NCCHC, a group comprised of 22 national service and professional organizations and service agencies related to correctional health, accredits correctional health systems. Accreditation is based on adherence to specific sets of standards for adult or juvenile correctional facilities (Bell, 2004). Some of the areas addressed by the juvenile standards were presented on page 729. Similar areas are addressed in the standards for adult correctional facilities.

The first standards for nursing practice in correctional settings were promulgated by the ANA in 1985. These standards were revised in 1995 and are currently undergoing subsequent revision. They address the scope of nursing practice in correctional settings as well as standards of care. Nursing standards for correctional settings are summarized on page 742. The standards of care reflect the expected level of care to be provided to individual clients in the correctional setting as well as system-wide program development reflective of the aggregate focus of community health nursing.

Some of the standards differentiate between basic and advanced nursing practice in correctional settings. Basic nursing primarily involves provision of care to individuals and families. The advanced practice nurse, on the other hand, can execute all of the responsibilities of the basic nurse but is also engaged in formulation of policy and in the development, implementation, and evaluation of programs of care for client groups, again incorporating more of the practice of community health nursing. The responsibilities of basic nursing practice include disease prevention and health promotion, recognition

TABLE 26-2 Focus Areas of the American Public Health Association *Standards for Health Services in Correctional Institutions*

Focus Area	Considerations	Focus Area	Considerations
Organizing principles of care	• Contribution to community health • Access to care • Ethical and legal issues	Specific clinical issues and services (cont.)	• Tobacco cessation • Sexuality • Dental health • Vision services • Pharmacy services • Distance-based medicine • Food services and nutrition • Palliative care • Hospice care • End-of-life decision making
Organizational principles	• Information systems • Quality improvement • Staffing and organization of health services • Reference libraries • Health care facilities • Health records		
Continuum of clinical services	• Initial medical screening and medical examination • Prisoner-initiated care (sick call) • Follow-up care • Specialty consultation • Urgent and emergency treatment • Hospital and infirmary care • Periodic health assessment • Transfer and discharge	Specific populations	• Women • Children and adolescents • Frail-elderly or disabled persons • Segregation • Transgendered persons
		Restraint	• Physical restraint • Medication as behavioral restraints
Chronic care management	• Identification of inmates with chronic disease • Management and follow-up • Continuity of care • Discharge planning	Wellness promotion and health education	• Injury prevention (intentional and unintentional) • Occupational health • Health education and promotion (mental health, substance abuse, tobacco, safety, nutrition, family life, disease prevention and control, prenatal care, personal hygiene, physical fitness, dental health, discharge planning) • Health maintenance and exercise
Mental health services	• Diagnostic and therapeutic services for acute and chronic psychiatric illnesses • Voluntary services • Separation of health care and custodial functions • Confidentiality • Comprehensive range of services • Suicide prevention • Specialized training for health care and corrections personnel • Institutional mental health promotion	Environmental health	• Grounds and structures • Services and utilities (e.g., temperature, lighting, laundry, waste disposal, water supply, vermin control, etc.) • Facilities (recreational, hygiene, etc.) • Safety (fire safety, disaster planning, noise, etc.) • Hygiene and personal requirements (bedding, space, toileting facilities) • Inspections, personnel, and supervision
Specific clinical issues and services	• Communicable disease control and treatment • Drug and alcohol detoxification and treatment		

Data from: American Public Health Association. (2003). Standards for health services in correctional institutions. Washington, DC: Author.

and treatment of disease and injury, and counseling. Those of the advanced practice nurse involve supervision of the practice of others, advanced clinical practice (e.g., treatment of minor illness by nurse practitioners), management, and evaluation of the effects of correctional health care programs (ANA, 1995).

Ethical Concerns in Correctional Nursing

There are several ethical considerations that are particularly relevant to nursing in a correctional facility. The right to health care is an ethical as well as legal issue that has already been addressed. Other ethical issues include confidentiality and appropriate use of health

care personnel, refusal of care, abuse of prisoners, and advocacy. Many of these issues are addressed in the various sets of standards discussed above, and readers should review the APHA (2003) and NCCHC (Bell, 2004) documents for information on the positions of these organizations with respect to these issues. Confidentiality issues may be a source of conflict in correctional settings when health care providers have access to information that may be of use in criminal proceedings against inmates. Health professionals in correctional institutions may be pressured to divulge client information or to assist with procedures designed to provide evidence for criminal proceedings (e.g., body cavity searches, blood alcohol levels). When these procedures

SPECIAL CONSIDERATIONS

CORRECTIONS NURSING: SCOPE AND STANDARDS

Standard 1. Assessment: The corrections nurse collects comprehensive data pertinent to the patient's health and condition or the situation.

Standard 2. Diagnosis: The corrections nurse analyzes the assessment data to determine the diagnoses or issues.

Standard 3. Outcomes Identification: The corrections nurse identifies expected outcomes for a plan individualized to the patient or the situation.

Standard 4. Planning: The corrections nurse develops a plan that prescribes strategies and alternatives to attain expected outcomes.

Standard 5. Implementation: The corrections nurse implements the identified plan.

> **Standard 5a: Coordination of Care:** The corrections nurse coordinates care delivery.
>
> **Standard 5b: Health Teaching and Health Promotion:** The corrections nurse employs strategies to promote health and a safe environment.
>
> **Standard 5c: Consultation:** The advanced practice registered nurse and the nursing role specialist provide consultation to influence the identified plan, enhance the abilities of others and effect change.
>
> **Standard 5d: Prescriptive Authority and Treatment:** The advanced practice registered nurse uses prescriptive authority,

procedures, referrals, treatments, and therapies in accordance with state and federal laws and regulations.

Standard 6. Evaluation: The corrections nurse evaluates progress towards attainment of outcomes.

Standard 7. Quality of Practice: The corrections nurse systematically enhances the quality and effectiveness of nursing practice.

Standard 8. Education: The corrections nurse attains knowledge and competency that reflects current nursing practice.

Standard 9. Professional Practice Evaluation: The corrections nurse evaluates one's own nursing practice is relation to professional practice standards and guidelines, relevant statutes, rules, and regulations.

Standard 10. Collegiality: The corrections nurse interacts with and contributes to the professional development of peers and colleagues.

Standard 11. Collaboration: The corrections nurse collaborates with patient, family and others in the conduct of nursing practice.

Standard 12. Ethics: The corrections nurse integrates ethical provisions in all areas of practice.

Standard 13. Research: The corrections nurse integrates research findings into practice.

Standard 14. Resource Utilization: The corrections nurse considers factors related to safety, effectiveness, cost, benefits, and impact on practice in the planning and delivery for nursing services.

Standard 15. Leadership: The corrections nurse provides leadership in the professional practice setting and the profession.

Reprinted with permission from American Nurses Association. (in press). Corrections nursing: Scope and standards of practice. Silver Spring, MD: Nursesbooks.org.

need to be performed by trained personnel (e.g., venipuncture), they should be the task of personnel hired specifically for these types of responsibilities to prevent conflict of interest for health care providers and to avoid jeopardizing a relationship of trust between provider and client. Similarly, health care professionals should not be called on to engage in security measures or to participate in disciplinary decisions or in execution by lethal injection (ANA, 1995). Assuring appropriate use of personnel in the correctional setting may also mean making sure that nonprofessionals (including inmates) are not allowed to perform medical tasks or dispense medications.

Confidentiality, particularly with respect to HIV status, may be more difficult to achieve in a correctional environment. The intensive nature of treatment and the need for multiple doses of medication may serve to label inmates as infected, even when official confirmation of disease is not provided. This potential for lack of confidentiality may act as a deterrent to HIV testing and noncompliance with treatment in infected individuals. Another potential conflict related to confidentiality is the question of whether security personnel should be alerted to inmates' HIV-infection status to ensure their use of universal precautions.

In addition to maintaining confidentiality, nurses may be called on to support an inmate's refusal of care, including forcible administration of psychotherapeutic medications. Inmates have the right to refuse care unless they are determined to be legally incompetent to make that decision. Inmates' right to refuse care, however, must be balanced against state interests in four areas: preserving and protecting life, preventing suicide, protecting the interests of third parties, and maintaining security. Decisions regarding abrogation of the right to refuse treatment should be based on facts in the individual situation, including the inmate's medical condition, prognosis, benefits and burdens of treatment, and the impact of refusal on other inmates. Refusal of care should be carefully documented, including the nature of the care refused, the inmate's stated reason for refusal, the date and time of refusal, provision of education on the possible consequences of refusal, and the inmate's signature or initials (Vogt, 2005).

Aggressive or potentially suicidal inmates may be subjected to physical restraint if they are deemed a danger to themselves or to others. This includes the use of medical isolation when clients suspected of infectious diseases refuse screening procedures or treatment. Medical isolation may also be legitimately employed to protect inmates with symptomatic AIDS from opportunistic

GLOBAL PERSPECTIVES

*I*n 1992, a survey was conducted to determine how health was addressed in European prisons (Gatherer, Moller, & Hayton, 2005). The results of that survey were published in *Prison Health: International Standards and National Practices in Europe*. This and other international corrections efforts led to the development of the World Health Organization's (WHO) Health in Prisons Project (HIPP) to improve health care delivery in prisons through policy change and the development of consensus recommendations on best practices. The underlying principles of HIPP include (a) the right of prisoners to health care at a level commensurate with what is available in the community, (b) the importance of the health of prisoners to society at large, (c) the recognition of the particular vulnerability of prisoners, and (d) the violation of prisoners' human rights with policies for mandatory HIV testing and lack of confidentiality.

HIPP has resulted in several consensus statements that have been accepted by a growing group of European nations. The first HIPP consensus statement focused on communicable disease control, particularly HIV, in prison settings (WHO/UNAIDS, 2001), and subsequent statements addressed mental health (WHO Health in Prisons Project, 2001) and substance abuse issues, including the issue of harm reduction in correctional settings (e.g., providing clean syringes for intravenous drug users) (WHO Regional Office for Europe, 2002). Additional consensus statements have dealt with the needs of minority prisoners, incarcerated youth, and prison health as an aspect of public health practice (Gatherer et al., 2005). Do you think such consensus on best practices in correctional health care could be achieved among correctional systems in the United States? Why or why not?

infection. Although the U.S. Supreme Court has upheld segregation of HIV-infected inmates, many health care professionals suggest that segregation actually increases the potential for the spread of communicable diseases such as tuberculosis (National Center for HIV, STD, and TB Prevention, 2000). For example, segregation may foster the belief that all others in the institution are uninfected and may lead to high-risk activities. Segregation also breaches confidentiality and denies segregated inmates access to programs, such as work release and other programs, available to other inmates. In addition, segregation may contribute to exacerbation of psychoses or depression (Hills et al., 2004).

Because of the imbalance of power inherent in a correctional setting, there is always the potential for abuse of inmates in the name of punishment. For example, pepper spray is occasionally used as a means of forcing compliance among inmates. Punitive use of such chemicals over and above necessary use for subduing violence has been described as constituting torture and falls within the Eighth Amendment proscription of cruel and unusual punishment (Cohen, 1997). Findings also suggest that juvenile inmates may be punished for exhibiting symptoms of mental illness (Coalition for Juvenile Justice, 2000). Preventing this and other forms of abuse of inmates (e.g., denial of health care services) is another ethical aspect of nursing in correctional settings.

Finally, nurse advocacy may be needed in the correctional setting. Advocacy may be required at the level

FOCUSED ASSESSMENT

Assessing Health and Illness in Correctional Settings

Biophysical Considerations

- What is the age, gender, and ethnic composition of the correctional population (inmates and staff)?
- What communicable and chronic health problems are prevalent among inmates? Among staff?
- What is the prevalence of pregnancy among inmates?
- What are the immunization levels in the population?

Psychological Considerations

- What procedures are in place for dealing with suicidal ideation or attempts? Are these procedures followed?
- What is the psychological effect of incarceration? Does the individual inmate exhibit signs of depression? Does the inmate express thoughts of suicide?
- What is the extent of sexual assault among inmates? What are the psychological effects of assault?
- Are there inmates in the setting under sentence of death? If so, what psychological effects does this have? Are there terminally ill inmates in the population?
- What is the prevalence of mental illness among inmates?

Physical Environmental Considerations

- Are there health or safety hazards present in the correctional facility?
- Is there potential for disaster in the area? Is there a disaster plan?

Sociocultural Considerations

- What are the attitudes of health and correctional personnel toward inmates?
- What is the attitude of the surrounding community to the correctional facility and to the inmates?
- What family concerns influence the health of inmates?
- Are there intergroup conflicts within the population? Do these conflicts result in violence?
- What is the extent of mobility in the population?
- Are inmates employed in the correctional setting? Are they employed outside? What health hazards, if any, are posed by the type of work done?
- How do security concerns affect the ability of health care personnel to provide services?

Behavioral Considerations

- Are there inmates with special nutritional needs? How well are they being met? What is the nutritional quality of food served in the correctional setting?

Continued on next page

FOCUSED ASSESSMENT (*continued*)

- What are the health-related behaviors of the correctional population? How do they affect health?
- How are medications dispensed in the correctional setting? Are there procedures in place to prevent inmates from selling medications or accumulating them for use in a suicide attempt?
- What is the extent of sexual activity in the correctional setting? To what extent do inmates engage in unsafe sexual practices? What is the availability of condoms?

Health System Considerations

- What health services are offered in the correctional setting? Are they adequate to meet needs?

- Are there isolation procedures in place for inmates with communicable diseases? Are these procedures followed?
- How are health care services funded? Is funding adequate to meet health needs? Are inmates charged a fee for health care services?
- What is the quality of interaction between internal and external health care services?
- What is the extent of emergency response capability of the correctional facility (e.g., to myocardial infarction, stab wound)?
- What provisions are made for continuity of care after release from the correctional facility?

---

of the individual client to ensure that rights are upheld and that appropriate health care services are received or at the aggregate level to assure adequate health care delivery systems in correctional institutions.

Assessing Health and Illness in Correctional Settings

Features of the correctional setting that influence health are assessed by the community health nurse and used to derive nursing diagnoses. The community assessment guide included in Appendix G on the Companion Website can be used to assess correctional populations. In addition, a comprehensive tool for assessing the health status of correctional populations is provided in the *Community Assessment Reference Guide* designed to accompany this book. Assessment tips for use with correctional populations are provided on page 743.

The age, gender, and ethnic composition of the correctional population can be derived from system records. Information on existing health conditions, on the other hand, is best derived from a combination of intake assessment data and sick call trends, as well as agency records on the types of treatment provided and the kinds of referrals made for outside care. Incidence and prevalence trends in specific conditions, including pregnancy, should also be noted. Information regarding immunizations can be obtained in intake interviews or early health status assessments. However, in many instances, it may be appropriate to assume that vaccination levels are low in the general population and offer immunization to all inmates. Screening data for specific conditions (e.g., TB and HIV infection) can also provide information on the incidence and prevalence of these diseases in the population.

Assessment of considerations in the psychological dimension should include the prevalence of mental illness determined in intake interviews as well as requests for psychotropic medications during sick call. Triage personnel should also be alert to evidence of mental health problems including mental retardation and psychiatric illness during sick call. Institutional records can

provide information about the incidence of sexual assault and completed or attempted suicides in the population, as well as identifying inmates who are under sentence of death. Assessment in this area should also consider the adequacy of protocols for suicide prevention and for addressing psychiatric emergencies.

Physical environmental conditions in the correctional setting are probably best assessed by observation. Information on accidental injuries brought forward in sick call or treated as emergencies may also highlight environmental safety hazards. The potential for disaster and the extent of institutional disaster preparation should also be assessed by identifying disaster risks in the larger community and discussing them with institutional administration.

Information about many sociocultural factors influencing inmate and staff health can be gleaned from observation or knowledge about the surrounding community, particularly in local correctional settings. For example, if the economic level of the surrounding community is low, the same is probably true of the majority of inmates housed in a local jail. Educational levels are likely to be low in the population overall, but community health nurses working in correctional settings should not assume that all inmates have low levels of education. Intake assessments may or may not address educational and other socioeconomic factors, but health care assessment should include these factors and aggregate data can be derived from such individual assessments. Intragroup conflicts may surface in observations of inmates or of interaction between inmates and correctional personnel. Assessment of sociocultural factors should also consider the extent to which inmates are transferred within settings or among correctional settings and the possible health consequences of these transfers. Information about family issues will probably need to be derived directly from inmates themselves. Experience in the setting will give nurses some idea of how security concerns and procedures promote or interfere with effective health care delivery.

Information about special dietary needs and substance use and abuse should be obtained in intake or health care assessments and aggregate data developed on the incidence and prevalence of such behaviors as smoking and drug use and the need for special diets. Corrections nurses should also assess how medications are dispensed and managed in the correctional setting, particularly for inmate subgroups who require multiple medications. Provisions for directly observed therapy for HIV infection and TB should also be identified. Information related to sexual activity can be interpolated from data on sexually transmitted diseases, but can also be derived from interviews with inmates.

Assessment considerations related to the health system dimension include the adequacy of internal and external systems to meet health care needs identified in the population. Nurses should determine what priority is given to health promotion and illness prevention initiatives and to providing treatment for long-term conditions such as chronic diseases and substance abuse. The extent of funding for correctional health services can be obtained from administrative personnel, and both inmates and health care personnel can provide information on the quality of interaction between internal and external health care services. For example, local health department staff may have insights into the effectiveness of discharge planning for inmates with HIV infection or TB. Morbidity and mortality rates are one indication of the effectiveness of emergency response capabilities. Finally, the nurse should assess the policies and procedures to promote continuity of care on release from the correctional setting, as well as the effectiveness of those processes.

Diagnostic Reasoning and Care of Clients in Correctional Settings

Based on information obtained in assessing the dimensions of health, the nurse in the correctional setting formulates nursing diagnoses. Diagnoses should be validated with the client, significant others, or other health care providers when possible. Community health nurses working in correctional settings determine nursing diagnoses for individual clients as well as diagnoses related to the health needs of the total population of inmates and staff. For example, an individual diagnosis might be "uncontrolled diabetes mellitus due to substance abuse." A diagnosis related to the population group might be "increased potential for violence due to racial tensions and unrest." This second diagnosis would affect facility personnel as well as inmates since all might be involved in any violence that occurs.

Planning and Implementing Health Care in Correctional Settings

Planning to meet identified health problems in correctional settings may be accomplished by the nurse him- or herself or in conjunction with other personnel within and outside the institution. Interventions may take place at the primary, secondary, or tertiary level of prevention.

Primary Prevention

Primary prevention in correctional settings involves both health promotion and illness prevention. Health promotion emphases include adequate nutrition, rest and exercise, health education, prenatal care, and contraceptive services. Preventive efforts center on prevention of communicable diseases, suicide prevention, and violence prevention.

HEALTH PROMOTION Health promotion in correctional settings differs from that in other settings in a number of ways. First, the general purpose of health promotion in correctional settings is to protect the health of others rather than to enhance the health of the particular inmate. Second, group health promotion efforts may be hampered by the compulsory nature of inmates' presence in the institution. For example, inmates may be resistant to health education because they perceive themselves as a "captive audience" with little option regarding participation. Third, the great majority of offenders are men who tend not to be as highly motivated with respect to health promotion as women. Health promotion in correctional settings often needs to focus less on information transmission than on attitude development or change, and behavioral change may not be as easy within the constraints of the correctional setting as in the outside world. In addition, the correctional emphasis on punishment for crimes may result in political interference with health promotion efforts. Finally, given the extensive health problems encountered in this population, there may be little time or few resources available for health promotion efforts, which may receive lower priority than curative activities.

Nutritional intake in correctional settings may be far from adequate. NCCHC recommendations include the initiation of heart-healthy diets as a routine aspect of correctional settings (NCCHC, 2003). The nurse in this setting may need to monitor the diet of inmates and may need to influence administrative decisions regarding the nutritive value of meals served. There may also be a need to suggest changes in food served to facility personnel if meals are provided for them as well. In addition, the nurse may need to make arrangements to meet the special dietary needs of specific inmates based on their health status. Examples include a diabetic diet or a liquid diet for an inmate recuperating from a broken jaw.

Attention should also be given to provisions for adequate rest and exercise by inmates. Nurses may need to advocate for adequate space and facilities for sleeping in inmate housing units. In addition, the nurse should work to assure that time and facilities are provided for inmates to obtain exercise. In some instances, this may mean curtailing certain activities that place inmates at risk because of existing health problems. Nurses can also educate both inmates and staff on the benefits of exercise and suggest forms of exercise congruent with health status and available opportunities.

Both inmates and facility staff may be in need of a variety of health education efforts. Areas of importance include the elimination of risk factors for disease. Education programs that may be planned and implemented by nurses may include smoking cessation campaigns or stress management classes. Nurses can also advocate for access to smoking cessation assistance and aids such as nicotine patches. Education regarding problem solving and positive coping strategies may also benefit both staff and inmates.

Prenatal care is a significant health promotion activity for pregnant female inmates. The NCCHC (2003) recommendations include provision of pregnancy screening to all women inmates and further screening of pregnant women for HIV and other STDs. Areas to be addressed in prenatal care include adequate nutrition, the effects of smoking and other substances on the fetus, parenting skills, discomforts of pregnancy, and planning for childcare if the child is delivered while the client is still in custody. HIV prevention education is another area of importance among incarcerated women (and men) who are often at high risk for infection (McClelland, Teplin, Abram, & Jacobs, 2002). Contraceptive education may benefit both pregnant and nonpregnant inmates. There may also be a need for treatment for HIV- or HBV-infected women or those with other STDs. The NCCHC (2003) recommendations also include collaboration between correctional facilities and community health agencies to provide HBV immunization for infants born to mothers with evidence of HBV infection. Similar collaborative efforts should be undertaken to treat the infants of HIV-infected women.

ILLNESS AND INJURY PREVENTION Preventing the spread of communicable diseases in correctional settings is an important primary prevention activity. The concern for public health issues arising in correctional populations has led to the development of a series of "pocket guidelines" for prevention and control of specific diseases in correctional settings. These guidelines are intended to "introduce sheriffs, correctional administrators, correctional health care practitioners, public health leaders, and those who make critical public policy and funding decisions to specific guidelines and recommendations arising out of the interface of public health and corrections" (American Correctional Health Services Association [ACHSA], n.d., p. 1). Guidelines developed as of mid-2006 included TB prevention and control, prevention and control of disease outbreaks, STD prevention, HIV prevention, control of methicillin-resistant *Staphylococcus aureus*, and prevention and control of viral hepatitis. The guidelines are available from the ACHSA Web site at http://www.achsa.org/displaycommon.cfm?an=1&suba rticleebbr=23. These guidelines are congruent with the NCCHC (2003) recommendation to the U.S. Congress that correctional health care services make use of nationally accepted evidence-based clinical guidelines.

Possible approaches to illness prevention include the use of universal precautions in the handling of blood and body fluids (see Chapter 21 ∞ for a discussion of universal precautions), isolation of infected persons when appropriate, immunization, and education on condom use during sexual encounters (Bauserman et al., 2003). Isolation is appropriate for diseases spread by airborne transmission such as measles and influenza. Isolation of HIV-infected individuals is not generally recommended. Immunization is particularly recommended for HBV (Division of Viral Hepatitis, 2004a), but other immunizing agents may be needed as well, depending on the incidence of specific diseases in the general community. For example, measles immunizations may be warranted for all inmates and staff during a measles outbreak in the community, and hepatitis A vaccine is recommended for inmates at risk for hepatitis A (e.g., inmates who engage in oral-anal intercourse). Corrections staff, particularly health care personnel, should also receive HBV immunization. Condom use and substance abuse education on harm reduction strategies can also help to prevent the spread of hepatitis B and C in correctional populations (Weinbaum, Lyerla, & Margolis, 2003). Because correctional settings house a large proportion of inmates who are infected with or at risk for hepatitis, provision of HBV vaccine is a good way to minimize disease prevalence within correctional settings and in the larger community (Division of Viral Hepatitis, 2004b). Community health nurses in correctional settings may be actively involved in providing immunizations and advocating their availability to inmates.

Recommended tuberculosis control measures in correctional settings include screening of all inmates for infection, isolation of suspected and confirmed cases, and treatment of persons with active or latent TB infection. Preventing the spread of tuberculosis may also employ engineering controls related to adequate ventilation systems, air filtration, and irradiation of areas where infected persons are housed (Centers for Disease Control and Prevention [CDC], 2004). **TB prophylaxis** is the treatment of persons with reactive tuberculin skin tests but without evidence of active tuberculosis (in other words, those with latent infection), to prevent their development of disease. Prophylactic treatment is also recommended for persons with HIV infection even in the absence of

Think Advocacy

In October 2004, the *San Diego Union Tribune*, the major newspaper in the San Diego area, published an Associated Press story on citizens who were irate that prisoners were being given influenza immunizations when vaccine shortages prevented community members from obtaining protective immunization (Flu shots for inmates, 2004). Who do you think should receive priority access to a limited supply of vaccine? Why? What actions might you take to advocate for access to vaccines for the group you think should receive priority?

evidence of tuberculosis. Corrections personnel with positive skin tests should also receive prophylaxis. In addition, all inmates and personnel should be educated on infection control procedures and universal precautions. Community health nurses are often responsible for providing directly observed TB therapy and in monitoring its effectiveness. They also monitor clients receiving therapy for potential adverse reactions to medication.

Other more mundane avenues for preventing communicable diseases include routine skin screening for infectious lesions and effective wound infection control procedures. Promotion of inmate hygiene, use of alcohol-based hand rubs for handwashing, and effective laundry procedures can also prevent the spread of MRSA infections (Tobin-D'Angelo et al., 2003).

Other avenues for illness and injury prevention include suicide prevention and prevention of violence. The primary mode of suicide prevention is identification of inmates at risk for suicide. Those at risk for suicide should be closely monitored and receive timely referrals for psychiatric services. Suicide assessment involves obtaining information regarding past personal or family history of suicide attempts, the extent of life stress and social support, presence of suicidal ideation, and presence of mental illness (White, 2001). According to the NCCHC, components of an effective suicide prevention plan include identification of inmates at risk, staff training, inmate assessment by qualified mental health professionals, appropriate housing, and referral to needed mental health services. Other elements of effective plans include adequate communication between corrections and health care staff, immediate intervention for a suicide attempt or suicide in progress, and notification and documentation protocols and processes. Finally, an effective plan includes administrative data review and identification of plan weaknesses and improvement processes (Hills et al., 2004).

Suicide prevention may include four levels of monitoring for inmates at risk for suicide. The first level involves continuous observation of an inmate who has made a recent suicide attempt. Level-two observation is for those at high risk and involves placement in a safe room with active observation by staff every 5 to 15 minutes. Level-three observation is used with inmates who are judged to have a moderate risk of suicide or are moving away from level one or two and involves observation every 10 minutes while awake and every 30 minutes while asleep. At level four, inmates have a significant risk history (e.g., history of recent loss) but are not actively suicidal. Inmates at level four are observed every 30 minutes awake or asleep (Hills et al., 2004).

Violence prevention activities may need to be directed to both inmates and corrections staff. The purpose of such activities is to teach alternative behavioral responses to violence. Recommended components of violence prevention programs in correctional settings include incorporation of violence assessment (including prior exposure to violence) in intake screening, referral of inmates with a history of personal violence or violence exposure for counseling, education on alternative responses to potentially violent situations for both inmates and corrections staff, and referral of inmates for continued counseling on release. Primary prevention emphases in correctional health care are summarized in Table 26-3◆.

Secondary Prevention

Secondary prevention activities in correctional health settings focus on screening and diagnostic and treatment activities.

SCREENING Standards related to screening have been described as some of the more important standards for correctional health care. Screening has a threefold purpose: identifying and addressing the health needs of inmates, promoting early identification of key problems prior to more comprehensive assessments, and identifying and isolating potentially communicable inmates (Stanley, 2004b).

Screening activities in correctional settings typically center on communicable diseases (e.g., hepatitis, HIV infection, other STDs, and TB) and suicide risk. NCCHC (2003), however, also recommends screening of all inmates for hypertension, asthma, obesity, and seizure disorder. Women inmates should also be screened for pregnancy, as noted earlier. Other recommended screening procedures include Papanicolaou smears, mammography, and colorectal cancer screening (Binswanger, White, Perez-Stable, Goldenson, & Tulsky, 2005). However, some authors note that it may be difficult for inmates from minority groups to request such screening procedures that are not conducted routinely

TABLE 26-3	Primary Prevention Foci and Related Activities in Correctional Settings
Focus	**Related Activities**
Health promotion	• Provision of adequate nutrition • Provision of opportunities for adequate rest and exercise • Health education for self-care, risk factor elimination, stress reduction, etc. • Prenatal care for pregnant inmates • Contraceptive education • Advocacy for available health promotion services in correctional settings
Illness and injury prevention	• Control of communicable diseases • Immunization • Isolation of persons with infectious diseases • Use of universal precautions for blood and body fluids • TB prophylaxis • Education for safe sex • Suicide prevention • Violence prevention • Advocacy for illness and injury prevention service availability

due to the need to make written requests for services in English. Similarly, emergency care needs may receive higher priority than such screening procedures, making them hard to access (Magee, Hult, Turalba, & McMillan, 2005). Community health nurses can be particularly helpful in advocating for routine health screening activities for inmates in keeping with the recommendations of the U.S. Preventive Services Task Force (2005).

As we saw earlier, assessment for suicide risk should be an integral part of every intake interview. Screening for certain communicable diseases may also be warranted based on client health status and the incidence and prevalence of specific conditions in the surrounding community. Screening for tuberculosis has been identified as a need for all employees and new inmates. Inmates who will be in custody long enough for the test to be read (48 to 72 hours) should be given a Mantoux skin test (see Chapter 28∞ for information on tuberculin skin tests), whereas a chest x-ray is recommended for those in short-stay units. Because of the tendency for HIV-infected individuals to have negative TB skin tests even with active disease, it has been suggested that chest x-ray, anergy testing, and sputum collections may be more appropriate for persons known to be HIV-positive and for those whose HIV status is unknown in areas with high prevalence rates of multi-drug-resistant tuberculosis infection (National Center for HIV, STD, and TB Prevention, 2000).

Screening for HIV infection is also recommended. Voluntary screening programs have not been very effective due to the multiple barriers to screening encountered in correctional settings. These include fear of disclosure and discrimination if HIV status becomes known, isolation, inability to access programs and services available to noninfected inmates, prohibition of conjugal visits, and so on (Braithwaite & Arriola, 2003). For these reasons, routine screening for all inmates on admission to state and federal prison has been recommended. Use of oral screening measures for HIV infection have been found to increase screening acceptability among inmates, particularly those in high-risk groups (Bauserman et al., 2001).

There is also some debate about the advisability of targeted or routine screening for other diseases. For example, one study indicated that targeting HCV screening to inmates with risk factors such as IDU missed 65.5% of infected male inmates and 44.2% of infected women (Macalino, Dhawan, & Rich, 2005), suggesting that routine screening of all inmates might be more appropriate. Nurses in correctional settings are often responsible for conducting routine screenings and interpreting their results for inmates.

Specific screening approaches have also been recommended for juvenile offenders. For example, the Office of Juvenile Justice and Delinquency Prevention (OJJDP) has suggested screening of all incarcerated youth for substance abuse and mental disorders and further assessment of youth with identified problems

(NCCHC, 2005c). The OJJDP has also published a document entitled *Screening and Assessing Mental Health and Substance Abuse Disorders among Youth in the Juvenile Justice System: A Resource Guide for Practitioners*, which includes 42 assessment and screening tools for use with youth. These tools encompass screening for substance abuse; specific psychiatric disorders; psychosocial problems, strengths, and needs; and cognitive ability (OJJDP, 2004). This document is available on the OJJDP Web site at http://www.ncjrs.gov/pdffiles1/ojjdp/204956.pdf.

Screening for mental health problems is another important element of secondary prevention in correctional settings. Mental health screening is needed to identify inmates at risk for harm to themselves or others, determine inmates' functional capabilities, identify the need to transfer inmates to a specific mental health unit, and determine the inmate's potential to benefit from treatment (Hills et al., 2004).

Suggested elements of mental health assessment in correctional settings include an inmate's psychiatric history, current use of psychotropic medications, presence of suicidal ideation, and a history of suicide attempt. Other relevant screening information includes drug and alcohol use, history of violence or victimization, history of special education placement, and history of traumatic brain injury. Assessment also includes evaluation of the inmate's response to incarceration and evidence of developmental disability (Hills et al., 2004).

Data sources for identifying juveniles with mental health problems include self-report, family history, screening measures, observation, collateral information sources (e.g., prior treatment records), and behavior symptom checklists (Boesky, 2003). Similar sources of information may serve to identify mental health problems in adult inmates. Community health nurses working in correctional settings will employ these data sources to identify inmates with mental health problems. They may also assess inmates' readiness and motivation for treatment. Motivational assessment would consider the inmate's perceptions regarding the seriousness of mental health problems (including substance abuse problems), perceived importance of treatment, desire to change alcohol and drug use behaviors, if any, and past attempts to address mental health problems or substance abuse (Hills et al., 2004).

DIAGNOSIS AND TREATMENT Diagnosis and treatment may be required for medical conditions, mental illness, or substance abuse. Correctional nurses may be actively involved in the diagnosis and treatment of existing medical conditions. Many minor illnesses are handled exclusively by nurses working under medical protocols. In other instances, nurses are responsible for implementing medical treatment plans initiated by physicians or nurse practitioners. This may involve giving medications or carrying out treatment procedures. Treatment procedures would be handled in much the same way as in any health care facility. Dispensing medications in a correctional setting, however, requires that the nurse directly observe the client taking the medication, and often only a single dose is dispensed at a time rather than giving the client several doses of medication to be taken at prescribed times. This precaution is necessary because of the potential for inmates to sell medications to other inmates or to stockpile certain medications for use in a suicide attempt. The U.S. courts have upheld the practice of corrections personnel dispensing medications, but significant safeguards must be in place to ensure that corrections personnel dispense medications correctly and accurately document dispensing (NCCHC, 2001a). In some instances (e.g., syphilis outbreaks and epidemics of other communicable diseases) mass treatment of the entire correctional population or subpopulation in a given setting may be warranted (Chen, Callahan, & Kerndt, 2002).

Treatment for tuberculosis and HIV infection in correctional settings is complicated by the long-term nature of the therapies. Inmates with tuberculosis (except those also infected with HIV) should be placed in respiratory isolation in negative-pressure rooms until they are no longer communicable. If negative-pressure rooms are not available in the correctional facility, arrangements should be made to transport the inmate to a local hospital with such facilities. Respiratory isolation should also be instituted for all inmates with respiratory symptoms suspicious of TB. Tuberculosis treatment should involve a multi-drug regimen, particularly when exposure to multi-drug-resistant infection is suspected. Drug susceptibility testing should be carried out on all inmates with active TB, and treatment should rely on directly observed therapy (DOT).

HIV/AIDS therapy is also difficult in correctional settings because of the number of factors that promote noncompliance. As noted earlier, having to receive multiple doses of medication each day may "tag" inmates as infected and leave them open to discrimination and assault. Security practices such as lockdowns and search and seizure may interfere with dispensing of medications or attendance at support group or education programs. A **lockdown** occurs when inmates are locked in their cells at times when they would ordinarily have greater freedom to come and go throughout the facility, usually in response to a security incident or to permit a search for contraband items (drugs, alcohol, weapons) or a **search and seizure** procedure. During search and seizure, all medications are taken away, so clients in some facilities where self-medication is permitted may have their medications removed and be unable to take doses as directed.

Strategies that can increase compliance with HIV/AIDS treatment regimens include simplifying the regimen to include fewer doses or combining medications into a single pill, protecting confidentiality, using medications with fewer side effects, and dealing with those side effects that occur. DOT has also been found to be effective in promoting compliance with highly active antiretroviral

therapy (HAART) for inmates with HIV/AIDS (NCCHC, 2005b). Treatment is also more effective if provided by health care professionals who have expertise with HIV/AIDS. In larger systems, inmates with HIV infection may be moved to facilities with this expertise or where this expertise is available in the community.

Treatment may also be needed for a variety of chronic health problems experienced by correctional populations. Again, community health nurses working in correctional settings may provide treatment and monitor treatment effectiveness under approved protocols. They may also be responsible for making referrals for specialty services to outside health care agencies. This may require particular advocacy on the part of community health nurses to assure that outside appointments are kept when they are jeopardized by security concerns or lack of security personnel to escort inmates to community facilities.

Treatment should also be available for substance abuse and mental health problems. There are a number of sound reasons for mental health care in correctional settings. Among these are the need to reduce the disabling effects of mental illness and to maximize the ability of inmates to participate in rehabilitation programs. A second reason is to minimize the suffering of the inmates themselves. Finally, treatment of inmates with mental illness and substance abuse problems promotes the safety of all, both within the correctional setting and in the community when the inmate is released (Hills et al., 2004).

The American Psychiatric Association recommends several aspects of treatment for mental illness and substance abuse in correctional settings. These aspects include:

- Crisis intervention programs with residential beds for stays of 10 days or less
- Acute inpatient care programs for inmates able to care for themselves

EVIDENCE-BASED PRACTICE

*H*ills, Siegfried, and Ickowitz (2004) noted that there is significant research to demonstrate that substance abuse services decrease repeated incarceration. For example, one Federal Bureau of Prisons study indicated that only 3% of prisoners who received treatment were rearrested within 6 months of release, compared to 12% of untreated prisoners. Research also indicates that programs that begin in prison but also include aftercare components are more effective than those that include only in-house treatment. For example, a program in Texas state correctional facilities includes a 9- to 12-month therapeutic community program in prison, followed by 3 months in a residential facility after release and another 9 to 12 months of outpatient therapy. Unfortunately, few correctional systems provide such comprehensive programs for substance abuse. What evidence can you find that supports the effectiveness of such programs? How would you use this evidence to promote such a program in your own state?

- Chronic care programs in housing units for the chronically mentally ill who cannot function in the general population
- Outpatient care programs
- Consultation with other correctional personnel
- Discharge and transfer planning (Hills et al., 2004)

Additional mental health services that should be present in correctional settings, based on the NCCHC standards for correctional health programs, include screening by qualified personnel within 24 hours of admission; information regarding available services; a complete health appraisal, including mental health assessment, within 7 days of admission; and mental health evaluation within 14 days of admission for inmates exhibiting signs of mental disorders. Care should also include development of appropriate treatment plans for inmates with serious mental illness and provision of care by qualified mental health professionals within 48 hours of a request for non-emergent services. Correctional health care systems should also include provisions for dealing with psychiatric emergencies and suicide attempts (Hills et al., 2004).

Treatment modalities can include a broad variety of approaches, including the use of psychotropic medications, individual and group psychotherapy, and family interventions. Another possible approach is therapeutic communities, which are a comprehensive set of interventions in a residential setting separated from the general inmate population, intended to engender lifestyle changes that foster mental health in inmates (Peters & Matthews, 2003). Relapse prevention skills and self-help groups such as Alcoholics Anonymous may also be helpful for inmates with substance abuse problems. It is recommended that substance abuse treatment also include frequent random urine screening for drugs. Mental health care for women inmates should provide an integrated approach to dealing with problems of mental illness, substance abuse, and the frequent history of psychological and physical trauma (Hills et al., 2004).

Methadone maintenance is a special area of consideration in treatment for substance abuse. For many opiate abusers, methadone may be an important step in treatment for addiction. Approximately 10% of persons enrolled in methadone treatment programs will be arrested during their enrollment, yet few correctional settings make provision for continuing methadone treatment except for pregnant inmates. Involuntary cessation of methadone leads to painful withdrawal symptoms and risk of death, as well as relapse to opiate use and subsequent rearrest. Studies have indicated that only 56% of correctional systems ask about opiate addiction during intake. As much as 85% of systems do not continue methadone treatment, and 77% do not use appropriate protocols for methadone detoxification. Further, only 27% of systems routinely contact community methadone programs regarding care of inmates enrolled in those programs. Study recommendations included development of

a uniform national policy regarding methadone use with inmates, better coordination between community methadone treatment programs and correctional systems, better education of corrections personnel regarding methadone, and less restrictive regulation of methadone use in correctional settings (Fiscella, 2005).

The Mentally Ill Offender Treatment and Crime Reduction Act of 2004, also known as the Second Chance Act, authorized $50 million per year for mental health programming and services in U.S. correctional facilities and community settings (Bell, 2005). Unfortunately, in spite of the availability of this funding, provision of mental health services in correctional settings is often hampered by variables related to correctional systems, personnel, and inmates (Holton, 2003). System-level variables include limited fiscal allocations for services, privatization of correctional facilities, the institutional climate, and limitations in access to care posed by inmate classification systems. Hopefully, the Second Chance Act will address fiscal barriers to care. Privatization of correctional settings (government contracting with private corporations for operation of correctional facilities) often leads to cost cutting to remain competitive, and cost cutting may eliminate services, such as mental health services, that are considered "nonessential." In addition to entire correctional systems run by private for-profit companies under contract to government agencies, health care services in correctional settings may also be privatized. For example, a county sheriff's department may contract with a private firm for health care personnel and services within the correctional setting rather than hiring health care personnel as county employees. Government service contracts are usually given to the lowest bidder, providing an incentive to decrease the quality or frequency of services in the interests of cost containment. In addition, privatization may lead to less official oversight of correctional facilities and the quality of care provided. On the other hand, privatization has the advantage of services provided by people who have a health care perspective rather than a custodial focus.

The institutional climate is frequently one of punishment rather than treatment, so inmates may not receive needed mental health services. Finally, classification of inmates as security risks may put them at risk for isolation, exacerbation of mental health problems, and lack of access to many services available to other inmates.

Personnel variables that affect mental health treatment services in correctional settings include staff attitudes to mentally ill inmates and training of correctional and health care personnel relative to mental health needs. Cultural diversity and differences between correctional personnel and inmates may make identification of mental health problems more difficult (Holton, 2003). Cultural factors related to mental health and illness are discussed in more detail in Chapters 9 and 30∞.

Inmate-related variables include mental health treatment history, a slower response to medication among inmates than in the general population due to the prevalence of substance abuse, and peer pressure within the setting not to appear weak or vulnerable. In addition, the nuisance side effects associated with psychotropic medications may lead many inmates to be noncompliant with treatment plans (Holton, 2003).

One approach to treatment of mentally ill inmates and those with substance abuse diagnoses is diversion. **Diversion** is the practice of moving mentally ill or substance-abusing offenders from the criminal justice system and placing them in treatment facilities. Diversion may occur prior to booking (before arrest or before criminal charges have been filed) or post-booking (after arrest or conviction). Diversion relies on intersectoral collaboration between legal and mental health care systems to address factors that contribute to **recidivism** (rearrest, reincarceration, or frequent rehospitalization) among mentally ill and substance-abusing inmates. Issues that need to be addressed, in addition to mental health or substance abuse treatment needs, include continuity of public assistance, housing support, and the need for social service referrals and treatment of other medical conditions. In one study of correctional systems, 34% of local jails had some kind of diversion program, but only 18% of them met criteria for true diversion to address recidivism (Broner et al., 2002).

Research has indicated that treatment of substance abuse while an inmate is in prison reduces the likelihood of rearrest and reduces the return to previous drug use patterns. For example, evaluation of one 28-day detention and treatment program in a local jurisdiction demonstrated fewer arrests within 5 years in the treatment group than in a control group (77% versus 60%) (Kunitz et al., 2002). Similarly, youth who receive structured, meaningful, and sensitive treatment for mental illness exhibit 24% less recidivism than those who are not treated (Coalition for Juvenile Justice, 2000), and in-house residential programs of 6 to 12 months have demonstrated a 9% to 18% reduction in criminal recidivism and a 15% to 35% reduction in drug relapse. Unfortunately, only about 60% of mentally ill inmates receive adequate treatment while incarcerated, half receive psychotropic medications, and 44% receive some counseling. Similarly, only a fourth of parole systems include mental health programs (Travis et al., 2001). Community health nurses working in correctional systems can advocate for the availability of adequate mental health and substance abuse programs as well as provide care in such programs.

When physical or mental health services needed by inmates are not available within the correctional health care setting, community health nurses are often responsible for arranging appointments with outside consultants or providers. In addition to arranging for appointments, correctional nurses usually have to arrange transportation and security supervision. This often means that scheduling of appointments can be extremely complicated. Once inmates have been seen by outside providers, correctional nurses also need to follow through on recommendations for treatment. Because many outside providers do not understand the constraints of correctional systems, nurses may need to be creative in promoting treatment compliance. For example, in some small rural jails, there are no facilities for warm soaks to injuries, and special diets may also be difficult to arrange. Other recommendations that pose security hazards may not be able to be fulfilled (e.g., metal braces that can be converted to weapons) (Johnson, 2006). Community health nurses may need to advocate for treatments that are not typically used in the setting, or may need to explain to outside providers why a particular treatment option is not feasible in a correctional setting.

Nurses will also be involved in emergency response to life-threatening situations. Emergency situations likely to be encountered include seizures, cardiac arrest, diabetic coma or insulin reaction, attempted suicide, and traumatic injury due to inmate violence. The nurse would respond to these situations with actions designed to relieve the threat to life and stabilize the client's condition prior to transportation to a hospital facility either within or outside the correctional system. Correctional nurses may also find themselves involved in emergency care of large numbers of persons injured in human-caused or natural disasters involving the correctional facility. Major foci in secondary prevention in correctional settings are summarized in Table 26-4◆.

TABLE 26-4	Secondary Prevention Foci and Related Activities in Correctional Settings
Focus	**Related Activities**

Screening	• Screening for communicable diseases
	  • Tuberculosis
	  • HIV infection
	  • Hepatitis B
	  • Sexually transmitted diseases
	• Routine screening for chronic conditions
	  • Asthma, hypertension, obesity, seizure disorder
	  • Mammography
	  • Papanicolaou smear
	  • Colorectal cancer
	• Provision of specialized screening services for inmates at risk (e.g., diabetes)
	• Screening for suicide risk
	• Screening for pregnancy
	• Screening for mental illness and substance abuse
	• Screening for treatment motivation
	• Advocacy for availability of routine and specialized screening services

Diagnosis and treatment	• Provision of diagnostic services relevant to inmate needs • Treatment of existing acute and chronic conditions • Treatment of mental illness and substance abuse • Methadone maintenance for opiate users • Emergency care for accidental and intentional injuries • Care for psychiatric emergencies • Emergency care in the event of a disaster • Advocacy for effective and available diagnostic and treatment services in correctional settings

Tertiary Prevention

Tertiary prevention in correctional settings focuses on areas similar to that in any setting, preventing or dealing with complications of disease and preventing problem recurrence when possible. Tertiary prevention directed toward preventing complications of existing health problems depends on the conditions experienced by inmates. For example, tertiary prevention for the inmate with diabetes will be directed toward preventing circulatory changes, diabetic ketoacidosis, and hypoglycemia. For the client with arthritis, tertiary prevention will focus on pain management and prevention of mobility limitations. Community health nurses may also help inmates deal with the long-term consequences of chronic conditions. An example might be providing a walker to an inmate with mobility limitations. Tertiary preventive activities may also be directed toward preventing the recurrence of problems once they have been resolved. For example, the nurse may educate an inmate who has been treated for gonorrhea on the use of condoms to prevent reinfection.

In addition, there are three special considerations in tertiary prevention in correctional settings: long-term care planning, reentry planning, and end-of-life care. Each of these major foci will be addressed briefly.

LONG-TERM CARE PLANNING With the aging of the correctional population throughout the world, there is a need to engage in long-term care planning for elderly inmates and those with chronic conditions. Correctional systems have taken a variety of approaches to long-term care planning for these subpopulations. Older inmates or those with disabilities related to chronic illness may be transferred to appropriate facilities or housing conditions separate from the general inmate population. Usually such facilities have an infirmary where exacerbations of chronic conditions requiring hospitalization can be addressed in-house. In other instances, inmates may be transferred to assisted living facilities that provide assistance with the activities of daily living.

ETHICAL AWARENESS

Fazal (2005) reported that many states and the federal government have regulations that permit seriously ill or disabled inmates to obtain "medical release" or "medical parole." Many of these regulations exclude those with life sentences or execution orders, sex offenders, or those under 70 years of age. Regulations may also require inmates to have served a certain portion of their sentences and may revoke parole if the inmate's condition improves. Health care coverage for many inmates who receive medical parole is provided under Medicare or Medicaid. Unfortunately, Fazal noted that few jurisdictions employ these laws, even where they exist, to assist seriously ill inmates. Who do you think should be eligible for medical parole? What criteria do you think should be used to determine eligibility? How might you go about advocating for medical parole for an inmate with a serious health condition?

Terminally ill inmates may be transferred to specialized hospice units or to community hospices. Alternatively, hospice services can be provided to inmates housed in the general population, at least until inmates become severely debilitated. Finally, some correctional systems provide continuing care retirement communities for older and disabled inmates similar to comparable institutions in the community, but incorporating the custodial functions of correctional facilities (NCCHC, 2002).

When inmates with chronic illnesses or disability are housed in the general population, correctional systems may provide "home care" services and case management to address their long-term care needs. In such systems, nurses might go to inmate housing units to provide care in the same way that they would provide home care in community settings. Another alternative is to have other inmates function as "personal care attendants" for disabled inmates, assisting them with certain activities of daily living (e.g., bathing). Other systems may create adult day care programs in which inmates with long-term care needs are housed in the general population, but spend a portion of each day in an area of the facility, frequently an infirmary, where these needs can be addressed (NCCHC, 2002).

Other tertiary prevention activities related to long-term care include providing assistive devices, monitoring the status of chronic conditions and treatment compliance, monitoring for adverse effects of treatment, and providing support in dealing with the emotional and physical consequences of long-term physical or mental illness. Community health nurses may be involved in providing these interventions or in advocating their availability in the correctional setting. They may also need to advocate for access to these kinds of services for specific inmates.

REENTRY PLANNING Approximately 98% of the 8 million people admitted annually to correctional settings will ultimately be released back into the community (Conklin, 2004). Annual turnover rates are as high as 800% in jails and 50% in federal and state prisons (Discharge Planning, 2002). In a large metropolitan correctional system like that of Los Angeles County, the inmate population changes completely every 44 days (Inmate Infections Spread, 2005). Many of these inmates reenter the larger society as probationers or parolees. A **probationer** is an adult offender who has been remanded to community-based supervision, often as an alternative to incarceration. Probationers usually are held in correctional facilities for only a short time until their case has been tried in court. A **parolee** is an adult released from a correctional system to community supervision after serving all or part of his or her sentence. Both probationers and parolees are subject to reincarceration if they violate the terms of probation or parole. At the end of 2004, there were 4.9 million U.S. men and women under federal, state, or local probation and 765,400 on parole. Approximately 75% of these former inmates are under active supervision by correctional systems (BJS, 2005g).

The dual process of incarceration and reentry, labeled by some authors as "coercive mobility" (Golembeski & Fullilove, 2005), has been cited as a public health opportunity. In the words of two authors, "Given the inevitability of reentry, every prisoner should be viewed as a future member of free society. Accordingly, the period of time in prison should be viewed as an opportunity to provide health interventions that will yield better health outcomes not only in prison but, equally importantly, after the prisoner's release" (Travis & Sommers, 2004, p. 19). Unfortunately, little planning may be initiated toward meeting inmates' reentry needs. One of the purposes of the federal Second Chance Act is to strengthen community reentry services for released inmates (Pogorzelski, Wolff, Pan, & Blitz, 2005). However, reentry planning should begin, ideally, at admission to a correctional facility, not at the time of or after release (Hills et al., 2004).

Reentry, in the correctional context, is defined as "the process of leaving prison and returning to society" (Travis et al., 2001, p. 1). Two challenges inherent in reentry are protecting the public and promoting effective reintegration into the community. Reentry also poses risks for the spread of communicable diseases within the general population if inmates have not been effectively treated.

Released inmates often have limited job skills and social support networks, so many of them have difficulty reintegrating into the larger community. They may have difficulty finding employment and housing due to the stigma attached to incarceration (Cooke, 2004). At the same time, the social capital or infrastructure of communities that reabsorb large numbers of released inmates are often stretched beyond their capacity. Studies indicate that a small number of communities, and an even smaller number of neighborhoods within those communities, receive the bulk of released inmates. Given the lack of support services, resources, and opportunities for legitimate employment, many released inmates are reintroduced to criminal activities (Golembeski & Fullilove, 2005). An estimated two thirds of inmates released in any given year will be rearrested for a felony or serious misdemeanor within three years of release (Travis & Sommers, 2004). Research, however, indicates that inmates, particularly those with substance abuse problems, who receive health insurance and employment assistance are less likely to return to drug use and be rearrested (Freudenberg, Daniels, Crum, Perkins, & Richie, 2005).

Reentry planning begins with the development of systematic discharge protocols to be used with all inmates to be released from a correctional setting. Such protocols are most effective when they are developed with input from the communities to which inmates will be released (Golembeski & Fullilove, 2005). Community health nurses can be active advocates for reentry planning for all inmates. They can also advocate community involvement in the development of reentry planning protocols and in designing community infrastructures to support reentry.

Planning considerations related to individual inmates are based on an individualized needs assessment and include issues related to health care and social and financial needs. The American Public Health Association (2003) noted a need to provide inmates with a complete copy of their health records, a sufficient supply of medications, referrals (and possibly actual appointments) for physical and mental health services in the community, and assistance with health insurance coverage. This may mean advocacy on the part of community health nurses to get Medicaid, Medicare, or Veteran's Administration benefits reinstated, or assisting inmates to find low-cost health care services. Advocacy may also be required to ensure that inmates have a sufficient supply of necessary medications until they can find employment and purchase medications on their own. This is particularly important for inmates who are receiving long-term therapy for HIV/AIDS or TB. Community health nurses may also need to advocate for continuing therapy for mental illness or substance abuse. There is a particular need for effective communication between the correctional system and community health agencies. Too often, inmates are discharged with ongoing health needs (e.g., HIV/AIDS or TB treatment) without local health authorities being notified. In addition to making referrals and links to community services, community health nurses in correctional settings should also develop systems for monitoring service continuation and its effects on inmate health status.

Reentry planning should also address a variety of social and financial needs of released inmates. For example, many inmates have alienated family members and may not be able to find shelter with their families. In this case, community health nurses may need to assist in arranging housing for former inmates. Referrals may also be needed for employment assistance or job training. Unfortunately, federal spending on employment training in correctional settings was cut by 50% in the 1990s and has never been reinstated (while overall corrections costs escalated by 521%) (Golembeski & Fullilove, 2005). Community health nurses may need to advocate at the societal level for job training programs for inmates and others with low levels of employability. They may also need to advocate for relaxation of restrictions on financial and other assistance benefits for people who have been incarcerated.

For some inmates, reentry planning may entail assistance with family reintegration. Community health nurses may assist families to deal with concerns about bringing a released inmate back into the family constellation, particularly if the inmate was incarcerated for a crime involving family violence. There are also some instances in which inmates should not return to families if their presence may put family members at risk of harm.

END-OF-LIFE CARE End-of-life care for inmates with terminal illnesses may be similar to that on the outside. For example, community health nurses may need to discuss advance directives with inmates and help those who wish to execute advance directives. Community health nurses may also need to advocate adherence to advance directives when they have been executed by an inmate. According to the NCCHC (2005a) data, discussions of advance directives have been undertaken with less than 1% of inmates. In some cases, seriously ill inmates have chosen not to execute advance directives, possibly out of a fear of being abandoned as they are dying. In addition to discussing advance directives with inmates, correctional health care personnel need to develop policies regarding the timing of advance directives, communicating information about advance directives when inmates are transferred to outside hospitals or hospice settings, and addressing effective pain control for seriously ill inmates (NCCHC, 2005a). Correctional health systems also need to develop policies for notifying family members and significant others of imminent death (APHA, 2003).

Just as in the general population, referral for hospice care may be appropriate for terminally ill inmates. Some correctional facilities have in-house hospice units, and others may transfer inmates to community hospices when there is no security risk to the public (NCCHC, 2002). Whether in a hospice setting, in an infirmary, or in the general correctional population, terminally ill inmates are likely to need assistance in setting their affairs in order. For some inmates, there may also be a need to reconcile with family members. Community health nurses can be instrumental in facilitating these end-of-life activities. For example, they may advocate with family members for reconciliation or assist inmates to obtain legal assistance in settling any assets they may have on their heirs. Symptom control and palliative care are also important aspects of end-of-life care in correctional settings.

There are also two unique aspects to end-of-life care that need to be addressed in correctional settings. The first is the concept of "compassionate release" or "medical parole." **Medical parole** is the release of a seriously ill or disabled inmate back into the community (Fazal, 2005) to receive needed health care services from community agencies and, often, to permit time with family members. Medical parole is most often used for terminally ill inmates. As noted in Table 26-5◆, community health nursing advocacy may be required to initiate or support a medical parole decision. In addition to advocating for medical parole when appropriate,

community health nurses will assist with arranging for follow-up care after release.

The second unique aspect of end-of-life care in correctional settings relates to inmates who have been sentenced to death. In 2002, more than 3,500 inmates were facing the death penalty (U.S. Census Bureau, 2005). These inmates have the same needs for psychological end-of-life care as those with terminal illnesses, but their care is often complicated by feelings of hopelessness and attendant security measures (e.g., the use of handcuffs and shackles and constant supervision) (Boisaubin, Duarte, Blair, & Stone, 2004). Aspects of tertiary prevention in correctional settings are summarized in Table 26-5◆.

TABLE 26-5	Tertiary Prevention Foci and Related Activities in Correctional Settings
Focus	**Related Activities**
Long-term care planning	• Transfer to appropriate facility as needed • Provision of "home care" in general population • Assistance by a personal care attendant • Use of assistive devices as needed • Adult day care services • Continued monitoring of the status of chronic conditions • Monitoring treatment compliance • Monitoring for adverse effects of treatment • Provision of support in dealing with long-term consequences of chronic illness • Advocacy for effective long-term care service availability
Reentry	• Development of systematic discharge protocols • Development of individual discharge plan • Provision for continuity of health care • Arrangement for a supply of necessary medications on discharge • Arrangement for health insurance coverage • Provision for housing and financial assistance needs • Assistance with job training and employment as needed • Assistance with family reintegration as needed • Coordination of community health care and correctional activities • Advocacy for effective prerelease planning for all inmates • Advocacy for development of community infrastructure to support reentry • Advocacy for civil rights of released inmates
End-of-life care	• Development of advance directives as desired by inmates • Symptom control and palliative care • Advocacy for medical parole and arrangement for follow-up care • Advocacy for use of advance directives by personnel • Provision of emotional and spiritual support to inmates and significant others • Referral to hospice care • Assistance with setting life in order • Assistance with family reconciliation as needed

Evaluating Health Care in Correctional Settings

The principles that guide the evaluation of health care in correctional settings are the same as those applied in other settings. The nurse evaluates the outcomes of care for individual clients in light of identified goals. Correctional nurses may also be involved in evaluating health outcomes for groups of inmates or for the entire facility population, including staff. In addition, the nurse examines processes of care and makes recommendations for improvements in terms of quality, efficiency, and cost-effectiveness.

Correctional facilities present a useful setting in which community health nurses can engage in health-promotive and illness-preventive activities with clients who may have little knowledge of these activities. Clients in correctional settings may be less motivated than those in other settings, but can realize substantial health benefits through the efforts of community health nurses during incarceration and in promoting follow-up on release. Community health nursing efforts in correctional settings also help to prevent the flow of health problems back into the larger population, thereby benefiting society as a whole.

Case Study

Nursing in the Correctional Setting

You are the only nurse on the night shift in a county jail housing 150 male inmates. A new inmate is admitted to the jail for driving under the influence of alcohol. During your initial history and physical, the inmate tells you that he is on kidney dialysis and missed his last dialysis appointment, which was yesterday. It is Sunday night and your facility does not have dialysis capabilities. The dialysis unit at the local hospital does not function on Sundays except in the case of emergencies. The inmate appears to be in no immediate distress and has normal vital signs and no evidence of edema. He is appropriately alert and oriented despite the odor of obvious alcohol consumption. The watch commander tells you he has no one to spare to transport the inmate to the hospital, and if he goes it will have to be by private ambulance. Your back-up physician is out of town for the weekend and the on-call physician is tied up with an emergency.

1. What are the biophysical, psychological, physical environmental, sociocultural, behavioral, and health system factors operating in this situation?
2. What are your nursing diagnoses? How would you prioritize those diagnoses?
3. What action would you take in this situation? Why?

Test Your Understanding

1. What are the implications, for inmates and for the general public, of providing health care in correctional settings? (pp. 727–728)

2. Describe some of the ethical considerations facing nurses in correctional settings. What values are in conflict in each of these areas? (pp. 726, 741–744)

3. How do basic and advanced nursing practice in correctional settings differ? (pp. 740–741)

4. What are some of the biophysical, psychological, physical environmental, sociocultural, behavioral, and health system factors that influence health in correctional settings? How might these factors differ for inmates and correctional staff? (pp. 728–740)

5. What are the major aspects of primary prevention in correctional settings? What activities might nurses perform in relation to each? (pp. 745–747)

6. What are the main aspects of secondary prevention in correctional settings? How might community health nurses be involved in each? (pp. 747–751)

7. Discuss considerations and community health nursing involvement in tertiary prevention in correctional settings. (pp. 752–754)

EXPLORE MediaLink

http://www.prehall.com/clark
Resources for this chapter can be found on the Companion Website.

Audio Glossary
Appendix G: Community Health Assessment and Intervention Guide
Exam Review Questions
Case Study: Penitentiary Nursing

MediaLink Application: Puppetry in Prison (video)
MediaLink Application: Interview with Author of *Acres of Skin* (video)
Media Links

Challenge Your Knowledge
Update *Healthy People 2010*
Advocacy Interviews

References

Abrahams, N., & Jewkes, R. (2005). Effects of South African men's having witnessed abuse of their mothers during childhood on their levels of violence in adulthood. *American Journal of Public Health, 95*, 1811–1816.

American Academy of Pediatrics. (2001). Health care for children and adolescents in the juvenile correctional care system. *Pediatrics, 107*, 799–803.

American Correctional Health Services Association. (n.d.). *Pocket guide series.* Retrieved March 30, 2006, from http://www.achsa.org/displaycommon.cfm?an=1&subarticlenbr=23

American Nurses Association. (1985). *Standards of nursing practice in correctional facilities.* Kansas City, MO: Author.

American Nurses Association. (1995). *Scope and standards of nursing practice in correctional settings.* Washington, DC: Author.

American Public Health Association. (2003). *Standards for health services in correctional institutions.* Washington, DC: Author.

Bauserman, R. L., Richardson, D., Ward, M., Shea, M., Bowlin, C., Tomoyasu, N., et al. (2003). HIV prevention with jail and prison inmates: Maryland's prevention case management program. *AIDS Education and Prevention, 15*, 465–480.

Bauserman, R. L., Ward, M. A., Eldred, L., & Swetz, A. (2001). Increased voluntary HIV testing by offering oral tests in incarcerated populations. *American Journal of Public Health, 91*, 1226–1229.

Bell, C. C. (2004). *The sanity of survival: Reflections on community mental health and wellness.* Chicago: Third World Press.

Bell, C. C. (2005). Mentally ill offender law brings help . . . and hope. *Correct Care, 19*(1), 3.

Binswanger, I. A., White, M. C., Perez-Stable, E. J., Goldenson, J., & Tulsky, J. P. (2005). Cancer screening among jail inmates: Frequency, knowledge, and willingness. *American Journal of Public Health, 95*, 1781–1787.

Boesky, L. M. (2003). Identifying juvenile offenders with mental health disorders. In T. J. Fagan & R. K. Ax (Eds.), *Correctional mental health handbook* (pp. 167–198). Thousand Oaks, CA: Sage.

Boisaubin, E. V., Duarte, A. G., Blair, P., & Stone, T. H. (2004). "Well enough to execute": The health professional's responsibility to the death row inmate. *Correct Care, 18*(4), 8.

Braithwaite, R. L., & Arriola, K. R. J. (2003). Male prisoners and HIV prevention: A call for action ignored. *American Journal of Public Health, 93*, 759–763.

Braithwaite, R. L., Treadwell, H. M., & Arriola, K. R. J. (2005). Health disparities and incarcerated women: A population ignored. *American Journal of Public Health, 95*, 1679–1681.

Brodie, J. (2000). Caring—The essence of correctional nursing. *Correct Care, 14*(4), 1, 15, 18.

Broner, N., Borum, R., & Gawley, K. (2002). Criminal justice diversion of individuals with co-occurring mental illness and substance use disorders: An overview. In G. Landsberg, M. Rock, L. K. W. Berg, & A. Smiley (Eds.), *Serving mentally ill offenders: Challenges and opportunities for mental health professionals* (pp. 83–106). New York: Springer.

Brunswick, M. (2005). "Meth mouth" plagues many state prisoners. Reprinted from *Star Tribune*, Minneapolis-St. Paul in *Correct Care, 19*(1), 7.

Bureau of Justice Statistics. (2003a). *Prevalence of imprisonment in the U.S. population, 1974–2001.* Retrieved March 30, 2006, from http://www.ojp.usdoj.gov/bjs/abstract/piusp01.htm

Bureau of Justice Statistics. (2003b). *Reentry trends in the United States.* Retrieved March 30, 2006, from http://www.ojp.usdoj.gov/bjs/reentry/reentry.htm

Bureau of Justice Statistics. (2005a). *Crime characteristics.* Retrieved March 30, 2006, from http://www.ojp.usdoj.gov/bjs/cvict_c.htm

Bureau of Justice Statistics. (2005b). *Criminal victimization.* Retrieved March 30, 2006, from http://www.ojp.usdoj.gov/bjs/cvictgen.htm

Bureau of Justice Statistics. (2005c). *Jail statistics.* Retrieved March 30, 2006, from http://www.ojp.usdoj.gov/bjs/jails.htm

Bureau of Justice Statistics. (2005d). *Prison and jail inmates at midyear 2004.* Retrieved March 30, 2006, from http://www.ojp.usdoj.gov/bjs/pub/pdf/pjim04.pdf

Bureau of Justice Statistics. (2005e). *Prison statistics.* Retrieved March 30, 2006, from http://www.ojp.usdoj.gov/bjs/prisons.htm

Bureau of Justice Statistics. (2005f). *Prisoners in 2004.* Retrieved March 30, 2006, from http://www.ojp.usdoj.gov/bjs/pub/pdf/p04.pdf

Bureau of Justice Statistics. (2005g). *Probation and parole statistics.* Retrieved March 30, 2006, from http://www.ojp.usdoj.gov/bjs/pandp.htm

Centers for Disease Control and Prevention. (2004). Tuberculosis transmission in multiple correctional facilities—Kansas, 2002–2003. *Morbidity and Mortality Weekly Report, 53*, 734–738.

Chen, J. L., Callahan, D. B., & Kerndt, P. R. (2002). Syphilis control among incarcerated men who have sex with men: Public health response to an outbreak. *American Journal of Public Health, 92*, 1473–1475.

Coalition for Juvenile Justice. (2000). *Handle with care: Serving the mental health needs of young offenders.* Retrieved June 2, 2001, from http://www.juvjustice.org

Cohen, M. D. (1997). The human health effects of pepperspray—A review of the literature and commentary. *Journal of Correctional Health Care, 4*, 73–88.

Conklin, T. (2004). Medicaid a must for new releasees. *Correct Care, 18*(3), 3.

Conklin, T., Lincoln, T., Wilson, R., & Gramarossa, G. (2003). Innovative model puts public health services into practice. *Correct Care, 17*(3), 1, 14–15.

Cooke, C. L. (2004). Joblessness and homelessness as precursors of health problems in formerly incarcerated African American men. *Journal of Nursing Scholarship, 36*, 155–160.

Coolman, A., & Eisenman, D. (2003). Sexual assault: A critical health care issue. *Correct Care, 17*(4), 3.

Cuellar, A. E., Kelleher, K. J., Rolls, J. A., & Pajer, K. (2005). Medicaid insurance policy for youths involved in the criminal justice system. *American Journal of Public Health, 95*, 1707–1711.

Cutler, D. L., Bigelow, D., Collins, V., Jackson, C., & Field, G. (2002). Why are severely mentally ill persons in jail and prison? In P. Backlar & D. L. Cutler (Eds.), *Ethics in community mental health care: Commonplace concerns* (pp. 136–154). New York: Kluwer Academic/Plenum.

Discharge planning: Reintegrating inmates living with HIV/AIDS into the community. (2002). *HIV Inside, 4*(1), 1–11.

Division of Viral Hepatitis. (2004a). Hepatitis B vaccination of inmates in correctional facilities—Texas, 2000–2002. *Morbidity and Mortality Weekly Report, 53*, 681–683.

Division of Viral Hepatitis, National Center for Infectious Diseases. (2004b). Incidence of acute hepatitis B—United States, 1990–2002. *Morbidity and Mortality Weekly Report, 53*, 1252–1254.

Division of Viral Hepatitis. (2004c). Transmission of hepatitis B virus in correctional facilities—Georgia, January 1999–June 2002. *Morbidity and Mortality Weekly Report, 53*, 678–681.

Durose, M. R., Harlow, C. W., Langan, P. A., Motivans, M., Rantala, R. R., & Smith, R. L. (2005). *Family violence statistics: Including statistics on strangers and acquaintances.* Washington, DC: Bureau of Justice Statistics.

Fagan, T. J. (2003). Mental health in corrections: A model for service delivery. In T. J. Fagan & R. K. Ax (Eds.), *Correctional mental health handbook* (pp. 1–19). Thousand Oaks, CA: Sage.

Fazal, S. (2005). Medical parole: With safeguards, a practical solution. *Correct Care, 19*(3), 19.

Fiscella, K. (2005). Methadone treatment absent in many jails. *Correct Care, 19*(1), 1, 14.

Fiscella, K., Pless, N., Meldrum, S., & Fiscella, P. (2004). Alcohol and opiate withdrawal in US jails. *American Journal of Public Health, 94*, 1522–1524.

Flu shots for inmates upset people seeking vaccine. (2004, October 20). *San Diego Union Tribune*, A9.

Francis J. Curry National Tuberculosis Center and National Commission on Correctional Health Care. (2003). *Corrections tuberculosis training and education resource guide, 2004–2005.* Chicago: Authors.

Freudenberg, N., Daniels, J., Crum, M., Perkins, T., & Richie, B. E. (2005). Coming home from jail: The social and health consequences of community reentry for women, male adolescents, and their families and communities. *American Journal of Public Health, 95*, 1725–1736.

Fry, R. L. (2003). Transsexualism: A correctional, medical or behavioral health issue? *Correct Care, 17*(1), 1, 20.

Fulco, S. D. (2001). Babies behind bars: The rights and liabilities of babies and mothers. *Correct Care, 15*(1), 6.

Gatherer, A., Moller, L., & Hayton, P. (2005). The World Health Organization European Health in Prisons Project after 10 years: Persistent barriers and achievements. *American Journal of Public Health, 95*, 1696–1700.

Gershon, R. R. M., (2002). Infectious disease risk in correctional health care workers. *Correct Care, 16*(3), 3.

Golembeski, C., & Fullilove, R. (2005). Criminal (in)justice in the city and its associated health consequences. *American Journal of Public Health, 95*, 1701–1706.

Hammett, T. M., Harmon, M. P., & Rhodes, W. (2002). The burden of infectious diseases among inmates of and releasees from US correctional facilities, 1997. *American Journal of Public Health, 92*, 1789–1794.

Hayes, L. M. (2004). Juvenile suicide study finds gaps in prevention. *Correct Care, 18*(4), 13.

Head, G., Kelly, P. J., Bair, R. M., Baillargeon, J., & German, G. (2000). Risk behaviors and the prevalence of chlamydia in a juvenile detention facility. *Clinical Pediatrics, 9*, 521–527.

Heines, V. (2005). Speaking out to improve the health of inmates. *American Journal of Public Health, 95*, 1685–1688.

Hills, H., Siegfried, C., & Ickowitz, A. (2004). *Effective prison mental health services: Guidelines to expand and improve treatment.* Retrieved March 30, 2006, from http://www.nicic.org/misc/URLshell.aspx?SRC=Catalogue&REFF=http://nicic.org/library/018604&ID=018604&Type=PDF&URL=http://nicic.org/pubs/2004/018604.pdf

Holton, S. M. B. (2003). Managing and treating mentally disordered offenders in jails and prisons. In T. J. Fagan & R. K. Ax (Eds.), *Correctional mental health handbook* (pp. 101–122). Thousand Oaks, CA: Sage.

Inmate infections spread. (2005). *NurseWeek, 18*(1), 7.

Johnson, D. (2006). Don't let outside consultations be a liability minefield. *Correct Care, 20*(1), 9.

Kahn, A. J., Simard, E. P., Bower, W. A., Wurtzel, H. L., Kristova, M., Wagner, K. D., et al. (2005). Ongoing transmission of hepatitis B virus infection among inmates at a state correctional facility. *American Journal of Public Health, 95*, 1793–1799.

Kim, S., & Crittenden, K. S. (2005). Risk factors for tuberculosis among inmates: A retrospective analysis. *Public Health Nursing, 22*, 108–118.

Kunitz, S. J., Woodall, G., Zhao, H., Wheeler, D. R., Lillis, R., & Rogers, E. (2002). Rearrest rates after incarceration for DWI: A comparative study in a southwestern US county. *American Journal of Public Health, 92*, 1826–1831.

Kushel, M. B., Hahn, J. A., Evans, J. L., Bangsberg, D. R., & Moss, A. R. (2005). Revolving doors: Imprisonment among the homeless and marginally housed population. *American Journal of Public Health, 95*, 1747–1752.

Macalino, G. E., Dhawan, D., & Rich, J. D. (2005). A missed opportunity: Hepatitis C screening of prisoners. *American Journal of Public Health, 95*, 1739–1740.

Macalino, G. E., Vlahov, D., Sanford-Colby, S. Patel, S., Sabin, K., Salas, C., et al. (2004). Prevalence and incidence of HIV, hepatitis B virus, and hepatitis C virus infections among males in Rhode Island prisons. *American Journal of Public Health, 94*, 1218–1223.

MacNeil, J. R., Lobato, M. N., & Moore, M. (2005). An unanswered health disparity: Tuberculosis among correctional inmates, 1993 through 2003. *American Journal of Public Health, 95*, 1800–1805.

Magee, C. G., Hult, J. R., Turalba, R., & McMillan, S. (2005). Preventive care for women in prison: A qualitative community health assessment of the Papanicolau test and follow-up treatment at a California state women's prison. *American Journal of Public Health, 95*, 1712–1717.

Maruschak, L. M., & Beck, A. J. (2001). *Medical problems of inmates.* Retrieved June 2, 2001, from http://www.ojp.usdoj.gov/bjs

McClelland, G. M., Teplin, L., Abram, K. M., & Jacobs, N. (2002). HIV and AIDS risk behaviors among female jail detainees: Implications for public health policy. *American Journal of Public Health, 92*, 818–825.

Mertens, D. J. (2001). Pregnancy outcomes of inmates in a large county jail setting. *Public Health Nursing, 18*, 45–53.

Meyer, J. A. (2003). Improving men's health: Developing a long-term strategy. *American Journal of Public Health, 93*, 709–711.

Morgan, R. (2003). Basic mental health services: Services and issues. In T. J. Fagan & R. K. Ax (Eds.), *Correctional mental health handbook* (pp. 59–71). Thousand Oaks, CA: Sage.

Murray, O. (2006). Hurricane Rita leaves lessons in its wake. *Correct Care, 20*(1), 3.

National Center for HIV, STD, and TB Prevention. (2000). Drug-susceptible tuberculosis outbreak in a state correctional facility—South Carolina, 1999–2000. *Morbidity and Mortality Weekly Report, 49*, 1041–1044.

National Center for HIV, STD, and TB Prevention. (2005). *What is the difference between jail and prison?* Retrieved March 30, 2006, from http://www.cdc.gov/nchstp/od/cccwg/difference.htm

National Commission on Correctional Health Care. (1999). A summary guide to revisions in the 1999 Standards for Health Services in Juvenile Detention and Confinement Facilities. *Correct Care, 13*(2), 18–19.

National Commission on Correctional Health Care. (2001a). COs passing meds passes court—but wise wardens will mandate controls. *Correct Care, 15*(2), 6.

National Commission on Correctional Health Care. (2001b). Study released on health needs of detained youth. *Correct Care, 15*(1), 19.

National Commission on Correctional Health Care. (2002). Long-term care planning needed, say PA researchers. *Correct Care, 16*(2), 15.

National Commission on Correctional Health Care. (2003). Policy recommendations for better health care. *Correct Care, 17*(1), 17–18.

National Commission on Correctional Health Care. (2004a). CMS asks states to maintain Medicaid enrollment for inmates. *Correct Care, 18*(2), 15.

National Commission on Correctional Health Care. (2004b). Hasta la vista, cigs! *Correct Care, 18*(3), 7.

National Commission on Correctional Health Care. (2005a). Advance directives study shows room for improvement. *Correct Care, 19*(4), 15.

National Commission on Correctional Health Care. (2005b). DOT for HAART shows promise. *Correct Care, 19*(1), 15.

National Commission on Correctional Health Care. (2005c). Guidance on tools to screen, assess youth mental health. *Correct Care, 19*(1), 13.

Newkirk, C. F. (2003). The unique needs of incarcerated women. *Correct Care, 17*(1), 3.

Norman, A., & Parrish, A. (2000). Prison health care. *Nursing Management, 7*(8), 26–29.

Office of Juvenile Justice and Delinquency Prevention. (2004). *Screening and assessing mental health and substance use disorders among youth in the juvenile justice system: A resource guide for practitioners.* Retrieved April 12, 2006, from http://www.ncjrs.gov/pdffiles1/ojjdp/204956.pdf

Paris, J. E. (2005). New thinking on "appropriate" approaches to HIV care. *Correct Care, 19*(3), 3.

Patterson, G. T. (2002). Overview: The law enforcement response to social problems: Mental health as a case in point. In G. Landsberg, M. Rock, L. K. W. Berg, & A. Smiley (Eds.), *Serving mentally ill offenders: Challenges and opportunities for mental health professionals* (pp. 47–50). New York: Springer.

Peters, R. H., & Matthews, C. O. (2003). Substance abuse treatment programs in prisons and jails. In T. J. Fagan & R. K. Ax (Eds.), *Correctional mental health handbook* (pp. 73–99). Thousand Oaks, CA: Sage.

Pogorzelski, W., Wolff, N., Pan, K.-Y., & Blitz, C. L. (2005). Behavioral health problems, ex-offender reentry policies, and the "Second Chance Act." *American Journal of Public Health, 95*, 1718–1724.

Porter, J. (2005). Clearing the air on tobacco use in corrections. *Correct Care, 19*(2), 1, 22.

Reisig, M. D., Holtfreter, K., & Morash, M. (2002). Social capital among women offenders. *Journal of Contemporary Criminal Justice, 18*, 167–186.

Restum, Z. G. (2005). Public health implications of substandard correctional health care. *American Journal of Public Health, 95*, 1689–1691.

Richardson, L. (2003). Other special offender populations. In T. J. Fagan & R. K. Ax (Eds.), *Correctional mental health handbook* (pp. 199–216). Thousand Oaks, CA: Sage.

Shimkus, J. (2004a). Corrections copes with health care for the aged. *Correct Care, 18*(3), 1, 16.

Shimkus, J. (2004b). Juveniles in jails: Different models, similar outcomes. *Correct Care, 18*(1), 9.

Snyder, H. N. (2004). *Juvenile arrests 2002.* Retrieved March 30, 2006, from http://www.ncjrs.gov/html/ojjdp/204608/contents.html

Stanley, J. A. (2004a). Teamwork vital to meeting the medical autonomy standard. *Correct Care, 18*(4), 16.

Stanley, J. A. (2004b). The most important standard: Receiving screening. *Correct Care*, *18*(3), 20–21.

Stringer, H. (2001). Prison break. *NurseWeek*, *14*(6), 13–14.

Teplin, L. A., Abram, K. M., McClelland, G. M., Washburn, J. J., & Pikus, A. K. (2005). Detecting mental disorder in juvenile detainees: Who receives services? *American Journal of Public Health, 95*, 1773–1780.

Teplin, L. A., Mericle, A. A., McClelland, G. M., & Abram, K. M. (2003). HIV and AIDS risk behaviors in juvenile detainees: Implications for public health policy. *American Journal of Public Health, 93*, 906–912.

Thigpen, M. L., Hunter, S. M., & Watson, B. P. (2002). *Services for families of prison inmates: Special issues in corrections.* Longmont, CO: National Institute of Corrections Information Center.

Tobin-D'Angelo, M., Arnold, K., Lance-Parker, S., La Marre, M., Bancroft, E., Jones, A., et al. (2003). Methcillin-resistant *Staphylococcus aureus* in correctional facilities—Georgia, California, and Texas, 2001–2003. *Morbidity and Mortality Weekly Report, 52*, 992–995.

Travis, J., Solomon, A. L., & Waul, M. (2001). *From prison to home: The dimensions and consequences of prisoner reentry.* Retrieved September 25, 2003, from http://www.urban.org/URL.cfm?ID=410098

Travis, J., & Sommers, A. (2004). New perspectives foster better health outcomes. *Correct Care, 18*(1), 1, 19.

Treadwell, H. M., & Ro, M. (2002). Poverty, race, and the invisible men. *American Journal of Public Health, 92*, 705–706.

U.S. Census Bureau. (2005). *Statistical abstract of the United States: 2004–2005.* Retrieved May 12, 2005, from http://www.census.gov/prod/2004pubs/04statab

U.S. Preventive Services Task Force. (2005). *The guide to clinical preventive services, 2005.* Retrieved August 13, 2005, from http://www.ahrq.gov/clinic/pocketguide.htm

Vogt, R. P. (2002). Inmate co-pay finds support in the courts. *Correct Care, 16*(3), 8.

Vogt, R. P. (2005). When an inmate refuses medical care. *Correct Care, 19*(3), 8.

Wagaman, G. L. (2003). Managing and treating female offenders. In T. J. Fagan & R. K. Ax (Eds.), *Correctional mental health handbook* (pp. 123–143). Thousand Oaks, CA: Sage.

Wakeen, R., & Roper, J. (2002). Good eatin': Sensible guidelines for medical diets. *Correct Care, 16*(2), 17.

Weinbaum, C., Lyerla, R., & Margolis, H. (2003). Prevention and control of infections with hepatitis viruses in correctional settings. *Morbidity and Mortality Weekly Report, 52* (RR-1), 1–36.

Weiskopf, C. S. (2005). Nurses' experiences of caring for inmate patients. *Journal of Advanced Nursing, 49*, 336–343.

White, T. W. (2001). Assessing suicide risk: Taking it step by step is your best bet. *Correct Care, 15*(3), 1, 21.

Wolfe, M. I., Xu, F., Patel, P., O'Cain, M., Schlinger, J. A., St. Louis, M. E., et al. (2001). An outbreak of syphilis in Alabama prisons: Correctional health policy and communicable disease control. *American Journal of Public Health, 91*, 1220–1225.

World Health Organization Health in Prisons Project. (2001). *Consensus statement on mental health promotion in prisons.* Retrieved July 10, 2006, from http://www.hipp-europe.org/events/hague/0040.htm

World Health Organization Regional Office for Europe. (2002). *Prison, drugs and society: A consensus statement on principles, policies, and practices.* Retrieved July 10, 2006, from http://www.hipp-europe.org/downloads/England-prisonsanddrugs.pdf

World Health Organization/UNAIDS. (2001). *HIV in prisons.* Retrieved July 10, 2006, from http://www.euro.who.int/document/E77016.pdf

Care of Clients in Disaster Settings

CHAPTER OBJECTIVES

After reading this chapter, you should be able to:

1. Describe ways in which disaster events may vary.
2. Describe the elements of a disaster.
3. Describe two aspects of disaster-related assessment.
4. Identify biophysical, psychological, physical environmental, sociocultural, behavioral, and health system considerations to be assessed in relation to a disaster.
5. Describe two aspects of primary prevention related to disasters.
6. Discuss the principles of community disaster preparedness.
7. Identify the component elements of an effective disaster response plan.
8. Analyze the role of community health nurses in primary, secondary, and tertiary prevention related to disaster situations.

KEY TERMS

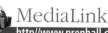

MediaLink
http//www.prenhall.com/clark

Additional interactive resources for this chapter can be found on the Companion Website. Click on Chapter 27 and "Begin" to select the activities for this chapter.

Advocacy in Action

Mobilizing the Hispanic Community for Disaster Preparedness

U.S. public health officials face the challenge of disaster preparedness and response, particularly for ethnically diverse populations. A graduate nursing student, fluent in Spanish, developed a much-needed "risk communication plan" for the local Hispanic population.

The student completed a targeted assessment of needs and resources in the Hispanic community and noted that approximately two thirds of the population needed assistance in speaking and reading English. Key informant interviews, focus groups, and surveys were conducted to determine important sources of news and emergency information for Hispanic community members. The student also contacted local Hispanic radio and television stations for ideas about disseminating emergency information.

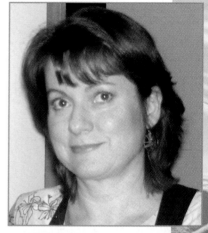

Veronica Vogt

Three goals for risk communication were formulated: (a) raising community awareness, (b) conveying disaster preparedness information to Hispanic community members, and (c) promoting development of a disaster plan in every Hispanic family. The communication plan addressed precrisis and crisis response phases. Components of the precrisis plan included establishing collaborative relationships with local Spanish radio stations and selecting and disseminating printed preparedness materials in church bulletins and at local Hispanic markets. Crisis response plan elements included training interpreters, updating Spanish media sources, disseminating specific messages in Spanish, enlisting trusted community

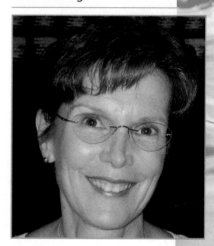

Pamela A. Kulbok

spokespersons to assist with communication, and utilizing a Spanish information call-in line with prerecorded messages. The importance of word-of-mouth and cell phone communication was emphasized in both phases of planning.

This project was conducted in the true spirit of advocacy. A comprehensive assessment was conducted in partnership with members of the Hispanic community, and the resulting plan, developed to reflect the diverse voices of community members, was reviewed by key stakeholders prior to being finalized.

Veronica Vogt, Graduate Student

Pamela A. Kulbok, DNSc, APRN, BC

Associate Professor of Nursing

University of Virginia/Charlottesville

*O*ne can hardly open a newspaper today without reading of a disaster that has occurred somewhere in the world. In the last 25 years, the United States has witnessed more than 442 natural disasters and 902 disaster declarations. The top 10 U.S. disasters in the previous century caused more than 16,500 deaths and adversely affected 2.3 million people (Bissell, Pinet, Nelson, & Levy, 2004), and these figures do not reflect the devastating effects of Hurricanes Katrina and Rita in 2005.

A **disaster** has been defined by the American Red Cross as "an occurrence, either natural or man-made, that causes human suffering and creates human needs that victims cannot alleviate without assistance" (as quoted in Langan & James, 2005, p. 4). This definition highlights the difference between an emergency and a disaster. An **emergency** is a serious threatening event that falls within the coping abilities of the individual, family, or community. A house fire, for example, is an emergency. A disaster, on the other hand, cannot be addressed with usual procedures and requires assistance beyond the ordinary. The wildfire that destroyed more than 300 homes and caused 16 deaths in San Diego in 2003 is an example of a fire-related disaster.

DISASTER TRENDS

Disasters seem to be occurring with greater frequency than ever before. In part this may be due to more extensive news coverage of catastrophic events around the world. It is clear, however, that disasters are having more horrendous effects than in the past. For example, Hurricane Katrina in 2005 was the deadliest hurricane since 1928 and the most costly natural disaster ever to occur in the United States (Daley, 2006b). The December 24, 2004, tsunami that arose in the Indian Ocean resulted in more than 230,000 deaths in India, Indonesia, the Maldives, Somalia, Sri Lanka, and Thailand. In addition, 500,000 people were displaced in Northern Sumatra, Indonesia, and more than 37,000 people were missing and presumed dead (Widyastuti et al., 2006).

Between August 2004 and October 2005, Florida experienced eight major hurricanes (Kay et al., 2006), and 2005 was the first season in recorded history that four hurricanes made landfall in the United States in one year (Daley, 2006b). Table 27-1◆ provides information on some of the more notable disaster events in recent years.

The increasing severity of disaster effects is due to a number of societal changes. Human populations are more densely concentrated and increasingly found in areas with high disaster potential (Landesman, 2005). For example, the majority of deaths related to Hurricane Katrina occurred when New Orleans levees were breached, allowing flooding of portions of the city constructed below sea level (Daley, 2006a, 2006b).

Global climate changes are also altering weather patterns, creating more severe storms with resulting damage. In addition, technological advances increase the potential for human-caused disasters such as toxic leaks, transportation disasters, and massive electrical power outages. Finally, recent events have demonstrated the willingness of some radical groups to engineer massive disasters to achieve their political goals through terrorism.

TYPES OF DISASTERS

Disasters are typically classified as natural or human-caused. Natural disasters result from some force of nature such as major storms (hurricanes, tornadoes, severe thunderstorms, blizzards), floods, earthquakes, wildfires, drought, famine, and eruptions (Langan & James, 2005). Naturally occurring epidemics of communicable diseases are another example of a natural disaster (Vale & Campanella, 2005). Epidemics that affect major segments of the world are called **pandemics**. The World Health Organization (WHO) has identified a cyclic sequence of phases of a pandemic. Phase zero is the interpandemic stage and occurs at four levels, as indicated in Table 27-2◆. In phase one, confirmed outbreaks have occurred in one country with spread to other countries. Phase two is characterized by outbreaks and epidemics in multiple countries and the potential for significant morbidity and mortality. Phase three encompasses the end of the first wave of cases and may be followed by a subsequent resurgence of infection in phase four. The pandemic ends with phase five as a result of increasing immunity levels within the population due to disease or vaccination. The cycle then returns to the zero phase (U.S. Department of Health and Human Services [USDHHS], 2004). Table 27-2◆ summarizes the phases and levels of a pandemic.

Human-caused or **technological disasters** are "complex emergencies, technological disasters, material sources, and other disasters not caused by natural hazards" (Langan & James, 2005, p. 4) that arise from human activity. Human-caused disasters may be accidental or intentional. Categories of unintentional human-caused disasters include hazardous materials releases and other industrial accidents (e.g., an explosion in a coal mine), transportation disasters, and technological disasters such as major power outages or interference with communication systems. Some of the same categories of disasters may also be deliberately caused. Two additional types of intentional disasters are civil conflict (e.g., war, rioting) and terrorism. War may include civil or international conflict, and terrorism may take a variety of forms, as discussed below. Urban renewal, with its consequent displacement of low-income populations, has also been considered a category of human-caused disaster by some authors (Vale & Campanella, 2005). Table 27-3◆ presents types and subtypes of disaster events.

TABLE 27-1 Selected Recent Disasters and Their Effects

Disaster	Year	Selected Effects
Earthquake, Indonesia	2005	▪ Second earthquake after major tsunami ▪ 300 deaths; thousands displaced ▪ Hampered tsunami relief operations
Florida hurricanes	2004	▪ 124 deaths ▪ 20% of homes sustained at least some damage
Freight train collision, North Carolina	2005	▪ 11,500 gallons of chlorine gas released ▪ Nine deaths; 529 people received medical treatment
Hurricane Katrina	2005	▪ 400,000 persons displaced from New Orleans ▪ 500 evacuation centers established in 18 states ▪ Estimated 1,000 deaths in Louisiana, 200 in Mississippi, 20 in Florida, Alabama, and Georgia ▪ 80% of New Orleans flooded ▪ 1,037 injuries/illnesses among rescue personnel
Multiple terrorist attacks	2003	▪ 208 events (190 international events) ▪ 307 deaths, 1,593 injured
Tsunami, India Ocean	2004	▪ Estimated 225,000 deaths in eight countries on two continents ▪ 120,514 deaths, 897 missing, and 403,428 displaced persons in Banda Aceh ▪ 80% of health care workers in Banda Aceh killed
War in Darfur, Sudan	2003	▪ 1 million internally displaced persons ▪ 200,000 refugees in camps in Chad ▪ Limited access to food, water, sanitation, shelter, and health care
World Trade Center attack	2001	▪ 2,726 related deaths as of August 16, 2002 ▪ 343 New York firefighters killed; 240 sought emergency treatment in the first 24 hours after the attacks

Data from: Banauch, G., McLaughlin, M., Horschorn, R., Corrigan, M., Kelly, K., & Prezant, D. (2002). Injuries and illness among New York City fire department rescue workers after responding to the World Trade Center attacks. Morbidity and Mortality Weekly Report, 51 (Special issue), 1–5; Bailey, M. A., Glover, R., & Huang, Y. (2005). Epidemiologic assessment of the impact of four hurricanes—Florida, 2004. Morbidity and Mortality Weekly Report, 54, 693–696; Daley, W. R. (2006). Public health response to Hurricanes Katrina and Rita—Louisiana, 2005. Morbidity and Mortality Weekly Report, 55, 29–30; Daley, W. R. (2006). Public health response to Hurricanes Katrina and Rita—United States, 2005. Morbidity and Mortality Weekly Report, 55, 229–231; Henry, C., Belflower, A., Drociuk, D., Gibson, J. J., Harris, R., Horton, D. K. et al. (2005). Public health consequences from hazardous substances acutely released during rail transit—South Carolina, 2005; Selected states, 1999–2004. Morbidity and Mortality Weekly Report, 54, 64–67; Joyce, N. (2005). Health care after the tsunami: From the front lines in Banda Aceh. Retrieved March 15, 2005, from http://www.medscape.com/viewarticle/500462; Pinto, A., Saeed, M., El Sakka, M., Rashford, A., Colombo, A., Valenciano, M. et al. (2005). Setting up an early warning system for epidemic-prone diseases in Darfur: A participative approach. Disasters, 29, 310–322; Schwartz, S. P., Li, W., Berenson, L., & Williams, R. D. (2002). Deaths in the World Trade Center terrorist attacks—New York City, 2001. Morbidity and Mortality Weekly Report, 51(Special issue), 16–18; Thai Ministry of Public Health. (2005). Health concerns associated with disaster victim identification after a tsunami—Thailand, December 26, 2004–March 31, 2005. Morbidity and Mortality Weekly Report, 54, 349–352; Toprani, A., Ratard, R., Straif-Bourgeois, S., Sokol, T., Averhoff, F., Brady, J. et al. (2006). Surveillance in hurricane evacuation centers—Louisiana, September–October 2005. Morbidity and Mortality Weekly Report, 55, 32–35; U.S. Department of State. (2004). Patterns of global terrorism, 2003. Retrieved November 22, 2004, from http://www.state.gov/s/ct/rls/pgtrpt/2003/c12153.htm; Widyastuti, E., Silaen, G., Pricesca, A., Handoko, A., Blanton, C., Handzel, T. et al. (2006). Assessment of health-related needs after tsunami and earthquake—Three districts, Aceh Province, Indonesia, July–August 2005. Morbidity and Mortality Weekly Report, 55, 93–97; Williams, W., Guarisco, J., Guillot, K., Wales, J., Revels, C., Barre, G. et al. (2005). Surveillance for illness and injury after Hurricane Katrina–New Orleans, Louisiana, September 8–25, 2005. Morbidity and Mortality Weekly Report, 54, 1018–1021.

Terrorism is a form of intentional disaster that is of significant concern in today's world. Terrorism was defined in Chapter 6∞, and according to the Federal Emergency Management Agency (FEMA, 2006c) involves the "use of force or violence against persons or property in violation of the criminal laws of the United States for purposes of intimidation, coercion, or ransom" (p. 1). Another definition is the "deliberate creation and exploitation of fear for bringing about political change" (Hoffman, as quoted in Langan & James, 2005, p. 5). This latter definition embodies the four elements that characterize terrorism: inducement of fear, use or threat of extraordinary violence, premeditation in the use of violence, and a political motivation (Brauer, 2002).

There are several possible avenues for terrorism, as indicated in Table 27-3◆. Biologic terrorism makes use of biological threats or "organisms or toxins that can kill or incapacitate people, livestock, or crops" (FEMA, 2006a, p. 1). When biologic organisms are directed against plants or animals intended as food, the term *agroterrorism* is used (Cupp, Walker, & Hillison, 2004). The Centers for Disease Control and Prevention (CDC) has defined biologic terrorism as "the use or threatened use of biologic agents against a person, group, or larger population to create fear or illnesses for the purposes of intimidation, gaining an advantage, interruption of normal activities, or ideologic activities" (Nolte et al., 2004, p. 3).

Biological agents are categorized by the CDC (2004) on the basis of their potential for destruction. Category A agents are those that have high priority for preparedness activity due to the threat posed to national security based on their ease of dissemination or high interpersonal communicability, high rates of mortality

TABLE 27-2   Phases and Characteristic Features of a Pandemic

Phase	Features
Zero	Interpandemic phase ▪ Level 0: No human cases of infection have been found. ▪ Level 1: One case has been identified in a human being. ▪ Level 2: Two or more cases have been identified, but there is no documented person-to-person spread. ▪ Level 3: Pandemic alert; person-to-person spread has been documented and there has been an outbreak in one country lasting two or more weeks.
One	An outbreak has been confirmed in one country with spread of infection to other countries and potential for serious morbidity and mortality.
Two	Outbreaks and epidemics have occurred in multiple countries, with widening global spread of infection.
Three	End of the first wave of infection
Four	Subsequent seasonal wave of infection
Five	End of the pandemic as a result of increasing herd immunity due to disease or vaccination.

Data from: U.S. Department of Health and Human Services. (2004). Pandemic influenza preparedness and response plan. *Washington, DC: Author.*

and potential for major public health impact, high potential for panic and social disruption, and requirements for special public health preparedness efforts. Category A agents include anthrax, botulism, plague, smallpox, tularemia, viral hemorrhagic fevers (e.g., Ebola virus infection), and adenoviruses. Category B agents are given the second-highest priority for action because of their moderate ease of dissemination, moderate morbidity and low mortality, and requirements for enhanced, but not totally different, diagnostic and surveillance capabilities on the part of the CDC. Category B agents include brucellosis, epsilon toxin of *Clostridium perfringens*, food safety threats (e.g., salmonellosis, shigellosis, *E. coli*), glanders, melioidosis, psittacosis, Q fever, Ricin

TABLE 27-3   Disaster Types and Subtypes

Natural	Human-Caused
▪ Storms	**Accidental**
▪ Floods	▪ Transportation disaster
▪ Earthquakes	▪ Technological disaster
▪ Wildfires	▪ Hazardous materials release
▪ Drought	▪ Industrial accident
▪ Famine	**Intentional**
▪ Volcanic eruptions	▪ Civil conflict
▪ Epidemics	• War
	• Rioting
	▪ Terrorism
	• Agroterrorism
	• Assassination
	• Bioterrorism
	• Chemical terrorism
	• Explosions
	• Hostage taking
	• Nuclear/radiological terrorism

toxin, staphylococcal enterotoxin, typhus fever, viral encephalitis, and water safety threats (e.g., cholera). Category C agents are those assigned third-highest priority for preparation and consist of emerging pathogens, such as *Nipah* and hantaviruses, that could be readily available and easily produced and disseminated. Biologic agents have been identified as the most significant type of terrorist threat because of the small quantities needed to create extensive morbidity, their low cost, strategic impact, and insidious nature. Another factor in the significance of biologic agents is the existence of weak international controls on biologic materials and ease of access to them (Horton, 2003).

Chemical terrorism employs poisonous aerosols, vapors, liquids, or solids to damage people, plants, or animals (FEMA, 2006b). Types of chemical agents include nerve agents that affect central nervous system function, vesicants that cause chemical burns on epithelial membranes of the skin and respiratory tract, and pulmonary agents that cause pulmonary edema. Additional chemical agents include blood agents and cyanides and riot control agents such as tear gas, which can be toxic in large doses. The effects of chemical attacks are influenced by the duration of the hazard and the persistence of the chemical in the environment as well as the route of entry (e.g., respiratory tract versus skin) and the ambient temperature, which may increase the volatility of chemicals and enhance respiratory inhalation (Spanjaard & Khabib, 2003). Chemical releases may be either overt or covert. In an overt release the nature of the event reveals itself as intentional. A covert release may go unrecognized until large numbers of people have been affected (National Center for Environmental Health, 2003).

Explosive devices such as conventional bombs, nuclear weapons, and radiological dispersion devices may also be used for terrorist purposes. Nuclear weapons create intense heat and light as well as damaging pressure waves and widespread radioactivity. Nuclear blasts may also cause electromagnetic pulses (EMPs) that act like lightning to damage electrical devices. Although the level of electrical impulse generated is probably insufficient to harm most humans, EMPs can destroy computers, communication systems, appliances, and vehicle ignitions within 1,000 miles of a high-altitude nuclear detonation. They can also interfere with pacemaker conductivity (FEMA, 2006d). A radiological dispersion device (RDD) uses conventional explosives to disperse dangerous amounts of radioactive material. RDDs are also known as "dirty nukes" or "dirty bombs" (FEMA, 2006e; Sutton & Gould, 2003).

CHARACTERISTICS OF DISASTERS

Disasters vary with respect to a number of characteristics, including their frequency, predictability, preventability, imminence, and duration. Disasters also vary in terms of the extent of their effects.

Some disasters occur relatively frequently in certain parts of the world. Consequently, people in those areas have some knowledge of what to expect and what can be done to minimize the effects of the event. For example, earthquakes occur periodically in California, and residents in earthquake-prone areas are encouraged to be prepared in the event of a large quake. Similarly, hurricanes and other severe storms are frequently experienced during certain seasons in other parts of the country.

Some disaster events are predictable. In general, the probability of destructive tornadoes increases from April through June in the United States. Similarly, many rivers are known to flood periodically with heavy spring rains. Severe blizzards can also be predicted, allowing people to stockpile food supplies, medications, or fuel for heating in case they are isolated by the storm. Other events, such as a plane crash, a fire in a chemical plant, or a terrorist attack are not predictable.

Some types of disasters are more easily prevented than others. For example, periodic flooding can be prevented by rerouting waterways or by building dams. Others, such as earthquakes and severe winter storms, cannot be controlled or prevented. Increased security measures are one attempt to prevent disasters resulting from terrorist activities, but their effectiveness remains to be seen.

Disasters also vary with respect to their imminence in terms of their speed of onset and may have a period of forewarning before striking. Some disasters provide evidence of their imminent occurrence and allow time for preparation prior to impact. For example, blizzards, hurricanes, and other severe storms can be tracked and their probable path determined. People along that path usually have sufficient warning to take preventive actions that minimize the potential for death and destruction. Other disasters such as fires and explosions occur instantaneously, with no prior warning. In some cases, the disaster event itself is of short duration, as in the case of an earthquake or a transportation disaster. At other times, the disaster event lasts some time. Examples of prolonged disasters are epidemics, famine, and war. Disasters such as hurricanes and blizzards have an intermediate duration.

Finally, disasters vary in terms of their impact and their destructive potential. Some disasters are fairly limited in scope, affecting a small geographic area or a relatively small number of people. For example, the effects of a mine cave-in are generally restricted to the area where the mine is located. The effects of war or famine, on the other hand, may be more far-reaching. The extent of disaster effects will be discussed in more detail later in this chapter.

THE ROLE OF THE PUBLIC HEALTH SYSTEM IN A DISASTER

Disasters are events that have significant effects on the health of the public. It is not surprising, then, that the public health system should play a major role in planning for and responding to a wide variety of disaster occurrences. Public health systems have responsibilities before, during, and after a disaster event. Before a disaster, members of the public health care system should be involved in identifying disaster risks and populations particularly vulnerable to their effects. They should then educate those populations regarding disaster prevention and preparedness. In addition, they should cooperate with other agencies in the use of public health science to develop plans to prevent disasters when possible and to limit the morbidity and mortality of disasters that cannot be prevented. They can also assist in the identification of resources available for disaster response. This may include the recruitment and training of volunteer health professionals to deal with the potential health effects of a disaster. Finally, public health professionals, including community health nurses, can advocate for and help develop public policies that reduce the potential for and effects of disasters (Landesman, 2005). For example, they might advocate for building codes that create structures that will withstand major earthquakes, or brush removal ordinances in fire-prone areas.

During a disaster event, public health professionals will assess and communicate information regarding health-related effects to relevant government agencies. They will also coordinate the provision of needed emergency and routine health care immediately after the disaster. They will also advise and assist in the prevention of injury and promotion of food and water safety, vector control, and control of communicable diseases. They may also be involved in inspecting shelter sites for health risks (Landesman, 2005).

Following a disaster, public health professionals would be involved in assuring that follow-up care is available to disaster victims with continuing needs. They would also participate in a collaborative evaluation of the disaster response and subsequent redrafting of response plans for future disasters (Landesman, 2005).

The public health system also has a similar role in responding to the health consequences of terrorist activities. Responsibilities center on prevention, preparedness, and response (Levy & Sidel, 2003). Public health activities to prevent terrorism may include reducing access to biological agents. In addition, public health professionals should assure that a balance is maintained between terrorism preparedness and addressing other public health issues and between preventing terrorism and protecting individual civil rights. Both of these latter responsibilities may require concerted advocacy initiatives on the part of public health professionals, particularly community health nurses. Several public health authorities have cautioned that preparedness, in particular, should not lead to inappropriate responses that infringe on civil rights or that draw resources from other elements of terrorism preparedness or other important public health initiatives (Berkowitz, 2002; Cohen, Gould, & Sidel, 2004; Levy & Sidel, 2003).

ELEMENTS OF A DISASTER

Disaster literature typically addresses three main elements of a disaster occurrence: the temporal element, the spatial element, and the role element. In this chapter, we will also address a fourth element, the effects element.

The Temporal Element: Stages of Disaster Response

Disaster experts characterize disasters as cyclic phenomena unfolding in five stages: the nondisaster or interdisaster stage, the predisaster stage, the impact stage, the emergency stage, and the recovery stage (Langan & James, 2005).

The Nondisaster Stage

The nondisaster stage, also referred to as the interdisaster phase, is the period of time before the threat of a disaster materializes. This period should be a time of planning and preparation. During this stage, communities should engage in such activities as identifying potential disaster risks and mapping their locations in the community. Vulnerability assessment and capability inventory are other features of this stage in which the community assesses the potential consequences of disasters likely to occur within the community and its ability to cope with these consequences. **Vulnerability assessment** involves predisaster identification of groups within the population who would be particularly vulnerable to the adverse effects of a disaster. Elderly persons are an example of a highly vulnerable population. The extent and location of vulnerable populations should be determined and plans made for meeting their unique needs in the event of a disaster. Capability inventory involves determination of the adaptive capacity of the community through inventory of resources that are likely to be needed in the event of specific types of disasters and their availability in the community.

During the nondisaster stage, the community should also engage in prevention, preparedness, and mitigation activities. **Mitigation** is action taken to prevent or reduce the harmful effects of a disaster on human health or property (Bissell et al., 2004). Mitigation is sometimes referred to as "hard" or "soft." Hard mitigation involves construction of the built environment to withstand the force of natural hazards (Lichterman, 2000). Retrofitting or reinforcing major highway overpasses is an example of hard mitigation being used in California to prevent the collapse of highways and bridges in the event of an earthquake. Soft mitigation is intended to minimize the adverse effects of disasters that cannot be prevented, for example, developing communication strategies that enhance the capability of multiunit response to major brush fires.

The final area of activity in the nondisaster planning period is the education of both professionals and the public regarding disaster prevention and preparation. Unfortunately, many communities deny the need for disaster planning when they are not faced with the direct threat of a disaster. Even when disaster planning occurs, if the plan is not widely disseminated, disaster response can be impeded.

The Predisaster Stage

The predisaster stage occurs when a disaster event is imminent but has not yet occurred. This stage may also be referred to as the warning or threat stage. Major activities during this stage are warning, preimpact mobilization, and, in some cases, evacuation. Warning involves apprising members of the community of the imminence of a disaster event and of the actions that should be taken to minimize its consequences. For example, storm warnings are broadcast in many areas when there is potential for a severe storm, but people do not immediately go to a storm cellar or leave the area, because the possibility remains that the storm will bypass the area.

For recurrent disasters, such as hurricanes, warnings may occur in four stages (Holland, 2003). The first stage involves routine reminders of the upcoming hurricane (or tornado, fire, etc.) season and the need to take general precautions. The second stage is an early warning stage in which the public is notified of a possible threat. The third stage involves a direct warning of the likelihood of imminent disaster and danger. The fourth level of warning involves an ongoing update on the development of the disaster conditions and effects as they occur.

Just as communities may accept or deny the need for disaster planning, members of the community may respond positively or negatively to warnings of possible disasters. Several factors can influence a person's response, including the source, content, and mechanism for warning, and individual perceptions and beliefs. Warning messages that are clear, practical, and relevant or that originate from credible sources are more likely to be acted on than vague or impractical warnings. Warnings need to specify the exact nature of the threat and provide specific recommendations for action. For example, vague warnings of the potential for additional terrorist activities following the September 11, 2001, attacks provided little direction for action. Specific guidelines on how to handle mail potentially contaminated with anthrax spores, on the other hand, were more effective in promoting action. Warnings should also contain sufficient information to allow people to decide on an appropriate course of action. It is sometimes erroneously believed that detailed information about a disaster will cause panic. In effect, failure to provide information usually leads to failure to act on warnings; providing information does not seem to contribute to panic among individual citizens. On occasion, overwarning, particularly for predictable disasters such as hurricanes, has resulted in unnecessary activity and expense (Pielke, 2003).

Response to a warning is also affected by each individual's perceptions about the possibility of disaster. These perceptions arise from past experiences with disaster, psychological traits, and sociocultural factors. For example, if people have previously been only on the fringes of a hurricane path, they may not perceive a hurricane as a very frightening event, and they may ignore storm warnings. Similarly, if the individual has a fatalistic attitude that one's own actions will not make much difference in the outcome of an event, he or she might not act in response to warnings. Such an attitude may be the result of an individual personality trait or a sociocultural norm in the group.

Warning confirmation also influences the way people respond. Warnings tend to be believed if the source of the warning is official, if the probability of the event is increasing, and if one is in close geographic proximity to the area where the disaster is likely to occur. For example, people who live on a recognized geological fault line are more likely to take warnings about potential earthquakes seriously than those who do not live on a fault.

Belief also influences action with respect to warnings. Again, belief in the potential for disaster is enhanced if the source of the warning is an official agency and if that agency has credibility. For example, if there have been numerous false alarms in the past, people are less likely to pay attention to warnings. Belief is also enhanced if the medium of the warning is personal rather than impersonal. People are more likely to evacuate their homes if someone comes to their door to warn them than if they hear a warning on the radio. Previous experience also influences the likelihood of belief. If one has experienced the full force of a hurricane before, one is more likely to believe and act on a hurricane warning than would otherwise be the case.

The frequency with which the warning is received also influences belief, as do observable changes in the situation. For example, if people see evidence of flames on a nearby hill, they are more likely to believe in the imminence of danger posed by a brush fire. Perceived behavior of others can influence belief either positively or negatively. When others act in response to the warning, belief is enhanced. If others appear to be ignoring the warning, however, belief is less likely. Factors influencing responses to disaster warnings are summarized in Table 27-4◆.

Preimpact mobilization is action aimed at averting the disaster or minimizing its effects. Activities involved in this stage might include efforts to prevent the disaster or its effects, seeking shelter from the effects of the disaster, evacuating people from areas threatened by the disaster, and implementing plans to deal with the effects of a disaster. For example, in the threat of a flood, people may sandbag riverbanks to divert floodwaters from a town, or board up windows and tie down equipment when a hurricane is forecast. People may seek shelter from tornadoes or other storms by moving to a basement, a storm cellar, or an interior room of a house. Preimpact mobilization might also involve evacuating people from an area threatened by fire, radiation, or chemical leakage. Finally, the initial phases of a disaster response plan may be implemented. For example, off-duty health care personnel may be recalled to health facilities in preparation for treating anticipated casualties.

EVIDENCE-BASED PRACTICE

Lasker (2004) reported a study of the American public that explored their potential response to two terrorist scenarios, smallpox dissemination and release of a "dirty bomb" with radioactive materials. Recommended actions in the scenarios were receipt of vaccination for smallpox at a public mass immunization site and staying indoors, respectively. Only two fifths of those surveyed reported they would comply with the smallpox recommendation, and three fifths would shelter in place. Reasons for intended noncompliance related to other priorities such as fear of exposure to smallpox in a public venue, fear of vaccine consequences, and concerns related to family members' safety. Lack of trust in public officials also influenced intentions to comply with the recommendations. What are the implications of these findings for planning public health responses to these two possible terrorist activities? How might these findings be used to guide response planning? How might community health nurses be involved in research to determine public perspectives on disaster preparedness in a particular jurisdiction?

TABLE 27-4	Factors Influencing Response to Disaster Warnings
Warning Feature	**Influencing Factors**
Warning message	▪ Clarity ▪ Practicality ▪ Relevance ▪ Informativeness
Individual perceptions	▪ Past experience with disasters ▪ Psychological traits ▪ Sociocultural attitudes
Warning confirmation	▪ Official source ▪ Increasing evidence and probability of disaster ▪ Geographic proximity to the expected disaster location
Beliefs	▪ Credibility of warning sources ▪ Personal rather than impersonal contact ▪ Previous experience of disaster ▪ Observable changes in the situation ▪ Frequency of warning ▪ Belief and action by others

The Impact Stage

In the impact stage of a disaster, the disaster event has occurred and its immediate effects are experienced by the community. One major activity in this stage is the assessment of the impact of the disaster with an inventory of the immediate needs of the community. Inventory is a rapid assessment of the damage to buildings and the type and extent of injuries suffered. This information is used to determine actions needed in carrying out the efforts of the emergency stage.

The Emergency Stage

The focus of the emergency stage of a disaster is on saving lives through rescue efforts, first aid, and emergency treatment (Landesman, 2005). The emergency response to a disaster usually begins with community members because there has not been time for assistance to arrive from outside sources. If the community is geographically isolated or access to the community is impeded by the disaster, this isolation period will be prolonged. Later, relief assistance is provided from sources outside of the area affected by the disaster. The activities performed are essentially the same, although performed by different agents in the two phases, and include search and rescue operations, first aid, emergency medical assistance, establishment or restoration of modes of communication and transportation, surveillance for public health effects of the disaster (e.g., infectious diseases, mental health problems), and, in some cases, evacuation of community members from affected areas.

The Recovery Stage

In the recovery stage, the focus is on returning the community to equilibrium. This stage can be divided into substages of restoration and actual reconstruction and ends in reconstitution. Mitigation may also occur in the recovery stage with efforts to prevent a recurrence of a disaster or to enhance preparedness and response capabilities.

Restoration is the reestablishment of a basic way of life and occurs within the first 6 months of a disaster. Activities of this stage include returning to homes or seeking alternative shelter, removing debris, and replacing lost or damaged property. At the community level, restoration involves reestablishing community services that may have been disrupted by the disaster (Landesman, 2005). After a flood, for example, people may return to their homes, clean up the mud, and replace water-damaged furniture. Schools reopen, and residents return to work. If a prominent community official was killed in the flood, someone is appointed to fill that post until an election can be held.

Reconstruction involves the rebuilding and reordering of the physical and social environments (Landesman, 2005). Homes, schools, businesses, and other structures may need to be rebuilt. Dams or levees may be constructed to prevent future flooding. Reconstruction may also entail alterations in the social environment. For example, terrorist activity has led to enhanced security provisions in airports, at international borders, and even in educational institutions, which are now required to more closely account for the activities of foreign students.

Reunification is a special instance of reconstruction for refugee families who have often been separated during their travels in search of safety. Immigration restrictions in permanent host countries may result in lengthy separations of family members as portions of families migrate in sequence. Refugee literature has identified three stages of separation and reunification for families—before the separation, during separation, and afterwards—each of which creates an imbalance in family function and challenges families' abilities to function effectively (Rousseau, Rufagari, Bagilishya, & Measham, 2004).

Reconstitution occurs when the life of the community has returned, as far as possible, to normal. This return to normal may take from several months to several years, depending on the degree of damage sustained in the disaster. It may take several years after a flood, for example, to restore the landscape of the community to its former state or to replenish the city treasury after disaster costs have depleted it. It may also take some time for individuals to adjust to the loss of loved ones or for the community government to be reconstituted. In extreme disasters, full reconstitution may never occur. For example, many people believe that life in the United States was completely changed by the terrorist attacks on September 11, 2001, and the full effects of that disaster are not yet known. The extent to which New Orleans will achieve full reconstitution following Hurricane Katrina may also be in question.

The final stage of recovery after a disaster is mitigation, which involves future-oriented activities to prevent subsequent disasters or to minimize their effects. For example, a community that has experienced a flood may take engineering action to prevent the likelihood of subsequent floods, or a community that was unprepared for disaster may develop a disaster response plan. Increased security measures and irradiating mail are other examples of efforts aimed at preventing subsequent terrorist activities and their effects. These activities cycle the community back into the nondisaster stage. Stages and related activities in the development of and response to a disaster are summarized in Table 27-5◆.

The Spatial Element

The spatial elements of a disaster refer to the extent of its effects on specific geographic regions. These regions include the area of total impact, the area of partial impact, and outside areas (Figure 27-1).

TABLE 27-5	Stages and Activities in Disaster Occurrence and Response
Disaster Stage	**Related Activities**
Nondisaster/ interdisaster stage	▪ Identification of potential disaster risks ▪ Vulnerability analysis ▪ Capability inventory ▪ Prevention and mitigation ▪ Response planning and plan dissemination ▪ Stockpiling necessary supplies ▪ Public and professional education
Predisaster stage	▪ Warning ▪ Preimpact mobilization ▪ Evacuation
Impact stage	▪ Damage inventory ▪ Injury assessment
Emergency stage	▪ Search and rescue ▪ First aid ▪ Emergency medical assistance ▪ Restoration of communication and transportation ▪ Public health surveillance ▪ Further evacuation, as needed
Recovery stage	▪ Restoration of functional capabilities ▪ Reconstruction of physical and social environments ▪ Reunification of families ▪ Reconstitution ▪ Mitigation of future disaster events

The area of total impact is the zone where the most severe effects of the disaster are found. In an earthquake, for example, this would include the area where the greatest damage to buildings has occurred and where the greatest number of injuries was sustained.

In the area of partial impact, evidence of the disaster can be seen but the effects are not of the magnitude of those in the total impact area. Using the earthquake example, windows may be broken or objects shaken from shelves in the partial impact area, but buildings are intact. Injuries, if any, are infrequent and relatively minor, or only telephone and electrical services might be disrupted in the partial impact area.

The outside area is not directly affected but may be a source of assistance in response to the disaster. Areas immediately adjacent to the disaster area are called on first to provide assistance, with further outlying areas being involved later as needed. In a major disaster, the federal government may be called on to provide assistance. This occurs once the area affected has been declared an official disaster area. Figure 27-2 depicts the process by which a presidential declaration of a major disaster or emergency is initiated and federal assistance is provided. As indicated in the figure, when a disaster occurs, local emergency personnel respond and assess the magnitude of the disaster. They inform local government officials of the extent of the problem and the need for outside assistance. Local officials request assistance from the state governor. The governor may initiate

further damage assessment or make an immediate request to the U.S. Department of Health and Human Services (USDHHS). The Secretary of Health and Human Services reviews the request and makes a recommendation for a presidential emergency disaster declaration. Once the President of the United States has made the official declaration, the USDHHS response plan is implemented and federal disaster assistance is provided to the local jurisdiction (FEMA, 2003).

Spatial elements of a disaster vary greatly from event to event. For example, the total and partial impact areas affected by a nuclear accident would be far larger than those affected by a fire at an industrial chemicals plant. The area from which assistance might be requested would also be larger given the greater magnitude of the problem, the number of victims involved, and the damage sustained.

Spatial elements of a potential disaster can also be explored prior to a disaster event. The World Health Organization (2004) suggested the creation of hazard maps to identify and locate potential disaster hazards in a country. At the community level, community risk maps and community resource maps are used to help delineate spatial dimensions in disaster planning. **Community risk maps** pinpoint the locations of disaster risks within the community. Risk maps also delineate probable areas of effect for different types of disasters. Figure 27-3 is an example of a community risk map. Two primary disaster risks are identified in the community risk map in the figure: a dam and reservoir that could result in flooding and a chemical manufacturing plant on the south side of the river. In addition, this community is in an area that experiences periodic tornadoes. The community risk map delineates the areas of the community likely to be affected by a flood (along the river) and a fire or explosion at the chemical plant. The area affected by a tornado would depend on where the tornado touched down. The map also indicates several pockets of particularly vulnerable populations in areas likely to be affected by disasters. These include residents of a nursing home, prison inmates, and schoolchildren in the vicinity of the chemical plant. These same groups, along with patients at the hospital at F and North River Streets and children in the school just north of the river, would be at risk in the event of a flood on the river.

Community resource maps indicate the locations of resources likely to be needed in the event of each of the types of disasters for which the community is at risk. Notations on a community resource map include, for example, potential shelter locations, designated command headquarters (and alternates if advisable), storage places for supplies, areas where heavy equipment is available, health care facilities, and proposed emergency morgue areas for the dead. Resource maps also indicate primary and alternate evacuation and transportation routes. Figure 27-4 is a sample resource map related to the community risks identified in Figure

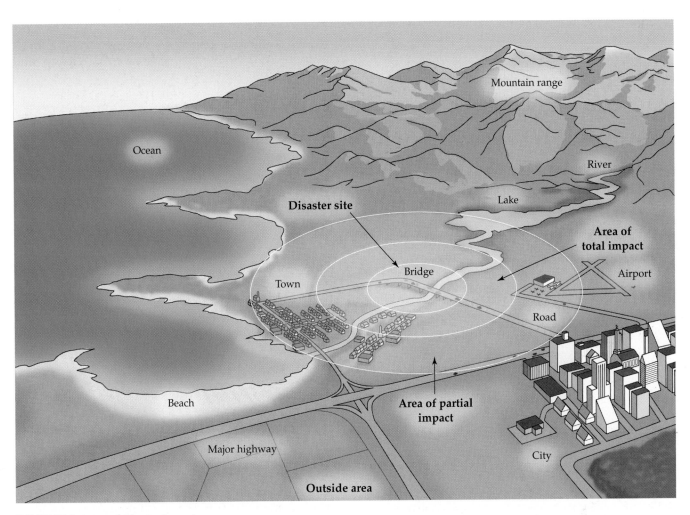

FIGURE 27-1 Areas of Disaster Impact

27-3. Looking at Figure 27-4, we see that city hall is adjacent to the river and likely to be affected by a flood. Therefore, the command headquarters has been situated at the television station in the northern part of town. It was believed that placement at the station would facilitate communication because of the equipment available there. A southern command post has also been established in the event that both bridges are impassable and response operations on the two sides of the river cannot be coordinated. Because of the potential for splitting the community and lack of access across the river, potential shelter sites have been established and supplies have been stored on both sides of the river. Health services are also available on both sides even if the hospital at F and North River Streets has to be evacuated due to flooding. Rescue operations for people stranded along the river would have to be handled from the north side of the river because that is where the boat docks are located. Personnel and supplies can be brought in from other towns in several different directions and could be brought directly to tent shelter sites if necessary. Only the road from Phildon is likely to be impassable if flooding reaches that far from the reservoir. Both the community risk and resource maps allow disaster planners to

visualize what is likely to occur in a disaster event and to plan the most effective response to a disaster.

The Role Element

The third element of a disaster is its role element. Two basic roles for people involved in a disaster are *victim* and *helper roles*.

Six levels of disaster victims have been identified in the disaster literature (Taylor & Frazer, as identified in Langan & James, 2005). Primary victims are those who experience maximum exposure to the disaster event. Secondary victims are not themselves directly affected by the disaster but are indirectly affected as friends and family of primary victims. Third-level victims include first responders and health care personnel involved in rescue and recovery efforts. Fourth-level victims are other community members who offer help or share the grief and loss experienced by the primary victims. Fifth-level victims are those who are not directly affected by the disaster, but who suffer psychological upset as a result. Sixth-level victims are those who are indirectly or vicariously affected by the disaster. In the case of the terrorist attacks of September 11, 2001, those who died or

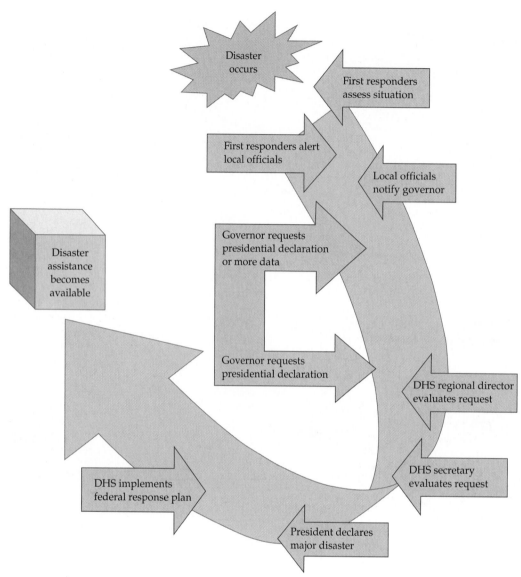

FIGURE 27-2 The Federal Process of Disaster Declaration

were injured in the collapse of the World Trade Center towers and those who survived the collapse uninjured were the primary victims of the disaster. Their friends and family members and other close associates (e.g., colleagues of the fire and rescue personnel who died) were secondary victims. Rescue and health personnel who attempted to meet the needs of those trapped in the rubble or injured were third-level victims. Other residents of lower Manhattan or members of church congregations who lost members to the disaster are examples of fourth-level victims. Fifth-level victims included people who developed post-traumatic shock disorder as a result of watching the disaster on television as well as people whose existing mental health problems were exacerbated by news of the disaster. Finally, most Americans could be considered sixth-level victims in terms of the indirect effects on feelings of security and curtailment of individual rights. Members of ethnic minority

groups who were accosted or threatened in retaliation for perceived responsibility for the attacks were a specific subcategory of sixth-level victims.

Refugees and internally displaced persons are special categories of primary victims of disasters. **Internally displaced persons (IDPs)** are those who are forced by the disaster to leave their homes but relocate in another part of their own country. Displacement may occur for a variety of reasons, including destruction of one's home, temporary hazardous conditions, and war, and may persist for varying periods. New Orleans residents displaced by Hurricane Katrina in 2005 relocated at least temporarily in as many as 18 different states. Refugees are a subgroup of displaced persons defined as those who have fled their own country "because of fear of persecution due to their belonging to a particular social, political, or religious group" (Steele, Lemieux-Charles, Clark, & Glazier, 2002, p. 118). Another group of

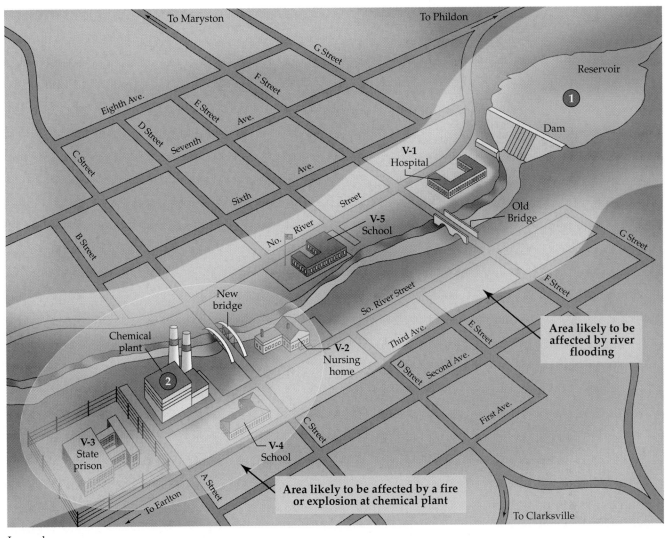

FIGURE 27-3 Sample Community Risk Map

Legend:

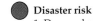 **Disaster risk**
1. Dam and reservoir: potential for flooding
2. Chemical plant: potential for explosion/fire

V Vulnerable populations
1. Hospitalized patients
2. Nursing home residents
3. State prison inmates
4. School children
5. School children

displaced people are *economic refugees*, those who have fled due to poverty, famine, or natural disaster rather than war or persecution. Economic refugees are not recognized by the United Nations and are often not eligible for the kinds of assistance provided to designated refugee populations. Refugee populations are often at higher risk for multiple health, environmental, and social problems than the general public. For example, in one study of Cuban refugee children, 31% suffered some sort of infectious disease, and 23% had lead poisoning (Entzel, Fleming, Trepka, & Squicciarini, 2003). Similarly, among 200,000 refugees from Darfur, Sudan, relocated in refugee camps in Chad, only 39% had access to food assistance and fewer yet had access to clean water,

sanitation, or health care services (Pinto et al., 2005). Many refugees have also been subjected to torture or other abuse. In one study, for example, the prevalence of torture experiences among Somali and Oromo refugees ranged from 25% to 69% among both men and women, and those who had experienced or witnessed torture were more likely than other refugees to experience PTSD and other mental health problems (Jaranson et al., 2004).

One of the ways in which the role aspect of a disaster influences disaster response lies in the actions taken by those affected by the disaster. As we will see later, disaster planning needs to take into consideration the likely response of people to the occurrence of a

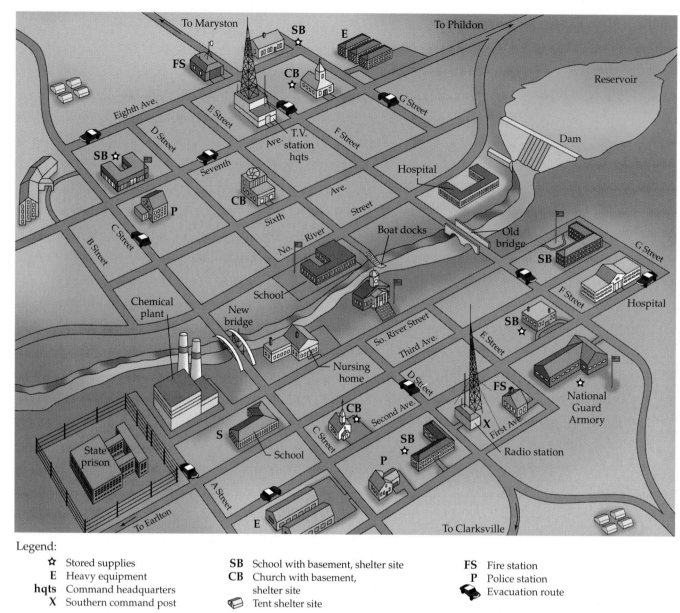

Legend:

☆	Stored supplies	**SB**	School with basement, shelter site	**FS**	Fire station
E	Heavy equipment	**CB**	Church with basement,	**P**	Police station
hqts	Command headquarters		shelter site		Evacuation route
X	Southern command post		Tent shelter site		

FIGURE 27-4 Sample Community Resource Map

disaster. Disaster planning can be completely ineffective if it fails to account for public response. As a case in point, a recent study was conducted to gauge potential public response to recommendations in two terrorist scenarios (Barclay, 2004). A sample of the U.S. public were asked if they would attend public immunization sites in the event of a smallpox epidemic or remain indoors as recommended with the detonation of a "dirty bomb." Results indicated that only 40% of the public would go to a mass immunization site due to fears of being exposed to disease at the site or fear of adverse consequences from the vaccine. Similarly, only 60% indicated that they would remain indoors in the event of a dirty bomb, citing concerns about the safety of family members as a reason for leaving refuge (Lasker, 2004).

Clearly the activities of disaster victims, whether positive or negative, will influence the effectiveness of disaster response.

The second aspect of the role element of a disaster involves persons that play helper roles. As we saw earlier, helpers have been identified as one level of disaster victim, but their role in the disaster is a different one than that of primary victims. Helpers include designated rescue and recovery personnel as well as community members who help provide care or who assist in the provision of necessities such as food, shelter, and clothing. Victim and helper roles may overlap, and rescue and recovery personnel or other community helpers may themselves have suffered injury or loss as a result of the disaster.

Both victims and helpers are under stress as a result of the disaster. Stressors for victims may be quite obvious and include injury and the loss of loved ones or property. Additional stressors for helpers during the rescue and recovery periods include encounters with multiple deaths that are frequently of a shocking nature, experiencing the suffering of others, and role stress. Frequently, the overwhelming nature of role demands or needs for assistance by victims leads to feelings of helplessness and depression. Other sources of role stress include communication difficulties, inadequacies in terms of resources or staff, lack of access to people needing assistance or resources to help them, bureaucratic difficulties, exhaustion, uncertainties regarding role or authority, and intragroup or intergroup conflicts. Stress may also arise from conflicts between the demands of the helper's family members and the needs of victims, and between the demands of one's regular job and one's disaster role.

The Effects Element

The final element of a disaster is the effects element. We have already discussed the geographic distribution of disaster effects in the spatial element of a disaster, but there are also various categories of effects that may result from disasters.

Many experts distinguish between primary or direct and secondary or indirect effects of disasters (Paul, 2005). Primary disaster effects are the immediate effects of the disaster event itself, such as the extent of death, injury, and destruction of property. Rapid-onset natural disasters, such as earthquakes, often have severe primary effects. Secondary disaster effects are those that occur indirectly as a result of the disaster. Examples include malnutrition due to disruption of food supplies, psychological problems such as post-traumatic stress disorder, and the disruption of the U.S. economy following the World Trade Center attack. Disaster effects may also be tangible or intangible. Tangible effects are usually those that can be measured in economic costs. Intangible effects are those that cannot be measured in terms of monetary losses, such as death and suffering (Paul, 2005).

Disasters also vary in terms of the severity of their effects. Some disasters cause moderate loss of life or property and result in only temporary inability to function, whereas others are devastating. The destructive potential of a nuclear explosion, for example, is far greater than that of a single plane crash.

Another way of categorizing the effects of disasters is into physical and mental health effects, economic effects, structural effects, and social effects. Physical health effects may arise as a direct result of the disaster itself (e.g., deaths or injuries) or as secondary effects (e.g., an epidemic of diarrheal disease among shelter residents). Mental health effects may be seen immediately after a disaster or surface days, weeks, or months later. Structural effects include homes, roads, and other structures destroyed by the disaster, and economic effects include the cost of rebuilding these structures as well as the economic costs of lost productivity, lost income, and care for disaster victims. Finally, social effects may occur that are either positive or negative. An example of a positive social effect might be an increased sense of community cohesion, whereas distrust and scapegoating of persons believed responsible for a disaster would be a negative effect. Change in the health care delivery system is another example of a social effect of a disaster. Each of these categories of disaster effects will be addressed in more detail in the discussion of disaster assessment later in this chapter.

COMMUNITY HEALTH NURSING AND DISASTER CARE

As public health professionals, community health nurses have a significant role to play in both disaster preparedness and response. Their involvement parallels the stages of the nursing process and involves collaboration in assessment, diagnosis, and disaster response planning, implementation, and evaluation.

Disaster-related Assessment

The assessment activities of community health nurses with respect to disaster care have two major aspects, the types of assessment conducted and specific assessment considerations.

Types of Assessment
Assessment with respect to disaster preparation and response occurs in two stages, before and after a disaster occurs. Community health nursing involvement in predisaster assessment involves assessing the potential for disaster and response capabilities within a specific community. Assessment during a disaster focuses on identification of disaster effects and related health needs.

ASSESSING DISASTER RISK AND CAPACITY Earlier we discussed the need to create community risk and resource maps. Because of familiarity with communities and their physical and social features, community health nurses are often in a prime position to identify potential disaster risks in a community. Not only are they aware of the types of industries in a community that may pose disaster hazards, but they may also recognize early signs of pending civil unrest among segments of the population that they serve. Identifying the potential for disaster in a particular community involves forecasting the types of disasters possible and the likelihood of their occurrence. The possible types of disasters, of course, vary from community to community. Disaster potential and the probable effects can be systematically assessed by examining factors related to each of the six dimensions of health. The dimensions-of-health perspective can also be used to assess the effects of an actual disaster. Both of these aspects of disaster assessment are discussed below in the section on assessment considerations.

Assessment of response capability is another aspect of predisaster assessment. This is closely tied to an assessment of the degree of disaster preparedness in the community and community attitudes to disaster planning. The community health nurse should assess the attitudes of community members toward disaster preparedness. To what extent are individuals and families in the area prepared for potential disasters? Have families in an earthquake-prone region, for example, gathered supplies that will be needed in the event of an earthquake and placed them in an accessible location? Have emergency escape routes from homes, schools, and other buildings been identified? Have families discussed an emergency contact person who can relay messages for and about family members separated in a disaster? Or are these types of preparation largely ignored?

Community health nurses also have knowledge of resources that might be brought to bear in a disaster situation. For example, they may be aware of community residents who should be involved in disaster response planning, or they may have a better grasp of potential public response to proposed disaster response initiatives than others involved in disaster planning. Again, specific categories of response capability are addressed in the discussion of the dimensions of health as they result to a disaster presented below.

POSTDISASTER RAPID ASSESSMENT Following the occurrence of an actual disaster event, community health

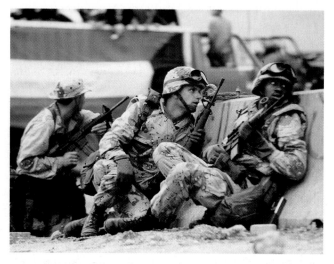

War causes multiple adverse health effects. (Charles Piatiau)

nurses will be actively involved in rapid assessment of disaster effects. Rapid assessment involves determination of the extent of damage caused by the disaster as well as the number of deaths, injuries, and/or illnesses resulting from the disaster. Community health nurses may be involved in identifying and reporting the extent of health-related disaster effects.

Assessment Considerations

Both risk and capacity assessment and assessment of the health-related effects of an actual disaster can be framed in terms of the dimensions of health as they influence a disaster situation.

BIOPHYSICAL CONSIDERATIONS One determinant in forecasting potential disasters is that of human biology. Certain groups of people are more likely than others to be affected by a disaster. For example, if the anticipated disaster is an epidemic of influenza, those most likely to be severely affected are the very young and the elderly; however, there also will be illness among the health care workforce that may impede efforts to halt the spread of disease. On the other hand, if there is potential for an explosion in a local chemical plant, those affected are likely to be company employees and persons in surrounding buildings. Again, this might include children if there is a school nearby. In disasters requiring evacuation, the elderly and disabled are at particular risk because of potential mobility limitations. The elderly and disabled are also the most likely groups to have necessary health care services disrupted and quality of life diminished by a disaster (Little et al., 2004).

Human biology is also a factor in predicting the types of effects expected as a result of the disaster. In the case of an influenza epidemic, illness potentially accompanied by dehydration and electrolyte imbalance may be expected. In an earthquake, many deaths result from injuries due to falling debris. Earthquakes may also result in a high incidence of *crushing syndrome*, a condition in which extensive injury to muscle tissue results in the release of endotoxins that lead to kidney failure (Doctors Without Borders, 2005b). In the classic 1906 San Francisco earthquake, however, the majority of damage was caused by the ensuing fires and rupture of city water mains (Rozario, 2005). Floods result primarily in drownings, but the floodwaters in New Orleans after Hurricane Katrina also led to clusters of diarrheal disease, wound infections, and skin infestations from working in contaminated water (Jablecki et al., 2005). Terrorist dissemination of anthrax spores, on the other hand, may result in cutaneous, inhalation, or intestinal forms of disease with related symptoms and complications (CDC, 2006).

The overall health status of the community also influences disaster planning requirements. For example, if hypertension is prevalent in the community, provisions need to be made in a disaster plan for ongoing treatment of hypertension or other prevalent diseases. It has been suggested that people with disabilities and other complex chronic conditions establish "go packs" that can be ready in case of the need for evacuation. Go packs should contain essential medication for at least 7 days, easily accessible assistive devices (e.g., canes), food and water for guide animals, and emergency health information. People with chronic conditions should also know where to evacuate so their own particular needs can be met (Landesman, 2005). Among households in evacuation centers in San Antonio, Texas, after Hurricane Katrina, 42% had at least one family member with a chronic illness that required ongoing health care (Rogers et al., 2006).

Clients with conditions such as tuberculosis (TB) and HIV infection are in particular need of continuing therapy following a disaster, and response plans should include mechanisms for locating these clients and continuing their treatment. For example, 195 persons in the Alabama, Louisiana, and Mississippi counties most affected by Hurricane Katrina were on TB medications at the time of the disaster (Jablecki et al., 2005). In New Orleans alone, 130 clients were undergoing active TB therapy when Katrina struck. Within 6 weeks, concerted community health efforts had relocated all 130 people and enabled reinitiation of treatment (DeGraw et al., 2006).

In the event of disaster, the community health nurse assesses the physiologic effects of the event on human biology. The most catastrophic effect of disasters is, of course, death. Disaster-related deaths may be of three types: direct deaths, indirect deaths, and disaster-related natural deaths (Jones et al., 2004). Direct deaths are those caused by the disaster itself. For example, fires directly cause death through burns and smoke inhalation. Indirect deaths are due to circumstances caused by the disaster. For example, starvation is indirectly attributable to drought and famine. Disaster-related natural deaths are the result of existing conditions that are exacerbated by the disaster. For example, a death due to myocardial infarction during a hurricane would most likely be a disaster-related naturally caused death. The terrorist attacks of September 11, 2001, actually led to development of a new category of mortality and morbidity in both the World Health Organization *International Classification of Diseases, Tenth Revision* (ICD-10) and the U.S. ICD-9, clinical modification to classify deaths and injuries related to terrorist activities (CDC, 2002).

The nurse appraises the extent of injuries incurred by victims and relief workers and may also assess other needs for health care. For example, the nurse might need to assess the health status of a disaster relief worker with diabetes or of a child with a fever. The nurse assists in assessing the health status of groups of people including both victims and rescue workers. For example, nearly a third of rescue workers and volunteers, including nonsmokers, exposed to the stress and

environmental toxins caused by the World Trade Center collapse on September 11, 2001, had abnormal spirometry readings (Levin et al., 2004), and 21% of surviving New York fire and EMS personnel were treated for respiratory irritation (Banauch et al., 2002). Other people not immediately affected by the disaster may also develop disaster-related illnesses. For instance, 27% of adults in the general Manhattan population reported worsening asthma following the WTC attacks (Fagan, Galea, Ahern, Bonner, & Vlahov, 2002). Similarly, high school and college personnel within 5 miles of the WTC were significantly more likely than those further away to report eye, nose, and throat irritation (Bernard et al., 2002). Possible biophysical effects of several types of disasters are presented in Table 27-6◆.

PSYCHOLOGICAL CONSIDERATIONS Components of the psychological dimension can also influence the effects of a disaster on health. As noted earlier, a number of psychological factors can affect the way people respond to a warning of disaster. For example, interviews with people who escaped from the World Trade Center indicated that four factors influenced their decision to leave the building. These factors included a perceived ability to walk down multiple flights of stairs and prior experience in evacuating one of the towers, including knowledge of stairwell locations and where they led. A third factor that impeded the decision to evacuate was concern over leaving the work area without supervisory permission. Finally, dissemination of information on what was happening, what floors were affected, and what to do influenced decisions (Gershon, Hogan, Qureshi, & Doll, 2004).

Similarly, four factors have been identified that influence the psychological response of communities to disaster. The first factor is the occurrence of extreme and widespread property damage in the area affected, and the second is the realization of serious and ongoing economic problems in the community. A high incidence of deaths and traumatic injuries is another influencing factor, and the last factor is the perception of human carelessness or intent as the cause of the disaster (Patterson, 2005). For individuals, influencing factors include bereavement or injury to self or loved ones, threat to life, panic during the disaster, separation from family members (especially for children), extensive property loss, and relocation or displacement. The effects of these factors on psychological response to a disaster seem to be additive; the more factors experienced, the greater the likelihood of psychological problems arising after a disaster (Patterson, 2005). Generally speaking, communities and persons with good coping skills usually respond more effectively in a disaster situation than those who have poor coping skills.

As noted earlier, both victims and relief workers may experience stress related to a disaster, and the nurse should be alert to signs of emotional distress in both

TABLE 27-6 Potential Biophysical Effects of Selected Disasters

Type of Disaster	Potential Biophysical Effects
All disasters	Greater loss of life and injury among the elderly, young children, and chronically ill and disabled persons
Avalanches	Asphyxiation Frostbite and other effects of exposure to cold Fractures or other forms of trauma
Bioterrorism	Widespread communicable disease, death, and disability
Chemical spills or chemical terrorism	Chemical burns of the skin Respiratory irritation and illness Poisoning, with a variety of symptoms depending on the chemical involved Eye irritation
Earthquakes	Crushing injuries and fractures from falling bricks, masonry, and other objects; may also cause *crushing syndrome* Burns suffered in fires and explosions due to ruptured natural gas mains Waterborne diseases because of ruptured water mains and lack of safe drinking water Electrocutions from fallen power lines
Epidemics	Communicable diseases with a variety of symptoms depending on the disease involved
Explosions	Burns due to associated fires Fractures or crushing injuries due to explosion impact or falling masonry, bricks, and other debris
Famine	Developmental delay in young children Failure to thrive in nursing infants because of inadequate lactation by mothers Protein-energy malnutrition and other nutritional deficiencies
Fire	Minor to severe burns Respiratory problems due to inhalation of smoke and hazardous fumes from burning objects
Floods	Drownings Waterborne and insect-borne diseases from contaminated water supplies and insect breeding grounds
Nuclear attacks or radiation leakage	Radiation burns or radiation sickness Later cancer Later infertility, spontaneous abortion, or fetal defects
Storms	Crushing injuries due to windblown objects and debris Minor to severe lacerations due to flying glass from broken windows
Transportation disasters	Crushing injuries and other trauma Burns from associated vehicle fires Drownings or asphyxiation if disasters occur over water or in tunnels Exposure to the elements if disaster occurs in a remote area
Volcanic eruptions	Toxic gas or radiation exposure, respiratory or eye irritations

groups. The immediate response to a traumatic event is an attempt to answer five questions, the answers to each of which promote adaptation. The first question is "What happened?" Discussion of this question helps people to verbalize their experiences and discharge some of the fear and anxiety generated by their experience. The second question, "Why did it happen to me?" may assist survivors to find meaning in the event and to address perceptions of personal guilt. The question "What did I do during and right after the disaster?" helps people examine their own behavior and the circumstances and emotions that motivated that behavior. A fourth question, "Why have I acted as I have since the

disaster?" may help people identify areas where help is needed to deal with the psychological effects of the disaster. Finally, an affirmative answer to the last question, "Will I be able to cope if it happens again?" helps to strengthen self-confidence and coping abilities (Figley & Figley, 2002).

Types of immediate psychological responses to disasters range along a continuum from calm, collected action to confusion and hysteria. Plans should be made for services to address each level of response. Health care providers should also keep in mind that psychological responses may change with time and with the progression of the disaster event. Psychological recovery occurs for most people within 6 to 12 months of the disaster, but a small segment of the population may exhibit ongoing problems and require therapy. For example, 3% of New York fire and rescue personnel experienced acute stress reactions within 24 hours of the September 11 attacks (Banauch et al., 2002), and 13% of rescue and recovery workers at the World Trade Center developed PTSD, four times the incidence seen in the general population (Smith et al., 2004). Similar incidence rates were noted for high school staff in schools close to the WTC compared to those of schools further away (Bernard et al., 2002). Another study found that 13% of residents in Hancock County, Mississippi, experienced mental health concerns 2 weeks after Hurricane Katrina (McNeil et al., 2006).

Community health nurses working in disaster situations can assess the extent and severity of psychological reaction in individual clients (victims, rescue personnel, and others) and population groups. They can use this information to make appropriate referrals for individual assistance and to help in the development of services to address identified mental health needs in the population.

PHYSICAL ENVIRONMENTAL CONSIDERATIONS Many disasters arise out of features of the physical environment. For example, the presence of a river near the community and the likelihood of heavy rainfall both contribute to the potential for flooding, as does the construction of homes and businesses on floodplains. A geological fault, a nuclear reactor, and a chemical plant are other examples of factors in the physical environment that may increase the potential for a disaster.

Elements of the physical dimension can either help or hinder efforts to control the effects of a disaster. For example, limited traffic access to the part of town where an explosives plant is located could hinder movement of emergency vehicles in the event of a fire or explosion. Similarly, the physical isolation of a mountain community may impede rescue efforts in the event of a forest fire or flood. For example, during the recent severe earthquake in India and Pakistan, many of the villages most seriously affected could only be reached on foot (Doctors Without Borders, 2005b). On the other hand, such isolation might spare the community from the effects of an epidemic in the surrounding area.

In conducting a community assessment, the community health nurse identifies physical environmental factors that might contribute to the occurrence of a disaster. The nurse also determines whether the community is prepared for potential disasters. When the community is not prepared, the nurse would advocate the planning activities described later in this chapter.

The nurse also identifies factors that might impede the community's response in the event of a disaster. The nurse can then share these observations with others involved in disaster planning, and interventions to modify or circumvent these factors can be incorporated

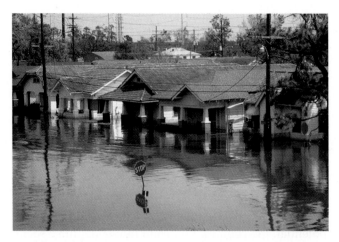

Flooding after Hurricane Katrina left major portions of New Orleans uninhabitable. (© Wesley Bocxe/The Image Works)

into the community's disaster response plan. Unfortunately, many environmental factors, such as blocked escape routes, stairway congestion, and lack of familiarity with building layout, impeded effective evacuation of the WTC towers (Gershon et al., 2004).

Disasters may also contribute to a wide variety of environmental health hazards. For example, Hurricane Katrina gave rise to many wound infections with methicillin-resistant *Staphylococcus aureus* and other pathogens due to exposure to floodwaters (Engelthaler et al., 2005; Jablecki et al., 2005; Sniffen et al., 2005). Flooding may also contaminate drinking water supplies, whereas fires and explosions result in exposure to smoke and other air pollutants. Extensive growth of a variety of molds was another environmental result of the flooding in New Orleans during Hurricane Katrina, and the failure of residents and workers to use respiratory protection led to respiratory health issues (Ratard et al., 2006). Mosquito infestations were another result of the extensive flooding (McNeil et al., 2006). Community health nurses can be actively involved in educating the public to prevent health effects of environmental hazards arising from disasters.

Crowding and congregate living in shelters, as well as lack of access to adequate sanitary facilities and facilities for bathing, washing clothes and bedding, and washing dishes, may also contribute to health problems for survivors (Jablecki et al., 2005). Community health nurses can identify poor shelter conditions and assist in planning to improve environmental conditions in shelters and refugee camps.

Finally, community responses to disaster conditions may give rise to environmental conditions that imperil health. For example, power outages following several hurricanes led residents to use portable generators as a power source, contributing to deaths and illness related to carbon monoxide (CO) poisoning (Kay et al., 2006). After Hurricane Katrina, for instance,

MediaLink   Student Nurses in the   Aftermath of Katrina (video)

51 cases of CO poisoning were reported in three affected states, all of which were related to use of portable generators or other gasoline-powered devices (Hampson et al., 2005). Many people connected portable generators to central electrical panels, not only creating the potential for CO poisoning but also placing utility personnel working on power lines at risk for electrocution (Tucker et al., 2006). Community health nurses can advocate for safe use of such equipment and help educate residents on the hazards of portable generators and their safe use based on the client education tips provided below.

SOCIOCULTURAL CONSIDERATIONS In assessing disaster potential, the community health nurse identifies social factors that might influence the way people respond to a disaster or even give rise to one. For example, the presence of racial tensions could trigger outbreaks of violence in some communities. War is another disaster arising out of social environmental conditions. For example, a report by Medact, the United Kingdom affiliate of the International Physicians for the Prevention of Nuclear War and the U.S. Physicians for Social Responsibility, estimated that the U.S. war in Iraq and the subsequent 3 months resulted in 48,000 to 260,000 deaths. They predicted that civil war in Iraq would result in another 20,000 directly caused deaths and an additional 200,000 postwar deaths due to indirect consequences. This number could rise to 3.9 million if nuclear weapons were used. In addition, war, like other disasters, has economic costs. The report estimated possible total U.S. costs of the war in Iraq at $150 to $200 billion dollars, more than $50 billion for the war itself and $5 to $20 billion each year for occupying forces (Salvage, 2002).

Terrorism, like war, arises out of sociocultural factors. Perceptions of the United States as arrogant, decadent, and indifferent to the plight of others fuel terrorist activity. Similarly, terrorism is often a strategy used by those who lack political or military power to address what they perceive as social wrongs. Poverty is another sociocultural factor that motivates terrorist activity, particularly in the face of affluence in other segments of society. Environmental justice issues, such as loss of biodiversity or perceived highjacking of natural resources without consideration for others who depend on them for their livelihood, also fuel terrorist initiatives (Easley & Allen, 2003). These and other politically motivated terrorists are generally motivated by a single issue, which if addressed may defuse terrorist activity (Simon, 2002).

Terrorism also has roots in religious beliefs and may surface in conflicts between religious groups at the national or international level or in the bombing of U.S. abortion clinics. It has been noted that religiously inspired terrorists may have fewer psychological constraints than others against killing or injuring large numbers of people (Simon, 2002). Concepts of national honor and shame may also motivate terrorist activity (Easley & Allen, 2003)—for example, in response to perceptions that adoption of Western values is corrupting women or youth. Ethnic/nationalist conflicts may have a religious component to them, but there is often a long history of intolerance of social and cultural differences outside of religious belief (Simon, 2002). Finally, terrorism may arise out of general *Occidentalism*, a rejection of all Western values (Easley & Allen, 2003).

Sociocultural factors may also contribute to the ability of terrorists to achieve their goals. Media attention to terrorist attacks, for example, provides perpetrators with the public attention to their position that they need. Some authors have described terrorism as a Western phenomenon dependent on a free press. Media coverage can be controlled in countries without a free press, thereby denying terrorists the showcase for their political ideology that is one of the major intents of terrorism (Brauer, 2002). The same may be true of media coverage of other disasters in what is termed *disaster pornography*, designed to promote giving or to highlight specific political perspectives (Martone, 2002). Treating disaster victims as individuals with dignity rather than as objects of disaster pornography is one of the tenets of the *Code of Conduct for the International Red Cross and Red Crescent Movement and Non-Governmental Organizations*, discussed on page 779.

Media coverage of disasters may also have beneficial effects. For example, news coverage of the September 11, 2001, attacks on the WTC and the Pentagon provided the comfort of familiar faces and an avenue to reduce public panic and provide information on what to do or not do. Media coverage also created a renewed connection between press and public when the press dropped its usual cynical stance and did not sensationalize or pursue reluctant victims for commentary. Finally, media coverage facilitated dialogue regarding Islam and may have prevented more scapegoating than actually occurred. One major disadvantage was that the

---

CLIENT EDUCATION | **Preventing Carbon Monoxide (CO) Poisoning**

- Do not use portable generators or other gasoline-powered tools indoors.
- Place gasoline-powered equipment away from doors, windows, and air intakes.
- Do not use gasoline-powered equipment in enclosed spaces (e.g., garage, basement, carport).
- Open windows and fans are not enough to prevent CO buildup.
- Leave the area and seek medical help if symptoms of CO poisoning are noted (headache, fatigue, dizziness, nausea, vomiting, loss of consciousness).

Data from: Hampson, N. B., et al. (2005). Carbon monoxide poisoning after Hurricane Katrina—Alabama, Louisiana, and Mississippi, August–September 2005. Morbidity and Mortality Weekly Report, 54, 996–998.

ETHICAL AWARENESS

The International Conference of the Red Cross and Red Crescent in 1995 adopted a *Code of Conduct for the International Red Cross and Red Crescent Movement and Non-Governmental Organizations* intended to guide international relief efforts (Hilhorst, 2005). Many organizations, however, have political objectives in addition to humanitarian aid purposes, leading to what has been called the "politicization of aid." Drafters of the Code of Conduct have argued that humanitarian organizations should maintain a strict policy of neutrality. The code consists of 10 articles that support four basic principles of humanitarian aid: humanity, impartiality, neutrality, and independence. The articles are as follows:

- The humanitarian imperative takes precedence over other objectives.
- Aid is provided without distinction with respect to race, creed, nationality, or other characteristics of recipients.
- Aid should not be used to promote a particular political or religious view.
- Humanitarian agencies should strive not to be used as instruments of government policy.
- Humanitarian agencies should respect the culture and customs of beneficiaries.
- Disaster response should be built on local capabilities.
- Program beneficiaries should be involved in the management of aid.
- Relief activities should reduce future vulnerabilities as well as meet basic needs.
- Aid agencies should be accountable to both recipients and donors.
- Information, publicity, and advertising activities should treat disaster victims with respect and dignity rather than as hopeless objects.

Data from: Hilhorst, D. (2005). Dead letter or living document? Ten years of the Code of Conduct for disaster relief. Disasters, *29, 351–369.*

repeated airing of scenes of horror increased the psychological trauma of viewers (Nacos, 2002).

Other social purposes to be achieved by terrorism include establishing the legitimacy of the terrorist group with its target audiences, demonstrating weakness on the part of the victim nation or organization, creating fear, and possibly undermining civil liberties and creating domestic unrest (Nacos, 2002). Terrorism appears to occur in cycles that promote achievement of these purposes. Significant terrorist events result in increased security, which leads to a lull in activities. When attention wanes and security becomes less strict, terrorist activity increases (Brauer, 2002).

Other aspects of society may lend themselves to terrorism. For example, dependence on mass-produced foods makes the United States more vulnerable to agroterrorism. Widespread destruction of food crops or animals would have significant effects on the health of the population as well as on national economics. For example, in California alone, 89,000 farms and ranches, 10,000 food processors, and 200,000 retail facilities provide ample opportunity for contamination of food supplies (Little Hoover Commission, 2003). Similarly, dis-

ruptions in electrical power or telecommunications could bring much of everyday life to a halt. Access to the Internet and other technological advances also make information on weapons that can be used for terrorist activity readily available to the general public (Simon, 2002).

Elements of the sociocultural dimension also may increase or limit the effects of a disaster on a community. For example, the economic status of community members and of the community at large may limit the ability of people to prepare for potential disasters or to recover after a disaster event. Language barriers may hamper evacuation or rescue efforts. Strong social networks in the community that can be tied into disaster planning aid in effective disaster response, whereas intragroup friction hampers response effectiveness. The nurse identifies social and cultural factors present within the community that may decrease the effectiveness of the community's response to a disaster and participates in planning efforts to modify these factors. The nurse also identifies social factors that enhance the community's ability to respond effectively in the event of a disaster. Planning groups could then capitalize on these factors in designing an effective disaster plan. For example, well-established cooperative relationships between groups and agencies in the community are an asset in designing and implementing a disaster plan, whereas the presence of relatively isolated cultural groups may impede planning and response efforts.

Occupational factors are another element of the sociocultural dimension that contribute to the potential for disaster in a community and should be assessed by the nurse. Occupational disasters are events related to a particular business or industry in which more than five deaths occur. The community health nurse should be aware of industries in the area that pose hazards related to fire or explosion. The potential for radiation exposure or leakage of toxic chemicals in the community should also be determined. The nurse may also want to appraise the extent to which local industries adhere to safety regulations related to hazardous conditions. Community health nurses working in industrial settings would be particularly likely to have access to this type

BUILDING OUR KNOWLEDGE BASE

Different cultural groups may have different perspectives on the need for and advisability of disaster preparedness as well as what constitutes effective preparedness. Cultural differences may also influence disaster response. How would you design a study to examine the cultural influences on disaster preparedness and response in your community? What would be the most appropriate approach to developing local knowledge on which to base community disaster planning? Whom would you ask to participate in your study and how would you obtain data?

CULTURAL COMPETENCE

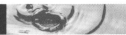

You live and work in a highly ethnically diverse community in which residents come from multiple different cultural backgrounds and where 38 different languages are spoken. Major sources of disaster potential in the area include the possibility of earthquakes and brush fires. How would you design community notification systems related to evacuation in the event of a major fire, accounting for the language barriers to communication and the fatalistic attitudes of some cultural groups in the area?

of information. Other community health nurses may need to advocate regular inspection of industrial conditions by the appropriate authorities.

The community health nurse also identifies occupational factors that may enhance a community's abilities to respond effectively in the event of a disaster. The nurse and others involved in disaster planning would explore the adequacy of rescue services and personnel for dealing with potential disasters. Is the number of firefighters in the community, for example, adequate to deal with an explosion and fire in a local chemical plant? Do fire-fighting units possess the equipment needed to deal with such an event? Planners also assess the existence of other occupational groups that may assist with disaster response. For example, are there construction companies in the community that could supply heavy equipment that might be needed for rescue operations?

In the event of an actual disaster, the nurse might also assess sociocultural factors influencing the community's disaster response. For example, the nurse might identify growing intergroup tensions in shelters for disaster victims or disorganization in efforts to reunite families separated by the disaster. Other areas for consideration include the degree of cooperation among groups providing disaster relief and, following the disaster, the availability of recovery assistance to individuals and families. Failure of government agencies and other organizations to interact effectively may be a sociocultural factor that hampers adequate disaster response. For example, some authors have noted that lack of agreement over jurisdiction, absence of conflict resolution mechanisms, and difficulty integrating a response over several sectors of society hampered rescue efforts at the WTC on September 11, 2001 (Klitzman & Freudenberg, 2003). Similarly, lack of coordination between local, state, and federal agencies delayed control of the San Diego wildfires in 2003, resulting in increased loss of life and extensive property damage.

Another social response to disasters, particularly those caused by terrorist activities, may include anger and hostility toward groups deemed responsible for the disaster. These emotions may be demonstrated in prejudice, discrimination, and attacks on innocent parties

believed to be related to the perpetrators. In a study conducted after the 2001 terrorist attacks in Washington, D.C., and New York, 29% of respondents favored establishing internment camps for legal immigrants from hostile nations (The Pew Research Center for the People and the Press, 2001). News media also reported a variety of unprovoked attacks against Muslims and other ethnic minority groups. Community health nurses may need to be involved in advocacy to prevent discrimination and violence against such groups.

Even well-intentioned social responses to disaster may have adverse effects. For example, food aid provided to countries experiencing famine may do as much harm as good. Famine has been described as "a disaster for the poor, but an opportunity for the rich" (Martone, 2002, p. 39). Potential negative effects of food aid include undermining the local economy and promoting black market sales of food goods. For example, in one instance an influx of food aid resulted in a 75% decrease in prices for locally grown produce. In addition, when food aid cuts into the revenue of profiteers, aid workers may be subjected to threats or violence. Other effects may include promoting rural to urban migration of people seeking relief assistance. Foreign aid may also create national dependency rather than promoting self-sufficiency. Misuse of supplies is also a problem. For example, people have eaten grain intended for planting that has been coated with pesticides, contributing to cases of poisoning. In addition, the costs and problems of shipping, storage, and dissemination of food supplies exhaust funds that could be used more effectively to promote local economies and infrastructures that prevent disaster. A balance of food and economic aid is recommended to promote the ability of developing countries to address their own needs while meeting the current survival needs (Martone, 2002).

Another element of assessment of sociocultural considerations in a disaster involves the social effects of the disaster for specific groups. For example, the effects of a disaster on family dynamics should be explored. Families most at risk for adverse consequences of disasters include the homeless, the poor, the elderly, single-parent families, and refugee families (Langan & James, 2005). Community health nurses can help identify families experiencing difficulties that are interfering with adequate family function and make referrals for assistance. They can also advocate for the availability of such assistance. Other sociocultural effects of disasters that are often overlooked in planning and response include the economic costs of business disruption (especially for small businesses) and the cost to individuals of resulting health and safety expenses (e.g., the expense of evacuation or preparation for a disaster) (Myers & White, 2003). Again, those with the fewest resources will have the most difficulty in adequately preparing for or responding to a disaster.

Think Advocacy

Many segments of society do not have the financial resources to comply with recommendations for disaster preparedness. This is particularly true of homeless individuals. How might you go about assuring that the disaster response plans address the special needs of homeless populations in your area?

One particular social group that needs to be considered in disaster response planning is jail and prison inmates. Evacuation of these populations poses special considerations related to public safety and security. Correctional officials may need to be able to safely relocate major inmate populations to multiple locations. For example, during Hurricane Rita, more than 10,000 inmates needed to be evacuated from 10 Texas prisons. In addition to planning for evacuation and continued efforts to meet the survival and health needs of inmates, there is a need to consider the transfer of medical and other records (Murray, 2006).

Health responses to disaster effects may also have social consequences. For example, isolation of disaster victims with communicable diseases may be difficult when families already traumatized by loss are faced with further enforced separation to prevent the spread of disease (Palacio et al., 2005). Finally, assessment of sociocultural considerations in a disaster setting includes exploration of the availability and adequacy of basic social services. Areas to be addressed include the availability of shelter, transportation, financial assistance, communication networks, and other goods and services. For example, more than 726,000 people were without power following Hurricane Isabel in 2003, which affected their access to food, water, and medical care. Two days after the hurricane, 65% of households in affected areas were without power, 4% had no access to water, and 21% were without access to a working land or cellular telephone (Morrow et al., 2004). Similarly, 93% of homes in Charlotte County, Florida, were damaged by Hurricane Charley in 2004; 19% of homes in DeSoto County were uninhabitable; and 54% of Desoto County homes were without adequate sanitation (Little et al., 2004). After Hurricane Katrina in 2005, 53% of households surveyed in Hancock County, Mississippi, had no telephone service; 37% had no working indoor toilet; 21.5% were without running water; and 26% had no access to transportation (McNeil et al., 2006). Community health nurses can help in the rapid assessment of postdisaster conditions, making referrals for assistance, and planning to assure that assistance is available to those in need.

BEHAVIORAL CONSIDERATIONS Behavioral factors related to consumption patterns and even leisure pursuits can influence the occurrence of disasters and their effects on the health of community members. Consumption patterns such as smoking, drinking, and drug use can contribute to disasters. Smoking, for example, is often the cause of residential fires and forest and brush fires that result in loss of life as well as extensive property damage. Drinking and drug abuse have both been known to contribute to transportation disasters, and they may also contribute to industrial disasters when the abuser is working in a setting with disaster potential. For example, if a person responsible for monitoring the safety of a nuclear reactor is intoxicated, he or she is unlikely to recognize or respond appropriately to signs of danger. The community health nurse assesses the extent of smoking and substance abuse in the community in relation to the potential for disaster. The nurse may also want to assess (or encourage others to assess) the effectiveness of substance abuse policies in transportation services and industries where there is potential for disaster. Another area for assessment is the extent of safety education in regard to smoking (e.g., not smoking in bed) that occurs in the community. Community health nursing advocacy may be needed to assure attention to these concerns.

Consumption patterns may also intensify the effects of a disaster on the health of a population. A community whose members are poorly nourished, for example, is at greater risk for consequences of disaster such as communicable diseases. Substance abuse may limit one's potential for appropriate behavior in an emergency and lead to injury and even death due to failure to respond appropriately. For example, intoxication may prevent someone from fleeing a burning building.

Consumption patterns and their effects are particularly relevant in disasters involving famine and large displaced or refugee populations. Famine is a population-wide condition involving substantial mortality from malnutrition. Common nutritional effects of famine among refugee populations include *protein-energy malnutrition (PEM)*, a severe state of undernutrition that may be either acute or chronic, and deficiencies of specific micronutrients such as vitamin A, iron, vitamin C, niacin, and thiamine. In some cases, famine is less a function of lack of food than of the inability of some segments of the population to afford what food is available (Martone, 2002). Technological advances that have resulted in a new product to treat severe malnutrition at home rather than in in-patient settings have increased survival rates of malnourished children in Niger to 85% to 90% (Doctors Without Borders, 2005a). Those in need, however, must have access to this new therapy.

Lack of exercise in the population can limit the ability to engage in strenuous labor that might be demanded in a disaster situation. Unaccustomed activity may result in exhaustion or heart attack. The nurse assesses the levels of exercise engaged in by the general population. Community health nurses in occupational settings may also be responsible for determining the physical fitness of personnel who would be involved in rescue operations in the event of a disaster (e.g., firefighters).

The leisure pursuits of community members may, on occasion, contribute to the occurrence of a disaster event. Careless campers, for example, could ignite a forest fire, or skiers might trigger an avalanche. Fires can be started by sparks from recreational vehicles. The community health nurse and others involved in disaster planning assess the extent of such leisure pursuits in the community, the existence of safety regulations related to these pursuits, and the degree of adherence to safety regulations. Advocacy may also be required for the development or enforcement of such regulations.

Leisure pursuits can also enhance the community's response to a disaster event, and the nurse assesses the presence of leisure pursuits that may have this effect. For example, the existence of a group with an interest in wilderness survival may be an advantage in the event of an avalanche or a plane crash in a remote area, or people with citizens-band radios may assist with communications in the event of an emergency.

Another behavioral consideration related to disasters is the extent of disaster preparedness among members of the population. For example, following Hurricane Katrina, 17% of households in Hancock County, Mississippi, did not have the recommended 3-day supply of food and water available (McNeil et al., 2006). Finally, disasters may affect consumption patterns other than dietary intake. For example, alcohol consumption among women, but not men, increased as a result of September 11, 2001, and the increase was further compounded by stress experienced by women in the work setting (Richman, Wislar, Flaherty, Fendrich, & Rospenda, 2004). In another study, 21% of people surveyed in Connecticut, New Jersey, and New York reported smoking more and 3% reported drinking more alcohol as a result of the attacks (Melnik et al., 2002). A similar study among New York City high school students found that increased smoking was not directly associated with the WTC attacks, but was associated with increased incidence of PTSD following the attacks (Wu et al., 2006). Drug and alcohol abuse may be seen as a means of coping with the negative psychological effects of a disaster.

HEALTH SYSTEM CONSIDERATIONS The adequacy of the health care system's response capability in the event of a disaster influences the extent to which a disaster affects a community and the health of its members. Assessing the ability of the health care system to respond to a disaster includes examining facilities and personnel as well as the organizational framework in which they operate. A community that has a variety of health care facilities joined in a cooperative network can respond more effectively to the health care demands of a disaster situation than can a community with limited facilities or no existing system for coordinating efforts.

The nurse and other disaster response planners identify the types of health care facilities available in the community and the number and type of health care personnel that could be called on in the event of a disaster. Categories of health-related personnel included in federal disaster response planning include Disaster Medical Assistance Teams (DMATs), National Nurse Response Teams (NNRTs), National Pharmacy Response Teams (NPRTs), Veterinary Medical Assistance Teams (VMATs), and Disaster Mortuary Operational Response Teams (DMORTs) (Landesman, 2005).

Planners might also determine the existence and adequacy of disaster plans developed by health care facilities. For example, has a local hospital developed a plan for evacuating patients if the hospital is affected by the disaster? Is there a plan for handling mass casualties of various types in the event of a disaster? In one study by the National Association of County and City Health Officials (2001), only 20% of hospitals surveyed were prepared for bioterrorist attacks, 56% were developing response plans, and 24% were not prepared at

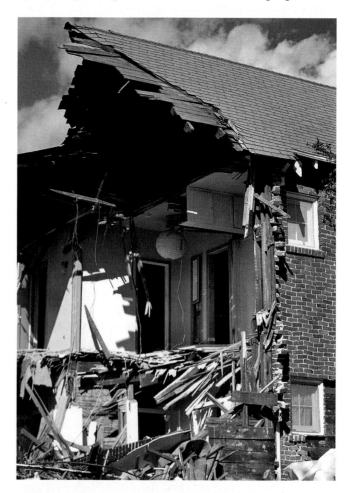

Earthquakes and other disasters destroy health care capacity as well as homes and businesses. (© Joe Sohm/The Image Works)

all. Similarly, 15% of countries responding to a 2001 survey indicated that they had bioterrorism response plans (Sandhu, Thomas, Nsubuga, & White, 2003). From 2001 to 2003, 100% of U.S. state health departments hired personnel specifically to develop surveillance for terrorist agents and infectious diseases, 98% had hired personnel to train public health workers regarding terrorist threats, and 91% were engaged in training health care providers (CDC, 2003). By 2004, however, only 38% of state and territorial health departments reported full or almost full capacity to deal with bioterrorism and emergency preparedness (Boulton, Abellera, Lemmings, & Robinson, 2005). A 2003 study of hospital preparedness indicated that 87% of metropolitan and 62% of nonmetropolitan hospitals had plans for dealing with major fires or explosions, but only 30% and 8% of the reporting hospitals conducted disaster drills related to their plans (National Center for Health Statistics, 2005).

Health care systems need to assess the likelihood of specific disasters in the area and prepare accordingly. As several authors have concluded, however, preventive measures for bioterrorist activities should be placed in priority with other existing public health needs and resources allocated based on those priorities (Geiger, 2003; Cohen, Gould, & Sidel, 2004; Sidel, Cohen, & Gould, 2001). For example, from 2002 to 2006, bioterrorism preparedness funding varied from $1.4 million to $1.7 million, averaging 22% of CDC's entire annual budget, and some public health proponents have decried the use of these funds that could be better spent addressing health problems with a higher probability of affecting the health of the public, such as obesity (Dowling & Lipton, 2005). Others have made the point that one-time funding does not markedly increase the capability of the system for dealing with everyday emergencies, much less disasters, and does not address the ongoing training needs to prepare health care professionals to recognize health effects resulting from bioterrorist or chemical attacks or other disaster effects (Scipioni, 2002).

In 2000, CDC published guidelines for preparedness for and response to biological and chemical terrorism. Acts of chemical terrorism are likely to be overt because their effects tend to be immediate and obvious. Some chemical agents are capable of covert dissemination in food and water, however. Biological terrorism tends to be covert in that its effects are more insidious and occur over sometimes extended incubation periods.

The two main facets of state and local public health preparedness to be assessed by community health nurses and other disaster response planners are the existence of surveillance systems capable of identifying unusual disease patterns and the availability of expertise and resources needed to respond to chemical or biological terrorist attacks. Specific preparation for biological attacks includes:

- Enhancing surveillance and response capabilities
- Providing for diagnostic services
- Establishing effective communication systems
- Educating health care providers on recognition and treatment of diseases caused by bioterrorism
- Educating the general public
- Obtaining and storing needed drugs and vaccines
- Supporting development of diagnostic tests, vaccines, and appropriate treatments (Centers for Disease Control and Prevention Strategic Planning Workgroup, 2000)

These guidelines were expanded by the National Center for Infectious Diseases (2001) to encompass the specific roles of health care providers in the recognition, reporting, and treating of high-priority biological agents. Laboratory personnel are also advised to test findings on cultures that would normally be discarded as contaminants when they occur in suspicious circumstances (e.g., febrile illness in a previously healthy person) and to be alert to unusual clusters of laboratory results. Laboratory precautions for handling suspected contaminants are also addressed, and unusual specimens should be sent to specialty laboratories as appropriate.

State health departments are charged with reeducating health care providers to recognize unusual diseases. For example, many U.S. providers will never have seen a case of smallpox and will need to be reminded of typical signs and symptoms of this disease. State health departments also need to remind providers of reporting requirements and procedures, improve capacities for immediate response to suspected bioterrorism, investigate unusual illness clusters, and develop and implement plans for collecting and transporting specimens to appropriate laboratory facilities and reporting suspected release of biological agents to CDC.

Guidelines for public health agency preparation for chemical attacks have also been provided by CDC (Centers for Disease Control and Prevention Strategic Planning Workgroup, 2000). Public health responsibilities in this area include developing capabilities for detecting and responding to chemical attacks, educating first responders and health care personnel regarding chemical terrorism, and obtaining and storing supplies of chemical antidotes (Spanjaard & Khabib, 2003). Additional responsibilities include developing diagnostic processes for chemical injuries and educating the public about potential effects and actions to be taken in the case of chemical attacks. Community health nurses and others assessing disaster preparedness should determine the extent to which state and large local public health agencies (e.g., those in large metropolitan areas) are capable of carrying out these responsibilities.

Assessment of potential avenues for obtaining health care personnel is also important. For example, local professional organizations might serve as a means of contacting and organizing health care providers, or area educational programs for health care professionals may provide a source of personnel. Retired or otherwise inactive nurses have been suggested as a group who could be trained to provide disaster response capabilities in addition to those of nurses and other health care professionals employed by health care agencies (Fothergill, Palumbo, Rambur, Reinier, & McIntosh, 2005). Prior to a disaster, training needs for health professional responses to disaster situations should be determined and appropriate education undertaken. Such training may include monitoring hazards, risks, resources, and capabilities; needs assessment; disaster management and coordination; information management; and the development of crisis response standards (WHO, 2004).

In the event of an actual disaster there is also a need to assess the effects of the disaster on the health care system and its ability to respond effectively. For example, are facilities badly damaged or unusable for other reasons? In some instances, health care facilities have collapsed in earthquakes or become inaccessible due to floodwaters or highway damage. After the 2004 tsunami, 80% of health care workers in Banda Aceh, one of the hardest hit areas, were killed, severely impairing the local response to disaster-related illness and injury (Joyce, 2005). Similarly, more than 6,000 physicians were displaced by Hurricane Katrina in 2005, many of them from the central areas of New Orleans. Losses included not only their homes and offices, but also their patient records (Arias, 2005).

Damage to the health system, as well as to other elements of the community infrastructure that permit access to health care services (e.g., roads, electricity, communication networks), can have negative consequences for the population's health. For example, 2 weeks after Hurricane Katrina, 29% of people surveyed in Hancock County, Mississippi, were unable to get prescriptions refilled (McNeil et al., 2006). Disasters may also have long-term consequences for health care delivery systems. For example, Hurricane Floyd, which affected significant portions of North Carolina in 1999, led to subsequent increases of $13.3 million in Medicaid expenditures due to increased emergency department, outpatient, and pharmacy services (Domino, Fried, Moon, Olinick, & Yoon, 2003).

An example of an organized and systematic response to a national disaster can be seen in the response of the Thai Ministry of Health–US CDC Collaboration (2005) to the 2004 tsunami. The Ministry of Public Health mobilized 100 emergency clinical teams within 24 hours of the disaster. Less than a week after the tsunami struck, area hospitals' caseloads had returned to normal and extra staff were allowed to return to their normal duties. In the 2 weeks following the disaster, response teams had treated 90,000 people.

Rapid assessment and action to prevent spread of disease limited the incidence of diarrheal disease to 2,950 cases per 100,000 people, compared to 87,000 to 120,000 per 100,000 population in prior disasters (Thai Ministry of Health–US CDC Collaboration, 2005).

In part, the effectiveness of Thailand's response lies in the development of a national preparedness plan. WHO (2004) has developed guidelines for preparedness plans for the national health sector. Based on these guidelines, such a plan would include the entire health sector, providing guidance for health sector involvement in disaster prevention, mitigation, preparedness, response, and recovery. Plans should also employ a multihazard approach rather than having specific plans for specific types of disasters. Finally, the health care sector should collaborate and coordinate with other sectors in disaster response planning. Health sector disaster planning should include contingency planning, response drills, and simulations. As much as possible, plans should be standardized across organizations and agencies so that all hospitals are responding in similar ways, and so on. Planning should also include mechanisms for minimizing the effects of a disaster on health facilities (e.g., structural design, engineering controls) (WHO, 2004).

Questions for assessing disaster potential and the health-related effects of a disaster are included in the focused assessment provided on page 785. A complete assessment tool to guide assessment in disaster situations is included in the *Community Assessment Reference Guide* 📋 designed to accompany this textbook.

Diagnostic Reasoning and Care of Clients in Disaster Settings

Based on the assessment of biophysical, psychological, physical environmental, sociocultural, behavioral, and health system factors, the nurse derives nursing diagnoses related to disaster care. These diagnoses may reflect the potential for disaster occurrence, the adequacy of disaster preparation, or the extent of effects in an actual disaster. A diagnosis related to disaster forecasting is "potential for major earthquake damage and injury due to community location on a geological fault." A diagnosis of "inadequate disaster planning due to fragmentation of planning efforts among community agencies" is a possible nursing diagnosis related to disaster preparedness. A diagnosis derived from information about the effects of an actual disaster is "need for additional shelter sites due to destruction of planned shelters by fire."

In the event of an actual disaster, nursing diagnoses might relate to individual clients as well as to the status of the overall community. For example, individual diagnoses include "grief due to loss of husband" and "pain due to leg fracture suffered in building collapse." Nurses may derive diagnoses related to disaster

FOCUSED ASSESSMENT

Disaster-related Assessment Considerations

Biophysical Considerations

- What is the age, gender, and ethnic composition of the population involved in the disaster? Are the effects of the disaster likely to be worse for some subgroups than others?
- What is the extent of injury or disease resulting from the disaster?
- What existing health problems are prevalent among those involved in the disaster?
- Are there pregnant women involved in the disaster?

Psychological Considerations

- How does the population respond to disaster warnings? What is the public's attitude to disaster preparedness?
- What is the extent of community/individual ability to cope with the disaster?
- What is the extent of existing mental illness among those involved in the disaster?
- What is the extent of damage or loss of life involved in the disaster?
- Does the disaster present the potential for continuing damage or loss of life?
- What is the effect of the disaster on rescue workers? On victims? What are the long-term psychological effects of the disaster on the community?

Physical Environmental Considerations

- What physical features of the community create the potential for disaster? What types of disasters are likely to occur?
- What structures are likely to be threatened by a disaster? To what extent are vital structures likely to withstand a disaster?
- What structures could be used as emergency shelters?
- Will weather conditions influence the effects of the disaster?
- Are there elements of the physical environmental dimension that will hinder response to the disaster (e.g., blockage of roads)?
- Have buildings been structurally damaged? Is there potential for additional structural damage? Does structural damage pose further risk to victims? To rescuers?
- Is there a need for sources of shelter for persons displaced by the disaster?
- Is there a safe water source available to victims of the disaster?
- To what extent are animals involved in the disaster? What health effects might this have?

Sociocultural Considerations

- Do relationships in the community have the potential to create a disaster (e.g., civil strife, war)?
- How cohesive is the community? Are community members able to work together for disaster planning? What level of priority is given to disaster planning by official agencies? By private organizations and individuals?
- What provisions have been made for reuniting families separated by disaster?
- What is the extent of social support available to disaster victims?
- What is the extent of collaborative interaction among relief agencies involved in the disaster?

- Has the community disaster plan been communicated to residents? How are disaster warnings communicated to residents? Are there language barriers that impede communication in the disaster setting? What is the effect of disaster on normal channels of communication?
- What community groups are responsible for disaster planning? Who is available to provide leadership in responding to the disaster? What is the level of credibility of leaders among those affected by the disaster?
- What community industries pose disaster hazards? What type of hazards are present? To what extent do local industries adhere to safety procedures that would prevent a disaster? Is adherence monitored by regulatory bodies?
- What occupational groups in the community are available to respond to the disaster?
- What is the extent of property damage and loss resulting from the disaster?
- What is the economic status of those affected by disaster? Do they have economic resources available to them? What is the effect of the disaster on the local economy?
- What is the effect of the disaster on transportation?
- What is the effect of the disaster on community services? What community services are available to assist with recovery?
- Is equipment needed to deal with the disaster available and in good repair?

Behavioral Considerations

- To what extent do consumption patterns (e.g., drugs or alcohol) create the potential for disaster in the community?
- Do community members engage in leisure pursuits that pose a disaster hazard? To what extent do community members engage in recreational safety practices that can prevent disasters? What leisure pursuits by community members could enhance the community's disaster response?
- What is the availability of food and water to disaster victims? To rescuers? Are there special dietary needs among those affected by the disaster? What provisions have been made to meet these needs?
- To what extent have psychological effects of the disaster increased the incidence or prevalence of substance abuse?

Health System Considerations

- How well prepared are health service agencies to respond to a disaster?
- What health care facilities are available to care for disaster victims? What are their capabilities? What health care personnel are available to meet health needs in a disaster? How can they best be mobilized?
- What is the extent of basic first aid and other health-related knowledge in the community?
- What is the effect of a disaster on health care facilities? On health care services?
- What physical and mental health care services are needed as a result of disaster? Are available services adequate to meet the need?

helpers as well as victims, such as "role overload due to need to rescue disaster victims and care for own family" and "stress related to constant exposure to death."

Planning: Disaster Preparedness

Activities related to disaster care take place in several areas. Two of these areas, prevention and minimization of adverse effects, involve primary prevention. The third area of activity, the actual emergency response, reflects secondary prevention, whereas recovery, the fourth area of activity, involves tertiary prevention (Levy & Sidel, 2003).

Primary Prevention: Mitigation

Primary prevention is geared toward preventing the occurrence of a disaster or limiting consequences when the event itself cannot be prevented. Activities to prevent or minimize the effects of a disaster take place during the nondisaster and predisaster stages of disaster response.

PREVENTING DISASTERS Community health nurses may be involved in identifying and eliminating factors that may contribute to disasters to the extent that they identify these factors and report their existence to the appropriate authorities. For example, the community health nurse working in an occupational setting may note that an employee who is responsible for monitoring pressure levels in a boiler may be drinking heavily. This employee's drinking problem may lead to lack of attention to rising pressures and an explosion and fire in the plant. In such a case, the nurse would call the employee's drinking behavior to the attention of a supervisor.

Community health nurses may also become politically active to ensure that risk factors for potential disasters present in the community are eliminated or modified. For example, the nurse might campaign for stricter building codes or barriers such as sea walls or dams (Myers & White, 2003) or serve as a mediator in an attempt to defuse social unrest in the community. Community health nurses can also advocate for maintenance and repairs of structures to promote disaster resistance or the creation of surveillance systems to identify covert biological or chemical terrorism (Scipioni, 2002). There may also be a need for advocacy regarding identification of potential terrorist targets or for strategies to minimize terrorist resources (Brauer, 2002). For example, there may need to be stricter controls on access to agents that can be used for biological or chemical terrorism. Safeguards should be developed related to production, storage, transport, and use of such substances (Little Hoover Commission, 2003). International treaties and national regulation of the sale of weapons and the production, distribution, storage, and use of biological, chemical, and nuclear agents may also be of some help in preventing international terrorist activities (Levy & Sidel, 2003).

As a general policy, hazardous materials should be routed away from highly populated areas during transport, and employees who work with these materials should be educated on appropriate responses to leaks and spills. Preventive maintenance for equipment and vehicles used in transporting hazardous materials can also help to prevent accidental releases (Henry et al., 2005). Similarly, steps can be taken to minimize the risk of agroterrorism through research that increases biodiversity and crop resistance to biological agents and improved veterinary education to recognize unusual disease in animals (Cupp et al., 2004). Community health nurses can engage in political advocacy to promote these preventive interventions as appropriate.

Buildings can also be protected from biological and chemical attacks by increasing the difficulty of introducing agents through security measures for air intake grills and restricting access to building systems and design information. Similarly, development of effective filter capabilities and emergency response capabilities for building ventilation and water systems can help minimize dispersal of hazardous substances. Increasing the ability to prevent terrorist access through building security may also be warranted (National Institute for Occupational Safety and Health [NIOSH], 2002). NIOSH recommendations for protecting buildings from terrorist attacks are available at http://www.cdc.gov/niosh.

Immunization is another primary preventive measure for epidemics of communicable disease that might occur naturally or result from biological terrorism. Community health nurses can educate the public regarding routine immunization as well as immunization for selected bioterrorism agents. For example, the Advisory Committee on Immunization Practices (ACIP) has recommended preexposure vaccination for populations at risk for anthrax (ACIP, 2002). In 2003, smallpox vaccine was administered to more than 39,000 health care workers in preparation for a possible bioterrorist attack (Smallpox Vaccine Adverse Events Coordinators, 2004). Vaccines are also available for plague and tularemia, two of the other Category A biological agents (Nolte et al., 2004).

Community health nurses are often involved in educating the public about how to prevent disasters and minimize their consequences. This may involve planning education for individuals, families, or groups of clients on home safety practices to prevent fires and explosions, how to prepare for a possible community disaster, and what to do in the event of a disaster situation.

The nurse would plan to acquaint clients with whom he or she works with the types of disasters possible in their community and actions they can take to minimize the consequences should an emergency arise. The nurse can also guide clients to resources that help them prepare for the possibility of a disaster. A variety of government agencies publish literature containing guidelines for emergency preparation by individual citizens. One such publication, *In Time of Emergency: A Citizen's Handbook*, is published by the Federal Emergency Management Agency. The American Red Cross publishes the *Family Disaster Plan and Personal Survival Guide*. These and similar publications offer general guidelines for emergency preparation as well as more specific recommendations for certain common types of disasters. Potential topics for family disaster education are presented below.

MINIMIZING DISASTER EFFECTS Community health nurses can also assist in the development of community-as-resource strategies for disaster response. These strategies consist of a series of training programs for disaster preparedness at the individual, neighborhood, and advanced level. Individual-level programs focus on basic family preparedness, reduction of household hazards, preparation of family emergency kits and plans, and developing family notification systems. The second level involves training and development of neighborhood response teams to carry out immediate response activities. Advanced training prepares local residents to augment the efforts of public response personnel such as police and firefighters (Lichterman, 2000).

Community health nurses educate people to prevent problems after the occurrence of a disaster. As we saw earlier, nurses can educate people on the safe use of portable generators and can encourage the placement of CO monitors in all homes (Tucker et al., 2006). Public education with respect to response to nuclear or radiological attacks would include staying indoors, limiting consumption of milk and locally produced food, and use of potassium iodide prophylaxis following exposure (Sutton & Gould, 2003). Community health nurses may need to advocate for the availability of prophylactic antidotes for a variety of potentially hazardous substances depending on the disaster potential in the community.

Postdisaster primary prevention may also involve use of personal protective equipment (PPE) for those working in disaster-affected areas. For example, those working in floodwaters should wear heavy boots and other protective gear to avoid wound exposure to contaminated water (Engelthaler et al., 2005). PPE (e.g., respirators) should also be used in disasters such as fires and the collapse of buildings in which smoke and lingering particulate matter pose health hazards for rescue and clean-up workers. PPE should be standardized across agencies when possible, and all responders, including volunteers, should be adequately trained in its use (Prezant et al., 2002). Similarly, work to identify the dead poses risks for morgue personnel, who should use PPE during examinations and arrange for appropriate disposal of bodies and autopsy fluids and samples. In the wake of the December 2004 tsunami, for example, the bodies of people from more than 30 countries had to be identified, and many were buried or cremated without identification in affected countries such as India (Thai Ministry of Public Health, 2005).

CLIENT EDUCATION   Disaster Preparedness

- Install and maintain smoke detectors in homes.
- Bolt bookcases and cabinets to walls in areas with earthquake potential.
- Seek shelter in a reinforced area (e.g., a doorway) during an earthquake and face away from windows. Stay indoors.
- Seek shelter from hurricanes or tornadoes in basements or inner rooms without windows.
- Seek high ground in the event of a flood.
- Drop to the ground and roll about to extinguish flaming clothing, or smother flames with a rug.
- Close doors and windows to prevent the spread of a fire, and place wadded fabric beneath doors to prevent smoke inhalation.
- Determine avenues of escape from the home or other buildings.
- Install fire escape ladders as needed at upper windows.
- Keep stairways and doors free of obstacles to permit an easy way out.
- Identify a place for family members to meet after escape from the home.
- Designate a person living outside the area as a family contact if family members are separated during a disaster.
- Learn community disaster warning signals and their meaning.
- Keep a battery-operated radio and extra batteries available (replace batteries periodically).

- Collect and store, in an accessible location, sufficient emergency supplies for one week, including:
    - Nonperishable foods (including pet foods)
    - Drinking water
    - Warm clothing
    - Bedding (blankets or sleeping bags)
    - Tent or other type of shelter
    - Source of light (flashlights or lanterns)
    - Chlorine bleach for treating suspect water supplies to prevent infection
    - First-aid supplies and first-aid manual
    - Medications needed by family members
- Replace stored food, water, and medications periodically.
- Know where natural gas and water valves are located and how to turn them off. Attach a wrench close to valves.
- Determine what valuables are to be taken if evacuation is required.
- Assign activities related to evacuation (e.g., designate the person responsible for taking the baby or family pets).
- Know the general plan and designated routes for evacuating the community.
- Know where proposed shelters will be located.
- Know what actions should be taken when warning is given.
- Know where to seek additional information.

GLOBAL PERSPECTIVES

*W*hat factors might influence the extent of and elements included in disaster response planning in different countries? Explore disaster preparedness in another country. How does it differ from the elements of disaster preparedness recommended for the United States as presented in this chapter? What are some of the reasons for any differences found?

Postdisaster immunization campaigns (e.g., for hepatitis A, influenza, varicella) may be warranted in shelter settings depending on conditions such as crowding, poor sanitation, or contamination of food and water (Jablecki et al., 2005). The federal pandemic avian influenza response plan calls for mass immunization to prevent the spread of disease, once an effective vaccine has been developed (USDHHS, 2004).Vaccination may also be needed for autopsy workers and mortuary personnel and their families in the event of disease outbreaks with multiple deaths (Nolte et al., 2004). Community health nurses may be involved in the design of immunization campaigns and their implementation and in educating the public about the need for immunization. Table 27-7◆ presents some of the specific activities of community health nurses related to primary prevention in disaster settings.

Secondary Prevention: Response Planning

Secondary prevention involves the response to a disaster occurrence. Disaster response is based on disaster planning that occurs in the nondisaster stage. In discussing disaster response, we will address purposes and principles of disaster preparedness, general considerations in planning, and specific elements of a disaster response plan.

PURPOSES OF DISASTER PREPAREDNESS Disaster preparedness has been defined by WHO as "the set of measures that ensure the organized mobilization of personnel, funds, equipment, and supplies within a safe environment for effective relief" (Bissell et al., 2004, p. 193). The general intent of disaster preparedness is to limit the morbidity and mortality resulting from a disaster and to decrease the population's vulnerability to the effects of a disaster. A second general purpose of disaster planning is to ensure that resources are available for effective response in the event of a disaster. This aspect of planning involves determining procedures that will be employed in response to a disaster event and obtaining material and personnel that will be required to implement the disaster plan.

The Working Group on "Governance Dilemmas" in Bioterrorism Response (2004) has identified five objectives of response to bioterrorism that have relevance for

TABLE 27-7	Primary Prevention Activities by Community Health Nurses in Disaster Settings
Primary Prevention Focus	**Related Nursing Activities**
Disaster prevention	▪ Assist in the identification of disaster risks. ▪ Advocate for the elimination or modification of disaster risks. ▪ Advocate for appropriate controls on the production, transport, storage, and use of hazardous materials. ▪ Advocate for measures to promote human dignity and prevent civil unrest. ▪ Advocate for effective building codes, maintenance, and security. ▪ Provide immunization services and educate the public on the need for immunization. ▪ Educate the public regarding disaster preparedness.
Minimizing disaster effects	▪ Assist in communicating community disaster response plans to the public. ▪ Educate the public to support "community-as-resource" strategies. ▪ Advocate for the availability and use of PPE by disaster responders. ▪ Educate responders on the use of PPE. ▪ Initiate postdisaster immunization campaigns and educate the public regarding the need for immunization.

other disasters as well. The first objective is to limit death and suffering through preventive, supportive, and curative care. The second objective is to maintain preparedness while defending civil liberties, using the least restrictive interventions possible. A third objective involves preserving economic stability. The fourth objective is not relevant to all disasters, but only to those caused by human error or intention, and deals with discouraging scapegoating and hate crimes. The final objective is to promote individual and community ability to rebound from a disaster while providing mental health support for those in need.

PRINCIPLES AND CHALLENGES OF DISASTER PREPAREDNESS Effective disaster planning is based on several principles that include the following:

- Response plans should be flexible enough to fit the needs of a given disaster situation (Langan & James, 2005). Plans also need to be easy to change if circumstances warrant (Landesman, 2005). In addition, plans should include contingencies most likely to arise in the types of disasters most likely to occur (Langan & James, 2005). Planning may take one of two approaches: agent-specific planning, which addresses the specific types of disaster most likely to occur in a locality, and all-hazards planning, which develops a general plan that can encompass most categories of hazards (Landesman, 2005). The World Health Organization (2004) recommends an all-hazards approach as the most effective way to plan for disaster response. When separate plans exist for different types of disasters, there is potential for confusion regarding roles and responsibilities in any particular situation.

- Disaster plans should be based, as much as possible, on everyday working methods and procedures. This eliminates the need for personnel to learn new procedures and prevents confusion about which procedure is applicable in a given situation.
- Disaster plans should include provisions for extended authority. Time is often a critical factor in effective disaster response and decision latitude should be given to people at the lowest levels of organization to permit immediate response to situations when delaying for higher approval may be costly in terms of lives or property damage (Landesman, 2005; Langan & James, 2005).
- Response plans should be based on knowledge of how people generally behave in emergency situations or how they would behave in specific situations (e.g., in response to an epidemic or a fire) (Landesman, 2005). Unless response plans are developed from a public perspective, members of the target population are unlikely to comply with its provisions, leading to ineffective disaster response (Lasker, 2004). Plans also need to be adjusted to people's needs and not vice versa. If a large portion of the population does not speak English, for example, it is unreasonable to issue disaster warnings only in English in the hope that someone will be available to translate the message.
- Disaster response should be locally focused, with support as needed from state and federal authorities (Landesman, 2005). As much as possible, communities should develop the capabilities to meet their own needs in the event of a disaster. This will prevent delays in response waiting for outside support. Depending on the extent of a particular disaster, federal and state resources may be stretched to the point that little is left to meet the needs of a specific community. For example, one of the reasons for the extensive damage in the 2003 San Diego wildfires was the fact that many local and state fire response units were already engaged in combating wildfires in another county. It may also be helpful to link the disaster plan for one area with those of surrounding areas to allow coordination of efforts in the face of widespread catastrophe. Conversely, when help is needed from surrounding areas, that help will better complement local efforts if plans are coordinated.
- Response plans should enlist the support and coordinate the efforts of the entire community. Major components of the community that would be involved in a disaster response should be involved in developing the response plan. Some of those that might be involved include police and fire departments, local governing bodies, major health care facilities, and large corporations. Predisaster incorporation of these sectors of the community limits confusion with respect to authority and direction for disaster-related activities and enhances the smooth operation of a disaster effort.
- Disaster plans should specify responsible persons by position or title rather than by name. This prevents a need to revise the plan when one person leaves and another takes over the position. For example, the plan may specify that the chief of police be notified of the emergency situation and put the disaster plan into effect. Then, whoever happens to be chief of police will know that it is his or her responsibility to mobilize personnel in the event of a disaster.
- Disaster response plans need to be acceptable to those who will implement them (Landesman, 2005). As is the case with the general public, compliance with elements of the plan can be undermined if the plan is not acceptable to those charged with its implementation.
- Disaster plans should include provisions for casualty distribution to prevent overloading certain health care facilities (Langan & James, 2005).
- Disaster response plans need to make provision for resource acquisition and management, including management of volunteers, donations, and crowd control as well as supplies and equipment (Langan & James, 2005).
- Response plans need to account for the mental as well as physical health needs of both victims and helpers (Langan & James, 2005).
- Disaster response plans must be widely disseminated to the general public and should be communicated by one or two trusted spokespersons (Langan & James, 2005).
- Finally, disaster response plans should be implemented in disaster drills to determine their potential effectiveness in real-life situations (Langan & James, 2005). Evaluations of drills should be used to revise the plan as needed before an actual disaster occurs.

Disaster preparedness, particularly as it relates to responses to bioterrorist threats, poses several challenges. These include preventing disaster (e.g., the spread of disease) without unduly infringing on individual freedom, supporting economic stability in the face of security controls that may disrupt commerce, supporting and restoring social bonds in the face of suspicion and uncertainty, and alerting the public to the occurrence of a crisis without creating fear and panic. Additional challenges include earning public confidence and support regarding the use of resources in responding to the disaster, maintaining credibility in situations in which information on which to base sound decisions is lacking, and promoting collaboration among multiple social sectors to promote effective response (Working

Group on "Governance Dilemmas" in Bioterrorism Response, 2004).

Community health nurses should be actively involved in disaster response planning and can help to assure that principles of effective planning are incorporated and that the challenges are met. For example, community health nurses might advocate for collection of community perspectives prior to developing a response plan or might help to assure that civil liberties are protected as much as possible. Similarly, community health nurses might advocate for a response plan that meets the needs of diverse segments of the community (e.g., non-English-speaking residents or those who cannot afford recommended disaster preparation activities).

GENERAL CONSIDERATIONS IN DISASTER RESPONSE PLANNING General considerations in planning the response to a disaster event include designating authority, developing communication mechanisms, providing transportation, and developing a record-keeping system.

Authority An effective disaster response plan designates a central authority and delineates the responsibilities that are delegated to specific persons and organizations. For example, if it is clear that evacuation decisions are made by the mayor and implemented by members of a local military installation, while police have the responsibility for keeping roads open, there will be less confusion, and evacuation efforts will be carried out more smoothly. Central authority may be assigned to several people in a hierarchical order so that in the absence of the first person designated, the second person has authority to implement the plan. In this individual's absence, a third person would assume that authority, and so on.

As we saw earlier, authority for on-the-spot decisions should be delegated to persons at the scene of a disaster to avoid time-consuming delays in response to an emergency situation. At the same time there needs to be a balance between immediate response and overall coordination of activities. Areas in which authority will be needed should be identified and responsibility designated. Gaps in authority should be prevented since this results in inability to engage in timely response. For example, one of the policies that prevented effective response to the San Diego wildfires in 2003 was the routine grounding of U.S. Forest Service helicopters half an hour before sundown. There was no one with local authority to invalidate this policy and allow at least one flight with fire retardant chemicals that could have helped contain the fires. Pilots of one helicopter that was already en route had to return to base even though they believed they could safely drop their load of chemicals before flight conditions became too dangerous.

Communication Communication is critical to the effective implementation of a disaster response plan. Effective communication serves a number of purposes. First, it increases the likelihood of appropriate action by responders and the general public. Second, it reduces anxiety and unnecessary action by segments of the population that are not threatened by the disaster. Third, and most important, effective communication facilitates relief efforts (Wray, Kreuter, Jacobsen, Clements, & Evans, 2004).

Modes of communication should be established, and disaster personnel and the general public should be familiarized with them. Specific considerations in this area include how warnings of an imminent disaster will be communicated, how communication between various emergency teams and facilities will be handled, and how communication with the outside world will be facilitated. It is important to remember that normal means of communication may be disrupted during an emergency, and that there is a need for "redundant communication systems" using multiple modes of communication from and to multiple locations (Klitzman & Freudenberg, 2003).

Some consideration should also be given to facilitating communication among members of the community. For example, there may be a central bulletin board where messages can be left or a specific agency that is responsible for handling personal communications that permit family members separated by a disaster to locate each other. There should also be two-way communication between authorities and the public so disaster response best meets community needs (Klitzman & Freudenberg, 2003). This may be facilitated by emergency information systems that collect data about disaster effects during impact, response, and recovery phases (Landesman, 2005).

Disaster-related communication should be factual, positive, and reassuring whenever possible (Landesman, 2005), and should convey information about risks and recommended courses of action. Communication mechanisms and messages may need to be targeted to specific audiences, which may necessitate developing ongoing relationships with public media prior to a disaster. For example, ethnic radio and television stations can broadcast warnings and instructions in a variety of languages, but specific contacts should be established before a disaster event occurs. Development of media dissemination plans will support disaster-related communication with the public. Specific messages should be developed based on communication and behavioral theory to promote positive responses, and messages should be accurate, clear, consistent, and timely in their delivery (Wray et al., 2004). Another consideration is the need for interoperable communication systems between response agencies that interface well. In addition, plans should be made to accommodate communication between and among fixed and mobile locations. There is also a need for emergency alert systems that will be easily understood by the general public (e.g., the air raid sirens designed to warn of enemy attack in the 1940s and 1950s). Other aspects of communication include designating reporting sites for rescue and health care personnel and mechanisms for identifying who these people are. For example, color-coded vests might be used to distinguish health care providers from rescue workers (Langan & James, 2005).

Communication components of a disaster response plan should consider three possible scenarios and develop contingency plans for each. In the first scenario, normal communication channels remain intact and can be used for disaster response purposes. In the second scenario, some normal channels are intact, but others have been incapacitated. In the third scenario, there is little intact communications technology and other means of communication need to be employed.

Communication considerations in disaster response planning must also include dissemination of the plan to the general public, the scientific and professional community, and other stakeholders to permit them to take appropriate action regarding their own preparation for and response to a disaster. Again, these communications should be targeted to specific audiences and be delivered by trusted spokespersons. Spokespersons play specific roles in a disaster context (Hooke & Rogers, 2005). These roles include removing psychological barriers to action, promoting public support for appropriate public health response to disaster, building trust and credibility for response organizations, and ultimately motivating people to actions that will reduce disaster-related illness, injury, and death. Because of their credibility in the community, community health nurses may function in this role or may help to identify others who can serve as spokespersons for specific segments of the community. Community health nurses can also help to identify appropriate mechanisms for communicating with community members and in drafting meaningful messages.

A final, highly specialized consideration with respect to disaster communication is how notification regarding the death of a family member will be handled. Protocols should be developed regarding how significant others will be notified of deaths and may necessitate coordination with mental health personnel (Landesman, 2005).

Transportation General plans for the provision of necessary transportation must also be considered in disaster response planning. There will be a need to transport personnel and equipment to the disaster site as well as to transport victims away from the site. There will also be a need to move personnel to areas where they are most needed. Another consideration with respect to transportation is keeping access roads open so that emergency vehicles can pass. There is a need to provide alternate transportation routes, especially for evacuating people from a high-risk area, in case first-choice routes are blocked.

Records Records are needed prior to a disaster regarding the availability of supplies and equipment and areas where they are stored. This information should be updated on a regular basis, and a systematic process for its updating should be established. Local institutions such as schools and businesses should be encouraged to keep records of all those present at any given time so that everyone can be accounted for and those missing can be identified as early as possible. Institutional records may also include emergency contact and health-related information that will facilitate reunification of families or meeting ongoing health needs (Lewis & Bear, 2002).

During the disaster itself, a variety of other types of records are needed. Victims must be identified and their condition and treatment documented. Deaths should also be recorded. Records are also needed of the use of supplies and equipment so that additional materials can be obtained if required. Records of the deployment of rescue personnel are needed to ensure the most effective use of personnel. It would be difficult to develop systematic record-keeping systems during an actual disaster, so it is important that such systems be in place before a disaster occurs.

ELEMENTS OF A DISASTER RESPONSE PLAN A comprehensive disaster plan should address notification, warning, control, coordination, evacuation, and rescue. Additional elements of the plan should specify protocols for immediate care, supportive care, recovery, and evaluation. These last two elements will be discussed under tertiary prevention, and the others will be briefly examined here.

Notification An effective disaster response plan specifies in a systematic fashion the means of notifying the person or persons who can set the plan in motion. Persons who might be in a position to have advance warning of a disaster (e.g., local weather service personnel) should have a clear understanding of who should be apprised of the potential for disaster. There must also be specific plans for notifying personnel and organizations involved in the disaster response. Notification should always include the fact of occurrence of a disaster, the type of disaster involved, and the extent of damage as far as it is known at the time. Notification should also convey any other relevant information that is known about the situation.

Warning The disaster plan should also spell out the procedures for disseminating disaster warnings to the general public. Procedures should specify the content of warnings, who will issue the warnings, and the manner in which warnings will be communicated. For example, the plan might specify that warnings include the type of disaster involved, the area affected, and specific directions on actions to be taken by community members. Warnings may be issued by local radio and TV stations and by police vehicles with loudspeakers, or sirens may be used to alert people if they have been informed beforehand of the meaning of the siren and where to turn for more information. If warnings are to be communicated by media personnel, the plan should specify contact persons at radio and TV stations. Plans for warning need to achieve a balance between waiting too long for appropriate action to be undertaken and overwarning that leads to unnecessary action (Landesman, 2005; Pielke, 2003).

Control A disaster plan also specifies how the effects of a disaster are to be controlled. Different control efforts are required for different types of disasters, and a community should be prepared to implement a variety of control activities. In the case of an earthquake, for example, control measures are directed at preventing and extinguishing fires before further damage is caused. Again, the procedures, materials, and personnel needed to carry out control measures must be specified in the plan.

Logistical Coordination Another element of a community disaster plan deals with logistical coordination. **Logistical coordination** is the coordination of attempts to procure, maintain, and transport needed materials. The disaster plan specifies where and how supplies and equipment will be obtained, where these will be stored, and how they will be transported to the disaster site.

Traffic control is another aspect of logistical coordination. The disaster plan should specify personnel and procedures for controlling access to the disaster site. Traffic control procedures should also specify means by which access to the disaster site is ensured for rescue vehicles and vehicles carrying personnel, supplies, and equipment.

Evacuation An effective disaster plan also specifies evacuation procedures. The plan should indicate how those to be evacuated will be notified, what they can take with them, and how the evacuation will be accomplished. The plan may need to specify several contingency evacuation procedures, depending on the type of disaster.

The disaster response plan also provides for the logistics of evacuation, including the personnel needed to carry out the evacuation, how they are to be recruited and assigned, and how they will be notified. The plan also specifies the forms of transportation to be used during evacuation, where appropriate vehicles can be obtained, and how they will be refueled.

Rescue The response plan should specify the process to be used to assess rescue needs and who is responsible for carrying out the assessment. Once the assessment is made, procedures should be in place for obtaining the appropriate personnel and equipment. For example, in the event of an earthquake, heavy construction equipment and operators are needed, whereas fire department personnel are needed in a fire-related disaster.

The rescue operation should focus on removing victims from hazardous conditions and providing first aid as needed. **Rescue chains** are the logistical component of emergency health services and reflect plans for moving injured persons to appropriate health care facilities. Rescue personnel should refrain from providing other forms of care as much as possible. This care can be provided by others, thus freeing rescue personnel to carry out the rescue operation.

Immediate Care Provision of immediate care is another consideration detailed in a disaster response plan. *Immediate care* is care required on the spot to ensure a disaster victim's survival or a disaster worker's continued ability to function. Plans for providing immediate care in four areas in the vicinity of the disaster site should be detailed in the disaster response plan (Figure 27-5). Immediate care begins at the actual site of the disaster, with a rapid initial assessment of all victims by the first health care provider on the scene. This phase of immediate care is geared to correcting any life-threatening problems.

The second area of immediate care is the triage area. **Triage** is the process of sorting casualties on the basis of urgency and their potential for survival to determine priorities for treatment, evacuation, and transportation. Triage decisions are intended to maximize the number of survivors of a disaster event. When victims are easily accessible, triage can take place at the site of the disaster. Victims are then removed to treatment areas based on their triage priority. In a disaster occurring in an enclosed environment (e.g., in a mine or in a building), victims may not be easily accessible and will probably need to be removed to a more distant triage area as they are found.

The triage process usually involves placing color-coded tags on victims. Typically, black tags are attached to victims who are already dead. Red tags indicate top priority and are attached to victims who have life-threatening injuries but who can be stabilized and who have a high probability of survival. Priority is automatically given to injured rescue workers, their family members, hysterical persons, and children. Yellow tags, indicating second priority, are assigned to victims who have injuries with systemic complications that are not yet life threatening and who are able to withstand a wait of 45 to 60 minutes for medical attention. Yellow tags are also assigned to victims with severe injuries who have a poor chance of survival. Green tags indicate victims

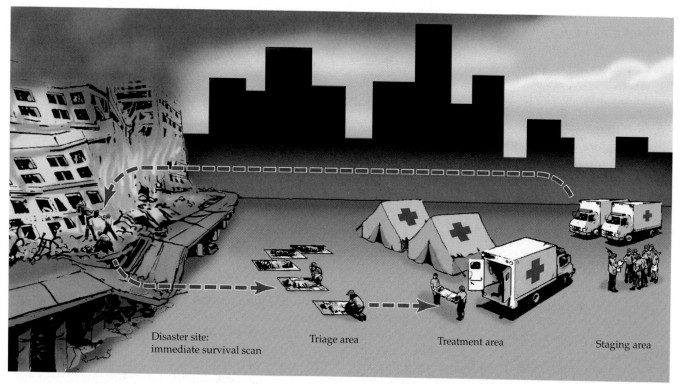

Disaster site:
immediate survival scan

Triage area

Treatment area

Staging area

FIGURE 27-5 Areas of Operation in Immediate Care

with local injuries without immediate systemic complications who can wait several hours for treatment.

The third area of immediate care at the disaster site is the treatment area to which victims are removed after triage. In this area, medical stabilization, temporary care, and emergency surgical stabilization are provided as needed. There may also be a need for psychological first aid at this point. The final area at the site of the disaster is the staging area. It is here that immediate care operations are coordinated and vehicles and personnel are directed to areas of greatest need. The disaster plan should specify the procedures for setting up and operating each of the four areas of immediate care. The plan should also address the supplies, equipment, and personnel needed in each area, how they will be obtained, and how they will be transported to the area.

Another aspect of immediate care that should be addressed in the disaster plan is care of the dead. Plans should be included for procedures to identify bodies and transport them to a morgue of some sort. Records of deaths should be kept, and procedures for rapid disposal of bodies should be specified should contagion be a problem. Plans should also include where and how body bags and identification tags will be obtained.

Plans should be made for casualty distribution and transport of persons with specific types of health problems to specific facilities (Langan & James, 2005). Casualty distribution plans prevent overloading health care facilities closest to the disaster, and may be based on the specific capabilities of certain health care facilities.

For example, victims with severe burns may be sent directly to a facility with a burn unit, whereas physical trauma patients are taken to other facilities.

Supportive Care Supportive care is another component of an effective disaster response plan. Supportive care includes providing food, water, and shelter for victims and disaster relief workers. Other considerations in this area are sanitation and waste disposal, providing medications and routine health care, and reuniting families separated by the disaster.

Shelter is required for those who are evacuated from their homes or whose homes are damaged in the disaster. The disaster response plan should specify which community buildings can be used to shelter victims and how victims are to be transported to shelters. There may also be a need to use the homes of private citizens to shelter victims if public shelters are insufficient. When such is the case, the plan should specify how to notify concerned citizens of the need to place victims in their homes and how placement is to be handled. It is helpful to have a list of people willing to provide shelter to others should a disaster occur. In the case of large groups of displaced persons, refugee camps may be set up. Potential camp sites should be carefully selected in relation to possible physical hazards or water runoff.

Within the shelter, there is a need for supplies to sustain daily living. Shelters should have adequate sanitation and sleeping facilities. There should be plans for heating shelters and cooking food if area gas and electrical power systems are disrupted. Mechanisms should also be specified for governance and security within the shelter, particularly if the shelter will be in use for some time. Shelter leaders can be appointed or elected, and persons within the shelter should have a means of providing input into governance in long-term shelter situations.

Food supplies should be planned and obtained prior to a disaster. There should also be a mechanism for obtaining more food and other supplies from outside the community in the event of damage to stores and stockpiled supplies. A source of clean water is needed, and the disaster plan should identify how and where water will be supplied. Equipment and supplies for water purification should be stored in case of need. Considerations that need to be addressed in planning to feed large groups, in addition to the availability of food supplies, include toilet and handwashing facilities, dishwashing facilities, waste storage and removal (both liquid and solid), cooking and refrigeration facilities, serving dishes and utensils, and food preparation personnel and equipment. Rodent control and food safety information for preparers are other elements of this part of the disaster response plan (Landesman, 2005).

Victims may have other health care needs unrelated to the disaster that need to be met, so plans for providing basic health care in shelters should also be specified. These plans should include stores of medications most likely to be needed by the general public and critical to survival. For example, diabetics will continue to need insulin or oral hypoglycemics, whereas individuals with heart conditions may need a variety of medications. Priority should be given to medications required for serious illnesses rather than for minor conditions. Because communicable diseases spread more rapidly in a debilitated population following a disaster, antibiotics and vaccines should be stored in case of need.

Actions to meet population health needs after a disaster are dependent on identification of those needs. Such identification can occur through early warning systems or syndromic surveillance. **Early warning systems** are planned surveillance systems designed to alert health care personnel of potential large-scale health problems resulting from a disaster. For example, an effective early warning system would identify early cases of communicable disease in a refugee camp, permitting immunization or other control measures to prevent an epidemic. Local surveillance for cases of anthrax or smallpox is another example of an early warning system. The success of early warning systems is dependent on timely reporting and investigation of case reports of specific conditions, pattern recognition, and monitoring of new types of data that can suggest disease outbreaks (e.g., work absence patterns) (Buehler, Hopkins, Overhage, Sosin, & Tong, 2004).

Syndromic surveillance is a special form of early warning system in which data are collected regarding specific clusters of symptoms or syndromes from a variety

of sources. Syndromic surveillance was employed in New York City following the WTC attacks to monitor potential bioterrorism. Syndromes for which incidence data were collected included gastrointestinal syndromes, respiratory syndromes, sepsis, rash, neurological syndromes, botulism-like weakness, and unexplained death with fever (Scipioni, 2002). In 2003, syndromic surveillance identified an outbreak of diarrheal disease from eating spoiled foods following a major power outage in New York City (Marx et al., 2006). Surveillance activities in the case of chemical releases or nuclear attacks may include environmental sampling (Sutton & Gould, 2003).

Specific screening activities may also be needed in a postdisaster situation. For example, TB screening may be warranted in extended shelter situations such as refugee camps. Similarly, screening for scabies or other infestations might be needed when outbreaks occur in sheltered populations. Screening may also be undertaken to identify people with mental health problems arising from the disaster.

Health care providers may need to be educated to recognize covert releases of biological or chemical agents. Covert releases are often difficult to recognize because initial symptoms of exposure might be mild or nonexistent or might be similar to those of other conditions. In addition, health care providers may not be familiar with symptoms of diseases or chemical exposures that are not often seen in their practice. Finally, cases of diseases may occur over a long period of time in various locations, making it difficult to identify any particular patterns (Patel et al., 2003). Epidemiologic cues that suggest covert chemical releases include an increase in the number of people presenting specific symptoms, unexplained deaths in healthy young people, clients emitting unusual odors, and clusters of illness in people that display common characteristics. Other potential signs of covert release include rapid onset of symptoms following exposure to potentially contaminated media, unexplained wildlife deaths, and symptoms suggestive of syndromes associated with chemical exposures (National Center for Environmental Health, 2003).

Secondary prevention will also include treatment for conditions identified. As noted earlier, antidotes for potential chemical and radiological agents should be readily available and providers should know how to administer them. Treatments for chemical exposures should be based on syndrome categories (e.g., respiratory effects) rather than on specific agents to minimize time spent in identifying specific agents (Patel et al., 2003). Appropriate treatment should also be provided for diseases caused by biological agents as well as for existing illness in the population affected by the disaster (e.g., hypertension, diabetes, HIV/AIDS, TB).

Supportive care also includes psychological counseling for those who are not coping adequately with the situation. Counseling may be required by both victims and disaster workers, and plans should be made to provide crisis intervention services during the response stage of the disaster. Psychological support can be provided by comforting and consoling those in distress and by protecting them from the ongoing disaster threat. Disaster response plans should include mechanisms for identifying those in need of counseling and providing them with the services required. For example, following the World Trade Center and Pentagon terrorist attacks, an online self-assessment was established for identifying persons with severe depression related to the attacks (National Mental Health Association, 2001). In another study, 75% of people surveyed in New York, Connecticut, and New Jersey reported some emotional problems after the attacks. Unfortunately, only 12% of them reported receiving help (Melnik et al., 2002), in spite of programs like the Green Cross Project initiated in New York City to address psychological reactions to the attacks. The objectives of the project, which are relevant to psychological care in any disaster setting, were to provide immediate crisis-oriented services, create a referral network of providers, and educate providers regarding "compassion fatigue" and the need to care for themselves as well as their clients (Figley & Figley, 2002).

Generally speaking, people pass through a series of phases in their psychological response to a disaster. The first phase occurs during disaster impact and is characterized by feelings of shock. This is followed by a period of defensive retreat and then by an acceptance of the reality of the event. Eventually, most people will enter a phase characterized by resolution, adaptation, and change (Langan & James, 2005). When people do not progress normally through these stages, they require supportive care.

Individual responses to a disaster occurrence and the need for care are influenced by a number of factors. These factors include one's perception of the event, one's physical and emotional status at the time of the event, and one's general coping abilities. Other factors that may influence people's response to a disaster include prior experience of similar situations and successful coping in those situations, the aspects of the situation itself, cultural influences, and the availability and response of one's support network (Langan & James, 2005).

Elements of psychological intervention that should be incorporated into disaster response planning include mental health triage, emergency psychological first aid and crisis intervention, provisions for meeting physical health needs, and establishment of a calm, stable environment that provides a sense of safety and protection. Other considerations include interventions to assist people to develop feelings of belonging, connection, mastery, and empowerment (Langan & James, 2005).

Disaster victims may require goal orientation and guidance, and they can be directed to perform specific tasks that help them achieve a sense of control. Support is needed for those who must identify loved ones among the dead. Expression of feelings should be fostered, and victims should be encouraged to make use of available support networks. Immediate referral to mental health personnel may be required in some instances. Structuring the environment and regularizing schedules, particularly in shelters, can also help to reestablish a sense of security.

Some relief from psychological stress can frequently be obtained if victims can be assured that family members are safe. Disaster plans should therefore include mechanisms for locating people and reuniting families. Names of persons admitted to shelters or health care facilities should be recorded and communicated to a central location where others can check for word of loved ones. Deaths should also be reported if the dead can be identified, and information should be kept on the assignment of disaster workers to specific areas. It is helpful if institutions, such as schools and businesses, compile the names of those who were present prior to a disaster so that they can be accounted for afterward.

Aside from advocacy for and participation in the development of disaster response plans, community health nursing involvement in secondary prevention in disaster response lies primarily in the areas of immediate care and supportive care. Community health nurses may be involved in triage activities and immediate first aid for disaster victims or rescue workers. Community health nurses may also be responsible for shelter supervision and action to meet the supportive care needs of the population after a disaster. They will most likely be involved in assessing health care needs in shelters and addressing those needs directly or making referrals to needed physical and psychological health services. Community health nurses can also advocate for participation in shelter governance by those housed there and help to address areas of conflict among shelter residents.

Community health nurses will also be involved in surveillance activities, and, because of their interactions with disaster victims, may be among the first to recognize signs of disease outbreaks. They may also identify symptoms in the general population suggestive of covert biological or chemical terrorism. If specific screening activities are warranted in shelter situations, community health nurses will probably be involved in developing and implementing screening programs. Finally, community health nurses may be involved in educating the public and other health care providers regarding recognition and treatment of health conditions related to the disaster. Secondary prevention activities by community health nurses in disaster situations are presented in Table 27-8◆.

MediaLink Case Study: Disaster Care

TABLE 27-8	Secondary Prevention Activities by Community Health Nurses in Disaster Settings
Secondary Prevention Focus	**Related Nursing Activities**
Immediate care	**Triage** ▪ Assess disaster victims for extent of injuries/illness. ▪ Determine priority for treatment, evacuation, and transportation. ▪ Place appropriate colored tag on victim depending on priority. **Treatment of injuries** ▪ Render first aid for injuries. ▪ Provide additional treatment as needed in definitive care areas.
Supportive care	**Shelter supervision** ▪ Coordinate activities of shelter workers. ▪ Oversee records of those admitted and discharged from shelters. ▪ Promote effective interpersonal and group interactions among shelter residents. ▪ Promote independence and involvement of those housed in the shelter. **Surveillance and screening** ▪ Participate in specific surveillance activities. ▪ Recognize evidence of disaster-related health effects. ▪ Recognize other health needs in the disaster population. ▪ Educate health care providers and others regarding recognition and treatment of disaster-related health effects. **Treatment** ▪ Provide treatment as needed for disease and injury under medically approved protocols. ▪ Refer for additional medical or psychological treatment as needed.

TABLE 27-9	Tertiary Prevention Activities by Community Health Nurses in Disaster Settings
Tertiary Prevention Focus	**Related Nursing Activities**
Follow-up care for injuries	▪ Provide continued care for people injured as a result of the disaster or during rescue operations. ▪ Monitor response to treatment.
Follow-up care for psychological problems resulting from the disaster	▪ Provide counseling for those with psychological problems resulting from the disaster. ▪ Refer clients for counseling as needed. ▪ Monitor progress in resolving psychological problems.
Recovery assistance	▪ Refer clients for financial assistance. ▪ Provide assistance in finding housing.
Prevention of future disasters and their consequences	▪ Advocate measures to prevent future disasters. ▪ Educate the public about disaster preparation to minimize the effects of subsequent disasters. ▪ Advocate protection of civil liberties while promoting national security.

Tertiary Prevention: Recovery

Tertiary prevention with respect to a disaster has two major goals. The first is recovery of the community and its members from the effects of the disaster and return to normal. The second aspect of tertiary prevention is preventing a recurrence of the disaster. During the recovery period, there may be a need to reestablish medical care and other services in the community.

Community health nurses have responsibilities in both community recovery and prevention of subsequent disasters. Nurses may be called on to provide sustained care to both victims and disaster workers following the disaster. They may also be involved in identifying health and psychosocial problems that require further assistance. Community health nurses should plan to provide counseling or referral for persons with psychological problems stemming from their experiences during the disaster. There may also be a need to refer disaster victims to continuing sources of medical care. Community health nurses may also need to plan referrals for clients

in need of social and financial assistance. For example, disaster victims may require help in finding housing or in getting financial aid to rebuild homes or businesses.

Community health nurses may also provide input into interventions designed to prevent future disasters or to minimize their effects. For example, if the disaster involved rioting by members of oppressed groups, the community health nurse might advocate measures to meet the needs of minority group members to prevent further rioting; or the nurse might campaign for stronger building codes to prevent the collapse of buildings in subsequent earthquakes. Community health nurses can also help to educate the public on disaster preparedness to minimize the effects of subsequent disasters. A particular challenge following disasters resulting from terrorist activities involves protection of civil liberties while promoting national security (Geiger, 2003). Tertiary prevention foci in disaster settings and related community health nursing activities are summarized in Table 27-9◆.

Implementing Disaster Care

Prior to the occurrence of a disaster, the community health nurse may be involved in activities preliminary to implementing a disaster plan, particularly in disseminating the plan to others. Dissemination needs to occur among persons and agencies who will have designated responsibilities during a disaster. Community health nurses participating in disaster planning are responsible for communicating elements of the plan to members of their employing agency. They may also ensure that the plan is disseminated to nursing organizations in the area (e.g., to members of a district nurses' association). The nurse who assumes this responsibility should be sure that the general plan, as well as the specific part to be played by members of the agency or organization, is understood.

The essential features of the community's disaster response plan should also be communicated to the general public so residents will be prepared to follow the plan in the event of a disaster. The community health nurse may be involved in helping to communicate the plan to the public by apprising clients with whom he or she works of relevant aspects of the plan. The public should be alerted to mechanisms that will be used to inform them of a disaster and where to go for additional information. Community members should also know the general procedures to be followed in terms of caring for disaster victims and setting up shelters. They should also be informed of the locations of proposed shelters. Finally, community members should be told of specific disaster preparations that should be undertaken by individuals and families.

When a disaster occurs, community health nurses will be actively involved in implementing the disaster plan. Some of the activities involved in implementation were discussed earlier in the section on secondary prevention in the disaster setting.

Advocacy in Action

After Katrina

From September 1 to 5, 2005, 12 senior BSN students, three faculty members, and one graduate nurse had the unique opportunity to practice disaster nursing during one of the worst natural disasters of our time—Hurricane Katrina. The students themselves initiated the trip to Hattiesburg, Mississippi, with the goal of providing immediate care to the victims of Hurricane Katrina. Although Hattiesburg is located 65 miles inland, the winds from the category 4 hurricane caused tremendous damage to the community.

Wesley Medical Center (WMC) in Hattiesburg was the only fully functioning hospital within 100 miles of the Gulf Coast, and was inundated by patients requiring medical attention. Upon arrival, we divided into teams, working in the emergency room, labor and delivery, and a medical-surgical unit. The ER was divided into a clinic and an acute side, which treated chainsaw injuries, gunshot wounds, seizures, and other emergent conditions. We took vital signs, acted as escorts, gave medications, assisted physicians and nurses, and consoled distraught patients. One student fed a patient who had waited hours for something to eat; another sat with a suicidal patient; others worked feverishly to save lives. Not only did Hurricane Katrina bring death and destruction, she induced the arrival of new lives. In labor and delivery, we fed, rocked, changed, and bathed babies and cared for laboring mothers. During deliveries, we assisted the nurses to calm anxious mothers and families. In what would normally be a joyous occasion, fear and worry remained constant emotions. One new mother had her older child staying in the room with her, as there was nowhere else for the child to go. Fourteen babies in the nursery were transported from the neo-natal intensive care unit across town when its generators failed. Those precious babies fighting for survival stole our hearts.

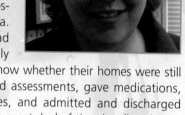

On the medical-surgical unit, many of the adults were evacuees from a hospital in Slidell, Louisiana. Most of the patients had not heard from family members and did not know whether their homes were still standing. We performed assessments, gave medications, started intravenous lines, and admitted and discharged patients. We also spent a great deal of time just listening to the concerns of those under our care.

The atmosphere at WMC was not that of a usual hospital setting: the hospital was in lockdown, with the only entrance/exit through the emergency room, and was guarded at all times. People lined up for hours outside waiting to get in out of the heat, or to get food or water. We, as well as health care workers from other facilities, were housed in the hospital's Wellness Center, sleeping on the gymnasium floor and taking 3-minute showers to conserve water.

Our stay at WMC lasted only 5 days, but in those 5 days we were able to meet needs that would have gone unmet if we had not been there. Troy University students and faculty worked in the hospital around the clock for the duration of the visit, donating approximately 800 hours of labor. Our patients were very grateful for the care they received, and we were grateful for the experience of advocating for individuals, families, and groups of people caught in an unimaginable situation. Many tears were shed as we left the patients, staff, and place we had grown to love during our stay. It was an honor to practice the nursing art of advocacy in its truest form, and under such deserving conditions.

Amy Spurlock, RN, PhD
Troy University School of Nursing

Evaluating Disaster Care

The final responsibility of community health nurses with respect to disaster care is evaluating that care. Nurses and others involved in the disaster participate in evaluative activities outlined in the disaster plan. Evaluation focuses on the adequacy of the plan for curtailing the disaster and meeting the needs of those involved in it. Evaluation of disaster response is sometimes referred to as "after-action analysis" (Scipioni, 2002).

In this effort it may be helpful to examine the disaster response in light of the six dimensions of health. Did the plan adequately provide for the needs of the people affected and the kinds of health problems that resulted? Did physical environmental, psychological, or sociocultural dimension factors impede implementation of the plan or limit its effectiveness? What influence did behavioral factors have on plan implementation, if any? Were health care services adequate to meet the health needs posed by the disaster itself as well as those encountered in the period after the disaster? Data obtained in the evaluative process are used to assess the adequacy of the community disaster plan and to guide revisions of the plan to better deal with future disasters.

The effectiveness of care provided to individual disaster victims should also be assessed. Evaluation in this area focuses on the degree to which individual needs were met and the extent to which problems resulting from the disaster were resolved.

Two specific sets of guidelines that may be used to evaluate the effectiveness of disaster response planning are the United Nations (UN) High Commissioner for Refugees' *Handbook for Emergencies* (2000) and the Sphere Project's *Humanitarian Charter and Minimum Standards in Disaster Response* (2004). The UN document addresses areas for emergency response related to emergency management, contingency planning, initial assessment and immediate response, operations planning, coordination and organization, and external relations. The guidelines also address provision of food, water, health care, and sanitation services; supplies and transport; voluntary repatriation of displaced persons; and commodity distribution systems for food relief. These guidelines are available from the High Commissioner for Refugees' Web site at http://www.unhcr.org/cgi-bin/texis/vtx/publ/opendoc/pdf?tbl=PUBL&id=3bb2fa26b.

The Sphere Project (2004), a group of humanitarian nongovernmental agencies and Red Cross and Red Crescent Societies, has also developed a handbook to address international disaster response. The handbook incorporates eight standards and related key indicators that can be used to evaluate the effectiveness of disaster response. Guidance notes, points to consider in applying the standards, are also included. The Sphere Project standards and related considerations are presented in Table 27-10◆. The full standards document can be

TABLE 27-10	The Sphere Project Standards and Related Considerations
Standard	**Related Considerations**
Participation	Beneficiary populations should participate in the assessment, design, implementation, monitoring, and evaluation of assistance programs.
Assessment	Assessment is required to provide an understanding of the situation and resulting threats to life and health; assessment helps determine whether or not outside aid is needed; assessment addresses all areas of need (e.g., water, food, sanitation, security, etc.); assessment data should be disaggregated by subgroup if possible.
Response	Outside response is required when local authorities are unable or unwilling to respond to the needs of the population.
Targeting	Aid should be targeted to all those in need and delivered equitably and impartially.
Monitoring	Program effectiveness and changes in situation are monitored to facilitate program changes or discontinuation as needed.
Evaluation	There is a need for systematic and impartial evaluation of aid programs.
Aid worker competencies and responsibilities	Relief workers should have the necessary qualifications, attitudes, and experience for working in the situation.
Personnel supervision, management, and support	Workers are effectively supervised and supported.

Data from: The Sphere Project. (2004). Humanitarian charter and minimum standards in disaster response. Retrieved May 1, 2006, from http://www/sphereproject.org/handbook/hdbkhtm/hdbkhtml

obtained from the project Web site at http://www/spherepro ject.org/handbook/hdbkhtm/hdbkhtml. Either set of standards or a combination of both can be used to evaluate the effectiveness of disaster response. Community health nurses would participate in using the standards to engage in action analysis related to a particular disaster. In addition, community health nurses would advocate for the evaluation of disaster services from the perspective of service recipients (Rutta et al., 2005). One further consideration in disaster evaluation is the cost of the disaster response and mechanisms to decrease the cost of future responses (Landesman, 2005).

Although disasters occur infrequently in community health practice, community health nurses should be prepared to respond effectively when they do occur. They should also be instrumental in assuring that individual clients and families, as well as communities, are prepared to respond effectively in the event of a disaster.

Case Study

Nursing in the Disaster Setting

Two commuter trains have collided in a tunnel at rush hour. Both trains derailed and one of them struck the side of the tunnel, causing it to collapse on two of the derailed cars. There were approximately 300 passengers on the two trains, and 50 or more people are trapped in the two buried cars. The accident occurred approximately one-quarter mile from the west end of the tunnel and two miles from the east end. The largest portions of both trains lie on the west side of the collapsed portion of the tunnel.

One of the passengers is a community health nurse. The nurse was not injured in the accident and was able to get out of the wreckage to the west end of the tunnel, where most of the survivors are gathered.

1. What are the biophysical, psychological, physical environmental, sociocultural, behavioral, and health system factors that may be influencing this disaster situation?
2. What role functions might the community health nurse carry out in this situation?
3. What primary, secondary, and tertiary preventive activities might be appropriate in this situation? Why?

Test Your Understanding

1. In what ways do disaster events vary? What are the implications of these variations for disaster preparedness? (pp. 763–764)

2. What are the four elements of a disaster? How does each influence disaster response? (pp. 765–773)

3. What are the purposes of disaster preparedness? (p. 788)

4. How might biophysical, psychological, physical environmental, sociocultural, behavioral, and health system considerations influence a disaster or a community's response to a disaster? (pp. 774–784, 785)

5. What are the principles of community disaster preparedness? (pp. 788–789)

6. What are the elements of an effective disaster plan? (pp. 791–795)

7. What is the role of the community health nurse in primary, secondary, and tertiary prevention related to disaster situations? (pp. 786–796)

EXPLORE MediaLink

http://www.prenhall.com/clark
Resources for this chapter can be found on the Companion Website.

Audio Glossary
Exam Review Questions
Case Study: Disaster Care

MediaLink Application: Student Nurses in the
  Aftermath of Katrina (video)
Media Links

Challenge Your Knowledge
Advocacy Interviews

References

Advisory Committee on Immunization Practices. (2002). Use of anthrax vaccine in response to terrorism: Supplemental recommendations of the Advisory Committee on Immunization Practices. *Morbidity and Mortality Weekly Report, 51*, 1024–1026.

Arias, D. C. (2005, December). Katrina displaced thousands of doctors. *The Nation's Health*, p. 13.

Bailey, M. A., Glover, R., & Huang, Y. (2005). Epidemiologic assessment of the impact of four hurricanes—Florida, 2004. *Morbidity and Mortality Weekly Report, 54*, 693–696.

Banauch, G., McLaughlin, M., Horschorn, R., Corrigan, M., Kelly, K., & Prezant, D. (2002). Injuries and illness among New York City fire department rescue workers after responding to the World Trade Center attacks. *Morbidity and Mortality Weekly Report, 51*(Special issue), 1–5.

Barclay, L. (2004). Public perceptions should be considered in terrorism planning: A newsmaker interview with Roz D. Lasker, MD. *Medscape Medical News*. Retrieved September 30, 2004, from http://www.medscape.com/viewarticle/489704

Berkowitz, B. (2002). Preserving our mission. *Public Health Nursing, 19*, 319–320.

Bernard, B. P., Baron, S. L., Mueller, M. S., Driscoll, R. J., Tapp, L. C., Wallingford, K. M., et al. (2002). Impact of September 11 attacks on workers in the vicinity of the World Trade Center—New York City.

Morbidity and Mortality Weekly Report, 51(Special issue), 8–10.

Bissell, R. A., Pinet, L., Nelson, M., & Levy, M. (2004). Evidence of the effectiveness of health sector preparedness in disaster response: The example of four earthquakes. *Family and Community Health, 27*, 193–204.

Boulton, M. L., Abellera, J., Lemmings, J., & Robinson, L. (2005). Terrorism and emergency preparedness in state and territorial public health departments—United States, 2004. *Morbidity and Mortality Weekly Report, 54*, 459–460.

Brauer, J. (2002). On the economics of terrorism. *Phi Kappa Phi Forum, 82*(2), 38–41.

Buehler, J. W., Hopkins, R. S., Overhage, J. M., Sosin, D. M., & Tong, V. (2004). Framework for evaluating public health surveillance systems for early detection of outbreaks: Recommendations from the CDC working group. *Morbidity and Mortality Weekly Report, 53*(RR-5), 1–13.

Centers for Disease Control and Prevention. (2002). New classification for deaths and injuries involving terrorism. *Morbidity and Mortality Weekly Report, 51*(Special issue), 18–19.

Centers for Disease Control and Prevention. (2003). Terrorism preparedness in state health departments—United States, 2001–2003. *Morbidity and Mortality Weekly Report, 52*, 1051–1053.

Centers for Disease Control and Prevention. (2004). *Bioterrorism agents/diseases*. Retrieved April 25, 2006, from http://www.bt/cdc/gov/agent/agentlist-category.asp

Centers for Disease Control and Prevention. (2006). *Anthrax: What you need to know.* Retrieved May 5, 2005, from http://www.cdc.gov/anthrax/needtoknow.asp

Centers for Disease Control and Prevention Strategic Planning Workgroup. (2000). Biological and chemical terrorism: Strategic plan for preparedness and response. *Morbidity and Mortality Weekly Report, 49*(RR-4), 1–14.

Cohen, H. W., Gould, R. M., & Sidel, V. W. (2004). The pitfalls of bioterrorism preparedness: The anthrax and smallpox experiences. *American Journal of Public Health, 94*, 1667–1671.

Cupp, O. S., Walker, D. E. II, & Hillison, J. (2004). Agroterrorism in the US: Key security challenges for the 21st century. *Biosecurity and Bioterrorism, 2*(2), 97–105.

Daley, W. R. (2006a). Public health response to Hurricanes Katrina and Rita—Louisiana, 2005. *Morbidity and Mortality Weekly Report, 55*, 29–30.

Daley, W. R. (2006b). Public health response to Hurricanes Katrina and Rita—United States, 2005. *Morbidity and Mortality Weekly Report, 55*, 229–231.

DeGraw, C., Kimball, G., Adams, R., Misselbeck, T., Oliveri, R., Plough, J., et al. (2006). Tuberculosis control activities after Hurricane Katrina—New Orleans, Louisiana, 2005. *Morbidity and Mortality Weekly Report, 55*, 332–335.

Doctors Without Borders. (2005a). Innovation in care of malnourished saves thousands. *Alert, 9*(3), 8–9.

Doctors Without Borders. (2005b). MSF responds to the earthquake in Pakistan and India. *Alert, 9*(3), 2–3.

Domino, M. E., Fried, B., Moon, Y., Olinick, J., & Yoon, J. (2003). Disasters and the public health safety net: Hurricane Floyd hits the North Carolina Medicaid program. *American Journal of Public Health, 93*, 1122–1127.

Dowling, K. C., & Lipton, R. I. (2005). Bioterrorism preparedness expenditures may compromise public health. *American Journal of Public Health, 95*, 1672.

Easley, C. E., & Allen, C. E. (2003). Exploring the roots of terrorism. In B. S. Levy & V. W. Sidel (Eds.), *Terrorism and public health: A balanced approach to strengthening systems and protecting people* (pp. 335–350). Oxford: Oxford University.

Engelthaler, D., Lewis, K., Anderson, S., Snow, S., Gladden, L., Hammond, R. M., et al. (2005). *Vibrio* illnesses after Hurricane Katrina—Multiple states, August–September 2005. *Morbidity and Mortality Weekly Report, 54*, 928–931.

Entzel, P. P., Fleming, L. E., Trepka, M. J., & Squicciarini, D. (2003). The health status of newly arrived refugee children in Miami–Dade County, Florida. *American Journal of Public Health, 93*, 286–288.

Fagan, J., Galea, S., Ahern, J., Bonner, S., & Vlahov, D. (2002). Self-reported increase in asthma severity after the September 11 attacks on the World Trade Center—Manhattan, New York, 2001. *Morbidity and Mortality Weekly Report, 51*, 781–784.

Federal Emergency Management Agency. (2003). *Federal response plan, Interim*. Retrieved April 27, 2006, from http://www.ohsep.louisiana.gov/olans/frp2003.pdf

Federal Emergency Management Agency. (2006a). *Biological threats*. Retrieved March 21, 2006, from http://www.fema.gov/hazard/terrorism/bio/index.shtm

Federal Emergency Management Agency. (2006b). *Chemical threats*. Retrieved March 21, 2006, from http://www.fema.gov/hazard/terrorism/chem/index.shtm

Federal Emergency Management Agency. (2006c). *General information about terrorism*. Retrieved March 21, 2006, from http://www.fema.gov/hazard/terrorism/info.shtm

Federal Emergency Management Agency. (2006d). *Nuclear blast*. Retrieved March 21, 2006, from http://www.fema.gov/hazard/terrorism/rad/index.shtm

Federal Emergency Management Agency. (2006e). *Radiological dispersion device*. Retrieved March 21, 2006, from http://www.fema.gov/hazard/terrorism/nuclear/index.shtm

Figley, C. R., & Figley, K. R. (2002). The Green Cross Project: A model for providing emergency mental-health aid after September 11. *Phi Kappa Phi Forum, 82*(2), 42–45.

Fothergill, A., Palumbo, M. V., Rambur, B., Reinier, K., & McIntosh, B. (2005). The volunteer potential of inactive nurses for disaster preparedness. *Public Health Nursing, 22*, 414–421.

Geiger, H. J. (2003). Protecting civil liberties. In B. S. Levy & V. W. Sidel (Eds.), *Terrorism and public health: A balanced approach to strengthening systems and protecting people* (pp. 322–334). Oxford: Oxford University.

Gershon, R. R. M., Hogan, E., Qureshi, K. A., & Doll, L. (2004). Preliminary results from the World Trade Center Evacuation Study—New York City, 2003. *Morbidity and Mortality Weekly Report, 53*, 815–817.

Hampson, N. B., Lai, M. W., McNeil, M., Byers, P., Ratard, R., Patel, M., et al. (2005). Carbon monoxide poisoning after Hurricane Katrina—Alabama, Louisiana, and Mississippi, August–September 2005. *Morbidity and Mortality Weekly Report, 54*, 996–998.

Henry, C., Belflower, A., Drociuk, D., Gibson, J. J., Harris, R., Horton, D. K., et al. (2005). Public health consequences from hazardous substances acutely released during rail transit—South Carolina, 2005; Selected states, 1999–2004. *Morbidity and Mortality Weekly Report, 543*, 64–67.

Hilhorst, D. (2005). Dead letter or living document? Ten years of the Code of Conduct for disaster relief. *Disasters, 29*, 351–369.

Holland, G. (2003). A century after Galveston, 1900. In R. Simpson (Ed.), *Hurricane! Coping with disaster: Progress and challenges since Galveston, 1900* (pp. 317–334). Washington, DC: American Geophysical Union.

Hooke, W. H., & Rogers, P. G. (Eds.). (2005). *Public health risks of disasters: Communication, infrastructure, and preparedness workshop summary*. Washington, DC: National Academies Press.

Horton, R. (2003). Bioterrorism: The extreme politics of public health. In R. Beaglehole (Ed.), *Global public health: A new era* (pp. 209–225). Oxford, UK: Oxford University.

Jablecki, J., Norton, S. A., Keller, R., DeGraw, C., Ratard, R., Straif-Bourgeios, S., et al. (2005). Infectious disease and dermatologic conditions in evacuees and rescue workers after Hurricane Katrina—Multiple states, August–September 2005. *Morbidity and Mortality Weekly Report, 54*, 961–964.

Jaranson, J. M., Butcher, J., Halcon, L., Johnson, D. R., Robertson, C., Savik, K., et al. (2004). Somali and Oromo refugees: Correlates of torture and trauma history. *American Journal of Public Health, 94*, 591–598.

Jones, K. T., Grigg, M., Crockett, L. K., Conti, L., Blackmore, C., Ward, D., et al. (2004). Preliminary medical examiner reports of mortality associated with Hurricane Charley—Florida, 2004. *Morbidity and Mortality Weekly Report, 53*, 385–387.

Joyce, N. (2005). Health care after the tsunami: From the front lines in Banda Aceh. Retrieved March 15, 2005, from http://www.medscape.com/viewarticle/500462

Kay, R. S., Hopkins, R. S., Blackmore, C., Johnson, D., Schauben, J. L., Weisman, R., et al. (2006). Monitoring poison control center data to detect health hazards during hurricane season—Florida, 2003–2005. *Morbidity and Mortality Weekly Report, 53*, 426–428.

Klitzman, S., & Freudenberg, N. (2003). Implications of the World Trade Center attack for the public health and health care infrastructures. *American Journal of Public Health, 93*, 400–406.

Landesman, L. Y. (2005). *Public health management of disasters: The practice guide* (2nd ed.). Washington, DC: American Public Health Association.

Langan, J. C., & James, D. C. (2005). *Preparing nurses for disaster management*. Upper Saddle River, NJ: Pearson Prentice Hall.

Lasker, R. D. (2004). *Redefining readiness: Terrorism planning through the eyes of the public.* Retrieved September 28, 2004, from http://www.cacsh.org/eptpp.html

Levin, S. M., Herbert, R., Moline, J. M., Todd, A. C., Stevenson, L., Landsbergis, P., et al. (2004). Physical health status of World Trade Center rescue and recovery workers and volunteers—New York City, July 2002–August 2004. *Morbidity and Mortality Weekly Report, 53,* 807–812.

Levy, B. S., & Sidel, V. W. (2003). Challenges that terrorism poses to public health. In B. S. Levy & V. W. Sidel (Eds.), *Terrorism and public health: A balanced approach to strengthening systems and protecting people* (pp. 3–18). Oxford: Oxford University.

Lewis, K. D., & Bear, B. J. (2002). *Manual of school health* (2nd ed.). Philadelphia: Saunders.

Lichterman, J. D. (2000). A "community as resource" strategy for disaster response. *Public Health Reports, 115,* 262–265.

Little, B., Gill, J., Schulte, J., Young, S., Horton, J., Harris, L., et al. (2004). Rapid assessment of the needs and health status of older adults after Hurricane Charley—Charlotte, DeSoto, and Hardee Counties, Florida, August 27–31, 2004. *Morbidity and Mortality Weekly Report, 53,* 837–840.

Little Hoover Commission. (2003). *To protect & prevent: Rebuilding California's public health system.* Sacramento, CA: State of California.

Martone, G. (2002). Rethinking responses to hunger. *American Journal of Nursing, 102*(10), 36–42.

Marx, M. A., Rodriguez, C. V., Greenko, J., Das, D., Heffernan, R., Karpati, A. M., et al. (2006). Diarrheal illness detected through syndromic surveillance after a massive power outage: New York City, August 2003. *American Journal of Public Health, 96,* 547–553.

McNeil, M., Goddard, J., Henderson, A., Phelan, M., Davis, S., Wolkin, A., et al. (2006). Rapid community needs assessment after Hurricane Katrina—Hancock County, Mississippi, September 14–15, 2005. *Morbidity and Mortality Weekly Report, 55,* 234–236.

Melnik, T. A., Baker, C. T., Adams, M. L., O'Dowd, K., Mokdad, A. H., Brown, D. W., et al. (2002). Psychological and emotional effects of the September 11 attacks on the World Trade Center—Connecticut, New Jersey, and New York, 2001. *Morbidity and Mortality Weekly Report, 51,* 784–786.

Morrow, J., Norman, E., Dickens, R., Garrison, H., Morris, T., Henderson, K., et al. (2004). Rapid community health and needs assessment after Hurricanes Isabel and Charley—North Carolina, 2003–2004. *Morbidity and Mortality Weekly Report, 53,* 840–842.

Murray, O. (2006). Hurricane Rita leaves lessons in its wake. *Correct Care, 20*(1), 3.

Myers, M. F., & White, G. F. (2003). Social choices in dealing with hurricanes. In R. Simpson (Ed.), *Hurricane! Coping with disaster: Progress and challenges since Galveston, 1900* (pp. 141–153). Washington, DC: American Geophysical Union.

Nacos, B. (2002). Terrorism, the mass media, and the events of 9–11. *Phi Kappa Phi Forum, 82*(2), 13–19.

National Association of County and City Health Officials. (2001). Assessment of local bioterrorism and emergency preparedness. Retrieved December 20, 2001, from http://www.naccho.org

National Center for Environmental Health. (2003). Recognition of illness associated with exposure to chemical agents—United States, 2003. *Morbidity and Mortality Weekly Report, 52,* 938–940.

National Center for Health Statistics. (2005). Percentage of hospitals having plans or conducting drills for attack by explosion or fire, by urbanization of area—United States, 2003. *Morbidity and Mortality Weekly Report, 54,* 1084.

National Center for Infectious Diseases. (2001). Recognition of illness associated with the intentional release of biologic agents. *Morbidity and Mortality Weekly Report, 50,* 893–897.

National Institute for Occupational Safety and Health. (2002). Protecting building environments from airborne, chemical, biologic, or radiologic attacks. *Morbidity and Mortality Weekly Report, 51,* 78–91.

National Mental Health Association. (2001). *Depression screening.* Retrieved September 24, 2001, from http://www.depression–screening.org

Nolte, K. B., Hanzlick, R. L., Payne, D. C., Kroger, A. T., Oliver, W. R., Baker, A. M., et al. (2004). Medical examiners, coroners, and biologic terrorism: A guidebook for surveillance and case management. *Morbidity and Mortality Weekly Report, 53*(RR-8), 1–36.

Palacio, H., Shah, U., Kilborn, C., Martinez, D., Page, V., Gavagan, T., et al. (2005). Norovirus outbreak among evacuees from Hurricane Katrina—Houston, Texas, September 2005. *Morbidity and Mortality Weekly Report, 54,* 1016–1018.

Patel, M., Schier, J., Belson, M., Rubin, C., Garbe, P., & Osterloh, J. (2003). Recognition of illness associated with exposure to chemical agents—United States, 2003. *Morbidity and Mortality Weekly Report, 52,* 938–940.

Patterson, K. (2005). Psychological triage. *NurseWeek, 18*(20), 26.

Paul, B. K. (2005). Evidence against disaster-induced migration: The 2004 tornado in north-central Bangladesh. *Disasters, 29,* 370–385.

The Pew Research Center for the People and the Press. (2001). Overwhelming support for Bush, military response, but American psyche reeling from terror attacks? Retrieved September 24, 2001, from http://www.people–press.org

Pielke, R. A. (2003). Reducing vulnerability. In R. Simpson (Ed.), *Hurricane! Coping with disaster: Progress and challenges since Galveston, 1900* (pp. 165–173). Washington, DC: American Geophysical Union.

Pinto, A., Saeed, M., El Sakka, M., Rashford, A., Colombo, A., Valenciano, M., et al. (2005). Setting up an early warning system for epidemic-prone diseases in Darfur: A participative approach. *Disasters, 29,* 310–322.

Prezant, D., Kelly, K., Jackson, B., Peterson, D., Feldman, D., Baron, S., et al. (2002). Use of respiratory protection among responders at the World Trade Center site—New York City, September, 2001. *Morbidity and Mortality Weekly Report, 51*(Special issue), 6–8.

Ratard, R., Brown, C. M., Ferdinands, J., Callahan, D., Dunn, K. H., Scalia, M. R., et al. (2006). Health concerns associated with mold in water-damaged homes after Hurricanes Katrina and Rita—New Orleans area, Louisiana, October 2005. *Morbidity and Mortality Weekly Report, 55,* 41–44.

Richman, J. A., Wislar, J. S., Flaherty, J. A., Fendrich, M., & Rospenda, K. M. (2004). Effects on alcohol use and anxiety of the September 11, 2001 attacks and chronic work stressors: A longitudinal cohort study. *American Journal of Public Health, 94,* 2010–2015.

Rogers, N., Guerra, F., Suchdev, P. S., Chapman, A. S., Plotinsky, R. N., Jhung, M., et al. (2006). Rapid assessment of health needs and resettlement plans among Hurricane Katrina evacuees, San Antonio, Texas, September 2005. *Morbidity and Mortality Weekly Report, 55,* 242–244.

Rousseau, C., Rufagari, M., Bagilishya, D., & Measham, T. (2004). Remaking family life: Strategies for re-establishing continuity among Congolese refugees during the family reunification process. *Social Science & Medicine, 59,* 1095–1108.

Rozario, K. (2005). Making progress: Disaster narratives and the art of optimism in modern America. In L. J. Vale & T. J. Campanella (Eds.), *The resilient city: How modern cities recover from disaster* (pp. 27–54). Oxford: Oxford University.

Rutta, E., Williams, H., Mwansasu, A., Mung'ong'o, F., Burke, H., Gongo, R., et al. (2005). Refugee perceptions of the quality of healthcare: Findings from a participatory assessment in Ngara, Tanzania. *Disasters, 29,* 291–309.

Salvage, J. (2002). *Collateral effects: The health and environmental costs of war on Iraq.* Retrieved March 20, 2003, from http://www.medact.org/tbx/docs/Medact%20Iraq%20report_final3.pdf

Sandhu, H. S., Thomas, C., Nsubuga, P., & White, M. E. (2003). A global network for early warning and response to infectious diseases and bioterrorism: Applied epidemiology and training programs, 2001. *American Journal of Public Health, 93,* 1640–1642.

Schwartz, S. P., Li, W., Berenson, L., & Williams, R. D. (2002). Deaths in the World Trade Center terrorist attacks—New York City, 2001. *Morbidity and Mortality Weekly Report, 51*(Special issue), 16–18.

Scipioni, L. (Ed.). (2002). Health system preparedness: Fine tuning communication, coordination, and care in a new era. *The Pfizer Journal, 6*(4), 1–35.

Sidel, V. W., Cohen, H. W., & Gould, R. M. (2001). Good intentions and the road to bioterrorism preparedness. *American Journal of Public Health, 91,* 716–718.

Simon, J. D. (2002). The global terrorist threat. *Phi Kappa Phi Forum, 82*(2), 10–12.

Smallpox Vaccine Adverse Events Coordinators, National Immunization Program. (2004). Update: Adverse events following civilian smallpox vaccination—United States, 2003. *Morbidity and Mortality Weekly Report, 53,* 106–107.

Smith, R. P., Katz, C. L., Holmes, A., Herbert, R., Levin, S., Moline, J., et al. (2004). Mental health status of World Trade Center rescue and recovery workers and volunteers—New York City, July 2002–August 2004. *Morbidity and Mortality Weekly Report, 53*, 812–815.

Sniffen, J. C., Cooper, T. W., Johnson, D., Blackmore, C., Patel, P., Harduar-Morano, L., et al. (2005). Carbon monoxide poisoning from hurricane-associated use of portable generators—Florida, 2004. *Morbidity and Mortality Weekly Report, 54*, 697–670.

Spanjaard, H., & Khabib, O. (2003). Chemical weapons. In B. S. Levy & V. Sidel (Eds.), *Terrorism and public health: A balanced approach to strengthening systems and protecting people* (pp. 199–219). Oxford: Oxford University.

The Sphere Project. (2004). *Humanitarian charter and minimum standards in disaster response.* Retrieved May 1, 2006, from http://www/sphereproject.org/handbook/hdbkhtm/hdbkhtml

Steele, L. S., Lemieux-Charles, L., Clark, J. P., & Glazier, R. H. (2002). The impact of policy changes on the health of recent immigrants and refugees in the inner city. *Canadian Journal of Public Health, 93*, 118–122.

Sutton, P. M., & Gould, R. M. (2003). Nuclear, radiological, and related weapons. In B. S. Levy & V. W. Sidel (Eds.), *Terrorism and public health: A balanced approach to strengthening systems and protecting people* (pp. 220–242). Oxford: Oxford University.

Thai Ministry of Health–US CDC Collaboration. (2005). Rapid health response, assessment, and surveillance after a tsunami—Thailand, 2004–2005. *Morbidity and Mortality Weekly Report, 54*, 61–64.

Thai Ministry of Public Health. (2005). Health concerns associated with disaster victim identification after a tsunami—Thailand, December 26, 2004–March 31, 2005. *Morbidity and Mortality Weekly Report, 54*, 349–352.

Toprani, A., Ratard, R., Straif-Bourgeois, S., Sokol, T., Averhoff, F., Brady, J., et al. (2006). Surveillance in hurricane evacuation centers—Louisiana, September–October 2005. *Morbidity and Mortality Weekly Report, 55*, 32–35.

Tucker, M., Eichold, B., Lofgren, J. P., Holmes, I., Irvin, D., Villanacci, J., et al. (2006). Carbon monoxide poisonings after two major hurricanes—Alabama and Texas, August–October, 2005. *Morbidity and Mortality Weekly Report, 55*, 237–239.

United Nations High Commissioner for Refugees. (2000). *Handbook for emergencies.* Retrieved May 1, 2006, from http://www.unhcr.org/cgi-bin/texis/vtx/publ/opendoc/pdf?tbl=PUBL&id=3bb2fa26b

U.S. Department of Health and Human Services. (2004). *Pandemic influenza preparedness and response plan.* Washington, DC: Author.

U.S. Department of State. (2004). *Patterns of global terrorism, 2003.* Retrieved November 22, 2004, from http://www.state.gov/s/ct/rls/pgtrpt/2003/c12153.htm

Vale, L. J., & Campanella, T. J. (2005). Introduction: The cities rise again. In L. J. Vale & T. J. Campanella (Eds.), *The resilient city: How modern cities recover from disaster* (pp. 3–23). Oxford: Oxford University.

Widyastuti, E., Silaen, G., Pricesca, A., Handoko, A., Blanton, C., Handzel, T., et al. (2006). Assessment of health-related needs after tsunami and earthquake—Three districts, Aceh Province, Indonesia, July–August 2005. *Morbidity and Mortality Weekly Report, 55*, 93–97.

Williams, W., Guarisco, J., Guillot, K., Wales, J., Revels, C., Barre, G., et al. (2005). Surveillance for illness and injury after Hurricane Katrina—New Orleans, Louisiana, September 8–25, 2005. *Morbidity and Mortality Weekly Report, 54*, 1018–1021.

The Working Group on "Governance Dilemmas" in Bioterrorism Response. (2004). Leading during bioattacks and epidemics with the public's trust and help. *Biosecurity & Bioterrorism, 2*(1), 25–40.

World Health Organization. (2004). *Strengthening health systems' response to crises: Towards a new focus on disaster preparedness.* Retrieved May 5, 2006, from http://www.who.int/document/e87920.pdf

Wray, R. J., Kreuter, M. W., Jacobsen, H., Clements, B., & Evans, R. G. (2004). Theoretical perspectives on public communication preparedness for terrorist attacks. *Family and Community Health, 27*, 232–241.

Wu, P., Duarte, C. S., Mandell, D. J., Fan, B., Liu, X., Fuller, C. J., et al. (2006). Exposure to the World Trade Center attack and the use of cigarettes and alcohol among New York City public high school students. *American Journal of Public Health, 96*, 804–807.

Population Health Issues

Advocacy in Action

An HIV Story

One of the best examples of nurse advocacy happened to me personally. When my brother Matthew was dying from AIDS in 1985, our family was immobilized with grief. We knew he had very little time left to live, and one of the nurses caring for him talked with my mom about making funeral arrangements ahead of time so we wouldn't have to face making all those decisions after he'd passed. My mother told her we would probably use the funeral home near us that had been used by many of our friends. The nurse politely warned us that most funeral homes wouldn't bury HIV-infected patients and that we should be ready for that response if it happened. She also supplied us with a list of funeral homes that were taking people who had died from HIV/AIDS. It was a short list.

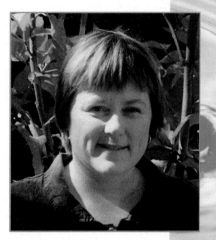

This nurse, through her advocacy for my family, spared us the pain, humiliation, and rage we would have experienced, at the worst of times, if we had been told our chosen funeral home wasn't willing to bury our beloved Matthew. Thankfully, times have changed, and this discrimination is less common. I remember few of the details of my brother's care. Yet the advocacy this nurse undertook on our behalf was something I will never forget.

Linda Robinson, PhD, RN

Associate Professor

Hahn School of Nursing and Health Science

University of San Diego

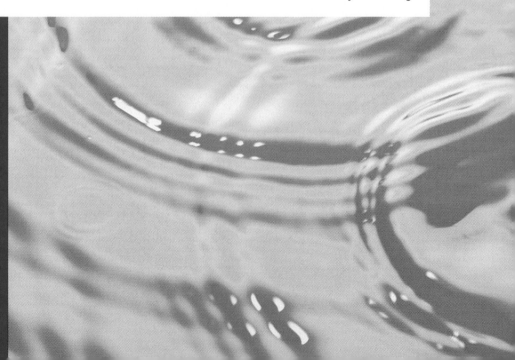

Communicable Diseases

CHAPTER OBJECTIVES

After reading this chapter, you should be able to:

1. Analyze major trends in the incidence of communicable diseases.
2. Identify the modes of transmission for communicable diseases.
3. Describe the influence of biophysical, psychological, physical environmental, sociocultural, behavioral, and health system factors on communicable diseases.
4. Analyze the potential effects of epidemics due to bioterrorist activity.
5. Analyze the role of community health nurses in controlling communicable diseases as it interfaces with those of other health professionals.
6. Provide examples of approaches to primary prevention of communicable diseases.
7. Describe major considerations in secondary prevention for communicable diseases.
8. Discuss tertiary prevention of communicable diseases.

KEY TERMS

anergy **823**
chain of infection **811**
co-infection **810**
communicable diseases **806**
contact notification **830**
cross-immunity **814**
directly observed therapy (DOT) **840**
endemic disease **807**
epidemic **807**
immunity **813**
incubation period **813**
induration **836**
infectious diseases **806**

isolation **843**
mass screening **835**
mode of transmission **811**
nosocomial infection **824**
opportunistic infections (OIs) **816**
outbreak **807**
prodromal period **813**
quarantine **843**
selective screening **835**
social distancing **844**
superinfection **810**
zoonoses **817**

MediaLink
http://www.prenhall.com/clark

Additional interactive resources for this chapter can be found on the Companion Website. Click on Chapter 28 and "Begin" to select the activities for this chapter.

*H*uman beings are subject to a variety of illnesses caused by pathogenic microorganisms. Although all of these illnesses can be considered infectious illnesses, not all of them are communicable diseases. **Infectious diseases** are those illnesses that result from the growth of pathogenic microorganisms in the body. **Communicable diseases**, on the other hand, are diseases caused by pathogens that are transmitted directly or indirectly from one person to another. Bacterial otitis media and wound infections are infectious diseases. Measles, hepatitis A, and HIV infection are examples of diseases that can be transmitted from one person to another and are communicable diseases.

Communicable diseases affecting humans arise from both human and animal sources. In fact, it has been suggested that domestication of wild animals and living in close proximity to them might have been the origin of infectious diseases in human beings (Watts, 2003). For instance, there is evidence of tuberculosis (TB) of the spine in Neanderthal man and in ancient Egypt, and it is believed that TB may have originated in the bovine form and been passed to human beings through cow's milk (Udwadia, 2000). More recently, sudden acute respiratory syndrome (SARS) appears to have been transmitted from civet cats to humans, and avian influenza, of course, originated in birds (Huey, 2004). At present, avian influenza is considered an infectious disease, because there has been only rare transmission from person to person. The current fear, however, is that the H5N1 virus that causes avian influenza will undergo mutation that allows it to be easily transmitted from one human to another, possibly leading to a pandemic (Trust for America's Health, 2005). Over the centuries, communicable diseases have continued to "plague" humanity, and communicable disease terminology, such as the word *plague*, has come to represent ongoing adversity in human language.

Historical events and human migrations have led to the spread of communicable diseases. For example, although smallpox is known to have existed as early as 1,000 B.C.E. in Egypt and was found in ancient China, India, and North Africa, it was not mentioned by European chroniclers until the 6th century (Graeme, 2005). There is no evidence that diseases such as measles and smallpox existed in the Western Hemisphere until after colonization by Europeans (Flight, 2002). Conversely, travel from the new world was probably responsible for the introduction of syphilis in Europe. It is hypothesized that members of Columbus's crew became infected with yaws in the Americas and that the causative spirochete mutated into the agent that causes syphilis on the voyage back to Europe (Watts, 2003). Similarly, it is believed that TB spread to Europe during the Indo-European invasion and migration into India, western Asia, Greece, and western Europe about 1500 B.C. (Udwadia, 2000).

In the last century and a half, immunization has enabled control of a number of communicable diseases. Incidence of vaccine-preventable diseases has decreased by 99% from peak incidence rates prior to vaccine availability. In 2004, however, an estimated 2 million U.S. 2-year-olds were missing at least one dose of recommended vaccines (Centers for Disease Control and Prevention [CDC], 2004), and new diseases continue to emerge to challenge human ingenuity. In spite of the remarkable decline in mortality due to communicable diseases in the United States and other developed nations, these conditions continue to exact a toll in worldwide suffering, death, and economic costs. Communicable diseases account for approximately one fourth of worldwide mortality, contributing to more than 15 million deaths each year (Kieny, Excler, & Girard, 2004).

TRENDS IN COMMUNICABLE DISEASE OCCURRENCE AND EFFECTS

As noted above, overall mortality from communicable diseases has declined significantly in some parts of the world, but these trends are not universal. Because of the potential for rapid spread of disease throughout the world, community health nurses need to be aware of trends in communicable disease incidence, prevalence, and mortality in their local areas as well as nationally and internationally. Communicable disease incidence also varies among geographic areas within the United States and among ethnic groups. Generally speaking, most communicable diseases have higher incidence rates among ethnic minority groups than among Caucasians, due to a number of social conditions such as poverty and lack of access to care.

One communicable disease, smallpox, has been completely eradicated from the world, although there is potential for its reintroduction through bioterrorism. The goal of the World Health Organization (WHO) is the elimination of several diseases, with their eventual eradication throughout the world. As noted in Chapter 6∞, eradication involves eliminating the causative organism of a disease from nature. Elimination, on the other hand, is more circumscribed and may involve eliminating a disease from a single country or region or controlling manifestations of the disease so it is no longer a public health problem.

Poliomyelitis has been targeted for eradication and has been eliminated in several areas, and measles has been targeted for elimination in major segments of the world. Prior to the advent of an effective vaccine, poliomyelitis caused paralysis in 13,000 to 20,000 people each year in the United States alone. The last U.S. case of indigenously acquired poliomyelitis due to wild polio virus occurred in 1979 (CDC, 2005a). In 2003, 1,270 cases of polio were reported in the six WHO regions, with more than half of those cases occurring in the African region (WHO, 2005b). Currently, three WHO regions have been certified as polio-free: the Americas, the Western Pacific, and Europe (Division of Viral and Rickettsial Diseases, 2005). Most of the world's remaining polio cases are concentrated in only a few countries, and as of April 2006 polio was considered endemic in only four countries—Afghanistan, India, Nigeria, and Pakistan (Polio Eradication Group, 2006). From 2002 to 2005, however, 21 previously polio-free countries reported cases of poliomyelitis imported from endemic countries (Division of Viral and Rickettsial Diseases, 2006). Only one case occurred in the United States in 2005 (CDC, 2006e), and it involved a woman exposed during international travel (Landaverde et al., 2006).

Although great strides have been made in preventing new cases of poliomyelitis, there has been a resurgence in disease effects among people who were infected 10 to 40 years earlier. Many former polio victims are experiencing post-polio syndrome (PPS), a neuromuscular disease characterized by the recurrence of motor symptoms of polio. Some of the effects of PPS are muscle pain, weakness and fatigue, memory loss, difficulty breathing, sleep disturbances, impaired swallowing, cold intolerance, urinary problems, and emotional stress (Kramasz, 2005). Community health nurses should be alert to the advent of these symptoms in clients with a history of poliomyelitis and refer them for diagnosis and treatment. Nurses may also need to help these clients deal with the long-term effects of their disease or advocate for needed services to assist them.

An **endemic disease**, as defined by CDC, is one that demonstrates a consistent chain of transmission from person to person for 12 months or more in a particular geographic area (Epidemiology and Surveillance Division, 2005). Prior to the advent of adequate sanitation, a wide variety of diarrheal diseases were endemic in the United States and remain endemic in many developing nations. Endemic diseases contrast with those that occur with epidemic frequency. An **epidemic** involves the occurrence of a great number of cases of a disease, far beyond what would ordinarily be expected in a given population. Earlier in U.S. history, for example, periodic epidemics of cholera swept the country. At that time, cholera was generally an endemic disease, with low incidence rates most of the time. Influenza epidemics continue to occur with some frequency in the United States, and there have also been periodic epidemics of pertussis when incidence rates far exceed those normally seen in a given year. A disease **outbreak** is an increased number of cases in the population that does not approach epidemic proportions. Disease outbreaks may be defined differently for different diseases depending on the usual number of cases of a disease typically encountered in the population. For example, a particular city might experience an outbreak of diarrheal disease when drinking water has been accidentally contaminated by sewage. As we saw

in Chapter 27∞, a pandemic is the simultaneous experience of extensive disease outbreaks or epidemics in several parts of the world. The worst pandemic of the 20th century occurred with the "Spanish flu" in 1918, which resulted in 500,000 U.S. deaths and 50 million deaths worldwide (Trust for America's Health, 2005).

A number of endemic and epidemic diseases besides poliomyelitis have been targeted for worldwide eradication or elimination. Dracunculiasis, a condition caused by the Guinea worm that results in ulcerative skin lesions, is a disease that has been targeted for worldwide eradication. People are exposed to dracunculiasis by ingestion of or standing in contaminated water. In 1986, WHO called for eradication of "Guinea worm disease." At that time, an estimated 3.5 million cases occurred each year and 120 million people were at risk for the disease. As of the end of 2004, Asia had been declared free of the disease, and incidence had decreased by 50% in Africa, where all of the remaining countries with endemic dracunculiasis lie (The Carter Center, 2005).

Rubella, another childhood vaccine-preventable disease, has been slated for eradication in the Americas by the Pan American Health Organization (PAHO). The target date for eradication is 2010. Past successes in eliminating communicable diseases such as polio and measles in the WHO region of the Americas have largely been the result of government commitment from all of the nations involved to effective immunization campaigns (de Quadros, 2004). Community health nurses are often involved in planning and implementing such campaigns and in advocating for governmental policies to support them.

The incidence of vaccine-preventable childhood diseases is diminishing in areas where vaccination coverage is high. For example, prior to the availability of measles vaccine, more than 400,000 cases of measles occurred each year in the United States. In 2004, only 37 U.S. cases were reported, for an all-time low incidence of less than 1 case per million people. Seventy-three percent of those cases were imported by U.S. residents traveling abroad or foreign nationals who entered the United States while infected. Most of those who acquired measles were unimmunized. The 37 cases included 9 children from China adopted by U.S. families (Dayan et al., 2005). In 2005, a total of 62 cases of measles occurred in the United States, an increase over the previous year, but still far lower than the number of cases prior to the advent of measles vaccine during the 1950s (CDC, 2006e). With the advent of widespread vaccine use, worldwide measles incidence declined by 48% from 1999 to 2004, and immunization coverage increased from 71% to 76% of the world's children (WHO, 2006b).

Slight increases in the number of actual cases of some vaccine-preventable diseases were noted in the United States between 2004 and 2005. For example, a total of 262 cases of mumps occurred in 2005, compared

MediaLink Old Bugs, New Threats (video)

to 239 in 2004 (CDC, 2006e). Mumps incidence remains below the *Healthy People 2010* objective of fewer than 500 cases per year (Hopkins et al., 2005). On average, 265 cases have been reported each year since 2001. In the first 3 months of 2006, however, 219 cases occurred during an outbreak among young adults in Iowa. Surprisingly, 65% of those for whom immunization status was known had received two doses of mumps vaccine (Quinlisk, Harris, Thornton, & Flamigni, 2006), suggesting a vaccine failure. A similar but more extensive epidemic occurred in the United Kingdom in 2004 and 2005 with more than 56,000 cases, again many in young adults. In this epidemic, many of those infected had not received mumps vaccination due to a vaccine shortage during their childhood (Savage, White, Brown, & Ramsay, 2006).

The number of U.S. cases of rubella increased from 10 to 17 between 2004 and 2005 (Kellenberg et al., 2005). Overall, however, the annual number of reported cases has remained fewer than 25 since 2001, compared to 12.5 million U.S. cases during the last rubella epidemic (1962 to 1965). Based on these figures, rubella is no longer considered endemic in the United States (Epidemiology and Surveillance Division, 2005). In 2003, only seven confirmed cases of rubella were reported in the United States, and the overall U.S. incidence rate was zero cases per 100,000 population (Hopkins et al., 2005). From 2001 to 2004, only four U.S. cases of congenital rubella syndrome (CRS) were reported but an estimated 100,000 infants are born with CRS each year throughout the world. In 2005, one case of CRS was reported in the United States in a child born to Liberian refugee parents, and rubella vaccination is recommended for women of childbearing age immigrating to the United States from countries where rubella remains endemic (Kellenberg et al., 2005).

Routine immunization with varicella vaccine has been recommended in the United States since 1996. By 2004, 44 states had implemented varicella immunization requirements for elementary school or preschool entry. From 1995 to 2003, the number of cases of varicella in the United States declined by 85%, and hospitalizations for complications of varicella decreased by 70%, largely as a result of increasing immunization rates. In 2003, the incidence rate for varicella was 7.27 per 100,000 population (Hopkins et al., 2005). During 2003 and early 2004, however, eight varicella-related deaths occurred in the United States (Klein et al., 2005), indicating a need for continued efforts to immunize susceptible people. In addition, an outbreak of varicella occurred in a Nebraska school in 2004. Although some previously immunized children developed varicella, the attack rate among immunized children was only one fifth that of unimmunized children, and immunized children had milder illnesses. Overall varicella vaccine has been found to be 80% to 85% effective in preventing disease and more than 95% effective in preventing serious illness (Huebner et al., 2006).

The number of cases of tetanus in the United States decreased from 27 to 19 from 2004 to 2005 (CDC, 2006e). From 1990 to 2004, a total of 624 cases of tetanus were reported, most of them occurring in adults and 3% in adolescents (Broder et al., 2006), and in 2003 U.S. tetanus incidence was less than 0.01 cases per 100,000 population (Hopkins et al., 2005). Although neonatal tetanus resulting from infection of the umbilical stump continues to occur in underdeveloped countries, only three cases were reported in the United States from 1990 to 2004 (Broder et al., 2006). No cases of diphtheria were reported in either 2004 or 2005 (CDC, 2006e), and one fatal case was reported in 2003 (Hopkins et al., 2005). Only seven U.S. cases were reported from 1998 to 2004 (Broder et al., 2006).

In spite of the slight increases in the number of cases of the diseases discussed above, incidence rates remain at less than 1 per 100,000 population. Pertussis, on the other hand, remains an endemic disease in the United States, and epidemics occur every 3 to 5 years in spite of the availability of an effective vaccine since the 1920s and its routine use since the 1940s (Bryant et al., 2005; Hopkins et al., 2005). From 1934 to 1943, more than 200,000 cases of pertussis were reported each year. Following the advent of an effective vaccine, the number of cases reached a low of 1,010 in 1976, but has been steadily increasing since then, particularly among adolescents and young adults. The number of pertussis cases in the United States averaged 9,431 each year from 1996 to 2003 for an average annual incidence rate of 3.3 per 100,000 population (Bryant et al., 2005). The 2003 incidence rate for pertussis was 4.04 per 100,000 people, 63% higher than the 1993 rate of 2.55 per 100,000 (Hopkins et al., 2005). In 2004, 22 outbreaks of pertussis occurred in the United States, and nearly 26,000 cases were reported (Broder et al., 2006) for an overall incidence rate of 8.5 cases per 100,000 population, the highest rate since 1959 (Tiwari, Murphy, & Moran, 2005). Outbreaks of pertussis have occurred in aggregate settings including sports facilities, summer camps, schools, and hospitals. The increase in pertussis incidence has occurred largely in infants too young to be fully immunized or people over age 7 due to waning immunity within 5 to 10 years of completing the initial immunization series (Bryant et al., 2005). Until 2005, however, there was no pertussis vaccine licensed for use with adolescents and adults. Currently tetanus toxoid, reduced diphtheria toxoid, and acellular pertussis (Tdap) vaccines are available to foster continued immunity in adolescents and adults (Broder et al., 2006), and Tdap is recommended for these populations.

Increasing trends in incidence and prevalence are also noted for other communicable diseases. For example, in 2003, more than 1 million people in the United States were infected with HIV. Approximately 25% of infected persons are not aware of their infection. Improved treatment with highly active antiretroviral therapy (HAART) has resulted in longer life for those infected and has decreased the potential for progression to AIDS (Espinoza, Hall, Campsmith, & Lee, 2005). From 2001 to 2004, more than 157,000 HIV/AIDS diagnoses were made in the 33 states that employ confidential, name-based reporting (Espinoza et al., 2005). In 2003, only three states (California, Florida, and New York) reported 11 or more pediatric AIDS cases. Only 14 U.S. states, the District of Columbia, Puerto Rico, and the Virgin Islands reported adult AIDS incidence rates of more than 15 cases per 100, 000 population. In 1993, the rate of new cases of AIDS was 40.2 per 100,000 population in the United States. By 2003, the incidence of new diagnoses had decreased to 15.36 (Hopkins et al., 2005). Worldwide, more than 40 million people are HIV-infected and 5 million new infections occur each year, including 800,000 infections among children (UNAIDS, 2005).

HIV prevalence rates are significantly higher in some parts of the world than in North America. In 2003, prevalence rates were highest in the African region of WHO at 7.1% of the population. The lowest prevalence rates were in the Western Pacific region (0.2%), with the region of the Americas slightly higher at 0.7% (WHO, 2005b). HIV/AIDS prevalence figures for developing nations may be somewhat inaccurate since diagnosis is often based on symptom presentation rather than laboratory diagnosis. The lack of sophisticated diagnostic capabilities in many parts of the world makes assessment of HIV/AIDS incidence and prevalence difficult, and community health nurses can be actively involved in advocating for funding to develop such services in underserved areas.

AIDS mortality rates decreased 65% from 1995 to 1999 and declined an average of 3% per year from 1999 to 2003 (Hopkins et al., 2005), primarily due to advances in treatment options. In 2004, AIDS resulted in an estimated 15,798 deaths, 99% of which occurred among adults and adolescents. The cumulative number of deaths due to AIDS in the United States, as of the end of 2004, was more than 529,000, with 5,515 deaths among children less than 13 years of age (CDC, 2006b). AIDS continues to be a significant cause of mortality in the rest of the world, with an estimated 3.1 million deaths in 2005 (UNAIDS, 2005). More than 25 million people have died worldwide since AIDS was first recognized in 1981.

Generally speaking, incidence rates for sexually transmitted diseases (STDs) have declined in the United States. In 1999, the CDC launched a campaign to eliminate syphilis from the United States. Elimination in this instance means a lack of sustained transmission, or transmission to other people, within 90 days of the report of an imported case of syphilis (Division of Sexually Transmitted Diseases Prevention, 2001). In 2003, the incidence rate for primary and secondary syphilis was 2.5 per 100,000 persons, a 75% decrease from 1993. Only four states, the District of Columbia, and New York City had incidence rates greater than 4 per 100,000 (Hopkins et al., 2005).

The incidence of congenital syphilis (CS) (syphilis passed from an infected mother to her unborn infant) declined an average of 17% per year from 1991 to 2004, and from 2003 to 2004 incidence decreased another 17.8% to a rate of 8.8 cases per 100,000 live births. In spite of these declines, however, 31 states still had CS rates above the *Healthy People 2010* target of 1 case per 100,000 births (Division of STD Prevention, 2005b).

Like the rates for syphilis, the overall incidence rate for gonorrhea declined significantly, dropping from 172.4 per 100,000 population in 1993 to 116.37 in 2003. Gonorrhea incidence in five states (all in the Southeast) and the District of Columbia, however, exceeded 200 cases per 100,000 population, and 17 states reported 100 to 200 cases per 100,000 (Division of STD Prevention, 2005b).

Incidence rates for *Chlamydia trachomatis* show the greatest increase among STDs, with an estimated 2.8 million infections occurring each year. This figure is most probably an underrepresentation of the extent of chlamydial disease since many health care providers do not report the disease, nor is it a reportable disease in many states. In addition, approximately 28% of cases do not receive adequate follow-up and reporting is often too late to permit contact notification and treatment before disease occurs (Matyas et al., 2005). In 2003, 15 states, the District of Columbia, and New York City reported chlamydia incidence rates among women of more than 500 cases per 100,000 population. The overall incidence in U.S. women for 2003 was 466.9 per 100,000 (Hopkins et al., 2005).

Incidence rates for cases of hepatitis vary with the causative agent. In 2003, for example, the incidence rate for hepatitis A virus (HAV) infection was 2.66 per 100,000 people, down from 9.4 per 100,000 in 1993. Hepatitis B (HBV) incidence decreased by almost half between 1993 and 2003 (Hopkins et al., 2005), yet 1 to 1.3 million people in the United States have chronic HBV infection, and 5,000 die each year of HBV-related cirrhosis or liver cancer (Willis, Ndiaye, Hopkins, & Shefer, 2005). Worldwide, HBV results in 600,000 deaths each year, 69% of which occur in people who were infected perinatally or as young children (Gacic-Dobo et al., 2003). The prevalence of chronic HBV infection in Africa, Asia, and the Western Pacific is as high as 8% of the population, compared to only 2% of the North American population (Poynard, 2004).

Approximately 1.8% of the U.S. population exhibit hepatitis C (HCV) antibodies (Al-Saden, 2004). The 2003 HCV incidence rate (0.38 per 100,000) represented an 80% decline from 1993 (Hopkins et al., 2005). Despite the decreasing incidence of these three diseases, they continue to cause mortality. In 2003, for example, HAV contributed to 83 deaths and HBV to 769 deaths. HCV, however, is the biggest contributor to hepatitis-related deaths, causing more than 4,600 deaths in 2003 (Hopkins et al., 2005), and contributing to 22% of hepatocellular carcinomas (Al-Saden, 2004).

Hepatitis also contributes to significant health care costs, with hepatitis A costing approximately $200 million per year in medical care and lost work time and hepatitis B accounting for $700 million per year (National Center for Infectious Diseases, 2000a, 2000b). The annual cost for HCV-related liver disease is estimated at $600 million (Al-Saden, 2004).

Hepatitis D (HDV) and E (HEV) virus infections occur far less frequently than hepatitis A, B, or C. Hepatitis D occurs only in conjunction with hepatitis B as a co-infection or as a superinfection. **Co-infection** means that the two diseases occur simultaneously, in the case of hepatitis B and D, usually as a result of injection drug use (IDU). **Superinfection** exists when infection with hepatitis D occurs in a person with existing chronic hepatitis B virus infection (National Center for HIV, STD, and TB Prevention, 2006b). Hepatitis E occurs primarily in areas of poor sanitation and, in the United States, is usually diagnosed in travelers returning from endemic areas such as South Asia and North Africa (National Center for HIV, STD, and TB Prevention, 2006c).

Two other communicable diseases of interest to community health nurses are tuberculosis (TB) and influenza. After several years of declining incidence, a resurgence of tuberculosis was noted in the United States with the influx of refugee populations from endemic areas of the world. In 2005, the U.S. incidence rate for TB was 4.8 per 100,000 population, and 42% of all cases occurred in foreign-born persons, who had incidence rates 8.7 times those of the native-born population. This figure, however, represents a decline of 36% in the rate of infection among foreign-born persons in the United States (Pratt, Robison, Navin, & Hlavsa, 2006). From 1993 to 2003, overall U.S. TB incidence decreased by 44% and is at a historic low. The Advisory Council for the Elimination of Tuberculosis has set a goal of eliminating TB in the United States; however, a 2000 study by the Institute of Medicine indicated that achieving this goal would take more than 70 years at the present rate of decline. In response to this report, CDC, in conjunction with the American Thoracic Society and the Infectious Diseases Society of America (American Thoracic Society, CDC, & Infectious Diseases Society of America, 2005), established a new set of recommendations for TB control.

Worldwide, TB affects 8 million people and causes 2 million deaths. As much as 90% of the world's TB occurs in developing nations, and 75% occurs among the most economically productive age groups. In 1993, the World Health Organization declared TB an international public health emergency, and in 2006 an international Patient's Charter for Tuberculosis Care was developed to delineate the rights and responsibilities of people with tuberculosis (World Care Council, 2006). In spite of concerted efforts to detect and treat persons with TB, however, it is estimated that only 45% of new cases of TB occurring in 2003 were actually diagnosed (Rusen & Enarson, 2006). Figures for 2003 indicate that TB incidence was highest in the WHO South-East Asia region at 85 cases per 100,000 population. Incidence was also high in the African region at 74 per 100,000, compared to only 19 cases per 100,000 population for the Americas and 22 per 100,000 for the European region (WHO, 2005b).

As noted earlier, the 1918 influenza pandemic resulted in millions of deaths worldwide. Since then, influenza has caused an average of 114,000 hospitalizations and 20,000 deaths per year in the United States (Willis et al., 2005). Although rates of infection are highest in the young, the elderly are at particular risk for complications and death (Bridges et al., 2003).

Currently, public health officials are concerned about the potential for an avian influenza pandemic. If it occurs, a pandemic will probably result from a mutation of the H5N1 virus that causes avian influenza, but it could result from other pathogens. Pandemics typically occur in waves of illness that may be separated by a few months in time. Rather than occurring during the winter months as annual influenza outbreaks tend to do, pandemic influenza might occur at any time. It is expected that a pandemic might affect as much as 50% of the population and be associated with much more severe illness and greater mortality than typical influenza. It is also likely that young adults would be the most seriously affected, in contrast to the higher risk among children and the elderly in annual influenza outbreaks. Because the viral strain that might cause an influenza pandemic is not yet known, it is probable that an effective vaccine would not be developed until several months into the pandemic. There is similar uncertainty about the effectiveness of antiviral drugs for any particular strain of virus that might cause a pandemic (Trust for America's Health, 2005). All of these factors explain the level of concern engendered by the possibility of a pandemic of avian influenza and the preparedness activities currently being undertaken by public health departments and other agencies responsible for the health of the public. Pandemic preparedness will be discussed in more detail later in this chapter.

Pneumococcal disease causes approximately 3,500 deaths, 3,000 cases of meningitis, 50,000 cases of bacteremia, and 500,000 cases of pneumonia each year. Despite the fact that pneumococcal vaccine is 65% to 75% effective in preventing disease, immunization rates are low, particularly among people aged 18 to 64. Among those with conditions for whom immunization is recommended, only 19% received pneumococcal vaccine in 2002 (Willis et al, 2005).

The diseases discussed here are not the only communicable diseases to affect the health of populations. Each year, new emerging and reemerging diseases occur due to a variety of circumstances. The World Health Organization estimates that as many as 30 new pathogens have been identified in the last 30 years (Huey, 2004). In addition, diseases once thought controlled are becoming more frequent and harder to treat due to development of antimicrobial-resistant strains of microorganisms. Changes in food preparation and distribution processes are spreading foodborne diseases in much wider geographic areas than in the past. Similarly, environmental changes are increasing human exposures to new pathogens (e.g., hantavirus).

The number of cases of tickborne diseases such as Rocky Mountain spotted fever is also increasing. In studies in the southeastern and south central United States, 22% of children were found to have serologic evidence of exposure to two pathogens transmitted by tick bites: *R. rickettsii*, which causes Rocky Mountain spotted fever, and *E. chaffensis*, which causes ehrlichiosis, a disease that may result in neurological damage or deafness (Chapman, 2006). From 1993 to 2003, Rocky Mountain spotted fever incidence more than doubled from 0.18 per 100,000 population to 0.38. Lyme disease is another tickborne condition for which incidence rates have more than doubled in the United States (Hopkins et al., 2005).

Other diseases caused by insect bites include malaria and West Nile virus (WNV) infection, both of which are transmitted primarily through mosquito bites. West Nile virus infection is the leading cause of insect-transmitted encephalitis, and in 2005, a total of 2,744 cases of WNV infection were reported in the United States. This represents an increase of more than 16% from 2004 figures. WNV infection is asymptomatic in 80% of cases; 20% of infected persons develop West Nile fever, and 1% of cases result in West Nile virus neuroinvasive disease (Smith, Hayes et al., 2005).

Another condition of growing concern is methicillin-resistant *Staphylococcus aureus* (MRSA) infection. Staphylococci are present in healthy people, and an estimated 25% to 30% of the population demonstrates *Staphylococcus aureus* in the nose. Most *Staphylococcus aureus* infections involve minor skin lesions that respond rapidly to antibiotic therapy. Recently, however, there has been an increase in the incidence of *Staphylococcus aureus* infections that are resistant to methicillin, one of the most commonly used therapeutic agents. MRSA occurs in both hospital-associated and community-associated infections. Hospital-associated infection (HA-MRSA) occurs in the context of procedures and other health care provided in health care settings. Community-associated infections (CA-MRSA), on the other hand, occur in otherwise healthy people who have no recent history of hospitalization or medical procedures. CA-MRSA frequently occurs in athletes, military recruits, MSM, and correctional inmates who have close contact or share personal items that may be contaminated, and among some ethnic minority groups (e.g., Pacific Islanders, Alaska Natives, and Native Americans) (CDC, 2005b, 2005c).

Modern building ventilation systems have spawned and spread diseases such as Legionnaires' disease. Recent outbreaks of Legionnaires' disease have also been reported on cruise ships (Joseph et al., 2005) and from drinking water in a Maryland hotel (Goeller et al., 2005). Medical advances, such as transfusions, have increased transmission of bloodborne diseases such as hepatitis C (National Center for HIV, STD, & TB Prevention, 2006a), and medical treatments for some conditions (e.g., steroids) produce immunosuppression and susceptibility to communicable diseases. There is also the potential for epidemics of communicable diseases due to bioterrorism as noted in Chapter 27∞. In spite of the advances made in controlling communicable diseases to date, there remains considerable work to be done.

GENERAL CONCEPTS RELATED TO COMMUNICABLE DISEASES

Several communicable disease concepts must be understood before control efforts can be undertaken. These include concepts related to the "chain of infection," such as modes of transmission and portals of entry and exit, and the concepts of incubation and prodromal periods.

Chain of Infection

In communicable diseases, epidemiologic factors related to the biophysical, psychological, physical environmental, sociocultural, behavioral, and health system dimensions create what may be termed a chain of infection. A **chain of infection** is a series of events or conditions that lead to the development of a particular communicable disease. The "links" in the chain are the infected person or source of the infectious agent, the reservoir, the agent itself, the mode of transmission of the disease, the agent's portals of entry and exit, and a susceptible new host. The concepts of reservoir, agent, and host were introduced in Chapter 4∞. This discussion focuses on the remaining links in the chain: modes of transmission and portals of entry and exit.

Modes of Transmission

The **mode of transmission** of a particular disease is the means by which the infectious agent that causes the disease is transferred from an infected person or animal to an uninfected one. Communicable diseases may be spread by any of several modes of transmission: airborne transmission, fecal–oral (gastrointestinal) transmission, direct contact, sexual contact, direct inoculation, insect or animal bite, or via inanimate objects or soil.

Airborne Transmission

Airborne transmission occurs when the infectious organism is present in the air and is inspired (inhaled) by a susceptible host during respiration. Diseases transmitted by the airborne route include the exanthems (diseases characterized by a rash, such as measles and chickenpox), infections of the mouth and throat (such as streptococcal infections), and infections of the upper and lower respiratory system (such as tuberculosis, pneumonia, influenza, and the common cold). Certain systemic infections are also products of airborne transmission. Examples of these are meningococcal meningitis and pneumococcal pneumonias, hantavirus pulmonary infections, coccidioidomycosis, anthrax, and smallpox. In the case of anthrax and smallpox, disease may also be transmitted by aerosolized dissemination of microorganisms.

Fecal–Oral Transmission

Fecal–oral transmission of an infectious agent may be either direct or indirect. Direct transmission occurs when the hands or other objects (fomites) are contaminated with organisms from human feces and then put into the mouth. Indirect transmission occurs via contaminated food or water. For example, a person with hepatitis A may defecate, fail to wash his or her hands properly, and then prepare a sandwich for someone else. The second person would ingest the virus with the sandwich and, if susceptible, might develop hepatitis A. Additional examples include *Salmonella-* or *Shigella-*caused diarrheas. Botulism is another disease in which the causative organism is ingested with contaminated food or water. Contamination usually occurs by accident through inadequate canning and preserving processes, but could potentially occur as a result of bioterrorist activity. Ingestion anthrax may also result from the intentional introduction of spores into food supplies.

Direct Contact

Direct contact transmission involves skin-to-skin contact or direct contact with mucous membrane discharges between the infected person and another person. Diseases typically spread by this route include infectious mononucleosis, impetigo, scabies, and lice. Smallpox may also be transmitted by contact with the lesions of infected persons. Scabies, lice, and other parasitic diseases also may be transmitted through contact with clothing and other items containing the eggs of the parasites. Similarly, the cutaneous form of anthrax is transmitted by handling contaminated objects (CDC, 2003a).

Sexual Transmission

Transmission of diseases via sexual contact is a special instance of direct contact transmission. Diseases spread by this mode of transmission are usually referred to as sexually transmitted diseases (STDs) or sexually transmitted infections (STIs). Diseases spread during sexual intercourse include (but are not limited to) HIV/AIDS, gonorrhea, syphilis, genital herpes, and hepatitis B, C, and D. These diseases may also be spread by other modes of transmission. For example, hepatitis B, C, and D and AIDS may be spread by direct inoculation.

Transmission by Direct Inoculation

Direct inoculation occurs when the infectious agent (a bloodborne pathogen) is introduced directly into the bloodstream of the new host. Direct inoculation can occur transplacentally from an infected mother to a fetus, via transfusion with infected blood or blood products, through the use of contaminated hypodermic equipment, or through a splash of contaminated body fluid to mucous membrane or nonintact skin. With the advent of several screening tests for blood donors, transmission via transfusion has been significantly decreased. Health care workers are particularly at risk for several communicable diseases caused by bloodborne pathogens. Diseases commonly spread by direct inoculation include HIV/AIDS and hepatitis B, C, and D.

Transmission by Insect or Animal Bite

Insect and animal bites can also transmit infectious agents. For example, the bite of the *Anopheles* mosquito is the mode of transmission for malaria, a disease that is widespread in much of the world. West Nile virus infection is another disease that is primarily transmitted by mosquitoes. Rabies frequently is transmitted via a bite from infected, warm-blooded animals such as dogs, skunks, and raccoons. Incidence of diseases such as rabies is low in the United States, due to widespread immunization of pets. From 1980 to 2004, 54 cases of rabies were reported in the United States; 64% of cases were the result of bat bites. In 2005, only one case of rabies was reported, and the source of infection was a bat. Rabies can also be transmitted from one person to another, however, and this one case resulted in a need for postexposure treatment of 32 health care workers who cared for the client (Palmer et al., 2006). Lyme disease and Rocky Mountain spotted fever are transmitted by the bite of infected ticks, and plague can be transmitted by fleas on infected rodents. Human encroachment into wildlife areas is increasing the potential for exposure to diseases caused by insect and animal bites.

Transmission by Other Means

Some communicable diseases are transmitted through contact with spores present in the soil or with inanimate objects. For example, exposure to the bacillus that causes tetanus frequently occurs through a dirty puncture wound. Modes of transmission and typical diseases most often transmitted by each mode are summarized in Table 28-1◆.

Portals of Entry and Exit

Communicable diseases also differ in terms of the portals through which the infectious agent that causes the disease enters and leaves an infected host. Portals of entry include the respiratory system, the gastrointestinal tract, and the skin and mucous membranes.

TABLE 28-1 Modes of Disease Transmission and Typical Diseases

Mode of Transmission	Diseases Transmitted
Airborne	Measles, mumps, rubella, poliomyelitis, *Haemophilus influenzae* type B (HiB) infection, tuberculosis, influenza, scarlet fever, diphtheria, pertussis, hantavirus, respiratory anthrax, coccidioidomycosis, smallpox, plague (pneumonic form)
Fecal–oral/ingestion	Hepatitis A and E, salmonellosis, shigellosis, typhoid, polio (in poor sanitary conditions), botulism, ingestion anthrax
Direct contact	Impetigo, scabies, lice, smallpox, cutaneous anthrax
Sexual contact	Chlamydia, gonorrhea, hepatitis B, C, and D, HIV infection, herpes simplex virus (HSV) infection, syphilis
Direct inoculation	Syphilis, hepatitis A, B, C, and D, HIV infection
Insect or animal bite	Malaria, rabies, Lyme disease, plague (bubonic form)
Other means of transmission	Tetanus, hookworm

Portals of exit also differ among communicable diseases. Infectious agents may leave an infected host through the respiratory system or through feces passed from the gastrointestinal tract. Blood and other body fluids such as semen, vaginal secretions, and saliva are the portals of exit for infectious agents causing diseases such as HIV/AIDS, gonorrhea, and hepatitis B. The skin acts as a portal of exit as well as a portal of entry for conditions such as impetigo, cutaneous anthrax, and syphilis. Portals of entry and exit and related modes of disease transmission are summarized in Table 28-2◆.

Incubation and Prodromal Periods

The **incubation period** of a communicable disease is the interval from exposure to an infectious organism to development of the symptoms of the disease (Friis & Sellers, 2003). The length of the incubation period for a particular disease may influence the success of efforts to halt the spread of the disease. Some diseases, such as influenza and scarlet fever, have incubation periods of less than a week. Others typically require incubation periods of one to two weeks (gonorrhea, measles, pertussis, and polio), two to three weeks (rubella, chickenpox, and mumps), or months (viral hepatitis, syphilis). In some diseases, such as AIDS, the incubation period can be years.

The **prodromal period** of a communicable disease is the period between the first symptoms and the appearance of the symptoms that typify the disease. For example, prior to the appearance of the jaundice that is characteristic of viral hepatitis, the client may experience prodromal symptoms of nausea, fatigue, and malaise. Similarly, a cough, runny nose, and watery eyes are prodromal symptoms for measles. In many diseases, the prodromal period is the time of greatest ability to infect others.

Immunity

Immunity is another concept of great importance in the control of communicable diseases. **Immunity** is a state of nonsusceptibility to a disease or condition. Physiologic immunity is based on the presence of specific antibodies to disease and is described as passive or active depending on the role of the host in developing those antibodies. In *active immunity*, the host is exposed to antigens, substances related to the disease-causing microorganism, that prompt the host's immune system to create antibodies that render the antigen harmless. Exposure to the antigen may occur as a result of having the disease or through immunization with active antigens (e.g., bacterial toxins such as tetanus or diphtheria toxoid or portions of live viruses that cause diseases such as measles and mumps). Active immunity is relatively long lasting, waning over

TABLE 28-2 Portals of Entry and Exit for Each Mode of Disease Transmission

Mode of Transmission	Portal of Entry	Portal of Exit
Airborne	Respiratory system	Respiratory system
Fecal–oral/ingestion	Mouth	Feces
Direct contact	Skin, mucous membrane	Skin, mucous membrane
Sexual contact	Skin, mouth, urethra, rectum	Skin lesions, vaginal or urethral secretions
Direct inoculation	Across placenta, bloodstream	Blood
Animal or insect bite	Wound in skin	Blood, saliva
Other means of transmission	Wound in skin, intact skin	Animal feces, soil

several years if at all. In *passive immunity*, externally produced antibodies are provided to the host by way of immunization (e.g., immune serum globulin from someone who has had a specific disease and developed active immunity) or transfer (e.g., from a mother with active immunity to her fetus across the placenta).

Cross-immunity occurs when immunity to one microorganism or disease also confers immunity to a related disease-causing agent. Cross-immunity was the basis for the smallpox vaccine developed by Edward Jenner. Jenner inoculated people with material from cowpox lesions to prevent smallpox after noticing that milkmaids who developed cowpox from exposure to infected cows did not develop smallpox.

Herd immunity is another concept related to physiologic immunity that has particular relevance for population groups. Herd immunity is generalized resistance to a particular disease within the population that arises because the majority of people have developed specific immunity to the condition. Herd immunity decreases the potential for exposure to the disease among those few people who do not have immunity.

THE EPIDEMIOLOGY OF COMMUNICABLE DISEASES

The development and effects of any communicable disease are influenced by factors in each of the six dimensions of health. Community health nurses concerned with control of a communicable disease should be familiar with factors in each dimension that influence the disease. Such knowledge provides guidance for interventions to prevent the disease, deal with it when it occurs, and prevent further spread in the population.

Biophysical Considerations

Biophysical considerations such as age, gender, race/ethnicity, and physiologic health status influence the development of many communicable diseases. In the case of some diseases, age may influence susceptibility to a disease or its effects. Tuberculosis seems to occur most often in the very young and the very old. In 2003, for example, TB incidence was highest among people 65 years of age and older. Young children, on the other hand, are among the most likely group to progress from latent tuberculosis infection (LTBI) to active disease (American Thoracic Society et al., 2005). In addition, young children are more likely to develop severe forms of TB, such as TB meningitis (Fitzpatrick et al., 2005).

Young children are often at greater risk for complications of many communicable diseases. For example, children under 2 years of age are at greater risk for hospitalization due to influenza than older children and are one of the target groups for influenza immunization (Santibanez, Singleton, Santoli, Euler, & Bridges, 2006). From October 2005 to January 2006, 11 influenza-associated deaths occurred in the United States in people under age 18 (CDC, 2006f). For hepatitis A virus infection (HAV), on the other hand, the highest fatality rates occur among people 40 to 50 years of age (Wise & Sorvillo, 2005).

The elderly are most at risk for tetanus in the United States because they are the least likely to have been immunized. In addition, older persons seem to develop more severe cases of tetanus and are at higher risk of death (National Immunization Program, 2002). In developing countries with unsafe delivery conditions, neonates are at high risk for tetanus fatality.

Neonates are also at risk for diseases that can be passed from mother to child perinatally. Such diseases include congenital rubella syndrome (CRS), HIV infection, syphilis, and hepatitis B and C. For example, a total of 23 cases of CRS were reported in the United States between 1998 and 2000. From 2001 to 2004, however, only four cases of CRS were reported (Epidemiology and Surveillance Division, 2005). The number of new diagnoses of HIV/AIDS in U.S. children under age 13 in 2003 was 802, and children accounted for less than 1% of all HIV/AIDS diagnoses. Similarly, people over age 65 comprised only 1.5% of those diagnosed in 2003, whereas people 25 to 34 years of age accounted for 29% of new diagnoses and people aged 35 to 44 accounted for 36% (Selik, Glynn, & McKenna, 2004).

Vertical transmission of HIV (from mother to child) occurs in approximately 25% of pregnancies involving HIV-infected women (County of San Diego Health and Human Services Agency, 2004). In highly endemic countries, the risk of vertical transmission occurs in approximately 35% to 40% of babies born to mothers with HIV infection, but decreases to 5% to 10% with prenatal HIV screening and treatment. With effective antiretroviral therapy, the risk of transmission can be reduced to less than 1% of infants born to HIV-infected women (Seipone et al., 2004). For example, the number of infants with perinatally transmitted HIV infection declined from a peak of 1,650 in the early 1990s to 144 to 236 in 2002 as a result of maternal testing and treatment programs (Fenton & Valdiserri, 2006). In 2004, only 48 cases of perinatally acquired AIDS were diagnosed, a 95% decline from 1992 (Mofenson et al., 2006).

Prior to the availability of hepatitis B vaccine, approximately 30% to 40% of chronic HBV infection occurred in infants and young children of HBV-infected mothers. Without treatment, 90% of infected infants and 30% of children under age 5 will develop chronic HBV infection. These children were at higher risk for cirrhosis and hepatocellular carcinoma than people without chronic infection. People over age 60 are also at higher risk for HBV-associated death (Mast et al., 2005).

Age may also affect the symptoms with which some communicable diseases present. For example, approximately 70% of children with hepatitis A are asymptomatic (Dembek et al., 2005). Similarly, elderly persons with pneumococcal pneumonia may not present with classic symptoms of cough and fever, but may instead exhibit gastrointestinal symptoms.

Age also influences one's chances of exposure to some communicable diseases. For example, STDs and hepatitis B, C, and D occur more frequently in younger than older people because of their propensity to engage in high-risk sexual behaviors and injection drug use. As we saw earlier, pertussis and mumps incidence have increased in adolescents and young adults, largely because of waning immunity from initial immunizations (Broder et al., 2006; Quinlisk et al., 2006). During 2004, for example, 34% of reported U.S. cases of pertussis occurred among adolescents for an incidence rate of 30 per 100,000. Another 13% of cases occurred in infants less than a year of age; 21% among those age 1 to 10 years, and 19% in adults age 19 or older (Broder et al., 2006).

Communicable disease incidence and prevalence also vary by gender and by race/ethnicity, although differences are more likely to be the result of differential levels of exposure and other behavioral and sociocultural factors than of differences in inherent susceptibility. For example, disparities in tuberculosis incidence among some groups may reflect crowded living conditions, and increased incidence of other diseases (e.g., pertussis) in some ethnic minority populations may be a result of lack of access to health-promotive and illness-preventive knowledge and resources. Although disparities do not arise because of gender or ethnic minority group membership per se, community health nurses should be aware of gender and racial/ethnic differences in communicable disease incidence in order to be able to target intervention strategies to those most in need of them. Approximately 73% of HIV/AIDS cases from 2001 to 2004, for example, occurred among men, suggesting a need to tailor interventions specifically to this target group. At the same time, HIV/AIDS incidence among women increased from 15% of cases from 1981 to 1995 to 27% of cases in the 2001 to 2004 time period. These data suggest a need for increased attention to strategies to decrease HIV infection among women (Schneider, Glynn, Kajese, & McKenna, 2006).

Racial disparities in HIV/AIDS are particularly pronounced. From 2001 to 2004, for example, Blacks accounted for 51% of all HIV/AIDS diagnoses, 68% of diagnoses among women, and 69% of cases of perinatal transmission in 33 states that report confidential name-based statistics (Prejean, Satcher, Durant, Hu, & Lee, 2006). Whites accounted for 29%, Hispanics for 18%, Asian/Pacific Islanders for 1%, and American Indian/Alaska Natives for less than 1% of infections (Espinoza et al., 2005). Blacks were overrepresented in all transmission categories, including cases among men who have sex with men (MSM), injection drug use, and high-risk heterosexual contact (Prejean et al., 2006). The prevalence of HIV infection is also increasing among Latina women much faster than among non-Hispanic White women. Latinas comprise 20% of all AIDS diagnoses among women, and HIV/AIDS is the fourth leading cause of death for U.S. Latinas 25 to 44 years of age. The majority of HIV infections (64%) in Latinas occur in the context of heterosexual activity, with another 34% resulting from injection drug use. Latino men also have high incidence rates—approximately three times those of non-Hispanic White men (Zambrana, Cornelius, Boykin, & Lopez, 2004).

Disparities are also noted with respect to TB incidence. For example, in 2005, U.S. Asians had TB incidence rates 19.6 times higher than those for Whites, and Blacks and Hispanics had rates 8.3 and 7.3 times higher, respectively (Pratt et al., 2006). Table 28-3◆ provides comparative racial/ethnic incidence rates for selected diseases based on 2002 figures (the most recent comparative data available).

HAV is another disease that demonstrates large racial disparities in incidence, occurring with greater frequency among American Indians and Alaska Natives (AI/AN) than in other racial/ethnic groups. From 1990 to 1996, for instance, HAV incidence among AI/AN

TABLE 28-3	Racial/Ethnic Disparities in Incidence for Selected Communicable Diseases, United States, 2002 (rates per 100,000 population)			
Disease	White	Black	Asian/ Pacific Islander	American Indian/ Alaska Native
Chlamydia	90.2	905.9	108	512.1
Gonorrhea	23.6	570.4	18.3	96.1
Hepatitis A, acute	2.3	2.0	2.3	4.2
Hepatitis B, acute	1.5	3.9	2.2	5.6
Hepatitis C, acute	0.5	0.4	0.1	0.8
Measles	-	-	0.1	-
Mumps	0.1	0.1	0.4	-
Pertussis	3.7	1.6	1.0	4.2
Syphilis, primary and secondary	1.1	9.4	0.8	2.3

Data from: Adekoya, N., & Hopkins, R. S. (2005). Racial disparities in nationally notifiable diseases—United States, 2002. Morbidity and Mortality Weekly Report, 54, 9–11.

populations was 3.5 to 10.2 times higher than that for the overall U.S. population. With the advent of an effective vaccine, however, incidence among AI/AN peoples declined twentyfold from 1997 to 2001 (Bialek et al., 2004), reinforcing the concept that it is not ethnicity per se that is the influencing factor, but lack of access to services for some ethnic minority groups that contributes to many disparities in communicable disease incidence.

The presence of other physical health conditions may also influence one's propensity to develop certain communicable diseases. For example, children and adolescents who have certain high-risk medical conditions or who are taking aspirin on a regular basis are at higher risk than the general population for complications of influenza (Santibanez, Singleton et al., 2006). Similarly, HIV infection increases one's risk of a variety of opportunistic infections. **Opportunistic infections (OIs)** are diseases caused by organisms that either do not usually cause illness in humans or that usually cause only mild disease. For example, HIV infection increases the incidence of tuberculosis as well as the rate of progression to active disease (American Thoracic Society et al., 2005). In Southeast Asia, 25% to 40% of HIV-infected persons with TB die, five to ten times as many as those with TB who do not have HIV infection. Deaths also tend to occur rapidly after TB diagnosis (Vannarith et al., 2005). In addition, diabetes, chronic renal failure, low body weight, organ transplant, and other physiologic conditions increase the risk of progression from latent tuberculosis infection (LTBI) to active TB disease (Jensen, Lambert, & Iademarco, 2005). Use of agents such as tumor necrosis factor alpha (TNF-α) antagonists to treat autoimmune-related conditions (e.g., Crohn's disease and rheumatoid arthritis) has also been shown to increase the potential for progression to active TB (American Thoracic Society et al., 2005). Screening for LTBI is recommended prior to beginning TNF-α therapy. Because autoimmune diseases may decrease tuberculin skin test sensitivity, some experts suggest treating clients with TB risk factors for LTBI before initiating TNF-α therapy. TNF-α use may also increase susceptibility to other communicable diseases, such as candidiasis and histoplasmosis, particularly in clients who are already immunocompromised (Costamagna et al., 2004).

Conversely, the presence of other STDs increases the potential for HIV infection. This is particularly true for STDs that cause lesions, such as secondary syphilis and herpes simplex virus (HSV) infection, but also occurs with inflammatory STDs such as gonorrhea, Chlamydia, and trichomonas infections (Fox et al., 2001). Syphilis infection may also speed progression from HIV infection to AIDS (Division of STD Prevention, 2004b). The presence of several of these diseases also increases one's risk of hepatitis B, particularly among MSM (Remis et al., 2000).

Another biophysical consideration with respect to communicable diseases relates to the effects of the diseases themselves. Most childhood diseases are relatively mild and self-limiting. On occasion, diseases such as measles, varicella, and mumps result in death. The overall case fatality rate for untreated tetanus in unimmunized individuals, however, is 10% (National Immunization Program, 2002). As noted in Chapter 4∞, the case fatality rate is the number of persons who have a disease who will die as a result of it. Hepatitis B, C, and D often result in chronic liver disease, with 1% to 5% of HCV infections resulting in death (National Center for HIV, STD, & TB Prevention, 2006a). HCV is a primary factor in liver transplants (Al-Saden, 2004). Persons with hepatitis B are also at high risk of cirrhosis and liver cancer, and those with HDV superinfection have a greater risk of developing chronic liver disease than those with HBV alone (National Center for HIV, STD, & TB Prevention, 2006b). Possible questions for assessing biophysical factors contributing to communicable disease incidence in the population are included in the focused assessment provided below.

Psychological Considerations

Psychological considerations may play a part in the development of some communicable diseases. For example, stress has been shown to contribute to the development of active tuberculosis in persons with latent infection. Psychological factors may lead to risk-taking behaviors such as unprotected sexual activity or injection drug use that increase the risk of STDs, HIV infection, and hepatitis B, C, and D.

Communicable diseases may also have psychological consequences for those infected. This is particularly true for conditions that have long-term consequences (e.g., HSV infection, HIV infection, or chronic hepatitis C) or require changes in lifestyle and behavior. In addition, clients with HIV/AIDS may develop dementia, which alters behavior and makes them difficult to care for.

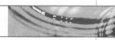

FOCUSED ASSESSMENT

Biophysical Considerations in Assessing Communicable Disease Risk

- What age groups are most likely to develop the disease? Are there differences in disease effects among age groups?
- Are there racial or gender differences in disease incidence?
- What physiologic conditions, if any, increase the risk of disease?
- Does treatment for existing physiologic conditions increase the risk of disease?
- What are the signs and symptoms of the disease?
- What are the physiologic effects of the disease? What is the effect of the disease in pregnancy?
- What is the mode of disease transmission? What are the physiologic portals of entry and exit?

Depression may also be a significant consequence of stigmatizing diseases such as HIV infection or tuberculosis in some cultural groups. Depression was associated, in one study, with greater HIV mortality among women. Conversely, mental health service use by HIV-infected women was associated with decreased mortality (Cook et al., 2004). Similarly, HIV infection has been associated with the prevalence of substance abuse, intimate partner violence, childhood sexual abuse, and depression among MSM (Stall et al., 2003).

Depression and subsequent high-risk sexual behaviors may be a result of exposure to violence and trauma. In one study in Los Angeles, for example, HIV-infected women were significantly more likely to report experience of adult sexual abuse regardless of race or ethnicity than those without infection. Among African American women, HIV infection was also associated with intrafamilial childhood sexual abuse. In addition, the greater the overall history of trauma (adult or child sexual abuse and relationship violence), the more likely the woman was to be HIV positive (Wyatt et al., 2002). The focused assessment questions provided below can assist the community health nurse to identify psychological factors related to communicable disease incidence in the population as well as in an individual client.

Physical Environmental Considerations

Physical environmental factors play a part in the development of diseases spread by airborne transmission and those transmitted by fecal–oral means. Overcrowding contributes to the incidence of such diseases as measles, mumps, rubella, polio, diphtheria, pertussis, and varicella. Crowded living conditions also enhance the spread of tuberculosis and influenza. Wind factors are an element of the physical environment that would influence the spread of aerosolized pathogens in the event of a terrorist attack.

Sanitation and disposal of both human and animal feces are other factors in the physical environmental dimension that affect the development of communicable diseases, particularly hepatitis A, tetanus, and polio. The organism causing tetanus is found on a variety of surfaces and is more common in areas where there is animal excrement. In addition, home delivery and poor hygiene on the part of untrained midwives in developing countries and some parts of the United States contribute to the development of tetanus in neonates and, occasionally, in postpartum women.

In developing countries, poor environmental sanitation contributes to the incidence of diseases such as hepatitis A and E and poliomyelitis. Sanitation is a less likely factor in the development of these diseases in the United States; however, contaminated food and water supplies have been implicated in several disease outbreaks related to *Escherichia coli*, hepatitis A, botulism, and other enteric pathogens.

Exposure to tick-bearing animals such as white-tailed deer, elk, and wild rodents in recreational areas or during outdoor work increases the risk of tickborne diseases such as Rocky Mountain spotted fever, ehrlichiosis, and human granulocytotropic anaplasmosis (HGA), a condition that affects neutrophil function and may lead to immunopathologic changes and opportunistic infections (Dumler et al., 2005). Household pets may also be infested by ticks and pose a risk of exposure to humans.

Animals serve as a source of human infection for many diseases. In fact, there are approximately 250 **zoonoses**, diseases that can be transmitted from animals to human beings (Huey, 2004). Rabies and bubonic plague are two examples of zoonoses. In the case of these diseases, prevention of infection in human beings often depends on disease control in animals. Community health nurses can help educate the public regarding zoonoses and actions that will prevent their spread to people. For example, routine vaccination of pets against rabies has led to marked decreases in the incidence of human rabies. Community health nurses can educate people on the need to immunize their pets and to avoid wild animals that may have rabies. Similarly, nurses can educate the public about the danger of eating raw eggs, which are often contaminated by pathogens such as *Salmonella*.

Because of differences in physical environmental conditions by region and by season, there are geographic and seasonal differences in the incidence of some communicable diseases. For example, more than 30% of cases of West Nile virus infections in 2005 occurred in California, but seasonal transmission also occurred in the Midwest and other areas of the country (Smith, Hayes, et al., 2005). Tickborne diseases are also most likely to occur in seasons when people are outdoors for recreational and occupational activities (Chapman, 2006).

Environmental contamination of food and water supplies may also result in exposure to pathogens that cause communicable diseases. For example, each year more than 5 billion pounds of fresh tomatoes are eaten

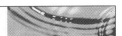

FOCUSED ASSESSMENT

Psychological Considerations in Assessing Communicable Disease Risk

- Does exposure to stress increase the risk of disease?
- Do psychological factors increase the risk of exposure to disease?
- What effect, if any, do psychological factors have on high-risk behaviors that contribute to disease?
- Is past trauma associated with the risk of disease?
- Does the presence of mental illness (e.g., depression) increase the risk of disease?
- Does the disease have potential psychological consequences (e.g., suicide risk)?

in the United States. In 2004, three outbreaks of *Salmonella* infections in the United States and Canada were attributed to eating Roma tomatoes. Contamination of the tomatoes may have occurred during growth in contaminated soil or during processing in tomato-packing houses (Corby et al., 2005). Bacterial contamination of produce is common, particularly produce grown in countries that use human excrement as fertilizer (Epidemiology Program Office, 2003). Similarly, a number of waterborne disease outbreaks occur each year in the United States, as discussed in Chapter 10∞.

The physical environment of health care settings may also contribute to the spread of communicable diseases. For example, one study of computer keyboards in various areas of a major in-patient facility found that 50% of keyboards were contaminated with pathogenic organisms including staphylococci and diphtheroids (Rutala, White, Gergen, & Weber, 2006). As we will see in the section on health system considerations, contaminated equipment and supplies in health care settings have been implicated in cases of communicable disease.

Physical environmental conditions may also complicate treatment for some communicable diseases that require long-term therapy such as TB and HIV infection. As we saw in Chapter 27∞, Hurricane Katrina led to interruptions in TB treatment for those affected by the hurricane. CDC has recommended that all TB control programs should plan for continued treatment of clients in the event of a disaster. Based on experience gained with Hurricane Katrina, Texas and Louisiana implemented contingency strategies in advance of Hurricane Rita that included developing lists of clients on therapy in the areas most likely to be affected, giving clients a 2- to 4-week supply of medication, providing clients with information on reestablishing contact with the health department if evacuated, providing backup copies of client records to share with other jurisdictions if needed, and moving essential supplies and medications to safer areas. These activities contributed to continued therapy for those clients affected by Hurricane Rita (DeGraw et al., 2006). Similar strategies could be used to support continued treatment for clients with chronic hepatitis or HIV/AIDS, and community health nurses caring for clients with these conditions may need to advocate for contingency planning in the event of a disaster. The focused assessment questions above right can assist the community health nurse in identifying physical environmental factors influencing communicable disease incidence in the community.

Sociocultural Considerations

A variety of social and cultural factors influence the development and course of communicable diseases. For example, congregating with large groups of people indoors during the winter facilitates the spread of airborne diseases, and poverty and poor nutrition increase

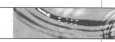

FOCUSED ASSESSMENT

Physical Environmental Considerations in Assessing Communicable Disease Risk

- What effect, if any, do crowded living conditions have on the incidence of the disease?
- Do elements of the physical environment serve as sources of contamination and exposure to disease (e.g., computer keyboards, contaminated ventilation systems)?
- Can the disease be transmitted to humans by animals or insects?
- What environmental factors increase the risk of human exposure to animal or insect sources of disease (e.g., standing water where mosquitoes breed)?
- Is the disease spread by contaminated food or water?
- Does poor sanitation affect disease incidence?
- Are there seasonal variations in disease incidence? If so, when is the disease most likely to occur? What environmental factors are present at that time that contribute to disease incidence?
- Do environmental factors impede access to diagnostic or treatment services?

susceptibility to a variety of diseases, particularly tuberculosis. Congregate living in institutional settings also contributes to the spread of disease. For example, TB outbreaks frequently occur in correctional settings, particularly among HIV-infected inmates (Jensen et al., 2005). Many inmates are also at risk for HBV transmission prior to and during incarceration (Khan et al., 2005). For example, 29% of all new U.S. HBV infections in 2001 occurred in people who had been previously incarcerated (Kelley et al., 2004). College campuses and military installations experience frequent outbreaks of measles, mumps, pertussis, and meningococcal meningitis among young adults in close quarters who are not immunized or whose levels of immunity have declined over time.

Poverty and unemployment, with consequent loss of health insurance, are social factors that may limit the ability of parents to have their children immunized or to provide prompt medical care when illness does occur, resulting in more serious consequences of disease. Pregnant women with low incomes might not receive prenatal care and are thus denied the opportunity to obtain screening and counseling for syphilis and HIV infection or susceptibility to rubella.

Lower socioeconomic status (SES) is associated with a variety of communicable diseases, including TB. TB is also associated with lower SES occupational groupings and unemployment (American Thoracic Society et al., 2005). Research has also suggested that it is not just personal income that affects TB incidence. In one California study, for example, higher incidence of pediatric TB was noted in census tracts with lower median incomes and larger ethnic and racial minority and immigrant populations. In this particular study, in contrast to others, overcrowding and unemployment were not found to be related to TB incidence (Myers, Westenhouse,

Flood, & Riley, 2006). Community health nurses will need to function as political advocates to assure the availability of communicable disease services for all segments of the population, particularly those of low SES.

Other sociocultural factors that influence TB incidence and prevalence include homelessness and incarceration. In 2003, more than 6% of persons diagnosed with TB were homeless during the previous year, and the incidence rate for TB among homeless persons is estimated to be five times that of the general population. Similarly, jail and prison inmates account for approximately 3% of U.S. TB diagnosed annually and have an incidence rate of 200 cases per 100,000 population (American Thoracic Society et al., 2005). In large part, the high incidence of TB in these populations is the result of a greater number of risk factors for disease, including behaviors such as drug and alcohol use, increased prevalence of HIV disease, and poor nutritional status. In working with these populations, community health nurses may need to advocate for screening and treatment services. They may also educate clients in these settings regarding disease prevention. At the aggregate level, they may advocate for policies that prevent the spread of disease (e.g., routine TB screening at the time of incarceration or in homeless shelters).

Language barriers, cultural beliefs and values, and lower education levels among some ethnic and socioeconomic groups may impede awareness of the need for immunization or other preventive measures for communicable diseases. In addition, the beliefs of some religious groups prohibit immunizations, thus increasing the size of the susceptible population among their members and in the community at large. Because of reduced herd immunity, the presence of these unimmunized individuals increases the potential for the spread of disease throughout the community. Community health nurses may need to advocate for the availability of immunization services for low-income populations as well as educate them on the need for immunization. They may also be involved in the development of culturally and linguistically appropriate immunization services.

CULTURAL COMPETENCE

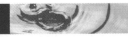

You are an international community health nurse who has been hired to develop and implement a national immunization campaign in India. You know from your study of other cultures that many Hindus, a primary cultural group in India, believe that immunization will anger the goddess Devi, who is responsible for bringing illness, and may actually bring about disease rather than prevent it. You are also aware that many parents have discontinued the vaccine series because of local inflammation at the injection site. How will you design your immunization campaign to account for these factors? Might these factors influence the immune status of Asian Indian immigrants to the United States? How would you determine the influence of these factors in the U.S. immigrant population to avoid stereotyping Asian Indian immigrants?

Gender socialization may also play a part in risk factors that promote STDs, particularly among women. In one study of Black women in North Carolina, for instance, many women with HIV infection were unemployed, had multiple lifetime sexual partners, and engaged in high-risk sexual behaviors. Reasons given for these behaviors included financial dependence on male partners, feelings of invincibility, low self-esteem and a need to feel loved, and alcohol and drug use. In spite of these behaviors, many of the women believed themselves to be at low risk for HIV infection (Leone et al., 2005). Similarly, traditional gender socialization, lack of knowledge, limited sex education, and limited parental communication regarding sexuality are some of the reasons given for the increasing rates of heterosexually acquired HIV infection in Latinas (Zambrana et al., 2004). In working with these women, community health nurses can help them find educational and employment opportunities that decrease their dependence on men. They can also help them develop assertiveness skills to negotiate condom use and other preventive measures with their partners.

Occupational factors are another part of the sociocultural dimension that may contribute to communicable diseases. Employees in the adult film industry, for example, are at increased risk for HIV infection and other STDs such as Chlamydia and gonorrhea as a result of failure to use condoms and frequent prolonged contact with multiple sexual partners (Division of STD Prevention, 2005a). Worldwide, sex workers who do not use barrier protection increase the spread of HIV infection and other STDs (Lee & Zwi, 2003). Community health nurses can help to educate sex workers regarding their vulnerability to STDs and the need for preventive measures. People who work with animals that transmit zoonoses to humans may also require education regarding prevention of exposure or recognition of symptoms of disease.

Health care workers and "first responders" (e.g., emergency personnel) are at increased risk for blood-borne diseases, and health care workers are frequently exposed to a variety of other communicable diseases. Health care workers have the potential for both exposure to and transmission of diseases such as influenza, yet vaccine coverage among health care personnel is low (less than 50%) (Pearson, Bridges, & Harper, 2006). Health care workers also represent approximately 3% of U.S. cases of TB (American Thoracic Society et al., 2005). The average risk of HIV infection after percutaneous exposure among health care workers has been estimated at 0.3%, whereas the risk of infection resulting from mucous membrane and intact skin exposures is far lower. Health care workers who experience occupational exposures to HIV infection should receive preventive treatment with antiretroviral agents (Panlilio, Cardo, Grohskopf, Heneine, & Ross, 2005). Community health nurses can help to educate other health care personnel and first responders regarding disease prevention, particularly with respect to universal precautions for bloodborne diseases.

As another example, hepatitis B and hepatitis C infections occur in health care workers after occupational exposures. HBV and HCV exposures may occur in the context of more than 800,000 sharps injuries that occur in health care settings each year (Al-Saden, 2004). When these injuries involve equipment contaminated by the blood of clients with HBV or HCV infection, health care workers have the potential for developing these diseases. Employees and children are at risk for hepatitis A when outbreaks occur in childcare settings, but risk for hepatitis A infection among health care workers is minimal. Certain occupations may contribute to the spread of disease as well as increased potential for exposure. For example, food service personnel may spread hepatitis A, and health care workers may expose clients to a number of communicable diseases.

Social stigma is another aspect of the sociocultural dimension that influences exposure to communicable diseases and attitudes to people who have them. Stigma may derive from fear of people who are different or from fear of exposure to disease, and affects people with communicable diseases in several ways. For example, stigma may increase the personal burden experienced by those with the disease or prevent them from seeking health care when stigmatized diseases are suspected. Stigma may also attach to professionals and community volunteers who provide services to those with certain communicable diseases. Finally, stigma may result in considerable financial loss if people avoid potential sources of exposure. For example, fears of exposure to severe acute respiratory syndrome (SARS) and avian influenza have decreased tourism to some parts of the world, severely affecting local economies (Des Jarlais, Galea, Tracy, Tross, & Vlahov, 2006).

The extent of stigma and its effects on people with specific communicable diseases are influenced by other socioeconomic and psychological factors. For example, research has indicated that people with greater personal resources, higher education levels, and better mental health were less likely to be concerned about exposure to HIV/AIDS and SARS and less likely to stigmatize people with these diseases (Des Jarlais et al., 2006). In one study in South Africa, families hid HIV-infected family members from health care providers, denying them needed care because of the stigma of having a family member with HIV/AIDS. In other instances, families disowned members who died of AIDS, refusing to collect their bodies or belongings or never acknowledging the cause of death. Churches and schools were also found to undermine HIV prevention efforts by refusing to provide education that might "encourage youth to sin" (Campbell, Foulis, Maimane, & Sibiya, 2005). In other settings, however, religious emphasis on abstinence has contributed to low rates of HIV infection. Other research has also suggested that providing quality health care services for people with these diseases minimizes the stigma attached to them (Castro & Farmer, 2005).

Stigma attached to communicable diseases exists within symbolic, politicoeconomic, and cultural contexts. In the symbolic context, having a particular disease is linked to negatively valued behaviors (e.g., IDU, sexual promiscuity, or homosexuality) or groups. An historical example of the latter is the variety of terms used for syphilis in the 19th and early 20th centuries. The English labeled it "the French disease" and vice versa, each nation linking the disease to its greatest enemy.

The general contexts of poverty and disempowerment also play a part in perceptions of stigma. The poor and disenfranchised, who are often the ones most affected by communicable diseases, are devalued in society. Factors in the cultural context include attitudes to sexuality and sex education that lead to perceptions of high-risk behaviors as sinful. Some authors note that when a group has little in the way of economic or political power and limited access to material goods, disparaging people with communicable diseases is one of the few means of claiming respectability open to them. Finally, stigmatization may arise out of poor responses of health care professionals to people with specific communicable diseases or the lack of resources to respond. The perceived lack of concern by health care providers may lead to a societal failure to acknowledge responsibility for the care of people with stigmatizing diseases. If having a disease is a result of unsanctioned behavior, then the rest of society does not have to acknowledge the problem or attempt to do anything about it (Campbell et al., 2005).

Social norms that contribute to high-risk behaviors also foster the spread of some communicable diseases. For example, relaxed sexual mores have led to greater sexual promiscuity and increased risk of exposure to HIV infection, STDs, and some forms of hepatitis. Similarly, a social environment in which it is relatively easy to obtain drugs for injection drug use promotes infection with HIV, syphilis, and hepatitis B, C, and D.

Other social factors that can increase the incidence of communicable diseases include homelessness and other forms of social upheaval and media communications. The fatigue, malnutrition, exposure to cold and crowding, and general debilitation associated with homelessness have contributed to increased pertussis, influenza, and other communicable diseases in homeless populations.

Immigration is another social factor that influences communicable diseases. As we saw earlier, nearly half of TB cases in the United States occur in foreign-born individuals (Pratt et al., 2006). Although legal immigrants are screened for active tuberculosis on entry into the country, those with positive screening tests and no evidence of disease are rarely provided with prophylactic treatment. The stresses of immigration and possible poor living conditions in their adoptive countries put

BUILDING OUR KNOWLEDGE BASE

Lobato, Cegielski, and the Tuberculosis Along the U.S.–Mexico Border Work Group (2001) have noted the need for international cross-border research between the United States and Mexico to reduce the spread of tuberculosis across the border.

- What potential research questions might be appropriate?
- How would you design a study to answer one or more of the questions you have generated? What type of research methodology would be appropriate to the study? Why?
- How would you select your sample?
- What data would you collect? How would you go about collecting it?

members of immigrant populations at higher risk for developing active tuberculosis than the general public. Community health nurses can advocate for follow-up and prophylactic treatment for this population to promote their health status and protect the overall population. Importation of disease into previously polio-free countries is another example of the effects of immigration. Because of the potential for rapid international spread of communicable diseases, there is a need to develop cooperative international control programs, particularly between countries that share borders such as Mexico and the United States.

Large population movements may result in sanitation problems or tax the capabilities of local health services to provide immunizations or diagnostic and treatment services. This is particularly true of large influxes of refugee populations in times of war or civil strife. Increased incidence of communicable diseases is also a consequence of war, in part due to social conditions that promote disease (e.g., malnutrition), but also as a result of the dismantling of public health capabilities that often occurs as a result of war.

Media coverage of adverse vaccine reactions has led some people to refuse immunization for their children. A similar effect was noted with respect to immunization for smallpox among health care workers and anthrax in military personnel as a precaution against possible bioterrorism. Finally, media attention to the effectiveness of HIV therapy has reduced adherence to safe sexual practices in some segments of the population. Media presentations of sexual activity as desirable behavior have also contributed to the incidence of STDs. Portrayals of popular heroes and heroines as "sexy" and sexually active have fostered imitative behavior, particularly among adolescents.

Political unrest that leads to bioterrorism is another possible factor in the development of communicable diseases. As indicated in Chapter 27∞, CDC has designated three categories of biological agents with differing degrees of potential use in biological terrorist activities. Category A organisms are those that would most easily lend themselves to intentional dissemination. Category B

organisms would be slightly less easily disseminated, and category C pathogens have potential for development as biological weapons. (See Appendix E on the Companion Website for more information about these diseases.)

In addition to social factors that contribute to disease, communicable diseases may have social effects. For example, congenital rubella syndrome and congenital syphilis lead to long-term consequences in newborns that have extensive costs for society. Similarly, treatment of persons with chronic hepatitis or HIV infection imposes a costly burden on society, and care of children orphaned by parental death due to AIDS poses another social dilemma. On the other hand, social conditions may have positive effects on the incidence and prevalence of communicable diseases. For instance, raising the taxes on alcohol and increasing the age for legal consumption have been associated with lower incidence of gonorrhea. Alcohol lowers inhibitions to risky sexual behaviors, so control of alcohol use can minimize such behaviors (Division of Sexually Transmitted Diseases Prevention, 2000). Sociocultural factors influencing communicable disease incidence in the community can be identified using the focused assessment questions provided below.

FOCUSED ASSESSMENT

Sociocultural Considerations in Assessing Communicable Disease Risk

- Does society condone behaviors that increase the risk of disease (e.g., sexual activity)?
- Does social interaction increase the risk of the spread of disease?
- Is the disease spread easily in congregate living situations? What factors in congregate living situations contribute to the spread of disease?
- What are societal attitudes to the disease? Do they hamper control efforts? Is there social stigma attached to having the disease?
- What effect do media messages have on attitudes to the disease? On behaviors that contribute to disease? On willingness to seek care for the disease?
- Do occupational factors influence the incidence of the disease?
- Does socioeconomic status affect risk for the disease? Consequences of the disease?
- Is the disease more common in the homeless population?
- What effect, if any, do language and cultural beliefs and behaviors have on the incidence of the disease?
- What effect does education level have on disease incidence?
- To what extent does gender socialization contribute to disease incidence?
- Is the disease more common in immigrant populations?
- What effects do war and social unrest have on disease incidence, if any?
- What are the social effects of having the disease for the individual or of increased incidence of the disease for the population?
- Does the disease have potential as a biological weapon?

Behavioral Considerations

The major behavioral dimension factors that influence the development of communicable disease are related to diet, sexual activity, and drug use. Malnutrition makes people more susceptible to a number of diseases, particularly TB and childhood diseases in unimmunized populations. Malnutrition may also contribute to more severe disease and a greater chance of complications.

Sexual activity obviously increases the risk of STDs, but hepatitis B and D are also spread by sexual activity (Mast et al., 2005; National Center for HIV, STD, and TB Prevention, 2006b). The role of sexual intercourse in the transmission of hepatitis C is not a significant one, and screening of sexual partners of clients with HCV infection is not recommended unless there is a history of IDU (National Center for HIV, STD, and TB Prevention, 2006a).

Certain sexual behaviors increase one's risk of disease over and above just engaging in sexual intercourse. For instance, multiple sexual partners and unprotected intercourse increase exposure to disease. Sexual activity among adolescents may also include high-risk behaviors, particularly in some subsegments of the adolescent population. In one study of incarcerated youth, for instance, more than 90% of adolescent boys and 87% of girls were sexually active, and 37% of boys and 5% of girls reported more than three sexual partners in the previous 3 months. More than one in five boys and one in ten girls reported sexual intercourse with a high-risk partner, and more than two thirds of boys and half of girls reported having sexual intercourse while drunk or high (Teplin, Mericle, McClelland, & Abram, 2003). According to the 2003 Youth Risk Behavior Survey (YRBS), nearly 47% of U.S. high school students had ever had sexual intercourse, and 34% were currently sexually active. Fourteen percent of this population reported four or more sexual partners in their lifetime. Nearly 88% had received some education about HIV infection in school, but only 63% of currently sexually active students reported condom use at their last sexual encounter (CDC, 2003b).

Men who have sex with men (MSM) frequently engage in either receptive or insertive anal sex without the use of a condom, increasing their potential for HIV, HBV, and HDV infection. Research suggests that HCV infection, on the other hand, is not usually transmitted sexually in MSM except in the context of IDU (Alary et al., 2005). Oral–genital intercourse increases the potential for spread of syphilis, particularly in the presence of secondary lesions (Division of STD Prevention, 2004b). Increases in the incidence of both syphilis and rectal gonorrhea have been noted among MSM (Koblin et al., 2003).

Early in the HIV epidemic, many MSM adopted safer sexual practices, but more recent data indicate a return to unprotected anal intercourse. One study conducted in six U.S. cities found that 48% of MSM engage in unprotected receptive anal intercourse and 55% had unprotected anal intercourse within the previous month (Koblin et al., 2003). In another study, a quarter of Black MSM engaged in high-risk sexual practices (Hart, Peterson, & the Community Intervention Trial for Youth Team, 2004). Similar findings have been noted among HIV-infected women. In one study, for example, women receiving HAART were less likely to report multiple sexual partners after initiating therapy but were more likely to engage in unprotected sexual intercourse than before (Wilson et al., 2004). Even among the general public, the percentage of people who view AIDS as a significant public health problem has declined, leading to decreased motivation to adopt safe sexual behaviors, receive HIV screening tests, or seek diagnostic and treatment services (Fenton & Valdiserri, 2006).

Among men diagnosed with HIV infection between 2001 and 2004, 61% were exposed through male-to-male sexual activity; 16% of cases were related to high-risk heterosexual activity (e.g., intercourse with someone with known HIV infection or risk factors for HIV infection). Another 16% of cases were related to injection drug use (IDU). The majority of women with HIV infection diagnosed in the same time period (76%) were exposed through high-risk heterosexual activity. Another 21% of women were exposed through IDU (Espinoza et al., 2005).

MSM in some parts of the world are also at risk for lymphogranuloma venereum (LGV), a sexually transmitted disease caused by a strain of *Chlamydia trachomatis* not typically seen in industrialized countries. During 2003 and 2004, for example, an outbreak of 92 cases of LGV was reported in the Netherlands. The lesions caused by LGV infection also increase the potential for HIV infection and other bloodborne diseases (van de Laar et al., 2004).

Another behavior that increases the potential for HIV exposure is the failure of infected persons to disclose their status to sexual partners. In one study, for example, 42% of gay or bisexual men, 19% of heterosexual men, and 17% of women with HIV infection reported sexual intercourse with at least one partner without disclosing their infection. Most nondisclosure among gay or bisexual men occurred in the context of casual relationships. Nondisclosure among heterosexual men and women was equally likely in nonexclusive and exclusive partnerships (Ciccarone et al., 2003). Willingness to disclose one's HIV status may become more widespread with recent court rulings that persons who know, or even should know based on high-risk behaviors, that they are HIV-infected can be held responsible for infecting others. On July 3, 2006, for example, the California Supreme Court ruled that people who should have known that they were HIV-infected and infect others without disclosing their possible status are liable for "negligent HIV infection" (Elias, 2006).

Use of condoms is a behavioral factor that can protect against exposure to STDs. Unfortunately, the prevalence of condom use by sexually active persons waxes and wanes. Among adolescents, access to condoms may influence their use, but many people are reluctant to provide condoms to sexually active young people out of a fear of promoting sexual activity. At least one study, however, has indicated that the availability of condoms and instruction in their use was actually associated with less sexual activity among adolescents than nonavailability. Sexually active adolescents in schools where condoms were available were twice as likely to use them regularly as those in schools where condoms were not available (Blake et al., 2003). Community health nurses may educate sexually active clients, particularly adolescents, in the use of condoms. They may also need to advocate for condom availability to those who are sexually active.

Breast-feeding is another behavioral factor in vertical transmission of HIV infection from mother to infant. Approximately one third to one half of perinatal transmission of HIV infection in breast-feeding populations internationally has occurred as a result of breast-feeding, and avoidance of breast-feeding is recommended when other alternatives are available (Mofenson et al., 2006). WHO recommends replacement feeding for infants of HIV-infected mothers when it is safe, acceptable, affordable, feasible, and sustainable. In developing countries, however, replacement feeding brings other mortality risks for newborns. Statistical modeling has indicated that exclusive breast-feeding for the first 6 months would decrease overall mortality in infants of HIV-infected mothers, but that replacement feeding is probably safer after 6 months of age (Ross & Labbok, 2004). Community health nurses should encourage those HIV-infected women whose babies are born without infection to refrain from breast-feeding, particularly in countries where replacement feeding is safe and easily available.

Research with male-to-female (MTF) transgender persons also indicates a high incidence of multiple risk behaviors (Clements-Nolle, Marx, Guzman, & Katz, 2001). Some of the reasons for this return to high-risk behaviors include optimism regarding available treatment for HIV, the potential for postexposure treatment, and the possibility of a vaccine to prevent HIV infection (Wolitski, Valdiserri, Denning, & Levine, 2001). In addition, many MSM are experiencing what has been termed "fatigue" with messages about safe sexual practices to the point where they are often ignored (Fox et al., 2001). Because of the resulting changes in sexual behavior, there is also an increasing incidence of gonorrhea and syphilis among MSM (Wolitski et al., 2001).

Drug use is another behavioral factor that influences the incidence of several communicable diseases. For example, TB is more than 17 times more common in injection drug users (IDUs) than in nonusers, and the overall prevalence of TB in IDUs may be as high as 31% (Kim & Crittenden, 2005). Injection of methamphetamines increases the risk of both HCV and HIV infection (Boddiger, 2005). Drug use also increases one's risk of

hepatitis B, C, and D (National Center for HIV, STD, and TB Prevention, 2006a, 2006b, 2006c). IDU and use of crack cocaine may also increase one's risk for TB (Jensen et al., 2005). Finally, the incidence of tetanus is increasing among IDUs, and injection of black tar heroin has been associated with an increased risk of wound botulism (Division of Bacterial and Mycotic Diseases, 2003). Drug abuse, particularly opiate use, may also result in anergy, reducing the validity of tuberculin tests as a screening tool in this high-risk population. **Anergy** is an inability to react to antigens commonly used in tuberculosis skin testing due to suppression of cellular immunity. Anergy also occurs in the presence of HIV infection, making it more difficult to diagnose TB in HIV-infected individuals.

Smoking, as a behavioral risk factor, also plays a small part in the development of communicable diseases. For example, tobacco use is thought to play a part in TB incidence (Jensen et al., 2005). Failure to complete a standard course of treatment for TB also contributes to increased prevalence of the disease as well as the development of multi-drug-resistant TB (American Thoracic Society et al., 2005). The focused assessment below includes questions that can assist the community health nurse to identify behavioral factors influencing communicable disease incidence in population groups or individuals.

Health System Considerations

Factors related to the health care system may also influence the development and course of communicable diseases. For example, charging fees for immunizations may limit the ability of people in lower socioeconomic groups to become adequately immunized. Similarly, missed opportunities for immunizations and provider failure to give immunizations because of mythical contraindications also increase the risk of communicable diseases.

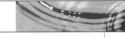

FOCUSED ASSESSMENT

Behavioral Considerations in Assessing Communicable Disease Risk

- Does diet play a part in the incidence of the disease (e.g., malnutrition as a risk factor for TB)? Does nutritional status influence the consequences of the disease?
- Does alcohol or drug use contribute to the incidence of the disease?
- Does sexual activity increase the risk of the disease? Do specific sexual behaviors increase or decrease the risk of the disease?
- Are people with the disease likely to disclose their infection to others? What barriers to disclosure exist? What effect does willingness to disclose have on controlling spread of the disease?
- Does breast-feeding increase the risk of infection in young children?
- Does smoking increase the risk of disease?
- Does noncompliance with treatment recommendations increase the risk of developing drug resistance in the organisms causing the disease? If so, what are the factors contributing to noncompliance?

Health care providers may also fail to provide screening or health education related to communicable diseases. Even among providers caring for clients with communicable diseases, the frequency of preventive counseling may be low. For example, in a study of HIV physicians in four U.S. cities, 60% reported counseling clients with newly diagnosed HIV infection, but only 14% routinely provided counseling to established clients (Metsch et al., 2004). In another national study of U.S. physicians, less than one third of physicians routinely screened their clients for STDs. In addition, although reporting of HIV/AIDS is mandatory in all states, only slightly more than half of physicians (57%) routinely reported cases diagnosed. The percentages of physicians reporting other STDs were even lower—37% for Chlamydia, 44% for gonorrhea, and 53% for syphilis. Finally, few physicians routinely notify sexual partners of clients with STDs of their exposure. Most of the physicians responding to the survey instructed clients to notify partners themselves (82% to 89%) or to contact the health department (25% to 34%) (St. Lawrence et al., 2002).

When health care providers do educate clients, however, their efforts appear to be effective. For example, in one study of voluntary HIV screening, 28% of men and 18% of women reported being tested on the recommendation of their health care provider or a friend. Similarly, 90% of people with a recent diagnosis of HIV infection reported a change in their sexual behaviors, presumably based on counseling by providers (Division of HIV/AIDS Prevention—Surveillance and Epidemiology, 2000). The availability of community-based HIV prevention programs may also influence high-risk behaviors. In one study, for instance, bisexual men in regions with HIV prevention programs were less likely to engage in unprotected intercourse with other men than those in regions without such programs. Unfortunately, the presence or absence of prevention programs did not seem to affect the frequency of unprotected heterosexual activity (Leaver, Allman, Meyers, & Veugelers, 2004).

Health care providers may also fail to recognize atypical forms of illnesses or emerging or reemerging diseases and treat them effectively. For example, because of its relative infrequency in modern society, providers may lack clinical experience with pertussis or fail to consider it as a possible diagnosis. Similarly, they may fail to consider a diagnosis of HIV in a client with no known risk factors. Health care providers who are unfamiliar with the symptoms of anthrax or other rarely seen conditions may misdiagnose them, leading to inappropriate treatment and greater spread of disease.

Health system factors may also contribute more actively to communicable diseases and their effects. For example, **nosocomial infection**, disease spread as a result of exposure in a health care setting, in hospitals and physicians' offices is a significant factor in the spread of varicella. As many as 2 million health-care-associated infections occur in hospitals alone each year, resulting in 88,000 deaths and $4.5 billion in unnecessary health care costs (CDC, 2005i). As an example, in 2003, a nurse working in a newborn nursery and maternity ward exposed more than 1,500 mothers and babies to active TB. The nurse had been diagnosed with LTBI 11 years earlier, but declined treatment that would have decreased her risk of developing active disease (Fitzpatrick et al., 2005).

Even routine health care interventions such as immunization may result in unintended illness. For example, in 2005 a young woman on a trip to Costa Rica developed paralytic poliomyelitis. Exposure resulted from virus shed by an infant in the home where she was staying who had recently been immunized with OPV. In this case, health system factors (immunization of the child) combined with sociocultural factors (lack of immunization of the young woman on religious grounds) to result in disease (Landaverde et al., 2006). Although the risk of vaccine-induced disease occurs, it is lower than the risk of exposure through travel to endemic areas, and immunization prior to travel is recommended.

Other medical treatment interventions have also been associated with communicable diseases in their recipients. For example, an estimated one of every 1,000 to 3,000 units of platelets have bacterial contaminants, and in 2004, platelet transfusions led to two deaths from transfusion-associated sepsis. From 1990 to 1998, transfusion-associated bacterial sepsis accounted for 17% of deaths related to transfusions. Although transfusion-related viral infection receives more attention, the risk of bacterial sepsis is actually higher (Arendt et al., 2005). Organ donation has also resulted in transmission of communicable diseases. For example, three of four recipients of organs from a single donor in 2005 developed West Nile virus infection (Teperman et al., 2005). WNV infection has also been transmitted via transfusion and possibly in dialysis units (Caglioti et al., 2004; Smith et al., 2004). Worldwide spread of HIV infection has occurred through the use of infected blood products as well as limited international access to screening, diagnostic, and treatment technologies in many parts of the world (Lee & Zwi, 2003).

Medical treatment for conditions such as asthma and autoimmune diseases that require immunosuppressive therapy places individuals at greater risk for complications of influenza. In addition, inappropriate prescription of antimicrobials by health care providers has led to the development of antibiotic-resistant strains of several microorganisms. For example, *Neisseria gonorrhoeae*, the causative organism for gonorrhea, began exhibiting resistance to penicillin and tetracycline in the 1980s. More recently, fluoroquinolone-resistant *N. gonorrhoeae* (QRNG) has become more prevalent, particularly in some parts of the United States (e.g., California and Hawaii) (Whiticar et al., 2002). MSM are also three times more likely than heterosexual men to develop QRNG, and the incidence of QRNG among MSM is nearly 5%.

Rates of QRNG are also high among people who acquire gonorrhea in Asia, the Pacific Islands, England, and Wales (Division of STD Prevention, 2004a).

Four strategies have been suggested to slow the development of drug-resistant microorganisms (Huey, 2004). First and foremost, providers should avoid unnecessary use of antimicrobials and should promote their use as directed. Failure of clients to complete an entire course of medication offers opportunities for development of drug-resistant strains of microorganisms. Second, local providers should establish guidelines for the use of antimicrobial agents based on local epidemiology and patterns of drug resistance. Third, testing should be available and routinely used to identify drug resistance, and finally, antimicrobials should be used in combinations and strengths best suited to eliminate susceptible organisms.

Provider attitudes to persons with stigmatizing diseases may also influence care. Potential questions for exploring health system factors in the development of communicable diseases are presented in the focused assessment below. A communicable disease risk inventory for assessing the risk of communicable diseases in population groups is included in the *Community Assessment Reference Guide* designed to accompany this text.

FOCUSED ASSESSMENT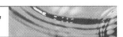

Health System Considerations in Assessing Communicable Disease Risk

- What primary preventive measures are available for the disease? Are they widely used?
- To what extent do health care providers educate the public on primary prevention of the disease?
- Is there a vaccine available for the disease?
- Is there a screening test for the disease? If so, are persons at risk for the disease screened?
- How is the disease diagnosed?
- To what extent are health care providers conversant with the signs and symptoms of the disease?
- To what extent do health care providers report cases of the disease? Do they engage in contact notification?
- To what extent do health care settings or provider behaviors contribute to the development of disease? What is the extent of nosocomial infection in the community?
- To what extent do routine medical interventions contribute to the incidence of communicable disease?
- Is there an effective treatment for the disease? Are diagnostic and treatment services for the disease available and accessible to infected persons?
- To what extent do health care providers engage in practices that might lead to the development of drug-resistant microorganisms?
- What are the attitudes of health care providers to persons with the disease? How do these attitudes affect willingness to seek diagnostic and treatment services? To what extent do they affect the quality of care provided?

COMMUNITY HEALTH NURSING AND CONTROL OF COMMUNICABLE DISEASES

Community health nurses play a variety of roles in controlling communicable diseases in individual clients and in population groups. These roles are incorporated into the nursing process and include assessing factors contributing to communicable diseases as well as the presence and extent of communicable disease in the individual or population, planning and implementing control strategies for communicable diseases, and evaluating the effectiveness of communicable disease interventions. In some official health agencies, community health nurses may be responsible for administering entire communicable disease programs.

Assessing Risk Factors for Communicable Diseases

Factors in each of the six dimensions of health influence the development of communicable diseases in individuals and in population groups, and the community health nurse assesses factors related to each dimension. The nurse may assess factors related to the development of communicable diseases in individual clients or in the population at large.

In the biophysical dimension, a community health nurse may recognize symptoms of an existing communicable disease in an individual client. Recognition of communicable disease in specific clients is an element of the case finding role of the community health nurse discussed in Chapter 1 ∞. At the community or aggregate level, the community health nurse may become aware of the development of outbreaks of disease in the population.

Community health nurses may also assess individuals or populations for risk factors for communicable disease in each of the six dimensions of health. For example, the nurse might assess the adequacy of sanitary facilities at a summer camp, or explore the extent of condom use among sexually active adolescents or correctional inmates. Similarly, the nurse would collect information on the extent of injection drug use in the population or by an individual. Nurses might also explore the attitudes of health care providers to specific communicable diseases and the extent to which they engage in preventive education with their clients.

Diagnostic Reasoning and Control of Communicable Diseases

The community health nurse may derive a variety of nursing diagnoses related to communicable diseases. These diagnoses may reflect the health needs of individuals, families, or population groups. Diagnoses may also reflect the potential for infection or the presence of active disease. For example, the nurse working with a family may diagnose "inadequate immunization status due to poor knowledge of children's immunization needs." A nursing diagnosis related to an individual client is "potential for infection with tetanus due to increased risk of occupational injury and lack of recent immunization," or "failure to obtain routine immunizations due to lack of transportation." A diagnosis related to the presence of active disease might be "probable tuberculosis as evidenced by cough, weight loss, and night sweats and recent travel to an endemic area."

Nursing diagnoses related to communicable diseases may also be derived for population groups. Diagnoses at the community level may reflect the current incidence of disease or the potential for spread of infection. Examples of such diagnoses are "increased incidence of HCV due to injection drug use" and "potential for increased transmission of HIV infection due to widespread use of unsafe sexual practices among MSM."

Nursing diagnoses may also reflect the presence of risk factors that affect the development of communicable diseases in individuals or population groups. For example, the nurse may diagnose an "increased risk of hepatitis A due to shellfish contamination in local waters" or "increased risk of tuberculosis transmission from refugees emigrating from endemic areas."

Planning and Implementing Control Strategies for Communicable Diseases

Many previously known as well as emerging communicable diseases contribute to a significant worldwide burden of disease, death, and suffering. Control of communicable diseases rests on an understanding of the factors that lead to their development and knowledge of interventions to prevent or treat them. Communicable disease experts have suggested that the recent SARS outbreaks throughout the world have highlighted four general considerations in controlling disease outbreaks (Huey, 2004). The first consideration is identifying the problem. For existing diseases, this may mean taking note of increased incidence of the disease. For emerging diseases, identification may involve recognition of a new disease entity and identifying causative factors. Because community health nurses often encounter people before they seek medical care for symptoms of disease, nurses may be among the first to identify potential outbreaks of existing diseases or to recognize symptoms suggestive of new diseases.

The second and third considerations are controlling the spread of disease through knowledge of modes of transmission and developing effective therapies. Epidemiologic investigations are needed to develop knowledge of a specific disease, how it is spread, its effects, and how it can best be controlled. Research may also be needed to develop effective therapies for existing and emerging diseases. Unfortunately, pharmaceutical research for new drugs to combat communicable

diseases is not very profitable (Huey, 2004). Unlike chronic disease therapies, which often extend over a lifetime, medications for communicable diseases have a time-limited utility. Once someone is cured, they no longer require medication (except for chronic infections such as HIV/AIDS and chronic hepatitis). Community health nurses may be involved in epidemiologic research to identify factors contributing to disease or may be active advocates for drug development research.

The final general consideration in controlling communicable diseases, which is particularly relevant to new diseases, is that health care workers need support in dealing with mysterious outbreaks. Fear of being exposed to or developing a poorly understood disease can greatly limit the effectiveness of health system response and further jeopardize the health of the public.

Addressing these four considerations may involve interventions at the primary, secondary, or tertiary levels of prevention. Community health nursing interventions related to each level of prevention are discussed below.

Primary Prevention

Primary prevention of communicable diseases is directed toward preventing the occurrence of disease. Major emphases in preventing communicable diseases include immunization, postexposure prophylaxis, and other preventive measures specific to particular communicable diseases.

IMMUNIZATION Immunization is the most effective method of preventing the occurrence of communicable diseases. The modern concept of immunization originated with William Jenner, and the first smallpox vaccine was developed in 1796, but its use did not become widespread for more than 100 years. Similarly, four other vaccines (rabies, cholera, typhoid, and plague) were developed between 1885 and 1897 but were not widely used (National Immunization Program, 1999). Based on U.S. immunization recommendations, discussed in Chapter 16∞, children should receive a total of 23 doses of vaccine before the age of 2 years. These immunizations are intended to protect them from 12 different diseases (CDC, 2005h). Immunization with selected vaccines is also recommended for adults, as noted in Chapters 17, 18, and 19∞, and for members of specific groups at high risk for infection. For example, people in certain occupational categories (e.g., health care providers) are at high risk for exposure to a variety of pathogens, and inmates in correctional settings are at increased risk for diseases such as HIV/AIDS, TB, and hepatitis (see Chapters 24 and 26∞ for more in-depth discussion of immunization needs in these populations).

Widespread use of vaccines is a 20th-century phenomenon, but barriers still exist to the use of immunization services. Some of these barriers include lack of access to services (e.g., due to cost), lack of knowledge regarding the need for immunization, parental concerns regarding the discomfort associated with administration of some vaccines (e.g., localized swelling with DTaP), and health system limitations such as differences in school entry requirements across jurisdictions, poor enforcement of immunization requirements, and poor data management. Other system barriers are the failure of providers to encourage immunizations other than those required for school entry and missed opportunities for immunization in the course of providing other services. Community health nurses can advocate for the availability of immunization services to all segments of the population and can educate the public and providers on the need for immunization.

Several of the 2010 national health objectives are related to increasing immunization coverage for a variety of communicable diseases (CDC, 2005f)◆. Some of these objectives with baseline data, current status, and 2010 targets are presented later in this chapter. Additional objectives may be viewed on the *Healthy People 2010* Web site at http://wonder.cdc.gov/data2010.

The problem of data management has also been addressed in the objectives with the recommendation to develop population-based immunization information systems (IISs) to consolidate records and generate reminders of subsequent immunization needs. IISs record and consolidate confidential information regarding immunizations given by multiple providers. As of 2004, approximately 48% of children under age 6 were enrolled in an IIS, and 76% of public and 39% of private immunization providers were submitting data to an IIS (Urquhart, Kelly, & Rasulnia, 2005). Community health nurses can advocate for the development of local IISs where they do not already exist and for health care provider participation in existing IISs.

The extent of vaccination coverage varies among specific communicable diseases. In 2003, approximately 27.5% of U.S. children 19 to 35 months of age lacked at least one or more doses of recommended vaccines (CDC, 2005h). Since 1994, childhood immunization for pertussis in the United States has exceeded 90%, the 2010 target objective (Brown et al., 2005). U.S. immunization rates for other childhood diseases are also high but rates are quite variable throughout the rest of the world.

In 2000, changes were made to U.S. recommendations for poliomyelitis immunization due to the incidence of vaccine-associated disease with oral polio vaccine (OPV). Current U.S. recommendations specify that all four doses of polio vaccine are to be given with inactivated polio vaccine (IPV) (CDC, 2006d). OPV continues to be used in endemic areas of the world because of its ease of administration. IPV is recommended for adults traveling to endemic areas, laboratory workers handling specimens potentially containing poliovirus, those providing care to persons with polio, and unvaccinated adults whose children receive OPV (Prevots, Burr, Sutter, & Murphy, 2000). As of April 2006, an estimated 80% of infants worldwide had received three doses of polio vaccine (Polio Eradication Group, 2006). In 2003, measles immunization rates ranged from a high of 93% of 1-year-olds in the region of the Americas to 63% in the African region. Similar differences were noted for coverage with three doses of DTP vaccine (the Americas—91%, Africa—61%) and hepatitis B (77% and 29%, respectively) (WHO, 2005b). Varicella immunization rates in the United States and elsewhere lag behind those for other immunizable childhood diseases, but may improve with the advent of a combined vaccine that immunizes against measles, mumps, rubella, and varicella with a single vaccine (CDC, 2005g). Recommendations for routine immunization for children and adolescents were presented in Chapter 16∞.

HBV vaccine is recommended for all U.S. children under 19 years of age, and in 1992, WHO recommended that all countries incorporate HBV vaccine into their routine childhood immunization schedules by 1997. By 2001, 66% of WHO member states had universal HBV childhood immunization programs, and approximately 32% of children less than 1 year of age were immunized in those countries (Gacic-Dobo et al., 2003). Immunization is particularly important for infants born to women who are HBsAg positive, and can even be given to premature infants within a month after birth or hospital discharge (Mast et al., 2005). In 2004, approximately 35% of adults aged 18 to 49 years had ever received HBV vaccine, with women slightly more likely than men to be immunized. A slightly higher percentage (45%) of people at high risk had been immunized (Weinbaum, Billah, & Mast, 2006).

Adolescents should also receive certain immunizations as indicated in Chapter 16∞. These include Tdap, a booster dose of MMR, and varicella vaccine if not previously immunized. Additional recommendations for adolescents include pneumococcal vaccine if not previously immunized and meningococcal vaccine (CDC, 2006d). In 2005, ACIP recommended that routine meningococcal vaccination of all adolescents at age 11 be implemented by 2008. Meningococcal immunization is particularly recommended for previously unimmunized college students living in dormitories (Bilukha & Rosenstein, 2005), and community health nurses may need to advocate for initiation and enforcement of immunization requirements for this population.

Think Advocacy

A local university does not require proof of immunization from incoming students. The university administration is afraid that requiring evidence of immunization will deter students from registering for courses. How might you go about convincing the administration that immunization status should be validated before students are allowed to register?

Persons younger than 29 years of age in the United States are unlikely to have been immunized against smallpox because vaccination was discontinued in 1972. In the event of a terrorist attack using variola virus, which causes smallpox, this age group would receive priority for use of limited vaccine supplies. It is likely that previously immunized persons, although probably not completely safe, might still have some level of immunity. In fact, in one smallpox outbreak in 1902–1903, 93% of people vaccinated as long as 50 years earlier were protected (Cohen, 2001). In the event of a vaccine shortage, priority would also be given to persons at greatest risk of exposure (e.g., health care providers) or essential personnel (e.g., public safety personnel).

Adult vaccine coverage for many of these diseases, however, lags behind child coverage. For example, many adults have not had recent tetanus and diphtheria boosters, and many older adults have never been immunized for tetanus and are at high risk for disease. Unimmunized women of childbearing age or those with waning immunity increase the risk of congenital rubella syndrome or neonatal tetanus in their infants. Similarly, many adults and adolescents are at risk for varicella and should be immunized. Adult immunization for some diseases, such as poliomyelitis, is recommended only for those traveling to areas where the disease continues to occur (Landaverde et al., 2006). Immunization is particularly recommended for diseases such as mumps among college students, whose initial immunity may be waning (Quinlisk et al., 2006). Rubella immunization is also recommended for susceptible women of childbearing age, particularly those emigrating from countries with endemic rubella (Kellenberg et al., 2005).

Vaccines are also available for hepatitis A and B, tuberculosis, and influenza, although many people at risk for these diseases are not adequately immunized. Hepatitis A vaccine became available in 1995 and its use is routinely recommended for all children in 11 states with average annual incidence rates of 20 cases of HAV per 100,000 population (Fiore, Bell, Barker, Darling, & Amon, 2005), travelers to endemic areas, those with clotting factor disorders or chronic liver disease, and those who encounter occupational risk for infection. In the 11 states with recommendations for routine immunization, coverage rates for at least one dose of vaccine among children 24 to 35 months of age averaged 50.9%. Coverage rates in six other states with relatively high rates of HAV incidence averaged 25%. In states with no HAV immunization recommendation, only 1.4% of children received at least one dose of vaccine (Fiore et al., 2005).

HBV immunization is recommended for all infants and persons at risk. Research has indicated that infants who receive the first dose of HBV vaccine at birth are more likely to complete the series than those who receive their first dose at 1 to 2 months of age (Yusuf, Daniels, Smith, Coronado, & Rodewald, 2000). In another study, 96% of prison inmates and 54% of jail inmates completed an HBV immunization series when it was offered in the correctional setting. Since inmates are at high risk for HBV, routine immunization in correctional settings has been recommended. Unfortunately, some of the immunization programs initiated have been discontinued due to lack of funds (Kelley et al., 2004). Unimmunized adolescents, who are at high risk for HBV infection from both sexual and drug use behaviors, should also receive HBV vaccine. HBV vaccine is also recommended for MSM, but a study of vaccine coverage in several U.S. cities indicated that only about 9% of persons in this group had been immunized. Similarly, only 6% of injection drug users in another study and 75% of occupationally exposed health care workers have been immunized (Willis et al., 2005).

Bacille Calmette–Guerin (BCG) vaccine is used for TB prevention in some parts of the world, but has been found to be only partially effective. In addition, use of BCG vaccine causes tuberculin skin tests to become reactive and invalidates skin tests as a screening measure for tuberculosis. New vaccines for TB are being developed, and several are currently being tested in animals, so a more effective vaccine may be available in the future.

Influenza vaccine has been shown to be highly effective in preventing disease or mitigating its severity when the vaccine is developed for strains of virus prevalent in a given year. In fact, immunization is 70% to 90% effective among healthy people under 65 years of age. Influenza vaccine is also cost-effective, with an estimated average savings of $13.66 per year per person immunized. Influenza vaccine must be received annually and is recommended for all persons over 65 years of age, people at increased risk for complications due to chronic illness, pregnant women who will be in the second or third trimester of pregnancy during influenza season, people in institutional settings, and people who live with or care for persons in high-risk groups (Harper, Fukuda, Uyeki, Cox, & Bridges, 2005). Community health nurses can advocate for available immunization services for vulnerable populations. They may also need to engage in political advocacy to assure an adequate supply of vaccine each year.

Health care workers, in particular, should receive influenza vaccine to minimize their potential for developing the disease and transmitting it to vulnerable clients and to minimize absenteeism in periods where hospital censuses are high (Pearson et al., 2006). Unfortunately, many people do not receive influenza immunizations. During the 2003 influenza season, for example, only 8.4% of children aged 6 to 23 months received the vaccine (Santibanez, Singleton, et al., 2006). Similarly, less than 68% of White non-Hispanic elderly U.S. residents were immunized in 2003, and immunization rates were even lower in other racial/ethnic groups (Black non-Hispanic—48%, Hispanic—45.4%) (Youngpairoj, Euler, Lu, Bridges, & Wortley, 2005). During the 2004–2005 influenza season, approximately 63% of people over age 65, 36% of health care workers, and 25.5% of people aged 18 to 64 with high-risk conditions received influenza immunization (Division of Adult and Community Health, 2005).

The extent of vaccine coverage in a population is affected by a number of variables, including perceptions of vaccine effectiveness and fear of possible adverse consequences of immunization. For example, in 2003, misunderstandings and misrepresentations about the safety of polio vaccine led leaders in part of one country to reject polio immunization campaigns. This response resulted in widespread disease as well as the reintroduction of polio into several previously polio-free nations (Aylward & Heymann, 2005). Vaccination coverage is also influenced by vaccine availability and distribution. For example, in periods of vaccine shortage, children served by public immunization clinics, those in rural areas, and those in the southeastern United States have been found to have less extensive vaccine coverage than other child populations, suggesting inequitable distribution of available supplies of vaccine (Santibanez, Santoli, & Barker, 2006). Similarly, American Indian/Alaska Native children served by Indian Health Service centers were less likely to receive needed immunizations than children in other settings (Groom, Cheek, & Bryan, 2006).

At present, there are no vaccines for most STDs; for hepatitis C, D, or E; or for HIV infection. In 2006, however, a vaccine was approved to prevent human papillomavirus (HPV) infection, which causes genital warts and contributes to cervical cancer. Because hepatitis D can only occur in the presence of HBV infection, HBV immunization is an effective prevention measure. There is also some potential for development of a vaccine for HIV infection, although development is complicated by the ease with which the virus mutates and the fact that it is not inherently containable by the human immune system as other vaccine-preventable diseases

are. Like HIV, development of a vaccine for HCV infection is hampered by rapid mutation of the virus (Des Jarlais & Schuchat, 2001).

Community health nurses educate the public regarding the need for immunizations. They are also frequently involved in planning, implementing, and evaluating immunization campaigns and in giving immunizations to susceptible individuals. When nurses actually provide immunizations, they are also involved in educating clients regarding normal reactions to vaccines and comfort measures that may be taken to address them (e.g., non-aspirin antipyretics for fever or pain following DTP immunization) as well as signs of potential adverse reactions. In addition, nurses should also caution parents of children who receive oral polio vaccine regarding the potential for shedding live polio virus and infecting immunocompromised family members.

Community health nurses may also advocate for access to immunization services for all segments of the population and may be involved in the enactment and enforcement of immunization policies designed to protect the general public. For example, community health nurses might advocate requirements that college entrants provide evidence of measles immunity or that varicella immunization be required for preschool or elementary school entry.

POSTEXPOSURE PROPHYLAXIS (PEP) AND CONTACT NOTIFICATION Postexposure prophylaxis (PEP), or the use of medications to prevent the onset of disease in exposed individuals, is another primary preventive measure for communicable diseases. When individuals are prevented from developing symptomatic disease, they are usually also prevented from spreading the disease to others.

PEP usually occurs in the context of contact identification and notification. Contact identification involves interviewing a person with a specific communicable disease to elicit names and contact information for other people who might have been exposed to the disease. Identification is based on the period of incubation and communicability of the disease as well as the mode of transmission and specific vulnerable populations. For example, a client with rubella would be asked to identify any pregnant women with whom he or she had been in contact in the week before or after development of the characteristic rash. A client with primary syphilis, on the other hand, would be interviewed to elicit all sexual contacts or injection drug partners in the 3 months prior to diagnosis. Community health nurses are often involved in both contact identification and notification. In some jurisdictions, however, contact identification may be undertaken by public health investigators who may follow up with contact notification or transmit contact information to community health nurses for follow-up. In other jurisdictions, community health nurses may elicit contact information that

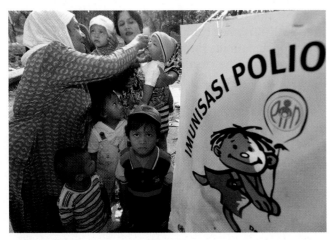

Immunization is one approach to preventing some communicable diseases. (2005 AFP)

is then transmitted to public health investigators. Finally, public health investigators may engage in both identification and notification of contacts and refer them to the community health nurse or other provider for diagnostic and treatment services.

Contact notification is the process of identifying persons who have been exposed to a communicable disease, informing them of exposure, testing them for the particular disease, and offering PEP to prevent them from becoming symptomatic and exposing others. In the context of sexually transmitted diseases, contact notification is referred to as *partner notification* and is defined as a "process whereby sex partners of patients (index cases) who have an STD or HIV diagnosed are informed of their exposure to infection and the need to seek medical evaluation" (Division of HIV Prevention, 2004, p. 129).

Contact notification can be carried out in one of two ways: client referral and provider referral. In client referral, individuals who are known to have a communicable disease notify their contacts themselves and refer them for testing and possible treatment. In provider referral, designated health care personnel solicit names of contacts from infected persons and notify the contacts of potential exposure. When given the option, many people with communicable diseases select provider referral as the preferred mechanism of contact notification. In other instances, they may prefer to notify their contacts themselves. Studies have indicated, for example, that approximately 20% of people notified through provider referral of exposure to HIV infection are themselves infected (Division of HIV/AIDS Prevention, 2003b), so contact notification is an effective means of preventing the spread of disease to others. Similarly, two thirds of contacts to persons with active infectious TB in one large study had reactive tuberculin skin tests and 2% had active TB (American Thoracic Society et al., 2005). Contact notification is one of the primary mechanisms for controlling the spread of TB, and specific guidelines for investigation of contacts have been developed by the National Tuberculosis Controllers Association and CDC (2005). Considerations in TB contact notification are presented at right. These considerations could be adapted to contact notification for many communicable diseases.

Community health nurses are frequently involved in the provider referral approach to contact notification. The process used is systematic and begins with an interview of the client with a communicable disease. In this interview, the community health nurse explains the need for notification, testing, and possible treatment of contacts, and then elicits names, addresses, and other information that will allow contacts to be located and informed of their exposure. Depending on how the notification system is organized, this same nurse may follow up on contacts whose names were elicited or communi-

SPECIAL CONSIDERATIONS

CONTACT NOTIFICATION FOR TB DISEASE

- Determine priorities for contact investigation based on the disease site, sputum smear and nucleic acid amplification assay (NAA) results (used to indicate infection caused by *M. tuberculosis* versus other less communicable strains of mycobacteria), and chest radiography findings. Priority should be given to notification of contacts of persons with:
  - Pulmonary TB (versus extrapulmonary forms of TB that are less communicable)
  - Positive acid fast smear results
  - Cavitation noted on chest x-ray (presence of cavities in lung tissue due to TB damage)
- Define the period of infectiousness (e.g., the time during which contact with the infected person would most likely have led to exposure to TB).
- Review medical records for transmission risk and infectiousness.
- Interview the infected person for names and locator information for close contacts and locations frequented by the infected person (e.g., workplace, church, etc.) where others might have had consistent and prolonged exposure to the client.
- Notify contacts of their exposure and arrange for tuberculin testing.
- Assess contacts for signs and symptoms of TB disease.
- Identify and make referrals to sources of health care.
- Identify additional contacts.
- Educate contacts about PEP.
- Assess contact's psychosocial needs that might interfere with follow-up compliance.
- Reinforce confidentiality.
- Arrange for treatment of contacts with LTBI or active disease and other high-risk contacts (e.g., family members).
- Conduct contact investigations among special populations as needed (e.g., homeless shelter residents, school personnel and students, inmates).

Data from: American Thoracic Society, CDC, and Infectious Diseases Society of America. (2005). Controlling Tuberculosis in the United States: Recommendations from the American Thoracic Society, CDC, and the Infectious Diseases Society of America. Morbidity and Mortality Weekly Report, *54(RR-12), 1–81.*

cate this information to another health care provider (frequently another community health nurse) who will get in touch with the individuals named. The identity of the client with the communicable disease from whom the names were elicited is not included in the information communicated.

Nurses involved in contact follow-up may make home visits or approach contacts at work or any other place where they can be located. When they approach contacts, nurses should speak to them in a setting that ensures privacy and inform them that they have been exposed to a communicable disease. Nurses frequently need to exercise creativity to prevent others from knowing why the person is being contacted by a nurse.

The nurse who approaches the contact never divulges information about the source of the exposure, but explains that the person has potentially been exposed to a communicable disease. In addition to notifying the contact regarding the exposure, the nurse educates the client about the potential for developing the disease and for spreading it to others and refers the client for testing and treatment for the condition as needed.

The purpose of contact notification is to identify persons who may be infected or in need of PEP. PEP is available for tuberculosis, gonorrhea, syphilis, hepatitis A and B, measles, *Haemophilus influenzae* type B (HiB) infection, diphtheria, tetanus, and rabies. PEP is also warranted for people exposed to HIV infection and other diseases such as anthrax and rabies. Approaches to PEP for communicable diseases include booster vaccination or immediate immunization for unimmunized contacts, immune globulins, antibiotics or antiviral medications, and provision of antitoxins. Community health nurses may actually provide PEP for some conditions (e.g., hepatitis, gonorrhea, and syphilis) under treatment protocols. More often, however, they will refer persons who have been exposed to communicable diseases to other private health care providers or public clinics for screening and PEP services.

Immediate postexposure immunization should be given to people exposed to pertussis, and may be given after exposure to polio, mumps, or rubella, although its efficacy in these three diseases is unknown. Booster immunizations should be given to previously immunized persons exposed to diphtheria, tetanus, and pertussis, and in the case of smallpox exposure. Postexposure varicella immunization is also recommended for people exposed to varicella virus with no contraindications for vaccination (CDC, 2006a).

Immune globulin (IG) is an effective prophylactic measure in measles, tetanus, and varicella, and following exposure to HAV or HBV infection (Mast et al., 2005). Hepatitis B IG may also be effective in preventing hepatitis D by virtue of preventing HBV infection, which must be present for HDV to occur. Hepatitis A IG may be given prophylactically either prior to exposure (e.g., prior to travel to endemic areas) or postexposure (National Center for Infectious Diseases, 2000a). IG administration does not appear to affect development of diseases such as rubella, mumps, HCV infection, or HEV infection. In February 2006, an investigational varicella zoster immune globulin product was made available. Its use is recommended for people in certain high-risk categories including immunocompromised clients; neonates born to mothers with symptoms of varicella at the time of delivery; premature infants born after 28 weeks gestation whose mothers do not demonstrate immunity; infants born prior to 28 weeks gestation or with birth weights less than 1,000 grams, regardless of the mothers' immune status, who are exposed to varicella in the neonatal period; and pregnant women (CDC, 2006a).

Antibiotics and antivirals are used to prevent disease after exposure to diphtheria, pertussis, HiB, HIV, TB, many STDs (e.g., gonorrhea, syphilis, and Chlamydia), anthrax, and influenza. TB prophylaxis should be given to all close contacts of persons with TB as well as persons with reactive tuberculin skin tests without evidence of active disease. These people are considered to have latent tuberculosis infection (LTBI). An estimated 9.6 to 14.9 million U.S. residents have LTBI, and those at highest risk of progression to active TB disease should be treated with antituberculin agents. Prophylaxis for TB is also recommended for persons with HIV infection, the homeless, foreign-born persons, and detainees and prisoners at high risk for disease. Unfortunately, it is estimated that only approximately half of contacts at risk for TB infection complete PEP (American Thoracic Society et al., 2005).

TB prophylaxis may be complicated by sociocultural factors such as illegal immigration. For example, many undocumented immigrants in the United States have LTBI with high risk of developing active TB due to poor health status and crowded living conditions. Unfortunately, fear of deportation may lead illegal immigrants to use multiple identities or for several people to share one identity, making contact notification and PEP treatment difficult (Kim et al., 2003).

Treatment with HAART has been shown to be effective in preventing vertical transmission of HIV infection from mother to infant. In 2005, the U.S. Department of Health and Human Services recommended PEP with a 28-day course of HAART initiated within 72 hours of nonoccupational exposure to blood, genital secretions, or other potentially infectious body fluids of someone known to have HIV infection (Smith, Grohskopf, et al., 2005). The CDC has developed specific guidelines for the prevention of common opportunistic infections in HIV-infected individuals (Kaplan, Masur, & Holmes, 2002).

Antiviral agents, such as amantadine, rimantadine, zanamivir, or oseltamivir, may be used in conjunction with influenza vaccine for prophylaxis. Use of these agents is recommended for persons immunized after the influenza season has started, for caretakers of persons at high risk for complications due to influenza, and in persons with diminished immune function (Bridges et al., 2003). Finally, tetanus antitoxin may be given as PEP for tetanus. Community health nurses are often involved in referring clients for PEP and may provide PEP themselves under established treatment protocols. For example, many community health nurses employed in official public health agencies administer IG to persons exposed to hepatitis A and B or monitor TB prophylaxis for people with LTBI.

Health care workers are often the recipients of PEP after occupational exposures to a variety of organisms. PEP is highly recommended for health care workers with LTBI and for those with HIV exposures. PEP following occupational exposure to HIV infection depends on the type and extent of exposure and the communicability of the source case. For example, in people with severe percutaneous exposures to HIV-positive clients with symptomatic infection, AIDS, or a known high viral load, a three-drug regimen is recommended. A basic two-drug regimen is recommended for less severe percutaneous exposures to clients who are known to be HIV positive but are asymptomatic or have low known viral loads. For mucous membrane and intact skin exposures, a two-drug regimen is recommended for large-volume exposures to clients with symptomatic infection, and may be considered for small-volume exposures to asymptomatic clients. Generally, no PEP is recommended when exposure is to the blood or body fluids of someone who is HIV negative or when HIV status is unknown, but a two-drug regimen may be considered when the source of exposure has risk factors for HIV infection (Panlilio et al., 2005). Community health nurses may need to advocate for effective PEP policies for specific vulnerable populations (e.g., homeless persons or inmates in correctional settings). They may also need to advocate for funding for and development of easily accessible services for the general public.

The issue of PEP is of particular concern with respect to bioterrorist-initiated exposure to pathogenic microorganisms. Because of probable drug shortages, PEP will need to be reserved for people who have experienced actual or probable exposure rather than provided to the general public. Community health nurses will be actively involved in educating the public regarding who should obtain PEP and dissuading those who are not candidates for PEP from overburdening the health care delivery system. They and other public health professionals will help to educate the public and health care providers in the private sector regarding indications for PEP and priorities for dispensing PEP in a given bioterrorist situation.

OTHER PRIMARY PREVENTION MEASURES Other primary prevention measures for communicable diseases may be directed toward the mode of transmission of specific diseases. Primary prevention for tetanus due to puncture wounds, for example, involves educating clients on the use of protective clothing (e.g., gloves, boots) to prevent injuries and the need for adequate cleansing of wounds with soap and water when injuries do occur. Effective wound care is also critical in preventing rabies after animal bites (Palmer et al., 2006). Disinfection of equipment, including computer keyboards, in health care settings also helps to prevent the spread of communicable diseases (Rutala et al., 2006).

For STDs, refraining from sexual activity is the most effective means of preventing diseases. For those who are sexually active, however, use of condoms and refraining from unsafe sexual practices may limit exposure to disease. Making condoms available to sexually active adolescents, in particular, may decrease the spread of STDs

(Blake et al., 2003). MSM and others who engage in high-risk sexual behaviors (e.g., with multiple partners, anal receptive intercourse) should also be encouraged to use condoms. Community health nurses can advocate for condom use with sexually active clients who engage in high-risk behaviors. They may also educate clients on the correct use of condoms or may advocate for condom availability to special groups like adolescents or correctional inmates. Community health nurses can also inform clients who engage in oral–genital intercourse as a mode of contraception that they continue to be at risk for STD transmission.

Use of microbicides may also provide some protection against STDs, including HIV infection. Unlike condoms, microbicide use is a strategy that can be used by women independent of their partners, providing an avenue for protection for women who are unable to negotiate condom use with their partners. In one study in four African and Asian countries, 73% of women indicated willingness to use microbicides. Willingness to use microbicides approached 100% in African nations where HIV infection rates are highest (Bentley et al., 2004). Research has indicated, however, that some microbicides (e.g., nonoxynol-9) are not effective in preventing HIV infection (Nielsen & Bartlett, 2004), but there are approximately 60 other products in development that may prove effective (Bentley et al., 2004). Again, community health nurses can encourage microbicide use by clients who are at risk for STD exposure and can educate them in their use. They may also be involved in advocacy to assure that microbicides are available to those in need of them. For example, they may work to include microbicides under health insurance coverage or to provide access to microbicides to women of low socioeconomic status.

Given the great disparities in HIV/AIDS incidence, targeted interventions that involve multisectoral participation should be developed. For example, partnerships among governmental agencies, community organizations,

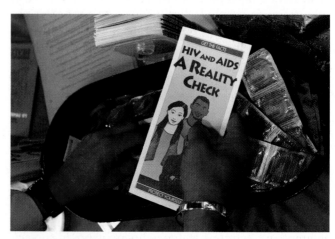

Condoms are an effective means of preventing sexually transmitted diseases. (Joe Raedle/Getty)

educational institutions, and faith-based groups have been suggested to address these disparities by targeting interventions to high-risk groups such as Blacks, Hispanics, and MSM (Prejean et al., 2006). Community health nurses can assist in these endeavors by helping with coalition building as discussed in Chapter 13∞. Because of their knowledge of communities and their connections with various segments of the community, nurses can motivate participation by diverse groups in community-wide initiatives.

Primary prevention for bloodborne diseases such as HIV/AIDS and hepatitis B, C, and D involves prevention of drug use or promotion of harm-reduction strategies such as needle exchanges and education on safer drug use procedures. Because these strategies are often not acceptable to the general public or to health policy makers, community health nurses may be involved in advocacy to establish needle exchange programs and other harm-reduction strategies. Infection through occupational exposure to bloodborne diseases can be prevented by means of universal precautions for the handling of blood and other bodily secretions and excretions. Unfortunately, many persons in these occupations fail to use universal precautions, increasing their risk of disease. Screening of blood and tissue donors for HIV and for hepatitis B, C, and D has virtually eliminated transmission of these diseases by means of transfusion.

For hepatitis A and E, control measures are aimed at improving sanitation, protecting food and water from contamination, and promoting adequate handwashing. Washing fruits and vegetables before eating, boiling contaminated water, and discouraging use of human waste as fertilizer may also serve to prevent both diseases in developing countries. Community health nurses can educate people regarding adequate hygiene and the need to wash fruits and vegetables before eating them, particularly those imported from other countries. They can also discourage consumption of shellfish retrieved from contaminated waters and promote environmental policies that prevent contamination of shellfish beds. In addition, nurses can advocate for effective sanitation and enforcement of food processing techniques that minimize the potential for bacterial contamination.

Community health nurses may also collaborate with environmental specialists to address issues of food or water contamination with pathogens. For example, the nurse might alert water authorities regarding a sudden increase in diarrheal diseases in a particular neighborhood, suggesting that water sources may be contaminated. Or the nurse might identify unsanitary conditions in a restaurant and notify the appropriate inspectors. The roles and functions of other public health personnel are described in more detail in Chapter 22∞.

Prevention of crowding and promotion of adequate nutrition are control measures for conditions such as TB and influenza. Other primary prevention measures include the use of adequate ventilation and ultraviolet light in areas that increase the risk of TB transmission. For example, areas in which aerosol sputum specimens are collected provide an environment conducive to the spread of disease that can be modified using these measures. Providing appropriate facilities for isolating infectious clients in hospitals and other institutions also minimizes the risk of transmission to health care personnel. Community health nurses can work with environmental engineers to address such problems or collaborate with housing authority personnel to address housing conditions conducive to diseases.

Prevention of tickborne diseases involves use of tick repellents, avoidance of tall grass and other vegetation, and use of protective clothing. Frequent inspections of people and pets for ticks is also recommended. Wearing light-colored clothing may make ticks more visible. Ticks should be removed as soon as possible by grasping them with tweezers close to the skin and exerting steady pressure to gently detach them from the skin. Ticks should not be crushed between the fingers after removal to prevent contamination, and hands and bite wounds should be carefully washed with soap and water and disinfected (Chapman, 2006).

Environmental measures for preventing exposure to tickborne diseases include use of pesticides on lawns, removal of brush and leaf litter from around homes, and creating buffer zones of wood chips or gravel between wooded or brushy areas and human habitations (Division of Vector-borne Infectious Diseases, 2004). Similarly, removal of standing water and other breeding grounds for mosquitoes can help prevent mosquito-borne diseases such as WNV infection. Pregnant women, in particular, should avoid mosquito exposure, use insect repellent, wear long sleeves and long pants, and avoid being outdoors at dawn and dusk to minimize the risk of WNV infection for themselves and their infants (Division of Birth Defects and Developmental Disabilities, 2004). Community health nurses often work with environmental specialists and veterinarians to address diseases transmitted from animals to humans.

Other measures that aid in the control of communicable diseases include legislation requiring screening for specific diseases in high-risk groups, mandatory reporting of cases of communicable disease with contact notification and follow-up, and regulation of potential vehicles of transmission such as insects. Community health nursing involvement in other control measures for communicable diseases generally lies in educating the public and individual clients regarding prevention and in identifying and helping to eliminate risk factors for exposure and disease.

PANDEMIC AND BIOTERRORISM PREPAREDNESS One further aspect of primary prevention related to communicable disease addresses preparation for a possible pandemic or bioterrorist event. As we saw in Chapter 27∞, community health nurses are actively involved in identifying the potential for and probable community effects of such disasters. For example, they would identify risk factors for infection in the population in the event of a pandemic (e.g., segments of the population with poor nutritional status that puts them at particular risk for serious disease). They would also be involved in planning for community response to a pandemic or bioterrorist attack. In addition, community health nurses would be actively involved in informing the public regarding preventive measures or other appropriate responses to the threat of a pandemic or bioterrorist event.

Bioterrorism and pandemic preparedness are important not only because of the potential for significant morbidity and mortality resulting from either event, but also because of other population effects that might occur. For example, either a pandemic or a bioterrorist-caused epidemic might cause severe economic effects as a result of business closures to prevent spread of the disease. Availability of food and other essential goods might also be impaired if production and transportation systems are severely affected. Short-term educational effects might also be noted if schools are closed for extended periods of time. One of the most serious effects might be the burden placed on an already overburdened health care system if health care personnel become ill in significant numbers. There is also the problem of inadequate facilities and supplies (including drugs and vaccines) needed to address widespread communicable disease incidence. Preparedness will help to mitigate these potential effects, although it is unlikely that they can be prevented altogether. Primary prevention strategies for communicable diseases, including pandemic and bioterrorism preparedness, are summarized in Table 28-4◆.

TABLE 28-4	Community Health Nursing Interventions in Primary Prevention of Communicable Diseases
Focus	**Community Health Nursing Interventions**
Immunization	▪ Educate clients and the public regarding the need for immunizations.
	▪ Refer clients for immunization services.
	▪ Provide immunization services.
	▪ Advocate for access to immunization services for all segments of the population.
Contact notification	▪ Educate providers regarding the legal requirements for reporting communicable diseases.
	▪ Interview clients with communicable diseases for names and locating information for close contacts.
	▪ Inform contacts of their exposure to a communicable disease.
	▪ Refer contacts for testing and PEP as needed.
	▪ Educate clients regarding preventive measures and the need to prevent the spread of disease to others.
	▪ Advocate for and plan effective contact notification services.
	▪ Promote contact notification by other health care providers and educate them regarding contact notification.
Postexposure prophylaxis	▪ Refer clients for PEP services as needed.
	▪ Provide PEP under established protocols.
	▪ Monitor and promote compliance with PEP among contacts.
	▪ Monitor for adverse effects and side effects of PEP and refer for medical evaluation if needed.
	▪ Advocate for the availability of PEP for clients in need.
Other primary prevention measures	▪ Promote adequate nutrition, rest, and other facets of good health.
	▪ Educate clients and the public regarding effective wound care.
	▪ Educate clients and the public on safe sexual practices, use of condoms, etc.
	▪ Prevent drug abuse or refer clients for drug abuse treatment.
	▪ Promote harm-reduction strategies to prevent infection among IDUs.
	▪ Promote use of universal precautions for bloodborne diseases.
	▪ Promote adequate handwashing, washing of produce, etc.
	▪ Advocate for adequate sanitation.
	▪ Advocate for policies and processes that prevent contamination of food and water supplies.
	▪ Promote adequate housing to prevent crowding and allow for adequate ventilation.
	▪ Promote use of ultraviolet light in settings where exposure to pathogens is common.
	▪ Advocate for preventive education and services.

Continued on next page

TABLE 28-4	Community Health Nursing Interventions in Primary Prevention of Communicable Diseases *(continued)*
Focus	**Community Health Nursing Interventions**
Pandemic and bioterrorism preparedness	▪ Assist in identifying the potential for a pandemic or bioterrorist event.
	▪ Assist in identifying particularly vulnerable populations and factors influencing their vulnerability.
	▪ Participate in planning community response to a pandemic or bioterrorist event.
	▪ Educate the public and other health care providers regarding prevention of illness or self-care during a pandemic or bioterrorist event.
	▪ Educate the public regarding the signs and symptoms of disease resulting from a pandemic or bioterrorist event and sources of treatment.

Secondary Prevention

Secondary prevention activities in relation to communicable diseases include case finding and surveillance, screening, diagnosis and reporting, and treatment.

CASE FINDING AND SURVEILLANCE Because they serve large segments of the population who may not receive care from other health care providers, community health nurses are in a unique position to identify possible cases of communicable diseases. Once a person with a potential communicable disease has been identified, the community health nurse may make a referral for further diagnosis and treatment. In some cases, the nurse may be involved in diagnosing and treating communicable diseases on the basis of medically approved protocols. The case finding function of the community health nurse was discussed in general in Chapter 1∞.

To identify a possible case of a communicable disease, community health nurses need to be familiar with the signs and symptoms of communicable diseases commonly seen in their area. They should also be familiar with the signs and symptoms of diseases that may result from bioterrorist activities. Signs and symptoms and other information regarding specific communicable diseases are described in Appendix E on the Companion Website.

Case finding at the population level contributes to surveillance. As we saw in Chapter 27∞, surveillance involves the gathering and analysis of data that reflect trends in disease incidence and prevalence as well as information on the effects of disease within the population. Community health nurses may collect surveillance data or identify cases of disease that are reported to local epidemiologists for inclusion in surveillance systems. Analysis of surveillance data is usually undertaken by epidemiologists or health information system specialists and the results of the analysis conveyed to public health officials and other health policy makers.

SCREENING Screening is presumptive identification of asymptomatic persons with disease. Screening may involve either selective or mass screening. **Selective screening** is directed toward persons exhibiting risk factors for a particular disease. **Mass screening** involves screening an entire population regardless of the level of risk among individuals (Friis & Sellers, 2003).

Screening is not generally done for communicable diseases that have a short incubation period such as measles, rubella, influenza, and so on. Screening tests are available, however, for diseases such as HIV/AIDS, hepatitis A, B, and C, TB, and STDs such as gonorrhea, syphilis, Chlamydia, and HSV infection.

Screening for HIV infection is recommended for all pregnant women at entry into prenatal care, and a second test during the third trimester of pregnancy is recommended for women with elevated risk for infection. The availability and acceptability of rapid testing have even made screening at the time of delivery feasible for women of unknown HIV status or those with high levels of risk (Mofenson et al., 2006). Screening is also recommended for other persons at risk for infection including injection drug users, men who have sex with men, and those with multiple sexual partners. In the 2005 HIV testing component of the National HIV Behavioral Surveillance (NHBS) system, 25% of MSM tested were infected with HIV; of these, 48% were not aware of their infection. As a result of these and similar findings, it is recommended that MSM should be screened for HIV infection at least annually (Sifakis et al., 2005). Overall, an estimated 250,000 people in the United States may have HIV infection without being aware of it. One strategy that has been suggested to improve identification of those with undiagnosed HIV infection is social networking. A social network strategy involves using HIV-infected clients and those at high risk for infection to recruit people from their social, sexual, and drug-use networks for HIV screening, counseling, and referral for treatment, if needed (Emerson et al., 2005). Because of widespread promotion of HIV testing, greater numbers of people are being screened. In 2002, for example, about half the people in the United States aged 15 to 45 years reported having a test for HIV infection at some time (Fenton & Valdiserri, 2006).

It has also been suggested that routine HIV screening should take place in the context of other services and in specific settings. For example, routine HIV screening in urgent care centers in Massachusetts has been shown to be an effective approach to identifying people with HIV infection (Massachusetts Department of Public Health, 2004; Walensky et al., 2005). Similarly, screening has been suggested for high-risk populations such as correctional inmates and injection drug users or people seeking

MediaLink Appendix E: Selected Communicable Diseases

treatment for other STDs. Routine screening for syphilis in the context of treatment for gonorrhea and Chlamydia has also been suggested as a mechanism for identifying those infected, particularly during an outbreak (Rosenman et al., 2004). Screening of all sexually active women under 26 years of age and pregnant women of all ages for *Chlamydia trachomatis* infection is also recommended (Shih et al., 2004). Community health nurses can advocate for screening of sexually active women for a variety of STDs during routine health promotion visits. They may also be involved in educating other health care providers regarding the need for screening.

Because of the close relationship between TB and HIV infection, persons with TB and their close contacts may also benefit from HIV screening (Division of Tuberculosis Elimination, 2000). Conversely, TB screening is recommended by the World Health Organization after HIV diagnosis, before initiation of HAART, and periodically during routine follow-up care of clients with HIV infection. In Cambodia, for example, TB screening is required as a precondition for HAART. It is also suggested that integrating TB and HIV services will increase TB screening rates and promote better control of both diseases (Vannarith et al., 2005).

Two concerns with respect to HIV screening are confidentiality and the length of time before results are known. MSM may be particularly concerned about confidentiality issues because of the twofold potential for stigmatization related to homosexual behavior and to HIV infection. Confidentiality concerns may deter people from being tested or encourage them to use anonymous testing. Anonymous testing, however, makes it impossible to notify persons with positive tests who do not return for their results. For this reason, screening tests that provide same-day results are preferred, particularly for pregnant women, to ensure prompt initiation of treatment for HIV infection (Cohen et al., 2003).

Pregnant women and persons at risk should also be screened for STDs and HBV (Mast et al., 2005). Emergency departments and correctional settings have been recommended as sites for STD screening because of the high incidence of STDs in these settings. For example, some authors have suggested screening all correctional inmates for HCV, not only those with a history of IDU. In one study, 66% of male inmates who were HCV positive did not give any history of IDU, suggesting that many cases would be missed if screening is targeted only to those with identified risk factors (Macalino, Dhawan, & Rich, 2005). Screening for TB should also be a routine procedure in correctional settings and among injection drug users, and community health nurses may need to actively advocate for screening as a regular practice in correctional and drug treatment settings. TB screening is cost-effective in high-risk groups. For example, targeted screening of foreign-born children in public school systems in Maryland has been found to be effective in identifying children with LTBI as well as a few with active

EVIDENCE-BASED PRACTICE

*R*esearch suggests that voluntary HIV screening should be implemented with specific high-risk population groups, such as pregnant women, correctional inmates, and people who seek treatment for STDs. To what extent are these recommendations incorporated in prenatal, correctional, and STD services in your area? What are the barriers to implementing this approach to evidence-based practice? How might these barriers be overcome?

TB. Approximately 90% of children found to have LTBI completed prophylactic treatment, and based on program results, it was estimated that every dollar spent on screening saved two dollars in lifetime costs of disease treatment (Chang, Wheeler, & Farrell, 2002).

Drug users should be screened for HIV infection as well as hepatitis B and C. Routine screening for HCV is not warranted for health care personnel or first responders unless other risk factors are present. Screening should occur with exposure to HCV-infected blood, however. Another population that should be screened for HCV is recipients of transfusions prior to 1992, when blood donors began to be tested for HCV. Although attempts have been made to contact recipients who received blood from donors known to be infected with HCV, many people have not been located and may be unaware of their risk for disease (Buffington, Rowell, Hinman, Sharp, & Choi, 2001). (See Appendix E on the Companion Website for information on screening for selected communicable diseases.)

Tuberculosis screening is recommended for health care workers as well as persons in congregate settings such as prisons, long-term-care facilities, and residential settings (e.g., university dormitories) (Pratt et al., 2006). Screening of health care workers may employ tuberculin skin tests (TSTs) or whole-blood interferon gamma release assays such as QuantiFERON®-TB Gold Test (QFT-G), a blood assay for *M. tuberculosis* (BAMT). A two-step screening process is recommended in settings using TSTs when those tested have not had a tuberculin test within 12 months. In the two-step test, a TST is given and read within 48 to 72 hours. If the test result is negative, a second TST is administered 1 to 2 weeks later. A two-step process helps to increase the accuracy of results in persons with prior mycobacterial infections, exposure to BCG vaccine, early TB infection, or depressed cell-mediated immunity (e.g., persons with HIV infection) (Campos-Outcalt, 2005). The initial test helps to "boost" the body's response to the tuberculin derivative used in the skin test and results in a positive second test. Two-step testing prevents "boosted" reactions from being interpreted as new infections (Francis J. Curry National Tuberculosis Center, 2004). A positive or significant reaction to TST is based on the degree of induration that results (American Lung Association, 2005). **Induration** is a palpable, hard, raised area around the injection site with clearly defined margins.

Induration does not refer to redness around the injection site. In a person with normal immune function, an area of induration of 15 mm or greater is considered a significant reaction. For health care providers or persons with underlying kidney disease or diabetes, 10 mm or more induration is considered positive, and 5 mm is considered a significant reaction for someone who is immunocompromised (Shiel, 2005). A positive tuberculin skin test is shown in the picture below. The area of induration in the picture is demarcated with ink on all four sides.

Based on CDC recommendations, TB surveillance among health care workers should include all those who have face-to-face contact with persons who have suspected or confirmed TB disease. This includes not only health care providers, but also transport staff, administrators, custodial staff, and others who may come in contact with TB-infected clients (Jensen et al., 2005). Community health nurses may need to advocate for screening among ancillary personnel as well as direct providers of care.

The frequency of TB screening among health workers is determined by the degree of exposure risk in the setting (low or medium). Risk is a function of the size of the clientele (e.g., bed size of a hospital) and the number of TB diagnoses made in the previous year. For example, an inpatient setting with fewer than 200 beds and more than three TB patients would be classified as a medium-risk setting, and health care workers should be screened at employment and annually thereafter. The cutoff for low risk in a larger institution (more than 200 beds) would be six TB patients. Health care workers in low-risk settings should be screened at the time of employment, but negative screening results need not be repeated unless exposure occurs (Jensen et al., 2005).

TB screening is also recommended for immigrants from countries with high TB incidence rates because of the prevalence of TB among foreign-born persons in the United States. As noted earlier, nearly half of U.S. TB occurs among foreign-born persons. Additional recommendations include treating immigrants with latent TB infection and coordinating control efforts across the U.S.–Mexico border and between immigration authorities and local health departments. Finally, screening, diagnostic, and treatment capabilities should be enhanced in host countries and areas where immigrants are evaluated (Pratt et al., 2006).

Community health nurses may refer individuals at risk for disease to appropriate screening resources. Many community health nurses may also be involved in conducting screening examinations and tests and in counseling clients regarding test results and their implications. Community health nurses may also need to advocate for the availability of screening services and for follow-up and treatment (therapeutic or prophylactic) of persons with positive screening tests.

DIAGNOSIS AND REPORTING Diagnosis of many communicable diseases relies on serologic evidence of disease markers or the actual presence of causative organisms. For example, diagnostic tests for syphilis and hepatitis A, B, C, and D rely on the presence of specific antibodies in the blood of infected persons. More sophisticated tests for syphilis, on the other hand, are based on demonstration of the presence of the actual causative organism in the bloodstream and are used when antibody-based tests are inconclusive. Similarly, tests for gonorrhea involve cultures of urine or urethral, vaginal, anal, or pharyngeal specimens for growth of *Neisseria gonorrhoeae*, and diagnostic tests for Chlamydia infection include culture of specimens for *Chlamydia trachomatis*. Diagnosis of many childhood diseases is based on physical signs and symptoms, with laboratory confirmation for some diseases (e.g., pertussis, diphtheria, tetanus, etc.). Information on specific diagnostic tests for selected communicable diseases is presented in Appendix E on the Companion Website.

Community health nurses may refer suspected cases of communicable diseases for diagnostic confirmation. In addition, nurses may educate clients regarding the types of diagnostic procedures likely to be used. Community health nurses may also be involved in conducting some diagnostic tests for communicable diseases. For example, community health nurses in some agencies routinely draw blood for diagnostic tests for syphilis, collect urine samples for gonorrhea testing, and provide tuberculin skin tests under approved protocols.

Diagnosis of TB is of particular concern worldwide, and the Tuberculosis Coalition for Technical Assistance (2006), a group composed of several national and international agencies, has developed *International Standards for Tuberculosis Care*, which address diagnostic and treatment standards. The diagnostic standards address the following:

- Evaluation of all persons with an unexplained productive cough
- Use of sputum specimens for all people suspected of having TB, including children capable of producing sputum

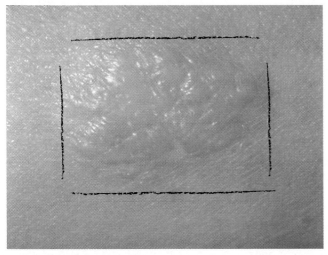

A significant TB skin test showing induration. (National Medical Slide)

MediaLink | Appendix E: Selected Communicable Diseases

- Collection of other appropriate specimens from people suspected of having extrapulmonary TB
- Use of sputum specimens to confirm diagnoses of people with x-ray findings suggesting TB
- Use of gastric washing or other means of specimen collection in children suspected of having TB who cannot expectorate sputum (Tuberculosis Coalition for Technical Assistance, 2006)

The standards also address the necessity for providers who diagnose cases of TB to report their findings to appropriate health authorities and to assure appropriate follow-up for close contacts.

Effective control of communicable diseases requires that diagnoses of many communicable diseases, including TB, be reported to local public health authorities. These reports are then forwarded to state and federal agencies. In the case of some diseases, national agencies report diagnosed cases to WHO. The list of reportable diseases varies somewhat from one jurisdiction to another (usually at the state level), and community health nurses should inform themselves regarding the reportable diseases in their own locale. Laboratories are required to report positive test results for reportable diseases to official public health agencies, and health care providers who make the actual diagnosis are also required to submit a disease notification report. Reports are usually completed by the physician, nurse practitioner, or other health care provider who makes the diagnosis, but in some settings, reports may be made by community health nurses or other nurses.

There are two categories of communicable disease reports: case reports and outbreak reports. Case reports are those related to the diagnosis of individual cases of a particular disease (e.g., measles or HIV infection). Outbreak reports address an increased incidence in the number of cases of a particular disease above that normally expected in the population. Outbreak reports may include diseases that are not normally officially reportable in a given jurisdiction or diseases of unknown etiology in the case of emerging infectious diseases (Heymann, 2004). Outbreak reports of five cases of *Pneumocystis carinii* pneumonia in 1981 led eventually to the identification of AIDS (Fenton & Valdiserri, 2006). Similarly, outbreak reports of an unusual respiratory disease among people attending a Legionnaires' convention in Philadelphia led to the identification of Legionnaires' disease.

Five categories are generally recognized for reporting of communicable diseases (Heymann, 2004). Class 1 diseases are reportable internationally to the World Health Organization under the *International Health Regulations* (IHR). Currently, only cholera, plague, and yellow fever are covered under the IHR. In 2005, however, the IHR were revised to include mandatory reporting of "all events that may constitute a public health emergency of international concern (PHEIC)" (WHO, 2005a, p. 1).

A PHEIC is defined as "an extraordinary public health event which constitutes a public health risk to other states, through the international spread of disease, and may require a coordinated international response" (WHO, 2005a, p. 1). The revised IHR also require nations to respond to requests for information regarding such events and to designate an IHR focal point and contact person to interface with WHO. Additional requirements include development of basic public health capacities to detect, report, and respond to potential public health emergencies and to implement control measures at airports and other international border points. Individual WHO member states have an opportunity to accept or reject the revised IHR or maintain certain reservations with respect to their implementation that are not rejected by other member states. Nonmember states may also accept the regulations, and regulations are legally binding on member and nonmember states that accept them beginning in June 2007 (WHO, 2006a).

For class 2 diseases, a case report is required wherever the disease is diagnosed, and would include all of the officially reportable diseases in a given jurisdiction. For example, the Centers for Disease Control and Prevention (CDC, 2006c) lists 61 disease categories as reportable at the national level. The State of California (2005), on the other hand, mandates reporting for 88 diseases. Class 3 diseases are required to be reported in selected endemic areas (e.g., schistosomiasis, or "snail fever," a blood fluke infestation with worms often carried by certain varieties of snails). Class 4 diseases are required to be reported in the instance of outbreaks only (e.g., diarrheal diseases due to contaminated food), and reporting of individual sporadic diagnoses is not required. Finally, class 5 diseases are not ordinarily reportable because they are uncommon or not directly transmissible from person to person or because reporting does not enhance the potential for controlling the spread of disease (e.g., the common cold) (Heymann, 2004).

TREATMENT Many communicable diseases are treated with antibiotics or antiviral medications, but some diseases such as varicella and uncomplicated measles are treated symptomatically. Antimicrobial treatment is recommended for tickborne diseases as well as for TB, HIV, hepatitis, sexually transmitted diseases, and influenza. Pertussis is another disease for which treatment is available (Tiwari et al., 2005). Treatment for selected communicable diseases commonly encountered by community health nurses is presented in Appendix E on the Companion Website. Other sources of information include federal treatment guidelines such as *Guidelines for Preventing Opportunistic Infections among HIV-infected Persons, 2002* (Kaplan et al., 2002), *Sexually Transmitted Diseases Treatment Guidelines, 2002* (Workowski & Levine, 2002), and *Guidelines for Using Antiretroviral Agents among HIV-infected Adults and Adolescents* (Dybul, Fauci, Bartlett, Kaplan, & Pau, 2002).

Some disease-causing agents are becoming resistant to some of the antimicrobials used in treatment. Experts suggest that some level of drug resistance begins to be noted within 3 years of the introduction of a new drug (Huey, 2004). During the 2005–2006 influenza season, 91% of influenza A viruses tested demonstrated resistance to amantadine and rimantadine, two of the antiretroviral medications most commonly used for PEP and treatment of influenza. Based on these findings, CDC recommended that neither be used for the remainder of the influenza season (Bright et al., 2006). Similarly, a growing proportion of tuberculosis is caused by multi-drug-resistant (MDR) strains. A WHO survey of international laboratories indicated that from 2000 to 2004 24% of tuberculosis isolates were multi-drug-resistant and 2% were extensively drug-resistant (XDR), meaning that they were also resistant to second-line drugs used to treat MDR TB. In the United States, 4.5% of drug-susceptibility testing results indicated strains of *Mycobacterium tuberculosis* resistant to three or more second-line drugs. People with XDR TB are more likely to die during therapy than clients with disease caused by nonresistant microbes (Wright et al., 2006). Fortunately, six new TB drugs that show promise in treating MDR and XDR TB will soon be tested in human beings (Pratt et al., 2006). Antibiotic resistance is fostered by inappropriate use of antibiotics, and community health nurses can be actively involved in educating the general public and health care providers to minimize inappropriate use. They can also advocate for completion of recommended antibiotic therapies (e.g., for TB) to prevent development of resistant microorganisms.

The *International Guidelines for Tuberculosis Care* (Tuberculosis Coalition for Technical Assistance, 2006) includes nine standards for treatment of tuberculosis. The standards address the health care providers' responsibility to provide appropriate treatment and monitor client compliance with treatment, the use of specific drug regimens for initial and continuation treatment at internationally recommended doses, the use of a patient-centered and mutually acceptable approach to treatment that addresses the needs of individual clients, and the need to monitor clients' responses to therapy through follow-up sputum cultures. Additional standards highlight the need for accurate documentation of treatment, bacteriologic effectiveness, and adverse reactions; routine HIV counseling and testing for clients with TB in areas with high rates of HIV infection; assessment of the need for concurrent antiretroviral and anti-tuberculin treatment in clients with both TB and HIV infection and use of cotrimoxazole to prevent other opportunistic infections; assessment of the likelihood of drug resistance and drug susceptibility testing as indicated; and use of specialized treatment regimens for clients with drug-resistant strains of TB.

Treatment of HIV infection with HAART has demonstrated its effectiveness in preventing progression to AIDS, reducing AIDS-related morbidity and mortality, and decreasing communicability (Division of HIV/AIDS Prevention, 2003a). Lack of access to HAART has been a continuing issue in developing nations. As of December 2004, less than 5% of those with HIV infection in WHO's Eastern Mediterranean region were receiving antiretroviral therapy. Rates for therapy were at 10% or less of the HIV-infected population in all regions except the Americas, which had a treatment rate of 65% (WHO, 2005b).

Use of HAART in the United States is also lower than one would wish in some segments of the population. For example, one study of women who were medically eligible for HAART found that one fourth of the women were not using it. Nonuse of HAART has been associated with depression, prior or current alcohol or drug use (particularly crack cocaine and heroin), minority group membership, and a history of physical or sexual abuse. Conversely, appropriate use of HAART is associated with mental health treatment and care from HIV specialists (Cohen et al., 2004). Community health nurses can advocate for the elimination of barriers to HAART use and for the availability of HAART for all segments of the population affected by HIV infection.

Effective treatment of HIV infection is dependent on several factors, including timely identification of

GLOBAL PERSPECTIVES

Lack of access to highly active antiretroviral therapy (HAART) in many developing nations has been highlighted as one of the major deterrents to international HIV/AIDS control. Several international agencies, including the World Bank; the Global Fund to Fight AIDS, Tuberculosis, and Malaria; the Gates and Clinton Foundations; and the World Health Organization, have spearheaded efforts to improve antiretroviral therapy access around the world. McCoy et al. (2005) have noted several pitfalls and dangers associated with such efforts that must be avoided if these initiatives are to have lasting effects. One of the possible effects of such initiatives is the diversion of energy and resources away from other equally important public health issues such as general maternal and child health. It is also feared that a focus on HIV treatment (secondary prevention) may diminish emphasis on primary prevention activities.

A second pitfall is that, in an effort to provide extensive coverage with HAART, other infrastructure elements may be compromised. For example, drug supplies may be insufficient to treat large numbers of people, leading to interruptions in treatment and potential for the development of resistant strains of HIV virus. Widespread efforts may also fail to provide for adequate training of health care providers.

Finally, targeted treatment programs may result in inappropriate "vertical" structures separate from other public health programs. These separate programs may further weaken the public health infrastructure of recipient nations by attracting needed public health personnel into better-paying jobs in private-sector endeavors. There is also the potential for profiteering by private for-profit health care systems that would undermine the accomplishment of program goals. What strategies might be employed to improve access to HAART without succumbing to the pitfalls described here? What kinds of resources would be needed to implement these strategies?

people in need of treatment through effective screening and diagnostic services, suppression of viral replication through use of HAART, and adherence to treatment regimens. Adherence should be promoted with measures to minimize drug toxicity and deal with drug side effects as well as provision of psychosocial support for people with HIV infection (Nielsen & Bartlett, 2004). Community health nurses may be actively involved in supervising HIV therapy and in motivating client compliance. In addition, nurses monitor clients on HAART for adverse effects of medications and assist them to deal with side effects. They may also advocate for the availability of HAART for HIV-infected clients and make referrals to appropriate services for those in need of care.

The International Treatment Preparedness Coalition (2005), an international alliance of HIV/AIDS treatment activists, identified several other barriers that impeded successful implementation of the World Health Organization's *3 by 5* initiative to provide HAART to 3 million people by 2005, which fell one million people short of its goal. The coalition noted that these barriers must be addressed if the subsequent goal of universal access to HAART is to be achieved by the 2010 target date. Barriers identified included:

- Failure of national governments to dedicate sufficient resources to implement HAART programs
- Global systems that create bottlenecks for dissemination of therapeutic services
- Inadequate and uncertain program funding
- Bureaucratic delays in allocation of resources to treatment programs
- Logistical challenges in procurement and dissemination of HAART
- Failure to address pervasive stigma attached to HIV/AIDS that prevents people from initiating therapy

Community health nurses can be active in advocating national policies that support international HAART treatment initiatives. For example, U.S. nurses can advocate for federal assistance to international AIDS endeavors. In addition, nurses may be involved in the efforts of non-governmental organizations to support HIV therapy through their churches or other social organizations. Nurses involved at the international level can assist in the development of policies and procedures that address some of the concerns noted above. In the United States, community health nurses can be involved in research that tests various approaches to providing HAART that may have implications for international implementation.

In addition to assisting with treatment of communicable diseases with antimicrobial agents, community health nurses may provide supportive care for clients with self-limiting diseases that have no specific treatment. Supportive care may include educating clients and families about measures to reduce fever or enhance

comfort until the disease has run its course. For example, parents should be informed of the dangers in giving aspirin for fever in children. Other supportive measures may include encouraging a low-fat diet in hepatitis A to deal with nausea.

TB treatment, and to a lesser extent HIV therapy, rely on a process called directly observed therapy. In **directly observed therapy (DOT)**, a client takes his or her medication in the presence of a nurse or other health care provider. In 2003, treatment success with DOT ranged from 91% of clients in WHO's Western Pacific region to 73% in the African region. The rate of DOT treatment success for TB in the Americas was 81% (WHO, 2005b). Community health nurses are actively involved in supervising DOT and in motivating clients to continue compliance with therapy. In addition, community health nurses are often involved in locating clients who are noncompliant and encouraging them to continue therapy. Promoting continued compliance often requires that community health nurses assist clients to deal with factors that interfere with compliance. For example, they may assist a homeless client in his or her search for shelter or employment to eliminate life circumstances that impede DOT compliance. They may also need to be actively involved in promoting access to DOT or to other needed services that support DOT compliance.

Treatment of communicable diseases is complicated by noncompliance and by the development of drug-resistant microorganisms, which is fostered by noncompliance. One approach to improving compliance with treatment for communicable diseases such as HCV infection and HIV is to treat correctional inmates. Because of their incarceration, they may be more open to messages encouraging treatment while incarcerated. In addition, DOT is much easier to implement in a controlled setting like a jail or prison than in the general community (Farley et al., 2005). Some studies have found, however, that inmates with TB were less likely than people in the general population to complete a full course of treatment in spite of the availability of DOT (MacNeil, Lobato, & Moore, 2005). On the other hand, provision of DOT during and after incarceration has been shown to increase compliance with HIV treatment (National Commission on Correctional Health Care, 2005).

Community health nurses may provide treatment for some communicable diseases under medical protocols, but are more likely to be involved in educating

ETHICAL AWARENESS

Some authors have suggested treating injection drug users who have hepatitis C only after they have ceased using drugs for at least 6 months (Des Jarlais & Schuchat, 2001). Do you think this is appropriate? Why or why not?

clients about treatment and promoting compliance. The role of community health nurses in treating communicable diseases may also involve political activity and advocacy. For example, the nurse might be actively engaged in efforts to assure access to health care for persons with AIDS or to change policies for providing treatment to drug users with chronic HCV infection. Emphases in secondary prevention of communicable diseases are summarized in Table 28-5◆.

Tertiary Prevention

Tertiary prevention of communicable diseases may occur with individual clients or with population groups. At the individual level, emphasis is on preventing complications and long-term sequelae, monitoring treatment compliance and effects, monitoring treatment side effects and assisting clients to deal with them, and providing assistance in dealing with long-term consequences of some communicable diseases.

Community health nurses can educate clients to prevent complications of communicable diseases with their attendant long-term sequelae. For example, clients with influenza can be encouraged to rest and to refrain from resuming normal activities until they are recovered. Similarly, parents can discourage scratching in children with varicella to prevent secondary infection in lesions and encourage clients with hepatitis to refrain from alcohol use to prevent further liver damage.

Community health nurses should also monitor clients with HIV infection for signs and symptoms of opportunistic infections and refer them for treatment when OIs are suspected. Nurses may also be involved in assisting clients with prophylactic regimens to prevent opportunistic infections. Clients with HIV infection may also experience a number of nutritional difficulties that may require nursing intervention. For example, weight loss and wasting may occur as a result of reduced food or calorie intake due to anorexia, nausea and vomiting, changes in taste or smell, fatigue, or painful oral or esophageal lesions. Weight loss, loss of muscle mass, and vitamin deficiencies may also result from malabsorption due to lactose or fat intolerance, gastrointestinal infection, malignancies, and so on. Finally, HIV-infected clients may experience metabolic alterations due to HIV, medications, and other circumstances (Keithley, Swanson, Murphy, & Levin, 2000). Community health nurses

TABLE 28-5	Community Health Nursing Interventions in Secondary Prevention of Communicable Diseases
Focus	**Community Health Nursing Interventions**
Case finding and surveillance	■ Recognize symptoms of communicable diseases in clients and refer them for diagnostic and treatment services as needed.
	■ Educate the public regarding signs and symptoms of specific communicable diseases.
	■ Recognize signs of disease outbreaks in the population.
	■ Collect surveillance data regarding communicable disease incidence, prevalence, contributing factors, and effects.
Screening	■ Recognize and refer possible cases of communicable diseases.
	■ Educate clients and the public regarding the need for screening for communicable diseases.
	■ Provide selective screening services.
	■ Plan and implement mass screening programs.
	■ Advocate for screening availability for populations at risk for communicable diseases.
Diagnosis and reporting	■ Refer clients for diagnostic procedures as needed.
	■ Educate clients regarding diagnostic procedures.
	■ Provide diagnostic services.
	■ Interpret diagnostic test results and counsel clients accordingly.
	■ Advocate for the availability of needed diagnostic services.
	■ Report cases of communicable diseases in accord with local, state, or national regulations.
	■ Educate other health care providers regarding reporting requirements.
	■ Follow up on reports of communicable diseases to obtain relevant epidemiologic information.
Treatment	■ Provide antimicrobial therapies.
	■ Educate clients regarding antimicrobial therapy.
	■ Supervise DOT.
	■ Educate clients and their families for supportive care.
	■ Educate health care providers, clients, and the public to prevent inappropriate use of antimicrobials and development of drug-resistant organisms.
	■ Advocate for the availability of needed treatment services for all segments of the population.

engaged in tertiary prevention would assist clients to overcome these nutritional deficiencies through nutritional counseling, promoting food and water safety, dealing with medication side effects, and suggesting complementary and alternative nutritional therapies such as the use of nutritional supplements. Community health nurses may also work closely with public health social workers and mental health counselors to address the tertiary prevention needs of clients with HIV/AIDS and other conditions (e.g., hepatitis C). Community health nurses may need to engage in political advocacy to assure the availability of tertiary preventive services for clients with these diseases. This may include services needed to address psychosocial as well as physical consequences of disease (e.g., unemployment, housing, discrimination).

Another issue related to HIV infection that requires tertiary prevention activity involves resumption of high-risk sexual or drug use behaviors. Again, because many people perceive HAART to be a "cure" for HIV infection, treatment may lead to continuation or reinitiation of behaviors that may transmit the disease to others (Fenton & Valdisseri, 2006). Resumption of unsafe sexual practices may be the result of several factors. Treatment may lead to improved health and functional status, increasing sexual activity as well. In addition, treatment may give rise to unrealistic expectations regarding the potential for disease transmission, leading those with HIV infection to be less cautious in their sexual practices (Wilson et al., 2004). Approximately one third to one fourth of people with HIV infection may maintain high-risk behaviors. Prevention case management, however, has led to a decrease in transmission risk behaviors. Prevention case management involves providing follow-up counseling and educational services to clients as well as assistance in dealing with other psychosocial effects of HIV infection (Gasiorowicz et al., 2005). Preventing resumption of high-risk sexual behaviors that may spread HIV infection is particularly important in light of the fact that in 2006 there were an estimated 1 million to 1.2 million people in the United States living with HIV (Wolitski et al., 2006).

Community health nurses also monitor communicable disease treatment compliance and treatment effects, particularly in diseases such as tuberculosis and HIV infection that require long-term therapy. Treatment of chronic hepatitis B, C, or D may also involve prolonged use of medications. In addition, community health nurses monitor the occurrence of adverse effects of treatment. For example, antituberculin drugs may result in hepatitis or visual disturbances, and the nurse should be alert to signs and symptoms of adverse effects.

Similarly, long-term highly active antiretroviral therapy (HAART) has a variety of complications that are only now beginning to manifest in many HIV-infected clients. For example, HAART has been associated with lipodystrophy (redistribution of body fat), hypercholesterolemia, hypertriglyceridemia, insulin resistance and diabetes, and mitochondrial toxicity that may lead to cardiomyopathy, peripheral neuropathy, pancreatitis, and lactic acidosis (*HIV Inside*, 2000). Many of these complications may have life-threatening consequences, and the nurse should closely observe clients receiving HAART for their occurrence.

Treatment for chronic HCV infection may also have multiple side effects such as fatigue, muscle aches, headache, nausea and vomiting, irritability, depression, reversible hair loss, skin rashes and itching, and nasal stuffiness. More serious adverse effects of therapy may also occur. Promoting treatment adherence in the face of multiple side effects can be difficult. Some strategies that may be effective in promoting compliance include reducing side effects where possible, simplifying the regimen to include fewer doses and fewer pills, establishing client trust in the efficacy of treatment, and tailoring therapy to fit the client's lifestyle whenever possible. Additional approaches may include clarifying treatment instructions and making sure that clients understand them, simplifying distribution systems (e.g., providing easy access to medication refills), and providing frequent follow-up.

Rehabilitation may be required following some communicable diseases. For example, rehabilitation may be needed to strengthen affected muscles or to promote individual and family adjustment to permanent disabilities from paralytic poliomyelitis. Active and passive range of motion may help restore muscle strength and prevent contractures. Maintaining skin integrity for clients with braces or those confined to bed or wheelchair is also important. Observation for recurrent disease (even many years later) is also needed. Families may also require assistance in financing rehabilitative care and procuring needed equipment and appliances, and community health nurses may collaborate with public health social workers in efforts to address these needs. In addition, community health nurses may need to be involved in political advocacy to assure that needed services are available to clients and their families.

Community health nurses may also need to help clients deal with the long-term consequences of communicable diseases. For example, children with anomalies or mental retardation due to congenital rubella syndrome or congenital syphilis will need ongoing care, and their families will need emotional support and assistance in finding resources to deal with their children's disabilities. Support may also be needed for long-term behavior changes required to prevent infecting others with HIV or hepatitis. Community health nurses may also need to function as advocates to prevent stigmatization and discrimination and to foster clients' integration into the community to the extent permitted by their health status. For example, nurses may need to educate those who interact with HIV-infected clients about how HIV infection is and is not transmitted. Similarly, when working with children with AIDS, advocacy by the community health nurse may necessitate planning activities that foster normal growth and development in each child.

Assistance may also be needed in dealing with the financial impact of HIV infection and other diseases that have long-term treatment needs. The community health nurse can help in this respect by referring clients and their families to sources of financial assistance. Advocacy by community health nurses may be required to ensure client eligibility for financial assistance programs. This may involve political advocacy for health policy changes at state or national levels.

For a few communicable diseases, tertiary prevention with individual clients entails preventing reinfection. This does not apply to the majority of the diseases discussed in this chapter because they result in immunity. For example, hepatitis A confers immunity against reinfection with hepatitis A, but does not provide immunity to other forms of hepatitis. Similarly, varicella, measles, and mumps usually confer immunity, and clients do not become reinfected. Some diseases, however, do not produce immunity, and reinfection is possible and even likely if clients do not change risk behaviors. For example, clients may be reinfected with gonorrhea or Chlamydia as a result of continued unprotected sexual activity. Similarly, reinfection with syphilis is possible unless the disease has progressed to the point of immunity, by which time the risk for long-term complications is quite high. Community health nurses need to educate clients about the potential for reinfection and the need for behavior changes to reduce the risk of reinfection. For example, nurses might educate clients about the need for condoms during sexual intercourse or educate IDUs on harm-reduction strategies such as not sharing needles or other drug paraphernalia.

Health systems must also be in place to meet the tertiary prevention needs of clients with communicable diseases. At the level of public policy, community health nurses may need to engage in political advocacy to assure necessary funding for assistance programs for clients experiencing long-term needs related to the effects of communicable diseases.

Tertiary prevention at the community level is directed toward preventing the spread of disease and providing access to long-term care services. Measures to prevent the spread of disease in the population include many primary prevention measures for individuals such as immunization and identification, notification, and prophylactic treatment of contacts. Changes in risk behaviors among persons who are chronic carriers of infection can also serve to prevent dissemination of disease.

Isolation or quarantine of infected or exposed persons may also prevent further spread of some communicable diseases within the community (Quinlisk et al., 2006). **Isolation** is the process of limiting the movement and interactions of people who have a communicable disease to prevent the spread of the disease to others. **Quarantine**, on the other hand, restricts the movements

of healthy people who have been exposed to a particular disease (CDC, 2005d). In both strategies, people who have the disease or have been exposed to it are kept separated from the well population.

Both isolation and quarantine may be voluntary procedures in which people who are infected or exposed self-limit their activities to prevent the spread of the disease to others. Staying home from work or school when one is ill is a simple example of voluntary isolation. Isolation or quarantine may also be mandated by legal authority at local, state, or national levels (CDC, 2005e). In 2003, an executive order from the U.S. president added SARS to the list of diseases for which quarantine might be imposed under federal law. Other diseases covered under federal regulations include cholera, diphtheria, infectious TB, plague, smallpox, yellow fever, and viral hemorrhagic fevers (White House Office of the Press Secretary, 2003).

As we saw in Chapter 3∞, quarantine was initiated as a strategy for containing the spread of epidemics from one population to another. The length of the period of quarantine varies from disease to disease, but generally is for a period of time equal to the farthest limits of the incubation period for the disease. For example, the incubation period for diphtheria is 2 to 5 days. Adults who work with unimmunized children or handle food are restricted from work for 7 days or until treated and found not to be carriers by means of nose and throat cultures (Heymann, 2004). In other instances, quarantine may only be imposed until people exposed to a microorganism such as aerosolized anthrax spores can be *decontaminated* through a shower and a change of clothes (Wikimedia Foundation, 2006). Quarantine and isolation may also be imposed on a long-term basis for certain diseases. For example, people with communicable TB who refuse treatment may be forcibly isolated from others.

Community health nurses may need to be advocates for long-term isolation of people who pose a risk of communicable disease to the public and initiate isolation procedures when absolutely necessary. At the same time, they need to be advocates for those with communicable diseases to be sure that mandatory isolation and quarantine procedures are warranted, that designated legal processes are followed, and that neither process is used to discriminate against vulnerable population groups. For example, community health nurses have been actively involved, with other civil rights activists, in resisting proposed efforts to quarantine or isolate people with HIV/AIDS.

Quarantine was believed by many people to be no longer essential with the advent of antimicrobial drugs. The recent SARS outbreaks, however, led to the reinstitution of quarantine procedures in many countries. Until other control measures become available for emerging diseases, quarantine remains a viable intervention for preventing the spread of diseases that are highly transmissible from person to person (Cava, Fay, Beanlands, McCay, & Wignall, 2005).

Outbreak response is another strategy for controlling the spread of communicable diseases in the population. Outbreak response is the corollary to epidemic or bioterrorism preparedness discussed in relation to primary prevention and is initiated once an outbreak has occurred. The two facets of a response to an outbreak of communicable disease are the management of those with the disease (secondary prevention) and interrupting disease transmission in the population (tertiary prevention). Steps in an outbreak response include verifying the diagnosis, confirming the existence of an outbreak, identifying those affected and factors contributing to their illness, defining the population at risk, identifying the source and factors contributing to the spread of the disease, and containing the outbreak (Heymann, 2004). Verification of diagnosis may involve the collection of specific specimens from those believed to have a particular disease. For example, community health nurses may collect stool specimens from neighborhood residents who exhibit diarrhea. The existence of an outbreak is confirmed by examining incidence figures in light of past trends in disease incidence. This step in the response to an outbreak is most often carried out by public health officials or epidemiologists rather than community health nurses.

Community health nurses are often involved, however, in obtaining case histories of those affected to determine factors contributing to disease. They may also be actively involved in identifying additional cases of disease. For example, nurses may go door-to-door asking about family members who have recently experienced diarrhea in an outbreak of diarrheal disease. The data gathered from these disease investigations can then be used by epidemiologists and others to identify persons at risk for the disease and to assist in the determination of the source of infection and factors influencing its spread. Community health nurses may be involved in identifying the source of the infection by collecting samples of suspected food or water sources and conveying them for laboratory testing.

Community health nurses are also actively involved in strategies to control the disease. Control may include managing cases of illness in those affected, and community health nurses are involved in educating people regarding disease management and referring them for medical care as needed as part of secondary prevention. They are also involved in educating the public on measures to prevent the spread of disease or on the need for mass immunization or PEP if available. Community health nurses may also be involved in surveillance for evidence of disease among people at risk, with follow-up care for those who become symptomatic.

Social distancing is a third approach to preventing the spread of communicable diseases within the population. **Social distancing** involves voluntarily limiting one's interactions with others in order to prevent potential exposure to pathogenic microorganisms (Lofgren,

2005). Social distancing measures taken by individuals (e.g., avoiding crowded places during an epidemic or disease outbreak, not sharing food or beverages or personal items with others, wearing a mask in public places, washing hands) would be a form of primary prevention. Some people may also choose to engage in *reverse* quarantine, in which well persons may choose to avoid contact with others as much as possible.

Social distancing measures taken at the population level would be tertiary prevention interventions aimed at preventing the spread of existing disease in the community. Population-based examples of social distancing include closing schools and businesses or restricting access to certain places. For example, hospitals might be closed to all but essential personnel in the event of an avian influenza epidemic, minimizing the exposure of well people to those who are ill. Canceling public events that would promote interaction among groups of people is another example of social distancing at the population level (GlobalSecurity.org, 2005). Community health nurses can educate individuals regarding relevant social distancing strategies to prevent exposure to disease. They may also participate in policy decisions related to population-level social distancing activities when these are warranted by the mode of transmission of a particular disease. They can also help to avoid excessive response to the threat of communicable diseases by educating the public and policy makers regarding factors influencing disease transmission. For example, participation in the gay bar scene has been associated with increased risk of HIV infection, but closing gay bars would not be an appropriate social distancing strategy for preventing the spread of HIV infection in the gay population. Strategies for tertiary prevention of communicable diseases, including social distancing, are summarized in Table 28-6◆.

Evaluating Communicable Disease Control Strategies

Evaluating primary prevention related to communicable diseases with individual clients is based on the prevention of occurrence of disease. If drug users educated for harm reduction do not develop HBV or HIV infection, intervention has been successful. At the community level, the effectiveness of primary prevention of communicable diseases is reflected in declining incidence and prevalence rates.

The effectiveness of secondary prevention is reflected in communicable disease mortality and continued morbidity. For example, HAART for HIV infection has decreased HIV/AIDS-related mortality and prolonged survival time for infected persons. Similarly, the effectiveness of TB therapy is reflected in the number of clients whose TB has been cured.

Evaluation of tertiary preventive measures focuses on the extent to which complications of communicable diseases have been prevented, the extent to which

TABLE 28-6 Community Health Nursing Interventions in Tertiary Prevention of Communicable Diseases

Focus	Community Health Nursing Interventions
Monitoring compliance	▪ Monitor client compliance with therapy.
	▪ Promote compliance with treatment regimens.
	▪ Locate noncompliant clients and promote reinitiation of therapy.
Monitoring treatment effects	▪ Monitor side effects and adverse effects of therapy and refer for medical evaluation as needed.
	▪ Monitor treatment effects by referring clients for follow-up testing as needed.
Dealing with consequences	▪ Prevent complications of communicable diseases.
	▪ Refer clients with complications to rehabilitation services as needed.
	▪ Promote adjustment to long-term consequences.
	▪ Advocate for the availability of long-term services as needed.
Preventing reinfection	▪ Educate clients and the public regarding safe sexual practices.
	▪ Refer clients for drug abuse treatment, as needed.
	▪ Promote/advocate for harm-reduction strategies for IDUs.
Preventing the spread of disease	▪ Plan and conduct mass immunization campaigns.
	▪ Engage in contact notification.
	▪ Promote screening of blood and tissue donors.
	▪ Advocate for and provide screening and treatment for infected pregnant women.
	▪ Promote behavior change to decrease subsequent exposure risks.
	▪ Promote isolation/quarantine of infected persons when required and educate them regarding the need for quarantine.
	▪ Prevent the use of isolation and quarantine as discriminatory procedures against vulnerable populations.
	▪ Advocate for and participate in effective response to disease outbreaks, including case identification and investigation, specimen collection, source identification, disease management, and control strategies.
	▪ Educate the public regarding social distancing strategies to prevent exposure to disease.
	▪ Participate in decisions regarding population-based social distancing strategies and educate policy makers regarding their advisability and utility in specific diseases.

reinfection occurs for those diseases where reinfection is possible, and the extent of disability and adverse consequences resulting from communicable diseases. Evaluation of each of the three levels of prevention is also reflected in the national objectives related to communicable diseases discussed earlier in this chapter. The current status of some of these objectives is presented below◆.

Although remarkable progress has been made in controlling communicable diseases, they remain significant contributors to morbidity and mortality in the United States and throughout the world. Community health nurses can be actively involved in preventing communicable diseases and in identifying and treating them when they do occur.

HEALTHY PEOPLE 2010
Goals for Population Health

OBJECTIVE	BASELINE	MOST RECENT DATA	TARGET
▪ 13-1. Reduce new AIDS cases among adolescents and adults (per 100,000 population over age 13)	19.5	18.6	1
▪ 13-6. Increase the proportion of sexually active persons who use condoms	23%	NDA	50%
▪ 13-11. Increase the proportion of adults with TB tested for HIV	55%	58%	85%
▪ 13-13d. Increase the proportion of HIV-infected persons who receive HAART	40%	73%	95%
▪ 13-14. Reduce HIV deaths (per 100,000 population)	5.3	4.9	0.7

Continued on next page

HEALTHY PEOPLE 2010 *continued*

■ 14-1. Reduce cases of vaccine-preventable diseases			
a. con genital rubella syndrome	7	1	0
b. diphtheria	1	0	0*
c. *Haemophilus influenzae* type b	163	187	0#
d. hepatitis B	708	159	9
e. measles	74	26	0
f. mumps	666	253	0
g. pertussis (children under 7 years of age)	3,417	4,109	2,000#
h. wild virus poliomyelitis	0	0	0
i. rubella	364	10	0
j. tetanus (persons under 35 years of age)	14	6	0
k. varicella	2.2 mil	1.15 mil	400,000
■ 14-6. Reduce new cases of hepatitis A (per 100,000 population)	11.2	2.9	4.5*
■ 14-8. Reduce new cases of hepatitis C (per 100,000 population)	2.5	1.4	1
■ 14-11. Reduce new cases of tuberculosis (per 100,000 population)	6.8	5.8	1
■ 14-12. Increase the proportion of people with TB who complete treatment within 12 months	74%	80%	90%
■ 14-13. Increase the proportion of TB contacts and high-risk persons with TB infection who complete prophylactic treatment	62.2%	NDA	85%
■ 14-22. Increase the proportion of vaccination coverage among children 19 to 35 months of age for universally recommended vaccines	43%–93%	81%–95%	90%
■ 14-26. Increase the proportion of children in population-based immunization information systems	21%	45%	95%
■ 14-28. Increase hepatitis B vaccine coverage in			
a. hemodialysis patients	35%	58%	90%
b. men who have sex with men	9%	NDA	60%
c. occupationally exposed workers	67%	NDA	98%
■ 14-29. Increase the proportion of adults over 65 years of age vaccinated against			
a. influenza (annually)	64%	66%	90%
b. pneumococcal disease (in lifetime)	63%	56%	90%#

NDA – No data available

* Objective has been met

 # Objective moving away from target

Data from: Centers for Disease Control and Prevention. (2005). Healthy people data. Retrieved September 5, 2005, from http://wonder.cdc.gov/data2010

Case Study

A Communicable Disease

Jane is an 18-year-old college student. She lives in the dorm with her roommate, Sally. Shortly after Jane returned from Christmas vacation, she developed a fever and a rash. She didn't feel too bad, but Sally persuaded her to see a doctor. Because it was Saturday, Jane went to the emergency department (ED) of the local hospital. The physician there made a diagnosis of rubella. Later that night, he and the nurses in the ED became very busy with victims of a multivehicle accident. As a result, no one completed the health department form reporting Jane's rubella until 2 days later.

By the time a community health nurse contacted Jane to complete a rubella case report, Sally and several other girls in Jane's dorm had also developed rubella. Sally gave it to her boyfriend, who exposed those in his classes. One of the women in his English class is pregnant.

1. Based on the information presented in the case description, what biophysical, psychological, physical environmental, sociocultural, behavioral, and health system factors are operating in this situation? What additional factors in these dimensions might influence the situation? How might you assess for the presence or absence of these factors?

2. What primary preventive measures could have been employed to prevent this situation? What primary prevention measures are appropriate at this point?

3. What secondary and tertiary measures by the community health nurse are appropriate at this time?
4. What roles will the community health nurse perform in dealing with this situation? What other public health personnel

might the community health nurse collaborate with in addressing the situation?
5. How would you evaluate the effectiveness of interventions in this situation?

Test Your Understanding

1. What are some of the major trends in communicable disease incidence in the United States? How do these trends differ from those worldwide? What factors are influencing those trends? (pp. 806–811)

2. What are the major modes of transmission of communicable diseases? What effects has technology had on disease transmission? (pp. 811–812)

3. How do biophysical, psychological, physical environmental, sociocultural, behavioral, and health system factors influence the incidence and control of communicable diseases? (pp. 814–825)

4. What effects might a pandemic or widespread bioterrorist attack have on the population? (pp. 833–834)

5. What are the major approaches to primary prevention of communicable diseases? Give an example of an intervention related to each approach. (pp. 826–835)

6. What are the major considerations in secondary prevention of communicable diseases? What interventions might be employed with respect to each consideration? (pp. 835–841)

7. What are the foci of tertiary prevention in the control of communicable diseases? What interventions might be employed in relation to each focus area? (pp. 841–844)

8. What roles do community health nurses play in the control of communicable diseases? (pp. 826–844, 845)

9. What other public health professionals are involved in communicable disease control? How does the role of the community health nurse interface with the roles of these other professionals? (pp. 829–830, 831, 832, 833, 835, 838, 842, 844)

EXPLORE MediaLink

http://www.prenhall.com/clark
Resources for this chapter can be found on the Companion Website.

Audio Glossary
Appendix E: Information on Selected Communicable Diseases
Exam Review Questions

Case Study: TB, a Communicable Disease
MediaLink Application: Old Bugs, New Threats (video)
Media Links

Challenge Your Knowledge
Update *Healthy People 2010*
Advocacy Interviews

References

Adekoya, N., & Hopkins, R. S. (2005). Racial disparities in nationally notifiable diseases—United States, 2002. *Morbidity and Mortality Weekly Report, 54*, 9–11.

Alary, M., Joly, J. R., Vincelette, J., Lavoie, R., Turmel, B., & Remis, R. S. (2005). Lack of evidence of sexual transmission of hepatitis C virus in a prospective cohort of men who have sex with men. *American Journal of Public Health, 95*, 502–505.

Al-Saden, P. C. (2004). Hepatitis C: An update for occupational health nurses. *AAOHN Journal, 52*, 210–217.

American Lung Association. (2005). *TB skin test fact sheet.* Retrieved July 25, 2006, from http://www.lungusa.org/site/pp.asp?c=dvLUK9O0E&b=35813

American Thoracic Society, CDC, and Infectious Diseases Society of America. (2005). Controlling Tuberculosis in the United States: Recommendations from the American Thoracic Society, CDC, and the Infectious Diseases Society of America. *Morbidity and Mortality Weekly Report, 54*(RR-12), 1–81.

Arendt, A., Carmean, J., Koch, E., Rolfs, R., Mottice, S., Strausbaugh, L., et al. (2005). Fatal bacterial infections associated with platelet transfusions—United States, 2004. *Morbidity and Mortality Weekly Report, 54*, 168–170.

Aylward, R. B., & Heymann, D. L. (2005). Can we capitalize on the virtues of vaccines? Insights from the polio eradication initiative. *American Journal of Public Health, 95*, 773–778.

Bentley, M. E., Fullem, A. M., Tolley, E. E., Kelly, C. W., Jogelkar, N., Srirak, N., et al. (2004). Acceptability of a microbicide among women and their partners in a 4-country phase 1 trial. *American Journal of Public Health, 94*, 1159–1164.

Bialek, S. R., Thoroughman, D. A., Hu, D., Simard, E. P., Chattin, J., Cheek, J., et al. (2004). Hepatitis A incidence and hepatitis A vaccination among American Indians and Alaska Natives, 1990–2001. *American Journal of Public Health, 94*, 996–1001.

Bilukha, O. O., & Rosenstein, N. (2005). Prevention and control of meningococcal diseases: Recommendations of the Advisory Committee on Immunization Practices. *Morbidity and Mortality Weekly Report, 54*(RR-7), 1–21.

Blake, S. M., Ledsky, R., Goodenow, C., Sawyer, R., Lohrmann, D., & Windsor, R. (2003). Condom availability programs in Massachusetts high schools: Relationships with condom use and sexual behavior. *American Journal of Public Health, 93*, 955–962.

Boddiger, D. (2005). Methamphetamine use linked to rising HIV transmission. *The Lancet, 365*, 1217–1218.

Bridges, C. B., Harper, S. A., Fukuda, K., Uyeki, T. M., Cox, N. J., & Singleton, J. A. (2003). Prevention and control of influenza: Recommendations of the Advisory Committee on Immunization Practices. *Morbidity and Mortality Weekly Report, 52*(RR-8), 1–34.

Bright, R. A., Shay, D., Bresee, J., Klimov, A., Cox, N., & Ortiz, J. (2006). High levels of adamantine resistance among influenza A (H3N2) viruses and interim guidelines for use of antiviral agents—United States, 2005—2006 influenza season. *Morbidity and Mortality Weekly Report, 55*, 44–46.

Broder, K. R., Cortese, M. M., Iskander, J. K., Kretsinger, K., Slade, B. A., Brown, K. H., et al. (2006). Preventing tetanus, diphtheria, and pertussis among adolescents: Use of tetanus toxoid, reduced diphtheria toxoid and acellular pertussis vaccines: Recommendations of the Advisory Committee on Immunization Practices (ACIP). *Morbidity and Mortality Weekly Report, 55*(RR-3), 1–43.

Brown, K., Cortese, M. M., Iqbal, K., Moran, J. S., Murphy, T. V., Sneller, V. P., et al. (2005). Pertussis—United States, 2001–2003. *Morbidity and Mortality Weekly Report, 54,* 1283–1286.

Bryant, K., Brothers, K., Humbaugh, K., Kistler, W., Stites, S., Jahre, J. A., et al. (2005). Outbreaks of pertussis associated with hospitals—Kentucky, Pennsylvania, and Oregon, 2003. *Morbidity and Mortality Weekly Report, 54,* 67–71.

Buffington, J., Rowell, R., Hinman, J. M., Sharp, K., & Choi, S. (2001). Lack of awareness of hepatitis C risk among persons who received blood transfusions before 1990. *American Journal of Public Health, 91,* 47–48.

Caglioti, S., Tomasulo, P., Raschke, R., Rodarte, M., Sylvester, T., Diggs, A., et al. (2004). Transfusion-associated transmission of West Nile virus—Arizona, 2004. *Morbidity and Mortality Weekly Report, 53,* 842–844.

Campbell, C., Foulis, C. A., Maimane, S., & Sibiya, Z. (2005). "I have an evil child at my house." Stigma and HIV/AIDS management in a South African community. *American Journal of Public Health, 95,* 808–815.

Campos-Outcalt, D. (2005). When, and when not, to use the interferon-gamma blood test. *Journal of Family Practice, 54.* Retrieved July 25, 2006, from http://www.jfponline.com/Pages.asp?AID=2769&UID

The Carter Center. (2005). Progress toward global eradication of dracunculiasis, January 2004–July 2005. *Morbidity and Mortality Weekly Report, 54,* 175–177.

Castro, A., & Farmer, P. (2005). Understanding and addressing AIDS-related stigma: From anthropological theory to clinical practice in Haiti. *American Journal of Public Health, 95,* 53–59.

Cava, M. A., Fay, K. E., Beanlands, H. J., McCay, E. A., & Wignall, R. (2005). Risk perception and compliance with quarantine during the SARS outbreak. *Journal of Nursing Scholarship, 37,* 343–347.

Centers for Disease Control and Prevention. (2003a). *Anthrax: What you need to know.* Retrieved May 20, 2006, from http://www.bt.dcd.gov/agent/anthrax/needtoknow.asp

Centers for Disease Control and Prevention. (2003b). *YRBSS: Trends in the prevalence of sexual behaviors.* Retrieved May 20, 2006, from http://www.cdc.gov/HealthyYouth/yrbs pdfs/trends-sex.pdf

Centers for Disease Control and Prevention. (2004). National Infant Immunization Week, April 25–May 1, 2004. *Morbidity and Mortality Weekly Report, 53,* 290.

Centers for Disease Control and Prevention. (2005a). 50th anniversary of the first effective polio vaccine—April 12, 2005. *Morbidity and Mortality Weekly Report, 54,* 335–336.

Centers for Disease Control and Prevention. (2005b). *Community-associated MRSA information for clinicians.* Retrieved July 27, 2006, from http://www.cdc.gov/ncidod/dhqp/ar_mrsa_ca_clinicians.html

Centers for Disease Control and Prevention. (2005c). *Community-associated MRSA information for the public.* Retrieved July 27, 2006, from http://www.cdc.gov/ncidod/dhqp/ar_mrsa_ca_public.html

Centers for Disease Control and Prevention. (2005d). *Fact sheet on isolation and quarantine.* Retrieved July 27, 2006, from http://www.cdc.gov/ncidod/sars/isolationquarantine.pdf

Centers for Disease Control and Prevention. (2005e). *Fact sheet on legal authorities for isolation and quarantine.* Retrieved July 27, 2006, from http://www.cdc.gov/ncidod/sars/factsheetlegal.pdf

Centers for Disease Control and Prevention. (2005f). *Healthy people data.* Retrieved September 5, 2005, from http://wonder.cdc.gov/data2010

Centers for Disease Control and Prevention. (2005g). Licensure of a combined live attenuated measles, mumps, rubella, and varicella vaccine. *Morbidity and Mortality Weekly Report, 54,* 1212–1214.

Centers for Disease Control and Prevention. (2005h). National infant immunization week—April 24–30, 2005. *Morbidity and Mortality Weekly Report, 54,* 361.

Centers for Disease Control and Prevention. (2005i). Publication of guidance on public reporting of healthcare-associated infections. *Morbidity and Mortality Weekly Report, 54,* 464.

Centers for Disease Control and Prevention. (2006a). A new product (VariZIG™) for post-exposure prophylaxis of varicella available under an investigational new drug application expanded access protocol. *Morbidity and Mortality Weekly Report, 55,* 209–210.

Centers for Disease Control and Prevention. (2006b). *HIV/AIDS basic statistics.* Retrieved May 20, 2006, from http://www.cdc.gov/hiv/topics/surveillance/basic.htm

Centers for Disease Control and Prevention. (2006c). *Nationally notifiable diseases—United States, 2006.* Retrieved July 27, 2006, from http://www.cdc.gov/EPO/dphsi/phs/infdis2006.htm

Centers for Disease Control and Prevention. (2006d). Recommended childhood and adolescent immunization schedule—United States, 2006. *Morbidity and Mortality Weekly Report, 54*(51 & 52), Q1–Q4.

Centers for Disease Control and Prevention. (2006e). Summary of provisional cases of selected notifiable diseases, United States, cumulative, week ending December 24, 2005 (51st week). *Morbidity and Mortality Weekly Report, 54,* 1309.

Centers for Disease Control and Prevention. (2006f). Update: Influenza activity—United States, January 15–21, 2006. *Morbidity and Mortality Weekly Report, 55,* 103–105.

Chang, S., Wheeler, L. S. M., & Farrell, K. P. (2002). Public health impact of targeted tuberculosis screening in public schools. *American Journal of Public Health, 92,* 1942–1945.

Chapman, A. S. (2006). Diagnosis and management of tickborne rickettsial diseases: Rocky Mountain spotted fever, ehrlichioses, and anaplasmosis—United States: A practical guide for physicians and other health-care and public health professionals. *Morbidity and Mortality Weekly Report, 55*(RR-4), 1–29.

Clements-Nolle, K., Marx, R., Guzman, R., & Katz, M. (2001). HIV prevalence, risk behaviors, health care use, and mental health status of transgender persons: Implications for public health intervention. *American Journal of Public Health, 91,* 915–921.

Ciccarone, D. H., Kanouse, D. E., Collins, R. L., Miu, A., Chen, J. L., Morton, S. C., et al. (2003). Sex without disclosure of positive HIV serostatus in a US probability sample of persons receiving medical care for HIV infection. *American Journal of Public Health, 93,* 949–954.

Cohen, J. (2001). And now the good news about smallpox. Retrieved October 30, 2001, from http://www.content.health.msn.com

Cohen, M. H., Olszewski, Y., Robey, M., Love, F., Branson, B., Jamieson, D. J., et al. (2003). Rapid point-of-care testing for HIV-1 during labor and delivery—Chicago, 2002. *Morbidity and Mortality Weekly Report, 52,* 866–868.

Cohen, M. H., Cook, J., Grey, D., Young, M., Hanau, L. H., Tien, P., et al. (2004). Medically eligible women who do not use HAART: The importance of abuse, drug use, and race. *American Journal of Public Health, 94,* 1147–1151.

Cook, J. A., Grey, D., Burke, J., Cohen, M. H., Gurtman, A. C., Richardson, J. L., et al. (2004). Depressive symptoms and AIDS-related mortality among a multisite cohort of HIV-positive women. *American Journal of Public Health, 94,* 1133–1140.

Corby, R., Lanni, V., Kistler, V., Dato, V., Weltman, A., Yozviak, C., et al. (2005). Outbreaks of *Salmonella* infections associated with eating Roma tomatoes—United States and Canada, 2004. *Morbidity and Mortality Weekly Report, 54,* 235–238.

Costamagna, P., Furst, K., Tully, K., Landis, J., Moser, K., Quach, L., et al. (2004). Tuberculosis associated with blocking agents against tumor necrosis factor-alpha—California, 2002–2003. *Morbidity and Mortality Weekly Report, 53,* 683–686.

County of San Diego Health and Human Services Agency. (2004). *Standards of care for the prevention of perinatal HIV transmission in San Diego County.* San Diego: Author.

Dayan, G., Redd, S., LeBaron, C., Rota, P., Rota, J., & Bellini, W. (2005). Measles—United States, 2004. *Morbidity and Mortality Weekly Report, 54,* 1229–1231.

DeGraw, C., Kimball, G., Adams, R., Misselbeck, T., Oliveri, R., Plough, J., et al. (2006). Tuberculosis control activities after Hurricane Katrina—New Orleans, Louisiana, 2005. *Morbidity and Mortality Weekly Report, 55,* 332–335.

Dembek, Z. F., Hadler, J. L., Castrodale, L., Funk, B., Fiore, A. E., Openo, K., et al. (2005). Positive test results for acute hepatitis A virus infection among persons with no recent history of acute hepatitis—United States, 2002–2004. *Morbidity and Mortality Weekly Report, 54,* 453–456.

de Quadros, C. A. (2004). The century of vaccines. *American Journal of Public Health, 94,* 910.

Des Jarlais, D. C., Galea, S., Tracy, M., Tross, S., & Vlahov, D. (2006). Stigmatization of newly emerging infectious diseases: AIDS and SARS. *American Journal of Public Health, 96,* 561–567.

Des Jarlais, D. C., & Schuchat, A. (2001). Hepatitis C among drug users: Deja vu all over again? *American Journal of Public Health, 91,* 21–22.

Division of Adult and Community Health. (2005). Estimated influenza vaccination coverage among adults and children—United States, September 1, 2004–January 31, 2005. *Morbidity and Mortality Weekly Report, 53,* 304–307.

Division of Bacterial and Mycotic Diseases. (2003). Wound botulism among black tar heroin users—Washington, 2003. *Morbidity and Mortality Weekly Report, 52,* 885–886.

Division of Birth Defects and Developmental Disabilities, National Center on Birth Defects and Developmental Disabilities. (2004). Interim guidelines for the evaluation of infants born to mothers with West Nile virus during pregnancy. *Morbidity and Mortality Weekly Report, 53,* 154–157.

Division of HIV/AIDS Prevention—Surveillance and Epidemiology. (2000). Adoption of protective behaviors among persons with recent HIV infection and diagnosis—Alabama, New Jersey, and Tennessee, 1997–1998. *Morbidity and Mortality Weekly Report, 49,* 512–515.

Division of HIV/AIDS Prevention, National Center for HIV, STD, and TB Prevention. (2003a). HIV/STD risks in young men who have sex with men who do not disclose their sexual orientation—Six U.S. cities, 1994–2000. *Morbidity and Mortality Weekly Report, 52,* 81–88.

Division of HIV/AIDS Prevention, National Center for HIV, STD, and TB Prevention. (2003b). Partner counseling and referral services to identify persons with undiagnosed HIV—North Carolina, 2001. *Morbidity and Mortality Weekly Report, 52,* 1181–1184.

Division of HIV Prevention, National Center for HIV, STD, and TB Prevention. (2004). Using the internet for partner notification of sexually transmitted diseases—Los Angeles County, California, 2003. *Morbidity and Mortality Weekly Report, 53,* 129–131.

Division of Sexually Transmitted Diseases Prevention. (2000). Alcohol policy and sexually transmitted disease rates—United States, 1981–1995. *Morbidity and Mortality Weekly Report, 49,* 346–348.

Division of Sexually Transmitted Diseases Prevention. (2001). Primary and secondary syphilis—United States, 1999. *Morbidity and Mortality Weekly Report, 50,* 113–117.

Division of STD Prevention, National Center for HIV, STD, and TB Prevention. (2004a). Increases in Fluoroquinolone-resistant *Neisseria gonorrhoeae* among men who have sex with men—United States, 2003, and revised recommendations for gonorrhea treatment, 2004. *Morbidity and Mortality Weekly Report, 53,* 335–338.

Division of STD Prevention, National Center for HIV, STD, and TB Prevention. (2004b). Transmission of primary and secondary syphilis by oral sex—Chicago, Illinois, 1998–2002. *Morbidity and Mortality Weekly Report, 53,* 966–968.

Division of STD Prevention, National Center for HIV, STD, and TB Prevention. (2005a). HIV transmission in the adult film industry—Los Angeles, California, 2004. *Morbidity and Mortality Weekly Report, 54,* 923–926.

Division of STD Prevention, National Center for HIV, STD, and TB Prevention. (2005b). *Sexually transmitted disease surveillance, 2004 supplement: Syphilis surveillance report.* Retrieved May 14, 2006, from http://www.cdc.gov/std/Syphilis2004/SyphSurv/Supp2004.pdf

Division of Tuberculosis Elimination. (2000). Missed opportunities for prevention of tuberculosis among persons with HIV infection—United States, 1996–1997. *Morbidity and Mortality Weekly Report, 49,* 685–687.

Division of Vector-borne Infectious Diseases, National Center for Infectious Diseases. (2004). Lyme disease—United States, 2001–2002. *Morbidity and Mortality Weekly Report, 53,* 365–368.

Division of Viral and Rickettsial Diseases. (2005). Progress toward poliomyelitis eradication—India, January 2005–May 2005. *Morbidity and Mortality Weekly Report, 54,* 655–659.

Division of Viral and Rickettsial Diseases. (2006). Resurgence of wild poliovirus type 1 transmission and consequences of importation—21 countries, 2000–2005. *Morbidity and Mortality Weekly Report, 55,* 145–150.

Dumler, J. S., Choi, K.-S., Garcia-Garcia, J. C., Barat, N. S., Scorpio, D. G., Garyu, J. W., et al. (2005). Human granulocytic anaplasmosis and *Anaplasma phagocytophilum*. *Emerging Infectious Diseases, 11,* 1828–1834.

Dybul, M., Fauci, A. S., Bartlett, J. G., Kaplan, J. E., & Pau, A. K. (2002). Guidelines for using antiretroviral agents among HIV-infected adults and adolescents: Recommendations of the Panel on Clinical Practices for Treatment of HIV. *Morbidity and Mortality Weekly Report, 51*(RR-7), 1–54.

Elias, P. (2006). Calif. court rules on responsibility for HIV infection. Retrieved July 4, 2006, from http://signonsandiego

Emerson, C., Brown, T., Illemsky, S., Jean-Jaques, L. Boyles, R., Simpson, G., et al. (2005). Use of social networks to identify persons with undiagnosed HIV infection—Seven U.S. cities, October 2003–September, 2004. *Morbidity and Mortality Weekly Report, 54,* 601–605.

Epidemiology and Surveillance Division. (2005). Elimination of rubella and congenital rubella syndrome—United States, 1969–2004. *Morbidity and Mortality Weekly Report, 54,* 279–282.

Epidemiology Program Office. (2003). Hepatitis A outbreak associated with green onions at a restaurant—Monaca, Pennsylvania, 2003. *Morbidity and Mortality Weekly Report, 52,* 1155–1157.

Espinoza, L., Hall, H. I., Campsmith, M. L., & Lee, L. M. (2005). Trends in HIV/AIDS diagnoses—33 states, 2001–2004. *Morbidity and Mortality Weekly Report, 54,* 1149–1153.

Farley, J., Vasdev, S., Fischer, B., Haydon, E., Rehm, J., & Farley, T. A. (2005). Feasibility and outcome of HCV treatment in a Canadian federal prison population. *American Journal of Public Health, 95,* 1737–1739.

Fenton, K. A., & Valdiserri, R. O. (2006). Twenty-five years of HIV/AIDS—United States, 1981–2006. *Morbidity and Mortality Weekly Report, 55,* 585–589.

Fiore, A., Bell, B., Barker, L., Darling, N., & Amon, J. (2005). Hepatitis A vaccination coverage among children aged 24–35 months—United States, 2003. *Morbidity and Mortality Weekly Report, 54,* 141–144.

Fitzpatrick, F., Purswani, M., Fazal, B., Burrowes, A., Granville, K., Driver, C., et al. (2005). *Mycobacterium tuberculosis* transmission in a newborn nursery and maternity ward—New York City, 2003. *Morbidity and Mortality Weekly Report, 54,* 1280–1283.

Flight, C. (2002). *Smallpox: Eradicating the scourge.* Retrieved July 25, 2006, from hppt://www.bbc.co.uk/history/british/empire_seapower/smallpox_01.shtml

Fox, K. K., del Rio, C., Holmes, K. K., Hook III, E. W., Judson, F. N., Knapp, J. S., et al. (2001). Gonorrhea in the HIV era: A reversal in trends among men who have sex with men. *American Journal of Public Health, 91,* 959–964.

Francis J. Curry National Tuberculosis Center. (2004). *Why perform two-step tuberculin skin testing?* Retrieved July 25, 2006, from http://www.nationaltbcenter.edu/resources/tbcontrol_faqs/1_why_perform_2step_tst.pdf

Friis, R. H., & Sellers, T. A. (2003). *Epidemiology for public health practice* (3rd ed.). Boston: Jones and Bartlett.

Gacic-Dobo, M., Birmingham, M., Kane, M., Hadler, S. C., Perilla, M. J., Shaw, F. E., et al. (2003). Global progress toward universal childhood hepatitis B vaccination, 2003. *Morbidity and Mortality Weekly Report, 52,* 868–870.

Gasiorowicz, M., Llanas, M. R., Di Franceisco, W., Benotsch, E. G., Brondino, M. J., Catz, S. L. et al. (2005). Reductions in transmission risk behaviors in HIV-positive clients receiving prevention case management services: Findings from a community demonstration project. *AIDS Education and Prevention, 17*(Suppl. A), 40–52.

GlobalSecurity.org. (2005). *Flu pandemic mitigation—Social distancing.* Retrieved July 27, 2006, from http://www.globalsecurity.org/security/ops/hsc-scen-3_flu-pandemic-distancing.htm

Goeller, D., Blythe, D., Davenport, M., Blackburn, M., Flanner, B., Lucas, C., et al. (2005). Legionnaires disease associated with potable water in a hotel—Ocean City, Maryland, October 2003–February 2004. *Morbidity and Mortality Weekly Report, 54,* 165–168.

Graeme, K. (2005). *Smallpox's history in the world.* Retrieved July 25, 2006, from http://www.graemekennedy.name/science/2/immunoweb/bad/invaders/viruses/smallpox/history

Groom, A. V., Cheek, J. E., & Bryan, R. T. (2006). Effect of a national vaccine shortage on vaccine coverage for American Indian/Alaska Native children. *American Journal of Public Health, 96,* 697–701.

Harper, S. A., Fukuda, K., Uyeki, T. M., Cox, N. J., & Bridges, C. B. (2005). Prevention and control of influenza: Recommendations of the Advisory Committee on Immunization Practices (ACIP). *Morbidity and Mortality Weekly Report, 54*(RR-8), 1–41.

Hart, T., Peterson, J., & the Community Intervention Trial for Youth Team. (2004). Predictors of risky sexual behavior among African American men who have sex with men. *American Journal of Public Health, 94,* 1122–1123.

Heymann, D. L. (Ed.). (2004). *Control of communicable diseases manual* (18th ed.). Washington, DC: American Public Health Association.

HIV Inside. (2000). Complications associated with long-term antiretroviral therapy, 2(1), 1, 3–4, 7–8.

Hopkins, R. S., Jajosky, R. A., Hall, P. A., Adams, D. A., Connor, F. J., Sharp, P., et al. (2005, April 22). Summary of notifiable diseases—United States, 2003. *Morbidity and Mortality Weekly Report, 52*(54), 1–85.

Huebner, D., Smith, S., Safranek, T., O'Keefe, A., Lopez, A., & Marin, M., et al. (2006). Varicella outbreak among vaccinated children—Nebraska, 2004. *Morbidity and Mortality Weekly Report, 55,* 749–752.

Huey, F. L. (2004). Emerging crisis in infectious diseases: Challenges for the 21st century. *The Pfizer Journal, V*(2), 1–40.

International Treatment Preparedness Coalition. (2005). *Missing the target: A report on HIV/AIDS treatment access from the frontlines.* Retrieved February 22, 2006, from http://www.aidstreatmentaccess.org/itpcfinal.pdf

Jensen, P. A., Lambert, L. A., & Iademarco, M. F. (2005). Guidelines for preventing the transmission of *Mycobacterium tuberculosis* in health-care settings, 2005. *Morbidity and Mortality Weekly Report, 54*(RR-17), 1–141.

Joseph, C., van Wijngaarden, J., Fix, A. M., Genese, C. A., Johnson, G. S., Kacica, M., et al. (2005). Cruise-ship-associated Legionnaires disease, November 2003–May 2005. *Morbidity and Mortality Weekly Report, 54,* 1153–1155.

Kaplan, J. E., Masur, H., & Holmes, K. K. (2002). Guidelines for preventing opportunistic infections among HIV-infected persons—2002: Recommendations of the U.S. Public Health Service and the Infectious Diseases Society of America. *Morbidity and Mortality Weekly Report, 51*(RR-8), 1–52.

Keithley, J. K., Swanson, B., Murphy, M., & Levin, D. G. (2000). HIV/AIDS and nutrition: Implications for disease management. *Case Management, 5*(2), 1–9.

Kellenberg, J., Buseman, S., Wright, K., Modlin, J. F., Talbot, E. A., Montero, J. T., et al. (2005). Imported case of congenital rubella syndrome—New Hampshire, 2005. *Morbidity and Mortality Weekly Report, 54,* 1160–1161.

Kelley, M., Linthicum, L., Spaulding, A., Billah, K., Weinbaum, C., & Small, R. (2004). Hepatitis B vaccination of inmates in correctional facilities—Texas, 2000–2002. *Morbidity and Mortality Weekly Report, 53,* 681–683.

Khan, A. J., Simard, E. P., Bower, W. A., Wurtzel, H. L., Kristova, M., Wagner, K. D., et al. (2005). Ongoing transmission of hepatitis B virus infection among inmates at a state correctional facility. *American Journal of Public Health, 95,* 1793–1799.

Kieny, M. P., Excler, J.-L., & Girard, M. (2004). Research and development of new vaccines against infectious diseases. *American Journal of Public Health, 94,* 1931–1935.

Kim, D.Y., Ridzon, R., Giles, B., Mireles, T., Garrity, K., Hathcock, A. L., et al. (2003). A no-name tuberculosis tracking system. *American Journal of Public Health, 93,* 1637–1639.

Kim, S., & Crittenden, K. S. (2005). Risk factors for tuberculosis among inmates: A retrospective analysis. *Public Health Nursing, 22,* 108–118.

Klein, R., Erbart, L., Gladden, L., Hammer, M., Snow, S., Zucker, J. R., et al. (2005). Varicella-related deaths—United States, January 2003–June 2004. *Morbidity and Mortality Weekly Report, 54,* 272–274.

Koblin, B. A., Chesney, M. A., Husnik, M. J., Bozeman, S., Celum, C. L., Buchbinder, S., et al., (2003). High risk sexual behaviors among men who have sex with men in 6 US cities: Baseline data from the EXPLORE study. *American Journal of Public Health, 93,* 926–932.

Kramasz, V. C. (2005). Polio patients take a second hit. *RN, 68*(11), 33–37.

Landaverde, M., Salas, D., Humberto, M., Howard, K., Walker, R., Everett, S., et al. (2006). Imported vaccine-associated paralytic poliomyelitis—United States, 2005. *Morbidity and Mortality Weekly Report, 55,* 97–99.

Leaver, C. A., Allman, D., Meyers, T., & Veugelers, P. J. (2004). Effectiveness of HIV prevention in Ontario, Canada: A multilevel comparison of bisexual men. *American Journal of Public Health, 94,* 1181–1185.

Lee, K., & Zwi, A. (2003). A global political economy approach to AIDS; Ideology, interests, and implications. In K. Lee (Ed.), *Health impacts of globalization: Towards global governance* (pp. 13–32). New York: Palgrave Macmillan.

Leone, P., Adimora, A., Foust, E., Williams, D., Buie, M., Peebles, J., et al. (2005). HIV transmission among black women—North Carolina, 2004. *Morbidity and Mortality Weekly Report, 54,* 89–92, 94.

Lobato, M. N., Cegielski, J. P. & the Tuberculosis Along the U.S.–Mexico Border Work Group. (2001). Preventing and controlling tuberculosis along the U.S.–Mexico border. *Morbidity and Mortality Weekly Report, 50*(RR-1), 1–27.

Lofgren, J. P. (2005). *Decreasing the risk of pandemic influenza by increasing social distance.* Retrieved July 27, 2006, from http://www.socialdistancing.org/background

Macalino, F. E., Dhawan, D., & Rich, J. D. (2005). A missed opportunity: Hepatitis C screening of prisoners. *American Journal of Public Health, 95,* 1739–1740.

MacNeil, J. R., Lobato, M. N., & Moore, M. (2005). An unanswered health disparity: Tuberculosis among correctional inmates, 1993 through 2003. *American Journal of Public Health, 95,* 1800–1805.

Massachusetts Department of Public Health. (2004). Voluntary HIV testing as part of routine medical care—Massachusetts, 2002. *Morbidity and Mortality Weekly Report, 53,* 523–526.

Mast, E. E., Margolis, H. S., Fiore, A., Brink, E. W., Goldstein, S. T., Wang, S. A., et al.

(2005). Comprehensive immunization strategy to eliminate transmission of hepatitis B virus infection in the United States. *Morbidity and Mortality Weekly Report, 54*(RR-16), 1–32.

Matyas, B., Bertrand, T., Tang, Y., Dumas, B., Ratelle, S., & DeMaria, A. (2005). Reporting of chlamydial infection—Massachusetts, January–June, 2003. *Morbidity and Mortality Weekly Report, 54,* 558–560.

McCoy, D., Chopra, M., Loewenson, R., Aitken, J.-M., Ngulube, T., Muula, A., et al. (2005). Expanding access to antiretroviral therapy in Sub-Saharan Africa: Avoiding the pitfalls and dangers, Capitalizing on the opportunities. *American Journal of Public Health, 95,* 18–22.

Metsch, L. R., Pereyra, M., de Rio, C., Gardner, L., Duffus, W. A., Dickinson, G., et al. (2004). Delivery of HIV prevention counseling by physicians at HIV medical care settings in 4 US cities. *American Journal of Public Health, 94,* 1186–1192.

Mofenson, L., Taylor, A. W., Rogers, M., Campsmith, M., Ruffo, N. M., Clark, J., et al. (2006). Reduction in perinatal transmission of HIV infection—United States, 1985–2005. *Morbidity and Mortality Weekly Report, 55,* 592–597.

Myers, W. P., Westenhouse, J. L., Flood, J., & Riley, L. W. (2006). An ecological study of tuberculosis transmission in California. *American Journal of Public Health, 96,* 685–690.

National Center for HIV, STD, and TB Prevention. (2006a). *Viral hepatitis C: Fact sheet.* Retrieved May 14, 2006, from http://www.cdc.gov/ncidod/diseases/hepatitis/c/fact.htm

National Center for HIV, STD, and TB Prevention. (2006b). *Viral hepatitis D: Fact sheet.* Retrieved May 14, 2006, from http://www.cdc.gov/ncidod/diseases/hepatitis/d/fact.htm

National Center for HIV, STD, and TB Prevention. (2006c). *Viral hepatitis E: Fact sheet.* Retrieved May 14, 2006, from http://www.cdc.gov/ncidod/diseases/hepatitis/e/fact.htm

National Center for Infectious Diseases. (2000a). *Viral hepatitis A—Fact sheet.* Retrieved June 13, 2000, from http://www.cdc.gov/ncidod/diseases/hepatitis/a/fact

National Center for Infectious Diseases. (2000b). *Viral hepatitis B—Fact sheet.* Retrieved June 13, 2000, from http://www.cdc.gov/ncidod/diseases/hepatitis/b/fact

National Commission on Correctional Health Care. (2005). DOT for HAART shows promise. *Correct Care, 19*(1), 15.

National Immunization Program. (1999). Impact of vaccines universally recommended for children—United States, 1990–1998. *Morbidity and Mortality Weekly Report, 48,* 243–248.

National Immunization Program. (2002). *Tetanus—In short.* Retrieved May 20, 2006, from http://www.cdc.gov/nip/diseases/tetanus/vac-chart.htm

National Tuberculosis Controllers Association & Centers for Disease Control and Prevention. (2005). Guidelines for the investigation of contacts of persons with infectious tuberculosis. *Morbidity and Mortality Weekly Report, 54,* 1–47.

Nielsen, N. D., & Bartlett, J. A. (2004). HIV infection and AIDS. In R. S. Kirby, C. C. Carson, M. G. Kirby, & R. N. Farah (Eds.), *Men's health* (2nd ed., pp. 459–474). London: Taylor & Francis.

Palmer, A., McVey III, E., McNeill, K. M., Hand, S., Rupprecht, C. E., Hanlon, C. A., et al. (2006). Human rabies—Mississippi, 2005. *Morbidity and Mortality Weekly Report, 55*, 207–208.

Panlilio, A. L., Cardo, D. M., Grohskopf, L. A., Heneine, W., & Ross, C. S. (2005). Updated U.S. Public Health Service guidelines for the management of occupational exposures to HIV and recommendations for postexposure prophylaxis. *Morbidity and Mortality Weekly Report, 54*(RR-9), 1–17.

Pearson, M. L., Bridges, C. B., & Harper, S. (2006). Influenza vaccination of health-care personnel: Recommendations of the Health Care Infection Control Practices Advisory Committee (HICPAC) and the Advisory Committee on Immunization Practices (ACIP). *Morbidity and Mortality Weekly Report, 55*(RR-2), 1–16.

Polio Eradication Group, World Health Organization. (2006). Progress toward interruption of wild poliovirus transmission—Worldwide, January 2005–March 2006. *Morbidity and Mortality Weekly Report, 55*, 458–462.

Poynard, T. (2004). Hepatitis B and C. In R. S. Kirby, C. C. Carson, M. G. Kirby, & R. N. Farah (Eds.), *Men's health* (2nd ed., pp. 475–489). London: Taylor & Francis.

Pratt, R., Robison, V., Navin, T., & Hlavsa, M. (2006). Trends in tuberculosis—United States, 2005. *Morbidity and Mortality Weekly Report, 55*, 305–308.

Prejean, J., Satcher, A. J., Durant, R., Hu, X., & Lee, L. M. (2006). Racial/ethnic disparities in diagnoses of HIV/AIDS—33 states, 2001–2004. *Morbidity and Mortality Weekly Report, 55*, 121–125.

Prevots, D. R., Burr, R. K., Sutter, R. W., & Murphy, T. V. (2000). Poliomyelitis prevention in the United States: Updated recommendations of the Advisory Committee on Immunization Practices. *Morbidity and Mortality Weekly Report, 49*(RR-5), 1–22.

Quinlisk, P., Harris, M., Thornton, T., & Flamigni, L. (2006). Mumps epidemic—Iowa, 2006. *Morbidity and Mortality Weekly Report, 55*, 366–368.

Remis, R. S., Dufour, A., Alary, M., Vincelette, J., Otis, J., Mâsse, B., et al. (2000). Association of hepatitis B virus infection with other sexually transmitted diseases in homosexual men. *American Journal of Public Health, 90*, 1570–1574.

Rosenman, M. B., Kraft, S. K., Harezlak, J., Mahon, B. E., Katz, B., Wang, J., et al. (2004). Syphilis testing in association with gonorrhea/chlamydia testing during a syphilis outbreak. *American Journal of Public Health, 94*, 1124–1126.

Ross, J. S., & Labbok, M. H. (2004). Modeling the effects of different infant feeding strategies on infant survival and mother-to-child transmission of HIV. *American Journal of Public Health, 94*, 1174–1180.

Rusen, I. D., & Enarson, D. A. (2006). FIDELIS—Innovative approaches to increasing global case detection of tuberculosis. *American Journal of Public Health, 96*, 14–16.

Rutala, W. A., White, M. S., Gergen, M. F., & Weber, D. J. (2006). Bacterial contamination of keyboards: Efficacy and functional impact of disinfectants. *Infection Control and Hospital Epidemiology, 27*, 372–377.

St. Lawrence, J. S., Montano, D. E., Kasprzyk, D., Phillips, W. R., Armstrong, K., & Leichliter, J. S. (2002). STD screening, testing, case reporting, and clinical and partner notification practices: A national survey of US physicians. *American Journal of Public Health, 92*, 1784–1788.

Santibanez, T. A., Santoli, J. M., & Barker, L. E. (2006). Differential effects of DTaP and MMR vaccine shortages on timeliness of childhood vaccination coverage. *American Journal of Public Health, 96*, 691–696.

Santibanez, T. A., Singleton, J. S., Santoli, J., Euler, G., & Bridges, C. B. (2006). Childhood influenza vaccination coverage—United States, 2003–04 influenza season. *Morbidity and Mortality Weekly Report, 55*, 100–103.

Savage, E., White, J. M., Brown, D. E. W., & Ramsay, M. E. (2006). Mumps epidemic—United Kingdom, 2004–2005. *Morbidity and Mortality Weekly Report, 55*, 173–175.

Schneider, E., Glynn, M. K., Kajese, T., & McKenna, M. T. (2006). Epidemiology of HIV/AIDS—United States, 1981–2005. *Morbidity and Mortality Weekly Report, 55*, 589–592.

Seipone, K., Ntumy, R., Smith, M., Thuku, H. Mazhani, L., Creek, T., et al. (2004). Introduction of routine HIV testing in prenatal care—Botswana, 2004. *Morbidity and Mortality Weekly Report, 53*, 1083–1086.

Selik, R. M., Glynn, M. K., & McKenna, M. T. (2004). Diagnoses of HIV/AIDS—32 states, 2000–2003. *Morbidity and Mortality Weekly Report, 53*, 1106–1110.

Shiel, W. C. (2005.). *Tuberculosis skin test (PPD skin test)*. Retrieved July 25, 2006, from http://www.medicinenet.com/tuberculosis_skin_test/article.htm

Shih, S., Scholle, S., Irwin, K., Tao, G., Walsh, C., & Tun, W. (2004). Chlamydia screening among sexually active young female enrollees of health plans—United States, 1999–2001. *Morbidity and Mortality Weekly Report, 53*, 983–985.

Sifakis, F., Flynn, C. P., Metsch, L., LaLota, M., Murrill, C., Bingham, T., et al. (2005). HIV prevalence, unrecognized infection, and HIV testing among men who have sex with men—Five U.S. cities, June 2004–April 2005. *Morbidity and Mortality Weekly Report, 54*, 597–601.

Smith, C. E., Jenkins, J. M., Staib, D., Newell, P. J., Mertz, K. J., Lance-Parker, S., et al. (2004). Possible dialysis-related West Nile virus transmission—Georgia, 2003. *Morbidity and Mortality Weekly Report, 53*, 738–739.

Smith, D. K., Grohskopf, L. A., Black, R., Auerbach, J. D., Veronese, F., Struble, K. A., et al. (2005). Antiretroviral postexposure prophylaxis after sexual, injection drug use, or other non-occupational exposure to HIV in the United States: Recommendations from the U.S. Department of Health and Human Services. *Morbidity and Mortality Weekly Report, 54*(RR-2), 1–20.

Smith, T. L., Hayes, E. B., O'Leary, D. R., Nasci, R. S., Komar, N., Campbell, G. L., et al. (2005). West Nile virus activity—United States, January 1–December 1, 2005. *Morbidity and Mortality Weekly Report, 54*, 1263–1265.

Stall, R., Mills, T. C., Williamson, J., Hart, T., Greenwood, G., Paul, J., et al. (2003). Association of co-occurring psychosocial health problems and increased vulnerability to HIV/AIDS among urban men who have sex with men. *American Journal of Public Health, 93*, 939–942.

State of California. (2005). *Title 17, California code of regulations (CCR), §2500, §2593, §2641–2643, and §2800–2812 reportable diseases and conditions*. Retrieved July 27, 2006, from http://www.dhs.ca.gov/dcdc/izgroup/pdf/title17.pdf

Teperman, L. W., Diflo, T., Fahmy, A., Morgan, G. R., Wetherbee, R. E., Ratner, L., et al. (2005). West Nile virus infections in organ transplant recipients—New York and Pennsylvania, August–September, 2005. *Morbidity and Mortality Weekly Report, 54*, 1021–1023.

Teplin, L. A., Mericle, A. A., McClelland, G. M., & Abram, K. M. (2003). HIV and AIDS risk behaviors in juvenile detainees: Implications for public health policy. *American Journal of Public Health, 93*, 906–912.

Tiwari, T., Murphy, T. V., & Moran, J. (2005). Recommended antimicrobial agents for the treatment and postexposure prophylaxis of pertussis: 2005 CDC guidelines. *Morbidity and Mortality Weekly Report, 54*(RR-14), 1–15.

Trust for America's Health. (2005). *It's not flu as usual*. Washington, DC: Author.

Udwadia, F. E. (2000). *Man and medicine: A history*. Oxford: Oxford University.

Tuberculosis Coalition for Technical Assistance. (2006). *International Standards for Tuberculosis Care (ISTC)*. Retrieved July 27, 2006, from http://www.stoptb.org/resources_center/assets/documents/listc_report.pdf

UNAIDS. (2005). *AIDS epidemic update: December, 2005*. Retrieved May 22, 2006, from http://www.unaids.org/epi/2005/doc/EPIupdate2005_pdf_en/epi-update2005_en.pdf

Urquhart, G., Kelly, J., & Rasulnia, B. (2005). Immunization information system progress—United States, 2004. *Morbidity and Mortality Weekly Report, 54*, 1157–1158.

van de Laar, M. J. W., Götz, H. M., de Zwart, P., van der Meijden, W. I., Ossewaarde, J. M., Thio, H. B., et al. (2004). Lymphogranuloma venereum among men who have sex with men—Netherlands, 2003–2004. *Morbidity and Mortality Weekly Report, 53*, 985–988.

Vannarith, C., Kanara, N., Qualls, M., Varma, J., Laserson, K., & Wells, C. (2005). Screening HIV-infected persons for tuberculosis—Cambodia, January 2004–February 2005. *Morbidity and Mortality Weekly Report, 54*, 1177–1181.

Walensky, R. P., Losina, E., Malatesta, L., Barton, G. E., O'Connor, C. A., Skolnik, P. R., et al. (2005). Effective HIV case identification through routine HIV screening at urgent care centers in Massachusetts. *American Journal of Public Health, 95*, 71–73.

Watts, S. (2003). *Disease and medicine in world history*. New York: Routledge.

Weinbaum, C., Billah, K., & Mast, E. E. (2006). Hepatitis B vaccination coverage among adults—United States, 2004. *Morbidity and Mortality Weekly Report, 54*, 509–511.

White House Office of the Press Secretary. (2003). *Executive order: Revised list of quarantinable communicable diseases*. Retrieved July 27, 2006, from http://www.cdc.gov/ncidod/sars/pdf/executiveorder040403.pdf

Whiticar, P. M., Ohye, R. G., Lee, M. V., Bauer, H. M., Bolan, G., Wang, S. A., et al. (2002). Increases in Fluoroquinolone-resistant *Neisseria gonorrhoeae*—Hawaii and California, 2001. *Morbidity and Mortality Weekly Report, 51*, 1041–1044.

Wikimedia Foundation. (2006). *Quarantine*. Retrieved July 27, 2006, from http://en.wikipedia.org/wiki/Quarantine

Willis, B. C., Ndiaye, S. M., Hopkins, D. P., & Shefer, A. (2005). Improving influenza, pneumococcal polysaccharide, and hepatitis B vaccination coverage among adults aged <65 years at high risk: A report on recommendations of the Task Force on Community Preventive Services. *Morbidity and Mortality Weekly Report, 54*(RR-5), 1–11.

Wilson, T. E., Gore, M. E., Greenblatt, R., Cohen, M., Minkoff, H., Silver, S., et al. (2004). Changes in sexual behavior among HIV-infected women after initiation of HAART. *American Journal of Public Health, 94*, 1141–1147.

Wise, M. E., & Sorvillo, F. (2005). Hepatitis A-related mortality in California, 1989–2000: Analysis of multiple cause-coded death data. *American Journal of Public Health, 95*, 900–905.

Wolitski, R. J., Henny, K. D., Lyles, C. M., Purcell, D. W., Carey, J. W., Crepaz, N., et al. (2006). Evolution of HIV/AIDS prevention programs—United States, 1981–2006. *Morbidity and Mortality Weekly Report, 55*, 597–603.

Wolitski, R. J., Valdiserri, R. O., Denning, P. H., & Levine, W. C. (2001). Are we headed for a resurgence of the HIV epidemic among men who have sex with men? *American Journal of Public Health, 91*, 883–888.

World Care Council. (2006). *The patients' charter for tuberculosis care: Patients' rights and responsibilities*. Retrieved July 27, 2006, from http://www.stoptb.org/resources_center/assets/documents/listc_charter.pdf

World Health Organization. (2005a). *The international health regulations (2005)*. Retrieved July 27, 2006, from http://www.who.int/csr/ihr/one_page_update_new.pdf

World Health Organization. (2005b). *World health statistics, 2005*. Retrieved September 21, 2005, from http://www.who.int/healthinfo/statistics/whostat2005en1.pdf

World Health Organization. (2006a). *Frequently asked questions about the international health regulations*. Retrieved July 27, 2006, from http://www.who.int/crs/ihr/howtheywork/faq/en/print.html

World Health Organization. (2006b). Progress in reducing global measles deaths, 1999–2004. *Morbidity and Mortality Weekly Report, 55*, 247–249.

Workowski, K. A., & Levine, W. C. (2002). Sexually transmitted diseases treatment guidelines. *Morbidity and Mortality Weekly Report, 51*(RR-6), 1–78.

Wright, A., Bai, G., Barrena, L., Boulahbal, F. Martin-Casabona, N., Gilpin, C., et al. (2006). Emergence of *Mycobacterium tuberculosis* with extensive resistance to second-line drugs—Worldwide, 2000–2004. *Morbidity and Mortality Weekly Report, 55*, 301–305.

Wyatt, G. E., Myers, H. F., Williams, J. K., Kitchen, K. R., Loeb, T., Carmona, J. V., et al. (2002). Does a history of trauma contribute to HIV risk for women of color? Implications for prevention and policy. *American Journal of Public Health, 92*, 660–665.

Youngpairoj, S., Euler, G. L., Lu, P. J., Bridges, C. B., & Wortley, P. M. (2005). Influenza vaccination levels among persons ≥ 65 years and among persons aged 18–64 years with high-risk conditions—United States, 2003. *Morbidity and Mortality Weekly Report, 54*, 1045–1049.

Yusuf, H. R., Daniels, D., Smith, P., Coronado, V., & Rodewald, L. (2000). Association between administration of hepatitis B at birth and completion of the hepatitis B and 4:3:1:3 vaccine series. *Journal of the American Medical Association, 284*, 978–983.

Zambrana, R. E., Cornelius, L. J., Boykin, S. S., & Lopez, D. S. (2004). Latinas and HIV/AIDS risk factors: Implications for harm reduction strategies. *American Journal of Public Health, 94*, 1152–1158.

Chronic Physical Health Problems

CHAPTER OBJECTIVES

After reading this chapter, you should be able to:

1. Describe personal and population effects of chronic physical health problems.
2. Identify biophysical, psychological, physical environmental, sociocultural, behavioral, and health system factors that influence the development of chronic physical health problems.
3. Describe strategies for primary prevention of chronic physical health problems and analyze the role of the community health nurse related to each.
4. Identify the major aspects of secondary prevention of chronic physical health problems and analyze community health nursing roles with respect to each.
5. Analyze community health nursing roles in tertiary prevention of chronic physical health problems.

KEY TERMS

activity limitations **855**
cancer survivors **890**
caregiver burden **888**
chronic disease **855**
decision support systems **882**
disability **855**
impairment **855**
participation restrictions **855**
risk markers **862**
self-management **883**
stigmatization **887**

MediaLink
http://www.prenhall.com/clark

Additional interactive resources for this chapter can be found on the Companion Website. Click on Chapter 29 and "Begin" to select the activities for this chapter.

Advocacy in Action

Diapers

A man in his mid-50s lived downtown by himself on public assistance because of his low income and spinal disease. He was suffering from incontinence and needed to wear diapers. The city office provided 120 diapers per month for free. The diapers were flat and did not work well for him because he was an active and outgoing person. He could not walk, although he could ride a bicycle.

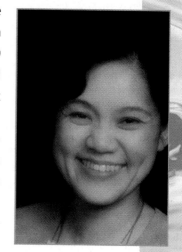

A public health nurse newly employed by the local public health center was assigned the district in which this client lived. She visited his house with the previously assigned public health nurse and heard his story. She had graduated from an interdisciplinary education program and had a unique network. One of her fellow alumni was working for a big textile goods company that had recently started a venture business in care-giving products. She asked her colleague to send some samples of new products. He collected and sent her several types of three-dimensional-shaped diapers and other new products, which she brought to the client's house and examined with him.

Her client found a diaper that met his needs and wanted to change from the flat diapers to the new product. The nurse went to the city hall and negotiated a policy change to allow recipients of diapers to choose the type of diaper that best meets their needs. Because of her work, the public services system was changed to better meet the needs of this particular client and others who receive similar services.

Ariko Noji
Niigata College of Nursing
Joetsu City, Niigata, Japan

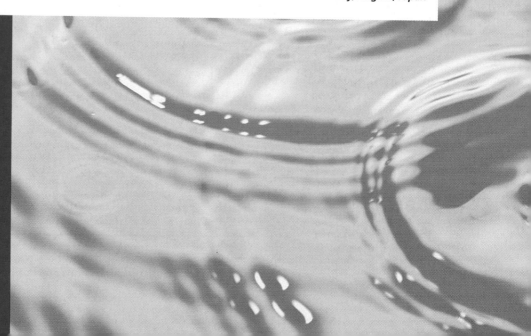

*B*ecause of the effectiveness of control measures developed for many previously fatal communicable diseases, chronic health problems have largely replaced communicable diseases as the leading causes of death and disability in the United States and elsewhere in the world. Each year, millions of people worldwide experience the suffering and the economic costs associated with chronic health problems, and many die as a result. An estimated 90 million people in the United States experience at least one chronic disease (Sitzman, 2004), and chronic diseases account for three fourths of U.S. health care expenditures each year (Bodenheimer, Wagner, & Grumbach, 2002a). On the plus side, the onset of many chronic diseases is occurring later in life than in the past. In spite of these gains, half of the U.S. population is expected to have at least one chronic condition and nearly one quarter will experience more than one (Plese, 2005b).

A **chronic disease** has been defined as "a condition that requires ongoing medical care, limits what one can do, and is likely to last longer than one year" (Partnership for Solutions, 2002, p. 1). Chronic conditions include diseases, injuries with lasting consequences, and other enduring abnormalities.

Chronic health problems may be either physical or emotional, and both types of chronic conditions are addressed in the national health objectives developed for the year 2010 (Centers for Disease Control and Prevention [CDC], 2005b). These objectives and current levels of achievement may be viewed at the *Healthy People 2010*◆ Web site at http://wonder.cdc.gov/data2010. In this chapter, we address chronic physical health problems. Chronic emotional conditions are addressed in Chapter 30∞.

GLOBAL PERSPECTIVES

*T*he World Health Organization (2005) has identified several misconceptions related to chronic diseases that hamper worldwide efforts to achieve control of these conditions:

- Everyone dies of something; it might as well be a chronic disease.
- Not everyone who has risk factors for a chronic disease will die of it.
- Prevention and control of chronic diseases is too expensive.
- Chronic diseases can't be prevented.
- Chronic diseases result from unhealthy lifestyle choices and are the fault of the people affected.
- Chronic diseases affect mostly men.
- Chronic diseases affect mostly older people.
- Chronic diseases affect mostly rich people.
- Middle- and lower-income countries should control infectious diseases before worrying about chronic conditions.
- Chronic diseases affect mostly affluent nations.

To what extent do you think these misconceptions exist in the United States? How would you go about countering these misconceptions to promote greater attention to prevention of chronic health problems?

THE EFFECTS OF CHRONIC PHYSICAL HEALTH PROBLEMS

Chronic health problems can arise from a variety of sources. For example, some people are born with chronic health problems. Conversely, a person might develop a chronic disability as a result of a serious accident or because of a disease such as arthritis, cardiovascular disease, chronic respiratory diseases, or cancer. Some chronic conditions, such as some cancers, may result in death. Others, although not fatal, cause persistent pain and disability.

The effects of chronic health conditions are not only experienced by individuals. Population groups and society at large are also affected by the consequences of chronic health problems.

Personal and Family Effects

The advent of a chronic condition has many personal effects for individual clients. Possible consequences of disease and injury include pain and suffering, impairment, and disability. Other consequences are family stress and economic burden. According to the International Classification of Functioning, Disability, and Health adopted by the World Health Organization (WHO) in 2001, **impairment** refers to "problems in body function and structure such as significant deviation or loss" (WHO as quoted in Kearney & Pryor, 2004, p. 165). Impairment may result in limitations in activity or restrictions in participation. **Activity limitations** are defined as "difficulties an individual may have in executing activities" in the domains of learning and applying knowledge, general tasks and demands, communication, mobility, self-care, domestic life, interpersonal interactions and relationships, major life areas (e.g., employment, school), and community, social, or civic life (Kearney & Pryor, 2004, p. 165). **Participation restrictions** are "problems an individual may experience in life situations" (p. 165) and may occur in the same domains as activity limitations.

Disability, on the other hand, is a "multidimensional phenomenon resulting from the interaction between people and their physical and social environment" (WHO, as quoted in Kearney & Pryor, 2004, p. 166). Disability results when health conditions and their interaction with contextual factors interfere with one's ability to function in ways that are expected or desired. For example, a person in a wheelchair whose workplace accommodates his or her mobility limitations is not disabled. The same person, however, might be considered disabled in another country where buildings have not been designed to facilitate wheelchair access.

Disability is a culturally defined concept that differs from one group of people to another. Some authors, however, make the point that the concept itself connotes difference from the norm that is heightened by societal *ableism* in which ideas, practices, institutions, and social relationships are predicated on presumptions of ablebodiedness (Gesler & Kearns, 2002). People with disabilities are often perceived and treated as different or socially undesirable, and community health nurses may need to educate the public and advocate changes in perceptions of people with disabilities.

Overall, 54 million Americans (more than 20% of the population) exhibit some form of disability (Carmona, 2005), and nearly 6% require the use of special equipment as a result of chronic health problems (Jiles et al., 2005). In 2003, 35 million Americans with disabilities were receiving Medicare benefits (U.S. Census Bureau, 2005).

Some chronic health conditions may make a greater contribution to disability than others. For example, 47% of people with epilepsy in one study reported disability compared to only 18% of the population without this disease, and those taking medication for epilepsy reported disability more than three times as often as those without (Ferguson et al., 2005). In July 2005, the U.S. Surgeon General issued a *Call to Action to Improve the Health and Wellness of Persons with Disabilities*. The four goals of this initiative are to (a) promote public understanding of disability and the capabilities of persons with disability, (b) increase the capability of health care providers to provide holistic care to persons with disabilities, (c) assist persons with disabilities to promote their own health, and (d) enhance access to the care and services required to promote independence among those with disabilities (Office of the Surgeon General, 2005). Community health nursing intervention and advocacy will be required to accomplish these goals. For example, community health nurses may need to advocate for holistic care for people with disabilities that meets more than physical health needs. Political advocacy may also be needed to assure access to needed services or to promote environmental changes that limit the disabling effects of chronic conditions.

In addition to a diminished quality of life, the presence of disability may impede other health-related behaviors. For example, women with disabilities in one California study were less likely than those without

BUILDING OUR KNOWLEDGE BASE

There is no standard definition of the word *disability*. In fact, there are more than 67 definitions of disability in federal legislation (Office of the Surgeon General, 2005). Some authors argue that a standard definition of disability should be developed to facilitate comparison of the findings of different research studies. Others suggest that since disability is often defined on the basis of the perceptions of the person experiencing it, continued research using different definitions of the term provides more meaningful information from the perspectives of those who experience the phenomenon.

- What are the advantages and disadvantages of each position?
- Which position would you adopt? Why?
- If you were planning to conduct a study related to disability, how would you define this variable?

disabilities to have received a Papanicolaou smear in the prior 3 years or a mammogram in the previous 2 years. Similarly, men with disabilities were less likely to report a prostate-specific antigen test in the prior 2 years. In addition, women with disabilities were less likely than those without to have received a provider recommendation for cervical cancer screening (Ramirez, Farmer, Grant, & Papachristou, 2005).

Activity limitations often require a change in lifestyle. Individuals with arthritis, for example, may need to adjust to their inability to do some things that they have done in the past or may need to learn to use special implements to accomplish everyday tasks like closing a zipper or buttoning a shirt. Similarly, clients with chronic respiratory conditions may find that they are less able to engage in vigorous activity than in the past and may require more frequent rest periods. The client seriously injured in an automobile accident may need to adjust to using a wheelchair. Frequently, such physical limitations make it necessary to rely on others to perform routine tasks of daily living. This enforced dependence on others may, in turn, adversely affect an individual's self-image.

Even when activities are not restricted, the presence of a chronic health problem usually requires lifestyle adjustments. For the person with diabetes or a heart condition, for example, changes in diet are required. The person with diabetes may also need to make changes in eating patterns. This might mean not skipping meals or not eating on the run.

Pain also accompanies a number of chronic conditions and is often unremitting. The client with arthritis or cancer, for example, may have to endure a long period of pain despite the continued use of analgesics. It is estimated that 42% of U.S. adults experience daily pain and that 89% experience pain at least one day a month (Vallerand, Fouladbakhsh, & Templin, 2003). In the 2002 Behavioral Risk Factor Surveillance System (BRFSS) survey, approximately one fourth of respondents in 18 states and the District of Columbia reported at least one day of difficulty with activity related to pain in the prior month. Pain was associated with obesity, increased smoking, decreased physical activity, and symptoms of depression and anxiety (Strine, Hootman, Chapman, Okoro, & Balluz, 2005). The constant battle with chronic pain can be disheartening and can lead to depression and possible suicide. Community health nurses can advocate for effective management of chronic pain and promote the use of appropriate pharmacologic and nonpharmacologic management strategies. Pain management with respect to chronic health problems is addressed in more detail later in this chapter.

The pain, lifestyle changes, decreased activity levels, and impaired mobility associated with chronic conditions can contribute to social isolation. The chronically ill individual may be less able to interact with others in familiar patterns or be unable to engage in activities that friends and family enjoy. Consequently, this person may

ETHICAL AWARENESS

Many chronic conditions involve considerable pain that is frequently only lessened but never eliminated. Other conditions result in significant disabilities that severely diminish clients' quality of life. How would you respond to a client who tells you he is considering assisted suicide because he can no longer live with the consequences of his condition? Would your response be different if he were considering euthanasia for a family member in intractable pain, rather than for himself? Why or why not? What are the legal ramifications of his planned course of action in your state? Is your response influenced by the legal ramifications? Why or why not?

feel left out unless concerted efforts are made to incorporate him or her into family and community life.

Chronic health problems have effects on families as well as on the individual affected. Family members with chronic conditions may no longer be able to fulfill their normal family roles, necessitating role reallocation and possibly role overload for other family members. Restructuring of family roles may also affect relationships among family members, changes in self-image and anger for the member with a chronic disease, and increased stress for other family members (Strunin & Boden, 2004). Family members may also have to give up work to care for a disabled member, limiting both the opportunity for respite and family income.

Finally, chronic health problems often entail considerable financial burden for both individuals and families. Most chronic conditions require the individual to take prescribed medications for the rest of his or her life, and the cost can escalate rapidly. Add to this the cost of frequent visits to health care providers to monitor the condition and the effects of therapy. Moreover, many individuals with chronic conditions require expensive special equipment or services. Disabled individuals have been found to be more than twice as likely as those who are not disabled to put off needed health care because of costs and are four times more likely to have health needs that are not covered by health insurance. Disabled individuals are also three times more likely to live in poverty than those without disability (National Organization on Disability, 2004). Community health nurses may need to advocate for services and financial assistance for families affected by chronic health conditions.

Population Effects

Chronic conditions also affect the general population. These effects are reflected in financial costs to society, morbidity, and mortality.

Societal Costs

Chronic health problems cost society millions of dollars each year, and the annual costs of disability related to chronic health conditions amount to $170 billion (Churchill, 2005). Overall, chronic diseases account for

75% of health care expenditures in the United States (National Center for Chronic Disease Prevention and Health Promotion, 2002). Societal costs of chronic health conditions include the direct medical costs of care, the indirect medical costs (e.g., home modification, special education), and other indirect costs such as productivity losses due to the inability of many of those affected to work, limitations on work ability, or premature death (National Center on Birth Defects and Developmental Disabilities [NCBDDD], 2004). Societal costs due to lost productivity may also apply to family caretakers who cannot be employed because of their caretaking responsibilities (Huey, 2001). For instance, asthma and allergies result in workplace productivity losses of more than $1.4 million each month for a total loss of more than $17 million per year (Institute for Health and Management Productivity, 2002). Family care of chronically ill children also results in considerable lost productivity and amounts to $155 billion to $279 billion each year (Wilson et al., 2005).

Similarly, heart disease accounted for 13% of U.S. hospitalizations in 2003 (National Center for Health Statistics [NCHS], 2005b), and total costs for heart disease in 2006 were expected to be more than $258 billion in the United States alone (Division for Heart Disease and Stroke Prevention, 2006a). Direct and indirect costs for diabetes amounted to $132 million in 2002 (CDC, 2005c). This figure is probably an underestimate of the true costs because it does not account for care provided by unpaid family members (American Diabetes Association, 2003b). In 2005, costs for stroke in the United States were nearly $57 billion (Division for Heart Disease and Stroke Prevention, 2006b).

Accidental injuries also contribute a major portion of societal costs related to chronic conditions and account for more than 10% of all medical expenditures in the United States, with treatment costs amounting to $64.7 billion a year. These costs do not even begin to account for costs related to lost productivity, property damage, litigation, and long-term mental health consequences (National Center for Injury Prevention and Control, 2004). The annual direct and indirect costs of epilepsy are estimated at $15.5 billion (CDC, 2006b), and arthritis results in $60 billion in lost productivity each year (Plese, 2005b). Overall disability costs amount to more than $300 billion each year, or roughly 5% of the gross domestic product (Office of the Surgeon General, 2005). It would seem clear from these cost figures alone that the United States can no longer bear the burden of chronic disease and must take steps to control these and other chronic conditions.

Morbidity

Societal costs of chronic health conditions are measured not only in dollars but also in terms of the extent of morbidity resulting from these conditions. Although some progress has been made in preventing mortality due to chronic conditions, their prevalence has been increasing over the years. Because the reporting of chronic health conditions is not mandatory, however, prevalence figures probably grossly underrepresent the extent of these conditions in the population.

Although effective treatment has been available for more than 50 years, hypertension continues to affect approximately 50 million people in the United States (CDC, 2002a). A median of 25% of respondents to the 2003 BRFSS survey reported that they had been told by a physician that they had high blood pressure (Jiles et al., 2005). Unfortunately, only 45% of people with hypertension in the United States receive treatment (Ayala et al., 2006), and only 29% of those being treated have achieved good control of their disease (Glover, Greenlund, Ayala, & Croft, 2005). Hypertension contributes to both stroke and heart disease. During 2006, 700,000 U.S. residents are expected to experience a stroke. Approximately 22.5% of these people will die and 15% to 30% will have some level of permanent disability (CDC, 2006d).

Various forms of heart disease affect major segments of the U.S. population as well. Cardiovascular disease is the leading cause of work-related disability in

U.S. men. Congestive heart failure (CHF) is also prevalent, with 4 million people affected in the United States and an estimated 400,000 new cases diagnosed each year. CHF is the most frequent reason for hospital admission among Medicare enrollees (Ranjan, Tarigopula, Srivastava, Obasanjo, & Obah, 2003). At the global level, ischemic heart disease is the greatest physical health contributor to disability-adjusted life years (DALYs) in developed countries, accounting for 6.7% of DALYs each year. Cerebrovascular disease accounts for another 4.9%, followed by Alzheimer's disease (4.3%), motor vehicle accidents (3.1%), lung cancer (3%), osteoarthritis (2.7%), chronic obstructive pulmonary disease (COPD) (2.5%), and adult onset hearing loss (2.5%). For developing nations, ischemic heart disease, cerebrovascular disease, and motor vehicle accidents are the seventh, ninth, and tenth top causes of DALYs, together accounting for 9.2% of DALYs (Bonita & Mathers, 2003). As described in Chapter 6∞, DALYs are a measure of the years of disability-free healthy life lost to disease.

Although overall cancer incidence rates declined by 4% from 1990 to 2002 (NCHS, 2005a), cancer remains a serious concern in the United States and worldwide. From 1973 to 1998, for example, the incidence of malignant melanoma increased more than 150% (Glanz, Saraiya, & Wechsler, 2002). Colorectal cancer is the second leading cause of cancer death in the United States (Brouse et al., 2003), and breast and ovarian cancer are the second and fifth leading causes of cancer death among U.S. women (Jacobellis et al., 2004). For men, prostate cancer is the second most common cause of cancer deaths after lung cancer (Calabrese, 2004).

Survival rates have improved for most cancers. Survival rates reflect the number of people with a diagnosed condition who are still alive after a given period of time (usually 5 or 10 years for most cancers). For example, 64% of adults diagnosed with cancer between 1995 and 2000 were expected to be alive 5 years later. One of the *Healthy People 2010*◆ objectives is to increase overall 5-year cancer survival rates to 70% of those diagnosed. This objective has already been achieved for children with cancer, among whom 79% of those diagnosed between 1991 and 2000 would be expected to be alive 5 years later and 75% at 10 years. In 2001, 14% of all people in the United States living with cancer had been diagnosed more than 20 years previously. Reasons for increased survival rates include earlier diagnosis as a result of cancer screening programs, the availability of more effective therapies, prevention of secondary disease among persons with cancer, and a decrease in mortality from other causes, leading to longer survival with cancer (Division of Cancer Prevention and Control, 2004). Care of cancer survivors will be addressed in more detail later in this chapter.

Approximately 18.2 million individuals in the United States have diabetes mellitus, a third of whom

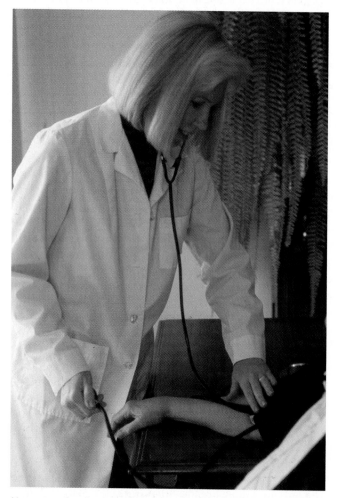

Hypertension is one of the most prevalent chronic health conditions. (Patrick J. Watson)

are not aware of their disease (U.S. Department of Health and Human Services [USDHHS], 2003b). In 2003, a median of 7.2% of the population of U.S. states and territories reported doctor-diagnosed diabetes (Jiles et al., 2005). Each year, roughly 1.3 million new diagnoses of diabetes are made in U.S. adults (American Diabetes Association, 2003c), and diabetes incidence is expected to double by 2050 (USDHHS, 2003b).

Diabetes is a significant contributor to disability in the United States. According to National Health and Nutrition Examination Survey (NHANES) data for 1999 through 2002, people over 40 years of age with diabetes were nearly twice as likely to report mobility limitation as those without diabetes (Eberhard, Saydah, Paulose-Ram, & Tao, 2005).

Asthma affects about 20.7 million U.S. adults and 8.9 million children (NCHS, 2006a). Asthma prevalence increased 74% from 1980 to 1996, then dropped slightly from 1997 to 1999. During this time, the rate for outpatient and emergency department visits for asthma increased, but hospitalization rates decreased (Mannino et al., 2002). As noted in Chapter 16∞, asthma accounts for more school absences than any other condition. In 2003, nearly one fifth of high school students reported a diagnosis of asthma and 16% had asthma at the time of the Youth Risk Behavior Survey. Of these students, nearly 38% had experienced an asthma attack during the prior year (Division of Environmental Hazards and Health Effects, 2005).

Asthma is also a significant problem in the workplace. In one study, one fifth of employees reported being affected by asthma or having a dependent with asthma. Six percent of employees with asthma reported

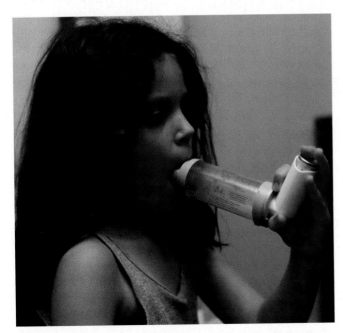

Morbidity and mortality due to asthma are increasing each year. (Patrick J. Watson)

average work absences of 3 days in the previous month due to their condition, and 11% reported missing partial workdays (Institute for Health and Management Productivity, 2002).

Arthritis is another chronic condition with significant health effects experienced by 43 million people or one fifth of the U.S. population (Hootman et al., 2005). Based on data from the 2003 BRFSS, the median prevalence of provider-diagnosed arthritis was 27%, and ranged from a low of 17.9% in Hawaii to 37.2% in West Virginia (Steiner, Hootman, Langmaid, Bolen, & Helmick, 2006). In 2002, possible arthritis was reported by an additional 17% of respondents (Division of Adult and Community Health, 2004b). In 2005, an estimated 58% of the U.S. population was affected by arthritis. Given the current rate of incidence, the percentage of people affected is expected to drop slightly to 58% by 2030, but the actual number of people with arthritis will nearly double (Division of Adult and Community Health, 2003). Arthritic conditions include osteoarthritis, rheumatoid arthritis, gout, ankylosing spondylitis, and juvenile rheumatoid arthritis. Arthritis is the leading cause of disability in the United States, and contributed to activity limitation in a median of 9.9% of people in states participating in the BRFSS (Steiner et al., 2006).

Epilepsy is another chronic condition that contributes to morbidity and mortality in the United States and elsewhere. An estimated 2.7 million persons in the United States have epilepsy, and about 10% of people will experience a seizure at some point in their lives (CDC, 2006b). An additional 200,000 new cases of epilepsy are diagnosed each year, including 45,000 children under 15 years of age (Epilepsy Foundation, n. d.). Epilepsy has been linked to social stigma, lost productivity, and decreased quality of life for those affected (CDC, 2004a).

Accidental injuries are another source of chronic disability, and their long-term consequences constitute chronic health conditions of concern to community health nurses. In 2000, for example, more than 16% of the entire U.S. population required treatment for at least one injury (National Center for Injury Prevention and Control, 2004). Accidents also contribute to 1.4 million traumatic brain injuries each year and to resulting long-term disability for 80,000 to 90,000 people (Coronado, Johnson, Faul, & Kegler, 2006). Community health nurses can help to educate the public regarding injury prevention. They can also advocate for environmental changes that minimize the potential for injury.

Some of the increase in incidence and prevalence figures for chronic health problems is attributable to better diagnosis as well as to the ability to prevent deaths due to these conditions. These and similar figures for other chronic conditions, however, indicate that Americans are making little progress in the primary prevention of chronic health problems.

Mortality

Many chronic health conditions contribute to increased mortality and loss of productive years of life among the population. As with morbidity figures, mortality figures provide only a partial picture of the extent of chronic health problems within the population; however, they can provide information on patterns and trends in chronic conditions over time. Table 29-1◆ presents the top 10 causes of death for developed and developing nations, highlighting some of the differences in mortality.

In the United States, chronic diseases cause 70% of all deaths (National Center for Chronic Disease Prevention and Health Promotion, 2002), and five of the six top causes of death in 2002 were chronic conditions (1st—diseases of the heart, 2nd—malignant neoplasms, 3rd—cerebrovascular diseases or stroke, 4th—chronic lower respiratory diseases including chronic obstructive pulmonary disease [COPD], and 6th—diabetes mellitus). The fifth cause of disease, unintentional injuries, also contributes to extensive morbidity in addition to being a significant cause of mortality (NCHS, 2005a).

Heart disease accounts for 29% of all U.S. deaths and for nearly 17% of mortality in people over 65 years of age (Division of Adult and Community Health, 2004a). From 1960 to 2002, overall cardiovascular disease mortality declined 32.5%. During the same period, the stroke mortality rate dropped more than 300% (U.S. Census Bureau, 2005). Unfortunately, stroke remains the third leading cause of death in the United States (Harris, Ayala, & Croft, 2006).

After several years of increasing cancer mortality rates, cancer deaths decreased by 22% between 1990 and 2002 (U.S. Census Bureau, 2005). Mortality due to malignant melanoma, on the other hand, increased by 44% from 1973 to 1998 and continues to rise (Glanz et al., 2002). The U.S. age-adjusted mortality rate for all forms of cancer was 194 per 100,000 population in 2002. Some forms of cancer are greater contributors to mortality than others. For example, cancers of the trachea, bronchus, and lungs remain the foremost cause of cancer mortality, with a mortality rate of 55.1 deaths per 100,000 population in 2002. Colorectal cancer was a distant second at 19.7 deaths per 100,000 (U.S. Census Bureau, 2005), but still accounted for more than 56,000 deaths in 2002 (Seeff, King, Pollack, & Williams, 2006). The breast cancer mortality rate for 2002 was 25.6 per 100,000 women, down by nearly 25% from 1950 (NCHS, 2005a).

Other chronic conditions also contribute to mortality figures for the nation. Diabetes mellitus, for example, accounted for 25.4 deaths per 100,000 population in 2002 (U.S. Census Bureau, 2005). This figure somewhat underrepresents the extent of the problem, as diabetes may contribute to death without being reported on death certificates. Overall, adults with diabetes have 2.6 times the risk of death as those without diabetes (Tierney et al., 2001).

COPD is the fourth leading cause of death in the world, and by 2020 is expected to be the fifth leading contributor to societal disease burden (Kara, 2005). The 2002 U.S. mortality rate for chronic lower respiratory diseases, including COPD, was 43.5 per 100,000 population (an increase of nearly 54% from 1980 (NCHS, 2005a). The asthma mortality rate for 2002 was 1.5 deaths per 100,000 population (NCHS, 2006a). Chronic liver disease and cirrhosis caused 9.3 deaths per 100,000 people in 2002 (U.S. Census Bureau, 2005), and accidents were the fourth leading cause of death for all age groups and the leading cause of death under 35 years of age (National Center for Injury Prevention and Control, 2004).

THE EPIDEMIOLOGY OF CHRONIC PHYSICAL HEALTH PROBLEMS

Factors related to the biophysical, psychological, physical environmental, sociocultural, behavioral, and health system dimensions can increase the risk of an individual or a

TABLE 29-1 Causes of Death in Developed and Developing Nations

Developed Nations		Developing Nations	
Cause of Death	Percent of Deaths	Cause of Death	Percent of Deaths
Ischemic heart disease	22.6%	Ischemic heart disease	9.1%
Cerebrovascular disease	13.7%	Cerebrovascular disease	8.0%
Cancer of the trachea, bronchus, or lungs	4.5%	Lower respiratory infection	7.7%
Lower respiratory infection	3.7%	HIV/AIDS	6.9%
COPD	3.1%	Perinatal conditions	5.6%
Colon/rectal cancer	2.6%	COPD	5.0%
Stomach cancer	1.9%	Diarrheal diseases	4.9%
Self-inflicted injury	1.9%	TB	3.7%
Diabetes mellitus	1.7%	Malaria	2.6%
Breast cancer	1.6%	Motor vehicle accidents	2.5%

Data from: Bonita, R., & Mathers, C. D. (2003). Global health status at the beginning of the twenty-first century. In R. Beaglehole (Ed.), Global public health: A new era (pp. 24–53). Oxford, UK: Oxford University.

population group with respect to a particular chronic condition. Conversely, the presence of a chronic health problem might affect factors in each of these areas.

Biophysical Considerations

Human biological factors related to age, sex, race and ethnicity, specific genetic inheritance, and physiologic function can increase one's risk of developing several chronic health problems. Factors in each of these areas will be addressed here.

Maturation and Aging

Many people think of chronic health problems as occurring primarily among the elderly, despite the fact that 7.8% of U.S. children experience some form of disability related to a variety of chronic conditions (Office of the Surgeon General, 2005), many of which were discussed in Chapter 16∞. An estimated 29% of people age 50 to 64 have one or more chronic health conditions (Immunization Services Division, 2003), and both the incidence and prevalence of chronic illness rise with increasing age. In one study, chronic conditions with disabilities and functional limitations were found in 6% of people age 65 to 74, 32% of those between 74 and 85 years of age, and 44% of people over age 85 (Committee on Rapid Advance Demonstration Projects, 2003). One fourth of people over 65 years of age experience four or more chronic conditions (Bodenheimer et al., 2002a).

Both the young and the elderly are at higher risk for accidental injuries and resulting disabilities. In part, this increased risk is due to maturational events of childhood and aging. The inability of a young infant to roll over or support his or her head contributes to suffocation as the leading cause of accidental death and disability in this age group. Similarly, normal toddler development involves a great deal of experimentation that may lead to accidental injury and disability if close supervision and safety precautions are not employed. The risk taking and feelings of invulnerability characteristic of preadolescent and adolescent development place young people at risk for motor vehicle and firearms accidents. Among the elderly, death and disabilities due to fires and falls are of the greatest concern. In 2002, for example, people over 75 years of age were hospitalized for traumatic brain injury twice as often as those in other age groups (264 per 100,000 population). They were followed by those aged 15 to 24 years at 103 hospitalizations per 100,000 people (Coronado et al., 2006). Typical causes of accidental injury and disability for selected age groups are presented in Table 29-2◆. Community health nurses can help to educate families and the general public regarding age-appropriate safety measures to prevent injuries. They can also engage in political advocacy to promote safe living and working conditions (e.g., legislation mandating functioning smoke alarms in all residences).

Young children and the elderly are also at higher risk for epilepsy than other age groups. By age 80, for instance, 3% of the U.S. population will have a diagnosis of epilepsy (CDC, 2006b).

Some chronic conditions and their effects are more prevalent in adults. For example, despite the popular belief that people with arthritis are elderly, most cases of arthritis have their onset in the fourth decade of life. For women over age 45, for example, arthritis is the major cause of activity limitation. Older persons do, however, tend to experience greater disability as a result of this condition. The prevalence of COPD tends to increase dramatically in the fifth through the seventh decades of life. The incidence of malignant neoplasms, in general, also increases with advancing age, and 60% of all new cancer diagnoses occur in people over age 65. Older people also represent 61% of all cancer survivors (Division of Cancer Prevention and Control, 2004). Diabetes prevalence is more than two times higher in people over age 60 than in younger people (National Center for Chronic Disease Prevention and Health Promotion, 2003), with 60% of the over-60 age group (8.6 million people) affected compared to 206,000 people under 20 years of age (American Diabetes Association, 2003a, 2003c).

Although a stroke can occur at any age, the incidence of stroke doubles for each decade after age 65, and three fourths of all strokes occur in people over 65 years of age (Division for Heart Disease and Stroke Prevention, 2006b).

Gender

Gender can also influence the risk of developing a variety of chronic health conditions. Women, for example, have lower incidence rates for hypertension, and those who do have hypertension are more likely than men to have their blood pressure under control. Men are more than twice as likely as women to die of chronic liver disease and unintentional injuries, and about one and one-half times more likely to die of heart disease or malignant neoplasms than women. Similarly, men have higher risks for death from stroke, COPD, and diabetes (NCHS, 2005a); however, arthritis prevalence for women exceeds that for men at all ages (Division of Adult and Community Health, 2004b). Estrogen seems to have a cardioprotective effect, so premenopausal and perimenopausal women have a lower incidence of heart

TABLE 29-2	Typical Causes of Injury and Disability
Age Group	Typical Causes of Injury and Disability
Infants (birth–1 year)	Suffocation, aspiration of food and other objects, fire, drowning
1–9 years	Motor vehicle accidents, drowning, poisoning, fires
10–14 years	Motor vehicle accidents, drowning, firearms, fires
15–64 years	Motor vehicle accidents, occupational injury, falls, fires
Over 65 years	Falls, fires

disease than men, but the incidence of heart disease in women increases considerably after menopause (Division of Adult and Community Health, 2004a). Women also survive cancer more often than men, primarily because lung cancer, which has a poorer prognosis than other forms of cancer, is more common in men than in women. Women more often have highly detectable and treatable cancers (Division of Cancer Prevention and Control, 2004).

Race and Ethnicity

For many chronic conditions, ethnic or racial factors function as risk markers rather than risk factors. **Risk markers** are factors that help to identify persons who may have an elevated risk of developing a specific condition but that do not themselves contribute to its development. For many chronic diseases, race and ethnicity are probably markers for differences in health behaviors, access to health care, and other factors that contribute to the development of disease (Division of Adult and Community Health, 2004a). For example, when socioeconomic status and the prevalence of risk factors are controlled, there is very little difference in mortality rates for cardiovascular disease between Black men and their White counterparts (Thomas, Eberly, Davey Smith, Neaton, & Stamler, 2005).

For some diseases, race may actually be a risk factor for disease. For example, darker skin color among Blacks is believed to decrease melanoma risk (Glanz et al., 2002). Conversely, sickle cell disease is more common in Blacks than in Whites. For hypertension, however, even though more prevalent among Blacks, skin pigmentation seems to have less influence than socioeconomic status (Gravlee, Dressler, & Bernard, 2005). Among Native Americans in the southwestern United States, as much as 27% of the population has diabetes, and incidence among American Indians and Alaska Natives is 2.2 times that of non-Hispanic Whites (American Diabetes Association, 2003c).

For the most part, the marked disparities noted in the incidence, prevalence, and effects of chronic physical health problems among racial/ethnic groups are associated with differences in socioeconomic status, access to care, and health-related behaviors. For example, in one study of American Indian/Alaska Native populations, these groups were more likely than others to report fair or poor health status and had worse scores on every health-related behavior measure (e.g., more smoking, less physical activity, fewer screening procedures) (Denny, Holtzman, & Cobb, 2003). Similarly, only 35% of Mexican Americans in one study received treatment for hypertension, compared to 49% of non-Hispanic Whites (Ayala et al., 2006). Among Latinas, who have lower rates of breast cancer survival and later stage at diagnosis, access to care and the quality of care received were associated with cancer screening rates, but ethnicity per se was not (Abraído-Lanza, Chao, & Gammon, 2004). Although overall U.S. breast cancer mortality declined

from 1980 to 2002, rates actually increased for Blacks, Native American/Alaska Natives, and Asian/Pacific Islanders (NCHS, 2005a).

Based on National Health Interview Survey data for 2000 and 2001, Black stroke survivors reported greater activity limitation in all areas than White survivors. Stroke incidence also showed an interaction between race and age, education, and income level, with Blacks being more likely than Whites to have a stroke before age 65, to have less than a high school education, and to be poor (McGruder, Greenlund, Croft, & Zheng, 2005). Stroke mortality in people under age 75 is higher in Blacks than in other racial/ethnic groups. In 2002, for instance, Blacks had a stroke mortality rate of 76.3 per 100,000 population, compared to 54.2 for Whites, 41.3 for Hispanics, 37.5 for American Indian/Alaska Natives, and 29.4 for Asians/Pacific Islanders (Harris, Ayala, Dai, & Croft, 2005).

With respect to hypertension, Blacks are more likely than Whites or Hispanics to have hypertension and more likely to be under current treatment for the disease, but have similar rates of blood pressure control as Whites (29.8%). Hispanics, on the other hand, are less likely than Blacks or Whites to have hypertension, but also less likely to be under treatment, and far less likely to have their blood pressure under control (Glover et al., 2005). In 2002, age-adjusted mortality for heart disease was 30% higher in African Americans than in Whites (Division for Heart Disease and Stroke Prevention, 2006a)

Diabetes is another chronic health problem that exhibits differential effects for different racial and ethnic groups. African Americans and Latinos, for example, have 50% to 100% greater diabetes-related illness and mortality than Whites and are twice as likely to develop blindness. Native Americans, Mexican Americans, and African Americans are also four to six times more likely than Whites to develop kidney disease as a result of diabetes, and ethnic and racial minority groups have a higher incidence of lower extremity amputations (Two Feathers et al., 2005).

Health-related behaviors also contribute to racial and ethnic disparities in chronic disease incidence and prevalence. For example, approximately 33% of Native Americans smoke, compared to 22% and 20% of the White and Black non-Hispanic populations, respectively, 15% of Hispanics, and 11% of Asian Americans (Maurice et al., 2005). Similarly, 39% of Native American men and 37.5% of women are obese, compared to 3% and 4% of Asian/Pacific Islander men and women, respectively. Members of ethic minority groups also tend to eat fewer than the recommended number of fruits and vegetables daily and engage in less physical activity (Liao et al., 2004).

Provider recommendations for healthy behaviors may also vary among racial and ethnic groups. For example, the findings of one study indicated that Hispanics and African Americans were less likely than

Whites to have been counseled by providers about smoking (Houston, Scarinci, Person, & Greene, 2005). Similar findings are noted for recommendations for routine cancer screening. Community health nurses can be actively involved in advocating and providing health promotion education and access to health care services to minimize racial and ethnic disparities in the incidence of chronic health problems.

Genetic Inheritance

Some chronic diseases seem to be associated with genetic predisposition. Thus, community health nurses should obtain a family history of chronic diseases to help determine the individual client's risk for these conditions. Genetic inheritance is thought to be a major contributing factor for some cancers, for diabetes, and for cardiovascular disease. For example, a family history of malignant melanoma in a first-degree relative has been associated with an eightfold increase in risk (Glanz et al., 2002). Specific genetic mutations have even been identified and screening tests developed for inherited breast (BRCA1) and ovarian (BRCA2) cancers. For example, having a sister with a BRCA1 mutation gives a woman a 50% risk of having the same genetic mutation (Jacobellis et al., 2004). Similarly, nearly 9% of children with mothers who have epilepsy and 2.4% of those whose fathers are affected will develop the disease (Epilepsy Foundation, n.d.).

Clients may not be knowledgeable regarding family history of disease. In the 2004 Family HealthStyles Survey, for example, more than 96% of people believed information about family history to be important to personal health, yet less than 30% of those surveyed had collected relevant family history information (Yoon et al., 2004). Community health nurses can educate the public regarding the need for family health history information and guide them in its collection.

Physiologic Function

Assessment of physiologic factors related to chronic conditions focuses on three areas: presence of physiologic risk factors, physiologic evidence of existing chronic health problems, and evidence of physiologic consequences of chronic conditions.

Physiologic traits over which one has little control may predispose one to certain chronic illnesses. For example, having fair skin, red or blonde hair, or a tendency to sunburn easily increases one's risk for skin cancers (Saraiya et al., 2003). Preventive interventions (e.g., staying out of the sun, use of sunscreen) can, however, mitigate the effects of these risks.

Certain physiologic conditions may predispose one to develop some chronic health problems. Activity limitations and impaired balance and mobility, for example, may contribute to injuries with long-term consequences, particularly in elderly individuals, whereas hypertension, elevated serum cholesterol, and diabetes

are all physiologic factors in the development of cardiovascular disease (Division of Adult and Community Health, 2004a). Diabetes also tends to increase the risk of stroke. Low birth weight and preterm birth have been associated with childhood asthma (Jaakkola & Gissler, 2004). Stroke and Alzheimer's disease increase the risk of epilepsy, with 22% of people who have had a stroke and 10% of those with Alzheimer's affected (Epilepsy Foundation, n.d.).

Obesity is a physiologic factor that can contribute to heart disease and diabetes, and coexistent hypertension may increase the risk of diabetic complications such as blindness. Obesity also places greater strain on joints and may exacerbate the effects of arthritis on affected joints. In fact, the risk of obesity-related arthritis has increased in successive cohorts of U.S. adults (Leveille, Wee, & Iezzoni, 2005). Obesity has even been linked to risk for death due to motor vehicle accidents among men (Zhu et al., 2006).

Obesity is also associated with increased disability among people with chronic illnesses. One study in eight states and the District of Columbia found that 27% of persons with disability were obese compared to 16.5% of the general population over 18 years of age (Division of Human Development and Disability, 2002). Obesity rates in the United States doubled from 1976 to 1980, then doubled again from 1990 to 2000 (Morabia & Costanza, 2005). In 2003, a median of 60% of people in the 50 states and U.S. territories were overweight, and the median prevalence of obesity was 23% (Jiles et al., 2005).

Past infection may also be implicated in the development of some chronic conditions. For example, viral infection is suspected as a contributing factor in both cancer and diabetes. A history of recurrent respiratory infections, particularly a history of severe viral pneumonias early in life, has been found to be associated with COPD. Respiratory allergy and asthma may also be predisposing physiologic factors in COPD, whereas viral infection may be a predisposing factor in childhood asthma. Human papillomavirus (HPV) infection in the form of genital warts has been linked to cervical cancer (Frieden, 2004). Viral infections have also been implicated in the development of some forms of lymphoma, Kaposi's sarcoma, nasopharyngeal cancers, and hepatocellular carcinoma (Perkins, 2005). Other physiologic conditions may be complicated by the existence of chronic illnesses. For example, diabetes places both the pregnant woman and her child at increased risk of adverse outcomes. Conversely, pregnancy complicates diabetes control.

People with chronic health problems may also develop secondary conditions as a result of their illnesses, and community health nurses caring for these clients should be alert to the development of signs of secondary conditions. For example, a client in a wheelchair may develop pressure ulcers, or a client with diabetes might develop diabetic retinopathy. Similarly, diabetes is the primary cause of end stage renal disease (ESRD), and the prevalence of ESRD among people with diabetes increased 162% from 1990 to 2002. ESRD incidence is higher in men than in women and in Blacks than in Whites (Burrows, Wang, Geiss, Venkat Narayan, & Engelgau, 2005).

Diabetes also increases the risk of lower extremity disease, often leading to amputation. Between 1999 and 2000, for example, 30% of U.S. adults with diabetes developed lower extremity disease, compared to 18% of those without diabetes (NCHS, 2005d). Similarly, based on 2002 data, people with diabetes were nearly twice as likely as those without to have glaucoma or some other type of vision impairment, and one and a half times more likely to report cataracts (Saaddine et al., 2004). Diabetes has also been linked to increased risk for preterm birth and cesarean section in women of all racial and ethnic groups and for low birth weight in Asians, Hispanics, and Whites, but not for Blacks (Rosenberg, Garbers, Lipkind, & Chiasson, 2005).

Other examples of secondary conditions include pain, sleep disturbances, fatigue, weight gain or loss, respiratory infections, and falls or injuries. When the nurse identifies the presence of secondary conditions, he or she will refer the client for appropriate medical therapy. In one study, as many as 86% of clients with disabilities had at least one secondary condition resulting from their disability (Kinne, Patrick, & Doyle, 2004). Community health nurses can advocate for effective care for health problems to prevent the development of these and other secondary conditions.

Tips for assessing the influence of biophysical factors on chronic health problems in the population are included in the focused assessment questions provided below.

Psychological Considerations

The major psychological factor contributing to chronic health problems is stress. Stress can result in carelessness and contribute to accidents that lead to chronic

disability. Similarly, stress has been implicated as a contributing factor in the development of cancer and cardiovascular disease. Stress may also lead to poor compliance with control measures in persons with diabetes, resulting in diabetic complications. Depression and anxiety have also been associated with the onset of cardiovascular disease and with coronary heart disease survival. Conversely, myocardial infarction increases one's risk for major depressive disorder. According to the National Heart Foundation of Australia (Bunker et al., 2003), there is compelling evidence that depression, social isolation, and poor-quality social support have a causal influence on coronary heart disease.

Psychological distress has also been found to play a part in exacerbation of symptoms among people who have asthma. For example, after the World Trade Center attacks in 2001, 27% of people with asthma in lower Manhattan reported a worsening of symptoms. In part, symptom increases resulted from increased smoke and debris in the air, but were also more common among those who reported greater psychological distress as a result of the attacks (Fagan, Galea, Ahern, Bonner, & Vlahov, 2002). Asthma was also linked in one study to suicide ideation and suicide attempts among adults. These findings were not explained by either the incidence of major depression or asthma treatment, although previous studies have shown an association between asthma and major depression (Goodwin & Eaton, 2005).

Some chronic conditions have also been found to have effects on mental and emotional function. Alzheimer's disease comes most easily to mind, but traumatic brain injury may also contribute to personality changes and increased aggressiveness. Similarly, insufficient blood circulation to the brain in congestive heart failure has been suggested as an explanation for mental effects such as memory deficit, diminished learning ability, poor executive function, and decreased psychomotor speed (Bennett, Suave, & Sahw, 2005).

Psychological effects of chronic and debilitating conditions also occur in response to perceived loss. In one study, people with epilepsy were more than twice as likely as those without to report mentally unhealthy days, and those taking medication for epilepsy were nearly three times more likely to experience mental health effects (Ferguson et al., 2005). Epilepsy has also been associated with low self-esteem, perceptions of stigma, and feelings of shame, fear, and worry (Pedroso de Souza & Barioni Salgado, 2006).

Diabetes, hypertension, and asthma have also been associated with increased incidence of serious psychological distress. In one study in New York City, for example, more than 10% of people with diabetes reported serious psychological effects (McVeigh, Mostashari, & Thorpe, 2004). Chronic illness has also been found to contribute to loneliness, both among those affected and their spouses (Kara & Mirici, 2004). Psychological resources available to clients in the form

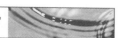

FOCUSED ASSESSMENT

Assessing Biophysical Factors Affecting Chronic Physical Health Problems

- What age groups are most likely to develop the problem? What age groups will be most seriously affected?
- Are there racial or gender differences in disease incidence? What factors influence these differences?
- Is there a genetic predisposition to the problem?
- Are there other physiologic conditions that increase the risk of developing the problem?
- What are the signs and symptoms of the problem?
- What are the physiologic effects of the problem? Does the problem limit functional abilities?

FOCUSED ASSESSMENT

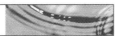

Assessing Psychological Factors Affecting Chronic Physical Health Problems

- Does exposure to stress increase the risk of the problem?
- Do existing psychological problems increase the risk for the chronic physical health problem? If so, in what way does this influence occur?
- Do existing psychological problems complicate control of physical health problems? If so, how?
- What are the typical psychological effects of the problem? Are there psychological effects for family members as well as for the person affected by the problem?
- What is the extent of adaptation to the problem? What factors or conditions facilitate or impede adjustment?

Think Advocacy

Exposure to pesticides and other chemicals used in agriculture increases the risk of chronic health problems for agricultural workers. Although OSHA regulations control use of such chemicals in large farming operations, they are not applicable to farms with only a few employees. In working in an area with many small family-operated farms that may employ two or three nonfamily members, you become aware of an increase in pesticide-related neurological conditions. How would you go about advocating for more effective control measures for pesticide use in the area? Who else would you involve in your advocacy efforts?

of a supportive partner and high levels of self-esteem, mastery, and self-efficacy tend to buffer the effect of chronic illness on emotional status (Bisschop, Kriegsman, Beekman, & Deeg, 2004). Community health nurses can assist clients to identify personal psychological resources or to bolster them through referral to support groups and other similar interventions. They can also advocate for access to psychological counseling, as needed, to help with adjustment to a chronic health problem.

Questions for exploring psychological considerations influencing chronic physical health problems in the population are included in the focused assessment provided above. Aspects of loss and considerations in dealing with them are addressed in the discussion of tertiary prevention of chronic physical health problems.

Physical Environmental Considerations

Physical environmental factors contribute to chronic health problems such as long-term sequelae of accidents, cancer, and COPD. Road conditions, weather, dangerous conditions for swimming, and other physical safety hazards can contribute to accidents that result in permanent physical disability, and the nurse assesses the existence of these types of hazardous conditions in the community.

The community health nurse also assesses the environment for pollutants that may be carcinogenic. Air pollution, in particular, contributes to COPD and asthma. Other environmental factors that may influence chronic respiratory conditions, particularly those with an allergic basis, include house dust, mites, molds, tobacco smoke, and occupational exposures to respiratory irritants. Increases in particulate matter and sulfur dioxide have been associated with increases in systolic blood pressure (Ibald-Mulli, Stieber, Wichman, Koenig, & Peters, 2001). Similarly, cumulative exposure to environmental tobacco smoke at work has been associated with a twofold increase in asthma risk, and in-home exposure produces an asthma risk 4.7 times higher than that for people with

no exposure (Jaakkola, Piipari, Jaakkola, & Jaakkola, 2003). Low-level exposures to arsenic in drinking water from private wells have been linked to hypertension and circulatory problems and the incidence of coronary bypass surgery (Zierold, Knobeloch, & Anderson, 2004). The effects of environmental pollution on health were addressed in more detail in Chapter 10∞.

Global climate changes also affect chronic health problems such as asthma. It is anticipated, for example, that global warming will increase the growth of plant allergens and may prolong periods of seasonal asthma related to pollens. Climate changes have also been found to increase overall pollen production and the actual allergenic content of pollen (Natural Resources Defense Council, 2004).

Seasonal variations have also been noted with respect to blood pressure levels, with higher blood pressures in winter months. In addition, the incidence of stroke and myocardial infarction increases during the winter (Rosenthal, 2004). Seasonal variations in blood pressures may need to be taken into account in the treatment of hypertension, and community health nurses can alert clients to the possibility of these changes and the need to consider modification of their treatment regimens.

Other aspects of the physical environment may contribute to chronic health problems. For example, night shift work has been linked to coronary heart disease, and breast cancer incidence has been found to be higher in nurses who work rotating night shifts for long periods of time (Schernhammer et al., 2001). One possible explanation for this last association is exposure to light during the night when protective processes that occur in darkness would normally occur (Davis, Mirick, & Stevens, 2001). Conversely, increased exposure to sunlight, being closer to the equator, higher elevation, the presence of light cloud cover, and the presence of reflective materials (water, concrete) increase the risk of melanoma (Glanz et al., 2002). The U.S. Preventive Services Task Force (2003) has indicated, however, that intermittent or intense exposure to sunlight increases melanoma risk, but chronic sun exposure seems to decrease risk.

Distance to treatment services has also been advanced as a possible explanation for increased cancer mortality among Native Americans. For example, in a 10-state area served by three Indian Health Service centers, Native American cancer mortality rates were 40% higher than that of the overall U.S. population. Travel distances to treatment facilities ranged from 5 to 215 miles per person, with a median of 109 miles, and 37% of clients traveled more than 300 miles round trip (Rogers & Petereit, 2005). Community health nurses can advocate for the development of necessary services within a reasonable distance of those in need of them. Political advocacy will also be needed to assure adequate funding for such services.

Community health nurses should also be concerned with the concept of environmental justice. Many environmental hazards are located in low-income neighborhoods, further increasing the effects of poverty and other social factors on health. Advocacy is required to prevent the location of hazardous industries in low-income residential areas and to promote elimination of existing hazards.

The other aspect of the physical environment related to chronic health problems is its effect on the functional abilities of persons with existing chronic conditions. The *disablement process* is influenced by a variety of factors, including the pathology of disease and the environmental conditions that lead to disability in someone with a chronic health problem. For example, substandard housing conditions can lead to fear of falling in older persons with mobility limitations, resulting in social isolation and disability. Similarly, lack of adequate heat increases the growth of molds, exacerbating respiratory problems for people with asthma and other chronic conditions (Clarke & George, 2005). Community health nurses examine personal and community environmental factors that promote disability in persons with chronic health problems. They may also need to educate clients on dealing with these environmental conditions or advocate for modification of conditions that contribute to chronic disease and/or disability in the population.

The focused assessment below provides tips for exploring physical environmental considerations as they affect the incidence, prevalence, and effects of chronic health problems in the population.

FOCUSED ASSESSMENT

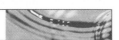

Assessing Physical Environmental Factors Affecting Chronic Physical Health Problems

- Do environmental pollutants contribute to the problem?
- What effect, if any, do weather conditions have on the problem?
- What influence, if any, do elements of the built environment have on the problem?
- Does the problem necessitate environmental changes (e.g., installation of ramps for a wheelchair)?

Sociocultural Considerations

The sociocultural dimension contributes to the development of chronic health problems primarily in terms of social support for unhealthful behaviors and factors that enhance or impede access to health care. Social norms that condone or promote behaviors such as smoking, drinking alcohol, and a sedentary lifestyle contribute to the development of a variety of chronic health problems.

Social factors also include role modeling of healthful behaviors. Sociocultural dimension factors may promote health and healthy behaviors and impede the development of chronic health problems. For example, social pressures to quit smoking may motivate many smokers to abandon their habit. Similarly, no-smoking policies in work settings have led to an overall decrease in smoking in many instances. Much of California's decrease in lung cancer deaths has been attributed to tobacco control initiatives and the prohibition of smoking in all public venues (Office on Smoking and Health, 2000), and community health nurses can advocate for similar no-smoking policies in other states or in local areas. The existence of strong social support networks has also been shown to reduce the risk of cardiovascular disease.

Media messages are another sociocultural factor that influences health-related behaviors. For example, "truth" antismoking advertisements that expose tobacco company marketing practices targeting youth have been associated with a significant reduction in smoking prevalence in this population (Farrelly, Davis, Haviland, Messeri, & Healton, 2005). Community health nurses can advocate with local and national media for support of health-promoting rather than illness-promoting messages. They may also engage in political advocacy regarding media messages. For example, community health nurses in one community were actively involved in the development of a local ordinance prohibiting billboards advertising tobacco products within a specified distance of elementary and secondary schools.

Culture may play a role in the extent of support for healthy or unhealthy behaviors that influence the development of chronic health conditions. For example, in many cultures, use of alcohol is discouraged, so the risk of chronic liver disease due to alcohol intake is reduced. Conversely, nondrinkers would not benefit from the potential positive effects of moderate alcohol intake on cardiovascular disease risk. Cultural factors such as language may influence knowledge of risk factors and health-promoting activity. For example, reading and speaking a language other than English, or more fluently than English, has been linked to decreased use of breast and cervical cancer screening services (Jacobs, Karavolos, Rathouz, Ferris, & Powell, 2005).

Cultural factors may also influence compliance with treatment regimens for chronic conditions. For example, in some cultural groups, health care providers

CULTURAL COMPETENCE

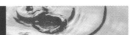

*T*he concept of chronic diseases is difficult for members of many cultural groups to understand. It is particularly difficult for some people to grasp the concept of needing to take medication for the rest of one's life, as is the case with many chronic diseases. Select a cultural group in your own area whose members believe that with treatment a condition should be cured. How would you convey to them, in culturally congruent terms, the need for lifelong therapy?

are expected to provide remedies that resolve a problem immediately and group members have difficulty conceiving of conditions that require life-long use of medications. Similarly, as discussed in Chapter 9∞, traditional cultural remedies may counteract or potentiate the effects of medications prescribed for chronic health conditions.

Social participation has also been found to have an influence on the development of chronic disease. In one study, for example, low social participation was associated with increased risk of coronary heart disease (Sundquist, Lindström, Malmström, Johansson, & Sundquist, 2004). Conversely, disability due to chronic disease may limit clients' ability to engage in social participation, resulting in social isolation.

Social environmental factors such as low income, low education levels, and unemployment may prevent access to health care for persons who have existing chronic conditions (Division of Diabetes Translation, 2002). Lack of care leads to the development of complications that might be averted if adequate treatment and monitoring were available. Even when care is available, low-income populations may be less compliant with therapeutic recommendations due to cost. In one study, for example, 18% of people had cut back on medication use during the previous year because of inability to afford medications, and 14% cut back on medications at least one time a month (Piette, Heisler, & Wagner, 2004). These types of socioeconomic factors explain some of the differences in survival rates for members of different ethnic groups who have cancer, and particularly explain the poor survival rates of African Americans with cancer. Income may also affect health behaviors. For example, a sedentary lifestyle has been shown to be inversely related to income levels, with those at lower levels engaging in less physical activity.

Certain specific factors in the sociocultural dimension may increase the risk for or effects of particular chronic diseases. For example, increased exposure to violence in the environment has been associated with greater frequency of asthma symptoms (Wright et al., 2004). Similarly, perceived neighborhood problems (e.g., traffic, noise, litter, odors, and smoke) have been linked to poorer quality of life, poorer physical function, and more depressive symptoms among people with asthma (Yen, Yelin, Katz, Eisner, & Blanc, 2006).

Occupational factors are another element of the sociocultural dimension that can contribute to the development of chronic health problems. As noted in Chapter 24∞, safety hazards in the work environment can result in accidents that lead to chronic disability. Clients' occupations may also increase their potential for exposure to various carcinogens found in the workplace. Repetitive movements involved in some jobs can lead to joint injuries and subsequent arthritis. Occupations involving exposure to organic and inorganic dusts or noxious gases increase the probability of COPD, with employment in plastics factories and cotton mills particularly associated with increased incidence of COPD. Work-related stress has also been shown to increase the risk of some chronic health problems, and working while ill has been linked to increased risk of serious coronary events (Kivimaki et al., 2005).

Health-related policies in the workplace also influence risk factors for chronic health problems. These policies may be directed at individuals or at the entire employee population. Policies with the latter focus may be more effective, however. For example, enforcement of workplace smoke-free policies have been shown to be approximately nine times more cost-effective in promoting smoking cessation than providing free nicotine replacement therapy to employees who smoke (Ong & Glantz, 2005). Other studies have also indicated that smoke-free workplace policies reduced cigarette consumption and increased the rate of smoking cessation among employees (Bauer, Hyland, Li, Steger, & Cummings, 2005). Community health nurses can be actively involved in promoting smoke-free workplace policies and in the development of other policies that promote health and prevent illness and injury in occupational settings.

Legislation is another sociocultural factor that influences chronic illness. For example, legislation mandating helmet use by motorcyclists and bicycle riders helps to prevent traumatic brain injury. Similarly, smoke-free indoor air laws not only reduce exposure to secondhand smoke but also lead to decreased cigarette consumption and increased rates of smoking cessation. Unfortunately, some states have passed legislation that prohibits local governments from enacting ordinances that are more stringent than those of the state. In 2004, for instance, 19 states had such *preemptive* legislation permitting smoking in such designated places as government worksites, private-sector worksites, or restaurants (Lineberger et al., 2005). In 2004, only seven states had legislation mandating smoke-free private-sector worksites; eight mandated smoke-free restaurants; and four mandated smoke-free bars (Chriqui et al., 2005). Taxing tobacco sales is another legislative measure that has greatly reduced tobacco consumption in some states (Sung, Hu, Ong, Keeler, & Sheu, 2005).

Tips for assessing the relationship of sociocultural factors to chronic health problems in the community are included in the focused assessment provided on page 868.

FOCUSED ASSESSMENT

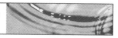

Assessing Sociocultural Factors Affecting Chronic Physical Health Problems

- Do social norms support behaviors that increase the risk of developing the problem (e.g., smoking)?
- What are societal attitudes to the problem? Do they hamper control efforts? Is there social stigma attached to having the problem? What social support systems are available to people with the problem?
- Do occupational factors influence the incidence of the problem?
- Does socioeconomic status influence the development or effects of the problem?
- What effect, if any, do cultural beliefs and behaviors have on incidence of the problem? On treatment of the problem?
- What effect, if any, does legislation have on risk factors for the problem?

Behavioral Considerations

Behavioral factors are the major contributors to the development of most chronic health problems. Behavioral considerations to be assessed by the nurse include consumption patterns, exercise, and other behaviors.

Consumption Patterns

Consumption patterns that play a role in the development and course of chronic health problems include diet and the use of tobacco and alcohol. Dietary consumption has increased significantly in the United States. In 2004, for instance, each person ate 1,775 pounds of food, compared to only 1,497 pounds in 1970, an increase of 18.5% (Newman, 2004). Poor dietary patterns contribute to chronic diseases such as diabetes and cardiovascular disease and to obesity, which is a risk factor for both of these conditions. According to figures from the 2003 BRFSS, the median prevalence of overweight in the United States was 60%, and the median state prevalence of obesity was 23% (Jiles et al., 2005). Some experts have suggested that the prevalence of overweight is, in part, a response to health-related messages to decrease fat consumption. When the American public decreased fat intake, they increased carbohydrate consumption (Newman, 2004).

Cholesterol consumption patterns are well-known correlates of cardiovascular disease, and excess blood cholesterol is a prevalent problem throughout the United States. A large percentage of the fat consumed by Americans comes from animal sources known to be high in cholesterol. In 2003, a median of 33% of people in states participating in the BRFSS reported being told that they had elevated blood cholesterol levels (Jiles et al., 2005). In addition, as the percentage of calories derived from fat increases, intake of more healthful foods such as fruits, vegetables, and dietary sources of vitamins A and C, folates, and fiber decreases. As a result, not only does increased fat intake contribute to obesity and thereby to chronic disease, it may also contribute to a variety of dietary deficiencies. In the 2003 Youth Risk Behavior Survey (YRBS), only 22% of the youth surveyed reported eating five or more fruits and vegetables a day (Grunbaum et al., 2004).

Diet has also been implicated in the development of some forms of cancer. Baseline data for the national health objectives for 2010 indicate that only 28% of the U.S. population eats two or more servings of fruit a day, and only 36% consume less than 10% of their calories as saturated fat. Similarly, only 46% of the population meets daily dietary recommendations for calcium intake, a preventive measure for osteoporosis (CDC, 2005b). Other nutrients may also have protective effects. For example, diets high in fiber, fruit, and vegetables and low in fat seem to lower the risk of colorectal cancer. Conversely, high-fat, high-calorie, low-calcium, and low-folate diets, as well as meat and alcohol consumption, have been associated with increased risk (Kather, 2005).

There is a growing body of evidence to suggest that vitamin D deficiency contributes to some forms of cancer, particularly colon, breast, ovarian, and prostate cancers. Although vitamin D is naturally synthesized by the skin with exposure to sunlight, synthesis is greatly reduced in the northeastern United States from November to March, indicating a need for dietary supplementation. Even during sunny weather, use of high-level sunscreen products blocks vitamin D formation in the skin (Garland et al., 2006). Community health nurses can encourage use of vitamin D fortified dairy products and exposure to sunlight without the use of sunscreen for up to 15 minutes a day as a means of improving vitamin D levels in the population and increasing the protective effects against cancer.

Use of tobacco is another consumption pattern highly correlated with the development of a variety of chronic health problems. Worldwide, more than 1.3 billion people smoke (Donohoe, 2005), and tobacco use is expected to result in 450 million deaths in the next 50 years (Costa de Silva et al., 2005). In the United States, smoking contributed to more than 438,000 deaths and accounted for 3.3 million years of productive life lost (YPLL) for men and 2.2 million YPLL for women each year from 1997 to 2001. Annual productivity losses due to smoking during this period were $61.9 billion for men and $30.5 billion for women (Armour, Woolery, Malarcher, Pechacek, & Husten, 2005). Annual per capita costs of smoking in the United States amount to $550 per person (Donohoe, 2005). Smoking contributed to 71% of all cancer deaths, 63.5% of deaths due to respiratory illnesses, and 13% of cardiovascular disease deaths (Armour et al., 2005).

Smoking has also been found to influence the incidence of cardiovascular disease and complications of diabetes and COPD. The association between smoking and cardiovascular disease is supported by findings that people who quit smoking reduce their risk of coronary heart disease by about half after a year of abstinence from tobacco. Smoking cessation also markedly reduces the risk of premature death in persons with existing cardiovascular disease. Smoking has been found to interact with diabetes to result in greater risk of complications. Smoking is also the primary contributing factor in the development of COPD. In addition to being the single most significant factor in the development of this disease, smoking interacts with all other contributing factors to increase the potential for COPD. Maternal smoking during pregnancy contributed to 9% of perinatal infant deaths (Armour et al., 2005) and has also been associated with increased risk of childhood asthma (Jaakkola & Gissler, 2004).

Based on the 2004 National Health Interview Survey, 20.9% of U.S. adults reported current smoking, and the prevalence of heavy smoking was 12%, down from 19% in 1993 (Maurice et al., 2005). Unfortunately, more than 27% of adolescents responding to the 2003 YRBS reported current tobacco use (Grunbaum et al., 2004). Similarly, more than 13% of middle-school students reported tobacco use in the 2002 National Youth Tobacco Survey (Marshall et al., 2006).

Alcohol use also contributes to the development of certain chronic health problems and their consequences. For example, alcohol is implicated in motor vehicle accidents, bicycling accidents, fires, falls, and boating accidents, many of which result in chronic disability. Alcohol abuse also contributes to mortality due to chronic liver disease, but moderate alcohol use appears to have a protective effect for coronary heart disease.

Use of complementary and alternative therapies (CAT) is another consumption pattern that should be considered in chronic disease risk and management. In one study, for example, 76% of participants reported using CAT for relief of pain, and 28% reported use of herbals and dietary supplements (Vallerand et al., 2003). Community health nurses should assess the use of these therapies in terms of their interaction with medications prescribed for chronic diseases and educate clients and the public in their safe use. They can also advocate for and conduct research regarding the effectiveness of CAT in controlling chronic health problems.

Exercise and Leisure Activity

Exercise, or the lack of it, can influence the development and course of some chronic conditions. Exercise may enhance the control of diabetes or contribute to hypoglycemic reactions. Physical exercise improves control of arthritis and limits its disabling effects. Both aerobic and strengthening exercises have been linked to improved physical function and decreased disability (CDC, 2006c). Physical activity has also been shown to be directly related to the incidence of heart disease. Several studies have documented that adults with active lifestyles have significantly lower risk of developing heart disease than their less active contemporaries. A sedentary lifestyle, on the other hand, is closely associated with obesity, a risk factor for cardiovascular disease. In the 2003 YRBS, 11.5% of U.S. adolescents had no vigorous physical activity in the prior week. Only 28% of the high school students surveyed engaged in physical education activities 5 days a week (Grunbaum et al., 2004). Among adults, a median of 23% of people in states participating in the BRFSS reported no leisure-time physical activity (Jiles et al., 2005), and only 46% engaged in the recommended amount of physical activity (Sapkota, Bowles, Ham, & Kohl, 2005).

Television viewing is frequently a component of a sedentary lifestyle and has been shown to be associated with obesity. Watching television is the third most time-consuming activity in the United States, and in 2003 adolescents watched more than 3 hours of television a day. As viewing time increases, physical fitness declines.

As we saw in Chapter 10∞, elements of the built environment may foster or impede physical activity for the general public. The same is true for individuals with existing chronic illness. For example, some walking trails have exercise stations that promote movement of other muscles than those used in walking. Fewer such trails, however, have activities or facilities designed to promote exercise for someone in a wheelchair or with other limitations. Similarly, one study of 35 health and fitness clubs found, at best, only moderate accessibility for persons with disabilities. Facilities were designed to accommodate neither persons with mobility limitations nor those with visual impairments (e.g., raised buttons on exercise equipment) (Rimmer, Riley, Wang, & Rauworth, 2005). Community health nurses may need to actively advocate for opportunities for physical activity for all segments of the population, including those with disabilities.

Other Behaviors

Other lifestyle behaviors that might influence the development and course of chronic diseases include the use of safety devices and precautions. The use of safety devices and safety precautions can prevent accidents that may result in chronic disability. For example, seat belt use is an important behavioral factor in preventing motor vehicle fatalities. Other safety factors to be considered include the use of bicycle or motorcycle helmets, occupational safety equipment, and so on. Community health nurses would also explore the presence or absence of legislation mandating their use and the extent to which such legislation is enforced.

Other behaviors can contribute to or prevent skin cancer. For example, reducing direct exposure to sunlight (particularly from 10 A.M. to 4 P.M.), using sunscreen protection, and wearing a broad-brimmed hat and other protective clothing can minimize the risk of malignant melanoma. According to some studies, only one third of adults use sunscreen, seek shade, or wear protective

FOCUSED ASSESSMENT

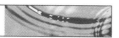

Assessing Behavioral Factors Affecting Chronic Physical Health Problems

- Do dietary factors influence the incidence of the problem? Does having the problem necessitate dietary changes?
- Does alcohol or drug use contribute to the incidence of the problem? What effect does alcohol or drug use have on the course of the problem?
- What effect does physical activity have on the incidence of the problem?
- Does smoking contribute to the incidence of the problem?
- Does the problem necessitate regular medication use or other disease management behaviors (e.g., glucose monitoring)?
- What effects do self-care behaviors have on the course of the problem?
- What effect do safety precautions have on the incidence of the problem? To what extent does the problem necessitate special safety precautions?

clothing, and across studies the median extent of use of protective clothing was 11% among adults and 25% among children (Saraiya et al., 2003).

Another aspect of the behavioral dimension of chronic physical health problems is their effect on client behaviors. Earlier we explored the relationships among chronic illness and functional limitations and disability. The presence of chronic disease may prevent or make it more difficult for people to engage in specific activities. One area that is often neglected is the effect of chronic disease on sexual function. People with asthma and other respiratory conditions may be particularly likely to report sexual limitations. In fact, in one study, 58% of people with asthma reported limitations in sexual functioning (Meyer, Sternfels, Fagan, & Ford, 2002). Other conditions that result in fatigue, such as cardiovascular disease and cancer, may also affect sexual function. Finally, as noted in Chapter 18∞, many medications used to treat chronic conditions may cause sexual dysfunction, particularly among men.

Questions to guide the examination of behavioral influences on the incidence and prevalence of chronic health problems in the population are included in the focused assessment above.

Health System Considerations

Health system factors may contribute to the development of chronic health problems or influence their course and consequences. Lack of access to care is an important contributing factor in the incidence and prevalence, as well as control, of chronic diseases. The Institute of Medicine (2002), noted that uninsured adults with chronic diseases are less likely to receive appropriate care than those with insurance. Uninsured adults are also less likely to continue with drug therapy for such

conditions as hypertension and are more likely to develop severe renal disease in the presence of diabetes.

The failure of health care professionals to educate their clients and the general public on the effects of diet, exercise, smoking, alcohol, and other factors in the development of chronic health problems contributes to the increased incidence of these conditions. To some extent this failure may be attributed to time constraints in today's health care system. For example, intensive lifestyle modification programs have been found to result in greater weight loss among persons with diabetes, yet no weight changes were observed in clients who were educated regarding lifestyle changes in the amount of time allotted for client education under Medicare reimbursement (Mayer-Davis et al., 2004). Community health nurses and others may need to advocate for changes to reimbursement policies to promote better education for self-management of chronic illnesses.

The extent of screening services for existing chronic conditions may influence their course and effects. It is estimated that diabetic screening programs, for example, detect only about half of the population affected by this disease (National Diabetes Information Clearinghouse, 2000). The extent to which low-cost screening procedures for various forms of cancer are available varies considerably throughout the country. Although screening services may be obtained from private health care providers, they are often costly, and many low-income people are prevented from taking advantage of them.

Provider factors may also affect screening prevalence in some populations. For example, although many people prefer to obtain health care services from a provider of the same ethnicity, in one study of Korean women in California, those with Korean primary care providers were less likely than those with non-Korean providers to have had a recent Papanicolaou smear, mammogram, or clinical breast examination, suggesting a need to educate some providers, as well as the general public, about the advisability of cancer screening procedures (Moskowitz, Kazinets, Tager, & Wong, 2004). Physician–client racial concordance, however, had little effect on patterns of hypertension care in another study, but continuity of care was associated with better diagnosis and treatment of hypertension (Konrad, Howard, Edwards, Ivanova, & Carey, 2005).

Health care system factors influence the availability and quality of treatment obtainable for persons with chronic conditions. For example, provider knowledge and expertise may affect the recognition and treatment of chronic health conditions. In one study of provider knowledge of the indications for genetic testing for breast and ovarian cancer risk, only 52% of providers were aware that genetic mutations for these cancers could be inherited from either parent and that having a sister with a known mutation increased a woman's risk of breast cancer (Jacobellis et al., 2004). Oncologists and obstetricians/gynecologists were more likely to be

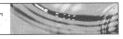

FOCUSED ASSESSMENT

Assessing Health System Factors Affecting Chronic Physical Health Problems

- Do health system factors contribute to the development of the problem?
- What primary preventive measures are available for the problem? Are they widely used? To what extent do health care providers educate the public regarding primary prevention of the problem?
- Is there a screening test for the problem? If so, are persons at risk for the problem adequately screened?
- How is the problem diagnosed? Are diagnostic and treatment services for the problem available and accessible to those who need them?
- Can the problem be controlled with conventional medical therapy? Are there alternative therapies that may contribute to the control of the problem? Do alternative therapies pose health risks themselves?
- What is the attitude of health care providers to persons with the problem?

knowledgeable about genetic risks, but they are often not women's primary care providers, suggesting a need for better education of primary care providers who may be the first to identify cancer risk. Community health nurses can assist in the education of both the public and providers regarding cancer risk factors and promote effective screening of high-risk populations.

The aggressiveness of treatment received also affects the outcome of chronic health conditions. Some studies, for example, suggest that poorer cancer survival rates among low-income populations may be related to reduced access to care. The quality of treatment received for diabetes may also vary widely and affect the consequences of this disease. Medical care, on the other hand, has greatly reduced mortality from cardiovascular and cerebrovascular diseases. This is largely due to a concerted effort to control hypertension, smoking, and diet. The focused assessment above provides questions to guide the examination of health system factors influencing chronic health problems in the population.

Risk factors related to the biophysical, psychological, physical environmental, sociocultural, behavioral, and health system dimensions all influence the development and outcomes of chronic physical health problems. Risk factors for selected chronic conditions are summarized in Appendix J on the Companion Website.

COMMUNITY HEALTH NURSING AND CONTROL OF CHRONIC PHYSICAL HEALTH PROBLEMS

Community health nurses are actively involved in efforts to control chronic physical health problems and their effects in individuals and population groups. These efforts involve assessment, diagnosis of chronic conditions, planning and implementation of control programs, and evaluation of their effectiveness.

Assessing for Chronic Physical Health Problems

Community health nurses use their assessment skills to assess for risk factors that contribute to chronic health problems and for existing chronic conditions and their effects. In addition to assessing individual clients for the presence of risk factors for chronic health problems, the community health nurse examines the incidence and prevalence of these risk factors in the general population to determine the potential for chronic health problems in the community. Nurses can also obtain family histories and construct genograms for specific families as described in Chapter 14∞. Positive findings related to chronic conditions with a genetic component direct the assessment to possible signs and symptoms of existing chronic health problems.

Community health nurses assess individual clients and groups of people for indications of existing chronic health problems. Finally, the nurse assesses clients with existing chronic conditions for evidence of related physical effects. Assessment considerations related to physiologic risk factors, signs and symptoms of existing chronic conditions, and evidence of physical problems related to selected conditions are summarized in Table 29-3◆.

In addition to assessing individual clients for levels and sources of stress and the adequacy of their coping mechanisms, the community health nurse assesses the psychological effects of chronic health problems on persons experiencing them. At the population level, the nurse would assess the extent of psychological effects among groups of people with chronic health problems. For example, the nurse might determine the extent of depression among people with asthma or epilepsy as a prelude to designing services to address both physical and psychological needs related to these conditions.

With respect to the physical environmental dimension of health, community health nurses assess for environmental risk factors that promote chronic illness or that contribute to illness-related disability. Nurses also assess the need to adapt the environment to accommodate the needs of clients with chronic conditions. For example, does the home have a shower to make personal hygiene easier for the person with arthritis who may have difficulty getting in and out of a bathtub? Or does the home of the person with cardiovascular disease or COPD have numerous stairs that cause the individual to become short of breath? Similarly, the nurse assesses for potential barriers that limit access to community services for persons with chronic disabilities. The long distances to health care facilities that are encountered in rural environments also place clients with chronic health problems at risk for deterioration of their conditions (Davis & Magilvy, 2000).

MediaLink Appendix J: Epidemiology of Selected Chronic Physical Health Problems

TABLE 29-3 Assessment Considerations Related to Selected Chronic Physical Health Problems

Condition	Physiologic Risk Factors	Signs and Symptoms	Potential Effects
Arthritis	Previous injury, obesity	Painful, swollen joints, limited range of motion	Contractures, mobility limitations, inability to perform activities of daily living (ADLs)
Cancer	Cervical dysplasia, viral infection	Weight loss, change in bowel or bladder habits, changes in voice quality, pain, skin changes, palpable lumps or growths, persistent cough, rectal bleeding or blood in stool	Debility, pain, death
Cardiovascular disease	Hypertension, hypercholesterolemia, diabetes, atherosclerosis, obesity, infection	Chest pain, shortness of breath on exertion, fatigue, arrhythmias, elevated blood pressure, cardiac enlargement, edema	Debility, myocardial infarction, death
Cerebrovascular disease	Hypertension, atherosclerosis, congenital anomaly, heart disease, diabetes, polycythemia	Headaches, confusion, vertigo, parasthesia of extremities, transient ischemic attacks, slurred speech, weakness	Paralysis, aphasia, incontinence, death
Chronic obstructive pulmonary disease	Asthma, respiratory allergy, frequent respiratory infections	Shortness of breath on exertion, cough, weakness, weight loss, diminished libido	Debility, inability to perform ADLs, heart failure
Diabetes mellitus	Obesity, viral infection	Polyuria, polydipsia, polyphagia, weight loss, frequent infections (especially monilia)	Ketoacidosis with nausea, anorexia, vomiting, air hunger, and coma; sensory neuropathy, diabetic retinopathy, poor wound healing and infection, amputation, sensory loss, postural hypotension, male impotence, nocturnal diarrhea, death
Hypertension	Atherosclerosis	Headache, blurred vision, dizziness, flushed face, fatigue, epistaxis, elevated blood pressure	Heart disease, stroke, death

In the sociocultural realm, community health nurses assess the jobs performed by individual clients and identify any risk factors for chronic health problems posed by the work environment or the work performed. Nurses also assess the community for potential occupational risk factors related to chronic health problems by determining the major employers and occupations present in the community and the types of products, services, and processes involved.

The community health nurse also assesses the social effects of chronic health problems on those clients experiencing them. For example, the nurse might note that the physical effects of arthritis or COPD may prevent clients from engaging in activities that provided them with opportunities for social interaction in the past, thus resulting in social isolation. Legislative factors can also influence health behaviors and consequent chronic health problems. For example, smoking has been shown to decrease when cigarette prices or taxes increase. Similarly, bicycle helmet use increases when use legislation is enforced.

In addition, the nurse should assess the adequacy of the client's social support network for dealing with the problems posed by chronic health problems. Areas to be considered include those who make up a client's social support network, the assistance provided by each, the adequacy of the network for meeting the client's needs, and the extent to which the network is appropriately used. For example, the nurse might note that the client's support network is not sufficiently broad to meet his or her needs or that the client is not using the existing network as fully as possible. At the population level, the nurse would assess community resources and social capital available for meeting the social support needs of people with chronic health problems. For example, is transportation available to meet the needs of disabled community members? Do community attitudes support independence for people with chronic and debilitating conditions?

In assessing the influence of consumption patterns on chronic health problems, the community health nurse identifies consumption patterns that place individuals at risk for chronic conditions. The nurse also determines the prevalence of high-risk consumption patterns in the community. In addition, the nurse explores unhealthful consumption patterns with clients who have existing chronic diseases and determines their effects on the course of the condition. For example, the nurse would determine whether a client with diabetes is adhering to a diabetic diet. The nurse also assesses for factors related to food preferences and modes of preparation that may impede adherence to special diets and the availability of healthy food at reasonable prices in the surrounding neighborhood.

The nurse assessing an individual client or a community for risk factors related to exercise or its lack would determine the extent of regular exercise obtained by the individual or the proportion of sedentary individuals who make up the population. The nurse would also assess the extent of the physical activity by clients with chronic diseases. For example, the nurse might assess a diabetic client's exercise in relation to his or her dietary intake and the amount of insulin taken.

The extent to which individual clients and their families practice safety measures is another aspect of assessment related to chronic health problems. Are there smoke detectors in the home? Are hazardous items, such as sharp objects and poisons, stored appropriately? Is there potential for falls owing to multiple obstacles in the homes of elderly persons? Do family members consistently use seat belts? The community health nurse also appraises the extent to which these and similar safety conditions and practices are found in the general population or in the work setting. Are smoke detectors and sprinkler systems present in public buildings or in businesses and industries? Is seat belt use mandatory in the jurisdiction and, if so, is it enforced? Are appropriate safety equipment and safety precautions employed in work settings?

In assessing individual and community risk for chronic health problems, the community health nurse determines the extent of preventive, diagnostic, and treatment services offered to community residents as well as their cost and accessibility. The nurse also assesses the extent to which available services are used and possible reasons for nonuse if indicated. A Chronic Disease Risk Factor Inventory to assist the community health nurse in assessing individual and population risk for chronic physical health problems is available in the *Community Assessment Reference Guide* 📋 designed to accompany this book.

Diagnostic Reasoning and Control of Chronic Physical Health Problems

Nursing diagnoses are derived from information collected relative to the incidence and prevalence of chronic health problems in the population and the factors contributing to these conditions. These diagnoses may relate to individual clients or to the general population. Examples of nursing diagnoses related to an individual client are "potential for cardiovascular disease due to smoking and sedentary lifestyle" and "uncontrolled diabetes due to inability to adhere to diabetic diet." At the group level, the nurse might derive diagnoses such as "increased prevalence of lung cancer due to smoking and occupational exposure to carcinogens." In each case, the nursing diagnosis contains a statement of the probable cause or etiology of the problem that directs interventions designed to resolve it.

Planning and Implementing Control Strategies for Chronic Physical Health Problems

Planning interventions related to chronic health problems for individual clients is based on the understanding of contributing factors derived from the assessment. It is particularly important to involve the client and his or her family or the community in planning solutions to chronic health problems because they will be responsible for implementing the plan or for using services designed. By involving the client/family or community, the nurse can tailor the plan of care to the specific circumstances influencing chronic disease. It is important to remember that the presence of a chronic health problem affects many facets of life. Effective planning accounts for these effects and minimizes the consequences of chronic illness for those affected.

Some authors have suggested that control of chronic disease at the community level should make greater use of traditional public health interventions including surveillance and reporting, environmental modification, regulation, effective clinical care, outbreak detection, case management and contact tracing, immunization, and health education (Frieden, 2004). Educational interventions and immunization reflect primary prevention. Regulation may also reflect primary prevention. Surveillance, reporting, and outbreak detection are elements of secondary prevention, as is effective clinical care. Case management reflects tertiary prevention of chronic disease, and environmental modification may encompass either primary or tertiary prevention. Each of these public health strategies will be discussed in the context of the relevant level of prevention.

In 2003, the U.S. Department of Health and Human Services (USDHHS, 2003d) established *Steps to a HealthierUS* initiatives to assist in the control of five chronic diseases that contribute significantly to morbidity and mortality in the United States. The initiatives are aimed at reducing the incidence and prevalence of asthma, cancer, diabetes, heart disease and stroke, and obesity. The basic elements of the steps initiatives are presented in Table 29-4◆. Specific action plans based on the steps initiative have been developed for diabetes (USDHHS, 2003c) and heart disease and stroke (USDHHS, 2003a) as well as the other target conditions. Community health nurses will be actively involved in achieving the goals of the steps initiatives as they relate to primary, secondary, and tertiary prevention of chronic physical health problems.

Primary Prevention

Nursing strategies for primary prevention of chronic conditions focus on two major areas: health promotion and risk factor modification. Both aspects of primary prevention can be applied to individual clients or to population groups.

TABLE 29-4 Elements of the *Steps to a HealthierUS* Initiatives

Promote health and wellness programs in schools, worksites, and faith- and community-based settings that

- provide environments and education to promote healthy eating, daily physical activity, and avoidance of tobacco, alcohol, and illicit drugs (primary prevention)
- engage in smoking cessation strategies (primary prevention)
- employ physical activity strategies (primary prevention)
- support, encourage, and assist people to obtain cancer screening services and navigate the health care system (secondary prevention)

Enact policies that promote healthy environments, such as

- safe walking and cycling trails (primary prevention)
- low-fat/high-fruit-and-vegetable menus (primary prevention)
- school incentives for physical education (primary prevention)
- smoke-free public places and workplaces (primary prevention)
- universal availability of 911 emergency services (secondary prevention)

Ensure access to quality health care services with

- improved access to effective screening and diagnostic services (secondary prevention)
- better education of health professionals in applying preventive interventions (primary prevention)
- public and private insurance coverage of chronic disease prevention, screening, and treatment services (primary and secondary prevention)
- training to empower clients to self-manage their conditions (secondary and tertiary prevention)

Eliminate racial, ethnic, and socioeconomic disparities through research to identify factors contributing to disparities and interventions to eliminate them.

Educate the public regarding health using approaches grounded in the findings of social marketing, health education, and consumer research.

Data from: U.S. Department of Health and Human Services. (2003). The power of prevention. Retrieved May 29, 2006, from http://www.healthierus.gov/steps/summit/prevportfolio/Power_of_ Prevention.pdf

HEALTH PROMOTION General health promotion is aimed at making people healthier and reducing their chances of developing a variety of health problems, including chronic conditions. Health promotion at both the individual and group levels involves promoting a healthier lifestyle, political activity to create conditions that promote health, and immunization for selected conditions.

Promoting Healthy Lifestyles Strategies to promote healthy lifestyles as a means of preventing chronic health problems focus on diet, exercise, and coping skills. The nurse employs the principles of health education discussed in Chapter 11∞ to educate both individual clients and the general public on basic nutrition and specific nutritional requirements based on age and activity level. For example, to prevent obesity the nurse would teach parents about the nutritional needs of infants and young children and encourage a well-balanced diet with minimal amounts of junk food. Similarly, the nurse would teach a pregnant woman, a nursing mother, or a physically active person about their specific nutritional needs. The nurse would also try to inform the general public about proper nutrition, including the need for adequate vitamin D in the diet or limited exposure to sunlight (Garland et al., 2006).

Access to healthy foods has also been associated with healthier diets. Access to foods such as fruits and vegetables is often related to socioeconomic level. For example, in one study, low-income minority and racially mixed neighborhoods in three states had four times as many small grocery stores and half as many supermarkets as higher-income areas. Low-income areas also tended to have fewer fruit and vegetable stores and natural food stores, but more liquor stores (Moore & Diez Roux, 2006). In another study, stores in more affluent neighborhoods were more likely to carry foods recommended for people with diabetes than those in lower-income neighborhoods (Horowitz, Colson, Hebert, & Lancaster, 2004). Healthy foods tend to be more expensive when purchased at small neighborhood stores than at supermarkets, thus lessening the ability of low-income families to afford them. Community health nurses may advocate for access to healthy foods in neighborhood stores and may assist local families in cooperative buying to decrease prices. In some areas, nurses may help communities to establish community gardens to improve consumption of fresh produce.

Exercise is another area in which health education may be required, and nurses would plan to inform both individual clients and the general public about the need for regular physical activity. The nurse might also assist clients to plan ways to incorporate physical activity into their daily routine or develop plans for exercise programs in the community or for employees of local businesses. For example, a simple means of motivating people to climb stairs is to display posters at stairwell entries encouraging use of stairs rather than elevators. Similar messages posted on stair risers have been found to be even more effective in motivating stair use (Webb & Eves, 2005).

Exercise is also beneficial for people with existing chronic illnesses. For example, people with arthritis can reduce their risk of physical activity limitation by 32% with regular physical activity. Unfortunately, 44% of people with arthritis in the United States are physically inactive (Steiner et al., 2006). Community health nurses can help people with arthritis and other chronic conditions to identify avenues for physical activity that are within their capabilities. For certain conditions, such as cardiovascular disease, nurses may suggest a thorough medical evaluation prior to undertaking a rigorous exercise regimen.

Teaching general coping skills is another way for community health nurses to promote health and prevent

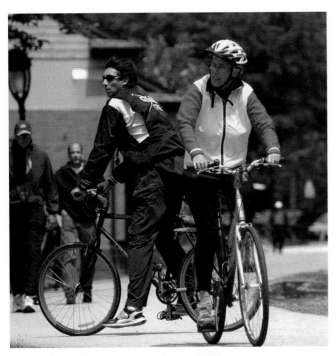

Exercise is a primary prevention measure for cardiovascular disease and obesity. (Patrick J. Watson)

chronic health problems that are influenced by stress. In this respect, the nurse might assist a harried mother of several small children to develop ways of coping with stress, or the nurse might assist school personnel to develop a program to teach basic coping skills as part of elementary and secondary school curricula. Another approach might be to plan a program to foster adequate coping among employees of local businesses.

Technology provides new avenues for promoting healthy lifestyles among the general public and in clients with chronic diseases. Experts have identified several points at which clients may turn to the Internet for information related to their health. Many people seek information on basic health promotion and health maintenance activities. When symptoms arise, people may seek information on the possible meaning of symptoms, or they may seek to validate a treatment regimen as the appropriate option after diagnosis. Clients may also use the Internet to search for information about their conditions or about specific treatment regimens or options, to identify possible side effects, or to participate in support groups (Ziebland et al., 2004). Community health nurses can make active use of Internet technology to educate clients for health-promoting lifestyles and to educate clients for self-care when illness occurs. Nurses can also refer clients to credible sources of information and educate them regarding mechanisms for evaluating the credibility of information retrieved from Internet sources.

Political Activity   Sometimes educational interventions are aimed at informing health policy makers and promoting legislative and regulatory strategies to control chronic illness in the population. Political activity related to primary prevention focuses on measures to promote access to preventive health services and to create a healthful environment. Nursing involvement in efforts at this level includes the planning strategies to influence health policy making discussed in Chapter 7∞. For example, community health nurses might campaign for better access to prenatal care for pregnant women or legislation to prevent or reduce pollution so as to prevent its contribution to chronic respiratory conditions and other chronic health problems.

Political activity by community health nurses might also be required to establish and enforce policies and legislation that foster healthful behaviors. For example, failure to enforce laws related to the sale of tobacco products to minors has enabled youngsters to purchase tobacco. Conversely, enforcement of seat belt legislation has significantly reduced motor vehicle accident fatalities.

Immunization   Although immunization is generally considered a primary preventive measure for communicable diseases, it can also serve to prevent some chronic conditions and their effects. For example, immunization of persons at risk for hepatitis B can eliminate this risk factor for chronic liver disease and cirrhosis. Those clients with existing liver disease should receive pneumococcal vaccine and annual immunizations for influenza, as should persons with diabetes and COPD. In 2003, however, the median state coverage for influenza vaccine among those over age 65 was 70%, and only 64% of this population had received pneumococcal vaccine. Among people 18 to 64 years of age, influenza vaccine coverage was only 34% for those with asthma and 49% for those with diabetes. Only 37% of people with diabetes had received pneumococcal vaccine (Bardenheir, Wortley, & Euler, 2004). In the future, vaccines for human papillomavirus infection may help to prevent cervical cancer (Frieden, 2004). At least one vaccine currently available has a 100% efficacy against the strain of HPV most often implicated in the development of cervical cancer (Moyer, 2004), and in June 2006 the HPV vaccine Gardasil was approved by the Food and Drug Administration for general use in girls and women 9 to 26 years of age. The vaccine protects against two strains of HPV that contribute to approximately 70% of cervical cancer and two additional strains that cause 90% of genital warts. The vaccine is not yet approved for use with men and boys who frequently transmit HPV to their sexual partners. Recommendations include administration of the vaccine before girls become sexually active (DeNoon, 2006). Community health nurses may be involved in educating individual clients and the general public about the need for and availability of vaccines or in designing and providing immunization services. They may also need to advocate for accessible immunization services and coverage of routine immunization under health insurance plans.

RISK FACTOR MODIFICATION Activities designed to eliminate or modify risk factors include quitting smoking, reducing weight, controlling hypertension, using safety and protective devices, and creating environments free of hazards. Additional problem-specific risk factor modification strategies include the use of aspirin to prevent cardiovascular events (U.S. Preventive Services Task Force, 2002), calcium supplementation to prevent osteoporosis, and exercise to prevent cardiovascular disease and obesity. Use of metformin and other pharmacologic agents has also been shown to delay the onset of diabetes in clients with prediabetic glucose intolerance (Ullom-Minnich, 2004). Community health nurses can educate both individual clients and the general public about the elimination or modification of risk factors for chronic health problems that are amenable to personal control. They can also advocate for access to pharmacologic interventions for clients at risk for such diseases as diabetes. Finally, they can advocate for the modification or elimination of environmental risk factors (e.g., air pollution) that are beyond individual control. Approaches to modifying risk factors such as smoking, obesity, hypertension, and safety and environmental hazards are presented below.

Smoking Some progress has been made in eliminating smoking as a risk factor for chronic health problems. Smoking cessation even as late as age 65 has been shown to add as much as 2 years of life for men and 3.7 years for women. Quitting smoking at age 35 increases longevity by as much as 8.5 years for men and 7.7 years for women (Taylor, Hasselblad, Henley, Thun, & Sloan, 2002).

Two general approaches have been used in decreasing smoking incidence and prevalence: personal efforts and public activity. Personal efforts are designed to prevent smoking initiation and to encourage smokers to quit. Among adults, these efforts have been relatively successful, and as of 2004, less than 21% of the adult population in the United States were smokers (Maurice et al., 2005). Unfortunately, the prevalence of tobacco use among adolescents is somewhat higher, at 27% in 2003 (Grunbaum et al., 2004). As noted earlier, some ethnic minority groups also have higher rates of tobacco use.

Overall, an estimated 70% of U.S. smokers desire to stop smoking (CDC, 2005a). Community health nurses can educate smokers regarding the hazards of smoking and direct them to sources of assistance in smoking cessation. In addition, the community health nurse can provide support and encourage family members to support the smoker's efforts to quit. Nurses can also educate young people regarding the hazards of smoking and develop programs that discourage them from initiating the habit. Finally, nurses can educate individual clients and groups of people to eliminate other forms of tobacco use such as snuff and chewing tobacco. There is some data to suggest, however, that health care providers, including nurses, are not prepared to counsel clients on

smoking cessation. In the Global Health Professionals study (Costa de Silva et al., 2005) conducted in 10 countries (not including the United States), 87% to 99% of third-year students in dentistry, medicine, nursing, and pharmacy believed that health professionals should engage in such counseling, but only 5% (Argentina) to 37% (Philippines) had received formal training to support smoking cessation. In addition, more than 20% of the students surveyed smoked themselves. Based on similar findings in the United States, the National Action Plan for Tobacco Cessation has recommended inclusion of specific tobacco cessation counseling competencies in medical and other health disciplines curricula (Geller et al., 2005). Community health nurses may need to actively educate themselves and other providers on how to counsel clients for smoking cessation.

Community involvement in anti-smoking education can be an effective means of conveying the message. For example, children from the Boys and Girls Club of Rochester, Minnesota, created a memorial wall with stories of actual people who died as a result of cigarette smoking (Plese, 2003). Such involvement provides a graphic picture of the real-life effects of smoking far better than brochures, billboards, or other media approaches.

Community health nurses may also be involved in political activity to limit smoking. Legislative and regulatory activities to control smoking can be of two types: legislation controlling smoking in public places and taxation of tobacco sales. In Great Britain, for example, prohibitively high taxes on cigarettes and other forms of tobacco have greatly reduced tobacco use. Legislation has also been effective in controlling smoking behavior by limiting smoking in public places (Office on Smoking and Health, 2000). Another area of public effort to reduce smoking lies in workplace restrictions, and community health nurses can be active in promoting no-smoking policies in business and industry and in public places.

Public smoking bans and smoke-free workplace policies not only affect smoking behaviors but also limit exposure to *secondhand* or *involuntary* smoking (also called environmental tobacco smoke). In 2006, the U.S. Surgeon General's report, *The Health Consequences of Involuntary Exposure to Tobacco Smoke* (USDHHS, 2006), made it clear that there is no risk-free level of exposure to secondhand smoke and that providing special areas for smokers and air filtration or ventilation systems does not eliminate secondhand smoke exposure. The report advocates creating completely smoke-free environments in homes and public places. Community health nurses can advocate for policies and legislation that promote smoke-free environments. They can also educate the public on the dangers of involuntary smoking and advocate for access to smoking cessation assistance for those who desire to stop smoking.

Obesity Control efforts for obesity have been less extensive than those for smoking. Health education related to caloric intake and fat consumption, particularly saturated fats, is required, and community health nurses should educate individual clients about the need to consume fewer calories and to reduce fat consumption. Dietary recommendations related to the year 2010 health objectives◆ include reducing fat intake to less than 30% and saturated fat to less than 10% of total caloric intake (CDC, 2005b). Community health nurses can educate clients about reading package labels to determine the fat and calorie content of various foods. They can also inform clients about foods that are low in saturated fats and about food preparation methods that minimize fat consumption.

Development of modified food products also assists in controlling fat intake. Community health nurses can encourage the food industry to pursue research on food modification. They can also campaign for legislation to require accurate labeling of food packages and disclosure of food contents.

Regular exercise can also be emphasized as a control strategy for obesity, as well as a means of counteracting the effects of a sedentary lifestyle, itself a risk factor in many chronic conditions. Community health nurses can encourage overweight or sedentary clients to incorporate more exercise into their daily routine. Nurses may also be involved in planning exercise programs for groups of overweight or sedentary clients in the community or in work settings.

Prevention of obesity and diet modification can also help to prevent the onset of other chronic health problems. For example, decreased fat consumption and lower blood cholesterol are two of several factors contributing to the decline in cardiovascular disease mortality. Prevention of obesity, weight loss, and supervised exercise programs may also help to decrease the incidence and disabling effects of arthritis (Health Care and Aging Studies Bureau, 2001).

Screening for high blood cholesterol is one means of identifying people in need of dietary modification to prevent obesity and cardiovascular disease. From 1991 to 2003, the percentage of people over age 65 reporting blood cholesterol screening in the previous 5 years increased from 82.5% to 89.3%. Similar increases were noted for people in younger age groups. Only Massachusetts and the District of Columbia, however, achieved the *Healthy People 2010*◆ target of 80% screening prevalence (Saddlemire et al., 2005). Community health nurses can advocate for and refer clients for cholesterol screening and weight control services. They can also advocate for weight control and nutrition counseling as a mandatory insurance benefit.

Hypertension In addition to being a chronic condition itself, hypertension is a risk factor for several other chronic health problems and their complications. For this reason, efforts to control hypertension constitute primary prevention for cardiovascular and cerebrovascular

diseases as well as for complications of diabetes. In fact, reductions of diastolic blood pressure by 5 to 6 mm Hg has been found to reduce stroke incidence by 35% and occurrence of myocardial infarction by 16% (Goldsmith, 2000). Hypertension control is particularly important in some segments of the population with continuing high rates of mortality from cardiovascular diseases.

Community health nurses should educate individual clients and the general public regarding the effects and signs and symptoms of hypertension. They can also identify people with hypertension and be involved in planning hypertension screening programs or in referring clients with elevated blood pressures for further evaluation and treatment.

The second aspect of hypertension control is encouraging behaviors that promote control of existing hypertension. Community health nurses can educate hypertensive clients on the appropriate use of antihypertensive medications and potential side effects. In addition, nurses should convey to clients the need to continue with therapy and to report any adverse effects of treatment to their primary care providers.

Safety Precautions and Environmental Modification The use of safety devices and other safety precautions can modify risk factors for accidents that may lead to chronic disability. Community health nurses can encourage clients to install smoke detectors in residences, provide adequate supervision for small children, store hazardous items appropriately, and remove hazards that contribute to falls in the elderly. They can also promote the use of seat belts in vehicles and campaign for legislation that makes seat belt use mandatory in all vehicles (e.g., school buses). Community health nurses can promote use of safety devices and safety precautions in the work setting to prevent accidental injury. Programs to prevent sports and occupational injuries will also help to prevent arthritis (Health Care and Aging Studies Bureau, 2001). Fall prevention through balance training, correcting visual impairment, limiting medication side effects, and environmental changes can also help to prevent injury, particularly in older populations (National Center for Injury Prevention and Control, 2004). Finally, community health nurses can motivate clients to use sunscreen, sunglasses, and protective clothing to prevent melanoma and cataracts. Staying indoors is another effective means of limiting sun exposure, but the U.S. Preventive Services Task Force (2003) has cautioned that remaining indoors may reduce both physical activity and vitamin D production, resulting in other health problems.

Modifications of environmental conditions that contribute to chronic health problems may also help to control them. For example, community health nurses can advocate for enforcement of clean-air legislation and promote measures that prevent contamination of drinking water by heavy metals and other agents that cause chronic health problems. Control of environmental conditions, such as radon emissions and air pollution, are particularly important in preventing some forms of cancer. Similarly, nurses and others can campaign for traffic control measures that minimize motor vehicle accidents and subsequent disability. Nurses can also advocate for environmental designs that promote physical activity.

Control of environmental working conditions for nurses themselves is of growing concern to the profession. Control of communicable disease exposures in health care settings was discussed in Chapter 28∞. Injury prevention is another facet of primary prevention of chronic health problems for nurses. A survey of nurses conducted by the American Nurses Association (ANA) found that 38% of nurses experience back pain related to work injuries severe enough to require time off work, and 12% of nurses leave the profession as a result of back pain (de Castro, 2004a). Nurses' aides, orderlies, and attendants rank second only to truck drivers in their risk of occupational strains and sprains, and registered nurses rank sixth (de Castro, 2004b). These and other similar findings led to the development of the ANA *Handle with Care* campaign to change conditions in health care settings to prevent musculoskeletal injury to nurses and related personnel. Specific elements of ergonomic safety programs for preventing injury to nurses can be adapted to prevent injury for family caretakers of people with disabling chronic conditions. Elements of ergonomic safety and their adaptation for family caretaking are presented in Table 29-5◆. Primary prevention goals in the control of chronic physical

health problems and related community health nursing activities are summarized in Table 29-6◆.

Secondary Prevention

Secondary prevention activities in the control of chronic illness are aimed at dealing with chronic health problems once they have occurred. The National Asthma Education and Prevention Program has identified four key strategies for asthma control that can be adapted for use with other chronic health problems: assessment and monitoring, control of factors contributing to the disease and its severity, pharmacotherapy, and education of clients and providers for partnerships in care (Williams, Schmidt, Redd, & Storms, 2003). These strategies and related interventions are summarized in Table 29-7◆. As noted in the table, the strategies involve both secondary and tertiary prevention. Here we will address the three major foci of secondary prevention: screening for existing chronic conditions, early diagnosis, and prompt treatment. Tertiary prevention strategies are discussed later in this chapter.

SCREENING Although the prevalence of many chronic conditions in the population has been increasing, there is less evidence of both upper and lower body limitations that may lead to disability. In all likelihood, this improvement in health status despite increased incidence of disease is due to earlier diagnosis and more effective disease management (Freedman & Martin, 2000). Screening is the first step in early diagnosis of many chronic health problems.

Screening tests are available for several chronic health problems. Pap smears, for example, are used to

---

TABLE 29-5 Elements of Ergonomics Safety Programs for Nurses and Adaptation for Family Caretakers

Elements of Injury Prevention for Nurses*	Adaptations for Family Caretakers
▪ Create an ergonomics committee to develop, implement, and monitor a comprehensive ergonomics program.	▪ Collaborate with client, family, and other caretakers to develop strategies for preventing caretaker injury.
▪ Analyze injury data, conduct a walk-through, and survey employees.	▪ Identify risks for injury in caring for a disabled family member (e.g., lifting or twisting in transfer activities). ▪ Assess the physical constraints of the caretaking situation (e.g., crowded bedroom, type of bed).
▪ Assess risky patient-handling tasks.	▪ Identify caretaking tasks that pose a risk for injury.
▪ Assess patient dependency levels.	▪ Assess client dependency levels and degree of assistance needed from caretakers.
▪ Develop and adopt a safe patient-handling policy.	▪ Develop and implement safe strategies for assisting the disabled family member.
▪ Evaluate patient-handling equipment and devices.	▪ Identify needed equipment and devices and assist family in obtaining them.
▪ Provide staff training on injury prevention measures, policies, and equipment.	▪ Educate caretakers regarding injury prevention strategies, use of assistive equipment, etc.
▪ Encourage reporting of injuries.	▪ Ask caretakers about injuries and refer for treatment as needed.
▪ Track injuries and evaluate the program.	▪ Document caretaker injuries, contributing factors, and effectiveness of injury prevention strategies.

*Data from: de Castro, A. B. (2004). Actively preventing injury: Avoiding back injuries and other musculoskeletal injuries among nurses. American Journal of Nursing, 104 (1). Retrieved July 28, 2006, from http://nursingworld.org/ajn/2004/jan/health.htm

TABLE 29-6 Goals for Primary Prevention and Related Community Health Nursing Interventions in the Control of Chronic Physical Health Problems

Primary Prevention Goal	Nursing Interventions

1. Health promotion
  a. Provide prenatal care.
	1. Promote client health.
	  a. Educate clients and public about the need for prenatal care. Refer to or provide prenatal care.

b. Maintain appropriate body weight through adequate nutrition.
    ▪ Breast-feed infants.
    ▪ Delay introduction of solid foods.
    ▪ Avoid use of food as pacifier or reward.
    ▪ Establish healthy food habits from childhood.
	b. Educate clients and public about adequate nutrition.
	    ▪ Obtain diet history and identify poor food habits.
	    ▪ Assist with breast-feeding.
	    ▪ Assist with menu planning and budgeting.
	    ▪ Refer for food-supplement plans as needed.
	    ▪ Encourage use of nonfood reward systems.

c. Engage in graduated program of exercise.	c. Educate public about need for exercise. Assist clients to plan appropriate exercise programs.
d. Develop coping skills.	d. Teach coping skills.
e. Immunize against communicable diseases that contribute to chronic health problems.	e. Educate clients and public regarding the need for immunizations. Refer for or provide immunization services. Advocate for accessible immunization services.

2. Risk factor modification
  a. Quit smoking and prevent initiation of smoking.
	2. Screen for risk factors. Educate public regarding risk factors.
	  a. Foster self-help groups for smokers.
	    ▪ Educate nonsmokers about the hazards of smoking.
	    ▪ Promote no-smoking policies in public places and in the workplace.

b. Decrease dietary intake of saturated fats, cholesterol, sodium, and alcohol.	b. Educate and help clients plan adequate nutritional intake. Foster self-help groups for overeaters.

c. Identify and treat existing health problems that are risk factors for chronic illness (hypertension, obesity).	c. Screen for and refer clients with existing conditions.
	    ▪ Educate clients regarding therapy for existing disease.
	    ▪ Adjust therapy to client's situation when possible.
	    ▪ Monitor for compliance, therapeutic effects, and side effects.

d. Eliminate environmental pollutants contributing to chronic conditions.	d. Educate public about pollution. Become politically active on environmental legislation.

e. Decrease exposure to sources of radiation (x-ray, sunlight).	e. Educate public about risks of radiation.
	    ▪ Discourage sunbathing.
	    ▪ Encourage use of sunscreen and protective clothing.

f. Eliminate occupational exposure to hazardous substances.	f. Monitor occupational safety conditions.
g. Prevent occupational and sports injuries.	g. Promote occupational safety and use of protective sports equipment.
h. Prevent caretaker injury.	h. Identify caretaker injury risk factors and plan appropriate interventions. Educate caretakers for injury prevention. Refer for help in obtaining client management equipment and assistive devices. Advocate for funding to provide needed caretaker assistance to prevent injuries.
i. Eliminate or modify effects of emotional stress. Avoid stressful situations when possible.	i. Assist clients to identify stressful situations. Explore with clients ways of decreasing stress.
j. Engage in other behaviors to modify risk factors.	j. Promote other risk modification behaviors (e.g., promote use of aspirin and antioxidants)

screen women for cervical cancer, and clinical breast examination and mammography assist in early detection of breast cancer. In 2002 and 2003, nearly 85% of U.S. women 50 to 69 years of age received Pap smears and 82% received a mammogram. Women without health insurance coverage were less likely to receive screening services than those with insurance (NCHS, 2005c). Community health nurses can refer women for these screening examinations as needed. They may also need to advocate for access to such services for women of all economic levels.

Early detection of colorectal cancers is assisted with annual fecal occult blood tests and digital rectal examinations. Additional screening tests that have been recommended for colorectal cancer include lower endoscopy examinations (flexible sigmoidoscopy every 5 years or colonoscopy every 10 years) (U.S. Preventive Services Task Force, 2005). In 2004, just over 57% of U.S. adults reported fecal occult blood testing and/or lower endoscopic examination in the previous year (Seeff et al., 2006). Screening for prostate cancer has been recommended annually for men over 50 years of age either on a routine basis or based on provider determination of need (U.S. Preventive Services Task Force, 2005). Dermatologic screening for skin cancers and hypertension and diabetes screenings are readily available and easily accessible in most areas.

Members of the public can be educated to recognize early signs of myocardial infarction and stroke. The Client Education tips on page 880 can assist clients

TABLE 29-7	Strategies for Control of Chronic Physical Health Problems
Strategy	**Clinical Activities**
Assessment and monitoring	■ Establish the diagnosis (secondary prevention). ■ Classify the severity of disease (secondary prevention). ■ Schedule routine follow-up care (tertiary prevention).
Control of factors contributing to disease severity	■ Recommend measures to control severity (tertiary prevention). ■ Treat or prevent comorbid conditions (tertiary prevention).
Pharmacotherapy	■ Prescribe appropriate pharmacotherapeutic agents (secondary prevention). ■ Monitor use of prescribed medications (tertiary prevention).
Education for partnership in care	■ Develop a disease management plan (secondary/tertiary prevention). ■ Educate clients on self-management (secondary/tertiary prevention).

Data from: Williams, S. G., Schmidt, D. K., Redd, S. C., & Storms, W. (2003). Key clinical activities for quality asthma care: Recommendations of the National Asthma Education and Prevention Program. Morbidity and Mortality Weekly Report, 52(RR-6), 1–8.

in recognizing the warning signs of stroke. According to CDC (2004b), only 17% of U.S. adults in 2004 recognized all of the warning signs and knew to call 911 for emergency assistance, yet there is a strong correlation between stroke education and care-seeking behavior (York, 2003). Research also suggests that stroke education should be targeted to people without a history of chronic illness as well as to those with risk factors for stroke such as high cholesterol levels (Robinson & Merrill, 2003).

Another aspect of screening related to chronic health problems involves a process similar to the traditional process of contact notification for communicable diseases. Although contacts of people with chronic health problems do not develop disease as a direct result of exposure, they may share similar genetic, environmental, and lifestyle factors (Frieden, 2004). Contact notification for chronic health problems could help to identify people with significant risk factors and promote

risk factor modification prior to or early in the development of disease, thus improving control and minimizing disease effects.

Although available, screening is not routinely recommended for conditions such as coronary heart disease. In fact, the U.S. Preventive Services Task Force (2004) has recommended against screening for coronary heart disease with resting electrocardiography, exercise treadmill tests, or electron-beam computerized tomography. In addition, the task force found insufficient evidence to recommend for or against the routine use of these tests to screen for coronary heart disease in adults at increased risk of disease. Similarly, screening of the general public for diabetes is not recommended, although screening is suggested for those at increased risk for maculovascular changes due to hypertension (Ullom-Minnich, 2004).

Community health nurses play an important role in screening for chronic illness. They are conversant with the prevalence of various risk factors in the community and can plan screening programs to detect conditions related to the most prevalent risk factors. They may also plan to motivate client participation in screening by educating the public regarding the need for screening. Knowledge of risk factors alone does not motivate the general public to seek screening opportunities, so motivational activities must go beyond educational campaigns. For example, community health nurses may be actively involved in referring clients for screening services and linking disease prevention to other goals valued by clients (e.g., the ability to continue working).

Interpretation of test results and referrals for further diagnosis and treatment of suspected conditions are also functions of community health nurses in secondary prevention of chronic health problems. (See Chapter 16∞ for recommendations for routine screening tests for children, Chapters 17 and 18∞ for screening recommendations for men and women, respectively, and Chapter 19∞ for recommendations for older adults.) In addition to routine screening recommendations, persons with specific risk factors for chronic conditions should be screened as needed.

At the population level, community health nurses may need to advocate for available and accessible screening services for underserved segments of the population. For example, lack of health insurance and presence of fee-for-service insurance (as opposed to managed care enrollment) have been associated with lack of cancer screening in women under 65 years of age. Conversely, the combination of Medicare and supplemental insurance has been linked to cancer screening in older women (Hsia et al., 2000). Community health nurses may also need to educate and motivate providers to recommend screening procedures to their clients since provider recommendation has been shown to be a strong predictor of prostate screening in men and

CLIENT EDUCATION — Warning Signs of Stroke

■ Sudden confusion, trouble speaking or understanding
■ Numbness or weakness of the face, arms, or legs (especially unilaterally)
■ Trouble seeing
■ Trouble walking, dizziness, or loss of balance
■ Severe headache without cause

Data from: Centers for Disease Control and Prevention. (2004). National stroke awareness month—May, 2004. Morbidity and Mortality Weekly Report, 53, 359.

cervical cancer screening in women (Epidemiology Program Office, 2000; Gill & McClellan, 2001).

EARLY DIAGNOSIS The effects of many chronic health conditions can be minimized when they are diagnosed and treated early in the course of the disease. Positive screening test results are always an indication of a need for further diagnostic testing. Persons with obvious symptoms associated with chronic diseases should also be referred for diagnostic evaluation.

Community health nurses frequently engage in case finding with respect to chronic diseases, identifying community members with possible symptoms of disease and referring them for diagnosis and treatment as appropriate. Community health nurses are also active in educating clients and the general public regarding signs and symptoms of chronic diseases and the need for medical intervention. Community health nurses who are nurse practitioners may also be involved in making medical diagnoses of chronic illnesses.

At the population level, early diagnosis may also involve surveillance for increasing incidence of specific chronic diseases and detection of "outbreaks" in particular populations. Some authors have suggested a mandatory reporting system, similar to that used for many communicable diseases, to assist in chronic disease surveillance (Frieden, 2004). Current cancer registries are one example of this type of reporting. Surveillance and reporting permit public health professionals, including community health nurses, to monitor trends in disease incidence and prevalence and to identify factors contributing to disease. Community health nurses may be involved in data collection for chronic disease registries or in advocating their development. They may also need to advocate for available and accessible low-cost diagnostic services for chronic health problems.

PROMPT TREATMENT The third aspect of secondary prevention in the control of chronic health problems is the treatment of existing conditions. The primary public health role in this area lies in promoting and monitoring treatment standards for chronic disease in the personal health care sector (Frieden, 2004). Treatment considerations in chronic conditions include stabilizing the client's condition as rapidly as possible, establishing a medical treatment regimen, promoting self-management, and preventing progression of the disease by monitoring treatment effectiveness. Unfortunately, many people with chronic illnesses do not receive effective clinical services. As many as three fourths of some populations with chronic illnesses have been found to lack access to care, and 74% had difficulty obtaining medications (Committee on Rapid Advance Demonstration Projects, 2003). For example, only 54% of people reporting a diagnosis of asthma in the 2002 BRFSS had visited a regular health care provider in the previous year, 18% had been seen in an emergency department (ED), and 28.5% were

seen in urgent care centers, suggesting a lack of ongoing care (National Center for Environmental Health, 2004). Emergency department use by people with asthma is linked to insurance status. In 2003, for example, 30% of medical visits by people with asthma who were uninsured occurred in the ED, compared to only 6% by those with health insurance (NCHS, 2006b).

Effective treatment of chronic illness can be facilitated with disease management and decision support systems. According to the Disease Management Association of America (2006), disease management involves developing "a system of coordinated health care interventions and communication for populations with conditions in which patient self-care efforts are significant" (p. 1). Disease management emphasizes prevention and client-provider collaboration. Evaluation of clinical, humanistic, and economic outcomes of care is an essential feature of disease management, which includes the following components: identification of affected populations; use of evidence-based practice guidelines; collaborative practice including the physician, client, and other health care professionals; education of clients for self-management; process and outcomes evaluation; and routine feedback to providers and clients. Disease management has been shown to result in better client health outcomes for several chronic health problems, but its effects on the cost of care are not yet clear. For example, disease management in the Kaiser Permanente health system decreased the number of visits to physicians but increased visits to other health care providers (e.g., dieticians), and overall costs for care increased. There was some suggestion, however, that the costs of care would have increased even more without disease management (Fireman, Bartlett, & Selby, 2004).

Disease management has been shown to be particularly effective in the control of diabetes. Diabetes management may be undertaken by primary health care providers or through specialized diabetes management programs. Services provided are comprehensive and should address the *National Performance Measures for Diabetes Mellitus Care*. Elements of diabetes case management addressed in the standards include periodic HbA_{1c} evaluation, lipid management, urine protein testing, annual dilated ophthalmologic examination, foot examination, blood pressure management, influenza immunization, and periodic provider visits to monitor health status (Akinci, Coyne, Healy, & Minear, 2004). Additional aspects of effective diabetes management include medical nutrition therapy, promotion of exercise, medication management (Lewis, 2004), and attention to psychosocial issues posed by the disease and its treatment (e.g., financing of care, changes in self-image). Similar disease management programs have been developed for other chronic diseases such as asthma, cardiovascular disease, and COPD.

Bodenheimer and associates (2002a) have identified a chronic care model that can be used to guide the care of clients with chronic physical health problems. The model envisions care that occurs in three overlapping areas: the provider organization, the health care system, and the community. Six elements comprise the model and make possible effective care of persons with chronic illnesses: community resources and policies, health care organization and structure, support for self-management, delivery system design, provider decision support, and clinical information systems.

Effective chronic illness care requires community resources and policies that link clients to needed services (e.g., exercise programs, self-help groups). Health care systems must view chronic care as a priority and must be designed to reward quality care if optimal control of chronic health problems is to be achieved. In chronic illness, clients provide the bulk of their own care, but systems of care must provide support for effective self-management, which will be discussed in more detail later in this chapter. The delivery system design element of the model refers to the need for care by practice teams that incorporate multiple disciplines in the care of clients with chronic illnesses. Decision support for providers is reflected in the use of clinical practice guidelines that are evidence-based. Finally, computerized information systems or decision support systems permit population-level surveillance regarding the incidence and prevalence of disease in the community as well as generating clinical practice reminders for providers and providing feedback on the effectiveness of care (Bodenheimer et al., 2002a). Several studies of the use of selected elements of the chronic care model with clients with diabetes have indicated the model's utility. Similar findings have been noted for its use in congestive heart failure and asthma (Bodenheimer, Wagner, & Grumbach, 2002b).

Decision support systems employ a public health perspective to manage chronic illness. Decision support systems are characterized by

- the use of a chronic care model as an organizing framework for disease management
- daily data input from laboratories and other data sources
- automated test interpretation based on consensus guidelines to guide treatment decisions
- use of communication mechanisms to report indicator findings to providers and clients
- report formats that are helpful to providers and clients alike (MacLean, Littenberg, & Gagnon, 2006)

Community health nurses can use the model to help design effective care systems for populations with selected chronic illnesses. They may also need to advocate for the availability of needed community resources and effective interdisciplinary care for chronic illness.

Stabilizing the Client's Condition   Community health nurses may need to provide emergency care to stabilize clients who are experiencing some chronic conditions. For example, a client having a heart attack may need cardiopulmonary resuscitation (CPR); emergency care is also required for the client in a diabetic coma. Community health nurses may actually provide emergency care in situations of this type or may educate clients and the public in emergency care procedures. Once the client has been stabilized, the nurse would refer the client to an appropriate source of medical care.

Establishing a Treatment Regimen   The medical treatment regimen for a chronic health problem may involve medication, radiation, chemotherapy, surgery, or other types of therapy. Although nurse practitioners may be involved in providing some of these forms of care, most community health nurses are not. They are, however, involved in preparing clients for treatments both physically and psychologically, and they provide supportive measures as needed during therapy. For example, the nurse may administer intravenous pain medication to clients in the terminal stages of cancer or help clients deal with the side effects of radiation or chemotherapy.

Nurses also educate clients about their treatment and motivate them to engage in self-care. For example, community health nurses can educate clients with hypertension about antihypertensive medications and their effects and side effects as well as about diet, weight loss, and the need for continued medical supervision.

At the community level, community health nurses may be politically involved in efforts to assure the presence and accessibility of prompt treatment for chronic conditions. They may also be involved in planning health care programs for the treatment of a variety of chronic health problems, using the principles of health program planning discussed in Chapter 15∞.

Motivating Compliance   Many persons with chronic conditions are noncompliant in following prescribed recommendations. Reasons for noncompliance include inability to understand recommendations, inconvenience of required actions, disruption of lifestyle, financial or situational constraints, and lack of belief in the severity of the problem or the efficacy of treatment.

Monitoring client compliance with therapy for chronic conditions is an important community health nursing function. Identifying and eliminating factors in a client situation that promote noncompliance may foster compliance instead. Clients may be physically or mentally unable to comply with recommendations. Clients who cannot remove the childproof cap or cannot remember to take their medication will not be compliant because of sheer inability. These are some of the considerations the nurse must make when planning to enhance client compliance with the recommended treatment plan. This is also further reason for incorporating the client and/or family members in the design of the treatment plan.

Other clients may be noncompliant because treatment requires too great an alteration in lifestyle. In this case the nurse can plan adjustments in the treatment plan to more closely fit the client's lifestyle. For example, the nurse can assist the client who has diabetes to incorporate culturally preferred foods into a diabetic diet. Research has indicated that clients themselves modify treatment regimens to better fit their lives (Koch, Jenkin, & Kralik, 2004). To do so safely and effectively, they need knowledge about areas that can reasonably be modified and areas where modifications are hazardous. People with chronic diseases may also tend to rely on medication for disease control, ignoring recommendations for behavior change intended to accompany medication use. Clients may also alter medication regimens without consulting their health care providers or be quite irregular in their use of medications.

Situational constraints can also lead to noncompliance. Clients who cannot afford to purchase their medication will not take it. Lack of running water may make warm soaks difficult for the arthritic client. The effort of bringing water from a well and heating it on the stove may be more detrimental to inflamed joints than doing nothing. The nurse plans measures to eliminate situational barriers to clients' compliance with treatment plans. For example, the nurse may plan a referral to assist a client to obtain Medicaid coverage to help pay for medical expenses, or help the client plan for other ways to provide moist heat to arthritic joints.

Noncompliance may also result when the client has a vested interest in being ill. The rare client who uses illness to get attention or qualify for disability benefits is unlikely to comply fully with a treatment program. In such cases, community health nurses must identify the goal of the client's noncompliance. They may then be able to help the client plan other means of achieving that goal and motivate greater compliance.

Finally, lack of motivation can contribute to noncompliance. Clients may lack motivation owing to a poor self-concept or because of discouragement. The nurse, family members, and friends can help improve the client's self-concept by encouraging independence, helping the client accomplish short-term goals, and positively reinforcing accomplishments. Discouragement can be abated through realistic goal setting and achievement of short-term goals. Emotional support by the nurse, provided through opportunities for the client to express feelings of fear and frustration, as well as positive reinforcement of accomplishments can help to alleviate discouragement and foster compliance. Another way to deal with this type of noncompliance is referral to an appropriate self-help group.

Promoting Self-Management **Self-management** of chronic health problems involves handling the day-to-day treatment of the disease and its effects. Two approaches to self-management are found in the health care literature. The first approach focuses on the ability of the individual client to control his or her own behavior relative to care of the disease. The second approach, called an ecological approach, considers both the skills and choices of the individual and the availability of resources and supports that promote effective self-care (Fisher et al., 2005). The classical example of individual client self-management is the alteration of insulin dosage based on blood glucose levels, presence of illness, and so on. Clients with diabetes also engage in self-management when they increase caloric intake to cover periods of intense physical activity. Clients with other chronic conditions may also engage in self-management. For example, clients with cardiovascular disease and COPD may regulate periods of rest and physical activity on the basis of symptoms of fatigue or overexertion. Similarly, clients and/or family members may regulate use of pain medication based on need in cases of terminal illness due to cancer. Clients with arthritis or other conditions causing chronic pain may also engage in self-management of pain relief.

Qualitative research has identified three models of self-management of chronic illness (Koch et al., 2004). In the medical model of self-management, the focus is on client willingness and ability to carry out a provider-prescribed treatment regimen. This model is fostered by education to promote compliance on the part of the client. The collaborative model focuses on joint decision making for disease management by provider and client. Some studies, however, have indicated that even when providers intend to foster collaborative decision making, they exert pressure on clients to conform to their perspective of disease management and have failed to provide the resources necessary to permit clients to make informed decisions about their own care. Providers were also seen to discount the experiential knowledge of clients with chronic illnesses (Paterson, 2001a). In the third model of self-management, the self-agency model, clients made independent decisions regarding ways to deal with their chronic illness, relying on their own expertise after living with chronic illness for some time (Koch et al., 2004). Community health nurses can foster a true collaborative model of self-management tempered with the client's life experience and knowledge of his or her own condition. They can advocate for client involvement in decision making and provide clients with the information on which to base self-care decisions.

Self-management has been shown to be effective in dealing with diabetes and has significant potential in other chronic illnesses as well. The ecological approach to self-management of chronic disease includes six key elements: individualized assessment, collaborative goal setting, skill development, follow-up and support services, continuity of care, and access to resources (Fisher et al., 2005). Individualized assessment incorporates the client's personal perspective of the disease and its treatment as well as cultural influences and implications. Assessment may be supported by computer-based applications that tailor interventions to a specific client's situation and characteristics.

Self-management from an ecological perspective requires collaborative goal setting by client and provider. Self-management interventions that stress individual choices and responsibilities and that fit the client's personal goals are more effective than goals developed by the provider and imposed on the client. Effective self-management also requires knowledge and confidence on the part of clients that they can deal with most of their care themselves. This necessitates enhancement of clients' knowledge and skills. Clients need to know what needs to be done to manage their condition and how to do it. For example, clients with diabetes need to learn how to modify insulin dosages based on glucose levels and to conduct an examination of their feet. Clients also need to be able to determine when self-care is not appropriate and professional care is needed. Community health nurses can educate clients regarding self-management of disease and determination of the need for professional care. Nurses may also need to motivate clients to engage in self-management as appropriate.

Chronic disease self-management often requires changes in lifestyle and health-related behaviors. For this reason, another aspect of the ecological approach to self-management is the provision of follow-up and support for the changes made. Clients also need continuing assistance in refining their management skills. Support may be provided by health professionals via Internet or telephone interactions or by nonprofessional lay health workers as well as during visits to health care providers.

Self-management of chronic diseases also requires access to resources needed for daily life with a chronic illness. For example, people need to be able to access healthy foods or opportunities for physical activity. Community health nurses can help clients identify the resources available to them and can advocate for access to such resources for all segments of the population.

The final element of ecological self-management for chronic diseases is continuity of quality professional care (Fisher et al., 2005). For example, care of clients with diabetes should be based on consensus guidelines to include eye examinations and other follow-up measures to determine treatment effectiveness. Similarly, care for arthritis should include effective pain management as well as promotion of physical activity.

Monitoring Treatment Effects The nurse involved in secondary prevention for chronic health problems also monitors clients for the presence of side effects related to treatment. For example, the nurse may note that a client is experiencing postural hypotension due to antihypertensive medications and will then educate the client about the need to change position gradually and will

continue to monitor blood pressure levels to be sure that they do not drop too low.

At the same time, the nurse monitors the therapeutic effects of treatment. For instance, the nurse may obtain periodic blood pressure measurements for the client with hypertension. If the nurse determines that antihypertensive therapy has not noticeably affected the client's blood pressure, the nurse would make sure that the client is taking the medication appropriately and refer the client to his or her primary provider for further follow-up.

The goal of monitoring the therapeutic effectiveness of interventions may also require community health nurses to advocate for routine treatment-monitoring services. For example, although effective diabetes management includes annual dilated eye examinations, foot examinations, and glycosylated hemoglobin (HbA1c) determinations, clients with diabetes may not receive these services. In fact, between 2002 and 2004 only 43% of adult diabetics received these services. Those without insurance were even less likely to receive services (25%) (Mukhtar, Pan, Jack, & Murphy, 2005). Goals for secondary prevention of chronic physical health problems and related community health nursing interventions are summarized in Table 29-8.◆

Tertiary Prevention

The aim of tertiary prevention is to promote the client's optimal level of function despite the presence of a chronic health problem. This entails preventing further loss of function in affected and unaffected systems, restoring function, monitoring health status, assisting the client to adjust to the presence of a chronic condition, and providing end-of-life care as needed.

PREVENTING LOSS OF FUNCTION IN AFFECTED SYSTEMS
Chronic health problems frequently result in some loss of function in organ systems affected by the condition, and tertiary prevention activities should be planned to prevent further loss of function in these systems. Activities may be planned to minimize losses or to eliminate risk factors that might lead to adverse consequences of the condition. Such activities on the part of the community health nurse might include motivating client compliance with treatment recommendations and assisting clients to identify and change risk factors that may lead to further loss of function. For example, the client who has had a myocardial infarction may be assisted to plan a regimen of diet and exercise that will prevent future infarcts. In 2001, however, only 29.5% of all those in 29 U.S. states who survived a myocardial infarction received cardiac rehabilitation services (Ayala et al., 2003). Community health nurses can advocate for the development of and access to such services for those in need of them. In addition, nurses can promote clients' active participation in rehabilitation activities for myocardial infarction as well as for stroke, COPD, and other chronic health problems.

TABLE 29-8 Goals for Secondary Prevention and Related Community Health Nursing Interventions in the Control of Chronic Physical Health Problems

Secondary Prevention Goal	Nursing Interventions

1. Screening
  a. Perform periodic health examinations.
 	
  b. Periodically screen for chronic disease.
	1. Screen for existing chronic diseases.
	  a. Educate public about need for health examinations. Provide periodic examinations.
	  b. Educate public about need for periodic screening. Plan and implement screening programs for high-risk groups.

2. Early diagnosis	2. Educate public about warning signs and symptoms of chronic disease.
	  a. Engage in case finding and refer for diagnosis as appropriate.
	  b. Prepare client for diagnostic procedures (physically and emotionally).
	  c. Conduct diagnostic tests as appropriate.

3. Prompt treatment
  a. Stabilize condition as soon as possible.
 	
  b. Establish treatment regimen.
    ▪ Medication
    ▪ Radiation
    ▪ Chemotherapy
    ▪ Surgery
  c. Promote self-management.
  d. Prevent disease progression.
	3. Assist with management of chronic disease.
	  a. Provide emergency care as needed.
	    ▪ Educate public to provide emergency care (CPR).
	    ▪ Refer for further treatment.
	  b. Prepare client for treatment procedures (physically and emotionally).
	    ▪ Carry out treatment regimen.
	    ▪ Provide supportive measures during treatment (relief of pain).
	    ▪ Educate clients about medications: dosage, side effects, etc.
	    ▪ Encourage client compliance with treatment.
	  c. Educate and motivate clients for self-management.
	  d. Monitor therapeutic effects of treatment.
	    ▪ Monitor side effects.
	    ▪ Refer for follow-up as needed.

Clients with arthritis may be assisted to identify safety factors in the home that might contribute to falls, leading to further mobility limitation. Other interventions aimed at preventing further loss of function in people with arthritis include weight and physical activity counseling and education to address pain management and other problems leading to disability. Unfortunately, in 2003, only 37% of overweight or obese clients with arthritis received weight counseling. Similarly, only 55% of those with arthritis were counseled by health care providers regarding physical activity, and only 10% had participated in an arthritis education program, far short of the *Healthy People 2010◆* targets for these three interventions (Hootman et al., 2005). Community health nurses can provide counseling and education in these areas or refer clients for these services. Community health nurses may also advocate for access to these services by promoting coverage under health insurance plans or fostering the development of such services for the uninsured.

Pain management may be another intervention that helps to limit loss of function in both affected and unaffected body systems. Pain management will be discussed in more detail in the section on promoting adjustment to chronic health problems.

PREVENTING LOSS OF FUNCTION IN UNAFFECTED SYSTEMS

Chronic health problems may also result in loss of function in other physical and nonphysical systems not directly affected by the condition. For example, the client with arthritis may develop skin lesions due to limited mobility, or the client with COPD may become malnourished because meal preparation is too exhausting.

Nursing interventions will be directed toward preventing both physical and social disability. Physical complications of chronic conditions may be prevented by activities such as teaching breathing exercises to clients with COPD and providing good skin care and teaching foot care for clients with diabetes. Clients may also need help in managing fatigue, a frequent effect of chronic health problems, particularly COPD and asthma. Prevention of additional physical effects may also entail immunization. Clients with diabetes and COPD, for example, are in particular need of influenza and pneumonia immunizations. Other measures to prevent loss of function in people with diabetes include tight glycemic control, control of hypertension, and lipid management (Ullom-Minnich, 2004). Community health nurses will be actively involved in educating clients with diabetes regarding strategies to control hyperglycemia (e.g., medication use, diet, exercise, glucose monitoring) and prevention of hypoglycemic reactions. They will also assist in monitoring clients' blood pressure and referring them for treatment if needed. In addition, they will educate clients regarding dietary fat intake and treatment measures for hyperlipidemia if prescribed. Community health nurses also educate clients with diabetes regarding skin and foot care and appropriate footwear. Another new measure for preventing amputations involves twice-daily measurement of temperatures on the soles of the feet to identify changes suggestive of infection (Lavery et al., 2004), and community health nurses may educate clients on the use of this and similar technologies. Low-income populations, however, particularly those without insurance, may not be able to afford such technological innovations, so community health nursing advocacy may be required to assure the availability of these and other services to all segments of the population. Community health nurses can also refer clients to sources of services to prevent deterioration in other body systems.

Nurses can also help prevent social disability by encouraging clients to interact with others, assisting clients to maintain their independence as much as possible, assisting with necessary role changes within the family, and referring the client to appropriate self-help groups. At the group level, community health nurses can work to prevent social isolation of those with chronic illnesses by advocacy and political activities to assure access to services. They can also work to educate the public and to develop positive attitudes to persons with chronic or disabling conditions.

RESTORING FUNCTION The restoration aspect of tertiary prevention focuses on regaining as much lost function as is possible given the client's situation. Specific rehabilitation services are needed to offset the consequences of many chronic health conditions, including accidental injury, stroke, and myocardial infarction. Unfortunately, many clients in need of rehabilitation services do not receive them. For example, only about 20% of people with cardiovascular disease begin and maintain a cardiac rehabilitation program. In addition, research indicates that traditional rehabilitation programs often do not address clients' perceived needs. For instance, participants in one study were more interested in stress management than behavior modification in cardiac rehabilitation (Pâquet, Bolduc, Xhignesse, & Vanasse, 2005). Community health nurses can refer clients to rehabilitation programs or advocate for their accessibility to those in need. They can also help design programs that meet the perceived needs of the client population.

Particular areas to be addressed in rehabilitation programs include functional status related to activities such as positioning, range of motion, transfer abilities, dressing, bowel and bladder control, hygiene, locomotion, and eating. Other functional considerations include vision, hearing, speech, mental ability, and capacity for social interaction. The nurse, together with the client and his or her significant others, can foster renewed abilities to perform these functions. For example, the nurse may develop a plan and teach the client and family how to reestablish bowel control following a stroke, or the nurse might assist the client with passive and active range-of-motion exercises to restore function after a broken arm has healed. Other considerations include teaching stress management, dealing with the limitations imposed by a chronic condition, and addressing the financial burden of disease that may limit clients' abilities to regain function.

Restoring function for clients with COPD may involve teaching specific breathing techniques and promoting adequate nutrition. Community health nurses may make use of specific teaching aids for clients with COPD available from the Cleveland Clinic Health Information Center Web site at http://www.clevelandclinic.org.

Other interventions may necessitate referral to other health care providers. For example, clients may need physical therapy to regain lost function after a stroke. Clients may also need rehabilitation services following myocardial infarction or to minimize the effects of arthritis or stroke. Community health nurses may assist individual clients to obtain these services or advocate for their availability and accessibility in the community.

MONITORING HEALTH STATUS Another aspect of tertiary prevention in the control of chronic health problems is monitoring clients' health status. The nurse would be actively involved in periodic reassessment, being particularly alert to changes in circumstances that may affect health. For example, the nurse may note that termination of unemployment benefits will limit the client's capacity to pay for health care. In this case, a referral might be made for additional financial assistance.

The nurse monitors the client's overall health status as well as the status of the chronic condition. When warranted, the nurse refers the client for medical follow-up. For example, the nurse may note that a client disabled by a serious accident is developing pressure sores due to long periods in a wheelchair. In this case, the nurse would suggest interventions to heal the pressure sores and prevent their recurrence or refer the client for medical assistance for severe lesions. Periodic follow-up of clients with chronic diseases may also promote self-management. For example, clients in Hong Kong with diabetes who received biweekly telephone calls from nurses after early hospital discharge had a greater decrease in HbA1c, engaged in more exercise, and checked their blood pressure more often than those who received continuing care in the hospital. Net savings of HK$11,888 per patient were noted using telephone follow-up due to the shorter hospital stay (Wong, Mok, Chan, & Tsang, 2005).

PROMOTING ADJUSTMENT Clients may display one of two perspectives in their adjustment to the presence of a chronic physical health condition or may shift between them at different points in the disease experience (Paterson, 2001b). In the "illness in the foreground" perspective, the client focuses on the illness and the attendant loss, suffering, and burden that accompany the illness. This perspective may be beneficial when it assists the client to conserve energy and other resources, but is self-absorbing and may interfere with interpersonal interactions. The "wellness in the foreground" perspective permits the client to focus on the positive aspects of life and state of health, but may lead to ignoring symptoms of deterioration and the need to seek professional care. Areas for special consideration in promoting adjustment to chronic health problems include functional and psychological adjustment, pain management, and survivorship care.

Functional Adjustment   Adjustments to the presence of a chronic disease occur in both functional and psychological realms. Functional adjustments reflect changes in lifestyle necessitated by the illness. Such changes may involve diet, activity patterns, restrictions (e.g., limiting alcohol use or caloric intake), and the need to take medications. Some diseases necessitate learning special skills. For example, insulin-dependent diabetic clients need to learn to give themselves insulin injections, and hypertensive clients may need to learn how to take their blood pressure. In other chronic conditions, such as arthritis, there may be a need for special apparatus to assist in performing routine activities. The need for medication may also necessitate budgetary changes that the client must adjust to.

Adjustment in the work setting is a special consideration for many people with chronic conditions. Failure to provide workplace accommodations for people with chronic health conditions limits their ability to participate in the workforce and minimizes societal productivity (Wang, Bradley, & Gignac, 2004). Promoting adjustment in the work setting usually combines a variety of approaches. First, community health nurses in occupational settings can enhance the employee's personal ability to cope with illness. This might be accomplished through education regarding medication management or self-monitoring skills or other interventions. Second, the nurse can advocate for the support of management or colleagues for self-care activities (e.g., scheduling flexible breaks or meals) and advocate for working conditions that accommodate any limitations or special needs (e.g., redesign of work stations to prevent exacerbation of carpal tunnel syndrome, assuring wheelchair access to all areas of the work setting). Third, nurses can connect employees to support groups and services outside the work setting, and finally, the nurse can assure adequate access to care and advocate for insurance benefits to cover the costs of care (Sitzman, 2004). Case management is also an effective approach to keeping employees with chronic health problems on the job. Disease management programs such as those discussed earlier may also be helpful for groups of employees with similar conditions (Kalina, Haag, & Tourigian, 2004).

Psychological Adjustment   Psychological adjustments are also necessary. Psychological adjustment to a chronic condition may be required in a number of areas. Self-esteem is one of these areas. A chronic disease may make a client more dependent on others and less able to engage in activities that promote a positive self-image. For example, the client may need to stop working or begin to rely on others for assistance with basic functions such as eating and toileting. This dependence may

be demeaning to one who has been self-reliant. The nurse should encourage the client to maintain as many functions as possible and help families to see the client's need for independence.

Loss of independence also necessitates adjustments in one's sense of control. Clients may feel they are not in control of events when the food they eat or the activities they perform are dictated in part by the chronic health problem. For some clients, noncompliance with recommendations might be an attempt to regain control over their own lives. Nurses can help prevent noncompliance by providing the client with other avenues for exercising control. Ways of doing this include involving the client in planning interventions and providing, whenever possible, choices in which the client can exercise control over actions and outcomes. Community health nurses may also help clients obtain assistive technology devices (e.g., braces, chairlifts, railings, shower seat, grab bars), which have been shown to decrease dependence on assistance from other people (Hoenig, Taylor, & Sloan, 2003).

Guilt may also require adjustments in the way clients think about themselves. Because behavioral factors are widely known to make a significant contribution to the majority of chronic conditions, clients may feel guilty about behaviors that may have contributed to their current health problems. The nurse can help clients explore their feelings and assist them to turn from an irredeemable past to present behaviors that minimize the effects of health problems.

Another area that may require adjustment for clients with chronic conditions is that of intimacy. Among men, for example, some chronic conditions or their treatments may result in impotence. In other cases, pain or changes in self-image may limit a client's ability to maintain intimate relationships with others. Another potential problem may be the withdrawal of significant others. Clients and their families can be encouraged to discuss intimacy issues openly, and significant others can be assisted to find ways of fulfilling intimacy needs that are congruent with the presence of a chronic health problem.

Stigma is another psychological issue in adjustment to a chronic health problem. Many chronic health conditions are stigmatized by the general population. **Stigmatization** is a social process of attaching meaning to behavior and individuals on the basis of certain traits or characteristics. Stigmatization tends to occur in response to three types of attributes: physical deformities, character blemishes, and tribal stigma based on race or religion (Joachim & Acorn, 2000). Some chronic health conditions create visible physical evidence, such as the malformed joints often seen in arthritis or the need to use a wheelchair or other assistive devices. The presence of other conditions, such as seizure disorder or mental retardation, may be perceived as evidence of inferiority.

Clients with visible evidence of disease may attempt to deal with stigma by minimizing the perceived consequences of the disease or covering them up as much as possible while still acknowledging their existence. Those whose condition is invisible are faced with decisions of whether to disclose their chronic illness, how much to disclose, and to whom. Clients who fear rejection on the basis of stigma attached to the disease may attempt to pass themselves off as healthy, but then endure the stress of possible discovery and loss of credibility as well as rejection (Joachim & Acorn, 2000). Community health nurses can assist clients to deal with perceptions of stigma and to make decisions regarding disclosure. For clients suffering from the psychological effects of stigmatization, referrals for counseling services may be warranted. Nurses may also engage in public education campaigns to diminish the stigma attached to certain chronic conditions.

In caring for clients who have chronic illnesses, the nurse must plan to assist them to return to a normal level of functioning as far as this is possible. When return to a former level of function is not possible, nurses can help clients cope with their disappointment. For example, discharge from physiotherapy following a stroke has been viewed by some clients as distressful and provoking feelings of abandonment, particularly when they have not achieved their expected level of recovery (Wiles, Ashburn, Payne, & Murphy, 2004). Continued follow-up by community health nurses may help to alleviate the sense of abandonment and accompanying depression. In addition to the assistance of the nurse, it may be appropriate to refer the client to a relevant self-help group. Self-help groups can be particularly helpful in dealing with the psychosocial adjustments required by a chronic condition. Clients may be able to relate better to persons experiencing similar problems than to the authority figures represented by health care professionals.

Referral to self-help groups and other assistance may also be needed for family members who experience caregiver burden. **Caregiver burden** is the effect of the stress of caring for a family member with a physical or mental illness on those providing the care (Plese, 2005a). Caregiver burden can stem from the extent of care required or from behaviors exhibited by the family member receiving care. For example, caregiver burden may be increased when the person to whom care is given exhibits behavioral disturbances.

Community health nurses can refer clients and caregivers to self-help groups or other community agencies that provide assistance in dealing with problems arising from chronic health conditions. Community health nurses should determine the availability of such agencies within their own communities and identify the services provided and eligibility requirements for each type of service in order to make appropriate referrals. When self-help groups are not available in the local area, community health nurses may be involved in their development. Nurses may also advocate for the provision of

services to promote functional and psychological adjustment to chronic health problems. For example, they may advocate for funding for homemaker assistance to permit people with disabilities resulting from chronic health problems to remain in their homes. Or they may advocate for insurance coverage for psychological counseling for clients with chronic physical health problems.

Pain Management Pain management is an important component of tertiary prevention of chronic physical health problems. Studies indicated that 43% of U.S. households (44 million families) include at least one person who is experiencing chronic pain. In approximately one third of chronic pain sufferers, their pain is severe enough to impair functional ability and significantly diminish their quality of life (Partners Against Pain, 2005).

Effective pain management is important not only for improving the quality of life of individual clients, but also for decreasing the economic costs of chronic health problems for society in general. Annual U.S. health care and lost productivity costs resulting from chronic pain amount to more than $100 billion (Partners Against Pain, 2005). Chronic pain has been found to contribute to greater total costs than treatment for heart disease, hypertension, and diabetes. In one study, for example, 20% of people surveyed reported significant chronic pain, and 21% of them made ER visits for uncontrolled pain. Effective pain control, on the other hand, has been found to decrease unscheduled hospital admissions by as much as 80% for some conditions (Partners Against Pain, n.d.). Chronic pain may also lead to difficulty carrying out occupational responsibilities and consequent job loss and financial hardship for the persons affected and their families (Partners Against Pain, 2005).

Goals of pain management in chronic illness include preventing pain whenever possible, reducing the severity or frequency of pain, improving physical function, reducing psychological distress, and improving the overall quality of life (McCarberg, 2004). Health care providers often prescribe pharmacologic agents for pain management, but community health nurses may be able to assist clients to find other means of dealing with pain. For example, they can refer clients for acupuncture services, which have been shown to be effective in decreasing some types of chronic pain. Similarly, the use of guided imagery and progressive muscle relaxation has been linked to decreased pain and increased mobility in clients with arthritis (Baird & Sands, 2004). Community health nurses can refer clients for these services or assist them to develop skills in this area themselves. Community health nurses may also advocate for reimbursement for nonpharmacological pain management strategies under insurance coverage.

In 1999, the Joint Commission on Accreditation of Healthcare Organizations (JCAHO) developed standards for assessing pain management in hospital and home care settings. These standards can also be used to guide pain management by community health nurses working with clients with pain due to chronic health problems. The standards address recognition of clients' rights to effective pain management, the need for accurate pain assessment, safe medication practices and procedures, promotion of competence in pain management among health care providers, monitoring and reassessment of clients' pain status, client education regarding pain management, and the need to plan for pain management in discharge planning. The standards also address the need to collect information to monitor the effectiveness of pain management programs at the aggregate level as well as for individual clients (Partners Against Pain, n.d.).

Unfortunately, most clients with chronic pain report inadequate pain management. In one survey, for example, 58% of those responding indicated that their over-the-counter pain medication was not very effective, and 42% indicated that prescription pain medication was ineffective in addressing their pain (Partners Against Pain, 2005).

Six types of barriers to effective pain management have been identified, including barriers related to the health care system, documentation, health care professionals, laws and regulations, societal barriers, and clients and their families. Health system barriers include lack of clear policies and guidelines on pain management; lack of coordination across care settings, with pain management "falling through the cracks"; cost concerns related to aggressive pain management; and inconsistent reimbursement for pain management services and specific strategies. Documentation barriers include lack of accurate documentation of levels of pain, actions taken, and their effectiveness. Barriers related to health care providers include perceptions that clients are not appropriate judges of their level of pain, lack of knowledge regarding effective pain control strategies, failure to accurately assess clients' levels of pain, lack of clear accountability for pain management, and concerns about addiction, respiratory depression, and other medication side effects (Partners Against Pain, n.d.).

Barriers to effective pain management arising from laws and regulations include requirements for prescription of controlled substances, dosage limitations, lack of legislative knowledge about effective pain control, and concerns about misuse of controlled substances. Societal barriers reflect concerns for addiction and misuse of pain medications, lack of knowledge about the adverse effects of pain, and, in some religious and cultural groups, beliefs that pain is to be endured. Finally, clients and their families may pose barriers to effective pain management, such as desires to save "strong" medications for more severe pain, side effects (e.g., drowsiness, diminished alertness, difficulty concentrating), fears of addiction, lack of knowledge regarding pain control, and financial constraints (Partners Against Pain, n.d.).

Community health nurses can work to educate health policy makers, providers, legislators, clients and their families, and the general public regarding the need for effective pain control and appropriate pain management strategies. They can also advocate for changes in laws or insurance coverage to promote effective pain management. In addition, community health nurses can assess the pain management needs of individual clients with chronic illnesses. A number of good pain assessment tools are available. One such tool, the Patient Comfort Assessment Guide (Narcessian, n.d.), is available on the Partners Against Pain Web site at http://www.partnersagainstpain.com/printouts/pcag.pdf. The tool addresses the character, frequency, and intensity of pain; contributing factors; and the effectiveness of various interventions as well as the effects of the pain on the client's quality of life and ability to function. Community health nurses using pain assessment tools should make sure that they are culturally appropriate to the client being assessed and address facets of pain management relevant to holistic care of the client. For example, the effects of economic constraints on pain control should be assessed, as should cultural beliefs regarding pain and pain control.

Survivorship Care   As we noted earlier, many people with cancer are surviving for extended periods of time after diagnosis and treatment. An estimated 65% of people with cancer are expected to live at least 5 years after diagnosis (CDC, 2006a). The vast majority of cancer survivors will need some level of continuing care for the rest of their lives because of their increased risk for recurrent cancers. Survivors may also need assistance in dealing with the psychosocial effects of their diagnosis. The concept of survivorship care was developed to address these ongoing needs. Although the concept was developed in relation to cancer survivors, elements of survivorship care are relevant to other health conditions that threaten life and have long-term consequences for survivors (e.g., HIV/AIDS and severe traumatic injuries).

Survivorship care encompasses care provided not only to clients who survive life-threatening conditions, but also to families, friends, and caregivers who are affected by the condition (CDC, 2006a). Life for all of these people is irrevocably changed. Survivors and those around them who are affected by their condition are subjected to physical, emotional, social, spiritual, and financial issues that require long-term care. Additional needs may include dealing with pain or side effects of treatment, many of which may occur well after treatment is completed. Psychological issues of anxiety and depression may also need to be addressed. Cancer survivors may also have special nutritional needs (e.g., clients who have had a gastric resection for stomach cancer) (National Coalition for Cancer Survivorship, n.d.) or increased susceptibility to infection. Survivors also need information about health promotion activities such as exercise and weight control. For example, obesity has been linked to worse survival outcomes for women with breast cancer and possibly for men with prostate cancer (CDC, 2006a). Survivors also require ongoing surveillance and periodic screening for recurrent cancer, although the type and frequency of screening recommendations will vary with the type of cancer involved.

A 2006 report by the Institute of Medicine entitled *From Cancer Patient to Cancer Survivor: Lost in Transition* (Hewitt, Greenfield, & Stovall, 2006) noted that more than 10 million people in the United States have a prior history of cancer and are considered cancer survivors. The report further noted that the health care system is not equipped to adequately address their needs. The report included recommendations for four essential components of survivorship care:

- Prevention of recurrent and new cancers and late treatment effects
- Surveillance for recurrent or new cancer and medical or psychological effects of the cancer and its treatment
- Interventions to address the consequences of disease and treatment
- Coordination of care between oncology specialists and primary care providers to assure that all the health needs of survivors are met

Survivorship care should be grounded in a *survivorship care plan* that includes information about the cancer diagnosis, treatment received, and possible consequences; recommended follow-up interventions (e.g., screening for cancer recurrence, reconstructive surgeries, dietary recommendations); recommendations for health promotion; information on legal protections related to employment and health insurance; and referral for psychosocial services (e.g., financial assistance, job training) as needed (Hewitt et al., 2006).

Community health nurses can be instrumental in developing cancer survivorship plans for clients or for assuring that assistance in developing such plans is available. They may also need to advocate for insurance coverage for plan development services and services needed to implement the survivorship plan. There is also a need to develop clinical practice guidelines for survivorship care for specific types of cancer, and community health nurses can advocate for or conduct research in this area. Nurses may also need to engage in political advocacy to promote insurance reforms that prohibit denial of health insurance based on a past history of cancer and to include coverage of survivorship care as an integral part of cancer care. Recently, changes were made in the Medicaid program to provide coverage for cancer care for women with breast and cervical cancer, but these changes apply only to women diagnosed through CDC-supported programs (Hewitt et al., 2006). Community health nurses could be involved in

political advocacy to expand this coverage to all uninsured persons with cancer and to cover survivorship care as well as treatment. Similarly, legal provisions, such as those of the Women's Health and Cancer Rights Act that mandate insurance coverage of reconstructive surgery, prostheses, and care for complications of mastectomy, could be expanded to include aftercare for other forms of cancer (Hewitt et al., 2006).

Survivorship care may occur in a collaborative effort between primary care providers and specialists, through nursing case management, or in specialized survivorship clinics and programs. In addition, there is a need for population-level planning for surveillance of survivors and their needs, development of community resource guides, service needs assessments, provider education on survivorship care, provision of primary and secondary prevention services, and evaluation of the effectiveness of survivorship care at the population level (Hewitt et al., 2006). Community health nurses can be actively involved in developing or advocating for such population-based survivorship care systems. Policy changes may also be needed to address employment issues at the aggregate level. Nurses may also need to advocate for prohibition of employment discrimination for individual clients or refer clients for legal assistance with discrimination. Political advocacy may also be needed to assure funding for educational, counseling, and vocational rehabilitation services for survivors.

END-OF-LIFE CARE A few chronic physical health problems are terminal in nature, and community health nurses may be involved in providing care to clients who are facing death and to their families. Recent literature contends that nurses are often ill-prepared to provide end-of-life care and that certain core competencies are required for effective care of dying clients and their

EVIDENCE-BASED PRACTICE

The Division of Cancer Prevention and Control (2004) of the CDC has noted that advances in cancer therapy have resulted in many people with cancer having to live with what has now become a chronic disease rather than a fatal illness. A change in terminology has also been fostered so that people living with cancer are referred to as "survivors" rather than cancer "victims." **Cancer survivors** are defined as "all living persons who ever received a diagnosis of cancer" (Division of Cancer Prevention and Control, 2004, p. 526). Because of the recent change in perceptions about cancer, there is a need for research on the long-term effects of cancer for survivors. This body of literature is growing, but much remains to be learned. Select a fairly common cancer with a relatively high survival rate (e.g., prostate cancer or breast cancer) and examine the literature on its long-term effects on survivors. What conclusions can you draw, if any, as a foundation for evidence-based practice with this population? What gaps exist in the evidence? How might you design a study to fill one of these gaps?

TABLE 29-9 Goals for Tertiary Prevention and Related Community Health Nursing Interventions in the Control of Chronic Physical Health Problems

Tertiary Prevention Goal	Nursing Interventions
1. Prevent further loss of function in affected systems. Decrease risk factors for recurrence, exacerbation, or development of crises.	1. Motivate client to comply with treatment regimen. Assist client to identify risk factors amenable to change. Assist client to identify ways of decreasing risk factors.
2. Prevent loss of function in unaffected systems. a. Prevent physical disability. b. Prevent social disability.	2. Assist client to maintain function in unaffected systems. a. Prevent physical complications of illness through: • Breathing exercises • Skin care • Range-of-motion exercises and physical activity • Adequate nutrition and fluids Provide physical care as required. Refer for assistance with physical care as needed. b. Accept client as a unique person. Encourage interaction with others. Assist significant others to deal with feelings about client's illness. Assist client to maintain independence as much as possible. Assist with identification of need for changes in family roles. Work to change public attitudes toward the disabled. Promote legislation to aid chronically ill to maintain their independence.
3. Restore function.	3. Assist with planning and implementation of programs to regain function (bowel training, physical therapy). Teach client and others to carry out program and evaluate effects.
4. Monitor health status.	4. Monitor client health status. Identify changes in client situation that affect health. Refer for follow-up as appropriate.
5. Promote adjustment. a. Deal with feelings about disease. b. Adjust lifestyle to accommodate chronic disease and its effects. c. Adjust environment to meet changed needs. d. Adjust self-image. e. Adjust to expense of chronic care. f. Deal with stigma. g. Effectively manage pain. h. Meet survivorship care needs.	5. Assist client to adjust to presence of chronic disease. a. Accept client at his or her level of development and acceptance of disease. Encourage client to discuss fears and apprehensions. Refer to self-help groups as appropriate. b. Assist client to identify needed changes in lifestyle. Assist client to plan and carry out lifestyle changes. c. Identify need for self-help devices and help client obtain them. Identify environmental changes needed to foster independence. Assist client to make necessary environmental changes. d. Assist client to adjust to change in self-image. Refer for counseling as needed. e. Refer for financial aid as needed. f. Assist with decisions regarding disclosure. Assist client to cope with effects of stigma. Educate public to minimize stigma. g. Accurately assess client pain levels. Assist in identifying appropriate pharmacologic and nonpharmacologic approaches to pain control. Refer for pain management services, as needed. Educate clients, family, providers, and the public regarding effective pain control. Advocate for available and accessible pain management services and insurance coverage for services. Monitor the effectiveness of pain control strategies. h. Identify survivorship care needs and participate in developing a survivorship care plan. Refer clients and families for survivorship care services as needed. Advocate for insurance coverage of survivorship care planning and needed survivorship care. Conduct research to identify care needs and best practices in survivorship care.
6. Adjust to impending death.	6. Provide end-of-life care. a. Provide pain management. b. Provide comfort care. c. Provide palliative care. d. Encourage advance directives. e. Refer to hospice services as needed.

families (White, Coyne, & Patel, 2001). These competencies are summarized on page 892.

Palliative care is an important aspect of end-of-life care related to chronic health problems. Research has indicated that most clients want to die at home. This means that palliative care services should be made available in the home setting as well as in health care facilities. Some of the challenges identified by community health nurses involved in palliative care include

dealing with physical problems such as pain relief, shortness of breath, and fatigue. Other difficulties lie in dealing with the emotional reactions of family members (and clients), particularly anger; addressing issues of disclosure (or nondisclosure) of prognosis; and dealing with personal feelings in caring for the dying client. Provision of holistic care for clients and for their families is a hallmark of palliative end-of-life care, but many community health nurses find it difficult to talk with clients

SPECIAL CONSIDERATIONS

CORE COMPETENCIES FOR END-OF-LIFE CARE

- Ability to talk with clients and their families about dying
- Knowledge of effective pain control strategies
- Comfort care skills
- Palliative care skills
- Ability to recognize impending death
- Ability to deal with one's own feelings
- Ability to deal with anger expressed by clients and families
- Knowledge of legal and ethical issues in palliative care
- Knowledge of advance directives and their support
- Ability to incorporate religious and cultural beliefs and values
- Knowledge of hospice services

Data from: White, K. R., Coyne, P. J., & Patel, U. B. (2001). Are nurses adequately prepared for end-of-life care? Journal of Nursing Scholarship, 33, *147–151.*

and families about death (Dunne, Sullivan, & Kernohan, 2005).

Tertiary prevention related to individuals with chronic health problems focuses on assisting clients to adjust to their condition and on preventing additional problems. Tertiary prevention at the community level might involve planning and implementing programs to assist with client adjustment or political activity to ensure the availability of tertiary prevention programs. Tertiary prevention goals and related nursing interventions are summarized in Table 29-9◆.

Evaluating Control Strategies for Chronic Physical Health Problems

Evaluating control strategies for chronic health problems is done in terms of care outcomes. Care may be evaluated in relation to the individual client or to a population group. In the case of the individual client, the nurse evaluates the status of the chronic condition as well as the client's adjustment to having a chronic health

problem. If interventions, both medical and nursing, have been effective, the condition will be controlled or may even be improving. Failing improvement, the condition will provide the least disruption possible to the life of the client and his or her significant others. Evaluative criteria reflect both the client's physiologic status and his or her quality of life.

When the recipient of care is a community or population group, evidence of success in controlling chronic health problems lies primarily in changes in morbidity and mortality figures. Are there fewer cases of hypertension or cardiovascular disease in the population now than before the initiation of control efforts? Are there fewer disabilities due to accidental injuries? Do those individuals with diabetes live longer or have fewer hospitalizations for diabetic complications? Based on the evaluative data, decisions can be made regarding the need to attempt other control strategies or to continue with current measures.

Evaluation of population-based control strategies may focus on the status of national objectives for 2010 for selected chronic diseases◆. Baseline and target information and the current status of several of these objectives are presented below. As can be seen in the table, only one of the selected objectives has been met, and several are moving away from the target. These data suggest that considerable work is yet to be done in controlling chronic physical health problems in the United States.

Chronic physical health problems have largely replaced communicable diseases as the major contributors to death and disability in developed countries. Significant morbidity and mortality due to chronic physical conditions is also seen throughout the world. Community health nurses are actively involved in efforts to educate the public to prevent these diseases as well as in the design and implementation of programs to provide diagnostic, treatment, and support services for persons with existing disease.

HEALTHY PEOPLE 2010

Goals for Population Health

OBJECTIVE	BASELINE	MOST RECENT DATA	TARGET
2-2. Reduce the proportion of adults with chronic joint symptoms with limitation in activity	36%	NDA	30%
2-9. Reduce the overall number of cases of osteoporosis in adults	10%	NDA	8%
4-4. Reduce the rate of new cases of end-stage renal disease (per million population)	300	334	217#
4-7. Reduce kidney failure due to diabetes (per million population)	129	145	78#
5-2. Prevent diabetes (new cases per 1,000 population)	5.5	6.4	2.5#

Continued on next page

HEALTHY PEOPLE 2010 *continued*

5-5. Reduce the diabetes death rate (per 100,000 population)	77	78	45#
5-7. Reduce deaths from cardiovascular disease in persons with diabetes (per 100,000 persons with diabetes)	332	275	309*
6-4. Increase the proportion of adults with disabilities who participate in social activities	95.4%	60.5%	100%#
6-6. Increase the proportion of adults with disabilities reporting satisfaction with life	87%	80.5%	96%#
12-1. Reduce coronary heart disease deaths (per 100,000 population)	203	180	166
12-7. Reduce stroke deaths (per 100,000 population)	62	56	48
12-9. Reduce the proportion of adults with high blood pressure	28%	NDA	16%
12-10. Increase the proportion of adults with high blood pressure whose blood pressure is under control	18%	NDA	50%
12-14. Reduce the proportion of adults with high total blood cholesterol levels	21%	NDA	17%
19-1. Increase the proportion of adults who are at a healthy weight	42%	34%	60%#
22-1. Reduce the proportion of adults who engage in no leisure-time physical activity	40%	38%	20%
24-1. Reduce activity limitations among persons with asthma	20%	NDA	10%
24-9. Reduce the proportion of adults with activity limitations due to chronic lung and breathing problems	2.5%	2.5%	1.5%
27-1a. Reduce cigarette smoking by adults	24%	20%	12%
27-2b. Reduce cigarette smoking by adolescents	35%	22%	16%

NDA — No data available

* Objective has been met

 # Objective moving away from target

Data from: Centers for Disease Control and Prevention. (2005). Healthy people data. Retrieved September 5, 2005, from http://wonder.cdc.gov/data2010

Case Study

A Chronic Physical Health Problem

You have just started working as a community health nurse for the Wachita County Health Department in Mississippi. During your employment interview, the nursing supervisor mentioned that one of your responsibilities would be to participate in developing plans for dealing with the high rate of hypertension in the county. The incidence rate for hypertension here is three times that of the state and twice that of the nation. The population of the county is largely African American, with high unemployment rates and little health insurance. Folk health practices are quite common, one of them being drinking pickle brine for a condition called "high blood." Although this condition is not related to high blood pressure, the two terms are frequently confused by lay members of the community and professionals alike. Dietary intake is typical of the rural South, consisting of a variety of fried foods, beans and other boiled vegetables, and corn bread.

Few health services are available in the county itself, although there is a major hospital 50 miles away. There are two general practitioners in the area and one pediatrician. The health department holds well-child, immunization, tuberculosis, and family planning clinics regularly, and all are well attended. Transportation is a problem for many community residents.

1. What are the biophysical, psychological, physical environmental, sociocultural, behavioral, and health system factors influencing the incidence and prevalence of hypertension in this county?
2. Write two objectives for your efforts to resolve the county's problem with hypertension.
3. What primary, secondary, and tertiary prevention activities might be appropriate in dealing with the problem of hypertension? Which of these activities might you carry out yourself? Which would require collaboration with other community members? Who might these other people be?
4. How would you evaluate the outcome of your interventions?

Test Your Understanding

1. What are some of the personal/family effects and population effects of chronic physical health problems? (pp. 855–860)

2. What are some of the biophysical, psychological, physical environmental, sociocultural, behavioral, and health system factors that influence the development of chronic physical health problems? How do these factors differ among chronic diseases? (pp. 861–871)

3. What are the major strategies for primary prevention of chronic physical health problems? Give an example of an activity that a community health nurse might perform in relation to each. (pp. 873–878, 879)

4. Identify at least three aspects of secondary prevention for chronic physical health problems. What is the role of the community health nurse with respect to each? (pp. 878–884)

5. What are the major considerations in tertiary prevention of chronic physical health problems? How might a community health nurse be involved in each? (pp. 884–892)

EXPLORE MediaLink

http://www.prenhall.com/clark
Resources for this chapter can be found on the Companion Website.

Audio Glossary
Appendix J: Factors in the Epidemiology of
Selected Chronic Physical Health Problems
Exam Review Questions

Case Study: Health Promotion for the
Chronically Ill
MediaLink Application: Living with Crohn's
Disease (video)

Media Links
Challenge Your Knowledge
Update *Healthy People 2010*
Advocacy Interviews

References

Abraído-Lanza, A. F., Chao, M. T., & Gammon, M. D. (2004). Breast and cervical cancer screening among Latinas and non-Latina whites. *American Journal of Public Health, 94,* 1393–1398.

Akinci, F., Coyne, J., Healey, B., & Minear, J. (2004). National performance measures for diabetes mellitus care. *Disease Management Health Outcomes, 12,* 285–298.

American Diabetes Association. (2003a). *Diabetes statistics for seniors.* Retrieved April 27, 2004, from http://www.diabetes.org/diabetes-statistics.jsp

American Diabetes Association. (2003b). Economic costs of diabetes in the U.S. in 2002. *Diabetes Care, 26,* 917–932.

American Diabetes Association. (2003c). *National diabetes fact sheet.* Retrieved April 27, 2004, from http://www.diabetes.org/diabetes-statistics.jsp

Armour, B. S., Woolery, T., Malarcher, A., Pechacek, R. F., & Husten, C. (2005). Annual smoking-attributable mortality, years of potential life lost, and productivity losses — United States, 1997–2001. *Morbidity and Mortality Weekly Report, 54,* 625–628.

Ayala, C., Moreno, M. R., Minaya, J. A., Croft, J. B., Mensah, G. A., & Anderson, R. N. (2006). Hypertension-related mortality among Hispanic subpopulations — United States, 1995–2002. *Morbidity and Mortality Weekly Report, 55,* 177–180.

Ayala, C., Orenstein, D., Greenlund, K. J., Croft, J. B., Neff, L. J., & Mensah, G. A. (2003). Receipt of cardiac rehabilitation services among heart attack survivors — 19 states and the District of Columbia, 2001. *Morbidity and Mortality Weekly Report, 52,* 1072–1075.

Baird, C. L., & Sands, L. (2004). A pilot study of the effectiveness of guided imagery with progressive muscle relaxation to reduce chronic pain and mobility difficulties of osteoarthritis. *Pain Management Nursing, 5*(3), 97–104.

Bardenheir, B. H., Wortley, P. M., & Euler, G. (2004). Influenza and pneumococcal vaccination coverage among persons aged ≥65 years and persons aged 16–64 years with diabetes or asthma — United States, 2003. *Morbidity and Mortality Weekly Report, 53,* 1007–1012.

Bauer, J. E., Hyland, A., Li., Q., Steger, C., & Cummings, K. M. (2005). A longitudinal assessment of the impact of smoke-free worksite policies on tobacco use. *American Journal of Public Health, 95,* 1024–1029.

Bennett, S. J., Suave, M. J., & Sahw, R. M. (2005). A conceptual model of cognitive deficits in chronic heart failure. *Journal of Nursing Scholarship, 37,* 222–228.

Bisschop, M. I., Kriegsman, D. M. W., Beekman, A. T. F., & Deeg, D. J. H. (2004). Chronic diseases and depression: The modifying role of psychosocial resources. *Social Science & Medicine, 59,* 721–733.

Bodenheimer, T., Wagner, E. H., & Grumbach, K. (2002a). Improving primary care for patients with chronic illness. *JAMA, 288,* 1775–1779.

Bodenheimer, T., Wagner, E. H., & Grumbach, K. (2002b). Improving primary care for patients with chronic illness: The chronic care model, Part 2. *JAMA, 288,* 1909–1914.

Bonita, R., & Mathers, C. D. (2003). Global health status at the beginning of the twenty-first century. In R. Beaglehole (Ed.), *Global public health: A new era* (pp. 24–53). Oxford, UK: Oxford University.

Brouse, C. H., Basch, C. E., Wolf, R. L., Shmukler, C., Neugut, A. I., & Shea, S. (2003). Barriers to colorectal cancer screening with fecal occult blood testing in a predominantly minority urban population: A qualitative study. *American Journal of Public Health, 93,* 1268–1270.

Bunker, S. J., Colquhoun, D. M., Essler, M., Hickie, I. B., Hunt, D., Jelinek, V. M., et al. (2003). Stress and coronary heart disease: Psychosocial risk factors, National Heart Foundation of Australia position statement update. *MJA, 178,* 272–276.

Burrows, N. R., Wang, J., Geiss, L. A., Venkat Narayan, N. K., & Engelgau, M. M. (2005). Incidence of end-stage renal disease among persons with diabetes—United States, 1990–2002. *Morbidity and Mortality Weekly Report, 54,* 1097–1100.

Calabrese, D. A. (2004). Prostate cancer in older men. *Urological Nursing, 24,* 258–264, 268–269.

Carmona, R. H. (2005). Improving the health and wellness of persons with disabilities: A call to action. *American Journal of Public Health, 95,* 1883.

Centers for Disease Control and Prevention. (2002a). American heart month — February, 2002. *Morbidity and Mortality Weekly Report, 51,* 126.

Centers for Disease Control and Prevention. (2002b). National arthritis month — May, 2002. *Morbidity and Mortality Weekly Report, 51,* 374–375.

Centers for Disease Control and Prevention. (2004a). National epilepsy awareness month — November, 2004. *Morbidity and Mortality Weekly Report, 53,* 1023–1024.

Centers for Disease Control and Prevention. (2004b). National stroke awareness month — May, 2004. *Morbidity and Mortality Weekly Report, 53,* 359.

Centers for Disease Control and Prevention. (2005a). Great American smokeout — November 17, 2005. *Morbidity and Mortality Weekly Report, 54,* 1121.

Centers for Disease Control and Prevention. (2005b). *Healthy people data.* Retrieved September 5, 2005, from http://wonder .cdc.gov/data2010

Centers for Disease Control and Prevention. (2005c). National diabetes awareness month — November, 2005. *Morbidity and Mortality Weekly Report, 54,* 1097.

Centers for Disease Control and Prevention. (2006a). *Cancer — Basic information about cancer survivorship.* Retrieved July 28, 2006, from http://aaps.nccd.cdc.gov/EmailForm/print_table.asp

Centers for Disease Control and Prevention. (2006b). *Epilepsy.* Retrieved May 28, 2006, from http:www.cic.gov/epilepsy

Centers for Disease Control and Prevention. (2006c). National arthritis month — May 2006. *Morbidity and Mortality Weekly Report, 55,* 477.

Centers for Disease Control and Prevention. (2006d). National stroke awareness month — May 2006. *Morbidity and Mortality Weekly Report, 55,* 529.

Chriqui, J., O'Connor, H., Babb, S., Blair, N. A., Vaughn, G., & MacNeil, A. (2005). State smoking restrictions for private-sector worksites, restaurants, and bars — United States, 1998 and 2004. *Morbidity and Mortality Weekly Report, 54,* 649–653.

Churchill, R. E. (2005). Disabled or enabled? *American Journal of Public Health, 95,* 1887–1888.

Clarke, P., & George, L. K. (2005). The role of the built environment in the disablement process. *American Journal of Public Health, 95,* 1933–1939.

Committee on Rapid Advance Demonstration Projects: Health Care Finance and Delivery Systems. (2003). *Fostering rapid advances in health care: Learning from system demonstrations.* Washington, DC: National Academies Press.

Coronado, V. G., Johnson, R. L., Faul, M., & Kegler, S. R. (2006). Incidence rates of hospitalization related to traumatic brain injury — 12 states, 2002. *Morbidity and Mortality Weekly Report, 55,* 201–204.

Costa de Silva, V., Chauvin, J., Jones, N. R., Warren, W., Sama, S., & Pechacek, T. (2005). Tobacco use and cessation counseling — Global Health Professionals Survey pilot study, 10 countries, 2005. *Morbidity and Mortality Weekly Report, 54,* 505–509.

Davis, R., & Magilvy, J. K. (2000). Quiet pride: The experience of chronic illness by rural older adults. *Journal of Nursing Scholarship, 32,* 385–390.

Davis, S., Mirick, D. K., & Stevens, R. G. (2001). Night shift work, light at night, and risk of breast cancer. *Journal of the National Cancer Institute, 93,* 1557–1562.

de Castro, A. B. (2004a). Actively preventing injury: Avoiding back injuries and other musculoskeletal disorders among nurses. *American Journal of Nursing, 104.* Retrieved July 28, 2006, from http://nursingworld .org/ajn/2004/jan/health.htm

de Castro, A. B. (2004b). Handle with Care®: The American Nurses Association's campaign to address work-related musculoskeletal disorders. *Online Journal of Issues in Nursing, 19*(3), Manuscript 2. Retrieved July 28, 2006, from http://nursingworld.org / ojin/topic25/tpc25_2.htm

Denny, C. H., Holtzman, D., & Cobb, N. (2003). Surveillance for health behaviors of American Indians and Alaska Natives: Findings from the Behavioral Risk Factor Surveillance System, 1997–2002. *Morbidity and Mortality Weekly Report, 52*(SS-7), 1–13.

DeNoon, D. (2006). *Cervical cancer vaccine approved.* Retrieved July 28, 2006, from http://www.webmd.com/content/Article/123/115099.htm?printing=true

Disease Management Association of America. (2006). *DMAA definition of disease management.* Retrieved May 25, 2006, from http://www.dmss.org/definition.html

Division for Heart Disease and Stroke Prevention. (2006a). *Heart disease facts and statistics.* Retrieved May 23, 2006, from http://apps .nccd.cdc.gov/emailform/print_table.asp

Division for Heart Disease and Stroke Prevention (2006b). *Stroke facts and statistics.* Retrieved May 23, 2006, from http://apps .nccd.cdc.gov/emailform/print_table.asp

Division of Adult and Community Health. (2003). Projected prevalence of self-reported arthritis or chronic joint symptoms among persons aged ≥65 years — United States, 2005–2030. *Morbidity and Mortality Weekly Report, 52,* 489–491.

Division of Adult and Community Health, National Center for Chronic Disease Prevention and Health Promotion. (2004a). Disparities in premature deaths from heart disease — 50 states and the District of Columbia, 2001. *Morbidity and Mortality Weekly Report, 53,* 121–125.

Division of Adult and Community Health, National Center for Chronic Disease Prevention and Health Promotion. (2004b). Prevalence of doctor-diagnosed arthritis and possible arthritis — 30 states, 2002. *Morbidity and Mortality Weekly Report, 53,* 383–386.

Division of Cancer Prevention and Control, National Center for Chronic Disease Prevention and Health Promotion. (2004). Cancer survivorship — United States, 1971–2001. *Morbidity and Mortality Weekly Report, 53,* 526, 528–529.

Division of Diabetes Translation. (2002). Socioeconomic status of women with diabetes — United States, 2000. *Morbidity and Mortality Weekly Report, 51,* 147–148, 159.

Division of Environmental Hazards and Health Effects. (2005). Self-reported asthma among high school students — United States, 2003. *Morbidity and Mortality Weekly Report, 54,* 765–767.

Division of Human Development and Disability. (2002). State-specific prevalence of obesity among adults with disabilities — Eight states and the District of Columbia, 1998–1999. *Morbidity and Mortality Weekly Report, 51,* 805–808.

Donohoe, M. (2005). Cigarettes: The other weapons of mass destruction. *Medscape Ob/Gyn & Women's Health, 10*(1). Retrieved April 13, 2005, from http://www.medscape .com/viewarticle/501586

Dunne, K., Sullivan, K., & Kernohan, G. (2005). Palliative care for patients with cancer: District nurses' experiences. *Journal of Advanced Nursing, 50,* 372–380.

Eberhard, M. S., Saydah, S., Paulose-Ram, R., & Tao, M. (2005). Mobility limitation among persons aged ≥ 40 years with and without diagnosed diabetes and lower extremity disease — United States, 1999–2002. *Morbidity and Mortality Weekly Report, 54,* 1183–1186.

Epidemiology Program Office. (2000). Screening with prostate-specific antigen test — Texas, 1997. *Morbidity and Mortality Weekly Report, 49,* 818–820.

Epilepsy Foundation. (n.d.). *Epilepsy and seizure statistics.* Retrieved March 8, 2006, from http://www.efa.org/answerplace/statistics.cfm

Fagan, J., Galea, S., Ahern, J., Bonner, S., & Vlahov, D. (2002). Self-reported increase in asthma severity after the September 11 attacks on the World Trade Center — Manhattan, New York, 2001. *Morbidity and Mortality Weekly Report, 51,* 781–784.

Farrelly, M. C., Davis, K. C., Haviland, L., Messeri, P., & Healton, C. G. (2005). Evidence of a dose-response relationship between "truth" antismoking ads and youth smoking prevalence. *American Journal of Public Health, 95,* 425–431.

Ferguson, P. L., Selassie, A. W., Wannamaker, B. B., Dong, B., Kobau, R., & Thurman, D. J. (2005). Prevalence of epilepsy and health-related quality of life and disability among adults with epilepsy — South Carolina, 2003 and 2004. *Morbidity and Mortality Weekly Report, 54,* 1080–1082.

Fireman, B., Bartlett, J., & Selby, J. (2004). Can disease management reduce health care costs by improving quality? *Health Affairs, 23*(6), 63–75.

Fisher, E. B., Brownson, C. A., O'Toole, M. L., Shetty, G., Anwuri, V. V., & Glasgow, R. E. (2005). Ecological approaches to self-management: The case of diabetes. *American Journal of Public Health, 95,* 1523–1535.

Freedman, V., & Martin, L. G. (2000). Contribution of chronic conditions to aggregate changes in old-age functioning. *American Journal of Public Health, 90,* 1755–1760.

Frieden, T. R. (2004). Asleep at the switch: Local public health and chronic disease. *American Journal of Public Health, 94,* 2059–2061.

Garland, C. F., Garland, F. C., Gorham, E. D., Kipkin, M., Newmark, H., Mohr, S. B., et al. (2006). The role of vitamin D in cancer prevention. *American Journal of Public Health, 96,* 252–261.

Geller, A. C., Zapka, J., Brooks, K. R., Dube, C., Powers, C. A., Rigotti, N., et al. (2005). Tobacco control competencies for US medical students. *American Journal of Public Health, 95,* 950–955.

Gesler, W. M., & Kearns, R. A. (2002). *Culture/place/health.* London: Routledge.

Gill, J. M., & McClellan, S. A. (2001). The impact of a referral to a primary physician on cervical cancer screening. *American Journal of Public Health, 91,* 451–454.

Glanz, K., Saraiya, M., & Wechsler, H. (2002). Guidelines for school programs to prevent skin cancer. *Morbidity and Mortality Weekly Report, 51*(RR-4), 1–18.

Glover, M. J., Greenlund, K. J., Ayala, C., & Croft, J. B. (2005). Racial/ethnic disparities in prevalence, treatment, and control of hypertension — United States, 1999–2002. *Morbidity and Mortality Weekly Report, 54,* 7–9.

Goldsmith, C. (2000). Hypertension: Still the silent killer. *NurseWeek, 13*(5), 16–17.

Goodwin, R. D., & Eaton, W. W. (2005). Asthma, suicide ideation, and suicide attempts: Findings from the Baltimore Epidemiologic Catchment Area follow-up. *American Journal of Public Health, 95,* 717–722.

Gravlee, C. C., Dressler, W. W., & Bernard, H. R. (2005). Skin color, social classification, and blood pressure in southeastern Puerto Rico. *American Journal of Public Health, 95,* 2191–2197.

Grunbaum, J. A., Kann, L., Kinchen, S., Ross, J., Hawkins, J., Lowry, R., et al. (2004). Youth risk behavior surveillance — United States, 2003. *Morbidity and Mortality Weekly Report, 53* (SS-2), 1–96.

Harris, C., Ayala, C., & Croft, J. B. (2006). Place of death after stroke. *Morbidity and Mortality Weekly Report, 55,* 529–532.

Harris, C., Ayala, C., Dai, S., & Croft, J. B. (2005). Disparities in deaths from stroke among persons aged <75 years — United States, 2002. *Morbidity and Mortality Weekly Report, 54,* 477–481.

Health Care and Aging Studies Bureau. (2001). Prevalence of arthritis—United States, 1997. *Morbidity and Mortality Weekly Report, 50,* 334–336.

Hewitt, M., Greenfield, S., & Stovall, E. (Eds.). (2006). *From cancer patient to cancer survivor: Lost in transition.* Retrieved July 29, 2006, from http://nap.edu/openbook/0309095956/html/R1.html

Hoenig, H., Taylor, D. T., & Sloan, F. A. (2003). Does assistive technology substitute for personal assistance among the disabled elderly? *American Journal of Public Health, 93,* 330–337.

Hootman, J. M., Langmaid, R., Helmick, C. G., Bolen, J., Kim, I., Shih, M., et al. (2005). Monitoring progress in arthritis management —

United States and 25 states, 2003. *Morbidity and Mortality Weekly Report, 54,* 484–488.

Horowitz, C. R., Colson, K. C., Hebert, P. L., & Lancaster, K. (2004). Barriers to buying healthy foods for people with diabetes: Evidence of environmental disparities. *American Journal of Public Health, 94,* 1549–1554.

Houston, T. K., Scarinci, I. C., Person, S. C., & Greene, P. G. (2005). Patient smoking cessation advice by health care providers: The role of ethnicity, socioeconomic status, and health. *American Journal of Public Health, 95,* 1056–1061.

Hsia, J., Kemper, E., Kiefe, C., Zapka, J., Sofaer, S., Pettinger, M., et al. (2000). The importance of health insurance as a determinant of cancer screening: Evidence from the Women's Health Initiative. *Preventive Medicine, 31,* 261–270.

Huey, F. L. (2001). A global perspective on the human and economic burdens of chronic disease. *The Pfizer Journal, 11*(2), 10–16.

Ibald-Mulli, A., Stieber, J., Wichman, H. E., Koenig, W., & Peters, A. (2001). Effects of air pollution on blood pressure: A population-based approach. *American Journal of Public Health, 91,* 571–577.

Immunization Services Division, National Immunization Program. (2003). Influenza vaccination coverage among adults aged ≥50 years and pneumococcal vaccination coverage among adults aged ≥65 years — United States, 2002. *Morbidity and Mortality Weekly Report, 52,* 987–992.

Institute for Health and Management Productivity. (2002, January). Allergy and Asthma in the Workplace study reveals major work impact findings. *NEWS-line for Nurses,* 12.

Institute of Medicine. (2002). *Care without coverage: Too little, too late.* Retrieved August 13, 2002, from http://books.nap.edu/books/0309083435/html/R1.html

Jaakkola, J. K. K., & Gissler, M. (2004). Maternal smoking in pregnancy, fetal development, and childhood asthma. *American Journal of Public Health, 94,* 136–140.

Jaakkola, M. S., Piipari, R., Jaakkola, N., & Jaakkola, J. K. K. (2003). Environmental tobacco smoke and adult-onset asthma: A population-based incident case-control study. *American Journal of Public Health, 93,* 2055–2060.

Jacobellis, J., Martin, L., Engel, J., VanEenwyk, J., Bradley, L. A., Kassim, S., et al. (2004). Genetic testing for breast and ovarian cancer susceptibility: Evaluating direct-to-consumer marketing — Atlanta, Denver, Raleigh-Durham, and Seattle, 2003. *Morbidity and Mortality Weekly Report, 53,* 603–606.

Jacobs, E. A., Karavolos, K., Rathouz, P. J., Ferris, T. G., & Powell, L. H. (2005). Limited English proficiency and breast and cervical cancer screening in a multiethnic population. *American Journal of Public Health, 95,* 1410–1416.

Jiles, R., Hughes, E., Murphy, W., Flowers, N., McCracken, M., Roberts, H., et al. (2005). Surveillance for certain health behaviors among states and selected local areas — Behavioral Risk Factor Surveillance System, United States, 2003. *Morbidity and Mortality Weekly Report, 54*(SS-8), 1–116.

Joachim, G., & Acorn, S. (2000). Stigma of visible and invisible chronic conditions. *Journal of Advanced Nursing, 32,* 243–248.

Kalina, C. M., Haag, A. B., & Tourigian, R. (2004). What are some effective chronic disease management strategies that can be used in case management? *AAOHN Journal, 52,* 420–423.

Kara, M. (2005). Preparing nurses for the global pandemic of chronic obstructive pulmonary disease. *Journal of Nursing Scholarship, 37,* 127–133.

Kara, M., & Mirici, A. (2004). Loneliness, depression, and social support of Turkish patients with chronic obstructive pulmonary disease and their spouses. *Journal of Nursing Scholarship, 36,* 331–336.

Kather, T. A. (2005). Colorectal cancer: Guidelines for prevention, screening and treatment. *Advance for Nurses, 20*(5), 15–17.

Kearney, P. M., & Pryor, J. (2004). The International Classification of Functioning, Disability, and Health (ICF) and nursing. *Journal of Advanced Nursing, 46,* 162–170.

Kinne, S., Patrick, D. L., & Doyle, D. L. (2004). Prevalence of secondary conditions among people with disabilities. *American Journal of Public Health, 94,* 443–445.

Kivimaki, M., Head, J., Ferrie, J. E., Hemingway, H., Shipley, M. J., Vahtera, J., et al. (2005). Working while ill as a risk factor for serious coronary events: The Whitehall II study. *American Journal of Public Health, 95,* 98–102.

Koch, T., Jenkin, P., & Kralik, D. (2004). Chronic illness self-management: Locating the "self." *Journal of Advanced Nursing, 48,* 484–492.

Konrad, T. R., Howard, D. L., Edwards, L. J., Ivanova, A., & Carey, T. A. (2005). Physician–patient racial concordance, continuity of care, and patterns of care for hypertension. *American Journal of Public Health, 95,* 2186–2190.

Lavery, L. A., Higgins, K. R., Lanctot, D. R., Constantinides, G. P., Zamorano, R. G., Armstrong, D. G., et al. (2004). Home monitoring of foot skin temperatures to prevent ulceration. *Diabetes Care, 27,* 2642–2647.

Leveille, S. G., Wee, C. C., & Iezzoni, L. I. (2005). Trends in obesity and arthritis among baby boomers and their predecessors, 1971–2002. *American Journal of Public Health, 95,* 1607–1613.

Lewis, G. (2004). Diabetes management: An overview. *Viewpoint 26*(4), 3, 12–16.

Liao, Y., Tucker, P., Okoro, C. A., Giles, W. H., Hokdad, A. H., & Harris, V. B. (2004). REACH 2010 surveillance for health status in minority communities — United States, 2001–2002. *Morbidity and Mortality Weekly Report, 53*(SS-6), 1–35.

Lineberger, L., O'Connor, J., Blair, N. A., Babb, D., Jordan, J., Vaughn, G., et al. (2005). Preemptive state smoke-free indoor air laws — United States, 1999–2004. *Morbidity and Mortality Weekly Report, 54,* 251–253.

MacLean, C. D., Littenberg, B., & Gagnon, M. (2006). Diabetes decision support: Initial experience with the Vermont Diabetes Information System. *American Journal of Public Health, 96,* 593–595.

Mannino, D. M., Homa, S. M., Akinbami, L. J., Moorman, J. E., Gwynn, C., & Redd, S. C.

(2002). Surveillance for asthma — United States, 1980–1999. *Morbidity and Mortality Weekly Report, 51*(SS-1), 1–13.

Marshall, L., Schooley, M., Ryan, H., Cox, P., Easton, A., Healton, C., et al. (2006). Youth tobacco surveillance — United States 2001–2002. *Morbidity and Mortality Weekly Report, 55*(SS-3), 1–56.

Maurice, E., Trosclair, A., Merritt, R., Caraballo, R., Malarcher, A., Husten, C., et al. (2005). Cigarette smoking among adults — United States, 2004. *Morbidity and Mortality Weekly Report, 54*, 1121–1124.

Mayer-Davis, E. J., D'Antonio, A. M., Smith, S. M., Kirkner, G., Levin Martin, S., Parra-Medina, D., et al. (2004). Pounds Off With Empowerment (POWER); A clinical trial of weight management strategies for black and white adults with diabetes who live in medically underserved rural communities. *American Journal of Public Health, 94*, 1736–1742.

McCarberg, B. (2004). Contemporary management of chronic pain disorders. *The Journal of Family Practice, 53*(10 Suppl.), S11–S22.

McGruder, H. F., Greenlund, K. J., Croft, J. B., & Zheng, A. J. (2005). Differences in disability among black and white stroke survivors — United States, 2000–2001. *Morbidity and Mortality Weekly Report, 54*, 3–6.

McVeigh, K. H., Mostashari, F., & Thorpe, L. E. (2004). Serious psychological distress among persons with diabetes — New York City, 2003. *Morbidity and Mortality Weekly Report, 53*, 1089–1092.

Meyer, L. H., Sternfels, P., Fagan, J. K., & Ford, J. G. (2002). Asthma-related limitations in sexual functioning: An important but neglected area of quality of life. *American Journal of Public Health, 92*, 770–772.

Moore, L. V., & Diez Roux, A. V. (2006). Associations of neighborhood characteristics with the location and type of food stores. *American Journal of Public Health, 96*, 325–331.

Morabia, A., & Costanza, M. C. (2005). The obesity epidemic as harbinger of a metabolic disorder epidemic: Trends in overweight, hypercholesterolemia, and diabetes treatment in Geneva, Switzerland, 1993–2003. *American Journal of Public Health, 95*, 632–635.

Moskowitz, J. M., Kazinets, G., Tager, I. B., & Wong, J. (2004). Breast and cervical cancer screening among Korean Women — Santa Clara County, California, 1994 and 2002. *Morbidity and Mortality Weekly Report, 53*, 765–767.

Moyer, P. (2004). Vaccine against HPV strain protects against high-grade cervical neoplasia. *Medscape Medical News*. Retrieved November 12, 2004, from http://www.medscape.com/viewarticle/493010

Mukhtar, Q., Pan, L., Jack Jr., L., & Murphy, D. L. (2005). Prevalence of receiving multiple preventive-care services among adults with diabetes — United States, 2002–2004. *Morbidity and Mortality Weekly Report, 54*, 1130–1133.

Narcessian, E. J. (n.d.). *Patient comfort assessment guide*. Retrieved July 28, 2006, from http://partnersagainstpain.com/printouts/pcag.pdf

National Center for Chronic Disease Prevention and Health Promotion. (2002). *The burden of chronic diseases and their risk factors: National and state perspectives, 2002*. Retrieved June 23, 2002, from http://www.cdc.gov/nccdphp/burdenbook2002/preface.html

National Center for Chronic Disease Prevention and Health Promotion. (2003). Prevalence of diabetes and impaired fasting glucose in adults — United States, 1999–2000. *Morbidity and Mortality Weekly Report, 52*, 833–837.

National Center for Environmental Health. (2004). Asthma prevalence and control characteristics by race/ethnicity — United States, 2002. *Morbidity and Mortality Weekly Report, 53*, 145–148.

National Center for Health Statistics. (2005a). *Health United States, 2005, with chartbook on trends in the health of Americans*. Retrieved December 23, 2005, from http://www.cdc.gov/nchs/data/hus/hus05.pdf

National Center for Health Statistics. (2005b). Hospitalizations for heart disease by diagnosis and percentage distribution — United States, 2003. *Morbidity and Mortality Weekly Report, 54*, 704.

National Center for Health Statistics. (2005c). Percentage of U.S. and Canadian women aged 50–69 years who were screened in accordance with national screening guidelines for Papanicolau (Pap) tests and mammograms by country and health insurance status, 2002–2003. *Morbidity and Mortality Weekly Report, 54*, 879.

National Center for Health Statistics. (2005d). Prevalence of lower extremity disease (LED) among adults aged ≥ 40 years with and without diabetes — United States, 1999–2000. *Morbidity and Mortality Weekly Report, 54*, 332.

National Center for Health Statistics. (2006a). *Asthma*. Retrieved May 30, 2006, from http://www.cdc.gov/nchs/faststats/asthma.htm

National Center for Health Statistics. (2006b). Health-care visits for asthma, by medical setting and health-insurance status — United States, 2003. *Morbidity and Mortality Weekly Report, 55*, 405.

National Center for Injury Prevention and Control. (2004). Medical expenditures attributable to injuries — United States, 2000. *Morbidity and Mortality Weekly Report, 53*, 1–4.

National Center on Birth Defects and Developmental Disabilities. (2004). Economic costs associated with mental retardation, cerebral palsy, hearing loss, and vision impairment — United States, 2003. *Morbidity and Mortality Weekly Report, 53*, 57–59.

National Coalition for Cancer Survivorship. (n.d.). *Palliative care and symptom management*. Retrieved July 28, 2006, from http://www.canceradvocacy.org/resources/essential

National Diabetes Information Clearinghouse. (2000). Why November is National Diabetes Month: The disturbing statistics behind diabetes. *Gourmet Connection*. Retrieved April 22, 2001, from http://www.gourmetconnection.com

National Organization on Disability. (2004). *The 2004 N.O.D./Harris survey of Americans with disabilities*. Retrieved May 31, 2006, from http://www.nod.org

Natural Resources Defense Council. (2004). *Heat advisory: How global warming causes more bad air days*. Retrieved September 30, 2004, from http://www.nrdc.org/globalwarming/heatadvisory/heatadvisory.pdf

Newman, C. (2004, August). Why are we so fat? *National Geographic*, pp. 47–49.

Office of the Surgeon General. (2005). *The Surgeon General's call to action to improve the health and wellness of persons with disabilities, 2005*. Retrieved May 24, 2006, from http://www.surgeongeneral.gov/library/disabilities/calltoaction/calltoaction.pdf

Office on Smoking and Health. (2000). Declines in lung cancer rates—California, 1988–1997. *Morbidity and Mortality Weekly Report, 49*, 1066–1069.

Ong, M. K., & Glantz, S. A. (2005). Free nicotine replacement therapy programs vs implementing smoke-free workplaces: A cost-effectiveness comparison. *American Journal of Public Health, 95*, 969–975.

Pâquet, M., Bolduc, N., Xhignesse, M., & Vanasse, A. (2005). Re-engineering cardiac rehabilitation programmes: Considering the patient's point of view. *Journal of Advanced Nursing, 51*, 567–576.

Partners Against Pain. (n.d.). *Pain management: Tools for implementing JCAHO's new standards*. Retrieved July 28, 2006, from http://partnersagainstpain.com/content/PM_GUIDE/pmg_1.htm

Partners Against Pain. (2005). *Pain in America*. Retrieved July 28, 2006, from http://partnersagainstpain.com/indexhs.aspx?sid=24

Partnership for Solutions. (2002). *Multiple chronic conditions: Complications in care and treatment*. Retrieved October 7, 2004, from http://www.partnershipforsolutions.org

Paterson, B. (2001a). Myth of empowerment in chronic illness. *Journal of Advanced Nursing, 34*, 574–581.

Paterson, B. L. (2001b). The shifting perspectives model of chronic illness. *Journal of Nursing Scholarship, 33*, 21–26.

Pedroso de Souza, E. A., & Barioni Salgado, P. C. (2006). A psychosocial view of anxiety and depression in epilepsy. *Epilepsy & Behavior, 8*, 232–238.

Perkins, R. (2005). A new focus on cancer. *The Pfizer Journal, IX*(1), 1–40.

Piette, J. D., Heisler, M., & Wagner, T. (2004). Cost-related medication underuse among chronically ill adults: The treatments people forgo, how often, and who is at risk. *American Journal of Public Health, 94*, 1782–1787.

Plese, N. K. (2003). Heart disease: An all-out attack on risk. *The Pfizer Journal, VII*(4), 1–49.

Plese, N. K. (Ed.). (2005a). A profile of caregiving in America (2nd ed.). *The Pfizer Journal, IX*(4), 1–40.

Plese, N. K. (2005b). Global summit on the aging workforce. *The Pfizer Journal, IX*(3), 1–40.

Ramirez, A., Farmer, G. C., Grant, D., & Papachristou, T. (2005). Disability and preventive cancer screening: Results from the 2001 California Health Interview Survey. *American Journal of Public Health, 95*, 2057–2064.

Ranjan, A., Tarigopula, L., Srivastava, R. K., Obasanjo, O., & Obah, E. (2003). Effectiveness of the clinical pathway in the management of congestive heart failure. *Southern Medical Journal, 96*, 661–663.

Rimmer, J. H., Riley, B., Wang, E., & Rauworth, A. (2005). Accessibility of health clubs for people with mobility disabilities and visual impairments. *American Journal of Public Health, 95,* 2022–2028.

Robinson, K. A., & Merrill, R. M. (2003). Relation among stroke knowledge, lifestyle, and stroke-related screening results. *Geriatric Nursing, 24,* 300–305.

Rogers, D., & Petereit, D. G. (2005). Cancer Disparities Research Partnership in Lakota country: Clinical trials, patient services, and community education for the Ogalala, Rosebud, and Cheyenne River Sioux tribes. *American Journal of Public Health, 95,* 2129–2132.

Rosenberg, T. J., Garbers, S., Lipkind, H., & Chiasson, M. A. (2005). Maternal obesity and diabetes as risk factors for adverse pregnancy outcomes: Differences among 4 racial/ethnic groups. *American Journal of Public Health, 95,* 1544–1551.

Rosenthal, T. (2004). Seasonal variations in blood pressure. *American Journal of Geriatric Cardiology, 13,* 267–272.

Saaddine, J., Benjamin, S., Pan, L., Venkat Narayan, K. M., Tierney, E., Kanjilal, S., et al. (2004). Prevalence of visual impairment and selected eye diseases among persons aged ≥50 years with and without diabetes — United States, 2002. *Morbidity and Mortality Weekly Report, 53,* 1069–1071.

Saddlemire, A. E., Denny, C. H., Greenlund, K. J., Coolidge, J. N., Fan, A. Z., & Croft, J. B. (2005). Trends in cholesterol screening and awareness of high blood cholesterol — United States, 1991–2003. *Morbidity and Mortality Weekly Report, 54,* 865–870.

Sapkota, S., Bowles, H. R., Ham, S. A., & Kohl III, H. W. (2005). Adult participation in recommended levels of physical activity — United States, 2001 and 2003. *Morbidity and Mortality Weekly Report, 54,* 1208–1212.

Saraiya, M., Glanz, K., Briss, P., Nichols, P., White, C., & Sas, D. (2003). Preventing skin cancer: Findings of the Task Force on Community Preventive Services on reducing exposure to ultraviolet light. *Morbidity and Mortality Weekly Report, 52* (RR-15), 1–12.

Schernhammer, E. S., Laden, F., Speizer, F. E., Willett, W. C., Hunter, D. J., Kawachi, I., et al. (2001). Rotating night shifts and risk of breast cancer in women participating in the nurses' health study. *Journal of the National Cancer Institute, 93,* 1563–1568.

Seeff, L. C., King, J., Pollack, L. A., & Williams, K. N. (2006). Increased use of colorectal cancer tests — United States, 2002 and 2004. *Morbidity and Mortality Weekly Report, 55,* 308–311.

Sitzman, K. (2004). Coping with chronic illness at work. *AAOHN Journal, 52,* 264.

Steiner, B., Hootman, J., Langmaid, G., Bolen, J., & Helmick, C. G. (2006). State prevalence of self-reported doctor-diagnosed arthritis and arthritis-attributable activity limitation — United States, 2003. *Morbidity and Mortality Weekly Report, 55,* 477–481.

Strine, T. W., Hootman, J. M., Chapman, D. P., Okoro, C. A., & Balluz, L. (2005). Health-related quality of life, health risk behaviors, and disability among adults with pain-related activity difficulty. *American Journal of Public Health, 95,* 2042–2048.

Strunin, L., & Boden, L. I. (2004). Family consequences of chronic back pain. *Social Science & Medicine, 58,* 1385–1393.

Sundquist, K., Lindström, M., Malmström, M., Johansson, S.-E., & Sundquist, J. (2004). Social participation and coronary heart disease: A follow-up study of 6900 women and men in Sweden. *Social Science & Medicine, 58,* 615–622.

Sung, H.-Y., Hu, T.-W., Ong, M., Keeler, T. E., & Sheu, M.-L. (2005). A major state tobacco tax increase, the Master Settlement Agreement, and cigarette consumption: The California experience. *American Journal of Public Health, 95,* 1030–1035.

Taylor, D. H. Jr., Hasselblad, V., Henley, S. J., Thun, M. J., & Sloan, F. A. (2002). Benefits of smoking cessation for longevity. *American Journal of Public Health, 92,* 990–996.

Thomas, A. J., Eberly, L. E., Davey Smith, G., Neaton, J. D., & Stamler, J. (2005). Race/ethnicity, income, major risk factors, and cardiovascular disease mortality. *American Journal of Public Health, 95,* 1417–1423.

Tierney, E. F., Geiss, L. S., Engelgau, M., Thompson, T. J., Schaubert, D., Shirely, L. A., et al. (2001). Population-based estimates of mortality associated with diabetes: Use of a death certificate check box in North Dakota. *American Journal of Public Health, 91,* 84–92.

Two Feathers, J., Kieffer, E. C., Palmisano, G., Anderson, M., Sinco, B. Janz, N., et al. (2005). Racial and Ethnic Approaches to Community Health (REACH) Detroit partnership: Improving diabetes-related outcomes among African American and Latino adults. *American Journal of Public Health, 95,* 1552–1560.

Ullom-Minnich, P. (2004). Strategies to reduce complications of type 2 diabetes. *The Journal of Family Practice, 53,* 366–374.

U.S. Census Bureau. (2005). *Statistical abstract of the United States, 2004–2005.* Retrieved May 12, 2005, from http://www.census .gov/prod/2004pubs/04statab

U.S. Department of Health and Human Services. (2003a). *A public health action plan to prevent heart disease and stroke.* Retrieved July 25, 2003, from http://www.healthierus .gov/steps

U.S. Department of Health and Human Services. (2003b). *Preventing chronic diseases: Investing wisely in health.* Retrieved July 25, 2003, from http://www.healthierus .gov/steps

U.S. Department of Health and Human Services. (2003c). *Prevention strategies that work.* Retrieved July 25, 2003, from http://www .healthierus.gov/steps

U.S. Department of Health and Human Services. (2003d). *The power of prevention.* Retrieved May 29, 2006, from http://www .healthierus.gov/steps/summit/prevportfolio /Power_of_Prevention.pdf

U.S. Department of Health and Human Services. (2006). *The health consequences of involuntary exposure to tobacco smoke — Executive summary.* Retrieved July 28, 2006, from http://www.surgeongeneral.gov/library/se condhandsmoke/report/executivesummary .pdf

U.S. Preventive Services Task Force. (2002). *Aspirin for the primary prevention of cardiovascular events — chemoprevention.* Retrieved August 13, 2005, from http://www.ahrq .gov/clinic/uspstf/uspsasmi.htm.

U.S. Preventive Services Task Force. (2003). Counseling to prevent skin cancer: Recommendations and rationale of the U.S. Preventive Services Task Force. *Morbidity and Mortality Weekly Report, 52*(RR-15), 13–17.

U.S. Preventive Services Task Force. (2004). *Screening for coronary heart disease.* Retrieved August 13, 2005, from http://www.ahrq .gov/clinic/uspstf/uspsacad.htm

U.S. Preventive Services Task Force. (2005). *The guide to clinical preventive services, 2005.* Retrieved August 13, 2005, from http:// www.ahrq.gov/clinic/pocketgd.pdf

Vallerand, A. H., Fouladbakhsh, J. M., & Templin, T. (2003). The use of complementary/alternative medicine therapies for the self-treatment of pain among residents of urban, suburban, and rural communities. *American Journal of Public Health, 93,* 923–925.

Wang, P. P., Bradley, E. M., & Gignac, M. A. (2004). Perceived need for workplace accommodation and labor-force participation in Canadian adults with activity limitations. *American Journal of Public Health, 94,* 1515–1518.

Webb, O. J., & Eves, F. F. (2005). Promoting stair use: Single versus multiple stair-riser messages. *American Journal of Public Health, 95,* 1543–1544.

White, K. R., Coyne, P. J., & Patel, U. B. (2001). Are nurses adequately prepared for end-of-life care? *Journal of Nursing Scholarship, 33,* 147–151.

Wiles, R., Ashburn, A., Payne, S., & Murphy, C. (2004). Discharge from physiotherapy following stroke: The management of disappointment. *Social Science & Medicine, 59,* 1263–1273.

Williams, S. G., Schmidt, D. K., Redd, S. C., & Storms, W. (2003). Key clinical activities for quality asthma care: Recommendations of the National Asthma Education and Prevention Program. *Morbidity and Mortality Weekly Report, 52*(RR-6), 1–8.

Wilson, L. S., Moskowitz, J. T., Acree, M., Heyman, M. B., Harmatz, P., Ferrando, S. J., et al. (2005). The economic burden of home care for children with HIV and other chronic illnesses. *American Journal of Public Health, 95,* 1445–1452.

Wong, F. K. Y., Mok, M. P., Chan, T., & Tsang, M. W. (2005). Nurse follow-up of patients with diabetes: Randomized controlled trial. *Journal of Advanced Nursing, 50,* 391–402.

World Health Organization. (2005). *Preventing chronic diseases: A vital investment, Part 1, Overview.* Retrieved January 5, 2006, from http://www.who.int/chp/chronic_disease_ report/contents/part1.pdf

Wright, R. J., Mitchell, H., Visness, C. M., Cohen, S., Stout, J., Evans, R., et al. (2004). Community violence and asthma mortality: An inner-city asthma study. *American Journal of Public Health, 94,* 625–632.

Yen, I. H., Yelin, E. H., Katz, P., Eisner, M. D., & Blanc, P. D. (2006). Perceived neighborhood problems and quality of life, physical functioning, and depressive symptoms among adults with asthma. *American Journal of Public Health, 96*, 873–879.

Yoon, P. W., Scheuner, M. T., Gwinn, M., Khoury, M. J., Jorgensen, C., Hariri, S., et al. (2004). Awareness of family health history as a risk factor for disease — United States, 2004. *Morbidity and Mortality Weekly Report, 53*, 144–147.

York, K. (2003). Rural case management for stroke: The development of a community-based screening and education program. *Case Management, 8*(3), 98–114.

Zhu, S., Layde, P. M., Guse, C. E., Laud, P. W., Pintar, F., Nirula, R., et al. (2006). Obesity and risk for death due to motor vehicle crashes. *American Journal of Public Health, 96*, 734–739.

Ziebland, S., Chapple, A., Dumelow, C., Evans, J., Prinjha, S., & Rozmovits, L. (2004). How the Internet affects patients' experience of cancer: A qualitative survey. *BMJ, 328*, 564–569.

Zierold, K. M., Knobeloch, L., & Anderson, H. (2004). Prevalence of chronic disease in adults exposed to arsenic-contaminated drinking water. *American Journal of Public Health, 94*, 1936–1937.

Advocacy in Action

An Incompetent Client

A home health nurse was assigned to visit a senior citizen with both mental and physical illnesses who lived in a large, unfurnished house with a caretaker. On the initial nursing visit, Harry was dirty, unshaven, and improperly dressed for the weather and the temperature in the house. He was gaunt and seemed undernourished, and there were piles of dog feces in the living areas from the caretaker's two Dobermans. The nurse tried to engage the caretaker, but it became obvious that the woman was mentally ill. She became hostile when questioned about Harry's care although she expressed commitment to caring for him.

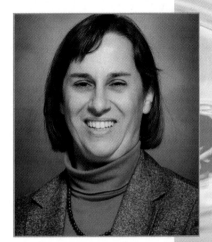

Harry had a foley catheter that was not draining properly and had to be reinserted. The on-call nurse was called nightly for several nights because the catheter had been pulled out. Eventually, the indwelling catheter was replaced with an external catheter to decrease trauma to the urethra. After several days of finding Harry wet or lying in feces, the nurse called the physician. The physician said there was nothing that could be done about the situation and the nurse's visits were to make sure conditions didn't deteriorate. The nurse, who thought this was an insufficient response, called the city's elder abuse line, and police were sent to the home. When the police asked Harry if he wanted to leave, he occasionally responded "yes" but more often, and under repeated questioning, said "no." The police said they had no grounds to remove Harry from the home because he did not want to go. When the nurse questioned Harry's competence to make such a decision, especially given his living conditions, the police replied that they had no formal determination that Harry was not competent, and thus could intervene no further.

After several similar interactions, the nurse contacted the state guardianship office and initiated proceedings to have Harry declared incompetent and removed from the home. The process took several months and, despite the nurse's calls, could not be expedited. The nurse continued to see Harry, trying to work with his caretaker and monitoring the situation. Harry was eventually evaluated by the State Guardianship office and court proceedings were scheduled, resulting in Harry's removal from this residence and placement in a protective long-term care facility.

Susan M. Swider, PhD, RNC

College of Nursing, Rush University Medical Center

Community Mental Health Problems

CHAPTER OBJECTIVES

After reading this chapter, you should be able to:

1. Analyze the personal, family, and societal impact of mental illness and mental health problems.
2. Analyze factors influencing the development of mental health problems.
3. Identify symptoms characteristic of common mental health problems.
4. Analyze the role of the community health nurse in strategies to prevent mental health problems.
5. Discuss approaches to community treatment of mental health problems and analyze the community health nurse's role in each.
6. Describe areas of emphasis in maintenance therapy for mental health problems and analyze the role of the community health nurse in maintenance.

KEY TERMS

community mental health problems **902**
dual diagnosis **910**
dysthymia **902**
ethnopsychopharmacology **922**
mental health **902**
mental health problems **902**
mental health promotion **918**
mental illness **902**
recovery **923**
resilience **918**
seasonal affective disorder (SAD) **912**
serious mental illness **902**
somatization **913**

 MediaLink

http://www.prenhall.com/clark

Additional interactive resources for this chapter can be found on the Companion Website. Click on Chapter 30 and "Begin" to select the activities for this chapter.

Mental illness is a growing problem throughout the world. Community health nurses may find themselves involved in efforts to promote mental health and prevent mental illness as well as activities required for the treatment of clients with mental illness. **Mental health** is the ability to successfully perform mental functions, to engage in productive activities and meaningful interpersonal relationships, and to adapt to change and cope with adversity. **Mental illness** or mental disorder, on the other hand, encompasses a wide variety of diagnosable mental disorders characterized by changes in thinking, mood, or behavior associated with stress or impaired function. **Serious mental illness** is defined as "a mental disorder . . . of such intensity that it disables people, preventing them from functioning adequately on the basis of their culture and background" (Sansbury Centre for Mental Health, as quoted in Askey, 2004, p. 12). **Mental health problems** involve signs and symptoms of mental distress that are of insufficient duration or intensity to qualify as mental disorders diagnosed on the basis of accepted criteria. **Community mental health problems** are those that occur with sufficient frequency in the community or population group to be of serious concern in the overall health status of the population. In this chapter we use the term *mental health problems* to refer to the composite of mental and emotional conditions that result in impaired function.

TRENDS IN COMMUNITY MENTAL HEALTH PROBLEMS

Overall, an estimated 20% to 29% of the U.S. population will experience some level of mental health problems in a given year, and 9% experience some disability related to mental health difficulties. For 7% of these people, symptoms will last more than a year, yet less than 15% of all those affected use mental health services (McLeer, 2004). During 2002 and 2003, 3.1% of U.S. adults experienced serious psychological distress (National Center for Health Statistics [NCHS], 2005a). The prevalence of serious psychological distress in the population is assessed on the basis of responses to six questions in the National Health Interview Survey, which address feelings of extreme sadness, nervousness, restlessness, hopelessness, and worthlessness, and perceptions that everything requires too much effort (NCHS, 2006). The prevalence of frequent mental distress in U.S. adults increased significantly from 1993 to 2001 (from 8.4% of the population to 10.1%) (Zahran et al., 2004).

In 2002, the rate for hospitalization in mental health facilities was 62.7 per 100,000 population, and more than 2.4 million inpatient episodes of care occurred (U.S. Census Bureau, 2006). At the international level, more than 450 million people have mental disorders, and one fourth of the world's population will experience mental health problems during their lives. In the United States, Canada, and Western Europe, mental health problems contribute to 25% of all disabilities (Marshall-Williams, Chapman, & Lando, 2005).

The National Institute of Mental Health (NIMH) addresses eight major categories of mental illness: attention deficit hyperactivity disorder (ADHD), depression, bipolar or manic-depressive disorder, schizophrenia, anxiety disorders, eating disorders, borderline personality disorders, and autism spectrum disorders. ADHD was discussed in Chapter 16∞. Each of the other categories of illness will be briefly discussed here before we turn to a discussion of the effects of mental health problems and the factors contributing to them.

Periodic depression, "feeling down" or "having the blues," is a common occurrence in all people, but major depression is not a normal phenomenon. In any given year, nearly 21 million U.S. adults or 9.5% of the population experience depressive illness (NIMH, 2000). In the next 10 years, depression is expected to become the second greatest cause of disability in the world (O'Malley, Forrest, & Miranda, 2003). Many people do not seek treatment for depression, but antidepressants are one of the most widely prescribed categories of medication in the United States. A milder, chronic, ongoing form of depressed mood that prevents one from functioning well or feeling good is called **dysthymia** (NIMH, 2005a).

In bipolar disorder, also known as manic-depressive disorder, people experience unusual shifts in mood, energy, and functional ability. Most people with bipolar disorder cycle through periods of depression alternating with periods of energy, excitability, and irritability called *mania*. Symptoms gradually flow through a continuum from severe mania and hyperactivity through hypomania, characterized by mild to moderate manic

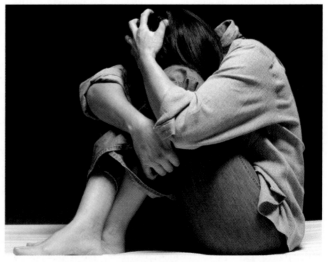

Depression affects physical health as well as quality of life. (Getty Images)

symptoms, followed by a normal mood state. Normal mood eventually shifts into mild depression and then into severe depression (NIMH, 2001c). Most people with bipolar disorder experience more depression than mania (75% to 90% of the time with altered mood symptoms) (Goldberg & Hoop, 2004). A few people with bipolar disorder experience symptoms of mania and depression simultaneously in a form of the disease called a *mixed* bipolar state. Bipolar disorder affects approximately 5.7 million U.S. adults or 2.6% of the population over 18 years of age (NIMH, 2001c). Both depression and bipolar disorder are risk factors for suicide. Symptoms of depression and mania are presented below.

Some experts argue that there is no specific disease of schizophrenia (Boyle, 2004). Reasons given for this position include the lack of specific diagnostic criteria similar to those used to diagnose physical illnesses such as diabetes or cardiovascular disease, but a menu of several signs and symptoms, and the wide variability of symptomatology among people with the same diagnosis. These experts also contend that what is perceived as schizophrenic behavior (e.g., hearing voices) is in some contexts perceived to be perfectly normal. For example, profound religious or bereavement experiences may involve hearing the voice of God or of a deceased loved one. These experts argue that rather than label such experiences as evidence of mental illness, society should expand its conception of what is normal.

Other authors argue that schizophrenia is a disease of abnormality in the brain and cite evidence of genetic alterations and structural and functional brain abnormalities demonstrable through technological measurement as rationale for their perspective (Agrawal & Hirsch, 2004). Whatever the validity of either argument, the fourth edition of the *Diagnostic and Statistical Manual of Mental Disorders-Text Revision* (DSM IV-TR) of the American Psychiatric Association (2000) lists schizophrenia as a specific category of disease with a set of diagnostic criteria. Based on these criteria, an estimated 1% of the world's population, including 2.4 million people in the United States, is affected by the conditions labeled as schizophrenia. Schizophrenia is characterized by three types of symptoms: positive symptoms, negative symptoms, and cognitive symptoms. Positive symptoms are unusual thoughts or perceptions that are not present in "normal" people. Negative symptoms are an absence of normal behaviors and emotional states, and cognitive symptoms reflect deficits in attention, memory, and executive functions that permit planning and organizing thoughts and behaviors (NIMH, 2005b). Positive, negative, and cognitive symptoms of schizophrenia are summarized below.

Anxiety disorders are a group of illnesses that result in chronic and overwhelming fear and anxiety that tend to grow progressively worse with time. More than 19 million U.S. adults are affected by these conditions

SPECIAL CONSIDERATIONS

CHARACTERISTIC SIGNS OF DEPRESSION AND MANIA

Depression

- Persistent sadness or despair
- Disturbances in sleep patterns
- Difficulty falling asleep
- Early morning awakening
- Difficulty waking up
- Alterations in eating habits
- Significant weight gain
- Significant weight loss
- Diminished energy level
- Decreased interest in sex
- Difficulty concentrating
- Social withdrawal

(The presence of one or more of these symptoms can indicate that a client is experiencing depression.)

Mania

- Persistent euphoria
- Grandiosity (inappropriately high self-esteem)
- Psychomotor agitation
- Decreased sleep
- Racing thoughts and distractibility
- Poor judgment and impaired impulse control
- Rapid or pressured speech

SPECIAL CONSIDERATIONS

POSITIVE, NEGATIVE, AND COGNITIVE SYMPTOMS OF SCHIZOPHRENIA

Positive Symptoms

- Hallucinations: Sensory experiences that occur without any sensory input (may occur in any sensory modality)
- Delusions: Distortions of inferential thinking that lead to misperceptions of experiences and erroneous beliefs
- Thought disorder: Unusual thought processes characterized by difficulty organizing thoughts or expressing them
- Disorders of movement: Clumsiness or lack of coordination, involuntary movements, or unusual mannerisms

Negative Symptoms

- Flat or blunt affect: Lack of emotional response, facial inexpressiveness, diminished body language
- Anhedonia: Inability to experience pleasure
- Diminished ability to plan and execute activity
- Infrequent speech

Cognitive Symptoms

- Poor executive function: Inability to process information and make decisions based on its interpretation
- Poor attention span: Inability to sustain attention
- Memory difficulties: Inability to retrieve and use recently learned information

Data from: National Institute of Mental Health. (2005). Depression: What every woman should know. Washington, DC: Author.

Data from: National Institute of Mental Health. (2005). Schizophrenia. Retrieved June 2, 2006, from http://www.nimh.hih.gov/publicat/schizoph.cfm

(NIMH, 2001a), and the estimated lifetime prevalence is 29% (Marshall-Williams et al., 2005). Phobias are the most common anxiety disorders. Other types of anxiety disorders are panic disorder, obsessive-compulsive disorder, post-traumatic stress disorder (PTSD), and general anxiety disorder. Phobias may be one of two types: social phobia and specific phobias. People with social phobia feel overwhelming anxiety, embarrassment, or humiliation that makes them incapable of interacting comfortably with others in social situations. Specific phobias are extreme and unreasonable fears of something that poses little real danger (e.g., heights, being closed in) (NIMH, 2001a).

Panic disorder is characterized by episodes of intense fear without any identifiable basis. Panic is manifested in cardiac, respiratory, and gastrointestinal symptoms of distress (e.g., shortness of breath, palpitations) or fear of dying. As noted in Chapters 17, 18, and 27∞, PTSD, another form of anxiety disorder, arises in response to experiencing or witnessing a traumatic event and is characterized by nightmares, flashbacks, irritability, depression, and poor concentration. Persons affected by obsessive-compulsive disorder are subject to repeated and unwanted thoughts (obsessions) or engage in repetitive behaviors that cannot be stopped or controlled (compulsions). Finally, general anxiety disorder is characterized by constant and excessive worry about everyday events. A given person may experience more than one type of anxiety disorder, and anxiety disorders frequently co-occur with other mental health problems such as depression, eating disorders, and substance abuse (NIMH, 2001a).

Eating disorders affect 0.5 to 5% of women in the population, with considerably lower incidence among men. Three types of eating disorders are common: anorexia nervosa, bulimia nervosa, and binge eating disorder. Anorexia nervosa is characterized by a strong resistance to maintaining a minimal weight for one's height and body type, by intense fear of gaining weight, and by a distorted body image that leads one to perceive oneself as fat even when significantly underweight. Anorexia nervosa results in mortality rates 12 times those of all other causes of death among young women 15 to 24 years of age. Bulimia nervosa is characterized by uncontrollable eating followed by compensatory purging or other behaviors to prevent weight gain that usually occur at least twice a week. Because of the compensatory behaviors, many people with bulimia are able to maintain a normal weight. Excessive overeating without compensatory purging and other behaviors is referred to as binge eating (NIMH, 2001e).

Borderline personality disorder (BPD) is characterized by rapidly changing moods and resulting difficulty with interpersonal relationships and an inability to function effectively in society. BPD affects approximately 2% of adults and, like eating disorders, occurs more often in women than men. People with BPD account for approximately 20% of all psychiatric hospitalizations in the United States. The characteristic mood changes of people with BPD occur rapidly, over a period of hours rather than days as is the case with depression or mania. The impulsivity that accompanies these mood changes may lead to self-injury or suicide, impulsive spending, or sudden shifts in attitudes toward others (e.g., from idealization to anger and dislike). People with BPD may see routine absences of significant others as evidence of rejection and abandonment and may resort to threats of self-harm or suicide in response (NIMH, 2001d).

Autism spectrum disorders (ASD), also called pervasive developmental disorders, tend to occur in young children and may be diagnosed as early as 18 months of age. They range from a relatively mild form called Asperger syndrome to the more severe autistic disorder to very severe and rare forms such as Rett syndrome and childhood disintegrative disorder. Severity of disease varies among those affected. ASD may be suspected in children who do not babble or engage in interactive behaviors such as pointing or speaking, do not respond to their names, fail to maintain eye contact, do not know how to play with toys, do not smile, and do not like to be cuddled. Children with ASD have difficulty learning to interpret social cues from others, which makes communication difficult. They may also under- or overreact to stimuli. Some children with ASD exhibit normal development at first, but begin to lose acquired interaction skills at some point in their development. Children with ASD have a higher risk of mental retardation, seizures (occurring in 25% of children with ASD), and tuberous sclerosis, a rare condition in which benign tumors grow in the brain (NIMH, 2004).

THE EFFECTS OF MENTAL HEALTH PROBLEMS

Mental health problems have burdensome effects for individuals and their families as well as for society as a whole. Some of these effects will be presented here.

Personal Effects

Suffering and disability are the two most prominent effects of mental health problems for the individuals they affect. There is no objective measure of the suffering endured, but measures of disability are discouraging. Depression and mental illness are the leading causes of disability and premature death in the United States (Dunlop, Song, Lyons, Manheim, & Chang, 2003). For example, a study by the National Alliance on Mental Illness (NAMI) found that 23% of people with mental illness needed help with activities of daily living, 74% needed help with community living skills, and 73% needed help with employment. An additional 60% and 68% of those affected needed assistance with illness and crisis management, respectively (McLeer, 2004). In another study, people with depression were 4.3 times more likely to exhibit inability to perform activities of daily living than those without depression (Dunlop, Manheim, Song, Lyons, & Chang, 2005).

Mental health problems not only result in mental disability but also cause physical and social impairments. Mental illness may result in worsening of physical health problems due to inability or lack of motivation for effective self-care (Dunlop et al., 2003). The NAMI study also found that 65% of people with serious mental illness required family assistance in their interactions with friends (McLeer, 2004).

Family Effects

Mental health problems also exact a toll on the families of people that experience them. The family costs of mental disorders are both economic and emotional. In Chapter 19∞, we reviewed the effects of caregiving on family members with Alzheimer's disease. Other chronic mental health problems also have family effects. For example, families with a member with schizophrenia may not progress through the normal stages of family development described in Chapter 14∞ due to the difficulty people with schizophrenia have with separating from home and becoming independent. Parents of a child with schizophrenia may find themselves extending the parental role indefinitely and delaying personal goals and plans for retirement (Jungbauer, Stelling, Dietrich, & Angermeyer, 2004).

Family members of persons with obsessive-compulsive disorder are also faced with dealing with dependence and bizarre behaviors in those affected, and may experience feelings of frustration, anger, and guilt. In addition, they often have to curtail personal activities to meet the needs of the affected family member. In one study, parents of adult children with obsessive-compulsive disorder experienced role changes and were faced with decisions about how to deal with compulsive behavior. Parents either supported the obsession or compulsion (e.g., engaging in the behavior themselves so the client would not need to) or opposed the behavior, and most parents questioned the correctness of their response. Parents were also concerned about concealing the illness to avoid for their child the social stigma attached to mental illness. Concealment, however, limited the social support available to parents because there were few people with whom they could discuss their concerns (Stengler-Wenzke, Trosbach, Dietrich, & Angermeyer, 2004).

Family members, particularly of persons with schizophrenia, may also perceive themselves as invisible participants in care undervalued by mental health professionals. In one study, for example, several parents of children with schizophrenia reported never being informed of the diagnosis. Parents were also engaged in a wide variety of activities to support their ill children. For example, they described "previsiting" facilities before attempting to motivate children to use them. They also voiced concerns regarding the difficulty in finding activities that could "normalize" life for their offspring and themselves and wanted health care professionals to take a more active role in advocating for such activities. In addition parents voiced a need for support and respite from the caregiver role (Sin, Moone, & Wellman, 2005). In another study, the level of client function, medication compliance, and client participation in a social rehabilitation program predicted caregiver burden for relatives of clients with schizophrenia (Koukia & Madianos, 2005).

Clients with mental illness may have difficulty holding a job because of the impairments resulting from their conditions. Unemployment and underemployment may lead to poverty for the individual and the family. In addition, family caretakers may be forced to take time from work or even stop working, further diminishing family income.

Major mental disorders may also prevent family members from carrying out their expected family roles. Mental illness in a family member often increases stress for the entire family and may contribute to family communication problems and perceptions of social stigma for both client and family (Draucker, 2005; Spencer & Chen, 2004).

Societal Effects

Mental illness and less severe mental health problems also pose a burden for society in general. Mental disorders are the leading cause of disability worldwide and account for a substantial portion of the global disease burden.

In addition to the burden of disability posed by mental disorder, society experiences considerable economic burden as well. As noted earlier, schizophrenia affects 1% of the world's population and accounts for 1.6% of the world's total health care budget (McCann, 2000). In 2000, for example, bipolar disease resulted in 55 days of work absence, $1,231 in short-term disability costs, and $554 in compensation costs for each U.S. employee affected. The estimated annual costs to employers for bipolar disease alone is $45.2 million (Matza, de Lissovoy, Sasane, Pesa, & Maus, 2004). In one study in the United Kingdom, the indirect costs of lost productivity resulting from mental illness was approximately four times higher than the direct costs (Frangou & Murray, 2000). In general, these figures indicate the magnitude of mental health problems as a community health issue.

The importance of chronic mental health problems in the United States is highlighted by the number of objectives related to these disorders in the national health objectives for the year 2010 (Centers for Disease

Control and Prevention [CDC], 2005). Some of these objectives are presented at the end of this chapter. The complete set of objectives for mental health and mental disorders can be viewed on the *Healthy People 2010*◆ Web page at http://wonder.cdc.gov/data2010.

THE EPIDEMIOLOGY OF MENTAL HEALTH PROBLEMS

Factors in each of the six dimensions of health of the dimensions model contribute to the development of mental health problems and their personal, family, and societal burden. Knowledge of factors in each of the dimensions will enable community health nurses to better contribute to control strategies for community mental health problems.

Biophysical Considerations

Biophysical factors influencing mental health problems include genetics and gender, maturation and aging, race and ethnicity, and physiologic function.

Genetics and Gender

Both genetics and gender appear to have differential effects on the incidence of specific mental health problems. Various studies of families, twins, and adopted children provide strong evidence that some people have a genetic predisposition to develop schizophrenia, and specific genes on almost every chromosome have been identified as potential contributors to the incidence of disease in a given individual or in the population (Keltner, 2005). The lifetime risk of developing schizophrenia for someone with one or more family members with schizophrenia is 10 times greater than for those with no family history of the disease (Frangou & Murray, 2000). Additional evidence of a genetic contribution to disease is seen in the incidence of schizophrenia in 50% of identical twins whose twin is affected, but in only 15% of nonidentical twins and 10% of nontwin siblings. Schizophrenia also occurs in approximately 35% of people whose parents both have schizophrenia. The fact that concordance is not perfect in identical twins, however, suggests the modifiability of genetic predisposition through environmental factors. Genetic factors may also influence the effectiveness of particular drugs in the treatment of schizophrenia (Keltner, 2005).

Genetic contributions to vulnerability are implicated in other mental health problems as well, including bipolar depression, early-onset depression, autism, ADHD, anorexia nervosa, panic disorder, and so on. It should be noted, however, that heredity plays a role in transmission of vulnerability to disease, not in transmission of disease itself. Furthermore, genetic research has indicated that it is not a single gene that causes most of these diseases, but a complex interaction of multiple genes with environmental factors (Keltner, 2005).

Genetic factors may even have differential effects in the development of a single mental disorder. For example, three basic genetic forms of familial schizophrenia have been identified: dopamine psychosis, neurodegenerative schizophrenia, and schizophrenia caused by genetic failure in neurological development during the second trimester of pregnancy (Flaskerud, 2000).

With respect to gender, NCHS data indicated that women were 70% more likely than men to report serious psychological distress (3.9% to 2.3%) (NCHS, 2005a), but this may be a function of men's reluctance to acknowledge feelings of distress (Zahran et al., 2004). Other possible reasons for lower incidence rates for depression in men include less willingness among providers to diagnose depression among men than women. Men are more likely than women with depression to attempt to self-medicate with alcohol or drugs than to seek treatment. Men with depression also have higher cardiovascular mortality than those without depression or women with depression. Successful suicides are also more common among depressed men than women (Monts, 2002).

Women have a lifetime prevalence of major depression nearly twice that of men (24% vs. 15%) (Eli Lilly and Company, 2004), but men and women have similar incidence rates for bipolar disorder. Women, however, may exhibit more depressive symptoms than men and experience more rapid cycling of the disease (Goldberg & Hoop, 2004). Some gender differences are also noted with schizophrenia, primarily in the age at onset. Schizophrenia occurs in young men in late adolescence and early adulthood and somewhat later in women. Borderline personality disorder and eating disorders are more common in women than in men. As we saw in Chapter 16∞, however, ADHD is two to three times more common in boys than in girls (NIMH, 2001b, 2001d, 2001e).

Maturation and Aging

All of the mental health problems discussed in this chapter tend to be life-long in their consequences, but they occur with different levels of frequency in different age groups. For example, 20% of children have mental health problems (Leighton, Worraker, & Nolan, 2003), an increase from 7% less than 20 years ago. By 2020, the worldwide prevalence of neuropsychiatric disorders among children is expected to increase by 50%, placing these disorders among the top five causes of morbidity, mortality, and disability in children (NAMI, 2002). An estimated 11% of children have resulting functional impairment, with 5% experiencing extreme impairment (American Academy of Pediatrics, 2004). Increasing problems in this age group are related to changes in family structure, family unemployment, loss of traditional community environments and supports, and poverty (Leighton et al., 2003). Among adults, the age group reporting the highest average percentage of serious psychological distress from 2002 to 2003 was those 45 to 54 years of age (4.2%). People over age 65 reported the least psychological distress (2.3%), with other age groups falling between these two levels.

Specific mental health problems tend to occur more frequently in some groups than in others. ASD, for example, is almost exclusively diagnosed in children, although those children affected and their families have to deal with its consequences into and through adulthood. Similarly, ADHD is most often diagnosed in childhood, but its effects persist into adulthood. Bipolar disorder typically develops in late adolescence or early adulthood (NIMH, 2001c), and tends to occur earlier than unipolar disorder (Goldberg & Hoop, 2004). Schizophrenia is rare in children, occurring in approximately one of every 40,000 children (NIMH, 2003) and seldom occurs after age 45 (NIMH, 2005b). In addition, the severity of symptoms of schizophrenia tends to decrease with age. Aging also results in a need for lower doses of antipsychotic medications due to diminished ability to detoxify drugs and higher incidence rates for extrapyramidal side effects in older people (Calandra, 2003). Eating disorders most frequently occur in adolescent and young adult women (NIMH, 2001e), as does BPD (NIMH, 2001d).

Depression occurs across the age spectrum, but is more common in older people than in younger ones. An estimated 15% to 20% of older adults are affected by depression (Weeks, McGann, Michaels, & Penninx, 2003), and as many as 44% of homebound elderly individuals are depressed (Loughlin, 2004). An additional 15% to 30% of older clients may have mild or subsyndromal depression. Depression in the elderly increases their risk for disability and exacerbates comorbid physical illnesses. Depression also increases caregiver burden and the risk of suicide in older clients with existing physical health problems (Antai-Otong, 2004). Predictors of depression in the elderly include disability and chronic illness, loneliness, and lack of satisfaction with family support (Loughlin, 2004; Tanner, 2004). Depression in the elderly is often misdiagnosed or inadequately treated. Depression in this population leads to increased health care use as well as functional decline and loss of independence. Depression in the context of physical health problems is often overlooked (Weeks et al., 2003).

Although not approaching the levels seen in older populations, depression is also prevalent among children and adolescents. Depression in the pediatric population was not a commonly recognized phenomenon until late in the 20th century (Miller, 2005). Today approximately 5% of U.S. children and adolescents experience episodes of depression at any given time (American Academy of Child & Adolescent Psychiatry [AACAP], 2004), and an estimated one third of children age 6 to 12 years with a diagnosis of major depression will go on to be diagnosed with bipolar disease within a few years (NAMI, n.d.). Increased stress, the experience of significant loss, and the presence of attentional, learning, conduct, and anxiety disorders increase the risk of depression in these age groups (AACAP, 2004). Runaway children and youth also have a high prevalence of depression, with as much as 80% of this population affected (NAMI, n.d.).

The presence of other chronic conditions may also contribute to depression in children and adolescents. For example, depression is frequently noted among children with severe asthma. In fact, in one outpatient sample, as many as one third of children with asthma had a comorbid diagnosis of depression. Depression has also been found to interact with asthma to result in worse school performance than occurs among children with asthma without depression (Galil, 2000). Similarly, several studies have found associations between obesity and psychopathology, particularly depression, in children and adolescents (Vila et al., 2004). The presence of comorbid depression also complicates treatment for physical disorders, often resulting in noncompliance and poor treatment outcomes (Galil, 2000; Miller, 2005).

Depression may manifest differently in children and adolescents than in adults. Common signs and symptoms of depression in youth include persistent sadness and crying, withdrawal from friends and previously enjoyed activities, boredom, irritability, low self-esteem and extreme reaction to failure or rejection, poor concentration and poor school performance, and indecision or forgetfulness. Other indicators of depression in children are anger and hostility, changes in eating or sleeping habits, and somatic complaints such as headache or stomachache. Depressed children and youth may also express thoughts of running away or committing suicide or other self-destructive behavior (e.g., self-injury) (AACAP, 2004; NAMI, n.d.). Community health nurses can educate parents, teachers, and the public regarding indications of depression in children and youth as well as make referrals and advocate for treatment services for those affected.

Although menopause is often perceived as a time of increased depression among women, studies show that the prevalence of depression actually decreases after menopause. Research has indicated that progression through natural menopause is not a risk factor for major depression, but that women who have a history of severe premenstrual syndrome or postpartum depression may be at higher risk for depression during perimenopause than other women. Conversely, depression prior to menopause may lead to earlier onset of menopause or to higher rates of cardiovascular disease and osteoporosis in postmenopausal women (Miller & Daniels-Brady, 2005).

Race and Ethnicity

Incidence of mental illness and mental health problems also varies among racial and ethnic groups. For example, an average of 9.7% of the American Indian/Alaska Native population reported serious psychological distress in the period from 2000 to 2004, compared to 3.5%

for White, 4.1% for Black, and 2.5% for Asian populations (NCHS, 2006). People of mixed racial heritage in 2000 and 2002 reported an even higher prevalence of distress, 7.3%, than most ethnic groups, perhaps reflecting the stress of belonging to two groups and being accepted by neither. People of Hispanic origin had a prevalence of serious psychological distress of 3.9%, slightly higher than that of White, African American, or Asian groups (NCHS, 2005a).

Based on data from the National Health and Nutrition Examination Survey (NHANES) III, major depression is more common among White Americans than African Americans or Mexican Americans. Conversely, dysthymic disorder is more prevalent among African and Mexican Americans than among Whites (Riolo, Nguyen, Greden, & King, 2005).

Physiologic Function

The interaction between mental health and physiologic factors is complex. The presence of physiologic conditions may increase one's risk for mental health problems. Conversely, mental health problems may pose risks for physiologic effects. Finally, the presence of either mental or physical conditions may complicate control of problems in the other realm.

There is considerable evidence that some mental health problems have a physiologic basis in brain chemistry and that neurophysiologic deficits are a major contributor to mental illness. Similarly, the presence of chronic physical illness, infection, malnutrition, and the effects of hormones and physical trauma have all been shown to play a part in the development of mental health problems. Infectious agents such as human immunodeficiency virus (HIV) and syphilis, for example, are implicated in the development of some forms of dementia. In a 2003 study in New Mexico, people with depression were found to report fair or poor health more than three and a half times as often as those without depression. Similarly, those with depression were 56% more likely to report diabetes and arthritis and 85% more likely to report asthma than those without depression. In addition, those with depression were three times more likely to report disability (Daniel et al., 2005). A similar study in New York found that adults with diabetes were twice as likely as those without diabetes to report serious psychological distress (McVeigh, Mostashari, & Thorpe, 2004). Depression has also been identified as a risk factor for hypertension and cardiovascular disease (Marshall-Williams et al., 2005) and for death among women with AIDS. Mental health services, on the other hand, were associated with decreased AIDS mortality (Cook et al., 2004).

Physiologic differences also account for differential effects of psychotropic drugs in different racial and ethnic groups. There is also some indication that biological markers for mental illness differ among racial ethnic groups. For example, African Americans have lower monoamine oxidase activity in schizophrenia than do Caucasians (Flaskerud, 2000).

Mental health problems may also increase one's risk for physical illness. For example, anxiety and depression have been shown to increase the risk for the onset of coronary heart disease (CHD) and to affect survival in persons with existing CHD. Conversely, people recovering from myocardial infarction are at increased risk for major depressive disorders. Depression may also be implicated in falls among the elderly, with abnormal gaits found more often in depressed than nondepressed clients. Treatment for depression may also increase fall risk and fallers may be prone to anxiety and depression (Turcu et al., 2004).

Complications of pregnancy and birth and exposure to influenza in the second trimester of pregnancy have been linked to the incidence of schizophrenia in adult children of affected women. Pregnancy does not seem to result in greater risk for rehospitalization among women with schizophrenia (as depression does), but schizophrenic women may have delusions regarding the pregnancy that are associated with high risk of complications due to noncompliance with prenatal care recommendations (Frangou & Murray, 2000).

Pregnancy, as a physiologic condition, has been found to influence the incidence of depression. Although pregnancy is often considered a joyful event and depression is more often associated with the postpartum period, an estimated 10% to 20% of women experience some level of depression during pregnancy. Depression during pregnancy is also known as antepartum depression. A woman's risk for antepartum depression is increased by relationship problems, a past history of depression (or family history of depression), prior pregnancy loss, and other stressful life events. Other contributing factors may include fertility treatments, pregnancy complications, and a history of abuse or trauma, particularly sexual abuse (American Pregnancy Association, 2006). Depression during pregnancy may be misinterpreted as hormonal imbalance, and community health nurses may need to educate pregnant women, health care providers, and the public about antepartum depression. They may also need to advocate for access to counseling and treatment services for those affected. For example, although many health insurance plans cover care for the pregnancy itself, they may not provide coverage for counseling services related to antepartum depression.

Depression in the postpartum period is more common and better recognized than antepartum depression and may occur in one of three forms: postpartum blues, postpartum depression, or puerperal or postpartum psychosis. Postpartum blues are a mild form of depression that affects 30% to 75% of women shortly after delivery. They are characterized by tearfulness and anxiety, are time-limited, and usually do not require treatment beyond emotional support (Registered Nurses Association of Ontario [RNAO], 2005).

Postpartum depression (PPD) occurs in 10% to 15% of pregnancies and is characterized by more severe emotions than postpartum blues. The fourth edition of the American Psychiatric Association's *Diagnostic and Statistical Manual of Mental Disorders (DSM-IV)* defined PPD as a major depressive disorder occurring within one month of delivery (Freeman et al., 2005), but the actual onset of PPD may occur anytime within one year of delivery, typically from 2 weeks to 3 months (Ugarriza & Schmidt, 2006). Several studies have indicated that women are more likely to be admitted to a psychiatric hospital in the first 4 weeks after delivery than at any other time in their lives (RNAO, 2005). Symptoms of postpartum depression are similar to those of other major depressive episodes, but may also include tearfulness, mood swings, feelings of guilt and inadequacy as a mother, and inability to cope with the demands of caring for an infant (Ugarriza & Schmidt, 2006).

Postpartum psychosis is relatively rare, occurring in 1 or 2 per 1,000 women after delivery. Its onset is rapid, often within 48 to 72 hours of delivery. Postpartum psychosis is characterized by mood fluctuations, disorganized behavior, and possible delusions or hallucinations (RNAO, 2005).

PPD is believed to be related to rapid hormonal changes following delivery, but other factors can increase a woman's risk of PPD. Major factors include antepartum depression and anxiety, past personal or family history of depression, and lack of social support (RNAO, 2005). Other factors that may contribute to an increased risk for PPD include physical trauma (e.g., rape), unresolved issues with parents or partners, perceptions of trauma during the birth experience (e.g., an unexpected cesarean section or exceptionally painful or prolonged labor) (Antares, 2005), incongruence between expectations and the reality of motherhood, loss of personal control and sense of self, and loneliness and isolation (RNAO, 2005).

Postpartum depression also occurs in men, but less often than among women, with 2% to 5% of new fathers affected. In men, PPD tends to occur later than in women, with higher incidence occurring toward the end of the first year after delivery. Men whose female partners are also experiencing PPD have a higher risk for PPD themselves (24% to 50%). Risk of PPD in men is also increased with a past history of depression, partner experience of antepartum depression, discrepancies between the expectations and reality of fatherhood, tendencies toward perfectionism or neuroticism, and poor social functioning or poor parental or spousal relationships. Other contributing factors include being part of a stepfamily, experiencing external social stresses (e.g., unemployment or job insecurity), and having a "blue collar" job (Strayer, 2005).

PPD in men may go unrecognized because of the tendency of many men to deny or hide emotional distress. In addition, men with PPD may exhibit symptoms

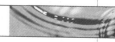

FOCUSED ASSESSMENT

Biophysical Considerations in Mental Health Problems

- Is there a family history of mental health problems?
- Are there any existing physical health conditions that may contribute to mental health problems? What effects do personal physical health conditions or those of family members have on mental health? Do physical health problems or their treatment cause signs and symptoms suggestive of mental health problems?
- Does the presence of a mental health problem complicate treatment of physical health conditions?

of anxiety rather than those more characteristic of depression (Strayer, 2005). Community health nurses can educate couples, health care providers, and the general public regarding signs and symptoms of PPD in both men and women and can advocate for access to treatment services as needed. Intervention is particularly needed in view of evidence that PPD in either parent may also have adverse effects on the infant. For example, infants of mothers with PPD are more likely than those whose mothers are not depressed to exhibit poor attachment, poor cognitive development, and later behavioral problems. In addition, parents with PPD are less likely to undertake routine preventive care for their infants (Freeman et al., 2005).

Mental health problems of all kinds may also interfere with treatment compliance for physical health conditions. The focused assessment above provides some questions for evaluating the contribution of biophysical dimension factors to community mental health problems.

Psychological Considerations

Psychological considerations to be addressed relative to community mental health problems include psychological risk factors, psychiatric comorbidity, coping skills, suicide potential, and characteristic manifestations of mental health problems for which the nurse would assess individual clients.

Psychological Risk Factors for Mental Health Problems

Personality traits, difficult temperament, experience of stressful life events, and below-average intelligence are some of the psychological factors that have been associated with the development of mental health problems. Some people's personalities appear to place them at increased risk for mental health problems. For example, people who are excessively critical or who have difficult temperaments may alienate others, receiving less social support for dealing with everyday sources of stress that we all encounter.

Psychological stress appears to play an important part in the development of mental disorders. Stress and an emotionally charged environment are also implicated in symptomatic relapses in clients with schizophrenia. Conversely, decreasing stress and increasing personal and interpersonal competencies appear to contribute to mental health and to control of existing mental health problems. Stressful life events may contribute to situational depression or exacerbate major depressive disorders.

Psychiatric Comorbidity

Clients with one mental disorder may concurrently experience other disorders. This co-occurrence of two mental disorders is referred to as psychiatric comorbidity. **Dual diagnosis** is the term commonly used to indicate the co-occurrence of a substance abuse disorder with one or more other psychiatric diagnoses (Vega, Sribney, & Achara-Abrahams, 2003). Several forms of comorbidity may occur. For example, depression frequently occurs with schizophrenia, panic disorder, and eating disorders (NIMH, 2000, 2001a, 2001c, 2005b). An estimated 25% of people with schizophrenia experience depression at any one time, and a large number of people with schizophrenia will experience depression prior to their first psychotic episode (Frangou & Murray, 2000). The presence of comorbidity complicates treatment for any given mental illness, and community health nurses working with clients with comorbid conditions or dual diagnosis may need to assure that clients receive treatment for all the disorders that they experience.

Coping Skills

The extent of an individual's coping abilities mediates the effect of stress on both physical and mental health. Coping strategies are culturally determined, and different cultural groups may display different approaches to coping with life's stress. Specific types of coping strategies have been linked to depression, with people who engage in emotion-focused coping more likely to exhibit depression than those who use task-oriented coping strategies. One study among youth, for example, found that substance use, emotional coping, and aggressive behavior as strategies for coping with anger were associated with an increased incidence of depression, but physical activity as a coping mechanism decreased depression risk (Goodwin, 2006). Negative thinking has been associated with an increased risk of depression in low-income single mothers (Peden, Rayens, Hall, & Grant, 2005). Negative thinking also mediated the relationship between low self-esteem and depression in these women (Peden, Rayens, Hall, & Grant, 2004). Other personal traits that increase the risk for depression include excessive worry and a sense of little control over one's life (NIMH, 2005a).

Some clients with mental health problems may turn to substance use or abuse as a coping strategy, which may contribute to the potential for dual diagnosis. Other clients may engage in other, more or less adaptive coping strategies for dealing with stress or with symptoms. Research has indicated, for example, that clients with schizophrenia have fairly well developed

BUILDING OUR KNOWLEDGE BASE

Stress is an acknowledged factor in the development of many mental health problems, including depression. Stress may also arise within the context of nursing education and practice. How would you conduct a study to examine the effects of specific types of coping behaviors used by nursing students on the incidence of depression in this population? What implications might your findings have, if any, for the development of depression in other populations?

coping skills for controlling their symptoms. Some of these coping strategies are healthier than others and can be encouraged by community health nurses working with clients with schizophrenia and their families. One category of coping skill displayed by schizophrenic clients dealt with behavior control by means of passive or active distraction (e.g., listening to music or reading versus playing an instrument or writing poetry), rest or physical activity (e.g., running), or indulgence (e.g., eating, drinking, or smoking). Other coping strategies included socializing with and talking to others, avoiding thinking about or ignoring misperceptions, shifting one's attention to other thoughts, engaging in future planning or problem solving, seeking medical care, prayer, and acceptance of symptoms. One final strategy, symptomatic behavior (e.g., telling voices to "shut up" or doing as told by voices) is a less healthy approach to dealing with symptoms of schizophrenia (Kingdon & Turkington, 2004).

Suicide Potential

Both the stress that contributes to the development of mental disorders and the hopelessness often associated with having a mental disorder place clients at increased risk for suicide, and community health nurses must be particularly alert to evidence of suicidal ideation in clients with mental health problems. Depression, in particular, whether due to major depressive, unipolar, or bipolar disorder or to situational factors, increases the potential for suicide (NIMH, 2000, 2001c). Suicide risk is also increased among people with schizophrenia (NIMH, 2005b). The nurse should explore with the client any suicidal tendencies or thoughts of suicide. Suicide tends to occur most frequently when clients are recovering from an episode of depression; this is because the severely depressed client probably does not have the energy to commit suicide. Suicide is addressed in more depth in Chapter 32∞.

Characteristic Manifestations of Selected Mental Health Problems

In their work with individual and family clients in the community, community health nurses are in a position to identify people with signs and symptoms suggestive of mental health problems. To effectively identify those individuals with problems, community health nurses

TABLE 30-1 Characteristic Features and Symptoms of Selected Mental Health Problems

Condition	Characteristic Features and Symptoms
Anxiety disorders ■ Panic disorder ■ Obsessive-compulsive disorder ■ Post-traumatic stress disorder (PTSD) ■ Phobias ■ General anxiety disorder	Features: Overall, occur in 1.3% of adults (phobias 8%, PTSD 3.6%, generalized anxiety disorder 2.8%, obsessive-compulsive disorder 2.3%, panic disorder 1.7%); create chronic overwhelming fear and anxiety Symptoms: ■ Feelings of fear/dread ■ Trembling, restlessness ■ Muscle tension ■ Rapid heart rate ■ Dizziness, lightheadedness ■ Increased perspiration ■ Cold hands and feet ■ Shortness of breath Treatment: Antidepressants (selective serotonin uptake inhibitors, benzodiazepines, beta-blockers), behavioral and cognitive behavioral therapy
Attention deficit hyperactivity disorder(ADHD)	Features: Affects 4.1% of 9- to 17-year-olds in a 6-month period; affects two to three times more boys than girls Symptoms: Inability to attend to a task to completion or to sit still; impulsivity Treatment: Controlled with medication (stimulants), behavior modification
Autism spectrum disorders (ASD) ■ Autistic disorder ■ Asperger syndrome ■ Rett syndrome ■ Childhood disintegrative disorder	Features: Autistic disorder affects 3 to 4 of every 1,000 children ages 3 to 10 years; may be seen as early as 18 months; others are much less frequent Symptoms: Deficits in social interaction and verbal and nonverbal communication, repetitive behaviors or interests, unusual response to sensory stimulation, delayed development Treatment: Variable, but applied behavior analysis has shown some promise, special education
Bipolar disorder	Features: Affects 2.6% of people over age 18 each year; typically develops in late adolescence; usually involves cycles through mania and depression but both may occur simultaneously in some people Symptoms: ■ Depressive stage: see *Special Considerations* box listing signs and symptoms of depression; diagnosis is based on the presence of five or more symptoms most of the time for 2 weeks or longer ■ Manic stage: see *Special Considerations* box listing signs and symptoms of mania; diagnosis is based on the presence of three or more symptoms most of the time for a week or longer Treatment: Mood stabilizers, counseling
Borderline personality disorder (BPD)	Features: Pervasive instability in moods and relationships Symptoms: Chronic instability of moods with intense anger, depression, and anxiety lasting only hours; may be accompanied by periodic aggression, self-injury, or substance abuse; frequent changes in life goals and plans; impulsivity Treatment: Group and individual psychotherapy, dialectical behavior therapy
Depression	Features: Affects 9.5% of U.S. adults Symptoms: see *Special Considerations* box listing signs and symptoms of depression Treatment: Antidepressants, counseling, stress management, and coping skills enhancement
Eating disorders ■ Anorexia nervosa ■ Binge eating ■ Bulimia nervosa	Features: Serious disturbance in eating behavior and perceptions of self; affects women far more often than men (anorexia nervosa—0.5% to 3.7% of women, bulimia—1.1% to 4.2% of women, binge eating—2% to 5% of U.S. adults) Symptoms: Intense fear of gaining weight; altered body image; infrequent menses; recurrent and uncontrolled eating followed by purging; misuse of laxatives, diuretics, enemas Treatment: Restoration to normal body weight, counseling for altered body image
Schizophrenia	Features: Affects 1% of the population worldwide; usually occurs in men in late teens and early twenties and mid-twenties to early thirties in women; rarely occurs before puberty or after age 45 Symptoms: Positive, negative, and cognitive symptoms of psychoses (see *Special Considerations* box listing signs and symptoms) Treatment: Antipsychotic medications, counseling

Data from: *National Institute of Mental Health, 2000; 2001a; 2001b; 2001c; 2001d; 2001e; 2004; 2005. (See References at the end of this chapter for full citations.)*

need to be conversant with signs and symptoms typical of the most commonly encountered mental disorders. Some of the signs and symptoms of serious mental illnesses were discussed earlier; others are included in Table 30-1◆. The fourth edition (text revised) of the *Diagnostic and Statistical Manual of Mental Disorders*

(DSM-IV-TR) of the American Psychiatric Association (2000) contains additional information on diagnostic criteria for major psychiatric illnesses. Signs and symptoms of substance abuse disorders are addressed in Chapter 31∞. Possible questions to assist community health nurses in identifying psychological factors

contributing to community mental health problems are included in the focused assessment below.

Physical Environmental Considerations

Physical environmental factors influence the development and course of some mental health problems. Chronic exposure to lead and other toxins may cause mental retardation and other forms of mental illness. For example, exposure to arsenic in well water has been associated with increased risk of depression in some populations (Zierold, Knobeloch, & Anderson, 2004). Evidence also suggests that schizophrenia may be triggered by neurotropic virus infections, anoxia, and radiation exposures in the environment (Flaskerud, 2000). Similarly, rehospitalization for serious mental illness has been associated with increased population density. Possible explanations for this association might be greater familiarity with the client and earlier identification of behavior changes preceding relapse by family and friends in areas of low population density or the increased stress that accompanies increased population density (Husted & Jorgens, 2000).

Seasonal changes may also contribute to mental health problems, as in the case of seasonal affective disorder. **Seasonal affective disorder (SAD)** is a form of depression that varies with the seasons, resulting in depression in the fall and winter when exposure to natural light is diminished and euthymia (positive mood) in spring and summer when natural light is more abundant (National Mental Health Association, 2006). The incidence of SAD increases at higher latitudes, and some people with SAD may experience a degree of mania in spring or summer (Watkins, 2002). People who work in enclosed environments without windows may experience symptoms at any time. A milder form of seasonal depression, called *winter blues*, is usually reduced with exercise and outdoor activity (Seasonal Affective Disorder, 2006). The occurrence of SAD may be mediated by cultural factors. In northern Norway, for example, which has extreme seasonal changes, SAD is uncommon. Possible explanations include cultural perceptions

that the changes in season are important, seasonal celebrations that promote connectedness with others, and rituals that assist one in coping with seasonal changes (Stuhlmiller, 1998). Physical environmental considerations in mental health problems are addressed in the focused assessment provided below.

Sociocultural Considerations

A number of sociocultural dimension factors influence risk for and treatment of mental health problems. These factors include societal disorganization, social and economic factors, family relationships, social support, culture, and societal attitudes to mental illness. As noted in Chapter 27∞, social upheaval such as war and disaster increases the incidence of mental health problems in the populations affected, particularly when the effects are long-lasting. Immigration, which may result from social upheaval, has also been linked with a high incidence of mental disorders (Frangou & Murray, 2000). Research has suggested that the coping strategies used by immigrants influence their psychological response to immigration. Immigrants who engaged in social, cultural, and country-related activities (e.g., interacting with other immigrants or with people in the host country through work, clubs, education, or information seeking about the new country) were able to adapt to immigration more successfully than those who used solitary strategies (e.g., reading, keeping busy, crafts) (Ward & Styles, 2005).

Mental health problems are also influenced by more contained social events. For example, the risk of depression increases with recent divorce or separation, unemployment, and bereavement. Inability to work and stresses associated with low income have also been associated with mental illness, as have overcrowding and living in an area with a high rate of disorganization.

Economic and employment factors may also influence one's mental status. For example, higher job status and job security have been linked to lower risk of depression in some populations. Recognition, adequate remuneration, and opportunity for socialization in the work setting have also been associated with decreased incidence of depression. Conversely, job-related conflict, higher physical demands on the job, and hazardous working conditions have been associated with greater

---

FOCUSED ASSESSMENT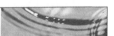

Psychological Considerations in Mental Health Problems

- What life stresses is the client experiencing? Does stress contribute to or exacerbate mental health problems? How does the client cope with stress?
- What signs and symptoms does the client exhibit that suggest the presence of mental health problems?
- What is the extent of adaptation to the mental health problem? How does the client cope with the problem?
- Is there existing psychiatric comorbidity? If so, what form does it take?
- Is the client at risk for suicide as a result of the mental health problem?

FOCUSED ASSESSMENT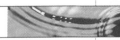

Physical Environmental Considerations in Mental Health Problems

- Are there seasonal fluctuations in the incidence or severity of particular mental health problems? If so, when do these fluctuations occur?
- Do environmental pollutants contribute to the incidence of mental health problems?

risk of depression. Similarly, the need to take an oppositional stance from coworkers and performing physically uncomfortable jobs have been found to increase the risk of depression in employees (Zimmerman, Christakis, & Vander Stoep, 2004).

With respect to economic factors, in 2002 and 2003 people living in poverty were nearly five times more likely to report serious psychological distress than the nonpoor. In addition, the near poor were three times more likely than the nonpoor to report serious distress. When poverty and race are considered together, poor Whites were more likely than poor African Americans or Hispanics to report distress (NCHS, 2005a).

Social mobility may also affect risk of mental health problems. For instance, in one study, families living in public housing in high-poverty areas that moved to low-poverty areas demonstrated less mental distress than those who remained in high-poverty areas. This finding was particularly true for young boys. In addition, there is evidence that neighborhood income levels as well as individual and family income influence mental health (Leventhal & Brooks-Gunn, 2003).

Family interactions may also influence the development and course of mental health problems. For example, research has linked schizophrenia with hereditary communication difficulties with one's parents, which compounds the disorientation experienced by the client with schizophrenia (Wuerker, 2000). High parental levels of expressed emotion conveying criticism, hostility, or stifling overinvolvement have been shown to be linked to relapse in clients with schizophrenia. High levels of negative emotional expression have also been associated with anorexia nervosa and depression. Conversely, warmth and positive family relationships may have a protective effect against mental health problems or assist family members to cope more effectively when problems do occur (Frangou & Murray, 2000).

Social support may assist clients to cope with the stresses of life and prevent mental health problems. Lack of social support, on the other hand, may increase the risk of mental illness, contributing to the feelings of isolation and poor social skills common among people with mental health problems.

The effects of culture on mental health are many and pervasive. Culture defines what constitutes mental illness for members of a group, and that definition may not always conform to the diagnostic criteria established in the *DSM-IV-TR*. What may be seen as abnormal behavior or feelings in one culture may be perfectly normal in another. Similarly, culture mediates one's experience of distress and how one expresses that distress. Culture, for example, creates what are known as "idioms of distress" or typical ways of expressing mental discomfort. In many cultural groups, for example, mental distress is expressed in terms of somatization (Liang, 2004). **Somatization** is the expression of mental or emotional distress in terms of physical symptoms.

Diagnostic criteria contained in the *DSM-IV-TR* are based on Western Anglo experience, and it is unclear how applicable diagnostic criteria are to members of other cultural groups. Some cultures also have recognized culture-bound syndromes generally reflecting concepts of mental illness that are culture-specific and fall outside Western psychiatric practice. Culture-bound syndromes were discussed in Chapter 9∞.

Cultural differences in diagnostic criteria, expressions of distress, and meanings and value attributed to different symptoms may result in misdiagnosis in cross-cultural encounters. Language barriers between provider and client also increase the potential for misdiagnosis, as do diagnostic measurements that are not linguistically or culturally sensitive (Flaskerud, 2000).

Culture also influences expectations regarding treatment that may enhance or impede compliance with therapy. Members of many cultural groups engage in the use of herbal remedies. For this reason, they may expect psychotropic medications to act rapidly, as most herbals do. The need to build effective blood levels of medications may be difficult for clients in these cultural groups to understand. Inability to see immediate results may lead to discontinuation of pharmacotherapy. Herbal therapies may also interact with prescription medications to impede or enhance their effects, contributing to therapeutic ineffectiveness or adverse reactions to medications (Flaskerud, 2000).

Culture also contributes to the way people view mental illness and to the degree of stigmatization encountered by those who experience mental illness. Stigmatization is characterized by bias, distrust, stereotyping, fear, embarrassment, anger, and avoidance. Stigmatization has the effect of reducing willingness to seek help and thereby reduces access to needed care. For example, personal and family perceptions of stigma attached to mental illness have been shown to reduce help-seeking for adolescents with depression (Draucker, 2005).

The response to perceived stigma is mediated by culture. For example, Asian Americans and Pacific Islanders are three times less likely to use mental health services than other ethnic groups (Spencer & Chen, 2004), often as a result of perceived stigma or because of perceived incongruence between group cultures and the Western mental health care system (Liang, 2004). Cultural barriers to obtaining mental health services include racial and cultural biases and inappropriate services, philosophical differences regarding disease causation or treatment, cultural attitudes to help seeking, language barriers, a lack of bilingual and culturally sensitive providers, and clients' lack of knowledge about available services. Clients from ethnic cultural groups may also be subjected to *language discrimination*, being treated unfairly because of language differences or accented speech. These barriers led, in one study, to a twofold increase in the propensity to seek help from

CULTURAL COMPETENCE

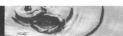

You are seeing Su-Chen, a 20-year-old single Chinese American woman who lives with her parents. Su-Chen is being treated for schizophrenia at the local mental health clinic after a referral from the student health center at the community college where she is enrolled. You have been asked to visit her because she has not been keeping appointments at the clinic. When you arrive at the home, Su-Chen tells you that her father will not allow her to continue to be seen at the clinic because he is afraid that their neighbors will find out that she is mentally ill. She is doing well and is free of symptoms at present, but she is almost out of her medications. The clinic will not authorize a refill unless she is seen by the provider. What cultural factors are operating in this situation? To what extent are these factors typical of traditional Chinese culture? How might acculturation affect the influence of these factors for another Chinese American woman? How will you address Su-Chen's needs?

informal caregivers, friends, and family rather than from professional mental health agencies (Spencer & Chen, 2004).

Stigmatization of the mentally ill may also decrease their access to needed resources and opportunities, such as those related to employment or housing. For the individual, stigma leads to low self-esteem, hopelessness, and social isolation. Clients with mental illness are faced with the same kinds of decisions regarding disclosure that were discussed in the context of chronic physical health problems in Chapter 29∞. At the population level, stigmatization influences public willingness to pay for services for the mentally ill or to locate treatment facilities in residential neighborhoods.

Stigma and the discrimination that results from belonging to a stigmatized group may also contribute to mental health problems. In one study, for example, workers who reported unfair treatment based on ethnicity or who were subjected to racial insults had higher risks for mental health disorders than those who did not experience discrimination (Bhui et al., 2005). Similarly, as we saw in Chapters 17 and 18∞, the stigma attached to nonheterosexual orientation has been associated with higher rates of suicide and depression.

A history of victimization has also been linked to mental illness. For example, in one study people with anxiety disorders had experienced more sexual assaults than those without illness. Similarly, people with schizophreniform disorders were subjected to more threatened and actual physical assaults than those without mental disorders (Silver, Arsenault, Langley, Caspi, & Moffitt, 2005).

Other evidence of societal attitudes toward mental illness lies in the number of the mentally ill who are incarcerated in correctional facilities. Mental illness may contribute to unlawful behaviors or to incarceration as an alternative to mental health care. For example, as many as three fourths of juvenile detainees exhibit one or

more psychiatric disorders (Teplin, Abram, McClelland, Washburn, & Pikus, 2005). Many of these youth are not guilty of any offense, but have been placed in juvenile justice systems for lack of any other means of obtaining care for mental health problems (Institute of Medicine [IOM], 2006). Similarly, an estimated 16% of state prison inmates have serious mental illness or have been previously hospitalized for a psychiatric condition (Hills, Siegfried, & Ickowitz, 2004). Although people with mental illness are often perceived as violent, research indicates that only a small percentage of this population actually engages in violent behaviors, and that violence is related to past victimization, substance abuse, and violence in the environment (Swanson et al., 2002). As noted in Chapter 26∞, correctional institutions are mandated to provide treatment for mental illness (unless refused by the client); however, there are few follow-up programs that ensure continuity of care on release. Focused assessment questions related to sociocultural dimension factors contributing to community mental health problems are provided below.

FOCUSED ASSESSMENT

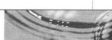

Sociocultural Considerations in Mental Health Problems

- What are the effects of mental health problems on social interactions (with family and others)?
- What are societal attitudes to the problem? Do they hamper control efforts?
- Is there social stigma attached to having the problem? What effect does stigma have on clients' willingness to seek care?
- What effect, if any, do cultural beliefs and behaviors have on mental health problems?
- Does the mental health problem contribute to the risk of homelessness for the client?
- What social support systems are available to persons with the mental health problem?
- How do social factors (e.g., unemployment) influence mental health problems?
- How does the mental health problem affect community members' ability to work?

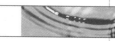

Behavioral Considerations

Personal behaviors also influence the development and course of mental health problems, but it is often difficult to determine the direction of influence. In some studies, for example, people with depression reported less physical activity, more smoking, more binge drinking, and higher rates of obesity than those without depression (Daniel et al., 2005). Depressed mood has also been found to predict initiation of marijuana use (Kelder et al., 2001). In other studies, depression has been linked to substance abuse and smoking. Major depressive disorders were three to four times more common among drug abusers than among nonabusers, and the extent of substance abuse and major depressive disorder comorbidity has been shown to be 20% to 30%, with depression antedating substance abuse by an average of 4.5 years (Kelder et al., 2001).

Physical activity and sexual activity are two other behavioral considerations in an assessment of mental health problems. For example, clients with mental illness have been shown to be less physically active and have a greater risk for obesity than those without illness. Barriers to physical activity among the mentally ill include symptoms of illness and apathy to other activities, medications and resulting weight gain, fear of discrimination, and safety concerns for those living in urban neighborhoods (McDevitt, Snyder, Miller, & Wilbur, 2006).

Sexual activity is an area that is often ignored in the care of clients with mental illness, and attention should be given to meeting sexual needs as well as to assessing high-risk sexual behaviors that may be exhibited by some mentally ill individuals. Sexuality issues are complicated by possible links with childhood sexual abuse, the sexual content of positive symptoms in clients with schizophrenia, sexual disinhibition in some conditions, and medication side effects such as diminished libido and disabling extrapyramidal effects that promote distancing and social isolation by other people. Use of safe sexual practices and contraception are other sexual behaviors that should be assessed (McCann, 2000). The focused assessment provided above right addresses behavioral dimension factors contributing to community mental health problems.

Health System Considerations

A report by the National Council on Disability (2002) noted that the use of the term *mental health system* with respect to care for mental health problems "is itself problematic. One of the primary problems is that states do not have a single system of mental health care, but a number of patchwork systems that are called upon to provide such care, often without a guiding vision of how to do so most effectively and frequently without the funding to actually deliver services and support to every eligible person" (p. 4). Mental health care actually

FOCUSED ASSESSMENT

Behavioral Considerations in Mental Health Problems

- Does alcohol or drug use influence the problem or its effects? Are alcohol or drugs used in an effort to self-manage symptoms?
- What effect, if any, does exercise have on the problem?
- Does smoking influence the problem?
- What effect does the problem have on self-care behaviors?

occurs in four arenas: the general medical or primary care sector, the specialty mental health care sector, the social services sector, and the volunteer support network sector (McLeer, 2004), all of which appear to be inadequate to meet the need for care. For example, in 2003, less than two thirds of children with definite or severe emotional or behavioral problems received mental health care from a mental health professional or general physician or through special education services (NCHS, 2005b). Similarly, from 2001 to 2003, only 40.5% of people in need of treatment for identified severe mental illness received care (IOM, 2006).

Mental health care has been perceived by some as improving over the last few years. In part, these improvements are credited to new, more effective medications with fewer side effects, the use of evidence-based practice guidelines, and changes in public attitudes toward mental health problems. However, in some segments of the population, access to services has declined as a result of the loss of public psychiatric hospital beds, Medicaid disenrollment, and increasing costs of care. Based on National Health Interview Survey data, for example, although the percentage of people receiving care from mental health professionals increased between 1997 and 2002, the percentage of people who did not receive care or medications due to cost also increased (Mojtabai, 2005). Other authors have noted that while access to mental health care has improved for people with serious mental illness, access for those with less serious conditions has actually decreased (Mechanic & Bilder, 2004).

A report by the Institute of Medicine (2006) indicated that many providers do not adhere to established clinical practice guidelines for such conditions as ADHD, anxiety disorders, dual diagnoses, depression, and schizophrenia. For example, in one study of general practitioners in Scotland and England, some providers did not adhere to depression guidelines because they did not agree with them and felt they were too rigid to permit application to a variety of clients. Other concerns voiced by providers included the number of guidelines received and the lack of time and resources needed for their effective implementation (e.g., lack of access to mental health professionals for referral) (Smith, Walker, & Gilhooly, 2004). A similar lack of adherence to treatment guidelines for schizophrenia and depression has been

GLOBAL PERSPECTIVES

Over the last few years, many Latin American countries have privatized many health care services, including mental health services. From 1952 until the 1980s, for example, Chile had a publicly funded national health service that provided universal health care coverage for its population. In the 1980s, however, legislation was passed to encourage development of private health insurance plans under which workers could choose to allocate their mandatory insurance contribution to public or private health care coverage. Many of the wealthier members of the population chose the private insurance system, depriving the public system of revenues from high-wage earners and leading to disparities in mental health care services between rich and poor segments of the population. Subsequent research has indicated that people with public insurance coverage display the greatest need for mental health services but the lowest rates of service utilization (Araya, Rojas, Fritsch, Frank, & Lewis, 2006). Has privatization of mental health services contributed to similar effects in the United States? Why or why not?

noted in the United States. Use of guidelines was found to be more common among mental health specialty providers than among primary care providers (Mechanic & Bilder, 2004).

Other problems in the U.S. mental health care system identified by the IOM included medication errors; excessive use of restraints and seclusion, resulting in 150 deaths each year; and "failure to provide *any* treatment for M/SU (mental/substance use) illness . . . even when people are receiving other types of health care and have financial and geographic access to treatment" (IOM, 2006, p. 5). Additional system flaws identified in the report are coercion of clients into treatment, a poorly developed structure for assessing treatment outcomes, limited use of information technology to coordinate care, and an educationally diverse workforce (IOM, 2006). Based on the report, the IOM has made two over-arching recommendations for strengthening the mental health care system in the United States:

- Health care for general, mental, and substance abuse problems and illnesses must be delivered with an understanding of the inherent interactions between the mind/brain and the rest of the body.
- The aims, rules, and strategies for redesign set forth in *Crossing the Quality Chasm* should be applied throughout M/SU health care on a day-to-day operational basis but tailored to reflect the characteristics that distinguish care for these problems and illnesses from general health care. (Institute of Medicine, 2006, pp. 9–10)

Other, more specific recommendations include support for client decision making; lack of coercion; dissemination of evidence-based practice information; development of quality assessment instruments and outcome measures; better linkages between health care organizations, providers, and systems; and coordination

of health and social services to best meet client needs. In addition, mental health care should be addressed as fully as care for physical health problems, and the Congress and state legislatures should mandate standard health insurance benefits that improve mental health care coverage. Computer technology should be used to standardize billing and information processes, and attention should be given to developing an adequate mental health workforce. The full recommendations can be viewed at http://www.nap.edu/openbook/o309100445/html/2.html.

Lack of adequate mental health care is apparent in other areas of the world as well as the United States. A 2001 World Health Organization report, for example, estimated that 30% of countries lack mental health programs. In addition, 40% of the world's nations lack effective mental health policy (Carty, Al-Zayyer, Arietti, & Lester, 2004).

Effective mental health care does not necessarily mean care provided by mental health specialists. Both psychotherapy and pharmacologic therapy for mental illness have proved to be effective when provided in primary care settings. Few such settings are equipped to provide this care, however. Neither primary care nor specialty mental health services are well equipped to address the mental health needs of minority group members, and cultural biases on the part of providers may lead to under- or overdiagnosis as well as inappropriate treatment. Research does suggest, however, that primary care physicians who provide comprehensive care that addresses behavioral and other aspects of health as well as physical health are more likely than others to ask clients about depressive symptoms (O'Malley et al., 2003). Similarly, it has been suggested that oncology nurses could effectively manage depression in clients with cancer (Strong et al., 2004).

Health system bias against those with mental illness is also seen in the relative level of expenditures for mental health care as compared to those for physical health care. In 2002, per capita expenditures for mental health services in the United States amounted to $119, far less than those for physical health care and less than the peak spending of $128 per person in 1994 (NCHS, 2005a). In 2002, total Medicaid costs were $29.1 billion for general hospitalization, compared to only $2.1 billion for mental hospital costs. The number of nonfederal psychiatric hospital admissions increased from 2.5 per 1,000 population in 1980 to 2.6 in 2003, but the number of days of hospitalization decreased by more than two thirds from 295 to 91 days per 1,000 people (U.S. Census Bureau, 2006).

Lack of insurance coverage for mental health impedes access to care. This lack of coverage is based on several assumptions: (a) mental health service costs are uncontrollable and unpredictable, (b) insurance coverage leads to unnecessary use of mental health services, (c) mental health care is not cost-effective, and (d) psychiatric treatment is not accountable enough to insurers

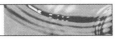

FOCUSED ASSESSMENT

Health System Considerations in Mental Health Problems

- What are the attitudes of health care providers to persons with mental health problems?
- Are health care providers alert to signs and symptoms of mental health problems?
- What treatment facilities are available to persons with mental health problems? How adequate are they? What types of therapy are available? How effective are they?
- Are diagnostic and treatment services available and accessible to persons with mental health problems?
- Does the client exhibit treatment side effects or adverse effects?
- Does treatment for other health problems cause or exacerbate the mental health problem?

(McLeer, 2004). Even when health insurance plans do cover mental health services, coverage is usually extremely limited and may include a lifetime limit on services provided. Community health nurses can be actively involved in political advocacy to reduce the disparities in insurance coverage for mental health services vis-à-vis physical health care. For example, they can campaign for state legislation making parity in mental health and physical health care coverage a state-mandated health insurance benefit. In addition, they can influence federal legislators to make similar changes in the Medicare and Medicaid programs.

One additional aspect of the health system that may influence mental illness recovery is the unintended effect of legitimizing the sick role and justifying a nonworking identity. Some authors, for example, have found that a diagnosis of depression may become an integral element in the self-identity of some clients, deterring a return to work even when the person is free of symptoms. These findings highlight the need to consider the meaning that a psychiatric diagnosis has for the individual and its significance in his or her life, particularly as it relates to employment (Millward, Lutte, & Purvis, 2005).

Tips for assessing health system factors influencing risk for mental health problems are presented in the focused assessment above. A tool for assessing the broad range of factors contributing to community mental health problems is included in the *Community Assessment Reference Guide* designed to accompany this text.

COMMUNITY HEALTH NURSING AND CONTROL OF MENTAL HEALTH PROBLEMS

As noted earlier, community health nurses may play a significant part in the control of mental health problems with individuals and with population groups. Effective control includes assessment of risks for and factors influencing mental health problems, as well as the planning, implementation, and evaluation of health care programs directed toward mental health.

Assessing Community Mental Health Status

Factors in each of the six dimensions of health influence the risk for and course of mental health problems for individuals and for communities. Community health nurses will be actively involved in assessing for these risks as well as for the presence of mental illness in individual clients and in the population as a whole. For example, community health nurses would assess the incidence and prevalence of specific mental health problems in the community by examining admission records of local mental health facilities. They might also examine police records of arrests for bizarre behavior or conduct surveys among the general public or targeted subgroups (e.g., youth or the elderly) to determine the prevalence of conditions such as depression. They would also examine the contribution of factors in the biophysical, psychological, physical environmental, sociocultural, behavioral, and health system dimensions that are contributing to mental health problems in the community.

In the biophysical dimension, information about the prevalence of chronic debilitating physical health problems in the community may help to identify people at risk for mental health problems. Such information might be available from local health department statistics or admission data for local health care facilities. Disease registries for conditions such as cancer may also help to determine the prevalence of some chronic conditions in the population. Absence data for schools or businesses might also shed light on the prevalence of chronic health problems in the community. Similarly, exploration of the effect of seasonal changes on the incidence of depressive episodes can assist nurses and others to plan effective strategies to deal with these seasonal effects. Again, admission information from local mental health facilities can help to identify trends in seasonal admissions.

Information about social sources of stress such as interracial conflict, violence, and unemployment can also identify factors contributing to mental illness in the community that are amenable to intervention. Social attitudes toward mental illness and their effect on treatment should also be explored. The nurse can survey community members or interview knowledgeable community informants to obtain information on attitudes toward mental health problems. Information on unemployment, poverty, and other social conditions can be obtained from local governments or census data for local census tracts. Police records and local newspapers can serve as sources of information on interracial conflict and violence in the community.

In the behavioral dimension, information about the incidence and prevalence of substance use and abuse can suggest the presence of dual diagnoses in the population and inform control strategies for both substance abuse and mental illness. The community health nurse would also determine the availability of mental health services in the community and the extent to which different segments of the community have access to those services. These data can be obtained from local treatment facilities as well as from other health care providers in the area. Community surveys may also provide information on insurance coverage and access to mental health services.

At the individual client level, the community health nurse would assess clients for evidence of mental health problems and for individual characteristics and circumstances that may be contributing to mental health difficulties. For example, the nurse might identify poor coping skills, unemployment, or family dysfunction as factors contributing to depression in a particular client.

Diagnostic Reasoning and Community Mental Health Problems

Community health nurses may make a variety of nursing diagnoses related to mental health problems. These diagnoses can reflect the health needs of an individual client, the client's family, or a population group. For example, the nurse might diagnose "impaired reality orientation due to schizophrenic episode" in an individual client or an "exacerbation of depression due to family stress." Another nursing diagnosis at this level might reflect "disruption of family function due to exhibition of symptoms of schizophrenia" on the part of one member.

Nursing diagnoses may also be made that reflect mental health problems affecting population groups. For example, the community health nurse might diagnose an "increased incidence of schizophrenia in the homeless population" or "inadequate treatment facilities for persons with chronic mental health problems due to reduced program funds."

Planning and Implementing Control Strategies for Community Mental Health Problems

The surgeon general's report on mental health (U.S. Public Health Service [USPHS], 1999) made several recommendations with respect to mental health care in the United States. These recommendations included the need to reduce the stigma attached to mental illness, improve public awareness of the availability of effective treatment for most mental health problems, assure the supply of providers and services for those in need, and ensure the use of state-of-the-art treatments. Additional recommendations addressed the need to tailor treatment to the age, gender, race, and culture of those

affected; to facilitate early entry into treatment; and to reduce financial barriers to treatment (USPHS, 1999). Although these recommendations were made a number of years ago, they remain relevant to efforts to control community mental health problems, and community health nurses can be actively involved in efforts to address these recommendations.

A 1994 study by the Institute of Medicine suggested that the public health concepts of primary, secondary, and tertiary prevention are not helpful in dealing with mental health problems and recommended that the concept of prevention be reserved for interventions designed to prevent a health problem from occurring (Mrazek & Haggerty, 1994). Difficulties also arise in the application of the secondary prevention elements of diagnosis and screening. Diagnosis of mental disorders is difficult in the absence of objectively verifiable signs of disease and specific diagnostic tests and the need to rely on subjective information from clients. In addition, the definitions of psychiatric disorders change over time, making diagnosis even more difficult. Also, there are few screening procedures for mental disorders, although some screening tools have been developed for identifying persons with depression. For this reason, the concepts of primary, secondary, and tertiary prevention, as used in other chapters of this book, have been recast as *prevention*, *treatment*, and *maintenance*. In this conceptualization, *prevention* is similar to primary prevention and involves preventing the occurrence of mental health problems. *Treatment* encompasses the identification and standard treatment of persons with mental illness or mental health problems, including prevention of co-occurring disorders. *Maintenance* incorporates some elements of secondary and tertiary prevention such as ongoing treatment and monitoring treatment effects. Each of these three levels of care will be discussed here.

Prevention

Prevention of mental health problems and mental disorders involves both promotion of protective factors and reduction of risk factors and is congruent with the concept of primary prevention as discussed elsewhere in this book. **Mental health promotion** has been defined as "the process of enhancing the capacity of individuals and communities to take control over their lives and improve their mental health. Mental health promotion uses strategies that foster supportive environments and individual resilience, while showing respect for equity, social justice, interconnections, and personal dignity" (Center for Health Promotion, quoted in Willinsky & Pape, 2002, p. 163). The goal of mental health promotion is to "increase people's ability to deal with life's challenges" (Willinksy & Pape, 2002, p. 167). Promotion of coping abilities and resilience can help prevent the development of mental health problems. **Resilience** is the ability to withstand chronic stress or to recover from traumatic and stressful events. Community health nurses can assist individual clients to develop coping skills that will increase their resilience in the face of adversity. In addition, nurses can be instrumental in developing programs that promote coping in school, work, or other settings. For example, an intervention aimed at reducing negative thinking reduced depressive symptoms in low-income single mothers with multiple stressors (Peden et al., 2005). Community health nurses might also organize stress management education programs as part of a school health curriculum or in a work setting.

Community health nurses are also actively involved in risk-reduction efforts. The support provided to clients with mental distress and efforts to ameliorate or eliminate sources of stress may prevent the occurrence of mental health problems. Community health nurses can assist individuals and families to identify sources of stress and plan strategies to eliminate or minimize them. For example, referral for financial assistance may alleviate economic stresses that can contribute to depression. The nurse may also refer clients experiencing situational stressors such as divorce or care of a chronically ill family member to support groups to help them deal with stress. Assisting clients and families to expand social support networks may also prevent mental health problems.

Community health nurses can also assist clients with chronic physical health problems to cope effectively with their illnesses and refer them for counseling when they are experiencing adjustment difficulties. Referral for family counseling may also help to prevent mental health problems arising out of poor family dynamics. Families can also be assisted by community health nurses to develop communication and interaction patterns that promote the mental health of family members.

At the population level, community health nurses can advocate for societal conditions that minimize stress and promote mental health. They can assist communities to identify and develop strategies to address existing sources of stress for community members. For example, community health nurses in one community were actively involved with other community members in advocating for a local ordinance mandating a living wage for people working for organizations that received city contracts to minimize the stress of poverty.

Interventions may also be undertaken to prevent postpartum stress. Community health nurses often work with pregnant women, so they are in an ideal position to take steps to prevent PPD. Interventions that may help to prevent PPD include good nutrition, development of social support networks, exercise, discussion of and education about parenting expectations, promoting coping skills, and assisting parents to seek the help of others in dealing with other household tasks (Antares, 2005; Strayer, 2005). Community health nurses can also engage in campaigns to change public perceptions of "good parents" to incorporate more realistic parenting

expectations and to change policies that require women to return to work soon after delivery. Cultural pressures to regain one's figure may also lead to excessive dieting, nutritional imbalance, and increased risk for PPD. Women may also need to have avenues for processing feelings about perceived birth trauma, and community health nurses may help to create groups or programs that allow this processing to occur. Supportive home visits by health professionals (not lay personnel) have also been shown to be helpful in preventing PPD (RNAO, 2005), and community health nurses can advocate for and create home visiting programs for all mothers, not just those with high-risk infants, where such services do not exist. Research suggests that preventive interventions for PPD are most effective when initiated after delivery and that prenatal interventions show little effect (RNAO, 2005).

There is also a need to promote health in clients with existing mental health problems. For example, second-generation antipsychotic medications increase the risk of weight gain and metabolic disorder, and people taking these drugs for schizophrenia need primary preventive interventions to control weight, such as diet instruction and encouraging physical activity (Ohlsen, Peacock, & Smith, 2005). Community health nurses can educate clients regarding the effects of psychotropic drugs and assist them to minimize these effects through counseling and structured physical activity programs.

At the population level, clients with mental health problems should have access to routine health promotion services tailored to meet their needs. For example, walk-in services may be needed for clients who, because of cognitive or emotional deficits, have difficulty making or keeping appointments. Conversely, routine health promotion and illness prevention services (e.g., influenza immunization) could be provided in the context of mental health services to promote ease of access. Community health nurses can assist in the development of mental health services that address health promotion and illness prevention as well as therapy for mental illness. They can also advocate for accessible health promotion services for people with mental illness.

Treatment

Treatment in the context of mental illness is analogous to secondary prevention. Early entry into treatment for mental disorders requires identification of those in need of treatment. Although there are no specific screening examinations for most mental illnesses as there are for some communicable diseases or chronic physical health problems, two aspects of screening are important in identifying clients who are in need of and will benefit from mental health services. The first aspect of screening is a mental health evaluation that includes a client's psychiatric history, use of current psychotropic drugs, presence of suicidal ideation or suicide attempt, drug and alcohol use, and a history of sex offenses,

ETHICAL AWARENESS

Some people have suggested that because people with serious mental illness are at higher risk and have higher incidence rates for HIV infection, HIV testing should be routinely incorporated into admission procedures in mental health treatment facilities. The suggestion has also been made that testing occur without a requirement for informed consent on the part of the client (Walkup, Satriano, Barry, Sadler, & Cournos, 2002). The rationale for this position is that, because of their illness, people with serious mental illness are not capable of making an informed choice regarding testing and that protection of the clients themselves and the general public warrants involuntary testing. What do you think of this proposal? Can it be justified on ethical grounds? If so, what is the justification?

victimization, or violence. Additional components of the mental health evaluation for an individual client include a history of special education placement, history of traumatic brain injury, incarceration, and evidence of mental retardation (Hills et al., 2004).

The second aspect of screening is assessment of a client's motivation for treatment. Areas to be considered include perceptions of the seriousness of mental health problems, desire for and perceived importance of treatment, and past attempts at treatment and their effects (Hills et al., 2004). Theories of motivation for change are discussed in Chapter 31 ∞ in the context of substance abuse. Once community health nurses have identified people in need of and desiring assistance with mental health problems, they can help them find appropriate treatment services. Treatment goals have been developed for treatment of depression in the elderly that can be adapted to treatment of other mental health problems in other populations (Antai-Otong, 2004). The first goal is to reduce suicide risk. For other conditions this goal might also encompass prevention of other personal and societal effects of mental health problems. The second goal is to improve the client's level of function, and the third goal is to improve the client's (and family's) quality of life.

Depression is one mental health condition for which screening tools are available, and community health nurses can use them to screen individuals for depression. They should make sure that any screening tools used are culturally and age appropriate to the populations with which they are used. For example, the best-practice guidelines for postpartum depression developed by the Registered Nurses Association of Ontario (2005) recommended the use of the Edinburgh Postnatal Depression Scale (EPDS) to identify mothers with postpartum depression. The EPDS has been shown to accurately identify women experiencing PPD and consists of a 10-item scale completed by the client. Use of the EPDS has been recommended as part of routine well-child visits to identify mothers who are experiencing

PPD (Freeman et al., 2005). The tool does not seem to be effective in screening for PPD in men because it does not address the symptoms of anxiety typically exhibited by men experiencing psychological distress (Strayer, 2005).

Projective drawings are another strategy that has been suggested for screening for mental health problems in children. One strategy employs the Human Figure Drawing (HFD) approach developed by Elizabeth Koppitz in which the child is asked to draw a picture of a person. Evaluation of the drawing centers on the inclusion of features appropriate to the child's developmental level and emotional indicators that suggest something about the child's feelings and perceptions. Interpretation of emotional indicators has been validated in a number of studies and has been shown to be valid and reliable as a basic screening to indicate children who are in need of further assessment. Like all screening tools, results are not intended to confirm a diagnosis of a mental health problem (Tielsch & Allen, 2005).

Community health nurses should be knowledgeable about and alert to signs and symptoms of mental illness. They can also educate the general public regarding signs and symptoms of conditions such as depression to promote self-screening or recognition of problems in friends or family members. Community health nurses also need to be conversant with the kinds of services available to the individual client and within the population. When appropriate services are not available, community health nursing intervention may focus on advocacy and assurance of access to needed services. For example, community health nurses may campaign for legislation to include mental health treatment as a mandatory health insurance benefit in their state or to eliminate time limits and other constraints on existing coverage.

Effective referral for services for clients in need of them requires that community health nurses have an understanding of the process of help seeking in mental illness identified in the 1999 publication *Mental Health: A Report of the Surgeon General* (USPHS, 1999). This process begins with the recognition of a problem and the determination that the problem is serious enough to seek care. The determination is then made as to the possible origin of the problem as either physical or mental in nature. At this point, the person needs to decide whether to seek help and, if so, where help should be sought. The decision to seek care is then followed by activities to obtain care. Once care has been obtained, there is the further decision of whether to continue with care or to adhere to care recommendations. Community health nurses may assist clients in making decisions throughout the process, as indicated in Table 30-2◆.

The 1999 surgeon general's report on mental illness in the United States stressed the availability of effective treatment for the majority of mental health problems and noted that, in many cases, clients have multiple options for treatment (USPHS, 1999). In general,

TABLE 30-2	Stages of the Help-Seeking Process and Related Community Health Nursing Interventions
Stage	**Possible Interventions**
Problem recognition	Inform client of problems observed by the nurse.
	Educate client regarding normal and abnormal findings.
Determination of seriousness	Review with the client the effects of the problem on client's life, family interactions, etc.
Determination of nature of problem as physical or mental	Explore the meaning of symptoms from the client's perspective.
	Explore with the client alternative explanations of the problem.
Choice to seek or not seek care	Review with the client possible consequences of seeking or not seeking care.
Choice to continue or not continue care	Review with the client probable consequences of continuing or not continuing care.

treatment for mental health problems is more cost-effective than nontreatment. Treatment can result in effectiveness rates comparable to those achieved for physical health problems such as heart disease. For example, angioplasty or atherectomy have success rates at or below 50%, comparable to those for serious mental health disorders such as schizophrenia, bipolar disorder, major depression, obsessive-compulsive disorder, and panic disorder (NAMI, 2002).

Not treating mental illness, on the other hand, poses significant costs for society. For example, people with mental illness are less likely than the general population to be insured, leading to poor access to health care for physical health conditions and more costly care when services are finally obtained. Similarly, lack of psychiatric inpatient beds and insufficient capacity of psychiatric emergency departments (EDs) lead to the extended use of general EDs by clients with psychiatric problems, resulting in costly care that could be provided with less expense in other settings. In addition, psychiatric treatment could prevent thousands of nonviolent crimes that are clogging the nation's criminal courts and jails and costing taxpayers an average of $9 billion each year. An additional cost of failing to treat people with mental health problems lies in school dropout rates and diminished productivity in a large segment of the population. Lack of education is also related to increased criminal activity and to unemployment, which place further drains on society. For example, approximately $25 billion is spent each year on Supplemental Security Income and Social Security Disability Insurance for people with severe mental illness who might be able to work and support themselves with adequate treatment. Effective treatment of mental illness would reduce

EVIDENCE-BASED PRACTICE

Goldman (2002) described a model for implementing evidence-based mental health practice that incorporates three key strategies. The first strategy is dissemination of best practices based on research findings through training and education of health care professionals. The second strategy involves enabling methods that promote use of best practices in mental health care settings. This strategy can be supported by the development of practice guidelines for use by clinicians. The third strategy is one of reinforcement of evidence-based practice through feedback on treatment effectiveness to mental health providers. This strategy might be supported by the use of case registries and computerized information systems that provide feedback to providers regarding the outcomes of care for their clients similar to those discussed in Chapter 29∞.

Choose one of these strategies and determine the extent to which it is being implemented. With respect to the first strategy, to what extent does your nursing education program include research-based information on best practices for the treatment of mental health problems? If you have chosen the second strategy, examine the treatment literature for a specific mental health problem to see the extent to which practice guidelines are available to clinicians. Examine the extent to which those guidelines are incorporated into mental health practice in your location. Finally, you might determine if there are any computerized information systems related to mental health and mental illness in your area. If so, to what extent do clinicians use available feedback to improve their practice?

homelessness and save at least a portion of the billions of dollars spent each year for emergency shelters and other services for the homeless mentally ill (NAMI, 2004).

Treatment for mental illness could also result in *cost offsets* for care of physical health problems. Mental illness may significantly impair compliance with recommended treatment of physical health conditions, leading to poor outcomes and higher treatment costs that could be *offset* by the increased compliance that might result from treatment of mental health problems (CIGNA Behavioral Health, 2006).

Several general approaches may be implemented for the treatment of mental illness. These approaches include pharmacotherapy, individual or group psychotherapy, family intervention, and use of self-help groups. Multimodal therapy involves a combination of approaches. It is beyond the scope of this book to discuss these therapeutic approaches in detail, but each will be addressed briefly.

Pharmacotherapy relies on the use of medications alone or in conjunction with other treatment approaches to mental illness. Most pharmacologic agents used in the treatment of mental disorders alter the action of neurotransmitters in the brain, either increasing or decreasing their activity. Major categories of pharmacotherapeutic agents include antipsychotics (neuroleptics), antidepressants, stimulants (used for ADHD), mood stabilizers, anxiolytics, and cholinesterase inhibitors (used for Alzheimer's disease) (USPHS, 1999). The role of community health nurses with respect to pharmacotherapy for mental disorders lies primarily in monitoring and motivating medication compliance, monitoring therapeutic effects, assisting with side effects, and identifying adverse effects. Community health nurses may also need to advocate for access to therapeutic drugs for clients without health insurance or those whose insurance does not cover prescription medications. For example, one community health nurse was able to convince the County Medical Services (CMS) division to cover psychiatric medications for a low-income client even though CMS services were usually reserved for addressing physical health needs rather than psychiatric illness. At the population level, community health nurses can advocate for changes to assistance programs to achieve parity for mental health conditions in comparison to physical health needs.

Community health nurses, as well as other providers who deal with clients with mental health problems, need an awareness of ethnopsychopharmacology. **Ethnopsychopharmacology** is the study of ethnic and cultural alterations in response to medication. These alterations reflect genetic differences in drug metabolism as well as cultural practices related to medication adherence, placebo effect, diet and its effects on medication absorption and effect, and the concomitant use of traditional therapies. Members of many ethnic groups have slowed drug metabolism compared to Caucasians, which may result in higher blood levels with typical dosages, leading to adverse effects (Flaskerud, 2000). Members of ethnic groups and others may also use herbal remedies for a variety of conditions that interfere with prescription medications or have other adverse effects. For example, St. John's wort is an herb frequently used for depression that has been found to affect metabolic pathways used by medications to treat conditions such as heart disease, cancer, and seizures and may interfere with treatment for these conditions (NIMH, 2005a). Community health nurses can educate clients, other health care providers, and the general public regarding ethnopsychopharmacologic implications and the potential for adverse drug effects. They can also engage in research to evaluate the effectiveness of ethnopsychopharmacologic approaches to mental health therapy.

Monitoring clients on psychotropic medications for side effects is an important role for community health nurses. Any of several different classes of antipsychotic drugs may be used in the initial treatment of clients with schizophrenia. Some clients will not respond to initial drug therapy or may experience adverse effects or annoying side effects that may limit compliance with the therapeutic regimen. In such cases, alternative drugs may be tried until the desired therapeutic effect is achieved, and community health nurses can assist clients to bring their concerns to the attention

of mental health providers so adjustments can be made. Nurses may also need to advocate for insurance coverage of particular medications when medications typically included in a health plan's formulary have not been effective.

Antidepressant medications are effective for major depression and may be used alone or in conjunction with other therapies. The use of antidepressants in bipolar disorder is more controversial because of the potential for mood destabilization and antidepressant-induced mania, particularly among clients with accompanying substance abuse or those who have been exposed to several different antidepressants (Goldberg & Hoop, 2004). Because depression and anxiety often go hand in hand, both symptoms can be treated pharmacologically. Several categories of antidepressant and antianxiety agents are commonly prescribed. Two classes of antidepressants have been prescribed since 1960: tricyclics such as amitriptyline (Elavil) and imipramine hydrochloride (Tofranil), and monoamine oxidase (MAO) inhibitors such as phenelzine sulfate (Nardil) and tranylcypromine sulfate (Parnate).

Although the reason for their effectiveness is not known, both types of antidepressants share one property: the ability to boost the action of serotonin and norepinephrine. While the tricyclics block reabsorption of these neurotransmitters, MAO inhibitors interfere with enzymes that break them down. When a client is started on a traditional tricyclic, he or she spends several weeks taking progressively larger doses. The health care provider uses blood tests to determine the effective serum concentration, which is different for each individual. Because an overdose of tricyclics can be extremely toxic, resulting in low blood pressure, heart disturbances, blurred vision, constipation, dizziness, sluggishness, and weight gain, many providers often prescribe too little. Because the therapeutic range is so narrow, too little medication is often ineffective. The MAO inhibitors can cause a hypertensive response to foods containing tyramine (e.g., liver, cheese, wines, etc.) (MedicineNet.com, 2005). Some people may choose to tolerate depression rather than experience these side effects.

The community health nurse caring for clients on antidepressant medications educates them about the medication and its therapeutic and toxic effects as well as potential side effects. Fluoxetine (Prozac) is one of the most commonly prescribed antidepressants in the United States. Prozac works like a tricyclic that focuses on serotonin. Although Prozac takes 3 weeks to become effective, there is no blood monitoring, because a dose of 20 to 40 mg is usually effective. There is less risk of overdose, and the most common side effects are nuisance effects such as headaches, nausea, insomnia, nervousness, weight loss, decreased sexual interest and loss or delay of orgasm, and a slight risk of seizures. In rare cases, suicidal thoughts and overtly violent behavior have been traced to Prozac. A small number of clients develop a "caffeine syndrome" in which they become restless and sometimes experience tremors.

Antianxiety agents, sedatives, and hypnotics are often prescribed when symptoms of anxiety are related to depression. These classes of drugs share similar pharmacologic properties, and they can be effective in small doses to relieve anxiety and in larger doses to induce sleep. The benzodiazepines are the most commonly used antianxiety agents. These include chlordiazepoxide hydrochloride (Librium) and diazepam (Valium), both of which are widely prescribed and widely abused. Other drugs in the benzodiazepine family include lorazepam (Ativan), alprazolam (Xanax), clonazepam (Klonopin), and triflupromazine (Vesprin). Drugs in the benzodiazepine family offer rapid, effective, and safe treatment for anxiety states. They have a low addiction potential and do not affect the metabolism of medications taken concurrently, although caffeine interferes with their effectiveness. The major side effect of the benzodiazepines is drowsiness, and community health nurses should warn clients not to drive when they feel drowsy.

The barbiturates (secobarbital [Seconal]) are a group of sedative–hypnotic drugs. These are often contraindicated in treating anxiety states because they are very addictive, used in suicide attempts, depress the central nervous and respiratory systems, and depress rapid eye movement (REM) sleep, possibly resulting in the insomnia these drugs are intended to control.

Lithium, one of the commonly used drugs in the control of mania, has a very narrow gap between therapeutic levels and toxic levels. For this reason, blood levels must be monitored frequently. When lithium is first prescribed, daily blood tests may be necessary, decreasing to weekly and, finally, to monthly checks during maintenance. Significant side effects are correlated with blood levels above 1.5 mEq/L. Community health nurses educate clients who are on lithium about the need to drink eight glasses of water a day, eat foods high in potassium (lithium can deplete potassium levels), and watch for early signs of toxicity. The nurse also monitors the client closely for signs of lithium toxicity, which are summarized above right, and refers the client back to the mental health provider if signs of toxicity are evident. The nurse also reinforces the need for periodic checks of blood levels of lithium to ensure early identification of toxic levels. Again, community health nurses may need to advocate for coverage of psychotropic medications for individual clients. They may also be involved in political advocacy to promote coverage of psychiatric services, including medication, as a mandated health insurance benefit on a par with coverage for physical illnesses.

Psychotherapy may be used with individual clients or with groups of people. The intent of psychotherapy is to develop an understanding of one's problems and ways of dealing with them. Several different

SPECIAL CONSIDERATIONS

SIGNS OF LITHIUM TOXICITY

Confusion	Seizures
Dizziness	Slurred speech
Hyperactive reflexes	Somnolence
Incontinence	Stupor
Nausea	Thirst
Polyuria	Tremor
Restlessness	Vertigo

approaches to psychotherapy are used, including psychodynamic therapy, behavior therapy, and humanistic therapy. A related therapy is psychoeducational intervention, which is directed toward teaching clients about their disorder and its signs and symptoms and helping to minimize the effects of stigmatization and promote medication compliance (Goldberg & Hoop, 2004). Psychotherapy may not be effective with clients from some cultural groups because it is incongruent with cultural norms of not dwelling on or thinking about problems.

Family intervention is directed toward alleviation of inappropriate family dynamics that promote stress and result in mental distress. The community health nurse's primary role with respect to psychotherapy and family interventions is referring clients for services.

Self-help groups are designed to promote mutual support, education, and personal growth among people who share similar kinds of mental health problems. Many self-help groups focus on the concept of recovery. **Recovery** involves restoration of a meaningful life rather than symptom relief, which is the emphasis in the medical model of care. In many cases, recovery does not imply a return to full function or the ability to discontinue medication use in chronic mental illnesses (USPHS, 1999). Self-help groups will be discussed in more detail in the context of substance abuse disorders in Chapter 31∞, but community health nurses may be actively involved in initiating and supporting self-help groups for clients with mental health conditions.

One other approach to treatment of bipolar disorder is the use of electroconvulsive therapy (ECT), or the use of low-level electric shock to stimulate the brain. Although previously discounted as a treatment for depression, newer technologies that deliver more focused stimulation that is not even consciously perceived by the client have shown an effectiveness rate of 50% to 100% in people with bipolar disorder. ECT has been suggested as most useful in clients with psychotic depression for whom medication is not appropriate (Goldberg & Hoop, 2004).

Treatment of postpartum depression often employs individual and group therapies similar to those used for other forms of depression. In addition to referring clients for these therapies, community health nurses

MediaLink Beyond the Black Hole of Depression (video)

may provide ongoing support to individual mothers (or fathers) experiencing PPD or design programs that promote weekly interactions with clients to help them deal with PPD. Nurses can also advocate with other family members for the kinds of emotional and material support that may be needed by a particular client or develop supportive services for new parents in the community (RNAO, 2005). One innovative approach to supportive care for mothers experiencing PPD involved telephone participation in a treatment program. Clients experiencing PPD are already stressed and the need to attend treatment sessions may further burden already overwhelmed parents. All of the women involved in a pilot study of the telecare program, even those who only participated in one session, exhibited a decrease in their levels of depression (Ugarriza & Schmidt, 2006).

Whatever the approach taken, community health nurses can be actively involved in promoting client empowerment in treatment for mental health problems. Because of their illnesses, people with mental-health-related diagnoses may be deemed incapable of participating in treatment decisions. However, as we know, clients can and do decide for themselves whether to comply with a provider-designated treatment plan. More effective care involves client participation in all aspects of treatment planning. A number of barriers to client empowerment have been identified, including stigma, impaired cognitive ability, medication effects, and lack of motivation, which may actually result from a history of disempowerment. Barriers to empowerment may also arise from health system factors such as funding sources and lack of time for providers to truly engage clients in treatment decisions (Finfgeld, 2004).

Empowerment may occur along a continuum, from simply participating in treatment activities designed by others, to choosing among alternatives, to client movement beyond their own personal needs to support and empower others, to a final level of empowerment characterized by equality between client, family, and provider and negotiation regarding the treatment plan (Finfgeld, 2004). Community health nurses can assist in client empowerment by addressing cognitive limitations and medication effects and framing treatment discussions in terms that clients can understand. Nurses can also arm clients with information about treatment options and an understanding of their rights and responsibilities. Community health nurses may also need to advocate for client empowerment and for acceptance of client choices even when providers think those choices may not be in the client's best interests.

Maintenance

Maintenance, in the context of mental health problems, is analogous to tertiary prevention as discussed in relation to other common community health problems. As was the case with the chronic physical health problems

discussed in Chapter 29 ∞, there is a need to focus on disease management rather than crisis-oriented care for chronic mental health problems. Maintenance involves long-term management of chronic mental illness and focuses on rehabilitating the client and preventing relapse. The goal of maintenance in chronic mental illness is to maintain the client's level of function and to prevent recidivism or frequent rehospitalization. Maintenance may include medications and a variety of other interventions. Community health nurses may be asked to follow clients with diagnoses of chronic mental illness to provide support, encourage compliance, and monitor the effects of treatment. Community health nurses can assist clients to plan regular lifestyles and to minimize sources of stress in their lives. For example, the nurse might help clients with bipolar disorder to reduce stress and to maintain regular sleeping and waking cycles to prevent relapses (Goldberg & Hoop, 2004).

Clients using pharmacologic agents should also be cautioned about potential interactions of medications and alcohol. The nurse can also help clients and their families to identify symptoms that signal a symptomatic relapse and to seek professional assistance when these symptoms are noted. For example, families should know that the annual prevalence of relapse for people with schizophrenia is approximately 35% and should be prepared to identify early signs of relapse (van Meijel, Kruitwagen, van der Gaag, Kahn, & Grypdonck, 2006). Community health nurses can educate clients and family members regarding signs of relapse and assist them to seek help when relapses occur.

Client and family involvement is an important aspect of maintenance in the control of chronic mental health problems. Some concerns voiced by clients include lack of involvement in treatment decisions, lack of information about nonpharmacological treatment options, and failure of health care providers to manage medication side effects (Gray, Rofail, Allen, & Newey, 2005). As noted earlier, community health nurses can promote client participation in clinical decision making as well as provide them with information on which to base decisions regarding treatment interventions. In addition, they can regularly monitor clients for medication side effects and offer suggestions for ameliorating them. If side effects cannot be effectively managed or threaten to undermine client compliance with treatment, community health nurses can advocate with mental health providers for a change in the treatment regimen to minimize side effects.

It is important that community health nurses learn to assess levels of depression and suicide risk and refer clients at risk to a mental health provider immediately if they are not already involved in ongoing therapy. Community health nurses are also using approaches such as diary writing and physical exercise to help individuals deal more effectively with depressive symptoms. For example, journaling may allow the client to identify triggers for depressive episodes or to recognize initial symptoms of depression so that medical assistance can be sought. Journaling may serve a similar function for clients with schizophrenia, allowing clients or family members to identify early signs of relapse and seek assistance. Open lines of communication are imperative among nurse, mental health provider, family, and client, particularly at times when the client is deeply depressed or actively suicidal.

Persons with chronic mental illness often have a high incidence of physical health problems and sometimes lack the capacity to seek health care in today's complex delivery systems. The community health nurse may be in the situation of following a person for a physical health problem who suddenly begins to show signs of mental illness. The nurse's role in this case is to refer the client for further diagnosis and treatment, as well as to assist in addressing the physical health problem. The community health nurse also refers clients who are exhibiting signs of exacerbation of their disorders.

Respite is another aspect of maintenance in the care of chronic mental illness. Respite has been shown to benefit both clients with serious mental illness and family caregivers (Jeon, Brodaty, & Chesterson, 2005). Community health nurses can refer clients and family members to existing respite services, which may be provided in the home or in specialized residential facilities. They may also be actively involved in advocating for the availability of respite for these families. Families and clients with mental illness may also benefit from participation in mutual support groups (Chien, Chan, Morrissey, & Thompson, 2005), and community health nurses can either make referrals to existing groups or work with clients and family members to establish such groups.

Many of the aspects of maintenance in the control of chronic mental health problems can be achieved through community health nursing case management. Case management services by community health nurses have been shown to reduce depressive symptoms in single parents and to promote social adjustment. In addition, case management services have been shown to be cost-effective. For example, in one study, although case management services did not reduce health care costs, they resulted in annual cost savings of $240,000 (Canadian) due to reduced social assistance use (Markle-Reid, Browne, Roberts, Gafni, & Byrne, 2002).

Evaluating Control Strategies for Mental Health Problems

Evaluation of mental health interventions occurs at the individual and family level as well as the population level. Evidence of effective intervention for the individual client may lie in diminished mental distress or a decrease in symptoms of a specific mental disorder. Similarly, effective family care may result in improved family dynamics or decreased disruption of family life by a mentally ill family member.

At the population level, evidence of effective primary prevention activities would lie in decreased incidence and prevalence of mental disorders as well as decreased reports of mental distress in the population. National health objectives for 2010◆ may also be used as guidelines for evaluating mental health care, particularly care related to secondary and tertiary prevention. Baseline data and 2010 targets for selected objectives are provided below.

Because of their presence in the community and familiarity with many community members experiencing adverse life situations, community health nurses are in a position to identify clients at risk for mental health problems. Nurses can engage in activities designed to ameliorate these risks and to promote resilience and coping. Community health nurses are also able to recognize clients with symptomatic mental illness and refer them for mental health services. Assisting clients with chronic mental illness to adjust to their conditions and live as normally as possible is another significant role for community health nurses. Finally, community health nurses may be actively involved in advocacy to assure that culturally appropriate preventive, diagnostic, and treatment services are available to those in need of them.

HEALTHY PEOPLE 2010
Goals for Population Health

OBJECTIVE	BASELINE	TARGET
■ 18-3. Reduce the proportion of homeless adults who have serious mental illness	25%	19%
■ 18-4. Increase the proportion of people with serious mental illness who are employed	42%	51%
■ 18-9. Increase the proportion of adults with serious mental disorders who receive treatment		
a. Adults 18–54 years of age with serious mental illness	47%	55%
b. Adults over 18 years with depression	23%	50%
c. Adults over 18 years with schizophrenia	60%	75%

Data from: Centers for Disease Control and Prevention. (2005). Healthy people data. Retrieved September 5, 2005, from http://wonder.cdc.gov/data2010

Case Study

Caring for a Client with Depression

You are the community health nurse assigned to see Donna for a well-baby visit several weeks after she delivered a healthy son. Donna is 39 and has been married to Jack, 48, for a year. Stephen is their first child. When you arrive at Donna's house, you note that she and her family live in a comfortable home in an upper-middle-class neighborhood. Donna answers the door, and you see that her eyes and nose are red as though she has been crying. You explain the purpose of your visit and examine the baby, who is in a freshly painted nursery with a bright mobile over the crib and plenty of stuffed animals and toys around. Stephen is neat, clean, and appears to be well fed, happy, and healthy.

When you finish with the baby, you ask how Donna is doing. Donna bursts into tears. She tells you that she has been feeling desperately unhappy since her pregnancy began. She has been feeling so depressed, she reports that she is not sure she will be able to get out of bed anymore to take care of her son. You say, "Tell me about this past year." Donna tells you that this is a first marriage for her and for Jack, and neither of them has children from previous relationships. In their discussions prior to marriage, she and Jack had never resolved their differences about having children. Donna was ambivalent about having a child; her husband was sure he did not want one. Because they are devout Roman Catholics, they used the rhythm method of birth control. When Donna told Jack she was pregnant after 2 months of marriage, he became very angry and blamed Donna for tricking him into having a baby. Although she had not tricked him, Donna felt guilty and blamed herself for becoming pregnant. Terrified that Jack would leave her if she told him how she felt, she kept all her own feelings of sadness, anger, and depression inside. She did not want to be a single parent. Abortion was never considered because of their religious beliefs.

During the pregnancy, Jack was emotionally withdrawn, depressed, and refused to take part in any activity related to the upcoming birth. Donna's sister attended Lamaze classes with her and coached her during the birth because Jack would not attend. Donna felt jealous of the women whose husbands were so attentive during these classes. Ever since her son's birth, Donna says

that she has had "postpartum depression." She has told no one how depressed she feels because she is afraid she will have to be hospitalized as she was several times in her late twenties and early thirties for episodes of clinical depression.

When you do a genogram with her, you discover a family history of depression. Both her grandmother and mother suffered bouts of deep depression, and her grandmother had been hospitalized for a year in a psychiatric institution following menopause. Donna's father is an emotionally withdrawn man whose only sister committed suicide when she was 40. Donna's sister has an eating disorder; she is bulimic.

Now that Donna has been home for 3 weeks with her son, she sees her sister twice a week. Jack is pleased that they have a son, and he is beginning to spend time after he comes home from work playing with Stephen. Donna cannot understand why it makes her angry instead of happy that Jack is becoming involved with their child. Because Jack has refused to support them in a manner that would allow Donna to stay home with Stephen, Donna must return to work after her 6-week maternity leave. She is afraid she will be unable to function at work and has yet to arrange childcare for Stephen. Donna worries about these things and has difficulty both falling asleep and getting up during the night to feed her son. She says she cries "at the drop of a hat" and has lost weight. She weighs less now than before she was pregnant. She has little interest in anything, including her baby, and she says that life does not really seem worth living anymore.

1. Does Donna have any typical signs of depression? If so, describe them.
2. How would you assess her potential for suicide?
3. Do you think Donna's depression is "normal" postpartum depression or clinical depression requiring psychiatric assessment and treatment? Why?
4. Based on your assessment, will you follow Donna yourself or refer her to a psychiatrist or mental health worker?
5. How will you involve Donna's husband and sister in the plan of care?
6. What other interventions might be warranted with this family?

Test Your Understanding

1. What are some of the personal, family, and societal effects of mental health problems? (pp. 904–906)

2. What are some of the factors that influence the development and progression of mental health problems? (pp. 906–917)

3. Describe symptoms characteristic of schizophrenia. Give an example of each. (pp. 903, 911)

4. What are the major strategies for preventing mental health problems? What is the role of the community health nurse with respect to each? (pp. 918–919)

5. What are the major approaches to treatment of mental health problems? How might community health nurses be involved in each? (pp. 919–924)

6. What are the areas of emphasis in maintenance therapy for mental health problems? Give an example of community health nursing involvement in each. (pp. 924–925)

EXPLORE MediaLink

http://www.prenhall.com/clark
Resources for this chapter can be found on the Companion Website.

Audio Glossary
Exam Review Questions
Case Study: Providing Nursing Care for the
  Mentally Ill

MediaLink Application: Beyond the Black
  Hole of Depression (video)
Media Links

Challenge Your Knowledge
Update *Healthy People 2010*
Advocacy Interviews

References

Agrawal, N., & Hirsch, S. R. (2004). Schizophrenia: Evidence for conceptualizing it as a brain disease. *Journal of Primary Prevention, 24*, 437–444.

American Academy of Child & Adolescent Psychiatry. (2004). *The depressed child.* Retrieved August 7, 2006, from http://www.aacap.org/page.ww?name = TheDepressed + Child&section = Facts + for + Families

American Academy of Pediatrics. (2004). Policy statement: School-based mental health services. *Pediatrics, 113*, 1839–1845.

American Pregnancy Association. (2006). *Depression during pregnancy.* Retrieved August 8, 2006, from http://www.american pregnancy.org/pregnancyhealth/depression duringpregnancy.html

American Psychiatric Association. (2000). *Diagnostic and statistical manual of mental disorders* (4th ed., Text Revision). (*DSM-IV-TR*). Washington, DC: Author.

Antai-Otong, D. (2004). Antidepressants and older adults. *Advance for Nurses, 1*(7), 15–17.

Antares, A. (2005, Winter). Reducing the risk of postpartum depression. *Midwifery Today* (76), pp. 40–41.

Araya, R., Rojas, G., Fritsch, R., Frank, R., & Lewis, G. (2006). Inequities in mental health care after health care system reform in Chile. *American Journal of Public Health, 96*, 109–113.

Askey, R. (2004). Case management: A critical review. *Mental Health Practice, 7*(8), 12–16.

Bhui, K., Stansfeld, S., McKenzie, K., Karlsen, S., Nazroo, J., & Weich, S. (2005). Racial/ethnic discrimination and common mental disorders among workers: Findings from the EMPIRIC study of the ethnic minority groups in the United Kingdom. *American Journal of Public Health, 95*, 496–501.

Boyle, M. (2004). Preventing a non-existent illness?: Some issues in the prevention of "schizophrenia". *Journal of Primary Prevention, 24*, 445–469.

Calandra, J. (2003). Mental health & older adults: Mental illness in later life. *NurseWeek, 16*(25), 21–22.

Carty, R. M., Al-Zayyer, W., Arietti, L. L., & Lester, A. S. (2004). *Journal of Professional Nursing, 20*, 251–259.

Centers for Disease Control and Prevention. (2005). *Healthy people data.* Retrieved September 5, 2005, from http://wonder.cdc.gov/data2010

Chien, W. T., Chan, S., Morrissey, J., & Thompson, D. (2005). Effectiveness of a mutual support group for families of patients with schizophrenia. *Journal of Advanced Nursing, 51*, 595–608.

CIGNA Behavioral Health. (2006). *The cost offset of psychiatric care.* Retrieved August 8, 2006, from http://www.cignabehavioral.com/web/basicsite/bulletinBoard/realBenefitMH Programs.jsp

Cook, J. A., Grey, D., Burke, J., Cohen, M. H., Gurtman, A. C., Richardson, J. L., et al. (2004). Depressive symptoms and AIDS-related mortality among a multisite cohort of HIV-positive women. *American Journal of Public Health, 94*, 1133–1140.

Daniel, J., Honey, W., Landen, M., Marshall-Williams, S., Chapman, D., & Lando, J. (2005). Health risk behaviors and conditions among persons with depression—New Mexico, 2003. *Morbidity and Mortality Weekly Report, 54*, 989–991.

Draucker, C. B. (2005). Processes of mental health service use by adolescents with depression. *Journal of Nursing Scholarship, 37*, 155–162.

Dunlop, D. D., Manheim, L. M., Song, J., Lyons, J. S., & Chang, R. W. (2005). Incidence of disability among preretirement adults: The impact of depression. *American Journal of Public Health, 95*, 2003–2008.

Dunlop, D. D., Song, J., Lyons, J. S., Manheim, L. M., & Chang, R. W. (2003). Racial/ethnic differences in rates of depression among preretirement adults. *American Journal of Public Health, 93*, 1945–1952.

Eli Lilly and Company. (2004). *Depression facts and figures.* Retrieved August 13, 2005, from http://www.lilly.com/products/health_women/depression/facts_figures.html

Finfgeld, D. L. (2004). Empowerment of individuals with enduring mental health problems: Results from concept analyses and qualitative investigations. *Advances in Nursing Science, 27*(1), 44–52.

Flaskerud, J. H. (2000). Ethnicity, culture, and neuropsychiatry. *Issues in mental health nursing, 21*, 2–29.

Frangou, S., & Murray, R. M. (2000). *Schizophrenia* (2nd ed.). London: Martin Dunitz.

Freeman, M. P., Wright, R., Watchman, M., Wahl, R. A., Sisk, D. J., Fraleigh, L., et al. (2005). Postpartum depression assessments at well-baby visits: Screening feasibility, prevalence, and risk factors. *Journal of Women's Health, 14*, 929–935.

Galil, N. (2000). Depression and asthma in children. *Current Opinion in Pediatrics, 12*, 331–335.

Goldberg, J. F., & Hoop, J. (2004). *Bipolar depression: Long-term challenges for the clinician.* Retrieved September 30, 2004, from http://www.medscape.com

Goldman, H. H. (2002). Improving access to evidence-based services: Translating need into supply and demand. In M. Hager (Ed.), *Modern psychiatry: Challenges in educating health professionals to meet new need* (pp. 93–114). New York: Josiah Macy, Jr. Foundation.

Goodwin, R. (2006). Association between coping with anger and feelings of depression among youths. *American Journal of Public Health, 96*, 664–669.

Gray, R., Rofail, D., Allen, J., & Newey, T. (2005). A survey of patient satisfaction with and subjective experiences of treatment with antipsychotic medication. *Journal of Advanced Nursing, 52*, 31–37.

Hills, H., Siegfried, C., & Ickowitz, A. (2004). *Effective prison mental health services: Guidelines to expand and improve treatment.* retrieved March 30, 2006, from http://www.nicic.org/misc/URLshell.aspx?SRC=Catalogue&REFF=http://nicic.org/library/018604&ID=018604&Type=PDF&URL=http://nicic.org/pubs/2004/018604.pdf

Husted, J., & Jorgens, A. (2000). Population density as a factor in the rehospitalization of persons with serious and persistent mental illness. *Psychiatric Services, 51*, 603–605.

Institute of Medicine. (2006). *Improving the quality of health care for mental and substance-use conditions.* Retrieved February 22, 2006, from http://www.nap.edu/openbook/0309100445/html/2.html

Jeon, Y.-H., Brodaty, H., & Chesterson, J. (2005). Respite care for caregivers and people with severe mental illness: Literature review. *Journal of Advanced Nursing, 49*, 297–306.

Jungbauer, J., Stelling, K., Dietrich, S., & Angermeyer, M. C. (2004). Schizophrenia: Problems of separation in families. *Journal of Advanced Nursing, 47*, 605–613.

Kelder, S. H., Murray, N. G., Orpinas, P., Prokhorov, A., McReynolds, L., Zang, Q., et al. (2001). Depression and substance use in minority middle-school students. *American Journal of Public Health, 91*, 761–766.

Keltner, N. L. (2005). Genomic influences on schizophrenia-related neurotransmitter systems. *Journal of Nursing Scholarship, 37*, 322–328.

Kingdon, D. G., & Turkington, D. (2004). *Cognitive-behavioral therapy of schizophrenia.* New York: Guilford Press.

Koukia, E., & Madianos, G. (2005). Is psychosocial rehabilitation of schizophrenic patients preventing family burden? A comparative study. *Journal of Psychiatric and Mental Health Nursing, 12*, 415–422.

Leighton, S., Worraker, A., & Nolan, P. (2003). School nurses and mental health: Part 1. *Mental Health Practice, 7*(4), 14–16.

Leventhal, T., & Brooks–Gunn, J. (2003). Moving to opportunity: An experimental study of neighborhood effects on mental health. *American Journal of Public Health, 93*, 1576–1582.

Liang, S. L. (2004). Overcoming stigma in Asian American mental health. *Medscape Psychiatry & Mental Health, 9*(2). Retrieved November 12, 2004, from http://www.medscape.com/viewarticle/419353

Loughlin, A. (2004). Depression and social support: Effective treatments for homebound elderly adults. *Journal of Gerontological Nursing, 20*(5), 11–15.

Markle-Reid, M., Browne, G., Roberts, J., Gafni, A., & Byrne, C. (2002). The 2–year costs and effects of a public health nursing case management intervention on mood-disordered single parents on social assistance. *Journal of Evaluation in Clinical Practice, 8*(1), 45–59.

Marshall-Williams, S., Chapman, D., & Lando, J. (2005). The role of public health in mental health promotion. *Morbidity and Mortality Weekly Report, 54*, 841–842.

Matza, L., de Lissovoy, G., Sasane, R., Pesa, J., & Maus, J. (2004). The impact of bipolar disorder on work loss. *Drug Benefit Trends, 16*, 476–481.

McCann, E. (2000). The expression of sexuality in people with psychoses: Breaking the taboos. *Journal of Advanced Nursing, 32*, 132–138.

McDevitt, J., Snyder, M., Miller, A., & Wilbur, J. (2006). Perceptions of barriers and benefits to physical activity among outpatients in psychiatric rehabilitation. *Journal of Nursing Scholarship, 38*, 50–55.

McLeer, S. V. (2004). Mental health services. In H. S. Sultz & K. M. Young (Eds.), *Health care USA: Understanding its organization and delivery* (4th ed., pp. 335–366). Sudbury, MA: Jones and Bartlett.

McVeigh, K. H., Mostashari, F., & Thorpe, L. E. (2004). Serious psychological distress among persons with diabetes—New York City, 2003. *Morbidity and Mortality Weekly Report, 53*, 1089–1092.

Mechanic, D., & Bilder, S. (2004). Treatment of people with mental illness: A decade-long perspective. *Health Affairs, 28*(4), 84–95.

MedicineNet.com. (2005). MAO inhibitors—oral. Retrieved October 20, 2006, from http://www.medicinenet.com/script/main/art.asp?articlekey=43919&ph=3&page=2

Miller, B. D. (2005). Mood disturbance: A complicating factor in the care of pediatric patients. *Current Opinion in Pediatrics, 17*, 605–606.

Miller, L. J., & Daniels-Brady, C. (2005). Depression during perimenopause. *Menopause Management, 14*(5), 10–16.

Millward, L. J., Lutte, A., & Purvis, R. G. (2005). *Journal of Psychiatric and Mental Health Nursing, 12*, 565–573.

Mojtabai, R. (2005). Trends in contacts with mental health professionals and cost barriers to mental health care among adults with significant psychological distress in the United States: 1997–2002. *American Journal of Public Health, 95*, 2009–2014.

Monts, R. (2002). Men don't seek treatment for depression. *Community Health Forum, 3*(5), 53–54.

Mrazek, P. J., & Haggerty, R. J. (Eds.). (1994). *Reducing risks for mental disorders: Frontiers for preventive intervention research.* Washington, DC: National Academy Press.

National Alliance on Mental Illness. (n.d.). *Early onset depression.* Retrieved August 8, 2006, from http://www.nami.org/Content/ContentGroups/Helpline1/Facts_About_Childhood_Depression.htm

National Alliance on Mental Illness. (2002). *Policy maker's fact sheet on the mental health system.* Retrieved August 8, 2006, from http://www.nami.org/Template.cfm?Section=Policy_Research_Institute&Template=/ContentManagement/ContentDisplay.cfm&ContentID=5143

National Alliance on Mental Illness. (2004). *Spending money in all the wrong places.* Retrieved August 8, 2006, from http://www.nami.org/Template.cfm?Section=policy_research_institute&Template=/ContentManagement/ContentDisplay.cfm&ContentID=14596

National Center for Health Statistics. (2005a). *Health, United States, 2005, with chartbook on trends in the health of Americans.* Retrieved December 23, 2005, from http://www.cdc.gov/nchs/data/hus/hus05.pdf

National Center for Health Statistics. (2005b). Percentage of children aged 14–17 years with emotional or behavioral difficulties who used mental health services, by type of service—United States, 2003. *Morbidity and Mortality Weekly Report, 54*, 852.

National Center for Health Statistics. (2006). Percentage of adults with self–assessed symptoms of serious psychological distress, by sex and race—United States, 2000–2004. *Morbidity and Mortality Weekly Report, 55*, 801.

National Council on Disability. (2002). *The well being of our nation: An intergenerational vision of effective mental health services and supports.* Retrieved January 30, 2003, from http://www.ncd.gov/newsroom/publications/pdf/mentalhealth.pdf

National Institute of Mental Health. (2000). *Depression.* Retrieved June 2, 2006, from http://www.nimh.nih.gov/publicat/depression.cfm

National Institute of Mental Health. (2001a). *Anxiety disorders.* Retrieved June 2, 2006, from http://www.nimh.nih.gov/publicat/NIMHadfacts.htm

National Institute of Mental Health. (2001b). *Attention deficit hyperactivity disorder.* Retrieved June 2, 2006, from http://www.nimh.nih.gov/publicat/NIMHhelpchild.pdf

National Institute of Mental Health. (2001c). *Bipolar disorder.* Retrieved June 2, 2006, from http://www.nimh.nih.gov/publicat/bipolar.cfm

National Institute of Mental Health. (2001d). *Borderline personality disorder.* Retrieved June 2, 2006, from http://www.nimh.nih.gov/publicat/bpd.cfm

National Institute of Mental Health. (2001e). *Eating disorders: Facts about eating disorders and the search for solutions.* Retrieved June 2, 2006, from http://www.nimh.nih.gov/publicat/eatingdisorders.cfm

National Institute of Mental Health. (2003). *Childhood-onset schizophrenia: An update from the NIMH.* Retrieved March 8, 2006, from http://nimh.nih.gov/publicat/schizkids.cfm

National Institute of Mental Health. (2004). *Autism spectrum disorders (pervasive developmental disorders).* Retrieved June 2, 2006, from http://www.nimh.nih.gov/publicat/autism.cfm

National Institute of Mental Health. (2005a). *Depression: What every woman should know.* Washington, DC: Author.

National Institute of Mental Health. (2005b). *Schizophrenia.* Retrieved June 2, 2006, from http://www.nimh.nih.gov/publicat/schizoph.cfm

National Mental Health Association. (2006). *Seasonal affective disorder.* Retrieved June 7, 2006, from http://nmha.org/infoctr/factsheets/27.cfm

Ohlsen, R. I., Peacock, G., & Smith, S. (2005). Developing a service to monitor and improve physical health in people with serious mental illness. *Journal of Psychiatric and Mental Health Nursing, 12*, 614–619.

O'Malley, A. S., Forrest, C. B., & Miranda, J. (2003). Primary care attributes and care for depression among low-income African American women. *American Journal of Public Health, 93*, 1328–1334.

Peden, A. R., Rayens, M. K., Hall, L. A., & Grant, E. (2004). Negative thinking and the mental health of low-income single mothers. *Journal of Nursing Scholarship, 36*, 337–344.

Peden, A. R., Rayens, M. K., Hall, L. A., & Grant, E. (2005). Testing an intervention to reduce negative thinking, depressive symptoms, and chronic stressors in low-income single mothers. *Journal of Nursing Scholarship, 37*, 268–274.

Registered Nurses Association of Ontario. (2005). *Nursing best practice guideline: Interventions for postpartum depression.* Retrieved August 7, 2006, from http://www.rnao.org/Storage/11/6000_BPG_Post_Partum_Depression.pdf

Riolo, S. S., Nguyen, T. A., Greden, J. F., & King, C. A. (2005). Prevalence of depression by race/ethnicity: Findings from the National Health and Nutrition Examination Survey III. *American Journal of Public Health, 95*, 998–1000.

Seasonal Affective Disorder. (2006). Retrieved June 7, 2006, from http://en.wikipedia.org/wiki/Seasonal_affective_disorder

Silver, E., Arsenault, L., Langley, J., Caspi, A., & Moffitt, T. E. (2005). Mental disorder and violent victimization in a total birth cohort. *American Journal of Public Health, 95,* 2015–2021.

Sin, J., Moone, N., & Wellman, N. (2005). Developing services for the careers of young adults with early-onset psychosis—listening to their experiences and needs. *Journal of Psychiatric and Mental Health Nursing, 12,* 589–597.

Smith, L., Walker, A., & Gilhooly, K. (2004). Clinical guidelines on depression: A qualitative study of GPs' views. *Journal of Family Practice, 53,* 556–561.

Spencer, M. S., & Chen, J. (2004). Effect of discrimination on mental health service utilization among Chinese Americans. *American Journal of Public Health, 94,* 809–814.

Stengler–Wenzke, K., Trosbach, J., Dietrich, S., & Angermeyer, M. (2004). Coping strategies used by the relatives of people with obsessive–compulsive disorder. *Journal of Advanced Nursing, 48,* 35–42.

Strayer, D. (2005). *Postpartum depression in fathers.* Retrieved August 7, 2006, from http://0-imagesrvr.epnet.com.sally.sandiego .edu/embimages/cin20/2006/5000001254.pdf

Strong, V., Sharpe, M., Cull, A., Maguire, P., House, A., & Ramirez, A. (2004). Can oncology nurses treat depression? A pilot study. *Journal of Advanced Nursing, 46,* 542–548.

Stuhlmiller, C. M. (1998). Understanding seasonal affective disorder and experiences in northern Norway. *Image: Journal of Nursing Scholarship, 30,* 151–156.

Swanson, J. W., Swartz, M., Essock, S. M., Osher, F. C., Wagner, R., Goodman, L. A., et al. (2002). The social-environmental context of violent behavior in persons treated for severe mental illness. *American Journal of Public Health, 92,* 1523–1531.

Tanner, E. (2004). Chronic illness demands for self-management in older adults. *Geriatric Nursing, 25,* 313–317.

Teplin, L. A., Abram, K. M., McClelland, G. M., Washburn, J. J., & Pikus, A. K. (2005). Detecting mental disorder in juvenile detainees: Who receives services? *American Journal of Public Health, 95,* 1773–1780.

Tielsch, A. H., & Allen, P. J. (2005). Listen to them draw: Screening children in primary care through the use of human figure drawings. *Pediatric Nursing, 31,* 320–326.

Turcu, A., Toubin, S., Mourey, F., D'Athis, P., Manckoundia, P., & Pfitzenmeyer, P. (2004). Falls and depression in older people. *Gerontology, 50,* 303–308.

Ugarriza, D. N., & Schmidt, L. (2006). Telecare for women with postpartum depression. *Journal of Psychosocial Nursing, 44*(1), 37–45.

U.S. Census Bureau. (2006). *Statistical abstract of the United States, 2006.* Retrieved June 5, 2006, from http://www.census.gov/prod/ 2005pubs/06statab

U.S. Public Health Service. (1999). *Mental health: A report of the surgeon general.* Washington, DC: Author.

van Meijel, B., Kruitwagen, C., van der Gaag, M., Kahn, R. S., & Grypdonck, M. H. F. (2006). An intervention study to prevent relapse in patients with schizophrenia. *Journal of Nursing Scholarship, 38,* 42–49.

Vega, W. A., Sribney, W. M., & Achara-Abrahams, I. (2003). Co-occurring alcohol, drug, and other psychiatric disorders among Mexican-origin people in the United States. *American Journal of Public Health, 93,* 1057–1064.

Vila, G., Zipper, E., Dabbas, M., Bertrand, C., Robert, J. J., Ricour, C., et al. (2004). Mental disorders in obese children and adolescents. *Psychosomatic Medicine, 66,* 387–394.

Walkup, J., Satriano, J., Barry, D., Sadler, P., & Cournos, F. (2002). HIV testing policy and serious mental illness. *American Journal of Public Health, 92,* 1931–1939.

Ward, C., & Styles, I. (2005). Culturing settlement using pre- and post-migration strategies. *Journal of Psychiatric and Mental Health Nursing, 12,* 423–430.

Watkins, C. E. (2002). *Seasonal affective disorder: Winter depression.* Retrieved June 7, 2006, from http://www.ncpamd.com/seasonal.htm

Weeks, S. K., McGann, P. E., Michaels, T. K., & Penninx, B. W. J. H. (2003). Comparing various short-form geriatric depression scales leads to the GDS-5/15. *Journal of Nursing Scholarship, 35,* 133–137.

Willinsky, C., & Pape, B. (2002). Mental health promotion. In L. E. Young & V. E. Haynes (Eds.), *Transforming health promotion practice: Concepts, issues, and applications* (pp. 162–173). Philadelphia: F. A. Davis.

Wuerker, A. K. (2000). The family and schizophrenia. *Issues in Mental Health Nursing, 21,* 127–141.

Zahran, H. S., Kobau, R., Moriarty, D. G., Zack, M. M., Giles, W. H., & Lando, J. (2004). Self-reported frequent mental distress among adults—United States, 1993 to 2001. *Morbidity and Mortality Weekly Report, 53,* 963–966.

Zierold, K. M., Knobeloch, L., & Anderson, H. (2004). Prevalence of chronic disease in adults exposed to arsenic-contaminated drinking water. *American Journal of Public Health, 94,* 1936–1937.

Zimmerman, F. J., Christakis, D. A., & Vander Stoep, A. (2004). Tinker, tailor, soldier, patient: Work attributes and depression disparities among young adults. *Social Science & Medicine, 58,* 1543–1553.

Advocacy in Action

Mandated Drug Testing

As a community health nursing student returning for my baccalaureate degree, I received a request to visit Debbie, a 20-year-old woman who had just delivered her first child. Debbie was referred to the health department for follow-up because of a positive drug screen at the time of delivery. In order to be allowed to take her baby home from the hospital, Debbie signed an agreement with the Child Protective Services (CPS) Division to have weekly drug screening tests.

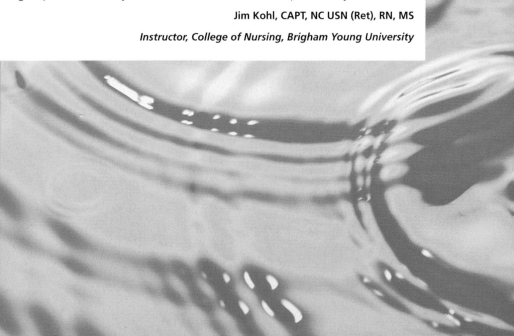

When I first visited Debbie, she and the baby were doing well, and she did not think she needed any assistance. I gave her information on how to reach me at the health department if she had questions. About a month later, Debbie called me to say that CPS was threatening to take the baby away because she had not been having the drug screens done. Her car had broken down. She couldn't afford to get it fixed, and she had no way to get to the laboratory. I checked on bus services, but the area of town where Debbie lived had no bus route.

Debbie assured me that she was "clean," and I did not notice any evidence of drug use in my visits to her. I called the CPS case worker, who informed me there was nothing they could do; Debbie would have to find transportation to the lab or the baby would be placed in foster care. I called another agency in town that provided court-mandated parenting classes for abusive parents. The staff there told me that the court system could issue taxi vouchers for Debbie to comply with the drug screening requirement. After numerous telephone calls to locate the right office, I was finally able to obtain taxi vouchers for Debbie. Debbie fulfilled the court's screening requirements, stayed clean, and was able to keep her baby.

Jim Kohl, CAPT, NC USN (Ret), RN, MS

Instructor, College of Nursing, Brigham Young University

Substance Abuse

CHAPTER OBJECTIVES

After reading this chapter, you should be able to:

1. Identify signs and symptoms of psychoactive substance dependence.
2. Distinguish between psychoactive substance dependence and abuse.
3. Identify substances that lead to dependence and abuse.
4. Analyze personal, family, and societal effects of substance abuse.
5. Analyze biophysical, psychological, sociocultural, behavioral, and health systems factors that influence substance abuse.
6. Discuss aspects of community health nursing assessment in relation to substance abuse.
7. Identify major approaches to primary prevention of substance abuse and analyze the role of the community health nurse with respect to each.
8. Describe the components of the intervention process in secondary prevention of substance abuse.
9. Identify general principles in the treatment of substance abuse.
10. Describe treatment modalities in substance abuse control and analyze the role of the community health nurse in their implementation.
11. Analyze the role of the community health nurse in tertiary prevention of substance abuse.
12. Discuss harm reduction and its role in control of substance abuse.

KEY TERMS

MediaLink
http://www.prenhall.com/clark

Additional interactive resources for this chapter can be found on the Companion Website. Click on Chapter 31 and "Begin" to select the activities for this chapter.

Most drugs are used appropriately for medicinal purposes. Even when used appropriately, however, drugs may result in substance-related disorders. Substance-related disorders are one of 17 diagnostic categories included in the fourth edition of the *Diagnostic and Statistical Manual of Mental Disorders (Text Revision) (DSM-IV-TR)* of the American Psychiatric Association (2000). **Substance-related disorders** are defined as "disturbances of behavior, cognition, and/or mood . . . caused by the taking and/or abuse of a drug, alcohol, or tobacco; the side effects of medication; or exposure to toxins" (McLeer, 2004, p. 341). In this chapter, we are concerned with substance-related disorders resulting from inappropriate use of psychoactive substances. **Psychoactive substances** are drugs or chemicals that alter ordinary states of consciousness, including mood, cognition, and behavior (Insel, Roth, & Price, 2005).

Substance abuse is a growing world problem. The illegal drug trade is big business, and the fact that many substances with the potential for abuse also have legitimate uses has made control of substance abuse difficult. **Drug use** is the taking of a drug in the correct amount, frequency, and strength for its medically intended purpose. **Drug abuse** or misuse, on the other hand, is the deliberate use of a drug for other than medicinal purposes in a manner that can adversely affect one's health or ability to function.

In the United States, the abuse of alcohol and other drugs and the use of tobacco products are of particular concern. For example, more than 1 million people in the United States sought substance abuse treatment in 2003 (U.S. Census Bureau, 2006). The magnitude of concern for problems of substance use and abuse is also seen in the development of more than 40 national health promotion and disease prevention objectives for the year 2010 related to tobacco use and the abuse of alcohol and other drugs (Centers for Disease Control and Prevention [CDC], 2005). These objectives can be reviewed on the *Healthy People 2010* Web site at http://wonder.cdc.gov/data2010◆. Baseline data, targets, and current data for selected objectives are provided at the end of this chapter.

In this chapter, perspectives on causes of abuse and trends in substance use and abuse are examined. Risk factors contributing to all forms of substance abuse, signs and symptoms of specific types of abuse, and community health nursing interventions in the control of substance abuse are addressed.

PSYCHOACTIVE SUBSTANCES: DEPENDENCE AND ABUSE

Substance abuse involves the inappropriate use of psychoactive substances. Research suggests that many drug abusers who begin drug use by their early 20s discontinue use without treatment; those who do not become dependent on the abused substances (Price, Risk, & Spitznagel, 2001). The *DSM-IV-TR* recognizes abuse of several substances under umbrella diagnoses of psychoactive substance dependence and psychoactive substance abuse. The **psychoactive substance dependence syndrome** is a cluster of cognitive, behavioral, and physiologic symptoms that indicate impaired control over the use of a psychoactive substance and continued use despite adverse consequences (American Psychiatric Association, 2000).

GLOBAL PERSPECTIVES

*I*ncreasing rates of alcohol consumption have been closely linked to higher rates of homicide in Russia, particularly after the dissolution of the Soviet Union. In fact, research has suggested that for every 1% increase in alcohol consumption, there is a 0.25% increase in homicide rates. Researchers have suggested that it is the culture surrounding alcohol consumption, as well as the lack of formal and informal social controls on drinking, that contributes to this relationship. The primary drink of choice in Russia is vodka, a form of distilled spirits that is often drunk in binges in unregulated settings. Although consumption of alcohol in public places is increasing, most consumption occurs in the home or other private setting with family members and friends. In such settings there is little control over consumption levels such as might be provided in a more public setting. Binge drinking of vodka leads to disinhibition, which may contribute to aggressive behavior and violence compounded by lack of any formal controls on behavior (e.g., police intervention or a bar bouncer), thus culminating in a higher frequency of homicide when violence escalates (Pridemore, 2002). Are there similar interrelationships that affect the societal effects of substance abuse in the United States or other countries? What factors are involved in these interrelationships? How might these factors be controlled? What approaches do other countries take to public health issues related to substance abuse? How effective are these approaches? Would these approaches be appropriate in the United States? Why or why not?

SPECIAL CONSIDERATIONS

SIGNS AND SYMPTOMS OF PSYCHOACTIVE SUBSTANCE DEPENDENCE

- Increasing amounts of substance used, or use extending over a longer period than intended
- Persistent desire for the substance or one or more unsuccessful attempts to control its use
- Increased time spent in obtaining, using, or recovering from the effects of the substance
- Frequent symptoms of intoxication or withdrawal interfering with obligations
- Elimination or reduction of important occupational, social, or recreational activities as a result of substance use
- Continued use of the substance despite recurrent problems caused
- Increased tolerance to the substance
- Experience of characteristic withdrawal symptoms
- Increased substance use to decrease withdrawal symptoms

Diagnosis of psychoactive substance dependence is based on the signs and symptoms presented on page 932.

Psychoactive substance abuse involves maladaptive patterns of substance use that do not meet the criteria for dependence. Criteria for a diagnosis of abuse include continued use of a substance (or substances) despite persistent or recurrent physical, psychological, or social problems related to its use, or recurrent use of the substance in physically dangerous situations (e.g., driving while intoxicated). Because substance abuse is a precursor to dependence, the term *substance abuse* is used throughout this chapter in discussing the role of the community health nurse in its prevention and control.

PERSPECTIVES ON CAUSATION IN SUBSTANCE ABUSE

The trajectory of substance abuse usually begins with occasional use and may progress to regular use. In some people, changes in brain metabolism and activity lead to the compulsive, uncontrollable use that characterizes abuse and dependence (National Institute on Drug Abuse [NIDA], 2005d). Not every user, however, progresses from initial experimentation to dependence. What explains progression to abuse and dependence in some people and not in others?

At present, there is no definitive answer to this question. An important trend to be noted, however, is the changing historical perspective on abusive disorders. For many years, society perceived substance abuse, particularly drunkenness, as a character defect and a vice. This view was largely supplanted in the 20th century by the biomedical concept of substance abuse and dependence as disease. This model, however, does not effectively address the current propensity for recreational use of drugs (Lennings, 2000). The most recent genre of theories of causation in substance abuse, biopsychosocial theory, suggests that abuse is a product of the interaction of multiple genetic, psychological, and environmental factors (NIDA, 2003). These factors will be discussed later in this chapter.

PSYCHOACTIVE SUBSTANCES AND THEIR USE

Psychoactive substances are abused because of their desirable initial effects. Some of these effects and the drugs associated with them are presented in Table 31-1◆. Unfortunately, many psychoactive drugs with potential for abuse have rebound effects that are usually the opposite of their initial effects and lead to repeated use to eliminate the undesirable symptoms created by the rebound. These adverse effects are discussed later in this chapter. Because of the phenomenon of tolerance, the user requires larger and larger doses of many drugs to

combat rebound effects and to achieve the desired pleasurable effect. **Drug tolerance** is an adaptation of the body to a substance such that previous doses do not have the desired effect. Psychoactive substances commonly involved in either dependence or abuse are presented below.

Alcohol

The alcohol contained in alcoholic beverages is ethyl alcohol created by the fermentation of grain mixtures or the juice of fruits and berries. After ingestion, alcohol is rapidly absorbed into the bloodstream through the gastrointestinal tract and functions as a central nervous system (CNS) depressant.

Although moderate alcohol intake has been found to have positive health effects, alcohol abuse remains a serious problem in the United States and elsewhere in the world. Alcohol use is the third leading cause of death in the United States, contributing to more than 100,000 deaths each year (Nelson, Naimi, Brewer, Bolen, & Wells, 2004). Alcohol abuse is the leading cause of chronic liver disease and cirrhosis, which resulted in more than 17,400 deaths among U.S. men in 2002 (National Center for Health Statistics [NCHS], 2005).

In 2003, 50% of the U.S. population age 12 and older reported current alcohol use and 22.6% reported binge drinking (more than five alcoholic drinks on a single occasion) (U.S. Census Bureau, 2006). According to the 2005 Behavioral Risk Factor Surveillance System (BRFSS) survey, this figure had declined to 14.4%, with 4.9% of the U.S. population reporting heavy drinking (more than two drinks per day for men or more than one drink a day for women) (National Center for Chronic Disease Prevention and Health Promotion [NCCDPHP], 2006a). Among young adults, nearly 32% of 35-year-old men and 13% of women reported heavy drinking (Merline, O'Malley, Schulenberg, Bachman, & Johnston, 2004).

SPECIAL CONSIDERATIONS

SUBSTANCES COMMONLY INVOLVED IN SUBSTANCE ABUSE OR DEPENDENCE

- Alcohol
- Sedatives, hypnotics, and anxiolytics
- Opioids
- Cocaine
- Amphetamines
- Hallucinogens
- Cannabis
- Inhalants
- Steroids
- Nicotine

TABLE 31-1 Selected Psychoactive Substances, Street Names, Typical Routes of Administration, and Effects Promoting Abuse

Substance	Street Names	Typical Route of Administration	Effects Promoting Abuse
Alcohol	Beer, wine, spirits, booze, various brand names	Orally ingested	Relaxation, decreased inhibitions, increased confidence, euphoria
Sedatives, hypnotics, and anxiolytics		Orally ingested, injected	Calming effect, decreased nervousness and anxiety, improved sleep, relaxation, mild intoxication, loss of inhibition
Barbiturates			
Amytal	Blues, downers		
Nembutal	Yellows, yellow jackets		
Phenobarbital	Phennie, purple hearts		
Seconal	Reds, F-40s, Redbirds		
Tuinal	Rainbows, tooies		
Quaalude	Ludes, 714s, Q's, Quay, Quad, mandrex		
Tranquilizers (minor)	Tranks, downs, downers, goof balls, sleeping pills, candy		
Dalmane			
Equanil/Miltown	Muscle relaxants, sleeping pills		
Librium			
Valium			
Serax			
Opioids		Orally ingested	Pain relief, euphoria
Codeine	Schoolboy	Orally ingested	
Demerol	Demies, dolls, dollies, Amidone	Injected	
Dilaudid	Little D, Lords	Injected	
Heroin	Smack, junk, downtown, H, black tar, horse, stuff	Injected, smoked, sniffed	
Methadone	Meth, dollies	Injected	
Morphine	M, Miss Emma, morph, morpho, tab, white stuff, monkey	Injected	
Opium	Blue velvet, black stuff, Dover's powder, paregoric	Orally ingested, smoked, injected	
Percodan	Perkies	Orally ingested	
Cocaine	Coke, snow, uptown, flake, crack, bump, toot, c, candy	Snorted, injected, smoked	Increased alertness, confidence, euphoria, reduced fatigue
Amphetamines		Orally ingested	Increased alertness, confidence, decreased fatigue, euphoria
Benzedrine	Bennies, pep pills, uppers, truck drivers		
Biphetamine	Black beauties		
Desoxyn	Co-pilots		
Dexedrine	Dex, speed, dexies		
Methedrine	Meth, crank, speed, crystal, go fast		
MDMA	Ecstasy		
Hallucinogens		Orally ingested, smoked, injected	Altered perceptions, mystical experience
Phencyclidine	Angel dust, krystal, DOA, hog, PCP, peace pill	Smoked, orally ingested, injected	Dreamlike state producing hallucinations
LSD	Acid, microdot, cubes		
MDA	The love drug		
Mescaline	Cactus, mesc		
Peyote	Buttons		
Psilocybin	Magic mushrooms, shrooms, sacred mushrooms		
Cannabis		Smoked, orally ingested	Relaxation, euphoria, altered perceptions
Hashish	Kif, herb, hash		
Hashish oil	Honey, hash oil		

Continued on next page

TABLE 31-1	Selected Psychoactive Substances, Street Names, Typical Routes of Administration, and Effects Promoting Abuse *(continued)*		
Substance	**Street Names**	**Typical Route of Administration**	**Effects Promoting Abuse**
Marijuana	Grass, ganja, weed, dope, reefer, Thai sticks, pot, Acapulco gold, roach, loco weed, Maui wowie, joint, Mary Jane		
Inhalants		Inhaled	Relaxation, euphoria, intoxication
Amyl nitrate	Poppers		
Butyl nitrate	Locker room, rush		
Nitrous oxide	Laughing gas		
Nicotine	Various brand names of tobacco products	Smoked, chewed	Relaxation, mild stimulation

Alcohol use is also prevalent among U.S. youth. The 2005 Youth Risk Behavior Surveillance (YRBS) survey, for example, indicated that more than one fourth of high school students in participating states and cities had used alcohol before age 13, and 43% had had one or more drinks in the past month. In addition, 25.5% of the students engaged in periodic heavy drinking, 28.5% had ridden with a driver who had been drinking, and nearly 10% had themselves driven after drinking alcohol (Eaton et al., 2006). Another national study, conducted in 2004, indicated that a total of 71% of high school seniors had used alcohol in the prior year (Bureau of Justice Statistics [BJS], 2005b). Overall, nearly 8% of the U.S. population (18.2 million people) meet diagnostic criteria for alcohol dependence or abuse (Substance Abuse and Mental Health Services Administration [SAMHSA], 2006a), indicating a serious public health problem.

Sedatives, Hypnotics, and Anxiolytics

A second group of drugs frequently abused is sedatives, hypnotics, and anxiolytics. Sedatives are used to calm nervousness, irritability, and excitement, whereas hypnotics induce sleep. Many drugs have sedative effects in lower doses and hypnotic effects in higher doses. Anxiolytics (also known as antianxiety agents or minor tranquilizers) are used to reduce anxiety and tension and promote sleep. All three types of drugs are CNS depressants.

These drugs are frequently prescribed for symptoms of nervousness, anxiety, or difficulty sleeping. Unfortunately, their prescription for legitimate use often creates dependence. In low doses, these drugs produce a mild state of euphoria, reduce inhibitions, and create feelings of relaxation and decreased tension. Their major pharmacologic action is CNS depression. Drugs involved in this category of substance abuse include tranquilizers such as chlordiazepoxide hydrochloride (Librium) and diazepam (Valium); barbiturate sedatives; nonbarbiturates such as hydroxyzine hydrochloride (Atarax) and meprobamate (Equanil); and hypnotics

such as methaqualone hydrochloride (Quaalude) and diphenhydramine hydrochloride (Nytol, Sleep-eze, Sominex). Because of their widespread use for both legitimate and illegitimate reasons and their easy availability, precise figures on the abuse of these drugs are difficult to obtain. However, an estimated 7% of the U.S. men and 8% of women in their 30s reported misuse of prescription drugs such as these (Merline et al., 2004).

Opioids

Opioids are also CNS depressants and are derived naturally from the opium poppy or created synthetically. Opioids bind to CNS cell receptors to mimic the action of naturally produced endorphins that relieve pain. In addition to relief of pain, opioids create a psychological euphoria that prompts continued use.

Chronic heroin use occurs in approximately 810,000 people in the United States (Goldsmith, 2000a). In 2003, the prevalence of current heroin use among persons aged 12 years and older was less than 1% (U.S. Census Bureau, 2006), but 3.3% of high school students reported ever using heroin (Grunbaum et al., 2004). By 2005, this figure had declined to 2.4% (Eaton et al., 2006).

Opioid use is increasing in other parts of the world as well. For example, opium and heroin are the drugs of choice in a growing epidemic of substance abuse in China. Opium is smoked in a pipe and its use probably arrived in the United States with travelers from the Far East. Heroin use in China may involve smoking heroin-laced cigarettes, inhaling vapors (called "chasing the dragon"), or intravenous injection. Injection drug use increased from 13.5% of heroin users in 1988 to 53.3% in 1999. Sharing of drug paraphernalia, including needles, syringes, or smoking equipment, is common, increasing the spread of HIV infection in the IDU population (Wu, Detels, Zhang, Li, & Li, 2002).

There is growing concern regarding abuse of the synthetic opioid oxycodone (or Oxycontin). Oxycontin is a time-release form of oxycodone intended for extended relief of pain. Street drug users have found, however, that crushing and inhaling the tablets invalidates the time-release mechanism, resulting in a rapid and powerful high similar to that achieved with morphine (Weiner, 2005). In six U.S. states that record opiate deaths, 40% of deaths due to opiate misuse were the result of oxycodone, hydrocodone, and methadone (SAMHSA, 2006c). Deaths also occur in response to intentional or unintentional adulteration of heroin with clenbuterol, a drug abused as an alternative to anabolic steroids (Hoffman et al., 2005).

Cocaine

Cocaine is a stimulant derived from the leaves of the coca plant. Its use produces euphoria and a sense of competence. Other desired effects include increased energy and clarity of thought. Unlike many of the other drugs presented here, the pleasurable effects of cocaine are extremely short acting (approximately 30 minutes) and are followed by an intense letdown and craving for another dose.

Use of cocaine may be accompanied by the practice of "freebasing." Normally, to maintain its stability, cocaine is combined with a hydrochloride base, creating a substance that is usually only about 25% cocaine. **Freebasing** involves the use of heat and ether to free the cocaine from its hydrochloride base, thus creating a purer product that produces a more intense effect. Because of the combination of heat and the highly volatile and explosive ether, freebasing is an extremely dangerous practice. To eliminate the need for freebasing, drug dealers created **crack**, a stable form of cocaine without the hydrochloride base that can be smoked rather than inhaled, for a more rapid and more intense effect.

Next to alcohol, cocaine is the abusive substance of greatest concern because of the rapid escalation in its use and its severe adverse effects. In 2003, 1% of persons over 12 years of age in the United States reported current cocaine use (U.S. Census Bureau, 2006). In the 2005 YRBS, 7.6% of high school students reported ever using cocaine, and 3.4% reported current use (Eaton et al., 2006). Among people over 35 years of age, 0.6% reported current cocaine use (U.S. Census Bureau, 2006).

Amphetamines

Amphetamines are CNS stimulants that are manufactured chemically. Amphetamines have, on occasion, been prescribed to assist weight loss and relieve fatigue, but they are not recommended for either condition. Amphetamines and similar drugs produce feelings of euphoria, energy, confidence, increased ability to concentrate, and improved physical performance. They are sometimes used by truck drivers and students who wish to stay awake to study or by athletes desiring to improve their performance.

Amphetamines lend themselves to chemical modifications to create "designer" or "club" drugs. **Designer drugs** are modifications of legal drugs whose use in their original form is restricted. Club drugs are used at group activities known as *raves*, all night parties with techno music (Weiner, 2005), and include 3,4-methylenedionymethamphetamine (MDMA), better known as "ecstasy"; ketamine; gamma-hydroxybutyrate (GHB); and Rohypnol (a tranquilizer), the so-called date rape drug (Vo, 2000). Club drugs may cause brain damage and coma as well as long-term effects on memory and learning abilities, seizures, malignant hyperthermia, paranoia, and hostility. The low cost of drugs like Rohypnol makes them popular with adolescents (Weiner, 2005).

Methamphetamine is a drug of particular concern because it is highly addictive and can be produced with inexpensive materials readily available to most people. *Crystal* is a crystalline form of methamphetamine hydrochloride that can be smoked. Other forms of methamphetamine may be taken orally, snorted nasally, or injected intravenously. Effects of methamphetamine include wakefulness, increased physical activity, diminished appetite, increased respiration, and euphoria. Additional central nervous system effects include confusion, anxiety, irritability, and insomnia. Users may also experience paranoia, hallucinations, delusions, and mood disturbances, and exhibit aggressive behavior. Binge use may include injection of as much as a gram of methamphetamine every 2 to 3 hours. Death may occur as a result of hyperthermia and convulsions. Withdrawal from methamphetamine does not produce physical symptoms but may result in depression, anxiety, fatigue, aggression, paranoia, and intense cravings (NIDA, 2005a, 2005b). Chronic methamphetamine use can result in brain damage similar to that caused by Alzheimer's disease or stroke (Office of National Drug Control Policy, 2006).

Production of methamphetamine occurs in makeshift laboratories using highly corrosive, explosive, and toxic materials, posing a significant fire and explosion hazard. Production employs easily available ingredients, so "meth" labs can be set up almost anywhere. Community health nurses should be alert to the following signs of a methamphetamine laboratory and alert local law enforcement personnel:

- Unusual chemical odors (e.g., ether, ammonia, acetone, urine)
- Excessive amounts of trash, particularly coffee filters, duct tape, red-stained cloth, containers from cold remedies that contain ephedrine or pseudoephedrine, or bottles of sulfuric, muriatic, or hydrochloric acid
- Glass cookware or frying pans with a powdery residue
- Extensive use of camp fuel, paint thinner, acetone, or drain cleaners

- Multiple lithium batteries
- Consistently covered windows
- Evidence of chemical waste dumping
- Frequent visitors at unusual times
- Extensive privacy or security measures
- Residents who go outside to smoke (although this could be an innocent measure to limit secondhand smoke inhalation for family members)
- Secretive or unfriendly occupants (Cooper, Rice, Wilburn, Horton, & Rossiter, 2005; U.S. Drug Enforcement Administration, n.d.)

Although exact figures on the use of these drugs is not known, one 2004 study found that 10% of high school seniors engaged in stimulant use (BJS, 2005b). From 1993 to 2003, the rate of substance abuse treatment for amphetamine use in people over age 12 more than quadrupled (SAMHSA, 2006e). In 2004, lifetime methamphetamine use was reported by nearly 5% of those participating in the National Survey on Drug Use and Health, with 1.4 million people reporting use in the previous year and 583,000 in the previous month (Office of National Drug Control Policy, 2006).

Hallucinogens

Phencyclidine (PCP) was originally developed as an anesthetic, but its use was discontinued because of its many adverse side effects. The effects of PCP are variable and may include stimulation or depression of the CNS or hallucinations. Its more desirable effects include heightened sensitivity to stimuli, mood elevation, a sense of omnipotence, and relaxation. Unfortunately, PCP has some serious adverse effects. PCP-induced psychosis constitutes a psychiatric emergency, and PCP use may lead to seizures, coma, and death.

Other hallucinogens or psychedelic drugs, such as *d*-lysergic acid diethylamide (LSD), mescaline, peyote, and psilocybin mushrooms, alter experience to create hallucinations. They also distort the distinction between self and the environment, making the user extremely vulnerable to environmental stimuli. Common effects of these drugs include changes in mood (euphoria or terror and despair), heightened sensation or synesthesia (merging of the senses so colors, for example, are experienced as odors or vice versa), changes in perceptions of time and objects, and changes in relationships, leading to depersonalization and feelings of merging with other people and objects.

In 2003, 14.5% of the U.S. population over the age of 12 reported ever having used hallucinogens. Current use of hallucinogens was reported by 0.4% of the population. More people reported ever having used LSD (10.3%) than PCP (3%), but data on current use of hallucinogens by type were not available (U.S. Census Bureau, 2006).

Cannabis

Cannabis species of plants are the source of marijuana and hashish. The primary psychoactive substance in these drugs is delta-9-tetrahydrocannabinol (THC). THC may be inhaled by smoking marijuana or hashish or ingested and produces relaxation, euphoria, and occasionally altered perceptions of time and space. Marijuana use may contribute to exacerbation of other mental health problems such as schizophrenia and depression.

Current marijuana use in the general population has declined from 9.7% in 1985 to 6.2% in 2003 (U.S. Census Bureau, 1999; 2006), but is higher among adolescents. In 2005, for example, 38% of high school students had ever used marijuana and 20% reported current use (Eaton et al., 2006). Among people over 35 years of age, 38.9% had ever used marijuana in 2003, and 3% were current users (U.S. Census Bureau, 2006).

Inhalants

Inhalants are abused by sniffing products such as airplane model glue, nail polish remover, gasoline, aerosols, and anesthetics such as nitrous oxide. They usually produce a sense of euphoria, loss of inhibition, and excitement. Inhalants are often used by people who do not have the financial resources to support more expensive drug habits. In addition to a variety of adverse physical effects such as kidney and heart damage, there is the potential for suffocation while inhaling these substances from a plastic bag. Because of their volatile nature, explosion is another hazard presented by inhalants.

Inhalant use is particularly common among adolescents. From 2002 to 2004, for example, an average of 598,000 youth initiated inhalant use in the previous year (SAMHSA, 2006b). Approximately 12% of adolescents reported ever having used inhalants in the 2005 YRBS (Eaton et al., 2006). Overall use in the United States in 2003 was reported at 0.2% of the population (U.S. Census Bureau, 2006).

Steroids

Most steroid use occurs under medical direction for treatment of a variety of conditions in which immunosuppression is a desired outcome (e.g., severe arthritis and other inflammatory conditions). Steroids are abused by a small segment of the population, however, particularly adolescents. For example, in 2004, 3.4% of high school seniors reported ever having used steroids for nonmedical reasons, and 2.5% reported use in the prior 30 days (NIDA, 2005c). Anabolic steroids may be used by adolescents and athletes because of their potential to increase strength and weight and to improve body image and athletic performance.

Prolonged use of anabolic steroids leads to acne, diminished breast size, ovulatory and menstrual difficulties, deepened voice, clitoral enlargement, and male-pattern baldness in women. In men, effects of prolonged use include continuing erections (priapism), difficult urination, gynecomastia, and impotence. Both men and women may experience liver impairment, urinary calculi, anemia, gastrointestinal problems (e.g., anorexia, nausea), and insomnia. Adolescents who take anabolic steroids before completing the typical adolescent growth spurt may permanently impede their growth (NIDA, 2005c).

Nicotine

Nicotine, the last of the abusive substances included in the *DSM-IV-TR* categories of psychoactive substance dependence and abuse, is the psychoactive substance present in tobacco smoke. Nicotine produces feelings of well-being, increases mental acuity and ability to concentrate, and heightens one's sense of purpose. Nicotine may also exert a calming effect on the smoker. Unfortunately, nicotine also contributes to a host of adverse physical effects, including heart disease, several forms of cancer, and chronic respiratory diseases.

Because of the highly addictive nature of nicotine and its adverse health effects, all forms of tobacco use should be discouraged. Unlike moderate alcohol use, even moderate smoking produces negative effects on health. Nicotine, unlike many other abused substances, has no medical applications.

Each year throughout the world nearly 5 million people die as a result of tobacco-related illnesses (Mochizuki-Kobayashi et al., 2006), and this figure is expected to double by 2020 (CDC, 2006d). According to the Global Youth Tobacco Survey, on average, 20% of all 13- to 15-year-olds used some form of tobacco between 1999 and 2005. Use is highest in the region of the Americas at more than 22%, followed by the European region (nearly 20%), and lowest in the Western Pacific (11%). Cigarette smoking was reported by nearly 9% of students worldwide (Mochizuki-Kobayashi et al., 2006).

Efforts to eliminate smoking in the U.S. population have been somewhat successful. For example, in 2005, 20.5% of people over 18 years of age smoked, compared to 39% in 1985 (NCCDPHP, 2006b; U.S. Census Bureau, 1999). Results of efforts to eliminate smoking among young people have been less effective. In 2003, for example, 22% of high school students reported current cigarette smoking. By 2005, this figure had increased to 23% (Office on Smoking and Health, 2006). More than 13% of high school students responding to the 2005 YRBS had engaged in daily smoking for a least one month in their lifetimes, and 8% were current users of smokeless tobacco products (Eaton et al., 2006). In 2002, 20.4 billion packs of cigarettes were sold in the United States, an average of 71.7 packs for every person in the nation (CDC, 2004).

EFFECTS OF SUBSTANCE ABUSE

Substance abuse contributes to adverse effects for the abusing individual, for his or her family, and for society at large.

Personal Effects

The effects of substance abuse on the individual are physical, psychological, and social. Physical effects include increased morbidity directly related to the effects of the drug or drugs abused, as well as increased potential for exposure to diseases such as AIDS and hepatitis when abuse involves use of contaminated needles or results in sexual promiscuity as a means of financing a drug habit or because of lowered inhibitions. The dual presence of HIV infection and injection drug use (IDU) also increases the risk of tuberculosis nearly eightfold over persons who are HIV negative, and injection drug users have a 17 times greater risk of TB than nonusers. Overall TB prevalence among injection drug users is estimated at 31% (Kim & Crittenden, 2005).

Other physical effects of substance abuse include unintentional injury, unintended pregnancy, and fetal alcohol syndrome (Nelson et al., 2004). Among the elderly, alcohol-related disease increases the risk of hip fracture almost threefold (Yuan et al., 2001). Substance use also contributes to a wide variety of other unintended injuries. An estimated 40% of residential fires, for instance, are related to alcohol use, and alcohol contributes to 25% to 50% of deaths related to water recreation (National Center for Injury Prevention and Control, 2006a, 2006b). Overall, alcohol use contributes to 30% to 40% of emergency department visits each year and to 50% of serious trauma (Saitz, 2005).

Some drugs, such as alcohol, nicotine, and barbiturates, also result in withdrawal symptoms when the drug is removed from the client's system. The **withdrawal syndrome** caused by these and other drugs is a complex of symptoms usually including severe discomfort, pain, nausea, vomiting, and, possibly, convulsions. Withdrawal is frequently seen in alcohol abusers, with up to 71% of those in need of detoxification exhibiting signs of withdrawal (Asplund, Aaronson, & Aaronson, 2004). A number of the drugs discussed, including cocaine, marijuana, methamphetamine, PCP, ecstasy, alcohol, and nicotine, can also lead to stroke and resultant death (Cabaniss, 2005). Some drugs also produce chromosomal changes that cause congenital malformations in children as well as increased potential for spontaneous abortion. Death is the ultimate adverse effect of drug use and may result from a drug overdose, from withdrawal, or from the long-term effects of drug use such as cirrhosis, cancer, cardiovascular disease, and stroke. Assessment for both short-term and long-term physical effects of specific substances is discussed later in this chapter.

In addition to the desired effects that promote drug use and abuse, psychological effects of drug abuse can include personality disturbances, anxiety, and depression. Organic mental disorders characterized by hallucinations, delusions, dementia, delirium, and disorders of mood or perception may also be caused by substance abuse. Aggressive behavior may also result from the use of some drugs (e.g., PCP, anabolic steroids) (NIDA, 2005c). In addition, substance abuse may trigger exacerbations of existing mental disorders.

Preoccupation with the abused substance can lead to a variety of social problems for the substance abuser. Relationships with family and friends may be impaired, or abusers may become incapable of or disinterested in performing their jobs and may be fired. Substance abuse may also lead to poor educational outcomes, limiting the abuser's employability. Unemployment can lead to difficulties in obtaining housing and can contribute to homelessness. Furthermore, the need to obtain money to support a drug habit or to obtain necessities may lead to criminal activity.

Family Effects

The effects of substance abuse on the family of the abuser can be many and severe. These families are characterized by frequent conflict, anger, ambivalence, fear, guilt, confusion, mistrust, and violence as a mode of conflict resolution. The family frequently becomes socially isolated in efforts to cover up the problem of abuse and so are not able to make use of sources of assistance that might be available to them (Grant, 2000). Substance abuse may also be a factor in poor parental role execution, leading to neglect and abuse of children (Ehrmin, 2001).

The effects of parental alcoholism on children have been widely studied. An estimated 11 million U.S. children under 18 years of age are exposed to alcohol abuse by family members, and the average school classroom has four to six students whose parents are chemically dependent. Children exposed to parental alcoholism have a four to six times higher risk of developing alcohol-related problems themselves than children whose parents do not abuse alcohol. They are also more likely to display eating disorders, depression, phobias, and anxiety disorders and to engage in antisocial behavior and have problems in interpersonal relationships. In addition, they have been shown to have a higher risk of asthma, hypertension, abdominal pain, headaches, gastrointestinal disorders, and allergies. In the school setting, they more often come late to class, have learning disabilities, and receive less help with homework than other children (Gance-Cleveland, 2004).

Family members may exhibit the phenomenon of co-dependence. A **co-dependent** is a person in a continuing relationship with the substance abuser, whose behavior enables the abuser to continue his or her drug-dependent existence (Insel et al., 2005). Co-dependents practice maladaptive behaviors to cope with the problem of abuse. Characteristics of co-dependents center on patterns of denial of feelings, low self-esteem, compliance with others' desires over personal interests, and control of others. A set of questions that addresses each of these patterns has been developed by Co-dependents Anonymous, a mutual-help group modeled on the 12-step program of Alcoholics Anonymous. These questions can be used to identify persons who are co-dependent and are available at http://www.coda.org/codapatt.htm.

Direct exposure of children to psychoactive substances has a variety of adverse physical and psychological effects. Children with perinatal exposure to alcohol, nicotine, or other drugs may be lower in birth weight, be particularly irritable and difficult to comfort, and experience poor school performance later in life. Drug use during pregnancy may also contribute to premature labor. Home exposure to tobacco smoke also affects the health status of children and may contribute to a variety of respiratory conditions as well as childhood cancers. The health effects of drug exposures for children are discussed in more detail later in this chapter.

Societal Effects

Societal effects of substance abuse include increased morbidity and mortality, higher economic costs, and increased crime. Physical morbidity related to psychoactive substance abuse was addressed in relation to the personal effects of substance abuse. At the societal level, abuse leads to increased incidence and prevalence of these conditions.

Mortality

As noted earlier, substance abuse leads to increased mortality, either directly as a result of drug overdose or withdrawal or indirectly due to other conditions related to abuse. The contribution of smoking to increased mortality was discussed in Chapter 29∞. Drug-related mortality rates decreased slightly from 9.0 per 100,000 population in 2002 to 8.7 per 100,000 in 2003. Alcohol-related mortality declined by a similar proportion during the same period, from 6.9 per 100,000 population to 6.6. Alcoholic liver disease contributed to more than 12,000 deaths in 2003 (4.1 deaths per 100,000 population) (U.S. Census Bureau, 2006).

Accidental mortality related to alcohol abuse is of particular concern. In spite of decreases in the number of alcohol-related motor vehicle fatalities, 39% of motor vehicle fatalities in 2004 involved alcohol (National Highway Traffic Safety Administration, 2006). Alcohol use is also implicated in other injury fatalities, including falls, drowning, and burns. In addition to accident fatalities, alcohol is a factor in other deaths, including homicide; suicide; deaths due to cancers of the lip, oral cavity, pharynx, esophagus, stomach, liver, and larynx; cardiovascular deaths; and deaths due to respiratory diseases, digestive diseases, and diabetes mellitus.

Cost

Substance abuse also affects society in terms of its economic costs. A 1992 study conducted for the National Institute on Drug Abuse (the most recent total cost estimates), indicated that the total economic cost for alcohol and drug abuse was $245.7 billion. This cost estimate included treatment and prevention costs as well as costs of lost productivity and criminal justice costs. The 1992 estimates represented a 50% increase in costs from 1985. Over half of these costs were the result of drug-related crime and criminal justice control (NIDA, 2006a). Law enforcement related to marijuana alone is estimated to cost $7.6 billion a year (Drug Reform Coordination Network, 2005), and the fiscal year budget allocation for the federal Drug Enforcement Administration is estimated at $2.2 billion (Office of Management and Budget, 2003). In addition, a 1995 study by the White House Office of National Drug Control Policy estimated that actual expenditures for drugs amounted to $57.3 billion from 1988 to 1995 (NIDA, 2006a). Estimated annual costs attributed to alcohol use amount to $185 billion (Saitz, 2005).

Without doubt, drug and alcohol abuse are costly public health problems that the nation can ill afford. Prevention of substance abuse, on the other hand, is cost-effective. NIDA (2003) estimates that every dollar invested in prevention of substance abuse in children and adolescents, for example, saves up to $10 in treatment costs. This figure does not even consider the reduction in costs for law enforcement and lost productivity.

Crime

One final social effect associated with the abuse of many substances (excluding nicotine) is increased crime. In 2004, there were 1.5 million drug-related arrests among adults and another 194,000 among juveniles in the United States. These figures represent a nearly fivefold increase in arrests among adults and more than a twofold increase for adolescents (BJS, 2005c). The 2003 arrest rate for drug abuse violations was 640.4 per 100,000 people. In 2003, the majority of juvenile arrests (84%) involved illegal possession of drugs, but 16% were related to the production and sale of illicit drugs. Similar proportions were noted for the breakdown of overall arrests. More than three fourths of arrests for drug possession by adolescents (78%) involved marijuana, 11% involved nonnarcotic drugs, 9% were for possession of heroin or cocaine, and 2.5% for possession of synthetic narcotics. In the general population, arrest rates were highest for nonnarcotic drugs (198.1 per 100,000 population) followed by marijuana (171.6 per

100,000) and heroin or cocaine (149.6 per 100,000). The lowest rate of arrests was for possession of synthetic drugs (18.9 per 100,000) (U.S. Census Bureau, 2006).

Drug and alcohol use have also been implicated in other crimes not strictly related to drugs. For example, 30% of violent crimes for which alcohol involvement was known were committed by people who had been drinking, and in 20% of cases the perpetrator had also been using drugs (BJS, 2005a). Among state prison inmates, 40% were using drugs or alcohol at the time they committed the crime for which they were incarcerated (Travis, Solomon, & Waul, 2001). Crimes may be committed as a result of the lowering of inhibitions caused by alcohol and other drugs. In other cases, crimes such as theft may be a means of supporting a drug or alcohol habit.

THE EPIDEMIOLOGY OF SUBSTANCE ABUSE

The epidemiology of substance abuse indicates that there are contributing factors in five of the six dimensions of health (biophysical, psychological, sociocultural, behavioral, and health system dimensions). Only the physical environmental dimension of health does not have a significant influence on substance abuse. Community health nurses should keep in mind that the interplay among factors in each of the five dimensions that leads to substance abuse is unique to each individual and to each population group. For this reason, nurses should assess the factors contributing to abuse in a given situation prior to developing interventions to address substance abuse in an individual or a population group.

Biophysical Considerations

Human biological factors influencing substance abuse and its effects include genetic inheritance, maturation and aging, and physiologic function.

Genetic Inheritance

A growing body of evidence suggests that substance abuse is associated with some form of genetic predisposition. Studies of adopted children, for example, indicate that alcohol abuse by one or both of the biological parents is associated with alcohol and drug abuse by the child, but no increased risk has been noted when adoptive parents drink. Further support for a genetic predisposition for substance abuse comes from the increased risk in the second twin if the first of monozygotic twins is substance dependent when compared with dizygotic twins (Uhl, Elmer, LaBuda, & Pickens, 2000). Meta-analysis of twin and adoptive studies has suggested that the heritability of alcohol abuse may be less than is suggested by individual studies and shows considerable variation by gender and other factors. For example, the genetic contribution to abuse seems to be stronger for men than for women (Walters, 2002). Although there has been some work on the identification of specific suspect genes (Edenberg et al., 2004), it seems safe to say at present that genetic factors interrelate in complex ways with other factors in their contribution to substance abuse (Uhl et al., 2000).

In assessing individuals and families for the level of risk for substance abuse, the community health nurse prepares a detailed genogram that includes information about the family history of substance abuse as well as the presence of physical and emotional illnesses with a genetic component. Community health nurses can also educate the public about the potential heritability of substance abuse and advocate for prevention among people who are at risk due to a family history of abuse.

Gender, race, and ethnicity are other factors that may influence substance abuse. For example, men were three times more likely than women to engage in binge drinking and somewhat more likely to report heavy drinking in the 2005 BRFSS. Women were also slightly less likely than men to be current smokers, with medians of 19.2% and 21.9%, respectively (NCCDPHP, 2006a, 2006b). With respect to racial or ethnic factors, Asians and African Americans are the ethnic groups most likely to abstain from alcohol use altogether. In 2003, the American Indian Service Utilization, Psychiatric Epidemiology, Risk and Protective Factors Project (AISUPERPFP) found that although U.S. men in general drank more often than American Indian men, American Indian men drank larger quantities of alcohol (Beals et al., 2003). In BRFSS surveys over several years, more American Indian men and women engaged in binge drinking than men and women in the general population (Denny, Holtzman, & Cobb, 2003). Community health nurses can initiate public education campaigns targeted and relevant to high-risk groups. For example, prevention campaigns among Native American groups should be culturally relevant and address the myriad social factors that may contribute to abuse as well as the physiologic differences in drug metabolism that influence development of substance-related problems.

Maturation and Aging

Age influences one's risk of exposure to tobacco, alcohol, and other drugs through social factors. For example, young people are more likely to be exposed to peer influence for drug use or smoking than are older people. Adolescents and preadolescents are particularly vulnerable to this type of influence because of their developmental need to conform to peer expectations and to be part of a group. Often, being part of the group depends on engaging in behaviors that place the individual at risk, such as sexual activity, smoking, and drug and alcohol use. Younger age at onset of alcohol, tobacco, and marijuana use has been linked to greater risk of progression to hard drugs (Golub & Johnson, 2001). Risk for

dependence also increases with younger age at initiation of use. Early initiation of substance use is also associated with an increased risk of psychiatric illness. For instance, the prevalence of young-adult alcohol dependence among those who were regular alcohol users during middle school was three times higher than for those who abstained from alcohol use. Marijuana dependence was nearly four times more common among those who initiated use during middle school (Gil, Wagner, & Tubman, 2004).

In 2005, the Youth Risk Behavior Surveillance (YRBS) survey found that nearly 74% of high school seniors had ever used alcohol, 43% were current users, and 25.5% engaged in episodic heavy drinking. More than one fifth of students (20.2%) reported current marijuana use, and nearly 8% reported ever using cocaine, with current cocaine use by 3.5% of students. Lifetime use of inhalants, steroids, and hallucinogens was reported by 12%, 4%, and 8.5% of students, respectively. In addition, 2.4% of students reported ever having used heroin, and 6% reported lifetime use of methamphetamines or ecstasy (Eaton et al., 2006).

Community health nurses working with young people should assess their level of maturity and their ability to resist pressure to conform. Fortunately, the majority of young people who experiment with drugs appear to "grow out of" their use. As noted by some authors, "As midlife begins, and individuals assume more personal, familial, and societal responsibilities, the incentives and the opportunities to use substances generally subside, and concerns regarding health risks and negative consequences of substance use tend to increase" (Merline et al., 2004, p. 96). Alcohol consumption has also been shown to decrease with increasing age, but recent age cohorts have shown a slower decline in consumption, suggesting greater potential for alcohol-related health effects as these cohorts age (Moore et al., 2005).

The elderly have lower levels of substance abuse than other age groups, but an estimated 7% of women over age 59 abuse alcohol, and misuse of benzodiazepines is relatively common. Approximately one third of older women who misuse drugs and alcohol initiate use after age 60. Aging results in diminished ability to metabolize alcohol because of reduced liver and kidney function. Increased body fat in some older persons also slows the excretion of alcohol. Older women have alcohol-related mortality rates 50% to 100% higher than those in older men (Finfgeld-Connett, 2004). Older people are also more likely than younger ones to experience health effects from smoking (Andrews, Heath, & Graham-Garcia, 2004). Substance abuse problems in older clients may not be diagnosed because health care providers are not alert to signs and symptoms of abuse in this age group.

Perinatal exposures to drugs and alcohol have a variety of adverse effects on the fetus. Some psychoactive substances, such as alcohol, amphetamines, and cocaine, have teratogenic effects when taken during pregnancy. **Teratogenic substances** are those that cause physical defects in the developing embryo. Other drugs do not affect fetal development per se, but have other adverse health effects for the neonate or long-term effects for the child. For example, fetal alcohol exposure may result in prenatal and postnatal growth deficits, CNS abnormality, and delayed psychomotor development. Fetal, neonatal, and developmental effects of selected psychoactive substances are presented in Table 31-2◆.

Worldwide fetal alcohol syndrome (FAS) prevalence ranges from 0.2 to 1.5 cases per 1,000 live births. An estimated 4 million infants are exposed to alcohol in utero each year, and 1,000 to 6,000 of these exposed babies will develop FAS (Bertrand, Floyd, & Weber, 2005). During 2002, 2% of pregnant U.S. adult women reported binge drinking, and 11% smoked during the pregnancy (National Center on Birth Defects and Developmental Disabilities, 2004a, 2004b).

Community health nurses are often involved in assisting either biological or foster parents to care for these children. As noted in Chapter 16∞, FAS is a condition resulting from maternal alcohol consumption during pregnancy and is characterized by growth retardation, facial malformations, and CNS dysfunctions that may include mental retardation. An estimated 5,000 infants are affected each year in the United States (CDC, 2004). Long-term effects of FAS include inability to hold down a job, impulsivity, social withdrawal, poor judgment, and mental retardation.

Even those infants exposed to moderate amounts of alcohol during pregnancy may have long-term effects. It is estimated that four times as many infants have fetal alcohol spectrum disorders (FASDs) as have FAS. FASDs are disorders caused by fetal alcohol exposure that do not have all of the features of FAS (National Center on Birth Defects and Developmental Disabilities, 2005).

In working with newborns and young children, the community health nurse is alert to signs of perinatal drug exposure. He or she also assesses for risk factors that would make the child or older person particularly vulnerable to substance abuse and its effects.

Physiologic Function

The relationship between substance abuse and physiologic function is bidirectional. Persons with chronic physical health problems or disability may abuse drugs or alcohol as an escape from pain, depression, or stress related to the disability. Substance abuse may stem from a desire for gratification when other avenues are denied or as a method of regaining control over one's choices and actions. In working with disabled clients, community health nurses assess clients' responses to disability and their vulnerability to substance abuse as a means of coping with disability.

Conversely, substance abuse may result in a variety of physiologic health problems. For example, substance abuse disorders increase the risks of death and disability due to cirrhosis, heart disease, hepatocellular carcinoma, and stroke. Injection drug users also have a

TABLE 31-2	Fetal, Neonatal, and Developmental Effects of Perinatal Psychoactive Substance Exposure		
Substance	**Fetal Effects**	**Neonatal Effects**	**Developmental Effects**
Alcohol	Growth deficiency, microcephaly, stillbirth, low birth weight (LBW), joint and facial anomalies, cardiac and kidney anomalies	Acute withdrawal with sedation, seizures, poor feeding	Developmental delay, low IQ, hyperactivity
Sedatives, hypnotics	Sedation at delivery	Tremors, hypertonicity, poor suck, high-pitched cry	Unknown
Opioids	Intrauterine growth retardation, microcephaly, prematurity, hyperactivity	Withdrawal with tremors, hypertonicity, poor feeding, diarrhea, seizures, irritability	Increased rate of sudden infant death syndrome (SIDS)
Cocaine	Spontaneous abortion	Tremors, hypertonicity, muscle weakness, seizures	Developmental delay, increased rate of SIDS
Amphetamines	Intrauterine growth retardation, biliary atresia, transposition of great vessels	Stillbirth, LBW, cardiac anomalies, withdrawal	Poor school performance
Hallucinogens	Agitation at delivery, microcephaly	Irritability, poor fine-motor coordination, sensory input problems	Unknown
Cannabis	Bleeding problems in delivery	Sedation, tremors, excessive response to light	Unknown
Inhalants	Unknown	Unknown	Unknown
Nicotine	Intrauterine growth retardation, microcephaly	Jitteriness, poor feeding	Poor school performance, increased rate of SIDS

high risk of impairment due to drug impurities and infection. As we saw in Chapter 28∞, injection drug use is associated with high incidence of HIV infection and hepatitis B, C, and D. Tetanus and abscesses at the injection site also occur with injection drug use. One major metropolitan hospital, for instance, spends more than $18 million per year to treat drug-related abscesses (Goldsmith, 2000a), and botulism wound infections have been linked to intravenous or subcutaneous injection of black tar heroin contaminated in the cutting process (Division of Bacterial and Mycotic Diseases, 2003). As noted earlier, substance use and abuse may also contribute to long-term physical consequences related to accidental injury. Smoking is the greatest contributor to premature death in the world. Half of those who smoke die in middle age, with an average loss of 20 to 25 years of life expectancy. Those who smoke two packs of cigarettes a day have a 25-fold increase in the risk of death compared to nonsmokers. Exposure to secondhand smoke also results in more than 3,000 lung cancer deaths each year (Andrews et al., 2004). Biophysical factors contributing to or resulting from substance abuse can be identified using the focused assessment questions provided below.

Psychological Considerations

Both personality traits and the presence of psychopathology may contribute to problems of substance abuse. There seem to be some commonalities in the personalities of substance abusers regardless of the type of substance abused. Personality traits that may place one at risk for substance abuse include rebelliousness and nonconformity that may lead to substance abuse as an expression of defiance or as an escape from the constraints and expectations of the adult world. Other common traits in abusers are a greater tolerance of deviant behavior, a poor self-concept, and passive surrender to belief in their own inevitable failure in life. Abusers of psychoactive substances also tend to be impulsive, be unable to value themselves, and have poor tolerance for

frustration and anxiety. They may also have difficulty in acknowledging their feelings and in developing interests and deriving pleasure from them. In addition, people who abuse psychoactive substances frequently feel alienated from those around them and are socially isolated. They may also feel powerless, and they usually have poor coping skills.

Substance abusers also tend to display a common set of defense mechanisms that include denial, projection, rationalization, and conflict minimization and avoidance. Abusers frequently deny that they have a problem with substance abuse and assert that they can change their behavior. They may exhibit inability to accept responsibility for their own behavior in other areas as well, and they frequently project or transfer the blame for their own behavior onto others. They also rationalize their behavior without developing true insights into the reason for that behavior. They tend to try to avoid conflict, and may turn to substance abuse as a means of escaping from the stress generated by conflict rather than engaging in positive modes of conflict resolution. Their thinking is characterized by an all-ornothing quality, and they often make decisions that are inflexible and narrow in scope.

The presence of definite psychopathology also places many people at increased risk of substance abuse, and substance abuse is frequently an attempt to relieve or mask the symptoms of underlying psychiatric disorders. Substance abuse may also reduce the effectiveness of treatment for psychiatric problems such as schizophrenia. For instance, people with schizophrenia are far more likely than the general population to develop nicotine addiction, and smoking has been shown to interfere with the effectiveness of antipsychotic drugs. In addition, smoking cessation may make the symptoms of schizophrenia worse, at least temporarily (National Institute of Mental Health, 2006).

Psychological factors are also implicated in tobacco use. For example, depression has been linked to smoking as well as to initiation of drug and alcohol use in adolescents (Kelder et al., 2001). Smokers do not tend to display the psychopathology, alienation, or defense mechanisms typical of other substance abusers; however, young people who begin smoking in the face of current social pressures not to smoke may be exhibiting the defiance that is typical of those who abuse other substances. Smoking may also be a mechanism for coping with stress (Andrews et al., 2004).

Substance abuse may have psychological consequences as well. For example, depression is more common among heavy drinkers than moderate drinkers and life-time abstainers (Paschall, Freisthler, & Lipton, 2005). More serious psychological consequences such as paranoia have been associated with the use of the club drug ketamine as well as with PCP. Guilt associated with substance abuse and its effects on family members, particularly children, may contribute to relapse after drug

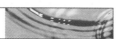

FOCUSED ASSESSMENT

Biophysical Considerations in Substance Abuse

- Are there existing physical health problems contributing to substance abuse? What effects does substance abuse have on efforts to control existing physical health problems (e.g., diabetes)?
- Is there a family history of substance abuse?
- Does the client exhibit signs of intoxication or withdrawal? Does the client exhibit long-term effects of substance use or abuse?
- What influence, if any, does age have on the effects of substance abuse?
- Is the client pregnant? What effects will substance abuse have on the fetus?

treatment unless clients are assisted to deal with their feelings of guilt (Ehrmin, 2001). Questions to help identify psychological dimension influences on substance abuse in the community are included in the focused assessment below.

Sociocultural Considerations

Factors in the sociocultural dimension may also contribute to problems of substance abuse. These factors can exist within the family unit, one's peer group, or society at large. Within the family, research indicates that perceived disapproval of marijuana as well as perceived risks of harm can influence use in adolescents. Reductions in perceived harm and disapproval have been linked to recent increases in use (U.S. Department of Health and Human Services [USDHHS], 2002). Similarly, the use of alcohol or drugs by parents or older siblings may influence drug use by children. Families with low cohesion, high levels of conflict, few shared interests and activities, poor coping strategies, and marital dissatisfaction increase the risk of substance abuse in their members. Families who encounter multiple stressors and have inadequate resources are also at risk. Episodes of violence within the family can also lead family members to abuse substances as a means of escape from family tensions. Good parent–child communication, maternal use of reasoning with children, and adequate supervision of children, on the other hand, have been associated with lower rates of binge drinking among adolescents (Guilamo-Ramos, Jaccard, Turrisi, & Johansson, 2005). Similarly, family cohesion, family involvement in religious activities, and the mother's negative attitude toward substance use by minors are associated with negative attitudes toward substance abuse among adolescents (Pilgrim, Abbey, & Kershaw, 2004). Conversely, excessive unsupervised free time has been associated with initial use of drugs by adolescents (Al-Kandari, Yacoub, & Omu, 2001). Community health nurses should assess families for conditions that may contribute to substance abuse by family members.

Peer influence is another factor in the social environment that may contribute to substance abuse. In adolescents and preadolescents in particular, pressure from peers to smoke, drink, or use other psychoactive drugs is a powerful motivator for initiating these behaviors. In working with young people, in particular, the nurse carefully assesses peer attitudes toward substance use and abuse as well as the degree to which the individual feels a need to conform to peer-dictated norms.

Social factors such as poverty, unemployment, and discrimination may create a sense of hopelessness and powerlessness that leads to substance abuse as an escape or to enhance one's own feelings of competence. These factors might explain the higher prevalence of some forms of substance abuse among members of minority groups and the poor. For example, neighborhoods with large percentages of minority residents and low education levels have been associated with adolescent initiation of injection drug use. No similar association was found for Whites in neighborhoods with low percentages of minority residents and high education levels (Fuller et al., 2005).

Some sociocultural factors that might be considered positive may also contribute to drug use. For example, higher alcohol consumption rates are found among employed people with higher incomes and higher educational levels and among smokers in the United States, suggesting that the ability to afford alcohol has an influence on the extent of consumption (Moore et al., 2005). At least in part, however, differing patterns of excessive alcohol consumption were noted in the Netherlands, where people with lower education levels were more likely to initiate excessive alcohol consumption than those with higher education levels. The authors explained their findings by association with exposure to financial stressors and low social support that accompanied lower education levels (Droomers, Schrijvers, & Mackenbach, 2004).

Societal attitudes toward drug use and abuse also influence the extent of substance abuse in the population. For example, attitudes that promote incarceration rather than treatment are not only ineffective but more costly than substance abuse treatment (Drug Reform Coordination Network, 2005). Societal action to restrict access to drugs, on the other hand, may be more effective. For example, increasing the minimum legal drinking age has decreased motor vehicle accident fatalities among adolescents. Ease of access to drugs and alcohol, on the other hand, increases the potential for substance abuse. In one study in New Hampshire, for example, 30% of adolescent attempts to purchase alcohol were successful (Division of Adult and Community Health, 2004). The ready availability of amphetamines in southern California, where methamphetamine labs abound, make this a drug of choice in the area and increase its abuse relative to other psychoactive substances.

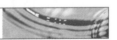

FOCUSED ASSESSMENT

Psychological Considerations in Substance Abuse

- Does the client have a poor self-image?
- What are the client's life goals? Are they realistic?
- Does the client exhibit poor impulse control? What is the client's level of frustration tolerance?
- What life stresses is the client experiencing? What is the extent of the client's coping abilities? What defense mechanisms does the client display?
- Is there underlying psychopathology contributing to substance abuse?

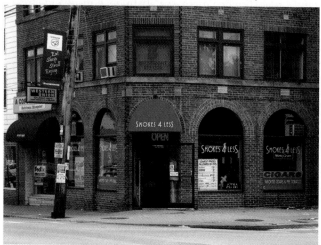

Tobacco continues to be one of the most significant drugs of abuse in its health effects. (Patrick J. Watson)

Social attitudes are often reflected in legislation. For example, no-smoking legislation in California has led to decreased cigarette consumption in the state. Legislation may also have negative effects. For example, lowering the minimum age for purchasing alcohol in New Zealand increased alcohol-related motor vehicle crashes by 12% among 18- to 19-year-old men and 51% among women. The legislative change also contributed to a 14% increase in alcohol-related accidents among men aged 15 to 17 years and a 24% increase among women (Kypri et al., 2006). Conversely, U.S. states with strong alcohol control policies have lower prevalence rates of binge drinking among college students as well as in the general population (Nelson, Naimi, Brewer, & Wechsler, 2005).

Perhaps the classic example of legislation related to substance use and abuse was the enactment of the Eighteenth Amendment and its enforcing legislation, the Volstead Act, which prohibited the manufacture or sale of alcoholic beverages (with a few exceptions) in the United States in the early 20th century. Prohibition, as it is usually known, was later repealed in 1933. Although prohibition was successful in decreasing the consumption of alcohol in general, it had several unintended consequences, including diminished access to care for habitual drunkards and movement of drinking behavior from taverns and saloons to the home, which led to increased public drinking among women. Prohibition also increased criminal activity related to illegal liquor supply and sale and virtually eliminated previously legitimate businesses such as distilleries and breweries. In addition, prohibition had an adverse effect on American ocean liners that were unable to compete for transatlantic business with European companies due to their "dry" status. The lessons learned from the experiment in prohibiting alcohol consumption suggest a need to carefully examine the potential consequences of legislative attempts to control behaviors (Block, 2006).

Culture also seems to play a part in the development of alcohol abuse. Cultural attitudes and modes of introducing alcohol use to young people can either contribute to or impede the development of alcohol abuse. Religion is an aspect of culture that may strongly influence drug use. Cultural factors also influence when drug use behaviors are accepted and when they are not. For example, smoking and use of hallucinogenics are part of traditional religious rituals in some Native American groups. Alcohol use also varies among cultural groups in terms of when and where it occurs, who drinks, levels of alcohol use considered acceptable, what is drunk, and how and why people drink. For example, use of alcohol in many cultures is celebratory in nature; in others it is part of normal dietary patterns (e.g., in France and Italy). Similarly, in some cultural groups alcohol is used by only certain segments of the population (e.g., adults), whereas in others it is consumed by all. Cultures in which alcohol use is generally disapproved may create a mystique that promotes inappropriate use among the young (e.g., among some conservative Protestant groups in the southern United States). When alcohol use is perceived as manly or desirable, it is embraced; when it is perceived as stupid or disgusting, it tends to be avoided (Heath, 2000). For example, in many Latino cultures and among the Irish, drinking is perceived as related to manly adulthood, and youngsters may begin alcohol use to demonstrate adult behaviors.

In today's world, cultural attitudes toward specific behaviors may be strongly influenced by media messages. For example, media portrayals of drinking and smoking as desirable behaviors influence use of alcohol and tobacco. Media are also being used to send messages to discourage inappropriate use of drugs and alcohol. In fact, some of these media messages are being generated by firms that produce alcoholic beverages. For example, distilleries and breweries such as Anheuser-Busch (2006) have mounted extensive advertising and community-based program initiatives to discourage irresponsible use of alcoholic beverages. Such

CULTURAL COMPETENCE

*A*mong some cultural groups, drinking is considered evidence of adulthood. Because of this perception, young people in these cultural groups may engage in alcohol use, thinking it makes them appear older and more sophisticated.

- What cultural attitudes toward alcohol are found in your area? Do different groups hold different attitudes toward alcohol use? Who holds these attitudes?
- How do cultural attitudes influence alcohol use in your community?
- How do cultural attitudes toward alcohol use in your community influence treatment for alcohol abuse?

initiatives include a guide for parents in discussing alcohol use with their children, training for alcohol retailers to recognize false identification cards, and other alcohol awareness activities. Information regarding these activities is available from Anheuser-Busch at http://www.familytalkonline.com/docs/AboutUs.htm.

Occupation is another sociocultural dimension factor that may contribute to substance abuse. Some occupational groups may be at increased risk for substance abuse, particularly those who are expected to entertain clients who drink. Similarly, substance abuse may occur among health care providers because of easy access to controlled drugs.

Employer attitudes toward and sanctions for alcohol, drug, and tobacco use also influence the extent of use among employees. As we saw in Chapters 24 and 29∞, smoke-free workplaces lead to reduced smoking among employees as well as decreased exposure to secondhand smoke for nonsmoking employees. Some businesses and industries also perform drug testing at the time of employment or periodically throughout employment. Unemployment and attendant stress and hopelessness may contribute to substance abuse. The effects of unemployment are also seen in the aftermath of substance abuse among recovering substance abusers who experience difficulty obtaining work.

Although many homeless individuals have substance abuse problems, the nature of the relationship between homelessness and substance abuse is not clear. Findings that link homelessness to substance abuse have been called into question because of the tendency to survey people who are chronically homeless and frequent shelter residents. In addition, studies often do not distinguish between current substance use and lifetime measures of use and abuse. Competition for scarce housing may put those with substance dependence at a disadvantage because of their low earning potential, increasing the possibility of homelessness. Conversely, substance use may help the homeless cope with their situation or be a means of self-medication for those who have concurrent psychiatric disorders. Finally, lack of a fixed residence makes substance abuse treatment more complex among the homeless than in the general population (National Coalition for the Homeless, 2005). In addition, the prevalence of substance abuse in the homeless population changes over time, so strategies are needed to account for changing prevalence rates as well as changes in contributing factors (North, Eyrich, Pollio, & Spitznagel, 2004).

For those substance abusers who are homeless, the constant effort to seek out shelter and food often interferes with participation in substance abuse treatment programs (Milby, Schumacher, Wallace, Freedman, & Vuchinich, 2005). Some authors contend that the restriction of shelter services to homeless substance abusers who remain sober prevents them from obtaining shelter when they have little access to substance abuse treatment

(National Coalition for the Homeless, 2005). Conversely, some research suggests that providing housing contingent on abstinence increases abstinence more effectively than providing housing without a requirement for sobriety or providing no housing assistance at all (Milby et al., 2005).

Substance abuse may also lead to other socially stigmatized behaviors. For example, drug abusers may engage in prostitution to support their drug habit (Ehrmin, 2001). Questions for exploring sociocultural dimension influences on substance abuse are included in the focused assessment provided below.

Behavioral Considerations

Recreational activities can contribute to the use of psychoactive substances in that alcohol and tobacco use is a frequent adjunct to such activities. People tend to drink and smoke when they socialize with others. Friday or Saturday night binges are a relatively common phenomenon, when people can "let go" and drink because they know they will have time to recover before returning to work on Monday. Next to alcohol, marijuana is the most widely used recreational drug, but cocaine is also used recreationally and has the connotation of high status, glamour, and excitement. PCP and the club drugs are also used for recreational purposes.

Among men who have sex with men (MSM), methamphetamine and other drug use during "circuit parties" has been linked to greater incidence of HIV infection. Methamphetamine and other drug use has also been associated with high-risk sexual activity, particularly among MSM (Boddiger, 2005; Thiede et al., 2003). IDU contributed to roughly one fourth of all AIDS cases diagnosed by December 2000, but the incidence of

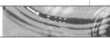

FOCUSED ASSESSMENT

Sociocultural Considerations in Substance Abuse

- To what extent do social mores contribute to substance abuse?
- What effect does legislative activity have on substance abuse?
- Do peer networks support substance use and abuse? Is substance use a regular part of social interaction?
- Does the client's family exhibit characteristics of co-dependence?
- What cultural or religious values or practices influence substance abuse?
- Has the client been a victim or perpetrator of family violence?
- What social factors (e.g., unemployment) contribute to substance abuse?
- How readily available are abused substances?
- What contribution, if any, does occupation make to substance abuse? What is the effect of substance abuse on the client's ability to work?
- What is the contribution of substance abuse to criminal activity? To homelessness?
- What is the extent of substance abuse among homeless individuals?

HIV infection in IDUs decreased by 42% from 1994 to 2000 (Division of HIV/AIDS Prevention, 2003).

Certain high-risk behaviors associated with substance abuse increase the potential for long-term consequences. The most common form of comorbidity is polydrug use. Combining alcohol with drug use also increases one's risk of morbidity and mortality, and certain drugs are more likely to be used in combination with alcohol than others.

Sharing of needles and other drug apparatus is a high-risk behavior that increases the risk of infection in IDUs. Research has indicated that some drug users engage in selective sharing only with members of a close-knit group. When local prevalence of infectious diseases such as HIV infection and hepatitis is low, selective sharing can minimize the risk of infection. However, frequent group turnover increases the potential for introduction of disease that, once introduced, progresses rapidly through the group (Valente & Vlahov, 2001). IDUs may also share cigarette filters used to strain drugs prior to injection. Since these filters are not fine enough to eliminate bacteria and viruses, they, too, are a potential source of infection (Caflish, Wang, & Zbinden, 1999). Behavioral considerations in substance abuse can be examined using the questions provided in the focused assessment below.

Health System Considerations

Many of the psychoactive substances with abuse potential originated within the health care system. Opioids were widely used for pain control even during the American Civil War and are still the drug of choice for relief of severe pain. Cocaine and PCP were first used as surgical anesthetics, and marijuana may have some medical use in the treatment of glaucoma and chronic pain. Sedatives and hypnotics are widely used for controlling anxiety, and amphetamines were originally developed as diet aids, although they no longer have any accepted medical use.

Several aspects of the U.S. health care system have contributed to the growing problem of substance abuse. Lack of attention to educating clients and the public about the hazards of substance abuse and failure to identify clients with substance abuse problems have impeded efforts to control abuse. In one study, 37% of primary care physicians caring for the elderly described a lack of time to address substance abuse issues with their clients. At the same time, some health care providers have actively fostered drug abuse by prescribing psychoactive drugs inappropriately or by not monitoring the extent of clients' use of these drugs (Finfgeld-Connett, 2004).

The health care system also impedes control of substance abuse by failing to provide adequate treatment for persons affected. Physicians in one study reported lack of coverage of substance abuse treatment by health insurance plans, particularly managed care plans, as a barrier to effective care. For example, Medicare only covers hospital-based detoxification and severely limits outpatient care coverage. Approximately 44% of people who receive treatment for alcohol or drug abuse pay for at least a portion of their treatment out-of-pocket (SAMHSA, 2006d). Coverage for smoking cessation is also lacking. In 2000, for example, only 71% of Medicaid programs covered at least one form of treatment for tobacco dependence, and four offered treatment only for pregnant women (Office on Smoking and Health, 2004).

Provision of adequate treatment of substance abuse may be further impeded by negative feelings on the part of health care providers toward those who abuse psychoactive substances. Studies have indicated, for example, that despite knowledge of the effectiveness of harm reduction strategies and the prevalence of periodic relapse during substance abuse treatment, many programs expel clients who revert to drug use during treatment (Lennings, 2000). Many clients in need may not have access to services. For example, many shelters for the homeless refuse abusers despite the fact that a large proportion of homeless individuals abuse alcohol and other drugs. It may also be difficult for pregnant abusers or women with children to find appropriate treatment programs.

The health care system may pose additional barriers to care that are particularly burdensome for some population groups. For instance, most treatment programs are geared toward the needs of younger people and may not recognize the unique needs of the elderly substance abuser. Certainly Medicare, in the implementation of the DRG (diagnosis-related group) system, does not take note of the extended time needed to safely detoxify the elderly substance abuser. In addition, because older people are often considered nonproductive members of society, priority for placement in treatment facilities may be given to younger people. Tips for assessing health system factors influencing substance abuse in individuals and in the population are included in the focused assessment on page 948. A Substance Abuse Risk Factor Inventory is provided in the *Community Assessment Reference Guide* 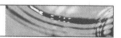 designed to accompany this book.

FOCUSED ASSESSMENT

Behavioral Considerations in Substance Abuse

- What substances are abused? Is there evidence of multisubstance abuse?
- Are abused substances used recreationally? Is substance use associated with leisure activities?
- To what extent does the client engage in other high-risk behaviors (e.g., driving while intoxicated, high-risk sexual activity)?

FOCUSED ASSESSMENT

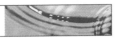

Health System Considerations in Substance Abuse

- What is the attitude of health care providers toward clients with substance abuse problems?
- Are health care providers alert to signs and symptoms of substance abuse?
- To what extent do health care providers educate clients about substance abuse?
- What health system factors contribute to substance abuse (e.g., inappropriate prescription of psychoactive drugs)?
- What treatment facilities are available to substance abusers? To special populations of substance abusers (e.g., pregnant women, adolescents)?
- How is substance abuse treatment financed?

COMMUNITY HEALTH NURSING AND CONTROL OF SUBSTANCE ABUSE

Control of substance abuse in the population requires use of the nursing process. Community health nurses assess the factors contributing to substance abuse as well as the incidence and prevalence of abuse in the population. They then collaborate with others to plan, implement, and evaluate control strategies for abuse.

Assessment

Assessment in the control of substance abuse problems occurs at two levels: the population or community level and the level of the individual client. Assessment at each of these levels will be discussed.

Community Assessment

The World Health Organization (WHO) has developed guidelines for the rapid assessment of communities and other population groups with respect to substance use and abuse. Rapid assessment is intended to increase timely response capabilities in dealing with health issues related to public behaviors. In 1998, the WHO rapid assessment approach was recast as rapid assessment and response (RAR) to emphasize its focus on action to resolve health problems. Evaluation of the RAR approach has indicated its utility in developing strategies to resolve substance abuse problems (Fitch, Stimson, Rhodes, & Poznyak, 2004; Stimson et al., 2006).

RAR is "a means of undertaking comprehensive assessment of a public health issue in a particular study area, including the characteristics of the health problem, population groups affected, settings and contexts, health and risk behaviors, and social consequences. It identifies existing resources and opportunities for intervention, and helps plan, develop and implement interventions" (WHO, 2003, Chapter 2, p. 1). RAR is intended for use with complex public health issues that are influenced by individual and group behavior and provides a structured framework for guiding assessments of

these issues. A specific RAR may focus on a particular problem, a specific population, or a particular risk or health-related behavior. RAR is intended not only to gather data, but to support rapid response to address the health problem or issue, and an RAR report would address: (a) the nature and extent of the problem or issue, (b) its adverse health and social consequences, (c) protective factors against adverse consequences, and (d) intervention proposals. The RAR guidelines encompass eight assessment modules for gathering data for the rapid issue assessment: initial consultation with the target population, a profile of the study area, a contextual assessment, a population and setting assessment, a health issue assessment, a health risk and behavior assessment, a social consequences assessment, and an intervention assessment. Each module addresses key areas and topics for the assessment, key questions to be addressed, potential data sources and methods, and how to use the resulting data to generate an intervention action plan.

Within the context of an RAR, an intervention is defined as "any action that is taken to help reduce a public health problem, help an affected population, change a particular setting, or change a health or risk behavior" (WHO, 2003, Chapter 2, p. 4). Because of the focus on developing relevant interventions, an RAR is only undertaken once the decision to intervene has been made. RAR interventions may occur at structural, community, or individual levels, or, more often, a combination of all three. Structural factors are those factors contributing to the health problem that are generally beyond the control of the individual or community affected by it. Structural factors include many of the elements of the sociocultural dimension discussed earlier, such as social, economic, political, legal, religious, and cultural factors. Legislation, taxes, health system development, and health system financing approaches are examples of structural interventions.

Community-level interventions address factors that are external to the individual but contained in the immediate environment, such as social networks, local norms, values and beliefs, and so on. Examples of community-level interventions are health education and media campaigns related to the issue and changes in communities and organizations. For example, development of a local needle exchange program would address community factors related to injection drug use. Individual-level interventions address the knowledge, attitudes, and behavior of individuals in the population. Treatment for substance abuse for those affected would be an example of an individual intervention. General guidelines for conducting an RAR are available from the WHO Web site at http://www.who.int/docstore/hiv/Core. Guidelines are also available or are being developed for conducting RARs for specific health issues such as youth tobacco use, HIV prevention for MSM (and youth), injection drug use, psychoactive substance use among vulnerable youth, and substance use and sexual behavior.

Individual Assessment

To control problems of substance abuse, community health nurses must identify those persons and groups at risk for substance abuse and its adverse effects, as well as those who are actually experiencing problems of abuse. The nursing process provides a framework for identifying these people and for planning, implementing, and evaluating interventions to assist them in controlling substance abuse. Assessment of individual clients may include assessing for risk factors, for signs of abuse and dependence, for intoxication, for signs of withdrawal, and for long-term physical and psychological effects of substance abuse. Because of the negative connotations associated with substance abuse, the nursing assessment must be conducted with tact and with an accepting and nonjudgmental, nonthreatening approach. Nurses must first examine their own attitudes toward substance abuse and work through any negative feelings that may interfere with nurse–client interactions.

ASSESSING FOR RISK FACTORS Community health nurses assess individual clients for risk factors for substance abuse in each of the five dimensions of health discussed earlier. For example, the nurse would be alert to physical illness that might lead to the use of alcohol or other drugs as a mechanism of escape or for existing mental illness and substance use for purposes of self-medication. Sociocultural factors such as unemployment, discrimination, marital conflict, or family dysfunction may also suggest increased risk for substance abuse. Cultural factors might be protective against risk or increase risk, and religious factors tend to be protective against the development of substance abuse problems.

Behavioral factors that influence substance abuse are related to consumption patterns and leisure activities. The community health nurse assesses individual and family consumption patterns related to tobacco, alcohol, and medications. The nurse should ascertain the frequency and amount of substance use as well as the appropriateness of its use. For example, the nurse might determine whether sedatives are in fact being used as prescribed, whether they are kept away from young people in the home, and whether they are ever used in conjunction with alcohol. Nurses should also determine the extent of alcohol use by families. Many people, for example, do not consider taking medications with an alcohol base as drinking, but may be receiving a hefty dose of alcohol through repeated use. Similarly, Mexican American families might return to Mexico to obtain medications such as paregoric (an opioid preparation used for diarrhea) without realizing their potential for abuse. The nurse also asks about medicinal uses of alcohol, particularly with children, such as giving alcohol for teething pain or to quiet a fretful child.

Evidence of other high-risk behaviors, such as high-risk sexual activity or failure to wear seat belts might suggest a risk for substance abuse as well. Finally, the nurse would explore the client's level of participation in and access to the health care system, including having health insurance and a regular provider of care.

ASSESSING FOR SIGNS OF SUBSTANCE ABUSE In addition to assessing individuals, families, and communities for risk factors that may contribute to substance abuse, the nurse should assess individual clients for general indications of existing abuse. Such assessment is particularly needed for clients with psychiatric disorders because of the high rates of dual diagnosis. General indicators that a person has a problem with abuse of a psychoactive substance include frequent intoxication, preoccupation with obtaining and using the substance, binge use, changes in personality or mood, withdrawal, problems with family members related to use of the substance, problems with friends or neighbors, problems on the job (absenteeism, poor performance, interpersonal difficulties), and conflicts with law enforcement officials. Assessing for signs of abuse would also include collecting information on patterns of alcohol or drug use including age at initiation, behaviors associated with use, administration methods, the presence of tolerance effects, history of uncontrolled use such as binge use or overdose or of prior attempts to stop use. Other signs of abuse to which the community health nurse would be alert include use of substances to self-medicate, attempts to hide use, physical signs of use (e.g., needle marks), and a history of positive drug tests (Hills, Siegfried, & Ickowitz, 2004).

T-ACE is a short, easily used screening tool that has been suggested to identify high-risk alcohol use in older clients and pregnant women (Stevenson & Masters, 2005). The tool consists of four questions that address drug tolerance, annoyance with others' comments on the extent of use, attempts to decrease use, and early-morning drinking. Copies of the tool may be obtained for clinical use from the Project Cork Web site at http://www.projectcork.org/clinical_tools/html/T-ACE.html. The CAGE questionnaire and the Alcohol Use Disorders Identification Test (AUDIT) are similar tools that can be used to assess for unhealthy alcohol use in other populations (Saitz, 2005).

ASSESSING FOR INTOXICATION Another aspect of the community health nurse's assessment related to substance abuse is assessing individuals for signs of intoxication. **Intoxication** is a state of diminished physical or mental control that occurs as a result of the current use of psychoactive drugs. Intoxication with different drugs may be reflected in differing symptoms. For example, cocaine intoxication is characterized by disinhibition,

TABLE 31-3 Signs of Intoxication with Selected Psychoactive Substances

Substance	Typical Indications of Intoxication
Alcohol	Decreased alertness, impaired judgment, slurred speech, nausea, double vision, vertigo, staggering, unpredictable emotional changes, stupor, unconsciousness, increased reaction time
Sedatives, hypnotics, anxiolytics	Slurred speech; slow, shallow respiration; cold and clammy skin; nystagmus; weak and rapid pulse; drowsiness, blurred vision, unconsciousness; disorientation; depression; poor judgment; motor impairment
Opioids	Sedation, hypertension, respiratory depression, impaired intellectual function, constipation, pupillary constriction, watery eyes, increased pulse and blood pressure
Cocaine	Irritability, anxiety, slow weak pulse, slow shallow breathing, sweating, dilated pupils, increased blood pressure, insomnia, seizures, disinhibition, impulsivity, compulsive actions, hypersexuality, hypervigilance, hyperactivity
Amphetamines	Sweating, dilated pupils, increased blood pressure, agitation, fever, irritability, headache, chills, insomnia, agitation, tremors, seizures, wakefulness, hyperactivity, confusion, paranoia
Hallucinogens	Dilated pupils, mood swings, elevated blood pressure, paranoia, bizarre behavior, nausea and vomiting, tremors, panic, flushing, fever, sweating, agitation, aggression, nystagmus (PCP)
Cannabis	Reddened eyes; increased pulse, respirations, and blood pressure; laughter; confusion; panic; drowsiness
Inhalants	Giddiness, drowsiness, increased vital signs, headache, nausea, fainting, stupor, fatigue, slurred speech, disorientation, delirium
Nicotine	Headache; loss of appetite; nausea; increased pulse, blood pressure, and muscle tone

impaired judgment and impulsivity, grandiosity, and compulsively repeated actions. Other common symptoms include hypersexuality, hypervigilance, and hyperactivity. Nicotine intoxication, on the other hand, is characterized by increased blood pressure, heart rate, and muscle tone. Signs of intoxication with selected psychoactive substances are presented in Table 31-3◆.

ASSESSING FOR WITHDRAWAL The physiologic dependence engendered by some psychoactive substances leads to a withdrawal or abstinence syndrome when the substance is withheld. A withdrawal syndrome is a complex of symptoms that accompany abstinence from

a psychoactive substance, usually characterized by severe discomfort, pain, nausea, vomiting, and possibly convulsions. The severity of withdrawal may vary with the abusive substance and the degree of dependence experienced by the client. The community health nurse working with clients who may abuse psychoactive substances assesses the client for signs of withdrawal. Typical withdrawal symptoms for selected psychoactive substances are presented in Table 31-4◆.

Withdrawal can be extremely dangerous and may even be life threatening, especially for vulnerable clients. Withdrawal is a particularly serious event for pregnant women, when both mother and fetus are at

TABLE 31-4 Indications of Withdrawal from Selected Psychoactive Substances

Substance	Indications of Withdrawal
Alcohol	Anxiety, insomnia, tremors, delirium, convulsions
Sedatives, hypnotics, anxiolytics	Anxiety, insomnia, tremors, delirium, convulsions (may occur up to 2 weeks after stopping use of anxiolytics)
Opioids	Restlessness, irritability, tremors, loss of appetite, panic, chills, sweating, cramps, watery eyes, runny nose, nausea, vomiting, muscle spasms, impaired coordination, depressed reflexes, dilated pupils, yawning
Cocaine	*Early crash:* agitation, depression, anorexia, high level of craving, suicidal ideation
	Middle crash: fatigue, depression, no craving, insomnia
	Late crash: exhaustion, hypersomnolence, hyperphagia, no craving
	Early withdrawal: normal sleep and mood, low craving, low anxiety
	Middle and late withdrawal: anhedonia, anxiety, anergy, high level of craving exacerbated by conditioned cues
	Extinction: normal hedonic response and mood, episodic craving triggered by conditioned cues
Amphetamines	Fatigue, hunger, long periods of sleep, disorientation, severe depression
Hallucinogens	Slight irritability, restlessness, insomnia, reduced energy level, depression
Cannabis	Insomnia, hyperactivity, decreased appetite
Inhalants	None reported
Nicotine	Nervousness, increased appetite, sleep disturbances, anxiety, irritability

risk, and for the elderly. The community health nurse should be alert in assessing these clients for signs of withdrawal. Interventions during the withdrawal phase are addressed later in this chapter.

The physical and psychological discomfort and the deep depression that may occur with withdrawal from psychoactive drug use may lead to suicide. The community health nurse assessing clients for withdrawal symptoms should also carefully assess them for potential suicide. Clients should be monitored carefully and asked about suicidal thoughts. Assessment of suicide risk is addressed in more detail in Chapter 32∞.

ASSESSING FOR LONG-TERM EFFECTS OF SUBSTANCE ABUSE In addition to assessing clients for signs and symptoms of intoxication and withdrawal, community health nurses should also assess individual clients for symptoms of long-term effects of substance abuse. These effects can be physical or psychological and vary with the psychoactive substance. For example, long-term effects of alcohol abuse include malnutrition, cirrhosis, and liver cancer, and typical effects of phencyclidine abuse are psychoses and insomnia. Typical long-term effects that should be considered with specific substances are presented in Table 31-5◆. The community health nurse assessing the health of population groups assesses morbidity and mortality related to these long-term effects of substance abuse in the population.

Diagnostic Reasoning and Control of Substance Abuse

Community health nurses make nursing diagnoses related to substance abuse at two levels. The first level is diagnoses related to individuals who have problems of substance abuse and their families. For example, the nurse might make a diagnosis for the individual client of "increased risk of substance abuse due to family history of alcohol abuse" or "abuse of sedatives due to increased life stress and poor coping skills." Nursing diagnoses related to the family of a substance abuser might include "co-dependency due to family feelings of guilt related to daughter's cocaine abuse" and "school behavior problems due to children's anxiety over mother's alcoholism."

At the second level, the community health nurse might make diagnoses of community problems related to substance abuse. For example, the nurse might diagnose an "increased incidence of motor vehicle fatalities due to driving under the influence of psychoactive drugs," or "increased prevalence of drug abuse among minority group members due to discrimination and feelings of powerlessness." Another community-based diagnosis is "increased prevalence of fetal alcohol syndrome due to alcohol use by pregnant women."

Planning and Implementing Control Strategies for Substance Abuse

Strategies for controlling problems of substance abuse can involve primary, secondary, or tertiary prevention.

Primary Prevention

There are three major goals for primary prevention of substance abuse: (a) to prevent nonusers from initiating use of psychoactive substances, (b) to prevent progression from experimentation to chronic use, and (c) to prevent expansion to the use of other substances. Using smoking as an example, primary prevention may be aimed at preventing the initiation of smoking in the first place, preventing movement from occasional smoking to regular use of tobacco, and preventing movement from tobacco use to the use of other drugs such as marijuana. Primary prevention efforts to control substance abuse usually focus on two approaches: education and risk factor modification.

TABLE 31-5	Long-Term Effects Associated with Abuse of Selected Psychoactive Substances
Substance	**Long-term Effects of Abuse**
Alcohol	Malnutrition; impotence; ulcers; cirrhosis; esophageal, stomach, and liver cancers; organic brain syndrome; deafness
Sedatives, hypnotics, anxiolytics	Potential for death due to overdose from increasing doses due to tolerance, impaired sexual function
Opioids	Lethargy, weight loss, sexual disinterest and dysfunction, increased susceptibility to infection and accidents, constipation
Cocaine	Damage to nasal tissue, high blood pressure, weight loss, muscle twitching, paranoia, hallucinations, disrupted sleeping and eating patterns, irritability, liver damage
Amphetamines	Depression, paranoia, hallucinations, weight loss, impotence
Hallucinogens	Memory loss, inability to concentrate, insomnia, chronic or recurrent psychosis, flashbacks
Cannabis	Chromosome changes, reduced sperm count, impaired concentration, poor memory, reduced alertness, inability to perform complex tasks
Inhalants	Organic brain syndrome, liver and kidney damage, bone marrow damage, anemia, hearing loss, nerve damage
Nicotine	Cardiovascular disease, lung cancer, bladder cancer, chronic disease, diabetic complications

EDUCATION Education usually focuses on acquainting the public, particularly young people, with the hazards of substance abuse. Both general public education campaigns and school-based education programs have shown moderate success in limiting the use of psychoactive substances; however, they tend to be more effective in moderating the effects of substance abuse, such as preventing drug-related motor vehicle fatalities. One of the criticisms of school-based programs is that they may not be reaching groups at greatest risk for substance abuse, those with a family history of abuse or who display characteristics associated with potential abusers. Merely providing information on the consequences of substance use and abuse has been shown to be insufficient to curb use. Instead, education programs should emphasize the development of life skills related to decision making, refusal, and critical analysis that affect substance use decisions. In addition, education should address interpersonal communication, problem solving, and stress management to provide practical approaches to factors that promote substance use and abuse.

One school-based program to educate middle-school children to prevent drug use initiation, project ALERT, was found to be effective in reducing cigarette and marijuana use in eighth grade students, but did not help committed smokers to quit. A moderate effect in preventing alcohol use was also noted, but disappeared by eighth grade. A revised program was able to decrease cigarette and marijuana use, minimize regular smoking, and prevent alcohol misuse, but did not have any noticeable effect on drinking per se (Ellickson, McCaffrey, Ghosh-Dastidar, & Longshore, 2003). Community-based programs involving village leaders, teachers, women, and youth leaders in the development of community and school-based activities were found to be effective in decreasing drug use initiation among youth. Other program effects included better knowledge of HIV/AIDS, attitudes toward disease, and community recognition of drug problems (Wu et al., 2002).

Community health nurses may be involved in educating individual clients and families or in providing substance abuse education for groups of people. In either case, the nurse would employ the principles of teaching and learning discussed in Chapter 11 ∞.

RISK FACTOR MODIFICATION Risk factor modification can occur with individuals, families, or society at large. Community health nurses may assist individuals to modify factors that put them at increased risk for substance abuse. For example, the nurse might assist clients experiencing stress to eliminate or modify sources of stress in their lives, or the nurse can assist clients and families to develop more effective coping skills.

In addition, the nurse may make referrals for social services to eliminate financial difficulties and other sources of stress. Or, the nurse might assist a harried single parent to obtain respite care. Nurses can also assist families to plan means of enhancing family communication and cohesion to minimize the risk of substance abuse among children. Preventing alcohol use and/or promoting contraceptive use among childbearing women can help to reduce the incidence of FAS (Sobell et al., 2003).

At the societal level, community health nurses can engage in political activity to control access to and limit the availability of psychoactive substances as well as to modify societal factors that contribute to abuse. For example, the nurse might advocate enforcement of laws restricting the sale of alcohol and tobacco to minors, or the nurse might work to reduce discrimination against members of minority groups or to ensure a minimal income for all families.

Effective prevention of substance abuse among young people usually involves both education and risk factor modification. In a national study of 46 prevention programs, the most effective programs were characterized by the inclusion of strong emphases on life skills development, team building and interpersonal skills, and self-reflection and introspection and by intense contact between program staff and participants. Programs with these characteristics tended to show long-term effects in deterring substance use behaviors in at-risk youth (Springer et al., 2004). Community health nurses can be actively involved in designing and implementing prevention programs that incorporate these characteristics.

The National Institute on Drug Abuse (2003) has developed a research-based guide for preventing drug abuse in children and adolescents. The prevention guide is based on a series of principles that include the following:

- Prevention should emphasize enhancing protective factors against substance abuse and reducing risk factors.
- Prevention should address all forms of drug abuse.
- Prevention should address specific types of drug abuse problems in the community, targeting modifiable risk factors and strengthening protective factors.
- Prevention should address risks specific to the population.
- Family-based prevention should enhance parenting skills and family bonding.
- Prevention should begin as early as preschool to address risk factors for abuse (e.g., poor interaction skills, aggressive behavior).
- Prevention in elementary school settings should address both academic and social-emotional learning related to risk factors for abuse (e.g., self-control, communication, problem solving, and academic support).

- Prevention in middle or junior high school settings should address continued development of academic and social skills.
- Prevention should be targeted to times of transition (e.g., from elementary to middle school).
- Prevention should combine several approaches to enhance effectiveness (e.g., family-based and school-based programs).
- Prevention messages should reach audiences in multiple settings and include consistent information.
- Prevention should be adapted to address community needs, norms, and cultures, but should retain core elements related to structure, content, and delivery based on evidence-based interventions.
- Prevention should be a long-term focus with repeated interventions to reinforce desired goals.
- Prevention should incorporate teacher training in classroom management to foster positive behavior and school achievement.
- Prevention should employ interactive techniques that encourage active involvement by participants.
- Prevention is cost-effective. (NIDA, 2003)

Secondary Prevention

Secondary prevention is employed when there is an existing problem with substance abuse. The goal in secondary prevention is early intervention aimed at those who have not yet developed irreversible pathological changes due to substance abuse. Elements of secondary prevention include screening, intervention, and treatment.

SCREENING Secondary prevention begins with screening for excessive or inappropriate use of psychoactive substances. Routine screening should be undertaken in multiple settings in which clients are seen. For example, universal screening for alcohol use is recommended for all women of childbearing age, not only those who are pregnant. Brief intervention is recommended for those who have evidence of high-risk drinking, and pregnant women should be advised to discontinue alcohol use altogether (Bertrand et al., 2005). The U.S. Preventive Services Task Force (2004) has recommended screening all adults for alcohol misuse, but found insufficient evidence to recommend routine screening among adolescents. Possible tools for use in screening individual clients for alcohol misuse were discussed earlier. Community health nurses may also be involved in the development of programs to screen populations for alcohol and other drug abuse.

Once screening indicates a substance use problem, planning secondary prevention necessitates mutual goal setting by the nurse, the client, and the family of the person experiencing the problem. Goals relate to intervention, treatment for substance abuse, and harm reduction.

INTERVENTION Intervention, in the context of substance abuse, is the act of confronting the substance abuser with the intent of making a referral for assistance in dealing with the abuse. The goal of the intervention is to elicit an agreement from the individual involved to be evaluated for a possible problem with substance abuse.

Community health nurses may facilitate intervention by families of individual abusers but are not usually the interveners themselves. In this respect, the family, rather than the abuser, is the community health nurse's client.

Many families may not see themselves as clients, and the community health nurse may need to reinforce the idea that substance abuse is a family disorder to motivate family members to engage in intervention. To this end, the first step in preparing for intervention is providing the family or significant others with basic information about substance abuse and the defense mechanisms used by both the abuser and his or her significant others. In this way, family members can be helped to see their role as co-dependents or enablers of the abusive behavior. The nurse also educates family members about the intervention process, their responsibility for that process, and some of the feelings they may experience during intervention.

In assisting family members to prepare for intervention, the nurse aids them to determine who should be involved. Some members may not be able to follow through with confronting the individual with his or her behavior and should be asked not to participate in the intervention. Individuals who should be involved in the intervention include those who are close to and concerned for the abuser, those who may be able to influence the abuser's behavior in a positive way, and those who are able to engage in the intervention.

Next, the nurse assists those who will be involved in the intervention to identify in writing the causes for their concern and to describe how they felt when significant events related to substance abuse occurred. Areas that the group should plan to address during the intervention are the problem as they perceive it, statements about the individual's behavior that indicate a problem of substance abuse, effects of the abuse problem, and their concern for the individual.

Prior to the intervention, the group should arrange an appointment for an evaluation for substance abuse to take place immediately after the intervention session, as it is wise to follow through on the referral as soon as possible while the individual is motivated to seek help. It is suggested that appointments be made in more than one facility so the individual can exercise some choice in the matter and feel less coerced.

The group planning the intervention should also consider potential roadblocks to the success of the effort. For example, the individual might be concerned about the cost of care or about the need for child care while he or she is in treatment. If anticipated, these difficulties can be circumvented.

The nurse can also assist family members to plan their response to the individual's possible refusal to comply with a request for evaluation for substance abuse. If the wife plans to threaten divorce if the husband does not seek help, will she be able to carry through this threat in the face of his refusal? The nurse can help the family plan for these contingencies and work through feelings created by the proposed intervention by helping group members practice the intervention (who will say what, when, and so on). Practice should also include who will sit nearest the individual (those with the greatest influence) and between the abuser and the door and who will initiate the intervention.

Once the group is ready for the intervention, the individual should be brought to the place selected and the intervention initiated. Just prior to the intervention, while waiting for the individual to arrive, the nurse may remind family members why they are there and what is planned. The nurse is present to keep the intervention moving, but is not otherwise an active participant.

If the individual agrees to be evaluated, one or more of the group members should accompany him or her to the evaluation appointment to prevent a potential suicide attempt. While this is occurring, the nurse may meet with the other members of the group to discuss their feelings about the process and its outcome. If the intervention has not been successful, the nurse can reassure group members and assist them to plan a subsequent intervention.

TREATMENT Treatment for substance abuse is based on several general principles that are discussed below. It also employs several different treatment modalities and should incorporate early treatment where possible as well as measures for managing withdrawal and cravings.

General Principles of Substance Abuse Treatment Treatment for problems of substance abuse varies somewhat depending on the type of substance involved. In 1999, however, the National Institute on Drug Abuse identified several general principles that guide treatment for substance abuse. These principles are still relevant to substance abuse treatment today. More recently, NIDA (2006b) published a related set of principles for the treatment of substance abuse in correctional populations. Both sets of principles are summarized below.

Treatment Modalities for Substance Abuse Treatment modalities that may be employed include biological methods, psychosocial methods, sociotherapies, and self-help and mutual-help approaches, and effective therapy usually encompasses several modalities. Biological methods use medication or other physiologically based therapies (such as acupuncture) to help the abuser deal with the symptoms of withdrawal or to handle cravings for the substance

SPECIAL CONSIDERATIONS

PRINCIPLES OF TREATMENT FOR SUBSTANCE ABUSE
General Principles

- No single treatment is appropriate for all individuals.
- Treatment must be readily available to all those in need.
- Effective treatment addresses multiple needs, not just those related to substance abuse.
- The treatment plan must be assessed constantly and modified as needed to meet changing needs.
- Completion of treatment is critical for effectiveness.
- Counseling and other behavioral therapies are important components of treatment.
- Medications, in conjunction with other therapies, are also important in treating substance abuse.
- Persons with dual diagnoses of substance abuse and psychiatric disorders should receive integrated treatment for both conditions.
- Medical detoxification is only the first stage of treatment for substance abuse and does little alone to change drug use behaviors.
- Treatment does not need to be voluntary to be effective.
- The potential for drug use during treatment must be closely monitored (e.g., with urinalysis or other tests).
- Treatment programs should also include screening and prevention for HIV, hepatitis, tuberculosis, and other diseases common among substance abusers.

- Multiple episodes of treatment may be necessary during recovery from substance abuse.

Data from: National Institute on Drug Abuse. (1999). Principles of drug addiction treatment. Retrieved August 9, 2006, from http://www.nida.gov/PDF/PODAT/ PODAT.pdf

Additional Principles of Treatment in Correctional Populations

- Drug addiction is a brain disease that affects behavior.
- Recovery requires treatment and management over time.
- Treatment must last long enough to result in sustainable changes.
- Treatment begins with assessment.
- Treatment services should be tailored to meet the needs of the individual affected.
- Treatment should address factors associated with criminal behavior.
- Criminal justice supervision should include drug abuse treatment plans, and mental health providers should be aware of correctional supervision requirements.
- Continuity of care is essential on reentry into the community.
- Effective treatment includes a balance of rewards and sanctions.

Data from: National Institute on Drug Abuse (2006). Principles of drug abuse treatment for criminal justice populations. Retrieved August 9, 2006, from http://www.nida.nih.gov/PDF.PODAT_CJ/PODAT_CH.pdf

involved. Pharmacologic management of substance abuse disorders may be used to address the immediate problems of intoxication and withdrawal, decrease the effects of an abused substance, create an aversion to the abused substance, substitute a less dangerous substance for a more dangerous one, or treat psychiatric comorbidity that is contributing to or complicating the substance abuse problem (Bailey, 2004). Medications such as benzodiazepines (e.g., Valium and Librium) are often used to treat the physical symptoms of withdrawal, and narcotic antagonists such as naloxone (Narcan) may be used to address life-threatening effects of opioid use such as respiratory depression. Beta-blockers such as propanolol have also been used in conjunction with benzodiazepines in alcohol withdrawal, and antipsychotic medications may be warranted for clients withdrawing from alcohol who experience delirium, delusions, or hallucinations (Bailey, 2004). Disulfiram (Antabuse), acamprosate (Campral), and naltrexone may also be used in long-term therapy for alcohol abuse to promote abstinence from alcohol. Use of naltrexone may precipitate alcohol withdrawal, so it should only be used after a few days of abstinence (Saitz, 2005).

Methadone or naloxone may be used as narcotic substitutes in the long-term treatment of opioid addictions. Methadone may also be used during detoxification. Buprenorphine (Subutex) or buprenorphine in combination with naloxone (Suboxone) is a newer drug that is used for maintenance therapy in opiate addiction (Bailey, 2004). In the past, methadone treatment for opiate addiction was permitted only in specially licensed facilities. Because of its higher safety profile and lower level of physical dependence, however, recent legislation has permitted private physicians to use buprenorphine in the treatment of narcotics abusers, thus expanding access to treatment and potentially reducing the attached stigma. It is hoped that this change may foster a perception of substance abuse treatment as similar to therapy for other chronic conditions (Sporer, 2004). Like naltrexone, buprenorphine may precipitate withdrawal and should only be initiated when withdrawal is already being experienced. Methadone, however, remains the treatment of choice for opiate abuse, with buprenorphine available as an alternative option (Srivastava & Kahan, 2006).

Community health nurses may refer clients for medical management of substance abuse. They may also be involved in monitoring treatment compliance or in providing long-term medication in maintenance programs. At the population level, community health nurses can advocate for available services and for prescription medication coverage for substance abuse treatment. They may also be involved in the development of treatment programs and in advocating for adequate funding for treatment services.

Psychosocial methods of treatment include individual, group, and family therapy; behavior modification; contracting; and aversion or relaxation therapies. Several behavioral therapies fit into this category of treatment. Contingency management is an approach that creates incentives for behavioral change. Incentives used may be cash, goods and services, or vouchers for goods and services. Long-term effects of contingency management may not continue when rewards are withdrawn unless the behavior change has been internalized and the client has created intrinsic rewards for maintaining the behavior (e.g., having less family conflict due to decreased drug use). Cognitive behavioral therapy focuses on an understanding of the triggers for and beliefs that support drug abuse and attempts to change the underlying causes. Family therapy focuses on the dynamics of family interaction and may attempt to change family structure to a hierarchical pattern with parents in charge and boundaries that promote closeness but also maintain individuality. Reframing, or positive thinking, is another usual component of family therapy (Racioppo, 2005).

Sociotherapy involves participation in therapeutic communities and residential programs where clients learn new lifestyles consistent with sobriety. Self-help therapies usually involve use of publications and educational materials that help people identify triggers for substance use and suggest specific strategies for curtailing use. Finally, mutual-help groups consist of people who are abusers of the same substance and who provide for each other understanding and support in conquering their substance abuse habit (Saitz, 2005). For example, Alcoholics Anonymous is a mutual-help group for alcohol abusers, and Potsmokers Anonymous is a mutual-help group for marijuana abusers. Mutual-help groups are discussed in more detail in the context of tertiary prevention later in this chapter. Unless community health nurses have a psychiatric background, they are not usually involved in behavioral therapies for substance abuse. They do, however, refer clients for existing services and may provide supportive care during treatment, monitoring treatment effects and assisting clients to make needed changes in their lifestyles to enhance the success of treatment. At the population level, community health nurses can identify the need for treatment services in the community and advocate for their availability and accessibility to all those in need. Treatment modalities typically used for specific types of substance abuse are indicated in Table 31-6◆.

Some complementary therapies have also been used for treating substance abuse. For example, hypnosis has been used successfully to assist some clients with smoking cessation and alcohol abuse. Similarly, drumming and participation in drum circles has been shown to promote substance abuse recovery possibly as a result

TABLE 31-6	Treatment Modalities Typically Used for Selected Forms of Psychoactive Substance Abuse
Substance	**Typical Treatment Modalities**
Alcohol	Detoxification, psychotherapy, group therapy, family therapy, mutual-help groups (Alcoholics Anonymous, Al-Anon), pharmacologic therapy (disulfiram, short-term use of tranquilizers or antidepressants), residential programs, referral for vocational rehabilitation and social services as needed
Sedatives, hypnotics, anxiolytics	Detoxification, psychotherapy and group therapy (for underlying psychiatric disorders)
Opioids	Pharmacologic therapy (methadone, opioid antagonists); therapeutic communities (Synanon, Odyssey House, Daytop, Phoenix House); group therapy; assistance with social skills, vocational training, and job placement; family therapy; mutual-help groups (Narcotics Anonymous, Chemical Dependency Anonymous); psychotherapy
Cocaine	Hospitalization, mutual-help groups, contingency contracting (client agreement to urinary monitoring and acceptance of aversive contingencies for positive results), pharmacologic therapy (tricyclic antidepressants)
Amphetamines	No established treatment guidelines; may be similar to treatment for cocaine abuse
Hallucinogens	Detoxification, psychotherapy (for underlying psychiatric disorders), group therapy, residential programs
Cannabis	Same as for hallucinogens; mutual-help groups
Inhalants	Psychosocial interventions, psychotherapy (for underlying psychiatric disorder), sociodrama, vocational rehabilitation, family therapy, social support services
Nicotine	Aversive conditioning, desensitization, substitution, hypnotherapy, group therapy, relaxation training, supportive therapy, abrupt abstinence

of enhanced relaxation and theta-wave production and brain-wave synchronization that produce altered states of consciousness similar to those achieved in meditation (Winkelman, 2003). Community health nurses can refer clients to sources of complementary therapy or recommend their involvement in drum circles or other forms of therapy.

Treatment for dual diagnosis of substance abuse and other psychiatric disorders may take one of three approaches: parallel, sequential, or integrated. In the parallel approach, the client receives treatment for both disorders simultaneously, but from different providers. This approach has distinct disadvantages when treatment for one condition interacts negatively with treatment for the other. In sequential treatment, the client receives treatment for one condition followed by treatment for the other. This is often ineffective because the substance abuse disorder and the psychiatric disorder may be extensively intertwined. For example, substance abuse may be a form of self-medication for a psychiatric disorder and cannot be addressed until the psychiatric disorder is addressed. At the same time, a psychiatric disorder such as depression may make detoxification more dangerous. The most effective approach to treatment of dual diagnoses is integrated therapy, in which the client receives treatment for both conditions simultaneously from the same treatment team. This approach permits attention to all of the factors that are interfering with optimal mental health and has a greater success rate in treating both substance abuse and mental illness (Hills et al., 2004).

Community health nurses may be involved in treatment for substance abuse in a number of ways.

First, nurses might identify cases of substance abuse and plan to refer clients and their families to treatment resources in the community. Nurses may also educate the general public on the signs and symptoms of substance abuse as well as the availability of treatment facilities. In addition, community health nurses can monitor the use of medications during withdrawal (if this is done on an outpatient basis) or on a long-term basis (e.g., methadone maintenance).

Community health nurses might also be involved in psychosocial therapies by referring clients to sources of group, individual, or family therapy, or the nurse might reinforce contracts made for reducing the use of substances. This is particularly true in measures to help clients stop smoking. In this instance, community health nurses may initiate behavioral contracts with clients to enable them to gradually cut down on tobacco consumption or quit smoking for gradually lengthened periods.

BUILDING OUR KNOWLEDGE BASE

Some evidence suggests that complementary therapies may be effective in the treatment of substance abuse. For example, drumming has been found to enhance substance abuse recovery. Examine the literature related to this or another complementary or alternative approach to substance abuse treatment. What does the evidence indicate regarding the effectiveness of the therapy selected? How would you conduct a study to determine the effectiveness of the therapy in treating nurses with substance abuse problems? What kinds of substance abuse would you include in your study? Why? How would you measure the effects of the therapy?

Community health nurses' involvement with therapeutic communities and mutual-help groups usually occurs in the form of referrals for these types of services. In some instances, however, community health nurses are actively involved in initiating support groups.

At the community level, nursing efforts to control substance abuse might include political activity to support the development of adequate treatment facilities, especially those geared to the needs of currently underserved population groups such as pregnant women, the homeless, and the elderly. Community health nurses might also be involved in political activity and advocacy to encourage insurance coverage of treatment for substance abuse.

The goals of treatment for substance abuse include intervening early for persons who have not yet become abusers but who use psychoactive substances and managing withdrawal and cravings for the substance involved. Treatment is also indicated for infants subjected to prenatal alcohol exposure and should be a part of routine newborn services for those in need. Other emphases in treatment of FAS include improved parent–child interaction, caregiver education, and developmental services. These services should also be made available to infants in adoptive or foster home settings (Bertrand et al., 2005).

Early Treatment   For some psychoactive substances, such as cocaine, use at any level frequently leads to abuse because of the vicious rebound cycle that occurs. For other substances, such as alcohol, sedatives, and tranquilizers, moderate use may be acceptable when these substances are used appropriately. Some authors suggest early intervention with people using these substances to allow them to use the substance in moderation. To this end, brief treatment is undertaken to stabilize and to moderate use of the substance in question so that it does not reach the level of abuse. **Brief intervention** involves time-limited, direct strategies to reduce substance use in nondependent users whose consumption rates put them at risk for problems associated with substance use (Finfgeld-Connett, 2004). A brief intervention usually takes 10 to 15 minutes and includes exploring the consequences of drinking, setting goals to reduce the amount of alcohol consumed, and planning for follow-up contact (Saitz, 2005). For example, in a brief intervention a college student who admits to binge drinking would be reminded of the potential for and consequences of alcohol-related motor vehicle accidents and helped to explore reasons for his or her drinking behavior as well as safer means of meeting the goals of the behavior. Brief intervention programs involve teaching clients skills for self-control and for decision making about responsible behavioral choices.

Research has suggested that nurses are not comfortable counseling clients about high-risk drug use.

Nurses who saw themselves as more competent in this area were more likely to engage in frequent counseling with clients who make excessive use of alcohol (Willaing & Ladelund, 2005). The A-FRAMES model has been developed to guide brief intervention in client–provider interactions. The model involves the following components:

A — Assessment: Identification of problem substance use

F — Feedback: Client education regarding the risks of substance use or potential impairment

R — Responsibility: Client is given the responsibility for decisions to change or not change use behaviors

A — Advice: Provision of assistance in goal development

M — Menu: Discussion of options for change in use behaviors

E — Empathy: Understanding of client viewpoints and concerns

S — Self-efficacy: Emphasis on the ability to change use behavior if desired (Finfgeld-Connett, 2004)

A similar model, the five As model, has been developed to assist clients with smoking cessation. Steps of the model include: (a) asking clients about smoking behaviors, (b) advising them of the adverse consequences of smoking, (c) assessing their willingness to stop smoking, (d) assisting them to develop cessation strategies based on the desire to stop, and (e) arranging follow-up. Follow-up is suggested within a short time after the intervention (e.g., within a week) with periodic follow-up thereafter (Andrews et al., 2004).

A concept similar to brief intervention has been used in the correctional system to modify drinking behavior among people with a first sentence for driving while impaired (DWI). A 28-day detention and treatment program was found to reduce the probability of repeat arrest within the next 5 years by nearly 28% (Kunitz et al., 2002).

Another strategy in the early treatment of substance abuse behaviors involves use of the transtheoretical model of change to identify the stage of change exhibited by a particular client or population group. According to the model, behavior change progresses in a series of stages of readiness to act from precontemplation, through contemplation, preparation, and action, to maintenance (Prochaska et al., 2004). In the precontemplation stage, the client or population group is unaware of the problem, denies the problem, or considers it of no importance, and does not plan to take any action. For example, an individual might think his or her drinking behavior is not out of line, or a university administration may not acknowledge the extent of drinking or drug use on campus. In the contemplation stage, the individual or group recognizes some advantages to changing the current situation but experiences ambivalence because the disadvantages of changing are overestimated. The individual or group generally intends to act sometime within the next 6 months. People in the preparation stage have decided to take action and may even have made some small efforts at change. In the action stage, people are actively engaged in changing individual behavior or, in the case of the university, modifying conditions that promote the unhealthful behavior. In the maintenance stage, the behavior change has been sustained for at least 6 months and the focus is on preventing a relapse to the previous behavior.

Different intervention strategies are appropriate at each stage of readiness for change. Prochaska and colleagues (2004), who originated the model, noted that externally imposed change during the precontemplation and contemplation stages may result in resistance and defensiveness and actually impede change. Strategies that are appropriate in these early stages include consciousness raising, dramatic relief (graphic representation of the possible consequences of behavior), and self- and environmental reevaluation. Self-reevaluation might emphasize how the current behavior is incongruent with one's perception of oneself as intelligent or independent or other valued self-conceptualizations. Environmental reevaluation might highlight the ability to afford a better apartment with the money saved by stopping smoking or differences for the family if the individual were to stop drinking or using drugs. In later stages of the change process, appropriate strategies are more behavioral in nature. For example, in the action stage, exercise might be substituted for smoking behavior, or nicotine patches might be purchased, whereas in the maintenance stage, the individual might stop frequenting places where other people smoke, or the university might extend no-smoking bans to sports and other events.

Community health nurses can help individual clients and population groups identify where they are in the change process and can design intervention strategies that promote movement through the stages of change. They can also design community-based programs that are grounded in an understanding of the stages of change. In addition, they can foster in the client or group a sense of self-efficacy for enacting the change and work to alter the balance of perceived advantages and disadvantages to the change until the client or group is ready and willing to take action (Prochaska et al., 2004).

Managing Withdrawal and Cravings For clients who have already reached a level of substance abuse that does not admit to moderate use or with substances for which there is no level of moderate use, the goal of treatment is abstinence and long-term sobriety (Goldsmith, 2000b). The first step to abstinence is detoxification, which often involves supporting the client through withdrawal. Community health nurses may be involved in referring clients to detoxification facilities and in supporting them during detoxification.

Persons who are at risk for serious consequences of withdrawal should always go through detoxification under medical supervision. Care in an outpatient setting can be used for clients with mild to moderate symptoms of alcohol withdrawal and no significant comorbidity. Moderate withdrawal will usually require the use of benzodiazepines to relieve symptoms and prevent seizures. Other interventions used to stabilize the client's condition include correction of electrolyte and nutritional imbalances. Anticonvulsants may also be required (Asplund et al., 2004). Of particular concern are pregnant women and the elderly. Many of the drugs used to mitigate the adverse symptomatology of withdrawal from psychoactive substances are contraindicated in pregnancy. For example, benzodiazepines such as Valium and Librium, both of which may be used to combat the anxiety and sleeplessness that often accompany withdrawal, may be teratogenic and should not be given to the pregnant substance abuser. Similarly, detoxification procedures may need to be modified for older adults because of their tendency to be overmedicated by relatively small doses of medication.

Community health nurses may monitor medication use during withdrawal or on a long-term basis, and they should be alert to the potential for use of medications for suicide purposes and to the potential for abuse of some of the substances used (e.g., Valium, methadone). The nurse should assess clients on medications for suicide potential and should monitor mood changes closely. The nurse should also educate clients and their families as to the adverse effects of combining medications with alcohol or other psychoactive drugs. Because disulfiram (Antabuse), in particular, is contraindicated in both pregnant women and clients with cardiac arrhythmias and pulmonary disease, the nurse should monitor clients for evidence of these conditions.

Other nursing considerations related to withdrawal and craving include maintaining levels of hydration and nutrition. Hydration is particularly important for the client who abuses alcohol because of its diuretic effects. Nutrition is important for most drug abusers because substance abuse frequently leads to a disinterest in food in favor of consumption of the abusive substance. Decreased intake of stimulants such as caffeine is also advisable. Treatment can also be enhanced by a regular program of exercise that will improve self-esteem, prevent excessive weight gain, and stimulate the release of endorphins. Community health nurses can educate clients on the need for hydration and nutrition and suggest exercise. Vigorous aerobic exercise should not be undertaken before a thorough medical assessment of cardiovascular status has been conducted. In the interim, however, the nurse can suggest a program of stretching exercises.

Tertiary Prevention

Tertiary prevention is aimed at preventing a relapse into prior substance-abusing behaviors by the individual or into enabling behaviors by family members and significant others. Additional purposes in tertiary prevention include dealing with the consequences of abuse, building a foundation for recovery, and harm reduction.

RELAPSE PREVENTION The emphasis in relapse prevention is elimination of personal triggers for substance use and abuse (Hills et al., 2004). Relapse prevention is based on the perspective that drug use behavior is reinforced by external cues that have become linked with rewards (e.g., the positive effects of drugs) and that these cues must be avoided to promote abstinence. Such cues may include people, places, drug use paraphernalia, or sensations previously associated with drug use. Relapse may also be precipitated by stress (Hyman, 2005). Other factors that may contribute to relapse include inadequate skills to deal with pressures to return to substance use, poor skills in dealing with interpersonal conflict, and a desire to test personal control over behavior. Because of the chronic nature of substance abuse, recovery requires long-term commitment to changes in attitudes and behaviors, with significant potential for relapse into using behavior. Relapse prevention usually entails assessment of prior relapses and contributing factors, development of strategies to modify contributing factors, and ongoing treatment (Treatment Improvement Exchange, 2002b).

Recovery and relapse prevention tend to occur in stages. The first stage involves abstinence from drugs and alcohol, which is followed by separation from people, places, and objects that promote substance use and development of networks that support recovery. The third stage focuses on eliminating self-defeating behaviors that prevent awareness of painful feelings and irrational thoughts. For example, if guilt over the death of a friend in an automobile accident is a contributing factor in alcohol abuse, the abuser can face the guilt and work through it to minimize its influence on behavior. In the fourth stage, the abuser learns to manage feelings and emotions in healthy ways that do not include use of drugs. Abusers must also learn to change addictive thinking patterns that are self-defeating (e.g., thinking that they are incapable of overcoming their substance abuse problem). Finally, abusers identify and change mistaken beliefs about themselves and their world that contribute to substance use (Treatment Improvement Exchange, 2002a).

Several principles have been identified that guide relapse prevention. The first principle deals with self-regulation. When people are capable of self-regulating thoughts, emotions, memory, and judgment, they are less likely to relapse into abusive behaviors. Self-regulation is supported by stabilizing physical and psychological states through detoxification, resolving immediate stresses (e.g., unemployment, family conflict), learning skills to manage withdrawal and drug preoccupation (e.g., exercise), and developing a healthy daily routine (Treatment Improvement Exchange, 2002a).

Integration is the second principle of relapse prevention. Integration involves conscious understanding and acceptance of situations, including previous relapses. Integration is facilitated by self-assessment and exploration of substance use behaviors and contributing factors, warning signs of relapse, and problems that have contributed to relapse in the past (Treatment Improvement Exchange, 2002a).

The third principle addresses the need for understanding the causes of relapse and is facilitated by education regarding causes and strategies for preventing relapse. Self-knowledge is the fourth principle. When people are able to recognize personal warning signs of relapse, the potential for relapse decreases. Coping skills reflect the fifth principle. The risk of relapse decreases as coping abilities increase. Specific coping skills must be developed to address the warning signs of relapse as they occur. Coping includes avoidance of situations that trigger warning signs, resolution of irrational thoughts and unmanageable feelings that accompany warning signs, and resolution of underlying issues that contribute to warning signs (Treatment Improvement Exchange, 2002a).

The sixth principle is change and involves the development of specific strategies or recovery activities related to each warning sign. Awareness is the seventh principle and reflects use of a daily inventory to check for the presence of warning signs. Use of the inventory includes development of daily goals, a to-do list related to goals, and an assessment of goal completion (Treatment Improvement Exchange, 2002a).

Principle eight addresses the need to incorporate significant others into recovery and relapse planning. For example, the abuser might enlist family members or counselors to help identify and intervene when warning signals of relapse are noted. The final principle is maintenance and underscores the need to update the relapse prevention plan on an ongoing basis (initially monthly, then quarterly, and then every 6 months) during the first 3 years of recovery. An update would include a review of the identified warning signs and management strategies, assessment of their effectiveness, identification of additional warning signs and strategies, and development of new recovery activities or elimination of those that are no longer needed (Treatment Improvement Exchange, 2002a). Principles and strategies for relapse prevention are summarized in Table 31-7◆.

Community health nurses can assist clients with substance abuse problems to identify triggers for relapse and to develop strategies for dealing with them. They can also assist in the development of relapse prevention groups that provide clients with the support of

TABLE 31-7	Relapse Prevention Principles and Related Strategies
Principle	**Related Strategies**
Self-regulation	Physical and psychological stabilization
Integration	Self-assessment of substance use history, contributing factors, and warning signs of relapse
Understanding	Education regarding causes and prevention of relapse
Self-knowledge	Identification of warning signs that signal impending relapse
Coping skills	Development of strategies to manage warning signs when they occur
Change	Development of a schedule of recovery activities that address warning signs for relapse
Awareness	Completion of a daily inventory of goals, activities, and their accomplishment
Significant others	Involvement of significant others in recognizing and dealing with warning signs of relapse
Maintenance	Periodic update of the relapse-prevention plan

Data from: Treatment Improvement Exchange. (2002). Counselor's manual for relapse prevention with chemically dependent offenders. Retrieved August 10, 2006, from http://tie.samsha.gov/TAPS/TAPS19/TAP19part2.html

others in dealing with their relapse issues. They may also help to motivate family members and significant others to participate in relapse prevention, educating both clients and significant others about relapse, its causes, and prevention strategies.

One approach that community health nurses may take to assisting clients with relapse prevention includes the use of relapse prevention maps. **Relapse prevention maps** are graphic representations of the factors that contribute to relapse into substance-abusing behaviors drawn by the client with the assistance of a nurse or counselor. For example, the relapse prevention map of a college student with an alcohol problem might include a drawing of the university to represent the stress of making good grades; an endless circle among classrooms, the library, and work representing excessive demands on the student; and the bar where the student stops to relax every night on the way home from class. Other elements of the map might include a demanding employer or girlfriend or friends who encourage drinking. Relapse prevention maps can help clients with substance abuse problems identify factors that contribute to relapse and suggest strategies for dealing with them (e.g., making new friends, cutting back on work, or going to school part-time). Similar maps can also be used during the early recovery stage to help identify factors that contribute to substance abuse behaviors (Weegmann, 2005).

Community health nurses can also contribute to tertiary prevention efforts by providing emotional support to recovering abusers and their families and by linking them with other sources of support. Other tertiary prevention measures might include efforts to eliminate or modify stressors that contribute to relapse. For example, assisting the recovering abuser to find work can alleviate the stress of unemployment and financial worries.

The nurse can also reinforce the individual's motivation to abstain from drug use by commending and highlighting successes and periods of sobriety.

Development of positive coping skills may also prevent relapse. Other tertiary prevention needs may involve providing information on resources, providing respite from onerous burdens of care, or helping individuals plan time for themselves.

At the population level, community health nurses may be involved in planning and implementing tertiary prevention services for people with substance abuse problems (e.g., initiating a mutual-help group or a relapse prevention group). They may also need to participate in political advocacy to assure the availability of tertiary prevention services or to mandate their coverage as a routine health insurance benefit.

DEALING WITH CONSEQUENCES OF ABUSE Substance abuse may lead to a variety of physical, psychological, and social consequences with which community health nurses need to assist clients. Community health nurses may provide treatment for physical consequences of substance abuse and assist clients to deal with psychological and social consequences. For example, they may treat abscesses due to injection drug use or refer clients for treatment if necessary. Other examples include assisting clients in recovery to deal with the feelings of guilt engendered by their behavior and its effects on loved ones, or helping them to regain custody of children placed in foster care.

Community health nurses may also need to help family members deal with the consequences of substance abuse in the family. For example, group interventions for schoolchildren whose parents have substance abuse disorders have been shown to reduce feelings of isolation and to improve problem solving, conflict resolution, and social skills as well as enhance academic skills. In addition, such programs provide a sense of personal safety and belonging, and program staff can engage in advocacy for appropriate care of these children (Gance-Cleveland, 2004). Community health nurses can be actively involved in developing these and similar programs. They can also engage in political activity to assure access to and funding for these types of programs. Political advocacy may also be needed to assure insurance coverage for health services to deal with the physical and emotional consequences of abuse for both abusers and their family members.

BUILDING A FOUNDATION FOR RECOVERY Treatment for substance abuse is more than a matter of detoxification and modification of cravings for the drug in question. It is usually a total program of modification that results in changes in modes of thinking and acting. This may be achieved through professional therapy as discussed above, participation in mutual-help groups, changes in environment and lifestyle, self-image enhancement, and development of new coping skills and new patterns of family interaction.

Mutual-help groups have been shown to be quite effective in dealing with many health problems. The effectiveness of these groups stems from several assumptions. First, the emotional support of others with similar problems reduces the social isolation experienced by many clients with substance abuse problems. Second, a collective self-identity emerges through group participation, allowing group members to develop new personal self-concepts. Third, group participation permits sharing of experiential knowledge and practical suggestions for coping with problems encountered. Finally, group participation fosters a more active orientation to health, greater reliance on individual and group support systems, and less dependence on health care providers.

Alcoholics Anonymous (AA) is a highly successful mutual-help group for alcohol abusers. AA groups are available in most communities and are often focused on specific segments of the population (e.g., adolescents, professionals). Some authors have noted, however, that AA has its foundation in religious tenets and may not be appropriate for all clients with alcohol abuse problems. A similar group, Al-Anon, assists family members of alcohol abusers, and Adult Children of Alcoholics

provides similar assistance for adults with lingering issues related to an alcohol-abusing parent. Other mutual-help groups include Narcotics Anonymous for narcotics abusers and Dual Recovery Anonymous for clients with dual diagnoses (Hills et al., 2004). Co-dependents Anonymous for co-dependent family members and others was discussed earlier.

Community health nurses may be involved in the initiation of mutual-help groups or in subsequent support of such groups. Nurses also refer individual clients to existing groups as appropriate. Nurses should function as facilitators of the group process, not as "leaders" or active participants in the group, unless they also experience the condition involved.

Community health nurses can facilitate the work of mutual-help groups in several ways. These include monitoring and directing active involvement by group members, encouraging the sharing of experiences and solutions to common problems, encouraging provision of mutual aid, and encouraging utilization of professional assistance as needed. Other facilitative measures include emphasizing personal responsibility for and control over events, maintaining positive pressure for behavior change, and emphasizing the need for positive coping strategies. Finally, the nurse should facilitate group interaction by providing the least amount of personal input possible.

Nurses can also assist clients to plan changes in their environment to minimize stresses that may contribute to substance abuse. For example, the nurse can refer a client for help with financial difficulties or for respite from the care of a handicapped child or elderly parent. Socially isolated older persons who abuse substances can be linked to sources of social support, and unemployed persons can be assisted to find employment or to learn skills that enhance their employability.

Community health nurses can also help clients develop stronger self-images by reinforcing their successes and helping them realistically examine their failures and their expectations for themselves. In addition, nurses can help clients who abuse psychoactive substances to develop alternative ways of coping with stress by taking action to modify stressors or changing their perceptions of and responses to stressors.

Treatment efforts are also needed for members of the abuser's family to enable them to recover from co-dependence. Goals in the care of families of substance abusers include stabilizing the family system, making changes in family interactions, and developing mechanisms for maintaining those changes. Family stabilization may be achieved by linking families to needed support services and engaging in the crisis intervention strategies described in Chapter 14∞. The nurse can also make referrals for marital or family therapy as needed and can assist families to identify their use of defense mechanisms similar to those used by the substance abuser.

Think Advocacy

Most State Board of Nursing disciplinary actions involve substance abuse by nurses. State Boards of Nursing and Medicine often have very different perspectives on substance abuse by members of the two professions. Among physicians, problems of abuse are often handled by physician addiction specialists outside of the licensing board, and cases often are not referred to the board if they can be handled at this peer counseling level (Haack & Yocom, 2002). What are the policies for dealing with substance abuse by nurses and physicians in your state? Are they the same? If there are differences, how might you go about advocating for equitable treatment for substance abuse problems between the two professions?

The community health nurse might also provide families with anticipatory guidance about the negative effects of life change events and help them deal with these events without resorting to substance abuse. Family members may also need help in working through resentment related to substance abuse and subsequent behaviors by the abuser.

Building positive experiences in the life of the family also fosters cohesion and helps to stabilize the family. The community health nurse can assist the family to plan activities in which all members can participate. It is particularly important to integrate the substance-abusing member into these occasions, if possible, to prevent further alienation.

The community health nurse can also assist families to develop new patterns of interaction. For example, the nurse might help the family realign members into the more usual husband–wife coalition rather than parent–child coalitions by improving family communication and developing joint problem-solving skills. The nurse can also assist family members to identify and express feelings and learn negotiating strategies.

HARM REDUCTION An alternative approach to the control of substance abuse is based on the philosophy of harm reduction. Traditionally, the goal of policy development and implementation related to substance abuse has been a reduction in drug use. It has been suggested that a more appropriate focus would be to reduce the harm to society resulting from drug abuse. **Harm reduction** is an approach to drug use that focuses on moderation of substance use and minimization of its harmful effects (Lennings, 2000). Approaches to harm reduction include provision of methadone to heroin users, needle exchange programs, provision of syringe filters, initiation of outpatient wound clinics for injection abscesses, and wound care programs at needle exchange sites. Provision of Narcan, a narcotic antagonist, to opiate addicts has even been suggested as a means of preventing deaths from overdose (Goldsmith, 2000a).

Methadone treatment substitutes controlled use of methadone, a drug that has psychological effects similar to those of heroin, for uncontrolled use of the more dangerous heroin. When used as prescribed, methadone has been found effective in reducing heroin use among abusers. Methadone use has also been suggested as early treatment for people who sniff heroin to prevent their transition from sniffing to injecting the drug, thus preventing some of the consequences of IDU such as wound infections and septicemia (Kelley & Chitwood, 2004).

Needle exchange programs for injection drug users are one of the more common forms of harm reduction advocated in controlling substance abuse (McKnight et al., 2005). An offshoot of needle exchange programs involves the creation of safer injection facilities, where IDUs can use preobtained drugs under the supervision of a nurse. At least one study has documented reductions in public drug use and needle sharing as a result of such facilities (Wood et al., 2006). Needle exchange programs also provide an opportunity to screen participants for bloodborne diseases such as HIV/AIDS and hepatitis and to refer clients with positive tests for further diagnosis and treatment (Pratt, Paone, Carter, & Layton, 2002).

Although needle exchange programs have demonstrated the ability to decrease high-risk injection behaviors and the incidence of bloodborne disease in IDUs, their effectiveness may be affected by other factors. For example, in one study, intensive street-level law enforcement efforts to disrupt drug sales on targeted street corners close to needle exchange program locations led to a significant reduction in the use of the needle exchange program. The explanation given for the decrease was fear of arrest or search for carrying syringes, as well as police harassment of those participating in the exchange programs (Davis, Burris, Kraut-Becher, Lynch, & Metzger, 2005). Community health nurses can work to change the attitudes of public officials and the general public regarding the effectiveness of needle exchange programs in preventing some of the more drastic consequences of injection drug use. They may also be involved in developing and implementing such programs and in motivating injection drug users to take advantage of existing programs. Community health nurses working in needle exchange programs can also work to motivate participants to seek treatment for their drug abuse problems. In addition, they can assist these clients to address other issues such as physical illness or infection, homelessness, and unemployment.

ETHICAL AWARENESS

One of the recent developments in harm reduction strategies for substance abuse is the provision of safe facilities where IDUs can inject previously obtained illicit drugs under the supervision of a nurse, who can help prevent overdose, use of contaminated equipment, and other adverse effects of injection drug use (Wood et al., 2006). Do you think it is appropriate for nurses to participate in a behavior such as drug use that is harmful to clients? Why or why not? What are the conflicting values operating in this ethical dilemma? How would you prioritize these values to decide on an appropriate course of action for a nurse in this situation?

EVIDENCE-BASED PRACTICE

Review the literature related to a particular approach to harm reduction. Is there sufficient evidence for the effectiveness of harm reduction strategies to warrant a change in policy regarding public health efforts to control substance abuse? To what extent are harm reduction strategies used in your local area? What is the response of local law enforcement personnel to the concept of harm reduction in your area? What factors promote or impede the use of harm reduction strategies in the area?

Wound and abscess clinics are another approach to harm reduction for injection drug users. Injection drug use often leads to wound infections that may result in cellulitis, septicemia, and necrotizing fasciitis. The prevalence of such infections has been found to be as high as 32% in some populations of IDUs. A wound and abscess clinic held in conjunction with a syringe exchange program was able to provide care at an average of $5 per person, compared to estimated hospital-based treatment costs of $185 to $360 per person excluding the costs of physician services and medications. Provision of wound care also offered an additional opportunity to encourage safer injection practices and to identify abusers interested in substance abuse treatment (Grau, Arevalo, Catchpool, & Heimer, 2002). Community health nurses can provide wound care to individual clients in such clinics as well as educate them regarding safe shooting techniques to prevent future infections. In the context of the clinic, community health nurses can engage in assessment of clients' motivation for change and employ strategies to move them through the stages of change discussed earlier. Nurses can also educate the drug-using population regarding infection prevention. Finally, they can be active advocates for the availability of wound clinics and funding for the services provided. Table 31-8◆ lists primary, secondary, and tertiary prevention goals and related nursing interventions in the control of substance abuse.

Evaluating Control Strategies for Substance Abuse

Evaluating interventions with individual substance abusers and their families focuses on the extent to which problems of substance abuse have been resolved. Has

TABLE 31-8	Primary, Secondary, and Tertiary Prevention Goals and Related Community Health Nursing Interventions in the Control of Substance Abuse	
Goal of Prevention	**Nursing Interventions (Individual/Family)**	**Nursing Interventions (Community)**
Primary Prevention		
1. Positive coping skills	1. Teach coping skills.	1. Advocate for incorporation of coping skills in school curricula; develop and implement programs to teach coping skills to the general public.
2. Strong self-image	2. Foster and reinforce development of strong self-image.	2. Promote societal attitudes and conditions that foster development of healthy self-images in members of the public; work to change social attitudes toward stigmatized groups that might foster substance abuse.
3. Knowledge of the hazards of substance abuse	3. Educate clients about the hazards of substance abuse; educate clients for moderate use of substances as appropriate (e.g., not tobacco, cocaine, etc.).	3. Conduct public education campaigns on the contributing factors in and consequences of substance abuse; advocate for substance education in school curricula; advocate for funding for public education campaigns.
4. Policies and programs to prevent abuse		4. Engage in political activity and advocacy for legislation and other policies to modify factors that contribute to substance abuse.
Secondary Prevention		
1. Early detection of persons with substance abuse problems	1. Engage in case finding; educate individuals and families on the signs and symptoms of substance abuse.	1. Assess populations for the extent of use of various substances and the prevalence of abuse of specific substances; design and conduct education campaigns to alert members of the public to signs and symptoms of substance abuse; advocate for funding for public education campaigns.
2. Early intervention for persons with problems related to substance abuse	2. Assist families to plan and carry out intervention; engage in brief intervention for persons with excessive substance use.	
3. Treatment of substance abuse	3. Refer client for treatment. Monitor client during treatment.	3. Advocate for the availability and accessibility of substance abuse treatment for all those in need.
4. Provision of treatment facilities		4. Engage in political activity to support treatment facilities and programs.

Continued on next page

TABLE 31-8 Primary, Secondary, and Tertiary Prevention Goals and Related Community Health Nursing Interventions in the Control of Substance Abuse *(continued)*

Goal of Prevention	Nursing Interventions (Individual/Family)	Nursing Interventions (Community)
5. Insurance coverage for treatment		5. Engage in political activity and advocacy to assure inclusion of substance abuse treatment in all health insurance plans, including Medicare and Medicaid and other government programs.
Tertiary Prevention		
1. Support for abusers	1. Provide emotional support and encouragement; refer to support groups; assist with reintegration into family and society; refer for assistance with employment and other sources of support.	1. Advocate for development of and access to support services for all substance abusers, including prescription medication, social services, etc.
2. Identification of relapse warning signs	2. Assist with identification of warning signs and strategies for dealing with them; assist with development of a relapse prevention plan.	2. Initiate relapse prevention support groups.
3. Lifestyle changes that discourage abusive behavior and prevent relapse	3. Assist with lifestyle changes; help to identify and eliminate triggers for substance abuse.	
4. Modification of stressors that contribute to substance abuse	4. Assist with modification of stressors.	4. Advocate for societal changes that eliminate stressors that contribute to substance abuse.
5. Treatment for consequences of substance abuse	5. Refer for or provide assistance in dealing with physical, psychological, and social consequences of abuse.	5. Advocate for available and accessible services for dealing with physical and social consequences of substance abuse; develop and implement programs to provide treatment services for consequences of substance abuse; advocate for changes in social attitudes toward substance abusers.
6. Harm reduction	6. Educate substance-abusing clients on specific harm reduction strategies; provide harm reduction services (e.g., wound care for IDUs).	6. Advocate for the use of harm reduction strategies; educate the public and policy makers on the need for harm reduction; develop harm reduction programs.

the abuser been able to remain sober for extended periods? Have stresses contributing to substance abuse been modified?

At the level of the community, the nurse could evaluate the effects of intervention programs on the incidence and prevalence of substance abuse as well as indicators of morbidity and mortality related to abuse. The nurse evaluating the effects of programs directed at substance abuse might examine the extent to which national health promotion and disease prevention objectives have been met in the community. Evaluative information on efforts to meet the national objectives for 2010◆ is presented on page 965.

Another source of evaluative information on the overall effectiveness of criminal justice approaches to the control of substance abuse lies in the Office of Management and Budget (OMB) assessment of the federal Drug Enforcement Administration (DEA). In a 2003 assessment, the OMB gave the DEA a rating of 26% for program results and accountability, citing its minimal achievement of long-term and annual performance goals and lack of independent evidence of program achievement. It would seem clear that drug enforcement activities are not having a significant effect on the problem of substance abuse in the United States, and that other strategies are needed.

HEALTHY PEOPLE 2010

Goals for Population Health

OBJECTIVE	BASELINE	MOST RECENT DATA	TARGET
▦ 26-1. Reduce deaths and injuries due to alcohol-related motor vehicle crashes			
a. Deaths (per 100,000 population)	5.9	NDA	4
b. Injuries (per 100,000 population)	113	NDA	65
▦ 26-2. Reduce cirrhosis deaths (per 100,000 population)	9.6	9.4	3
▦ 26-3. Reduce drug-induced deaths (per 100,000 population)	6.8	9.0	1#
▦ 26-4. Reduce drug-related hospital emergency visits	542,544	NDA	350,000
▦ 26-9. Increase the proportion of adolescents who remain alcohol and drug free			
c. Alcohol	19%	23%	29%
d. Illicit drugs	46%	49%	56%
▦ 26-11. Reduce the proportion of people engaging in binge drinking in the last month			
a. High school seniors	32%	28%	11%
c. Adults	16.6%	NDA	6%
▦ 26-12. Reduce average annual alcohol consumption (gallons per person)	2.18	NDA	2
▦ 26-13. Reduce the proportion of adults who exceed guidelines for low-risk drinking			
a. Females	72%	NDA	50%
b. Males	74%	NDA	50%
▦ 26-14c. Reduce steroid use by 12th graders	1.7%	2.1%	0.4%#
▦ 26-15. Reduce inhalant use by adolescents	2.9%	NDA	0.7%
▦ 26-17. Increase the proportion of adolescents who perceive great risk associated with substance abuse			
a. Alcohol	47%	NDA	80%
b. Marijuana	31%	NDA	80%
c. Cocaine	54%	NDA	80%
▦ 26-20. Increase the number of admissions to treatment for injection drug use (per year)	167,960	NDA	200,000
▦ 27-1a. Reduce cigarette smoking by adults	24%	20%	12%
▦ 27-2a. Reduce tobacco use by adolescents	40%	27%	21%
▦ 27-4. Increase the age of first use of tobacco			
a. By adolescents	12	NDA	14
b. By young adults	15	NDA	17
▦ 27-5. Increase smoking cessation attempts by adults	41%	42%	75%
▦ 27-6. Increase smoking cessation during pregnancy	14%	17%	30%
▦ 27-8. Increase insurance coverage for treatment of nicotine dependence in			
a. Managed care programs	75%	NDA	100%
b. Medicaid programs	24%	NDA	51%
▦ 27-10. Reduce the proportion of nonsmokers exposed to environmental tobacco smoke	88.1%	53.0%	45%
▦ 27-11. Increase tobacco-free environments in schools	37%	45%	100%
▦ 27-12. Increase the proportion of worksites with formal smoking policies	79%	NDA	100%

NDA — No data available

* Objective has been met

Objective moving away from target

Data from: Centers for Disease Control and Prevention. (2005). Healthy people data. Retrieved September 5, 2005, from http://wonder.cdc.gov/data2010.

Case Study

Caring for the Client with a Substance Abuse Problem

You have been working with the Schumacher family for the last several months. The youngest child, who is 18 months old, has multiple physical handicaps and has been in and out of the hospital numerous times for surgery. He is currently enrolled in physical and occupational therapy programs to promote his development. You have been following this child and working with the family to meet his needs. On your most recent home visit, Mrs. Schumacher voiced concern about her husband's drinking.

Since the birth of the baby, Mr. Schumacher has gone on periodic drinking binges. Initially, these occurred about once a month, but lately he has been getting drunk almost every weekend. This week Mrs. Schumacher had to call her husband's office, where he is employed as a civil engineer, to tell his employer that her husband was ill. Actually, he was too hungover to go to work. She has tried to talk to her husband about his drinking, but he becomes angry and storms out of the house. When he returns, he is drunk. Each time, after he sobers up, he is repentant and promises not to drink again. Mrs. Schumacher thinks her husband's drinking is the result of his worry about financial problems.

Since Mr. Schumacher's drinking problem has escalated, the older children have been reluctant to bring friends home because they are embarrassed by their father's drunken behavior. They have begun to ask Mrs. Schumacher rather pointed questions about their father, such as "Is Daddy an alcoholic?" They know that their grandfather, Mr. Schumacher's father, died of cirrhosis stemming from alcoholism. Mrs. Schumacher says she has told the children their father is not an alcoholic but is just tired and has been under a lot of stress at work.

Mr. Schumacher has always been a successful provider for the family and did not drink much before the baby was born. He did well in school, completing a master's degree in engineering, and was promoted to a new position with his engineering firm about 2 years ago. His job pays relatively well, but because their health insurance did not cover the baby when he was born, they have had to pay all of the new infant's medical expenses out of pocket. Mrs. Schumacher says they have exhausted their savings and indicates that they are having some difficulty meeting mortgage payments on their house. She would like to work but would have trouble finding someone to care for the baby, who has a tracheostomy and requires periodic suctioning. She has discussed her willingness to work with her husband, but he insists that he is not going to have his wife working when the children need her at home and that he will take care of things.

1. What are the biophysical, psychological, sociocultural, behavioral, and health system factors influencing the health of this family?
2. What are the health problems evident in this situation? Develop several nursing diagnostic statements related to these problems.
3. What evidence of co-dependence is present in this family situation?
4. What client care objectives would you set in working with this family?
5. What primary, secondary, and tertiary intervention strategies should be employed with this family? Why?
6. What community resources might you refer this family to? Why have you selected these resources?
7. How would you evaluate the effectiveness of your interventions with the Schumacher family? What evaluative criteria would you use? How would you obtain the evaluative data needed?

Test Your Understanding

1. What are the criteria for diagnosing psychoactive substance dependence? Give examples of behaviors that might demonstrate these criteria. (p. 932)

2. Distinguish between psychoactive substance dependence and abuse. (pp. 932–933)

3. What are the psychoactive substances that most often lead to dependence and abuse? (pp. 933–938)

4. Describe some of the personal, family, and societal effects of substance abuse. (pp. 938–940)

5. What are some of the biophysical, psychological, sociocultural, behavioral, and health system factors that influence substance abuse? (pp. 940–948)

6. Discuss the use of the WHO Rapid Assessment and Response guidelines in assessing substance abuse in a population. (pp. 948–949)

7. What are the five aspects of community health nursing assessment of an individual client in relation to substance abuse? (pp. 949–951)

8. What are the major approaches to primary prevention of substance abuse? How might community health nurses be involved in each? (pp. 951–953)

9. What are the components of the intervention process in secondary prevention of substance abuse? What might be the role of the community health nurse in the intervention process? (pp. 953–954)

10. What are the general principles in the treatment of substance abuse? (p. 954)

11. What are the major treatment modalities in substance abuse? What is the role of the community health nurse with respect to each? (pp. 954–958)

12. What are the major emphases in tertiary prevention of substance abuse? How might the community health nurse be involved in each? (pp. 958–963)

13. What is harm reduction and how does it relate to control of substance abuse? (pp. 962–963)

EXPLORE MediaLink

http://www.prenhall.com/clark
Resources for this chapter can be found on the **Companion Website**.

Audio Glossary
Exam Review Questions
Case Study: The Effects of Substance Abuse

MediaLink Application: Overcoming
    Addiction: Combined Therapies (video)
Media Links

Challenge Your Knowledge
Update *Healthy People 2010*
Advocacy Interviews

References

Al-Kandari, F. H., Yacoub, K., & Omu, F. (2001). Initiation factors for substance abuse. *Journal of Advanced Nursing, 34*, 78–85.

American Psychiatric Association. (2000). *Diagnostic and statistical manual of mental disorders* (4th ed., text revision) (DSM-IV-TR). Washington, DC: Author.

Andrews, J. O., Heath, J., & Graham-Garcia, J. (2004). Management of tobacco dependence in older adults. *Journal of Gerontological Nursing, 30*(12), 13–24.

Anheuser-Busch. (2006). *Family talk: Helping parents talk with their children about underage drinking.* Retrieved June 7, 2006, from http://www.familytalkonline.com/docs/AboutUs.htm

Asplund, C. A., Aaronson, J. W., & Aaronson, H. E. (2004). 3 regimens for alcohol withdrawal and detoxification. *Journal of Family Practice, 53*, 545–554.

Bailey, K. P. (2004). Pharmacological treatments for substance abuse disorders. *Journal of Psychosocial Nursing, 42*(8), 14–20.

Beals, J., Spicer, P., Mitchell, C. M., Novins, D. K., Manson, S. M., & the AI-SUPERFP Team. (2003). Racial disparities in alcohol use: Comparison of 2 American Indian reservation populations with national data. *American Journal of Public Health, 93*, 1683–1685.

Bertrand, J., Floyd, L., & Weber, M. K. (2005). Guidelines for identifying and referring persons with fetal alcohol syndrome. *Morbidity and Mortality Weekly Report, 54*(RR-11), 1–14.

Block, J. S. (2006). Did prohibition really work? Alcohol prohibition as a public health innovation. *American Journal of Public Health, 96*, 233–243.

Boddiger, D. (2005). Methamphetamine use linked to rising HIV transmission. *The Lancet, 365*, 1217–1218.

Bureau of Justice Statistics. (2005a). *Crime characteristics.* Retrieved March 20, 2006, from http://www.ojp.usdoj.gov/bjs/cvict_c.htm

Bureau of Justice Statistics. (2005b). *Drug use.* Retrieved June 9, 2006, from http://www.ojp.usdoj.gov/bjs/dcf/du.htm

Bureau of Justice Statistics. (2005c). *Estimated arrests for drug abuse violations by age group, 1970–2003.* Retrieved June 9, 2006, from http://www.ojp.usdoj.gov/bjs/glance/tables/drugtab.htm

Cabaniss, R. (2005). Strokes related to drug use. *Advance for Nurses, 2*(13), 17–19.

Caflish, C., Wang, J., & Zbinden, R. (1999). The role of syringe filters in harm reduction among injection drug users. *American Journal of Public Health, 89*, 1252–1254.

Centers for Disease Control and Prevention. (2004). Indicators for chronic disease surveillance. *Morbidity and Mortality Weekly Report, 53*(RR-11), 1–114.

Centers for Disease Control and Prevention. (2005). *Healthy people data.* Retrieved September 5, 2005, from http://wonder.cdc.gov/data2010

Centers for Disease Control and Prevention. (2006a). *Behavioral risk factor surveillance system: Prevalence data: Alcohol consumption, Binge drinkers.* Retrieved August 9, 2006, from http://apps.nccd.cdc.gov/brfss/sex.asp?cat=AC&yr=2005&qkey=7306&state=US

Centers for Disease Control and Prevention. (2006b). *Behavioral risk factor surveillance system: Prevalence data: Alcohol consumption, Heavy drinkers.* Retrieved August 9, 2006, from http://apps.nccd.cdc.gov/brfss/sex.asp?cat=AC&yr=2005&qkey=4413&state=US

Centers for Disease Control and Prevention. (2006c). *Behavioral risk factor surveillance system: Prevalence data: Tobacco use.* Retrieved August 9, 2006, from http://apps.nccd.cdc.gov/brfss/sex.asp?cat=TU&yr=2005&qkey=4396&state=US

Centers for Disease Control and Prevention. (2006d). World No Tobacco Day—May 31, 2006. *Morbidity and Mortality Weekly Report, 55*, 553.

Cooper, D., Rice, N., Wilburn, R., Horton, D. K., & Rossiter, S. (2005). Acute public health consequences of methamphetamine laboratories —16 states, January 2000–June 2004. *Morbidity and Mortality Weekly Report, 54*, 356–359.

Davis, C. S., Burris, S., Kraut-Becher, J., Lynch, K. G., & Metzger, D. (2005). Effects of an intensive street-level police intervention strategy on syringe exchange program use in Philadelphia, PA. *American Journal of Public Health, 95*, 233–236.

Denny, C. H., Holtzman, D., & Cobb, N. (2003). Surveillance for health behaviors of American Indians and Alaska Natives: Findings from the Behavioral Risk Factor Surveillance System, 1997–2002. *Morbidity and Mortality Weekly Report, 52*(SS-7), 1–13.

Division of Adult and Community Health, National Center for Chronic Disease Prevention and Health Promotion. (2004). Alcohol use among adolescents and adults—New Hampshire, 1991–2003. *Morbidity and Mortality Weekly Report, 53*(SS-2), 1–96.

Division of Bacterial and Mycotic Diseases. (2003). Wound botulism among black tar heroin users—Washington, 2003. *Morbidity and Mortality Weekly Report, 52*, 885–886.

Division of HIV/AIDS Prevention, National Center for HIV, STD, and TB Prevention. (2003). HIV diagnoses among injection-drug users in states with HIV surveillance—25 states, 1994–2000. *Morbidity and Mortality Weekly Report, 52*, 634–636.

Droomers, M., Schrijvers, C. T. M., & Mackenbach, J. P. (2004). Educational differences in starting excessive alcohol consumption: Explanations from the longitudinal GLOBE study. *Social Science & Medicine, 58*, 2023–2033.

Drug Reform Coordination Network. (2005). *Marijuana law enforcement costs more than $7 billion a year—And doesn't work.* Retrieved June 13, 2006, from http://stopthewar.org/chronicle/739/report1.shtml

Eaton, D. K., Kann, L., Kinchen, S., Ross, J., Hawkins, J., Harris, W. A., et al. (2006). Youth risk behavior surveillance—United States, 2005. *Morbidity and Mortality Weekly Report, 55*(SS-5), 1–108.

Edenberg, H. J., Dick, D. M., Xuei, X., Tian, H., Amasy, L., Bauer, L. O., et al. (2004). Variations in *GABRA2*, encoding the α subunit of the GABA$_A$ receptor, are associated with alcohol dependence and with brain oscillations. *American Journal of Human Genetics, 74,* 705–714.

Ehrmin, J. T. (2001). Unresolved feelings of guilt and shame in the maternal role with substance-dependent African American women. *Journal of Nursing Scholarship, 33,* 47–52.

Ellickson, P. L., McCaffrey, D. F., Ghosh-Dastidar, B., & Longshore, D. L. (2003). New inroads in preventing adolescent drug use: Results from a large-scale trial of Project ALERT in middle-schools. *American Journal of Public Health, 93,* 1830–1836.

Finfgeld-Connett, D. L. (2004). Treatment of substance misuse in older women: Using a brief intervention model. *Journal of Gerontological Nursing, 30*(8), 30–37.

Fitch, C., Stimson, G. V., Rhodes, T., & Poznyak, V. (2004). Rapid assessment: An international review of diffusion, practice and outcomes in the substance use field. *Social Science & Medicine, 59,* 1819–1830.

Fuller, C. M., Borrell, L. N., Latkin, C. A., Salea, S., Ompad, D. C., Strathdee, S. A., et al. (2005). Effects of race, neighborhood, and social network on age at initiation of injection drug use. *American Journal of Public Health, 95,* 689–695.

Gance-Cleveland, B. (2004). Qualitative evaluation of a school-based support group for adolescents with an addicted parent. *Nursing Research, 53,* 379–386.

Gil, A. G., Wagner, E. F., & Tubman, J. G. (2004). Associations between early-adolescent substance use and subsequent young-adult substances use disorders and psychiatric disorders among a multiethnic male sample in South Florida. *American Journal of Public Health, 94,* 1603–1609.

Goldsmith, C. (2000a). The new face of heroin: Nurses seeing younger users. *NurseWeek, 13*(13), 13.

Goldsmith, C. (2000b). Tough lessons: Alcohol treatment programs debate abstinence vs. moderation. *NurseWeek, 13*(20), 28–29.

Golub, A., & Johnson, B. D. (2001). Variation in youthful risks of progression from alcohol and tobacco to marijuana and to hard drugs across generations. *American Journal of Public Health, 91,* 225–232.

Grant, B. F. (2000). Estimates of US children exposed to alcohol abuse and dependence in the family. *American Journal of Public Health, 90,* 112–115.

Grau, L. E., Arevalo, S., Catchpool, C., & Heimer, R. (2002). Expanding harm reduction services through a wound and abscess clinic. *American Journal of Public Health, 92,* 1915–1917.

Grunbaum, J. A., Kann, L., Kinchen, S., Ross, J., Hawkins, J., Lowry, R., et al. (2004). Youth risk behavior surveillance—United States, 2003. *Morbidity and Mortality Weekly Report, 53*(SS-2), 1–96.

Guilamo-Ramos, V., Jaccard, J., Turrisi, R., & Johansson, M. (2005). Parental and school correlates of binge drinking among middle school students. *American Journal of Public Health, 95,* 894–899.

Haack, M. R., & Yocom, C. J. (2002). State policies and nurses with substance use disorders. *Journal of Nursing Scholarship, 34,* 89–94.

Heath, D. B. (2000). *Drinking occasions: Comparative perspectives on alcohol and culture.* Philadelphia: Brunner/Mazel.

Hills, H., Siegfried, C., & Ickowitz, A. (2004). *Effective prison mental health services: Guidelines to expand and improve treatment.* Retrieved March 30, 2006, from http://www.nicic.org/misc/URLshell.aspx?SRC=Catalogue&REFF=http://nicic.org/library/018604&ID=018604&Type=PDF&URL=http://nicic.org/pubs/2004/018604.pdf

Hoffman, R. S., Nelson, L. S., Chan, G. M., Halcomb, S. E., Bouchard, N. C., Ginsburg, B. Y., et al. (2005). Atypical reactions associated with heroin use—Five states, January–April 2005. *Morbidity and Mortality Weekly Report, 54,* 793–796.

Hyman, S. E. (2005). Addiction: A disease of learning and memory. *American Journal of Psychiatry, 162,* 1414–1422.

Insel, P., Roth, W. T., & Price, K. (2005). *Core concepts in health* (10th ed.). New York: McGraw-Hill.

Kelder, S. H., Murray, N. G., Orpinas, P., Prokhorov, A., McReynolds, L., Zhang, Q., et al. (2001). Depression and substance use in minority middle-school students. *American Journal of Public Health, 91,* 761–766.

Kelley, M. S., & Chitwood, D. D. (2004). Effects of drug treatment for heroin sniffers: A protective factor against moving to injection? *Social Science & Medicine, 58,* 2083–2092.

Kim, S., & Crittenden, K. S. (2005). Risk factors for tuberculosis among inmates: A retrospective analysis. *Public Health Nursing, 22,* 108–118.

Kunitz, S. J., Woodall, G., Zhao, H., Wheeler, D. R., Lillis, R., & Rogers, E. (2002). Rearrest rates after incarceration for DWI: A comparative study in a southwestern US county. *American Journal of Public Health, 92,* 1826–1831.

Kypri, K., Voas, R. B., Langley, J. D., Stephenson, S. C. R., Begg, D. J., Tippetts, S., et al. (2006). Minimum purchasing age for alcohol and traffic crash injuries among 15- to 19-year-olds in New Zealand. *American Journal of Public Health, 96,* 126–131.

Lennings, C. J. (2000). Harm minimization or abstinence: An evaluation of current policies and practices in the treatment and control of intravenous drug using groups in Australia. *Disability and Rehabilitation, 22*(1/2), 57–64.

McKnight, C. A., Des Jarlais, D. C., Perlis, T., Krim, M., Auerbach, J., Purchase, D., et al. (2005). Update: Syringe Exchange Programs—United States, 2002. *Morbidity and Mortality Weekly Report, 54,* 673–676.

McLeer, S. V. (2004). Mental health services. In H. S. Sultz & K. M. Young, *Health care USA: Understanding its organization and delivery* (4th ed., pp. 335–366). Sudbury, MA: Jones and Bartlett.

Merline, A. C., O'Malley, P. M., Schulenberg, J. E., Bachman, J. G., & Johnston, L. D. (2004). Substance use among adults 35 years of age: Prevalence, adulthood predictors, and

impact of adolescent substance use. *American Journal of Public Health, 94,* 96–102.

Milby, J. B., Schumacher, J. E., Wallace, D., Freedman, M. D., & Vuchinich, R. E. (2005). To house or not to house: The effects of providing housing to homeless substance abusers in treatment. *American Journal of Public Health, 95,* 1259–1265.

Mochizuki-Kobayashi, Y., Fishburn, B., Baptiste, J., El-Awa, F., Nokogosian, H., Peruga, A., et al. (2006). Use of cigarettes and other tobacco products among students aged 13–15 years—Worldwide, 1999–2005. *Morbidity and Mortality Weekly Report, 55,* 553–556.

Moore, A. A., Gould, R., Reuben, D. B., Greendale, G. A., Carter, K., Zhou, K., et al. (2005). Longitudinal patterns and predictors of alcohol consumption in the United States. *American Journal of Public Health, 95,* 458–465.

National Center for Chronic Disease Prevention and Health Promotion. (2006a). *Alcohol consumption—2005.* Retrieved June 13, 2006, from http://www.nccd.cdc.gov/brfss/index.asp

National Center for Chronic Disease Prevention and Health Promotion. (2006b). *Four level smoking status.* Retrieved June 13, 2006, from http://www.nccd.cdc.gov/brfss/index.asp

National Center for Health Statistics. (2005). *Health, United States, 2005 with chartbook on trends in the health of Americans.* Retrieved December 23, 2005, from http://www.cdc.gov/nchs/data/hus/hus05.pdf

National Center for Injury Prevention and Control. (2006a). *Fire deaths and injuries: Fact sheet.* Retrieved June 12, 2005, from http://www.cdc.gov/ncipc/factsheets/fire.htm

National Center for Injury Prevention and Control. (2006b). *Water-related injuries: Fact sheet.* Retrieved June 12, 2005, from http://www.cdc.gov/ncipc/factsheets/drown.htm

National Center on Birth Defects and Developmental Disabilities. (2004a). *ADHD: Attention-deficit/hyperactivity disorder.* Retrieved June 16, 2005, from http://www.cdc.gov/ncbddd/adhd/injury.htm

National Center on Birth Defects and Developmental Disabilities. (2004b). Alcohol consumption among women who are pregnant or might become pregnant—United States, 2002. *Morbidity and Mortality Weekly Report, 53,* 1178–1181.

National Center on Birth Defects and Developmental Disabilities. (2005). *Fetal alcohol spectrum disorders.* Retrieved June 13, 2006, from http://www.cdc.gov/ncbddd/factsheets/FAS.pdf

National Coalition for the Homeless. (2005). *Addiction disorders and homelessness.* Retrieved November 29, 2005, from http://www.nationalhomeless.org/publications/facts

National Highway Traffic Safety Administration. (2006). *Traffic safety facts 2004.* Retrieved June 12, 2006, from http://www-nrd.nhtsa.dot.gov/pdf/nrd-30/NCSA/TSFann.TSF2004.pdf

National Institute of Mental Health. (2006). *Schizophrenia*. Retrieved March 8, 2006, from http://www.nimh.nih.gov/public/schizoph.cfm

National Institute on Drug Abuse. (1999). *Principles of drug addition treatment*. Retrieved August 9, 2006, from http://www.nida.gov/PDF/PODAT/PODAT.pdf

National Institute on Drug Abuse. (2003). *Preventing drug abuse among children and adolescents: In Brief* (2nd ed.). Retrieved June 13, 2006, from http://www.drugabuse.gov/pdf/prevention/InBrief.pdf

National Institute on Drug Abuse. (2005a). *NIDA infofacts: Methamphetamine*. Retrieved August 9, 2006, from http://www.nida.nih.gov/infofacts/methamphetamine.html

National Institute on Drug Abuse. (2005b). *Research report series: Methamphetamine abuse and addiction*. Retrieved August 9, 2006, from http://www.nida/nih.gov/ResearchReports/Methamph/methamph3.html

National Institute on Drug Abuse. (2005c). *Steroids (Anabolic-Androgenic)*. Retrieved June 13, 2006, from http://www.nida/nih.gov/infofacts/steroids.html

National Institute on Drug Abuse. (2005d). *Understanding drug abuse and addiction*. Retrieved June 13, 2006, from http://www.nida.nih.gov/infofacts/understand.html

National Institute on Drug Abuse. (2006a). *Costs to society*. Retrieved June 13, 2006, from http://www.nida.nih.gov/infofacts/costs.html

National Institute on Drug Abuse (2006b). *Principles of drug abuse treatment for criminal justice populations*. Retrieved August 9, 2006, from http://www.nida.nih.gov/PDF.PODAT_CJ/PODAT_CH.pdf

Nelson, D. E., Naimi, T. S., Brewer, R. D., Bolen, J., & Wells, H. E. (2004). Metropolitan-area estimates of binge drinking in the United States. *American Journal of Public Health, 94*, 663–671.

Nelson, D. E., Naimi, T. S., Brewer, R. D., & Wechsler, H. (2005). The state sets the rate: The relationship among state-specific college binge drinking, state binge drinking rates, and selected state alcohol control policies. *American Journal of Public Health, 95*, 441–446.

North, C. S., Eyrich, K. M., Pollio, D. E., & Spitznagel, E. L. (2004). Are rates of psychiatric disorders in the homeless population changing? *American Journal of Public Health, 94*, 103–108.

Office of Management and Budget. (2003). *Drug Enforcement Administration Assessment*. Retrieved June 13, 2006, from http://www.whitehouse.gov/omb/expectmore/detail.10000170.2005.html

Office of National Drug Control Policy. (2006). *Methamphetamine: Overview*. Retrieved August 9, 2006, from http://www.whitehousedrugpolicy.gov/drugfact/methamphetamine/index.html

Office on Smoking and Health. (2006). Cigarette use among high school students—United States, 1991–2005. *Morbidity and Mortality Weekly Report, 55*, 724–726.

Office on Smoking and Health, National Center for Chronic Disease Prevention and Health Promotion. (2004). State Medicaid coverage for tobacco dependence treatments—United States, 1994–2002. *Morbidity and Mortality Weekly Report, 53*, 54–57.

Paschall, M. J., Freisthler, B., & Lipton, R. I. (2005). Moderate alcohol use and depression in young adults: Findings from a national study. *American Journal of Public Health, 95*, 453–457.

Pilgrim, C., Abbey, A., & Kershaw, T. (2004). The direct and indirect effects of mothers' and adolescents' family cohesion on young adolescents' attitudes toward substance abuse. *Journal of Primary Prevention, 24*, 263–283.

Pratt, C.-C. N. U., Paone, D., Carter, R. J., & Layton, M. C. (2002). Hepatitis C screening and management practices: A survey of drug treatment and syringe exchange programs in New York City. *American Journal of Public Health, 92*, 1254–1256.

Price, R. K., Risk, N. K., & Spitznagel, E. L. (2001). Remission from drug abuse over a 25-year period: Patterns of remission and treatment use. *American Journal of Public Health, 91*, 1107–1113.

Pridemore, W. A. (2002). Vodka and violence: Alcohol consumption and homicide rates in Russia. *American Journal of Public Health, 92*, 1921–1930.

Prochaska, J. M., Prochaska, J. O., Cohen, F. C., Gomes, S. O., Laforge, R. G., & Eastwood, A. L. (2004). The transtheoretical model of change for multi-level interventions for alcohol abuse on campus. *Journal of Alcohol and Drug Education, 47*(3), 34–50.

Racioppo, M. (2005). *Substance abuse: Effective treatments*. Retrieved June 9, 2006, from http://www.nimh.nih.gov/outreach/partners/raciopp2005.cfm

Saitz, R. (2005). Unhealthy alcohol use. *New England Journal of Medicine, 352*, 596–607.

Sobell, M. B., Sobell, L. C., Johnson, K., Velasquez, M. M., Mullen, P. D., von Sternberg, K., et al. (2003). Motivational intervention to reduce alcohol-exposed pregnancies—Florida, Texas, and Virginia, 1997–2001. *Morbidity and Mortality Weekly Report, 52*, 441–444.

Sporer, K. A. (2004). Buprenorphine: A primer for emergency physicians. *Annals of Emergency Medicine, 43*, 580–584.

Springer, J. F., Sale, E., Hermann, J., Sambrano, S., Kasim, R., & Nistler, M. (2004). Characteristics of effective substance abuse prevention programs for high-risk youth. *Journal of Primary Prevention, 25*, 171–194.

Srivastava, A., & Kahan, M. (2006). Buprenorphine: A potential new treatment option for opioid dependence. *Canadian Medical Association Journal, 174*, 1835–1836.

Stevenson, J. S., & Masters, J. A. (2005). Predictors of alcohol misuse and abuse in older women. *Journal of Nursing Scholarship, 37*, 329–335.

Stimson, G. V., Fitch, C., Des Jarlais, D., Poznyak, V., Perlis, T., Oppenheimer, E., et al. (2006). Rapid assessment and response studies of injection drug use: Knowledge gain,

capacity building, and intervention development in a multisite study. *American Journal of Public Health, 96*, 288–295.

Substance Abuse and Mental Health Services Administration. (2006a). *Alcohol dependence or abuse—2002, 2003, & 2004*. Retrieved June 9, 2006, from http://oas.samhsa.gov/2k6/alcDepend/alcDepend.cfm

Substance Abuse and Mental Health Services Administration. (2006b). *Characteristics of recent adolescent inhalant initiates*. Retrieved June 9, 2006, from http://oas.samhsa.gov/2k6/inhalants/inhalants.cfm

Substance Abuse and Mental Health Services Administration. (2006c). *Opiate-related drug misuse deaths in 6 states, 2003*. Retrieved June 9, 2006, from http://oas.samhsa.gov/2k6/opiateDeaths.cfm

Substance Abuse and Mental Health Services Administration. (2006d). *Sources of payment for substance abuse treatment*. Retrieved June 9, 2006, from http://oas.samhsa.gov/2k6/pay/pay.cfm

Substance Abuse and Mental Health Services Administration. (2006e). *Trends in methamphetamine/amphetamine admissions to treatment, 1993–2003*. Retrieved June 9, 2006, from http://oas.samhsa.gov/2k6/methTX/methTX.cfm

Thiede, H., Valleroy, L. A., MacKellar, D. A., Celentano, D. D., Ford, W. L., Hagan, H., et al. (2003). Regional patterns and correlates of substance abuse among young men who have sex with men in 7 urban areas. *American Journal of Public Health, 93*, 1915–1921.

Travis, J., Solomon, A. L., & Waul, M. (2001). *From prison to home: The dimensions and consequences of prisoner reentry*. Retrieved September 25, 2003, from http://www.urban.org/URL.cfm?ID=410098

Treatment Improvement Exchange. (2002a). *Counselor's manual for relapse prevention with chemically dependent offenders*. Retrieved August 10, 2006, from http://tie.samhsa.gov/TAPS/TAP19/TAP19part2.html

Treatment Improvement Exchange. (2002b). *Treatment for alcohol and other drug dependence: Opportunities for coordination*. Retrieved August 10, 2006, from http://tie.samhsa.gov/Taps/Tap11/tap11chap9.html

Uhl, F. R., Elmer, G. I., LaBuda, M. C., & Pickens, R. W. (2000). *Human substance abuse vulnerability and genetic influences*. Retrieved August 9, 2006, from http://www.acnp.org/g4/GN401000174/CH170.htm

U.S. Census Bureau. (1999). *Statistical abstract of the United States, 1999* (119th ed.). Washington, DC: Author.

U.S. Census Bureau. (2006). *Statistical abstract of the United States, 2006*. Retrieved June 5, 2006, from http://www.census.gov/prod/2005pubs/06statab

U.S. Department of Health and Human Services. (2002). Household survey finds millions of Americans are in denial about drug abuse. *Prevention Report, 17*(1), 7–9.

U.S. Drug Enforcement Administration. (n.d.). *Clandestine laboratory indicators*. Retrieved August 9, 2006, from http://www.dea.gov/concern/clandestine_indicators.html

U.S. Preventive Services Task Force. (2004). *Screening for alcohol misuse*. Retrieved August 13, 2005, from http://www.ahrq.gov/clinic/uspstf.uspsdrin.htm

Valente, T. W., & Vlahov, D. (2001). Selective risk taking among needle exchange participants: Implications for supplemental interventions. *American Journal of Public Health, 91*, 406–411.

Vo, K. (2000). The party's never over. *Nurse-Week, 13*(4), 33.

Walters, G. D. (2002). The heritability of alcohol abuse and dependence: A meta-analysis of behavior genetic research. *American Journal of Drug and Alcohol Abuse, 28*, 557–584.

Weegmann, M. (2005). The road to recovery: Journeys and relapse risk maps. *Drugs and Alcohol Today, 5*(3), 42–45.

Weiner, S. M. (2005). Perinatal substance abuse. *Advance for Nurses, 2*(9), 19–21.

Willaing, I., & Ladelund, S. (2005). Nurse counseling of patients with an overconsumption of alcohol. *Journal of Nursing Scholarship, 37*, 30–35.

Winkelman, M. (2003). Complementary therapy for addiction: "Drumming out drugs." *American Journal of Public Health, 93*, 647–651.

Wood, E., Tyndall, M. W., Qui, Z. Zhang, R., Montaner, J., & Kerr, T. (2006). Service uptake and characteristics of injection drug users utilizing North America's first medically supervised safer injecting facility. *American Journal of Public Health, 96*, 779–783.

World Health Organization. (2003). *Rapid Assessment and Response technical guide.* Retrieved June 7, 2006, from http://www.who.int/docstore.hiv/Core

Wu, Z., Detels, R., Zhang, J., Li, V., & Li, J. (2002). Community-based trial to prevent drug use among youths in Yunnan, China. *American Journal of Public Health, 92*, 1952–1957.

Yuan, Z., Dawson, N., Cooper, G. S., Einstadter, S., Cebul, R., & Rimm, A. A. (2001). Effects of alcohol-related disease on hip fracture and mortality: A retrospective cohort study of hospitalized Medicare beneficiaries. *American Journal of Public Health, 91*, 1089–1093.

Societal Violence

CHAPTER OBJECTIVES

After reading this chapter, you should be able to:

1. Compare types of societal violence.
2. Analyze the influence of biophysical, psychological, physical environmental, sociocultural, behavioral, and health system factors on societal violence.
3. Identify major foci in primary prevention of societal violence.
4. Describe approaches to the secondary prevention of societal violence.
5. Discuss considerations in tertiary prevention of societal violence.
6. Analyze the role of community health nurses with respect to societal violence.

KEY TERMS

battering **974**
child maltreatment **973**
critical incident stress **988**
elder maltreatment **975**
emotional abuse **973**
family violence **973**
intimate partner violence (IPV) **974**
neglect **974**
physical abuse **973**
psychological battering **974**
sexual abuse **973**
shaken baby syndrome **978**
violence **973**

MediaLink

http://www.prenhall.com/clark

Additional interactive resources for this chapter can be found on the Companion Website. Click on Chapter 32 and "Begin" to select the activities for this chapter.

Advocacy in Action

A Question of Neglect

Students and faculty working in a weekly "clinic" in a church basement had developed some credibility in the community when they were asked by a Child Protective Services (CPS) social worker to work with a family that had been reported for child neglect. The family was somewhat nontraditional in that the husband was approximately three times as old as the wife. Their marriage had been strongly opposed by the wife's family.

The couple had a 3- or 4-month-old child, and family members had reported them to CPS for child neglect because they were feeding the child raw eggs. The CPS worker did not view this as neglect, but did not have the staff to work with the family. The worker made a referral to the clinic during the summer when no students were available, so follow-up was initiated by a faculty member. During a home visit, the faculty member discovered that the parents knew that eggs were a nutritious food but were unaware of the potential for bacterial contamination in raw eggs and for egg allergies in young children. They thought they were helping the child by putting raw eggs into his formula.

The community health nurse began by educating them about basic child nutrition, but also identified a number of other issues that needed to be addressed. For example, the mother weighed close to three hundred pounds and had remarkably poor hygiene, although the baby was always clean. The house was usually cluttered, with numerous objects on the floor that presented a choking hazard for the child. In addition, the father was disabled and unemployed and smoked heavily.

Over several months of working with the family and capitalizing on their desire to take good care of their child, the community health nurse faculty member was able to assist the mother to lose weight and to improve her own hygiene. The father stopped smoking and was helped to find a vocational training program that permitted him to work despite his disability. The child was thriving and the family was discharged from services.

Approximately a year later, the husband called the faculty member. There had been a fire in the apartment and the door was blocked with the mother and child inside. The mother was able to throw the baby out the second-story window to a bystander, but was still too heavy to fit through the window herself. She had second- and third-degree burns over much of her body and was taken to the local hospital to the intensive care unit. The husband was calling because the hospital wanted to send his wife to a burn unit at the other end of the state. Because she was on Medicaid, no closer unit would take her. After several phone calls, the nurse was able to arrange for transfer to a burn unit closer to the family's home. Unfortunately, the wife's injuries were such that she died, but at least the family was able to spend more time with her before her death than if she had been 500 miles away.

*V*iolence is a pervasive phenomenon in our society. In part, this is a function of the American heritage and the activities required to carve a nation from a wild and uncivilized land. Violence has historically been seen as a mode of resolving conflict and even of ensuring support of law and order. The vigilante approach to justice on the Western frontier is one example of the use of violence to protect society. Excessive attention to "national security" issues may also be used to justify societal violence and is an effect that community health nurses can help to guard against by advocating the protection of civil liberties. The World Health Organization defined **violence** as the "intentional use of physical force or power, threatened or actual, against oneself, another person, or against a group or community, that either results in or has a high likelihood of resulting in injury, death, psychological harm, maldevelopment, or deprivation" (Krug, Dahlberg, Mercy, Zwi, & Lozaro, 2002, p. 3).

In societies in which survival is subjected to physical threats that must be countered by physical force, violent behavior may be more or less of a necessity. Some authorities, however, contend that humankind has failed to adapt to changes in survival needs and has continued to exercise proclivities to violence that are not warranted in today's society. Societal violence has become a global as well as national concern.

Societal violence costs millions of dollars in hospital care alone and results in millions of days of lost work productivity. Add to this the personal costs of victimization as well as the mounting cost of police and other protective services and related court costs, and it becomes apparent that the United States cannot afford the current level of violence and must do something to contain it. Evidence of public concern for problems of societal violence is found in a number of objectives related to violence and injury prevention in the national objectives for 2010 (Centers for Disease Prevention and Control [CDC], 2005a). These objectives may be viewed on the *Healthy People 2010* ◆. Web site at http://wonder.gov/data2010.

Family violence, assault and homicide, and suicide are forms of violence that are of particular concern to society and, hence, to community health nurses who are charged with promoting the health of the population. Violence contributes to a variety of physical and psychological health problems that can be prevented by community health nursing efforts to modify factors that contribute to violence against self or others.

TRENDS IN SOCIETAL VIOLENCE

Societal violence seems to be escalating throughout the world. In part, the increasing frequency with which violence is reported may be a result of greater recognition of violent behaviors. Violent crime in the United States, on the other hand, reached an all-time low in 2004 (Bureau of Justice Statistics [BJS], 2005a). Trends in three forms of societal violence will be addressed here: family violence, assault and homicide, and suicide.

Family Violence

Family violence, also referred to as *domestic violence*, has been defined as "all types of violent crime committed by an offender who is related to the victim either biologically or legally through marriage or adoption" (Durose et al., 2005, p. 4). Overall rates of family violence in the United States declined from 5.4 per 1,000 population in 1993 to 2.1 in 2002. Unfortunately, however, 10% of violent victimization continues to occur within a family context, and family violence accounts for 11% of all violence in the United States. As many as 3.5 million incidents of family violence occur each year, 49% directed at spouses, 11% at children, and 41% against other family members. Most of this violence involves simple assault, with less than 0.5% of cases resulting in homicide (Durose et al., 2005). Most victims of reported family violence are women and most perpetrators are men, although, as we will see later, these figures may be a function of willingness to report violence rather than representing the actual incidence of gender-based family violence.

Family violence encompasses child and elder maltreatment and intimate partner violence (IPV). In many families, these forms of abuse are intertwined, creating an intergenerational pattern of violence in which children who are subjected to or witness violence in the family internalize violence as a mode of family interaction (Abrahams & Jewkes, 2005). These children may then become abusive or enter abusive relationships in adulthood. These abusive relationships may also carry over into care of aging parents, particularly if the parents were abusive themselves.

Child Maltreatment

Child maltreatment or abuse involves intentional physical or mental harm to a child by someone responsible for the child's welfare. Several different types of child abuse occur in the context of family–child interactions. These include physical abuse, emotional abuse, sexual abuse, and physical or emotional neglect (Massey-Stokes & Lanning, 2004). **Physical abuse** involves intentional injury of a child by a caretaker that may result in harm. **Emotional abuse** consists of either intentional verbal or behavioral actions that may have negative emotional consequences for the child. Constant belittling of a child is an example of emotional abuse. **Sexual abuse** is any involvement of a child in an act designed to provide sexual gratification to an adult and includes both sexual acts and sexual exploitation. Both child pornography and sexual intercourse with a child are examples of sexual abuse. According to the Centers for Disease Control and Prevention (CDC, 2004), 1 of every

6 U.S. women and 1 of every 33 men is subjected to sexual violence in childhood or as an adult. In addition, 2 of every 1,000 children were subjected to confirmed sexual abuse in 2003 (National Center for Injury Prevention and Control [NCIPC], 2006d). **Neglect** is failure to provide for a child's physical, educational, or emotional needs. In physical neglect, caretakers fail to provide the child with the material requirements for healthy growth. Physical neglect may include failure to feed or clothe a child appropriately or failure to provide needed medical attention. Finally, emotional or psychological neglect involves failure to provide a child with the love and affection needed for optimal emotional development.

In 2003, more than 1.5 million reports of maltreatment involving more than 787,000 children were made in the United States. Of these, 61% involved neglect, 19% involved physical abuse, 10% involved sexual abuse, 5% involved emotional abuse, and 2.3% involved medical neglect (U.S. Census Bureau, 2006). In 2002, approximately 1,500 deaths occurred among children as a result of abuse (NCIPC, 2006a), with 85% of fatalities occurring in children under age 5 (Massey-Stokes & Lanning, 2004).

Perpetrators of child abuse tend to be family members, typically parents. Other perpetrators include mothers' boyfriends, baby-sitters, and stepfathers. A very small percentage of children are abused by older siblings; however, approximately 10% of family homicides are perpetrated by siblings (Hoffman & Edwards, 2004).

Societal costs for child maltreatment are extensive. For example, direct judicial, law enforcement, and medical costs related to child abuse amount to more than $24 billion each year with another $69 billion in indirect costs (NCIPC, 2006a). In addition, abused children usually have longer hospital stays and charges (averaging $19,266 per child) twice those of children who are not abused. These additional charges are most often paid by Medicaid further increasing the societal burden of child maltreatment (Rovi, Chen, & Johnson, 2004).

Intimate Partner Violence

An estimated 29% of women and 22% of men in one national study had experienced intimate partner violence at some time in their lives, and 20% of nonfatal violence against women and 3% of violence against men occurs within a family context (NCIPC, 2006b). **Intimate partner violence (IPV)** refers to "any behavior within an intimate relationship that causes physical, psychological, or sexual harm to those in the relationship" (Krug et al., 2002, p. 89).

Nearly 5.3 million U.S. women and 3.2 million men experience IPV in a given year, although most incidents involve relatively minor actions such as pushing or slapping (NCIPC, 2006b). Each year, however, 1.5 million U.S. women and more than 835,000 men are raped or physically assaulted by an intimate partner (CDC, 2003a; Hahn et al., 2003a). Approximately 70% of rapes or sexual assaults of women are perpetrated by a family member or intimate partner (BJS, 2005a). Worldwide estimates of IPV range from 10% to 66% of women (Silverman, Mesh, Cuthbert, Slote, & Bancroft, 2004). These figures probably vastly underrepresent the true incidence and prevalence of IPV since only about 20% of sexual assaults, 25% of physical assaults, and 50% of stalkings are reported to authorities (NCIPC, 2006b).

Intimate partners include spouses, ex-spouses, boyfriends or girlfriends, or former boyfriends or girlfriends. Risk of severe violence may actually be higher once a relationship has been terminated than during the relationship (NCIPC, 2006b). Intimate partner violence includes "battering." **Battering** is chronic and continuing violence of one partner against another that is characterized by vulnerability, entrapment, and loss of control of one's life on the part of the abused partner. **Psychological battering** exists when there is no current physical or sexual abuse being perpetrated, but fear of potential abuse keeps the victim subservient (Coker, Smith, McKeown, & King, 2000). Psychological battering differs from psychological abuse in that it centers on the threat of actual physical or sexual abuse to control the behavior of another, whereas emotional abuse involves repeated verbal assaults on the victim's sense of self or self-worth. Battering is believed to occur in a predictable cycle that includes a period of growing tension in the batterer, culminating in a specific incident of battering followed by a period of remorse and forgiveness (Walker, 2000).

Based on 2003 dollars, the estimated annual costs for medical and mental health care and lost productivity due to IPV is $8.3 billion. Severe IPV results in the loss of nearly 8 million days of work productivity for employed women and 5.6 million days of lost household productivity (NCIPC, 2006b).

Intimate partner violence occurs throughout the world in all nations and in all social, economic, religious, and cultural groups. In more than 50 international studies, 10% to 50% of women reported physical abuse or threats of abuse by male partners at some time in their lives. IPV is often referred to as *gender-based violence* because in many cultures it arises in part from women's subordinate social status (Ahmed, van Ginneken, Razzaque, & Alam, 2004). Like child abuse, several different forms of IPV occur, including physical and sexual abuse, threats of physical or sexual violence, stalking, and emotional or psychological abuse. Other measures by which intimate partners exert coercive control include threats to children and control of financial assets.

Although most people think of IPV as occurring in heterosexual relationships, there is evidence to suggest that IPV also occurs in same-sex relationships and that IPV "occurs with the same or greater frequency in gay and lesbian communities" as in the general public (Freedberg, 2006, p. 15). For example, in one study of men who have sex with men (MSM) in four U.S. cities, 34% of respondents reported psychological or "symbolic" battering by their partners in the prior 5 years, 22% reported physical abuse, and 5% reported sexual abuse (Greenwood et al., 2002). As we saw in Chapters 17 and 18∞, other studies have also found IPV among same-sex couples. As many as 50,000 to 100,000 lesbians and 500,000 gay men may be subjected to IPV each year. However, reporting may be inhibited by perceptions of IPV as occurring in "mutual combat" and fear of one's same-sex orientation being "outed" by the sexual partner in retaliation for reporting abuse (Freedberg, 2006).

Intimate partner violence and child abuse tend to co-occur in families. Even when children are not themselves abused, witnessing family violence has profound psychological and social consequences that will be discussed later in this chapter. It is estimated that as many as 10 million children may witness family violence each year (Gomby, 2000).

Intimate partner violence also occurs outside the family constellation. In 2004, the prevalence rate for date rape was 1 per 1,000 population (BJS, 2005b). In the 2005 Youth Risk Behavior Surveillance (YRBS) survey, 9.2% of high school students reported experiencing dating violence and 7.5% were forced to have sexual intercourse (Eaton et al., 2006). In another study of 14-year-old to college-age women, 32% reported experiencing dating violence. Lifetime risk of dating violence is estimated at 15%, with a 9% risk of rape. In one study, women assaulted by dating partners in high school were found to be at higher risk for revictimization in college (Smith, White, & Holland, 2003).

Elder Maltreatment

Elder maltreatment or abuse is purposeful physical or psychological harm or exploitation of elderly persons (Jech, 2002). Elder abuse can occur within families or in institutional settings such as nursing homes and other residential facilities for the elderly. The focus of this chapter, however, is on abuse of older persons by family members.

An estimated 700,000 to 1.2 million older adults are abused each year in the United States (Fulmer, 2002). U.S. reports of elder maltreatment increased by 150% from 1986 to 1996, due in part to better recognition of the problem (Jech, 2002). Elder abuse also occurs throughout the world, even in countries where elders hold a cultural position of respect. In one study in Hong Kong, for example, 27.5% of elderly participants reported at lease one incident of abuse by a caregiver in the previous year. Most of this abuse (27%) was verbal, but physical abuse was reported by 2.5% of the elders, and violation of rights was reported by more than 5%. Similarly, abuse of older family members has been reported in Canada, Great Britain, Greece, and Australia (Yan & Tang, 2004).

Several forms of elder abuse occur, many of them similar to the types of abuse found among children and couples. Types of abuse that may be encountered by community health nurses working with elderly clients include physical and sexual abuse, neglect, emotional abuse, financial or material exploitation, violation of personal rights, and abandonment. Physical abuse of the elderly may include injury, inappropriate restraint, or overmedication. Neglect may involve failure to meet physical or emotional needs, failure to attend to medical needs, or self-neglect by the older person him- or herself. Emotional abuse may consist of verbal abuse or disrespect or social isolation. Older clients may also be financially exploited when their funds or material goods are appropriated by others rather than used to meet their needs. Older clients' personal rights may be violated if they are not allowed to participate in decisions regarding their lives when they are capable of making such decisions. Some older clients may be abandoned or deserted by those responsible for their care (Fulmer, 2002). Additional forms of elder abuse identified by the United Nations Economic and Social Council (2002) include loss of respect, systemic abuse, economic violence, scapegoating, and HIV/AIDS-related violence. In addition, community violence and political violence disproportionately affect the elderly as well as children. These and other forms of domestic violence are summarized in Table 32-1◆.

Perpetrators of elder maltreatment are usually family members or acquaintances (NCIPC, 2003), but older clients may also engage in self-neglect. *Self-neglect* has been defined as "behavior of an elderly person that threatens his or her safety" (Jech, 2002, p. 22), and as many as 100,000 cases may occur each year (Mouton et al., 2004). Institutional abuse of the elderly may also occur and is defined as "abuse and neglect that occurs in residential facilities that care for the elderly" (Jech, 2002, p. 23). Others may also take advantage of older persons to defraud them in financial scams (United Nations Economic and Social Council, 2002).

Older people who are physically or cognitively impaired or who have functional disabilities are at greater risk for abuse than those with better functional abilities. Women constitute 60% of abused elderly persons and 75% of those subjected to psychological abuse. Women are also more likely than older men to experience financial abuse (92% vs. 8%) (Jech, 2002). Consequences of abuse of older people include injury, medication and substance abuse, decreased immune response, malnutrition or eating disorders, depression, fear and anxiety, and suicide (United Nations Economic and Social Council, 2002). As is the case with child maltreatment and IPV, elder maltreatment may end in death. In 2002 and 2003, the U.S. homicide rate for people over age 65 was 2.82 per 100,000 men and 1.38 for women (NCIPC, 2005).

TABLE 32-1 Categories and Types of Family Violence and Their Descriptive Features

Category of Family Violence	Type of Violence	Descriptive Features
Child maltreatment	▪ Physical abuse	▪ Purposeful action that results in physical injury
	▪ Emotional abuse	▪ Chronic and purposeful belittling, demeaning, intimidation, or other actions that may impair a child's mental or emotional health
	▪ Sexual abuse	▪ Involvement of a child in meeting the sexual gratification needs of an adult; may include sexual intercourse, fondling, sexual exploitation (e.g., pornography)
	▪ Neglect	▪ Failure to meet a child's physical, emotional, educational, or health care needs
Intimate partner violence (IPV)	▪ Physical abuse	▪ Purposeful action that results in physical injury
	▪ Psychological abuse	▪ Consistent verbal denigration of one's partner that impairs his or her mental or emotional health
	▪ Sexual abuse	▪ Forced sexual intimacy; nonconsensual sexual activity; forcible rape; forced marriage or childbearing
	▪ Threats of violence	▪ Coercion through threats of injury to the partner, children, pets, or treasured possessions
	▪ Stalking	▪ Persistent forcing of one's attentions on someone who does not want them; may involve following and observation, unwanted telephone calls or visits, or other intrusive behaviors
	▪ Dating violence	▪ Physical, psychological, or sexual abuse in the context of a dating relationship
	▪ Denial of rights	▪ Forced social isolation; control of finances; restriction of activity; failure to permit seeking needed services
	▪ Economic discrimination	▪ Inequitable compensation for similar labor; restriction of property rights or inheritance rights
	▪ State violence	▪ Lack of protection of individual rights; inequitable access to goods and services or other resources to meet basic human needs (e.g., education, employment); inequitable treatment in legislative policies or judicial systems
	▪ Sexual enslavement	▪ Possession of another human being for purposes of sexual gratification
Elder maltreatment	▪ Physical abuse	▪ Actions that result in physical injury; inappropriate restraint or confinement
	▪ Emotional or psychological abuse	▪ Failure to respect an older person's privacy and belongings or to consider his or her wishes; denial of access to significant others; failure to meet social interaction needs; denigration
	▪ Sexual abuse	▪ Nonconsensual sexual contact
	▪ Financial exploitation	▪ Improper use or misappropriation of an older person's property or resources; forced changes to wills or other documents; denial of financial control; financial scams and schemes that defraud the elderly
	▪ Neglect	▪ Failure to provide adequate clothing, food, shelter, health care, and personal hygiene; denying social contact; not providing necessary assistive devices; failing to prevent physical harm or provide needed supervision
	▪ Self-neglect	▪ Failure of the older person to engage in effective self-care; failure to eat or maintain a clean, livable environment
	▪ Medication abuse	▪ Failure to administer medications or overuse of medications (e.g., for sedation)
	▪ Abandonment	▪ Failure of designated caretakers to provide needed care
	▪ Loss of respect	▪ Treatment of the older person in a disrespectful or insulting way
	▪ Systemic abuse	▪ Social and economic marginalization of older people; inequitable allocation of resources; discrimination in service provision; forced retirement
	▪ Economic violence	▪ Economic, social, and political structures that permit control of older person's assets by others
	▪ Scapegoating	▪ Blaming older people (particularly women) for community ills; frequently occurs in the context of witchcraft beliefs
	▪ Community violence	▪ Criminal violence in society and neighborhoods that may victimize older people or make them fearful for their safety
	▪ Political violence	▪ Failure to meet the needs of older clients displaced by civil conflict; marginalization in refugee camps
	▪ HIV/AIDS-related violence	▪ Burdening older people (particularly women) with the care of dying relatives or their orphaned children without adequate support systems; made worse by social stigma attached to HIV/AIDS in some groups

Assault and Homicide

Considerable societal violence also occurs outside of the family unit. Multiple forms of physical assault take place each day in the United States, with the most extreme form of assault resulting in homicide. Homicide rates have declined significantly in recent years, from 10.2 per 100,000 population in 1980 to 6 per 100,000 in 2003 (BJS, 2005b; U.S. Census Bureau, 2006). These figures are somewhat misleading in that part of the decline in homicide-related fatalities lies in better medical care for those who have been assaulted. Some authors believe a more accurate indicator of societal violence is the rate of aggravated assault. An aggravated assault is one in which a weapon is used or in which serious injury is inflicted (U.S. Census Bureau, 2006). In 2003, the U.S. rate for assault was 19.3 per 1,000 persons, indicating a decline in incidence from 37.6 per 1,000 in 1995. Other forms of assault have also declined but remain sources of societal problems. For example, the rate of forcible rape decreased from 36.8 per 100,000 people in 1980 to 32.1 in 2003 after a peak incidence of 41.1 in 1990 (U.S. Census Bureau, 2006). In 2000, 1.6 million people were treated for assault-related injuries in emergency departments, and nearly 64,000 of these assaults were sexual in nature (Division of Violence Prevention, 2002a).

Assault and homicide are also problems at the international level, with an estimated 520,000 homicides worldwide in 2000. Approximately 90% of these homicides occurred in low- to middle-income countries with high levels of poverty and significant income disparities between segments of the population (Mirabal, Rodriguez, Velez, Crosby, & Hoffman, 2006).

Although schools are often perceived as safe places for children, violence occurs in schools on a regular

Multiple forms of physical assault occur each day in the United States, with the most extreme resulting in homicide.

basis. From 1994 to 1996, for example, 126 school-related fatalities occurred as a result of homicide and suicide (Division of Violence Prevention, 2003a), and several events included both homicide and suicide (Division of Violence Prevention, 2003b).

Frequently, societal violence involves the use of weapons, which are readily available among the general public. Evidence of this is seen in the fact that nearly one fifth of California adolescents reported having access to firearms at home (Sorenson & Vittes, 2004). Similarly, 18.5% of high school students in the 2005 Youth Risk Behavior Surveillance (YRBS) survey admitted carrying a weapon in the last 30 days and 6.5% of students carried a weapon to school. In addition, nearly 8% of the students indicated that they had been threatened or injured with a weapon at school. Overall, more than 35% of the students reported being involved in a physical fight in the prior year and 3% reported being injured in a fight (Eaton et al., 2006).

Suicide

Suicide is another serious problem in the United States and worldwide. An estimated 4.5% of Americans attempt suicide at some point in their lives, and suicide is the 3rd leading cause of death for men aged 15 to 24 years (Sugrue, 2004) and the 8th leading cause for all U.S. men (NCIPC, 2006e). Worldwide suicide is the 13th leading cause of all deaths and the 11th leading cause in the United States (CDC, 2003b). Suicide rates are particularly high in Japan (about twice those for the United States) and lower than U.S. rates in countries such as China, Singapore, Italy, and the United Kingdom (Sung, Long, Boore, & Tsao, 2005).

In 2002, more than 132,000 people were hospitalized in the United States as a result of attempted suicide, and another 116,000 were treated in emergency departments and released (NCIPC, 2006e). Although suicide mortality is highest among elderly members of the population, the greatest monetary cost to society in terms of present value of lifetime earnings (PVLE) occurs among middle-aged Americans. In 2002, for example, 67% of the 1 million years of productive life lost (YPLL) occurred in this age group. Overall lost productivity costs related to PVLE amounted to $13 million. This does not reflect the societal costs of hospitalization after a suicide attempt, estimated at $581 million in 1994 (Knox & Caine, 2005).

THE EPIDEMIOLOGY OF SOCIETAL VIOLENCE

Factors in each of the six dimensions of health influence one or more of the forms of societal violence presented in this chapter. Generally speaking, violence results from a combination of predisposing, precipitating, and protective factors in several areas (Pirkis, Goldney, & Burgess, 2003). Predisposing factors are those that increase one's risk of violent victimization or perpetration of violence. Predisposing factors may be categorized as vulnerability factors or risk factors. In the context of violence, vulnerability factors increase one's risk of being a victim of violence; risk factors increase the potential that one will perpetrate violence on others. Precipitating factors are those that give rise to a specific incident of violence. Protective factors, on the other hand, decrease the risk of violence perpetration and victimization. For example, connectedness to school has been found to be a protective factor for youth violence (NCIPC, 2006d). Areas to be addressed in examining factors contributing to societal violence include biophysical, psychological, physical environmental, sociocultural, behavioral, and health care system considerations.

Biophysical Considerations

Biophysical considerations include both factors that contribute to violence and those that arise as a consequence of violence. Both contributing factors and consequences relate to considerations of age and physiologic status as well as gender and ethnicity.

Age and Physiologic Status

Age and physiologic status tend to interact in terms of their influence on family violence. For example, children with disabilities are nearly twice as likely to be abused as those without disabilities (Massey-Stokes & Lanning, 2004). Mental retardation in the child also increases the risk of maltreatment (NCIPC, 2006a). When physical difficulties in the child are combined with immaturity on the part of the parent (e.g., adolescent parents) the potential for abuse is even greater. Older clients made vulnerable by poor health and other forms of dependence are also at greater risk of abuse than those who are more independent and in better health. For example, dependence on caregivers and age were the most significant predictors of abuse in a study of elderly Chinese in Hong Kong, and similar influences are noted in the United States. According to the study, abuse was more likely to occur among elderly who lived with the perpetrators (Yan & Tang, 2004).

Younger children are more likely than older ones to experience serious injury or death as a result of maltreatment. For example, 38% of juvenile homicide victims are under age 5. Approximately 1,200 to 1,600 infants experience shaken baby syndrome each year, and death occurs in 25% to 30% of victims. **Shaken baby syndrome** is a constellation of signs and symptoms that result from violent shaking in an infant or child. Other effects include visual, motor, and cognitive impairment (NCIPC, 2006a).

Homicide victimization in children under 15 years of age is five times higher in the United States than in 25 other developed nations (Hahn et al., 2003b), and homicide is the 4th leading cause of death in children aged 5 to 14 years and the 2nd leading cause of death in

those 15 to 19 years of age (American Academy of Pediatrics, 2004). Homicide is also the 15th leading cause of death in infants, with the greatest risk of death occurring on the day of birth and 9% of deaths occurring in the first week of life (Division of Violence Prevention, 2002c). In 2003, more than 5,500 homicides occurred in people 10 to 24 years of age in the United States (NCIPC, 2006f). Overall, homicide causes 15% of deaths in the 10- to 24-year-old age group (Grunbaum et al., 2004), with higher rates of occurrence among African American, Hispanic, American Indian/Alaska Native and Asian/Pacific Islander youth than among White youth (NCIPC, 2006f).

Experience of abuse as a child has also been shown to lead to later risky sexual behavior and early pregnancy (Hahn et al., 2003a; Maman et al., 2002). Sexual abuse of women and adolescent girls may also result in pregnancy, with more than 32,000 pregnancies resulting from rape each year (NCIPC, 2006d).

Pregnancy itself may be a biophysical risk factor for abuse of women, although there is some difference of opinion regarding whether or not pregnancy increases a woman's risk of abuse. An estimated 4% to 8% of women are abused during pregnancy. Some research has indicated that violence against women usually begins before pregnancy and continues into the pregnancy rather than being initiated during pregnancy. Some studies have indicated an increase in emotional abuse of women during pregnancy, but a decrease in physical or sexual abuse (Castro, Peek-Asa, & Ruiz, 2003). Statewide surveys of new mothers have indicated that 5.3% experienced violence while pregnant and 7.2% in the year prior to pregnancy. In another study, more than 10% of pregnant women reported abuse, 8.9% during pregnancy and 4.9% in the 6 months after pregnancy. Nearly two thirds of the women were only abused during the pregnancy, 22% were abused repeatedly, and 17% were only abused after delivery (Koenig, Whitaker et al., 2006).

If pregnancy does indeed increase the risk of abuse, one suggested explanation lies in *evolutionary theory*. According to evolutionary theory, people innately attempt to successfully reproduce their own particular gene pattern. Women, because of their role in gestation and delivery, are sure that a given child is theirs. Men do not have that physiologic certainty, and men who raise someone else's child are not perpetuating their genetic pattern. According to evolutionary theory, men who are uncertain of paternity may be less invested in maintaining the health of either the pregnant woman or the child, increasing the possibility of IPV during pregnancy and later abuse of both mother and child. Proponents of this theory advance as evidence the relative response of men and women to marital infidelity, with men being twice as likely as women to perceive adultery as a reason for divorce (Burch & Gallop, 2004). Although evolutionary theory may explain some aspects of IPV during pregnancy, more research is needed to address this issue completely.

Sexual abuse also increases the risk of sexually transmitted diseases (STDs). Conversely, HIV infection may increase one's risk for abuse. For example, HIV-positive women in one study were 10 times more likely to report violence than those who were HIV negative (Maman et al., 2002).

Age differences are also noted with respect to suicide. Suicide rates are highest among the elderly and increase with age. For example, in 2002, the suicide rate for men 85 years of age and older was 51.1 per 100,000 population, more than twice that for men aged 65 to 69. Among women, peak suicide rates occurred in the 45-to-49 age group (8.02 per 100,000 women) (Knox & Caine, 2005). In 2002 and 2003, the suicide rate for people over 65 years of age was 27.23 per 100,000 population for men and 4.43 per 100,000 for women (NCIPC, 2005).

Suicide also occurs at lower, but still alarming, rates among adolescents and young adults, particularly men. For example, suicide is the 3rd leading cause of death among adolescents worldwide (Hindin & Gultiano, 2006), and from 1950 to 2004, the U.S. suicide rate among 10- to 24-year-olds tripled (Aseltine & DeMartino, 2004). In the 2005 YRBS, nearly 30% of high school students reported being sad or hopeless enough to stop their usual activities, 13.8% had considered suicide, 11.7% had developed a suicide plan, and 8.4% actually attempted suicide, with 2.3% of students requiring medical treatment for a suicide attempt (Eaton et al., 2006). Approximately half of all poisoning incidents among adolescents are due to suicide attempts (NCIPC, 2006c).

Age differences also occur in the method of suicide. For example, among elderly suicide victims in New York City, falling from a height, usually from one's own high-rise apartment building, was the preferred method of suicide. Among those 15 to 34 years of age, on the other hand, firearms were the most frequently used method of suicide (Abrams, Marzuk, Tardiff, & Leon, 2005). At the national level, 62% of youth used firearms to commit suicide, compared to 59% of adults, and Black and White youth were more likely to use firearms in suicide attempts than American Indian or Asian youth (Snyder & Swahn, 2004).

In addition to being victims of violence, youth also perpetrate societal violence. In 2002, for example, more than 2.2 million juveniles were arrested, more than 92,000 of them for violent offenses. This represents a significant drop in juvenile arrests for violent crime, and 2002 figures (the most recent data available) were the lowest since 1980. Even so, juveniles accounted for 12% of all violent crime in the United States, including 5% of murders, 12% of rapes, and 12% of aggravated assaults (Snyder, 2004). Firearms were even more likely to be used by youth for homicide than suicide (73% vs. 62%) (Snyder & Swahn, 2004).

Violence results in a variety of physiological effects for people of all age groups. For example, violence against women leads to twice as many health care visits and an 800% increase in mental health visits as well as increased risk of hospitalization compared to women who are not abused (Murdaugh, Hunt, Sowell, & Santana, 2004). Approximately 42% of physically abused women and 20% of men require medical care for injuries received. In addition, victims of IPV may experience chronic headaches, back pain, pelvic pain, sexually transmitted diseases, gastrointestinal disorders, and heart conditions. IPV directed at women may also result in injuries to children. For example, children of abused mothers have been found to be 57 times more likely to suffer maltreatment than children whose mothers were not abused (NCIPC, 2006b).

Child maltreatment results in a variety of physical health effects beyond immediate injury. For example, abused children are more likely to experience gastrointestinal problems, functional disabilities, and hospitalization than those who are not abused (Thompson, Kingree, & Desai, 2004). Abused children have also been found to be at higher risk for obesity than children who are not abused (NCIPC, 2006a). Childhood physical abuse has also been linked to increased incidence of gastrointestinal problems and migraine headaches in adults (Goodwin, Hoven, Murison, & Hotopf, 2003).

Victimization, in general, may increase the likelihood of certain physical health problems. For example, one study of high school students indicated that any experience of victimization or missing school because of fears for personal safety was associated with increased risk for asthma episodes (Swahn & Bossarte, 2006). Physical signs and symptoms, another aspect of the biophysical dimension, may also indicate the presence of current abuse. Physical and other indicators of child maltreatment are presented in Table 32-2◆. Indicators of intimate partner violence and elder maltreatment are presented in Tables 32-3 and Table 32-4◆.

Gender and Ethnicity

Generally speaking, child maltreatment occurs at similar levels for boys and girls, although young girls are four times more likely to be sexually abused than boys (Stokes-Massey & Lanning, 2004). For example, high school girls are nearly twice as likely as boys to report sexual assault (NCIPC, 2006d). Boys, however, are more likely than girls to die as a result of abuse, accounting for 64% of abuse-related fatalities (Snyder, 2004).

Among adults, women are more likely to experience victimization at the hands of a friend, acquaintance, or intimate partner, while men are more likely to be victimized by strangers (BJS, 2005a). Women experience more domestic violence and men are more often subjected to street violence which occurs in public places (Steen & Hunskaar, 2004). An estimated 85% of reported IPV is directed against women (Stinson & Robinson, 2006), and American Indian/Alaska Native women and men, African American women, and Hispanic women are at particular risk for IPV. Younger women, particularly poor

TABLE 32-2 Physical and Psychological Indications of Child Maltreatment

Type of Abuse	Physical Indications	Psychological Indications
Neglect	Persistent hunger Poor hygiene Inappropriate dress for the weather Constant fatigue Unattended physical health problems Poor growth patterns	Delinquency due to lack of supervision School truancy/poor school performance Begging or stealing food Behavior problems
Physical abuse	Bruises or welts in unusual places or in several stages of healing; distinctive shapes Burns (especially cigarette burns; immersion burns of hands, feet, or buttocks; rope burns; or distinctively shaped burns) Fractures (multiple or in various stages of healing, inconsistent with explanations of injury) Joint swelling or limited mobility Long-bone deformities Lacerations and abrasions to the mouth, lip, gums, eye, genitalia Human bite marks Signs of intracranial trauma Deformed or displaced nasal septum Bleeding or fluid drainage from the ears or ruptured eardrums Broken, loose, or missing teeth Difficulty in respirations, tenderness or crepitus over ribs Abdominal pain or tenderness Recurrent urinary tract infection	Wary of physical contact with adults Behavioral extremes of withdrawal or aggression Apprehensive when other children cry Inappropriate response to pain
Emotional abuse	Nothing specific	Overly compliant, passive, and undemanding Extremely aggressive, demanding, or angry Behavior inappropriate for age (either overly adult or overly infantile) Developmental delay Attempted suicide
Sexual abuse	Torn, stained, or bloody underwear Pain or itching in genital areas Bruises or bleeding from external genitalia, vagina, rectum Sexually transmitted disease Swollen or red cervix, vulva, or perineum Semen around the mouth or genitalia or on clothing Pregnancy	Withdrawn Engages in fantasy behavior or infantile behavior Poor peer relationships Unwilling to participate in physical activities Wears long sleeves and several layers of clothing even in hot weather Delinquency or running away Inappropriate sexual behavior or mannerisms

young women, are more likely to be victims of IPV than those who are older (NCIPC, 2006b). In 2003, the rate for IPV victimization among women was more than six times that for men (U.S. Census Bureau, 2006). Sexual assault, in particular, tends to be directed against younger women, with half of all rape victims under 18 years of age and 22% under 12 (NCIPC, 2006d). Sexual assault accounts for 8% of assaults on women and 1% of assaults on men, with a rate of reported sexual assault for women five times that for men (Division of Violence Prevention, 2002a).

Both men and women engage in violence within and outside of intimate relationships. Most perpetrators of sexual violence are men, even for male sexual victimization (NCIPC, 2006d). Women most often victimize other women, but much of female-to-female victimization has been found to occur in the context of mutual violence in fights over personal respect, gossip, and men (Hirschinger et al., 2003). In one study of assault victims seen in an emergency department, 74% of cases involved men assaulting other men, 21% involved

TABLE 32-3 Physical and Psychological Indications of Intimate Partner Violence

Physical Indications	Psychological Indications
Chronic fatigue Vague complaints, aches, and pains Frequent injuries Recurrent sexually transmitted diseases Muscle tension Facial lacerations Injuries to chest, breasts, back, abdomen, or genitalia Bilateral injuries of arms or legs Symmetric injuries Obvious patterns of belt buckles, bite marks, fist or hand marks Burns of hands, feet, buttocks, or with distinctive patterns Headaches Ulcers	Casual response to a serious injury or excessively emotional response to a relatively minor injury Frequent ambulatory or emergency room visits Nightmares Depression Anxiety Anorexia or other eating disorder Drug or alcohol abuse Poor self-esteem Suicide attempts

TABLE 32-4	Physical and Psychological Indications of Elder Maltreatment	
Type of Abuse	**Physical Indications**	**Psychological Indications**
Neglect	Constant hunger or malnutrition Poor hygiene Inappropriate dress for the weather Chronic fatigue Unattended medical needs Poor skin integrity or decubiti Contractures Urine burns/excoriation Dehydration Fecal impaction	Listlessness Social isolation
Emotional abuse	Hypochondria	Habit disorder (biting, sucking, rocking) Destructive or antisocial conduct Neurotic traits (sleep or speech disorder, inhibition of play) Hysteria Obsessions or compulsions Phobias
Physical abuse	Bruises and welts Burns Fractures Sprains or dislocations Lacerations or abrasions Evidence of oversedation	Withdrawal Confusion Fear of caretaker or other family members Listlessness
Sexual abuse	Difficulty walking Torn, stained, or bloody underwear Pain or itching in genital area Bruises or bleeding on external genitalia or in vaginal or anal areas Sexually transmitted diseases	Withdrawal
Financial abuse	Inappropriate clothing Unmet medical needs	Failure to meet financial obligations Anxiety over expenses
Denial of rights	Nothing specific	Hesitancy in making decisions Listlessness and apathy

women attacked by men, 4% involved women assaulting other women, and 2% involved men attacked by women (Steen & Hunskaar, 2004). Another study examined the gender of plaintiffs and defendants in requests for Abuse Prevention Orders, a civil court order to prevent domestic abuse. In this study, men and women were found to be equally abusive in terms of physical or psychological aggression. Male defendants were more likely than female defendants to have engaged in sexual assault. Both men and women were equally likely to threaten to kill or harm their partner. Most requests for orders were made by women (81%), but the author contended that this may be the result of perceptions of stigma attached to men who are abused by women. In addition, petitions by male victims were more likely to be denied than those made by female victims, and male victims were sometimes discouraged from filing a petition for an abuse prevention order. Court systems and community services tend to favor women, with few resources available to male victims of IPV. The author suggested that societal policies related to violence that are based on research that ignores IPV perpetrated by women may place male victims at a distinct disadvantage (Basile, 2004). Similar findings were noted by Busch and

Rosenberg (2004), who found that men and women were equally likely to subject their partners to serious violence and to inflict serious injuries, although women perpetrators were more likely than men to report mutual violence at the time of their arrest.

Suicide also displays gender differences. Approximately 85% of suicides in people over 65 years of age involve men (NCIPC, 2006e). Overall, completed suicide is four times more likely in men than in women, although women are more likely to engage in a suicide attempt (Monts, 2002). In 2000, for example, the rate of self-inflicted injury (60% of which was probable suicide attempts) was 107.7 per 100,000 population among

Think Advocacy

Several of the references cited in this chapter suggest that little attention has been given to intimate partner violence directed against men. Social stigma, legal system biases, and lack of support services are some of the factors that have been identified as mitigating against equitable treatment of male victims of IPV. How might you go about changing societal awareness of and attitudes toward IPV directed against men?

women and 83.6 for men (Division of Violence Prevention, 2002b). Male-female differences in rates of completed suicide lie primarily in the lethality of methods most often chosen by men.

Racial and ethnic disparities are also noted in the incidence of particular forms of societal violence. For example, suicide is the eighth leading cause of death for all U.S. men and for White, Asian/Pacific Islander, and Latino men, but sixth for American Indian/Alaska Native men. Similarly, homicide is the sixth leading cause of death among all African Americans, but fifth among African American men and sixth among American Indian/Alaska Native and Hispanic men. Among women, neither homicide nor suicide ranks in the top 10 causes of death for any racial or ethnic group (National Center for Health Statistics [NCHS], 2005). IPV directed at women is particularly prevalent among Latinas (nearly 55% of this group of women) (Murdaugh et al., 2004) and Asian immigrant women (Raj & Silverman, 2003). Among youth, White juveniles aged 7 to 17 years are 1.5 times more likely to commit suicide than to be murdered, but Black youth are 7 times more likely to be murdered than to commit suicide (Snyder & Swahn, 2004).

Although racial and ethnic variations in violence occur, studies have found that disparities are explained by a variety of socioeconomic factors, including marital and immigration status and neighborhood social context. These findings suggest that general interventions to improve social and economic factors affecting populations will help to reduce racial and ethnic disparities in the incidence and prevalence of violence (Sampson, Morenoff, & Raudenbush, 2005). For immigrant populations, the stresses arising from acculturation and language and economic barriers may contribute to abuse and could also be resolved by improvement in social conditions (Murdaugh et al., 2004). Community health nurses can be actively involved in advocacy to improve living conditions for both immigrant and nonimmigrant populations. Focused assessment questions related to biophysical considerations in societal violence are provided below.

FOCUSED ASSESSMENT

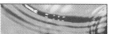

Biophysical Considerations in Societal Violence

- Are there physical considerations that place clients at risk for family violence or suicide (e.g., disability, pregnancy)? What is the extent of these conditions in the population?
- Is there physical evidence of abuse?
- What influence does age have on the incidence and prevalence of violence in the population? What is the age distribution among victims of specific types of violence? What is the age distribution among perpetrators of violence?
- Are there gender differences in victimization or perpetration of specific forms of violence in the population?
- What is the racial/ethnic distribution of violence victimization and perpetration in the population?

Psychological Considerations

As was the case with biophysical considerations, psychological factors serve as both contributors to and consequences of violence. For example, caregiver resentment, fatigue, family conflict, and personality traits have been found to contribute to elder abuse. Similarly, grief at the loss of a loved one may also contribute to abuse (Farella, 2000). The presence of psychiatric disorders also increases the potential for all forms of violence. For example, people with bipolar disorder have been found to have rates of completed suicide of 10% to 15% (Goldberg & Hoop, 2004). Similarly, persons with unipolar depression or schizophrenia have higher rates of suicide than the general population (National Institute of Mental Health, 2005a, 2005b).

Psychological factors that may contribute to family violence include poor coping skills, the emotional climate in the family, personality traits of the abuser or the victim, and the presence of psychopathology. The abuser's level of emotional intelligence has also been suggested as a factor influencing domestic violence. Emotional intelligence is defined as "an array of non-cognitive capabilities, competencies, and skills that influence one's ability to succeed in coping with environmental demands and pressures" (Bar-On, as quoted in Winters, Clift, & Dutton, 2004, p. 256). In one study, for example, perpetrators of IPV were found to score significantly lower on several components of emotional intelligence than the general population. Specifically, abusers had difficulties with emotional self-awareness, self-regard, assertiveness, independence, problem solving, flexibility, and impulsivity (Winters et al., 2004). Community health nurses can assist individual clients and families as well as population groups in the development of adequate coping skills. They can also advocate for including coping education in school curricula and in other settings (e.g., stress management education in the workplace).

Families with poor coping skills have difficulty dealing with situational stressors that create tension, resulting in violence. Constant family crises or upheavals indicative of poor coping abilities are frequently characteristic of abusive families. Types of coping used by victims of abuse may also influence the frequency and severity of violence. For example, some research has found that women who engage in avoidance coping mechanisms are subjected to more violence than women who use more active coping strategies. In addition, women subjected to severe abuse may encounter avoidance behaviors on the part of family and friends, further diminishing their sources of support (Waldrop & Resick, 2004).

The emotional climate in the family can also contribute to abuse. Families that exhibit increased emotional tension and anxiety, with little display of visible affection or emotional support, are considered emotionally impoverished and are at risk for violence. Similarly, family communication patterns that are nonnurturing, destructive, or ambiguous may also indicate risk for family violence. Couples that experience intimate partner violence have been found to have poorer communication skills and less satisfying relationships than other couples and often engage in mutual exchange of negative communication (McClellan & Killeen, 2000). These couples may also be characterized by poor conflict negotiation skills, poor problem-solving skills, and defensiveness on the part of both members (Lloyd, 2000; Tilley & Brackley, 2005). Community health nurses can assist families in the development of effective communication patterns and problem-solving abilities.

The distribution of power within the family is another element of the emotional climate that may lead to abuse. Abusive families are often characterized by autocratic decision making and power struggles between members. Abusers tend to abuse the power they have over other family members when they feel their power is threatened.

Personality traits of either the abuser or the victim can influence the incidence of family violence. Abusers and victims alike tend to have poor self-esteem. Abusers may also be emotionally immature, hostile, and unable to cope with problems in a healthy manner. They frequently feel personally insecure and inadequate, although they often appear successful to others.

Child abusers may exhibit unrealistic expectations of children, particularly as sources of warmth and love. When they are disappointed in these expectations, abuse may occur. For example, children who are irritable, who cry often, or who do not care to be cuddled may be perceived as rejecting the parent. For parents with low self-esteem, this perceived rejection can set the stage for abuse. Community health nurses can assist parents to develop age-appropriate expectations of their children and to recognize and foster normal child development.

Abused women may be dependent, passive, and reluctant to make changes. Some authors attribute these characteristics to feelings of learned helplessness in which the woman can no longer predict with any accuracy that any action she may take will have the desired effect, leading to loss of motivation for any action (Walker, 2000). Grief and guilt are other feelings frequently exhibited by victims of intimate partner violence. Community health nurses can assist clients who are victims of abuse to overcome feelings of hopelessness and guilt. They can also advocate for changes in societal perceptions of and attitudes toward victims of abuse to prevent feelings of guilt and diminished self-worth.

Youth violence is also believed to have strong associations with psychological problems. For example, it is estimated that 31% of initial involvement with the juvenile justice system and 28% of repeat involvement could be prevented with effective mental health services for youth in need (Foster, Qaseem, & Connor, 2004). Similarly, mental illness and substance abuse disorders have been identified as major risk factors for suicide (Institute of Medicine, 2006). Community health nurses can help to minimize crime and violence among youth by advocating for effective treatment for mental illness.

Mental illness may also be a risk factor for other forms of violence victimization. In one New Zealand study, for example, young people with anxiety disorders were more likely than those without mental disorders to experience sexual assault, and those with schizophrenia were at greater risk for physical assault. People with substance abuse disorders were also more likely than those with no mental health problems to be subjected to threatened or actual physical assault (Silver, Arsenault, Langley, Caspi, & Moffitt, 2005).

Psychological consequences of abuse are many and varied and may arise both from the experience of being abused and witnessing abuse. For example, childhood sexual abuse has been linked to depression, suicide, sleep disturbances, panic disorder, and attention deficit hyperactivity disorder (ADHD) (NCIPC, 2006a). Victims of sexual and other forms of abuse may also experience post-traumatic stress disorder (PTSD) as well as decreased ability to interact with others, depression, anxiety, low self-esteem, antisocial behavior, inability to trust men, and fear of intimacy (NCIPC, 2006b). Abused women have been found to be 3.6 times more likely to be hospitalized for psychiatric diagnoses and nearly five times more likely to attempt suicide than nonabused women (Kernic, Wolf, & Holt, 2000).

Psychological consequences of IPV for women appear to be mediated by perceptions of their ability to control violence, but the direction of effects is somewhat unusual. For example, in one study women who believed they should be able to control current violence were at greater risk for depression and low self-esteem than those who did not perceive themselves as able to control the abuse. Expectations of abilities to control future abuse, however, were linked to decreased risk for dysphoria and hopelessness and increased self-esteem (Clements, Sabourin, & Spiby, 2004). Community health nurses may help abused clients to see that abuse is not their fault but that they can control future abuse by taking steps to remove themselves from an abusive situation.

Consequences of witnessing abuse among children include emotional and behavioral problems, anxiety, poor school performance, low self-esteem, disobedience, nightmares, physical complaints, and aggression. Depression is a particularly common effect of witnessing parental domestic violence, especially among adolescents (Hindin & Gultiano, 2006). In some groups, boys who witnessed IPV against their mothers were more likely than other men to exhibit violence against their own partners as adults. Witnessing IPV against their mothers was also associated with other forms of

FOCUSED ASSESSMENT

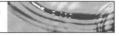

Psychological Considerations in Societal Violence

- What is the level of stress experienced by potential abusers or suicide victims? To what extent are stressors present in the population (e.g., unemployment) that might influence family violence or suicide? What coping strategies are employed by members of the population? By family members? How effective is coping by members of the population or family?
- Is there evidence of psychiatric disorder in the family? Depression? What is the extent of psychiatric illness in the population and what effect does it have on the incidence of societal violence?
- Do potential victims or perpetrators of violence exhibit poor self-esteem? Poor impulse control?
- Is there a negative emotional climate in the family that might contribute to violence? In the population (e.g., general hostility or feelings of frustration with life circumstances)?

public violence such as weapons violations and involvement in physical fighting (Abrahams & Jewkes, 2005). The focused assessment above includes questions that the community health nurse can use to examine psychological considerations influencing violence in a specific population group or family.

Physical Environmental Considerations

A few physical environmental factors influence the incidence and prevalence of societal violence. For example, IPV is believed to be more common in rural than urban areas because of the relative isolation of families and lack of available services. It has also been proposed that some abusers purposely choose rural locations because of their greater isolation from others (Murty et al., 2003). Urban settings, however, have higher rates of firearms homicides than rural areas, perhaps due to greater ease of access to firearms (Branas, Nance, Elliott, Richmond, & Schwab, 2004). Similarly, workplaces and other settings with limited visibility increase the potential for violent victimization. Urbanization, in general, has been found to be protective against suicide in Japanese men, but not in women (Otsu, Araki, Sakai, Yokoyama, & Voorhees, 2004). On the other hand, strong associations between homicide and urbanization and socioeconomic conditions have also been found (Cubbin, Pickle, & Fingerhut, 2000). One additional physical environmental factor that has been associated with increased societal violence is increased levels of lead in ambient air (Stretesky & Lynch, 2001), although further research is needed to confirm this association.

Sociocultural Considerations

Sociocultural factors play a considerable part in the occurrence of societal violence. Social disorganization theories of homicide, for example, suggest that the inability of communities to realize the common values

of their members and maintain social controls on behavior contribute to homicide. In other theoretical perspectives, homicide is an instrumental act designed to obtain money or property denied one because of economic hardship or lack of opportunity. A third perspective posits that homicide arises out of a subculture of violence in which violence is perceived as a legitimate means of conflict resolution (Cubbin et al., 2000).

Cultural themes also influence intimate partner violence. In many cultural groups, men are believed to have a right to control women. Norms granting financial and physical control of women lend themselves to multiple forms of abuse. Personal belief in strict gender roles is a risk factor for perpetration of IPV. For example, intimate partner violence in China has been found to be strongly associated with male patriarchal values. Even though Chinese culture has little value for the concept of privacy, IPV is considered a private family affair, and as many as 43% of Chinese women in one study reported IPV victimization at some time in their lives (Xu et al., 2005). Similarly, immigrant South Asian women have been found to be at higher risk than other women for IPV, perhaps in part due to the stresses of immigration and consequent social isolation (Raj & Silverman, 2003). Immigrant women may also be less likely to report IPV because of language barriers or fear of deportation (Dienemann, Glass, & Hyman, 2005). The risk for IPV may be particularly high when couples have differing cultural conceptions of the role of women in society. Cultural accommodations may need to be made by both parties, and this may be difficult if they do not recognize the influence of culture in their expectations (Locsin & Purnell, 2002).

Cultural attitudes that foster abuse of women are not confined to ethnic minority populations. For example, two studies of incarcerated men guilty of IPV found cultural themes consistent with prior literature. Both studies found that men provided cultural justifications for their abusive actions. Major justifications included perceptions that men have a right to control and discipline women and that violence is excused when women provoke it by failing to respect men's position of authority (Tilley & Brackley, 2005; Wood, 2004). Beliefs in men's responsibility to discipline their partners have also been found in a variety of other cultures (Gundersen, 2002). A second approach taken by the incarcerated men was to minimize their behavior and dissociate themselves from "real abusers," noting that they limited their abuse and did not do as much damage as they could have or that they did not enjoy the abuse as a real abuser would (Wood, 2004). An additional cultural theme—men perceiving themselves as protectors of women—provided some protection from extreme abuse. Unfortunately, abusive men who held this perspective justified their abuse by pointing out that it was never physical because a "real man doesn't hit women." The study author noted, however, that both themes are based on an underlying belief that men are dominant and superior to women (Wood, 2004). Also consistent with the concept of male control over women, U.S. women with higher educational levels than their partners have been found in some studies to be at greater risk for IPV than those with equal or lower education levels because they challenge male superiority (NCIPC, 2006b). It has been suggested that changing these cultural attitudes should be a major focus in the primary prevention of IPV and that interventions should be undertaken particularly with school-age children to change their perceptions of gender-appropriate roles and behaviors (Gundersen, 2002). Community health nurses can be instrumental in advocating and planning curricula that address appropriate gender socialization in school settings and other venues for youth.

Culture-based violence goes beyond the intimate partner context to encompass political and cultural practices that discriminate against and disadvantage women. According to the United Nations (1993), violence against women is defined as "any act of gender-based violence that results in, or is likely to result in, physical, sexual, or mental harm or suffering to women, including threats of such acts, coercion or arbitrary deprivation of liberty, whether occurring in public or private"(p. 1). Elements of culturally sanctioned violence against women include physical abuse (including female genital cutting, which was discussed in Chapter 16∞), mental abuse (including forced marriage or prostitution), economic discrimination, violation of human and reproductive rights, and "state violence," which may involve inhumane treatment of women in prisons or legal systems, failure to enact legal protection for women, or stereotyping them as evil and the cause of humanity's woes (El-Mouelhy, 2004). Other examples of cultural violence against women include traditions of *widow inheritance*, in which a woman may become the sexual partner or wife of her husband's brother at the husband's death, widowhood rites that punish widows as a sign of mourning, and sexual enslavement of young girls to religious leaders or others (Amoakohene, 2004). Culture-based violence against women has an ideologic base in patriarchal social structures in which women are considered inferior and subordinate to men (Ahmed et al., 2004). Violence in this cultural context has been described as "mundane" because of its pervasive and commonplace occurrence and acceptance as a normal fact of life in some population groups (Amoakohene, 2004).

Cultural factors may also influence other forms of societal violence or response to violence. For example, for adolescent boys in Hong Kong, self-direction was associated with diminished risk of suicide. For girls, however, adherence to traditional values of obedience and respect for elders was more protective against suicide (Lam et al., 2004). Willingness to report violence is also affected by culture-based perceptions of stigma. For example, stigma is one of the major barriers to seeking

CULTURAL COMPETENCE

Women in many cultural groups adhere to cultural norms that permit men to control their lives even when this control may be harmful to themselves and to their children. Among many Chinese women, for example, family rules and values may promote intimate partner violence. Chinese women are expected to display "three obediences" to men: first to their fathers, then to their husbands, and later to their sons. Some authors report that because of traditional Asian cultural beliefs, many women do not perceive themselves as victims of violence. Even when they do see themselves as being victimized, they may be reluctant to report abuse because of feelings of shame, embarrassment, or loss of face. Others may also feel guilt, believing themselves to be at fault for the abuse (Magnussen et al., 2004).

Women's rights have not always been supported in the dominant U.S. culture either. In 1877, for example, all states had passed legislation that prohibited women from voting, and the 14th amendment to the Constitution specifically defined "citizens" and "voters" as male. It was not until 1920 that the 19th amendment granted women the right to vote, but the amendment was not actually ratified by Mississippi until 1984. In 1839, Mississippi became the first state to allow women to own property in their own name (with their husband's permission), and in 1855, the Missouri court ruled that a Black woman was considered property and did not have the right to defend herself from rape by her master. Similarly, in 1873, the U.S. Supreme Court ruled that states could prohibit married women from practicing law (National Women's History Project, n.d.), and the Equal Pay Act was not passed until 1963 (Imbornoni, 2006). Based on the history of cultural attitudes to and legal and social restrictions on women, of which these are only a few examples, it is not surprising that many women may have internalized these perceptions.

What would you do if you were working with a woman who was being abused but refused to take action because of her cultural beliefs and values? Should you attempt to change her perspectives or those of the cultural group? Why or why not? If so, how would you go about trying to change cultural values that support violence against women?

---

help for depression in Asian populations, leading to high rates of suicide in countries like Japan (Liang, 2004).

Women's risk of IPV is increased by financial dependence on their partners, partners' relationships with other women, inability to negotiate condom use, lower levels of education and household income, and cohabitation or short-term relationships with multiple partners (Maman et al., 2002). Childlessness is also a risk for IPV against women in societies where childbearing is considered women's primary function (Koenig, Stephenson, Ahmed, Jejeebhoy, & Campbell, 2006). Cohabitation has also been associated with greater risk for child maltreatment and fatality (Giorgianni, 2003).

A World Health Organization study (WHO, 2005) found that many women surveyed accepted IPV as a reasonable response by the partner in specific circumstances. Female infidelity was the justification most often given for IPV, but not completing housework, refusing to have sexual intercourse, and disobeying the husband were also advanced as acceptable reasons for abuse. In some countries, 10% to 20% of women believed women were never justified in refusing to have sex, whatever the circumstances.

Family relationships and dynamics may increase the risk for child maltreatment or serve as protective factors. Family risk factors include social isolation, parental lack of understanding of child development, family disorganization, and lack of family cohesion. Negative parent–child interactions and parental stress levels may also contribute to family violence. Protective factors within families include supportive family relationships, nurturing parenting skills, stable family relationships, household rules, and adequate role models outside the family. Employment and adequate housing also influence interpersonal family violence (NCIPC, 2006a). Community health nurses can work with families to enhance protective factors against violence and to modify those that contribute to violence. For example, the nurse may teach parenting skills or assist with finding employment.

Other sociocultural factors have been shown to influence violence as well. For example, IPV is five times more common in households with annual incomes under $15,000 than in those with incomes over $50,000

GLOBAL PERSPECTIVES

Societal violence is of growing concern throughout the world. Each day, violence claims the lives of more than 4,500 people. Approximately half of these deaths result from suicide and one third from homicide; another 20% of violent deaths are caused by war. Estimated global homicide rates are 8.8 per 100,000, with considerably higher rates in the WHO African and Americas regions. Global suicide rates are approximately 50% higher than U.S. rates, with the highest rates occurring in the European and Western Pacific regions (Mercy, Krug, Dahlberg, & Zwi, 2003).

Worldwide, 10% to 69% of women in 48 countries report physical abuse by an intimate partner, compared to about 22% in the United States. The extent of sexual assault of women ranges from roughly 6% in Yokohama, Japan, to 47% in Cuzco, Peru, and forced first sexual intercourse is reported by 7% of women in New Zealand to 48% in the Caribbean. Physical abuse may affect as many as half of the children in some countries, and 20% of women and 5% to 10% of men worldwide report being victims of sexual abuse as children (Mercy et al., 2003). Similar variations were noted for violence among women in selected countries in a study conducted by the World Health Organization (WHO, 2005).

Some of the justification given for societal violence in its many forms include cultural traditions and social practices that promote violence. For this reason, preventive measures must take into account cultural norms. For example, public shaming of abusive men by other members of society has been found to be an effective deterrent to continued IPV in cultures in which the opinions and views of others are valued and respected (Gundersen, 2002; Mercy et al., 2003). Similarly, attention to income inequality and social justice may help to reduce the potential for violence (Mercy et al., 2003).

(Division of Violence Prevention, 2000a). Victims of IPV may also stay in abusive relationships because of limited resource availability and social isolation. Lack of social resources, both tangible social support and emotional support provided by friends and family, has also been linked to child abuse (NCIPC, 2006a). Economic factors and the cultural factor of ageism may contribute to abuse of elderly individuals. In addition, unemployment has been linked to increased risk of suicide (Voss, Nylen, Floderus, Diderichsen, & Terry, 2004). Widowhood is also associated with greater risk of suicide, particularly for young White and African American men and White women (Luoma & Pearson, 2002).

For youth, association with delinquent peers, gang involvement, and social rejection by peers may contribute to increased violence. At the community level, social disorganization, diminished economic opportunities, increased transience, and low levels of community participation have been linked to violence among youth. Conversely, religiosity, intolerant attitudes to deviance, family connectedness, high parental performance expectations, and parental supervision have been linked to decreased risk of youth violence, as have commitment to school and involvement in social activities (NCIPC, 2006f). Social factors associated with increased suicide potential among adolescents include poor school performance and long absences from school (Thompson, Eggert, Randell, & Pike, 2001), as well as lack of social connectedness and interpersonal conflict (NCIPC, 2006e).

The social response to violence also influences its occurrence. Cultural factors, for example, influence the willingness of persons outside the intimate relationship to take action when IPV is suspected. The incidence of abuse tends to be higher in cultures in which family matters are considered "private" and where community sanctions against IPV are weak (NCIPC, 2006b). Being a victim of certain forms of violence may carry with it a level of social stigma that may prevent victims from reporting the violence or taking action to escape it. For example, stigma was one of the most common reasons given for failure to report rape by as much as 84% of women in one study. The social stigma attached to rape is often the product of enduring myths such as perceptions that women lead men on, participate willingly in the violation, or make false accusations of rape for their own purposes (CDC, 2005b). Community health nurses can be involved in educating the public to change these perceptions and foster willingness to report and take action to prevent abuse.

Legislation prohibiting violence, protecting victims, and mandating sanctions for abusive behaviors is another social response to violence, particularly family violence. Although all U.S. states have legislation related to child abuse, fewer states have adequate legislation and policy addressing IPV and elder abuse. For example, the Family Violence Prevention Fund (2001) has evaluated state efforts with respect to domestic violence. Based on the state "report cards" in 2001, only one state, Pennsylvania, met all the criteria for an "A," indicating that the state has addressed each of six criteria related to training health professionals, screening, legislative protocols, reporting, and protections against health insurance discrimination on the basis of abuse victimization. Six additional states received grades of "B" for their legislative efforts related to domestic violence, and one state, Colorado, rated an "F." Unfortunately, no further study has been done to update this information.

Social responses to violence also include the development of support services for victims of violence, particularly family violence. In many U.S. cities, for example, there are safe houses and shelters for abused women, children, and elders. Use of shelters, of course, depends on the willingness of victims to leave an abusive situation. Even when shelters are used, the purpose for use may vary with specific victims. Some research has demonstrated two major purposes for shelter use among women subjected to IPV: respite and transition. In one study, for example, women who came to shelters for respite generally returned to an abusive situation after a period of time. Other women saw movement to a shelter as a point of transition from which they expected to make major changes in their lives. Women who viewed shelter residence as a time of transition were more likely than those who came for respite to engage in specific behaviors to limit future abuse (e.g., seeking a restraining order against the abuser, making a police report, or seeking counseling) (Krishnan, Hilbert, McNeil, & Newman, 2004).

Social attitudes concerning suicide seem to be changing somewhat, at least with respect to what has been termed *rational suicide* among persons with terminal illness. Some authors note that in the wake of the right-to-die movement, some people in American society have begun to perceive a "good death" as a personal right (Fontana, 2002). Rational suicide, as presented in health care literature, has certain requisite conditions. First, the person contemplating suicide must have a clear and realistic assessment of the situation. Second, the person must be capable of unimpaired mental processes to arrive at an informed decision. Finally, the rationale for the decision to commit suicide should be understandable to most people, and the decision should include family members whenever possible. The concept of rational suicide raises questions of the nurse's role as a client advocate and what constitutes care in the face of terminal illness (Fontana, 2002). For example, nurses may need to decide whether or not they can ethically advocate for rational suicide by an individual client or for policies and laws that permit rational suicide at the population level.

Legal alternatives open to victims may also influence response to violence. For example, women may be more likely to seek a restraining order or protection order (PO) against an abusive partner than to press criminal charges. POs entail automatic legal responses to their violation without the emotional and financial costs of lengthy court proceedings. POs also help to deter retaliation against the victim for taking action. An estimated 22% of abused women seek POs in the face of physical abuse (Division of Violence Prevention, 2000b). Most studies of the effectiveness of restraining or protection orders have indicated that they resulted in decreased threats, assaults, stalking, and worksite harassment whether or not the order was granted. Two studies, on the other hand, found that abuse increased after a request for a PO (McFarlane et al., 2004b).

Family violence frequently occurs in the context of divorce and child custody battles. Granting custody of children to men who have a history of IPV and/or child abuse and granting visitation rights to abusive parents or partners have been regular occurrences in U.S. courts that are viewed as violations of international human rights. Additional court-perpetrated violations of rights include the refusal to accept evidence of IPV or child abuse as relevant to cases reviewed (Silverman et al., 2004)

Social recognition of violence as a public health problem influences the level of resources that are allocated to its resolution. In both national and international arenas, recognition of specific aspects of violence is growing. For example, the United Nations has adopted the U.N. Convention on the Rights of Children, a formal international statement against child maltreatment (Silverman et al., 2004).

Social factors may also have protective effects against societal violence. For example, social connectedness is known to be inversely related to suicide, and social support and regular church attendance have been shown to be protective against abuse among Latino women (Lown & Vega, 2001). Similarly, having social power outside the family and intervention by family members have demonstrated protective effects in preventing the abuse of women.

Another social factor that influences societal violence is media attention. Some authors contend that unbalanced media attention to some types of homicide (e.g., of children or by children) provides the public with an inaccurate view of the problem that hampers their ability to engage in effective problem solving. Others suggest that exposure to media violence is a causal factor in homicide and suicide. For example, the claim is made that murder rates tend to double with the introduction of television into new areas and that "the data linking violence in the media to violence in society is superior to that linking cancer and tobacco" (Grossman, 2000, p. 12). The media no longer presents extensive coverage of youth suicides, for example, because of the known effect seen in cluster suicides. The contention is made that similar coverage of adolescent homicide creates inappropriate role models for vulnerable youth. In some counties, in fact, reporting of the names and images of juvenile criminals is prohibited in efforts to prevent "copycat" violence (Grossman, 2000).

The availability of lethal weapons, particularly guns, is another social factor that influences violence. U.S. firearms-associated homicides exceed those of 25 other developed nations (Hahn et al., 2003b). Firearms are used in approximately 67% of homicides and in 49% of suicides (Office of Statistics and Programming, 2003; U.S. Census Bureau, 2006). In one study, firearms were more likely to be found in homes of women subjected to IPV than in other households, and in two thirds of these homes, intimate partners had either threatened to shoot the women or had actually shot them (Sorenson & Weibe, 2004). Findings of another study indicated that the risk of IPV ending in homicide increased with perpetrator access to a gun and previous threats with a weapon (Campbell et al., 2003). At the community level, areas where household firearms ownership rates are high also have high rates of homicide (Miller, Azrael, & Hemenway, 2002). In the 2005 YRBS, 18.5% of high school students reported carrying a weapon, and more than 5% carried a gun (Eaton et al., 2006), attesting to the easy availability of weapons to U.S. youth.

Occupation is another social factor to be addressed in assessing contributions to societal violence. Assault, homicide, suicide, and intimate partner violence all occur in work settings. The National Institute for Occupational Safety and Health (NIOSH) has defined workplace violence as "violent acts, including physical assaults and threats of assault directed toward individuals at work or on duty" (as quoted in Anderson, 2004, p. 24). Each year more than 1 million workers are assaulted in the work setting, and workplace violence accounts for 15% of all violence affecting the U.S. population 12 years of age and over. Workplace violence results in 1.75 million work days lost each year at a cost of $55 million in lost wages. These figures exclude days lost as annual leave or sick days (Anderson, 2004). Workplace violence is most likely to occur among police

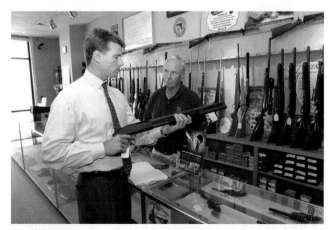

Availability of weapons increases the potential for societal violence. (Greg Mathieson/Mai)

officers, corrections officers, taxicab drivers, private security guards, and bartenders (BJS, 2005a).

In addition to violence among workers or perpetrated on workers in the process of a crime, IPV spills over from the home into the workplace (Malecha, 2003). Seventeen percent of workplace homicides with women victims are perpetrated by current or former husbands or boyfriends, and homicide is the leading cause of occupational death for women. More than 13,000 acts of workplace violence each year involve intimate partners. IPV in the work setting results in 175,000 missed workdays each year and costs $3 million to $5 million in the United States alone (Anderson, 2004).

Workplace policies, as well as setting, influence the incidence of violence in occupational settings. Some people have advocated allowing employees to have guns on the job for purposes of protection. In at least one study, however, homicides occurred five times more often in workplaces where guns were permitted than in those that prohibited guns (Loomis, Marshall, & Ta, 2005).

Nurses, as well as members of other occupational groups, may be at increased risk for both suicide and assault. In one German study, for example, 10% of health care workers, most of whom were nurses, required medical care after assault in the work setting. In addition to the physical effects of assault, many nurses experience long-term psychological consequences and as many as 14% suffer from severe PTSD (Needham, Abderhalden, Halfens, Fischer, & Dassen, 2005). U.S. surveys indicate that as much as 28% of nurses are subjected to violence in the work setting, increasing to 82% of emergency department (ED) nurses (Hemmila, 2003). Some of the reasons given for the level of violence encountered in the ED include the number of combative psychiatric patients, substance abusers, and adults with dementia who present to emergency departments for lack of any other source of care and the stress of illness and injuries that may exceed people's ability to cope (Bonifazi, 2003).

Suicide is the fifth most common cause of death among nurses, as high as six times the rate for the general population in some studies. Nurses are also more likely than the general public to be successful in suicide attempts due to their greater knowledge of the lethality of various methods. Increased suicide rates among nurses have been attributed to high job stress and "critical incident stress." **Critical incident stress** is the stress that accompanies experiencing or witnessing events that cause unusual emotional upset (Bellanger, 2000).

Schoolteachers have also been subjected to increasing levels of violence, and approximately 20% of teachers who leave the profession do so because of the dangers of the school environment. Teachers have the fourth highest rate of nonfatal occupational victimization, exceeded only by law enforcement personnel, mental health professionals, and retail sales clerks (Ruff, Gerding, & Hong, 2004). Occupation is also a factor in some assaults and homicides. Homicide is the second leading cause of occupational deaths in the United States. In addition to working in an occupation that has an intrinsically high risk for violence (e.g., police personnel), working at night or on Saturday, in a setting with only one employee, or in a setting with only male employees increases the risk of occupational homicide (Loomis, Wolf, Runyan, Marshall, & Butts, 2001).

Bullying is a form of societal violence that occurs in occupational as well as school settings. Research indicates that bullying occurs in every type of occupation, and that men and women are equally likely to be bullies, although women are more likely to be targets of occupational bullying. Unfortunately, bullying in the workplace is not prevented by law unless it can be linked to discrimination (Sitzman, 2004). Bullying also occurs with some frequency in school settings. Among students involved in suicide or homicide in school settings between 1994 and 1999, 14% were related to bullying by peers (Division of Violence Prevention, 2003a). In addition, more than 6% of high school students reported not going to school one or more days in the preceding month because of personal safety concerns. Despite the publicity given to school-associated homicides in the media, less than 1% of youth homicides are school-related (NCIPC, 2006f). Students who engage in bullying, however, have been found to be more likely than those who are bullied to engage in a variety of violence-related behaviors. For example, bullies in one study were more than 3 times more likely than those bullied to carry a weapon on a weekly basis and to engage in frequent fighting (Nansel, Overpeck, Haynie, Ruan, & Scheidt, 2003).

Exposure to violence as well as experiencing violence may have adverse health effects. For example, high levels of community violence have been associated with increased frequency of asthma symptoms among children. In at least one study, this link remained even when socioeconomic factors, family unemployment, education level, and housing deterioration were controlled, suggesting a direct association between levels of community violence and asthma (Wright et al., 2004). Similarly, local area deprivation has been associated with suicide, particularly in older people. Explanations given for this association include an increased sense of vulnerability to crime in deprived areas and the consequent fear of leaving home, leading to social isolation and depression (Walters et al., 2004).

War and civil conflict are other sociocultural settings for violence. Approximately 250 wars occurred during the 20th century. In prior eras most casualties of war were soldiers, but today as much as 90% of war-related violence involves civilians. Victims of war-related violence are often women who are frequently subjected to rape during invasion or in refugee camps. Rape of women and children may also accompany attempts at ethnic genocide, as was the case in the

"ethnic cleansing" of Bosnia or efforts at genocide in Rwanda (Donohoe, 2004). Community health nurses may be involved in helping refugee populations to deal with the long-term consequences of war and similar forms of violence.

Questions for exploring the sociocultural factors influencing societal violence are included in the focused assessment below.

Behavioral Considerations

Behavioral factors also contribute to societal violence. For example, alcohol abuse by a male partner was found to be the strongest correlate of intimate partner violence in one study (Coker et al., 2000). Similarly, alcohol and drug abuse by family members are risk factors for child maltreatment (NCIPC, 2006a). Some research suggests, however, that the association between substance use or misuse and violence is mediated by beliefs about substance use. For example, in one study, attitudes approving of marital aggression, perceptions of alcohol use as an excuse for abusive behavior, and expectations of aggressive behavior by someone who has been drinking were linked to IPV among people who drink. Drinkers without these attitudes were less likely to engage in IPV, suggesting that it was not alcohol use *per se* that contributed to IPV, but perceptions of alcohol use and its effects (Field, Caetano, & Nelson, 2004).

Behavioral factors such as smoking may also contribute to suicide. For example, nurses who smoke have been found to be 4 times more likely than nonsmokers

FOCUSED ASSESSMENT

Sociocultural Considerations in Societal Violence

- Do sociocultural norms support violence?
- What legislative approaches have been taken to prevent violence? To support victims of violence?
- Is there intergenerational evidence of violence in the family? In the population?
- Are family social interactions positive or negative? What is the quality of social interactions between various segments of the population?
- Do societal conditions contribute to stress (e.g., unemployment, homelessness)?
- Do cultural or religious values influence the risk of violence? Is this influence protective or does it support violence?
- Are there adequate social support networks available to family members? To members of society?
- Are there occupational risks for violence? If so, what occupations are most affected? What features of these occupations increase the risk for violence?
- What is the societal response to violence? What is the media response to violence?
- Is there a perception of social stigma attached to reporting or experiencing violence?
- Is there social unrest in the population that may contribute to increased violence (e.g., war or other social conflict)?

to commit suicide, whereas excessive caffeine intake appears to be associated with a decreased risk of suicide (Bellanger, 2000). Some studies have indicated that the link between smoking and suicide involves a dose response relationship, with former smokers 1.4 times more likely, light smokers 2.5 times more likely, and heavy smokers 4.3 times more likely to commit suicide than nonsmokers (Miller, Hemenway, & Rimm, 2000).

Significant numbers of women in treatment for drug abuse have a history of IPV. In fact, data suggest that 25% to 57% of women in treatment programs experienced IPV in the prior year, compared to 1.5% to 16% of women in the general population. Research indicates that the relationship between substance abuse and IPV is bidirectional, with substance abuse increasing risk for abuse and also resulting as a means of coping with abuse (El-Bassel, Gilbert, Wu, Go, & Hill, 2005).

Sexual orientation, most likely in combination with psychological and sociocultural factors, also contributes to risk for violent victimization. For example, gay and lesbian youth are two to three times more likely to have attempted suicide than heterosexual youth. In some studies, as much as 72% of gay and lesbian youth have contemplated suicide and as much as 42% have made a suicide attempt (Russell & Joyner, 2001). The increased risk for suicide in youth with a same-sex orientation seems to be greater for boys than girls, particularly when the same-sex couple are members of the same ethnic group (Pinhey & Millman, 2004). Similar findings of increased suicide risk are noted for older gay and bisexual men (Paul et al., 2002).

Experience of physical or sexual abuse by gay, lesbian, and bisexual adolescents has also been associated with increased risk of injection drug use and high-risk sexual behavior. Adolescents in the general population who are sexually abused or assaulted have also been found to be at high risk for early sexual debut, more unprotected intercourse, multiple partners, prostitution, and illicit substance use (Saewyc et al., 2006).

As noted earlier, a significant proportion of homicides occur in work settings (18%), but even more occur in the context of leisure pursuits (22%) (BJS, 2005a). Homicide risk is particularly high in recreational settings that involve heavy consumption of alcohol (e.g., bars and night clubs) or that occur in high crime areas.

Conversely, violence may lead to high-risk behaviors. For example, sexual abuse may contribute to high-risk sexual behaviors in victims, increasing the potential for unwanted pregnancy or STDs (NCIPC, 2006a). Intimate partner violence also contributes to substance abuse among victims (NCIPC, 2006b). Similarly, child abuse has been shown to increase later risk for smoking, alcohol and drug abuse, and eating disorders (NCIPC, 2006a). The focused assessment above right includes questions to identify behavioral dimension factors influencing societal violence.

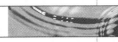

FOCUSED ASSESSMENT

Behavioral Considerations in Societal Violence

- Is there evidence of substance abuse in the family situation? What is the extent of substance abuse in the population? How does it influence societal violence?
- What is the extent of smoking among family members? In the general population?
- Is there evidence of high-risk sexual behavior by family members? In the general population?
- To what extent does sexual orientation contribute to risk for violence in the individual or population?
- To what extent do members of the population engage in other behaviors that might lead to violence (e.g., bullying, carrying weapons)?

Health System Considerations

Health system factors contributing to violence relate primarily to the failure of health care providers to identify clients at risk for or experiencing violence. Providers are generally able to deal with the physical effects of intimate partner violence or attempted suicide or homicide but may be less adept at dealing with underlying causes or addressing safety issues. As we will see, only a small percentage of health care providers routinely screen clients for risk for violence.

Even when abuse is suspected or confirmed, providers may be hesitant to report findings. Barriers to reporting abuse of older clients also exist. For example, some providers identify confidentiality issues, fear regarding the response of the abuser, desires to avoid involvement in court proceedings, distrust of the effectiveness of follow-up, and doubt of their own abilities to accurately recognize abuse as reasons for not reporting abuse. Community health nurses can help to educate providers about the need to identify and report abuse and can help them develop skills in intervening in abusive situations.

Health care providers also often fail to identify clients at risk for suicide. For example, most elderly people who commit suicide were seen by their primary provider a few weeks prior to their suicide, and a large number of them had recently been diagnosed with a first episode of depression. Older adults who commit suicide are also more likely than younger people to be affected by physical illness (NCIPC, 2006e). This suggests that better disease management for prevalent chronic illnesses could help to reduce suicide incidence among the elderly. Similar findings were noted for younger suicide victims in at least one study, with 34% to 76% being seen by a primary care provider in the month prior to suicide (Conner, Langley, Tomaszewski, & Connell, 2003).

In part, the lack of health care provider screening for societal violence may lie in lack of education

FOCUSED ASSESSMENT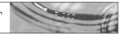

Health System Considerations in Societal Violence

- Are health care providers alert to risk for or evidence of violence?
- To what extent does the health care system provide for support and care of victims of societal violence? For perpetrators of violence?
- What is the response of health care providers to evidence of violence or potential for violence?

regarding issues of violence. Several studies have indicated that educational content in nursing and medical education programs encompassed fewer than 5 hours in a 4-year curriculum (Freedberg, 2006; Stinson & Robinson, 2006). Even with knowledge, however, providers may be reluctant to address issues of abuse and violence for a variety of reasons (e.g., unwillingness to become involved, discomfort in asking about abuse, lack of knowledge of resources for dealing with abuse). For example, one study of nurse practitioners indicated that nearly 78% had received information on IPV in their basic or advanced nursing education, but only 43% indicated that they routinely screened all female clients for IPV (Hinderliter, Doughty, Delaney, Pitula, & Campbell, 2003).

Numerous biophysical, psychological, sociocultural, behavioral, and health system factors contribute to the occurrence of violence in individual clients and families and in society at large. Tips for exploring health system factors involved in societal violence are presented in the focused assessment above. Tools for assessing risk for family violence and suicide are also provided in the *Community Assessment Reference Guide* designed to accompany this text.

COMMUNITY HEALTH NURSING AND SOCIETAL VIOLENCE

Community health nurses have an active role in responding to societal violence. In part, this role may be enacted in services to individual clients and families. Community health nurses may also be involved in planning and implementing interventions to control the problem of violence at the community or population level.

Assessing for Societal Violence

Community health nursing assessment related to societal violence may entail identification of risk factors at individual/family or population levels. For example, nurses working with families would assess them for factors in each of the six dimensions of health that increase their risk for family violence, suicide, or homicide. In addition, nurses would be alert to the signs and symptoms of actual family violence presented in Tables 32-2, 32-3, and 32-4◆ or signs of impending

suicide. At the community or population level, nurses would identify risk factors that lend themselves to high incidence and prevalence of societal violence. For example, they would identify unemployment or other causes of social stress (e.g., homelessness, racial/ethnic tension) as risk factors for social violence. Information on risk factors for and the incidence and prevalence of violence would be used to derive nursing diagnoses and to plan strategies to minimize or control societal violence.

Diagnostic Reasoning and Societal Violence

Nursing diagnoses may be derived from assessment data related to individual clients and families or population groups. An example of a nursing diagnosis for an individual client might be "potential for child abuse due to increased stress of single parenthood and care of a disabled child." A population-based diagnosis might be "increased potential for violence due to prevalence of weapons carrying among high school students."

Planning and Implementing Interventions for Societal Violence

Community health nurses are actively involved in planning intervention strategies for societal violence at primary, secondary, and tertiary levels of prevention. Some interventions at each level are discussed below.

Primary Prevention

There is growing recognition that little attention has been given to primary prevention of societal violence in the United States. For example, most interventions related to IPV have focused on secondary and tertiary prevention, addressing the treatment and rehabilitation needs of current victims and their abusers. This was a natural response when society first became aware of the existence and extent of IPV, but the problem of IPV cannot be resolved without attention to the cultural and other factors that contribute to it (Gundersen, 2002).

Primary prevention of all of the forms of societal violence discussed here focuses on three major approaches: increasing personal aversion to violence as a means of resolving conflict, increasing personal abilities to deal with stress, and eliminating or reducing factors that contribute to stress. These interventions may be targeted to one of three levels: universal prevention strategies, selective interventions, and indicated interventions (Knox, Conwell, & Caine, 2004). Universal interventions are directed toward the entire population and might include teaching effective coping, conflict resolution, and anger management strategies to all school-age children. Selective interventions are focused on specific target groups that do not yet exhibit risk factors for violence, but have the potential for developing them. An example might be assisting gay and lesbian youth in accepting and adjusting to their sexual orientation to prevent depression, which is a risk factor for suicide. Indicated interventions are targeted to people who exhibit immediate risk factors. Again, using suicide as an example, indicated interventions might focus on depressed adolescents or attempt to decrease the social isolation of the elderly population. Some authors add a fourth level of primary prevention related to suicide—clinical interventions with those who are actively suicidal (Pirkis et al., 2003).

One example of a school-based suicide prevention strategy is the SOS program designed to increase awareness of suicide risk, screen students for depression and other suicide risk factors, assist in recognition of suicide potential, and support action. The program employs an ACT strategy, in which A stands for acknowledgement and awareness of suicide potential, C reflects caring, and T stands for telling someone in authority about suicide potential in oneself or a classmate. Evaluations of the program indicated a decrease in suicide attempts and greater knowledge of and adaptive attitudes to depression (Aseltine & DeMartino, 2004).

Increasing aversion to violence may be accomplished by teaching alternative methods of conflict resolution and by imposing cultural and social sanctions against violent behavior. For example, in societies in which violence is not perceived as an acceptable approach to interpersonal conflict, less violence occurs. Similarly, strong religious convictions may deter attempted suicide. For example, a school-based intervention program called *Safe Dates* attempts to reduce dating violence by educating both potential victims and perpetrators. An evaluation of the program indicated that it was effective in reducing both physical and sexual dating violence perpetration and victimization, with demonstrated effects lasting as long as 4 years (Foshee et al., 2004). Community health nurses can be actively involved in teaching positive modes of conflict resolution, anger management, and coping strategies and in activity to change societal attitudes toward the acceptability of violence.

Community health nurses can also assist clients and families at risk to develop effective parent–child and intimate partner relationships by providing anticipatory guidance, assistance with communication, and so on. For instance, the nurse can educate new parents about child behavioral cues and appropriate parental responses as well as provide reinforcement for positive responses. In addition, the nurse can suggest activities that will enhance the bond between parents and child (e.g., reading to or playing with the child) and educate parents regarding appropriate forms of discipline.

Community health nurses can also help to remove or reduce factors that contribute to stress and the potential for abuse. For example, the nurse might refer caretakers of an elderly client or a child with disabilities for

respite services, assist an unemployed parent to find employment, or increase social support networks for socially isolated families. Treatment of substance abuse problems in the individual or family may also decrease the potential for violence. Crisis intervention and hotlines may also prevent suicide. Decreasing access to weapons has also been suggested as a primary prevention measure for violence, but the Task Force on Community Preventive Services found insufficient evidence that firearms control legislation prevents violence. The task force examined such approaches as bans on specific types of weapons, waiting periods before purchase, purchase restrictions, registration and licensing of firearms, prevention of child access to firearms, and zero tolerance policies in schools and found insufficient evidence to recommend any of them as major foci for violence prevention (Hahn et al., 2003b). Control of sales of ammunition to youth, on the other hand, has been effective in reducing access to ammunition, although the ultimate effects of such programs on youth violence are not yet known (Lewin et al., 2005).

Specific prevention of financial abuse of older clients may involve four options to safeguard their funds and property. These options include a financial representative trust, durable power of attorney, designation of a representative payee, and joint tenancy.

In a *financial representative trust*, the older person transfers to a trustee, selected by him- or herself, responsibility for managing his or her property. In this type of arrangement, the trustee is required to manage the older person's assets in a particular manner for the benefit of the older person or others designated (e.g., grandchildren).

A *durable power of attorney* is a written document in which the older person grants another person the authority to act in his or her stead. The durable power of attorney comes into force only when the older person (the "principal") chooses to relinquish control of his or her affairs to the designated person or when the principal becomes incapacitated.

A *representative payee* is a person or organization that receives payments as a substitute for the beneficiary. For example, an older person may make arrangements for his or her Social Security benefits to be paid to a specific family member who uses that money to meet the beneficiary's financial obligations. This type of arrangement is restricted to payments to veterans, recipients of Social Security and Supplemental Security Income, and retirees from railroad companies or state agencies. The agreement covers only that one source of the older person's income. The person receiving the money is required by law to use the funds for the care of the beneficiary, and the agency remitting the checks may demand an accounting of expenditures.

In *joint tenancy,* the older person is co-owner of the assets covered with one or more designated others. All parties involved have the use of funds or property covered under joint tenancy. In the event of the death of one party, ownership automatically devolves on other members of the joint tenancy agreement. Advantages and disadvantages of these four methods of preventing financial abuse of older people are summarized in Table 32-5◆. The community health nurse can assist older clients at risk for financial abuse to evaluate these financial management options and select those best suited to their needs. If the older person needs help in implementing the alternative suggested, the nurse could refer the individual to a source of assistance.

Societal-level interventions to prevent violence must address the needs of both victims and perpetrators. For example, assertiveness training, anger management, and promotion of coping strategies have all been found to be effective in preventing IPV. Similarly, societal interventions to deal with stresses contributing to violence are needed (e.g., strategies for dealing with unemployment, substance abuse, etc.). Community health nurses can be actively involved in advocating for such interventions and for social support systems that decrease the stresses that contribute to violence.

At the international level, WHO has developed a series of recommendations for decreasing the incidence of domestic violence against women. Similar strategies may be needed to prevent violence against men as well. The WHO recommendations include:

- Promoting gender equality and women's rights
- Engaging in multisectoral action plans to prevent violence against women
- Enlisting influential leaders in advocacy for the protection of women
- Developing systems for data collection related to violence and contributing factors
- Prioritizing family violence as a public health issue
- Coordinating violence prevention with HIV/AIDS prevention and adolescent health initiatives

- Creating safer physical environments for women (e.g., better lighting, greater police vigilance)
- Making schools safer for girls
- Developing responses to address the impact of violence against women
- Using reproductive health services as an entry point for interventions to prevent violence against women
- Strengthening formal and informal support available to abused women
- Sensitizing legal systems to the needs of abused women
- Supporting research on factors contributing to violence and effective interventions
- Increasing funding to programs that address violence against women (WHO, 2005)

Community health nurses may be involved in a variety of activities related to these recommendations. For example, they may conduct research on the extent of IPV against men and factors contributing to violence. Or they may develop and test interventions to reduce abuse by intimate partners. They may also plan and implement interventions designed to change adolescent attitudes and behaviors related to dating violence.

Secondary Prevention

Secondary prevention of family violence involves identification of abuse and treatment for its immediate effects. Many victims of abuse choose not to identify themselves or report the abuse for a variety of reasons. Female victims of IPV, for example, may fear additional violence. In other cases, victims may feel stigmatized or wish to protect the abuser. In one study of women in Ghana, failure to report abuse was justified by not wanting to be ridiculed for reporting normal husbandly behavior or not wanting to "air their dirty laundry in public" (Amoakohene, 2004).

TABLE 32-5 Advantages and Disadvantages of Financial Arrangements to Prevent Financial Abuse of the Elderly

Type of Financial Arrangement	Advantages	Disadvantages
Financial representative trust	Legal accountability for use of funds Ability to specify use of funds and beneficiaries	Cost of establishing and administering trust
Durable power of attorney	Financial needs met if older person becomes incapacitated Ability to designate person to control funds Retention of control of funds by older person until he or she chooses to relinquish it or becomes incapacitated	Limited measures to safeguard older person if designee does not use funds as intended
Representative payee	Limited control of funds by designated payee Legal responsibility to use funds for the benefit of the stated beneficiary Mechanism for demanding accounting of use of funds	Restrictions on types of funds covered
Joint tenancy	Ability of older person to designate recipient of funds Automatic right of survivorship eliminates inheritance taxes	Both parties have access to and use of property, and the joint tenant may use them for his or her own benefit and not that of the older person

Identification requires screening for those at risk for or experiencing abuse, and routine screening for abuse has been suggested in emergency departments, women's health clinics, and primary care settings. Workplace screening programs have also been suggested, and community health nurses can be involved in designing and implementing screening programs in the work setting and other venues. Requisites for workplace screening have been identified and are relevant to screening programs in other settings. They include:

- Policies related to IPV and IPV screening
- Education and training of health care providers regarding screening for and response to IPV
- Knowledge of community resources and development of referral networks
- Screening and intervention protocols that address documentation, support, and safety issues (Malecha, 2003)

A variety of screening tools have been developed for screening for IPV, most of them directed toward women. Three such tools are the Woman Abuse Screening Tool (WAST), the HITS tool, and the SAFE tool (Davis-Snavely, 2002). The tools all address the extent of physical violence in an intimate relationship, and some of them also address emotional abuse and the woman's response to abuse. The shortest of the three tools is SAFE, which addresses the quality of the *spousal* relationship, typical events or outcomes of an *argument* between partners, the effects of a *fight*, and the development of an *emergency* plan. Community health nurses can test and use these or similar tools to help identify women experiencing or at risk for IPV and assist them in obtaining assistance for dealing with problems of IPV.

As noted in Chapter 17∞, the U.S. Preventive Services Task Force has not found evidence that screening for IPV is effective in reducing the incidence and prevalence of abuse. Neither has the task force found evidence for the effectiveness of screening for abuse in older clients. The task force noted that existing studies primarily addressed screening among pregnant women, and methodological flaws have implications for their interpretation. Members of the task force found that the lack of evidence does not indicate that screening is ineffective but that little research has been conducted to evaluate the outcomes of screening programs (Nelson, Nygren, McInerney, & Klein, 2004). Until such studies are conducted to reveal a lack of effect, screening for IPV and elder abuse in emergency department and primary care settings makes sense. When screening is conducted, screening questions should be gender neutral to promote disclosure of IPV in same-sex relationships (Freedberg, 2006). Gender-neutral questions may also help to promote disclosure of IPV victimization by men and could be used to screen all clients in certain care settings (e.g., emergency departments, primary care). Potential gender-neutral questions might include:

- Have you been physically injured by anyone in the past year? If so, by whom?
- Do you feel safe in your current relationship?
- Does a previous intimate partner make you feel unsafe? (Freedberg, 2006)

One study of screening in an obstetrics and gynecology clinic found that 72% of women seen had documentation of screening for IPV (Scholle et al., 2003). Other studies have found that less than 10% of providers caring for adults routinely screen clients for IPV. Barriers to screening include lack of time, fear of offending clients, and lack of comfort with and resources to address IPV (Zink, Regan, Goldenhar, Pabst, & Rinto, 2004). It is estimated that health care providers identify only about 5% of women subjected to IPV (Murdaugh et al., 2004).

One study of women exposed to IPV delineated their expectations and desires when they disclosed IPV to health care providers (Dienemann et al., 2005). The women in the study wished to be treated with respect and concern and to be believed. They suggested that abused women were more likely to report abuse when providers asked about it directly. The women also wanted providers to maintain confidentiality and to protect them even when they did not specifically disclose abuse. For example, women felt that providers should be suspicious of partners who hovered and spoke for the woman and should attempt to speak with the woman alone and ask directly about abuse. They also wanted providers to make an initial response that included action to help them resolve the problem of abuse but wanted that action to be based on their own choices after health care professionals provided them with options. In addition, the women wanted to feel that they could return for assistance at a later time, even if help was initially refused. Finally, the women desired complete and accurate documentation of the evidence of abuse, including photographs that would be kept in their records (Dienemann et al., 2005). Areas that have been suggested by others for documenting IPV include a thorough description of injuries with photographs when possible, use of direct quotes to report the client's description of the abusive event with as much detail as possible, a description of the client's demeanor (e.g., crying, fearful, or calm), and the time of the examination with an indication of the time the abuse occurred (Malecha, 2003).

Some authors have suggested the use of administrative sanctions against health care providers who fail to screen for IPV as directed by agency protocols (Larson, Rolniak, Hyman, MacLeod, & Savage, 2000). Others, however, caution that failure to screen clients for IPV may reflect personal experiences with violence and, in the absence of effective occupational programs to help employees deal with the aftermath of violence, mandatory screening may do more harm than good (Johnson, 2001). Some jurisdictions have found that educating the public, including perpetrators of violence and those who know them, regarding the risk factors for and inappropriateness of violent behaviors has led to self-report of abusive behavior and initiation of treatment prior to filing of a criminal complaint. Similarly, parents have been found to report and seek assistance for teenage children with sexual behavior problems prior to major offenses as a result of public education campaigns (Division of Violence Prevention, 2001). Training for health care providers in the identification and assistance of victims of domestic violence has also improved provider attitudes toword screening for and assisting with IPV (Hamberger et al., 2004). Community health nurses may be involved in providing education programs for the general public and recognition and response training programs for other health care providers.

Once evidence of family violence has been detected, treatment focuses on assessing the client for immediate danger, providing appropriate care for the consequences of violence, documenting the client's condition, developing a safety plan, and making needed referrals to community services. Management of IPV may include the ABCDES approach in which

- The victim is assured that he or she is not *alone*.
- The nurse assures the victim of the nurse's *belief* that the victim is not at fault for the abuse.
- The victim is assured of *confidentiality* of information shared, making clear the limits of confidentiality mandated by applicable state laws.
- Injuries are accurately and thoroughly *documented*, with photographs if possible.
- The victim is *educated* regarding resources and options available.
- The victim is assisted to develop a *safety* plan and to recognize danger signs that would necessitate implementation of the plan. Development of a safety plan may depend on the victim's ability to deal with the psychological effects of abuse and may require referral for counseling. (Campbell & Furniss, 2002)

Elements of a safety plan should include hiding money and extra keys, establishing a secret code with friends or family members, asking neighbors to call the police in the event of an altercation, removing weapons from the home, and putting copies of important documents in a handy and secure location. Documents may include social security numbers (for the victim and children as well as the abuser), rent and utility receipts, birth certificates and marriage license if relevant, driver's license or other identification (e.g., a passport), bank account and insurance policy numbers, jewelry and other easily transported valuables, names and telephone numbers of important contacts, extra clothing, and

BUILDING OUR KNOWLEDGE BASE

Some authors have noted that mandatory reporting of abuse, particularly IPV, may result in increased risk, but that there is little research that examines the effects of mandatory reporting on the incidence and prevalence of abuse at the individual family or population level (Campbell & Furniss, 2002). How would you go about conducting a study to determine the effects (both positive and negative) of mandatory reporting of IPV?

essential toiletries (Malecha, 2003). Community health nurses can assist clients at risk for abuse in developing a safety plan and in identifying sources of assistance.

Intervention may include referring an abused family member to a shelter or removing a dependent victim from the abusive situation. Secondary prevention at this point also includes treatment for the perpetrator of violence and for family members who witness violence. Resources may need to be developed to address the needs of male as well as female victims of violence. In addition, criminal justice systems must provide equitable treatment for victims of abuse, whether they are men or women. Community health nurses can advocate for equitable enforcement of laws prohibiting violence as well as for legislation that protects victims from abuse and assures the availability of resources to both victims and abusers.

Secondary prevention also involves mandatory reporting of suspected child abuse and, in some jurisdictions, reporting of intimate partner violence or elder abuse. Reports are generally made initially by telephone to the appropriate agency and are followed, usually within 48 hours, by a written report. (Sample reporting forms are included in Appendix D∞.) In making a report, the community health nurse should be careful to focus on objective evidence that suggests abuse and to report exactly what he or she has seen or verbatim reports of those involved.

ETHICAL AWARENESS

Some states have passed legislation mandating reporting of physical abuse of women. Some authors, however, maintain that mandatory reporting may put women at risk for subsequent abuse, and some health care providers have indicated that they may not abide by the requirement if the woman herself does not agree to the report.

- Do you think that mandatory reporting should be legislated?
- What are the ethical implications of mandatory reporting of intimate partner violence?
- What are the conflicting values influencing this issue? How would you prioritize these values to arrive at an appropriate course of action?
- Do these implications differ for mandatory reporting of abuse of children or elderly persons? Why or why not?

When IPV involves sexual assault or rape, or when such events occur outside intimate relationships, community health nurses should refer victimized clients to a local emergency department for assessment. Most emergency departments have sexual abuse response teams (SART) that have extensive background in assessment and care of persons who have been sexually assaulted. SART members also have expertise in the collection of forensic evidence that may be used in criminal proceedings against the abuser. Community health nurses should encourage victims of sexual abuse and other intimate partner violence to report the event and to seek help in an emergency department. Clients should be particularly cautioned not to "clean themselves up" following the assault as this destroys physical evidence of the assault.

Programs to prevent violence by chronically delinquent youth have shown some success. Therapeutic foster care is one such program. Therapeutic foster care is an approach in which young people with a history of delinquent behavior are placed with a foster family with special training in providing a structured environment that fosters the development of social and emotional skills. Therapeutic foster care may be used as an alternative to incarceration or placement in residential treatment facilities. Based on evaluation of the effectiveness of therapeutic foster care, the Task Force on Community Preventive Services has recommended this intervention for use in preventing violence among youth (Hahn et al., 2004). Community health nurses may be involved in the establishment of therapeutic foster care programs or in providing support to foster parents and their young charges.

Much of the nursing research related to IPV and other forms of societal violence is directed toward identifying contributing factors and responses of and effects on victims or witnesses, with few controlled studies of the effectiveness of interventions. Interventions that have demonstrated some effectiveness, however, include periodic telephone contact with women experiencing IPV to educate them regarding safety-promoting behaviors. In one study, women who received the telephone intervention displayed more safety behaviors than other abused women who received care typically provided by the family violence unit of the local district attorney's office (McFarlane et al., 2004a). Safety-promoting behaviors addressed the elements of a safety plan described above. In another study, two interventions were found equally effective in decreasing the incidence of assault, work harassment, and risk of homicide: a wallet-sized card listing elements of a safety plan and IPV resources, and nurse case management addressing emotional support, anticipatory guidance regarding resources and the potential risks of using them, and referrals to needed services. Women in both groups also engaged in more safety-related behaviors after intervention than before, but also made less use of community

resources (McFarlane, Groff, O'Brien, & Watson, 2006). There is a continuing need to evaluate the effectiveness of both primary and secondary prevention interventions for all forms of societal violence.

Secondary prevention of societal violence also involves the early identification of persons who are contemplating suicide or homicide and intervention to prevent the act or limit the consequences. Nurses, teachers, and counselors may recognize the signs of impending suicide or escalating aggression and should take immediate action. Such action might include counseling, referral, or hospitalization if the danger appears imminent. Community health nurses may also be involved in educating individuals who work with young people, the elderly, and others at risk for suicide to recognize indicators of a potential suicide attempt. Indications of suicide risk are summarized in the focused assessment below.

FOCUSED ASSESSMENT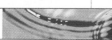

Indications of Suicide Risk

- Is there a family history of suicide? Of other forms of violence?
- Do family or cultural views support suicide? Do cultural beliefs lead to stigma and unwillingness to seek help for depression or other problems?
- Does the client hold religious beliefs that would protect against suicide?
- Is there a history of prior suicide attempt(s) by the client or by significant others?
- Is there a history of mental illness? Is the client exhibiting current symptoms of mental illness? Has the client experienced barriers to obtaining mental health services?
- Is there a history of substance abuse by the client or significant others?
- Does the client exhibit impulsive or aggressive behavior?
- Has the client experienced a recent serious loss (particularly in the last 6 months)?
- Does the client have a chronic illness that is severely affecting his or her quality of life?
- Does the client exhibit signs of depression?
- Does the client express feelings of hopelessness or helplessness?
- Does the client talk about wanting to die or express the wish that he or she were dead?
- Does the client express feelings of being a burden to others?
- Does the client express feelings of isolation?
- Does the client display evidence of anxiety, irritability, or panic?
- Does the client fail to refer to future goals or activities?
- Does the client express frequent or persistent thoughts of suicide?
- Has the client developed a carefully thought-out plan for suicide?
- Has the client chosen a lethal method for suicide with reduced likelihood of rescue?
- Does the client have easy access to lethal methods of suicide?
- Is suicide planned for the near future?
- Does the client exhibit behavior designed to "put one's house in order" (e.g., making a will, giving away prized possessions)?
- Does the client engage in behavior that would be likely to result in death (e.g., provoking fights with others, hazardous driving)?
- Has there been extensive media attention to recent suicides?

EVIDENCE-BASED PRACTICE

*H*allfors et al. (2006) evaluated the feasibility of population-based screening for suicide risk in high school students. On the basis of Suicide Risk Screen results, 29% of the students were rated at risk of suicide. Only about half of these students were later deemed to be at high risk for suicide, suggesting that routine suicide screening in school settings is not effective. The U.S. Preventive Services Task Force (2005) has also found insufficient evidence for the effectiveness of routine suicide screening in children and adolescents, although routine screening has been recommended for adults in practice settings in which follow-up care is available. Given the lack of effectiveness of population-based screening, what approaches have been described in the literature as effective in identifying adolescents at risk for suicide?

Tertiary Prevention

Tertiary prevention of societal violence involves dealing with the consequences of violence and preventing its recurrence. Interventions intended for the individual or family level include providing treatment for long-term physical or psychological effects of violence. For example, victims of IPV may need a referral for treatment for PTSD, or children who witness or experience abuse can be referred for counseling. Victims of abuse may also need assistance in finding coping strategies as alternatives to subsequent alcohol and drug abuse or high-risk sexual behaviors (Miller & Mancuso, 2004). Similarly, the loved ones of suicide or homicide victims may need assistance in dealing with their loss. Assistance needed may range from counseling to cope with the loss of a loved one to help with concrete tasks such as planning a funeral, filing claims for death benefits, settling the victim's estate, and dealing with the criminal justice system (Horne, 2003). Another tertiary prevention measure for suicide and homicide is control of media representations that promote copycat events.

Tertiary prevention of family violence also entails changing circumstances that promote violence. For example, the community health nurse may assist abusive parents to understand the needs and behavioral cues of their children or help caregivers of disabled children or elderly family members to find respite. Other potential tertiary strategies for elder maltreatment include providing alternatives to home care of the elderly and increasing community support services for persons who are caring for older family members.

Community health nurses may also be involved in the development of programs to assist the perpetrators of violence. For example, they may plan and implement anger management programs for people who see violence as a means of dealing with anger. They may also advocate for and assist in initiating treatment programs for abusers. One such program is the STOP program, a 13-week program designed to change the attitudes, perceptions, and behaviors of abusive men. STOP is an acronym for stopping to [S]urvey the situation, [T]hink about consequences, consider [O]ptions, and [P]revent violence (Wood, 2004). Another approach involves parenting classes for abusive parents and referral to Parents Anonymous, a mutual-help group for parents who have a history of or are at risk for child abuse.

Tertiary prevention with both abusers and victims of IPV and elder abuse and with child abusers should be geared to the stage of change in which the client (victim or abuser) finds him- or herself. The transtheoretical model of stages of change was addressed in Chapter 31 ∞ but is also relevant to societal violence. Identification of stages of change has been found to be helpful in predicting attrition among men involved in batterer treatment programs (Scott, 2004) as well as in decision processes for women involved in abusive situations (Burke, Denison, Gielen, McDonnell, & O'Campo, 2004). Research in IPV has suggested that abusive men further along in the change process are more successful in behavior change as a result of treatment programs and that such programs should consider the offender's stage of change and design strategies specifically to move the abuser through the various stages of change to reduce IPV (Eckhardt, Babcock, & Homack, 2004). As noted in Chapter 31 ∞, differing intervention strategies are warranted in early and later stages of readiness for change. In the precontemplation and contemplation stages of change, for example, community health nurses might engage in strategies to increase the awareness of batterers and victims that abuse is not a normal phenomenon. In the action stage, on the other hand, the nurse might assist the client to identify specific actions that can be taken to resolve the problem. For example, the nurse might help the victim of abuse identify a place of safety to which he or she could go or refer the abuser to a treatment plan.

Nurses may also assist family members to improve coping and communication skills as well as to improve self-esteem. This is particularly important for victims of child abuse if the intergenerational cycle of abusive behavior is to be broken. Research with women and children who have experienced or witnessed IPV has indicated that many families engage in a process labeled *regenerating family*. In this process, mother and children purposefully replace destructive interaction patterns with those that promote a predictable and respectful environment that fosters family members' emotional health. The process of regeneration also involves creating an atmosphere of teamwork and development of new expectations of family members based on ideals of how family interaction should occur. Regeneration is also fostered by paying attention to one's own behavior and that of others and reflecting on the underlying meaning of behavior. The family may also develop new standards of behavior and modes of communication and

Advocacy in Action

Escape

A community health nursing student was following an adolescent girl with a young child. The client was enrolled in a special continuation school in which young mothers brought their children to school while they completed their high school education. The children were cared for in a day care center on the high school campus, and periodically during the school day the mothers would come to the center to participate in the children's care. In this way, the girls were allowed to continue their education and also learned appropriate childcare skills and built support networks among themselves.

The particular girl that the student was working with was Hispanic, and the nursing student was African American. It took some time for the student to establish a climate of trust with her client. Several weeks into the semester, however, the client confided concerns about her own mother to the nursing student. The girl's mother was being verbally and physically abused by her husband. The nursing student offered to meet with the mother and discuss her options, but the mother was afraid to meet with her. Because of her cultural heritage, she was reluctant to leave the abusive situation. Her daughter had urged her to leave or to call the police, but the mother was reluctant to do either.

All the student could do was provide the adolescent with information about the location of safe houses in the community and what her mother should take with her if she decided to remove herself and her younger children from the home. Before the end of the semester, however, the mother made a decision to leave and called the police to take her to one of the safe houses. Because the nursing students were also working in the safe houses, the student was able to work with the mother to assure that she received the help she needed to make a permanent escape from an abusive situation.

work to maintain a balance between family connectedness and individual autonomy (Wuest, Merrit-Gray, & Ford-Gilboe, 2004). Community health nurses can assist families in this process of regeneration by helping them to clarify past interaction patterns and identifying appropriate changes in those patterns and mechanisms to achieve those changes.

Goals for primary, secondary, and tertiary prevention of societal violence and related community health nursing interventions are summarized in Table 32-6◆.

TABLE 32-6	Goals for Primary, Secondary, and Tertiary Prevention of Societal Violence and Related Community Health Nursing Interventions	
Goal of Prevention	Nursing Interventions (Individual/Family)	Nursing Interventions (Community)
Primary Prevention		
1. Development of effective coping skills	1. Teach coping skills and stress management skills to individuals and families.	1. Teach coping and stress management skills to population groups; advocate for inclusion of coping skills in school curricula.
2. Development of self-esteem	2. Foster self-image.	2. Advocate school programs to foster self-esteem in young people.
3. Development of realistic expectations of self and others	3. Educate parents on child development; educate caregivers on needs of the elderly; help clients recognize strengths.	3. Educate the public regarding developmental expectations; advocate for and initiate parenting education programs; develop caregiver education programs.
4. Development of effective parenting and interpersonal skills	4. Teach parenting skills; teach and role-model effective communication skills; refer families with communication difficulties for counseling assistance.	4. Advocate for communication education in school curricula; advocate for and implement parenting education programs; advocate for available counseling services to improve family communication.
5. Treatment of psychopathology or substance abuse	5. Refer for treatment.	5. Advocate for available and accessible treatment services.
6. Promotion of nonviolent conflict resolution	6. Teach nonviolent conflict management strategies.	6. Advocate for inclusion of conflict management content in school curricula and other education programs.
7. Provision of emotional and material support	7. Refer to sources of assistance as needed; assist in development or expansion of social support networks.	7. Advocate for supportive services for perpetrators and victims of violence; advocate for societal changes to minimize sources of stress contributing to violence.

Continued on next page

TABLE 32-6 Goals for Primary, Secondary, and Tertiary Prevention of Societal Violence and Related Community Health Nursing Interventions (continued)

Goal of Prevention	Nursing Interventions (Individual/Family)	Nursing Interventions (Community)
8. Reduction of risk behaviors	8. Encourage clients not to frequent places where homicides occur and not to use drugs and alcohol in circumstances in which interpersonal conflict is likely.	8. Educate the public on the influence of drugs and alcohol on violence; advocate for adequate police protection in high crime areas; advocate for societal mores that promote early intervention to prevent escalation of conflict to violent behaviors.
9. Decreased availability of weapons, drugs, and alcohol	9. Encourage removal of weapons from homes; encourage responsible alcohol use.	9. Engage in political activity to promote control of weapons and limit access to drugs and alcohol.
10. Change in societal attitudes toward violence	10. Teach nonviolent modes of conflict resolution; teach problem-solving and decision-making skills; discuss appropriate approaches to discipline.	10. Develop and implement campaigns to change cultural perceptions of violence as a means of conflict resolution.
11. Development of policies that discourage violence and protect potential victims		11. Engage in political activity and advocacy; promote positive attitudes toward the elderly and disabled; advocate for women's social rights.
Secondary Prevention		
1. Identification of persons at risk for violence	1. Engage in case finding; teach teachers and counselors to recognize signs of abuse or potential for violence; screen for evidence of abuse or potential for violence.	1. Educate the public regarding factors contributing to risk of violence; develop screening programs for risk for violence.
2. Provision of counseling for persons at risk for violence	2. Refer for counseling.	2. Advocate for availability of counseling services for those in need.
3. Provision of treatment for victims of violence	3. Refer for necessary services.	3. Engage in political activity and advocacy to assure adequate treatment facilities.
4. Identification of episodes of violence	4. Report instances of violence.	4. Monitor trends in societal violence to identify problem areas.
5. Provision of safe environments	5. Remove victims of abuse to safe environments as needed; plan with victims for achieving a safe environment; refer to a shelter as needed; initiate involuntary commitment proceedings if the person is a clear danger to self or others.	5. Advocate for available shelter and other resources for victims of violence.
6. Provision of treatment for violent persons	6. Refer for treatment; provide emotional support to both victims and perpetrators.	6. Advocate for availability of treatment services and facilities.
Tertiary Prevention		
1. Prevention of suicide clusters and copycat murders		1. Assist in the development of community response plans; advocate for control of media exposures to violence.
2. Provision of care to families of homicide and suicide victims	2. Assist family members to work through feelings of grief and guilt; assist families to find positive ways to cope with loss; refer for assistance with legal and other tasks as needed; refer for counseling as needed.	2. Advocate for support services for families of victims.
3. Treatment of consequences of violence	3. Refer for physical and psychological treatment services as needed.	3. Advocate for available services for victims and perpetrators of violence.
4. Reduction of sources of stress	4. Refer to sources of assistance; develop or expand social support networks; arrange for respite care as needed; assist with employment and other social needs.	4. Advocate for social changes to minimize sources of stress that contribute to violence; advocate for development of respite care and other support services.

Evaluating Control Strategies for Societal Violence

The effectiveness of control strategies for societal violence can be evaluated at the level of the individual client or family or at the population level. For example, the nurse might determine whether or not child abuse has been prevented in a family at high risk for abuse, or whether subsequent instances of abuse have been experienced by an older client or pregnant woman. At the population level, the community health nurse might look for changes in suicide or homicide rates or the frequency of reports to child protective services to evaluate the effectiveness of population-based interventions. As noted earlier, there is a great need for nursing research to examine the effectiveness of primary, secondary, and tertiary interventions to address societal violence. For example, nurses might study the effects of school curricula on culturally prescribed gender roles and their influence on IPV. Or they might contribute to the body of knowledge on the effectiveness of screening for suicide risk in decreasing the incidence of suicide among the elderly.

In assessing the effectiveness of strategies to reduce societal violence, community health nurses and others might evaluate the extent to which national objectives related to violence and suicide have been achieved◆. Baseline and target information for selected objectives are presented below. As can be seen in the table, only two of the objectives have been met, and four objectives are actually moving away from the target goals, suggesting the need for greater attention to violence control strategies in the United States.

HEALTHY PEOPLE 2010

Goals for Population Health

OBJECTIVE	BASELINE	MOST RECENT DATA	TARGET
■ 15-4. Reduce the proportion of people living in homes with firearms that are loaded and unlocked	19%	NDA	16%
■ 15-32. Reduce homicides (per 100,000 population)	6.0	6.1	3.0#
■ 15-33. Reduce			
a. Maltreatment of children (per 1,000 children)	12.6	12.4	10.3
b. Child maltreatment fatalities (per 100,000 children)	1.6	1.8	1.4#
■ 15-34. Reduce the rate of physical assault by current or former intimate partners (per 1,000 population)	4.4	2.6	3.3*
■ 15-35. Reduce the annual rate of rape or attempted rape (per 1,000 population)	0.8	0.7	0.7*
■ 15-36. Reduce sexual assault other than rape (per 1,000 population)	0.6	0.5	0.4
■ 15-37. Reduce physical assaults (per 1,000 population)	31.1	21.8	13.6
■ 15-39. Reduce weapon carrying by adolescents on school property	6.9%	6.1%	4.9%
■ 18-1. Reduce the suicide rate (per 100,000 population)	10.5	10.9	5.0#
■ 16-2. Reduce the rate of suicide attempts by adolescents requiring medical attention (12-month average)	2.6%	2.9%	1%#

NDA—No data available

* Objective has been met

\# Objective moving away from target

Data from: Centers for Disease Control and Prevention. (2005). Healthy people data. Retrieved September 5, 2005, from http://wonder.cdc.gov/data2010

Case Study

Caring for a Physically Abused Client

On a routine postpartum visit, your client, Mrs. Montanez, mentions that she is very concerned about her next-door neighbor, Mrs. Abood, who is pregnant. Mrs. Montanez tells you that she thinks Mr. Abood beat his wife last night. She heard shouting during the night, and this morning she noticed that Mrs. Abood had a black eye that she said she got when she ran into the bedroom door in the dark. Before leaving the apartment complex, you knock on the Aboods' door, but no one answers. You leave your card asking Mrs. Abood to call you.

When Mrs. Abood phones the next day, you explain that you were responding to the concern of a friend for her safety and ask if she is in need of assistance. Mrs. Abood tells you that there is nothing wrong. When you mention that Mrs. Montanez described some injuries, she denies that her husband is abusive. She states that she is receiving prenatal care from a private physician, will contact him if she has any problems with the pregnancy, and is not in need of your services. You accept her refusal of help, but you inform her that you are available and can be reached by phone if she needs assistance at some time in the future.

A month later you receive a call from Mrs. Abood, who asks to see you. She indicates that she is afraid to have you come to her home lest her husband return while you are there. She says that her husband has already been involved in physical fights with her brother over what he perceives as infringements on his authority over his wife. She agrees to meet you at the health department when she comes to get a copy of her daughter's immunization record for school entry.

When you see Mrs. Abood, she admits that her husband beat her the previous day. This is the second time he has assaulted her since she became pregnant. She has several bruises on her face and one particularly large bruise on her abdomen where her husband hit her. Mrs. Abood says that her husband is very jealous and does not believe the baby is his. She insists that she has been faithful to her husband and has tried to convince him of this. She says her husband gets angry because she "shows herself off to other men and gives them a come-on." She comments, "I guess he's right. I do wear shorts a lot, because they're comfortable in this hot weather. I really should try to respect his wishes more."

Mrs. Abood has tried to convince her husband that the baby is his. She has stopped going out with female friends and even tries to avoid talking to the mailman and other males who come to the house. She has not even been to see her family because her husband refuses to go with her and accuses her of meeting her lover on these excursions.

Since the beating yesterday, Mrs. Abood says she is afraid for her own safety as well as that of her unborn child. She says that her husband loves their 3-year-old daughter and would not hurt her.

Mrs. Abood has never worked, although she completed nursing school before she got married. She feels as though she should get away from her husband even though she still loves him; however, she has no money to support herself and her daughter. She

does not feel she can go to relatives because her husband would be able to find her there and bring her back home. She is also afraid that if she leaves him, her husband will attempt to get custody of their daughter.

1. What are the health problems evident in this situation? What are the biophysical, psychological, sociocultural, behavioral, and health system factors influencing these problems?
2. What considerations are important in planning care for Mrs. Abood?
3. What concerns might arise with respect to your own safety in this situation? How might you deal with these concerns?
4. What secondary prevention measures would be warranted to deal with existing health problems? Describe specific actions that you would take to resolve these problems.
5. What could be done in terms of tertiary prevention to prevent further consequences or recurrence of health problems in this situation?
6. What primary prevention measures might have prevented the development of the health problems in this situation? How might you, as a community health nurse, be involved in such measures?

Test Your Understanding

1. What are the major types of societal violence of concern to community health nurses? (pp. 973–977)

2. What biophysical, psychological, physical environmental, sociocultural, behavioral, and health system factors influence societal violence? In what ways are these influences similar among the types of violence described in the chapter? In what ways do they differ? (pp. 978–991)

3. What are the major foci in primary prevention of societal violence? What roles do community health nurses play in each? (pp. 991–993, 998–999)

4. What are the major approaches to secondary prevention of societal violence? Give an example of a community health nursing activity related to each approach. (pp. 993–996, 999)

5. What are the major considerations in tertiary prevention of societal violence? How might community health nurses be involved in tertiary prevention activities? (pp. 997–998, 999)

EXPLORE MediaLink

http://www.prenhall.com/clark
Resources for this chapter can be found on the Companion Website.

Audio Glossary
Exam Review Questions
Case Study: Violence and Teenagers

MediaLink Application: Raising Awareness
 of Domestic Abuse (video)
Media Links

Challenge Your Knowledge
Update *Healthy People 2010*
Advocacy Interviews

References

Abrahams, N., & Jewkes, R. (2005). Effects of South African men's having witnessed abuse of their mothers during childhood on their levels of violence in adulthood. *American Journal of Public Health, 95,* 1811–1816.

Abrams, R. C., Marzuk, P. M., Tardiff, K., & Leon, A. C. (2005). Preference for fall from height as a method of suicide by elderly residents of New York City. *American Journal of Public Health, 95,* 1000–1002.

Ahmed, M. K., van Ginneken, J., Razzaque, A., & Alam, N. (2004). Violent deaths among women of reproductive age in rural Bangladesh. *Social Science & Medicine, 59,* 311–319.

American Academy of Pediatrics. (2004). Policy statement: School-based mental health services. *Pediatrics, 113,* 1839–1845.

Amoakohene, M. I. (2004). Violence against women in Ghana: A look at women's perceptions and review of policy and social responses. *Social Science & Medicine, 59,* 2373–2385.

Anderson, D. G. (2004). Workplace violence in long haul trucking. *AAOHN Journal, 52,* 23–27.

Aseltine, R. H., & DeMartino, R. (2004). An outcome evaluation of the SOS suicide prevention program. *American Journal of Public Health, 94,* 446–451.

Basile, S. (2004). Comparison of abuse alleged by same- and opposite-gender litigants as cited in requests for abuse prevention orders. *Journal of Family Violence, 19,* 59–68.

Bellanger, D. (2000). Nurses and suicide: The risk is real. *RN, 63*(10), 61–64.

Bonifazi, W. (2003). Defusing emergency department violence: How you can make your ED safer. *Nursing Spectrum* (Western Edition), *4*(9), 8–10.

Branas, C. C., Nance, M. L., Elliott, M. R., Richmond, T. S., & Schwab, C. W. (2004). Urban-rural shifts in intentional firearm death: Different causes, same results. *American Journal of Public Health, 94,* 1750–1755.

Burch, R. L., & Gallup, G. G. (2004). Pregnancy as a stimulus for domestic violence. *Journal of Family Violence, 19,* 243–247.

Bureau of Justice Statistics. (2005a). *Crime characteristics.* Retrieved March 30, 2006, from http://www.ojp.usdoj.gov/bjs/cvict_c.htm

Bureau of Justice Statistics. (2005b). *Criminal victimization.* Retrieved March 30, 2006, from http://www.ojp.usdoj.gov/bjs/cvictgen.htm

Burke, J. G., Denison, J. A., Gielen, A. C., McDonnell, K. A., & O'Campo, P. O. (2004). Ending intimate partner violence: An application of the transtheoretical model. *American Journal of Health Behavior, 28,* 122–133.

Busch, A. L., & Rosenberg, M. S. (2004). Comparing women and men arrested for domestic violence: A preliminary report. *Journal of Family Violence, 19,* 49–57.

Campbell, J. C., & Furniss, K. K. (2002). *Violence against women: Identification, screening, and management of intimate partner violence.* Washington, DC: Association of Women's Health, Obstetric and Neonatal Nurses.

Campbell, J. C., Webster, D., Koziol-McLain, J., Block, C., Campbell, D., Curry, M. A., et al. (2003). Risk factors for femicide in abusive relationships: Results from a multisite case control study. *American Journal of Public Health, 93,* 1089–1097.

Castro, R., Peek-Asa, C., & Ruiz, A. (2003). Violence against women in Mexico: A study of abuse before and during pregnancy. *American Journal of Public Health, 93,* 1110–1116.

Centers for Disease Control and Prevention. (2003a). Domestic violence awareness month, October 2003. *Morbidity and Mortality Weekly Report, 52,* 942.

Centers for Disease Control and Prevention. (2003b). Suicide and attempted suicide. *Morbidity and Mortality Weekly Report, 53,* 471.

Centers for Disease Control and Prevention. (2004). Sexual Assault Awareness Month, April 2004. *Morbidity and Mortality Weekly Report, 53,* 189–190.

Centers for Disease Control and Prevention. (2005a). *Healthy people data.* Retrieved September 5, 2005, from http://wonder.cdc.gov/data2010

Centers for Disease Control and Prevention. (2005b). Sexual assault awareness month—

April, 2005. *Morbidity and Mortality Weekly Report, 54,* 311.

Clements, C. M., Sabourin, C. M., & Spiby, L. (2004). Dysphoria and hopelessness following battering: The role of perceived control, coping, and self-esteem. *Journal of Family Violence, 19,* 25–36.

Coker, A. L., Smith, P. H., McKeown, R. E., & King, M. J. (2000). Frequency and correlates of intimate partner violence by type: Physical, sexual, and psychological battering. *American Journal of Public Health, 90,* 553–559.

Conner, K. R., Langley, J., Tomaszewski, K. J., & Connell, Y. (2003). Injury hospitalization and risks for subsequent self-injury and suicide: A national study from New Zealand. *American Journal of Public Health, 93,* 1128–1131.

Cubbin, C., Pickle, L. W., & Fingerhut, L. (2000). Social context and geographic patterns of homicide among US black and white males. *American Journal of Public Health, 90,* 579–587.

Davis-Snavely, F. (2002, Spring). Universal screening for domestic violence. *Perinatal Care Matters,* pp. 2–3.

Dienemann, J., Glass, N., & Hyman, R. (2005). Survivor preferences for response to IPV disclosure. *Clinical Nursing Research, 14,* 215–233.

Division of Violence Prevention. (2000a). Intimate partner violence among men and women—South Carolina, 1998. *Morbidity and Mortality Weekly Report, 49,* 691–694.

Division of Violence Prevention. (2000b). Use of medical care, police assistance, and restraining orders by women reporting intimate partner violence—Massachusetts, 1996–1997. *Morbidity and Mortality Weekly Report, 49,* 485–488.

Division of Violence Prevention. (2001). Evaluation of a child sexual abuse prevention program—Vermont, 1995–1997. *Morbidity and Mortality Weekly Report, 50,* 77–78, 87.

Division of Violence Prevention. (2002a). Nonfatal physical assault-related injuries treated in hospital emergency departments—United States, 2000. *Morbidity and Mortality Weekly Report, 51,* 461–463.

Division of Violence Prevention. (2002b). Nonfatal self-inflicted injuries treated in hospital emergency departments—United States, 2000. *Morbidity and Mortality Weekly Report, 51,* 436–438.

Division of Violence Prevention. (2002c). Variation in homicide risk during infancy—United States, 1989–1998. *Morbidity and Mortality Weekly Report, 51,* 187–189.

Division of Violence Prevention. (2003a). School-associated suicides—United States, 1994–1999. *Morbidity and Mortality Weekly Report, 52,* 476–478.

Division of Violence Prevention. (2003b). Suicide attempts and physical fighting among high school students—United States, 2001. *Morbidity and Mortality Weekly Report, 52,* 474–476.

Donohoe, M. (2004). War, rape, and genocide: Never again? Retrieved October 26, 2004, from http://www.medscape.com/viewarticle/491147

Durose, M. R., Harlow, C. W., Langan, P. A., Motivans, M., Rantala, R. R., & Smith, R. L.

(2005). *Family violence statistics: Including statistics on strangers and acquaintances.* Washington, DC: Bureau of Justice Statistics.

Eaton, D. K., Kann, L., Kinchen, S., Ross, J., Hawkins, J., Harris, W. A., et al. (2006). Youth Risk Behavior Surveillance—United States, 2005. *Morbidity and Mortality Weekly Report, 55*(SS-5), 1–108.

Eckhardt, C. I., Babcock, J., & Homack, S. (2004). Partner assaultive men and the stages and processes of change. *Journal of Family Violence, 19,* 81–93.

El-Bassel, N., Gilbert, L., Wu, E., Go, H., & Hill, J. (2005). Relationship between drug abuse and intimate partner violence: A longitudinal study among women receiving methadone. *American Journal of Public Health, 95,* 465–470.

El-Mouelhy, M. (2004). Violence against women: A public health problem. *Journal of Primary Prevention, 25,* 289–303.

Family Violence Prevention Fund. (2001). *State-by-state report card on health care laws and domestic violence.* Retrieved June 19, 2006, from http://endabuse.org/statereport/list.php.3

Farella, C. (2000). Love shouldn't hurt: Understanding domestic violence. *Nursing Spectrum, 1*(2), 14–16.

Field, C. A., Caetano, R., & Nelson, S. (2004). Alcohol and violence related cognitive risk factors associated with the perpetration of intimate partner violence. *Journal of Family Violence, 19,* 249–253.

Fontana, J. S. (2002). Rational suicide in the terminally ill. *Journal of Nursing Scholarship, 34,* 147–151.

Foshee, V. A., Bauman, K. E., Ennett, S. T., Linder, G. F., Benefield, T., & Suchindran, C. (2004). Assessing the long-term effects of the Safe Dates Program and a booster in preventing and reducing adolescent dating violence victimization and perpetration. *American Journal of Public Health, 94,* 619–624.

Foster, E. M., Qaseem, A., & Connor, T. (2004). Can better mental health services reduce the risk of juvenile justice system involvement? *American Journal of Public Health, 94,* 859–865.

Freedberg, P. (2006). Health care barriers and same-sex intimate partner violence: A review of the literature. *Journal of Forensic Nursing, 2*(1), 15–24, 41.

Fulmer, T. (2002). Elder abuse and neglect assessment. *Try this: Best practices in nursing care to older adults.* New York: Hartford Geriatric Institute for Nursing.

Giorgianni, S. J. (Ed.). (2003). *How families matter in health: Challenges of the evolving 21st-century family.* New York, NY: Impact Communications.

Goldberg, J. F., & Hoop, J. (2004). Bipolar depression: Long-term challenges for the clinician. Retrieved September 30, 2004, from http://www.medscape.com

Gomby, D. S. (2000). Promise and limitations of home visitation. *Journal of the American Medical Association, 284,* 1430–1431.

Goodwin, R. D., Hoven, C. W., Murison, R., & Hotopf, M. (2003). Association between childhood physical abuse and gastrointestinal disorders and migraine in adulthood. *American Journal of Public Health, 94,* 1065–1067.

Greenwood, G. L., Relf, M. V., Huang, B., Pollack, L. M., Canchola, J. A., & Catania, J. A. (2002). Battering victimization among a probability-based sample of men who have sex with men. *American Journal of Public Health, 92,* 1964–1969.

Grossman, D. (2000). Teaching kids to kill. *National Forum, 80*(4), 10–14.

Grunbaum, J. A., Kann, L., Kinchen, S., Ross, J., Hawkins, J., Lowry, R., et al. (2004). Youth risk behavior surveillance—United States, 2003. *Morbidity and Mortality Weekly Report, 53* (SS-2), 1–96.

Gundersen, L. (2002). Intimate partner violence: The need for primary prevention in the community. *Annals of Internal Medicine, 136,* 637–640.

Hahn, R. A., Biluka, O. O., Crosby, A., Fullilove, M. T., Liberman, A., Moscicki, E. K., et al. (2003a). First reports evaluating the effectiveness of strategies for preventing violence: Early childhood home visitation: Findings from the Task Force on Community Preventive Services. *Morbidity and Mortality Weekly Report, 52*(RR-14), 1–9.

Hahn, R. A., Biluka, O. O., Crosby, A., Fullilove, M. T., Liberman, A., Moscicki, E. K., et al. (2003b). First reports evaluating the effectiveness of strategies for preventing violence: Firearms laws: Findings from the Task Force on Community Preventive Services. *Morbidity and Mortality Weekly Report, 52*(RR-14), 11–20.

Hahn, R. A., Lowry, J., Biluka, O., Snyder, S., Briss, P., Crosby, A., et al. (2004). Therapeutic foster care for the prevention of violence: A report of the recommendations of the Task Force on Community Preventive Services. *Morbidity and Mortality Weekly Report, 53*(RR-10), 1–8.

Hallfors, D. Brodish, P. H., Khatapoush, S., Sanchez, V., Cho, H., & Steckler, A. (2006). Feasibility of screening adolescents for suicide risk in "real world" high school settings. *American Journal of Public Health, 96,* 282–287.

Hamberger, L. K., Guse, C., Boerger, J., Minsky, D., Pape, D., & Folsom, C. (2004). Evaluation of a health care provider training program to identify and help partner violence victims. *Journal of Family Violence, 19,* 1–11.

Hemmila, D. (2003). In the line of fire: Hospitals and staff take precautions to guard against growing wave of violence in health care settings. *NurseWeek, 16*(3), 25–27.

Hinderliter, D., Doughty, A. S., Delaney, K., Pitula, C. R., & Campbell, J. (2003). The effect of intimate partner violence education on nurse practitioners' feelings of competence and ability to screen patients. *Journal of Nursing Education, 42,* 449–454.

Hindin, M. J., & Gultiano, S. (2006). Associations between witnessing parental domestic violence and experiencing depressive symptoms in Filipino adolescents. *American Journal of Public Health, 96,* 660–663.

Hirschinger, N. B., Grisso, J. A., Wallace, D. B., McCollum, K. F., Schwarz, D. F., Sammel, M. D., et al. (2003). A case-control study of female-to-female nonintimate violence in an urban area. *American Journal of Public Health, 93,* 1098–1103.

Hoffman, K. L., & Edwards, J. N. (2004). An integrated theoretical model of sibling

violence and abuse. *Journal of Family Violence, 19,* 185–200.

Horne, C. (2003). Families of homicide victims: Service utilization patterns of extra- and intrafamilial homicide survivors. *Journal of Family Violence, 18,* 75–82.

Imbornoni, A.-M. (2006). *Women's rights movement in the U.S.* Retrieved August 13, 2006, from http://www.infoplease.com/spot/womenstimeline1.html

Institute of Medicine. (2006). *Improving the quality of health care for mental and substance-use conditions.* Retrieved February 22, 2006, from http://www.nap.edu

Jech, A. J. (2002). Elder abuse: Mistreatment of older Americans on the rise. *NurseWeek, 15*(23), 22–23.

Johnson, R. M. (2001). Emergency department screening for domestic violence. *American Journal of Public Health, 91,* 651.

Kernic, M. A., Wolf, M. E., & Holt, V. L. (2000). Rates and relative risk of hospital admission among women in violent intimate partner relationships. *American Journal of Public Health, 90,* 1416–1420.

Knox, K. L., & Caine, E. D. (2005). Establishing priorities for reducing suicide and its antecedents in the United States. *American Journal of Public Health, 95,* 1898–1903.

Knox, K. L., Conwell, Y., & Caine, E. D. (2004). If suicide is a public health problem, what are we doing to prevent it? *American Journal of Public Health, 94,* 37–45.

Koenig, L. J., Whitaker, D. J., Royce, R. A., Wilson, T. E., Ethier, K., & Fernandez, M. I. (2006). Physical and sexual violence during pregnancy and after delivery: A prospective multistate study of women with or at risk for HIV infection. *American Journal of Public Health, 96,* 1052–1059.

Koenig, M. A., Stephenson, R., Ahmed, S., Jejeebhoy, S. J., & Campbell, J. (2006). Individual and contextual determinants of domestic violence in north India. *American Journal of Public Health, 96,* 132–138.

Krishnan, S. P., Hilbert, J. C., McNeil, K., & Newman, I. (2004). From respite to transition: Women's use of domestic abuse shelters in rural New Mexico. *Journal of Family Violence, 19,* 165–173.

Krug, E. G., Dahlberg, L. L., Mercy, J. A., Zwi, A. B., & Lozaro, R. (2002). *World report on violence and health.* Geneva, Switzerland: World Health Organization.

Lam, T. H., Stewart, S. M., Yip, P. S. F., Leung, G. M., Ho, L. M., Ho, S. Y., et al. (2004). Suicidality and cultural values among Hong Kong adolescents. *Social Science & Medicine, 58,* 487–498.

Larson, G. L., Rolniak, S., Hyman, K. B., MacLeod, B. A., & Savage, R. (2000). Effect of an administrative intervention on rates of screening for domestic violence in an urban emergency department. *American Journal of Public Health, 90,* 1444–1448.

Lewin, N. L., Vernick, J. S., Beilenson, P. L., Mair, J. S., Lindamood, M. M., Teret, S. P., et al. (2005). The Baltimore Youth Ammunition Initiative: A model application of local public health authority in preventing gun violence. *American Journal of Public Health, 95,* 762–765.

Liang, S. L. (2004). Overcoming stigma in Asian American mental health. *Medscape Psychiatry & Mental Health, 9*(2). Retrieved November 12, 2004, from http://www.medscape.com/viewarticle/419353

Lloyd, S. A. (2000). Intimate violence: Paradoxes of romance, conflict, and control. *National Forum, 80*(4), 19–22.

Locsin, R. C., & Purnell, M. J. (2002). Intimate partner violence, culture-centrism, and nursing. *Holistic Nursing Practice, 16*(3), 1–4.

Loomis, D., Marshall, S. W., & Ta, M. L. (2005). Employer policies toward guns and the risk of homicide in the workplace. *American Journal of Public Health, 95,* 830–832.

Loomis, D., Wolf, S., Runyan, C., Marshall, S., & Butts, J. (2001). Homicide on the job: Workplace and community determinants. *American Journal of Epidemiology, 154,* 410–417.

Lown, E. A., & Vega, W. A. (2001). Prevalence and predictors of physical partner abuse among Mexican American women. *American Journal of Public Health, 91,* 441–445.

Luoma, J. B., & Pearson, J. L. (2002). Suicide and marital status in the United States, 1991–1996: Is widowhood a risk factor? *American Journal of Public Health, 92,* 1518–1522.

Magnussen, L., Shoultz, J., Oneha, M. F., Hla, M. M., Brees-Saunders, Z., Akamine, M., et al. (2004). Intimate partner violence: A retrospective review of records in primary care settings. *Journal of the American Academy of Nurse Practitioners, 16,* 502–512.

Malecha, A. (2003). Screening for and treating intimate partner violence in the workplace. *AAOHN Journal, 51,* 310–316.

Maman, S., Mbwambo, J. K., Hogan, N. M., Kilonzo, G. P., Campbell, J. C., Weiss, E., et al. (2002). HIV-positive women report more lifetime partner violence: Findings from a voluntary counseling and testing clinic in Dar es Salaam, Tanzania. *American Journal of Public Health, 92,* 1331–1337.

Massey-Stokes, M., & Lanning, B. (2004). The role of CSHPs in preventing child abuse and neglect. *Journal of School Health, 74,* 193–194.

McClellan, A. C., & Killeen, M. R. (2000). Attachment theory and violence toward women by male intimate partners. *Journal of Nursing Scholarship, 32,* 353–360.

McFarlane, J., Malecha, A., Gist, J., Watson, K., Batten, E. Hall, I., et al. (2004a). Increasing the safety-promoting behaviors of abused women. *American Journal of Nursing, 104*(3), 40–50.

McFarlane, J., Malecha, A., Gist, J., Watson, K., Batten, E. Hall, I., et al. (2004b). Protection orders and intimate partner violence: An 18-month study of 150 black, Hispanic, and white women. *American Journal of Public Health, 94,* 613–618.

McFarlane, J. M., Groff, J. Y., O'Brien, J., & W son, K. (2006). Secondary preventi intimate partner violence: A ran controlled trial. *Nursing Research*

Mercy, J. A., Krug, E. G., Da Zwi, A. B. (2003). Violen United States in a *American Journal of*

Miller, A., & Man childhood victim drug problems: Imp *Journal of Primary Prev*

Miller, M., Azrael, D., & Hemenway, D. (2002). Rates of firearm ownership and homicide across US regions and states, 1988–1997. *American Journal of Public Health, 92*, 1988–1993.

Miller, M., Hemenway, D., & Rimm, E. (2000). Cigarettes and suicide: A prospective study of 50,000 men. *American Journal of Public Health, 90*, 768–773.

Mirabal, B., Rodriguez, I., Velez, C. N., Crosby, A., & Hoffman, J. (2006). Homicides among children and young adults—Puerto Rico, 1999–2003. *Morbidity and Mortality Weekly Report, 55*, 361–366.

Monts, R. (2002). Men don't seek treatment for depression. *Community Health Forum, 3*(5), 53.

Mouton, C. P., Rodabough, R. J., Rovi, S. L. D., Hunt, J. L., Talamantes, M. A., Brzyski, R. G., et al. (2004). Prevalence and 3-year incidence of abuse among postmenopausal women. *American Journal of Public Health, 94*, 605–612.

Murdaugh, C., Hunt, S., Sowell, R., & Santana, I. (2004). Domestic violence in Hispanics in the southeastern United States: A survey and needs analysis. *Journal of Family Violence, 19*, 107–115.

Murty, S. A., Peek-Asa, C., Zwerling, C., Stromquist, A. M., Burmeister, L. F., & Merchant, J. A. (2003). Physical and emotional abuse reported by men and women in a rural community. *American Journal of Public Health, 93*, 1073–1075.

Nansel, T. R., Overpeck, M. D., Haynie, D. L., Ruan, W. J., & Scheidt, P. (2003). Relationships between bullying and violence among US youth. *Archives of Pediatrics & Adolescent Medicine, 157*, 348–353.

National Center for Health Statistics. (2005). *Health United States, 2005 with chartbook on trends in the health of Americans.* Retrieved December 23, 2005, from http://www.cdc.gov/nchs/data/hus/hus05.pdf

National Center for Injury Prevention and Control. (2003). Nonfatal physical assault-related injuries among persons aged >60 years treated in hospital emergency departments—United States, 2001. *Morbidity and Mortality Weekly Report, 52*, 812–816.

National Center for Injury Prevention and Control. (2005). Homicide and suicide rates—National Violent Death Reporting System, six states, 2003. *Morbidity and Mortality Weekly Report, 54*, 377–380.

National Center for Injury Prevention and Control. (2006a). *Child maltreatment: Fact sheet.* Retrieved June 14, 2006, from http://www.cdc.gov/ncipc/factsheets/cmfacts.htm

National Center for Injury Prevention and Control. (2006b). *Intimate partner violence: Fact sheet.* Retrieved June 14, 2006, from http://www.cdc.gov/ncipc/factsheets/ipvfacts.htm

National Center for Injury Prevention and Control. (2006c). *Poisonings: Fact sheet.* Retrieved June 14, 2006, from http://www.cdc.gov/ncipc/factsheets/poisoning.htm

National Center for Injury Prevention and Control. (2006d). *Sexual violence: Fact sheet.* Retrieved June 14, 2006, from http://www.cdc.gov/ncipc/factsheets/svfacts.htm

National Center for Injury Prevention and Control. (2006e). *Suicide: Fact sheet.* Retrieved

June 14, 2006, from http://www.cdc.gov/ncipc/factsheets/suifacts.htm

National Center for Injury Prevention and Control. (2006f). *Youth violence: Fact sheet.* Retrieved June 14, 2006, from http://www.cdc.gov/ncipc/factsheets/yvfacts.htm

National Institute of Mental Health. (2005a). *Depression: What every woman should know.* Washington, DC: Author.

National Institute of Mental Health. (2005b). *Schizophrenia.* Retrieved June 2, 2006, from http://www.nimh.nih.gov/publicat/schizoph.cfm

National Women's History Project. (n.d.). *Timeline of legal history of women in the United States: A timeline of the women's rights movement 1848–1998.* Retrieved August 13, 2006, from http://www.legacy98.org/timeline.html

Needham, I., Abderhalden, C., Halfens, R. J. G., Fischer, J. E., & Dassen, T. (2005). Non-somatic effects of patient aggression on nurses: A systematic review. *Journal of Advanced Nursing, 49*, 283–296.

Nelson, H., Nygren, P., McInerney, Y., & Klein, J. (2004). Screening women and elderly adults for family and intimate partner violence: A review of the evidence for the U.S. Preventive Services Task Force. *Annals of Internal Medicine, 140*, 387–396.

Office of Statistics and Programming, National Center for Injury Prevention and Control. (2003). Methods of suicide among persons aged 10–19 years—United states, 1992–2001. *Morbidity and Mortality Weekly Report, 52*, 471–474.

Otsu, A., Araki, S., Sakai, R., Yokoyama, K., & Voorhees, A. S. (2004). Effects of urbanization, economic development, and migration of workers on suicide mortality in Japan. (2004). *Social Science & Medicine, 59*, 1137–1146.

Paul, J. P., Catania, J., Pollack, L., Moskowitz, J., Canchola, J., Mills, T., et al. (2002). Suicide attempts among gay and bisexual men: Lifetime prevalence and antecedents. *American Journal of Public Health, 92*, 1338–1345.

Pinhey, T. K., & Millman, S. R. (2004). Asian/Pacific Islander adolescent sexual orientation and suicide risk in Guam. *American Journal of Public Health, 94*, 1204–1206.

Pirkis, J., Goldney, R., & Burgess, P. (2003). Suicidality in the community. In P. Liamputtong & H. Gardner (Eds.), *Health, social change and communities* (pp. 328–339). Oxford: Oxford University Press.

Raj, A., & Silverman, J. G. (2003). Immigrant South Asian women at greater risk for injury from intimate partner violence. *American Journal of Public Health, 93*, 435–437.

Rovi, S., Chen, P., & Johnson, M. S. (2004). The economic burden of hospitalizations associated with child abuse and neglect. *American Journal of Public Health, 94*, 586–590.

Ruff, J. M., Gerding, G., & Hong, O. (2004). Workplace violence against K–12 teachers. *AAOHN Journal, 52*, 204–209.

Russell, S. T., & Joyner, K. (2001). Adolescent sexual orientation and suicide risk: Evidence from a national study. *American Journal of Public Health, 91*, 1276–1281.

Saewyc, E., Skay, C., Richens, K., Reis, E., Poon, C., & Murphy, A. (2006). Sexual orientation,

sexual abuse, and HIV-risk behaviors among adolescents in the Pacific Northwest. *American Journal of Public Health, 96*, 1104–1110.

Sampson, R. J., Morenoff, J. D., & Raudenbush, S. (2005). Social anatomy of racial and ethnic disparities in violence. *American Journal of Public Health, 95*, 224–232.

Scholle, S. H., Buranosky, R., Hanusa, B. H., Ranieri, L., Dowd, K., & Valappil, B. (2003). Routine screening for intimate partner violence in obstetrics and gynecology clinic. *American Journal of Public Health, 93*, 1070–1072.

Scott, K. L. (2004). Stage of change as a predictor of attrition among men in a batterer treatment program. *Journal of Family Violence, 19*, 37–52.

Silver, E., Arsenault, L., Langley, J., Caspi, A., & Moffitt, T. E. (2005). Mental disorder and violent victimization in a total birth cohort. *American Journal of Public Health, 95*, 2015–2021.

Silverman, J. G., Mesh, C. M., Cuthbert, C. V., Slote, K., & Bancroft, L. (2004). Child custody determinations in cases involving intimate partner violence: A human rights analysis. *American Journal of Public Health, 94*, 951–957.

Sitzman, K. (2004). Workplace bullying. *AAOHN Journal, 52*, 220.

Smith, P. H., White, J. W., & Holland, L. J. (2003). A longitudinal perspective on dating violence among adolescent and college-age women. *American Journal of Public Health, 93*, 1104–1109.

Snyder, H. N. (2004). *Juvenile arrests 2002.* Retrieved March 30, 2006, from http://www.ncjrs.gov/html/ojjdp/204608/contents.html

Snyder, H. N., & Swahn, M. H. (2004, March). Juvenile suicides, 1981–1998. *Youth Violence Research Bulletin.* Retrieved March 20, 2004, from http://www.ojp.usdoj.gov/ojjdp

Sorenson, S. B., & Vittes, K. A. (2004). Adolescents and firearms: A California statewide survey. *American Journal of Public Health, 94*, 852–858.

Sorenson, S. B., & Weibe, D. J. (2004). Weapons in the lives of battered women. *American Journal of Public Health, 94*, 1412–1417.

Steen, K., & Hunskaar, S. (2004). Gender and physical violence. *Social Science & Medicine, 59*, 567–571.

Stinson, C. K., & Robinson, R. (2006). Intimate partner violence: Continuing education for registered nurses. *Journal of Continuing Education in Nursing, 37*(2), 58–62.

Stretesky, P. B., & Lynch, M. J. (2001). The relationship between lead exposure and homicide. *Archives of Pediatrics & Adolescent Medicine, 155*, 579–582.

Sugrue, D. P. (2004). Men and suicide: Assessment, management and aftermath in a primary care setting. In R. S. Kirby, C. C. Carson, M. G. Kirby, & R. N. Farah (Eds.), *Men's health* (2nd ed, pp. 443–457). London: Taylor & Francis.

Sung, F.-K., Long, A., Boore, J., & Tsao, L.-I. (2005). Suicide: A literature review and its implications for nursing practice in Taiwan. *Journal of Psychiatric and Mental Health Nursing, 12*, 447–455.

Swahn, M. H., & Bossarte, R. M. (2006). The associations between victimization, feeling unsafe, and asthma episodes among US high school students. *American Journal of Public Health, 96,* 802–804.

Thompson, E. A., Eggert, L. L., Randell, B. P., & Pike, K. C. (2001). Evaluation of indicated suicide risk prevention approaches for potential high school dropouts. *American Journal of Public Health, 91,* 742–752.

Thompson, M. P., Kingree, J. B., & Desai, S. (2004). Gender differences in long-term health consequences of physical abuse of children: Data from a nationally representative survey. *American Journal of Public Health, 94,* 599–604.

Tilley, D. S., & Brackley, M. (2005). Men who batter intimate partners: A grounded theory study of the development of male violence in intimate partner relationships. *Issues in Mental Health Nursing, 26,* 281–297.

United Nations. (1993). *Declaration on the elimination of violence against women.* New York: Author.

United Nations Economic and Social Council. (2002). *Abuse of older persons: Recognizing and responding to abuse of older persons in a global context.* Retrieved June 19, 2006, from http://www.un.org/ageing/enc52002eng.pdf

U.S. Census Bureau. (2006). *Statistical abstract of the United States, 2006.* Retrieved June 5, 2006, from http://www.census.gov/prod/2005pubs/06statab

U.S. Preventive Services Task Force. (2005). *The guide to clinical preventive services, 2005.* Retrieved August 13, 2005, from http://www.ahrq.gov/clinic/pocketgd.pdf

Voss, M., Nylen, L., Floderus, B., Diderichsen, F., & Terry, P. D. (2004). Unemployment and early cause-specific mortality: A study based on the Swedish twin registry. *American Journal of Public Health, 94,* 2155–2161.

Waldrop, A. E., & Resick, P. A. (2004). Coping among adult female victims of domestic violence. *Journal of Family Violence, 19,* 291–302.

Walker, L. E. A. (2000). *The battered woman syndrome* (2nd ed.). New York: Springer.

Walters, K., Breeze, E., Wilkinson, P., Price, G. M., Bulpitt, C. J., & Fletcher, A. (2004). Local area deprivation and urban–rural differences in anxiety and depression among people older than 75 years in Britain. *American Journal of Public Health, 94,* 1786–1794.

Winters, J., Clift, R. J., & Dutton, D. G. (2004). An exploratory study of emotional intelligence and domestic abuse. *Journal of Family Violence, 19,* 255–267.

Wood, J. T. (2004). Monsters and victims: Male felons' accounts of intimate partner violence. *Journal of Social and Personal Relationships, 21,* 555–576.

World Health Organization. (2005). *Summary report: WHO multi-country study on women's health and domestic violence against women.* Retrieved February 22, 2006, from http://www.who.int/gender/violence/whomulti-country_study/summary_report_English2.pdf

Wright, R. J., Mitchell, H., Visness, C. M., Cohen, S., Stout, J., Evans, R., et al. (2004). Community violence and asthma morbidity: The Inner-city Asthma Study. *American Journal of Public Health, 94,* 625–632.

Wuest, J., Merritt-Gray, M., & Ford-Gilboe, M. (2004). Regenerating family: Strengthening the emotional health of mothers and children in the context of intimate partner violence. *Advances in Nursing Science, 27,* 257–274.

Xu, X., Zhu, F., O'Campo, P., Koenig, M. A., Mock, V., & Campbell, J. (2005). Prevalence of and factors for intimate partner violence in China. *American Journal of Public Health, 95,* 78–85.

Yan, E. C.-W., & Tang, C. S.-K. (2004). Elder abuse by caregivers: A study of prevalence and risk factors in Hong Kong Chinese families. *Journal of Family Violence, 19,* 269–277.

Zink, T., Regan, S., Goldenhar, L., Pabst, S., & Rinto, B. (2004). Intimate partner violence: What are physicians perceptions? Retrieved October 13, 2004, from http://www.medscape.com/viewarticle/489079

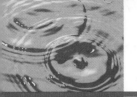

Appendix A

Quad Council PHN Competencies

DOMAIN 1 Analytic Assessment Skills	Generalist/Staff PHN		Manager/CNS/Consultant/ Program Specialist/Executive	
	Individuals & Families	Populations/ Systems	Individuals & Families	Populations/ Systems
1. Defines a problem	Proficiency	Knowledge	Proficiency	Proficiency
2. Determines appropriate uses and limitations of both quantitative and qualitative data	Knowledge	Awareness	Proficiency	Proficiency
3. Selects and defines variables relevant to defined public health problems	Knowledge	Knowledge	Proficiency	Proficiency
4. Identifies relevant and appropriate data and information sources	Proficiency	Knowledge	Proficiency	Proficiency
5. Evaluates the integrity and comparability of data and identifies gaps in data sources	Knowledge	Awareness	Proficiency	Proficiency
6. Applies ethical principles to the collection, maintenance, use, and dissemination of data and information	Proficiency	Knowledge	Proficiency	Proficiency
7. Partners with communities to attach meaning to collected quantitative and qualitative data	N/A (see Note 1)	Knowledge	N/A (see Note 1)	Proficiency
8. Makes relevant inferences from quantitative and qualitative data	Knowledge	Awareness	Proficiency	Proficiency
9. Obtains and interprets information regarding risks and benefits to the community	Knowledge	Knowledge	Proficiency	Proficiency
10. Applies data collection processes, information technology applications, and computer systems storage/retrieval strategies	Knowledge	Awareness	Proficiency	Proficiency
11. Recognizes how the data illuminates ethical, political, scientific, economic, and overall public health issues	Knowledge	Awareness	Proficiency	Proficiency

Definitions:

Awareness: Basic level of mastery of the competency. Individuals may be able to identify the concept or skill but have limited ability to perform the skill.

Knowledge: Intermediate level of mastery of the competency. Individuals are able to apply and describe the skill.

Proficiency: Advanced level of mastery of the competency. Individuals are able to synthesize, critique, or teach the skill.

Note 1 (applicable to Domains 1, 2, and 4): These competencies, because of their population- or system-focused language, do not apply at the individual/family level, but are applicable to the broader context of population-focused public health services and systems.

DOMAIN 2 Policy Development/Program Planning Skills

	Generalist/Staff PHN		Manager/CNS/Consultant/ Program Specialist/Executive	
	Individuals & Families	Populations/ Systems	Individuals & Families	Populations/ Systems
1. Collects, summarizes, and interprets information relevant to an issue	Knowledge	Awareness	Proficiency	Proficiency
2. States policy options and writes clear and concise policy statements	Awareness	Awareness	Proficiency	Proficiency
3. Identifies, interprets, and implements public health laws, regulations, and policies related to specific programs	Knowledge	Knowledge	Proficiency	Proficiency
4. Articulates the health, fiscal, administrative, legal, social, and political implications of each policy option	Awareness	Awareness	Proficiency	Proficiency
5. States the feasibility and expected outcomes of each policy option	Awareness	Awareness	Proficiency	Proficiency
6. Utilizes current techniques in decision analysis and health planning	Knowledge	Awareness	Proficiency	Proficiency
7. Decides on the appropriate course of action	Knowledge	Awareness	Proficiency	Proficiency
8. Develops a plan to implement policy, including goals, outcome and process objectives, and implementation steps	Knowledge	Awareness	Proficiency	Proficiency
9. Translates policy into organizational plans, structures, and programs	N/A (see Note 1)	Awareness	N/A (see Note 1)	Proficiency
10. Prepares and implements emergency response plans	Knowledge	Knowledge	Proficiency	Proficiency
11. Develops mechanisms to monitor and evaluate programs for their effectiveness and quality	Knowledge	Knowledge	Proficiency	Proficiency

Note 1 (applicable to Domains 1, 2, and 4): These competencies, because of their population- or system-focused language, do not apply at the individual/family level, but are applicable to the broader context of population-focused public health services and systems.

DOMAIN 3 Communication Skills

	Generalist/Staff PHN		Manager/CNS/Consultant/ Program Specialist/Executive	
	Individuals & Families	Populations/ Systems	Individuals & Families	Populations/ Systems
1. Communicates effectively both in writing and orally, or in other ways	Proficiency	Knowledge	Proficiency	Proficiency
2. Solicits input from individuals and organizations	Proficiency	Knowledge	Proficiency	Proficiency
3. Advocates for public health programs and resources	Proficiency	Knowledge	Proficiency	Proficiency
4. Leads and participates in groups to address specific issues	Proficiency	Knowledge	Proficiency	Proficiency
5. Uses the media, advanced technologies, and community networks to communicate information	Knowledge	Awareness	Knowledge*	Knowledge*
6. Effectively presents accurate demographic, statistical, programmatic, and scientific information for professional and lay audiences	Knowledge	Knowledge	Proficiency	Proficiency
7. Attitudes: Listens to others in an unbiased manner, respects points of view of others, and promotes the expression of diverse opinions and perspectives	Proficiency	Proficiency	Proficiency	Proficiency

* Reflects ability to determine need for and to utilize experts in these areas

DOMAIN 4	Cultural Competency Skills				
		Generalist/Staff PHN		Manager/CNS/Consultant/ Program Specialist/Executive	
		Individuals & Families	Populations/ Systems	Individuals & Families	Populations/ Systems
1.	Utilizes appropriate methods for interacting sensitively, effectively, and professionally with persons from diverse cultural, socioeconomic, educational, racial, ethnic and professional backgrounds, and persons of all ages and lifestyle preferences	Proficiency	Proficiency	Proficiency	Proficiency
2.	Identifies the role of cultural, social, and behavioral factors in determining the delivery of public health services	Knowledge	Knowledge	Proficiency	Proficiency
3.	Develops and adapts approaches to problems that take into account cultural differences	Proficiency	Knowledge	Proficiency	Proficiency
4.	Attitudes: Understands the dynamic forces contributing to cultural diversity	N/A (see Note 1)	Knowledge	N/A (see Note 1)	Proficiency
5.	Attitudes: Understands the importance of a diverse public health workforce	N/A (see Note 1)	Knowledge	N/A (see Note 1)	Proficiency

Note 1 (applicable to Domains 1, 2, and 4): These competencies, because of their population- or system-focused language, do not apply at the individual/ family level, but are applicable to the broader context of population-focused public health services and systems.

DOMAIN 5	Community Dimensions of Practice Skills				
		Generalist/Staff PHN		Manager/CNS/Consultant/ Program Specialist/Executive	
		Individuals & Families	Populations/ Systems	Individuals & Families	Populations/ Systems
1.	Establishes and maintains linkages with key stakeholders		Knowledge		Proficiency
2.	Utilizes leadership, team building, negotiation, and conflict resolution skills to build community partnerships		Knowledge		Proficiency
3.	Collaborates with community partners to promote the health of the population		Knowledge		Proficiency
4.	Identifies how public and private organizations operate within a community		Knowledge		Proficiency
5.	Accomplishes effective community engagements		Knowledge		Proficiency
6.	Identifies community assets and available resources		Knowledge		Proficiency
7.	Develops, implements, and evaluates a community public health assessment		Knowledge		Proficiency
8.	Describes the role of government in the delivery of community health services		Knowledge		Proficiency

DOMAIN 6   Basic Public Health Sciences Skills

	Generalist/Staff PHN		Manager/CNS/Consultant/ Program Specialist/Executive	
	Individuals & Families	Populations/ Systems	Individuals & Families	Populations/ Systems
1. Identifies the individual's and organization's responsibilities within the context of the Essential Public Health Services and core functions	Knowledge	Knowledge	Proficiency	Proficiency
2. Defines, assesses, and understands the health status of populations, determinants of health and illness, factors contributing to health promotion and disease prevention, and factors influencing the use of health services	Knowledge	Knowledge	Proficiency	Proficiency
3. Understands the historical development, structure, and interaction of public health and health	Knowledge	Knowledge	Proficiency	Proficiency
4. Identifies and applies basic research methods used in public health	Awareness	Awareness	Knowledge	Knowledge
5. Applies the basic public health sciences including behavioral and social sciences, biostatistics, epidemiology, environmental public health, and prevention of chronic and infectious diseases and injuries	Awareness	Awareness	Knowledge	Knowledge
6. Identifies and retrieves current relevant scientific evidence	Knowledge	Knowledge	Proficiency	Proficiency
7. Identifies the limitations of research and the importance of observations and interrelationships	Awareness	Awareness	Knowledge	Knowledge
8. Attitudes: Develops a lifelong commitment to rigorous critical thinking	Proficiency	Proficiency	Proficiency	Proficiency

DOMAIN 7   Financial Planning and Management Skills

	Generalist/Staff PHN		Manager/CNS/Consultant/ Program Specialist/Executive	
	Individuals & Families	Populations/ Systems	Individuals & Families	Populations/ Systems
1. Develops and presents a budget		Awareness		Proficiency
2. Manages programs within budget constraints		Knowledge		Proficiency
3. Applies budget processes		Awareness		Proficiency
4. Develops strategies for determining budget priorities		Awareness		Proficiency
5. Monitors program performance		Knowledge		Proficiency
6. Prepares proposals for funding from external sources		Awareness		Proficiency
7. Applies basic human relations skills to the management of organizations, motivation of personnel, and resolution of conflicts		Knowledge		Proficiency
8. Manages information systems for collection, retrieval, and use of data for decision making		Awareness		Proficiency
9. Negotiates and develops contracts and other documents for the provision of population-based services		Awareness		Proficiency
10. Conducts cost-effectiveness, cost-benefit, and cost utility analyses		Awareness		Proficiency

DOMAIN 8	Leadership and Systems Thinking Skills	Generalist/Staff PHN		Manager/CNS/Consultant/ Program Specialist/Executive	
		Individuals & Families	Populations/ Systems	Individuals & Families	Populations/ Systems
1.	Creates a culture of ethical standards within organizations and communities		Knowledge		Proficiency
2.	Helps create key values and shared vision and uses these principles to guide action		Knowledge		Proficiency
3.	Identifies internal and external issues that may impact delivery of essential public health services (i.e., strategic planning)		Knowledge		Proficiency
4.	Facilitates collaboration with internal and external groups to ensure participation of key stakeholders		Knowledge		Proficiency
5.	Promotes team and organizational learning		Knowledge		Proficiency
6.	Contributes to development, implementation, and monitoring of organizational performance standards		Knowledge		Proficiency
7.	Uses the legal and political system to effect change		Knowledge		Proficiency
8.	Applies theory of organizational structures to professional practice		Awareness		Proficiency

Source: Reprinted with permission of Quad Council of Public Health Nursing Organizations. Quad Council PHN Competencies, *2003.*

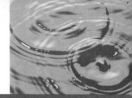

Appendix B

Cultural Influences on Health and Health-Related Behaviors

TABLE B-1	Selected Examples of Culture-Bound Syndromes	
CONDITION	**CULTURAL GROUPS**	**DESCRIPTION**
Aagwaschse	Amish	"Livergrown," condition characterized by crying and abdominal discomfort caused by a jostling, rough buggy ride
Abnemme	Amish	Failure to thrive in a child
Ataque de nervios or *Ataque*	Latino, Puerto Rican, Mediterranean, Caribbean	An attack of nerves, hyperkinetic activity, aggression, or stupor due to tension, stress, grief, uncontrollable shouting, crying, trembling, and heat in the chest
Amok	Malaysian, other Asian	Isolation and withdrawal followed by violence and aggression
Anorexia nervosa	United States	Eating disorder characterized by inaccurate perceptions of body size and shape and drastic measures to lose weight
Bad blood	African American, Appalachian	Sexually transmitted disease acquired through sexual promiscuity (not necessarily related to bacterial or viral infection) or blood contaminated by disvalued behavior
Bilis, colera, or *muina*	Latino	Rage resulting in tension, headache, trembling, screaming
Boufée délirante	East African, Haitian	Agitated aggressive behavior and confusion
Brain fag	West African	Brain fatigue resulting in poor memory, concentration, pain/pressure in the head, blurred vision, and feeling of "worms" in the head due to the stress of school
Caida de mollera	Latino	A depressed fontanel resulting from an infant being bounced too vigorously or having a nipple suddenly or forcefully withdrawn from the mouth
Ch'eena	Native American	Sadness experienced when leaving one's homeland
Coraje (rage)	Latino	Hyperactivity, screaming, or crying due to an extreme emotional reaction
Dhat or *Shen-kei*	Indian, Sri Lankan, Chinese, Taiwanese	Anxiety and hypochondria associated with discharge of semen, whitish urine, weakness, and exhaustion
Empacho	Latino	Adherence of a bolus of food to the walls of stomach or intestine
Espanto	Latino	Severe fright caused by witnessing supernatural beings or events
Falling out	Southern African American, Bahamian, Haitian	Sudden collapse, loss of vision with eyes open, inability to move, dizziness
Ghost sickness	Native American	Preoccupation with death, bad dreams, fear, fainting, appetite loss, hallucinations
High blood	African American, Appalachian	An excess of blood in the body or too much blood high in the body (not related to hypertension), or excessive sweetness in the blood
Herzinsuffizienz	German biomedicine	Cardiovascular condition
Hwa-Byung	Korean	Anger or fire illness with epigastric pain due to a mass in the throat or upper abdomen
Koro or *Suk-yeong*	Chinese, Assam, Thai, East Asian	Intense anxiety over genitals retracting into the body and causing death
Koucharang	Cambodian	Preoccupation with distressing thoughts and memories due to "thinking too much"
Latah	Siberian, Thai, Japanese, Filipino	Trancelike behavior due to hypersensitivity to sudden fear
Locura	Latino	Psychosis due to inherited vulnerability, incoherence, agitation, hallucinations, possible violence

Continued on next page

TABLE B-1	Selected Examples of Culture-Bound Syndromes *(continued)*	
CONDITION	CULTURAL GROUPS	DESCRIPTION
Low blood	African American, Appalachian	Too little blood (comparable to anemia), or excessive bitterness in the blood
Mal de cerebro ode la mente	Latino	Bad in the brain
Mal de ojo (evil eye)	Latino, Arab, Asian, Italian, Greek, Scottish, German, Jewish, Filipino	Disease caused by someone with the evil eye looking at, admiring, or envying the victim (may not be intentional)
Mal puesta	Latino	Unusual behavior caused by magic, voodoo
Pasmo	Puerto Rican	Paralysis due to an imbalance of hot and cold forces
Pibloktoq	Eskimo	Physical and verbal violence followed by convulsions and coma
Poison blood	African American, Appalachian	Septicemia or illness due to witchcraft
Pujos	Latino	Umbilical protrusion and grunting in an infant exposed to a menstruating woman
Qi-gong	Chinese	Psychotic reaction after practicing "exercise of vital energy" (time-limited)
Seasonal affective disorder (SAD)	North American biomedicine	Depression caused by diminishing natural light in winter
Serena	Latino	Upper respiratory symptoms caused by dampness, draft, or evil spirits
Shin-Byung	Korean	Anxiety and dissociation, somatic complaints due to possession by ancestral spirits
Susto	Latino	Magical fright resulting in soul loss
Taijin kyofusho	Japanese	Intense fear that bodily parts or functions displease or anger others
Thin blood	African American, Appalachian	Increased susceptibility to illness
Toa	Khmer	Extreme cold after childbirth leading to physical collapse
Tosca	Roma (gypsy)	A nervous disorder
Zar	North African, Middle Eastern	Spirit possession causing shouting, laughing, head banging

TABLE B-2	Selected Examples of Culturally Unacceptable Behavior
UNACCEPTABLE BEHAVIOR	RECOMMENDED APPROACH
Disrespect for elders and others in authority, especially men (Asian, African American, Latino, Appalachian, Native American, Gypsy, Arab)	Show respect for elders and those in authority, incorporate them in treatment decisions
	Give things to elders with both hands (Hmong, Japanese)
Using informal forms of address inappropriately (Asian, Latino, African American, European American)	Use appropriate forms of address (e.g., using formal mode of speech with older persons), ask about preferred form of address
	Use last name with Mexican American clients
	Use first name only with close African American friend
Using the titles of "Miss" or "Mrs." for women (dominant U.S.)	Use title "Ms."
Direct eye contact (Native American, Latino, Appalachian, Arab—sexual overture between sexes, Navajo—may cause soul loss, Asian—implies equality)	Look at the ground or to the side when speaking to others
Not maintaining eye contact (European, Filipino, dominant U.S.)	Maintain eye contact when speaking to others
Asking someone their name (Hmong)	Ask a third party, "Whose son (daughter, wife, etc.) is this?"
Assuming authority over others (Appalachian)	Avoid conflict
	Mind your own business
Arguing with authority figures (Asian, Latino, Appalachian)	Show respect and acceptance
	Avoid conflict
Competing with others (Native American, Appalachian)	Cooperate with others
Causing others to "lose face" (Asian)	Prevent others from losing face
Strong hand clasp (Native American)	Moderate grasp when shaking hands
	Lightly touch hand (Native American)
Weak hand clasp (European American)	Firm handshake
Writing a "life story" (Native American)	Display modesty and respect for privacy

Continued on next page

TABLE B-2	Selected Examples of Culturally Unacceptable Behavior (continued)
UNACCEPTABLE BEHAVIOR	**RECOMMENDED APPROACH**
Self-disclosure (Native American, Asian, Latino, Appalachian, Gypsy, Arab)	Use tact in obtaining health history
	Use trusted interpreters
	Provide for physical privacy
Overt discussion of sexuality (Asian, Latino, Arab, Hmong)	Discuss sexual matters without members of opposite sex present; ensure availability of same-sex health care provider
Aggressiveness or self-assertion (Native American, Latino, Asian, Appalachian)	Display humility and self-effacement
Lack of motivation or initiative (European American)	Display initiative in task accomplishment
Drawing attention to oneself (Native American, Asian)	Display humility and self-effacement
Expressing personal opinions (Asian)	
Ridiculing others, teasing (Asian, Appalachian)	Direct humor at self (especially with Appalachian clients)
Dependence on others, being a burden (Asian, Appalachian, European American)	Display self-reliance
Complaining (Asian, Filipino)	Accept without complaining
Displaying emotion (Asian, Native American, Appalachian)	Control emotions
Accepting things when first offered (Asian)	Repeat offers of food, pain medication
Giving negative information or disagreeing (Asian, Arab, Filipino)	Give a polite response (whether true or not)
Giving misinformation (dominant U.S.)	Tell the truth, however hurtful
Putting personal needs before family needs (Asian, Latino, Appalachian, Asian Indian)	Try to incorporate personal needs into family goals
Physical contact by opposite sex (Asian, Appalachian, Latino)	Avoid physical contact when possible
Physical contact with same sex (dominant U.S.)	Avoid physical contact when possible
Touching the head (Hmong, Vietnamese)	Avoid touching the head if possible
Pointing at others, especially with feet (Vietnamese, Asian Indian, Native American)	Avoid pointing objects at others
Being more successful than one's husband (Navajo, Arab)	Help with role conflict
Interrupting, chattering (Native American)	Maintain silence, do not interrupt
	Allow time to formulate answers
Failure to understand others (Asian—causes loss of face for teacher)	Validate client's understanding of information
Getting right down to business (Asian, Latino, Native American, Appalachian)	Observe social amenities before business
Wasting time (dominant U.S.)	Come to the point immediately
Saying no, refusing a request (Asian)	Graciously accept requests
Refusing hospitality (Asian, Appalachian, Arab, European American)	Graciously accept hospitality
Being late for an appointment or social event (dominant U.S.)	Arrive on time

TABLE B-3	Selected Cultural Beliefs and Behaviors Regarding Menstruation, Conception, and Contraception	
FOCUS	**BELIEF OR BEHAVIOR**	
General	The uterus is the center of female energy. (Hmong)	
	Sexuality should not be discussed between men and women. (Asian, Latino, Arab)	
Menstruation	Menstrual cramping can be alleviated by avoiding hot spicy food. (Appalachian, Latino)	
	Menstruation is a "hot" condition, so "cold" foods should be eaten. (Appalachian)	
	Menstruation opens one to infection. (African American)	
	Burning menstrual pads prevents them from being used to lay a hex. (African American)	
	Avoid sex during menstruation and wear shoes to keep poisons from entering the body. (African American)	
	A normal menstrual flow indicates health. Increased or decreased flow is not healthy. (African American)	
	The presence of a menstruating woman pollutes the environment and endangers living things, especially strong males and vulnerable persons (e.g., infants). (African American)	
	Exposure of an infant to a menstruating woman may cause an umbilical hernia. (African American, Latino)	
	Menstruating women are unclean and should never walk in front of a man. (Roma)	

Continued on next page

TABLE B-3	Selected Cultural Beliefs and Behaviors Regarding Menstruation, Conception, and Contraception *(continued)*
FOCUS	**BELIEF OR BEHAVIOR**
Contraception	Herbal preparations can be used to prevent pregnancy. They may be given as teas, suppositories, or douches; applied topically; or inhaled. (Latino)
	Pregnancy should be prevented by abstinence. (Chinese, Filipino, Latino, Roman Catholic)
	Oral contraceptives cause birth defects and ill health for the mother. (Appalachian)
	Oral contraceptives cause decreased menstrual flow, which is not healthy. (African American)
	Abortion can be caused by drinking ginger root tea, jumping from a height, or stepping over a rail fence. (Appalachian)
	A wife who asks her husband to use a condom marks herself as a prostitute. (Latino)
	Nine drops of turpentine taken nine days after intercourse will prevent conception. (Appalachian)
	Charms and ceremonies may prevent conception. (Native American)
	Contraception challenges the will of God. (Latino, Arab)
	An ice water and vinegar douche slows sperm and kills them. (African American)
	Holding one's breath during orgasm, standing up immediately after intercourse, or holding one's nose and blowing forcefully through the mouth can expel semen from the vagina and prevent pregnancy. (African American)
Conception	Childbearing allows one's ancestors to be reborn; barrenness is the greatest misfortune of a woman. (Ghanan)
	Herbs can be used to "heat" the womb to promote conception. (Latino)
	The fertile period for a woman is a few hours of a "heat cycle" midway between menstrual periods. (Appalachian)
	The child's sex is determined by the side the mother turns to after intercourse. (Appalachian)
	The right ovary produces "girl seeds"; the left produces "boy seeds." (Appalachian)
	Pregnancy is more apt to occur during one's menses. (African American)[a]
	One cannot conceive until after the first menses following delivery. (African American)[a]
	Infertility may be perceived as failure to fulfill family role expectations. (Chinese)[a]

[a]Potentially harmful beliefs or practices.

TABLE B-4	Selected Cultural Beliefs and Behaviors Regarding the Perinatal Period
FOCUS	**BELIEF OR BEHAVIOR**
Pregnancy	Childbirth is a natural event. (Appalachian)
	Children are a sign of a man's virility. (Latino)
	Wives should become pregnant as soon as possible after marriage. (Latino, Korean)
	A visible double pulse in the neck, dreaming of fish, or change in skin color indicates pregnancy. (African American)
	A pregnant woman is considered ill or weak. (Latino)
	Pregnancy is a time of danger for mother and child, but is not an illness. (Asian)
	Pregnant women should eat a balanced diet and avoid sweets and snacks. (Appalachian)
	Pregnancy is a "hot" condition, so meat should be avoided and sodium intake increased. (African American)
	"Hot" foods including protein foods should be avoided in pregnancy. (Latino)[a]
	"Cold" foods (many vegetables) should be avoided in pregnancy. (Chinese)[a]
	Red meat should be avoided during pregnancy to prevent "high blood." (African American, Appalachian)[a]
	Iron in the prenatal diet causes hardening of the bones and a difficult labor. (Asian)[a]
	Milk during pregnancy may result in a large baby and a hard labor. (Latino)[a]
	Soy sauce and shellfish should be avoided during pregnancy. (Asian)
	Unclean foods should be avoided during pregnancy. (Asian)
	Cravings should be satisfied to prevent a defect related to the food craved. (Appalachian, Latino)
	Ginseng tea will strengthen the pregnant woman. (Asian)
	Strong emotions during pregnancy will leave a mark on the baby. (Appalachian, Latino)
	Fright or surprise during pregnancy can injure the baby. (Latino, Appalachian)
	A pregnant woman's workload should be reduced. (Native American)
	Pregnant women should avoid raising their arms or hanging laundry to prevent knots in the umbilical cord. (Latino)
	Untying knots during labor will prevent knots in the umbilical cord. (Roma)
	Sitting cross-legged will cause knots in the umbilical cord. (Latino)
	Bathing should be encouraged during pregnancy. (Latino)

Continued on next page

TABLE B-4	Selected Cultural Beliefs and Behaviors Regarding the Perinatal Period *(continued)*
FOCUS	**BELIEF OR BEHAVIOR**
	Pregnant women should sleep on their backs. (Latino)
	Pregnant women should keep active. (Latino)
	Nausea and vomiting can be treated with a mixture of flour and water, lemon and water, or chamomile tea. (Latino)
	Violent purging herbs can be used for constipation in pregnancy. (Latino)[a]
	Prenatal care and delivery by a woman is preferred. (Appalachian, Asian)
	Pregnant women should be accompanied to the doctor by husbands or female family members. (Latino)
	Periodic massage during pregnancy can help fix the uterus in the correct position for delivery. (Latino)
	Baby showers should be held close to the time of delivery to prevent envy and the "evil eye." (Latino)
	Supplies should not be purchased for the baby until after delivery. (Navajo)
	Planning for the baby prior to delivery defies God's will. (Arab)
	Sexual activity should be continued throughout pregnancy to keep the birth canal lubricated. (Latino)
Delivery	There is a correlation between the hour of conception and time of delivery. (Appalachian)
	Labor can be stimulated by the use of herbal preparations. (Latino)
	Tea made of winter fat leaves and roots will enhance contractions. (Hopi) Raspberry leaf tea taken late in pregnancy will increase the strength of contractions. (European)
	Dates eaten during labor will strengthen uterine contractions. (Muslim)
	Wrapping warm cloths around the mother's ankles will speed delivery. (Appalachian)
	The presence of the father or an article of his clothing will speed delivery. (Appalachian)
	The father or one of his relatives should deliver the child. (Hmong)
	Husbands should not be present during labor and delivery. (other Asian, Latino, Arab)
	Husbands should be present during delivery. (dominant U.S.)
	One's sister-in-law should be present for delivery.
	Children should be excluded from delivery. (dominant U.S.)
	Physical exertion will initiate labor in women who go over term. (European American)
	The pregnant woman's mother-in-law should attend her during delivery. (Chinese)
	Birth attendants should be female. (Native American)
	Changes in the moon's phase may trigger labor. (African American)
	The person who delivers and "breathes life into" the baby has a special bond with the baby. (Native American)
	Pain speeds delivery so pain relief is to be avoided. (African American)
	It is inappropriate to exhibit pain during labor. (Asian, many European Americans)
	Emotional expression is expected during labor. (Arab, Italian)
	Labor pains can be "cut" by placing a sharp implement under the bed. (Appalachian)
	Aspirin given for pain will thin the blood and cause increased bleeding. (Appalachian)
	Recitation of certain biblical passages will stop hemorrhage. (Appalachian)
	The lithotomy position is most suitable for delivery. (biomedical)[a]
	A clean episiotomy promotes perineal healing. (biomedical)[a]
	An enema is required to create a "clean" environment for the birth. (biomedical)
	Women in labor should be kept NPO in case surgery is required. (biomedical)[a]
	Delivery should take place in a squatting position. (Asian)
	Delivery causes a loss of body heat that must be replaced. (Asian)
	Delivery is a "hot" condition, so no pork (a hot food) should be eaten afterward, also no penicillin, which is a hot medicine. (Latino)
	Delivery is a "cold" experience that may allow spirits to leave the body. (Hmong)
	Spinal anesthesia/epidural is dangerous. (Arab)
Postpartum	Castor oil or paregoric should be given to the woman after delivery. (Appalachian)[a]
	Boiled cedar tea should be drunk to cleanse the mother after delivery. (Native American)
	Cleansing rituals including washing, incense, or burning sage may be used after delivery. (Native American)
	Fresh fruit and other "cold" foods should not be eaten after delivery. (Appalachian, Asian, Hmong, Mexican)
	Incompatible "hot" and "cold" foods should be avoided during hospitalization after delivery. (Arab)
	A postpartum diet should include chicken, soup, nonsticky rice, and special herbs to "wash out" the uterus. (Hmong)

Continued on next page

TABLE B-4	Selected Cultural Beliefs and Behaviors Regarding the Perinatal Period *(continued)*
FOCUS	BELIEF OR BEHAVIOR
	Warm or hot fluids should be drunk after delivery. (Hmong, other Southeast Asian) Cold fluids should be avoided. (Asian). Cold water may make the blood solid or cause clots. (Southeast Asian)
	A heated rock on the abdomen can replace lost heat, prevent blood clots, and flatten the stomach. (Southeast Asian)
	Ginseng tea should be drunk after delivery to build the blood. (Chinese)
	Salads and sour foods cause postpartum incontinence. (Asian) Sour, spicy, oily, or greasy foods, seafood, beef, fruits, and juices should be avoided. Pork, chicken, soft noodles, and rice should be eaten. (Southeast Asian)
	Postpartum fluid intake should be decreased to prevent stretching the stomach. (Asian)[a]
	Beef and seafood cause itching at the episiotomy site. (Asian)
	Alcohol in rice wine causes bleeding. (Asian)
	Prolonged bed rest and avoidance of strenuous activity prevent complications after delivery. (Appalachian, Asian, Hmong, Chinese)
	Mothers should remain at home for the first month after birth (Chinese, Filipino, East and Southeast Asian). Mothers should observe *la cuarentena* (quarantine) for 40 days after birth. (Mexican)
	Failure to rest and stay warm may lead to premature aging or "urine coming down" in old age. (Southeast Asian)
	Bathing should be avoided after delivery. (Mexican)
	One's mother or mother-in-law should care for the mother and new baby. (Chinese)
	Outside visitors should be discouraged after delivery. (Korean)
	Strangers after delivery may steal the mother's milk. (Hmong)
	Postpartum pain can be relieved by whiskey or by hanging the husband's pants over the bedpost. (Appalachian)
	Herbal preparations can relieve afterpains. (Latino)
	Burning, burying, or salting the placenta will prevent harm to mother and child. (Appalachian, Hmong, African American)
	The placenta should be disposed of in the Rio Grande with a prayer ceremony. (southwestern Native American)
	Drinking cold water should be avoided after delivery. (Asian)
	No water should be drunk for 4 months after delivery; then water from the Rio Grande should be drunk. (southwestern Native American)
	Intercourse should be avoided 2 to 3 months after delivery to prevent disease. (Asian)
	Women are unclean after delivery due to 9 months' accumulation of menstrual blood during pregnancy. (African American) Women are unclean after birth until the baby is baptized. (Roma)
Infant	Infants should not be fussed over or cuddled or evil spirits may steal them. (Vietnamese)
	A beautiful baby may provoke envy and the evil eye, so praise should be given to the mother for her performance in delivery rather than to the baby. (Arab)
	Wearing of amulets and not mentioning the number 5 will protect against the evil eye. (Arab)
	Massage of the newborn by the mother promotes bonding. (Native American)
	Infants do not join human society until the third day after birth. No funeral is held if death occurs prior to the third day. (Hmong)
	The Shaman invokes a soul to be reborn in the infant. The infant should be given a silver necklace to prevent the soul from wandering. (Hmong)
	The father should whisper a prayer into the ear of his newborn child. (Muslim)
	The infant should not be named until it is brought home. (Vietnamese)
	An Indian name may be given at a traditional naming ceremony and a saint's name at baptism. (Native American)
	An infant's name may be given by an older relative or tribal leader. (Native American)
	An infant's name may be selected on the basis of his or her horoscope or personal characteristics. (Asian)
	Infants should be breast-fed for 2 years. (Muslim)
	Colostrum is "bad milk" and may make the infant ill; breast-feeding should not start until actual milk comes in. (Latino, Chinese) Breast-feeding during emotional upset may sour the milk. (Latino, dominant U.S.)
	Castor oil will seal the umbilical stump. (Appalachian)[a]
	A raisin on the umbilical stump will prevent air from entering the infant's body. (Latino)[a]
	Kohl should be put on the umbilical stump. (Arab, southwestern Native American)[a]
	Cobwebs or animal manure will seal the cord stump. (African American)[a]
	A belly band on the infant will prevent umbilical hernia or protuberant umbilicus. (Latino)
	Infants should be given a purge or tonic (may contain lead). (Asian, African American)[a]

Continued on next page

TABLE B-4	Selected Cultural Beliefs and Behaviors Regarding the Perinatal Period *(continued)*
FOCUS	BELIEF OR BEHAVIOR
	A second stillbirth can be prevented by placing a dead infant facedown in the coffin. (Appalachian)
	Infants should be warmly clothed and wrapped. (dominant U.S., Latino)
	Infants should not be cuddled too much to avoid spoiling them. (European American)
	Infants should be kept wrapped on a cradle board provided by the father. (Native American)
	The child should be kept physically close to the mother for the first year. (Mexican)
	Breast-feeding may continue for several years. (Asian)
	Males do not do child care. (Middle Eastern) Males do not carry children. (U.S. military)

aPotentially harmful beliefs or practices.

TABLE B-5	Selected Cultural Beliefs and Behaviors Regarding Death and Dying
FOCUS	BELIEF OR BEHAVIOR
General	Death is a normal part of life. (Native American, Asian)
	Death is passage from one realm of life to a better one. (African American, Appalachian)
	Death is passage into the next life. (Asian)
	No belief in an afterlife. (Native American)
	Flowers should not be given to the living because they are reserved for the dead. (Vietnamese)
	Visitation by a clergy member may be perceived as indicating imminent death. (Vietnamese)
Violent death	Violent death provokes stronger emotional outbursts than does a normal death. (African American)
	Violent death is punishment for misdeeds. (Lao)
	Violent death creates a ghost to wander forever. (Navajo, Cheyenne)
Suicide	Suicide should be concealed because of its shameful nature. (Latino, Filipino)
	Suicide may be used to restore family honor. (other Asian)
Time and place of death	Hospitalization means death is imminent. (African American, Asian, Native American, Appalachian)
	Death should occur at home. (Hmong, Vietnamese)
	Removal of life support should be postponed until an "auspicious" time. (some Asian)
Preparation and disposal of body	Touching a dead body may bring misfortune. (Navajo, Tlingit)
	Touching an animal struck by lightning can bring misfortune. (Navajo)
	Passing an ill child over a dead body may cure illness. (African American)
	The entire body must be disposed of together. Autopsy may be resisted. (Native American, Vietnamese)
	Bodies should be cremated. (Tlingit, Quechan)
	Bodies should be buried. (Pueblo tribes)
	Bodies should be exposed to air on a funeral platform. (Sioux)
	The dying person should be dressed in funeral clothes before death. (Tlingit)
	Family members should prepare the body for disposal. (Sioux)
	Bodies are prepared for burial by commercial mortuary. (Latino, European American)
	Bodies should be richly dressed and wrapped in new blankets. (Navajo)
	The clothing of a dead person may contain evil spirits. (Chinese)
	The hair of the dead person should be unraveled. (Navajo)
	The home of a dead person may contain evil spirits and should be sealed to prevent its future use. (Navajo)
	Touching articles belonging to a dead person may bring misfortune. (Navajo)
	The dead should be buried in family graveyards when possible. (Appalachian)
	Graveyards should be placed on hilltops to prevent the graves from being covered by water. (Appalachian)
	If a body is exhumed and reburied, the person will not go to heaven. (Appalachian)
	The body should be buried facing Mecca. (Arab)
	Organ donation is prohibited. (Arab)
Grief and mourning	Emotional grieving lasts 4 days, after which the name of the dead is never spoken. (Cheyenne, Quechan, Navajo)
	White should be worn during the mourning period. (Hmong)
	Black should be worn during the mourning period. (Latino, European American, dominant U.S.)

Continued on next page

TABLE B-5	Selected Cultural Beliefs and Behaviors Regarding Death and Dying *(continued)*	
FOCUS	**BELIEF OR BEHAVIOR**
	Social activities should be restricted during the mourning period. (Latino)
	The dead should be included in rituals commemorating ancestors. (Vietnamese)
	Homage paid to ancestral spirits will prevent illness. (Hmong, Vietnamese)
	The funeral and wake are a time to rejoice for the dead and comfort the living. (African American)
	Funeral Mass is preceded by saying the Rosary. (Latino)
	The first Monday after death begins 9 days of evening prayer for the dead. (Latino)
	Funerals should be followed by food. (European American, African American, Hmong)
	Condolences should be offered with a handshake and special phrases of consolation. (Arab)
	Bits of colored paper should be burned at the funeral to provide the deceased with money in the spirit world. (Hmong)
	Food and drink should be offered to the spirit of the deceased at the funeral. (Hmong)
	Gifts brought to the grieving family should include whiskey, a basket of lunch, and the liver of a pig or chicken. (Hmong)
Participation and knowledge	Dying clients should be protected from knowledge of impending death. (Latino, Chinese, Japanese, Arab, African American)
	Bad news should be mixed with an element of hope. (Hmong)
	Children should participate in the care of dying family members, funerals, and mourning. (Native American, Latino)
	The eldest son should be present at the death of a parent. (Chinese)
	Family members must be present for the spirit to leave the body. (Native American)

TABLE B-6	Selected Cultural Beliefs and Practices Related to Health Promotion and Illness Prevention	
FOCUS	**BELIEF OR BEHAVIOR**
General	Moving in a clockwise direction in the home maintains balance with the environment. (Navajo)
	A variety of herbal preparations can be used to promote health and prevent illness. (Asian, Latino, African American, Native American, Appalachian, European American)
	Periodic purges keep the system open and prevent disease. (African American)[a]
	Silver or copper bracelets worn by young girls warn of impending illness by turning the surrounding skin black. (African American)
	A *limpia* or cleansing ceremony may be used as a general preventive measure. (Otomi)
	Herbal remedies must be gathered at appropriate times to be effective. (Chinese, Appalachian)
	Avoid water after engaging in a "hot" activity. (Mexican)
	Sulfur and molasses rubbed on the back provide a spring tonic. (African American)
	Hanging garlic or onions in the home can prevent illness. (Native American)
	Burning refuse will prevent disease. (Native American, biomedical)
	Dressing warmly can prevent illness. (European American, Latino)
	Red pepper and urine in scrub water can protect the home against evil. (African American)
Diet	Children, pregnant women, convalescents, and the elderly should avoid red meat to prevent "high blood." (African American, Appalachian)[a]
	Pork, cabbage, instant coffee, "store tea," fish with scales, round-hoofed animals, oysters, potatoes, plums, grapefruit, cherries, cranberries, graham crackers, salt, and saccharin lead to waste buildup and illness and should be avoided. (Appalachian)
	A balance of "hot" and "cold" foods should be eaten. (Asian, Latino, Appalachian, Arab)
	"Hot" foods include beef, pork, potatoes, and whiskey. "Cold" foods include chicken, fish, fruit, and beer. (Pakistani)
	Eating three meals, including breakfast, promotes health. (African American, dominant U.S., biomedical)
	Eating a 1,000-year-old egg can prevent illness. (Chinese)
Lifestyle	Excess in food, drink, and activity should be avoided. (African American, Islam, biomedical)
	Keeping the body clean inside and out will prevent illness. (African American)
	Rest promotes health. (African American)
	Staying active promotes health. (Appalachian)

Continued on next page

TABLE B-6	Selected Cultural Beliefs and Practices Related to Health Promotion and Illness Prevention *(continued)*
FOCUS	BELIEF OR BEHAVIOR
Prayer and magic	Carrying a printed prayer on one's person will prevent mishap. (African American, Appalachian)
	Prayer and veneration of the relics of saints can prevent illness. (Latino, and other Roman Catholic)
	Blessing throats on St. Blaise's feast day (Feb. 3) can prevent choking. (Latino and other Roman Catholic)
	Wearing garlic on one's person wards off evil spirits. (African American)
	Charms made of the fat of a person who died a violent death can scare away evil spirits. (Lao)
	Amulets, chains, and tattoos prevent spirit invasion. (Khmer)
	A string on the wrist or neck protects the infant from evil spirits. (Hmong)
	Charms and fetishes will ward off evil. (Native American)
	Wearing religious medals or displaying religious statues in the home can prevent misfortune. (Latino, and other Roman Catholic)
	Carrying or wearing a medicine bundle can prevent illness. (Native American)
	Placing a red ribbon on a child can prevent illness. (Mexican)
	Prevent evil spirits by wearing amulets in the hair or in a red bag pinned to clothing or hanging them over doors, on walls, or on curtains. (Chinese)
	Jade charms bring health. If the charm dulls or is broken, misfortune follows. (Chinese)
	Tying a string on an arm, leg, or around the neck controls spirits. (Vietnamese)
	A gold ring on a red ribbon around the neck will prevent anxiety. (Latino)
	Keeping a black animal will prevent witchcraft. (Mexican)
	Wearing coral around the neck or wrist will prevent depression and "evil eye." (Latino)
	Touching a child while admiring him or her will prevent evil eye. (Mexican, Filipino)
	Moistening a finger with saliva and tracing a cross on a child's forehead can prevent evil eye. (Filipino)
	Charms can prevent the evil eye. (Mediterranean)
	Wearing copper or silver bracelets, necklaces, or anklets prevents soul loss by locking the soul into the body. (Hmong)
Specific prevention	Eating onions or baking soda will prevent "flu." (Appalachian)[a]
	Avoiding tomatoes will prevent cancer. (Appalachian)
	Immunization prevents smallpox. (ancient Chinese, biomedical)
	Asafetida, or rotten flesh, worn in a bag around the neck prevents communicable disease. (African American)
	Avoiding cutting infants' fingernails will prevent heart disease. (Asian)
	Nosebleeds can be prevented by not becoming overheated. (Latino)
	Prevent chills by not eating or drinking cold things when hot. (Latino)
	Not cutting one's hair will prevent loss of strength. (Native American)
	Avoid writing one's story to prevent loss of life spirit. (Native American)
	Isolation will prevent the spread of communicable diseases. (Native American, biomedical)
	Isolating ill persons will prevent their condition from becoming worse. (Native American, biomedical)
	Not going barefoot will prevent tonsillitis. (Latino)
	Chachayotel, a seed, tied around the waist will prevent arthritis. (Mexican)
	Cod liver oil prevents colds. (African American)
	Avoid sitting under a mango tree when hot to prevent kidney infection and back problems. (Puerto Rican)
	Avoid baby formula for infants because it causes rashes. (Puerto Rican)
	Avoid going into the coffee fields when hot to prevent respiratory illness. (Puerto Rican)
	Avoid drinking cold water when hot to prevent colds. (Puerto Rican)
	Black caraway seeds boost the immune system. (Islam)
	Garlic and onions prevent infection, cardiovascular disease, and diabetes. (Islam)
	Green tea, turtle, lin chee (dried mushroom), dandelion, shark bones, monkey head mushrooms, lotus, and snake tongue grass prevent cancer. (Chinese)

[a]Potentially harmful belief or practice.

TABLE B-7	Selected Cultural Beliefs and Practices Related to Diagnosis and Treatment of Illness
FOCUS	**BELIEF OR BEHAVIOR**
Diagnosis	Diagnosis is made by means of dreams, "hand tremblers," "star gazers," or "crystal gazers." (Native American)
	Diagnosis is made using techniques of inspection, listening, questioning, and palpation. (Chinese)
	Diagnosis of women should be made on the basis of pulses only. (Asian)
	Women may point to areas on an alabaster figure to indicate areas of complaint. (Chinese)
	Diagnosis is made by iridology, the condition of the iris. (Asian)
	Susceptibility to certain illnesses is determined by signs of the zodiac. (Appalachian)
General treatment	Exercise may be suggested as a remedy for illness. (Asian, biomedical)
	Herbal preparations are used to treat illness. (Asian, Native American, Latino, African American, Appalachian)
	Sweat baths may be used to treat illness. (Native American, Lao, Khmer)
	Massage may be used to treat illness. (Zuni, Otomi, Lao, Hmong, Chinese)
	Onions placed on the wall of a sickroom will absorb illness. (Appalachian)
	Signs of the zodiac should be consulted when planning surgery. (African American)
	Pressure on specific points on the foot (reflexology) may relieve illness. (Japanese)
	Medication should be discontinued when symptoms disappear. (Lao, other Asian, African American)
	Wounds should be covered to keep them clean. (Lao, dominant U.S., biomedical)
	Medicines are usually prepared by boiling herbs in a prescribed amount of water and taking all of the preparation. (Chinese, other Asian)[a]
	Scientific medicines are considered "hot" and may not be taken for a "cold" illness. (Otomi, Asian)[a]
	Scientific medicines are considered very strong, so clients may take only half the prescribed dose. (Vietnamese)[a]
	Everything has an opposite; every disease has a cure. (African American)
Diet	"Hot" foods should be taken to treat "cold" illnesses and "cold" foods taken to treat "hot" illnesses. (Asian, Latino, Appalachian)
	Treat "cold" illnesses such as diarrhea and fever with "hot" foods such as sweets, candies, and spices. Treat "hot" illnesses such as pimples, boils, and skin problems with "cold" foods such as vegetables and fruits and water. (Vietnamese)
	"Cold" foods used to treat "hot" illnesses include tropical fruit, dairy products, goat, fish, chicken, honey, cod, raisins, bottled milk, and barley water. "Hot" foods used to treat "cold" illnesses include chocolate, cheese, temperate-zone fruits, eggs, peas, onions, aromatic beverages, oils, beef, waterfowl, mutton, goat's milk, cereals, and chili peppers. (Mexican)
	Eating snake flesh improves vision. (Chinese)
	Use green vegetables and onions to treat respiratory disease. (Otomi)
	Use cooked onions to gain weight, raw onions to lose weight. (Otomi)
	Avoid spices, salt, and garlic when ill and eat plain food and soup. (Hmong)
	Treat constipation with vegetables, tea, honey, or prunes. (Chinese)
	Karo syrup added to the bottle will help constipation in an infant. (dominant U.S.)[a]
	Chicken soup stimulates recovery from illness. (Jewish, dominant U.S.)
	Jell-O water or flat soft drinks should be given to persons with diarrhea. (dominant U.S.)
Prayer and magic	Prayer may bring about cure of illness. (Latino, Native American, Filipino)
	Promises, visiting shrines, offering medals or candles, and prayer may help cure illness. (Mexican)
	Gather bark from the east side of a tree to appease the gods (Native American) or for greater potency. (Appalachian)
	Use cornmeal in healing rituals. (Native American)
	Gist, or medicine bundles, are used in healing rituals. (Native American)
	Like cures like. (African American, Appalachian)
	Use invocations to spirits accompanied by rattle or drum in healing rituals. (Native American)
	Prayers and laying-on-of-hands may cure illness. (African American, Appalachian)
	Songs or chants amplify the forces of good in their battle with evil. (Otomi, other Native American)
	A *limpia*, or cleansing of evil, may be accomplished by passing an object over the body to pick up evil spirits. (Otomi, Latino)
	Recital of the Twenty-third Psalm, reading Scripture, prayer, and positive reminiscences may cure illness caused by a hex. (African American)
	A *baci* ceremony may be used to placate spirits causing illness. (Lao)

Continued on next page

TABLE B-7	Selected Cultural Beliefs and Practices Related to Diagnosis and Treatment of Illness *(continued)*
FOCUS	**BELIEF OR BEHAVIOR**
	Small spirit cures (chants) may be used for minor problems. For major problems, large spirit cures are required to release demons. (Hmong)
	After releasing evil spirits in a place away from home, a chant should be sung to prevent the spirits from following the healer home. (Hmong)
Herbal treatments	"Hot" herbs or medicines used for "cold" illnesses include ginger, garlic, cinnamon, anise, penicillin, tobacco, vitamins, iron, cod liver oil, castor oil, and aspirin. "Cold" herbs or medicines include orange flower water, linden, sage, milk of magnesia, and sodium bicarbonate. (Mexican)
	Herbal teas may be used for fatigue, cold, sore throat, cough, chest ailments, and other conditions. (Appalachian)
	Sassafras is used for agues, lung fever, ulcers, stomach problems, skin conditions, sore eyes, catarrh, gout, dropsy, syphilis, and anemia (Appalachian) or for colds. (African American)
	Use goldenseal (an herb) for weak stomach, liver, or intestinal problems, hemorrhages, poor circulation, and "nerves." (Appalachian)
	Use ginseng for stomach and female problems, aging, sore eyes, asthma, poor appetite, rheumatism, longevity, and luck (Appalachian) or for anemia, colic, depression, indigestion, impotence, rheumatism, or as a sedative (cannot be prepared in any metal container). (Chinese)
	Any plant root or plant with a yellow cast can be used to treat jaundice. (Appalachian)
	A hot moist tea bag held in the mouth relieves canker sores. (European American)
	Oil of clove is good for a toothache. (European American)
	Whiskey rubbed on the gums will soothe a teething baby. (European American)[a]
	Horehound drops or honey and lemon are effective for sore throat. (dominant U.S.)
	Vicks VapoRub is useful for chest congestion and cough or stuffy nose. (dominant U.S.)[a]
	Use yellow root tea for sore throat, stomach upset, high blood pressure, canker sores, or tonic. (Appalachian)
	Treat diarrhea with boiled green persimmons. (Appalachian)
	Treat indigestion with chrysanthemum, crystal, ginseng, or other teas. (Chinese)
	Smoke jimson weed for asthma. (Appalachian)
	Use ginger to strengthen the heart and treat nausea and dyspepsia. (Asian)
	Grind up guava and put in the mouth to treat sores. (Otomi)
	Boiled banana peel or stems will stop heavy or prolonged menstrual bleeding. (Otomi)
	A tamarind bath can be used for the chronically fatigued child. (Otomi)
	Chopped garlic, onion, parsley, and water can be used as an expectorant. (African American)
	Onions applied to the feet wrapped in warm blankets will cure fever. (African American)
	Goldenrod tea is used for colds, sore throat, and cough. (Zuni)
	Thistle concoctions can be used for fever, gastrointestinal problems, or genitourinary infections (Zuni) or to treat worms. (Hopi)
	Blanket flower can be used to treat painful urination. (Hopi)
	A tea made from painted cup can be used for menstrual pain. (Hopi)
	Witch hazel or sweet flag is used for colds. (Oneida)
	Elderberry flowers can be used for diarrhea. (Oneida)
	Dried raspberry leaves can be used for mouth sores. (Oneida)
	Mustard plant can be used to treat headache or sunburn. (Zuni)
	Use sage to treat burns (Zuni) or on boils. (Hopi)
	Tansy and sage can be used to treat headache. (Oneida)
	Use a sunflower water bath for spider bites. (Hopi)
	Chew the root of a bladder pod plant and put it on a snake bite. (Hopi)
	Fleabane can be bound to the head or used in a tea for headache. (Hopi)
	Yucca stem can be used as a laxative.
	Raw potato soaked in vinegar may be placed on the forehead to treat headache. (Latino)
	Treat skin conditions with grated potato or tomato. (Latino)
	Oregano tea may be used for cough. (Latino)
	Earache is treated with a preparation of rue on cotton placed in the ear. (Latino)
	Hot tea or a dock (weedy plant) or saline gargle can be used to treat sore throat. (Latino) Or use comfrey. (Oneida)

Continued on next page

TABLE B-7	Selected Cultural Beliefs and Practices Related to Diagnosis and Treatment of Illness *(continued)*
FOCUS	**BELIEF OR BEHAVIOR**
	Fever may be treated with an enema of "malva leaves." (Latino)
	Chamomile tea (Latino) or garlic (Vietnamese) is good for high blood pressure.
	High blood pressure may be treated by eating pears, being tranquil, and eating garlic (to prevent stroke). (Latino)
	Put globe mallow on cuts and wounds. Chew the root for broken bones. (Hopi)
	Use cliff rose to wash wounds. (Hopi)
	Swab a baby's mouth with its own diaper to treat thrush. (African American)[a]
External treatments	Coining is used to treat pain, colds, vomiting, and headache (Khmer); heatstroke, indigestion, and colic (Chinese); colds, flu, and wind entering the body. (Vietnamese)
	Virgin olive oil can be used for dry skin and eczema. (Roma)
	Honey may be used to treat skin ulcers. (Roma)
	Maggots may be used to remove necrotic tissue. (biomedical)
	Leeches may be used to decrease swelling in reattached digits or muscle flap grafts. (biomedical)
	Pinching is used for headache and sore throat. (Vietnamese)
	Cupping is used to treat headache and body ache by removing noxious elements (Khmer); to treat arthritis, abdominal pain, abscess, and stroke paralysis (Chinese); to treat joint or muscle pain. (Vietnamese, also some Europeans)
	Moxibustion is used to treat mumps, convulsions, and nosebleed, and during labor and delivery. (Chinese)
	Balms and medicated plasters can be applied to the skin for bone and muscle problems. (Vietnamese)
	Treat pain with acupuncture, acupressure, blowing in the ear, painting with a purple spot, pinching, cupping, or coining. (Asian)
	Acupuncture may also be used to treat any "hot" illness. (Chinese)
	Sweat baths are useful for childbirth, opium withdrawal, mental disorder, and psychosomatic illness. (Lao)
	Warts can be removed with water from the rotted stump of a chestnut tree. (Appalachian)
Other treatments	Treat object intrusion with massage to draw the object up; then suck over the area. (Otomi, other Native American)
	Use "bluestone" powder in open wounds or for poison ivy. (African American)
	Use stale bread or sour milk or salt pork on lacerations. (African American)
	Use the skin from inside the shell of a raw egg for boils. (African American)
	Piñon sap is used to treat ulcers. (Zuni)
	Piñon gum may be used as an antiseptic and to keep air from wounds. (Zuni, Hopi, Navajo)
	Tape treated with camphor balm can be placed over the temples to treat headache. (Lao)
	Poultices may be used to treat heart pain (Otomi) or inflammation. (African American)
	Deer antler strengthens bones, improves potency, and eliminates nightmares. (Chinese)
	Rhino horn can be used for pus boils and snakebite. (Chinese)
	Turtle shell can be used to stimulate the kidneys and cure gallstones. (Chinese)
	Seahorses can be used to treat gout. (Chinese)
	Use quicksilver (mercury) to treat venereal disease. (Chinese)[a]
	Dissolve certain tree insects in the mouth to treat sores, or drink the juice of the insect. (Otomi)
	Purgatives should be used for "poison." (Otomi)
	Drink sugar and turpentine for worms; rub it into the skin for backache. (African American)
	Clay in a dark leaf can be wrapped around a sprained ankle. (African American)
	For stiff neck, place crossed pieces of silverware over the area. (African American)
	Fluid intake should be decreased with fever. (Khmer)[a]
	Anemia may be treated with blood pudding. (Latino)
	Greta or azarcon can be used to treat *empacho* (both have high lead content). (Latino)[a]
	Rattlesnake capsules may be used for a variety of chronic conditions. (Latino)[a]
	Use warmth to treat fever. (Japanese, other Asian, Latino, African American)

[a]Potentially harmful practice

Appendix C

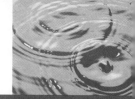

Nursing Interventions for Common Health Problems in Children

The interventions presented here are general guidelines that the community health nurse can use to educate parents for home care of health problems commonly encountered among young children.

ORGAN SYSTEM	PROBLEM	INTERVENTIONS
TABLE C-1	**Nursing Interventions for Common Health Problems in Children**	
Gastrointestinal	Spitting up	Burp baby more frequently.
		Keep infant upright for short time after feeding.
		Check size of nipple hole.
		Change to soy formula.
	Colic	Give small amounts of warm water.
		Exert gentle pressure on abdomen with infant's legs and thighs bent.
	Mild diarrhea or vomiting	Begin oral rehydration to prevent dehydration.
		Do not discontinue feedings.
		Seek medical help if condition continues or worsens.
	Constipation	Increase fluid intake.
		Add bulk to diet.
		Encourage regular toileting habits.
		Discourage postponing defecation.
		Avoid use of laxatives or enemas.
Respiratory	Mild respiratory infection	Increase fluid intake.
		Use a cold mist humidifier to ease breathing.
		Do not use Vicks or other aromatic substances.
		Seek medical help for severe or persistent cough, difficulty breathing, stridor, or nasal flaring.
Integumentary	Diaper rash	Wash diapers with mild soaps and rinse thoroughly.
		Add 3/4 cup vinegar to last rinse to remove ammonia.
		If using disposable diapers, use ones that allow air circulation.
		Change diapers frequently, thoroughly cleaning diaper area.
		Do not use powders or lotion in diaper area.
		Leave diaper area exposed when possible.
	Allergic dermatitis	Explore changes in foods or soaps.
		Eliminate possible causative substances.
		Seek medical help for severe rashes or secondary infection.
	Cradle cap	Scrub scalp with soap and soft washcloth during bath.
		Brush scalp with soft brush after bath.
		Do not use oil or lotion on scalp.
	Minor abrasions and lacerations	Wash with soap and water.
		Keep clean.
Urinary	Urinary tract infection	Seek medical assistance.
	Bedwetting	Limit fluid intake after dinner.
		Empty bladder before bed.
		Awaken child to urinate before parents go to bed.
		Do not make an issue of the problem.
		If problem is severe or continues beyond age 6, seek medical attention.

Continued on next page

TABLE C-1 Nursing Interventions for Common Health Problems in Children *(continued)*

ORGAN SYSTEM	PROBLEM	INTERVENTIONS
Musculoskeletal	Sprains and fractures	Perform basic first aid and immobilize injured area.
		Seek medical attention.
	Leg cramps	Increase calcium intake.
		If severe or persistent, seek medical attention.
Neurological	Headache	Give nonaspirin analgesic according to child's age and size.
		If severe or recurrent, seek medical attention.
	Hearing problem	Seek medical attention.
	Vision problem	Seek medical attention.
	Delayed speech	Discourage older children and parents from talking for child.
		Encourage child to verbalize needs before meeting them.
		Seek medical attention for prolonged delay.
	Speech defect	Seek medical attention.
Other	Fever	For temperature over 102°F, give nonaspirin antipyretic.
		For high or persistent fever, seek medical attention.
	Suspected abuse	Report to child protective services.
		Refer family to Parents Anonymous or other support groups.
	Night terrors	Use a night-light or leave bedroom door open.
		Use bedtime rituals of checking for "monsters" if helpful.
		Use a "guardian" stuffed animal to scare away monsters.
		Comfort the child after waking and stay until child returns to sleep.
		Seek assistance for persistent terrors or those related to a real traumatic event.
	Jealousy of new baby	Prepare siblings for birth of another child.
		Have child assist with care of newborn.
		Emphasize positive aspects of being older.
		Accept regressive behavior and do not belittle child.
		Spend time with just the older child.
		Encourage friends and relatives to pay attention to older child as well as new baby.
	Sibling rivalry	Mediate arguments.
		Encourage children to work out their own differences.
		Encourage compromise.
		Give reasons for differences in privileges.
		Use role-play with older children to give insight into feelings and behaviors of others.
	Tantrums	Ignore behavior if possible.
		Remove child to bedroom if disturbing others.
		Do not give in to child's demands.
	Bedtime	Complete bedtime rituals and put child in bed.
		Ignore crying for 15 to 20 minutes. If the child does not stop, see what is wrong.
		If child gets up, put him or her back to bed.
		Place several safe toys in bed with child and allow play until the child falls asleep.
	Poor self-esteem	Praise child for accomplishments.
		Correct mistakes without denigrating child.
		Help child identify and strengthen talents.
		Assist child to accept limitations.
		Seek assistance for severe depression or low self-esteem on the part of child.

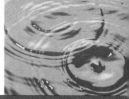

Appendix D

Suspected Abuse Report Forms

The forms included here are examples of the type used to report suspected abuse and violence. Generally, cases of suspected or confirmed abuse are reported immediately by telephone and followed with a completed reporting form with 24 to 48 hours. Whenever feasible, specific events leading to suspicion of abuse should be described as fully as possible, including information about specific behavior observed or exact words of those describing events. Community health nurses should become familiar with specific forms used in their local jurisdictions, including special forms for reporting spouse and elder abuse if required.

MEDICAL SERVICES
DOMESTIC VIOLENCE AND VIOLENT
INJURY REPORT

California Penal Code sections 11160 and 11161 require hospitals and physicians to report immediately, both by telephone and in writing, all injuries resulting from the use of a gun or knife or other deadly weapon, or otherwise inflicted in violation of the criminal law, whether by act of the patient or of another person. EXCEPTION: Any physical or psychological condition brought about solely by the voluntary self-administration of any narcotic or restricted dangerous drug is not reportable.

Time of call to police _____   By _____
                                                              Print name

REASON FOR REPORT

_____ Gunshot
_____ Knife wound (or from other deadly weapon)
_____ Injury from other criminal law violation

PATIENT'S NAME: _____

PATIENT'S ADDRESS: _____

PATIENT'S WHEREABOUTS: _____

_____

(Facility Name and Address)

_____ Other (specify) _____

NATURE AND EXTENT OF INJURY: _____

_____

_____

_____   _____
    Date/Time   Signature of Attending Physician
                                             (or other reporting party)

TELEPHONE REPORT GIVEN TO _____ *of* _____
                          Name/ID # of officer   Agency

                    _____   *by* _____
                          Date/Time   ED Staff

Original: Law Enforcement Agency
Yellow: Patient's Chart
Pink: District Attorney, Domestic Violence Unit

If officer does not respond, mail yellow and pink copies to the District Attorney, Domestic Violence Unit, 101 W. Broadway, San Diego, California 92101. Mail original to appropriate law enforcement agency with jurisdiction where the battery occurred.

SUSPECTED CHILD ABUSE REPORT
To Be Completed by Reporting Party
Pursuant to Penal Code Section 11166

A. CASE IDENTIFICATION *(TO BE COMPLETED BY INVESTIGATING CPA)*

VICTIM NAME: _____

REPORT NO./CASE NAME: _____

DATE OF REPORT: _____

B. REPORTING PARTY

NAME/TITLE

ADDRESS

PHONE ( )	DATE OF REPORT	SIGNATURE OF REPORTING PARTY

C. REPORT SENT TO

☐ POLICE DEPARTMENT   ☐ SHERIFF'S OFFICE   ☐ COUNTY WELFARE   ☐ COUNTY PROBATION

AGENCY	ADDRESS
OFFICIAL CONTACTED	PHONE ( )	DATE/TIME

D. INVOLVED PARTIES

VICTIM

NAME (LAST, FIRST, MIDDLE)	ADDRESS	BIRTHDATE	SEX	RACE

PRESENT LOCATION OF CHILD	PHONE (___)

SIBLINGS

NAME	BIRTHDATE	SEX	RACE	NAME	BIRTHDATE	SEX	RACE
1.				4.			
2.				5.			
3.				6.			

PARENTS

NAME (LAST, FIRST, MIDDLE)	BIRTHDATE	SEX	RACE	NAME (LAST, FIRST, MIDDLE)	BIRTHDATE	SEX	RACE
ADDRESS				ADDRESS			
HOME PHONE ( )	BUSINESS PHONE ( )			HOME PHONE ( )	BUSINESS PHONE ( )		

E. INCIDENT INFORMATION

IF NECESSARY, ATTACH EXTRA SHEET OR OTHER FORM AND CHECK THIS BOX. ☐

1. DATE/TIME OF INCIDENT	PLACE OF INCIDENT *(CHECK ONE)* ☐ OCCURRED ☐ OBSERVED

IF CHILD WAS IN OUT-OF-HOME CARE AT TIME OF INCIDENT, CHECK TYPE OF CARE:
☐ FAMILY DAY CARE   ☐ CHILD CARE CENTER   ☐ FOSTER FAMILY HOME   ☐ SMALL FAMILY HOME   ☐ GROUP HOME OR INSTITUTION

2. TYPE OF ABUSE: *(CHECK ONE OR MORE)* ☐ PHYSICAL ☐ MENTAL ☐ SEXUAL ASSAULT ☐ NEGLECT ☐ OTHER

3. NARRATIVE DESCRIPTION:

4. SUMMARIZE WHAT THE ABUSED CHILD OR PERSON ACCOMPANYING THE CHILD SAID HAPPENED:

5. EXPLAIN KNOWN HISTORY OF SIMILAR INCIDENT(S) FOR THIS CHILD:

SS 8572 (REV. 7/87)   **INSTRUCTIONS AND DISTRIBUTION ON REVERSE**

DO NOT submit a copy of this form to the Department of Justice (DOJ). A CPA is required under Penal Code Section 11169 to submit to DOJ a Child Abuse Investigation Report Form SS-8583 if (1) an active investigation has been conducted and (2) the incident is **not** unfounded.

Blue and Green Copies to: Social Services Dept.
P.O. Box 11341
San Diego, CA 92111

Police or Sheriff-WHITE Copy; County Welfare or Probation- BLUE Copy; District Attorney-GREEN Copy; Reporting Party-YELLOW Copy

Index

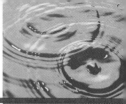

Page numbers followed by "f" indicate figures, and those followed by "t" indicate tables.

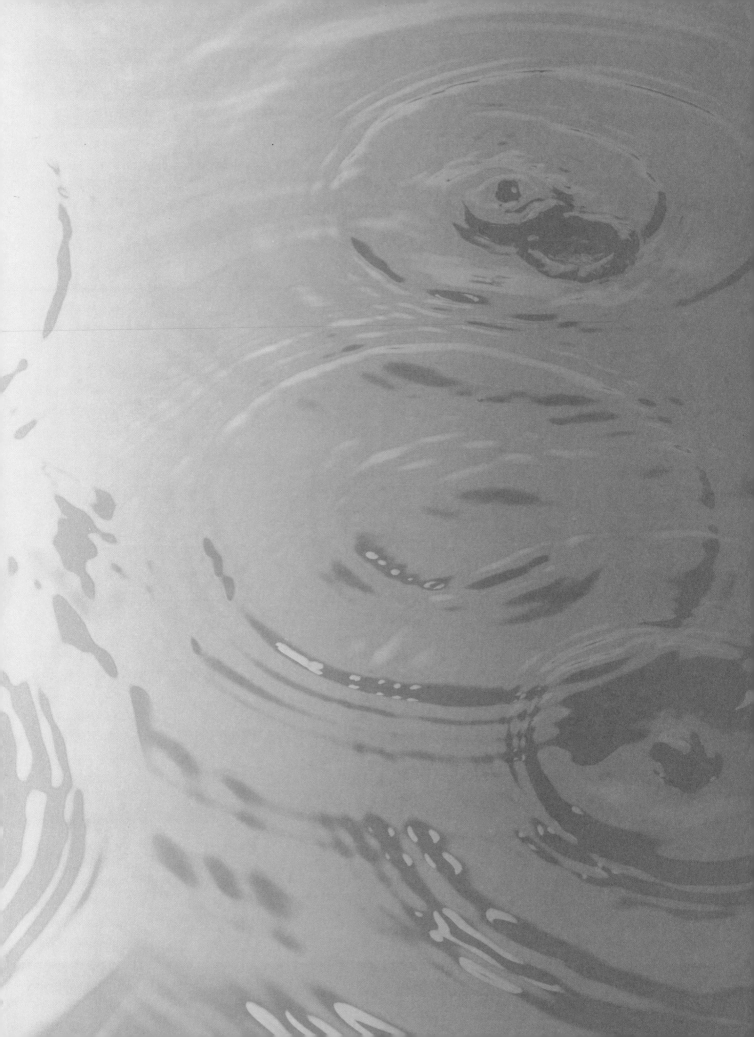

Excellence in Nursing Skills

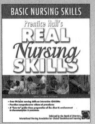
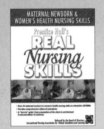
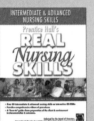
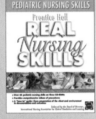
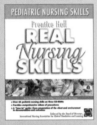
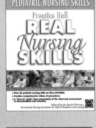
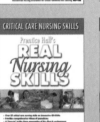
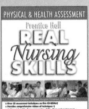
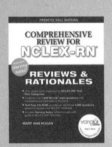

Prentice Hall's Real Nursing Skills on CD-ROMS

Prentice Hall Real Nursing Skills series offers you the complete foundation for competency in performing clinical skills. The CD-ROMS provide comprehensive procedures demonstrated in hundreds of videos, animations, illustrations, and photographs. These skills CD-ROMs are designed to help you visualize how to perform each skill and understand the concepts and rationales for each skill.

Basic Nursing Skills:
94 skills on 5 CD-ROMs. 2005, ISBN: 0-13-191526-6
Intermediate & Advanced Nursing Skills:
84 skills on 5 CD-ROMs. 2005, ISBN: 0-13-119344-9
Physical & Health Assessment Nursing Skills:
25 skills on 5 CD-ROMs. 2006, ISBN: 0-13-191525-8
Maternal-Newborn & Women's Health Nursing Skills:
24 skills on 2 CD-ROMs. 2005, ISBN: 0-13-191527-4
Pediatric Nursing Skills:
65 skills on 3 CD-ROMs. 2006, ISBN: 0-13-191524-X
Critical Care Nursing Skills:
35 skills on 2 CD-ROMs. 2005, ISBN: 0-13-119264-7

Excellence in NCLEX-RN® Review

Prentice Hall's Comprehensive Review for NCLEX-RN® is designed specifically to help you achieve nursing excellence by simplifying your review and making the most of your valuable study time. This review book is uniquely organized according to the April 2007 NCLEX-RN® Test Plan, providing you with both a comprehensive content review and practice questions in sections covering * Safe, Effective Care Environment * Health Promotion * Physiological Integrity, and * Psychosocial Integrity. Throughout this book, you will find:

2008, ISBN 0-13-119599-9

- **Memory Aids** that help you remember key concepts.
- **NCLEX® Alerts** that identify critical concepts you are likely to see on the NCLEX-RN®.
- **Check Your NCLEX® IQ** boxes that help you to assess your readiness for the NCLEX-RN® on the topics covered in the chapter.
- **Practice Tests** at the end of the chapter that review the concepts from that chapter and provide comprehensive rationales and test-taking strategies to help you find the right answers.

The **NCLEX-RN® Test Prep CD-ROM** that comes with your book simulates the test-taking environment by allowing you to practice questions on the computer. It contains all the questions in the book PLUS thousands of additional questions. You can choose to practice in Study, Quiz, or Exam modes, and you will receive detailed reports that will help you focus your preparation for NCLEX-RN®.